# *Varney's* Midwifery

## SEVENTH EDITION

**Julia Phillippi, PhD, CNM, FACNM, FAAN**
Professor of Nursing
Vanderbilt University, Nashville, Tennessee

**Ira Kantrowitz-Gordon, PhD, CNM, FACNM, FAAN**
Associate Professor
University of Washington, Seattle, Washington

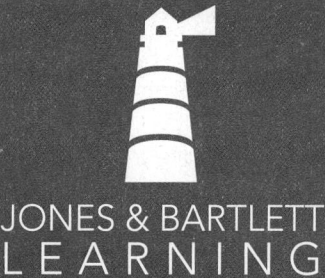

JONES & BARTLETT
LEARNING

*World Headquarters*
Jones & Bartlett Learning
25 Mall Road
Burlington, MA 01803
978-443-5000
info@jblearning.com
www.jblearning.com

Jones & Bartlett Learning books and products are available through most bookstores and online booksellers. To contact Jones & Bartlett Learning directly, call 800-832-0034, fax 978-443-8000, or visit our website, www.jblearning.com.

Substantial discounts on bulk quantities of Jones & Bartlett Learning publications are available to corporations, professional associations, and other qualified organizations. For details and specific discount information, contact the special sales department at Jones & Bartlett Learning via the above contact information or send an email to specialsales@jblearning.com.

**Production Credits**
Vice President, Product Management: Marisa R. Urbano
Vice President, Content Strategy and Implementation: Christine Emerton
Director, Product Management: Matthew Kane
Director, Content Management: Donna Gridley
Product Manager: Tina Chen
Content Strategist: Jessica Covert
Content Coordinator: Samantha Gillespie
Director, Project Management and Content Services: Karen Scott
Manager, Program Management: Kristen Rogers
Project Manager: John Fuller
Senior Content Services Specialist: Carolyn Downer
Senior Product Marketing Manager: Lindsay White
Content Services Manager: Colleen Lamy
Product Fulfillment Manager: Wendy Kilborn
Composition: S4Carlisle Publishing Services
Cover Design: Briana Yates
Senior Media Development Editor: Troy Liston
Rights & Permissions Manager: John Rusk
Cover Image (Title Page, Part Opener, Chapter Opener): © iPiCfootage.com/Shutterstock
Printing and Binding: LSC Communications

**Library of Congress Cataloging-in-Publication Data**
Names: Phillippi, Julia, editor. | Kantrowitz-Gordon, Ira, 1968- editor.
Title: Varney's midwifery / [edited by] Julia Phillippi, Ira Kantrowitz-Gordon.
Other titles: Midwifery
Description: Seventh edition. | Burlington, MA : Jones & Bartlett Learning, [2024] | Includes bibliographical references and index.
Identifiers: LCCN 2022050000 (print) | LCCN 2022050001 (ebook) | ISBN 9781284250565 (hardcover) | ISBN 9781284250572 (epub)
Subjects: MESH: Midwifery | Nurse Midwives | Obstetric Nursing | Pregnancy | Pregnancy Complications | BISAC: MEDICAL / Nursing / Maternity, Perinatal, Women's Health
Classification: LCC RG950 (print) | LCC RG950 (ebook) | NLM WY 157 | DDC 618.2--dc23/eng/20230429
LC record available at https://lccn.loc.gov/2022050000
LC ebook record available at https://lccn.loc.gov/2022050001

6048
Printed in the United States of America
28 27 26 25 24    10 9 8 7 6 5 4 3 2

# Dedication

For midwives, student midwives, and all those who provide person-centered, evidence-based health care. Our profession and our world are improved by your devotion.

# Brief Contents

# Contents

# Preface

In this edition, the lead editors, Julia Phillippi and Ira Kantrowitz-Gordon, worked closely with a team of section editors—Mary Barger (primary care), Melissa Avery (sexual, gynecologic, and reproductive health), Nicole Carlson (intrapartum), Pam Reis (newborn), and Tekoa King (anatomy and physiology)—to engage with new and established authors and update this foundational text to meet the needs of current midwifery learners.

The Hallmarks of Midwifery and the current needs of those persons seeking midwifery care have been forefront in our minds in preparing this edition. We have attempted to weave information about how structural and social determinants of health affect health outcomes. We have strived to incorporate an antiracism approach to promote health equity. Many of our examples focus on the experiences of Black women in the United States, as they have been subjected to widespread inequities across history, and immediate action is needed to improve health equity. More broadly, a thorough understanding of how structural and social forces affect the well-being and health of individuals is essential for providing midwifery care that is appropriately tailored to all clients. This framing is useful for recognizing and acting on health inequities locally and across the globe. Because of historical and current inequities, midwives need to listen and act on the health concerns of racialized and marginalized individuals.

In this edition, we provide learners with a wide variety of sources to explore the rich histories and contexts of midwifery. While we provide suggestions for starting sources to ground the learner, we want readers to be able to see the diversity of midwifery and find histories that resonate with their own identities and planned practice locations and populations.

Throughout this text, we have also moved toward gender-neutral language in this edition to be inclusive of all individuals receiving midwifery care. We have also infused content about care to individuals across the spectrum of gender expression and physical anatomy throughout the chapters and appendices. When reporting results from the literature, we have strived to accurately represent the populations studied. If a study included only women, it would be inaccurate to generalize the findings to all adults. Similarly, we have moved toward descriptive terms for anatomy and skills rather nomenclature focused on the names of individuals who first described the body part or skill in Western literature (e.g., *oviducts* or *uterine* tubes instead of *fallopian tubes*).

We have added a chapter on sexuality to this edition to better prepare learners to provide holistic midwifery care. This content is essential for providing comprehensive sexual and reproductive health care, as learners need information about the relationships between sexuality, sexual behaviors, and well-being. In addition, sexuality is often a component of family building and important in person-centered care, especially for fertility care and in supporting family and interpersonal relationships.

Clinical practice is rapidly evolving. Midwifery has always focused on person-centered care within the context of the individual, family, and community. We have worked to be more inclusive in supporting the health and self-identified needs of individuals across the lifespan. As midwifery has expanded, we have expanded the text's content on methods for mitigating clinician bias, fertility treatments, pregnancy loss, and abortion, among others. The knowledge, skills, and abilities needed by midwives have changed to meet the needs of individuals seeking midwifery care. In this new edition, we have attempted to demonstrate the great potential for midwifery to be inclusive and welcoming. We also recognize that midwifery and this text, despite their imperfections, continue to evolve. It is our hope that this text will give learners the knowledge and skills needed to enhance and enrich the lives of those whom they serve and the midwifery profession as a whole.

—*Julia C. Phillippi and*
*Ira Kantrowitz-Gordon*

# Acknowledgments

There is so much to acknowledge as each text, each edition, is a team effort, the result of the work of so many individuals and moments of growth and collaboration. First, I want to acknowledge my family, who encouraged my dreams; without them, entering into the midwifery profession would never have been a possibility for me. I am indebted to the wonderful midwives who midwifed me, holding my hands to catch babies (such as Jill Alliman), teaching me to mentor others (Margaret McGill and Mavis Schorn), and supporting me in writing and editing (Francie Likis and Tekoa King). I am so grateful you made room for me in this profession and work. The individuals I have served have taught me so much; it has been such an honor to be welcomed into your sacred moments. The students I have mentored have been a constant source of drive to present the most up-to-date and person-centered approaches to midwifery care: I cannot express how proud I am of the great care you provide. Working with the incredible editors and authors on this edition has been a highlight of my career. They have been so deliberate in working on this foundational text to improve our approach and advance our profession. And to David, August, Sarah, and Benjamin, I am grateful for your steadfast support and the myriad ways you propel and sustain me on our journeys.

—*Julia C. Phillippi*

My midwifery career has taken me in unexpected and exciting directions, yet I never imagined that I would one day help develop the next edition of *Varney's Midwifery*. I am fortunate to have worked with so many supportive, hard-working, and dedicated midwives and nurses over the course of my career and most recently during the long labor to birth this new edition. I am grateful to the midwives who shared their wisdom and patience when I was a student and throughout my career as a midwife. Among the many, a few deserve special mention: Marjorie Smith, who showed me how to provide quiet and gentle support while keeping the patient at the center; Aileen MacLaren, who believed in me as a student and as a colleague; and Tekoa King and Francie Likis, who mentored me as an author and editor. I am especially grateful to Sharona, who has been my support every step of the way, and to my children, Maayan, Moshe, Raquel, and Yael, who make it all worthwhile and never dull. My mother, Betty Kantrowitz, zichronah livracha, passed away before this edition was complete. As a high school mathematics teacher, she was a role model for excellence in teaching and engagement of students in active learning. I miss you every day.

—*Ira Kantrowitz-Gordon*

# Contributors

Amy Alspaugh, PhD, CNM
University of Tennessee
Knoxville, Tennessee

Alexis Dunn Amore, PhD, CNM, FACNM, FAAN
Emory University
Atlanta, Georgia

Melissa D. Avery, PhD, CNM, FACNM, FAAN
*Journal of Midwifery & Women's Health*
Silver Spring, Maryland

Victoria L. Baker, PhD, CNM, PhD, CPH
Nica Family Support, LLC
Arvada, Colorado

Ana Sofia Barber de Brito, MSN, CNM
Brown University
Providence, Rhode Island

Mary K. Barger, PhD, MPH, CNM, FACNM
University of California, San Francisco
San Diego, California

Tracey Bell, NNP-BC, DNP
Emory University
Atlanta, Georgia

Amanda D. Boys, DNP, CNM, WHNP-BC
Ascension St. Vincent
Anderson, Indiana

Heather M. Bradford, PhD, CNM, FACNM
Georgetown University
Kirkland, Washington
Vanderbilt University
Nashville, Tennessee

Jessica Brumley, PhD, CNM, FACNM
University of South Florida
Tampa, Florida

Rebecca Huffer Burpo, DNP, CNM, FACNM
Texas Tech University
Lubbock, Texas

Lucinda Canty, PhD, CNM, FACNM
University of Massachusetts Amherst
Amherst, Massachusetts

Nicole Carlson, PhD, CNM, FACNM, FAAN
Emory University
Atlanta, Georgia

Melody J. Castillo, MSN, CNM, FNP-C
Golden Valley Health Centers
Merced, California

Anne Z. Cockerham, PhD, CNM, WHNP-BC,
  CNE, FACNM
Frontier Nursing University
Versailles, Kentucky

Kathleen Danhausen, MSN, MPH, CNM
Vanderbilt University
Vanderbilt University Medical Center
Nashville, Tennessee

Katie DePalma, DNP, CNM, WHNP-BC, FACNM
Georgetown University
Washington, DC

Melissa G. Davis, DNP, CNM, FNP, FACNM
Vanderbilt University
Vanderbilt University Medical Center
Nashville, Tennessee

Stephanie DeVane-Johnson, PhD, CNM, FACNM
Vanderbilt University
Nashville, Tennessee

Hannah Diaz, DNP, CNM, FACNM
Vanderbilt University
Vanderbilt University Medical Center
Nashville, Tennessee

Debora M. Dole, PhD, CNM, FACNM
Georgetown University
Washington, DC

Meghan Eagen-Torkko, PhD, CNM, FACNM
University of Washington
Bothell, Washington
Public Health Seattle–King County
Seattle, Washington

Esther R. Ellsworth Bowers, MSN, MS, MEd,
    CNM, WHNP
North Country HealthCare
Flagstaff, Arizona
Georgetown University
Washington, DC

Debra A. Erickson-Owens, PhD, CNM, FACNM,
    FAAN
University of Rhode Island
Kingston, Rhode Island

Melicia Escobar, DNP, CNM WHNP-BC, FACNM
Georgetown University
Washington, DC

Jenifer O. Fahey, PhD, CNM, FACNM
University of Maryland
Baltimore, Maryland

Eva Fried, DNP, CNM, WHNP
University of Cincinnati
Cincinnati, Ohio

Vanessa R. Garcia, MSN, CNM, WHNP-BC,
    IBCLC
Enloe Medical Center
Chico, California
University of California at San Francisco
San Francisco, California

Ami L. Goldstein, MSN, CNM, FNP
University of North Carolina
Chapel Hill, North Carolina

Nikia D. Grayson, DNP, MPH, MA, CNM, FNP-C,
    FACNM
Choices Memphis Center for Reproductive Health
Memphis, Tennessee

Pandora T. Hardtman, DNP, CNM, FACNM
Jhpiego
Baltimore, Maryland

Sharon L. Holley, DNP, CNM, FACNM, FAAN
University of Alabama at Birmingham,
Birmingham, Alabama

Abigail Howe-Heyman, PhD, CNM
University of Pennsylvania
Philadelphia, Pennsylvania

Linda A. Hunter, EdD, CNM, FACNM
Brown University
Providence, Rhode Island
Journal of Midwifery & Women's Health
Silver Spring, Maryland

Deborah Karsnitz, DNP, CNM, CNE, FACNM
Frontier Nursing University
Versailles, Kentucky

Ira Kantrowitz-Gordon, PhD, CNM, FACNM,
    FAAN
University of Washington School of Nursing
Seattle, Washington
Journal of Midwifery & Women's Health
Silver Spring, Maryland

Amy Kayler, MSN, CNM, FNP
Pediatrix Medical Group
Atlanta, Georgia

Julia Lange Kessler, DNP, CM, FACNM
Georgetown University
Washington, DC

Tekoa L. King, MPH, CNM, FACNM
Oakland, California
University of California at San Francisco
San Francisco, California

Melissa E. Kitzman, MSN, CNM, WHNP
M Health Fairview
Minneapolis, Minnesota
Georgetown University
Washington, DC

Julie Knutson, DNP, CNM, WHNP, FACNM
Brown University
Providence, Rhode Island

Jan M. Kriebs, MSN, CNM, FACNM
Thomas Jefferson University
Philadelphia, Pennsylvania

Gwen Latendresse, PhD, CNM, FACNM, FAAN
University of Utah
Salt Lake City, Utah

**Jain Lattes, MSN, CNM, PMHNP**
Baystate Medical Center
University of Massachusetts
Springfield, Massachusetts

**Nigel Lee, PhD, CNM**
University of Queensland
St Lucia, Queensland, Australia

**Miriam E. Levi, DNP, CNM, FNP, WHNP, IBCLC, MBA**
Mayo Clinic
Rochester, Minnesota

**Amy Marowitz, DNP, CNM, CNE**
Frontier Nursing University
Versailles, Kentucky

**Lena B. Mårtensson, PhD, CNM**
University of Skövde
Skövde, Sweden
University of Queensland
Brisbane, Queensland, Australia

**Linda McDaniel, DNP, CNM, RNFA, FACNM**
Frontier Nursing University
Versailles, Kentucky

**Judith S. Mercer, PhD, CNM, FACNM**
University of Rhode Island
Kingston, Rhode Island

**Elizabeth G. Muñoz, DNP, CNM, FACNM**
University of Alabama at Birmingham
Birmingham, Alabama
Carle Midwifery Services
Urbana, Illinois

**Jeremy L. Neal, PhD, CNM, FACNM**
Vanderbilt University
Nashville, Tennessee

**Signey Olson, DNP, CNM, WHNP-BC, FACNM**
Georgetown University
Signey Olson Health, LLC
Washington, DC

**Kathryn Osborne, PhD, CNM**
Rush University
Chicago, Illinois

**Julia C. Phillippi, PhD, CNM, FACNM, FAAN**
Vanderbilt University
Nashville, Tennessee

**Bunny Pounds, DNP, FNP-BC**
Frontier Nursing University
Versailles, Kentucky

**Barbara J. Reale, DNP, CNM, FACNM**
Thomas Jefferson University
Philadelphia, Pennsylvania

**Pamela J. Reis, PhD, CNM, NNP-BC, FACNM**
East Carolina University
Greenville, North Carolina

**Leissa Roberts, DNP, CNM, FACNM**
University of Texas, UT Health
Houston, Texas

**Melissa A. Saftner, PhD, CNM, FACNM**
University of Minnesota
Minneapolis, Minnesota

**Bethany Sanders, PhD(c), CNM, FACNM**
Vanderbilt University Medical Center
Vanderbilt University
Nashville, Tennessee

**Alice R. Sattler, MSN, CNM**
Planned Parenthood of Greater Washington and
    North Idaho
Ellensburg, Washington

**Robyn Schafer, PhD, CNM, IBCLC, CNE, FACNM**
Rutgers University
Newark, New Jersey

**Mavis N. Schorn, PhD, CNM, CNE, FACNM, FNAP, FAAN**
Vanderbilt University
Nashville, Tennessee

**Julia S. Seng, PhD, CNM, FACNM, FAAN**
University of Michigan School of Nursing
Ann Arbor, Michigan

**Erin E. Sing, DNP, CNM, FACNM**
Texas Tech University
Lubbock, Texas

**Emily S. Slocum, MSN, CNM**
Vanderbilt University
Nashville, Tennessee

**Melan J. Smith-Francis, DNP, CNM, FNP-C**
Vanderbilt University
Nashville, Tennessee

**Ellen Solis, DNP, CNM, FACNM**
University of Washington
Seattle, Washington

**Lisa A. Spencer, MSN, CNM, WHNP**
University of Maryland
Baltimore, Maryland

**Stephanie Tillman, MSN, CNM, FACNM**
Feminist Midwife, LLC
Chicago, Illinois

**Shaughanassee Vines, DNP, CNM, CNE, FACNM**
Frontier Nursing University
Versailles, Kentucky

**Katie Ward, DNP, WHNP**
University of Utah
Salt Lake City, Utah

**Kate Woeber, PhD, MPH, CNM, FACNM**
University of Nevada
Las Vegas, Nevada

**Andrea Zengion, MS, ND, CNM, WHNP-BC, LAc**
Swedish Midwifery
Seattle, Washington
University of California at San Francisco
San Francisco, California

**Ruth E. Zielinski, PhD, CNM, FACNM, FAAN**
University of Michigan
Ann Arbor, Michigan

# About the Editors

**Julia C. Phillippi, PhD, CNM, FACNM, FAAN,** earned a bachelor of arts degree from Maryville College, a master of science degree from Vanderbilt University, and a PhD in nursing from University of Tennessee Knoxville. She has been active in midwifery practice, teaching, and research; over the course of her career, she has provided midwifery services in homes, birth centers, and hospitals in both rural and urban areas. She has been a midwifery educator for 18 years and currently serves as professor of nursing at Vanderbilt University School of Nursing. Her research has been funded by the Agency for Healthcare Research and Quality, the National Institute of Child Health and Human Development, and the National Institute of Nursing Research, among others. She has publications in a variety of perinatal journals and has made numerous presentations at midwifery and health services–related conferences. Her awards include the American College of Nurse-Midwives Foundation Excellence in Teaching and Kitty Ernst Awards, March of Dimes of Middle Tennessee Nurse Researcher of the Year, and Outstanding Peer Reviewer and Best Review Article from the *Journal of Midwifery & Women's Health*. She has been an associate editor for the *Journal of Midwifery & Women's Health* since 2019. She is a fellow of the American College of Nurse-Midwives and American Academy of Nursing.

**Ira Kantrowitz-Gordon, PhD, CNM, FACNM, FAAN,** earned a bachelor of science degree in biology from Brown University, a bachelor of science degree in nursing and a master's degree in nursing from University of Washington, and a PhD in nursing from Washington State University. He has been active in midwifery practice, teaching, and research for many years. He has been a midwifery educator for 14 years and is currently an associate professor of nursing at University of Washington School of Nursing. His research focuses on mindfulness interventions during pregnancy and early parenting, reducing the stigma of perinatal opioid disorder, and increasing workforce diversity in midwifery and biomedical science. He has published in midwifery, nursing, and multidisciplinary journals. His awards include the American College of Nurse-Midwives Foundation Excellence in Teaching and Outstanding Peer Reviewer from the *Journal of Midwifery & Women's Health*. He has been a deputy editor for the *Journal of Midwifery & Women's Health* since 2021 and is a member of the Maternal Mortality Review Panel for Washington State. He is a fellow of the American College of Nurse-Midwives and American Academy of Nursing.

## Section Editors

### Newborn

**Pamela J. Reis, PhD, CNM, NNP-BC, FACNM,** earned a bachelor of science degree in nursing from Duke University, a master of science degree in nursing and post-master's certificate in nurse-midwifery from East Carolina University, and a PhD in nursing from East Carolina University in Greenville, North Carolina. She was a neonatal nurse practitioner for 10 years and has been active in midwifery practice, teaching, and research for more than 30 years. Her research focuses on advanced practice nursing workforce issues, and she is the project director of a grant funded by the Health Resources Services Administration for a primary care training program for advanced practice registered nurses. She serves as an associate editor and peer reviewer for the *Journal of Midwifery & Women's Health*. Her awards include the American College of Nurse-Midwives Foundation Excellence in Teaching Award and the Dorothea Lang Pioneer Award. She is a fellow of the American College of Nurse-Midwives.

## Anatomy and Physiology

**Tekoa L. King, CNM, MPH, FACNM,** earned a bachelor of science degree from the University of California at San Francisco (UCSF), a master of public health degree from the University of California, Berkeley, and midwifery certification from Georgetown University. She was a member of an interprofessional collaborative practice with maternal–fetal medicine physicians at UCSF, where she practiced clinically and participated in teaching medical students and obstetric residents for many years. From 1985 to 2021, she was the co-chair of UCSF's annual Antepartum and Intrapartum Management continuing education conference. During her tenure at UCSF, she participated in the National Institute of Child Health and Human Development expert panels and subsequent publications on fetal heart rate monitoring and vaginal birth after cesarean section, and was a member of the Centers for Disease Control and Prevention working group that published national guidelines for group B *Streptococcus* prophylaxis from 1996 to 2010. She was the editor-in-chief of the *Journal of Midwifery & Women's Health* from 2001 to 2006, then deputy editor until 2021. She was also the senior editor of the fifth and sixth editions of *Varney's Midwifery* and co-editor of the first and second editions of *Pharmacology for Women's Health*. She has multiple publications, both peer-reviewed journals and book chapters, and has represented the American College of Nurse-Midwives as liaison to the American College of Obstetricians and Gynecologists (ACOG) Committee on Obstetric Practice, wherein she contributed to the development of several ACOG Committee Opinions. Her awards include the American College of Nurse-Midwives Lifetime Achievement Award, the *American Journal of Nursing* Book of the Year award, and Best Review Article from the *Journal of Midwifery & Women's Health*. She is a fellow of the American College of Nurse-Midwives.

## Intrapartum

**Nicole S. Carlson, PhD, CNM, FACNM, FAAN,** earned a bachelor of science degree in biology, anthropology and nursing from Emory University, a master of science degree from Oregon Health and Science University, and a PhD in nursing from University of Colorado Denver. She conducts research on the biological mechanisms of labor, and strategies for achieving optimal perinatal outcomes and decreasing racial disparities, including midwife-led care. She has received support for her research from the National Institutes of Health, the March of Dimes, and the American College of Nurse-Midwives (ACNM), and was awarded Best Research and Review article and Best Research Podium awards by ACNM and the *Journal of Midwifery & Women's Health*. She led a team of nurse-midwife scholars to produce the first ACNM Clinical Bulletin on labor induction and was the sole nurse and nurse-midwife technical expert for a systematic review on outpatient cervical ripening conducted by the Agency for Healthcare Research and Quality's Effective Health Care workgroup. Her work with large national data sets to reveal strategies for decreasing cesarean birth and postpartum maternal morbidity was recognized by awards from the Eunice Kennedy Shriver National Institute of Child Health and Human Development and citation in the Centers for Medicare and Medicaid Service's Recommendations for Maternal Health. She has practiced clinically for more than 20 years, serving birthing people in both hospital and birth center settings, and contributed to the education of many nurse-midwives over the past decade. She is a fellow of the ACNM and the American Academy of Nursing.

## Primary Care

**Mary K. Barger, PhD, MPH, CNM, FACNM,** earned a bachelor's degree in nursing from Stanford University, a master of public health in maternal–child health/nurse-midwifery from Johns Hopkins School of Public Health, and a doctorate in epidemiology from Boston University. Although recently retired, she practiced full-scope midwifery for more than 30 years, caring for a wide spectrum of patients. She has taught for 40 years in schools of public health, medicine, and nursing. Her research interests center on maternal morbidity and mortality and issues related to sleep and women's health. She has more than 40 peer-reviewed publications and published chapters in several textbooks. She has served on the American Midwifery Certification Board and the American College of Nurse-Midwives Fellows Board of Governors. Her awards include the American College of Nurse-Midwives Foundation's Excellence in Teaching and the Dorothea Lang Pioneer Awards, California Nurse-Midwives Association Pioneer and Research Awards, Outstanding Peer

Reviewer Award, and the Association of Teachers of Maternal and Child Health Loretta Lacey Award for Maternal and Child Health Academic Leadership.

## Sexual, Gynecologic, and Reproductive Health Care

**Melissa D. Avery, PhD, CNM, FACNM, FAAN,** earned her bachelor of science degree from Northern Illinois University, her master of science degree from the University of Kentucky, and her PhD in nursing at the University of Minnesota (UMN). She practiced full-scope midwifery for 25 years and directed the UMN nurse-midwifery education program for 24 years, leading funded projects to develop quality hybrid-distance education programs and simulation experiences. Her research has been funded by multiple agencies and examined exercise in pregnancy, breastfeeding, and confidence for physiological labor and birth. In addition to published articles, she has published two edited/co-edited books. Most recently, Dr. Avery was co-principal investigator of a nationally funded, multisite project launched by the American College of Nurse-Midwives (ACNM) and the American College of Obstetricians and Gynecologists, which aimed to develop resources and examine interprofessional education among midwifery students and obstetrics and gynecology residents. Her awards include the *American Journal of Nursing* Book of the Year Award, Maternal–Child Health Category (with co-author Linda Cole, DNP, CNM), and induction into the UMN Academic Health Center Academy of Excellence in the Scholarship of Teaching and Learning. Dr. Avery is currently Professor Emeritus at the UMN School of Nursing and editor-in-chief of the *Journal of Midwifery & Women's Health*. She is a fellow in ACNM and the American Academy of Nursing, and a past president of ACNM.

# I

# Midwifery

CHAPTER

# 1

# Context of Individuals Seeking Midwifery Care

LUCINDA CANTY

## Introduction

Midwives serve the full spectrum of humanity. They aim to provide care that is holistic, values individuals and their needs and preferences, and acknowledges the myriad factors that shape individuals' health and preferences for care. While midwives serve people as individuals, the influences on their health span beyond the clinical encounter. One of the most important influences on perinatal health is the society in which an individual is born, lives, and functions. Midwifery care involves going beyond the clinical aspects of care to understand and address the various social and structural factors that influence health outcomes.

All people are born into a larger society and environment that affects all aspects of their lives from the time they are conceived until their last breath. Midwives need to be aware that the health of the people whom they serve is intertwined with the effects of past and current societal and structural burdens. Midwives need to be knowledgeable and aware of the challenges and to understand how historically midwifery care addressed those challenges to improve the health and well-being of populations.

Many chapters in this text discuss factors that affect health. For example, the text includes chapters discussing nutrition, genetics, anatomy, exercise, and pathogens. While these topics are certainly integral to an understanding of perinatal health, this chapter focuses on the larger societal and structural factors that influence the health of individuals. Indeed, midwives across history have understood and acted on social determinants of health before this term was formally conceptualized. Midwives have a long history of providing care in communities that are marginalized, and plagued by racism, poverty, socioeconomic barriers, and structural barriers.

For midwives, our understanding of our identity as "midwife" allows us to situate ourselves into a position to address the healthcare needs of those who seek midwifery care and, more broadly, to improve health within the communities we serve. This text provides foundational knowledge for the essential role of midwives in our healthcare systems.

The topics presented in this chapter include some examples of well-known disparities in health care. Although it addresses just a few of the many social determinants of health, this content can serve as a foundation to help midwives identify learning needed to provide quality healthcare services to persons from all cultures and populations.

Midwives are integral to the communities they serve, and particularly to marginalized and vulnerable communities. Their knowledge of the culture, its history, and the challenges that influence healthcare delivery, utilization of healthcare services, and health outcomes is important to improve the healthcare system as a whole. The care midwives provide is shaped by their efforts to learn what individuals and communities need to maintain their health and wellness.

Familiarity with the various factors that create barriers and prevent individuals from maintaining their health, quality of life, and well-being is essential to midwifery practice. If midwives develop a thorough understanding of how social determinants of health and structural factors, such as racism and implicit bias, contribute to disparities in health outcomes, then they will be better equipped to address those barriers and promote health equity.

3

## Social and Structural Determinants of Health

The term *social determinants of health* (SDoH) is used to describe a wide range of factors that impact health. Over the last two decades, public health, medical, nursing, and midwifery researchers have made significant advances in understanding the effects of historical, social, political, and socioeconomic factors on individual and population health. The Centers for Disease Control and Prevention (CDC) defines SDoH as "conditions in the environments in which people are born, live, learn, work, play, worship, and age."[1] These factors can either promote good health or contribute to poor health. Research about SDoH has demonstrated that unequal distribution of power, money, and resources underlies the differences that contribute to disparities in health outcomes.[2] Because these forces are social, political, cultural, and economic in nature, clinical care alone cannot address the causes of these disparities. Consistent with the Hallmarks of Midwifery, attention to equity and justice in the context of policy, structure, and culture changes is required to address and eliminate these inequities.

As system-level factors, SDoH are deeply embedded in the larger society and shape the distribution of power and resources. The structural elements of society manifest as institutional policies and procedures, cultural norms, legal justice systems, and laws.[3] Thus, the structures that are currently in place have a long history and are manifestations of societal beliefs.

Emerging theoretical frameworks provide a broader understanding of SDoH by including structural determinants of health to elucidate the root causes of inequities. These frameworks reinforce the value of looking beyond the individual risk factors that cause racial disparities in maternal and infant health to understanding the "historical, systemic, structural, and political forces that created them."[3] Restoring Our Own Through Transformation (ROOTT), created by Jessica Roach in 2016, is an example of one such theoretical framework.[4] ROOTT explains the web of causation between structural and social determinants of health and their influences on maternal and infant health outcomes.[3,4]

It is essential for midwives to understand the root causes of health disparities and to position themselves to improve the quality of care they provide and use their power and privileges to create change and protect the most vulnerable members of society. These actions require midwives to recognize the influences of social and structural determinants as well as injustice, and to challenge these systems and provide care to women in spite of these injustices. Achieving the desired outcomes through action requires an understanding of SDoH so as to provide high-quality care to all persons, including those from underserved communities.[5] Facilitation of positive change also requires midwives to move beyond biologic and moral assumptions about groups of individuals, and to use research and community engagement to inform midwifery education and practice.[6]

Midwives have a long history of recognizing and addressing social and structural determinants of health. Long before the SDoH term was coined, midwives worked as general healers within their communities, with their services encompassing both public health and preventive health perspectives.[7]

While it is important to examine the influence of social and structural determinants of health in midwifery care, it is also crucial to examine the structures of oppression associated with health disparities, which all too frequently impact our most vulnerable communities.[3] Doing so requires midwives to move beyond making biologic and moral assumptions about groups of individuals and instead use research to inform midwifery education and practice.[6]

## Definitions of Race and Ethnicity

Race is a social construct; it has no genetic foundation. A person's race does not provide substantive genetic information about the individual, nor does it offer an account of the individual's ancestry or culture.[8,9] Race can be defined in multiple ways. In the United States, skin color is a physical trait often used to define race. Other categories are ambiguously defined based on the geographic location of ancestral origin. Migration of groups of people across time, however, means that this categorization has nebulous value.

To understand racial disparities, examination of the classification of race is foundational. *Merriam-Webster Dictionary* defines race as "any one of the groups that humans are often divided into based on physical traits regarded as common among people of shared ancestry."[10] Race has deep historical origins in the United States. Indeed, racial categories were established several hundred years ago and have long been used as criteria for discrimination.

Ethnicity is defined as a shared lifestyle informed by cultural, historical, religious, and/or national affiliations.[11] The U.S. Census recognizes only two ethnic categories: Hispanic and non-Hispanic. Other organizations around the world, such as those in Asia and Africa, often acknowledge more than 100 ethnic groups. A key problem that arises with reliance on limited ethnicity categories is erasure of ethnic identity when the available categories do not capture someone's identity.

An increasing number of people have genetic and cultural backgrounds that span multiple groups. Not everyone fits neatly into the narrowly defined categories, particularly those from multiple racial or ethnic groups. Many forms, such as the standard U.S. birth certificate, now allow individuals to select multiple categories when identifying their race and ethnicity.

Individuals should always be allowed to self-identify their race and ethnicity. In the past, individuals were often placed into racial or ethnic categories at the discretion of an observer. To *racialize* is to assign someone to a racial category based on their physical or historical characteristics. The (often erroneous) assignment of race and ethnicity to an individual without their input still occurs in many settings and is a component of explicit and implicit bias.

Both racial and ethnic categories are problematic ways to identify people. Currently, the primary value of these categories lies in grouping people according to their likely exposure to societal privilege or marginalization/racism. However, even this application has limitations that may obscure the overall impact of racism and xenophobia in the United States. For instance, Muslim women who cover their hair often experience bias and discrimination, yet they are often classified as non-Hispanic and white in terms of their race/ethnicity. Similarly, these categories do not allow differentiation of individuals with a genetic background from the Indian continent from those with ancestors from the area now known as China, but experiences of discrimination in the United States have clearly varied between these groups.

The current categorizations of individuals using census and birth certificate data on race and ethnicity are limited and do not reliably reflect either genetics or geographic origin. However, they are one of only a few widely collected markers available for measuring the effects of social and structural determinants of health. This text uses these terms when they have value in discussions

of health as measures of societal categorization, but not as signifiers of genetic characteristics. Midwives need to be careful with how race and ethnicity data are used because they could perpetuate stereotypes and misinformation about the causes or risk factors for certain health conditions or health outcomes.

### Racism

Racism has been described as "an organized social system in which the dominant racial group, based on an ideology of inferiority, categorizes, and ranks people into social groups called 'races' and uses its power to devalue, disempower, and differentially allocate valued societal resources and opportunities to groups defined as inferior."[12(p106)] In 2000, Dr. Camara Jones, a physician, epidemiologist, and antiracism activist, published the groundbreaking work *Levels of Racism: A Theoretic Framework and a Gardener's Tale*. In it, Jones noted, "The variable 'race' is not a biological construct that reflects innate differences, but a social construct that precisely captures the impacts of racism."[8(p1212)]

Four levels of racism can be distinguished in our society: personally mediated, internalized, institutional, and structural. *Personally mediated racism* involves prejudice and discrimination on the individual level. Prejudice is "differential assumptions about the abilities, motives, and intentions of others according to their race," whereas discrimination is "differential actions toward others according to their race."[8(p1212)] This level of racism encompasses conscious and unconscious or implicit bias, and often manifests as disrespect, devaluation, and dehumanization.

*Internalized racism* is defined as "acceptance by members of the stigmatized races of negative messages about their own abilities and intrinsic worth."[8(p1212)] Those who experience internalized racism accept negative stereotypes about their racial or ethnic group. Internalized racism can have a significant impact on health behaviors and individuals' perception of a lack of control over their treatment in the healthcare system.

*Structural/institutionalized racism* goes beyond personally mediated and internalized practices to the larger society and refers to the way racism becomes deeply embedded in society via laws, structures, and norms.[8,13] The structural/institutionalized forms of racism are "codified in our institutions of custom, practice, and law, so there need not to be an identifiable perpetrator"[8(p1212)] Structures operate daily and determine access to resources, power, and opportunities based on racialized identity. Thus, structural racism integrates levels of discrimination that have permeated everyday life structures in the United States, and that disadvantage people of color and place them at higher risk for poor health outcomes compared to their white counterparts.[13]

All forms of racism place individuals at risk for poor health outcomes and may have long-lasting effects on physical and mental well-being. Weathering is one concept believed to explain why Black women are at increased risk for poor maternal health outcomes compared to white women. This conceptual framework explains the effects of chronic stress related to social inequalities due to racism and the influence on perinatal health outcomes.[14,15] The process of weathering increases risk for poor infant health outcomes, such as low birth weight, preterm births, and infant mortality.[14,15]

If midwives focus on understanding the experience of racialized people in the healthcare system, they can start to understand the individual and structural factors that place people at increased risk for poor health outcomes. All individuals are at different stages of learning about and understanding racism and bias and how it impacts individuals and midwifery care. From the midwife's perspective, it is important to acknowledge that bias still exists within the healthcare system and continues to cause harm. This requires critical self-reflection and acknowledgment that personal and societal biases are embedded deep within our society and have long been part of both midwifery history and the U.S. healthcare system. When midwives have a deep understanding of racism, going beyond just the simple definition of this term, they can begin to change the structures that contribute to poor health outcomes for individuals of color.

Race can influence how individuals are viewed by healthcare providers and may play a role in the quality of care they receive. Notably, even when socioeconomic status (SES), onset of prenatal care, and comorbidities are controlled for, racial and ethnic disparities in maternal health continue to exist.[16-21] Racism has been shown to create power imbalances influencing health education, treatment options, and whether individuals feel vulnerable and traumatized by the care they received.[22-24] Racism exhibited by healthcare providers can leave individuals feeling unseen, afraid, disrespected, and in environments where they are unsafe, placing them at risk for poor health outcomes. Individuals of color are more likely than their white counterparts to experience maltreatment during childbirth, including violent behavior, such as yelling, being ignored, or being dismissed.[25] Black and Indigenous birthing people are more likely to "report high levels of mistrust, experiences of disrespect, and lack of autonomy when receiving prenatal care" as compared to white people.[26] Discrimination can decrease a person's sense of belonging, dissuade someone from utilizing healthcare services that they need, and result in resistance, mistrust, and distrust.[27]

Racialized identity is a significant factor in how individuals present and are treated in the healthcare system. Thus, it is inaccurate to assume that race alone places Black and Indigenous people at risk for dying from a pregnancy-related cause. Racism—not race—places birthing people of color at risk for poor maternal health outcomes.[28-31] Healthcare providers who do not critically examine the role of societal racism may blame racialized people for their own health outcomes.[32]

## Implicit Bias

Implicit bias, also known as unconscious bias, comprises learned stereotypes that are automatic, unintentional, and deeply ingrained, and that influence behavior.[33] These assumptions about social identities, even without our conscious awareness of them, shape our likes, dislikes, and judgments about a person or a community. Such assumptions arise due to a lifetime of repeated exposure to attitudes, images, and ideas about age, gender, race, ethnicity, religion, social class, sexuality, disability status, and nationality that are not based on factual or accurate information. They unconsciously influence our behavior during interactions with others and could be harmful and disruptive to establishing an excellent healthcare provider–patient relationship.[34]

Implicit bias reinforces stereotypes and contributes to disparities in healthcare delivery, resulting in unequal access to quality healthcare services and preventable poor health outcomes.[33] It can create an environment in which individuals feel they are not seen, heard, or valued, leading to feelings of distrust. Implicit bias can place individuals in midwifery care in unsafe situations and prevents them from receiving the care they need. Although implicit bias is unconscious, it can still cause harm and contribute to negative experiences in healthcare encounters and preventable complications.

Implicit bias can influence decisions made in the delivery of health care. For example, research has demonstrated racial disparities in pain assessment and treatment of pain during the postpartum period.[35,36] Specifically, white women had more documented pain assessments compared to Black and Hispanic women; Black and Hispanic women reported higher pain scores than white women and received fewer opioids compared to white women; and Black and Hispanic women were less likely to receive opioid prescriptions at discharge even after having a cesarean birth.[35,36] If the midwife unconsciously believes that someone does not understand or feel pain, they may not fully evaluate the person or counsel them about all possible treatment options.[35,36]

Implicit bias can have a harmful effect by influencing how individuals seek and utilize healthcare services. As an example, suppose a pregnant American Indian person enters the healthcare system for prenatal care. Although the individual does not have a history of alcohol use or substance misuse, the healthcare provider might ask them several times about the last time that they used drugs or drank alcohol, even examining their arms for signs of intravenous drug use.[37] The pregnant individual may feel as if their provider does not believe them, leading to feeling that they are not believed or valued by the healthcare provider. In consequence, they may not return for another prenatal visit to avoid being mistreated.

It may be challenging for midwives to recognize how implicit bias could impact the midwifery care they provide. Recognizing the existence of one's implicit biases is a useful starting point, but ongoing self-education about the nature of bias is key to minimizing the harmful effects of implicit bias.[33] Midwives can learn and evolve from their own biases. This process starts with midwives questioning their own assumptions about the individuals who seek midwifery care. Several resources are available that encourage self-reflection on biases, such as Project Implicit's Interactive-Race Implicit Association Test.[38]

## Health Disparities

Health disparities are differences in health outcomes and the determinants of those outcomes between groups within a population, as defined by social, demographic, environmental, and geographic attributes.[2] Health disparities can be seen in the prevalence of diseases, mortality rates, morbidity rates, and rates of survival. For example, infant mortality rates among American Indian/Native Alaskan populations are 2.7 times higher than white infants.[39]

Health disparities are complex because numerous social and structural conditions may potentially

| Table 1-1 | Factors Associated with Health Disparities |
|---|---|
| **Factors Linked with Health Disparities** ||

Education

Citizenship, immigration/refugee status

Geographic location (i.e., local neighborhood, rural-urban continuum, state policies)

Gender identity

Language

Race/ethnicity (i.e., exposure to racism and discrimination)

Religion

Sexual orientation

Socioeconomic status (i.e., income, nutrition, housing)

Violence and trauma exposure

influence health and health outcomes. Investigation of health disparities provides a lens into the factors that disproportionately impact one group versus another. **Table 1-1** shows some factors associated with health disparities.

While health disparities are complex, some known factors that contribute to health disparities could certainly be addressed in the delivery of healthcare services. The combined effects of SDoH, healthcare provider bias, racism, and discrimination form a potent force that creates and perpetuates health disparities. Healthcare providers are sometimes unaware of the historical context that contributes to these disparities and that puts vulnerable populations at risk.[3] Understanding these factors is important to develop interventions to improve health outcomes in the populations most strongly impacted by them. Health disparities should not just be cited to quantify health outcomes, but should also be considered as providing insights into the social and structural factors that can negatively influence the health of a population.[40,41]

### Racial Disparities in Perinatal Health Outcomes

Racial/ethnic health disparities in perinatal health continue to persist in our society. Women of color, and particularly Black and Indigenous women, continue to experience disproportionately higher rates of maternal mortality; sexually transmitted infections (STIs), including human immunodeficiency

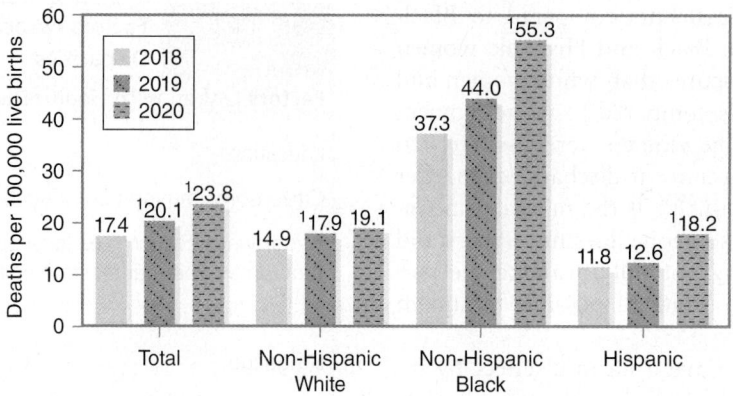

<sup>1</sup>Statistically significant increase in rate from previous year (p<0.05).
NOTE: Race groups are single race.
SOURCE: National Center for Health Statistics, National Vital Statistics System, Mortality

**Figure 1-1** Maternal mortality rates in the United States, 2019–2020.
Reproduced from Hoyert DL. Maternal mortality rates in the United States, 2020.
*NCHS Health E-Stats*. 2022. DOI: https://dx.doi.org/10.15620/cdc:113967.

virus (HIV); cervical cancer; and endometrial cancer mortality.[42,43]

Among the most noticeable disparities are racial disparities in maternal health outcomes, including maternal mortality ratios, rates of severe maternal morbidity, prematurity rates, and infant mortality. Black women are 3 to 4 times more likely to die from a pregnancy-related cause, and Indigenous women are 2 times more likely to die from such causes compared to white women. According to the CDC, the U.S. maternal mortality rate for 2020 was 23.8 deaths per 100,000 live births, up from 20.1 in 2019 (**Figure 1-1**).[44]

Some highlights of the 2019–2020 data follow: For white birthing people, the maternal mortality rate increased from 17.9 deaths per 100,000 in 2019 to 19.1 deaths per 100,000 in 2020. For Black birthing people, the rate increased from 44.0 per 100,000 in 2019 to 55.3 per 100,000 in 2020. For Hispanic birthing people, the rate increased from 12.6 per 100,000 in 2019 to 18.2 per 100,000 in 2020 (although as a group Hispanic individuals have the lowest maternal mortality rates, there was a significant increase in their rate after the start of the COVID-19 pandemic). The maternal mortality rate for American Indians has not been reported for 2020, but the rate for 2016–2018 was 26.5 deaths per 100,000 live births.[45]

Although this chapter describes just a few examples of health disparities, this content can serve as a foundation to help midwives identify learning needed to provide quality healthcare services to persons from all cultures and populations.

## What Midwives Can Do

Midwives are in a unique position to address racial and ethnic health disparities because of the way that they are situated both within the healthcare system and within the communities they serve. Social justice has a foundation in midwifery care. Midwifery focuses on bringing equitable care to some of the most vulnerable communities and improving health outcomes even when access to resources is limited.

Midwives should work to understand the larger societal and structural contexts of the individuals whom they serve. They need to be aware of the historical context that contributes to disparities and that places vulnerable populations at risk. Nevertheless, midwifery care can improve the health of individuals only when certain conditions are met. First, individuals must have access to healthcare services. Second, the care offered must be of high quality and based on evidence. Healthcare services are likely to be ineffective if the factors that affect access to and quality of care are not addressed.

Midwifery care has always been about more than just performing clinical skills: It also focuses on the physical, social, and emotional needs of the individual. Midwifery models of care that adopt a holistic approach have been shown to improve health outcomes and the experience of care among all birthing people, including those from vulnerable and marginalized communities.[46,47]

The relationship between the person seeking midwifery care and the midwife is a critical part of the experience of health care. Persons who seek midwifery care often want a meaningful relationship with their healthcare provider[48]—a relationship in which they are acknowledged and respected.[49,50] They want their healthcare provider to be attentive to their physical and emotional needs. In their experience of care, they want to feel safe and supported and trust their healthcare provider is providing care in their best interest.[23,25,51]

According to the American College of Nurse-Midwives (ACNM), the Hallmarks of Midwifery include empowering, listening to, and advocating for informed choice, shared decision making, and the right to self-determination for individuals receiving care.[5] Excellent communication is an essential component of this relationship. Midwives must arm themselves with the tools needed to provide care that meets the needs of the recipients of their care.

Provisions of health information tailored to meet the needs of the individual empowers that person to actively engage in decisions regarding their care and treatment options.[52] Part of that tailoring includes use of educational resources that are culturally appropriate in a language that is relevant to the population served.

Birthing people have reported being disrespected or even experiencing forms of violence during healthcare encounters.[51,53] Women have reported harm, such as threats, from healthcare providers when they declined treatments or procedures offered to them during childbirth.[53] In a study by Vedam and associates, 32% of Indigenous women, 25% of Hispanic women, and 22.5% of Black women reported experiencing mistreatment by healthcare providers during childbirth.[25] Women reported that care providers did not listen to them, doubted their perceptions and feelings, ignored their wishes, imposed their will on women, and made them feel guilty or like a failure.[25]

Midwives can ensure that individuals are treated with respect and dignity and receive care that addresses their healthcare needs. Person-centered care begins with learning and understanding the needs of those who seek midwifery services. Persons seeking midwifery care want to be seen as an individual; they want their experiences to be valued; and they want their culture to be acknowledged.[48,51] Midwives can provide care in environments that are free from racism and discrimination.

The ACNM's Hallmarks of Midwifery include the practice of incorporating evidence-based care into clinical encounters.[5] Midwives have a responsibility to seek knowledge that will inform clinical practice and address the unique needs of those receiving their care. A growing body of research from diverse researchers has amplified the experiences of those most impacted by health disparities and encourages development of interventions to address the needs of gender diverse individuals and communities of color. This research can be incorporated into midwifery education, practice, and health policies that influence midwifery care.

## Conclusion

Midwives have a long history of providing safe, competent, quality care to communities, particularly those that are marginalized and vulnerable. Historically, midwives understood social determinants of health and provided primary care even before those terms were formally conceptualized.

Today's midwives should understand the factors that place individuals at risk for poor health outcomes and recognize how midwifery care can address these factors. When doing so, they should be aware of their own implicit bias and aim to provide care that meets the needs of the individual at any given time.

Social and structural determinants of health are not new to midwifery, but require midwives to fully understand their role in providing care that can address factors, such as racism, that prevent individuals from receiving the midwifery care they need and that place individuals at risk. Midwives need to engage in ongoing self-reflection and evaluation of the care they provide.

Midwifery care involves empowering the individuals whom midwives serve and creating spaces where individuals feel safe, respected, listened to, and free from racism and discrimination. Midwives have the knowledge and skills to provide evidence-based and culturally appropriate care to individuals and their communities, and to create an environment that protects all community members from harm.

## Resources

| | |
|---|---|
| **American College of Nurse-Midwives (ACNM)**<br><br>Addressing Racism and Advancing Equity in Midwifery Education: A Program Content Toolkit for Action | Created by the Program Content Subgroup of the Racism in Midwifery Education Task Force. The toolkit is intended to provide faculty with resources for addressing the historical racism in American midwifery, and to prepare faculty and future midwives to be aware of racism and bias in themselves, in institutions, and in the healthcare system. |
| **ACNM History Webpage** | Contains information about ACNM's history and links to external resources. |
| **ACNM Midwives of Color Committee (MOCC) in consultation with SHIFT**<br><br>Unpacking Our Birth Bag: Anti-Racism Toolkit for Midwives | The "birth bag" is part of midwives' identity and a history inseparable from racism. This toolkit should be used to unpack racism and privilege from your "birth bag" in hopes of restoring culturally competent care and making the midwifery profession more inclusive to all. |
| **ACNM Position Statement: Racism and Racial Bias** | The ACNM is committed to eliminating racism and racial bias in the midwifery profession and race-based disparities in reproductive health care. |
| **Black Lives Matter: A Message and Resources for Midwives** | A collection of racism, antiracism, and racial equity resources for clinicians and educators, recommended by midwives of color. Resources to promote meaningful dialogue and action against racism, white supremacy, and the oppression of people of color. |
| **Black Mamas Matter Alliance (BMMA)** | A national network of Black women–led and Black-led, birth and reproductive justice organizations and multidisciplinary professionals, working across the full spectrum of maternal and reproductive health. |
| **Centers for Disease Control and Prevention**<br>HEAR HER Campaign | Resources for healthcare professionals to understand their role in eliminating preventable maternal mortality. Addresses the need to hear women's concerns during and after pregnancy and engage in an open conversation to make sure any issues are adequately addressed. |
| ***Journal of Midwifery and Women's Health***<br>Racism, Antiracism, and Racial Equity article library | This library contains articles published in *JMWH* that focus on racism, antiracism, and racial equity. |

## References

1. Centers for Disease Control and Prevention. Social determinants of health: what affects health. https://www.cdc.gov/socialdeterminants/index.htm. Published 2020. Accessed September 26, 2022.

2. Baciu A, Negussie Y, Geller A. *Communities in Action: Pathways to Health Equity*. Washington, DC: National Academies Press; 2017. doi:10.17226/24624.

3. Crear-Perry J, Correa-de-Araujo R, Lewis Johnson T, et al. Social and structural determinants of health inequities in maternal health. *J Womens Health*. 2021;30(2):230-235. doi:10.1089/jwh.2020.8882.

4. Roach J. ROOTT's theoretical framework of the web of causation between structural and social determinants of health and wellness—2016. Restoring Our Own Through Transformation (ROOTT). https://www.roottrj.org/web-causation. Published 2016. Accessed June 1, 2022.

5. American College of Nurse-Midwives. Core competencies for basic midwife practice. Basic Competency Section, Division of Advancement of Midwifery. http://www.midwife.org/acnm/files/acnmlibrarydata/uploadfilename/000000000050/ACNMCoreCompetenciesMar2020_final.pdf. Approved March 20, 2020. Accessed January 27, 2023.

6. McLemore MR, Asiodu I, Crear-Perry J, et al. Race, research, and women's health: best practice guidelines for investigators. *Obstet Gynecol*. 2019;134(2):422-423.

7. Niles PM, Drew, M. Constructing the modern American midwife: white supremacy and white feminism collide. Nursing CLIO. https://nursingclio.org/2020/10/22/constructing-the-modern-american-midwife-white-supremacy-and-white-feminism-collide/. Published 2020. Accessed January 27, 2023.

8. Jones CP. Levels of racism: a theoretic framework and a gardener's tale. *Am J Public Health.* 2000;90(8): 1212-1215.

9. Mwilu J. Race vs. racism: the eligibility of African American race as a risk factor. *Am J Nurs.* 2021;121(8). https://doi.org/10.1097/01.NAJ.0000767736 .82258.17.

10. *Merriam-Webster Dictionary.* Race. https://www .merriam-webster.com/dictionary/race. Published 2022. Accessed January 27, 2023.

11. Desmond M, Emirbayer M. *Race in America.* 2nd ed. New York, NY: W. W. Norton & Company; 2020.

12. Williams DR, Lawrence JA, Davis BA. Racism and health: evidence and needed research. *Annu Rev Public Health.* 2019;40(1):105-125. https://doi .org/10.1146/annurev-publhealth-040218-043750.

13. Nardi DN, Waite R, Nowak M, Hatcher B. Achieving health equity through eradicating structural racism in the United States: a call to action for nursing leadership. *J Nurs Scholar.* 2020;2(6):696-704.

14. Geronimus AT. The weathering hypothesis and the health of African-American women and infants: evidence and speculations. *Ethn Dis.* 1992;2(3): 207-221.

15. Geronimus AT. Understanding and eliminating racial inequalities in women's health in the United States: The role of the weathering conceptual framework. *J Am Med Womens Assoc.* 2001;56(4):133-136.

16. Aseltine RH Jr, Yan J, Fleischman S, et al. Racial and ethnic disparities in hospital readmissions after delivery. *Obstet Gynecol.* 2015;126(5):1040-1047. https://doi.org/10.1097/AOG.0000000000002937.

17. Gyamfi-Bannerman C, Srinivas SK, Wright JD, et al. Postpartum hemorrhage outcomes and race. *Am J Obstet Gynecol.* 2018;219(2):185e181-185e110. https://doi.org/10.1016/j.ajog.2018.04.052.

18. Howland RE, Angley M, Won SH, et al. Determinants of severe maternal morbidity and its racial/ ethnic disparities in New York City, 2008–2012. *Matern Child Health J.* 2019;23(3):346-355. https:// doi.org/10.1007/s10995-018-2682-z.

19. Leonard SA, Main EK, Scott KA, et al. Racial and ethnic disparities in severe maternal morbidity prevalence and trends. *Ann Epidemiol.* 2019;33:30-36. https://doi.org/10.1016/j.annepidem.2019.02.007.

20. Rosenberg D, Geller SE, Studee L, Cox SM. Disparities in mortality among high risk pregnant women in Illinois: a population based study. *Ann Epidemiol.* 2006;16(1):26-32. https://doi.org/10.1016/j.annepidem .2005.04.007.

21. Tangel V, White RS, Nachamie AS, Pick JS. Racial and ethnic disparities in maternal outcomes and the disadvantage of peripartum Black women: a multistate analysis, 2007–2014. *Am J Perinatol.* 2019;36(8):835-848. https://doi.org/10.1055/s-0038-1675207.

22. Altman MR, Oseguera T, McLemore MR, et al. Information and power: women of color's experiences interacting with health care providers in pregnancy and birth. *Soc Sci Med.* 2019;238:112491. https://doi.org/10.1016/j.socscimed.2019.112491.

23. Canty L. The lived experience of severe maternal morbidity among Black women. *Nurs Inquiry.* 2022:e12466. doi:10.1111/nin.12466.

24. Karbeah JM, Hardeman R, Almanza J, Kozhimannil KB. Identifying the key elements of racially concordant care in a freestanding birth center. *J Midwifery Womens Health.* 2019;64(5):592-597. https://doi .org/10.1111/jmwh.13018.

25. Vedam S, Stoll K, Taiwo TK, et al. The Giving Voice to Mothers study: inequity and mistreatment during pregnancy and childbirth in the United States. *Reprod Health.* 2019;16(1):77. doi:10.1186 /s12978-019-0729-2.

26. Attanasio LB, Hardeman RR. Declined care and discrimination during the childbirth hospitalization. *Soc Sci Med.* 2019;232:270-277. doi:10.1016/j .socscimed.2019.05.008.

27. Vo T. Cultural alienation: a concept analysis. *Nurs Forum.* 2020. doi:10.1111/nuf.12512.

28. Alhusen JL, Bower KM, Epstein E, Sharps P. Racial discrimination and adverse birth outcomes: an integrative review. *J Midwifery Womens Health.* 2016;61(6):707-720. doi:10.1111/jmwh.12490.

29. Beck AF, Edwards EM, Horbar JD, et al. The color of health: how racism, segregation, and inequality affect the health and well-being of preterm infants and their families. *Pediatr Res.* 2020;87(2):227-234. doi:10.1038/s41390-019-0513-6.

30. Bridgeman-Bunyoli AM, Cheyney M, Monroe SM, et al. Preterm and low birthweight birth in the United States: Black midwives speak of causality, prevention, and healing. *Birth.* March 11, 2022. doi:10.1111 /birt.12624.

31. Mileski MR, Shirey MR, Patrician PA, Childs G. Perceived racial discrimination in the pregnant c population: a concept analysis. *Adv Nurs Sci.* 2021;44(4):306-316. doi:10.1097/ANS.0000000000000392.

32. Scott KA, Britton L, McLemore MR. The ethics of perinatal care for Black women: dismantling the structural racism in "Mother Blame" narratives. *J Perinat Neonatal Nurs.* 2019;33(2):108-115. doi: 10.1097/JPN.0000000000000394.

33. Akparewa N. *The Clinician's Guide to Microaggressions and Unconscious Bias.* Baltimore, MD: Blurb; 2020.

34. Saluja B, Bryant, Z. How implicit bias contributes to racial disparities in maternal morbidity and mortality in the United States. *J Womens Health.* 2021;30(2):270-273. doi:10.1089/jwh.2020.8874.

35. Badreldin N, Grobman WA, Yee LM. Racial disparities in postpartum pain management. *Obstet Gynecol.*

2019;134(6):1147-1153.    https://doi.org/10.1097/AOG.0000000000003561.

36. Johnson JD, Asiodu IV, McKenzie CP, et al. Racial and ethnic inequities in postpartum pain evaluation and management. *Obstet Gynecol.* 2019;134(6):1155-1162. doi:10.1097/AOG.0000000000003505.

37. Chuck E, Assefa H. She hoped to shine a light on maternal mortality among Native Americans. Instead, she became a statistic of it. NBC News. https://www.nbcnews.com/news/us-news/she-hoped-shine-light-maternal-mortality-among-native-americans-instead-n1131951. Published February 8, 2020. Accessed January 27, 2023.

38. Project Implicit. Interactive-Race Implicit Association Test. https://implicit.harvard.edu. Published 2011. Accessed January 27, 2023.

39. Centers for Disease Control and Prevention. Infant mortality statistics from the 2018 period linked birth/infant death data set. *Natl Vital Stat Rep.* 2020;89(7): Table 2. https://www.cdc.gov/nchs/data/nvsr/nvsr69/NVSR-69-7-508.pdf. Accessed January 27, 2023.

40. Braveman P. The social determinants of health: it is time to consider the causes of the causes. *Public Health Rep.* 2014;129(suppl 2):19-31.

41. Chinn JJ, Martin IK, Redmond N. Health equity among Black women in the United States. *J Womens Health.* 2021;30(2):212-219. doi:10.1089/jwh.2020.8868.

42. Prather C, Fuller TR, Marshall KJ, Jeffries WLT. The impact of racism on the sexual and reproductive health of African American women. *J Womens Health.* 2016;25(7):664-671. doi:10.1089/jwh.2015.5637.

43. Valdez N, Deomampo D. Centering race and racism in reproduction. *Med Anthropol.* 2019;38(7):551-559. doi:10.1080/01459740.2019.1643855.

44. Hoyert DL. Maternal mortality rates in the United States, 2020. *NCHS Health E-Stats.* 2022. https://dx.doi.org/10.15620/cdc:113967.

45. Centers for Disease Control and Prevention. Pregnancy mortality surveillance system. https://www.cdc.gov/reproductivehealth/maternal-mortality/pregnancy-mortality-surveillance-system.htm. Last reviewed June 22, 2022. Accessed January 27, 2023.

46. Joseph J. The JJ Way: a patient-centered model of care. Commonsense Childbirth. https://commonsensechildbirth.org/the-jj-way/. Accessed May 28, 2022.

47. Niles PM, Vedam S, Witkoski Stimpfel A, Squires A. Kairos care in a Chronos world: midwifery care as model of resistance and accountability in public health settings. *Birth.* 2021. doi:10.1111/birt.12565.

48. Altman MR, McLemore MR, Oseguera T, et al. Listening to women: recommendations from women of color to improve experiences in pregnancy and birth care. *J Midwifery Womens Health.* 2020. doi:10.1111/jmwh.13102.

49. Lori JR, Yi CH, Martyn KK. Provider characteristics desired by African American women in prenatal care. *J Transcultural Nurs.* 2011;22(1):71-76. https://doi.org/10.1177/1043659610387149.

50. Tucker Edmonds B, Mogul M, Shea JA. Understanding low-income African American women's expectations, preferences, and priorities in prenatal care. *Fam Commun Health.* 2015;38(2):149-157. https://doi.org/10.1097/FCH.0000000000000066.

51. Jain J, Moroz L. Strategies to reduce disparities in maternal morbidity and mortality: patient and provider education. *Semin Perinatol.* 2017;41(5):323-328. doi:10.1053/j.semperi.2017.04.010.

52. McLemore MR, Altman MR, Cooper N, et al. Health care experiences of pregnant, birthing and postnatal women of color at risk for preterm birth. *Soc Sci Med.* 2018;201:127-135. doi:10.1016/j.socscimed.2018.02.013.

53. Niles PM, Stoll K, Wang JJ, et al. "I fought my entire way": experiences of declining maternity care services in British Columbia. *PLoS ONE.* 2021;16(6):e0252645.https://doi.org/10.1371/journal.pone.0252645.

CHAPTER

# 2

# Professional Foundations of Midwifery

JESSICA BRUMLEY, JULIA LANGE-KESSLER, AND AMANDA BOYS

## Introduction

Midwifery is recognized nationally and globally, with standards for education, practice, and regulation that make it a profession rather than an occupation or vocation. Safe midwifery practice requires skills, knowledge, and judgment in the provision of health care. However, being a safe, legal, independent, interdependent, and successful midwife requires much more than just clinical competence. This chapter provides an overview of the profession of midwifery in the United States and internationally. It reviews the myriad factors that influence midwives' ability to practice, the context in which midwives practice, the business of midwifery, and the breadth of opportunities for midwives.

## The Profession of Midwifery

To develop the professionalism of midwifery that has been fostered for decades, midwives have created standards for education and practice; they have also defined the scope of practice of midwives and determined how that scope has been adapted over time. It is important for midwives to be able to answer a critical question: What does it take to be a professional?

According to Ament, "[I]n the United States, the overall objective of protecting the public welfare . . . is accomplished through three interdependent mechanisms: 1) a prescribed, accredited course of study; 2) national certification; and 3) governmental, usually state or other jurisdiction, licensure."[1] In addition, healthcare professionals are expected to codify their body of knowledge in peer-reviewed journals and textbooks.

The American College of Nurse-Midwives publishes a peer reviewed journal, the *Journal of Midwifery & Women's Health*, established in 1955.[2] The primary textbook used in U.S. midwifery programs, *Varney's Midwifery*, was first published in 1980.[3] Through the years, several other books have been developed by midwives to support midwifery education.[4-6] In addition, midwifery leaders and healthcare policy makers are able to rely on the robust set of documents published by the American College of Nurse-Midwives (ACNM) and the Midwives Alliance of North America (MANA) that both define the profession of midwifery, as practiced by certified nurse-midwives (CNMs), certified midwives (CMs), and certified professional midwives (CPMs), and justify licensure.

There is a difference between being a member of a profession and being a "professional." As Kennedy stated, the "midwife's professionalism is a key factor in empowering women during the childbearing process."[7] Kennedy identified three dimensions of midwifery professionalism:

- The *dimension of therapeutics*, which illustrates how and why the midwife chooses and uses specific therapies when providing care
- The *dimension of caring*, which reflects how the midwife demonstrates that they care for the individuals seeking midwifery care
- The *dimension of the profession*, which examines how midwifery might be enhanced and accepted by "exemplary" practice

Kennedy divided the *dimension of therapeutics* into two qualities that must be held in balance: supporting the normalcy of birth, while simultaneously maintaining vigilance and attention to detail, intervening only when necessary. Kennedy's approach to support the normalcy of birth is often described as the "art of doing 'nothing'"—that is, appearing calm on the outside while inwardly being actively engaged in data collection and critical thinking.[7]

The *dimension of caring* is demonstrated by respecting the uniqueness of each individual, and by creating respectful settings.[7] Midwives explore and honor each individual's personal history and cultural context. These clinicians work in partnership with patients to achieve the goals of providing emotional support and strengthening their self-confidence. Although it is controversial to say that others can empower an individual, such support can increase self-confidence and facilitate empowerment.

Qualities identified by Kennedy as linked to the *dimension of caring* include "an unwavering integrity and honesty, compassion and understanding, the ability to communicate effectively, and flexibility."[7] Midwives are emotion-workers. For example, exemplary midwives are experts at creating physically and emotionally safe clinical settings; midwives who care for laboring individuals create a peaceful environment that is conducive to a healthy birth process, maternal satisfaction, and immediate postpartum bonding; and midwives providing contraceptive care use the time to develop a trusting relationship and a safe environment that supports disclosure of intimate topics.

The *dimension of the profession* focuses on "the delineation, promotion, and sustenance of midwifery as a professional role."[7] Midwives demonstrate this dimension through evidence-based practice, quality and peer review, continuing education, commitment to and passion for the profession, and nurturing and caring for themselves. The exemplary midwife's focus is not just on the individual; in addition, the midwife is driven to foster the midwifery profession as a whole and to advocate for improving exemplary health outcomes locally and globally.

Professional midwifery in the United States, as practiced by CNMs, CMs, and CPMs, is a dynamic profession. The transition from a focus on individual practice to a focus on the status of a profession within society resembles the evolution of midwifery around the world. In the United States, the scope of midwifery practice is broad, the core knowledge needed to provide safe care has grown at a rapid pace, and the need to promote interprofessional teamwork is well understood. Simultaneously, society has expanded its expectations for all healthcare professionals, and midwives have responded by adopting new standards for education and practice.

## Types of Midwives

While an increasing number of people are familiar with and choose care with midwives, most midwives have been asked the following questions about their profession: What is the difference between a CNM, a CM, and a CPM? What is a lay midwife? A direct-entry midwife? An Indigenous midwife? While the answers to these questions continue to evolve, they can be both confusing and controversial. An exploration of the similarities and differences, summarized in Table 2-1, among midwives is important to the profession.[8] The regulatory requirements and scope of practice described here were current as of the time of this text's publication. Laws pertaining to midwifery practice vary by state and will, like many other statutes, evolve as the political process reflects broader social and cultural changes.

Terms such as "lay midwife" and "direct-entry midwife" are defined more generally than the certified roles. A lay midwife is an individual who has no formal education as a midwife but may have been trained in an apprenticeship or have participated in self-study. A direct-entry midwife (DEM) is typically considered a midwife who has entered the profession without first becoming a nurse. DEMs may include CPMs, CMs, and any midwife who is not also a nurse. Each state has its own laws regarding the regulation of DEMs. Although many midwives complete degrees in nursing to enter a midwifery program, this pathway requires a large investment of time and money on the part of those who primarily want to be a midwife.

The CM was recognized by the ACNM in 1994 as a vehicle to open the profession to other pathways to midwifery. Nursing and midwifery are two separate professions; that is, one is not dependent on the other to engage in the practice of midwifery. While CMs enter midwifery directly, they are educated in the same programs that educate CNMs and they take the same national certification examination. CNMs and CMs have the same scope of practice and in many states have the same scope of prescriptive privileges. CMs practice in the same locations as CNMs—that is, hospitals, homes, and birth centers. The majority of CMs practice in hospitals. In some states, direct-entry midwife and licensed midwife are categories of licensure that bring together a variety of midwives and are distinct from the licensure of CNMs/CMs. In an optimal scenario, all midwives work together for the safety of their community, and they share resources to do so.

| Table 2-1 | Types of Midwives in the United States | | |
|---|---|---|---|
| **National Midwifery Credentials in the United States** | **Certified Nurse-Midwife** | **Certified Midwife** | **Certified Professional Midwife** |
| **Education** | | | |
| **Minimum degree required for certification** | Graduate degree required. | | Certification does not require an academic or graduate degree but is based on demonstrated competency in specified areas of knowledge and skills. |
| **Minimum education requirements for the admission to midwifery education program** | Bachelor's degree or higher from an accredited college or university AND Earn RN license prior to or within midwifery education program | Bachelor's degree or higher from an accredited college or university AND Successful completion of required science and health courses and related health skills prior to or within midwifery education program | High school diploma or equivalent. Prerequisites for accredited programs vary, but typically include specific courses such as statistics, microbiology, anatomy, and physiology, and experience such as childbirth education and doula certification. There are no specified requirements for entry to the North American Registry of Midwives' (NARM) Portfolio Evaluation Process (PEP) pathway, an apprenticeship process that includes verification of knowledge and skills by qualified preceptors. |
| **Clinical experience requirements** | Attainment of knowledge, skills, and professional behaviors as identified by the American College of Nurse-Midwives' (ACNM) Core Competencies for Basic Midwifery Education. Clinical education must occur under the supervision of an American Midwifery Certification Board (AMCB)–certified CNM/CM or other qualified preceptor who holds a graduate degree, has preparation for clinical teaching, and has clinical expertise and didactic knowledge commensurate with the content taught; more than 50% of clinical education must be under CNM/CM supervision. | | Attainment of knowledge and skills, identified in the periodic job analysis conducted by NARM. NARM requires that the clinical component of the educational process must be at least 2 years in duration and include a minimum of 55 births in three distinct categories. Clinical education must occur under the supervision of a midwife who must be nationally certified, be legally recognized, and have practiced for at least 3 years and attended 50 out-of-hospital births post-certification. CPMs certified via the PEP may earn a Midwifery Bridge Certificate (MBC) to demonstrate they meet the International Confederation of Midwives (ICM) standards for minimum education. |
| **Education Program Accrediting Organization** | | | |
| | The Accreditation Commission for Midwifery Education (ACME) is authorized by the U.S. Department of Education to accredit midwifery education programs and institutions. Midwifery education programs must be located within or affiliated with a regionally accredited institution. | | The Midwifery Education Accreditation Council (MEAC) is authorized by the U.S. Department of Education to accredit midwifery education programs and institutions. The scope of recognition includes certificate- and degree-granting institutions, programs within accredited institutions, and distance education programs. |

*(continues)*

| Table 2-1 | Types of Midwives in the United States (*continued*) | | |
| --- | --- | --- | --- |
| **National Midwifery Credentials in the United States** **Scope of Practice** | **Certified Nurse-Midwife** | **Certified Midwife** | **Certified Professional Midwife** |
| **Range of care provided** | Midwifery as practiced by certified nurse-midwives (CNMs) and certified midwives (CMs) encompasses the independent provision of care during pregnancy, childbirth, and the postpartum period; sexual and reproductive health; gynecologic health; and family planning services, including preconception care. Midwives also provide primary care for individuals from adolescence throughout the lifespan as well as care for the healthy newborn during the first 28 days of life. Midwives provide care for all individuals who seek midwifery care, inclusive of all gender identities and sexual orientations. Midwives provide initial and ongoing comprehensive assessment, diagnosis, and treatment. They conduct physical examinations; independently prescribe medications including, but not limited to, controlled substances, treatment of substance use disorder, and expedited partner therapy; admit, manage, and discharge patients; order and interpret laboratory and diagnostic tests; and order medical devices, durable medical equipment, and home health services. Midwifery care includes health promotion, disease prevention, risk assessment and management, and individualized wellness education and counseling. These services are provided in partnership with individuals and families in diverse settings such as ambulatory care clinics, private offices, telehealth and other methods of remote care delivery, community and public health systems, homes, hospitals, and birth centers. | | Midwifery as practiced by CPMs offers expert care, education, counseling, and support to women and their families throughout the caregiving partnership, including during pregnancy, birth, and the postpartum period. CPMs provide ongoing care throughout pregnancy and continuous, hands-on care during labor, birth, and the immediate postpartum period, as well as maternal and well-baby care through the 6- to 8-week postpartum period. CPMs provide initial and ongoing comprehensive assessment, diagnosis, and treatment. They are trained to recognize abnormal or dangerous conditions requiring consultation with and/or referral to other healthcare professionals. They conduct physical examinations, administer medications, use devices as allowed by state law, and order and interpret laboratory and diagnostic tests. |
| **Practice settings** | All settings—hospitals, homes, birth centers, and offices. The majority of CNMs and CMs attend births in hospitals. | | Homes, birth centers, and offices. The majority of CPMs attend births in homes and birth centers. |
| **Prescriptive authority** | All U.S. jurisdictions | New York, Rhode Island, Maine, Maryland, Virginia, and the District of Columbia | CPMs do not maintain prescriptive authority; however, they may obtain and administer certain medications in selected states. |
| **Third-party reimbursement** | Most private insurance; Medicaid coverage mandated in all states; Medicare; TRICARE | Most private insurance; Medicaid coverage in New York, New Jersey, Rhode Island, and the District of Columbia | Private insurance mandated in 6 states; coverage varies in other states; 13 states include CPMs in state Medicaid plans. |

| National Midwifery Credentials in the United States | Certified Nurse-Midwife | Certified Midwife | Certified Professional Midwife |
|---|---|---|---|
| **Certification** | | | |
| **Certifying organization** | American Midwifery Certification Board (AMCB) | | North American Registry of Midwives (NARM) |
| | AMCB and NARM are accredited by the National Commission for Certifying Agencies. | | |
| **Requirements prior to taking national certification examination** | Graduation from a midwifery education program accredited by the Accreditation Commission for Midwifery Education (ACME); AND Verification by program director of completion of education program AND Verification of master's degree or higher *CNMs must also submit evidence of an active RN license at time of initial certification.* | | Completion of NARM's Portfolio Evaluation Process (PEP) OR Graduation from a midwifery education program accredited by the Midwifery Education Accreditation Council (MEAC) OR AMCB-certified CNM/CM with at least 10 community-based birth experiences OR Completion of an equivalent state licensure program. All applicants must also submit evidence of current adult CPR and neonatal resuscitation certification or course completion. |
| **Recertification requirement** | Every 5 years | | Every 3 years |
| **Licensure** | | | |
| **Legal status** | Licensed in 50 states plus the District of Columbia and U.S. territories as midwives, nurse-midwives, advanced practice registered nurses, or nurse practitioners | Licensed in Colorado Delaware, Hawaii, Maine, Maryland, New Jersey, New York, Oklahoma, Rhode Island, Virginia, and the District of Columbia | Licensed in 35 states and the District of Columbia |
| **Licensure agencies** | Boards of Midwifery, Medicine, Nursing, Nurse-Midwifery, or Departments of Health | Boards of Midwifery, Medicine, Complementary Healthcare Providers, or Departments of Health | Boards of Midwifery, Medicine, Nursing, Complementary Healthcare Providers, or Departments of Health or Departments of Professional Licensure or regulation |
| **Professional Association** | | | |
| | American College of Nurse-Midwives (ACNM) | | National Association of Certified Professional Midwives (NACPM) |
| **Other Midwifery Organizations** | | | |
| | Midwives Alliance of North America (MANA) International Confederation of Midwives (ICM) | | |

Note: This table does not address individuals who are not certified and who may practice midwifery with or without legal recognition.

Reproduced and updated with permission from American College of Nurse-Midwives. Comparison of certified nurse-midwives, certified midwives, certified professional midwives clarifying the distinctions among professional midwifery credentials in the U.S. http://www.midwife.org/acnm/files/cclibraryfiles/filename/000000008494/20220418_CNM-CM-CPM%20Comparison%20Chart_FINAL.pdf. Accessed November 1, 2022.

The terms "traditional midwife," "community midwife," and "Indigenous midwife" acknowledge the individuals who follow traditional customs as they attend births in their community. These midwives typically work in areas where they have limited access to the formal education and well-staffed hospitals found in larger cities, but also explicitly value traditional ways of knowing. The World Health Organization uses the term "traditional birth attendant" (TBA) to describe individuals who have not received formal education and training prior to providing perinatal care. Traditional midwives often are, or have learned from, elders who are influential and trusted because they provide care in concert with local belief systems. The practice of Indigenous midwives includes an understanding of the impact of history and colonization on the communities they serve. These midwives use this knowledge to provide culturally safe, respectful care.

The CPM credential, which was first issued in 1994, was originally developed to provide competency-based certification for midwives who were primarily apprentice trained in out-of-hospital births. The natural consequences of creating the CPM certification examination were the obligation to ensure that those who take the examination meet common standards for education and practice, along with the creation of a structure within which to discipline those who do not perform in a manner consistent with the standards. Standards for education, certification, and practice for CPMs have been developed, and CPMs continue to seek to expand licensure in states that do not currently have CPM licensure statutes.[9]

At approximately the same time as the CPM credential was being developed, the board of directors of the ACNM endorsed the development of an alternative educational path to midwifery that did not require a nursing degree. This process led to the creation of the CM credential in 1991. Over the next 7 years, the requirements to accredit education programs and certify graduates who were not registered nurses were designed and tested to ensure that, after graduation and certification, one could not distinguish between the knowledge and skills of a CNM and a CM. The first CM credential, which required passing the same certification examination that is offered to nurse-midwives, was issued in 1998.

Although significant variations between CPMs, CNMs, and CMs still exist (Table 2-1), the collaborations between the three membership organizations for midwives—the ACNM, the MANA, and the National Association of Certified Professional Midwives (NACPM)—focus more on common values and goals than on differences.[10] In the United States, where the consumer may find it difficult to distinguish between the various types of midwives who have different credentials, each individual who uses the title "midwife" assumes responsibility for the image of the entire profession. Since the publication of the International Confederation of Midwives (ICM) standards on education and regulation, the professional organizations representing midwives in the United States have engaged in regular discussions about how to meet and support the ICM standards and increase access to high-quality midwifery care in a variety of settings. These discussions have sought to clarify the differences between CNMs, CMs, and CPMs. Over time, the differences may decrease.

Of course, very few of the midwifery profession's hard-won accomplishments would have moved from internal ideals to cultural norms without consumer support. From the Maternity Center Association (now known as the Childbirth Connection; a program developed by the National Partnership for Women and Families) to Citizens for Midwifery, consumers have provided inspiration, influence, and financial resources to promote and protect access to midwifery care.[11,12] The list of people who created a public demand for midwifery services and stood beside midwifery during some of the profession's difficult times is long and diverse. Families have also been essential to supporting the profession and the continued growth in the practice of midwifery.

## Core Competencies in the United States and Abroad

The Core Competencies for Basic Midwifery Practice is an ACNM standard-setting document that describes the fundamental knowledge, skills, and abilities of all new CNMs/CMs.[13] These competencies are utilized in the development of the American Midwifery Certification Board (AMCB) examination and serve as the curricular foundation for midwifery education programs accredited by the Accreditation Commission of Midwifery Education (ACME). Core competencies may also be used by regulatory agencies, policy makers, consumers, and employers.

ACNM is a member organization of ICM and therefore agrees to have core competencies that are inclusive of the ICM's Essential Competencies for Midwifery Practice.[14] This document is a fundamental part of the revision of the ACNM Core

Competencies, which are updated every 5 years in a process guided by a taskforce of ACNM members. The revision process includes a review of the current state of clinical practice through a survey of individuals who were certified by AMCB fewer than 5 years ago (AMCB Task Analysis), member feedback, and expert opinion. Through the years since the Core Competencies were first established, the scope of entry-level clinical practice has expanded to include primary care, and ACNM has clarified important core concepts such as cultural humility, advocacy for health equity, social justice, and—most recently—the midwife's role in the care of gender-diverse individuals.

The Core Competencies not only describe the clinical care and skills of entry-level midwives but also include the Hallmarks of Midwifery, which are considered the defining characteristics of the profession (**Table 2-2**). They identify the philosophical underpinnings of the profession and are considered by many to be unique aspects of the profession. Hallmarks include skills such as "Ability to provide safe and effective care across settings including home, birth center, hospital, or any other maternity care service." Some Hallmarks are knowledge based, such as "Incorporation of evidence-based integrative therapies." Others are value based, such as "Recognition, promotion, and advocacy of menarche, pregnancy, birth, and menopause as normal physiologic and developmental processes" and "Promotion of person-centered care for all, which respects and is inclusive of diverse histories, backgrounds, and identities."[13]

Midwives may occasionally find themselves in conflict with these values. Their place of employment may not easily facilitate continuity of care, or a review of current evidence may support an intervention to prevent instead of treating a complication. When in a state of cognitive dissonance, it can be helpful to complete a full review of the Hallmarks of Midwifery and discuss with others if the practice is in alignment with the Hallmarks, personal, and professional values.

## Ethics

Ethics is defined as a guiding set of principles that inform actions.[15] Midwives must be well versed in the ethics involved in all healthcare interactions.[16,17] Ethical guidelines encourage self-regulation, foster professional identity, protect midwives and clients, and serve as a measure of professional maturity.[18] An ethical framework for practice, beginning with the concept of accountability, is critical to the

| Table 2-2 | American College of Nurse-Midwives' Hallmarks of Midwifery |
|---|---|
| | 1. Recognition, promotion, and advocacy of menarche, pregnancy, birth, and menopause as normal physiologic and developmental processes |
| | 2. Advocacy of non-intervention in physiologic processes in the absence of complications |
| | 3. Incorporation of evidence-based care into clinical practice |
| | 4. Promotion of person-centered care for all, which respects and is inclusive of diverse histories, backgrounds, and identities |
| | 5. Empowerment of women and persons seeking midwifery care as partners in health care |
| | 6. Facilitation of healthy family and interpersonal relationships |
| | 7. Promotion of continuity of care |
| | 8. Utilization of health promotion, disease prevention, and health education |
| | 9. Application of a public health perspective |
| | 10. Utilizing an understanding of social determinants of health to provide high-quality care to all persons including those from underserved communities |
| | 11. Advocating for informed choice, shared decision making, and the right to self-determination |
| | 12. Integration of cultural safety into all care encounters |
| | 13. Incorporation of evidence-based integrative therapies |
| | 14. Skillful communication, guidance, and counseling |
| | 15. Acknowledgment of the therapeutic value of human presence |
| | 16. Ability to collaborate with and refer to other members of the interprofessional health care team |
| | 17. Ability to provide safe and effective care across settings including home, birth center, hospital, or any other maternity care service |

Used with permission from the American College of Nurse-Midwives. *Core Competencies for Basic Midwifery Practice.* Silver Spring, MD: American College of Nurse-Midwives, 2020.

continuation of midwifery as an independent and respected profession.[16,17] The subject of professional ethics in health care is complex, and the brief introduction presented here is not a comprehensive review of this important topic. Additional resources that address health literacy, health numeracy, values clarification, options counseling, the interface between legal and ethical issues, and ways to communicate risk are listed at the end of this chapter.

The *ACNM Code of Ethics with Explanatory Statements* provides an in-depth review of common ethical dilemmas faced by midwives and provides guidance for resolving these dilemmas.[18] As defined in the *ACNM Code of Ethics*, CNMs and CMs have three ethical mandates directed toward individual recipients of care, the public good, and the profession of midwifery. The *ACNM Code of Ethics* was first published in 1990, and the ICM ethical code was introduced in 1993. These documents, as well as MANA's *Statement of Values*, provide guidance for the ethical behavior of midwives in various roles, including provision of clinical care, education, research, public policy, business management, and financial organization of health services.[19,20]

## Ethical Principles

The original foundational ethical norms for clinical practice are to do good (benevolence) and not do harm (nonmaleficence). Over time, other principles have been adopted, such as autonomy, veracity, informed consent, confidentiality, and justice (Table 2-3).[21]

## Ethics of Care

These modern ethical principles imply an impartiality in decision making and an equality between midwife, client, and institution free of personal bias that is not truly feasible. The reality is that each of us exists within systems of power and decision making; in turn, we are inevitably influenced by how that power is used. One strategy for addressing these biases and power differentials between the midwife and the dependent client is to apply an ethic of care framework that focuses on attentiveness, responsibility, competence, and responsiveness.[22] This framework acknowledges that the relationship is unequal, that individuals seeking care are vulnerable, and that the midwife has a responsibility to demonstrate compassion.[23] An ethic of care can also be used to overcome the ethical dilemmas that occur when institutions prioritize the relationship of the midwife to the institution over the relationship of the midwife to the individual.[24]

## Reproductive Justice

A framework particularly relevant to ethical care in midwifery is the reproductive justice framework. It is based on the principles that all people with the capacity to reproduce have a fundamental human right to not have a child or to have a child, and to do so in a safe and healthy environment.[25] This framework addresses historical, social, cultural, and economic factors that contribute to discrimination, particularly in communities of color in the United States. Midwives aiming to provide ethical care to communities must understand how history informs the modern context in which sexuality and reproduction exist in our society. For example, when providing contraceptive care, it is equally important to understand modern laws regarding abortion access and funding for a full spectrum of contraceptive options as it is to understand the history of medical experimentation on enslaved women, forced sterilization, and coercive use of long-acting reversible contraceptives.

## Shared Decision Making

Midwives often encounter ethical dilemmas—that is, situations where they "must make a decision and

| Table 2-3 | Ethical Principles |
|---|---|
| Benevolence | To do good; to benefit patients and promote well-being. |
| Nonmaleficence | Do no harm; an obligation to consider both the potential benefit and the potential harm of an intervention, and to choose the options with the least likelihood for harm. |
| Autonomy | Each individual has worth and therefore the right to self-determination. |
| Veracity | Truth telling; the obligation to tell the patient all the information necessary to make a decision. |
| Informed consent | An extension of autonomy; requires that an individual be competent, receive full information, comprehend the information, be free from coercion, and provide consent. |
| Confidentiality | An obligation not to share confidential information with anyone outside of the care team without the patient's consent. |
| Justice | Fair and equitable treatment or distribution of resources. |

Based on Varkey B. Principles of clinical ethics and their application to practice. *Med Princ Pract.* 2021;30:17-28.

| Table 2-4 | Agency for Healthcare Research and Quality's SHARE Model | |
|---|---|---|
| | **Step** | **Sample Conversation Starter** |
| S | Seek the patient's participation. | "Now that we have identified the problem, it's time to think about what to do next. I'd like us to make this decision together." |
| H | Help the patient explore and compare treatment options. | "Let me tell you what the research says about the benefits and risks of the medicine/treatments that you are considering." |
| A | Assess the patient's values and preferences. | "When you think about the possible risks, what matters most to you?" |
| R | Reach a decision with the patient. | "So now that we had a chance to discuss your treatment options, do you have a preference for treatment? Which treatment do you think is right for you?" |
| E | Evaluate the patient's decision. | "Let's plan on reviewing this decision at our next appointment." |

Adapted from Agency for Healthcare Research and Quality. The SHARE approach. https://www.ahrq.gov/professionals/education/curriculum-tools/shareddecisionmaking/index.html. Published July 2014; reviewed February 2017. Accessed on December 10, 2021.

follow through with that decision by taking specific action, but the right action to take may be unclear."[26] Experts agree that ethics education in midwifery should include competencies in clinical ethical decision making such as respect, shared decisions, bias, effective communication, critical thinking, and research.[27] Shared decision making (SDM) is a model of communication in which clinicians and patients share the best available evidence to help explore the available options, and in which patients are supported in communicating an informed decision.[28] Use of an SDM model incorporates key ethical principles and acknowledges the interdependence of the midwife and the decision maker. The midwife is considered an expert who possesses knowledge of evidence related to the risks and benefits of the available options, and the client is the expert on their own personal values and priorities. SDM acknowledges that there is typically no one right decision, only the one that best fits the individual currently. It is important to acknowledge that the midwife exerts power and potential bias in how they present information, as well as that the midwife–client relationship and acknowledged levels of privilege can influence how information is shared.[29]

Several SDM models have been described to facilitate integration into clinical practice. For example, in the *Three Talk Model*, Team Talk, Options Talk, and Decision Talk are utilized in the setting of active listening and deliberation.[30] Team Talk refers to language that encourages active participation in decision making, such as "Let's work together." Options Talk refers to the process of describing available options and the risks and benefits of those options. Decision Talk refers to the

process of deciding together, including eliciting the patient's preferences and values. The use of decision aids—that is, tools that depict the options—has been demonstrated to lead to improved knowledge, greater confidence, and more active involvement in decision making.[31]

The Agency for Healthcare Research and Quality (AHRQ) describes a five-step model symbolized by the SHARE acronym (**Table 2-4**).[32] This acronym is a mnemonic intended to help practitioners remember the five-step process, but is not intended to imply a linear process. The steps should all be addressed but may be more of an iterative process.

Every SDM approach includes respectful communication, support for autonomy, and respecting the patient's decision to decline intervention even when the evidence clearly supports an intervention. This scenario can strain the midwife–client relationship, but open, honest communication that facilitates SDM can limit the risk of bias and coercion. Megregian and Nieuwenhuijze describe a common scenario in which a pregnant patient chooses to decline the recommended screening test for gestational diabetes.[33] This case study provides an example of how SDM and respectful communication can be utilized to benefit the midwife–client relationship in the setting of informed refusal.

### Ethical Dilemmas

Professional ethics dictates that a conflict between two or more moral obligations in a particular situation be addressed through deliberate ethical analysis and decision making, including weighing and balancing principles, and preferably involving and achieving consensus among all affected parties. For example, one healthcare provider's attempt to "do good," such as performing a cesarean section for a diagnosis of failure to progress, might be interpreted by the recipient of care as "doing harm"—in this case, performing surgery without adequate time waiting for a vaginal birth.

Equally challenging is the fact that midwifery is a field in which the professional attending a birth has two individuals for whom to provide care, the pregnant person and the fetus, whose interests may not be balanced (also known as being in equipoise). However, a person's right to autonomy does not change because they are pregnant. The consensus of modern ethics is that the duty owed to the fetus may be different from that owed to the pregnant individual, and the duty to both changes depending on the gestational age and maternal condition(s).[24]

Examples of ethical scenarios are presented in **Table 2-5** and **Table 2-6**.

| Table 2-5 | Ethical Scenario 1 |
|---|---|

A client who has had an uncomplicated pregnancy presents feeling "miserable" and requests an induction at 37 weeks' gestation. They state that they will go elsewhere for their care if the midwife will not induce their labor. The midwife validates the client's feelings and explains the risks of elective induction but supports the position that induction at 37 weeks is not recommended.

The midwife knows that the benefits to the pregnant person and fetus are maximized (beneficence) and harm is minimized (nonmaleficence) with labor later in gestation. This professional must weigh this information with the principle of autonomy, the person's right to make an informed decision about their body and fetus.

| Table 2-6 | Ethical Scenario 2 |
|---|---|

During the initial prenatal visit, a client tells the midwife that they are uninsured and do not have many financial resources. Typically, the midwife explains genetic testing options in pregnancy at the first visit. It becomes clear to the midwife during their conversation that the client would not be able to afford any of the costly genetic testing and wonders if counseling should be performed. The midwife decides to provide counseling in the same manner as any other client.

The midwife's decision to provide counseling regardless of ability to pay for genetic testing illustrates the principle of justice.

## Workforce Diversity in Midwifery

### Characteristics of the U.S. Midwifery Workforce

Descriptive data about members of ACNM have been collected through membership surveys for more than five decades. In 1963, 229 members were mailed a survey and 72% responded.[34] The results revealed a median age of 41 years, the existence of six educational programs, and a geographic distribution of practices primarily clustered on the East Coast. Several states or jurisdictions had laws prohibiting midwifery practice. In 2020, the Bureau of Labor Statistics reported an estimated 7120 CNMs/CMs. Most were employed by physician offices ($n = 3050$), outpatient care centers ($n = 1170$), and offices of other healthcare practitioners ($n = 580$). A small portion were employed by colleges, universities, or other professional schools ($n = 110$) and governmental agencies ($n = 80$).[35] The vast majority (99%) of the 13,409 AMCB-certified midwives in the United States are CNMs and only 1% were CMs.[36]

The 2019 ACNM Core Data Survey ($N = 1231$ respondents) found that midwives employed full-time had the following clinical care responsibilities: antepartum (86%), intrapartum (81%), postpartum (84%), and reproductive services (76%).[37] Primary care services were provided by almost half (49%), but fewer than one-fifth provided newborn care (15%). Midwives' nonclinical roles included midwifery education (29%), midwifery/other administrative work (27%), and research (10%). Most respondents attended births (78%). The primary birth setting was the hospital (89%), but CNMs/CMs also attended births in hospital birth centers (7%), freestanding birth centers (9%), and homes (8%).

The racial diversity of practicing midwives has not changed dramatically over the last half-century.[38,39] Racial disparities in perinatal and early childhood health outcomes have not improved despite a variety of attempts to increase access to and quality of care.[40] The population of the United States is increasingly racially diverse, yet racism, when institutionalized, often goes unrecognized by those not experiencing it. While the midwifery profession has a long history of serving women at risk for poor pregnancy outcomes, one solution remains a challenge for the profession—the evidence that race-concordant care can reduce racial health disparities.[41] While recent evidence shows an increase in the number of new CNMs/CMs who identify as people of color (14.5% in 2013), the ACNM membership remains disproportionally (more than 90%) white. In 2021, the American Midwifery

Certification Board (AMCB) reported that the vast majority of CNMs/CMs are white, non-Hispanic women aged 30 to 69 years.[36] Data collected about race show that only 7.3% of CNMs/CMs identify as Black or African American, 1.7% identify as Asian, and 0.61% identify as American Indian or Alaska Native. Ethnicity data reveal that 5% of CNMs/CMs identify as Hispanic/Latino.

### Racial and Ethnic Incongruence

In 2020, CNMs/CMs attended 372,991 births in the United States; in 14.24% of CNM/CM-attended births, the mother's race was identified as Black and in 22.9% of these births the mother's ethnicity was identified as Hispanic.[42] When compared to the AMCB data on CNM/CM race and ethnicity, it is clear that CNMs/CMs are not representative of the childbearing individuals whom they serve.

It is critical for midwives to understand how their own professional history has impacted the health of the communities they serve (see the *Resources on the History of Midwifery* appendix). Midwifery in the United States includes a history of Black granny midwives, Indigenous midwives, and parteras who cared for Black and Brown communities as well as serving white communities. Legislation such as the Sheppard Towner Act was used to eradicate the granny midwives and create public health professionals who laid the foundations for the nurse-midwives found in the United States today.[43] The founding years of the nurse-midwifery profession almost completely excluded Black and Brown individuals from midwifery education and leadership, thereby creating a culturally incongruent healthcare system.[44]

An Institute of Medicine[*] report, *In the Nation's Compelling Interest: Ensuring Diversity in the Health Care Workforce*, sought to bring attention to the importance of congruence among patient and provider race and ethnicity. It underscored the evidence showing that a racial and ethnically diverse workforce improves access to care for racialized patients, patient satisfaction, and educational experiences for learners.[45]

In 2010, the Patient Protection and Affordable Care Act included dozens of provisions with the potential to address health equity, including healthcare workforce funding intended to increase the supply and diversity of healthcare professionals, support the safety net and healthcare services provided in community settings, provide training in cultural competency, enable workforce evaluation and assessment, and support pipeline programs for diverse students. The actualization of these programs has been limited, and as of 2016 substantial progress toward implementation had been made on only 7 of 17 of these provisions.[46]

In 2021, the ACNM worked to help introduce the Midwives for Maximizing Optimal Maternity Services Act. If passed, this legislation would have established grants to establish or expand midwifery programs and prioritize funding for institutions that focus on increasing the number of midwives from underrepresented groups. It would have also promoted practice in areas with limited access to professional healthcare services. Finding mechanisms to financially support the work of diversifying the profession is a critical strategy for addressing health inequities.

In addition to workforce strategies, much work can be done to improve the ethical provision of care for Black/Indigenous/people of color (BIPOC) communities. Scott et al. present a framework for the ethical perinatal care of Black individuals that can be applied to many vulnerable populations, thereby dismantling the structural racism of the "Mother Blame" narrative.[47] Their framework describes how social and economic factors can influence behaviors and the physiology that affects health outcomes. The authors emphasize use of interventions known to optimize birth outcomes, such as universal preconception care, nurse–family partnership programs, group prenatal care, and kangaroo care.

In *Setting the Standard for Holistic Care of Black Women*, the Black Mamas Matter Alliance describes eight essential competencies that can be applied to the ethical perinatal care of Black women.[48] (1) "Listen to Black women" refers not only to individual care visits, but also centering the voice of Black women in the design of policy and research that target Black women. By recognizing the (2) "historical experiences and expertise of Black women and families," we have a context for Black women's experiences and interactions with midwives. When providing (3) "care through a reproductive justice framework," midwives can use relationship, collaboration, and prioritization of consent over provider bias. When midwives take the time to listen holistically to Black women and treat them as valuable, loved individuals instead of leaning on stereotypes, it is possible to (4) "disentangle care practices from the racist beliefs in modern medicine." The current healthcare system is often regimented and rushed, but through the implementation models of care that are centered on the

---

*The Institute of Medicine was renamed the National Academy of Medicine in 2015.

Black woman, and that provide information, access, and opportunities for relationship, we can (5) "replace white supremacy and patriarchy with a new care model." The SDM model addresses the next recommendation—to (6) "empower all patients with health literacy and autonomy." Doing so, however, takes time, trust, and complete honesty.

Some of the most successful models of prenatal care utilize a team model of care that aims to (7) "empower and invest in health paraprofessionals." Paraprofessionals are more likely to be culturally congruent with and socioeconomically like the patients being served. This allows for higher levels of trust and relatability and is an asset to quality health care. The final recommendation is to (8) "recognize that access does not equal quality care." Equitable care does not mean just access to care, but also access to resources that meet the client's needs. When clients are at higher risk of complications owing to race-related exposures, they need access to more supportive services (e.g., midwives, doulas, lactation support, community-based care) that are often not covered by insurance and whose costs may make them unattainable.

The preceding recommendations illustrate the need to address behaviors at the individual provider level and highlight the need to create system-level change. Midwives are perfectly positioned to address change from multiple angles. They are forging new systems of care through the creation of community-based, midwife-owned practices. They are also working within larger institutions lobbying for change, such as improved data collection, support for culturally congruent care providers and learners, awareness-building campaigns, implicit bias training, and social justice advocacy. Midwives are partnering with state perinatal quality associations to implement quality improvement initiatives with an equity focus. They are lobbying for legislative changes such as providing funding for midwifery students from underrepresented backgrounds, improving funding for midwifery care and patient-centered models of care, and increasing autonomous practice for midwives. Midwife researchers are centering their efforts on hearing the voices of Black women to identify areas of need.

## Diversity and Inclusion in Gender and Sexual Identity

There is growing awareness of the need for midwifery care to be inclusive and supportive of all who seek midwifery care. Improving care for lesbian, gay, bisexual, queer, and intersex (LGBTQI) individuals

is an important facet of improving perinatal care. The number of openly LGBTQI individuals in the United States is increasing, and this trend is likely to continue if individuals feel safe expressing their sexual and gender-related identities in society and healthcare settings. For example, the number of lesbian and same-sex couples accessing fertility treatment and maternity care has increased by as much as 20% each year in the last decade, making this population one of the fastest-growing groups to access fertility and maternity care.

Evidence shows that sexual orientation or gender identity can have a significant impact on physical, mental, and sexual well-being.[49] Transgender and nonbinary individuals (TNB) have a wide range of healthcare needs and face significant obstacles to obtaining needed healthcare services. Research indicates that TNB individuals experience high rates of discrimination and health disparities; however, gender-affirming clinical interventions have been demonstrated to have a positive impact on their physical and emotional well-being.[50-53] Many transgender individuals desire a future pregnancy or are parents already.[54]

Given that the Hallmarks of Midwifery include person-centered, evidence-based care with a focus on shared decision making, the midwifery profession is perfectly positioned to meet the healthcare needs of LGBTQI individuals by offering safe, inclusive care. An exclusive practice focus on care of women ignores transgender and gender-diverse individuals. The ACNM has affirmed that it is within the midwife's scope of practice to provide gender-affirming care such as respecting TNB individuals, becoming knowledgeable about their healthcare needs, advocating for inclusive respectful environments including the use of gender-inclusive language, and providing gender-affirming hormone therapy.[55]

Unfortunately, discrimination based on gender and sexual orientation still occurs in some perinatal healthcare environments, and is an obstacle to advancing the diversity of the midwifery workforce. Practice environments are often not welcoming or are openly discriminatory against midwives who have a gender identity, sexuality, or family structure that differs from the majority of others within the practice or institution. Only about 1% of midwives identify as male, and 0.33% identify as nonbinary; statistics describing the sexuality of midwives are not available in the ACNM Core Data Survey.[37] Improved educational and working environments that welcome diverse individuals and respect their contributions can improve both the midwifery profession and the health care offered to the patients whom midwives serve.

## Structures

### Practice Patterns

Improving the health of clients or patients is a personal, communal, and political responsibility, and midwives work wherever they are needed. While many midwives attend births and provide reproductive health services, they may also work as entrepreneurs, policy makers, and educators. In all of these positions, midwives collaborate with a variety of team members.

In clinical practice, midwives may work for large hospitals or healthcare systems in metropolitan areas, in small private practices in rural communities, and anywhere in between. Midwives may attend births in homes, freestanding birth centers, or hospitals. They may be self-employed in a private business, or they may be employees of physicians or healthcare organizations. CNMs/CMs can provide primary health care or limit their practice to specific populations or conditions, such as family planning, infertility, menopause, incontinence, or pelvic pain. CPMs are typically licensed exclusively to provide perinatal care.

Since the 1960s, the majority of CNMs, and now CMs, who attend births have done so in hospitals and freestanding birth centers, whereas the vast majority of CPMs have attended births in homes or freestanding birth centers. Although these trends may continue, the future may present more workplace opportunities for all midwives.

With so many opportunities, the typical midwife searches for an opportunity that is a good match to their experience, personality, skill set, and lifestyle. When considering an employment position, one of the first actions is for the midwife to perform a personal evaluation: Which work and lifestyle factors are important to the individual midwife? Which skills and talents would be important to stress to a prospective employer? What do employers in the area need or want? When evaluating the positives and negatives of any position, it is important to review various aspects of the business that may contribute to success or frustration—for example, availability of and relationship with physicians and other providers (e.g., dieticians, physical therapists), ancillary support (e.g., billing, office flow), reimbursement for professional expenses (e.g., licenses, certification, and continuing education), payment for malpractice premiums, availability of student loan payments, and retirement benefits. Understanding of certain core concepts and professional structures are necessary to be successful regardless of the setting.

### Scope of Practice

Midwifery has a long-standing reputation for focusing on a childbirth experience that honors the physiologic process of birth as well as the transformational power of the childbearing experience.[56] A midwife's scope of practice is determined by multiple factors, including professional practice standard–setting documents, legal jurisdiction, institutional policies, locations of care, collaborative practice agreements, and individual education and experience.[57] State laws and facility bylaws may define the clinical or professional relationship between a midwife and a consulting or collaborating physician. Scope of practice is complex and dynamic for an individual midwife's practice. For example, a midwife's scope of practice has some inflexible boundaries (e.g., the midwife cannot perform services that are prohibited by law) and some flexibility (e.g., advanced clinical skills such as first assisting for cesarean births, may be acquired as needed through a formal process).[58]

### Licensure

State laws governing midwifery practice vary. When consistent with the ACNM recommendations for legislation, state laws support the ability of CNMs and CMs to autonomously practice to the full extent of their education, training, and certification. At their most restrictive, state laws require direct physician supervision of midwives. The rules and regulations governing midwifery practice usually are available on state government websites. Professional organizations such as ACNM and MANA provide online summaries of all the states' midwifery laws, and political action groups work to change laws that do not permit midwives to practice to the full scope of their preparation. Figure 2-1 provides a synopsis of regulations on the practice of AMCB-certified midwives.

In many states, CNMs are licensed as advanced practice registered nurses (APRN). In 2008, through collaboration with more than 70 nursing organizations, a framework for APRN regulation was developed.[59] The Consensus Model for APRN Regulation: Licensure, Accreditation, Certification, and Education ("LACE Consensus Model") contains seven elements, covering APRN role recognition, title protection, licensure, education, certification, independent practice, and independent prescribing. Congruence of each individual state nurse practice act with these seven elements would allow APRNs licensed in a participating state to practice in other participating states.

In 2011, ACNM, AMCB, and ACME released a statement on specific points of the LACE Consensus

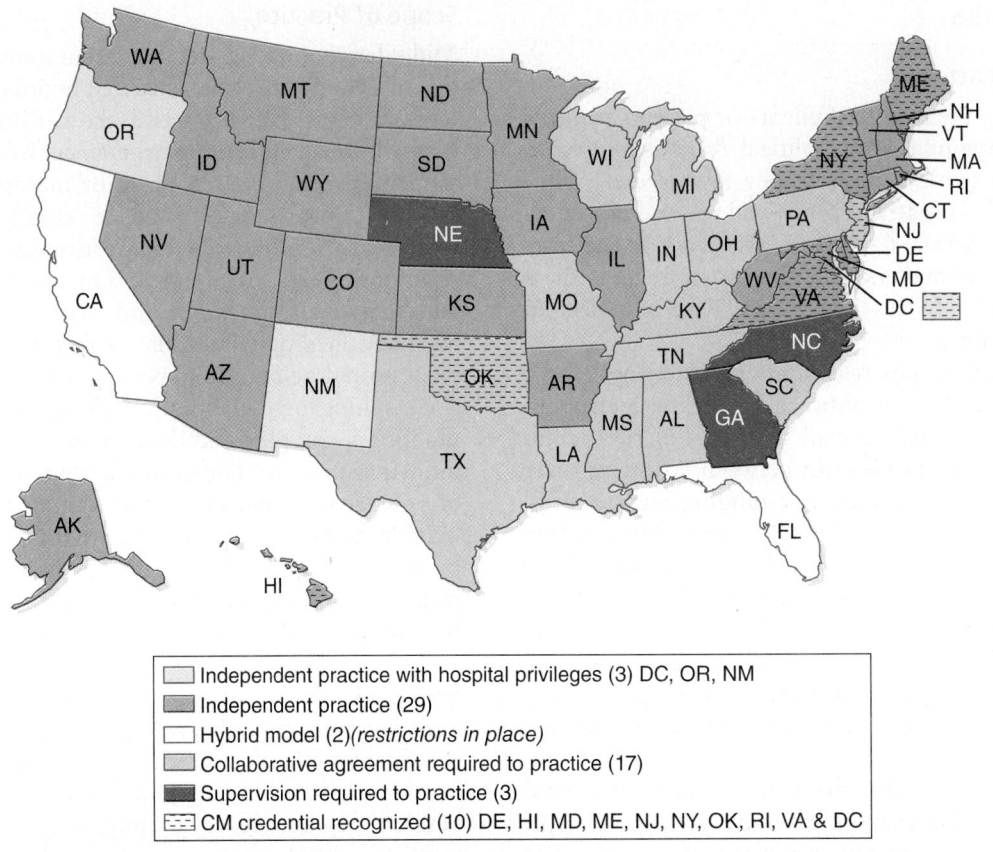

Legend:

☐ Independent practice with hospital privileges (3) DC, OR, NM
▨ Independent practice (29)
☐ Hybrid model (2) *(restrictions in place)*
▨ Collaborative agreement required to practice (17)
▨ Supervision required to practice (3)
▨ CM credential recognized (10) DE, HI, MD, ME, NJ, NY, OK, RI, VA & DC

**Figure 2-1** Practice environments for AMCB-certified midwives.
Modified with permission from American College of Nurse-Midwives. Practice environments for AMCB-certified midwives—April 2022. https://www.midwife.org/full-practice-authority-stad. Accessed November 27, 2022.

Model as they relate to midwifery.[60] To implement this model, state legislation eliminating mandates for supervision or collaboration would be necessary in many states. Elimination of these mandates has long been a legislative advocacy focus of ACNM state affiliate organizations.

The LACE Consensus Model requires that APRNs be educated in at least one of six population foci, including women's health/gender related. Although the document does describe the CNM scope of practice as including primary care of women and newborns, no one population focus describes the full scope of CNM practice, so concern exists that the full scope of midwifery care may not be included in future legislation. Given that recent updates to the ACNM Core Competencies and Scope of Practice include care of transgender and gender-nonconforming individuals, there are additional concerns that these populations may be omitted from the scope of midwifery care. This concern is likely valid, as other components of the LACE Consensus Model have been misinterpreted at the state level.

The LACE model recognizes that CNMs may be regulated by Boards of Midwifery or Boards of Nurse-Midwifery. This is an important caveat that would allow for the potential expansion of the CM credential into new states. However, the initial version of the LACE Consensus Model contains inconsistent language around education requirements. It describes a requirement for a graduate or postgraduate degree in nursing or nursing-related fields, but some parts of the document simply refer to nursing degrees. Some states have already implemented a requirement for a nursing master's degree. CNMs and CMs may earn graduate degrees in midwifery, public health, or health sciences and are equally prepared for certification, licensure, and practice. Overall, the LACE Consensus Model does provide an avenue to advocate for legislative changes that would be supportive of the goal to expand access to full-scope midwifery.

### Hospital Privileges and Credentialing

Midwives who attend births in hospitals and most birth centers are required to be credentialed and privileged by that healthcare facility. Credentialing refers to the process used to verify an individual's qualifications such as completion of an accredited program of study. Privileging refers to the specific tasks and procedures and patient care services that an individual is permitted to perform. Bylaws, established by the healthcare facility, define the requirements for obtaining privileges, the responsibilities of those who are granted privileges, specific procedures that may be performed by the individual providers, protections offered to those who are privileged, and grounds for removal of privileges. These bylaws may also specify the role and responsibilities of midwives in relation to collaborating physicians and the responsibilities of each party. All privileged providers are expected to adhere to institution bylaws, even if the bylaws are more restrictive than the state law.

The ability to be credentialed by a hospital dictates a midwife's ability to create a practice for hospital birth and to provide continuity of care to patients planning a community-based birth but requiring transfer. Institutional bylaws also determine whether a midwife has voting privileges and can serve on hospital or department committees. Serving on committees provides midwives with the ability to have a voice in facility policies.

Healthcare outcomes are optimized when midwives are fully integrated into the healthcare system. Access to full and independent credentialing and privileging is necessary for full integration. Almost all states have laws allowing midwives to admit patients to hospitals, and most have laws permitting midwives to be members of the hospital medical staff. Nevertheless, individual hospitals or medical staff boards may choose to not privilege midwives or may do so only with supervision or restrictions. In 2020, an ACNM survey of CNMs/CMs found that only 163 out of 435 had full medical privileges and about half (48.8%) had privileges only if they were employed by a physician.[61] In 2022, ACNM was working with members of Congress on the introduction of legislation to amend the Medicare statute and require hospitals to establish equitable procedures for the granting of clinical privileges for midwives, including admission of patients.

## The Business of Midwifery

### Midwifery Employment

Whether considering one or multiple job opportunities, midwives should analyze several factors that will influence their job satisfaction, some of which are listed in Table 2-7. This table describes factors important for midwives interested in joining an existing practice as an employee. The weight of any of the factors will vary based on the individual midwife's desires and needs. The factors are not presented in any specific order, nor is this an exclusive list.

If the prospective employer does not offer a formal contract, asking for a confirmation letter that puts the offered remuneration and job specifics in writing is wise. If the midwife is asked to sign a contract, consultation with an attorney is advised. Even if a contract is considered non-negotiable, the midwife should thoroughly understand the content prior to signing. Table 2-8 provides a list of topics that should be addressed prior to accepting a position or signing a contract.[62,63]

### Midwife Entrepreneurs

Most midwives consider midwifery to be a vocation. Thus, it can be challenging to think of midwifery as "a business"—yet all midwives need to understand the basic principles of running a successful business.

| Table 2-7 | Factors to Clarify When Considering Joining a Practice | |
|---|---|
| **Practice Characteristics** | **Compensation/Benefits** |
| Location | Salary |
| Philosophy | Productivity requirements |
| Clientele (volume, demographics, outcomes of care) | Requirements/bonuses/overtime |
| Practice providers (physicians, midwives, nurse practitioners, others, and culture of collaboration) | Payment/nonclinical responsibilities |
| | Ability to own part of the practice |
| Interaction with learners | Malpractice insurance (type, tail if needed) |
| Support staff (billing, assistants in office, marketing) | Vacation/paid time off |
| | Maternity/paternity leave (if appropriate) |
| Clinical hours | Other professional benefits (continuing education units, dues, licenses, parking, smartphone) |
| Environment (equipment, facilities, financial stability) | |
| Birth facility | Health insurance, retirement |
| Orientation plan | Student loan repayment |
| Time needed for credentialing, insurance networks | Opportunity to precept midwifery students |

| Table 2-8 | Topics Usually Found in a Contract |
|---|---|

Title of position

Responsibilities, including scope of practice, currency of credentials, expectations of volume and hours

Compensation and benefits, including bonuses, productivity, professional/business expenses, tuition reimbursement, health and malpractice insurance, and paid time off

Duration and requirement for renewal of employment/contract

Reason for termination by employer and/or employee

How to alter or update the contract

**Additional Topics That May Be Included**

Non-compete clause[a]

Partnership arrangements (buying in or out of a practice)

Termination without cause[a]

Formulae (for bonuses, productivity, quality-based, patient satisfaction, and profit-based)

Ownership of records upon dissolution/termination

[a] Not recommended but often included.

Based on Buppert C. *Nurse Practitioner's Business Practice and Legal Guide.* 6th ed. Burlington, MA: Jones & Bartlett Learning; 2018; Bryant C. *An Administrative Manual for Midwifery Practices.* 5th ed. Silver Spring, MD American College of Nurse-Midwives; 2022.

| Table 2-9 | Content for a Typical Business Plan |
|---|---|

Cover page with name of business and contact information

Description of practice

Services

Clientele

Relationships

Company strategies

Market research

Fiscal outlook

Plans (marketing, operating, and financial)

Anticipated team and schedule

Modified from Bryant C. *An Administrative Manual for Midwifery Practices.* 5th ed. Silver Spring, MD American College of Nurse-Midwives; 2022.

There is a growing need for midwives to become accomplished administrators and business managers.

Many midwives have, either independently or in groups, become business owners. The opportunity to avoid the limitations imposed by the business model or clinical guidelines developed by others, such as physicians, hospitals, and community clinics, can be very tempting, and in some cases, may be a necessity. For midwives who want to start their own business, the advice offered by successful entrepreneurs is consistent—namely, consult experts, invest in marketing, develop competence in billing, and collect and analyze data. Each of these aspects of running an independent midwifery practice is an important factor that can facilitate long-term success.

### Business Advice from Experts

It is unwise to open a business without seeking the expertise of, at a minimum, an attorney and an accountant. The legal structure of a midwifery business (e.g., sole proprietorship, partnership, or limited liability company) will have short- and long-term personal and financial consequences. Midwife business owners should be experts on the laws and regulations that govern midwifery practice, and should also know how the laws governing medical practice, the corporate practice of medicine, and pharmacy regulations might affect their plans. Midwives providing care during home and freestanding birth center births must comply with health department regulations, birth center requirements, building codes, and a variety of business regulations. Midwives who employ others must determine how they will compensate those employees and follow the relevant employment tax codes and antidiscrimination policies. Beyond malpractice insurance coverage, new business owners are often surprised to learn how many insurance policies need to be purchased and how many business contracts need to be finalized. In all of these areas, good advice can save money, protect investments, and enable midwives to provide high-quality care.

Preparing a business plan and seeking guidance from an accountant on the costs of doing business can provide clarity for all involved and are requirements when seeking loans to help establish a business. Common elements found in a business plan are listed in **Table 2-9**.[63] The time spent establishing a reporting system for revenues versus expenses is a good investment, as such a system provides a way to measure of financial success.

Given that independent business ownership is valued highly in the United States, many types of support exist for small business owners, including information on how to formulate business plans and where to apply for small business loans. Midwives who are business owners often agree to mentor a new entrepreneur. The Business Section of the ACNM Division of Standards and Practice is committed to sharing information, providing support to midwives interested in the business aspects of midwifery, and increasing the number of midwife-owned practices. The Business Section partners with ACNM to sponsor the annual conference Midwifery Works, and to publish the *Administrative Manual for Midwifery Practices*.[63] The American Association of Birth Centers also offers workshops on how to open a birth center, during which many of these concepts are covered in depth. Other business guides in areas outside of midwifery may provide additional useful information.[62]

## Midwifery Practices Within Institutions

Midwifery practices that are not independent businesses still have business and administrative work that must be addressed. No matter the number of employees, a midwifery service must reach an agreement on scheduling, compensation, records management, monitoring of financial statements, negotiation of collaborative agreements, peer review, and strategies to handle personal and professional adversity. While responsibilities for the success of the service are shared, there needs to be a designated leader or service director, who serves as the primary contact, assumes responsibility for participating in department- or corporate-level committees, is able to describe the success of the service in corporate terms, and knows how to move an agenda forward within the organization. Midwives place a high value on building relationships with their clients and on positive feedback from the individuals for whom they provide care. Those skills can be extrapolated into the business arena and will serve midwives well.

## Data Collection

Collection of data on outcomes for labor and birth has long been valued. Birth registries have been used to not only record births, but also address the impact of public health interventions.[64] In modern times, the ACNM has recognized the need to provide data that demonstrate the quality of care provided by practicing midwives. As early as 1982, recommendations were being made to promote national data collection.[65] Several readily accessible mechanisms for collecting and collating practice-specific and national data exist that can be used to describe the care provided by midwives. Members

of ACNM can join in the ACNM Benchmarking Project, which allows participants to examine their practices and compare them to other, like practices across the United States.[66] The MANA Division of Research, with its MANA Stats system, and the American Association of Birth Centers, with its Perinatal Data Registry (PDR), have developed web-based data collection tools that can be used by individuals to contribute data to a national database on the outcomes of midwifery care in all settings.[67,68]

## Marketing

Many advisors encourage early attention to a marketing plan when starting a new business. Without a coherent, consumer-friendly message about the services offered and an identified medium for reaching the target population, the business may not have enough clients to sustain itself. Not every practice can afford an extensive marketing campaign, but all midwives can develop marketing skills.

Today, using social media may be the most effective, and least expensive, marketing strategy. Clients expect practices to have an up-to-date website. Regular posts from midwives can provide reminders about healthy behaviors. To be successful, practices should engage with a variety of social media, while maintaining awareness of all their clients' privacy.[69,70]

Professional organizations are often a source of marketing advice and materials. Several organizations are involved in national marketing campaigns that can be adapted to local settings, such as the *ACNM Discover Midwives* consumer-facing PowerPoint presentation.[71]

## Billing for Services

A midwifery practice cannot continue to exist over the long term without financial stability. One of the first financial lessons in the healthcare business is that what is billed for a service is never what the insurance company will pay. Actual reimbursement rates are always lower—a factor that must be taken into consideration when calculating a budget. Whenever the services provided by midwives are billable, the services provided must be clearly documented and the billing process must be completed. The midwife is responsible for fulfilling the requirements for documentation that support the billing codes. For example, the amount paid for an examination will vary based on the intensity of the examination as measured by the number of systems included in the physical assessment, the types of problems identified, and the amount of time spent providing and coordinating care. If this content is not thoroughly documented in the healthcare record, payment may be reduced or even denied.

Regardless of how the billing is performed, the owner(s) of the practice is (are) responsible for establishing a system of checks and balances that monitors the accuracy and timeliness of the billing process and limits the opportunity for fraud. The time and money spent establishing a viable healthcare record and billing systems are necessary outlays to ensure the ongoing business success. Even midwives who are employees should be informed about the business revenue and expenses, so they will understand the financial stability of the practice.

## Malpractice Insurance Coverage

While the terms "medical malpractice insurance" and "professional liability insurance" are often used interchangeably, these types of insurance coverage are not the same. Medical malpractice insurance provides coverage for patient injury caused by healthcare professionals, including midwives and nurses. Professional liability insurance provides compensation for actual or alleged negligent injury resulting from professional services. Professional liability insurance offers the benefit of additional coverage for allegations such as slandering another healthcare provider or inadequately training an assistant. While medical malpractice insurance covers only injury to patients, professional liability insurance also covers acts, errors, and omissions in the provision of professional services in addition to patient injury.[72]

In a 2018 national survey of ACNM members, one-third of members reported being named in a lawsuit at some point in their professional careers[72]; 64.2% of these lawsuits pertained to care received in a hospital setting, 25.4% in a clinic setting, 8.7% in a freestanding birth center, and 2.0% in a home setting. Fetal assessment and shoulder dystocia remain the most common reasons for claims made during the intrapartum period, whereas claims made against home and birth center midwives most often involve transfer of care to a hospital.

It is recommended that all midwives carry professional liability insurance and familiarize themselves with their obligations, rights, and responsibilities under this insurance contract. Midwives should understand any exceptions to coverage listed by the insurance policy and be aware of when their practice is outside of the bounds of their contract coverage.[72]

Sources of professional liability insurance coverage include ACNM insurance services, self-insurance, joint underwriting associations, and the Federal Tort

Claims Act. ACNM insurance services include advice and sharing of information from colleagues, affiliates, and leadership of ACNM about insurance companies based on experiences within the midwifery community. Self-insurance occurs when individuals in similar situations and institutions purchase insurance coverage that is tailored to their circumstances. For example, a large hospital or university may offer its employed midwives insurance coverage through its self-insurance program. Self-insurance organizations set aside funds and invest the capital themselves, with the goal of accruing enough income to pay future claims.

Joint underwriting associations (JUAs) are chartered through state legislation to provide insurance when other sources are not obtainable. JUAs have been formed by several commercial insurance companies that are compelled by states to offer insurance. Texas, Minnesota, Pennsylvania, South Carolina, and Florida all have established JUAs through legislation.

Finally, midwives employed by federally qualified health centers and government institutions, such as military hospitals, often have professional liability insurance provided at no cost through the Federal Tort Claims Act. Under this act, claims that occur during the time of employment or coverage will be covered regardless of when the claim is filed.[72]

Types of insurance policies include occurrence policies, claims-made policies, slot policies, and shared limits policies (**Table 2-10**). Occurrence policies are the most comprehensive—and most expensive—type of insurance policies. Events that occur during the policy period are covered with such policies, regardless of the date of discovery or the date when the claim is filed. With occurrence policies, it does not matter if the claim is made years after the event occurred or if the midwife is no longer employed by that employer or no longer in practice.

Claims-made policies are less expensive, but more limited in scope than occurrence policies. Claims-made policies cover only claims that are made while the insurance policy is active. Once the policy ends, it no longer covers claims made that occurred during the time the policy was active. In such a case, the midwife may need to purchase tail coverage if they leave their place of employment or cease practicing. Tail coverage provides coverage for events that occur during the time the policy was in effect. Tail coverage does tend to be expensive, and the annual premium increases each year until the fifth year of coverage, when it will then remain stable. The length of the tail coverage can vary between

| Table 2-10 | Important Information When Purchasing Malpractice Coverage | |
|---|---|---|
| **Terms** | **Explanation** | **What the Midwife Needs to Know** |
| Indemnification | Large healthcare organizations can be self-insured, meaning they indemnify employees who are named in a malpractice lawsuit. Coverage typically does not extend to work settings not owned by the organization. | What are the payout limits of the policy? The midwife is covered only when their actions are consistent with the job description. Is the policy an occurrence or claims-made policy? Pros and cons of purchasing a second policy? |
| Malpractice policy | Purchased from private insurance companies. Individuals can purchase as an individual, and sometimes midwives are covered as an employee of a physician. Need to be clear regarding the circumstances when the policy will end. | Do I need and can I get prior-acts coverage? Do I need to have my own policy or am I named as an employee on a physician policy? Is this an occurrence policy or a claims-made policy? I have an occurrence policy now; can I purchase prior-acts coverage under my new policy? Can I purchase a tail when I no longer need the policy? If yes, how is that priced? |
| Claims-made coverage | More limited in scope and less expensive than occurrence policies. The insured has malpractice coverage only for claims that are made when the policy is in effect. The midwife will need to obtain tail coverage when a claims-made policy ends or upon leaving their position of employment. | Can I purchase a tail when I no longer need this policy? If yes, how is that priced and how long will the tail policy cover? |
| Occurrence coverage | Most comprehensive. The insured is covered during the policy period, regardless of the date of discovery or the date the claim is filed. Typically, the most expensive type of insurance. | If employment ends, coverage for future events ends but coverage is still in place for events that occurred when the policy was in place. Tail coverage should not be needed. |
| Going bare | The individual midwife decides to not carry malpractice insurance. | While some consider this approach unethical, the rising cost of premiums often brings up this discussion. Two major concerns need to be considered: (1) Your personal or family savings and property may be at risk and (2) if you apply for hospital privileges in the future, a period of clinical practice without malpractice coverage may lead to denial of privileges. |
| Limits of coverage | Professional liability policies have two sets of limits: a per-claim or per-incident limit and the aggregate limit that the insurer will pay during the policy period (usually 1 year). Example: $1 million per claim/$3 million per policy period | Do state law and/or hospital bylaws dictate the minimum coverage a midwife must carry? |

Data from Page K. *Midwives' Guide to Professional Liability.* 3rd ed. Silver Spring, MD: American College of Nurse-Midwives; 2020.

insurance companies. The statute of limitations for an adverse birth outcome is usually 2 years in most states, but some states permit claims for adverse birth outcomes to be filed as late as 21 years following birth. Therefore, it is important to know the length of coverage provided by the tail insurance.

Slot policies are a mixture of occurrence and claims-made policies. The employer purchases a certain number of "slots," and each full-time midwife in the practice is assigned to a slot, receiving an individual policy. In some cases, part-time midwives may share a single slot. When a midwife occupying one slot leaves the practice, no tail is due unless the practice closes the slot; then the normal tail rate applies. If the midwife leaving the practice is replaced, the new midwife now occupies the slot.

The previous midwife remains covered for the period during which the slot was occupied.

Finally, with shared limits policies, multiple midwives within a practice share a single policy with defined limits. The policy is priced depending on the size of the group and the risk of lawsuit. Tail coverage does not need to be purchased when a midwife leaves the practice.[72]

## Other Opportunities Within Midwifery

Midwives often engage in many types of activities at any one time. They can use their various skill sets to not only provide clinical care, but also support and advance the profession itself. These activities may include participation in policy making, education, and team development. Any or all of these roles may be assumed as a midwife in clinical practice or may be the primary area of expertise of a midwife not in clinical practice.

### Engagement in Policy

The building blocks of the midwifery profession (standards for education, certification, licensure, and practice) are key policy decisions with far-reaching influence. Federal, state, and institutional policies determine which healthcare services and birth settings are available to clients, as well as who will be reimbursed and at what rate. Which education programs receive government funding is also a matter of policy. Hospitals, clinics, and employers all write policies that influence access to and provision of midwifery care. With so much at stake for the profession and the clients cared for by midwives, every midwife needs to be knowledgeable about and engaged in policy-making processes. Table 2-11 lists ICM's tips for midwives participating in advocacy.[73]

Professional organizations remain dependent on work from members to keep policies relevant. Meeting the policy needs of the profession is a labor of love and shows determination to turn a vision into reality. Opportunities to engage in policy work with the professional association can be personally rewarding—and for some, may become a full-time endeavor. Many of the midwives who successfully work in policy making initially doubted their abilities or hoped someone else would do it.[74] The midwifery profession is filled with successful midwife role models, and guidance on how to make this transition is available (Table 2-12).

Social media, when used effectively, can help reach more people when advocating for new policies or policy change. Suggestions from the ICM about using social media for advocacy purposes appear in Table 2-13. While social media can be helpful in amplifying your message, comments to posts

| Table 2-11 | International Confederation of Midwives' Tips for Advocacy in Midwifery |
|---|---|

1. Take responsibility. Each person in a problematic situation must understand their responsibility in creating that problem. It is imperative that we take responsibility for our own part.
2. Never give up. While politicians and policymakers are knowledgeable, they need information. Keep it simple and precise.
3. Get the support of the persons for whom we provide care. The population midwifery serves need to know that midwifery exists and demand it. Build the grassroots base.
4. Be one team, with one voice. Join midwifery associations to combine efforts, knowledge, and skills.
5. Collaborate. Policy cannot be tackled alone! Develop relationships with key potential partners. Utilize social media platforms, raise awareness, and speak up!
6. Be convincing. Inform yourself well about maternal and newborn health issues in your community, state, nation, and world. Arm yourself with convincing facts and information.
7. Use evidence and stay positive. Collaboration, cooperation, the use of evidence, being politically astute, and being skilled in the use of media are all important factors in creating change.
8. Be strategic. Be specific; do not be too broad or too complex. Multiple small, effective campaigns are better than one great idea that is not concrete enough or too broad to get off the ground.
9. Stay focused on the population midwifery serves; let others see the commitment.
10. Be bold and speak without fear. Start with the desire and interest to make a change. Do not let fear be the barrier.

Modified from International Confederation of Midwives. ICM advocacy toolkit for midwives. https://www.internationalmidwives.org/assets/files/advocacy-files/2020/03/icm_midwivesadvocacytoolkit_final_2019.pdf. Published 2019. Accessed November 20, 2022.

need to be monitored and offensive content quickly removed. All social media posts should be sensitive to the need to protect patient identity.

In spite of many past successes, considerable policy work remains to be done in relation to midwifery. Some physician associations are opposed to laws that recognize advanced practice clinicians and midwives as independent providers; instead, they advocate for physician supervision. Many state laws governing the practice of midwifery need to be

| Table 2-12 | How to Influence the Policy-Making Process: Volunteer, Observe, and Practice |
|---|---|

**Institutional policies: Write policies for your midwifery practice, hospital, and/or local midwifery organization.**

- Is there a template to follow?
- What must be done to have the policy approved?

**Legislative policies: Observe legislative policy in action by attending a hearing that addresses a regulatory issue that affects your practice.**

- Who seems to be the most effective legislator and why?
- What is common etiquette and the standard for appearance and dress?
- Was the speaker effective? How did you know?
- How did the committee respond?

**Identify a mentor.**

- Get help preparing statements.

**Come prepared and speak a language the audience can understand.**

- Create the draft for discussion so others have to respond to your ideas.
- Stay on topic.

**Know your strengths.**

- Offer a lived experience.
- Be the voice of a midwife or support a client or family member who agrees to speak.

**Know your opposition and do not attend alone. Leave the door open for your return.**

- Make friends in the room.
- Defer to other experts.

**If you can't do policy, support your colleagues who can do this work, including financially.**

| Table 2-13 | Strategies for Utilizing Social Media for Advocacy |
|---|---|
| **Social Media Platform** | **Strategies** |
| Facebook | Use midwifery-themed photos as profile or cover photos |
| | Set up a page about your intended policy or event |
| | Post messages |
| | Share pictures and videos |
| | Invite friends to attend events |
| | Engage with followers by asking questions and sending messages |
| Twitter | Post messages using the hashtag #Midwives |
| | Share pictures |
| | Change the profile photo and header photo to midwife-themed photos |
| | Announce an event |
| | Share live and unfolding updates |
| | Post links to midwifery content such as blogs, articles, and videos |
| | Retweet, comment on, and like tweets about #Midwives |
| Instagram | Promote events through photos and videos |
| | Share high-quality photos and videos from events or activities |
| | Request engagement with your posts by asking questions |
| | Post messages using hashtags such as #Midwives, #GenderEquality, etc. |
| | Share midwifery messages, visuals, and videos |
| | Use a midwifery-themed profile photo |
| Blog posts | Typically short articles or editorials |
| | Often tell a personal story |
| | Can be used to respond in depth to current events or previously published information |

Modified with permission from Williams DR. We need to say in unison: we are midwives, and we do policy! [Editorial]. *J Midwifery Women's Health.* 2008;53(2):101-102. © 2008, with permission from Wiley.

Based on International Confederation of Midwives. ICM advocacy toolkit for midwives. https://www.internationalmidwives.org/assets/files/advocacy-files/2020/03/icm_midwivesadvocacytoolkit_final_2019.pdf. Published 2019. Accessed November 20, 2022.

changed to permit independent practice. The midwifery profession will also continue to adapt in response to federal and state legislation.

In addition, the midwifery profession has some major decisions looming. These include decisions about whether (1) CNMs should promote midwifery practice acts that are separate from nursing and include their CM colleagues or stay under the APRN umbrella; (2) CNMs/CMs and CPMs should be licensed under the same practice act; and (3) a doctoral degree should be required for CNM/CM certification.

### Education

All midwives are educators. Policy makers, potential employers, and consumers need to learn about the unique and valuable midwifery approach to care. Many clients seek out midwives because they want to learn more about how to care for their own bodies and how to safely prepare for puberty, pregnancy, menopause, and all the points in between. Consumer-oriented materials often are used for this purpose, and many materials are written by midwives. For example, the *Journal of Midwifery & Women's Health* publishes a health education handout series titled *Ask the Midwife*. These copyright-free handouts, targeted to midwifery clients, review important clinical topics using appropriate language and illustrations for all levels of health literacy. Some handouts are also available in Spanish.

Because many midwives are committed to precepting students, the midwifery profession continues to flourish. The legacy of midwifery depends on mentoring midwifery students as they enter into this role. For those who choose an academic career devoted to teaching midwifery students, there are more than 40 midwifery education programs accredited by ACME. Midwives who serve as faculty for schools of nursing and medicine have a unique opportunity to prepare the next generation of healthcare providers.

### Quality Improvement

The importance of data collection was discussed earlier in this chapter. Once data are collected, the question remains regarding what to do with these data. Benchmarking is an excellent means of comparing outcomes for similar-size practices to reward success and determine areas for improvement. Quality improvement science provides the tools for implementing and evaluating change. The Institute for Healthcare Improvement (IHI) is a resource for midwives worldwide to develop skills in the science of improvement.[75] The IHI process focuses on establishing a goal or aim, deciding how to define improvement, and producing concrete steps to create change. This is partnered with rapid tests of change in the form of plan–do–study–act cycles.

Midwives can serve as leaders and partners in implementing change in their practices and facilities. The Alliance for Innovation on Maternal Health, for example, has published patient safety bundles to assist perinatal care providers in improving the processes of care and patient outcomes.[76] ACNM members have served as authors of many of these patient safety bundles, and many ACNM state affiliates partner with state perinatal quality collaboratives to implement these bundles.

### Research and Research Implementation

Midwifery has a long tradition that includes learning by watchful waiting; sharing empirical knowledge via oral traditions; defining and protecting the physiologic birth process; and actively challenging "the evidence." These characteristics have served midwives well, especially when research has validated the midwifery approach to care. Examples where midwives have had a strong influence in the evolution of best practices include elimination of routine episiotomies,[77] redefinition of the Friedman labor curve,[78,79] promotion of early and prolonged breastfeeding for neonatal and maternal health,[80] delayed cord-clamping,[81,82] immediate skin-to-skin contact between mother and newborn,[83] water immersion during labor,[84] an alternative pain assessment tool for those in labor,[85] and nonpharmacologic methods of pain control.[86]

A 2017 American College of Obstetricians and Gynecologists (ACOG) Committee Opinion, *Approaches to Limit Intervention During Labor and Birth*, has the potential to improve labor management.[87] Acknowledging that "many common obstetric practices are of limited or uncertain benefit for low-risk women in spontaneous labor," this document makes 11 evidence-based recommendations intended to decrease unnecessary interventions and increase maternal and family satisfaction. These recommendations closely align with ACNM recommendations.[88]

In 2000, Sackett et al. concisely defined evidence-based practice (EBP) as the "integration of the best research evidence with clinical expertise and patient values."[89] Not all midwives need to actively conduct research, but all need to understand relevant research and implement evidence-based care. The call for systematic use of evidence in perinatal care is often credited to the 1989 publication of *Effective Care in Pregnancy and Childbirth*.[90] In this ground-breaking treatise, the authors carefully evaluated existing research and identified those clinical practices supported by research as well as those not based on evidence.

Several databases that summarize the most recent evidence on a multitude of clinical topics are available to sexual and reproductive and perinatal healthcare providers. One important evidence-based database is the Cochrane Library. Cochrane

Reviews are systematic reviews of primary research in human health care and health policy and are widely recognized for the quality of the reviews.[91] Other sources of research that midwives often use include PubMed, the Up-to-Date Database, and DynaMed.

When assessing research data and results, it is important to remember that not all evidence is equal. As detailed in *the Interpreting Published Research Data with a Clinical Midwifery Lens* appendix, evidence is evaluated to determine its strength.[92] Several rating criteria have been developed to evaluate the strength and quality of research. One of the most commonly used rating scales is that used by the U.S. Preventive Services Task Force, which is discussed in the *Health Promotion Across the Lifespan* chapter.

Systematic reviews of the literature have documented that midwifery-led care (care in which the primary provider is the midwife) for essentially healthy women is equivalent to the care provided by physicians. For several outcome measures, midwifery care has been found to be associated with improved outcomes compared to physician care. A 2008 Cochrane meta-analysis reviewed 11 trials including 12,276 women and found several statistically significant differences in outcomes for those women who received midwife-led care.[93] All of the studies included in this systematic review were randomized controlled trials; in addition, the studies were not limited to one country. The findings showed that midwife-led care resulted in fewer prenatal hospitalizations, less use of regional analgesia, fewer episiotomies, and fewer instrument deliveries. In addition, women who received midwife-led care were more likely to experience no intrapartum analgesia/anesthesia, spontaneous vaginal birth, feeling in control during childbirth, attendance at birth by a known midwife, and initiation of breastfeeding. Finally, the newborns of women who had midwife-led care were more likely to have a shorter length of hospital stay. The authors concluded that "most women should be offered midwife-led models of care, and women should be encouraged to ask for this option although caution should be exercised in applying this advice to women with substantial medical or obstetric complications."[93]

Similar results were highlighted in a 2011 systematic review that examined outcomes for APRNs in the United States. For the purposes of this study, the authors defined certified nurse-midwives as a type of APRN, and CNM birth outcomes from 1990 to 2008 were examined separately from those of other groups of providers who were not CNMs.[94]

This review summarized the results from all levels of studies, including observational studies, and studies were limited to the United States. A high level of evidence was found that patients of CNMs, as compared to patients of physicians, had lower rates of cesarean section birth, episiotomy, operative birth, labor analgesia, and perineal lacerations, and equivalent rates of labor augmentation, low Apgar scores, and low-birth-weight infants. The systematic review also demonstrated a moderate level of evidence that care by CNMs is associated with lower rates of epidural use and induction of labor, comparable or higher rates of vaginal births, comparable or lower rates of newborn intensive care unit admissions, and higher rates of breastfeeding than care from other professionals.[94]

In 2016, the Cochrane Pregnancy and Childbirth Group published a review comparing midwife-led continuity models and other models of care,[95] updating the 2008 systematic review conducted by Hatem et al.[93] Fifteen trials involving 17,674 women were reviewed. In all trials, the pregnant women were randomly assigned to midwife-led continuity models of care or other models of care. In short, women who received the midwife-led continuity model of care were less likely to experience interventions, were more likely to be satisfied with their care, and had at least comparable rates of adverse outcomes compared to women who received other models of care. The major findings from this review are summarized in Table 2-14.

Midwives do not work in isolation, but frequently collaborate with and refer to other perinatal healthcare professionals. In 2018, a multidisciplinary team analyzed data across 50 states examining midwifery practice and interprofessional collaboration.[96] Differences across states in scope of practice, autonomy, governance, and prescriptive authority, as well as restrictions that can affect patient safety, quality, and access to maternity providers across birth settings, were analyzed. The results showed that state regulatory environments that supported greater integration of midwives into the health system were significantly associated with greater access to maternity services, higher rates of spontaneous vaginal birth, vaginal birth after cesarean section (VBAC), and breastfeeding at birth and at 6 months, as well as lower rates of obstetric interventions, preterm birth, low-birth-weight infants, and neonatal death. In the state-by-state comparison, the best outcomes for mothers and babies occurred in states where all types of midwives were integrated into the healthcare system regardless of birth setting.[96] Furthermore, a *Lancet* analysis of

| Table 2-14 | Systematic Review of Midwife-Led Continuity of Care, 2016 | | |
|---|---|---|---|
| Outcome or Subgroup Title | Number of Studies; Quality of Evidence | Number of Participants | Relative Risk (95% Confidence Interval) |
| **Primary Outcomes: Significant Risk Reductions Found for Patients of Midwives** | | | |
| Regional anesthesia | 14; high quality | 17,674 | RR = 0.85 (0.78–0.92) |
| Instrumental vaginal birth | 13; high quality | 17,501 | RR = 0.90 (0.83–0.97) |
| Preterm birth: less than 37 weeks' gestation | 8; high quality | 13,238 | RR = 0.76 (0.64–0.91) |
| Less all fetal loss before and after 24 weeks' gestation plus neonatal death | 13; high quality | 17,561 | RR = 0.84 (0.71–0.99) |
| **Patients of Midwives Were More Likely to Experience** | | | |
| Spontaneous vaginal birth | 12; high quality | 16,687 | RR = 1.05 (1.03–1.07) |
| No difference between groups for cesarean birth and intact perineum. | | | |
| **Secondary Outcomes: Significant Risk Reductions Found for Patients of Midwives** | | | |
| Amniotomy | 4 | 3253 | RR = 0.80 (0.66–0.98) |
| Episiotomy | 14 | 17,674 | RR = 0.84 (0.77–0.92) |
| Fetal loss less than 24 weeks' gestation and neonatal death | 11 | 15,645 | RR = 0.81 (0.67–0.98) |
| **Patients of Midwives Were More Likely to Experience** | | | |
| No intrapartum analgesia or anesthesia | 7 | 10,499 | RR = 1.21 (1.06–1.37) |
| Longer length of labor | 3 | 3328 | RR = 0.50 (0.27–0.74) |
| Attended at birth by known midwife | 7 | 6917 | RR = 7.04 (4.48–11.08) |

Based on Sandall J, Soltani H, Gates S, et al. Midwife-led continuity models versus other models of care for childbearing women. *Cochrane Database Syst Rev.* 2016;4:CD004667. doi:10.1002/14651858.CD004667.pub5.

maternal health policy performed in 2014 revealed that countries with a sustained 20-year decrease in maternal mortality had increased country-wide access to health care through targeted investment in midwifery care.[97]

In addition to these large reviews, numerous other published research studies have focused on specific practices of midwives that may account for differences in maternal and neonatal outcomes. In 2019, ACNM updated a PowerPoint slide set titled "The Pearls of Midwifery," which communicates the evidence for midwifery care.[88] This presentation serves as a resource for sharing the evidence for midwifery practices such as continuous labor support and intermittent auscultation with both providers and families.

## Interprofessional Team Collaboration

All healthcare providers work within a healthcare system that includes professionals who have different scopes of practice, professional cultures, and professional roles. Being a team member in the healthcare system does not imply assumption of a subservient role: In some situations, a midwife is the team leader; in others, the midwife is a colleague on an interprofessional team. Factors that make interprofessional relationships work well are critically important when a patient develops complications or conditions that extend beyond the scope of midwifery practice. Although it has long been recognized that interprofessional teams provide better care than single-disciplinary groups for individuals

| Table 2-15 | Guiding Principles of Team-Based Care |
|---|---|

The patients and families are central to and actively engaged as members of the healthcare team.

The team has a shared vision.

Role clarity is essential to optimal team building and team functioning.

All team members are accountable for their own practice and to the team.

Effective communication is key to the creation of high-quality teams.

Team leadership is situational and dynamic.

Based on Jennings J, Nielsen P, Buck ML, et al. Executive summary: collaboration in practice: implementing team-based care: report of the American College of Obstetricians and Gynecologists' Task Force on Collaborative Practice. *Obstet Gynecol.* 2016;127(3):612-617.

with complex healthcare needs,[98,99] interprofessional collaboration and communication have only recently been the focus of research, education, and clinical initiatives.[100,101] Guiding principles of interprofessional team–based care are summarized in Table 2-15.

In 1999, a ground-breaking report from the Institute of Medicine, *To Err Is Human*, reported an estimated that 45,000 to 98,000 individuals die each year in U.S. hospitals due to healthcare errors.[102] Subsequent safety reports have highlighted poor communication and inadequate team coordination as the source of many of these errors. For example, a Joint Commission sentinel event analysis on preventing infant death and injury during birth identified communication problems as the root cause of the healthcare delivery error in 72% of the cases analyzed.[103] In the same analysis, 55% of the organizations studied cited organizational culture, including "hierarchy and intimidation, failure to function as a team, and failure to follow the chain-of-communication," as commonly encountered barriers to effective communication and teamwork.[103]

In the years following these publications, much work has been done to identify ways to foster and support teamwork in healthcare delivery. Successful interprofessional collaboration in care during pregnancy, for example, has been associated with improved outcomes, a high degree of client satisfaction, fewer cesareans, and lower costs.[104] According to the ICM's *Essential Competencies for Basic Midwifery Practice*, "The midwife . . . works collaboratively (teamwork) with other health workers to improve the

delivery of services to women and families."[14] Moreover, "[the] midwife has the skill and/or ability to . . . identify deviations from normal during the course of pregnancy and initiate the referral process for conditions that require higher levels of intervention."[14]

ACNM recognizes that midwives are independent practitioners who function within a complex healthcare system, which includes collaboration with multiple healthcare professionals, to ensure the health and safety of patients and their newborns.[105] The levels of collaborative management as defined by ACNM include consultation, collaboration, and referral. The definitions for each of these levels often serve as guidelines for similar language within state laws and hospital bylaws. While the ACNM definitions address the midwife–physician relationship, the expertise of many other healthcare professionals may be needed to provide the best care possible. It is imperative that all members of the team understand their role in caring for a specific patient (Table 2-16).[106]

The 2022 ACNM and ACOG *Joint Statement of Practice Relations Between Obstetrician-Gynecologists and Certified Nurse-Midwives/Certified Midwives* declares that "health care is most effective when it occurs in a system that facilitates communication across care settings and among clinicians."[106] NACPM and MANA have published documents that address the relationship between CPMs and physicians.[9,107] In these documents, midwifery practice is described as autonomous and CPMs are expected to collaborate, refer, and transfer care in critical situations. Essential components of communication and teamwork are summarized in Table 2-17.[108–110]

Teamwork and communication are skills that can be learned.[111–113] Although healthcare outcomes following simulation training have not yet fully been determined, it appears that simulation training improves teamwork, team coordination, and interprofessional communication.[114–116]

ACNM and ACOG, with funding from the Josiah Macy Jr. Foundation, have partnered in the development of interprofessional education models that aim to increase the number of midwives educated alongside obstetrician-gynecologist residents. Through this project, modules were created on topics such as guiding principles of team-based care, patient-centered care, roles of scopes of practice on midwives and obstetrician-gynecologists, collaborative practice, history of both professions, care transitions, and difficult conversations.[117] Learners participating in these modules have reported an overall improvement in their ability to collaborate and especially valued the team-based experiences.[118]

| Table 2-16 | The Continuum of Collaborative Management in Midwifery Care | | | | |
|---|---|---|---|---|---|
| Type of Collaborative Management | Definition | Primary Responsibility for Care | Midwife's Role | Collaborator's Role | Comments |
| **Consultation** | "The process whereby a CNM or CM seeks the advice or opinion of a physician or another member of the healthcare team." | Midwife | Primary provider | Advisor/ consultant | Prepare for the consultation.<br><br>Know the client's health history.<br><br>Review the basics for management of the diagnosis or problem.<br><br>Understand the social and psychosocial factors underlying their health.<br><br>Understand the practice setting and scope of practice.<br><br>Remember the Midwifery Management Process. |
| **Collaboration** | "The process whereby a CNM or CM and physician jointly manage the care of a patient or newborn who has become medically, gynecologically, or obstetrically complicated." | Collaborative management; depending on the severity of the complication, the midwife may remain the primary care provider | Normal processes, coordination of care, continuity with the individual | Care for the perinatal, gynecologic, or neonatal complications | Use interprofessional communication techniques such as SBAR and closed-loop communication.<br><br>Clearly delineate roles to ensure all aspects of the POC are considered.<br><br>Communicate with the client and their family about the relationship. |
| **Referral**[a] | "The process by which the CNM or CM directs the client to a physician or another healthcare professional for management of a particular problem or aspect of the client's care." | Physician or other referral provider | Coordination of care, timely and full transfer of care, continuity of services | Assumes the primary responsibility for care of the individual | Ensure that referral/transfer is the best POC for the individual.<br><br>Ensure that the client understands that they have been transferred to another provider's care and that they have access to appointment and contact information.<br><br>Consider the potential problem of abandonment of the client and/or "punting" of a difficult-to-care-for client.<br><br>Let the client and provider know if the client can return to midwifery care when/if the condition resolves.<br><br>Use interprofessional communication techniques within a formal handoff. |

Abbreviations: CM, certified midwife; CNM, certified nurse-midwife; POC, plan of care; SBAR, Situation, Background, Assessment, Recommendation.

[a]Referral in this continuum refers to transfer of care. Referral in the context of insurance is providing an individual with a reference to a specialty provider.

Based on the American College of Nurse-Midwives. Position statement: collaborative management in midwifery practice for medical, gynecologic, and obstetric conditions. https://www.midwife .org/ACNM/files/ACNMLibraryData/UPLOADFILENAME/000000000058/Collaborative-Mgmt-in-Midwifery-Practice-Sept-2014.pdf. Published September 2014. Accessed February 17, 2022.

| Table 2-17 | Essential Components of Successful Collaboration and Teamwork[a] |
|---|---|

Professional competence of each member of the team (common body of knowledge, shared language, similarities in treatment modalities)

Common orientation to the client or newborn as the primary unit of attention

Shared mental model: Every member of the team can anticipate the needs of the others

Recognition and acknowledgment of interdependence among all members of the team

Interprofessional respect and mutual trust

Formal system of communication between providers

Effective communication based on the goal of reaching consensus (an interest in solutions that maximize the contributions of all parties)

Mutual performance monitoring (identification of mistakes and provision of feedback within the team to facilitate self-correction)

Identified team leader for each situation

Situation monitoring and adaptability as the situation changes

Ability to shift work responsibilities as needed to under-utilized team members

[a] This list is compiled from different analyses of essential characteristics for teams in general and for teams in specific urgent or emergency situations. It is not designed to be complete or the components placed in rank order; rather, the intent is to identify some characteristics that are essential for successful interprofessional team function. Midwives are always members of interprofessional teams.

Based on Interprofessional Education Collaborative Expert Panel. *Core Competencies for Interprofessional Collaborative Practice: Report of an Expert Panel.* Washington, DC: Interprofessional Education Collaborative; 2011; Ivey S. A model for teaching about interdisciplinary practice. *J Allied Health.* 1988;17: 189-195; King TL, Laros RK, Parer JT. Interprofessional collaborative practice in obstetrics and midwifery. *Obstet Gynecol North Am.* 2012;39:411-422.

| Table 2-18 | Example of SBAR Used for a Consultation |
|---|---|

A midwife at an office is caring for a female patient who is at 33 weeks' gestation and was diagnosed earlier in the pregnancy with gestational diabetes. When reviewing their blood glucose log, the midwife observes that more than 20% of her values are high and calls the consulting maternal–fetal medicine physician and requests consultation using SBAR.

**S:** I want to consult with you about a female patient with uncontrolled gestational diabetes.

**B:** MG is a 24-year-old primigravida at 33 weeks by LMP consistent by 19-week ultrasound. Her 1-hour glucose tolerance test was 150 mg/dL and her 3-hour glucose tolerance test had two elevated values. She was sent to the diabetes education center, where she received diet and glucose monitoring education as well as information on regular exercise. Over the last 2 weeks, 20% of her values are out of range, with five fasting levels between 100 mg/dL and 110 mg/dL and five 2-hour postprandial levels higher than 150 mg/dL, the highest being 180 mg/dL. She had a reactive NST today, the fetus is size equal to dates, and her urinalysis was negative for glucose.

**A:** My concern is that the dietary changes and exercise have been inadequate to control glucose levels, and I believe she needs medication.

**R:** I would like to schedule her to see you for a consultation within the next few days.

Abbreviations: LMP, last menstrual period; NST, nonstress test; SBAR, Situation, Background, Assessment, Recommendation.

AHRQ has developed a series of materials and training curricula, collectively titled TeamSTEPPS, that can be used in healthcare settings to help foster successful teamwork.[119] The TeamSTEPPS curricula emphasize the development of four core competencies: communication, mutual support, situation monitoring, and leadership.

## Communication Techniques for Successful Collaboration

Direct and deliberate communication techniques include SBAR, closed-loop communication, and the handoff. SBAR—an acronym for Situation, Background, Assessment, and Recommendation— is a structured communication tool that has been shown to significantly improve the quality of communication between healthcare providers and to reduce errors.[112] The SBAR approach omits the nonessential elements of a patient's history, distills the most pertinent information, and clarifies what is needed. The midwife can use the SBAR approach to obtain a consultation from a specialist (**Table 2-18**) or to communicate during an emergency (**Table 2-19**).

In closed-loop communication, the midwife directs the message to a particular team member, the team member repeats the order or request aloud, and the midwife confirms that the team member heard correctly. This communication approach is particularly important during times of stress, as it allows the entire team to hear the orders and correct any errors before the orders are

| Table 2-19 | Example of SBAR Used in an Emergency Situation |
|---|---|

A midwife at a small community hospital is caring for a client who is bleeding heavily immediately after giving birth and has called for physician assistance from a provider in the next room. When the physician arrives, the midwife says:

**S:** M.T. is having a postpartum hemorrhage.

**B:** M.T. gave birth to her fifth child 15 minutes ago over an intact perineum. The total EBL is 800 mL. We gave 40 IU of oxytocin (Pitocin), 0.2 mg of ergonovine (Methergine), and 250 mcg of carboprost (Hemabate). The placenta appeared intact, and there are no clots in the lower uterine segment.

**A:** Severe uterine atony is present, and I think I feel some placental tissue in the anterior portion of the fundus.

**R:** I need you to put on gloves and assist me.

Abbreviations: EBL, estimated blood loss; SBAR, Situation, Background, Assessment, Recommendation.

| Table 2-20 | Sample Critical Elements for a Transfer Note from Community to Inpatient Care |
|---|---|

Record time and destination, method of transportation, and who is accompanying the birthing person/newborn when care is transferred.

Identify the birthing person/neonate and the transferring provider; as well as the receiving provider.

The critical elements are customized to the individual and the situation but generally include:

1. Risk factors for the current situation/disorder requiring transfer
2. Signs and symptoms indicating need for transfer
3. Care provided before transfer: procedures and results; laboratory results or if pending; medications (dosage, route, and time of last dose); response to treatment
4. Assessment/diagnosis of the situation
5. Summary of the rationale for the transfer
6. Statement on whether the person can return to midwifery care after the issue has resolved
7. Request for information about the treatment plan for follow-up

executed. Closed-loop communication tools such as the *call-out* and the *check-back* can be used to communicate critical information to all members of the team, thereby allowing them to anticipate what will be needed next. Use of such techniques also requires that team members communicate what they intend to do and have done with the information.

When a patient needs to be transferred to another provider for care, especially for a higher level of care, a formal note should be written in the health record and shared with the new provider. The goal of this communication is to give the new provider all the pertinent information needed to safely care for the patient and family. In several of the chapters in this text, *critical elements* are listed for conditions that typically require a transfer of care. In some situations, a midwife may receive a transfer from another provider. In that case, the midwife who receives the transfer should communicate, either verbally or in writing, with the referring provider to acknowledge that the patient has been seen and provide a summary of the course of care. Table 2-20 provides an overview of the content of a transfer or handoff note and the critical elements it should contain. Strategies for a safe transfer from a community-based setting to a hospital are described in the *Home Birth Summit: Best Practice Guidelines Transfer from Home Birth to Hospital*, and a companion resource includes model home birth transfer forms.[120,121]

Communication skills such as SBAR, closed-loop communication, and the handoff are like any clinical skill: They must be adapted to individual settings and practiced until they become second nature.

## The Midwifery Profession Globally

Midwives' commitment to providing personalized care that is responsive to each individual's needs and their significant improvements of communities' health outcomes has resulted in recognition of the value of midwives' role among the global community of healthcare professionals. This multi-layered approach—from the individual, to the profession, to evidence-based practice, to individuals wherever they need care—is reflected throughout this text.

For many years, midwives in the United States and many countries around the world were undervalued by the policy makers who designed and funded healthcare systems. Most would agree that this lack of recognition, and the accompanying low pay, was a direct reflection of the value that policy makers assigned to women, gender-diverse people, and sexual/reproductive health care. In a trajectory that closely follows the change in rights of women and gender-diverse individuals, midwives have found their collective voice, established professional standards for education and practice that compare favorably to those of their physician colleagues, and proved their value to modern society.

While public acceptance and legal recognition of midwives as professional and autonomous healthcare providers has varied by state in the United States as well as by country internationally, the global community of midwives is increasingly united around the need to earn and seek this recognition. The ICM is a global federation of midwifery associations that has worked for more than 100 years to support, represent, and strengthen professional associations of midwives throughout the world.

ICM initially provided a much-needed forum for midwives to learn from each other and expand access to midwifery care. Nevertheless, it was not until 1972 that the confederation agreed to set standards for who should be able to use the midwife title. The original focus of this organization—to increase the number of midwives—reflected an understanding that too many people were dying during childbirth because they were giving birth unattended. Over time, it became clear that a lack of common standards for the preparation and practice of midwives could also put the lives of women at risk.

Many midwives feared that setting standards for midwifery education and practice would isolate traditional midwives and decrease access to care. Others emphasized the value for midwives of setting their own standards and using these standards as the justification to fund education for midwives, especially in countries with limited resources. In 1972, the ICM published its first *Definition of a Midwife*; it was most recently updated in 2017. In 2010, ICM published the *Essential Competencies for Basic Midwifery Practice*; it was most recently updated in 2019.[14] In addition, ICM has highlighted the importance of Indigenous midwives to the health and well-being of Indigenous communities.[122] It recognizes the need to ensure that Indigenous midwives are legally recognized and to advocate for funding of Indigenous midwives who are educated and regulated to their community standards.

Between 2008 and 2011, the ICM accepted the difficult challenge of formally describing the three pillars of midwifery: education, regulation, and essential core competencies for midwifery practice. These core ICM documents have an important impact on midwifery in all nations.[14,123] For example, the Midwifery Education, Regulation, and Association work group,[124] a collaboration of the seven midwifery professional associations in the United States, has worked to adapt the ICM documents for midwifery in the United States. The 2015 publication of *Principles for Model U.S. Midwifery Legislation and Regulation* is one of the outcomes of this collaboration.[10] ICM now publishes multiple gap analysis tools and curriculum guidelines designed to assist midwifery associations and policy makers in actualizing their support for professional midwifery practice. ICM continues to evolve its support for midwifery globally. In 2021, ICM updated its Midwifery Framework to expand on the three pillars of midwifery, including an additional seven elements: the midwifery philosophy, essential competencies for midwifery, research, midwife-led continuity of care model of practice, leadership, enabling environment, and commitment to gender equality, justice, diversity, and inclusion.[125] Since its launch in the early 1900s, ICM has expanded to include, as of 2023, 140 midwifery associations from 119 countries, representing 1 million midwives globally.[125]

The ACNM has been a member of ICM since 1956. The ACNM and many CNMs/CMs have made significant contributions to ICM's mission by strengthening midwifery associations globally, publishing training materials for midwives such as the *Life-Saving Skills Manual for Midwives*[126] and *Home-Based Skills Manual for Midwives*,[127] and advocating for reduction of preventable pregnancy-related and neonatal deaths globally.

## Conclusion

In the twenty-first century, midwifery is an evolving profession with a strong, inspirational foundation; a mature infrastructure to promote policies that improve access to high-quality midwifery care; highly educated individuals who are defining best practice; and plenty of unfulfilled potential. Midwives have demonstrated their capacity to do the hard work of profession building, critically evaluate traditional models of care, challenge policies based on flawed research and practices, and pursue a more just healthcare delivery system. Future changes and growth in the profession will reflect the innovation and expertise of the next generation of midwives, what brings them to the profession, their educational experiences, and their desire to contribute to furthering the profession of midwifery and to partnering with their clients in creating a world where all persons receive the best care possible.

## Resources

### Midwifery and Related Organizations

| Organization | Description |
| --- | --- |
| American Association of Birth Centers (AABC) | A multidisciplinary membership organization dedicated to the birth center model of care. |
| American College of Nurse-Midwives (ACNM) | Professional organization for certified nurse-midwives and certified midwives in the United States. The Hallmarks of Midwifery can be found on its website. |
| American College of Obstetricians and Gynecologists (ACOG) | Founded in 1951, ACOG is the specialty's professional membership organization dedicated to the improvement of women's health. |
| American Nurses Association (ANA) | ANA advances the nursing profession and advocates on healthcare issues that affect nurses and the public. |
| American Public Health Association (APHA) | APHA works to strengthen the profession and to speak out for public health issues and policies supported by science. |
| Association of Women's Health, Obstetric, and Neonatal Nurses (AWHONN) | AWHONN works to improve and promote the health of birthing persons and newborns, and to strengthen the nursing profession. |
| Black Mamas Matter Alliance (BMMA) | BMMA is a Black women–led cross-sectoral alliance that centers Black mothers and birthing people to advocate, drive research, build power, and shift culture for Black maternal health, rights, and justice. |
| Childbirth Connection | Founded in 1918 as the Maternity Center Association, this organization is now a program in the National Partnership for Women and Families. It works to improve the quality and value of maternity care through consumer engagement and health system transformation. Childbirth Connection promotes safe, effective, and satisfying evidence-based maternity care and is a voice for the needs and interests of childbearing families. |
| Coalition for Quality Maternal Care (CQMC) | In April 2011, nine national professional, consumer, and human rights organizations announced the formation of this coalition to champion the urgent need for national strategies to improve the quality and value of maternal and newborn health care in the United States. |
| International Confederation of Midwives (ICM) | This global federation of midwifery associations has worked for more than 100 years to support, represent, and strengthen professional associations of midwives throughout the world. |
| Midwives Alliance of North America (MANA) | The mission of MANA is to unite, strengthen, support, and advocate for the midwifery community and to promote educational, economic, and cultural sustainability of the midwifery profession. |
| National Association of Certified Professional Midwives (NACPM) | Professional organization for CPMs in the United States. |
| National Association of Nurse Practitioners in Women's Health (NPWH) | NPWH works to ensure the provision of quality primary and specialty health care to women of all ages by women's health and women's health–focused nurse practitioners. |
| National Association to Advance Black Birth (NAABB) | NAABB's mission is to combat the effects of structural racism within maternal and infant health to advance Black birth outcomes. |
| National Birth Equity Collaborative (NBEC) | NBEC creates transnational solutions that optimize Black maternal, infant, sexual, and reproductive well-being. It aims to shift systems and culture through training, research, technical assistance, policy, advocacy, and community-centered collaboration. |

| Organization | Description |
|---|---|
| National Black Midwives Alliance (NBMA) | The mission of NBMA is to establish a representative voice at the national level that organizes, advocates, and brings visibility to the issues impacting Black midwives and the communities they serve. |
| National Partnership for Women and Families (NPWF) | Founded in 1971 as the Women's Legal Defense Fund, NPWF promotes fairness in the workplace, reproductive health and rights, access to quality, affordable health care, and policies that help individuals meet the dual demands of work and family. |
| National Women's Health Network (NWHN) | Feminist health activists who use policy analysis as a tool. Starting in 1940 with a protest about the risks of estrogen, NWHN has sought to bring the voice of people concerned about women's health to the decision makers who create and implement health policies. |
| White Ribbon Alliance | International organization with a mission to catalyze and convene advocates who campaign to uphold the right of all women to be safe and healthy before, during, and after childbirth. |

## References

1. Ament LA. *Professional Issues in Midwifery.* Sudbury, MA: Jones and Bartlett; 2007.

2. Shah MA, Barger MK, King TL. Editors choice: the first 25 years of *The Journal. J Midwifery Womens Health.* 2010;50(2):154-158.

3. Varney H. *Nurse-Midwifery.* Hoboken, NJ: Blackwell Science; 1980.

4. Dutton LA, Desmore JE, Turner MB. *A Pocket Guide to Clinical Midwifery: The Efficient Midwife.* Burlington, MA: Jones & Bartlett Learning; 2019.

5. Tharpe NL, Farley CL, Jordan RG. *Clinical Practice Guidelines for Midwifery and Women's Health.* Burlington, MA: Jones & Bartlett Learning, 2022.

6. Walsh L. *Midwifery: Community Based Health Care During the Childbearing Years.* Philadelphia, PA: WB Saunders, 2001.

7. Kennedy HP. A model of exemplary midwifery practice: results of a Delphi study. *J Midwifery Womens Health.* 2000;45(1):4-19.

8. American College of Nurse-Midwives. Comparison of certified nurse-midwives, certified midwives, certified professional midwives clarifying the distinctions among professional midwifery credentials in the U.S. http://www.midwife.org/Updated-CNM-CM-CPM-Comparison-Chart-October-2017. Published October 2017. Accessed January 18, 2022.

9. National Association of Certified Professional Midwives. Who are CPMs? https://www.nacpm.org/new-page-2#:~:text=A%20Certified%20Professional%20Midwife%20(CPM,birth%20and%20the%20postpartum%20periods. Accessed March 5, 2023.

10. U.S. Midwifery Education, Regulation, and Association. Principles for model US midwifery legislation & regulation. http://www.usmera.org/wp-content/uploads/2015/11/US-MERALegislativeStatement2015.pdf. Accessed March 5, 2023.

11. Childbirth Connection. Home page. http://www.childbirthconnection.org. Accessed February 18, 2022.

12. Citizens for Midwifery. Welcome to Citizens for Midwifery! https://www.citizensformidwifery.org. Accessed February 18, 2022.

13. American College of Nurse-Midwives. *Core Competencies for Basic Midwifery Practice.* Silver Spring, MD: American College of Nurse-Midwives; 2020. https://www.midwife.org/acnm/files/acnmlibrarydata/uploadfilename/000000000050/ACNMCoreCompetenciesMar2020_final.pdf. Accessed November 20, 2021.

14. International Confederation of Midwives. *Essential Competencies for Midwifery Practice.* https://www.internationalmidwives.org/our-work/policy-and-practice/essential-competencies-for-midwifery-practice.html. Accessed November 20, 2021.

15. Foster IR, Lasser J. *Professional Ethics in Midwifery Practice.* Sudbury, MA: Jones and Bartlett; 2011.

16. Thompson JB. A human rights framework for midwifery care. *J Midwifery Womens Health.* 2004;49(3):175-176.

17. Thompson JB, King TL. Resources for clinicians: a code of ethics for midwives. *J Midwifery Womens Health.* 2004;49(3):263-265.

18. American College of Nurse-Midwives. ACNM code of ethics with explanatory statements. http://www.midwife.org/ACNM/files/ACNMLibraryData/UPLOADFILENAME/000000000293/Code-of-Ethics-w-Explanatory-Statements-June-2015.pdf. Published June 2015. Accessed February 28, 2023.

19. Midwives Alliance of North America. Statement of values and ethics. https://mana.org/resources/statement-of-values-and-ethics. Accessed February 28, 2023.

20. Beauchamp TL, Childress JF. *Principles of Biomedical Ethics.* 5th ed. New York, NY: Oxford University Press; 2001.

21. Varkey B. Principles of clinical ethics and their application to practice. *Med Princ Pract.* 2021;30:17-28.

22. Tronto JC. *Moral Boundaries: A Political Argument for an Ethic of Care.* London, UK: Routledge; 1993.

23. MacLellan J. Claiming an ethic of care for midwifery. *Nurs Ethics.* 2014;21(7):803-811.

24. Newnham E, Kirkham M. Beyond autonomy: care ethics for midwifery and the humanization of birth. *Nurs Ethics.* 2019;26(7-8):2147-2157.

25. Ross L, Solinger R. *Reproductive Justice: An Introduction.* Berkeley, CA: University of California Press; 2017.

26. Butts JB, Rich KL. *Nursing Ethics: Across the Curriculum and Into Practice.* Burlington, MA: Jones & Bartlett Learning; 2016.

27. Megregian M, Low LK, Emeis C, et al. Essential components of midwifery ethics education: results of a Delphi study. *Midwifery.* 2021;96:102946.

28. Elwyn G, Coulter A, Laitner S, et al. Implementing shared decision making in the NHS. *BMJ.* 2010;341:c5146.

29. Altman MR, Oseguera T, McLemore MR, et al. Information and power: women of color's experiences interacting with health care providers in pregnancy and birth *Soc Sci Med.* 2019;238:112491.

30. Elwyn G, Durand MA, Song J, et al. A three-talk model for shared decision making: multistage consultation process. *BMJ.* 2017;359. doi:j4891.10.1136/bmj.j4891.

31. Stacey D, Légaré F, Col NF, et al. Decision aids for people facing health treatment or screening decisions. *Cochrane Database Syst Rev.* 2017;4:CD001431.

32. Agency for Healthcare Research and Quality. The SHARE approach. https://www.ahrq.gov/professionals/education/curriculum-tools/shareddecisionmaking/index.html. Published July 2014; reviewed February 2017. Accessed December 10, 2021.

33. Megregian M, Nieuwenhuijze M. Choosing to decline: finding common ground through the perspective of shared decision making. *J Midwifery Womens Health.* 2018;63(3):340-346. doi:10.1111/jmwh.12747.

34. American College of Nurse-Midwives. Descriptive data nurse-midwives—USA. *Bull Am Col Nurse-Mid.* 1963;8(1):30-37.

35. Bureau of Labor Statistics. Occupational employment and wages, May 2020. https://www.bls.gov/oes/current/oes291161.htm. Accessed February 18, 2022.

36. American Midwifery Certification Board. 2021 demographic report. https://www.amcbmidwife.org/docs/default-source/reports/demographic-report-2021.pdf?sfvrsn=cac0b1e8_2. Published 2021. Accessed February 19, 2022.

37. American College of Nurse Midwives. The ACNM Core Data Survey. https://www.midwife.org/acnm/files/cclibraryfiles/filename/000000008289/CDS_2019_Major%20Findings%20Final.pdf. Published 2019. Accessed February 19, 2022.

38. Kennedy HP, Erickson-Owens D, Davis JA. Voices of diversity in midwifery: a qualitative research study. *J Midwifery Womens Health.* 2006;51(2):85-90.

39. Holmes LJ. *Into the Light of Day: Reflections on the History of Midwives of Color Within the American College of Nurse-Midwives.* Washington, DC: LJH Consultancies; 2011.

40. Health Resources and Services Administration. The rationale for diversity in the health professions: a review of the evidence. http://docplayer.net/255577-The-rationale-for-diversity-in-the-health-professions-a-review-of-the-evidence.html. Published 2006. Accessed February 28, 2023.

41. Serbin J, Donnelly E. The impact of racism and midwifery's lack of racial diversity: a literature review. *J Midwifery Womens Health.* 2016;61(6):694-706.

42. U.S. Department of Health and Human Services, Centers for Disease Control and Prevention, National Center for Health Statistics, Division of Vital Statistics. Natality public use data 2016–2020, on WONDER online database, October 2021. https://wonder.cdc.gov/natality-expanded-current.html. Accessed November 30, 2021.

43. Niles P, Drew M. Constructing the modern American midwife: white supremacy and white feminism collide. Nursing CLIO. https://nursingclio.org/2020/10/22/constructing-the-modern-american-midwife-white-supremacy-and-white-feminism-collide/. Published October 22, 2020. Accessed February 18, 2022.

44. Luke J. *Delivered by Midwives: African American Midwifery in the Twentieth-Century South.* Jackson, MS: University Press of Mississippi; 2018.

45. Smedley L, Butler A, Bristow L . *In the Nation's Compelling Interest: Ensuring Diversity in the Health-Care Workforce.* Washington, DC: National Academies Press; 2004. https://doi.org/10.17226/10885.

46. Siddiqui NJ, Andrulis DP, Stelter A, et al. *Taking Stock: The Affordable Care Act's Progress Toward Advancing Health Equity.* Austin, TX: Texas Health Institute; 2016.

47. Scott KA, Britton L, McLemore MR. The ethics of perinatal care for Black women: dismantling the structural racism in "mother blame" narratives. *J Perinat Neonatal Nurs.* 2019;33(2):108-115. doi:10.1097/JPN.0000000000000394.

48. Black Mamas Matter Alliance. Setting the standard for holistic care of Black women. https://blackmamasmatter.org/wp-content/uploads/2018/04/BMMA_BlackPaper_April-2018.pdf. Published April 2018. Accessed February 18, 2022.

49. James SE, Herman JL, Rankin S, et al. The report of the 2015 U.S. Transgender Survey. https://transequality.org/sites/default/files/docs/usts/USTS-Full-Report-Dec17.pdf. Published 2016.

50. Hughto JMW, Gunn HA, Rood BA, et al. Social and medical gender affirmation experiences are inversely associated with mental health problems in a U.S. non-probability sample of transgender adults. *Arch Sex Behav*. 2020;49(7):2635-2647.

51. Turban JL, King D, Carswell JM, et al. Pubertal suppression for transgender youth and risk of suicidal ideation. *Pediatrics*. 2020;145(2):e20191725. doi:10.1542/peds.2019-1725.

52. de Vries AL, McGuire JK, Steensma TD, et al. Young adult psychological outcome after puberty suppression and gender reassignment. *Pediatrics*. 2014;134:696-704.

53. Grant JM, Mottet LA, Tanis J, et al. *Injustice at Every Turn: A Report of the National Transgender Discrimination Survey*. Washington, DC: National Center for Transgender Equality & National Gay and Lesbian Task Force; 2011. https://transequality.org/sites/default/files/docs/resources/NTDS_Report.pdf.

54. Tornello SL, Bos H. Parenting intentions among transgender individuals. *LGBT Health*. 2017;4(2):115-120. doi:10.1089/lgbt.2016.0153.

55. American College of Nurse-Midwives. Position statement: health care for transgender and gender non-binary people. http://www.midwife.org/acnm/files/acnmlibrarydata/uploadfilename/000000000326/ACNM--PS--Care%20for%20TGNB%20People-%20Final_1.pdf. Published 2021. Accessed February 18, 2022.

56. American College of Nurse-Midwives, Midwives Alliance of North America, National Association of Certified Professional Midwives, Supporting healthy and normal physiologic childbirth: a consensus statement by ACNM, MANA and NACPM. https://www.midwife.org/ACNM/files/ACNMLibraryData/UPLOADFILENAME/000000000272/Physiological%20Birth%20Consensus%20Statement-%20FINAL%20May%2018%202012%20FINAL.pdf. Accessed January 19, 2017.

57. Schuiling KD, Slager J. Scope of practice: freedom within limits. *J Midwifery Womens Health*. 2000;45(6):465-471.

58. American College of Nurse-Midwives. Expansion of midwifery practice and skills beyond basic core competencies. https://www.midwife.org/acnm/files/acnmlibrarydata/uploadfilename/000000000066/2022_ps_expansion-of-midwifery-practice-beyond-core-competencies.pdf. Published September 10, 2022. Accessed September 15, 2022.

59. APRN Consensus Work Group, National Council of State Boards of Nursing APRN Advisory Committee. Consensus model for APRN regulation: licensure, accreditation, certification & education. National Council of State Boards of Nursing. https://www.ncsbn.org/public-files/Consensus_Model_for_APRN_Regulation_July_2008.pdf. Published July 2008.

60. American College of Nurse-Midwives, Accreditation Commission for Midwifery Education, American Midwifery Certification Board. Midwifery in the United States and the Consensus Model. https://www.midwife.org/ACNM/files/ccLibraryFiles/Filename/000000001458/LACE_White_Paper_2011.pdf. Published 2011. Accessed February 28, 2023.

61. American College of Nurse-Midwives. 2020 privileging survey data. https://www.midwife.org/acnm/files/cclibraryfiles/filename/000000008226/ACNM%20Privileging%20Survey.pdf. Updated January 15, 2021. Accessed February 18, 2022.

62. Buppert C. *Nurse Practitioner's Business Practice and Legal Guide*. 6th ed. Burlington, MA: Jones & Bartlett Learning; 2018.

63. Bryant C. *An Administrative Manual for Midwifery Practices*. 5th ed. Washington, DC: American College of Nurse-Midwives; 2022.

64. Brumberg H, Dozor D, Golombek S. History of the birth certificate: from inception to the future of electronic data. *J Perinatol*. 2012;32:407-411. https://doi.org/10.1038/jp.2012.3.

65. Baxter L. Documenting nurse-midwifery outcomes. *J Nurse-Midwifery*. 1986;31(4):169-170.

66. American College of Nurse-Midwives. The ACNM Benchmarking Project. http://www.midwife.org/Benchmarking. Accessed November 10, 2022.

67. Midwives Alliance of North America. MANA Statistics Project. https://mana.org/research/about-manastats. Accessed November 10, 2022.

68. American Association of Birth Centers. AABC Perinatal Data Registry (PDR). http://www.birthcenters.org/PDR. Accessed November 10, 2022.

69. Demiris G. Consumer health informatics: past, present, and future of a rapidly evolving domain. *Yearb Med Inform*. 2016;suppl 1:S42-S47.

70. Arcia A. Facebook advertisements for inexpensive participant recruitment among women in early pregnancy. *Health Educ Behav*. 2014;41(3):237-241.

71. American College of Nurse-Midwives. Discover midwives presentation for consumers. http://www.midwife.org/discover-midwives-presentation-for-consumers. Accessed November 10, 2022.

72. Page K. *Midwives' Guide to Professional Liability*. 3rd ed. Silver Spring, MD: American College of Nurse-Midwives; 2020.

73. International Confederation of Midwives. ICM advocacy toolkit for midwives. https://www.international midwives.org/assets/files/advocacy-files/2020/03/icm_midwivesadvocacytoolkit_final_2019.pdf. Published 2019. Accessed November 20, 2022.

74. Williams DR. We need to say in unison: we are midwives and we do policy! [Editorial]. *J Midwifery Women's Health*. 2008;53(2):101-102.

75. Institute for Healthcare Improvement. Science of improvement. https://www.ihi.org/about/Pages/ScienceofImprovement.aspx. Accessed November 20, 2022.

76. Alliance for Innovation on Maternal Health. Patient safety bundles. https://saferbirth.org/patient-safety-bundles/#what-are-psbs. Accessed November 20, 2022.

77. Jiang H, Qian X, Carroll G, et al. Selective versus routine episiotomy for vaginal birth. *Cochrane Database Syst Rev*. 2017. http://onlinelibrary.wiley.com/doi/10.1002/14651858.CD000081.pub3/full.

78. Albers LL, Schiff M, Gorwoda JG. The length of active labor in normal pregnancies. *Obstet Gynecol*.1996;87:355-359.

79. Zhang J, Troendle JF, Yancey MK. Reassessing the labor curve in nulliparous women. *Am J Obstet Gynecol*. 2002;187:824-828.

80. Horta BL, Bahl R, Martines JC, et al. *Evidence on the Long-Term Effects of Breastfeeding: Systemic Review and Meta-analyses*. Geneva, Switzerland: World Health Organization; 2013. https://apps.who.int/iris/handle/10665/43623.

81. Mercer JS, Vohr BR, McGrath MM, et al. Delayed cord clamping in very preterm infants reduces the incidence of intraventricular hemorrhage and late-onset sepsis: a randomized, controlled trial. *Pediatrics*. 2006;117(4):1235-1242.

82. McDonald SJ, Middleton P, Dowswell T, et al. Effect of timing of umbilical cord clamping of term infants on maternal and neonatal outcomes. *Cochrane Database Syst Rev*. 2013;7:CD004074. doi:10.1002/14651858.CD004074.pub3.

83. Moore ER, Bergman N, Anderson, GC, et al. Early skin-to-skin contact for mothers and their healthy newborn infants. *Cochrane Database Syst Rev*. 2016;11. doi:10.1002/14651858.CD003519.pub4.

84. Cluett ER, Burns E, Cuthbert A. Immersion in water in labour and birth. *Cochrane Database Syst Rev*. 2018;2(5):CD000111. doi:10.1002/14651858.CD000111.pub4.

85. Roberts L, Gulliver B, Fisher J, et al. The coping with labor algorithm: an alternate pain assessment tool for the laboring woman. *J Midwifery Womens Health*. 2010;55:107-116.

86. Jones L, Othman M, Dowswell T, et al. Pain management for women in labour: an overview of systematic reviews. *Cochrane Database Syst Rev*. 2012;3:CD009234. doi:10.1002/14651858.CD009234.pub2.

87. American College of Obstetricians and Gynecologists. ACOG Committee Opinion No. 766: approaches to limit intervention during labor and birth. https://www.acog.org/clinical/clinical-guidance/committee-opinion/articles/2019/02/approaches-to-limit-intervention-during-labor-and-birth/. Published February 2019. Accessed February 28, 2023.

88. American College of Nurse-Midwives. Evidence-based practice: pearls of midwifery: a presentation by the American College of Nurse-Midwives, Washington, DC, 2019. https://www.midwife.org/Evidence-Based-Practice-Pearls-of-Midwifery. Accessed February 28, 2023.

89. Sackett DL, Straus SE, Richardson WS, et al. *Evidence-Based Medicine: How to Practice and Teach EBM*. 2nd ed. Edinburgh, UK: Churchill Livingstone; 2000.

90. Chalmer I, Enkin M, Marc JM, et al. *Effective Care in Pregnancy and Childbirth*. Oxford, UK: Oxford University Press; 1989.

91. *Cochrane Database of Systematic Reviews*. http://www.cochranelibrary.com. Accessed February 28, 2023.

92. U.S. Preventive Services Task Force. Grade definitions. https://www.uspreventiveservicestaskforce.org/uspstf/about-uspstf/methods-and-processes/grade-definitions. Published 2016. Accessed November 10, 2022.

93. Hatem M, Sandall J, Devane D, et al. Midwife-led versus other models of care for childbearing women. *Cochrane Database Syst Rev*. 2008;4:CD004667. doi:10.1002/14651858.CD004667.pub2.

94. Newhouse RP, Stanik-Hutt J, White KM, et al. Advanced practice nurse outcomes 1990–2008: a systematic review. *Nurs Econ*. 2011;29(5):230-250.

95. Sandall J, Soltani H, Gates S, et al. Midwife-led continuity models versus other models of care for childbearing women. *Cochrane Database Syst Rev*. 2016;4:CD004667. doi:10.1002/14651858.CO004667.pub5.

96. Vedam S, Stoll K, MacDorman M, et al. Mapping integration of midwives across the United States: impact on access, equity, and outcomes. *PLOS ONE*. 2018;13(2):e0192523. https://doi.org/10.1371/journal.pone.0192523.

97. Midwifery. *Lancet*. June 23, 2014. http://www.thelancet.com/series/midwifery.

98. Baldwin DC Jr. Some historical notes on interdisciplinary and interprofessional education and practice in health care in the USA. *J Interprof Care*.1996;21(suppl 1):23-37.

99. Avery M, Montgomery O, Brandl-Salutz E. Essential components of successful collaborative maternity care models. *Obstet Gynecol North Am*. 2012;39:423-434.

100. Waldman R, Kennedy HP, Kendig S. Collaboration in maternity care: possibilities and challenges. *Obstet Gynecol Clin North Am.* 2012;39:435-444.

101. Jennings J, Nielsen P, Buck ML, et al. Executive summary: collaboration in practice: implementing team-based care: report of the American College of Obstetricians and Gynecologists' Task Force on Collaborative Practice. *Obstet Gynecol.* 2016;127(3):612-617.

102. Kohn LT, Corrigan JM, Donaldson MS. *To Err Is Human: Building a Safer Health System.* Washington, DC: National Academy Press; 2000.

103. The Joint Commission. *Sentinel Event Alert: Preventing Infant Death and Injury During Delivery* (Issue No. 30). Oakbrook Terrace, IL: The Joint Commission; 2004. https://www.jointcommission .org/resources/sentinel-event/sentinel-event-alert -newsletters/sentinel-event-alert-issue-30-preventing -infant-death-and-injury-during-delivery/#. ZAS6kXbMLIU. Accessed March 5, 2023.

104. Jackson DJ, Lang JM, Swartz WH, et al. Outcomes, safety, and resource utilization in a collaborative care birth center program compared with traditional physician-based perinatal care. *Am J Public Health.* 2003;93:999-1006.

105. American College of Nurse-Midwives. Position statement: collaborative management in midwifery practice for medical, gynecologic, and obstetric conditions. https://www.midwife.org/ACNM/files/ACNM LibraryData/UPLOADFILENAME/000000000058 /Collaborative-Mgmt-in-Midwifery-Practice -Sept-2014.pdf. Published September 2014. Accessed February 17, 2022.

106. American College of Nurse-Midwives. Joint statement of practice relations between obstetrician-gynecologists and certified nurse-midwives/certified midwives. https://www.acog.org/clinical-information /policy-and-position-statements/statements-of -policy/2018/joint-statement-of-practice-relations -between-ob-gyns-and-cnms November 2022).pdf. Published November 2022. Accessed March 5, 2023.

107. Midwives Alliance of North America. The midwives model of care. https://mana.org/about-midwives /midwifery-model. Accessed February 28, 2023.

108. Interprofessional Education Collaborative Expert Panel. *Core Competencies for Interprofessional Collaborative Practice: Report of an Expert Panel.* Washington, DC: Interprofessional Education Collaborative; 2011.

109. Ivey S. A model for teaching about interdisciplinary practice. *J Allied Health.* 1988;17:189-195.

110. King TL, Laros RK, Parer JT. Interprofessional collaborative practice in obstetrics and midwifery. *Obstet Gynecol North Am.* 2012;39:411-422.

111. King H, Battles J, Baker DP, et al. TeamSTEPPS® 2.0: team strategies and tools to enhance performance and patient safety. In: Henriksen K, Battles JB, Keyes MA, et al., eds. *Advances in Patient Safety: New Directions and Alternative Approaches (Vol. 3: Performance and Tools).* Rockville, MD: Agency for Healthcare Research and Quality; August 2008. https://www.ncbi.nlm.nih.gov/books/NBK43686/. Accessed February 28, 2023.

112. Merien AER, van der Ven J, Mol BW, et al. Multidisciplinary team training in a simulation setting for acute obstetric emergencies: a systematic review. *Obstet Gynecol.* 2010;115(5):1021-1031.

113. Crofts JF, Ellis D, Draycott TJ, et al. Change in knowledge of midwives and obstetricians following obstetric emergency training: a randomized controlled trial of local hospital, simulation center and teamwork training. *BJOG.* 2007;114:1534-1541.

114. Robertson B, Schumacher L, Gosman, G, et al. Simulation-based crisis team training for multidisciplinary obstetric providers. *Simulation in Healthcare.* 2009;4(2):77-83.

115. Baker DP, Gustafson S, Beaubien J, et al. *Medical Teamwork and Patient Safety: The Evidence-Based Relation Literature Review.* Rockville, MD: Agency for Healthcare Research and Quality; 2005. https:// archive.ahrq.gov/research/findings/final-reports /medteam/medteamwork.pdf. Accessed February 28, 2023.

116. Miller LA. Patient safety and teamwork in perinatal care: resources for clinicians. *J Perinat Neonat Nurs.* 2005;19(1):46-51.

117. Avery MD, Jennings JC, Germano E, et al. Interprofessional education between midwifery students and obstetrics and gynecology residents: an American College of Nurse-Midwives and American College of Obstetricians and Gynecologists collaboration. *J Midwifery Womens Health.* 2020;65(2):257-264. doi:10.1111/jmwh.13057.

118. Avery MD, Mathiason M, Andrighetti T, et al. Improved self-assessed collaboration through interprofessional education: midwifery students and obstetrics and gynecology residents learning together. *J Midwifery Womens Health.* 2022;67(5):598-607. doi:10.1111/jmwh.13394.

119. Agency for Health Care Research and Quality. TeamSTEPPS 2.0 curricula. https://www.ahrq.gov /teamstepps/about-teamstepps/index.html. Accessed November 10, 2022.

120. Home Birth Summit. Best practice guidelines: transfer from planned home birth to hospital. https://www .homebirthsummit.org/wp-content/uploads/2014/03 /HomeBirthSummit_BestPracticeTransferGuidelines .pdf. Accessed February 18, 2022.

121. Home Birth Summit. Transfer guidelines model forms. https://www.homebirthsummit.org/best -practice-transfer-guidelines/transfer-guidelines -model-forms/. Accessed February 18, 2022.

122. International Confederation of Midwives. Position statement: partnership between Indigenous and non-Indigenous midwives. https://www.internationalmidwives.org/assets/files/statement-files/2021/09/ps2021_en_indigenous-and-non-indigenous-midwives.pdf. Published 2021. Accessed November 10, 2022.

123. International Confederation of Midwives. Global standards for midwifery regulation 2010; amended 2013. https://www.internationalmidwives.org/assets/files/general-files/2018/04/companion-guidelines-for-ed-standards-2011---amended-web-edition-june-2013.pdf. Published 2013. Accessed March 5, 2023.

124. International Confederation of Midwives. ICM professional framework for midwifery 2021. https://www.internationalmidwives.org/assets/files/general-files/2022/05/professional-framework-2022.pdf. Accessed November 10, 2022.

125. International Confederation of Midwives. Who we are. https://www.internationalmidwives.org/about-us/international-confederation-of-midwives/. Accessed March 5, 2023.

126. Marshall MA, Buffington ST, Beck DR, Clark PA. *Life-Savings Skills: Manual for Midwives.* 4th ed. Silver Spring, MD: American College of Nurse-Midwives; 2008. http://www.midwife.org/ACNM-Publications. Accessed November 11, 2022.

127. Buffington ST, Sibley LM, Beck R, Armbruster DA. *Home Based Life Saving Skills.* 2nd ed. Silver Spring, MD: American College of Nurse-Midwives; 2010. http://www.midwife.org/ACNM/files/ccLibraryFiles/Filename/000000000545/Book%201_Basic%20Information_print%20ready.pdf. Accessed March 5, 2023.

# A P P E N D I X

# 2A

# Interpreting Published Research Data with a Clinical Midwifery Lens

MARY K. BARGER

Midwives need to be savvy consumers of scientific literature so that they can utilize the most current evidence to inform their clinical practice and shared decision making with patients. This appendix presents an overview of how to interpret published research to find meaning for clinical practice. It is beyond the scope of this appendix to provide extensive knowledge of biostatistics or the interpretation of clinical research. Instead, the goal is to examine commonly used approaches to present research findings and to demonstrate how these findings can be translated into clinical practice with care.

## Brief Overview of Selected Statistics

### Statistical Terms

Statistics appearing in published literature fit within several basic categories: descriptive, inferential, and Bayesian. Descriptive statistics provide basic information about a set of data or numbers, including the average (mean or median) and range of values. Sometimes descriptive statistics show a rate of an outcome in a population (the ratio of the number of people with the outcome to the total number of people in the population). For example, birth rates are often reported as the number of births per 1000 population in a year.

The kind of descriptive statistic used to analyze information depends on the nature of the data—that is, whether it is continuous, such as age and weight, or in categories. Categorical, or nominal, variables can be dichotomous, (e.g., cesarean birth: yes or no), or several categories, such as race and ethnicity. Other data can be in discrete categories but have an implied ranking (ordinal), such as scores on a Likert-type scale. These types of data are commonly found in questionnaires that measure symptoms

such as depression and anxiety. When these types of questionnaires are scored, the result can be similar in appearance to a continuous variable. Relative risk (RR) and odds ratio (OR) are descriptive statistics that describe the ratio of an outcome between two or more groups.

Inferential statistics are a set of tests used to analyze data and test hypotheses about the relationships between sets of data. Inferential statistics are used when trying to infer information about a population using a representative subgroup of the population. For example, are the average scores on a test different between two population groups? Knowing the type of data reported in a study is important for evaluating the analytic statistics because the type of data determines the exact inferential test that needs to be used. The kinds of inferential statistics most commonly used to convey results in published studies are simple comparisons between two variables (bivariate) or sets of data, such as a $t$-test for a difference in means or a chi-square test for a difference in frequencies in categorical variables. For comparing more than two groups, analysis of variance (ANOVA) can be used for continuous data. When statistics are used to predict an outcome, regression analysis is commonly used. If adjustment for baseline differences is important, then multivariate regression modeling can be used. Basic statistic textbooks or Internet resources can provide details on the inferential statistics for different kinds of independent and dependent variables.

Bayesian analysis is a type of statistical analysis that begins with a statistical model based on prior knowledge and then uses observed data from the current research or testing to make probability statements about the likelihood of a particular outcome. In reproductive health care, it is used in noninvasive prenatal testing (NIPT) to make statements

| Table 2A-1 | Statistical Terms Found in Research Studies |
|---|---|
| **Term** | **Definition** |
| Absolute risk | The number of individuals with a condition as a proportion of the total population. |
| Analysis of variance (ANOVA) | A statistical test to determine whether means are different between two or more groups. When there are only two groups, ANOVA is equivalent to a *t*-test. |
| Chi-square | A statistical test to determine whether the frequency of a categorical outcome is different among groups. |
| Confidence interval | The possible range of a result based on chance. Often reported as 95% confidence, which corresponds to a *P*-value of 0.05. |
| Effect size | A relative measure of the strength of association between variables or characteristics. |
| Numbers need to treat (NNT) | The number of individuals who need to receive an intervention so as to result in an improved outcome for one individual. This number should be considered along with the risk of the intervention and the risk of not intervening. |
| Odds ratio (OR) | The ratio of the odds of a condition in two groups. Odds are calculated as the percentage of the sample with the condition divided by the percentage of the sample without the condition. If the prevalence of an outcome is 20% in group A and 10% in group B, the odds of the outcome in group A is 20%/80% = 0.25; the odds of the outcome in group B is 10%/90% = 0.11. The odds ratio is 0.25/0.11 = 2.27. Odds ratios tend to exaggerate the effect when compared to relative risk, unless the outcome is rare (< 10%). |
| *P*-value | Statistical likelihood that a result could have happened by chance instead of representing an actual difference. Values range between 0 and 1, but are never 0 or 1. Often a *P*-value of 0.05 is used as a cutoff for statistical significance. |
| Probability | How likely it is that a specific outcome has happened or will happen. |
| Relative risk (RR) | The ratio of absolute risk in two groups. An RR of 1 means the risk is the same in the two groups. If the prevalence of an outcome is 20% in group A and 10% in group B, then the relative risk is 20%/10% = 2.0. |
| *t*-test | A statistical test to determine whether means are different between two groups. |

about the likelihood that a particular fetus has a chromosomal abnormality.

Table 2A-1 provides definitions of commonly used statistical terms.

## Screening Test Statistics

Midwives order many screening tests for their patients, such as 1-hour glucose tolerance tests and chlamydia tests. The principles for screening, along with the screening test statistics and an excellent example from clinical practice, are presented in the *Health Promotion Across the Lifespan* chapter. Briefly, all screening tests have a measurable sensitivity (i.e., how good the test is at identifying the people with the condition), and specificity (i.e., how good the test is at excluding those without the condition). In practice, no screening test is both 100% sensitive and 100% specific. When developing a screening test, the cutoff point established for a positive test result tries to maximize these two statistics but also considers the risks of missing those individuals with the condition (false negatives) versus identifying too many without it (false positives).

Although test sensitivity and specificity are not affected by the prevalence of the condition in a population, if the baseline prevalence of the disease being screened for is very low, most of the positive tests in this population will be false positives even if the test has an excellent sensitivity and specificity. Therefore, clinical practices may perform different screening tests depending on the prevalence of the condition in their patient population. As explained in the *Health Promotion Across the Lifespan* chapter, chlamydia screening may be limited to younger individuals, as there is a higher incidence of the infection in this age group.

Another screening statistic that relates to the problem of false positives is the positive predictive value. From a patient's point of view, the positive predictive values indicates "What is the probability that my positive test result means I have the condition?" This statistic highly depends on the prevalence of the condition in the population being screened. Although it is a probability that most patients really want to know, unless the prevalence is known in the specific population, it may be more difficult to quantify. A related statistic is the likelihood ratio, which describes the likelihood that a given test result would be expected in a patient with the condition compared to the likelihood that that same result would be expected in a patient without the condition. When evaluating the utility of a screening test, especially a new one, it is crucial to know the population screened during the test's development and the prevalence of the condition in that population.

An important consideration for the use of screening tests is to have a plan of action for the result, whether it is positive or negative. If the result will not change the plan of care, then it may not be worth the time and expense of performing the test. Because screening tests only screen for disease, a positive test should be followed with a diagnostic test. Sometimes this diagnostic test is fairly noninvasive, such as a urine culture for a urine dipstick that tests positive for leukocytes and nitrites. At other times, a positive screening test can lead to a cascade of diagnostic tests, such as with a positive test for Ca-125, a cancer biomarker. Unfortunately, when it comes to cancer screening tests, patients frequently want tests that will make no difference to their longevity and can result in harmful interventions leading to premature death.[1,2]

## Absolute Versus Relative Risk

Shared decision making with patients often includes discussions about the risks of alternative treatment options. It is important to know over what period of time the risk is calculated. Many people know the statistic, "the risk of breast cancer in women is 1 in 8." However, this does not mean on any given day an adult woman has a 12% chance of getting breast cancer. In fact, the 10-year risk of breast cancer in the highest-risk group, 70-year-old women, is only 4%.[3] The "1 in 8" statistic simply means that 12% of all women will develop breast cancer by the age of 80. Therefore, it is crucial to put statistics into context for patients.

Another important distinction is the difference between an absolute risk (AR) and a relative risk (RR). Context is very important when it comes to discussing relative risk statistics. Relative risk compares incidence of an outcome in someone with a condition or disease versus someone without that condition or disease. A large relative risk may not convey a large absolute risk if the baseline incidence for the outcome is rare. For example, suppose a new oral contraceptive has few side effects, including minimal weight gain. However, studies begin to show it has a RR of 3 for myocardial infarction (MI). This seems alarming, but the baseline risk for MI in women of childbearing age is about 1 in 1 million. Thus, the new contraceptive increases the MI risk from 1 in 1 million to 3 in 1 million. If a person stops taking this contraceptive due to publicity about increased MI risk and becomes pregnant, their risk of dying in pregnancy in the United States is approximately 200 per 1 million live births, or 67 times greater than the risk of MI.[4] **Table 2A-2** provides another example of the difference between RR and AR, describing ectopic pregnancy related to contraceptive methods.[5] Unless baseline risk is accounted for, relative risk can overstate the risks of medication or intervention.

## Study Designs

### Randomized Controlled Trials

Randomized controlled trials (RCTs), also known as randomized trials, enroll individuals in a research study and then allocate them to groups randomly, rather than providing a treatment or an intervention based on the person's needs or preferences. While this approach provides the best evidence for whether an intervention leads to the desired outcome, it has several limitations.

RCTs have strict inclusion and exclusion criteria, which helps assure that study participants are similar to each other. Some of these criteria may mean the study population will not reflect the clinical population seen by practitioners. Those individuals who agree to participate in the study may be very different than all of those who meet the study's criteria, which can lead to bias. For example, in a set of RCTs of epidural analgesia, although age was not an inclusion criterion, nearly all participants were 24 or younger (mean, 20 years; standard deviation [SD], 4.0).[6] The studies did not mention the number of people who were approached about the study but refused to participate, but it is clear that older people refused to be randomized to either epidurals or patient-controlled opioids. The studies included only nulliparous women, which also limits the generalizability of findings to all laboring persons. Both the study inclusion criteria and who ends up participating can limit the generalizability of the study

| Table 2A-2 | Using Risk of Ectopic Pregnancy by Contraceptive Method as an Example of Putting Relative Risk Within the Context of Absolute Risk | | | |
|---|---|---|---|---|
| Method | If Become Pregnant, Risk of Ectopic Pregnancy<br>A | Relative Risk for Ectopic Pregnancy<br>B | 1-Year Pregnancy Risk with Typical Use<br>C | Absolute Ectopic Risk per 1000 Persons<br>(Col A × Col C) × 1000 |
| No contraception | 2% | Reference (1.0) | 85% | 17 |
| Hormonal contraception | 3.5% | 1.75 | 7 % | 2.45 |
| Hormone-releasing intrauterine device | 10% | 5 | 0.2% | 0.2 |
| Tubal ligation | 25% | 12.5 | 0.5% | 1.25 |

Data from Herrell H. Absolute risk versus relative risk: a clinical example. *Howardisms.* https://howardisms.com/obgyn/absolute-risk-versus-relative-risk-a-clinical-example/. Published December 8, 2015. Accessed March 1, 2023.

findings to the total population of birthing people, which is important for translating results to an individual practice site. At the time of those epidural studies, women 24 or younger accounted for only one-third of all births.[7]

RCTs can assess whether a drug or an intervention produces an effect under *ideal* conditions. It is important to remember that real-world clinical conditions rarely reflect those in a study where everyone is trained to know the study protocol and, ideally, follow the protocol of the assigned intervention(s). In addition, because participants in a study are closely monitored and know they are being monitored, their adherence to the intervention is likely to be higher than that of the typical patient. The same can be said of the clinicians carrying out an intervention in the context of an RCT; their practice within a research context may not reflect their "standard" practice. Therefore, the size of the effect observed in an RCT will nearly always be much larger than the effect observed in clinical practice.

Another issue is study protocol fidelity and adherence to assigned group interventions. Study protocol fidelity is typically not well described in many published studies, but it is key to having valid study results. An unfortunate example where protocol fidelity and adherence were problematic was a very large, multisite trial of fetal movement (FM) counting in England.[8] In some centers, the individuals were placed in groups by which side of the hallway their clinic room was on—those seen in rooms on one side of the hallways were given FM instructions and those on the other side of the hallway were not. However, no steps were taken to prevent participants

from sharing information in the waiting room or with friends. There was little data collection about whether a participant actually monitored FM and if so, how often, regardless of group assignment. For the FM group, no information was provided on providers' adherence to the protocol, including a review of the FM chart at each prenatal visit and provision of follow-up instructions on when to call in the event of decreased FM. This study, despite its large sample size of 68,000, showed no difference in outcomes between the groups, which many clinicians interpreted as meaning that FM counting was ineffective in preventing stillbirth. However, several prior studies—both RCTs and cohort studies—uniformly demonstrated a decreased stillbirth rate of at least 50% when FM was consistently asked about at each visit and instructions for decreased movement were clear.[9,10] Cross-over between interventions will bias results toward finding no difference.

Sometimes the study itself can make the groups different, thereby defeating the purpose of randomizing the study groups in the first place. For instance, participants might not be willing to receive the intervention because it takes a lot of time or the drug causes a lot of side effects. An *intention-to-treat* (ITT) analysis preserves the attempts to equalize baseline differences and accounts for issues related to feasibility or acceptability of the treatment by analyzing study participants in their randomly assigned group, whether or not they completed the intervention. If the researchers conducting an RCT do not perform an ITT analysis, the study groups are likely to be different from how they were at the study's beginning, which potentially makes the groups no longer comparable.

Another threat to the purpose of randomization is differential drop-out or "lost to follow-up" rates between groups. Drop-out rates greater than 20% should be a concern, especially if they occur more in one group than another.[11] At minimum, a well-done RCT that does not include an ITT analysis should present a table of the baseline characteristics of participants in the final analysis in each group.

### Translating RCT Results to Clinical Practice: ARRIVE Trial Example

A Randomized Trial of Induction Versus Expectant Management (ARRIVE) was a multi-site RCT of elective induction of labor at 39 weeks' gestation compared to expectant management, whose results were published and received much publicity in 2019.[12] This trial among low-risk nulliparous individuals with a singleton, vertex pregnancy found no statistical differences on a neonatal composite measure but a significantly lower cesarean birth rate in those persons induced at 39 weeks' gestation (18.6% versus 22.2%). The question, then, is should elective induction be offered to all low-risk nulliparous individuals?

First, among the 50,000 individuals screened, half were not "healthy" enough to be eligible for the study. Then, another 13% did not meet one inclusion criterion—namely, a relatively certain last menstrual period. Of all those meeting all study criteria, only 27% agreed to participate. Those who agreed to possible induction at 39 weeks were younger than the U.S. birthing population, with only 4% being age 35 or older. Also, participants were more likely to be people of color than all study-eligible people. Therefore, the study population might be very different from that encountered by a particular clinical practice. Without replication studies in a variety of settings, we cannot know whether these results would be similar in a different population.

A less tangible issue to assess in an RCT is provider bias. In the ARRIVE trial, both providers and participants knew the participants' group assignment. It would be conceivable that a provider who favored elective induction would give a participant assigned induction a longer time to progress than one assigned to the expectant management group, either consciously or unconsciously. This trial was conducted at a time when there was strong advocacy for elective induction, which was highlighted with a debate, "Why not induce everyone at 39 weeks?" at the national American College of Obstetricians and Gynecologists (ACOG) conference, and covered by the media.[13]

Additionally, the size of results achieved in an RCT are rarely as large when translated into actual clinical practice.[14] Therefore, the 3.6% difference in cesarean rates with 39-week induction is likely to be smaller when translated into clinical practice.

Given the potential biases, issues related to the applicability of the findings to the general population of birthing individuals, the size of the effect in terms of potential decreased cesareans, and no difference in neonatal outcomes, it seems that a policy change to elective induction of all "healthy," low-risk nulliparous individuals is not appropriate based on this single trial. The number needed to treat (NNT) from this study is 28; that is, 28 inductions would be needed to avoid one cesarean birth. In general, interventions in healthy populations are not deemed to be of health benefit if the NNT is greater than 15.[15] Understanding the statistics used in research and the limitations of a study is helpful in understanding which research is valuable for implementation into care.

### Observational Studies

Study design dictates statistical analysis techniques. In perinatal care, most clinically useful research comes from observational studies, such as case-control or cohort studies, which are considered a lower quality of evidence than RCTs. Such study designs are often used when it is not ethical to perform RCTs. For example, it would be both unethical and infeasible to assign some individuals to smoke during pregnancy and others to not smoke to assess pregnancy outcomes. Similarly, it would be challenging to randomly assign people to different contraceptive methods.

In some cases, we want to know about outcomes that are (fortunately) rare, such as maternal or infant mortality. Even large RCTs do not have enough statistical power to find a difference in rare outcomes or outcomes that take years to develop. To assess for rare or delayed outcomes, case-control studies are valuable and cost-effective.

An excellent example of this approach is the case-control study that investigated a rare vaginal cancer in young women, which strongly suggested that diethylstilbesterol (DES) exposure in utero was the cause.[16] Researchers found 8 young women with vaginal cancer. They matched the young women with cancer (cases) with 32 women (controls) born on the same day in the same hospital. A detailed history of their mothers' pregnancy, childhood, and adolescent exposures, including recently introduced oral contraceptives, revealed the only difference between the cases and controls was that 7 of those with vaginal cancer had been exposed to DES in utero. None of the 32 healthy women had been exposed to DES—an infinitely large RR of 7/0. This result, corroborated with animal studies, so strongly suggested that DES was the cause of this otherwise rare vaginal cancer that DES is no longer given to pregnant people.

Another issue is that RCTs may not be able to answer the planned study question because patients assigned to one treatment might also receive the alternative treatment. This was the case in RCTs of the effect of epidural analgesia on cesarean birth rates. From an ethical standpoint, those participants randomized to receive intravenous opioid analgesia had to be offered an epidural if the opioid did not manage their pain. Those randomized to epidural analgesia may not have received one because their labor progressed too rapidly. As noted earlier, analysis of results in RCTs typically uses an ITT analysis, in which comparisons are made between the groups as assigned, rather than groups based on the actual treatment received. Therefore, the study result was not comparing those persons who did and did not actually receive epidurals.

In an analysis of five RCTs of epidurals from a single institution, the cross-over rate (the percentage of participants who were assigned to one treatment but received the other treatment) was about 30%.[6] A high cross-over rate dramatically increases the sample size necessary to show a difference in outcomes. Without cross-over, an RCT would need 400 participants to reliably demonstrate a doubling of cesarean risk (RR = 2) from 10% to 20%. With 30% cross-over, the trial would need 2400 participants to demonstrate the same finding. However, observational data might help answer this question.

A clinical trial examined perinatal outcomes in patients randomized to active management of labor versus usual management, and found no difference in cesarean birth rates.[17] However, the researchers collected a lot of data on participants' baseline characteristics at the time of admission, such as cervical dilation, fetal station, and estimated fetal weight. They then grouped participants with similar probability for an epidural intervention based on admission and baseline characteristics, similar to the principle of randomization. This method is called propensity score matching. Almost uniformly, within each group from lowest to highest probability for an epidural, those who received an epidural had twice the risk of a cesarean birth compared to those who did not.[18]

This example demonstrates how a well-designed observational study can rigorously control for other influences to answer the study question. Single studies, however, cannot be relied upon to answer these types of clinical questions. For example, meta-analyses of multiple RCTs that compared epidural analgesia to no epidural analgesia have not shown an association between epidural analgesia and cesarean birth.[19]

Observational data are routinely collected about patient care and outcomes in research databases, electronic medical records, and vital statistics, such as birth certificates. These data, if used ethically, can be used in clinical research and quality improvement initiatives. Two good examples are cohort studies that used hospital electronic records to evaluate differences in pain scores and receipt of pain medication by race or ethnicity.[20,21] One study had a sample size of 9900 and was able to control for differences in baseline characteristics among race and ethnic groups using propensity score matching, as previously described.[20] Both studies found Hispanic and Black women received significantly less pain medication than their white counterparts, despite the fact that they had 1.3 to 3 times the number of high pain scores.[20,21] As these studies suggest, conscious or unconscious bias in provision of pain medication is best studied with an observational study design.

## Systematic Reviews and Meta-analyses

A systematic review is a review of the health literature that uses a systematic strategy to search for studies on a particular topic, appraise the research quality, and synthesize the findings to inform practice. Some systematic reviews use meta-analysis, a statistical method that combines the results of several existing studies, usually smaller ones, to increase the number of participants so as to achieve the statistical power necessary to observe if there is a "true" effect. Systematic reviews and meta-analyses are considered a higher level of evidence because they show how a treatment or intervention performs across studies and, ideally, across different populations.

Systematic reviews and meta-analyses are used to develop clinical guidelines and recommendations. Researchers conducting systematic reviews should apply strict criteria to thoroughly search the literature and identify all studies that meet the inclusion criteria for the aim of the review. When evaluating a systematic review, it is important to examine the search terms used and the thoroughness of the search (e.g., inclusion of literature outside of traditional commercial and academic databases). For example, two meta-analyses on the use of evening primrose oil for cervical ripening or induction were published at the same time using the same search criteria.[22,23]

One identified six studies and the other nine, but only three studies were included in both reviews.

Also, it is important to recognize that publication bias means studies that show no effect are less likely to be published, or might be presented only as conference abstracts. When systematic reviews make a real effort to find those studies, publication bias can be reduced.

Further, the language of the search may be important. Reviews of acupuncture that do not include studies published in Asian-language journals may exclude studies from geographic areas where acupuncture is more widely practiced.

Once studies are identified, authors assess their quality and the risk for bias in different aspects of their study design. Poorly done studies are not valid and should not be included.

Included studies typically have different populations, as well as differences in the frequency, duration, or type of intervention. For a meta-analysis to be meaningful, it is crucial that similar studies are compared. The way acupuncture is practiced in China may be very different from how it is practiced in the United States, for example, so meta-analysis results from studies in China may not be generalizable to the United States.[24] Another important consideration for meta-analysis is that all studies included need to measure the same outcome.

Meta-analyses often use a forest plot, a graphic representation of individual study findings along with the finding for the combination of studies, to illustrate their data. The forest plot shows the result for each study with the 95% confidence interval around the study measure of effect. Examination of the forest plot should determine (1) the number of studies included; (2) whether most of the study results appear on the same side of the plot; and (3) whether the combined results are dominated by one very large study. If one study was dominant, then that study should be scrutinized for its validity. The authors of a meta-analysis should do an analysis without the larger study to see if the meta-analysis result was similar. Typically, an $I^2$ statistic is presented that measures the heterogeneity among studies. Summary results with a very high $I^2$ value, such as more than 75%, should be interpreted cautiously since this may indicate that the included studies were too different from each other to provide a meaningful synthesis.[25]

## Meaningfulness of Results

When evaluating research findings, it is important to know whether the study results show a difference between groups and that the difference did not happen by chance. To evaluate for differences between groups, the vast majority of studies calculate a $P$-value, which is the probability of obtaining results at least as extreme as the observed results assuming there was no difference between groups (the null hypothesis). The $P$-value is simply a probability.

### P-Values Versus Confidence Intervals

At the start of the study, the researcher decides which $P$-value cutoff will designate statistical significance. The mathematical term *statistical significance* means the results were not due to chance. This value is the probability at which the researcher will say their data are not consistent with the null hypothesis (i.e., they reject the null hypothesis). Setting a statistically significant $P$-value at 0.05 is arbitrary but common practice. Another issue with $P$-values is that they are influenced by both effect size and sample size. Therefore, in large data sets, such as birth certificate data, nearly any result will have a small $P$-value, even if the effect size is very small.[26]

A more informative statistic, but one that has similar pitfalls to the $P$-value, is the confidence interval (CI). A CI, in combination with a measure of effect, lets the reader know the range of possible effects around the result. For example, a relative risk might be reported as follows: RR = 1.97 (95% CI, 1.55–2.33). In this case, the RR is almost double, with a 95% CI of 1.55 to 2.33. With a CI for relative risk, the number "1" is important. In this example, the 95% CI (1.55–2.33) does *not* include 1 (no effect or null hypothesis). Reporting a 95% CI is mathematically the same as a $P$-value of 0.05. Table 2A-3 provides an example comparing interpretations of $P$-values and OR.

Interpretation of an RR that is less than 1 can be confusing. Hanson and colleagues conducted a meta-analysis of the use of probiotics in pregnancy to decrease the risk of group B *Streptococcus* (GBS) infection.[27] They found a RR = 0.56 (95% CI, 0.34–0.92). The CI did not include 1, so $P < 0.05$. This result should be interpreted as follows: Those participants using probiotics had a 44% (1.00 − 0.56 = 0.44) decreased risk of a positive GBS test at the onset of labor.

### Magnitude of Effect

The effect size is a result that has more meaning than a simple $P$-value when assessing study results. As a midwife, it is important to know how large of an effect was observed in a study. Table 2A-4 shows the interpretation of effect sizes for different statistical tests.

| Table 2A-3 | The Information Provided by Results Presented as *P*-Values Compared to Odds Ratios with Confidence Intervals and Their Interpretation | | | |
|---|---|---|---|---|
| **Perinatal Outcome** | **No Coercion (*N* = 180)** *n* (%) | **Coercion (*N* = 17)** *n* (%) | ***P*-Value** | **Unadjusted Odds Ratio (95% CI)** |
| Low birth weight | 5 (3.1) | 3 (17.6) | 0.03 | 7.50 (1.62, 34.69) |
| Stillbirth/neonatal death | 9 (5.5) | 2 (11.8) | 0.28 | 2.53 (0.50, 12.81) |

Interpretation with just the *P*-value: Persons experiencing reproductive coercion had a statistically significant risk of having a low-birth-weight infant but there was no difference by coercion status for having a stillbirth or neonatal death.

Interpretation with odds ratio and 95% CI: Persons experiencing reproductive coercion had 7.5 times increased odds of having a low-birth-weight infant—but due to the small sample size, the 95% confidence intervals are wide, meaning this estimate could be as small as 1.62 or as high as 34.69. There was no difference by coercion status (the confidence interval includes 1.0) for stillbirth or neonatal death, but again the confidence interval is quite wide.

Abbreviation: CI, confidence interval.

Data from Fay KE, Yee LM. Birth outcomes among women affected by reproductive coercion. *J Midwifery Womens Health*. 2020;65(5): 627-633.

| Table 2A-4 | Qualitative Assessment of Calculated Effect Sizes for Common Statistical Tests | | | | |
|---|---|---|---|---|---|
| | | **Qualitative Assessment** | | | |
| **Statistical Test** | **Effect Estimator** | **Small** | **Medium** | **Large** | **Very Large** |
| *t*-test | Cohen's *d* | 0.2 | 0.5 | 0.8 | 2 |
| Analysis of variance (ANOVA) | Omega-squared (Partial) eta-squared | 0.01 | 0.06 | 0.14 | |
| Multiple linear regression | *R*-squared | 0.02 | 0.13 | 0.26 | |
| | Cohen's *f* | 0.14 | 0.39 | 0.59 | |
| Correlation | Correlation | 0.1 | 0.3 | 0.5 | 0.7 |
| Binominal regression | Relative risk | 1.2 | 1.9 | 3.0 | 5.7 |
| Randomized controlled trials | | 0.83 | 0.59 | 0.33 | 0.18 |
| Logistic regression | Odds ratio | 1.5–1.7 | 3.5 | 6.75 | 10 |
| Cohort studies | | 0.66 | 0.33 | 0.15 | 0.10 |
| Absolute difference | Risk difference | –7% points | –18% points | –30% points | –45% points |

Data from Watson P. Rules of thumb on magnitudes of effect sizes. University of Cambridge. https://imaging.mrc-cbu.cam.ac.uk/statswiki/FAQ/effectSize. Published 2021; Chen H, Cohen P, Chen S. How big is a big odds ratio? Interpreting the magnitudes of odds ratios in epidemiological studies. *Commun Stat Simul Comput*. 2010;39(4):860-864. doi:10.1080/03610911003650383.

The OR for the effect of reproductive coercion on low birth weight in Table 2A-3, which is equal to 7.50, would be considered a large effect. A midwife cannot change a person's history of reproductive coercion, but knowing this information might allow the midwife to encourage smoking cessation (also associated with low birth weight) as well as use of resources to decrease and optimize nutrition to decrease the overall risk of low birth weight in a particular patient.

The meta-analysis RR result for probiotic use and GBS, RR = 0.54, is an example of a medium effect.[27] However, even if the effect size were smaller, the intervention has few drawbacks and may have other positive effects beyond reducing GBS colonization that might make it a worthwhile intervention for patients who are at high risk for GBS or who are GBS-positive at their prenatal screen.[28] Altman and colleagues examined the use of resources by nurse-midwives compared to obstetricians in a cohort study of more 1400 low-risk women.[29] They found certified nurse-midwives (CNMs) had an adjusted 30% decreased odds for cesarean births (aOR = 0.39; 95% CI, 0.12–0.69), which is a medium effect size.

The previous examples were binary outcomes—the condition was either present or absent. There are fewer examples of continuous outcomes in the midwifery literature. An RCT found that nulliparous individuals using spontaneous pushing in second-stage labor versus a directed Valsalva maneuver pushed for 5.20 minutes less ($P = 0.001$), a large effect size (Cohen's $d = 0.79$), and the overall length of the second stage was 9.3 minutes shorter, a nearly medium effect size (Cohen's $d = 0.41$).[30] Given the previous caveats about translating RCT effects into clinical practice, the effect in practice would likely not be as large, but given the better neonatal outcomes found in this study, worth pursuing in clinical practice. Notably, meta-analyses on this topic failed to find differences in length of pushing or neonatal outcomes, but there was high heterogeneity among studies.[31,32]

A study in late pregnancy examined the correlation between anxiety, as measured by the State-Trait Anxiety Inventory, with the number of respiratory infections in infants. The researchers found correlations of 0.20, 0.36, and 0.12 for 30, 48, and 60 months of age, respectively; the effect sizes ranged from small to medium.[33] It is important to remember that although correlation studies cannot indicate causation, they do help establish a foundation for forming hypotheses for further studies.

Another measure of effect already cited is the number needed to treat (NNT) or the number needed to harm (NNH). This number indicates how many people need to undergo the intervention to achieve one outcome. It is the reciprocal of the absolute risk difference, so it is typically applied to RCTs, although it can be applied to other types of studies.[34] The most ideal outcome would be NNT = 1; that is, for every person treated, an improved outcome is achieved. Consensus varies on a cutoff for a health benefit, although NNT values of ≤15 and ≤9 for asymptomatic persons have been reported in the literature.[15,34] Again, much depends on the intervention and the consequences of both a benefit and any harm; thus, any findings must be put into a particular clinical context for a particular patient.

## Translating the Evidence into Patient-Centered Counseling and Midwifery Care

As indicated throughout this appendix, evidence must be tailored to meet an individual patient's personal characteristics as well as their preferences and personal perspective on what is important to them. Counseling a healthy nulliparous individual whose fetus is in good health about an elective induction at 39 weeks' gestation is a very different conversation than for a patient who has hypertension or cholestasis, two conditions that put the pregnant person and fetus at risk. Knowing the population studied and the limitations of trials or studies, especially those that receive a lot of publicity, is essential.

Midwifery care frequently cannot rely on just individual pieces of evidence, but needs different kinds of studies to ensure good care and good outcomes. Consider epidural analgesia, a form of pain relief used by approximately 70% of laboring people.[35] Some evidence suggest that the longer an epidural is in place during labor, the higher the risk of fever—which carries potential risks for the neonate, such as neonatal seizures.[36] Additionally, epidural analgesia increases the number of fetuses in occiput posterior position at birth, one cause for a longer second stage of labor.[37] How can midwives meet the needs of the persons in their care who want epidural analgesia while also decreasing potential complications? A prenatal discussion should include why the use of nonpharmacologic measures to cope with labor should be tried first and then progress to epidural use when these are not helping with coping, a strategy that can limit the opportunity for fever in labor and rotation into occiput posterior position. Once someone has an epidural, then the use of frequent position changes within the motor constraints of the epidural has been shown to be valuable.[38]

## Resources

Greenhalgh T. *How to Read a Paper: The Basics of Evidenced-Based Medicine and Healthcare.* 6th ed. Hoboken, NJ: Wiley-Blackwell; 2019.

Motulsky H. *Essential Biostatistics: A Nonmathematical Approach.* Oxford, UK: Oxford University Press; 2016.

## References

1. Scherer LD, Valentine KD, Patel N, et al. A bias for action in cancer screening? *J Exp Psych Applied.* 2019;25(2):149-161.

2. Schwartz LM, Woloshin S, Fowler FJ Jr, Welch HG. Enthusiasm for cancer screening in the United States. *JAMA.* 2004;291(1):71-78.

3. Institute NC. Breast cancer risk in American women. https://www.cancer.gov/types/breast/risk-fact-sheet. Updated December 16, 2020. Accessed February 23, 2022.

4. Hoyert D. Maternal mortality rates in the United States, 2019. *NCHS Health E-Stats.* 2021. doi:/10.15620/cdc:103855.

5. Herrell H. Absolute risk versus relative risk: a clinical example. Howardisms website. https://howardisms.com/obgyn/absolute-risk-versus-relative-risk-a-clinical-example/. Updated December 8, 2015. Accessed February 22, 2022.

6. Sharma SK, McIntire DD, Wiley J, Leveno KJ. Labor analgesia and cesarean delivery: an individual patient meta-analysis of nulliparous women. *Anesthesiology.* 2004;100(1):142-148; discussion 146A.

7. Martin JA, Hamilton BE, Sutton PD, et al. Births: final data for 2003. *Natl Vital Stat Rep.* 2005;54(2):1-116.

8. Grant A, Elbourne D, Valentin L, Alexander S. Routine formal fetal movement counting and risk of antepartum late death in normally formed singletons. *Lancet.* 1989;2(8659):345-349.

9. Moore TR, Piacquadio K. A prospective evaluation of fetal movement screening to reduce the incidence of antepartum fetal death. *Am J Obstet Gynecol.* 1989;160(5 pt 1):1075-1080.

10. Thomsen SG, Legarth J, Weber T, Kristensen J. Monitoring of normal pregnancies by daily fetal movement registration or hormone assessment: a random allocation study. *J Obstet Gynaecol.* 1990;10:189-193.

11. Bell ML, Kenward MG, Fairclough DL, Horton NJ. Differential dropout and bias in randomised controlled trials: when it matters and when it may not. *BMJ.* 2013;346:e8668.

12. Grobman WA, Rice MM, Reddy UM, et al. Labor induction versus expectant management in low-risk nulliparous women. *N Engl J Med.* 2018;379(6):513-523.

13. Marguiles M. Should pregnant women be induced at 39 weeks? *Washington Post.* June 27, 2016. Accessed February 21, 2022. https://www.washingtonpost.com/national/health-science/should-pregnant-women-be-induced-at-39-weeks/2016/06/27/e1bb9d16-27fe-11e6-b989-4e5479715b54_story.html.

14. Heneghan C, Goldacre B, Mahtani KR. Why clinical trial outcomes fail to translate into benefits for patients. *Trials.* 2017;18(1):122.

15. Chong CA, Tomlinson G, Chodirker L, et al. An unadjusted NNT was a moderately good predictor of health benefit. *J Clin Epidemiol.* 2006;59(3):224-233.

16. Herbst AL, Ulfelder H, Poskanzer DC. Adenocarcinoma of the vagina: association of maternal stilbestrol therapy with tumor appearance in young women. *N Engl J Med.* 1971;284(15):878-881.

17. Frigoletto FD, Lieberman E, Lang JM, et al. A clinical trial of active management of labor. *N Engl J Med.* 1995;333(12):745-750.

18. Lieberman E, Lang JM, Cohen A, et al. Association of epidural analgesia with cesarean delivery in nulliparas. *Obstet Gynecol.* 1996;88(6):993-1000.

19. Anim-Somuah M, Smyth RM, Cyna AM, Cuthbert A. Epidural versus non-epidural or no analgesia for pain management in labour. *Cochrane Database Syst Rev.* 2018;5(5):CD000331. doi:10.1002/14651858.CD000331.pub4.

20. Badreldin N, Grobman WA, Yee LM. Racial disparities in postpartum pain management. *Obstet Gynecol.* 2019;134(6):1147-1153.

21. Johnson JD, Asiodu IV, McKenzie CP, et al. Racial and ethnic inequities in postpartum pain evaluation and management. *Obstet Gynecol.* 2019;134(6):1155-1162.

22. Hemmatzadeh S, Mohammad Alizadeh Charandabi S, Veisy A, Mirghafourvand M. Evening primrose oil for cervical ripening in term pregnancies: a systematic review and meta-analysis. *J Complement Integr Med.* 2021. doi: 10.1515/jcim-2020-0314.

23. Moradi M, Niazi A, Heydarian Miri H, Lopez V. The effect of evening primrose oil on labor induction and cervical ripening: a systematic review and meta-analysis. *Phytother Res.* 2021;35(10):5374-5383.

24. Barger MK. Current resources for evidence-based practice, July/August 2020. *J Midwifery Womens Health.* 2020;65(4):567-573.

25. Guyatt GH, Oxman AD, Kunz R, et al. GRADE guidelines: 7. Rating the quality of evidence—inconsistency. *J Clin Epidemiol.* 2011;64(12):1294-1302.

26. Gómez-de-Mariscal E, Guerrero V, Sneider A, et al. Use of the *p*-values as a size-dependent function to address practical differences when analyzing large datasets. *Sci Rep.* 2021;11(1):20942.

27. Hanson L, VandeVusse L, Malloy E, et al. Probiotic interventions to reduce antepartum group B *Streptococcus* colonization: a systematic review and meta-analysis. *Midwifery.* 2022;105:103208.

28. Garcia VR. Impact of intrapartum antibiotic prophylaxis for group B *Streptococcus* on the term infant gut microbiome: a state of the science review. *J Midwifery Womens Health.* 2021;66(3):351-359.

29. Altman MR, Murphy SM, Fitzgerald CE, et al. The cost of nurse-midwifery care: use of interventions, resources, and associated costs in the hospital setting. *Womens Health Iss.* 2017;27(4):434-440.

30. Yildirim G, Beji NK. Effects of pushing techniques in birth on mother and fetus: a randomized study. *Birth.* 2008;35(1):25-30.

31. Lemos A, Amorim MM, Dornelas de Andrade A, et al. Pushing/bearing down methods for the second stage of labour. *Cochrane Database Syst Rev.* 2017;3(3):CD009124.

32. Prins M, Boxem J, Lucas C, Hutton E. Effect of spontaneous pushing versus Valsalva pushing in the second stage of labour on mother and fetus:

a systematic review of randomised trials. *BJOG.* 2011;118(6):662-670.

33. Zijlmans MAC, Beijers R, Riksen-Walraven MJ, de Weerth C. Maternal late pregnancy anxiety and stress is associated with children's health: a longitudinal study. *Stress.* 2017;20(5):495-504.

34. McAlister FA. The "number needed to treat" turns 20—and continues to be used and misused. *CMAJ.* 2008;179(6):549-553.

35. Butwick AJ, Bentley J, Wong CA, et al. United States state-level variation in the use of neuraxial analgesia during labor for pregnant women. *JAMA Netw Open.* 2018;1(8):e186567-e186567.

36. Morton S, Kua J, Mullington CJ. Epidural analgesia, intrapartum hyperthermia, and neonatal brain injury: a systematic review and meta-analysis. *Br J Anaesth.* 2021;126(2):500-515.

37. Lieberman E, Davidson K, Lee-Parritz A, Shearer E. Changes in fetal position during labor and their association with epidural analgesia. *Obstet Gynecol.* 2005;105(5 pt 1):974-982.

38. Hickey L, Savage J. Effect of peanut ball and position changes in women laboring with an epidural. *Nurs Womens Health.* 2019;23(3):245-252.

# APPENDIX

# 2B

# Reproductive Health Statistics

IRA KANTROWITZ-GORDON

*The editors acknowledge Mary C. Brucker and Tekoa L. King, who were authors of this appendix in the previous edition.*

Health statistics are an accepted measure of the effectiveness of a healthcare system and are widely used as indicators of a nation's health. Mortality statistics also illustrate how pregnant individuals and newborns fare both internationally and within the United States. There are striking differences in mortality and morbidity statistics between the United States, other developed nations, and low-resource nations. Within the United States, there are notable racial and ethnic disparities in maternal and infant health outcomes. This appendix briefly reviews definitions of health-related statistics and how they are used.

Vital statistics information is collected to document trends in the health status of individuals and populations during and after pregnancy as well as the health of their fetuses and newborns. These statistics are used extensively in healthcare research and by governments and institutions worldwide when deciding where to dedicate resources. In the United States, data on births and deaths of fetuses, newborns, and anyone who is pregnant or has been pregnant within the last year are collected by each state or jurisdiction and reported as vital statistics to the National Center for Health Statistics. The National Vital Statistics System is a partnership between the federal government, 50 states, 2 cities (Washington, DC, and New York City), and 5 territories (Puerto Rico, the Virgin Islands, Guam, American Samoa, and the Commonwealth of the Northern Mariana Islands).[1] The states and territories have the legal responsibility to register vital events. Although most jurisdictions use the standard U.S. forms for birth and death data, some variations are apparent between states and territories with regard to which data are collected. Thus, the data collected are not completely uniform across all jurisdictions.

Definitions of key reproductive statistics are presented in **Table 2B-1**, as typically used in the United States. Definitions may vary slightly in other countries and international comparisons. The definitions created by the Centers for Disease Control and Prevention (CDC) still use gendered terminology for pregnancy-capable individuals. The most recent infant mortality, fetal death, and pregnancy-related mortality ratios are presented in **Table 2B-2** and **Figure 2B-1**. More information about statistics describing contraceptive efficacy is presented in the *Fertility, Family Building, and Contraception* chapter.

## Fetal Death and Stillbirth

States have different reporting requirements for fetal death. Most report fetal deaths that are 20 weeks' gestation or greater and/or 350 grams or greater birth weight, and use 20 weeks' gestation as the gestational age threshold for distinguishing a stillbirth from the product of a miscarriage. A few states report all pregnancy losses as a fetal death regardless of the period of gestation. In 2020, the fetal death rate in the United States was approximately the same as the infant mortality rate (IMR), at 5.7 fetal deaths after 20 weeks' gestation per 1000 live births and fetal deaths combined (denominator).[2] The incidence varies by race/ethnicity and is highest in non-Hispanic Black individuals.

| Table 2B-1 | Selected Reproductive Health Indices |
|---|---|
| **Term** | **Definition and Explanations** |
| Fertility rate | Births per 1000 women aged 15 to 44. |
| Fetal death rate (see Stillbirth) | Spontaneous death of the fetus occurs prior to birth, irrespective of the duration of the pregnancy.<br>Fetal death is indicated by no signs of life after birth (e.g., heartbeats, umbilical cord pulsations, breathing, or voluntary muscle movement).<br>The fetal death rate is the number of fetal deaths at ≥ 20 weeks' gestation that occur during a year divided by the sum of live births plus fetal deaths during the same year, and expressed per 1000 live births plus fetal deaths. |
| Infant mortality rate (IMR) | Number of infants dying before reaching 1 year of life per 1000 live births in a given year. |
| Lifetime risk of pregnancy-related death (maternal death) | Risk of an individual dying from pregnancy or childbirth during their lifetime; calculated by multiplying the maternal mortality rate by 30, or the number of years of exposure to pregnancy between ages 15 and 44. Calculations are based on maternal mortality and fertility rates in the country. This method recognizes that women of high fertility or women lacking in universal access to effective family planning have an extremely high risk of dying as a result of pregnancy or childbirth, as they are repeatedly exposed to the risk of pregnancy. |
| Live birth | Complete expulsion or extraction of a product of human conception from a pregnant individual, irrespective of the duration of pregnancy, and the newborn shows any evidence of life (i.e., heartbeats, umbilical cord pulsations, breathing, or voluntary muscle movement), regardless of whether the umbilical cord has been cut or the placenta is attached. Heartbeats are distinguished from transient cardiac contractions, and breathing is distinguished from fleeting respiratory efforts or gasps. |
| Live birth rate | Number of live births per 1000 population. |
| Neonatal mortality rate | Number of deaths of newborns in the first 28 days of life per 1000 live births.<br>Early neonatal deaths are the number of neonatal deaths that occur during the first 7 days of life.<br>Late neonatal deaths are the number of neonatal deaths that occur between 7 and 27 days of age. |
| Perinatal mortality rate[a] | The sum of fetal deaths (more than 20 weeks' gestation) plus early neonatal deaths (within the first 7 days after birth) during a year divided by the sum of live births plus fetal deaths during that year. Expressed per 1000 live births plus fetal deaths. |
| Pregnancy mortality rate (maternal mortality rate) | An estimate of the number of deaths during pregnancy or within 42 days after completion of the pregnancy, per 100,000 pregnancy-capable people in a given year. This rate is difficult to obtain and often not used in low-resource countries, since births are more easily measured than the number of pregnancy-capable people. |
| Pregnancy-associated death | Death of a person occurring during or within 1 year of pregnancy but not causally related to pregnancy. |
| Pregnancy-related death | Death of a person while pregnant or within 1 year of the end of a pregnancy—regardless of the outcome, duration, or site of the pregnancy—from any cause related to or aggravated by the pregnancy or its management, but not from accidental or incidental causes. This includes a pregnancy complication, a chain of events initiated by pregnancy, or the aggravation of an unrelated condition by the physiologic effects of pregnancy. |

*(continues)*

| Table 2B-1 | Selected Reproductive Health Indices (*continued*) |
|---|---|
| **Term** | **Definition and Explanations** |
| Pregnancy-related mortality ratio (maternal mortality ratio) | An estimate of the number of deaths during pregnancy or within 42 days after completion of the pregnancy, for every 100,000 live births. This ratio is the method most commonly used to express trends within a country and to make international comparisons. In some jurisdictions, the ratio includes deaths up to 1 year after completion of pregnancy. Note: The pregnancy mortality *ratio* differs from the pregnancy mortality *rate* in that the denominator is births and not pregnancy-capable people of reproductive age. The rate is more difficult to measure, especially in countries with less sophisticated data gathering. |
| Stillbirth | Fetal death that occurs at ≥ 20 weeks' gestation. |

[a] There are several definitions of perinatal death rate in use today, including neonatal deaths within 7 days or within 28 days after birth; others use fetal deaths occurring with a gestation of more than 28 weeks.

Based on Centers for Disease Control and Prevention. Infant mortality. https://www.cdc.gov/reproductivehealth/maternalinfanthealth/infantmortality.htm. Accessed December 7, 2022; Centers for Disease Control and Prevention. Pregnancy Mortality Surveillance System. June 22, 2022. https://www.cdc.gov/reproductivehealth/maternal-mortality/pregnancy-mortality-surveillance-system.htm. Accessed December 7, 2022; National Center for Health Statistics. Fetal deaths. https://www.cdc.gov/nchs/nvss/fetal_death.htm. Accessed December 7, 2022; Valenzuela CP, Gregory ECW, Martin JA. *Decline in Perinatal Mortality in the United States, 2017–2019. NCHS Data Brief*, no. 429. Hyattsville, MD: National Center for Health Statistics; 2022. https://dx.doi.org/10.15620/cdc:112643; World Health Organization. Maternal mortality ratio. https://www.who.int/data/gho/indicator-metadata-registry/imr-details/26. Accessed December 7, 2022; World Health Organization. Neonatal mortality rate. https://www.who.int/data/gho/indicator-metadata-registry/imr-details/67. Accessed December 7, 2022.

| Table 2B-2 | Pregnancy, Fetal, and Infant Death Rates in the United States by Race/Ethnicity | | |
|---|---|---|---|
| **Race/Ethnicity** | **Pregnancy-Related Mortality Ratio: *n*/100,000 Live Births[a]** | **Fetal Mortality Rate: *n*/1000 Live Births and Fetal Deaths[b]** | **Infant Mortality Rate: *n*/1000 Live Births[c]** |
| Non-Hispanic Black | 55.3 | 10.3 | 10.6 |
| American Indian/Alaska Native | 26.5[d] | 7.8 | 7.9 |
| Hispanic | 18.2 | 4.9 | 5.0 |
| Non-Hispanic white | 19.1 | 4.7 | 4.5 |
| Asian | 14.1[e] | 3.9 | 3.4 |
| Native Hawaiian/Pacific Islander | 14.1[e] | 10.6 | 8.2 |
| Overall | 23.8 | 5.7 | 5.6 |

[a] 2020 data.

[b] 2020 data. Includes fetal deaths of at least 20 weeks' gestation.

[c] 2019 data.

[d] 2016–2018 data.

[e] 2016–2018 data for Asian and Native Hawaiian/Pacific Islander reported in aggregate.

Based on Hoyert DL. Maternal mortality rates in the United States, 2020. *NCHS Health E-Stats.* 2022. https://dx.doi.org/10.15620/cdc:113967; Centers for Disease Control and Prevention. Pregnancy Mortality Surveillance System. June 22, 2022. https://www.cdc.gov/reproductivehealth/maternal-mortality/pregnancy-mortality-surveillance-system.htm. Accessed November 4, 2022; Gregory ECW, Valenzuela CP, Hoyert DL. Fetal mortality: United States, 2020. *Natl Vital Stat Rep.* 2022;71(4). https://dx.doi.org/10.15620/cdc:118420; Ely DM, Driscoll AK. Infant mortality in the United States, 2019: Data from the period linked birth/infant death file. *Natl Vital Stat Rep.* 2021;70(14). https://dx.doi.org/10.15620/cdc:111053.

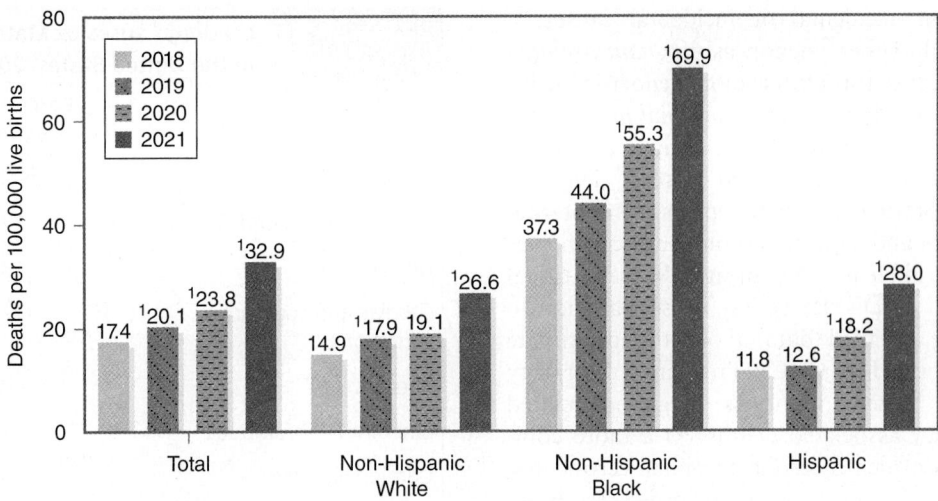

**Figure 2B-1** Maternal mortality rates, by race and Hispanic origin: United States, 2018–2021.

[1]Statistically significant increase in rate from previous year ($p < 0.05$).

Note: Race groups are single race consistent with data definitions.

National Center for Health Statistics, National Vital Statistics System. Mortality.

Reproduced with permission from Hoyert DL. Maternal mortality rates in the United States, 2021. *NCHS Health E-Stats.* 2023. https://dx.doi.org/10.15620/cdc:124678.

## Infant Mortality

In 2020, the overall IMR in the United States was 5.4 infant deaths per 1000 live births.[3] However, the IMR varies by geographic location and race/ethnicity, and is highest among non-Hispanic Black infants (Table 2B-2). The most common causes of infant death are congenital anomalies, low birth weight, sudden infant death syndrome (SIDS), unintentional injuries, and maternal complications of pregnancy.[3]

The IMR has historically been used as an indicator of the health of a population because the health of infants in the first year of life is heavily dependent on factors such as maternal health, quality of health care, socioeconomic conditions (e.g., nutrition, education, wealth), and public health practices (e.g., sanitation, preventive health services).[4] The IMR also has a high correlation with population health measures such as disability-adjusted life expectancy.[5] Despite spending larger amounts of money on healthcare services than many other countries, in 2020 the United States ranked 35th out of 36 developed member nations in the Organization for Economic Cooperation and Development (OECD), with an IMR that was approximately twice as high as that of most other developed nations.[6,7]

The reasons that the IMR in the United States remains high despite higher levels of healthcare spending are complex and not fully understood. International comparisons have found that the higher IMR can be largely attributed to increased rates of preterm birth and higher death rates in infants born after 37 weeks' gestation.[4]

The most modifiable etiology is likely preterm birth.[8] Many studies have explored strategies designed to decrease the risk of preterm birth, including investigation of environmental epigenetics, suggesting that improving social determinants of health can directly affect perinatal outcomes.[9] Methods for lowering the rate of preterm birth include interventions such as increasing breastfeeding/chestfeeding rates (which increases interpregnancy intervals), offering more parental support and education, and improving access to healthcare services.

## Pregnancy-Related Mortality

The CDC defines a pregnancy-related death as "the death of a woman while pregnant or within 1 year of pregnancy termination—regardless of the duration or site of the pregnancy—from any cause related to or aggravated by the pregnancy or its management, but not from accidental or incidental causes."[10] We refer to this phenomenon as *pregnancy-related mortality* because this term is more gender-inclusive than the commonly used term *maternal mortality*.

Pregnancy-related deaths are evaluated by three different systems in the United States.[10] The National Vital Statistics System reports the maternal mortality rate and ratio based on death certificates using the World Health Organization's International Classification of Disease codes. These statistics do not generate detailed data about the proximate cause of death. The CDC's Pregnancy Mortality Surveillance System monitors pregnancy-related and pregnancy-associated deaths via a more complex analysis of death certificates, birth certificates, and pregnancy data that are recorded on both. These statistics generate more detailed data about the causes of death. The third source of information comes from maternal mortality review committees that analyze pregnancy-related deaths in more detail at the local level. While international comparisons of pregnancy-related mortality include deaths up to 42 days after the end of pregnancy, national- and state-level data typically examine deaths up to 1 year after the end of pregnancy.

Pregnancy-related mortality is much less common than infant or fetal death and is reported as the ratio of pregnancy-related deaths for every 100,000 live births. A single individual dying in childbirth is a tragedy; an increase in the number of people dying is a societal catastrophe and national embarrassment. Despite advances in standard of living and healthcare technology, the number of women who die from a pregnancy-related causes has increased in the United States from 7.2 deaths per 100,000 live births in 1987 to a high of 32.9 deaths per 100,000 live births in 2021.[11] The pregnancy mortality rate in non-Hispanic Black individuals is more than 2.5 times higher than that in non-Hispanic white individuals (66.9 versus 26.6 deaths per 100,000 live births), which is one of the most striking perinatal health disparities in the United States today (Figure 2B-1).[11] There are also striking differences in pregnancy mortality by age: In 2021, the pregnancy mortality ratio was 138.5 per 100,000 live births for individuals age 40 and older, compared to 20.4 for those younger than age 25.[11] In 2020, the United States ranked last for maternal mortality among the 36 developed countries in the OECD.[7,12] It is estimated that approximately 80% of the U.S. pregnancy-related deaths are preventable.[13]

Historically, the most common causes of maternal mortality were hemorrhage, infection, hypertension, and anesthesia complications. As the

| Table 2B-3 | Leading Causes of Maternal Death in the United States, 2017–2019 |
|---|---|
| **Cause** | **Percentage of Pregnancy-Related Deaths** |
| Mental health conditions | 22.7 |
| Hemorrhage | 13.7 |
| Cardiac and coronary conditions | 12.8 |
| Infection | 9.2 |
| Embolism—thrombotic | 8.7 |
| Cardiomyopathy | 8.5 |
| Hypertensive disorders of pregnancy | 6.5 |
| Amniotic fluid embolism | 3.8 |
| Injury | 3.6 |
| Cerebrovascular accident | 2.5 |
| Cancer | 1.9 |
| Metabolic/endocrine conditions | 1.2 |
| Pulmonary conditions | 1.2 |

Based on Trost SL, Beauregard J, Njie F, et al. *Pregnancy-Related Deaths: Data from Maternal Mortality Review Committees in 36 US States, 2017–2019*. Atlanta, GA: Centers for Disease Control and Prevention, U.S. Department of Health and Human Services; 2022.

pre-pregnancy health status of pregnancy-capable individuals has changed over time, so have the causes of mortality and morbidity. The most common direct causes of pregnancy-related death during 2017 to 2019 are listed in Table 2B-3. Notably, mental health conditions have emerged as the most common cause of pregnancy-related death, including opioid overdose and suicide.[13]

## The Rising Trend of Pregnancy Mortality in the United States

Multiple studies have attempted to identify the reasons for the rising incidence of maternal death in the United States. Initially, the increase was deemed temporary and associated with changes in birth certificates, categorization of causes of death, or other record-keeping issues.[14,15] Nevertheless, these data collection factors do not explain changes in specific states. For example, the maternal mortality rate (MMR) doubled within a

2-year period in one state; such a rise was unexpected in the absence of war, natural disaster, or severe economic disaster.[15] This state and others have now initiated maternal mortality review committees (MMRCs), which are charged with directly examining records of individuals who have died. Such groups are not universally available across the country, however.[16] MMRCs also examine preventability, structural determinants of health, and racism at individual and systemic levels to develop policy recommendations to improve perinatal care and reduce death. MMRCs are multidisciplinary groups that can include midwives, nurse practitioners, physicians, nurses, pathologists, and community members.[17]

Many factors contribute to the racial and ethnic inequities in pregnancy mortality, including social determinants of health, longstanding structural racism in the United States, and ongoing discrimination and resulting distrust of the health system.[18] Racial disparities in pregnancy morbidity and mortality can also be attributed to variations in quality of care at the hospital level.[19,20]

Prominent among the potential etiologies of pregnancy-related deaths is the fact that care of pregnant individuals varies dramatically across the country by state, region, and institution. Drivers of system-level disparities include scarcities of resources in rural locations, funding of perinatal care, and integration of midwifery care in perinatal care. In many developed countries, best practices are shared and followed regardless of birth site. In the United States, there is no standard approach to treatment of complications of pregnancy or management of individuals experiencing an emergency in childbirth. This problem is currently the focus of many policy initiatives. For example, the California Maternal Quality Care Collaboration developed "bundles" or standard practice protocols that were disseminated throughout the state on topics such as postpartum hemorrhage.[21] These practice guidelines are a good example of how statistics drives research that first affects policy and then is translated into clinical practice.

## Pregnancy Morbidity

Pregnancy morbidity is much more common than pregnancy-related mortality. As difficult as it is to obtain accurate mortality data, however, morbidity data collection is even more elusive. Mortality data measure a single event or incidence. Morbidity data, by comparison, are much less likely to be recorded, suffer from a lack of standard case definitions, and frequently involve several comorbidities

(e.g., an individual with multiple conditions such as severe anemia, vesico-vaginal fistula, repeated urinary tract infections, and clinical depression). When data are collected in the health record, they are not publicly available for research.

Near-miss pregnancy mortality is a life-threatening event that could result in death. Recent efforts to define and track near-misses have been proliferating as a method to further assess the quality of health care and the effectiveness of interventions.[22] Early warning criteria are being instituted as part of patient safety bundles in an effort to decrease the incidence of maternal morbidity.[23]

## Reproductive Health: The Global Picture

Although pregnancy-related deaths in the United States are a critical concern nationally, approximately 99% of pregnancy deaths occur in low-resource nations. It is difficult to compare maternal mortality ratios across nations because of inconsistency in definitions and reporting. On a worldwide basis, many individuals never enter the healthcare system during pregnancy, even when gravely ill, so deaths and disabilities are not well captured in vital statistics, surveillance data, or other records.

Because the pregnancy-related mortality rate is difficult to obtain, the pregnancy-related mortality ratio (PMR) is used more frequently. When comparing countries, the pregnancy mortality ratio is the number of maternal deaths per 100,000 live births in a given period of time. The estimated worldwide PMR was 211 in 2017 (80% confidence interval, 199 – 243). There are large variations in the PMR, with the highest estimated PMRs in sub-Saharan Africa, ranging from 500 to 1150.[24] The largest number of deaths occurred in Nigeria and India, accounting for approximately 100,000 pregnancy-related deaths, or 35% of the world's pregnancy-related deaths.[24]

### Global Factors Associated with Maternal Mortality

The most common causes of maternal mortality in low-resource nations are hemorrhage, infection, hypertension, complications during birth, and unsafe abortion.[25] Betrán et al. reported findings of a systematic review of maternal mortality in 141 countries in 2005.[26] Using standard regression models, these authors found that (1) the proportion of births assisted by a skilled attendant, (2) the infant mortality rate, and (3) national per capita expenditures on health were three factors strongly related to maternal mortality worldwide.[26]

In addition, a phenomenon known as the "three delays" has been identified as a critical determinant of maternal mortality.[27] Once an emergency occurs in childbirth, its cause can be analyzed within the following framework, whose elements collectively prevent timely, high-quality care from reaching those most in need:

1. Delay in recognizing there is a problem and making the decision to seek care

2. Delay in reaching the appropriate level of care once the problem or complication has been recognized

3. Delay in receiving the appropriate care after arrival at the service site

### The Safe Motherhood Initiative

In an effort to address some of the global factors involved in maternal and infant mortality, the Safe Motherhood Initiative held its first meeting in 1987 in Africa.[28] Another group that was organized a few years later but has similar goals is the White Ribbon Alliance. The White Ribbon Alliance includes many of the same members as the Safe Motherhood group, but is broader based and includes international nongovernmental organizations (INGOs), government agencies, local nongovernmental organizations (NGOs), and community-based organizations in resource-limited countries. The general goals of the alliance members are to promote practices, protocols, and guidelines that help women obtain high-quality gynecologic, family planning, prenatal, delivery, and postpartum care, so as to achieve optimal health for the mother, fetus, and infant during the perinatal period.

## Conclusion

There are multiple complexities involved in the definition, collection, and reporting of vital statistics that make it difficult to rely on exact numbers. Nonetheless, trends in these numbers tell a powerful story. The United States spends more on health care than any other nation in world, and the IMR has decreased in recent years. Yet, the IMR in the United States remains higher than that in many other developed nations, pregnancy mortality and morbidity are increasing, and racial/ethnic disparities in maternal–child health are striking.

The link between national vital statistics and clinical care of individuals may seem remote but, in fact, these statistics play an important role in each clinical encounter. The underlying etiologies of morbidity and mortality are both social and biologic in nature; in turn, midwifery care of each individual must address social determinants of health as well as biologic indicators. Midwifery has a long and storied history of providing such care internationally, and today's midwives are charged with continuing that care.

### References

1. National Center for Health Statistics. About the National Vital Statistics System. https://www.cdc.gov/nchs/nvss/about_nvss.htm. Published January 4, 2016. Accessed December 7, 2022

2. Gregory ECW, Valenzuela CP, Hoyert DL. Fetal mortality: United States, 2020. *Natl Vital Stat Rep.* 2022;71(4). https://dx.doi.org/10.15620/cdc:118420.

3. Murphy SL, Kochanek KD, Xu JQ, Arias E. *Mortality in the United States, 2020. NCHS Data Brief,* no. 427. Hyattsville, MD: National Center for Health Statistics; 2021.

4. MacDorman MF, Mathews TJ, Mophangoo AD, Zeitlin J. International comparisons of infant mortality and related factors: United States and Europe, 2010. *Nat Vital Stat Rep.* 2014;63(5):1-10.

5. Reidpath DD, Allotey P. Infant mortality rate as an indicator of population health. *J Epidemiol Community Health.* 2003;57(5):344-346. doi:10.1136/jech.57.5.344.

6. United Health Foundation. America's health rankings: 2019 annual report. https://www.americashealthrankings.org/learn/reports/2019-annual-report/international-comparison. Accessed December 7, 2022.

7. Organization for Economic Cooperation and Development. Health status: maternal and infant mortality. https://stats.oecd.org/index.aspx?queryid=30116. Accessed December 7, 2022.

8. MacDorman MF, Gregory EC. Fetal and perinatal mortality: United States, 2013. *Natl Vital Stat Rep.* 2015;64(8):1.

9. Vick AD, Burris HH. Epigenetics and health disparities. *Curr Epidemiol Rep.* 2017;4(1):31-37.

10. St Pierre A, Zaharatos J, Goodman D, Callaghan WM. Challenges and opportunities in identifying, reviewing, and preventing maternal deaths. *Obstet Gynecol.* 2018;131:138-142.

11. Hoyert DL. Maternal mortality rates in the United States, 2021. *NCHS Health E-Stats.* 2023. https://dx.doi.org/10.15620/cdc:124678.

12. Gunja MZ, Seervai S, Zephyrin L, Williams RD II. Health and health care for women of reproductive age: how the United States compares with other high-income countries. Commonwealth Fund; April 2022. https://doi.org/10.26099/4pph-j894.

13. Trost SL, Beauregard J, Njie F, et al. *Pregnancy-Related Deaths: Data from Maternal Mortality Review Committees in 36 US States, 2017–2019.* Atlanta, GA: Centers for Disease Control and Prevention, U.S. Department of Health and Human Services; 2022.

14. Joseph KS, Lisonkova S, Muraca GM, et al. Factors underlying the temporal increase in maternal mortality in the United States. *Obstet Gynecol.* 2017;129(1):91-100.

15. MacDorman MF, Declercq E, Cabral H, Morton C. Recent increases in the U.S. maternal mortality rate: disentangling trends from measurement issues. *Obstet Gynecol.* 2016;128(3):447-455.

16. Centers for Disease Control and Prevention: Enhancing Reviews and Surveillance to Eliminate Maternal Mortality (ERASE MM). (2020). https://www.cdc.gov/reproductivehealth/maternal-mortality/erasemm/index.html.

17. Bradford H. The essential role of nurse practitioners and midwives on maternal mortality review committees. *Nurs Womens Health.* 2021;25(2):107-111. doi:10.1016/j.nwh.2021.01.005.

18. Collier AY, Molina RL. Maternal mortality in the United States: updates on trends, causes, and solutions. *Neoreviews.* 2019;20(10):e561-e574. doi:10.1542/neo.20-10-e561.

19. Howell EA, Egorova NN, Balbierz A, et al. Site of delivery contribution to Black–white severe maternal morbidity disparity. *Am J Obstet Gynecol.* 2016;215(2):143-152. doi:10.1016/j.ajog.2016.05.007.

20. Howell EA, Egorova NN, Janevic T, et al. Severe maternal morbidity among Hispanic women in New York City: investigation of health disparities. *Obstet Gynecol.* 2017;129(2):285-294. doi:10.1097/AOG.0000000000001864.

21. Main EK, Goffman D, Scavone BM, et al. National Partnership for Maternal Safety consensus bundle on obstetric hemorrhage. *J Midwifery Womens Health.* 2015;60:458-464.

22. Mhyre JM, D'Oria R, Hameed AB, et al. The maternal early warning criteria: a proposal from the National Partnership for Maternal Safety. *Obstet Gynecol.* 2014;124:782-786.

23. Zuckerwise LC, Lipkind HS. Maternal early warning systems: towards reducing preventable maternal mortality and severe maternal morbidity through improved clinical surveillance and responsiveness. *Semin Perinatol.* 2017;41(3):161-165. doi:10.1053/j.semperi.2017.03.005.

24. Trends in maternal mortality 2000 to 2017: estimates by WHO, UNICEF, UNFPA, World Bank Group and the United Nations Population Division. UNICEF. https://data.unicef.org/resources/trends-maternal-mortality-2000-2017/. Published September 2019. Accessed March 1, 2023.

25. Say L, Chou D, Gemmill A, et al. Global causes of maternal death: a WHO systematic analysis. *Lancet Global Health.* 2014;2(6):e323-e333.

26. Betrán AP, Wojdyla D, Posner SF, Gülmezoglu AM. National estimates for maternal mortality: an analysis based on the WHO systematic review of maternal mortality and morbidity. *BMC Public Health.* 2005;12(5):131-143.

27. Actis Danna V, Bedwell C, Wakasiaka S, Lavender T. Utility of the three-delays model and its potential for supporting a solution-based approach to accessing intrapartum care in low- and middle-income countries: a qualitative evidence synthesis. *Glob Health Action.* 2020;13(1):1819052. doi:10.1080/16549716.2020.1819052.

28. Islam M. The Safe Motherhood Initiative and beyond. *Bull WHO.* 2007;85(10):735.

# APPENDIX

# 2C

# Global Health: An Overview of Practicalities and Practice

PANDORA T. HARDTMAN

The core context of global health is shifting for the modern midwife considering this area as a career path. Gone are the days when simply "playing catch" in a foreign country was the entree to a lifelong passion. With ongoing efforts to decolonize global health, needs have shifted from simplistic service delivery to the need for midwife practitioners who can contribute to health systems strengthening at every level of the system, from bedside to boardroom, shifting the focus away from care offered by a provider to an individual to equitable population health. Considering the social, political, cultural, economic and environmental changes that will impact health, it is useful to remember that global health has its roots in public health nursing, with a distinct connection between the knowledge, skills, and attitudes required in this realm.

The American College of Nurse Midwives' (ACNM) *Global Health Competencies*,[1] developed by the Division of Global Engagement, is intended for members and midwives interested in global health. It aims to provide structure for their education experiences while identifying expertise essential for contributing to differing work streams in global health. Nine competencies are identified in the ACNM document, along with attendant suggested skills.

The Consortium of Universities for Global Health's *Global Health Education Competencies Toolkit*[2] is a comprehensive toolkit with annotated bibliographies for many of the competencies and other useful resources. This organization's website also has helpful resources for global health practitioners.

The Centers for Disease Control and Prevention's *10 Essential Public Health Services*[3] also provide a useful framework for public health. Its aim of protecting and promoting the health of all people in all communities is also applicable to international framing and practice. According to this framework, practitioners should prepare to:

1. Assess and monitor population health status, factors that influence health, and community needs and assets.
2. Investigate, diagnose, and address health problems and hazards affecting the population.
3. Communicate effectively to inform and educate people about health, factors that influence it, and how to improve it.
4. Strengthen, support, and mobilize communities and partnerships to improve health.
5. Create, champion, and implement policies, plans, and laws that impact health.
6. Utilize legal and regulatory actions designed to improve and protect the public's health.
7. Assure an effective system that enables equitable access to the individual services and care needed to be healthy.
8. Build and support a diverse and skilled public health workforce.
9. Improve and innovate public health functions through ongoing evaluation, research, and continuous quality improvement.
10. Build and maintain a strong organizational infrastructure for public health.

## Common Settings for Global Health Practice

### Volunteer Organizations

When choosing a volunteer organization from which to make a short-term contribution to global health, it is important to be familiar with the goals and objectives of the organization. Some key attributes to look for in organizations are a commitment to contributing to the long-term outcomes of the host organizations through a mutually beneficial and equitable partnership, a structured system for volunteer contributions that builds on past efforts, and a greater focus on teaching than on service delivery.[4]

### Academic Centers

Many universities operate global health programs and have long-established partnerships with host organizations and universities outside of the United States. The Consortium of Universities for Global Health has many resources and conferences for member universities.

### Implementing Agencies

Implementing agencies typically have contracts to carry out specific projects in specific settings, such as ACNM's Global Outreach Program. Terms commonly used to describe different kinds of organizations as well as the large organizations that are part of the United Nations system are provided later in this appendix.

## Common Asks of the Global Midwife in Practice

- Providing evidence-based methods for clinical and classroom-based instruction and evaluation to students, clinicians, or other learners emphasizing best practices
- Supporting formal and informal professional development and mentoring opportunities requested by partner-country faculty and clinicians
- Facilitating academic–clinical partnerships to develop practice improvement projects that strengthen care at the point of service and provide learning opportunities for students and clinical staff
- If appropriate, working with national (including ministries of health and education) nursing and midwifery organizations to assist in the planning, implementation, and/or evaluation of policies that support the enhancement of the professions of nursing and midwifery

## Historical "Should Know Abouts" That Have Shaped Global Health

The beginning of global health work can be traced to a series of formative events and documents that are still widely referenced today. A thorough understanding of these roots of global health will provide the foundational underpinnings for effective function in this arena.

### Alma Ata Declaration

The International Conference on Primary Health Care was held in 1978 at Alma Ata, Kazakhstan, and was cosponsored by the World Health Organization (WHO) and the United Nations Children's Fund (UNICEF). A major achievement of the conference was the adoption of a resolution, the Declaration of Alma-Ata,[5] aimed at attaining Health for All by the Year 2000.

## Universal Declaration of Human Rights

The Universal Declaration of Human Rights (UDHR)[6] was adopted by the United Nations General Assembly in December 1948 following the atrocities of World War II and is a basis for international human rights law. This document makes explicit those inalienable rights that are necessary for freedom, justice, and peace.

## Kinds of Global Health Organizations

Global or international organizations that employ midwives working within maternal–newborn health can generally be categorized as follows:

- *Multilateral organizations* cross several countries and borders, and receive funding from multiple organizations and sources. Examples of these organizations include the United Nations, the World Health Organization, the Pan American Health Organization, and the World Bank.
- *Bilateral global organizations* address country-specific needs through a single agency. Examples include the U.S. Agency for International Development (USAID) and the Swedish International Development Cooperation Agency. USAID's mission is to address extreme poverty globally and to promote democratic societies while preserving security and prosperity.

- *Nongovernmental organizations* (NGOs) and *international nongovernmental organizations* (INGOs) address global health needs across several technical areas. Examples of NGOs include Partners in Health, Doctors Without Borders, Medicines du Monde, Oxfam, and the International Red Cross. Jhpiego is an example of an INGO.
- *Faith-based organizations* (FBOs) are grassroots organizations whose values are based on faith and/or beliefs. The missions of FBOs are based on the social values of the particular faith but are not necessarily religious. FBOs draw on leaders, staff, and volunteers from a particular faith group at both the local and international scales. Funding for FBOs generally comes from member donations.

## The United Nations System

Maternal health influencers within the UN system include the following organizations.

The *World Health Organization* (WHO), established in 1946, focuses on international health needs. It has the comprehensive organization required of a health agency seeking to address the scope of the world's health problems and the design of initiatives aimed at mitigating these problems.

The *Pan-American Health Organization* (PAHO) is the oldest public health agency. It was established in 1902 to address the health of people who lived in the Americas and to develop partnerships to address health and quality of life. PAHO is identified as the Regional Office for the Americas of WHO and is a member of the UN system.

The *World Bank* is a multilateral agency whose mission is "to end extreme poverty" by lending money to resource-limited countries to address the health needs of populations. Health-related and environmental programs are funded to support health through the provision of electricity, access to safe water, communication systems, and programs focusing on sexual and gender-based violence.

The *United Nations Population Fund* (UNFPA) uses country population data to create policies and programs that aim to reduce poverty and to ensure that every pregnancy is wanted, every birth is safe, every young person is free of human immunodeficiency virus (HIV)/acquired immunodeficiency syndrome (AIDS), and every girl and woman is treated with dignity and respect.

Building upon the unfinished Millennium Development Goals (MDGs), the United Nations' Sustainable Development Goals (SDGs) are a call to action for all countries at every stage of human development to collaborate in global partnership to end poverty. The SDGs encourage all countries to work actively on strategies that improve health and education, reduce inequality, and enhance economic growth while tackling climate change, deforestation, and marine conservation.

## Essential Knowledge and Skill Upgrades for Midwives

Besides a strong grounding in contraception, sexual reproductive health, and gender-based violence, knowledge and skills related to the following topics are highly recommended for midwives working in the global health realm:

- Tropical medicine updates
- Malaria
- HIV/antiretroviral therapy (ART)/voluntary male medical circumcision (VMMC)
- Tuberculosis
- Helping Mothers Survive, a suite of learning modules to improve perinatal care; it includes Helping Babies Breathe, Bleeding After Birth, and Essential Care for Small Babies
- Case management
- Outreach/health promotion/disease prevention
- Demand generation
- Safe childbirth checklist
- Female genital mutilation (circumcision) and reinfibulation
- Midwife as first assistant skills
- Respectful Maternity Care (RMC)
- Kangaroo Mother Care (KMC)
- Maternal and Perinatal Surveillance Response (MDPSR)
- Mental Health and Psychosocial Support/Psychological First Aid (MHPSS)
- Water, Sanitation, and Hygiene (WASH)
- WHO Labor Care Guide
- Health Management Information System (HMIS) and relevant Demographic and Health Surveys (DHS)

Resources for learning about these topics include OpenWHO course catalogues and USAID's Global Health eLearning Center.

## Core Texts to Know Outside of *Varney's Midwifery*

- Marshall JE, Raynor MD, eds. *Myles Textbook for Midwives*. London, UK: Elsevier; 2020.
- Klein S, Miller S, Thomson F. *A Book for Midwives*. Berkeley, CA: Hesperian Health Guides; 2021.

## Safety and Security Considerations

Before embarking on any overseas assignment, make sure you have received a full briefing and have plans for the unexpected, including possible threats to life and health. Here are some tips to consider:

- Learn which medical services your health insurance will cover overseas. If your health insurance policy provides coverage outside the United States, remember to carry both your insurance policy identity card as proof of insurance and a claim form.
- Consider what your health insurance company will pay for, including hospital costs abroad.
- Learn about medical evacuation and mortal remains transport options back to the United States.
- Consider a short-term supplement to your insurance—for example, CIGNA Global.
- Sign up for field rescue, medical evacuation, destination reports, and event alerts, which are available on the Global Rescue website.
- Enroll in *Smart Traveler Enrollment Program* (STEP), a free service that allows U.S. citizens traveling or living abroad to receive the latest security updates from the nearest U.S. embassy or consular office.
- Keep a "go bag," containing items such as copies of all documents, essential contact phone numbers, a solar phone charger, visas/passports, medications, and legal currency to pay cash in full for an unexpected flight/transport.

## The Emotional Aspects of Working in Global Health

When tackling seemingly larger global health issues, such as high rates of morbidity and mortality, poverty, and hunger, there can be little space left for addressing mental health concerns. Few resources for mental health are generally available in low- and middle-income countries, and counseling needs for healthcare workers are an ongoing topic for capacity building.

Commonly occurring reactions to dealing with a medium- to long-term assignment include multiple manifestations of a prolonged stress response, such as changing sleep patterns and insomnia; a decline in motivation; severe mood swings; disassociation from friends, family, and colleagues; and an inability to disassociate oneself from work. It is not uncommon to find negative coping mechanisms among development workers, including high rates of alcohol and substance abuse.

A network of peers and recognition of the potential effects of the work are positive contributors to mental well-being in this sector. Health workers engaged in activities that directly affect the beneficiaries and involve high-risk work, such working with refugees, tend to view their work as a positive influence on their mental health. Before embarking upon an assignment, it is advisable to consult with your sponsoring agency about mental health support and resources.

Recommendations to support mental health and well-being in global health settings focus on building and reinforcing inner resilience. Practical suggestions include:

- Get adequate sleep or rest.
- Stay hydrated and eat nutritional foods.
- Exercise and practice good hygiene.
- Communicate with friends and family.
- Engage in mindfulness and meditation.
- Use symbols, ceremonies, or rituals that allow you to focus on stress reduction or honoring a memory of something positive.

### Resources

#### Websites and Organizations

| |
|---|
| International Confederation of Midwives (ICM) |
| International Council of Nurses (ICN) |
| United Nations Population Fund (UNFPA) |
| Joint United Nations Programme on HIV/AIDS (UNAIDS) |
| United Nations Children's Fund (UNICEF) |
| United Nations High Commissioner for Refugees (UNHCR) |

World Health Organization (WHO)

Helping Babies Breathe

Helping Mothers Survive (HMS)

International Committee of the Red Cross (ICRC)

International Medical Corps (IMC)

### *Resources for Self and Capacity Building*

WHO Mental Health Gap Action Programme

WHO Psychological First Aid for Field Workers

Psychological First Aid (Coursera)

### *Key Documents*

State of the World's Midwifery (SoWMY) 2021 (UNFPA)
(The 2014 and 2011 versions of the SoWMY Report may also be helpful.)

WHO Strategic Directions for Nursing and Midwifery 2021
(The 2015 version may also be helpful.)

International Confederation of Midwives Essential Competencies for Midwifery

WHO State of the World's Nursing 2020

WHO Midwifery Educator Core Competencies

### *Suggested Experiential Reading*

Holloway K. *Monique and the Mango Rains: Two Years with a Midwife in Mali*. Long Grove, IL: Waveland Press; 2006.

Fitzgerald L. *Those Who Eat Like Crocodiles*. London, UK: Unbound Digital; 2020.

Fadiman A. *The Spirit Catches You and You Fall Down: A Hmong Child, Her American Doctors, and the Collision of Two Cultures*. New York, NY: FSG Classics; 2012.

## References

1. American College of Nurse Midwives. Global health competencies and skills. https://www.midwife.org/acnm/files/cclibraryfiles/filename/000000007496/Global%20Health%20Competencies.pdf. Published 2018. Accessed June 15, 2022.

2. Consortium of Universities for Global Health Competency Sub-Committee. Global Health Education Competencies Toolkit. 2nd ed. https://www.cugh.org/online-tools/competencies-toolkit/. Published 2018. Accessed June 3, 2022.

3. Centers for Disease Control and Prevention. 10 essential public health services. https://www.cdc.gov/publichealthgateway/publichealthservices/essentialhealthservices.html. Revised 2020. Accessed June 3, 2022.

4. MacNairn E. Health volunteers overseas: a model for ethical and effective short-term global health training in low-resource countries. *Global Health Sci Pract*. 2019;7(3):344-354. doi:10.9745/GHSP_D_19-00140.

5. World Health Organization. Declaration of Alma Alta—September 1978. https://cdn.who.int/media/docs/default-source/documents/almaata-declaration-en.pdf?sfvrsn=7b3c2167_2. Accessed June 1, 2022.

6. United Nations. Universal Declaration of Human Rights. https://www.un.org/en/about-us/universal-declaration-of-human-rights. Accessed June 2, 2022.

# 2D

# Resources on the History of Midwifery

LUCINDA CANTY, IRA KANTROWITZ-GORDON, AND JULIA C. PHILLIPPI

*The editors would like to acknowledge the work of the authors of the ACNM Truth and Reconciliation Resolution, the ACNM Diverse History of Midwifery Reading and Resource List, and Black Lives Matter: A Message and Resources for Midwives. Liz Donnelly and Sharon Holley contributed references for this appendix. The editors also acknowledge Anne Z. Cockerham, Jyesha Wren Serbin, Simon Adriane Ellis, Elizabeth Donnelly, Kim Q. Dau, Betty Jane Watts Carrington, Heather Clarke, Carolyn Curtis, Nicolle L. Gonzales, Patricia O. Loftman, Felina M. Ortiz, M. Susan Stemmler, and Karline Wilson-Mitchell for their contributions to history-related chapters in the previous edition.*

Midwifery is one of the oldest professions: Midwives have been attending to pregnant, birthing, and postpartum people for millennia. In North America, midwifery's history is both rich and complex, and began long before the arrival of European colonists.

History provides the foundation for understanding the roots of the midwifery profession and appreciating how the profession can move forward. Knowledge of midwifery history plays a significant role in how we claim our identity as midwives and in understanding the challenges midwives had in the past and continue to have today. History also provides an understanding of past and present challenges within the healthcare system, the unique challenges faced by communities served by midwives, and the ways in which those challenges have impacted midwifery practice. Historical knowledge is essential to understanding current challenges such as lack of resources in a community and structural barriers that limit access to healthcare services. Midwives have long been able to overcome racial, economic, and cultural barriers to provide health care to individuals and families and demonstrate good perinatal outcomes. Historical knowledge can assist midwives at any stage in their career, whether they are current student midwives to retired midwives.

The origins of midwifery focus on holistic and person-centered care, and can be traced to midwives' strong connection to their communities. Historically, midwives were rooted deep within the communities they served. Midwives were often the only healthcare providers in their communities and were essential to the communities they served, particularly marginalized and vulnerable communities. In turn, the communities they served depended heavily on them. There was a sense of community and safety that was inherent in the care provided. Birthing persons trusted their midwives, who provided care during pregnancy and beyond childbearing to both individuals and families.

The midwifery approach to care developed as a consequence of situating care within communities. When the midwife cares for individuals during childbirth, birth is seen as a natural process, focusing on supporting during childbirth. Midwifery care does not only involve examination of the physical needs, but also involves awareness of the social factors that influence health outcomes. For example, grand midwives in the American South, such as Onnie Lee Logan, brought food and social support in addition to clinical care for their clients, who were living in poverty.[1] Midwives have a long history of providing care to vulnerable populations. For example, Maude Callen provided midwifery care and generalized public health care in Pineville, South Carolina; she served a rural Black community with a population of 10,000.[2]

In the twentieth century, when care during childbirth shifted from the home to the hospital, the competency of midwives, especially Black and immigrant midwives, was challenged. With increased rates of hospital births, mortality rates did not improve, especially for Black and Indigenous birthing people.[3,4] Disparities in maternal and infant mortality continue to the present day.

## Sources of Midwifery History

Midwifery has evolved and adapted to meet the needs of a changing society throughout history. Midwifery's history is rich with diverse midwives from all geographic areas and cultural communities. It is filled with a multitude of micro-histories, rather than forming a singular, objective, linear timeline. It is important to critically look at the context of the times to understand how midwives were able to provide care with limited resources and when systems were challenging their safety and value to the communities they served. Our intent is to acknowledge the depth of midwifery history and to understand the challenges that influenced healthcare delivery, utilization of health care, and health outcomes. Since midwifery practice was tightly embedded with the communities and people served, the history of midwifery needs to be contextualized in the community. Midwifery histories provide not only knowledge of the experience of midwives, but also information on the experiences of those who received midwifery care.

When exploring history, it is helpful to obtain primary sources generated by or with midwives themselves, if they are available, and to consider their narratives within the larger context of the cultural, societal, and structural pressures exerted on those individuals. Histories and interpretations of events, especially those from external (rather than insider) sources, can be presented from a single, and potentially erroneous, viewpoint and may contain or reinforce larger societal narratives or stereotypes. Examination of personal narratives and multiple viewpoints is helpful when studying midwifery history.

To obtain an inclusive history of American midwifery, it is essential to challenge narratives that exclude the contributions of traditional midwives and those known as healers who provided essential care to their communities.[5] Much of midwifery's history has been under-reported or suppressed; some narratives and histories are just now being documented, studied, and disseminated. Some areas of midwifery's history are not often discussed, such as the elimination of immigrant and traditional Black midwives.

The historical contributions of all midwives need to be acknowledged and incorporated into midwifery education. Historical knowledge is often incomplete, as many participants are not given the opportunity to tell their stories—and midwifery is no exception. As perinatal associations are becoming more open about issues of racism, including the need for diversity, inclusion, and equity, resources that profile the historical contributions of all midwives are becoming more readily available. To strengthen the profession and midwifery care, all stories and experiences of all midwives are needed. The history of all midwives is essential for taking on a midwifery identity that is inclusive, not colonizing, and not based on the medical model.

As part of this movement, it is important to consider who was providing midwifery care to Indigenous, Hispanic, Black, and immigrant populations. Often midwives providing care were cultural members of these communities. They had knowledge of the culture, spoke the language, and understood the social and structural factors that influenced health. An expanded awareness of the diverse history of midwifery will not only strengthen the profession, but can also improve the care that is provided to all communities.

It is beyond the scope of this text or appendix to provide all of the many histories of midwifery in North America; instead, an extensive list of articles, books, films, and blogs is offered to expand the reader's knowledge of midwifery's rich history/histories in North America. These sources provide multiple perspectives on the history of midwifery across many communities and times, although they cannot be considered comprehensive, given that not all communities have committed their histories to archivable forms. The sources are organized by time period and in alphabetical order by author. The *Truth and Reconciliation Resolution from the American College of Nurse-Midwives*[6] can serve as a starting point for understanding the need to explore deeply diverse histories of midwifery, and to recognize that not all historical accounts present full details of the time period, and many intentionally exclude individuals or cultural communities.

## Appendix Text References

1. Logan OL, Clark K. *Motherwit, an Alabama Midwife's Story.* New York, NY: Dutton; 1989.

2. *Angel in Twilight Maude Callen—Nurse-Midwife.* South Carolina Hall of Fame; 2013. https://youtu.be/m6gq8nMe1C8.

3. King CR. The New York Maternal Mortality Study: a conflict of professionalization. *Bull Hist Med.* 1991;65(4):476-502.

4. Thomasson MA, Treber J. From home to hospital: the evolution of childbirth in the United States, 1928–1940. *Explor Econ Hist.* 2008;45(1):76-99.

5. Niles PM, Drew M. Constructing the modern American midwife: white supremacy and white feminism collide. *Nursing CLIO.* October 22, 2020. https://nursingclio.org/2020/10/22/constructing-the-modern-american-midwife-white-supremacy-and-white-feminism-collide/. Accessed March 1, 2023.

6. Truth and Reconciliation Resolution from the American College of Nurse-Midwives. 2021. https://www.midwife.org/acnm/files/cclibraryfiles/filename/000000008234/ACNM_Truth_and_Reconciliation_Resolution-Apr2021.pdf. Accessed March 1, 2023.

## Midwifery History Resources

### Early Modern History (Pre-1700s)

Ehrenreich B, English D. *Witches, Midwives, and Nurses: A History of Women Healers.* 2nd ed. New York, NY: Feminist Press at the City University of New York; 2010.

### Mid-Modern History (1700s–1880s)

Leavitt JW. *Brought to Bed: Childbearing in America, 1750 to 1950.* 30th anniversary edition. Oxford, UK: Oxford University Press; 2016.

Manocchio RT. Tending communities, crossing cultures: midwives in 19th-century California. *J Midwifery Womens Health.* 2008;53(1):75-81. doi:10.1016/j.jmwh.2007.03.006.

McMillen SG. *Motherhood in the Old South: Pregnancy, Childbirth, and Infant Rearing.* Baton Rouge, LA: Louisiana State University Press; 1990.

Sessions PB, Smart DT. *Mormon Midwife: The 1846–1888 Diaries of Patty Bartlett Sessions.* Logan, UT: Utah State University Press; 1997.

Ulrich LT. *A Midwife's Tale: The Life of Martha Ballard, Based on Her Diary, 1785–1812.* 1st Vintage books edition. New York, NY: Vintage Books; 1991.

Vanderspank-Wright B. Caregiving on the periphery: historical perspectives on nursing and midwifery in Canada. Myra Rutherdale, ed. *Can Bull Med Hist.* 2012;29(2):415-416. doi:10.3138/cbmh.29.2.415.

Wilkie LA. *The Archaeology of Mothering: An African-American Midwife's Tale.* New York, NY: Routledge; 2003.

### Turn of the Twentieth Century (Circa 1880s–1930s)

Barney SL. *Authorized to Heal: Gender, Class, and the Transformation of Medicine in Appalachia, 1880–1930.* Chapel Hill, NC: University of North Carolina Press; 2000.

Bonaparte AD. *The Persecution and Prosecution of Granny Midwives in South Carolina, 1900–1940.* ProQuest Dissertations Publishing; 2007. https://etd.library.vanderbilt.edu/etd-07252007-122217_http://hdl.handle.net/1803/13563.

Bonaparte AD. Physicians' discourse for establishing authoritative knowledge in birthing work and reducing the presence of the granny midwife. *J Hist Sociol.* 2015;28(2):166-194. doi:10.1111/johs.12045.

Bonaparte AD. "The Satisfactory Midwife Bag": midwifery regulation in South Carolina, past and present considerations. *Soc Sci Hist.* 2014;38(1-2):155-182. doi:10.1017/ssh.2015.14.

Cooper Owens DB. *Medical Bondage: Race, Gender, and the Origins of American Gynecology.* Athens, GA: University of Georgia Press; 2017.

Fleming SE. *Seattle Pioneer Midwife: Alice Ada Wood Ellis: Midwife, Nurse & Mother to All: As Told by Her Great-Granddaughter.* 2nd ed. [Publisher not identified]; 2014.

Fraser GJ. *African American Midwifery in the South: Dialogues of Birth, Race, and Memory.* Cambridge, MA: Harvard University Press; 1998.

Goan MB. *Mary Breckinridge: The Frontier Nursing Service & Rural Health in Appalachia.* Chapel Hill, NC: University of North Carolina Press; 2008.

Hill JJ. *Birthing the West: Mothers and Midwives in the Rockies and Plains.* Lincoln, NE: Bison Books; 2022. doi:10.2307/j.ctv25wxd0g.

Luke JM. *Delivered by Midwives: African American Midwifery in the Twentieth-Century South.* Jackson, MS: University Press of Mississippi; 2018.

Morrison SM, Fee E. Nothing to work with but cleanliness: the training of African American traditional midwives in the South. *Am J Public Health.* 2010;100(2):238-239. doi:10.2105/AJPH.2009.182873.

Reagan LJ. *When Abortion Was a Crime: Women, Medicine, and Law in the United States, 1867–1973.* Berkeley, CA: University of California Press; 2022. doi:10.2307/j.ctv2kx88fq.

Shoemaker MT. *History of Nurse-Midwifery in the United States.* New York, NY: Garland; 1984.

Smith CC, Roberson MHB. *My Bag Was Always Packed: The Life and Times of a Black Virginia Midwife.* Bloomington, IN: 1stBooks; 2003.

Smith KC. *Orlean Puckett: The Life of a Mountain Midwife, 1844–1939.* Boone, NC: Parkway; 2003.

### Early Twentieth Century (Circa 1930s–1960s)

Association of American Medical Colleges under the auspices of the Georgia Dept. of Public Health. *All My*

*Babies: A Midwife's Own Story*. Image Entertainment; 2007. https://www.loc.gov/2017604960.

Bovard WL, Milton G. *Why Not Me? The Story of Gladys Milton, Midwife*. Summertown, TN: Book Publishing Co.; 1993.

Brown VO. *Mountain Midwife: Life and Times of Isabella Brown Neal*. Charleston, WV: Mountain Memories Books; 2010.

Campbell M. *Folks Do Get Born*. New York, NY: Rinehart & Company; 1946.

Craven C, Glatzel M. Downplaying difference: historical accounts of African American midwives and contemporary struggles for midwifery. *Feminist Stud*. 2010;36(2):330-358.

Dawley K. Origins of nurse-midwifery in the United States and its expansion in the 1940s. *J Midwifery Womens Health*. 2003;48(2):86-95. doi:10.1016/s1526-9523(03)00002-3.

Ferguson SR. *Birth Cry: A Personal Story of the Life of Hannah D. Mitchell, Nurse Midwife*. Bloomington, IN: West Bow Press; 2011.

Logan OL, Clark K. *Motherwit, an Alabama Midwife's Story*. New York, NY: Dutton; 1989.

Pelley R, O'Leary S. *Island Maid: Voices of Outport Women*. St. John's, Canada: Breakwater Books; 2010.

Roush RE. The development of midwifery—male and female, yesterday and today. *J Nurse-Midwifery*. 1979;24(3):27-37. doi:10.1016/0091-2182(79)90078-8.

Slaney Brown E. *Labours of Love: Midwives of Newfoundland and Labrador*. St. John's, Canada: DRC Publishing; 2007.

Smith CC, Roberson MHB. *Memories of a Black Lay Midwife from Northern Neck Virginia*. Lisle, IL: Tucker Publications; 1994.

Smith MC, Holmes LJ. *Listen to Me Good: The Life Story of an Alabama Midwife*. Columbus, OH: Ohio State University Press; 1996.

Smith SL. *Japanese American Midwives: Culture, Community, and Health Politics, 1880–1950*. Urbana, IL: University of Illinois Press; 2005.

Smith SL. White nurses, Black midwives, and public health in Mississippi, 1920–1950. *Nurs Hist Rev*. 1994;2:29-49.

Smith-Ledford S. *Etta "Granny" Nichols: Last of the Old-Timey Midwives*. Chapel Hill, NC: Professional Press; 1998.

South Carolina ETV. "Angel in Twilight' Maude Callen: Nurse-Midwife. South Carolina Hall of Fame 2013. https://www.youtube.com/watch?v=jZnveOj57F0. Accessed November 4, 2022.

Susie DA. *In the Way of Our Grandmothers: A Cultural View of Twentieth-Century Midwifery in Florida*. Athens, GA: University of Georgia Press; 1988.

Worth J, Coates T. *The Midwife: A Memoir of Birth, Joy, and Hard Times*. New York, NY: Penguin Books; 2009.

### Late Twentieth Century (Circa 1970s–Present)

Armstrong P, Feldman S. *A Midwife's Story*. New York, NY: Arbor House; 1986.

Burgess VD. *The Midwife: A Biography of Laurine Ekstrom Kingston*. Salt Lake City, UT: Signature Books; 2012.

Buss FL. *La Partera: Story of a Midwife*. Ann Arbor, MI: University of Michigan Press; 1980.

Cohen E. *Laboring: Stories of a New York City Hospital Midwife*. Createspace Independent; 2013.

Cole LJ, Avery MD, eds. *Freestanding Birth Centers: Innovation, Evidence, Optimal Outcomes*. New York, NY: Springer; 2017.

DeLibertis J. Shifting the frame: a report on diversity and inclusion in the American College of Nurse-Midwives. https://www.midwife.org/acnm/files/ccLibraryFiles/Filename/000000005329/Shifting-the-Frame-June-2015.pdf. Published 2015. Accessed November 4, 2022.

Ettinger LE. *Nurse-Midwifery: The Birth of a New American Profession*. Columbus, OH: Ohio State University Press; 2006.

Gaskin IM. *Spiritual Midwifery*. 5th ed., 8th print ed. Summertown, TN: Book Publishing Company; 2009.

Guerra-Reyes L, Hamilton LJ. Racial disparities in birth care: exploring the perceived role of African-American women providing midwifery care and birth support in the United States. *Women Birth*. 2017;30(1):e9-e16. doi:10.1016/j.wombi.2016.06.004.

Harman P. *The Blue Cotton Gown: A Midwife's Memoir*. Boston, MA: Beacon Press; 2008.

Holmes LJ, American College of Nurse-Midwives. *Into the Light of Day: Reflections on the History of Midwives of Color Within the American College of Nurse-Midwives*. Silver Spring, MD: Midwives of Color Committee of the American College of Nurse-Midwives; 2012.

Patruno P. *The American Dream: Birth in America for Black Mothers* [Film]. 2016. http://www.birthisadream.org/the-american-dream. Accessed November 4, 2022.

Lake R, Epstein A, Rossi L. *The Mama Sherpas: Midwives Across America*. Kino Lorber; 2015. https://kinolorber.com/product/the-mama-sherpas-dvd.

Lee V. *Granny Midwives and Black Women Writers: Double-Dutched Readings*. New York, NY: Routledge; 1996.

Leonard C. *Lady's Hands, Lion's Heart: A Midwife's Saga*. 2nd ed. Hopkinton, NH: Bad Beaver Publishing; 2010.

Muhlhahn C. *Labor of Love: A Midwife's Memoir*. New York, NY: Kaplan Publishing; 2009.

Nestel S. *Obstructed Labour: Race and Gender in the Re-emergence of Midwifery*. Vancouver, Canada: UBC Press; 2006.

Oparah JC, Arega H, Hudson D, et al. *Battling Over Birth: Black Women and the Maternal Health Care Crisis*. Amarillo, TX: Praeclarus Press; 2018.

Oparah JC, Bonaparte AD, eds. *Birthing Justice: Black Women, Pregnancy, and Childbirth*. New York, NY: Routledge; 2016.

Phillippi JC, Alliman J, Bauer K. The American Association of Birth Centers: history, membership, and current initiatives. *J Midwifery Womens Health*. 2009;54(5): 387-392. doi:10.1016/j.jmwh.2008.12.009.

Popova R, Levake C. *Midwife Memories: Tales of Amish and "English" Birth Culture*. [Independently published]. 2020.

Scrimshaw SC, Backes EP, Division of Behavioral and Social Sciences and Education, et al. *Birth Settings in America: Outcomes, Quality, Access, and Choice*. Washington, DC: National Academies Press; 2020.

Simkins G. *Into These Hands: Wisdom from Midwives*. Traverse City, MI: Spirituality & Health Books; 2011.

Vincent P. *BabyCatcher: Chronicles of a Modern Midwife*. New York, NY: Scribner; 2003.

Yarger L. *Lovie: The Story of a Southern Midwife and an Unlikely Friendship*. Chapel Hill, NC: University of North Carolina Press; 2016.

***Across History***

American College of Nurse-Midwives. Truth and Reconciliation Resolution from the American College of Nurse-Midwives. 2021. https://www.midwife.org/acnm/files /cclibraryfiles/filename/000000008234/ACNM_Truth _and_Reconciliation_Resolution-Apr2021.pdf.

Avery MD. The evolution of the Core Competencies for Basic Midwifery Practice. *J Midwifery Womens Health*. 2000;45(6):532-536. doi:10.1016/s1526-9523(00)00079-9.

Avery MD. The history and evolution of the Core Competencies for Basic Midwifery Practice. *J Midwifery Womens Health*. 2005;50(2):102-107. doi:10.1016/j.jmwh .2004.12.006.

Bourgeault IL, Benoit CM, Davis-Floyd R. *Reconceiving Midwifery*. Montréal, Canada: McGill-Queen's University Press; 2004.

Cockerham A. History of midwifery in the United States. In: King TL, Bruker MC, Osborne K, Jevitt CM, eds. *Varney's Midwifery*. 6th ed. Burlington, MA: Jones & Bartlett Learning; 2019:3-34.

Dawley K. The campaign to eliminate the midwife. *Am J Nurs*. 2000;100(10):50-56.

De Vries RG. *Making Midwives Legal: Childbirth, Medicine, and the Law*. 2nd ed. Columbus, OH: Ohio State University Press; 1996.

Dixon LZ. *Delivering Health: Midwifery and Development in Mexico*. Nashville, TN: Vanderbilt University Press; 2020.

Drew ML, Reis P. Black lives matter: a message and resources for midwives. *J Midwifery Womens Health*. 2020;65(4):451-458. doi:10.1111/jmwh.13155.

Goodwin M. The racist history of abortion and midwifery bans. https://www.aclu.org/news/racial-justice/the-racist -history-of-abortion-and-midwifery-bans. Published 2020. Accessed November 4, 2022.

Green LB, Summers M, eds. *Precarious Prescriptions: Contested Histories of Race and Health in North America*. Minneapolis, MN: University of Minnesota Press; 2014.

Greenfield E, Minter D. *The Women Who Caught the Babies: A Story of African American Midwives*. Carrboro, NC: Alazar Press; 2019.

Laako H, Sánchez Ramírez G. *Midwives in Mexico: Situated Politics, Politically Situated*. London, UK: Routledge; 2021.

Litoff JB. *American Midwives, 1860 to the Present*. Westport, CT: Greenwood Press; 1978.

McCool WF, McCool SJ. Feminism and nurse-midwifery. Historical overview and current issues. *J Nurse Midwifery*. 1989;34(6):323-334. doi:10.1016/0091-2182(89) 90006-2.

Ortiz FM. *El Espiritu de las Parteras* [Film]. 2005.

Ortiz FM. History of midwifery in New Mexico: partnership between curandera-parteras and the New Mexico Department of Health. *J Midwifery Womens Health*. 2005;50(5):411-417. doi:10.1016/j.jmwh.2004.12.001.

Phillippi JC, Avery MD. The 2012 American College of Nurse-Midwives core competencies for basic midwifery practice: history and revision. *J Midwifery Womens Health*. 2014;59(1):82-90. doi:10.1111/jmwh.12148.

Roberts DE. *Killing the Black Body: Race, Reproduction, and the Meaning of Liberty*. New York, NY: Pantheon Books; 1997.

Robinson SA. A historical development of midwifery in the black community: 1600–1940. *J Nurse Midwifery*. 1984;29(4):247-250. doi:10.1016/0091-2182(84)90128-9.

Rooks J. *Midwifery and Childbirth in America*. Philadelphia, PA: Temple University Press; 1997.

Shruti N. Birth justice denied: the continued marginalization of community birth settings and midwives. https:// www.yaledistilled.com/post/birth-justice-denied-the -continued-marginalization-of-community-birth-settings -and-midwives. Published 2021. Accessed November 4, 2022.

Thompson J, Walker J, Thomson A. *100 Years of the International Confederation of Midwives: Empowering Midwives and Empowering Women*. Wick, United Kingdom: Brown Dog Books; 2022.

Varney H, Thompson JB. *A History of Midwifery in the United States: The Midwife Said Fear Not*. New York, NY: Springer; 2016.

Washington HA. *Medical Apartheid: The Dark History of Medical Experimentation on Black Americans from Colonial Times to the Present*. New York, NY: Anchor Books; 2008.

Wertz RW, Wertz DC. *Lying-in: A History of Childbirth in America*. New York, NY: Free Press; 1977.

Wren Serbin J, Donnelly E. The impact of racism and midwifery's lack of racial diversity: a literature review. *J Midwifery Womens Health*. 2016;61(6):694-706. doi:10.1111/jmwh.12572.

## Competencies, Definitions, and Standards for Practice

| Organization | Document |
|---|---|
| **International** | |
| International Confederation of Midwives | *International Definition of the Midwife* (2005, 2011, 2017) <br> *Essential Competencies for Basic Midwifery Practice* (2010, 2019) |
| World Health Organization | *Sexual and Reproductive Health Core Competencies in Primary Care: Attitudes, Knowledge, Ethics, Human Rights, Leadership, Management, Teamwork, Community Work, Education, Counselling, Clinical Settings, Service, Provision* (2011) |
| **Canada** | |
| Canadian Midwifery Regulators Council | *Canadian Competencies for Midwives* (2019, 2020) |
| **Mexico** | |
| Asociación Mexicana de Parterí | *Essential Competencies for Midwifery Practice in Mexico* (2014) |
| **United States** | |
| American College of Nurse-Midwives | *Core Competencies for Basic Midwifery Practice* (1978, 1985, 1992, 2002, 2007, 2012, 2020) <br> *Definition of Midwifery and Scope of Practice of Certified Nurse-Midwives and Certified Midwives* (1992, 2004, 2011, 2012, 2021) <br> *Standards for the Practice of Midwifery* (2003, 2009, 2011, 2022). Formerly *Standards for the Practice of Nurse-Midwifery* (1987, 1993) and *Functions, Standards, and Qualifications* (1983). |
| Midwives Alliance of North America | *Standards and Qualifications for the Art and Practice of Midwifery* (2005) <br> *The Midwives Alliance Core Competencies* (1994, 2011, 2014) |
| National Association of Certified Professional Midwives | *Scope of Practice for the National Association of Certified Professional Midwives* (2004) <br> *Standards of Practice for NACPM Members* (2004) |
| National Black Midwives Alliance | *21-Point Black Midwives Care Model* (2021) developed by Jamarah Amani for the National Black Midwives Alliance, a project of the Southern Birth Justice Network. |

# II

P A R T

# Primary Care

### Section Editor
MARY K. BARGER

# II

# Primary Care

CHAPTER

# 3

# An Introduction to Sexual, Reproductive, and Primary Care

JAN M. KRIEBS

## Midwifery: Changing Scope, Enduring Philosophy

Midwifery is both art and science—and above all midwifery is care for people and their families. While the core of midwifery is often seen as associated with pregnancy and birth, the role of the midwife has always extended beyond birth, whether formally acknowledged or not. Midwifery in the United States has grown from local efforts to care for women with the few resources available into a well-respected profession that offers primary care, reproductive and sexual care, as well as pregnancy, birth, and newborn care.

This nation's first midwives were healers in their communities, and the first nurse-midwives were public health nurses; both provided elements of primary care as we know it today. Their scope of practice included general health and well-being for the whole family.[1] By the 1990s, competencies in primary care had been added to midwifery education and practice standards and were made even clearer in subsequent revisions.[2,3]

In the twenty-first century, midwifery has also acknowledged its role across gender boundaries, making it clear that all who seek midwifery care should be welcomed. Scope of practice can be understood on two levels. The first, defined by the American College of Nurse-Midwives, recognizes what any individual midwife can do within their practice.[3] The second level is the individual scope of a particular midwife. Not every midwife will provide colposcopy, intrauterine insemination, or community birth. Yet each of these skills is within the midwifery scope of practice writ large.

Midwives are autonomous practitioners, independent within their scope of practice. Midwifery services are provided using an interdisciplinary approach because midwives rely on the skills of gynecologists and obstetricians, nurses, social workers, and other health professionals, just as those professionals rely on midwives for their respective expertise. Key to understanding midwifery care is recognition of the interweaving of skills and knowledge from many sources, and the willingness to work with others to achieve the best possible health outcomes.

Evidence-based studies should be the foundation for the practice of midwifery. Unfortunately, relatively few of the guidelines on which clinicians rely have been drawn from high-quality research. In some situations, interventions have been adopted before large research studies were conducted to clarify their usefulness. The fact that guidelines are not consistently based on solid evidence has been acknowledged and there are ongoing discussions about widespread bias in research and practice.[4] For example, in 2011 the American College of Obstetricians and Gynecologists published data showing that fewer than one-third of its Practice Bulletins were based on "good and consistent" evidence.[5] Much of pregnancy care cannot be evaluated safely and ethically using the most rigorous types of research. Midwifery research continues to account for only a small percentage of the work being conducted in the area of sexual and reproductive health, although an increasing number of scholars are contributing knowledge in this area. Examples range from the development of CenteringPregnancy as a model of care to the research done on delayed cord-clamping after birth.[6,7] Deciphering the evidence, acknowledging the quality of information from which recommendations are made, and recognizing biases—both in midwives and in others—are all key components of midwifery care.

Midwifery is distinguished by characteristics that define it as a partnership with the people to whom midwives provide care. A willingness to listen; sensitivity to cultural, sexual, and generational differences; shared decision making; and the patience to be in partnership rather than dominating a relationship—all combine with professional behaviors to describe midwifery practice. This chapter addresses both clinical tasks and professional behaviors, and its goal is to identify those core skills needed to be a midwife.

Essential skills begin with an understanding of the midwifery management process. Developed by the midwifery education program in Mississippi in the early1970s,[5] the seven steps in this process serve as a guide to the process of care at an individual level and offer an opportunity to evaluate the effectiveness of care[8] (Table 3-1). As with other formats for organizing the process of collecting history, examining, making an assessment or diagnosis, and planning a course of care, the Midwifery Management Process described here serves as a framework for each patient encounter.

| Table 3-1 | The Midwifery Management Process |
|---|---|

1. Investigate by obtaining all necessary data for complete evaluation of the patient.

2. Accurately identify problems or diagnoses and healthcare needs based on correct interpretation of the data.

3. Anticipate other potential problems or diagnoses that might be expected because of the identified problems or diagnoses.

4. Evaluate the need for immediate midwife or physician intervention and/or for consultation or collaborative management with other healthcare team members, as dictated by the patient's condition.

5. Develop a comprehensive plan of care that is supported by explanations of the valid rationale underlying the decisions made and is based on the preceding steps.

6. Assume responsibility for the efficient and safe implementation of the plan of care.

7. Evaluate the effectiveness of the care given, cycling repeatedly and appropriately through the management process for any aspect of care that has been ineffective.

The midwifery management process emphasizes the midwife's responsibility as an autonomous care provider and is based on the scientific process. Even when other practitioners may be involved in care, the midwife assumes responsibility for ensuring the patient and their family receive adequate and prompt treatment and health education. The recognition of the interdependence of many disciplines in creating a holistic plan of care is inherent in midwifery.

The comprehensive plan noted in the management process focuses first on evidence-based treatment options that promote health and prevent morbidity and/or treat current conditions. These interventions encompass more than pharmaceuticals—they also comprise a plan of care customized to meet the patient's needs. Considerations in the design of such a plan include cost, accessibility, and convenience, among other factors.

The midwifery management process also acknowledges that most care is provided not in discrete sessions, but rather over time. Optimally, continuity over time is critical in improving quality of care.

## Culture, Race, Gender, and Identity

Midwives will, over time, meet individuals who are hesitant to share their health concerns because they have learned to distrust how their beliefs and identity may be received. What does this mean for the midwife in practice? Awareness of one's own cultural assumptions, as well as appreciation of one's personal biases and choices about practice parameters, is an essential first step for providing sensitive care to all patients. Unless midwives know themselves, they are at increased risk of manifesting unconscious offenses and implicit bias that may hinder the therapeutic relationship, increase reluctance to share important information, prevent a patient from seeking care, and, as a result, worsen outcomes.[9] This is a lifelong project. Few, if any, individuals come into adulthood fully sensitive to these topics.

It is important to remember that health care is a cultural construct as well—emerging from beliefs about the characteristics of disease and their impact on the human body. Consequently, culture is a primary factor in the provision of health care that influences both the provider and the receiver of care. This idea extends not only to the care provider, but also to structural and process aspects of care. Beyond considering culture as a way to identify beliefs or attitudes about health care, a midwife should consider the implications of racism, oppression, and societal inequity experienced by marginalized groups across socioeconomic groupings as obstacles to developing a more inclusive environment.[10,11]

One solution that has been examined is the benefits of racial concordance for health care. The racial disparities in healthcare outcomes are well known and have been recognized as salient concerns for decades. So has the effect of implicit bias among providers on those outcomes. One way to improve these disparities is to promote diversity among providers at all levels, by encouraging the growth of a more diverse work force.[12] The second is to ensure diversity within healthcare teams and leadership. Diversity benefits include increases in innovation and productivity, more accurate risk assessment, and increased likelihood that Black, Asian, and Latinx patients will come for preventive care visits.[13] There is also increasing evidence that cultural concordance and diverse teams contribute to better outcomes of care.[14]

Two concepts important to decreasing health inequities aggravated by providers' communication with patients are positionality and intersectionality. Positionality uses the lens of personal characteristics such as age, race, ethnicity, and social class to help individuals see the way in which their interactions might affect care.[15] Intersectionality is "the complex, cumulative way in which the effects of multiple forms of discrimination (such as racism, sexism, and classism) combine, overlap, or intersect especially in the experiences of marginalized individuals or groups."[16] Taken together, they open a path to consideration of what it will take to create a more equitable system of care. The various components of identity create levels of privilege in a relationship. For example, a white midwife might be disadvantaged next to their consultant physician (who may hold power over their ability to practice midwifery in the clinical setting), but will be privileged by race and profession compared to their Black or Latinx patient with Medicaid insurance. A full discussion of the issues of inequity and racism, and of the social justice movement, is beyond the scope of this chapter. Nevertheless, these basic ideas should give all midwives an opportunity to assess their own relationships with patients, other staff, and clinicians. Resources with which to explore the topic of equity further are listed at the end of this chapter.

Beyond race or ethnicity, another consideration for midwives is that of gender identity and diversity. Transgender and nonbinary people experience inequitable care in many settings. At the same time, insurance may not pay for gender-affirming care when such services are perceived as cosmetic.[17] Nonetheless, gender-affirming care can improve mental health and reduce body dysphoria (distress caused by a discrepancy between one's assigned gender at birth and one's gender identity). Examples of making a clinical space more inclusive include unisex bathrooms and forms that offer multiple gender identities rather than only male or female.[18] Other approaches to ensuring the provision of a more affirming site are discussed later, as they relate to many populations needing a safer space for care. Rabelais recommends a sequence of listening, believing, trusting, and reflecting as an approach to providing safe care.[17] Most clinicians will never share the experience of living as a transgender or nonbinary person, any more than they will share the experiences of a different ethnic group. Midwives can, however, provide a safe space for midwifery care. It is essential to understand that individuals have a wide range of cultural, sexual, and gender identities and expressions, as discussed in more detail in the *Context of Individuals Seeking Midwifery Care* chapter.

## Communication

Clear communication is an essential component of any therapeutic interaction and deserves conscious attention if it is to be effective. Several important variables influence the success of communication between a midwife and a patient who seeks healthcare services.

Many characteristics that contribute to a person's identity play an important role in the relationships between patients and their midwives. Cultural identity, sexual and gender identity, race and ethnicity, immigration status, and socioeconomic status are just a few examples of the factors that influence a person's interactions with others. Health literacy and health numeracy affect how well an individual understands medical communications. In addition, language itself can facilitate or be a barrier to comprehension.

### Health Literacy and Health Numeracy

The midwife should address the patient in language they can understand, with explanations that are clear and do not omit factual information that is important. Health literacy is defined by the Institute of Medicine (renamed the National Academy of Medicine in 2015) as "the degree to which individuals have the capacity to obtain, process, and understand basic health information and services needed to make appropriate health decisions."[19] Approximately half of the U.S. adult population has low health literacy.[20] This functional level of literacy permits understanding of health education and its use within clearly identified goals or plans. Nutbeam and Lloyd argue that higher levels of literacy can become a social determinant of health.[21] In contrast, low health literacy is associated with more hospitalizations and lower use of preventive services such as mammography and vaccinations. Although educational attainment frequently is used as a proxy for health literacy, many individuals actually read and—more importantly—comprehend at levels below their formal educational level. Be aware that lack of education is not equivalent to lack of common sense, nor is it a sign of lack of intelligence. Research is being conducted into the use of graphics, apps, and digital presentations as ways to share health information with individuals who are not highly literate.[22]

Health numeracy, which is the degree to which individuals understand quantitative and probabilistic health information, is an important component of health literacy.[23] Strategies to increase the likelihood that an individual will understand the probability of an event include using absolute numbers instead of percentages, relative risks, or risk ratios;[24] avoiding the words *rare*, *unlikely*, *uncommon*, and *unusual*, as these are imprecise concepts subject to individual interpretation; and using small denominators and whole numbers.[25] For example, "1 in 4" is more easily understood than "25 out of 100" or "25%." Studies of health literacy and health numeracy often portray these abilities as individual patient skills, but effective communication by the midwife is an equally important factor in ensuring understanding.[26,27] Resources for learning more about health literacy and health numeracy are included in the Resources Section at the end of this chapter.

### Use of Language

Learning to listen to one's own words and see one's physical position relative to others is a skill like any other. Both speech and body language affect the relationship between the midwife and the patient. Among other things, this means that word choice needs to be appropriate for the patient's educational and cultural background. The midwife must move to where the patient is in terms of understanding; by beginning there, both can move together to identify and discuss a problem. The language that any healthcare provider spends years mastering is not the common tongue.

Active listening is an essential skill. It requires the patience to allow someone to tell their own story where they wish to start it, with minimal interruptions or directive language. Asking open-ended questions encourages someone to put their concerns into their own words. When one listens actively, one focuses on what is being said, reflects back what one hears, and verifies that both participants in the conversation share understanding. Waiting silently to encourage additional information; paraphrasing an unclear statement by asking, "I think you mean ____; is that correct?"; reflecting back, such as by saying, "I hear you saying _____"; and providing reassurance that the patient's information is important are all critical tools. Validating understanding of a problem as described by the patient is essential—it is all too easy to misunderstand the actual concern. Further, every person needs to believe that what they say will be held in confidence, and that they may safely say anything they need to say.

Active listening also incorporates a nonverbal component, which in some cultures includes making eye contact, leaning toward a person rather than away, having an open body position that suggests acceptance, avoiding closed positioning (e.g., not crossing the arms), and maintaining a professional facial expression. Respectful, active listening behaviors vary by culture, and knowledge of best practices for the community served by the midwife is important.

Another instrument for assessing the effectiveness of one's listening is to consider how communication in a professional setting affects the patient's ability to hear what is being said. The midwife's words should answer the following four questions. These questions are based on similar concepts that have traditionally been attributed to various individuals and groups, such as the mystical Sufi tradition, Socrates, and, more recently, the Quakers. Although their origins may be murky, the concepts remain relevant today. The questions are appropriate when considering how communication in a professional setting affects the ability to hear what is being said. The midwife's words should answer the following four questions:

1. *Is it truthful?* If not, there is no need to say it.
2. *Is it kind?* Many topics that need to be discussed in a healthcare setting require kindness to make it possible for the listener to accept unpalatable advice. Kindness is using terminology and wording that is appropriate to the situation and respectful to the individual while not ignoring a problem, and not being patronizing. For example, there are many ways to talk about weight and health. Compare "You're obese and you need to eat less" with "We understand that there are

health risks associated with high body mass index. Would you like to discuss ways to improve your health?" Which of these statements will be more likely to encourage the patient to accept a referral to a nutritionist?

3. *Is it necessary?* Preventing damage from diabetes or hypertension in this example can hinge on the patient accepting the referral and actively participating in improving their health. Do not ask a question unless the answer changes the management plan, and always be able to explain why the question is needed.

4. *Is it appropriate?* In one sense, discussing weight management is always appropriate—but what if this individual has come to be treated for a sexually transmitted infection (STI)? Perhaps weight loss is not the concern they need to focus on today.

## Addressing Sensitive Concerns

Midwives deal with some of the most intimate and personal aspects of a person's life. The choice of partner, decisions about childbearing, and sexual experiences constitute just a few of the themes that impact the person's life. The risk for being exposed to violence, whether physically, sexually, or emotionally, is another theme. The choices individuals have made with regard to lifestyle or habits, exposure to infections, and whether they have basic necessities such as adequate food and shelter are all topics that can and will come up during midwifery care.

People may experience stigma for many reasons. When a person has been exposed to negative reactions in the community enough times, that individual tends to withdraw from interactions that might create new opportunities to be stigmatized. It is the midwife's job to create a safe environment, where questions can be asked and answered, and where help can be sought and offered. When greeting a person or a family in the office, when providing care, and when discussing choices, watch for physical or verbal cues that suggest that another topic needs to be addressed.

## The Midwifery Management Process

### Approaching the Patient

The first steps in any clinical encounter usually occur before the midwife and the patient meet. Somehow, the individual has found the practice, made an appointment, been checked in for a visit, and

possibly been seen by a nurse or medical assistant. They have observed whether the setting is professional and the furnishings are in good repair. They will notice whether they are greeted privately and respectfully by staff who have received training in working with diverse populations, and whether the organization itself is supportive.[28]

Aspects of the physical office environment that can affect a patient's sense of how they will be treated include having seating appropriate for all weights and using illustrations that show diversity with multiple races, different gender presentations, and ages.[18,28] Although it is not the purpose of this chapter to discuss specific practice management, all of these factors will have shaped impressions of the midwife and of midwifery.

Seemingly simple choices about work flow prior to the midwife entering the visit, such as whether the patient is seen first in an office or undressed on an examination table, say something about mutual respect. Just as when making a home visit, the midwife looks for clues about the patient's lifestyle and health of the family; likewise, the patient seeks clues about the midwife's practice and professionalism.

Before asking any questions, however, mutual introductions should take place. Think of the relationship forged during this encounter as a framework for the care that the patient will receive. The patient should be seated comfortably and with adequate personal space. The midwife's position should promote direct eye contact. An important initial question is to ask about the patient's preferred name, and how they would like their gender documented in the records. Documentation of gender identity and sexual orientation is actually a requirement for federally certified electronic records.[29] Next, asking "How are you today?" or "How are you feeling?" begins to establish concern for the patient as an individual. Listening to the answer assists the establishment of mutual trust and trust in midwifery care.

From a legal compliance or payment perspective, the order of the visit's elements encapsulates the essential components of care. In this context, *compliance* refers to legal requirements (such as Medicare regulations and not the patient's agreement with the management plan) and *payment* refers to what is required to receive compensation from insurers; both incorporate standards that must be met.

Some visits will be tightly problem focused; some will be comprehensive examinations. Both types of visits follow the same sequence. All begin with the same question: "Why have you come in to see us today?" The answer establishes the chief concern—that is, the reason for the visit. The terms "concern" and "reason for coming" are less value laden than "chief complaint," an older phrase used in documentation. Sometimes other, more pressing problems will become apparent during the conversation or examination, but asking about the initial reason for the visit is always the starting point.

The structural components of the visit include the following: chart review of previous records and test results, history, and review of systems; the examination and any office-based tests; the assessment and diagnosis; and decision making about future visits, tests, and treatment plus the discussion, teaching, and guidance offered. The *Standard and Airborne Precautions* appendix lists standard precautions that are an essential component of any healthcare visit.

## Obtaining Consent

Depending on the purpose of the visit, the midwife may ask for the patient's consent several times. When collecting the history, permission to ask questions about sexual behaviors and history should be given. Before the physical examination, when the examination advances to evaluation of the breast/chest, and again before positioning a patient for pelvic examination, ask for the patient's permission to proceed. When the patient believes that they have control of what happens to their body, it can help them relax, decreasing discomfort.

For anyone caring for adolescents, a different issue comes into play. The age at which a minor may give sexual consent, the age at which they may consent to sexual and reproductive health care, and the age at which they can consent for care to their own newborn of infant all vary by state.[30] These laws can and do change, so verifying the rules in one's own practice location is necessary.

## Collecting the Health History

When collecting a health history, the midwife first considers the purpose of the visit. If the patient has come for a comprehensive or general reason, the history obtained will be broader than if the visit is problem focused. Consider an initial prenatal visit, which will include a complete personal, social, and family history, as well as genetic risks. Contrast it with a triage visit for nausea and vomiting of pregnancy, which will focus on the current concern, asking about exposure to spoiled food and infectious contacts, allergies, gastrointestinal disorders, and problems with nausea in any prior pregnancies.

The general principle is to work from the least invasive questions to those that require more

personal exposure. When one question at a time is asked, and there is a pause to wait for each response, information is less likely to be confused or omitted. Establishing and maintaining an easy flow of dialogue and a nonjudgmental manner promotes open exchange of information. Patients should be advised that some questions are very personal, and that they are not required to answer ones that they do not wish to discuss. It may be necessary to ask particularly sensitive questions on more than one occasion before the patient is able to give a full answer. An example of a situation that may require such an approach is caring for a person who has experienced prior abuse, as discussed later in this chapter. As the health history is completed, it is wise to ask oneself if any questions are missing or any aspect was not considered. The *Collecting a Health History* appendix provides a review of the complete health history.

## Review of Systems

The review of systems (ROS) bridges the divide between prior health history and the current examination. It includes recent signs and symptoms the patient has noticed, such as burning on urination or a rash. The ROS, in combination with the history, can open up more extensive lines of questioning. In many practices, the ROS is a checklist provided in the waiting area to be completed before being seen. During a focused visit, the ROS may be part of the conversation during the examination. When questions are asked well, this part of the encounter can identify further areas of concern or topics for health education.

## The Physical Examination

Most examinations in midwifery offices are screening examinations, unless the midwife is serving as the primary care provider (PCP), and the history or ROS has identified additional potential health problems that need to be explored in depth. Screening-oriented physical examinations limit the details that can be elicited when every organ system is fully evaluated. *The Physical Examination* appendix outlines a comprehensive physical examination. A complete review is beyond the scope of this chapter, and interested readers can find multiple written and online resources that cover this topic.

By tradition, an initial health assessment, whether the patient is pregnant or not, is comprehensive, meaning that it includes all major organ systems. Individuals who see their midwife regularly and have another provider designated as a PCP can receive a single-system examination that targets and more completely evaluates the genitourinary and reproductive systems. In that case, the thyroid, breasts, abdomen, and pelvis are examined fully, but other systems are not addressed.

Reproductive systems care of any kind, whether during pregnancy or as part of primary care, is intimate care. Trauma-informed care makes the assumption that everyone may have had sexual trauma at some point, perhaps even at the present time. Using a trauma-informed approach that gives control over what is happening to the patient, rather than the provider, is always appropriate. This can include talking through the process before positioning a patient for an exam, explaining each step as it occurs, asking permission before beginning each component of the exam, and reminding the patient that they can always say no.[31]

A pelvic examination is required only when there are signs or symptoms of an abnormality or when cervical cancer screening is due. There is no evidence that routine examination of asymptomatic patients is necessary.[32] Pelvic examinations—even the external evaluation—can be difficult for individuals with a history of prior painful examinations, prior trauma, or negative experiences based on gender or sexual identity.[33] This component of the examination should be reviewed before the midwife begins examining the patient. Some patients will believe that a pelvic examination is standard practice; providers can use this as an opportunity for shared decision making.[34] Examples of reasons to perform a pelvic exam might include reported infection symptoms, desire for STI evaluation, collection of cervical cancer screening samples, or evaluation for preterm cervical dilation. In every case, it is important that directed counseling or forceful encouragement is avoided in favor of truly informed consent.

Because the breast/chest and pelvic examinations are key to a complete reproductive and sexual health assessment, these components of the physical examination are reviewed in the *Breast and Chest Examination* and *Pelvic Examination* **Appendices**.

### In-Office Laboratory Testing

A final part of the office examination is the completion of any in-office tests to be performed. Some tests are obtained and sent for analysis, whereas others are performed in the office and the results determined by the individual performing the test. The latter often are termed *point-of-care testing*. Among the point-of-care tests commonly performed in midwifery offices are urine dipstick; nasopharyngeal swabs for infection such as flu or *Streptococcus*;

saline and potassium hydroxide (KOH) slides to test for the presence of yeast, trichomoniasis, or bacterial vaginosis; and pregnancy tests (*Collecting Laboratory Specimens* appendix).

The Clinical Laboratory Improvement Amendments (CLIA) regulate tests performed in an office (42 CFR part 493).[35] The CLIA regulations are federal regulatory standards for all clinical laboratory tests done on humans in all settings except research protocols. They identify three categories of laboratory tests based on the complexity of the test methodology: (1) waived tests, (2) tests of moderate complexity, and (3) tests of high complexity. Waived tests are those that are accurate (i.e., the likelihood of erroneous results is negligible), pose little risk of harm if performed incorrectly, and have been cleared by the Food and Drug Administration (FDA) to be performed at home. Examples of waived tests and tests of moderate complexity are listed in Table 3-2.

Accurate results require correct performance of even the simplest test. When the Centers for Disease Control and Prevention (CDC) surveyed laboratories performing waived tests, high rates of errors in quality control and documentation were noted; a document regarding best practices in laboratory testing was subsequently published.[36]

If *only* waived tests will be performed in an office, then a Certificate of Waiver can be obtained to license the office laboratory. The Centers for Medicare and Medicaid Services (CMS) provides explanations of the waiver process and requirements on its website.[37] CLIA tests that are of moderate and high complexity require further registration and documentation. Provider-performed microscopy, for example, is considered a subcategory of moderate-complexity testing. Information on obtaining a license for an office laboratory can be found in the current CLIA regulations.[38]

### Establishing a Differential Diagnosis: Making an Assessment

When all the information available during the visit has been gathered, the midwife makes an assessment based on a differential diagnosis. The differential summarizes the various conditions, disorders, and health problems that might be the cause of each identified concern. It is sometimes very straightforward—for example, assuming someone has come for an annual examination, they are in good health, and the only questions were about choosing a birth control method, the assessment addresses normal examination findings and the contraceptive counseling or initiation of a method that is appropriate. At other times, the differential

| Table 3-2 | CLIA Testing Categories: Waived and Moderately Complex | |
|---|---|
| **CLIA Waived Tests** | **CLIA Tests of Moderate Complexity** |
| Dipstick or tablet reagent urinalysis (nonautomated) for bilirubin, glucose, hemoglobin, ketones, leucocytes, nitrates, pH, protein, specific gravity, and urobilinogen | Provider-performed microscopy: all direct wet-mount preparations for the presence or absence of bacteria, fungi, parasites, and human cellular elements |
| Fecal occult blood | All KOH preparations |
| Ovulation tests: visual color comparison tests for luteinizing hormone | Postcoital direct, qualitative examinations of vaginal or cervical mucus |
| Urine pregnancy tests: visual color comparison tests | Qualitative semen analysis (limited to the presence or absence of sperm and detection of motility) |
| Blood glucose by glucose monitoring devices cleared by the FDA specifically for home use | Fern tests |
| Diagnosis of STIs or vaginal conditions: trichomoniasis, bacterial vaginosis, rapid HIV | Pinworm examinations |
| | Urine sediment examinations |
| | Nasal smears for granulocytes |
| | Fecal leukocyte examinations |

Abbreviations: CLIA, Clinical Laboratory Improvement Amendments; FDA, U.S. Food and Drug Administration; HIV, human immunodeficiency virus; KOH, potassium hydroxide; STIs, sexually transmitted infections.

diagnosis can be complex. Right lower quadrant (RLQ) abdominal pain in a person in early pregnancy may be appendicitis, an ectopic pregnancy, a corpus luteum cyst, or any of many other possible disorders. Those conditions that create the highest risk for the patient's health are the first differentials considered, followed by those that are most common. The symptoms, history, and examination findings are considered to determine the most likely cause. Always document the considered differential, not just the final diagnosis.

Sometimes the initial differential diagnosis will be descriptive rather than diagnostic. In the earlier example of RLQ pain in a person in early pregnancy, ectopic pregnancy will always be the first condition considered, as it can cause irremediable harm to the patient.

The differential diagnosis suggests avenues for further testing or evaluation and helps to direct the plan. Continuing with the example of the individual with abdominal pain in early pregnancy, the initial diagnosis is descriptive: RLQ pain during pregnancy. The first tests ordered should be a pelvic ultrasound and a quantitative level of serum human chorionic gonadotropin (hCG).

## Designing a Plan

The plan should always include any lab work or procedures ordered, any medications prescribed, and the date of the next visit. For midwives, however, the plan never includes just these three items.

Among the *Hallmarks of Midwifery* are health education, counseling, and guidance.[2] Every plan for every patient includes documentation ensuring that these aspects of care were addressed. The reputation of midwifery rests in part on midwives' ability to be available for support, knowledge, and clarity of information. The education and counseling sometimes include just-in-time teaching, such as what a group B *Streptococcus* (GBS) screening culture is and why it is recommended at the 36-week prenatal visit. At other times, they consist of information that addresses long-term plans—for example, new cervical cytology screening guidelines and why the intervals are changing. The plan also includes information that will lead to shared decision making.

### Shared Decision Making

The midwife is responsible for providing evidence-based information; the patient is responsible for considering the alternatives, asking questions, and making the decision. There are only rare occasions where professional judgment can override a person's consent, most of which involve implied consent to care during potentially fatal emergencies requiring rapid action.[39] Even then, there are limitations on action—some decisions require consent of a family member, ethics committee consideration, or even court approval. Simply seeking care does not constitute consent.

Shared decision making is different from presenting risks and benefits. Patient-centered decision making can occur only when risks, benefits, and the range of available options are clearly communicated in a nondirected manner. When information is presented in this way, the individual is able to make a decision within the context of their personal values, beliefs, and preferences.

Midwives have the responsibility to verify that every patient is satisfied with the amount and type of information received, and feels that their needs have been addressed during the visit. *Informed consent* and *informed refusal* are the traditional terms for documenting agreement or disagreement with a procedure or plan of care, whereas *shared decision making* encompasses both types of informed decisions but does not imply that a plan of action is simply presented to the individual. The term "informed consent" remains commonly used in practice, however, and has been codified in several legal documents, especially those stating that the healthcare provider must legally and ethically obtain this type of consent before administering a treatment or procedure.[40,41]

Studies have concluded that care that incorporates evidence-based, shared decision making has the potential to improve quality and outcomes.[42,43] To obtain the most effective results, the care process should be thought of in terms of shared decision making, as such a process allows for the patient to question and decline treatment in whole or in part (i.e., make an informed consent or informed refusal). Providers need to again consider their privilege in relationship to individuals from marginalized communities at this point in the process. Evidence indicates that women who declined care were more likely to report negative experiences and discrimination if they were Black.[44] Equitable care demands that the provider take the time to support the patient through shifting from an assumption of dependency to confidence in participating in the decision.[45] Table 3-3 summarizes the essential components of informed decision making.

Ethical behavior requires that no harm be done (nonmaleficence), that the midwife acts for the good of the family or community involved (beneficence), that all persons are treated equitably (justice), and that the patient be able to make a choice (autonomy). It is sometimes difficult to accept the choice that a patient makes when it is not the one a midwife is comfortable with, or even an option under initial consideration.

When a midwife cannot or does not provide a requested service, the obligation is to advise the patient about resources in an unbiased manner.[46] The patient's ability to choose is impaired when the line

| Table 3-3 | Essential Elements to Make an Informed Decision |
|---|---|

The known or possible diagnosis

The nature and purpose of the proposed treatment or procedure

The benefits and risks associated with the recommended or usual plan

Complications and side effects (both common and severe)

The likelihood of success for this individual

Reasonable alternatives available, including no treatment

Benefits and risks associated with the alternatives

Possible consequences of not following the proposed plan of care

Assessment of the person's understanding and agreement

between the midwife's personal beliefs and their professional actions is not clearly drawn. No midwife should act in a way that violates their understanding of safety and evidence-based care. Likewise, no midwife should withhold information or care based on their personal beliefs. When a chosen action is outside the scope of midwifery care, whether because of its complexity or because of safety concerns, then the midwife is obligated to refer the patient to another provider. Boundaries in care provision are complex, embedded within institutional culture and broader systems, and include legal and ethical decision making. The choices that clinicians and systems make can impact patients when resources are not readily available elsewhere. Midwives should be advocates for change when decisions impact patient access to necessary health care.

## Conclusion

Expert midwives have mastered the skills of history taking, examination, diagnosis, and treatment. They have become comfortable teaching, guiding, and caring for individuals across the scope of sexual and reproductive health and providing appropriate primary care. Using solid evidence as a base for decisions and focusing on safety will have become second nature. Equally important, expert midwives have moved beyond simple performance of the necessary elements of care to a level where each person is seen both as an individual and as a member of their community and care is individualized to meet their needs.

## Resources

| Organization | Description |
|---|---|
| Centers for Disease Control and Prevention (CDC) | General information on health literacy |
| CDC TRAIN Learning Network | TRAIN is a national learning network that provides quality training opportunities for professionals who protect and improve the public's health. The course catalog includes many topics of interest to midwives, including communication, cultural competence, and sexual and reproductive health. |
| U.S Department of Health Resources and Services Administration (HRSA) | Culture, language, and health literacy: resources for recognizing and addressing the unique cultures, languages, and health literacy of diverse communities. |
| American Public Health Association | Health equity |
| Robert Wood Johnson Foundation | Health equity |

## References

1. Varney H, Thompson JB. *A History of Midwifery in the United States: The Midwife Said Fear Not.* New York, NY: Springer; 2016.

2. American College of Nurse-Midwives. The core competencies for basic midwifery practice: adopted by the American College of Nurse-Midwives, May 1997. *J Nurse Midwifery.* 1997;42(5):373-376.

3. American College of Nurse-Midwives. Definition of midwifery of and scope of practice for certified nurse-midwives and certified midwives. December 2021. https://www.midwife.org/acnm/files/acnmlibrarydata/uploadfilename/000000000266/Definition%20Midwifery%20Scope%20of%20Practice_2021.pdf. Accessed February 11, 2022.

4. Sniderman AD, Furberg CD. Why guideline-making requires reform. *JAMA.* 2009;301(4):429-431.

5. Wright JD, Pawar N, Gonzalez J, et al. Scientific evidence underlying the American College of Obstetricians and Gynecologists' Practice Bulletins. *Obstet Gynecol.* 2011;118(3):505-512.

6. Rising SS, Quimby CH. *The Centering Pregnancy Model.* New York, NY: Springer; 2017.

7. Mercer JS, Erickson-Owens DA, Collins J, et al. Effects of delayed cord clamping on residual placental blood volume, hemoglobin and bilirubin levels in term infants: a randomized controlled trial. *J Perinatol.* 2017;37(3):260-264.

8. Erwin DK, Hosford B. Demystifying the nurse-midwifery management process. *J Nurse Midwifery.* 1987;32(1):26-32. doi:10.1016/0091-2182(87)90053-X.

9. Hall WJ, Chapman MV, Lee KM, et al. Implicit racial/ethnic bias among health care professionals and its influence on health care outcomes: a systematic review. *Am J Public Health.* 2015;105(12):e60-e76. doi:10.2105/AJPH.2015.302903.

10. Smedley BD, Stith AY, Nelson AR, eds. *Unequal Treatment: Confronting Racial and Ethnic Disparities in Health Care.* Washington, DC: National Academies Press; 2002. doi:10.17226/12875.

11. Petersen EE, Davis NL, Goodman D, et al. Racial/ethnic disparities in pregnancy-related deaths—United States, 2007–2016. *MMWR.* 2019;68(35):762-765. doi:10.15585/mmwr.mm6835a3.

12. Effland K, Hays K, Ortiz F, Blanco B. Incorporating an equity agenda into health professions education and training to build a more representative workforce. *J Midwifery Womens Health.* 2020;65(1):149-159. doi:10.1111/jmwh.13070.

13. Ma A, Sanchez A, Ma M. The impact of patient–provider race/ethnicity concordance on provider visits: updated evidence from the Medical Expenditure Panel Survey. *J Racial Ethn Health Disparities.* 2019;6(5):1011-1020. doi:10.1007/s40615-019-00602-y.

14. Gomez LE, Bernet P. Diversity improves performance and outcomes. *J Natl Med Assoc.* 2019;111(4):383-392. doi:10.1016/j.jnma.2019.01.006.

15. Altman MR, Kantrowitz-Gordon I, Moise E, et al. Addressing positionality within case-based learning to mitigate systemic racism in health care. *Nurse Educ.* 2020;46(5):284-289. doi:10.1097/NNE.0000000000000937.

16. *Merriam-Webster Dictionary.* Intersectionality. https://www.merriam-webster.com/dictionary/intersectionality. Accessed February 14, 2022.

17. Rabelais E. Missing ethical discussions in gender care for transgender and non-binary people: secondary sex characteristics. *J Midwifery Womens Health.* 2020;65(6):741-744. doi:10.1111/jmwh.13166.

18. Selix NW, Rowniak S. Provision of patient-centered transgender care. *J Midwifery Womens Health.* 2016;61(6):744-751. doi:10.1111/jmwh.12518.

19. Institute of Medicine. *Health Literacy: A Prescription to End Confusion.* Washington, DC: National Academies Press; 2004. https://www.ncbi.nlm.nih.gov/books/NBK216032/. Accessed February 11, 2022.

20. Nelson W, Reyna VF, Fagerlin A, et al. Clinical implications of numeracy: theory and practice. *Ann Behav Med.* 2008;35(3):261-274.

21. Nutbeam D, Lloyd JE. Understanding and responding to health literacy as a social determinant of health. *Ann Rev Public Health.* 2021;42(1):159-173. doi:10.1146/annurev-publhealth-090419-102529.

22. Kim H, Xie B. Health literacy in the eHealth era: a systematic review of the literature. *Patient Educ Couns.* 2017;100(6):1073-1082. doi:10.1016/j.pec .2017.01.015.

23. Golbeck AL, Ahlers-Schmidt CR, Paschal AM, Dismuke SE. A definition and operational framework for health numeracy. *Am J Prev Med.* 2005;29(4):375-376.

24. Galesic M, Gigerenzer G, Straubinger N. Natural frequencies help older adults and people with low numeracy to evaluate medical screening tests. *Med Decis Making.* 2009;29(3):368-371. doi:10.1177/0272989X08329463.

25. Ancker JS, Kaufman D. Rethinking health numeracy: a multidisciplinary literature review. *J Am Med Informatics Assoc.* 2007;14(6):713-721.

26. Baker DW. The meaning and the measure of health literacy. *J Gen Intern Med.* 2006;21(8):878-883.

27. Edwards A, Elwyn G, Mulley A. Explaining risks: turning numerical data into meaningful pictures. *BMJ.* 2002;324(7341):827-830.

28. DeMeester RH, Lopez FY, Moore JE, et al. A model of organizational context and shared decision making: application to LGBT racial and ethnic minority patients. *J Gen Intern Med.* 2016;31:651.

29. Thompson HM, Kronk CA, Feasley K, et al. Implementation of gender identity and assigned sex at birth data collection in electronic health records: where are we now? *Int J Environ Res Public Health.* 2021;18(12):6599. doi:10.3390/ijerph18126599.

30. Guttmacher Institute. An overview of consent to reproductive health services by young people: as of January 1, 2022. https://www.guttmacher.org/state -policy/explore/overview-minors-consent-law. Accessed February 11, 2022.

31. Tillman S. Consent in pelvic care. *J Midwifery Womens Health.* 2020;65(6):749-758. doi:10.1111/jmwh.13189.

32. U.S. Preventive Services Task Force; Bibbins-Domingo K, Grossman DC, Curry SJ, et al. Screening for gynecologic conditions with pelvic examination: US Preventive Services Task Force recommendation statement. *JAMA.* 2017;17(9):947-953. doi:10.1001 /jama.2017.0807.

33. O'Laughlin DJ, Strelow B, Fellows N, et al. Addressing anxiety and fear during the female pelvic examination. *J Prim Care Community Health.* 2021;12:2150132721992195. doi:10.1177 /2150132721992195.

34. Chor J, Stulberg D, Tillman S. Shared decision-making framework for pelvic examinations in asymptomatic, nonpregnant patients. *Obstet Gynecol.* 2019;133(4):810-814. doi:10.1097/AOG .0000000000003166.

35. Centers for Disease Control and Prevention. Clinical Laboratory Improvement Amendments (CLIA). https://www.cms.gov/Regulations-and-Guidance/ Legislation/CLIA. Accessed February 11, 2022.

36. Centers for Disease Control and Prevention. Good laboratory practices for waived testing sites: survey findings from testing sites holding a certificate of waiver under the Clinical Laboratory Improvement Amendments of 1988 and recommendations for promoting quality testing. *MMWR.* 2005;54(RR-13):1-21.

37. Centers for Medicare and Medicaid Services. Clinical Laboratory Improvement Amendments (CLIA): how to obtain a CLIA Certificate of Waiver. https://www .cms.gov/Regulations-and-Guidance/Legislation /CLIA/Downloads/HowObtainCertificateofWaiver .pdf. Accessed February 11, 2022.

38. Centers for Disease Control and Prevention. Provider-performed microscopy procedures. https:// www.cms.gov/regulations-and-guidance/legislation /clia/downloads/ppmplist.pdf. Accessed February 11, 2022.

39. Pozgar GD. *Legal and Ethical Issues for Health Professionals.* 5th ed. Burlington, MA: Jones & Bartlett Learning; 2019.

40. Lipkin M. Shared decision making. *JAMA Intern Med.* 2013;173(13):1204-1205.

41. King JS, Moulton BW. Rethinking informed consent: the case for shared medical decision-making. *Am J Law Med.* 2006;32(4):429-501.

42. Moore JE, Titler MG, Kane Low L, et al. Transforming patient-centered care: development of the evidence informed decision making through engagement model. *Womens Health Issues.* 2015;25(3):276-282.

43. Moore JE. Women's voices in maternity care: the triad of shared decision-making, informed consent, and evidence-based practices. *J Perinat Neonatal Nurs.* 2016;30(3):218-223. doi:10.1097/JPN .0000000000000182.

44. Attanasio LB, Hardeman RR. Declined care and discrimination during the childbirth hospitalization. *Soc Sci Med.* 2019;232:270-277. doi:10.1016/j. socscimed.2019.05.008.

45. Altman MR, Oseguera T, McLemore MR, et al. Information and power: women of color's experiences interacting with health care providers in pregnancy and birth. *Soc Sci Med.* 2019;238:112491. doi:10.1016/j.socscimed.2019.112491.

46. Eagen-Torkko M, Levi AJ. The ethical justification for conscience clauses in nurse-midwifery practice: context, power, and a changing landscape. *J Midwifery Womens Health.* 2020;65(6):759-766. doi:10.1111 /jmwh.13170.

# APPENDIX

# 3A

# Standard and Airborne Precautions

JAN M. KRIEBS

Healthcare-associated infections (HAIs) are any infections that individuals acquire while receiving direct services. HAIs affect approximately 3% of all U.S. patients in hospital settings, even after years of efforts to reduce this risk.[1] Moreover, about half of all hospitalized patients each day are given an antimicrobial, increasing the risk that antibiotic resistance might develop.[1] Although activities designed to prevent HAIs were originally targeted toward protecting consumers, healthcare workers are also at risk for such infections. Therefore, knowledge and institution of standard precautions are core standards of practice to protect the patients and families for whom midwives provide care, as well as the midwives themselves.

Standard precautions are essential activities that should be employed by all healthcare workers in all healthcare settings for the purpose of preventing HAIs without regard to specific infection risks. They are the most basic level of infection control.

Standard precautions[2] are sometimes viewed as interfering with the close relationship valued by midwives and their patients. However, they are also the most effective method of preventing both parties from accidentally being exposed to infection. On some occasions, it is the midwife who is at greater risk when caring for a patient with an infection than the patient is. Standard precautions are not limited to the hospital environment, although some accommodations to precautions are observed in ambulatory settings.[3] For example, complete contact precautions are not always possible when a patient presents with an open lesion that was not previously disclosed. The following recommendations summarize the recommendations from the CDC[2]; additional droplet and contact precautions can be found in the Guidelines for Isolation Precautions.[3]

## Standard Precautions

### Hand Hygiene

1. During the delivery of health care, avoid unnecessary touching of surfaces in close proximity to the patient to prevent both contamination of clean hands from environmental surfaces and transmission of pathogens from contaminated hands to surfaces.

2. When hands are visibly dirty, contaminated with proteinaceous material, or visibly soiled with blood or body fluids, wash hands with either a nonantimicrobial soap and water or an antimicrobial soap and water.

3. If hands are not visibly soiled, or after removing visible material with nonantimicrobial soap and water, decontaminate hands in the clinical situations described next. The preferred method of hand decontamination is with an alcohol-based hand rub. Alternatively, hands may be washed with an antimicrobial soap and water. Frequent use of alcohol-based hand rub immediately following hand washing with nonantimicrobial soap may increase the frequency of dermatitis.

4. **Perform hand hygiene in the following clinical situations:**

   a. Before having direct contact with patients

   b. After contact with blood, body fluids or excretions, mucous membranes, nonintact skin, or wound dressings

   c. After contact with a patient's intact skin (e.g., when taking a pulse or blood pressure or lifting a patient)

d. If hands will be moving from a contaminated body site to a clean body site during patient care

e. After contact with inanimate objects (including medical equipment) in the immediate vicinity of the patient

f. After removing gloves

5. Wash hands with nonantimicrobial soap and water or with antimicrobial soap and water if contact with spores (e.g., *Clostridium difficile* or *Bacillus anthracis*) is likely to have occurred. The physical action of washing and rinsing hands under such circumstances is recommended because alcohols, chlorhexidine, iodophors, and other antiseptic agents have poor activity against spores.

6. Do not wear artificial fingernails or extenders if duties include direct contact with patients at high risk for infection and associated adverse outcomes (e.g., those in intensive care units or operating rooms).

   a. Develop an organizational policy on the wearing of non-natural nails by healthcare personnel who have direct contact with patients outside of the groups specified earlier.

### Personal Protective Equipment (PPE)

1. Observe the following principles of use:

   a. Wear PPE when the nature of the anticipated patient interaction indicates that contact with blood or body fluids may occur.

   b. Prevent contamination of clothing and skin during the process of removing PPE.

   c. Before leaving the patient's room or cubicle, remove and discard PPE.

### Gloves

1. Wear gloves when it can be reasonably anticipated that contact with blood or other potentially infectious materials, mucous membranes, nonintact skin, or potentially contaminated intact skin (e.g., of a patient incontinent of stool or urine) could occur.

2. Wear gloves with fit and durability appropriate to the task.

   a. Wear disposable medical examination gloves for providing direct patient care.

   b. Wear disposable medical examination gloves or reusable utility gloves for cleaning the environment or medical equipment.

3. Remove gloves after contact with a patient and/or the surrounding environment (including medical equipment) using proper technique to prevent hand contamination. Do not wear the same pair of gloves for the care of more than one patient. Do not wash gloves for the purpose of reuse since this practice has been associated with transmission of pathogens.

4. Change gloves during patient care if the hands will move from a contaminated body site (e.g., perineal area) to a clean body site (e.g., face).

### Gowns

1. Wear a gown, which is appropriate to the task, to protect skin and prevent soiling or contamination of clothing during procedures and patient care activities when contact with blood, body fluids, secretions, or excretions is anticipated.

   a. Wear a gown for direct patient contact if the patient has uncontained secretions or excretions.

   b. Remove the gown and perform hand hygiene before leaving the patient's environment.

2. Do not reuse gowns, even for repeated contacts with the same patient.

3. Routine donning of gowns upon entrance into a high-risk or intensive care unit is not indicated unless it is specific to communicable diseases.

### Mouth, Nose, and Eye Protection

1. Use PPE to protect the mucous membranes of the eyes, nose, and mouth during procedures and patient care activities that are likely to generate splashes or sprays of blood, body fluids, secretions, and excretions. Select masks, goggles, face shields, and combinations of each according to the need anticipated based on the task to be performed.

2. During aerosol-generating procedures (e.g., bronchoscopy, suctioning of the respiratory tract [if not using in-line suction catheters], endotracheal intubation) in patients who are not suspected of being infected with an agent

for which respiratory protection is otherwise recommended (e.g., *Mycobacterium tuberculosis*, severe acute respiratory syndrome [SARS], or hemorrhagic fever viruses), wear one of the following: a face shield that fully covers the front and sides of the face, a mask with attached shield, or a mask and goggles (in addition to gloves and gown).

### Respiratory Hygiene/Cough Etiquette

1. Educate healthcare personnel on the importance of source control measures to contain respiratory secretions to prevent droplet and fomite transmission of respiratory pathogens, especially during seasonal outbreaks of viral respiratory tract infections (e.g., influenza, respiratory syncytial virus [RSV], adenovirus, parainfluenza virus) in communities.

2. Implement the following measures to contain respiratory secretions in patients and accompanying individuals who have signs and symptoms of a respiratory infection, beginning at the point of initial encounter in a healthcare setting (e.g., triage, reception, and waiting areas in emergency departments, outpatient clinics, and physician offices).

   a. Post signs at entrances and in strategic places (e.g., elevators, cafeterias) within **ambulatory** and **inpatient settings** with instructions to patients and other persons with symptoms of a respiratory infection to cover their mouths and noses when coughing or sneezing, use and dispose of tissues, and perform hand hygiene after hands have been in contact with respiratory secretions.

   b. Provide tissues and no-touch receptacles (e.g., foot-pedal–operated lid or open, plastic-lined waste basket) for disposal of tissues.

   c. Provide resources and instructions for performing hand hygiene in or near waiting areas in **ambulatory** and **inpatient settings**. Provide conveniently located dispensers of alcohol-based hand rubs and, where sinks are available, supplies for hand washing.

   d. During periods of increased prevalence of respiratory infections in the community (e.g., as indicated by increased school absenteeism, increased number of patients seeking care for a respiratory infection), offer masks to coughing patients and other symptomatic persons (e.g., persons who accompany ill patients) upon entry into the facility or medical office and encourage them to maintain special separation, ideally a distance of at least 3 feet from others in common waiting areas.

### Patient-Care Equipment and Instruments/Devices

1. Establish policies and procedures for containing, transporting, and handling patient-care equipment and instruments/devices that may be contaminated with blood or body fluids.

2. Remove organic material from critical and semi-critical instrument/devices, using recommended cleaning agents before high-level disinfection and sterilization to enable effective disinfection and sterilization processes.

3. Wear PPE (e.g., gloves, gown), according to the level of anticipated contamination, when handling patient-care equipment and instruments/devices that are visibly soiled or may have been in contact with blood or body fluids.

### Care of the Environment

1. Establish policies and procedures for routine and targeted cleaning of environmental surfaces as indicated by the level of patient contact and degree of soiling.

2. Clean and disinfect surfaces that are likely to be contaminated with pathogens, including those that are in close proximity to the patient (e.g., bed rails, over-bed tables) and frequently touched surfaces in the patient care environment (e.g., door knobs, surfaces in and surrounding toilets in patients' rooms) on a more frequent schedule compared to that for other surfaces (e.g., horizontal surfaces in waiting rooms).

3. Use Environmental Protection Agency (EPA)–registered disinfectants that have microbiocidal (i.e., killing) activity against the pathogens most likely to contaminate the patient-care environment. Use in accordance with the manufacturer's instructions.

   a. Review the efficacy of in-use disinfectants when evidence of continuing transmission of an infectious agent (e.g., rotavirus, *C. difficile*, norovirus) may indicate resistance to the in-use product, and change to a more effective disinfectant as indicated.

4. In facilities that provide health care to pediatric patients or have waiting areas with toys for children, establish policies and procedures for cleaning and disinfecting the toys at regular intervals.
   a. Select play toys that can be easily cleaned and disinfected.
   b. Do not permit use of stuffed furry toys if they will be shared.
   c. Clean and disinfect large stationary toys (e.g., climbing equipment) at least weekly and whenever visibly soiled.
   d. If toys are likely to be mouthed, rinse with water after disinfection; alternatively, wash in a dishwasher.
   e. When a toy requires cleaning and disinfection, do so immediately or store in a designated labeled container separate from toys that are clean and ready for use.
5. Include multiuse electronic equipment in policies and procedures for preventing contamination and for cleaning and disinfection, especially those items that are used by patients, those used during delivery of patient care, and mobile devices that are moved in and out of patient rooms frequently (e.g., daily).
   a. No recommendation is made for use of removable protective covers or washable keyboards.

## Textiles and Laundry

1. Handle used textiles and fabrics with minimum agitation to avoid contamination of air, surfaces, and persons.
2. If laundry chutes are used, ensure that they are properly designed, maintained, and used in a manner to minimize dispersion of aerosols from contaminated laundry.

## Safe Injection Practices

The following recommendations apply to the use of needles, cannulas that replace needles, and intravenous delivery systems.

1. Use aseptic technique to avoid contamination of sterile injection equipment.
2. Do not administer medications with the same syringe to multiple patients, even if the needle or cannula on the syringe is changed. Needles, cannulas, and syringes are sterile, single-use items; they should not be reused for another patient or to access a medication or solution that might be used for a subsequent patient.
3. Use fluid infusion and administration sets (i.e., intravenous bags, tubing, and connectors) for one patient only, and dispose of them appropriately after use. Consider a syringe or needle/cannula to be contaminated once it has been used to enter or connect to a patient's intravenous infusion bag or administration set.
4. Use single-dose vials for parenteral medications whenever possible.
5. Do not administer medications from single-dose vials or ampules to multiple patients or combine leftover contents for later use.
6. If multidose vials must be used, both the needle or cannula and the syringe used to access the multidose vial must be sterile.
7. Do not keep multidose vials in the immediate patient treatment area, and store them in accordance with the manufacturer's recommendations. Discard the vials if their sterility is compromised or questionable.
8. Do not use bags or bottles of intravenous solution as a common source of supply for multiple patients.

## Infection Control Practices for Special Lumbar Puncture Procedures

Wear a surgical mask when placing a catheter or injecting material into the spinal canal or subdural space (i.e., during myelograms, lumbar puncture, and spinal or epidural anesthesia).

## Worker Safety

Adhere to federal and state requirements for protection of healthcare personnel from exposure to bloodborne pathogens.

## Airborne Precautions

1. Use airborne precautions as recommended for patients known or suspected to be infected with infectious agents that may be transmitted person-to-person by the airborne route.
2. **In ambulatory settings:**
   a. Develop systems (e.g., triage, signage) to identify patients with known or suspected infections that require airborne precautions upon entry into **ambulatory settings**.

b. Place the patient in an airborne infection isolation room (AIIR) as soon as possible. If an AIIR is not available, place a surgical mask on the patient and place them in an examination room. Once the patient leaves, the room should remain vacant for the appropriate time, generally one hour, to allow for a full exchange of air.

c. Instruct patients with a known or suspected airborne infection to wear a surgical mask and observe respiratory hygiene/cough etiquette. Once the patient is in an AIIR, the mask may be removed; the mask should remain on if the patient is not in an AIIR.

3. **Personnel restrictions.** Restrict susceptible healthcare personnel from entering the rooms of patients known or suspected to have measles (rubeola), varicella (chickenpox), disseminated zoster, or smallpox if other immune healthcare personnel are available.

4. **Use of PPE:**

   a. Wear a fit-tested National Institute for Occupational Safety and Health (NIOSH)–approved N95 or higher-level respirator for respiratory protection when entering the room or home of a patient when the following diseases are suspected or confirmed:

      i. Infectious pulmonary or laryngeal tuberculosis or when infectious tuberculosis skin lesions are present and procedures that would aerosolize viable organisms (e.g., irrigation, incision and drainage, whirlpool treatments) are performed.

      ii. Smallpox (vaccinated and unvaccinated). Respiratory protection is recommended for all healthcare personnel, including those with a documented "take" after smallpox vaccination, due to the risk of a genetically engineered virus against which the vaccine may not provide protection, or of exposure to a very large viral load (e.g., from high-risk aerosol-generating procedures, immunocompromised patients, or hemorrhagic or flat smallpox.

5. Discontinue airborne precautions according to pathogen-specific recommendations.

6. Consult CDC's "Guidelines for Preventing the Transmission of *Mycobacterium tuberculosis* in Health-Care Settings, 2005" and the "Guideline for Environmental Infection Control in Health-Care Facilities" for additional guidance on environmental strategies for preventing transmission of tuberculosis in healthcare settings. The environmental recommendations in these guidelines may be applied to patients with other infections that require airborne precautions.

## References

1. Centers for Disease Control and Prevention. HAI and antibiotic use prevalence survey. https://www.cdc.gov/hai/eip/antibiotic-use.html. Accessed February 11, 2022.

2. Siegel JD, Rhinehart E, Jackson M, et al. 2007 guideline for isolation precautions: preventing transmission of infectious agents in healthcare settings. Last updated July 2019. https://www.ncbi.nlm.nih.gov/pmc/articles/PMC7119119/. Accessed February 11, 2022.

3. Centers for Disease Control and Prevention, National Center for Emerging and Zoonotic Infectious Diseases Division of Healthcare Quality Promotion. Guide to infection prevention for outpatient settings: minimum expectations for safe care, version 2.3. https://www.cdc.gov/infectioncontrol/pdf/outpatient/guide.pdf. Accessed February 11, 2022.

APPENDIX

# 3B

# Collecting a Health History

JAN M. KRIEBS

In visits to a midwife, the chief concerns, or reasons for a visit, are frequently focused on reproductive or sexual concerns. This does not mean that the personal health or family history can be omitted. Overall health influences healthcare decision making, as prior illnesses and surgeries can affect which type of examination is indicated and which medications can be prescribed. Family history may open up a discussion about future health risks. For midwives with an active primary care practice, many general health concerns, elicited in the history and review of systems, may also be addressed during routine examinations.

Because the scope of practice for midwives is not gender based, an early question with any new patient is "What pronouns do you prefer to use?" While sexual and reproductive care is a broad topic, for certain aspects of care, the organ is the target of assessment, rather than the identified gender.

## History of the Present Illness

After determining the chief concern for a visit, the next step is to inquire about the history of the present illness (HPI). This term is often a misnomer—for example, the reason for a visit of "I need my Pap test and birth control pills" leads to an HPI that addresses how the patient is managing their contraception and satisfaction with their current method (and possibly to a discussion of screening recommendations). A chief concern that begins with abnormal uterine bleeding leads to the more traditional assessment of the current symptoms. A commonly used mnemonic for the questions asked

about a health problem is OLD CARTS (Onset, Location/radiation, Duration, Character, Aggravating factors, Relieving factors, Timing, and Severity). These questions can be followed by "What has changed now that made you come in?" or "How did you decide it was time to come in?"

## Past Health History

A past health history includes a review of all organ systems, mental health, common infections, blood transfusions, injuries and traumas, and surgeries including any complications (Table 3B-1). The list in Table 3B-1 is not comprehensive, but does include questions that are frequently or specifically germane in a reproductive health examination. Clearly, any other problems that are identified should also be investigated.

Some commonly asked questions include the following:

1. Have you ever had a major illness—for example, any breathing problems, stomach or liver problems, or any bladder infections?

2. Are there any other health problems generally you can think of?

3. Have you ever had to have any special tests or procedures?

4. Have you ever been admitted to the hospital because you were sick or injured? When was that? Why were you in the hospital?

5. Who has been taking care of you for (problem)? Have they suggested you see anyone else?

| Table 3B-1 | Past History |
|---|---|

| 1. Neurologic | 2. Skin | 3. Respiratory | 4. Cardiovascular |
|---|---|---|---|
| Migraine headaches | Chronic skin conditions | Asthma | Hypertension |
| Other types of headaches | | Tuberculosis | Hyperlipidemia |
| Epilepsy or seizure disorders | | | Cerebral vascular accident |
| Multiple sclerosis | | | Myocardial infarction |

| 5. Breast/Chest | 6. Gastrointestinal | 7. Genitourinary | 8. Musculoskeletal |
|---|---|---|---|
| Report of breast/chest self-examinations | Gastroesophageal reflux disease | Frequent urinary tract infections | Arthritis |
| Biopsy, cyst or adenoma removal | Chronic diarrhea or constipation | Pain or urgency of urination | Any limitations of motion |
| Breast enlargement, reduction, reconstruction, or removal of unwanted tissue | Cholecystectomy | Genital tract infections | |
| | Appendectomy | Sexually transmitted infections | |
| Other problems | Bariatric surgery | Hysterectomy, myomectomy, oophorectomy | |
| | | Post childbirth repair | |
| | | Cervical loop electrosurgical excision procedure (LEEP), cone biopsy | |
| | | In utero diethylstilbestrol (DES) exposure | |

| 9. Hematologic | 10. Endocrine | 11. Infections | 12. Psychological |
|---|---|---|---|
| Sickle cell disease, hemoglobinopathies | Thyroid disorders | Childhood infections | Depression |
| Anemia | Diabetes | Vaccinations, especially tetanus, diphtheria, acellular pertussis (TDaP) and influenza | Postpartum depression |
| Bleeding disorders | | Chronic illnesses: human immuno-deficiency virus (HIV), hepatitis B or C, herpes | Other mental disorders |
| | | Pelvic inflammatory disease | |
| | | Endometritis | |

| 13. Allergies | 14. Medications | 15. Other | |
|---|---|---|---|
| Drug | Prescription | Surgeries | |
| Environmental | Vitamins | Physical trauma | |
| Food | Over the counter | Injuries | |
| | Herbal, homeopathic, nutritional, or other supplements | | |

For the person who is seen on a regular basis, asking whether there has been any change in their health, and possibly reminding them of prior reports, can assist with time management during the visit.

## Social History

The social history, like the sexual history, brings up topics that can be embarrassing or even threatening to some individuals (Table 3B-2). Ask these questions in a quiet, professional tone, and respect the patient's need to avoid certain answers. Explaining why the information is needed often reassures the patient and can help the midwife feel comfortable asking for it. Obviously, if there is no reason for eliciting sensitive information, asking about it should be omitted. Relationship questions should be asked in a pattern that allows the individual to reveal relationships beyond "single" or "married with children."

| Table 3B-2 | Social History | | | |
|---|---|---|---|---|
| **Relationships** | **Diet** | **Substance use** | | **Access to resources** |
| Ask: What is your support system? At home, in the community? | Eating habits, history of eating disorders | Caffeine | | Whether they work for pay, volunteer, or go to school or any programs |
| If there is an intimate partner, what is their relationship with you? | Diet recall | Tobacco | | Whether lack of money, access to transportation, or child care makes keeping appointments difficult |
| | Any food restrictions—allergies, vegetarian or vegan, religious, cultural limitations | Alcohol | | |
| | | Marijuana | | |
| | | Illicit drugs | | |
| | | Use of others' prescriptions | | |
| **Hazardous exposures at work or home** | **Physical activity, types and frequency** | **Personal safety** | | **Guns or weapons in home** |
| | | Violence may be within the home from a partner or family member, or it may occur in other settings. It includes physical, sexual, or emotional abuse, and may be ongoing or a past experience. | | |
| **Seat belt use** | | | | |

## Sexual/Reproductive History

This area is a natural progression after the general history is taken, and some of the items mentioned previously need not be re-asked if the answer is already recorded. Listen for answers to questions not yet asked and note them (Table 3B-3).

## Sexual History

The CDC recommends obtaining a complete sexual history during an initial visit, as part of routine preventive examinations, and for anyone who presents for care of possible STIs.[1] The sexual history in Table 3B-4 is based on the CDC-recommended "5 P's"—partner, practices, protection from STIs, past history of STIs, and prevention of pregnancy—while adding questions that will support a more open discussion in a more affirming way. Begin with a statement that confirms these questions are asked of everyone, regardless of age, gender, or relationships. Then ask for permission to proceed. You might say: "May I ask you a few questions about your sexual health and sexual practices? I understand that these questions are personal, but they are important for your overall health." Follow up with a reminder that all health information is confidential unless someone is being harmed.[1,2] The *Sexuality* chapter provides a more nuanced approach to completing a sexual history than recommended by the CDC.

## Family History

Family histories assist in identifying risk factors and genetic concerns. Some concerns can be a disease or condition; other factors can relate to psychological or social concerns. The health histories of first- and second-degree relatives are most important. Minimum components include the elements listed in Table 3B-5 for parents, siblings, and grandparents.

The final question in the history taking should be some variant of "Is there anything else I should have asked you today?" or, alternatively, "Is there anything else I should know or that you want to share with me?"

## Review of Systems

The review of systems (ROS) acts as a bridge from the past to the present. It is a structured inquiry about current symptoms or concerns related to each body system. This part of the examination serves as a check for symptoms that the patient can be experiencing but has not yet mentioned. Table 3B-6 is an example of a self-administered ROS form that patients can complete while waiting for the visit with the midwife. In some practices, a standard screening tool for depression is also provided for patients to fill out privately before the visit. Alternatively, an ROS may be completed with the physical examination, asking the patient about symptoms as the examination progresses.

| Table 3B-3 | Sexual and Reproductive History | | |
|---|---|---|---|
| **For All Patients** | | | |
| **Cervical cytology screening (for patients with a cervix)**<br>Abnormal Pap test, any location<br>Colposcopy<br>Cervical treatment or surgery | **Age at onset of sexual activity**<br>Additional information in the sexual history in Table 3B-4 | **Contraceptive history**<br>Types<br>Duration of use<br>Any problems | **Other**<br>Infertility<br>Reproductive life plan (See the *Preconception Care* appendix) |
| **If This Individual Menstruates or Has Ever Menstruated** | | | |
| **Last menstrual period and last regular menstrual period** | **Age at menarche, timing of menstrual cycles**<br>Any irregularity of timing<br>Amount and duration<br>Premenstrual symptoms<br>Dysmenorrhea<br>Endometriosis | **Perimenopausal symptoms**<br>Age at menopause—surgical or natural<br>Use of hormone therapy | **Pregnancy (if ever pregnant)**<br>*G/P-TPAL*<br>• Gravida (number of pregnancies)<br>• Para (number of births); T: term; P: preterm; A: spontaneous or elective abortions; L: number of living children<br>Ectopic and multiple pregnancies<br>Problems with pregnancies, births, or recovery<br>Genetic testing<br>Postpartum depression |

| Table 3B-4 | Sexual History |
|---|---|
| **Before Proceeding, Ask About the Patient's Sexual Identity** | |

Are you attracted to men, women, or both?

How do you identify your sexual orientation?

Do you have any concerns related to sexual identity, sexuality, or gender?

**1. Partners**

Are you sexually active?

If no: Have you ever been sexually active? How recently?

If yes: Are your sexual partners men, women, or nonbinary? Keep in mind that if the partner is a trans woman or man, the answer will likely reflect the partner's gender identity, not their genital anatomy. (If the individual has sexual partners from multiple genders, ask the next questions about partners for each kind of partner.)

In recent months, how many sexual partners have you had?

Did they have a penis or a vagina?

Do you have any problems with your sexual partner, or does your sexual partner have any problems you want to discuss?

Has anyone ever forced themselves on you sexually, or touched you sexually without your permission?

**2. Practices**

Have you ever had oral sex, meaning mouth on penis or vagina sex? How many times have you had oral sex without a condom or dental dam? Do you have receptive oral sex, meaning your partner inserts their penis into your mouth?

Have you ever had vaginal sex, meaning any type of sex that involves insertion of penis or objects into the vagina? Which objects are inserted into the vagina? Are you the receptive partner in intercourse, meaning that your partner ejaculates while in your vagina? How many times have you had vaginal sex without a condom or safe sex practices?

Have you ever had anal sex, meaning penis or object in rectum/anus sex? Are you the receptive partner, meaning that your partner inserts their penis into your rectum? How many times have you had anal sex without a condom?

If the person or their partner(s) are using any kind of sex toy, ask about sharing and cleaning.

Are your sexual practices more painful than you would like?

If yes: Explore for sexual violence, dyspareunia, and other sources of pain.

### 3. Protection from Sexually Transmitted Infections

Do you use anything to protect yourself from STIs?

If no: Can you tell me the reason?

If yes: Which kind of protection do you use and how often do you use it?

Do you have any questions about methods to protect against STIs?

### 4. Past History of STIs

Have you ever had an STI?

If yes: When and/or how were you treated for it?

Have you ever been tested for HIV or other STIs? Would you like to be tested?

Have you had any recurring symptoms?

Has your current sexual partner or former partners ever had an STI, including HIV?

If yes: Were you tested at the same time?

### 5. Prevention of Pregnancy

Are you currently trying to conceive a child?

Are you concerned about getting pregnant or your partner getting pregnant?

Are you using any form of birth control? Do you need information about birth control?

### 6. Additional Questions

What other concerns about your sexual health or sexual practices would you like to discuss?

Do you have any other concerns or questions?

Thank the patient for being open. Offer praise for protective practices and/or discuss any concerns.

Abbreviations: HIV, human immunodeficiency virus; STI, sexually transmitted infection.

Adapted from Centers from Disease Control and Prevention. A guide to taking a sexual history. https://www.cdc.gov/std/treatment/sexualhistory.pdf. Accessed February 11, 2022; and Eckstrand KL, Ehrenfeld JM. *Lesbian, Gay, Bisexual, and Transgender Healthcare: A Clinical Guide to Preventive, Primary, and Specialist Care.* Springer; 2016. doi:10.1007/978-3-319-19752-4.

| Table 3B-5 | Family History (Three Generations) | |
|---|---|---|
| **1. Parents and Siblings** | **2. Chronic Disorders** | **3. Genetic Problems** |
| Living or dead | Heart disease—especially coronary artery disease | Birth defects |
| Age at death | Diabetes | Developmental delay |
| Cause of death | Cancer—especially breast, reproductive, or colon | Behavioral conditions |

| Table 3B-6 | Sample Review of Systems for Patient Self-Report |
|---|---|

Please mark any of the following that are bothering you now or have bothered you within the last 2 weeks.

**1. Constitutional**
- weight loss
- weight gain
- fatigue
- fever
- change in appetite

**2. Neurologic**
- dizziness
- seizures
- numbness
- trouble walking
- memory problems
- headaches
- fainting

**3. Skin**
- rash
- sore
- dry skin
- moles
- acne
- eczema

**4. Eyes**
- double vision
- vision changes
- spots before eyes
- glasses/contacts

**5. Ears, Nose, Throat**
- sinus problems
- hearing problems
- earaches
- ringing in ears
- sore throat
- mouth sores
- dental problems

**6. Respiratory**
- painful breathing
- wheezing
- short of breath
- chronic cough
- spitting up blood

**7. Cardiovascular**
- chest pain or pressure
- leg swelling
- difficulty breathing when active
- rapid or irregular heartbeat

**8. Breasts/Chest**
- pain
- lump or lesion
- nipple discharge
- discoloration

**9. Gastrointestinal**
- frequent diarrhea
- bloody stools
- nausea/vomiting
- constipation
- passing gas or stool involuntarily

**10. Genitourinary**
- blood in urine
- pain with urination
- frequent urination
- incomplete emptying of bladder
- unintended urine leaking
- leaking urine with cough or lifting
- abnormal vaginal/penile discharge
- pain with sex
- abnormal vaginal bleeding
- painful periods
- premenstrual symptoms (PMS)
- hot flashes

**11. Muscle and Skeletal**
- muscle weakness
- spasms
- muscle or joint pain
- frequent falls

**12. Hematologic and Lymphatic**
- frequent bruising
- enlarged lymph nodes
- cuts that do not stop bleeding

**13. Endocrine**
- hair loss
- heat/cold intolerance
- abnormal thirst
- hot flashes

**14. Mental Health**
- mood swings
- frequent crying
- anxiety
- trouble sleeping
- thoughts of hurting yourself or someone else

**15. Allergies**
- hay fever
- hives
- seasonal allergies
- latex allergy
- food allergies

## References

1. Centers for Disease Control and Prevention. A guide to taking a sexual history. https://www.cdc.gov/std/treatment/sexualhistory.pdf. Accessed February 11, 2022.

2. Eckstrand KL, Ehrenfeld JM. *Lesbian, Gay, Bisexual, and Transgender Healthcare: A Clinical Guide to Preventive, Primary, and Specialist Care*. Springer; 2016. doi:10.1007/978-3-319-19752-4.

**A P P E N D I X**

# 3C

---

# The Physical Examination

JAN M. KRIEBS

---

As with the health history, this description of the physical examination focuses on those aspects most significant for sexual and reproductive health. Be alert for any inconsistency between the history and the physical examination. This description is a summary intended for the clinician. For a discussion of a complete physical examination, the reader is directed to any of several available texts or online sites.

## Review of General Principles

1. As with every healthcare visit, hand washing is essential immediately prior to beginning the examination. Alcohol-based gels and/or foams are appropriate. Hand washing within the patient's vision may offer reassurance.

2. Ask the patient whether there is any specific body area in particular that is a concern.

3. Drape the patient in such a way that only the area being examined is exposed. This approach demonstrates respect for the patient's body as well as respect for their right to modesty and privacy.

4. The examination should progress from head to toe, and minimize the number of times the patient has to change position (Table 3C-1).

5. Talk as the examination proceeds, both to let the patient know what will happen next and to share reassuring findings. Alert the patient in advance if any part of the examination will be uncomfortable.

6. Use a touch that is as firm as needed to elicit accurate information.

7. Share the findings with the patient. If they are anxious about something that is normal, describe why the examination is normal.

8. Discuss physical changes that may be abnormal briefly during the examination and in more detail after the patient is dressed at the end of the visit.

| Table 3C-1 | Physical Examination |
|---|---|

| 1. Constitutional Findings | 2. Neurologic | 3. Skin |
|---|---|---|
| Measured height and weight, calculation of BMI | Orientation to time, place, and person | Normal tone and turgor |
| Vital signs: blood pressure, pulse, respiratory rate, temperature | Cranial nerves (visible alterations) | Rashes, boils, or lesions |
| General appearance, grooming, cleanliness | Mood and affect | Examination of the breast/chest region. See the *Breast and Chest Examination* appendix for details |
| | Depression score (if formal assessment done) | |
| **4. Head and Neck** | **5. Respiratory** | **6. Cardiovascular** |
| Eyes with PERRLA | Lung sounds | Heart rate and rhythm |
| Oral examination for dental care needed, lesions, early cancer signs | Respiratory effort | Audible murmurs or extra heart sounds |
| Thyroid | | Pulses |
| Enlargement of lymph nodes | | Varicosities |
| **7. Gastrointestinal** | **8. Genitourinary** | **9. Musculoskeletal** |
| Abdominal tone, guarding, rigidity | CVAT (as illustrated in *Common Conditions in Primary Care* chapter) | Spinal deformity |
| Bowel sounds | Suprapubic tenderness | Range of motion |
| Size of liver and spleen, masses | See the *Pelvic Examination* appendix for detailed examination | Deep tendon reflex |
| Hernias, inguinal lymph nodes | | Clonus (as described in detail in *Complications During Labor and Birth* chapter) |
| Rectum (hemorrhoids, fissure) | | Focal pain or weakness |

Abbreviations: BMI, body mass index; CVAT, costovertebral angle tenderness; PERRLA, pupils equal, round, and reactive to light and accommodation.

APPENDIX

# 3D

# Breast and Chest Examination

STEPHANIE TILLMAN

Clinical examination of the breasts and chest involves consideration of any disclosed concerns, new changes, relevant personal or family history, and review of any prior records or reports. Routine self-examination is no longer recommended, but rather has been replaced by "awareness" as a way to encourage people to recognize abnormal changes between clinical evaluations. There is no consensus about the frequency of clinical examinations.[1-3] Neither the American Cancer Society[2] nor the U.S. Preventive Services Task Force[3] recommends regular clinical examination for asymptomatic patients. The American College of Obstetricians and Gynecologists continues to recommend offering clinical examinations to patients at average risk for breast cancer every 1 to 3 years for those aged 25 to 39 years and annually starting at age 40 years.[1] Until more risk-based data exist for transgender and nonbinary individuals based on organs in situ and gender-affirming hormone therapy, cisgender guidelines can be reasonably followed for these populations.[4] In some cases, duration of hormone therapy may affect recommendations for screening.[5] More information on breast and chest evaluation and diagnosis can be found in the *Breast and Chest Conditions* chapter.

Breast/chest examination is considered an intimate healthcare examination. Depending on a patient's personal history, a breast/chest examination may be especially intimate or activating for previous life experiences, including trauma. Given the intimate nature of this examination, providers should consider the trauma-informed care framework to be the standard of care.[6] The midwife should review each step of the exam, guided by visual aids to support patient comprehension, while being attentive to offering inclusive images for all patient populations. Patients should be welcomed to share the language they use for their own body—an especially important step for queer patients, who may use verbiage specific to their identity, anatomy, and experience. The midwife should offer language for informed consent before and during the examination, and invite the patient to modify the language and their consent-based needs to individualize their care.[7] Since patients' activation during an intimate exam may mimic their reaction to an initial trauma, including responses such as verbal or physical paralysis for survivors of sexual violence, providers should consider offering myriad ways for patients to indicate either discomfort or their need to stop an exam. While language like "Stop" may be accessible to some patients, others may find raising their hand or covering their body to be most communicative. Providers should be attentive to these variations as well as aware of other nonverbal cues of trauma activation during intimate care.

## Procedure for Breast/Chest Examination

1. Wash hands prior to beginning the examination.
2. Maintain patient privacy by keeping all areas covered unless the area is actively being examined.
3. The patient should be seated on the examining table facing the examiner. Once both patient and provider are ready to begin the examination, ask the patient to open the gown or drape to visualize both sides of the breasts/chest.
4. Look at the breasts or chest in three positions: with arms first loose at the sides, then raised overhead, and finally with hands on

hips so that the elbows are extended 90 degrees from the plane of the abdomen. In this final position, ask the patient to lean forward to check that all aspects of the breast tissue or chest wall move freely.

a. With arms raised, the pectoral fascia is elevated. If a carcinoma has become attached to the fascia, the breast or chest may show an indentation in the contour or skin retraction. When hands are pressed on hips, the pectoral muscles contract; if a carcinoma is fixed to the underlying fascia, the breast or chest may elevate more than expected or skin dimpling or nipple deviation may occur. Similarly, when leaning over, the breasts or chest will normally move forward without pulling on the tissue, but may exhibit asymmetry or retraction if the fibrosis of a breast lesion is present.

b. Note any visible scars for documentation and palpation in subsequent positions.

5. Palpate the lymph nodes above and below the clavicle on both sides.

6. Suggest the patient replace the drape or gown covering until positioned for the next portion of the exam.

7. Next, when the patient is ready, ask that they lie reclined or supine on the examination table. Verbally guide them to raise their arm on the examining side and fold it so that they place their hand near the face or behind their head.

a. If there is a known concern or something visualized at the beginning of the exam, begin the examination on the opposite side of the chest or breast.

b. Ask for the patient to advise when they are ready to begin the exam.

8. Gently palpate the axillary lymph nodes. The palpating hand should be moved within the axilla to press anteriorly for the pectoral nodes, posteriorly for the subscapular nodes, along the upper arm for the lateral brachial nodes, and deep in the middle for the central axillary nodes (**Figure 3D-1**).

a. Small isolated lymph nodes that are superficially palpable may reflect irritation from shaving, a localized infection, or recent vaccination. They should be reevaluated within 1 month.

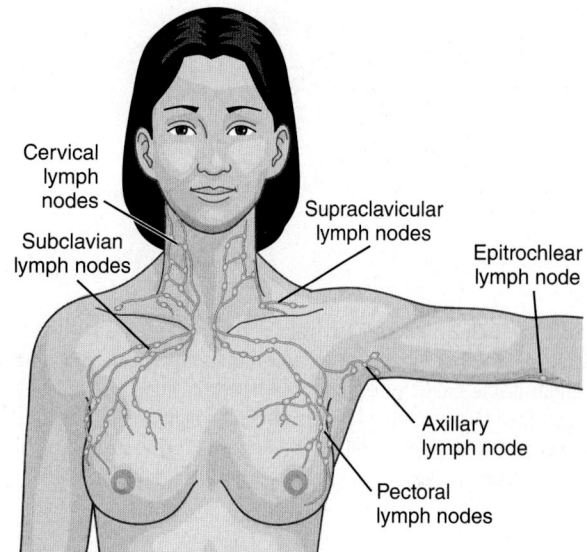

**Figure 3D-1** Lymph nodes in the superficial region of the chest and the axillary region.

9. Inspect the appearance of the nipples and areolae.

a. Nipples may be erect, flat, or inverted. The appearance changes with the reproductive cycle, active and previous pregnancy, breastfeeding/chestfeeding, and aging.

b. Spontaneous discharge, cracking, lesions, and bleeding are abnormal.

10. Inspect the appearance of the breasts.

a. Skin texture and appearance change over time.

b. Edema, redness, retracted or collapsed areas, visible sores, and masses are all abnormal observations.

11. The most effective pattern for clinical examination works up and down the breast or chest wall, beginning under the axilla and working toward the sternum, and from the clavicle to below the inframammary ridge (**Figure 3D-2**).

12. Palpate each breast or chest area for changes in texture and masses. Using the flat surface of the fingers, gently palpate each area being assessed, as illustrated in **Figure 3D-3**. A circular motion is used each time the fingers are placed on the breast. This should not be confused with an older method of breast examination in which the direction of palpation was circular—that method is no longer recommended. For larger breasts or dense

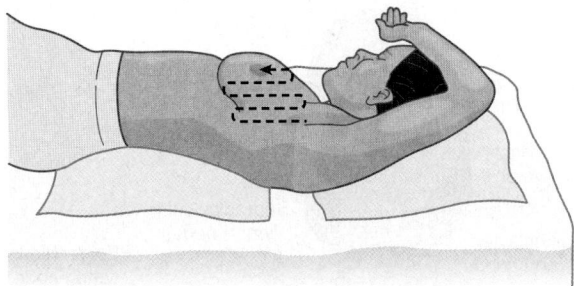

**Figure 3D-2** Direction of palpation for the clinical breast examination. Begin under the axilla and move the fingers down the length of the breast tissue from the clavicle to the inframammary ridge, then up the length of the breast tissue from the inframammary ridge to the clavicle, gradually moving toward the sternum until all the breast tissue has been palpated to three different levels of pressure.

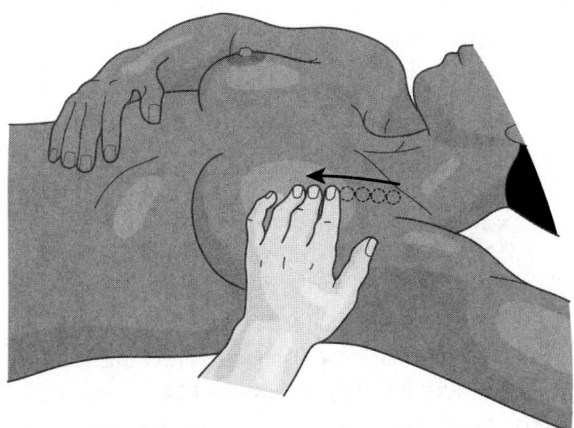

**Figure 3D-3** Palpation technique for clinical breast and chest examination.

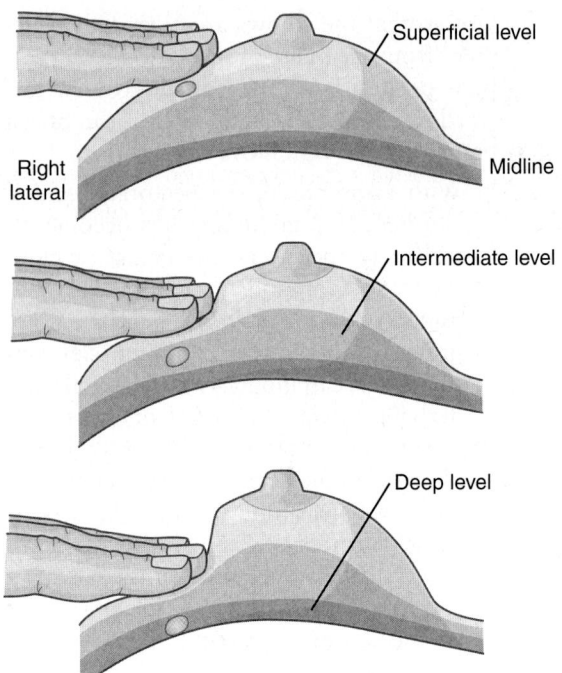

Apply pressure in a circular motion with the pads of your fingers to increasing levels, making three circles: superficial, intermediate, and deep pressure.

**Figure 3D-4** Palpating breast or chest tissue to three different levels of pressure.

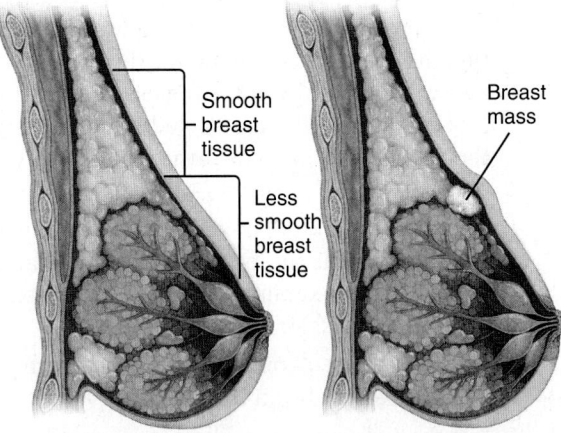

**Figure 3D-5** Nodular breast texture versus a mass.

tissue, if the typical pressure pattern does allow complete examination through the tissue to the chest wall, compress the breast or chest tissue between fingers on both hands to palpate to the complete depth.

13. Examine the full depth of the breast to the underlying rib cage (**Figure 3D-4**).

    a. Breast and chest tissues have texture. Normal variations depend on age, surgery, previous pregnancy, and breastfeeding/chestfeeding. This can range from smooth tissue to an all-over nodular texture. The texture of the breast should be consistent.

    b. Prior to menses, coarse nodularity or firmness may be more palpable.

    c. Palpable masses of any kind need to be evaluated further (**Figure 3D-5**).

14. While performing the breast or chest evaluation, the examiner describes what is being palpated and explains how the patient can recognize changes on their own. Providers can offer guidance on both breast/chest self-awareness and self-examination depending on the patient's history and examination findings.

Sample documentation of a breast/chest examination is provided in **Table 3D-1.**

| Table 3D-1 | Documentation of a Breast/Chest Examination |
| --- | --- |

*Note any patient-preferred language for anatomy.*

*Note any necessary modifications for patient comfort or for atraumatic care.*

Axillary and clavicular nodes not enlarged and nontender.

Breasts/chest wall symmetric, smooth, and nontender. No nodules, masses, retraction, dimpling, nipple deviation, asymmetry, or scars.

Areola without cracking, lesions, or bleeding.

Nipples erect bilaterally, without spontaneous or expressed discharge.

## References

1. American College of Obstetricians and Gynecologists. Practice Bulletin No. 179: breast cancer risk assessment and screening in average-risk women. *Obstet Gynecol.* 2017;130:e1-16. Reaffirmed 2021.

2. American Cancer Society. American Cancer Society recommendations for the early detection of breast cancer. https://www.cancer.org/cancer/breast-cancer/screening-tests-and-early-detection/american-cancer-society-recommendations-for-the-early-detection-of-breast-cancer.html. Revised January 14, 2022. Accessed June 19, 2023.

3. Siu AL, on behalf of U.S. Preventive Services Task Force. Screening for breast cancer: U.S. Preventive Services Task Force recommendation statement. *Ann Intern Med.* 2016;164:279-296.

4. Sterling J, Garcia MM. Cancer screening in the transgender population: a review of current guidelines, best practices, and a proposed care model. *Transl Androl Urol.* 2020;9(6):2771-2785. https://doi.org/10.21037/tau-20-954.

5. Deutsch MB. *Screening for Breast Cancer in Transgender Women.* UCSF Transgender Care; June 17, 2016. https://transcare.ucsf.edu/guidelines/breast-cancer-women. Accessed June 19, 2023.

6. Owens L, Terrell S, Low LK, et al. Universal precautions: the case for consistently trauma-informed reproductive healthcare. *Am J Obstet Gynecol.* 2022;226(5):671-677. https://doi.org/10.1016/j.ajog.2021.08.012.

7. Tillman S. Consent in pelvic care. *J Midwifery Women Health.* 2020;65(6):749-758. https://doi.org/10.1111/jmwh.13189.

# APPENDIX

# 3E

---

# Pelvic Examination

STEPHANIE TILLMAN

---

The overarching term "pelvic examination" typically refers to the external visual genital exam, vaginal speculum exam, and internal bimanual exam. Depending on a patient's anatomy, concerns, symptoms, or personal or family history, one or all of these components may be recommended. It is important to note that an indication for one type of exam does not immediately indicate another type—for example, not all speculum exams need to be followed by a bimanual examination. Midwives must be clear with patients which components of an examination are recommended, given the potential language and social confusion about distinctions between pelvic exams, cervical cancer screening, and other associated examinations and testing. Of note, at the time of this writing the bimanual examination should be conducted only if the patient has symptoms, which may be a significant shift in routine care or patient expectations. Midwives should be attentive to this conversation, as this is a newer revision to standard practice.[1]

Pelvic examinations are considered intimate healthcare examinations. Depending on a patient's personal history, a pelvic examination may be especially intimate or activating for previous life experiences, including trauma. Given the intimate nature of this examination, providers should consider the trauma-informed care framework to be the standard of care.[2] Prior to beginning the pelvic examination, the midwife should inquire as to the patient's prior experience with pelvic examinations, and welcome discussion of any concerns, questions, or history of discomfort or trauma during a pelvic examination.[3] The midwife should review each step of the exam, guided by visual aids to support patient comprehension, while being attentive to offering inclusive images for all patient populations. Patients should be welcomed to share the language they use

for their own body—an especially important step for queer patients, who may use verbiage specific to their identity, anatomy, and experience. The midwife should offer language for informed consent before and during the examination, and invite the patient to modify the language and their consent-based needs to individualize their care.[4] Since patients' activation during an intimate exam may mimic their reaction to an initial trauma, including responses such as verbal or physical paralysis for survivors of sexual violence, providers should consider offering myriad ways for patients to indicate either discomfort or their need to stop an exam. While language like "Stop" may be accessible to some patients, others may find raising their hand or closing their knees to be most communicative. Providers should be attentive to these variations as well as aware of other nonverbal cues of trauma activation during intimate care.

While this appendix offers a clear structure for the standard pelvic examination, increasing guidance on trauma-informed care, pelvic health care for sexual assault survivors, and queer-specific intimate care should be reviewed as it becomes available so that the midwife can offer the best individualized care for all patients. Progressive visits that begin with building rapport and then planning a subsequent examination, offering speculum self-insertion or self-swabbing, prescribing anxiolytics, and discussing coping mechanisms for trauma activation before, during, and after examinations are current best practices within this framework.[4]

Midwives must be well versed on variations in normal anatomy. This includes the size and shape of the labia and clitoris, hair pattern distribution, and hymenal structure including ring and tags. Awareness of variations related to intersex genital anatomy as well as neo-anatomy following gender-affirming surgical care is also crucial to patient-centered care. For some examinations the patient may be the best source to guide the midwife in learning their anatomy and needs, but in all circumstances the midwife should be well informed in genital anatomy for all patients.

During and after a pelvic examination, all words and facial expressions should be used with intention. A professional demeanor and approach are important throughout. Midwives must be attentive to both verbal and nonverbal cues of patient discomfort or needs to reassess consent. Therefore, body positioning during the pelvic examination should allow the patient and the midwife to visualize each other in an unobstructed manner throughout the procedure. Organizational guidance and practice policy may dictate the presence and role of chaperones, and midwives should obtain patient consent not only for chaperone presence but also for all student involvement. Additional extensions should be made for a patient-identified support person to be present.

1. All intake, counseling, and conversations about consent should occur while the patient is fully dressed in their own clothes. This practice is recommended to decrease physical vulnerability and mitigate the existing power dynamic between patient and midwife before an intimate exam begins.

2. Offer the patient the opportunity to use the bathroom before changing for the exam. Step out of the room or behind a curtain while the patient changes into a gown or drape. Minimize the amount of time the patient is waiting in a gown or drape in the clinic setting.

3. Wash hands, preferably in front of the patient for reassurance. Then assemble all necessary equipment prior to beginning the examination. This includes taking lids off containers and opening any packages needed.

4. Offer positioning options for the examination. These can include bent knees with feet resting on the examination table, foot rests, knee rests, or a reclined position in a chair. These positions should be offered for all patients regardless of perceived disability or disclosed trauma history. Once in a comfortable position, the midwife can verbally guide the patient into flattening their back into the examination table and tilting their pelvis upward, which will improve the positioning

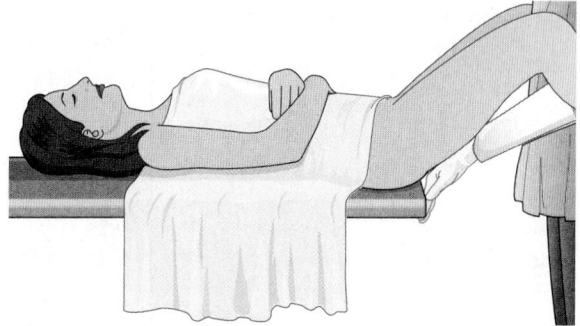

**Figure 3E-1** Positioning a patient for a pelvic examination.

of the cervix for the speculum or bimanual examination. While a traditional position includes the patient's pelvis resting at the end of the examination table (Figure 3E-1), consider this a general example that can be modified into other positions. Support the patient in adjusting the drape sheet or gown for their privacy. Only adjust the drape to visualize the genitalia when the patient verbalizes they are ready to begin the exam

   a. The midwife should conduct initial and ongoing consent throughout the examination. This includes assessing facial, verbal, and physical cues of discomfort or pain.

   b. Note that this is common positioning in North America. In Europe, providers often examine someone in a lateral position.[1]

   c. Trauma-informed care invites the patient to choose the position most comfortable or empowering for them, so midwives should be able to accommodate a variety of positions. This may be especially important for patients with a known physical disability or mental health diagnosis.

5. Organize all tools, including the chair and light, before donning gloves to maintain a clean environment.

   a. Place the speculum and any needed supplies for the examination on a clean surface. In some practices, the specula are placed on clean areas with heating pads beneath them to warm the instruments.

   b. It is important for the midwife to be continuously aware of hand cleanliness. Cross-contamination can occur easily, especially by touching equipment, the light, or the clean area on the table after

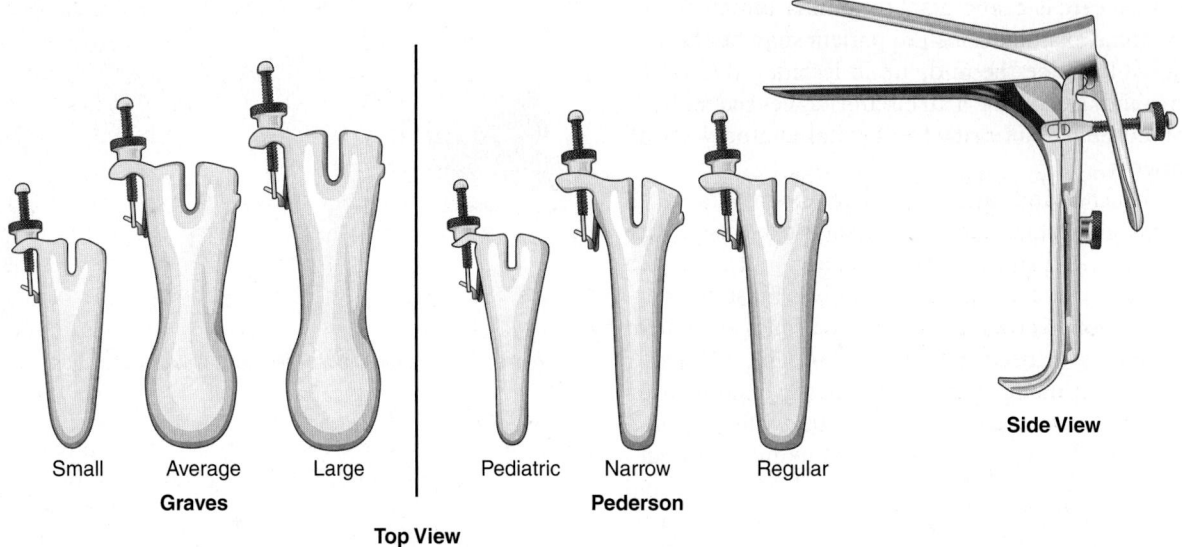

**Figure 3E-2** Common vaginal speculum types.

touching the genitalia. It is also helpful to be cautious with language and avoid using terms such as "clean" and "dirty" to designate the hand used for either equipment or direct contact with the patient. The word "dirty" can be heard as a commentary on the patient's body or symptoms. The following are the possible options for gloving to maintain a clean environment:

   i. Some midwives double-glove both hands and remove the outermost glove if it touches the patient or any secretions to avoid cross-contamination.

   ii. Others double-glove only the hand that will be used for external palpation or internal examination. The first glove is then removed after contact with the patient's body.

   iii. In the past, it was common to use one glove only, which was placed on the hand that performed the internal examination. However, with the advent of universal precautions, most midwives also glove the hand that performs the external/abdominal portion of the examination.

  c. The correct choice of a speculum can both facilitate visualization and decrease discomfort. The midwife should begin the examination with the smallest speculum necessary, and speculum size should never be assumed based on body habitus, weight, or pregnancy history. Specula come in many sizes and designs. Pederson specula are straight sided; Graves models have a "duck-billed" shape that increases visualization of the vaginal vault and fornices when lax musculature or submucosal fat impedes visualization of the upper vagina. Narrow specula and shorter pediatric specula are also available for use whenever conditions require a smaller device. Figure 3E-2 shows the variety of specula available. Disposable plastic specula are similar in shape to the Pederson metal specula and come in a variety of sizes.

## External Inspection of the Genitalia

1. Let the patient advise when they are ready to begin the exam. At that point, verbally guide them into their comfortable position before advising them when you will move the drape sheet or gown.

2. Once the patient is ready, let them know to drop their knees out to the sides or elevate the upper leg if in lateral position.

  a. Remind the patient that you will be engaging them about informed consent throughout the exam. Based on your pre-examination discussion, either encourage them to speak immediately in case of pain or if desiring the examination to pause or stop, or to use other approaches like raising their hand or closing their knees Always be attentive for nonverbal indications of discomfort or trauma activation.

b. If you visualize tension in the patient's vulvar muscles or pelvic floor, offer language to guide the patient to soften or drop the muscles downward to decrease their discomfort during the exam. This may also be a trauma activation response, so if this verbal guidance is ineffective, consider pausing the exam and reassessing consent, comfort, and support measures.

c. Gently place the back of the gloved dominant examining hand on the inside of the thigh before proceeding with vulvar palpation to slowly introduce the start of the exam.

3. Inspect the external genitalia (**Figure 3E-3**). To do so, advise the patient that you will next carefully separate the labia majora and inspect the labia minora. Then separate the labia minora and inspect the clitoris, the inside of the labia minora, vestibule, urethral orifice, and vaginal introitus. Inspect the perianal area for signs of infection, hemorrhoids, or trauma. For complete visualization, if the midwife needs the patient to adjust their pelvic position, or move obscuring tissue from the patient's inner thighs or buttocks, they should invite the patient to do so themselves or offer to help them to do so before the midwife physically does so. Note that if the midwife is using the word "inspect" while verbally guiding the patient through the exam, the midwife should be aware that even superficial touch can be unexpected and cause distress. If palpation is indicated, make sure to advise the patient *before* performing this step, and even then begin palpation only with explicit consent. Table 3E-1 lists observations to be noted. Midwives should assess for female genital mutilation (cutting or circumcision) when caring for patient populations where this is practiced (Figure 3E-4 and Table 3E-2).[5]

a. Visually inspect the paraurethal (Skene's) glands and urethra for irritation, swelling, lesions, redness, or discharge.

b. Inspect the greater vestibular (Bartholin's) glands for masses, fluctuation, redness, heat, or pain.

c. Inspecting these glands before performing the speculum examination increases the likelihood that any discharge will be noted, as it may otherwise be obscured by the clinical lubricant.

4. Now an uncommon component of the routine asymptomatic exam, palpation of the vulvar glands may be indicated if irritation, swelling, redness, odor, or discharge is noted. Notify the patient of these findings

**Figure 3E-3** External genitalia.

| Table 3E-1 | Observations of the External Genitalia |
|---|---|
| During examination of the external vulvar and perianal genitalia, many observed changes provide information of clinical significance. Assess the following: | |
| Pattern of hair growth | Discoloration or bruising |
| Size and shape of each area | Cysts, polyps, condyloma, or other growths |
| Appearance of the introitus | Lesions, fissures, rashes, ulcerations, or crusting |
| Clitoral enlargement | Adhesion of tissues |
| Inflammation or irritation | Fistula |
| Swelling or edema | Bladder, cervical, uterine, or rectal prolapse |
| Scarring | Varicosities |
| Piercing(s) | Hemorrhoids |

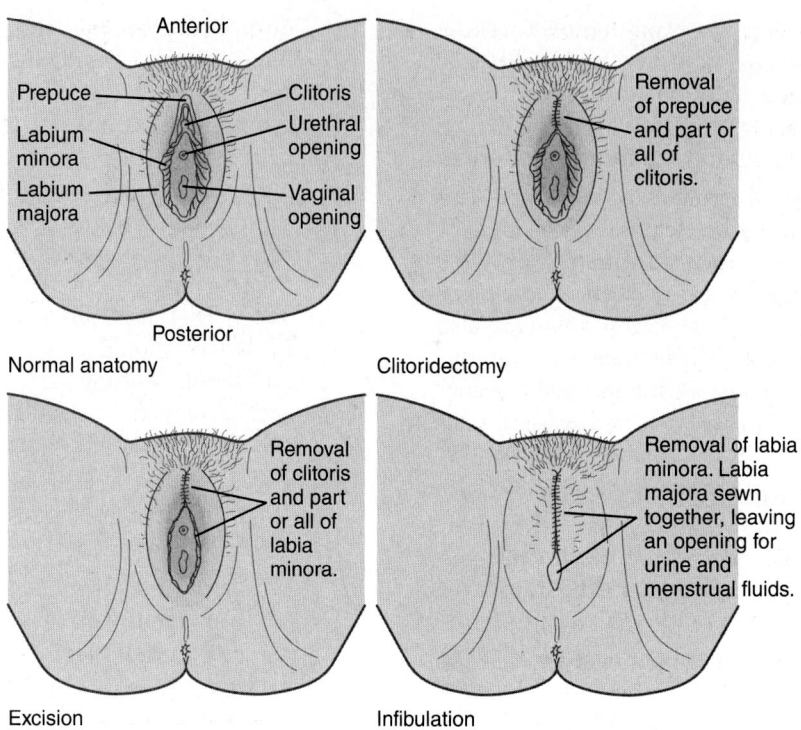

**Figure 3E-4** Female genital cutting.
Reproduced from Schuiling KD, Likis FE, eds. *Gynecologic Health Care*. 4th ed. Burlington, MA: Jones & Bartlett Learning; 2022.

| Table 3E-2 | Female Genital Cutting |
|---|---|

Female genital cutting, also called female circumcision and female genital mutilation, "comprises all procedures that involve partial or total removal of the external female genitalia, or other injury to the female genital organs for non-medical reasons."[6] There are four major types of female genital cutting.

| | |
|---|---|
| Type 1: clitoridectomy | Partial or total removal of the clitoris and/or the prepuce |
| Type 2: excision | Partial or total removal of the clitoris and the labia minora, with or without excision of the labia majora |
| Type 3: infibulation | Narrowing of the vaginal orifice through the creation of a covering seal, accomplished by cutting and repositioning the labia minora and/or the labia majora, with or without excision of the clitoris |
| Type 4: other | All other harmful procedures to the female genitalia for nonmedical purposes, such as pricking, piercing, incising, scraping, and cauterizing |

Long-term sequelae of female genital cutting include urinary problems, vaginal problems, menstrual problems, scar tissue, sexual problems, childbirth complications, need for later surgeries, and psychological problems.

Reproduced from World Health Organization. Female genital mutilation. https://www.who.int/news-room/fact-sheets/detail/female-genital-mutilation. Published January 31, 2023. Accessed June 19, 2023.

and consider palpation of these structures. This palpation should be performed only after receiving the patient's explicit consent to do so.

a. For the paraurethral glands: Separate the labia; insert one finger into the vagina, palm up; and sweep down the paraurethral glands at each side of the urethra toward the introitus. Pressing directly upward onto the urethra, again sweep from the apex of the vagina toward the introitus to elicit discharge from the urethra if present.

   b. For the greater vestibular glands: Separate the labia; place one finger in the vagina and the other fingers and thumb outside the vagina. Palpate the entire area, usually by gently palpating the tissue between the thumb and the index finger, both sides of the vaginal opening in turn. Pay particular attention to the posterolateral portion of the labia majora.

## Speculum Examination

1. Start with use of the hand to be designated for handling the equipment. Verify that the speculum previously chosen is appropriate in size and that it is warm (skin temperature). If not, discard the glove on the hand that palpated the external genitalia, correct the speculum size or temperature, and re-glove.

2. Check the speculum before using it to make sure the locking knobs (metal speculum) or latch (plastic speculum) works correctly.

3. Apply adequate lubrication to the entirety of the speculum blades.

4. While holding the speculum by the handle and securing the two blades together with the index finger across the top blade to avoid inadvertent opening and increasing the size/diameter of the device, use the opposite hand to separate the labia to fully visualize the introitus (Figure 3E-5).[5] Since the location of the introitus cannot be presumed by external visualization of closed labia, the exam should begin only when the introitus is fully visualized.

5. Provide gentle downward pressure as the speculum blades follow the patient's internal anatomy. The speculum should enter and be removed from the vagina at a 45-degree angle so the speculum avoids touching the sensitive anterior structures (e.g., pubic bone, urethra, clitoris).

6. Rotate the speculum to a horizontal position as it moves toward the posterior portion of the vagina. Do not open the blades until the speculum is fully inserted.

7. Maintaining downward pressure, withdraw the speculum slightly and open it only as much as is needed to visualize the cervix using the thumb piece.

   a. The most common cervical position is tilted slightly posterior, so placing the speculum behind the cervix and gently opening it is the technique most likely to identify the cervix with minimal discomfort.

8. When the cervix is visible, insert the speculum slightly deeper to stabilize and improve visibility, and then use the screws or latch (on a plastic speculum) to fix the open position of the speculum. The anterior blade of a metal speculum can be adjusted if a larger area needs to be created.

   a. Note any discharge, cysts, polyps, lesions or masses, vascularity, erosion, or eversion.

9. It is at this point that specimens are collected if needed.

After collecting specimens, gently remove the speculum from the cervix, noting if the cervix is pulling into the speculum on removal and modifying the technique as necessary to decrease added discomfort. Rotate the speculum to visualize the anterior and posterior walls of the vagina. Many midwives will perform this inspection as they slowly remove the speculum. Then, allow the vaginal walls to naturally close the speculum blades. The speculum should be rotated back at a 45-degree angle as it nears the vaginal introitus and then gently removed.

## Bimanual Examination

The bimanual examination is perhaps one of the most intimate examinations. Initial and ongoing informed consent and assessment of patient discomfort must be paramount throughout each step of the examination. If each part of this exam is conducted as outlined here, the patient should be aware of their engagement in bearing down, tightening muscles, or responding to assessments before the exam begins. Often a shorter version of the exam includes an internal assessment of the uterus and adnexa, unless other symptoms are present.

1. If necessary, discard gloves and don new ones. Apply water-based gel to the one or two fingers of the gloved hand that will be inserted into the vagina.

2. This portion of the examination is typically conducted with two fingers in the vagina, unless for patient comfort one examining finger is best.

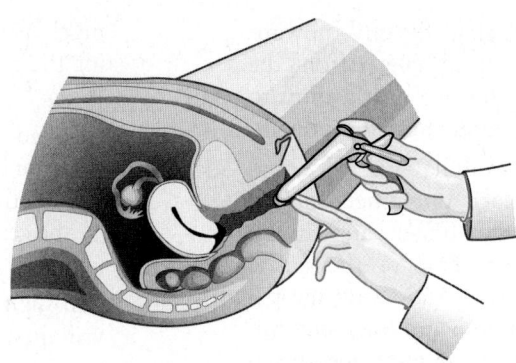

Note the speculum at an oblique angle and hand on perineum pushing down slightly.

**A**

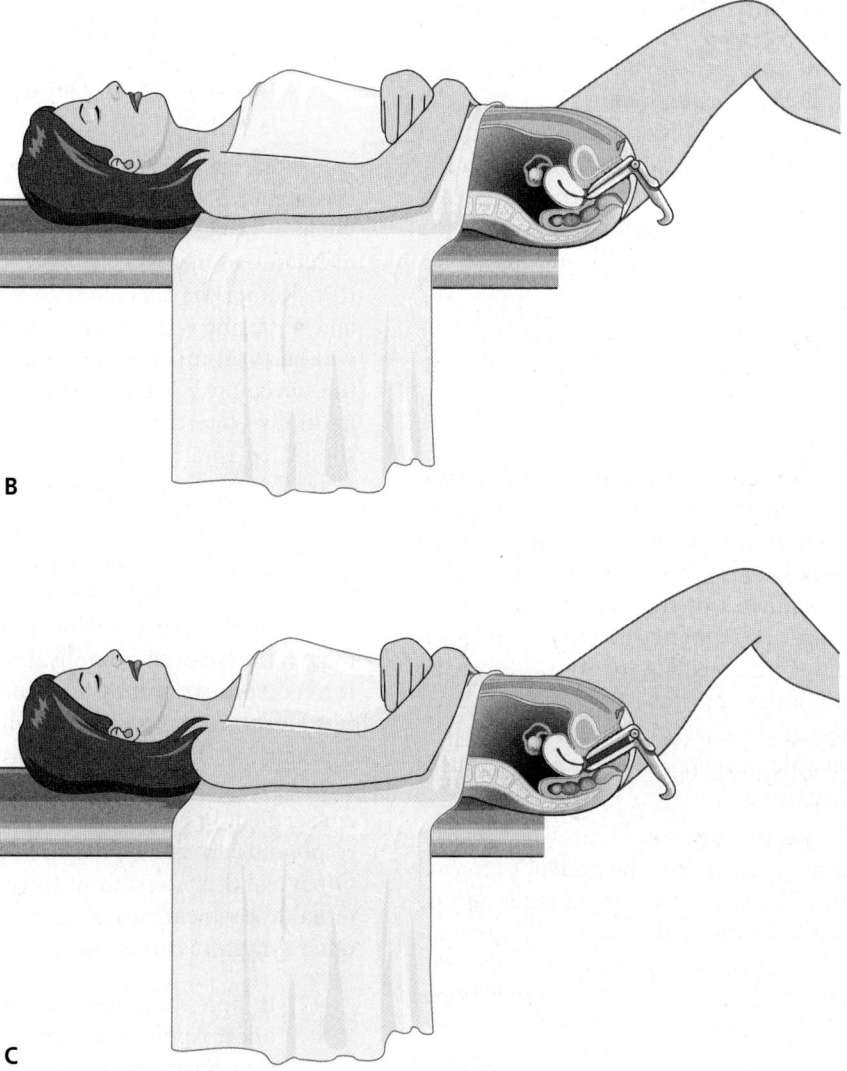

**B**

**C**

**Figure 3E-5** Speculum examination. **A.** Position of the hands and speculum at insertion (speculum at oblique angle). **B.** Speculum inserted along the posterior wall of the vagina. **C.** Speculum open to visualize cervix.

Modified from Schuiling KD, Likis FE, eds. *Gynecologic Health Care*. 4th ed. Burlington, MA: Jones & Bartlett Learning; 2022.

a. Keep the thumb of the examining hand tucked to one side or folded into the palm to avoid unintentional pressure on the clitoris and to allow the examining fingers to reach farther into the vagina.

3. Using the thumb and fourth finger of the examining hand, separate the labia to visualize the introitus.

4. Place the one or two examining fingers at the introitus. Pressing gently downward, insert the examining finger(s) along the posterior wall of the vagina.

5. Press downward to be able to observe for the bulge of a cystocele, urethrocele, or uterine descent associated with prolapse. If necessary, ask the patient to bear down and explain why.

6. Separate the examining fingers and repeat the process to visualize for any posterior bulging associated with a rectocele or enterocele.

7. Ask the patient to tighten their vaginal muscles around the examining fingers to assess for strength and normalcy. The midwife can teach common pelvic floor exercises at this point if needed, or after the visit is completed.

8. Advise the patient that the examining fingers will be inserted farther and will be moved along the internal vaginal walls to assess for health or abnormalities. Sweep the vaginal fingers around the walls to assess for masses or lesions such as cysts, polyps, or condyloma.

9. Advise the patient that now the examining fingers will be inserted to the end of the vagina. When the fingers reach the cervix, they should be moved circumferentially around the cervix.

   a. Assess for size, consistency, smoothness, shape, mobility, and dilation.

10. Advise the patient that you will be moving the cervix and lower part of the uterus and they should alert the midwife to any discomfort or pain. Move the cervix gently side to side between two fingers to assess for cervical motion tenderness.

11. Advise the patient that you will place your other hand on their abdomen to assess organs within the pelvis. Place the external hand above the symphysis and press downward and forward toward the vaginal hand with the palmar surface of the fingers. With the vaginal hand, lift upward directly against the cervix to bring the uterine fundus in contact with the hand on the abdomen. Press both hands together gently to outline an anteverted or anteflexed uterus. The uterus should move smoothly between the hands. If necessary, reposition the abdominal hand farther up the abdomen to locate the fundus.

12. Note the position of the uterus (anteverted, retroverted, anteflexed, retroflexed, midline). Also note the shape, size, consistency, mobility, tenderness, or presence of any masses.

13. If the uterus is not identified, advise the patient that you will be pressing on either side of the pelvis and the pressure or cramping sensation may change. Repeat the maneuver with the vaginal fingers on either side of the cervix (Figure 3E-6 illustrates uterine positions).[5]

14. If the uterine position is still not palpated, it may be in a midline or posterior position. With fingers in the vagina above and below the uterus, press inward with the external hand and assess as much of the lower portion of the uterus as is possible.

15. To assess the adnexa, place the external hand in the area between the iliac crest of the innominate bone and the abdominal midline midway between the level of the umbilicus and the symphysis pubis. Use the flats of the palmar surface of fingers on the abdomen to press deeply downward and obliquely toward the symphysis pubis and toward the fingers in the vagina.

16. With the internal hand in the vagina, the palm should face upward. Both of the examining fingers in the vagina are placed in the lateral vaginal fornix corresponding to the side (right or left) that the abdominal hand is positioned to examine. Press the fingers deeply inward and upward toward the abdominal hand as far as possible.

17. Palpate the entire area between the uterus and the pelvic sidewalls with a sliding, gentle, but firm touch, pressing the internal and abdominal hands toward each other as they synchronously move together from the abdominal area above the pelvic brim downward toward the symphysis.

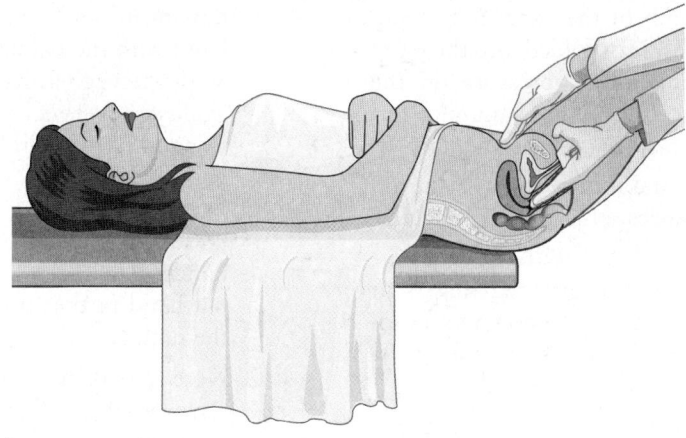

A

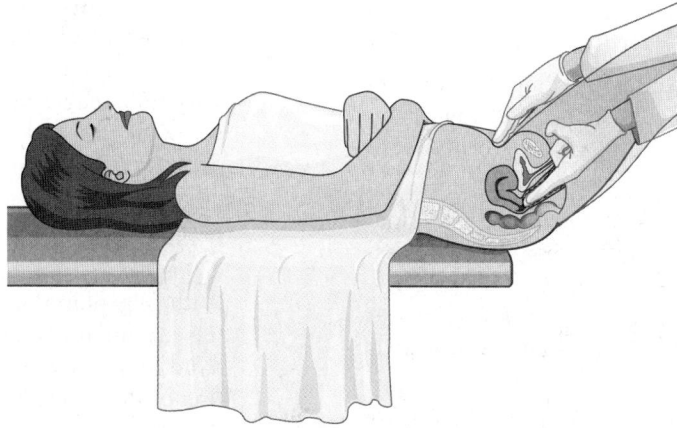

B

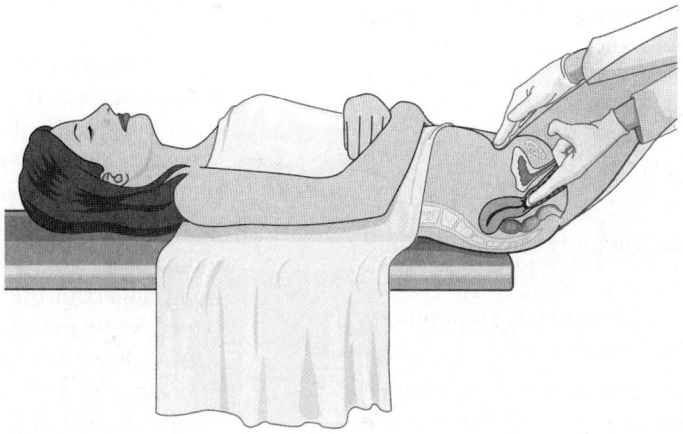

C

**Figure 3E-6** Uterine positions. **A.** Anteverted. **B.** Anteflexed. **C.** Retroverted.
Modified from Schuiling KD, Likis FE, eds. *Gynecologic Health Care*. 4th ed.
Burlington, MA: Jones & Bartlett Learning; 2022.

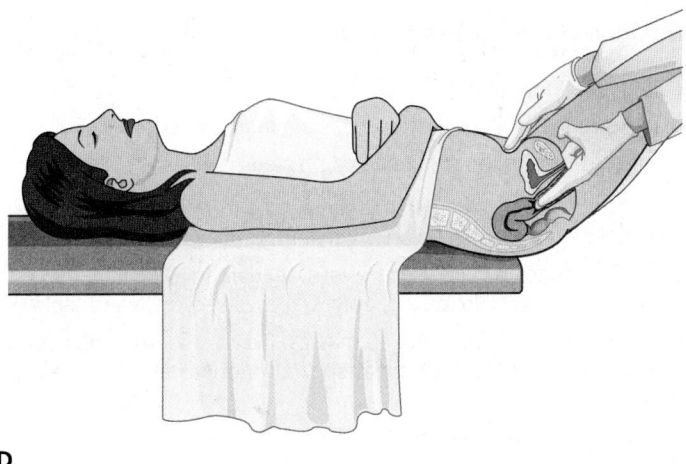

**D**

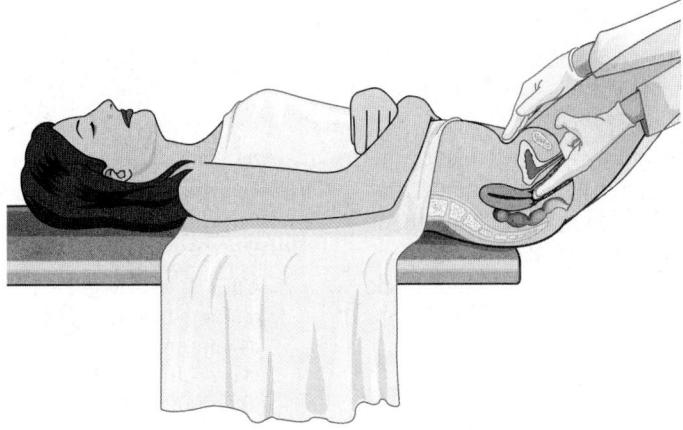

**E**

**Figure 3E-6** *Continued.* **D.** Retroflexed. **E.** Midline.

## Rectovaginal Examination

1. Not all regular examinations include a rectovaginal examination. If the need for this part of the examination is discovered as the pelvic exam proceeds, the midwife can assist the patient into a sitting position to explain why this examination is indicated—to further evaluate the uterus and adnexa or to check for a fistula and to explain what the next steps include.

2. Change the current gloves and lubricate the examining fingers.

3. Review the options for assessing the rectum. One option is to have the patient bear down (i.e., perform the Valsalva maneuver) to soften the pelvic muscles to decrease discomfort during the exam. Advise the patient before inserting any examining objects or tools, because doing so while the patient bears down can be disconcerting if not explicitly described beforehand. Another option is a slow insertion of the examining finger, allowing the patient to progressively soften the necessary muscles as they are able. Insert one gloved index finger into the vagina and insert the second finger into the rectum.

4. Palpate the area of the anorectal junction and superior to it. Ask the patient to tighten and soften the rectal sphincter.

   a. This position allows for assessment of sphincter tone and for internal hemorrhoids.

| Table 3E-3 | Documentation of a Pelvic Examination |
|---|---|

*Note any patient-preferred language for anatomy.*

*Note any necessary modifications for patient comfort or for atraumatic care.*

*Only necessary components of the examination should be completed.*

**External genitalia:** Typical hair distribution pattern. No erythema, lesions, masses, or tenderness. Paraurethral and greater vestibular glands without masses or discharge. Hymenal tissue/tags present at introitus.

**Speculum exam:** Vaginal walls pink, lubricated. No laxity, lesions, tenderness. No cystocele, rectocele, cervical or uterine prolapse. Cervix anterior, pink, moist, round. No lesions, polyps, growths, cysts. Non-friable with specimen collection.

**Bimanual exam:** Vaginal walls smooth, moderate tone, no masses. Cervix smooth, mobile, no CMT. Uterus anteverted, midline, mobile, nontender, normal size, shape, and consistency. Ovaries palpable bilaterally. No adnexal tenderness or masses.

**Perianal exam:** No external hemorrhoids, redness, irritation, lesions, or masses.

**Rectovaginal exam:** Anorectal junction with appropriate musculature. No hemorrhoids, fistula. Rectal wall without masses, fistula, or discomfort.

Abbreviation: CMT, cervical motion tenderness.

5. Advise the patient that you will insert the examining fingers in both the vagina and the rectum to allow for further assessment of the internal musculature. Palpate the rectal wall, sweeping the examining finger back and forth.

6. When a uterus is retroverted or retroflexed, the posterior side of the uterus may be palpated. Palpate as much of the posterior side of the uterus as possible with the rectal examining finger.

7. As the vaginal and rectal fingers are withdrawn, the other half of the rectal wall is examined as in Step 5.

8. Remove gloves and discard them. Perform hand hygiene.

9. Assist the patient to a sitting position and offer cleansing wipes and tissues with which to address any remnant lubricant.

10. Step out of the room or behind the curtain so the patient can dress.

11. Return to discuss the examination. Ask the patient which parts of the exam were helpful to them, and what they would need for a more comfortable future exam. Review any findings from the exam and the next steps.

Sample documentation of a pelvic examination is provided in **Table 3E-3**.

### References

1. Chor J, Stulberg DG, Tillman S. Shared decision-making framework for pelvic examinations in asymptomatic, nonpregnant patient. *Obstet Gynecol*. 2019;133(4):81014. doi:10.1097/AOG .0000000000003166.

2. Owens L, Terrell S, Low LK, et al. Universal precautions: the case for consistently trauma-informed reproductive healthcare. *Am J Obstet Gynecol*. 2022;226(5):671-677. https://doi.org/10.1016/j.ajog .2021.08.012.

3. William A, Williams M. A guide to performing pelvic speculum exams: a patient-centered approach to reducing iatrogenic effects. *Teach Learn Med*. 2013;25:383-391.

4. Tillman S. Consent in pelvic care. *J Midwifery Women Health*. 2020;65(6):749-758. https://doi.org /10.1111/jmwh.13189.

5. Schuiling KD, Likis FE, eds. Gynecologic Health Care. 4th ed. Burlington, MA: Jones & Bartlett Learning; 2022.

6. World Health Organization. Female genital mutilation. https://www.who.int/news-room/fact-sheets/detail /female-genital-mutilation. Published January 31, 2023. Accessed June 19, 2023.

# APPENDIX

# 3F

# Collecting Laboratory Specimens

LISA A. SPENCER

Specimens collected during pelvic, rectal, and/or pharyngeal examinations may be used to test for many health concerns, ranging from infections and cancer to risk of preterm labor or rupture of membranes. In all cases, standard precautions are used to prevent provider exposure to blood and body fluids.[1] The order of specimen collection is determined by the purpose and type of specimen collected and the preferences of the individual whose sample is being collected.

## General Principles for Specimen Collection

Cross-contamination should be carefully avoided—either of the equipment and supplies or of the patient and clinical specimens—by the appropriate use of gloves in either clean or sterile technique, and by attention to surroundings.

Avoiding the use of gel when collecting these specimens improves detection. The gel can interfere with testing by obscuring the collection site, altering the pH of a specimen, and making microscopy less accurate. Warm water may be used to moisten a speculum.

The common order of potential specimen collection is as follows:

1. Voided urine
2. Oral specimen collection:
   a. Pharyngeal swab for nucleic acid amplification tests (NAAT) or culture
3. Genital specimen collection:
   a. Bladder catheter collected urine
   b. Penile meatus collection
   c. Vaginal swab for NAAT or culture
   d. Vaginal swab for pH, saline, or KOH
   e. Endocervical swab for NAAT or culture
   f. Cervical cytology (Papanicolaou, "Pap") testing
4. Rectal specimen collection:
   a. Anal cytology (Papanicolaou, "Pap") testing
   b. Anal swab for NAAT or culture

## Procedure for Collecting Urine Specimens

Urine specimens can be used for urinalysis, urine culture, and NAAT for *Neisseria gonorrhoeae* and *Chlamydia trachomatis*.

1. Determine whether a catheterized specimen is necessary before collecting the specimen. Examples of times when this might be necessary are after rupture of the membranes, during the early postpartum period, when it will be difficult to adequately cleanse the area, or whenever a definitive measurement of urinary protein, leukocytes, or erythrocytes is necessary.
2. If performing a bladder catheter collection:
   a. Review the indications for and process of bladder catheter collection and obtain consent throughout.
   b. Open the sterile catheter using sterile technique and leave it in the sterile wrap.
   c. Don sterile gloves.
   d. Place the end of the catheter where the urine will drain from into a sterile collection device.

e. Apply a water-based lubricant to the tip of the catheter that will be placed through the urethra.

f. Holding the labia away from the urethra or with the urethra otherwise clearly exposed, cleanse the periurethral and surrounding area with soap (not disinfectant, which may interfere with culture). Wipe from front to back a total of three times, using a clean pad each time.

g. Using aseptic technique, insert the catheter into the urethra until urine is returned (usually 4–5 cm).

h. Slowly remove the catheter from the urethra when an adequate specimen is obtained or when urine no longer drains, depending on the indication for the procedure.

i. Cap the sterile collection device without contaminating the inside by touching it.

j. Remove gloves.

k. Label the sterile specimen.

3. Urine specimens as routine screening for *N. gonorrhoeae* and *C. trachomatis* via NAAT testing should be collected from a spontaneous void.

a. Review the indications for and process of collection and obtain consent.

b. The patient should not have voided within the last hour.

c. Do not cleanse the area immediately prior to voiding.

d. The patient should void an initial 20–30 mL of urine directly into a labeled urine collection container free of any preservative agents. Avoid greater quantities of urine, as this dilution decreases testing quality.

## Procedure for Collecting Penile Meatal Specimens

In some cases, sampling of the penile meatus may be used for the diagnosis of *N. gonorrhoeae*, *C. trachomatis*, *Mycoplasma genitalium*, or other infections. The sensitivity of urine screening is generally adequate when screening patients with a penis.[2]

1. Review the indications for and process of penile meatus collection and obtain consent throughout.

2. With the penile glans exposed, sample any exudate with a standard-size Dacron swab.

3. Clean the glans by wiping from the meatus outward with an appropriate skin cleanser.

4. Holding a mini-tip swab at the score line, place the mini-tip swab 2 cm into the urethra and rotate for 15 seconds.

5. Remove the swab and place it immediately into an appropriately labeled medium for transport.

## Procedure for Collecting Pharyngeal Specimens for *N. Gonorrhoeae* and *C. Trachomatis*

In cases of extragenital sexual contact and potential exposure to *N. gonorrhoeae* or *C. trachomatis*, pharyngeal testing may be appropriate. NAAT remains the testing modality of choice for adults, regardless of test site. If considering pharyngeal testing of children, *N. gonorrhoeae* culture can be considered. When collecting extragenital specimens for *N. gonorrhoeae* or *C. trachomatis* testing of any kind, ensure adequate technical support of your laboratory or testing agency.[2]

1. Review the indications for and process of pharyngeal collection and obtain consent throughout.

2. Hold the appropriate sterile swab between the first and second gloved fingers at the marked score line, being careful to avoid touching any area above the score line with your fingers or another object.

3. Gently sample the bilateral tonsils (when present) or side walls, and posterior pharyngeal wall for 10 seconds, or until the procedure is no longer tolerated.

4. Carefully withdraw the swab, avoiding contact with the tongue, teeth, gums, cheek, or lips.

5. Place the sample directly into the labeled transport medium.

## Procedure for Collecting and Interpreting Saline and Potassium Hydroxide Specimens for Vaginal Infections[1,3]

In the United States, microscopy for the diagnosis of infection or rupture of the amniotic membranes falls under the Clinical Laboratory Improvement

| Table 3F-1 | Use of the Optical Microscope |
|---|---|

- An optical microscope can be used to facilitate diagnosis in the clinical setting.
- Proper microscope maintenance—minimizing exposure to dust by covering the microscope when not in use, cleaning the eyepiece and objective lenses with compressed air and a lint-free paper wipe, and wiping down mechanical components with a microfiber or other lint-free cloth—will preserve the quality of the images.
- Prior to using a microscope for the first time, familiarity with the light source, adjustment of the fine- and coarse-focus knobs, technique for moving the slide on the mount, and the powers available for viewing a specimen are necessary.
- Most modern microscopes will have a 10× eyepiece lens and 4×, 10×, and 40× objective lenses. The oil immersion lens is not used for procedures discussed here.

Amendments of 1988 (CLIA). These federal regulations, which mandate improved quality controls, include requirements for competence in provider-performed microscopy. The Centers for Medicare and Medicaid Services is responsible for these regulations, which are published online through the Centers for Disease Control and Prevention.[4] As with any procedure that has the potential for exposure to blood or other body fluids, standard precautions are always observed. The first step is knowing how to use the microscope (Table 3F-1).

Saline specimens are used for the direct visualization of vaginal yeasts, trichomonads, and clue cells typical of bacterial vaginosis. Assessment of the presence or absence of lactobacilli and white blood cells can also aid diagnosis. Red blood cells or sperm can also be seen.

A sample placed in potassium hydroxide (KOH) is used to visualize yeasts. The KOH destroys the cell walls of bacteria and epithelial cells, but not the cell walls of fungi. A sample can also be collected for use in the "whiff" test; when a bacterial vaginosis specimen is exposed to an alkaline solution (KOH) it releases amines, which produce a strong odor.

1. Review the indications for and process of collection and obtain consent throughout.

2. Obtain dropper bottles of normal saline and KOH. Saline is preferred over distilled water to help maintain the living specimen throughout examination.

3. Determine the mode of collection.
   a. If a self-collected swab is appropriate and acceptable to the patient:
      i. Provide detailed instructions.
      ii. Either alone or with provider review, the patient may insert a sterile cotton swab about 2 inches into the vagina and rotate gently for 15–20 seconds.
      iii. The sample should be immediately returned to the provider to ensure living specimens are preserved for adequate evaluation.
   b. If a provider-collected swab is appropriate and acceptable to the patient:
      i. Don nonsterile gloves.
      ii. Lubricate a speculum with water, and insert it into the vagina to visualize the cervix.
      iii. As the speculum is inserted and positioned, note the appearance of structures, including the perineum, vaginal mucosa, cervical epithelium, and any discharge. Discharge is categorized by quantity, color, consistency, and odor.
      iv. Using a sterile cotton swab, collect a sample of fluid from the posterior fornix and/or from the vaginal wall. If necessary, a second swab may be used to obtain an adequate sample.
      v. Remove the speculum, discard the used gloves, and don clean gloves.
   c. Gently roll or blot the swab across a glass microscope slide. Repeat this on a second slide. The slide sample should avoid clumps and be generally thin.
   d. Consider retaining the sample cotton swab for a "whiff" test or repeat slide preparation, or discard as appropriate.
   e. If gloves are contaminated, discard and don a new set of nonsterile gloves.
   f. Place a single drop of saline onto one of the slide samples. Place a single drop of KOH solution onto the remaining slide sample. Separate slides are preferred to prevent contamination of KOH into the saline specimen.
   g. Cover each specimen with a cover slip by holding the coverslip by the edges at a 45-degree angle and lowering slowly from one side to the other (Figure 3F-1).

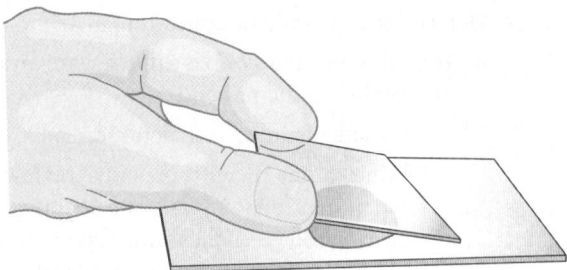

**Figure 3F-1** Cover slide placement.

h. Blot away excess fluid with a lint-free paper placed along the edge of the slide if the cover slip is floating.

i. Evaluate the saline slide first, followed by the KOH slide, when appropriate. If slides become confused and are unlabeled, saline slides will have epithelial cells visible. KOH slides will have only remnants of epithelial cells while yeast hyphae will remain visible.

j. Begin by focusing with the low-power lens (10×) at the edge of the cover slip using the coarse-focus knob. Then use the fine-focus knob to bring the specimen into clear view, being careful to avoid artifact from fingerprints, lint, or dust.

k. Examine several areas of the slide to ensure correct diagnosis, as the specimen may not be equally distributed across the slide.

l. Specimens of vaginal secretions are inspected under high power (40×). High power enables the differentiation of blood cells, bacteria, clue cells, trichomonas, yeast hyphae, and spores. Results are reported as positive/present or negative/absent (Figure 3F-2).[4] A more detailed discussion is found in the *Reproductive Tract and Sexually Transmitted Infections* chapter regarding the diagnosis of vaginal infections and STIs.

m. When evaluation of the sample is complete, lower the stage away from the optic, turn off the microscope light, clean surfaces, and properly discard the sample to complete the procedure.

n. In many settings, a separate log of the procedure is kept that includes patient identifiers, date, procedure completed, and results. Complete this as required by the site.

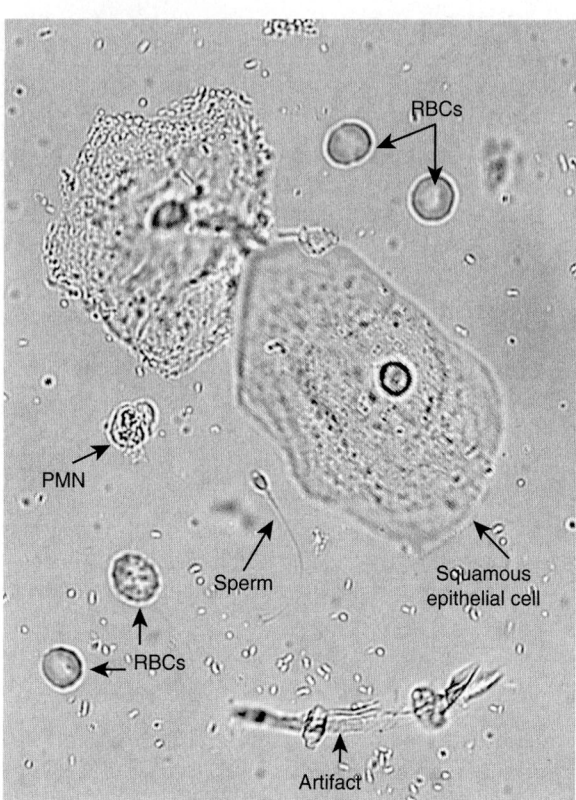

**Figure 3F-2** Vaginal slide prepared with saline. Abbreviations: PMN, polymorphonuclear; RBCs, red blood cells. Reproduced with permission from Centers for Disease Control and Prevention. CDC STI slide set. Used with permission from Seattle STD/HIV Prevention Training Center and Cindy Fennell, MS, MT, ASCP.

## Procedure for Collecting Vaginal or Cervical Specimens for *N. Gonorrhoeae, C. Trachomatis*, and Trichomoniasis

Most laboratories now use nucleic acid amplification tests (NAAT) or similar DNA-based testing for evaluation of mucopurulent cervicitis and for screening for *N. gonorrhoeae* and *C. trachomatis* infection.[5,6] These tests are the most sensitive available, and their specificity is similar to that of culture. If the product being used is approved for vaginal testing, these specimens are as accurate as cervical ones, and more accurate than urine specimens. A provider can collect vaginal swabs, or such samples may be self-collected by the patient. Vaginal trichomoniasis sampling is completed in the same fashion as vaginal *N. gonorrhoeae* and *C. trachomatis* sampling, and is often tested in the same collection specimen. Culture for *N. gonorrhoeae* is used as an alternative when NAAT tests are not available, when resistance testing is indicated,

when testing after a sexual assault in boys, or for oropharyngeal testing in children.[2] *Chlamydia* cultures have poor sensitivity and specificity and are not commonly used.

1. Review the indications for and process of specimen collection and obtain consent throughout.
2. Determine which collection process is appropriate for the clinical situation and acceptable to patient. This can include cervical collection with the use of a speculum, vaginal collection with or without the use of a speculum, and self-collection.
   a. For self-collected and provider-collected vaginal samples:
      i. Insert the Dacron swab approximately 2 inches into the vagina and gently rotate for 15–30 seconds.
      ii. Carefully remove the swab without allowing the cotton tip to touch skin or objects, and insert it immediately into the appropriate transport medium.
   b. For provider-collected samples:
      i. Don nonsterile gloves.
      ii. Insert a moistened speculum into the vagina and visualize the cervix.
      iii. Note the presence of any discharge or cervical irritation.
      iv. For a vaginal specimen, swab the upper vagina and posterior fornix for 15–30 seconds.
      v. For a cervical specimen, first remove any cervical mucus obscuring the os. Then insert the Dacron swab approximately 2 cm into the cervix and rotate for 5 seconds.
      vi. If collecting for cervical cytology, a single specimen is adequate for screening of chlamydia and gonorrhea.
      vii. Do not allow the cervical swab to touch the vaginal side walls while being removed.
      viii. Place the sample directly into the labeled transport medium.

## Procedure for Performing a Cervical Cytology Test

Liquid-based specimen collection (Papanicolaou, "Pap"), in which the specimen is collected at the cervix, has become the standard where available, due to the improved ability to interpret abnormalities it affords. This material can also be used for human papillomavirus (HPV) testing.[7] An extended-tip spatula plus endocervical brush technique or broom plus endocervical brush has been shown to provide the most accurate results, and should be used whenever available.[8,9] Self-collection of specimens for HPV testing can play an important role in improving access to screening for cervical cancer. This self-sampling is done in the same manner as described earlier for the self-collection of vaginal samples for *N. gonorrhoeae*, *C. trachomatis*, and trichomoniasis testing.

1. Discuss the indications for and process of cervical cytology testing and obtain consent throughout.
2. Don nonsterile gloves.
3. Insert a moistened speculum into the vagina and visualize the cervix.
4. If only a cytology test is being performed, a small amount of water-based gel can be used to lubricate the speculum.
5. Using a spatula or broom, sweep the cervix, rotating the spatula or broom 360 degrees to cover the entire ectocervix. An extended-tip spatula is the preferred device. If the squamocolumnar junction is visible, it should be included.
6. Remove the device without touching the vaginal sidewalls; rotate it gently in liquid medium to dislodge the cells, or roll it across a clean slide, depending on whether a liquid or dry collection method is used.
7. For dry specimens only: Place one flat side on the top half of the slide and stroke once to the end of the slide. Then turn the spatula or brush over and place the other flat side on the bottom half of the slide and stroke once to the end of the slide. If the specimen is too thick, take the edge of the device and, with a single light stroke down the slide, remove the excess.
8. Insert a cervical brush into the endocervix approximately 2 cm and rotate through 90 to 180 degrees.
9. Repeat the procedure for processing as in Steps 4 and 5.
10. If a dry technique is used, the specimen should immediately be fixed before transport to preserve cellular integrity.
11. This procedure should be performed on each cervix, if multiple cervices are present.

## Procedure for Performing an Anal Cytology Test or NAAT/Culture

When indicated, anal cytology testing may benefit some well-suited persons for cancer screening. In particular, persons who are HIV positive and who engage in receptive anal intercourse, have genital warts, or have a history of abnormal cervical cytology testing may benefit from such screening. However, there are currently no standardized guidelines on these tests' use. Anal cytology testing should be offered only in settings with adequate access to referral and follow-up as may be needed, including access to high-resolution anoscopy. For best results, use of douches, enemas, or anything in the anus should be avoided for the 24 hours prior to sampling.[10]

Unlike vaginal or cervical procedures, anal testing is commonly performed in a left-lateral position, with hips and knees flexed. From this position, the anal opening is visualized when the superior/right buttock is gently retracted.

1. Review the indications for and process of anal cytology testing and obtain consent throughout.

2. Don nonsterile gloves.

3. Moisten an appropriate Dacron or polyester-tipped swab with water and insert the swab 2–3 inches into the anus, so it is felt to be past the internal anal sphincter, and to the level of the squamocolumnar junction.

4. Rotate the swab around the 360 degrees of anal mucosa while applying firm lateral pressure, causing the swab to bow slightly; you may consider visualizing the sphincter as the fulcrum as you rotate the swab. Firm lateral pressure should enable the provider to sample the mucosa and avoid sampling rectal contents.

5. Slowly withdraw the swab over 15–30 seconds while continuing to rotate.

6. Promptly fix the sample as appropriate—onto a glass slide or agitated into a preservative-filled vial, as with cervical or vaginal testing.

### References

1. Centers for Disease Control and Prevention. STD prevention courses: national STD curriculum. https:// www.cdc.gov/std/training/courses.htm#train. Accessed February 11, 2022.

2. Centers for Disease Control and Prevention. Recommendation for the laboratory-based detection of *Chlamydia trachomatis* and *Neisseria gonorrhoeae* —2014. *MMWR.* 2014;63(RR02);1-19.

3. Lowe S, Saxe JM. *Microscopic Procedures for Primary Care Providers.* Philadelphia, PA: Lippincott Williams & Wilkins; 1999.

4. Centers for Disease Control and Prevention. CLIA law and regulations. https://wwwn.cdc.gov/CLIA/Regulatory/default.aspx. Accessed January 9, 2017.

5. Centers for Disease Control and Prevention. Sexually transmitted disease treatment guidelines, 2021. https://www.cdc.gov/std/treatment-guidelines/default.htm. Accessed August 17, 2022.

6. Association of Public Health Laboratories. Laboratory testing for *N. gonorrhea* and *C. trachomatis*. https://www.aphl.org/programs/infectious_disease/std/Pages/N-gonorrhoeae-and-C-trachomatis.aspx. Accessed August 4, 2022.

7. Hoda RS, Loukeris K, Abdul-Karim FW. Gynecologic cytology on conventional and liquid-based preparations: a comprehensive review of similarities and differences. *Diagn Cytopathol.* 2013;41(3):257-278. doi:10.1002/dc.22842.

8. Martin-Hirsch PL, Jarvis GG, Kitchener HC, Lilford R. Collection devices for obtaining cervical cytology samples. *Cochrane Database Syst Rev.* 2011;4.

9. Davis-Devine S, Day SJ, Anderson A, et al. Collection of the BD SurePath Pap Test with a broom device plus endocervical brush improves disease detection when compared to the broom device alone or the spatula plus endocervical brush combination. *CytoJournal.* 2008;6:4. doi:10.4103/1742-6413.45495.

10. University of California San Francisco Anal Dysplasia Clinic. Obtaining a specimen for anal cytology. *Anal Cancer Information,* 2014. https://analcancerinfo.ucsf.edu/obtaining-specimen-anal-cytology. https://analcancerinfo.ucsf.edu/obtaining-specimen-anal-cytology. Accessed September 22, 2021.

### Further Resources

William A, Williams M. A guide to performing pelvic speculum exams: a patient-centered approach to reducing iatrogenic effects. *Teach Learn Med.* 2013;25:383-391.

Schuiling KD, Likis FE, eds. *Women's Gynecologic Health.* 4th ed. Burlington, MA: Jones & Bartlett Learning; 2022.

CHAPTER

4

# Health Promotion Across the Lifespan

VICTORIA L. BAKER

*The editors acknowledge Kathryn Osborne*
*and Mary Ann Faucher, who were author of and contributor to this*
*chapter in previous editions.*

## Introduction

"Health is a state of complete physical, mental, and social well-being and not merely the absence of disease or infirmity."[1] This definition opens the Constitution of the World Health Organization (WHO), which was formed at the end of World War II, at a time when its founders might have been excused for some despondence and pessimism. They instead took a positive, holistic view of health—one that focuses on resilience and strengths, and one that shares a great deal with the midwifery view of pregnancy. Much as midwifery care assumes pregnancy is a healthy process, which midwives can support and promote, WHO defined health as a state of well-being, rather than as a series of diseases that need treatment.

This view of health opens the way for person-centered health promotion, rather than organization-centered disease treatment. Two decades later, the first international conference on the topic held by WHO defined health promotion as "the process of enabling people to increase control over, and to improve, their health."[2] Health promotion can be done with individuals and with populations, and this chapter addresses both approaches.

The levels of prevention are sometimes used to define where health promotion interventions operate. With this perspective, all care is preventive; even treatment aims to prevent further progression of existing disease. Where an intervention takes place in the timeline of disease progression defines whether the prevention is primary, secondary, or tertiary. Health promotion interventions fall earlier in that timeline and, therefore, are considered part of primary and secondary prevention (Table 4-1).[3]

## Clinical Health Promotion

### Components of Clinical Health Promotion

These definitions of the levels of prevention imply promoting health with individuals has related preventive clinical interventions:

- Counseling
- Screening
- Preventive medications
- Immunizations[4]

These interventions can provide the focus of a clinical encounter, such as in a screening physical examination or a pregnancy visit. Alternatively, health promotion interventions can be integrated into a problem-focused exam, such as a hypertension assessment, an asthma-related visit, or a dysuria concern.

### Counseling

#### Health Behavior Theories

Changing behavior is complex, and takes more than just knowing what must be done. Clinical health promotion includes counseling, which requires not only understanding the clinical content of healthy behaviors, but also having skills in using health behavior theory and cultural humility in helping persons to change behavior when they are ready to do so.

Health behavior models guide health promotion counseling.[5] One of the most useful is the Transtheoretical Model's Stages of Change (Table 4-2), which was developed and thoroughly studied in the 1990s, particularly in terms of addressing addictions.[6,7] The Stages of Change help clinicians intervene effectively, by addressing the needs of a person based on their stage. This theory is closely aligned with motivational interviewing techniques.[8] The theory and the techniques focus on meeting individuals where they are in their behavioral change journey and finding the right approach for their stage to help them meet healthy goals.

Other behavior theories also shed light on the process of behavior change and can guide the clinician in advising individuals about health decisions. When considering how to promote healthier behaviors, it can be easy to focus exclusively on the strengths and weaknesses of the *individual*. Social cognitive theory is salient in this setting because it includes the concept of reciprocal determinism, which highlights the *interaction* between the individual characteristics, the behavior, and the environment. Each of these factors contributes to the success or failure of an attempt to make a behavior change, and all must be accounted for in such attempts. Interventions should be considered in light of that interaction, as well as using the other useful concepts in the theory, shown in Table 4-3.[7]

Ecological models like Dahlgren and White's social determinants of health (SDoH)[9] bring out the many factors that can affect health behavior and outcomes that are not obvious in the clinical examination room (Figure 4-1). The characteristics at the center of the SDoH model are not modifiable, such as age and biologic sex. As you move into the outer shells, characteristics are modifiable, but less and less by the individual and more by larger and larger groups. Individual lifestyle factors include diet, sexual behaviors, addictions, physical activity, and coping skills. These behaviors are somewhat controlled by the individual, but are also very much affected by the outer shells. Social and community networks include churches, sports clubs, and the like. These resources are taken up (or not) by the individual, but offered by others. The outer shell, which comprises general socioeconomic, cultural, and environmental conditions, also has substantial

| Table 4-1 | Levels of Prevention |
| --- | --- |
| Primary prevention | Intervening before health effects occur, through measures such as vaccinations, altering risky behaviors (poor eating habits, tobacco use), and banning substances known to be associated with a disease or health condition |
| Secondary prevention | Screening to identify diseases in the earliest stages, before the onset of signs and symptoms, through measures such as mammography and regular blood pressure testing |
| Tertiary prevention | Managing disease after diagnosis to slow or stop disease progression through measures such as chemotherapy, rehabilitation, and screening for complications.[3] |

Centers for Disease Control and Prevention. *Prevention.* https://www.cdc.gov/pictureofamerica/pdfs/picture_of_america _prevention.pdf. Accessed December 10, 2022.

| Table 4-2 | Transtheoretical Model: Stages of Change | |
| --- | --- | --- |
| Stage | Definition | Potential Change Strategy |
| Precontemplation | Has no intention of taking action in the next 6 months | Increase awareness of need for change; personalize information about risks and benefits |
| Contemplation | Intends to take action in the next 6 months | Motivate; encourage making specific plans |
| Preparation | Intends to take action in the next 30 days and has taken some behavioral actions in this direction | Assist with developing and implementing concrete action plans; help set gradual goals |
| Action | Has changed behavior for less than 6 months | Assist with feedback, problem solving, social support, and reinforcement |
| Maintenance | Has changed behavior for more than 6 months | Assist with coping, reminders, finding alternative, avoiding slips/relapses (as applicable) |

National Cancer Istitute. *Theory at a Glance: A Guide for Health Promotion Practice.* 2nd ed. https://cancercontrol.cancer.gov/sites/default/files/2020-06/theory.pdf. Published 2005. Accessed December 10, 2022.

| Table 4-3 | Behavior Change Interventions Based on the Social Cognitive Theory | |
|---|---|---|
| **Concept** | **Definition** | **Potential Change Strategies** |
| Reciprocal determinism | The dynamic interaction of the person, the behavior, and the environment in which the behavior is performed | Consider multiple ways to promote behavior change, including making adjustments to the environment or influencing personal attitudes |
| Behavioral capability | Knowledge and skill to perform a given behavior | Promote mastery learning through skills training |
| Expectations | Anticipated outcomes of a behavior | Model positive outcomes of healthful behavior |
| Self-efficacy | Confidence in one's ability to take action and overcome barriers | Approach behavior change in small steps to ensure success; be specific about the desired change |
| Observational learning (modeling) | Behavioral acquisition that occurs by watching the actions and outcomes of others' behavior | Offer credible role models who perform the targeted behavior |
| Reinforcements | Responses to a person's behavior that increase or decrease the likelihood of reoccurrence | Promote self-initiated rewards and incentives |

Reproduced from National Cancer Institute. *Theory at a Glance: A Guide for Health Promotion Practice.* 2nd ed. https://cancercontrol .cancer.gov/sites/default/files/2020-06/theory.pdf. Published 2005. Accessed December 10, 2022.

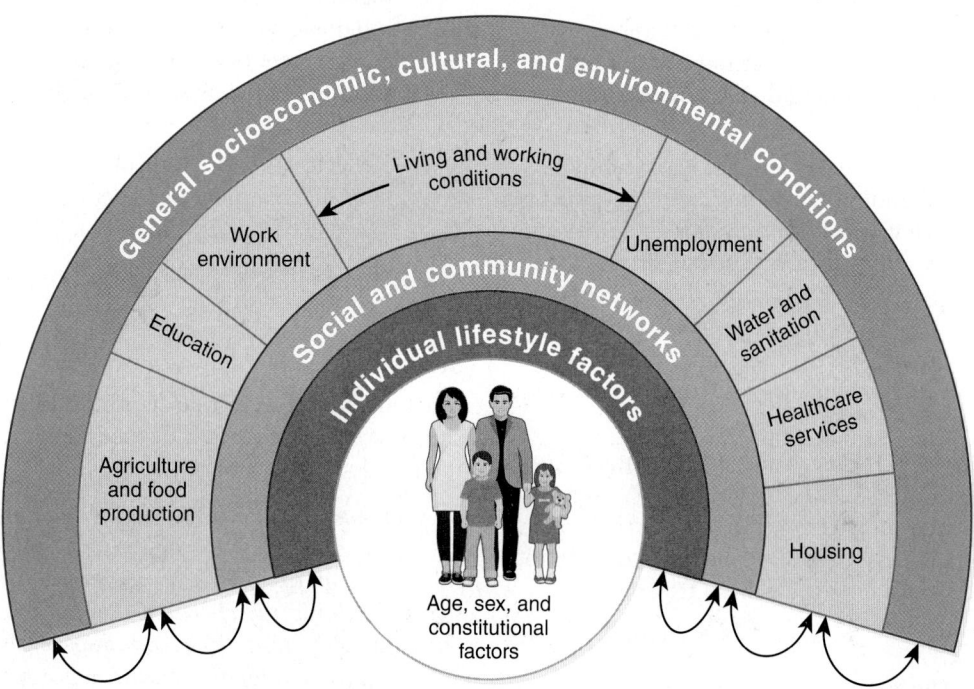

**Figure 4-1** The main determinants of health.
Reproduced with permission from Dahlgren G, Whitehead M. *European Strategies for Tackling Social Inequities in Health: Levelling Up (Part 2).* http://www.euro.who.int/__data/assets/pdf_file/0018/103824/E89384.pdf. Published 2006. Accessed December 10, 2022.

effects on health behavior and health outcomes. It includes conditions such as corn subsidies or taxes on sugary drinks, municipally subsidized recreation centers and walking trails, employer-sponsored

health centers, school lunches, and the like. These environmental characteristics change behavior in subtle ways. Clinicians can look beyond the examination room to help individuals become aware of the effects of SDoH and take advantage of the resources available to them. Using the SDoH framework helps a clinician remember to address factors that can either promote or detract from health, but that are not immediately apparent during a clinical examination. The Institute of Medicine urges all clinicians to take SDoH into account in delivering health care.[10]

### The 5 A's

Although this model was developed specifically for tobacco cessation counseling, the U.S. Preventive Services Task Force (USPSTF) recommends using the "5 A's" in any health behavior counseling.[11]

- **Assess:** Ask about and assess behavioral health risk(s) and factors affecting choice of behavior change goals and methods.
- **Advise:** Give clear, specific, and personalized behavior change advice, including information about personal health harms/benefits.
- **Agree:** Collaboratively select appropriate treatment goals and methods based on the patient's interest in and willingness to change the behavior.
- **Assist:** Using behavior change techniques (self-help and/or counseling), aid the patient in achieving agreed-upon goals by acquiring the skills, confidence, and social/environmental supports for behavior change, supplemented with adjunctive medical treatments when appropriate (e.g., pharmacotherapy for tobacco dependence, contraceptive drugs/devices).
- **Arrange:** Schedule follow-up contacts (in person or by telephone) to provide ongoing assistance/support and to adjust the treatment plan as needed, including referral to more intensive or specialized treatment.

### Cultural Humility

Cultural humility is the process of communication that supports "commitment and active engagement in a lifelong process that individuals enter into on an ongoing basis with patients, communities, colleagues, and with themselves."[12] This approach provides for more dynamic communication, focusing on interactions between individuals, rather than lists of the characteristics of groups. In addition, it incorporates the community context, allowing for a consideration of SDoH.

When primary care providers counsel patients about changing health behaviors, as in all health care, cultural humility plays an important role. For example, researchers have found that culturally tailored programs can improve outcomes in a wide range of behaviors, such as alcohol and other substance use,[13] mental health therapy,[14] counseling to increase physical activity,[15,16] and tobacco cessation.[17]

Cultural humility can be applied to individualized counseling using concrete action. The American Psychological Association has identified the following competencies for primary care psychologists, which are also applicable to midwives who provide counseling:[18]

- Asks about cultural identities, health beliefs, and illness history that impact health behaviors, and integrates and tailors diversity factors into treatment planning
- Demonstrates sensitivity to a variety of factors that influence health care (e.g., developmental, cultural, socioeconomic, gender, race, religious, sexual orientation and expression, gender identity and expression, disability, veteran status) as well as the intersections of these variables
- Reflects on own cultural identity and its impact on treatment of patients
- Modifies interventions for behavioral health change in response to a variety of social and cultural factors

### Screening

The long-standing, classic definition of screening for the prevention of chronic disease comes from a conference document from the 1950s:

*Screening is the presumptive identification of unrecognized disease or defect by the application of tests, examinations, or other procedures which can be applied rapidly. Screening tests sort out apparently well [emphasis added] persons who probably have a disease from those who probably do not. A screening test is not intended to be diagnostic. Persons with positive or suspicious findings must be referred to their physicians [sic] for diagnosis and necessary treatment.[19(p11)]*

Screening tests can take the form of lab tests, physical exams, or interviews. What they have in common is that they are indicated by the characteristics of the person, not symptoms; that is, screening is indicated by the population to which a person belongs, rather than by the concerns with which the person presents. Confusingly, sometimes the same tests are used for both screening and diagnosis. For example, an assessment for chlamydia is indicated when a person assigned female at birth has a vaginal discharge, but is also indicated for a 22-year-old person assigned female at birth at a routine visit. In the first case, the exam is diagnostic to determine the cause of vaginal discharge. In the second case, the chlamydia test is for screening as recommended for all sexually active persons assigned female at birth younger than 25 years. The same lab test is used in both cases—that is, for both screening and diagnosis.[20] For chlamydia, only the indication changes. Conversely, for tuberculosis, screening with the tuberculin skin test does not diagnose active tuberculosis. A positive result on the skin test requires further testing for diagnosis.[21]

Like the definition for screening, a common set of principles for when to screen a population has been universally accepted since the 1950s, and continues to underlie appropriate screening programs and clinical recommendations for screening.[22]

1. Screening should be for an important health problem with serious consequences. There is no point in screening for a problem with mild, short-term consequences for health.

2. Treatment for the condition screened should be effective or knowledge about the condition may be of use to a person. For example, genetic screening may offer valuable information for life planning even though no gene therapy is available.

3. Treatment for the condition screened should be available. There is no point in screening for a condition and then giving the person no options.

4. There should be a reasonable period of latency between when a screening test detects a condition and when signs or symptoms would appear. There is no point in screening if persons will be coming in shortly with concerns and asking for a diagnosis. Screening allows for an early start of treatment. Moreover, that early start should offer a chance for improved outcomes.

5. There should be a suitable test or examination. The test needs to be reliable and valid with acceptable sensitivity and specificity.

6. The screening test should be acceptable. There is no point in offering a test that no one will undergo.

7. The natural history of the condition, including its development from latent to actual disease, should be well understood.

8. What constitutes a diagnosis and who needs treatment should be clearly understood. When is a person considered to have diabetes? When should prostate cancer be treated? These are the kinds of questions that arise after positive screening test findings. Answers need to be clear before screening programs are undertaken.

9. Large population screening for chronic conditions such as hypertension and diabetes should be done at regular intervals—not just once, as in a single drive or fair. Most conditions will continue to come up, so a one-time screening program will not serve a population well.

10. The prevalence of the condition in a population needs to be high enough to warrant testing everyone in the group. Screening everyone for a rare condition will result in a larger proportion of false positives (discussed later in this section).

Screening has both risks and benefits, especially large public health screenings. Undertaking a screening program is a serious proposition, one that is expensive in terms of both money and the emotional burden imposed on those persons who are tested. It should not be undertaken without sufficient understanding of the likely outcomes and expected findings when a test is used on a large scale.

Most of these principles make sense to most clinicians. However, point 10 often needs more explanation. How can screening a population for a condition of low prevalence result in a higher proportion of false-positive test results? To some, this outcome is counterintuitive. Calculation of screening test values such as positive predictive value and negative predictive values are shown in Table 4-4. Grimes and Schultz do a superb job of explaining some of the harms of over-testing and the math behind population prevalence and false positives.[23]

To illustrate how this problem arises, Grimes and Schultz give the example of chlamydia screening for asymptomatic persons.[23] The screening test for chlamydia, polymerase chain reaction (PCR), is highly sensitive, correctly identifying those with disease 98% of the time, and highly specific, correctly identifying those without disease 97% of the time. Using typical prevalence statistics from populations at high versus low risk for sexually transmitted infections illustrates why *routine* chlamydia screening is not recommended universally. The examples here illustrate the risks of screening persons in a population with low prevalence for a disease compared to a higher prevalence. The chances of a true-positive result increase significantly with the higher prevalence population, from 13% to 57% (Table 4-5 and Table 4-6).[23] In populations where the prevalence is even higher, the chance of a true positive increases to 90% and greater. (The data used here differ somewhat from those used in the original article.)

There are potentially significant psychosocial implications of telling a person that they screened positive for chlamydia when they do not actually have this infection. What can a result like this mean to couples getting screened? It can mean one partner is certain that the other has had intercourse with someone else, when that has not been the case.

More is not always better. For other disease screenings, the follow-up diagnostic test may come with significant risks.

These examples make clear the importance of using evidence-based recommendations as the basis for recommending screening and of meeting the classic criteria for screening programs. Unfortunately, some screening tests become common practice even though they do not clearly meet these criteria. Grimes and Peipert give another example of how screening can be abused: Electronic fetal monitoring became a screening norm in labor even though it did not meet the standard criteria for a screening program.[24] Before performing a screening test, the clinician should ask, "Am I prepared to act on the information from this test?" If the answer is no, then the test probably does not meet the 10 principles of screening outlined earlier.

## Preventive Medications

When considering when to advise or prescribe preventive medications (i.e., chemoprophylaxis), just as with screening tests, an analysis of risks and benefits should be undertaken. Preventive medications can be used for primary prevention of disease—for example, prescribed medications such as statins, or vitamin and mineral supplements—or they can be used for secondary prevention—for example, chemoprophylactic drugs after breast cancer. Again, more is not always better. Just as not every screening test comes without risk, the same is true for potential preventive medications. For example, interactions with other therapeutic medications must be considered.

As with screening tests, risks and benefits of prescribing preventive medication change with the prevalence of disease in given populations. For example, the USPSTF recommendation for tamoxifen, raloxifene, or aromatase inhibitor for chemoprophylaxis in women older than 35 years supports use of these

| Table 4-4 | | Formulas for Calculating Screening Test Values | |
|-----------|--|-----------------------------|--|
| | | **True Disease State** | |
| | | **Positive** | **Negative** |
| **Test Results** | **Positive** | True positive a | False positive b |
| | **Negative** | c False negative | d True negative |

This table sets up the standard epidemiologic approach to calculating screening test values.

Sensitivity = a / (a + c)

Specificity = d / (b + d)

Positive predictive value = a / (a + b)

Negative predictive value = d / (c + d)

Data from Grimes DA, Schulz KF. Uses and abuses of screening tests. *Lancet.* 2002;359(9309):881-884. doi:10.1016/S0140-6736(02)07948-5.

| Table 4-5 | Calculating Screening Test Values in a High Prevalence Population | | |
|-----------|---------------------|---------------------|---------------------|
| **Test Results** | **Person Has Chlamydia** | **Person Does Not Have Chlamydia** | |
| Positive | 78 (True positive) | 38 (False positive) | 78/(78+38) = .67 Positive predictive value |
| Negative | 2 (False negative) | 1882 (True negative) | 1882/(2+1882) = .99 Negative predictive value |
| | 78/(78+2) = .98 Sensitivity | 1882/(38+1882)= .98 Specificity | |

These are the screening test values for a PCR chlamydia test in a population of 2000 persons with an 4% prevalence of chlamydia.

| Table 4-6 | Calculating Screening Test Values in a Low-Prevalence Population | |
|---|---|---|
| | **Presence of Chlamydia Population with 0.5% Prevalence** $n = 2000$ | |
| | **Positive** | **Negative** |
| **Test Results** **Positive** | True positive 10 a | False positive 40 b |
| **Negative** | c False negative 0 | d True negative 1950 |

These are the screening test values for a PCR chlamydia test in a population of 2000 persons with a 0.5% prevalence of chlamydia.

Sensitivity = a / (a + c) = 10 / (10 + 0) = 0.97 (1.00 with rounding)

Specificity = d / (b + d) = 1950 / (1950 + 40) = 0.98

Positive predictive value = a / (a + b) = 10 / (10 + 40) = 0.20

Negative predictive value = d / (c + d) = 1950 / (1950 + 0) = 1.00

Data from Grimes DA, Schulz KF. Uses and abuses of screening tests. *Lancet.* 2002;359(9309):881-884. doi:10.1016/S0140-6736(02)07948-5.

| Table 4-7 | Definitions Related to Immunity |
|---|---|
| Vaccination | The act of introducing a vaccine into the body to produce protection from a specific disease. |
| Immunization | A process by which a person becomes protected against a disease through vaccination. This term is often used interchangeably with vaccination or inoculation. |
| Community immunity | A situation in which a sufficient proportion of a population is immune to an infectious disease (through vaccination and/or prior illness), making the spread of that disease from person to person unlikely. Even individuals not vaccinated (such as newborns and those with chronic illnesses) are offered some protection because the disease has little opportunity to spread within the community. Also known as herd immunity.[27] |

Adapted from Centers for Disease Control and Prevention (CDC). Immunization: The basics. Published 2021. Accessed December 10, 2022. https://www.cdc.gov/vaccines/vac-gen/imz-basics.htm and Centers for Disease Control and Prevention. (2020, July 30). Vaccine glossary of terms. Retrieved December 10, 2022, from https://www.cdc.gov/vaccines/terms/glossary.html.

medications in those women with increased risk for breast cancer and recommends against them for those women not at increased risk.[25] Because of "convincing evidence" of risk for venous thrombolytic events, endometrial cancer, and other harms from these medications in older women, the population needs to be at higher risk for breast cancer for the supplements to offer enough benefit to warrant their use. Obviously, risks and benefits need to be discussed carefully with individuals before prescribing any medication or supplement for preventive purposes.

In other cases, midwives may recommend preventive medications without lengthy cost–benefit analysis discussions. For example, in the case of folic acid,[26] the adverse outcomes associated with taking this supplement appear to be minimal. Indeed, folic acid is a recommended daily nutrient. In addition, the benefits of folic acid supplementation for people who may become pregnant to protect against fetal neural tube defects are well established.

### Immunization

Table 4-7 defines important terms related to immunity. The definitions in Table 4-7 make it clear that vaccines are simply a preventive medication. However, community immunity concerns make the benefit–risk

analysis for a vaccination different than the analysis undertaken when an individual will be taking a medication. An individual can accrue the benefit of protection from infection via community immunity without assuming any risk associated with vaccination if the rest of the community gets vaccinated. Conversely, when an individual decides not to become vaccinated, that decision poses risks to more than their own health—that is, it creates the risk of infecting others.

In addition, because vaccinations prevent infectious disease, they often bring up public health and legal issues that spark controversy. They are treated separately from other preventive medication, both in clinical encounters and in public perceptions. By comparison, folic acid supplementation is not required in any workplace or school setting, so its use is less controversial. Recommendations for vaccinations are fairly complex and are made by the Centers for Disease Control and Prevention's (CDC's) Advisory Committee on Immunization Practices (ACIP).[28]

Since vaccine coverage affects population health, recommendations for their use can generate health policies and legal issues. All states require some vaccinations for children to attend school or daycare facilities, although all states do allow for some exemptions.[29] Some vaccinations are required for immigration into the United States,[30] or even to visit the United States.[31] These policies have been partly responsible for the very high rates of vaccination and very low rates of vaccine-preventable infectious diseases in the United States. Perhaps in part because of these conditions, impositions of vaccinations upon generations who have not experienced the targeted infections' morbidity and mortality often generate resistance. This resistance is called *vaccine hesitancy*, the "delay in acceptance or refusal of vaccines despite availability of vaccine services."[32]

Counseling for vaccine-hesitant individuals can be complicated. Fortunately, in view of the public health concerns raised by it, the issue of vaccine hesitancy has been intensely studied, with a wealth of information on the effectiveness of interventions being available to clinicians who seek to increase vaccine coverage among their patients.[32-35] In general, multipronged strategies work better than single-component approaches. So, the combination of dialogue in the clinical setting and community-based engagement (particularly religious or other community leaders) works better than either does alone. Passive interventions (reminders, posters) help mostly when the problem is not hesitancy but rather lack of information. Providing information routinely during encounters and providing information targeted to each person's concerns seems to work better than more general educational approaches. Community health workers may be able to decrease hesitancy. In summary, person-centered approaches and trust are key to addressing vaccine hesitancy.

## Evidence for Health Promotion Interventions

### U.S. Preventive Services Task Force

The USPSTF consists of a volunteer panel of experts in prevention and evidence-based health who conduct systematic reviews and produce recommendations graded on the basis of the evidence. The USPSTF is the most comprehensive and easily accessible source of systematic reviews evaluating health promotion interventions. It has published its reviews as more than 100 recommendations for counseling, screening, and preventive health care.[36] These recommendations influence whether the prevention interventions are reimbursed by Medicare and Medicaid, and other health insurers.[36] It should be noted that USPSTF is currently grappling with its use of sex and gender terms; going forward, specificity of the population will be discussed and the terms used to describe it will be decided on at the beginning of the guideline review or development process.[37]

Currently, guidelines use the term "woman," which in most instances is based on biologic effects of being born female.

Recommendations follow a specific format. They grade the strength of the evidence and whether it supports use of the intervention (Table 4-8).[38] All recommendations appear both online and in journals (previously the *Annals of Internal Medicine*, currently the *Journal of the American Medical Association*). Recommendations that relate to one another typically are published together, although the recommendations can earn different grades or address different interventions. Validated tools that help carry out interventions are also provided.

The USPSTF considers two questions in making health promotion counseling recommendations: "Do interventions in the clinical setting influence persons to change their behavior?" and "Does changing health behavior improve health outcomes with minimal harms?"[39] Many recommendations seem very reasonable to clinicians, fitting well with previous training. Others surprise clinicians. All merit careful review of the rationale, which is clearly and completely presented.

Midwives should know all the recommendations made by the USPSTF addressing the clinical population served in their practice and should use them in health promotion encounters. The USPSTF provides a free mobile application for use in clinical agencies, which is very helpful in the clinical setting[40] (see the Resources section at the end of this chapter).

### Centers for Disease Control and Prevention

The CDC also provides relevant screening guidelines and recommendations for the populations cared for by midwives. Specifically, it offers guidelines related to screening and treating sexually transmitted infections (discussed in the *Reproductive Tract and Sexually Transmitted Infections* chapter) as well as those related to vaccinations.

### Advisory Committee on Immunization Practices

National recommendations for immunization recommendations come from a panel of medical and public health professionals, ACIP, which advises the CDC on immunization recommendations.[28] The CDC reviews and publishes the recommendations. ACIP makes recommendations across the lifespan, including for adults, pregnant persons, and neonates.

The ACIP publishes childhood, adolescent, adult, and catch-up vaccination recommendations and schedules, which it updates annually and as needed. It also publishes numerous other resources

| Table 4-8 | United States Preventive Services Task Force Grade Definitions | |
|---|---|---|
| Grade | Definition | Suggestions for Practice |
| A | The USPSTF recommends the service. There is high certainty that the net benefit is substantial. | Offer or provide this service. |
| B | The USPSTF recommends the service. There is high certainty that the net benefit is moderate or there is moderate certainty that the net benefit is moderate to substantial. | Offer or provide this service. |
| C | The USPSTF recommends selectively offering or providing this service to individual patients based on professional judgment and patient preferences. There is at least moderate certainty that the net benefit is small. | Offer or provide this service for selected patients depending on individual circumstances. |
| D | The USPSTF recommends against the service. There is moderate or high certainty that the service has no net benefit or that the harms outweigh the benefits. | Discourage the use of this service. |
| I | The USPSTF concludes that the current evidence is insufficient to assess the balance of benefits and harms of the service. Evidence is lacking, of poor quality, or conflicting, and the balance of benefits and harms cannot be determined. | Read the clinical considerations section of the USPSTF recommendation statement. If the service is offered, patients should understand the uncertainty about the balance of benefits and harms. |

Abbreviation: USPSTF, U.S. Preventive Services Task Force.

U.S. Preventive Services Task Force. Grade definitions. https://www.uspreventiveservicestaskforce.org/uspstf/about-uspstf/methods-and-processes/grade-definitions. Accessed December 11, 2022.

for consumers and clinicians, and updates on vaccines shortages.[41]

Midwives in the United States should know all the recommendations for neonates, adolescents, and adults made by the ACIP. Vaccine-related counseling and recommendations are within the scope of midwifery practice. The ACIP provides a free mobile application that is very helpful.[42]

## Other Sources of Evidence

The American Academy of Family Practice's (AAFP's) Commission on Health of the Public and Science develops clinical preventive services recommendations.[43] This volunteer group of family physicians reviews the USPSTF recommendations and determines whether they agree with the conclusions reached based on the evidence presented. If they do not, they write separate conclusions and publish them on the AAFP website. In light of the occasionally controversial conclusions reached by the USPSTF, the AAFP Commission provides an interesting counterpoint.

The Women's Preventive Services Initiative (WSPI) publishes and updates guidelines every 5 years with support from the federal Health Resources and Services Administration.[44] At the time of writing, the WSPI had published 13 recommendations based

on systematic reviews of evidence, including the USPSTF recommendations.[45] The WSPI also reaches out to clinicians, including providing the Well-Woman Chart with a summary of its recommendations[46] (see the Resources section at the end of the chapter).

Naturally, maintaining current knowledge in the clinical practice of midwifery will include knowledge of health promotion interventions. This includes clinical bulletins from the American College of Nurse-Midwives and a subscription to the *Journal of Midwifery and Women's Health*. In addition, the American Academy of Pediatrics (AAP) makes its recommendations available through its website and also publishes them in *Pediatrics*. The American College of Obstetricians and Gynecologists (ACOG) provides clinical updates in the form of practice bulletins, practice advisories, and committee opinions in its journal *Obstetrics and Gynecology*. While not systematic reviews, ACOG provides uniformly well-researched clinical information that often address health promotion concerns. All three organizations work together on some screening recommendations, such as those related to group B streptococcal screening, which were published as an ACOG Committee Opinion.[47] The Midwives Alliance for North America publishes data on the safety of home births.

## Decision Making in the Face of Ambiguity

### General Approach to Decision Making in Health Promotion

*Stay person-centered.* Remember that the client makes the decision, usually with professional guidance. Use skills in cultural humility and behavioral change theories. Remember who makes the decisions about their own lives. Shared decision making includes both informed consent and informed refusal.[48]

*Practice consistently.* Practice partners should decide as a group which interventions they want to recommend to their clients—that is, which screening tests, preventive medications, and immunizations and the general content of counseling they will provide. If one partner is recommending one intervention at one visit and another makes different recommendations at the next, it creates unnecessary confusion for the patient and frustrating revisitation of decisions. When establishing a consistent approach, practices should consider evidence, the practice partners' concerns, and the populations commonly served, in terms of both cultural and common health concerns. Professional standards, such as the *Standards for the Practice of Midwifery*, call for this approach, requiring that "midwifery care is based upon knowledge, skills, and judgments which are reflected in written practice guidelines and are used to guide the scope of midwifery care and services provided to clients."[49]

*Use evidence.* Be ready to tell clients why a given intervention is recommended and on what evidence it is based. Be ready to share the details with those who want it, while keeping in mind the health literacy of the individual. An ACOG Bulletin written in technical language may not be understandable to lay persons.[50] Another excellent source of information for consumers is the *Share with Women* (now called *Ask the Midwife*) handouts produced by the *Journal of Midwifery and Women's Health,* which are regularly reviewed and updated. The CDC provides excellent consumer handouts for many health promotion topics on its website. In terms of time spent counseling, it is important to know whether evidence supports devoting time to counseling for this content in an ambulatory visit.

*Be ready for the individual patient.* Even when a practice has done all its homework and planned ahead, every encounter provides a new challenge. Be ready to apply evidence and clinical information to the person in front of you, whose needs may not fit the evidence or recommendations available.

### Official Disagreement in Recommendations

Clinicians do not always enjoy the luxury of clear guidance from recommendations made by reputable sources. For example, reputable sources have provided both clinicians and consumers with conflicting recommendations and generated controversy over reimbursement for breast cancer screening. Breast self-examination (BSE) was a mainstay of nursing education for many years. Then in 2010, the USPSTF released a D recommendation against it, along with an increase in the recommended age to begin mammograms from 40 to 50 years and a decrease in the recommended frequency of mammograms from 1 to 2 years.[51] Details about the data used to make these recommendations are beyond the scope of this text, but they focused on the ability of screening to detect cancer earlier and to decrease mortality. The American Cancer Society, ACOG, the American College of Radiology, and the Susan G. Komen Foundation all disagreed with the USPSTF mammogram recommendations and the effects they could have on reimbursement. These agencies created a national controversy over recommendations that rarely catch the attention of consumers, and successfully lobbied Congress to keep screening mammograms free for women in their 40s.[52,53] In 2016, after analyzing new research, the USPSTF made a C recommendation for mammography in women ages 40 to 49 years; it also withdrew the D recommendation for BSE in favor of a vaguer statement that women should be aware of bodily changes, including breast self-awareness, and report changes to their clinician.[54,55] Teaching breast self-awareness can be part of the midwifery philosophy to help people learn about their bodies and become experts for their body. However, in an environment of shorter visits, the midwife needs to decide which screening and counseling has the priority for *this* visit with *this* person.

Conflicting recommendations, no recommendations, or recommendations reporting insufficient evidence provide the clinician with opportunities for guiding clients through health information and health promotion decision making. How do midwives decide what is the right approach for patient counseling when the recommendations vary and lawmakers say they are making policies so individuals "can get mammograms if they and their doctors [sic] decide it's the right thing to do"?[53] Use of screening tests is not always the best choice for the reasons discussed previously, such as the health and psychological costs related to false-positive results and the follow-up tests and procedures needed to confirm they are indeed false positives. A thorough review for clinicians on the choices and accompanying risks and benefits for breast cancer screening approaches was done by Khan and Chollet.[56]

Even when the evidence is clear and agencies agree, recommendations do not always fit every individual person. Just as recommendations must be tailored to fit individual circumstances, so should clinicians tailor approaches to counseling about them. A person-centered approach means working as a partner with clients to help them make well-informed decisions about health promotion interventions. In addition, evidence from the Stages of Change model demonstrates that real behavior change happens when clinicians meet people where they are in their complicated, busy, and sometimes difficult lives.[6,57] Several shared decision-making models can help clinicians through the process[48] (see the Resources section for more information).

- When guidelines vary, some clients do not want to know about the controversy. The same is true when guidelines do not take the particular person's circumstances or characteristics in account. Some clients simply want to know the opinion of their own provider and to follow it. They trust their provider's expertise and want to use it. With those clients, it is fine to mention that not all agencies give the same recommendations, and to give the midwife's own choice along with a rationale.

- Other clients want to dive into the depths and decide for themselves. For these individuals, review the available choices in detail, including the pros and cons of each, preferably with a printed handout or an electronic link for home review.

- Many persons fall somewhere in between these extremes and want some help in making a decision of their own. Let each individual guide you on how much information they want.

It does not denote failure on the part of a clinician if their client chooses to follow a different recommendation than the clinician favors. Supporting clients in their decisions and helping them to see how they came to such choices supports them in their journey to health.[48]

## Insufficient Evidence for Official Recommendations

Many of the USPSTF recommendations earn a grade of "I" for insufficient evidence, denoting that either studies have not been done or the studies that have been done on the usefulness of the intervention have not yielded clear enough results to recommend its routine use. Many of these recommendations go even further, first giving an I grade to the general population and then offering epidemiologic information on which groups are at higher risk of the health condition of concern. It can be hard to decide what to do with these recommendations.

The 2020 I grade recommendation about screening for drug use (with interview questions) among adolescents provides a good example. The recommendation says evidence for screening adolescents for unhealthy drug use is "insufficient to assess the balance of benefits and harms."[58] A little further on in the recommendation under "Practice Considerations," the recommendation adds that "some factors are associated with a higher prevalence of unhealthy drug use [including] having a mental health condition, personality or mood disorder, or nicotine or alcohol dependence; a history of physical or sexual abuse, parental neglect, or other adversity in childhood; or drug or alcohol addiction in a first-degree relative." No change in the grade of the recommendation is given for these populations. What should a clinician do? Should midwives recommend this screening to persons from those populations? The authors of the recommendation do not give any guidance on this front; they simply pass on the epidemiologic information they gathered in their review of the evidence.

This question provides a good starting point for discussion among partners in a practice. Given the uncertainty of benefits and harms, which opportunities for health promotion do the partners hope this screening test will offer for this population? Which harms might accrue? Does the practice serve a substantial number of teens at higher risk? If so, are those the only teens who should be screened? Some of those risk factors are easy to miss—so maybe all teens should be screened? As noted earlier, coming to a practice-wide agreement on whether to routinely screen for a specific concern will reduce confusion among clients and reduce the chances of any particular person feeling singled out or confused by conflicting information.

## Official Recommendations That Are Counterintuitive

Some USPSTF recommendations repudiate previous training, and some clinicians find them difficult to implement. For example, the 2022 C grade recommendation for counseling related to diet and activity in primary care settings[59] recommends that clinicians individualize the decision to counsel on these topics to adults without a chronic disease in primary care settings. This includes during a screening examination, when this counseling was previously a staple component of the encounter. According to the USPSTF recommendation, studies have found that counseling in these encounters results in only a small amount of behavior change and any such change is short-lived. Time would be better spent, the authors report, on other activities.

When put in those plain terms, the recommendation does not seem quite so revolutionary. In fact, most people already know they should eat healthful food and get exercise. They hear it on the news, on talk shows, and at school. It does make some sense that if individuals do not have a chronic disease, a clinical provider might not be giving them any new information, or that in the absence of a chronic disease, they might not feel sufficient motivation to change their behavior due to clinical advice about diet and exercise. When considered in those terms, the study results fit well with what we know about the Stages of Change model and person-centered counseling. What is required of clinicians is to read each recommendation carefully to see what message it really brings, what evidence it compiles, and how that fits into a particular practice. Naturally, if an individual asks about healthy diet and exercise, clinical advice is definitely in order.

### No Official Recommendations Made

Many worthy topics related to health promotion have not been studied or had reviews on them published, particularly in terms of counseling and preventive medication. For example, for many health promotion topics, evidence has accrued that a behavior promotes health, but no evidence has surfaced that primary care counseling will promote increases in that healthy behavior. Many possible preventive medications have not been well studied for their effects or side effects. Moreover, the USPSTF and other agencies have not carried out systematic reviews on these topics. For example, USPSTF gives an I rating to seat belt use, but ACOG, AAP, and AAFP all have statements recommending population-specific counseling on seat belt and car seat safety.

Counseling on sleep habits provides another good example. Poor sleep, defined as either short duration or poor quality, is a highly prevalent and serious problem. Sleep deprivation and sleep disorders are associated with greater risk of heart attack, stroke, hypertension, diabetes, metabolic syndrome, obesity, depression, and mortality.[60] The American Academy of Sleep Medicine has summarized data showing the importance of sleep to cognition, safety-related performance, memory, mood, nociception, and brain metabolism. It recommends that adults get at least 7 hours of sleep for optimal health.[61] One-third of adults in the United States sleep less than this recommendation.[62] Sleep apnea may affect 10% of the population and has similar health associations.[63] Poor sleep in pregnancy is associated with increased rates of gestational diabetes, preeclampsia, preterm birth, and stillbirth.[64]

While recommendations for interventions to improve sleep exist, studies of their effectiveness vary in their results. Studies of brief counseling about these interventions demonstrate little or no effect on behavior change. One review identified interventions found useful in specific populations, such as hospitalized patients, children, and elderly persons.[65] This report found that reducing stimuli before retiring, cognitive-behavioral therapy, aromatherapy, relaxation techniques, and controlling the sleep environment all have some evidence to support their usefulness. The same report stated that sleep education had a modest effect on knowledge about healthy sleep, but no evidence for behavior change at follow-up. Pharmacologic treatments,[66] cognitive-behavioral therapy,[67] exercise,[67] and (perhaps) music[68] have all been found effective to treat insomnia. The CDC recommends some simple habits to improve sleep quality, known as sleep hygiene. These habits include going to bed and getting up at the same time consistently, being in bed at least 7 hours, keeping sleeping areas completely dark, and removing electronic devices from sleeping areas.[69] Providing this kind of sleep education for those clients who report poor sleep seems most feasible in an ambulatory patient encounter.

Sleep hygiene counseling and screening for most sleep disorders are topics that have not yet been addressed by the USPSTF. No recommendation gives a grade on whether counseling on sleep habits is likely to result in a change in behavior, or, more to the point, better health outcomes. The USPSTF provides an I grade recommendation for screening for sleep apnea and does not makes recommendations for screening for other sleep disorders.[63] This does not mean that neither screening nor counseling helps patients with sleep-related issues. Rather, it means that the clinician who wishes to screen for sleep duration, sleep quality, sleep apnea, or other sleep disorders, or who wishes to counsel about this topic routinely, does so without the support of a recommendation based on strong evidence. If better evidence were available, would it show that counseling on this topic is, like counseling on diet and physical activity, a grade C recommendation, apparently addressing something most people already know? Or, would sleep counseling turn out more like tobacco cessation, a grade A recommendation, where talking about it at an encounter has been found to help? Does screening constitute a good use of clinical time? There is not yet enough evidence to guide healthcare providers. It is up to clinicians to decide whether to discuss these interventions, perhaps based on the individuals or populations they serve and the amount of time they have in an encounter.

### Rapidly Changing Situations

Occasionally, evidence does not keep up with a changing situation. In those cases, clients depend on the expertise of their clinical providers more than ever to help interpret the data from myriad sources, not all of them trustworthy. COVID-19 provides a recent example of this situation.

The SARS-CoV-2 virus was novel enough that treatment for infection with it was difficult to design,[70] and both community-based and hospital-based infection reduction measures were hard to establish.[71,72] Initial death rates were astonishing and terrifying, both in the United States[73] and globally.[74] The speed with which several versions of a vaccine against the virus were designed and produced was unprecedented.[70] This very quickly changing clinical picture made it challenging to advise individuals about health promotion choices related to the virus. When the first COVID-19 vaccine became available in December 2020, the data were not clear about whether vaccination was the best choice for pregnant persons. COVID-19 in pregnancy was extremely dangerous, but the vaccine was not initially tested on this population.[75] Individuals had to decide what was more dangerous, the possibility of contracting the infection and its possible sequelae or the possible effect of the vaccine on the fetus or the pregnancy. Clinicians could not provide clear data to answer these questions.

In terms of advising a client, this presented a similar problem to the dilemma of conflicting official recommendations, although the issue was changing data in the case of COVID-19 vaccines. Individuals knew that no official recommendation had been issued for vaccinations for pregnant persons and no studies had been done in this population. Some persons might want to simply follow their clinician's recommendation. Some might ask for information and make their own decision. Most persons will fall somewhere in between. The main difference between this and other situations involving ambiguous recommendations is that the midwife has a clinical responsibility to stay current in a rapidly changing situation and be ready to pass on high-quality information and give its source.

## Health Promotion Topics

### Actual Causes of Death

Year after year, the leading causes of death in the United States include heart disease, cancer, and accidents.[76] But, for decades, scholars have explained that these causes of death—that is, what appears on death certificates—are not the *actual* causes of death. In 1979, the U.S. Surgeon General publicized findings that behavior (50%) and environment (20%) had a much larger effect on health outcomes than clinical services (10%) or genetics (20%).[77] In 1993, the *Journal of the American Medical Association* published a landmark study on the "Actual Causes of Death in the United States," which showed the top three to be tobacco use, diet and physical activity, and alcohol use.[78] By this, the authors meant that these modifiable behaviors were the actual causes of death, not what was directly reported on death certificates. As they pointed out, tobacco, diet, exercise, and alcohol are all implicated in heart disease and cancer, and alcohol is a prime etiology in injury deaths. These findings were replicated 7 years later.[79] Currently, opioids might find a place in the top three actual causes of death.

Both of the reports stressed the importance of preventive services, such as health promotion over curative treatments. An exception may be opioid deaths, which are fueled by a complex lack of mental health treatment resources as well as a lack of substance use disorder treatment facilities. Fortunately, these issues can be addressed with evidence-based interventions throughout the continuum of care provided by midwives.

### Tobacco

For the last three decades, scholars have recognized tobacco as the major cause of preventable mortality in the United States, accounting for about 480,000 deaths annually.[80] Tobacco causes death through its close links to cancers, cardiovascular and respiratory diseases, and diabetes, and it causes other lethal and nonlethal conditions as well.[80] Although the prevalence of adult smokers has decreased since the 1990s,[80] an estimated 19% of adults in the United States use tobacco products currently.[80] The vast majority of adult cigarette smokers started before they were 18 years old, making prevention among children particularly important.

Electronic cigarettes are a source of new concern in tobacco addiction. Most e-cigarettes contain nicotine, which is the addictive substance of cigarettes that can damage the developing brain of adolescents.[81] There is substantial evidence that e-cigarettes are addictive.[82] Since the 1990s, youth have smoked fewer cigarettes, but their use of e-cigarettes has increased.[81] Use of e-cigarettes in youth is associated with smoking cigarettes in adulthood.[83] In addition, the delivery system of e-cigarettes, vaping, has been associated with lung injuries.[83]

Recommendations are available for both tobacco prevention cessation and prevention. For children and adolescents, the USPSTF provides a B-grade recommendation to counsel against initiation of tobacco use, but an I-grade recommendation to screen for use and counsel on cessation.[82] The USPSTF gives its only A-grade counseling recommendation on tobacco: It calls for screening adults, including in pregnancy, about tobacco use and providing counseling on cessation to those who do.[82] It advises the use of the "5 A's" and a menu of other approaches to counsel adults about cessation of tobacco use. This includes physician or nurse advice, phone- and mobile app–based advice, counseling, and pregnancy-specific advice.

Although brief, individual counseling alone can be effective for tobacco cessation, longer-term counseling interventions and pharmacotherapy achieve the best results.[84] To achieve the best results, the brief intervention of the 5 A's will lead to referral for at least four to eight counseling sessions, along with use of pharmacologic agents such as bupropion hydrochloride sustained release, nicotine replacement, or varenicline. Many states have websites and telephone resources with information on where to get free pharmacotherapy and counseling (see the Resources section at the end of the chapter).

### Healthy Weight, Diet, and Physical Activity

Obesity is a severe problem for the United States, which affects more than 40% of adults[85] and almost 19% of children and adolescents. Obesity is associated with serious conditions, including heart disease, type 2 diabetes, respiratory diseases, and cancer as well as increased mortality.[86] Evidence indicates that increased physical activity and dietary changes can reduce both weight and the risk of the conditions associated with obesity.[86] See the *Skillful Communication to Mitigate Clinician Bias* appendix for an in-depth discussion of how to counsel with sensitivity.

The USPSTF provides B-grade recommendations to screen for obesity and offer referrals for comprehensive behavioral interventions to lose weight to obese children, adolescents, and adults.[86,87] These recommendations call for comprehensive behavioral interventions, lasting 1 to 2 years, often with core phases followed by support phases. For overweight adults, the recommendation is to "individualize the decision to provide or refer to behavioral counseling." For children, evidence suggests intensive interventions that last 2 to 12 months, shorter than for adults, but still over an extended course. These recommendations offer the opportunity to employ the 5 A's, which include assisting and arranging for these more intensive counseling interventions.

For adults with cardiovascular risk factors, the USPSTF provides a grade-B recommendation to counsel individuals to consume a healthful diet and engage in physical activity.[88] This recommendation defines risk for cardiovascular disease as adults with hypertension, dyslipidemia, or multiple risk factors leading to a 10-year risk equal to or higher than 7.5% using a risk assessment tool such as the Pooled Cohort Equations.[89] The intervention recommended is to counsel the individual to eat a diet low in saturated fats, salt, and sugar and high in fruits, vegetables, and whole grains. Counseling for physical activity should encourage the individual to engage in 90 to 180 minutes of moderate to vigorous physical activity over the course of a week. After that, individuals should be referred to more intensive counseling, with one-on-one time with a trained counselor over time. Family members may be included. Again, the 5 A's may be beneficial in an encounter of this sort.

The USPSTF recommendation for counseling on healthy diet[88] refers clinicians to federal guidelines on diet as an appropriate counseling resource (Figure 4-2; also see the Resources section). These guidelines suggest that individuals "start simple" by using the "MyPlate" tool, and offer some simple suggestions to increase their intake of fruits, vegetables, and whole grains and vary their sources of proteins. MyPlate tools include the use of the infographic shown in Figure 4-2 and smartphone applications that help with grocery shopping and meal planning. The *Dietary Guidelines for Americans*[90] go into more detail on how to achieve these behaviors, such as paying attention to portion size. (See the *Nutrition* chapter for further discussion.)

Counseling should also include encouragement of physical activity.[86–88] In addition to helping individuals maintain a healthy weight, it has many

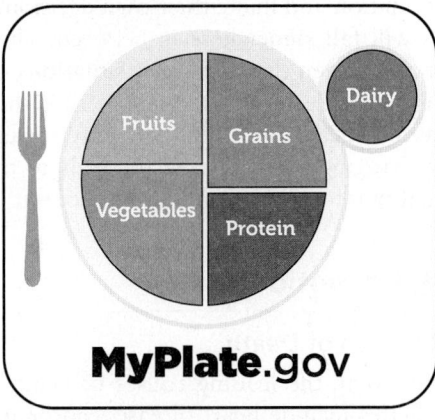

**Figure 4-2** MyPlate symbol of the five good groups.
Used with permission. MyPlate graphics. https://www.myplate.gov/resources/graphics/myplate-graphics.

other health benefits, such as bone health, cognition, protection against cancer, improved perinatal outcomes, fall reductions in the elderly, reduced mortality, and improved quality of life.[91,92] The *Physical Activity Guidelines for Americans* provide goals for people of different ages and with different conditions, including pregnancy, as well as some guidance for behavior change in this area.[92]

For adults of healthy weight without cardiovascular risk factors, the USPSTF does not recommend routinely discussing healthy diet and physical activity, a C-grade recommendation.[93] This seems counterintuitive to many clinicians. Doesn't an annual examination offer the opportunity for exactly that sort of discussion of healthy habits such as diet and exercise? The review for the recommendation presents evidence that unsolicited advice on diet and exercise provided in clinical encounters does not result in lasting changes in diet or exercise. However, midwives should provide such information to individuals who request it.

### Alcohol and Illicit Drugs

The United States has a "serious substance misuse problem"—that is, a problem with "the use of alcohol or drugs in a manner, situation, amount, or frequency that could cause harm to the user or to those around them."[94(p1-1)] In 2019, 26% of U.S. adults reported binge drinking in the previous month.[95] Approximately 5% (14.5 million persons) of all people in the United States 12 years and older have alcohol use disorder, including 2% of all adolescents. About 10% of U.S. children live with a parent who has alcohol use disorder.[96] Among persons 12 to 20 years old, approximately 2.2% report heavy alcohol use in the past month.[97] Emergency department visits have been on the rise and 19% of them are related to alcohol.[98] Annual mortality due to alcohol is about 95,000 persons in the United States.[95] Alcohol consumption, sometimes even small amounts, contributes to morbidity and mortality from both intentional and unintentional injuries including suicides.[99] In 2019, alcohol contributed to the 85,688 deaths from liver disease that occurred in the United States.[95] It also increases the risk of some cancers,[100] heart disease, depression, and stroke,[95] as well as fetal alcohol syndrome if used in pregnancy.[95] U.S. alcohol-related mortality doubled between 1999 and 2017.[101]

Substance misuse involving illicit drugs and prescription medications in the United States is associated with an equally bleak picture. Similar to the case with alcohol, individuals driving under the influence of drugs[102] have an increased risk of intentional and unintentional injuries.[94] The rate of

opioid overdose mortality in particular has skyrocketed over the two decades, increasing 345% between 2001 and 2016, from 33 to 131 deaths per million population.[103] Rates have continued to rise in more recent years, with adults between ages 25 and 45 most likely to die of this cause.[104]

Evidence supports screening adults for "risky or hazardous" drinking and then providing "brief behavioral interventions" as indicated in a primary care setting, a B-grade recommendation.[105] The screening tools recommended are short—one to three questions. One recommended tool is the Single Alcohol Screening Question (SASQ). A "yes" response can indicate a significant alcohol use disorder. The abbreviated Alcohol Use Disorders Identification Test–Consumption (AUDIT-C) has 10 questions, but only the first three apply to alcohol consumption (see Table 4-9 and the Resources section). Scores range from 0 to 12, with the cut-off for a positive screen being a score of 4 or greater in men and a score of 3 or greater in women.

| Table 4-9 | Screening Questions for Unhealthy Alcohol Use |
|---|---|

**Single Alcohol Screening Question (SASQ)[107]**

A single-question screener: "How many times in the past year have you had five or more drinks in a day (for males) or four or more drinks in a day (for females)?"

**Alcohol Use Disorders Identification Test–Consumption (AUDIT-C)[108]**

1. How often do you have a drink containing alcohol?

   *Never = 0; monthly or less = 1; 2–4 times/month = 2; 3–4 times/week =3; >4 times/week = 4*

2. How many drinks containing alcohol do you have on a typical day you are drinking?

   *0–2 = 0; 3–4 =1; 5–6 = 3; 7–9 =3; >10 =4*

3. How often do you have x (5 for males; 4 for females and for males older than age 65) or more drinks on one occasion?

   *Never = 0; monthly or less = 1; monthly = 2; weekly = 3; daily or almost daily = 4*

Based on Smith PC, Schmidt SM, Allensworth-Davies D, Saitz R. Primary care validation of a single-question alcohol screening test. *J Gen Intern Med.* 2009;24(7):783-788. doi:10.1007/s11606-009-0928-6 and Bush K, Kivlahan DR, McDonell MB, Fihn SD, Bradley KA. The AUDIT Alcohol Consumption Questions (AUDIT-C): An effective brief screening test for problem drinking. Ambulatory care quality improvement project (ACQUIP). Alcohol Use Disorders Identification Test. *Arch Intern Med.* 1998;158(16):1789-1795. doi:10.1001/archinte.158.16.1789.

Many clinicians use the Cut down, Annoyed, Guilty, Eyeopener (CAGE) tool, but it does not detect as wide a range of risky alcohol behaviors.[106] Both SASQ and AUDIT-C are supported by evidence that suggests they are effective in identifying unhealthy alcohol behaviors in adults.

Using the 5 A's to help individuals who screen positive for unhealthy alcohol use to find an evidence-based program fits well into the primary care role of midwives. For those individuals who screen positive, the USPSTF recommendation describes several evidence-based approaches to brief interventions that have evidence supporting their potential for reducing unhealthy alcohol behaviors in adults.[105] Many of these interventions are available on the Internet. Their time commitment is often from 30 minutes to 2 hours. Effective programs include such strategies as normative feedback (explaining how an individual's behavior fits in with recommended norms), personalized feedback, cognitive-behavioral therapy, diaries, action plans, and coping strategies.

The USPSTF did not find sufficient evidence for other counseling recommendations related to alcohol misuse and illicit drug use. Notably, the USPSTF issued an I-grade recommendation regarding screening and counseling adolescents on alcohol misuse.[105] The reviewers cited a dearth of studies on the outcomes of these interventions with this population. Likewise, the USPSTF assigned an I grade to counseling to prevent illicit drug use in children, adolescents, and young adults.[109] Again, reviewers pointed out that while some programs show promise, there is an overall lack of evidence for their effectiveness, particularly in terms of the need for replication studies. In addition, inconsistency in the outcomes measurements made results hard to evaluate. Finally, few studies addressed both benefits and harms, particularly legal and social harms.

While the USPSTF does not recommend screening and therefore any screening tool for illicit drug use, some tools have been studied and validated. The Substance Abuse and Mental Health Services Administration recommends use of the National Institute on Drug Abuse's (NIDA's) modified ASSIST questionnaire.[110,111] The Drug Abuse Screening Test is another screening interview tool for primary care settings with some evidence to support it[112] (see the Resources section). Remember that the decision on whether to screen should incorporate more considerations than just the strength of the tool. When making practice-specific screening decisions, always return to the characteristics of a good screening program.

## Reproductive Life Planning

Reproductive life planning (RLP) is a topic for health promotion that midwives frequently address. The *Preconception Care* appendix provides detailed preconception and interconception planning information, which addresses a part of RLP. A few of the lessons about health promotion counseling for RLP are highlighted here.

RLP and preconception care gained national attention in 2006 when the CDC issued a report supporting the intervention and giving 10 related recommendations.[113] The report explained that "a reproductive health plan reflects a person's intentions regarding the number and timing of pregnancies in the context of their personal values and life goals. This health plan might increase the number of planned pregnancies and encourage persons to address risk behaviors before conception, reducing the risk for adverse outcomes for both the mother and the infant."[113] In this report and in subsequent articles responding to its call, the topics of RLP and preconception care appeared together, at times almost interchangeably.[114–118] The idea was to encourage individuals to plan whether to have children or not, and to get the appropriate care for that decision, either preconception or contraception care.

Callegari and colleagues struck a different note, calling for a more person-centered approach.[119] They pointed out that not all individuals with childbearing potential have the same perspective on pregnancy planning: "Researchers in social science and medicine have long challenged the assumption that pregnancy intention is dichotomous and have suggested that, instead, it is a continuum shaped by a complex set of personal, social, and cultural factors."[119(p130)] Insisting that individuals decide on a definitive RLP at one point in time could hurt the clinical relationship, impair the understanding of information, evoke a sense of shame, or misdirect counseling. These authors recommend using open-ended questions, collaborating on strategies, recognizing that some individuals do not consider an unintended pregnancy a failure, and avoiding assumptions and judgments. Cultural humility and an assessment of the stages of change can be used productively here.

Both the CDC recommendations and Callegari and colleagues' approach are based on evidence, yet they came to different recommendations about RLP. The CDC looked at what is known about behaviors to improve outcomes. Callegari's group looked at qualitative and psychological data on responses to pregnancy and advice by persons assigned female at birth. It is important to keep in mind that evidence used to recommend a health behavior can come from differing perspectives and needs to be applied to an individual patient and an individual setting.

## Screening Exams

The screening or annual examination may be the most familiar health intervention we know. This examination is not initiated based on a specific health concern; it consists entirely of health promotion. This encounter often contains all the components taught to students as the basic physical examination: heart, lungs, reflexes, skin, pelvic examination, and so on. The usefulness of this kind of physical exam has been questioned for decades.[120] Rigorous testing in 17 randomized, controlled trials has not supported that it saves lives by reducing total mortality, cancer mortality, or cardiovascular mortality.[121] When these data first began appearing, some sources pointed out that periodic visits may promote relationships between clinicians and consumer, and this relationship also has importance in treating health conditions.[122]

The health promotion encounter does not have to be a complete screening physical examination. It often has been replaced by an encounter that includes more counseling and partnership, which can help develop the clinician–patient relationship. The most common interventions in a health promotion encounter include interviews, screening and lab tests, counseling, immunizations, and preventive medications. ACOG recommendations for a wellness visit and the adolescent first reproductive visit promote mainly counseling on recommended topics.[123,124] Not all patients are comfortable with this counseling-focused approach, which omits much of the physical exam and routine blood tests, or feel it is worth their time.[125] Nevertheless, evidence indicates that a counseling-focused approach offers the most effective use of clinical time, and it leaves individuals with more information to take home and use between visits.

## Social and Structural Determinants of Health

The ecological model described earlier in the chapter (Figure 4-1) makes clear to clinicians the risk and protective factors that are sometimes invisible in the examining room—that is, the social and structural determinants of health (SDoH). SDoH are "the conditions in which people are born, grow, work, live, and age, and the wider set of forces and systems shaping the conditions of daily life."[126] Starting in the 1970s,[77] and reinforced since then,[78] data have shown that SDoH have far more influence on health outcomes than does clinical care, with the environment estimated to be responsible for approximately 50% of the effect on outcomes and health care only approximately 10%. As time passes, increasing importance continues to be attributed to the effects of SDoH—not just on individuals' outcomes, but also on broader health inequities. The *Context of Individuals Seeking Midwifery Care* chapter offers more information on SDoH.

SDoH affect health outcomes and health equity in many ways. With such clear links drawn to these outcomes, it is not surprising that all health professionals need to learn about SDoH.[127] But, how does one move from the evidence of the importance of SDoH to clinical health promotion interventions? This is a question that many have asked in recent years, including the USPSTF in a very public way.[128,129] With few screening tests or counseling recommendations that address SDoH, the USPSTF analyzed barriers and opportunities in making such recommendations, as well as an analytic framework for moving forward.[129]

This framework subjects screening tests for SDoH to the same conditions as any other screening program, asking the same questions. The following is an expansion of the questions in this framework using the evidence from the USPSTF evidence report for screening for intimate partner violence (IPV) as an example.[130] Note all studies reviewed did not distinguish gender identification, and the report uses the terms "women" and "men."

1. Overall, the program recommended must show the characteristics of any screening program—that is, does the program result in improved quality or length of life for a population that participates in it? As noted previously, there are many aspects to consider for a universal screening, although IPV is more complex than most screenings because this problem includes both intergenerational and interpersonal aspects.[131] The USPSTF report identified four studies of screening among adult women followed by brief counseling, with no differences found in health or quality of life at 3 to 18 months.

2. Does the test accurately screen for an important SDoH in a population of sufficient prevalence? The USPSTF recommendation reports that 36% of women and 33% of men experience IPV in their lifetime, establishing

its importance. If midwives screen for IPV, does sufficient evidence show that a positive finding affects health outcomes? The recommendation statement reported three studies of ongoing (not brief) interventions that resulted in positive health outcomes.

3. What are harms associated with the test, and do they outweigh the benefits? The USPSTF statement included data on harms from screening in the section on research needs and gaps, so the statement did not meet this condition.

4. Is there treatment available to participants in the program? For example, if midwives screen for IPV, can they refer their clients to support programs? The USPSTF statement reported on programs that work. Several masked studies were cited in the statement showing that brief counseling did not make any difference. If a given agency does not have access to any programs, then screening should not be carried out. Instead, work should be done at the community level to develop programs.

5. What are the harms associated with treating the condition, and do they outweigh the benefits? Several studies were cited in the USPSTF statement indicating that screening did not seem to result in harms.

6. Is the treatment effective? As mentioned earlier, studies were reported in the statement that found longer-term treatments were effective, but not brief interventions.

7. Does an improvement in intermediate outcomes lead to improved health outcomes in the long term? The USPSTF statement summarized the randomized controlled trials included in the systematic review and found small improvements in only the perinatal programs, which were of longer duration. Brief interventions did not show differences in outcomes, for either pregnant or nonpregnant women.

This framework provides a good starting point for integrating SDoH into the USPSTF recommendations. It does well at applying the principles of screening tests, though it does not explicitly address issues specific to bringing SDoH into primary care. The USPSTF plans to address SDoH only when they are modifiable and only when they are modifiable by interventions by individuals. For example, the

USPSTF considers that community-based interventions (such as initiating an IPV support program) do not fall within the purview of the primary care provider. Sixteen existing recommendations have been identified, and new SDoH risk factors that meet those criteria could be reviewed for recommendations.[129]

## Population-Based Health Promotion

### Health Equity

With examination of the SDoH model (Figure 4-1), the need for population-based approaches to health promotion becomes glaringly obvious. Healthcare services directed toward individuals have an important role to play. Yet, the many other SDoH are where individuals spend most of their lives and have an enormous impact on their health. These conditions can be made better by interventions with a population focus.

Health inequity is a health issue that is revealed at the population level: "avoidable or remediable differences among *groups of people* [emphasis added], whether those groups are defined socially, economically, demographically, or geographically."[132] As a result, recommendations to reduce or eliminate health inequities tend to center on interventions at the system or population level. For example, a landmark report from the Institute of Medicine on healthcare inequities, *Unequal Treatment*,[133] made 20 recommendations, only one of which can be implemented by a clinician in their individual practice. The rest require implementation at the system level.

### U.S. Preventive Services Task Force

The USPSTF began to review systematically both its processes for developing recommendations and the content of its published recommendations in light of the long-standing history of systemic racism and resulting health inequities affecting Americans of color.[134] It found that while health disparities in risk factors or outcomes were frequently mentioned in the recommendation statements, the etiologic role of racism, which is well established in the literature, was mentioned in only one of these statements. Recommendations are applied to the general population, even when the studies with which evidence was developed included study participants who were not representative. As an example, only 1 out of every 7 people in the studies supporting a recommendation may be a person of color and only 1 out of the 7 may be a woman, yet the population targeted by the recommendation may be predominantly people of color and perhaps 4 out of 7 are women.[134] Although evidence frequently does not include studies that included a range of races and ethnicities in their samples, few statements call for more research to fill this gap in evidence. Answers to key questions for the Social Risk and Needs Framework should facilitate the development of recommendations that incorporate knowledge related to racism and its effect of the specific recommendation. One change planned at the USPSTF is to consistently address the representativeness of evidence in statement sections on gaps in evidence.

In the report's findings, the USPSTF identified several changes for future work.[134] It will use health equity frameworks to guide its work, prompting systematic incorporation of evidence on racism into reviews. In addition, it plans to use more consistent language to describe race, ethnicity, and culture. There are also ongoing efforts to foster a culture of diversity in membership, leadership, and values. Health equity will be added to the values used when considering new topics. The USPSTF plans to pilot inclusion of evidence for how recommendations may work differently in different populations or systems as part of its reviews. Statement sections on gaps in the evidence will be enhanced to address when evidence does not have a diversity of research study participants. Several new ideas are under consideration to address which populations were included in studies of the interventions. All of these changes were introduced by USPSTF in 2021 for pilot testing.

## Midwifery Contribution

Individual midwives can take many actions to join with others to promote health on the population level, which can have effects at the local, state, and national levels. Not only do midwives care for each individual and family ethically,[135–137] but they also enter into a social contract, agreeing as a profession to protect the public.[138] There are many ways to do this, incorporating the preferences and skills of each midwife.

### Local Level

At the local level, midwives can undertake quality improvement processes to ensure their provision of care is consistent with the relevant evidence. Quality improvement plans are aimed at improving the quality of care for all patients. However, they may unintentionally increase gaps in health outcomes.[139] This can occur if the improvement plan uses approaches that are more effective among advantaged versus less advantaged populations.[139] Therefore, it is essential that plans consider all populations whom they serve and the characteristics of these populations, so culturally and linguistically appropriate approaches are used.

Speaking at hearings offers an avenue for local, population-based health promotion. Nurses and midwives are trusted by the public and can use that trust when speaking publicly. Speaking at school board meetings, serving as an expert source for local organizations, and asking parents to provide healthy snacks for their children at school also all provide examples of population health promotion at the local level.

Community-based health promotion opportunities also present themselves in local agencies. Service to a health agency (hospital, birth center, clinic) to improve clinical protocols or on other committees offers an avenue of local work to promote health. Many midwives work in community organizations, carrying out community-based interventions for families, rather than clinical care.

### State Level

At the state level, avenues of population-based health promotion also abound. Service to the state affiliates of ACNM, the Midwives Alliance of North America, or other professional organizations can promote health by improving professional practice. Service on the board of nursing or midwifery, board of health, or maternal mortality review board often has an important influence on the health care delivered within a state. Many states have committees implementing safety bundles in hospitals, often focused on maternal mortality. The ACNM website has an advocacy section that details challenges and opportunities for improving the practice environment for midwives by state.

### National Level

Naturally, the national level has an even bigger effect on health. A variety of national entities welcome professional volunteers, such as The Joint Commission (for healthcare quality), the Accreditation Commission for Midwifery Education (for midwifery education quality), the National Quality Forum (on healthcare quality[140]), the USPSTF, and ACIP. Professional organizations organize member participation in lobbying efforts at the national level, such as occurred with a 2018 law that funded maternal mortality review boards across the nation.[141]

## Conclusion

Health promotion focuses on shared decision making and person-centered care, making it consistent with midwifery philosophy. Health promotion clinical interventions tend to fall into the primary and secondary levels of preventions. The components of a clinical health promotion encounter are counseling, screening, preventive medication, and immunization. While the evidence is sometimes contradictory or insufficient, guidelines for good counseling can enable clinicians to better help their clients. Today, screening exams have fewer physical exam components than they once did, but offer more opportunities for shared decision making. Social determinants of health represent a new area of screening and counseling. Health promotion at the population level might seem daunting, but health equity and obligations to the profession and the public require midwives to take the broader perspective and protect the public good at many levels.

## Resources

| Issue | Organization | Description |
|---|---|---|
| General health promotion | ACOG Well-Woman Preventive Services Initiative | Recommendations on well-women care, including the Well-Woman Chart |
| | American Academy of Family Practice (AAFP) | AAFP review of USPSTF clinical preventive services recommendations |
| | Centers for Disease Control and Prevention (CDC) | Complete listing of risk reduction, evidence-based interventions |
| | Guide to Community Preventive Services | Community-based preventive services recommendations based on systematic reviews |
| | *Theory at a Glance: A Guide for Health Promotion Practice* | Review of health promotion–related theories compiled by the National Cancer Institute |
| | U.S. Department of Health and Human Services (DHHS) | *Healthy People 2030* database of evidence-based, community-based, health promotion interventions |
| | U.S. Preventive Services Task Force (USPSTF) | Preventive health services graded recommendations based on systematic reviews |
| | U.S. Preventive Services Task Force (USPSTF) | Mobile device application for USPSTF recommendations |
| | Women's Preventive Services Initiative (WSPI) | Publishes and updates clinical preventive guidelines for women every five years |
| Addictions | Centers for Disease Control and Prevention (CDC) | Manual for clinicians planning to implement a brief intervention for risky alcohol use |
| | Centers for Disease Control and Prevention (CDC) | Screening tools for alcohol abuse |
| | Food and Drug Administrion (FDA) | The Real Cost Campaign; resources for tobacco prevention and cessation |
| | National Institutes of Health (NIH) | Tobacco quit lines and other tobacco addiction resources |
| | U.S. Department of Health and Human Services (DHHS) | DAST drug screening tool |
| | Substance Abuse and Mental Health Services Administration (SAMHSA) | NIDA-modified ASSIST drug screening tool |
| | U.S. Department of Health and Human Services (DHHS) | *Smoke-Free Women*: smoking-cessation resources for women |

| Issue | Organization | Description |
|---|---|---|
| Cervical cancer | American Society for Colposcopy and Cervical Pathology (ASCCP) | Cervical cancer screening guidelines |
| Diet | U.S. Department of Agriculture (USDA) | *Dietary Guidelines for Americans*; dietary guideline information and resources, including infographics, apps, and reports |
| Genetics | National Institutes of Health (NIH), National Human Genome Research Institute (NHGRI) | Genetic counseling services and resources for clinicians and women |
| Group B *Streptococcus* (GBS) screening | ACOG Committee Opinion with ACNM and AAP | Regularly updated guidelines on GBS screening in pregnancy |
| Immunization | Advisory Committee on Immunization Practices (ACIP) | Immunization recommendations across the lifespan |
| | Advisory Committee on Immunization Practices (ACIP) | Vaccine Schedules webpage |
| | Sage Working Group on Vaccine Hesitency | Report on factors creating vaccine hesitancy and how to create social norms to accept vaccination |
| Intimate partner violence (IPV) | Centers for Disease Control and Prevention (CDC) | Facts, screening, and programs related to IPV |
| Motor vehicle safety | Centers for Disease Control and Prevention (CDC) | Information about child safety seats for clinicians and parents |
| | National Highway Traffic Safety Administration (NHTSA) | Seat belt recommendations during pregnancy |
| Physical activity | Centers for Disease Control and Prevention (CDC) | Physical activity guidelines for individuals across the lifespan; resources for clinicians and women, including strategies for overcoming barriers |
| | U.S. Department of Health and Human Services (DHHS), Office of Disease Prevention and Health Promotion | Physical activity guidelines for different age groups, benefits, and behavior change strategies |
| Reproductive life planning | March of Dimes | Comprehensive interactive resources for individuals considering a pregnancy |
| Sexual violence | Centers for Disease Control and Prevention (CDC) | Sexual violence prevention strategies |
| Shared decision making | Agency for Healthcare Research and Quality (AHRQ) | Shared decision-making approach tools and training |
| | Ottawa Hospital Research Institute | Ottawa Decisional Support Framework tools and training |

## References

1. World Health Organization. *Constitution.* https://www.who.int/about/governance/constitution.Published 1947. Accessed December 10, 2022.
2. World Health Organization. *Ottawa Charter for Health Promotion 1986.* https://www.euro.who.int/__data/assets/pdf_file/0004/129532/Ottawa_Charter.pdf. Published 1986. Accessed December 10, 2022.
3. Centers for Disease Control and Prevention. *Prevention.* https://www.cdc.gov/pictureofamerica/pdfs/picture_of_america_prevention.pdf. Accessed December 10, 2022.
4. Harris RP, Helfand M, Woolf SH, et al. Current methods of the U.S. Preventive Services Task Force: a review of the process. *Am J Prev Med.* 2002;20(3S):21-35. https://doi.org/10.1016/j.amepre.2020.01.001.
5. Davis R, Campbell R, Hildon Z, Hobbs L, Michie S. Theories of behaviour and behaviour change across the social and behavioural sciences: a scoping review. *Health Psychol Rev.* 2015;9(3):323-344.

doi: 10.1080/17437199.2014.941722. Epub 2014 Aug 8. PMID: 25104107; PMCID: PMC4566873.

6. Prochaska JO, DiClemente CC, Norcross JC. In search of how people change: applications to addictive behaviors. *Am Psychol.* 1992;47(9):1102-1114. doi:10.1037//0003-066x.47.9.1102.

7. National Cancer Istitute. *Theory at a Glance: A Guide for Health Promotion Practice.* 2nd ed. https://cancercontrol.cancer.gov/sites/default/files/2020-06/theory.pdf. Published 2005. Accessed December 10, 2022.

8. Motivational Interviewing Network of Trainers. Understanding motivational interviewing. https://motivationalinterviewing.org/understanding-motivational-interviewing. Accessed March 9, 2021.

9. Dahlgren G, Whitehead M. *European Strategies for Tackling Social Inequities in Health: Levelling Up (Part 2).* http://www.euro.who.int/__data/assets/pdf_file/0018/103824/E89384.pdf. Published 2006. Accessed December 10, 2022.

10. National Academies of Sciences, Engineering, and Medicine. *A Framework for Educating Health Professionals to Address Social Determinants of Health.* Washington, DC: National Academies Press; 2016. doi:10.17226/21923.

11. Whitlock EP, Orleans CT, Pender N, Allan J. Evaluating primary care behavioral counseling interventions: an evidence-based approach. *Am J Prev Med.* 2002;22(4):267-284. doi:10.1016/s0749-3797(02)00415-4.

12. Tervalon M, Murray-García J. Cultural humility versus cultural competence: a critical distinction in defining physician training outcomes in multicultural education. *J Health Care Poor Underserved.* 1998;9(2):117-125. doi:10.1353/hpu.2010.0233.

13. Withy KM, Lee W, Renger RF. A practical framework for evaluating a culturally tailored adolescent substance abuse treatment programme in Molokai, Hawaii. *Ethn Health.* 2007;12(5):483-496. doi:10.1080/13557850701616920.

14. Soto A, Smith TB, Griner D, et al. Cultural adaptations and therapist multicultural competence: two meta-analytic reviews. *J Clin Psychol.* 2018;74(11):1907-1923. doi:10.1002/jclp.22679.

15. Murray KE, Ermias A, Lung A, et al. Culturally adapting a physical activity intervention for Somali women: the need for theory and innovation to promote equity. *Transl Behav Med.* 2017;7(1):6-15. doi:10.1007/s13142-016-0436-2.

16. Marutani M, Miyazaki M. Culturally sensitive health counseling to prevent lifestyle-related diseases in Japan. *Nurs Health Sci.* 2010;12(3):392-398. doi:10.1111/j.1442-2018.2010.00544.x.

17. Haddad LG, Al-Bashaireh AM, Ferrell AV, Ghadban R. Effectiveness of a culturally-tailored smoking cessation intervention for Arab-American men. *Int J Environ Res Public Health.* 2017;14(4). doi:10.3390/ijerph14040411.

18. American Pyschological Assocation. *Competencies for Psychology Practice in Primary Care: Report of the Interorganizational Work Group on Competencies for Primary Care Psychology Practice.* https://www.apa.org/ed/resources/competencies-practice.pdf. Published 2015. Accessed December 10, 2022.

19. CCI Conference on Preventive Aspects of Chronic Disease, 1951. Cited in Wilson JMG, Junger G. *Principles and Practices of Screening for Disease.* Geneva, Switzerland: World Health Organization; 1968.

20. U.S. Preventive Services Task Force. Chlamydia and gonorrhea: screening. https://www.uspreventiveservicestaskforce.org/uspstf/recommendation/chlamydia-and-gonorrhea-screening. Published 2014. Accessed March 9, 2021.

21. U.S. Preventive Services Task Force. Latent tuberculosis infection: screening. https://www.uspreventiveservicestaskforce.org/uspstf/recommendation/latent-tuberculosis-infection-screening. Published 2016. Accessed March 9, 2021.

22. Wilson JMG, Junger G. *Principles and Practice of Screening for Disease.* Geneva, Switzerland: World Health Organization; 1968. https://apps.who.int/iris/bitstream/handle/10665/37650/WHO_PHP_34.pdf?sequence=17. Accessed December 10, 2022.

23. Grimes DA, Schulz KF. Uses and abuses of screening tests. *Lancet.* 2002;359(9309):881-884. doi:10.1016/S0140-6736(02)07948-5.

24. Grimes DA, Peipert JF. Electronic fetal monitoring as a public health screening program: the arithmetic of failure. *Obstet Gynecol.* 2010;116(6):1397-1400. doi:10.1097/AOG.0b013e3181fae39f.

25. U.S. Preventive Services Task Force. Breast cancer: medication use to reduce risk. https://www.uspreventiveservicestaskforce.org/uspstf/recommendation/breast-cancer-medications-for-risk-reduction. Published 2019. Accessed April 9, 2021.

26. U.S. Preventive Services Task Force. Folic acid for the prevention of neural tube defects: preventive medication. https://www.uspreventiveservicestaskforce.org/uspstf/recommendation/folic-acid-for-the-prevention-of-neural-tube-defects-preventive-medication. Published 2017. Accessed April 9, 2021.

27. Centers for Disease Control and Prevention. Immunization: the basics. https://www.cdc.gov/vaccines/vac-gen/imz-basics.htm. Published 2021. Accessed April 9, 2021.

28. Centers for Disease Control and Prevention. Advisory Committee on Immunization Practices (ACIP): general committee-related information. https://www.cdc.gov/vaccines/acip/committee/index.html. Published 2020.

29. Centers for Disease Control and Prevention, Office for State, Tribal, Local, and Territorial Support. State school immunization requirements and vaccine exemption laws. https://www.cdc.gov/phlp/docs/school-vaccinations.pdf. 2017. Accessed December 10, 2022.

30. U.S. Citizenship and Immigraton Services. Vaccination requirements. https://www.uscis.gov/tools/designated-civil-surgeons/vaccination-requirements. Published 2020. Accessed April 9, 2021.

31. U.S. Department of State, Bureau of Consular Affairs. Vaccinations. https://travel.state.gov/content/travel/en/us-visas/immigrate/vaccinations.html. Accessed April 9, 2021.

32. Ryan J, Malinga T. Interventions for vaccine hesitancy. *Curr Opin Immunol*. 2021;71:89-91. doi:10.1016/j.coi.2021.05.003.

33. Sage Working Group on Vaccine Hesitancy. Report of the Sage Working Group on Vaccine Hesitancy. https://thecompassforsbc.org/sbcc-tools/report-sage-working-group-vaccine-hesitancy. Published 2014. Accessed December 10, 2022.

34. Dubé E, Gagnon D, MacDonald NE. Strategies intended to address vaccine hesitancy: review of published reviews. *Vaccine*. 2015;33(34):4191-4203. https://doi.org/10.1016/j.vaccine.2015.04.041.

35. Jarrett C, Wilson R, O'Leary M, et al. Strategies for addressing vaccine hesitancy: a systematic review. *Vaccine*. 2015;33(34):4180-4190. https://doi.org/10.1016/j.vaccine.2015.04.040/

36. U.S. Preventive Services Task Force. Recommendations. https://uspreventiveservicestaskforce.org/uspstf/topic_search_results?topic_status=P. Accessed May 9, 2022.

37. Caughey AB, Krist AH, Wolff TA, et al. USPSTF approach to addressing sex and gender when making recommendations for clinical preventive services. *J Am Med Assoc*. 2021;326(19):1953-1961. doi:10.1001/jama.2021.15731. [Published correction appears in *J Am Med Assoc*. 2021;326(23):2437.]

38. U.S. Preventive Services Task Force. Grade definitions. https://www.uspreventiveservicestaskforce.org/uspstf/about-uspstf/methods-and-processes/grade-definitions. Accessed December 10, 2022.

39. Curry SJ, Grossman DC, Whitlock EP, Cantu A. Behavioral counseling research and evidence-based practice recommendations: U.S. Preventive Services Task Force perspectives. *Ann Intern Med*. 2014;160:407-413. https://www.uspreventiveservicestaskforce.org/uspstf/about-uspstf/methods-and-processes/behavioral-counseling-research-and-evidence-based-practice-recommendations-us-preventive-services-task-force-perspectives. Accessed December 10, 2022.

40. U.S. Preventive Services Task Force. Prevention Task Force. https://www.uspreventiveservicestaskforce.org/apps/. Accessed December 10, 2022.

41. Centers for Disease Control and Prevention. Immunization schedules: resources for healthcare providers. https://www.cdc.gov/vaccines/schedules/hcp/resources.html. Published 2020. Accessed December 10, 2022.

42. Centers for Disease Control and Prevention (CDC). Immunization schedules: CDC vaccine schedules app for healthcare providers. https://www.cdc.gov/vaccines/schedules/hcp/schedule-app.html#download. Published 2021. Accessed December 10, 2022.

43. American Academy of Family Physicians. Overview of AAFP clinical preventive services recommendations. https://www.aafp.org/family-physician/patient-care/clinical-recommendations/aafp-cps/overview.html. Published 2021. Accessed December 10, 2022.

44. Women's Preventive Services Initiative. About WPSI. https://www.womenspreventivehealth.org/about/. Published 2018. Accessed December 10, 2022.

45. Women's Preventive Services Initiative. Recommendations. https://www.womenspreventivehealth.org/recommendations/. Published 2018. Accessed December 10, 2022.

46. Women's Preventive Services Initiative. Well-woman chart. https://www.womenspreventivehealth.org/wellwomanchart/. Published 2018. Accessed December 10, 2022.

47. Prevention of group B streptococcal early-onset disease in newborns: ACOG Committee Opinion, Number 797. *Obstet Gynecol*. 2020;135(2):e51-e72. doi:10.1097/AOG.0000000000003668. [Published correction appears in *Obstet Gynecol*. 2020;135(4):978-979.]

48. Megregian M, Nieuwenhuijze M. Choosing to decline: finding common ground through the perspective of shared decision making. *J Midwifery Womens Health*. 2018;63(3):340-346. doi:10.1111/jmwh.12747.

49. American College of Nurse-Midwives. *Standards for the Practice of Midwifery*. https://www.midwife.org/acnm/files/ACNMLibraryData/UPLOADFILENAME/000000000051/Standards_for_Practice_of_Midwifery_Sept_2011.pdf. Published September 2011. Accessed December 10, 2022.

50. Nutbeam D, Lloyd JE. Understanding and responding to health literacy as a social determinant of health. *Annu Rev Public Health*. 2021;42:159-173. doi:10.1146/annurev-publhealth-090419-102529.

51. U.S. Preventive Services Task Force. Screening for breast cancer: recommendation statement. *Am Fam Physician*. 2010;82(6):672-676.

52. Wise J. Women aged 50 to 74 should have mammogram every two years, say US guidelines. *BMJ Br Med J*. 2016;352. http://dx.doi.org/10.1136/bmj.i118.

53. Sun LH. New breast cancer screening guidelines at odds with Congress. *Washington Post*. https://www.washingtonpost.com/news/to-your-health/wp/2016/01/11/when-should-women-get-mammograms-congress-and-some-key-experts-disagree/. Published January 16, 2016. Accessed December 10, 2022.

54. Nelson HD, Tyne K, Naik A, et al. Screening for breast cancer: an update for the U.S. Preventive Services Task Force. *Ann Intern Med*. 2009;151(10):727-W242. doi:10.7326/0003-4819-151-10-200911170-00009.

55. U.S. Preventive Services Task Force. Breast cancer: screening. https://uspreventiveservicestaskforce.org

/uspstf/recommendation/breast-cancer-screening. Published 2016. Accessed December 10, 2022.

56. Khan M, Chollet A. Breast cancer screening: common questions and answers. *Am Fam Physician*. 2021;103(1):33-41. PMID: 33382554.

57. Prochaska JO, Butterworth S, Redding CA, et al. Initial efficacy of MI, TTM tailoring and HRI's with multiple behaviors for employee health promotion. *Prev Med*. 2008;46(3):226-231. https://doi.org/10.1016/j.ypmed.2007.11.007.

58. U.S. Preventive Services Task Force. Final recommendation statement: unhealthy drug use: screening. https://uspreventiveservicestaskforce.org/uspstf/recommendation/drug-use-illicit-screening. Published June 9, 2020. Accessed December 10, 2022.

59. U.S. Preventive Services Task Force. Healthful diet and physical activity for cardiovascular disease prevention in adults without known risk factors: behavioral counseling. https://uspreventiveservicestaskforce.org/uspstf/index.php/recommendation/healthy-lifestyle-and-physical-activity-for-cvd-prevention-adults-without-known-risk-factors-behavioral-counseling. Published 2017.

60. Institute of Medicine. *Sleep Disorders and Sleep Deprivation: An Unmet Public Health Problem*. Colten HR, Altevogt BM, eds. Washington, DC: National Academies Press; 2006. doi:10.17226/11617.

61. Panel CC, Watson NF, Badr MS, et al. Joint consensus statement of the American Academy of Sleep Medicine and Sleep Research Society on the recommended amount of sleep for a healthy adult: methodology and discussion. *Sleep*. 2015;38(8):1161-1183. doi:10.5665/sleep.4886.

62. Centers for Disease Control and Prevention. Sleep and sleep disorders: data and statistics. https://www.cdc.gov/sleep/data_statistics.html. Published 2017. Accessed July 2, 2022.

63. Bibbins-Domingo K, Grossman DC, Curry SJ, et al. Screening for obstructive sleep apnea in adults: US Preventive Services Task Force recommendation statement. *J Am Med Assoc*. 2017;317(4):407-414. doi:10.1001/jama.2016.20325.

64. Lu Q, Zhang X, Wang Y, et al. Sleep disturbances during pregnancy and adverse maternal and fetal outcomes. *Sleep Med Rev*. 2021;101436:1-14. doi:10.1016/j.smrv.2021.101436/.

65. Vézina-Im L-A, Moreno JP, Nicklas TA, Baranowski T. Behavioral interventions to promote adequate sleep among women: protocol for a systematic review and meta-analysis. *Syst Rev*. 2017;6(1):95. doi:10.1186/s13643-017-0490-y.

66. Rios P, Cardoso R, Morra D, et al. Comparative effectiveness and safety of pharmacological and non-pharmacological interventions for insomnia: an overview of reviews. *Syst Rev*. 2019;8(1):281. doi:10.1186/s13643-019-1163-9.

67. Alessi C, Vitiello MV. Insomnia (primary) in older people: non-drug treatments. *BMJ Clin Evid*. 2015;2015:2302. https://pubmed.ncbi.nlm.nih.gov/25968443. Accessed December 10, 2022.

68. Jespersen KV, Koenig J, Jennum P, Vuust P. Music for insomnia in adults. *Cochrane Database Syst Rev*. 2015;8:CD010459. doi:10.1002/14651858.CD010459.pub2.

69. Centers for Disease Control and Prevention. Tips for better sleep. https://www.cdc.gov/sleep/about_sleep/sleep_hygiene.html. Published 2016. Accessed November 12, 2021.

70. Tavilani A, Abbasi E, Kian Ara F, et al. COVID-19 vaccines: current evidence and considerations. *Metab Open*. 2021;12:100124. https://doi.org/10.1016/j.metop.2021.100124.

71. Fraser MR, Juliano C, Nichols G. Variation among public health interventions in initial efforts to prevent and control the spread of COVID-19 in the 50 states, 29 big cities, and the District of Columbia. *J Public Health Manag Pract*. 2021;27(suppl 1):S29-S38. doi:10.1097/PHH.0000000000001284.

72. Kampf G, Brüggemann Y, Kaba HEJ, et al. Potential sources, modes of transmission and effectiveness of prevention measures against SARS-CoV-2. *J Hosp Infect*. 2020;106(4):678-697. doi:10.1016/j.jhin.2020.09.022.

73. Wu J, Chiwaya N. Coronavirus deaths: U.S. map shows number of fatalities compared to confirmed cases. *NBC News*. https://www.nbcnews.com/health/health-news/coronavirus-deaths-u-s-map-shows-number-fatalities-compared-confirmed-n1166966. Published March 23, 2020. Accessed December 10, 2022.

74. World Health Organization. The true death toll of COVID-19. https://www.who.int/data/stories/the-true-death-toll-of-covid-19-estimating-global-excess-mortality. Published 2021. Accessed December 10, 2022.

75. Wainstock T, Yoles I, Sergienko R, Sheiner E. Prenatal maternal COVID-19 vaccination and pregnancy outcomes. *Vaccine*. 2021;39(41):6037-6040. https://doi.org/10.1016/j.vaccine.2021.09.012.

76. Centers for Disease Control and Prevention. Fast facts: leading causes of death. https://www.cdc.gov/nchs/fastats/leading-causes-of-death.htm. Published 2021. Accessed December 10, 2022.

77. Surgeon General of the United States. *Healthy People: The Surgeon General's Report on Health Promotion and Disease Prevention*. Washington, DC: U.S. Department of Health and Welfare; 1979. https://profiles.nlm.nih.gov/spotlight/nn/catalog/nlm:nlmuid-101584932X94-doc.

78. McGinnis JM, Foege WH. Actual causes of death in the United States. *J Am Med Assoc*. 1993;270(18):2207-2212. PMID: 8411605.

79. Mokdad AH, Marks JS, Stroup DF, Gerberding JL. Actual causes of death in the United States, 2000. *J Am Med Assoc.* 2004;291(10):1238-1245. doi:10.1001/jama.291.10.1238.

80. U.S. Department of Health and Human Services. *2014 Surgeon General's Report: The Health Consequences of Smoking—50 Years of Progress.* https://www.cdc.gov/tobacco/data_statistics/sgr/50th-anniversary/index.htm. Published 2014. Accessed December 10, 2022.

81. Owens DK, Davidson KW, Krist AH, et al. Primary care interventions for prevention and cessation of tobacco use in children and adolescents: US Preventive Services Task Force recommendation statement. *J Am Med Assoc.* 2020;323(16):1590-1598. doi:10.1001/jama.2020.4679.

82. Krist AH, Davidson KW, Mangione CM, et al. Interventions for tobacco smoking cessation in adults, including pregnant persons: US Preventive Services Task Force recommendation statement. *J Am Med Assoc.* 2021;325(3):265-279. doi:10.1001/jama.2020.25019.

83. National Academies of Sciences, Engineering, and Medicine. *Public Health Consequences of E-cigarettes.* Washington, DC: National Academies Press; 2018. doi:10.17226/24952.

84. Lancaster T, Stead LF. Individual behavioural counselling for smoking cessation. *Cochrane Database Syst Rev.* 2017;3(3):CD001292. doi:10.1002/14651858.CD001292.pub3.

85. Hales CM, Carroll MD, Fryar CD, Ogden CL. Prevalence of obesity and severe obesity among adults: United States, 2017–2018. *NCHS Data Brief.* 2020;360:1-8. PMID: 32487284.

86. Curry SJ, Krist AH, Owens DK, et al. Behavioral weight loss interventions to prevent obesity-related morbidity and mortality in adults: US Preventive Services Task Force recommendation statement. *J Am Med Assoc.* 2018;320(11):1163-1171. doi:10.1001/jama.2018.13022.

87. Grossman DC, Bibbins-Domingo K, Curry SJ, et al. Screening for obesity in children and adolescents: US Preventive Services Task Force recommendation statement. *J Am Med Assoc.* 2017;317(23):2417-2426. doi:10.1001/jama.2017.6803.

88. Krist AH, Davidson KW, Mangione CM, et al. Behavioral counseling interventions to promote a healthy diet and physical activity for cardiovascular disease prevention in adults with cardiovascular risk factors: US Preventive Services Task Force recommendation statement. *J Am Med Assoc.* 2020;324(20):2069-2075. doi:10.1001/jama.2020.21749.

89. American Heart Association, American College of Cardiology. *Prevention Guidelines Tool CV Risk Calculator.* http://static.heart.org/riskcalc/app/index.html#!/baseline-risk. Published 2018. Accessed December 10, 2022.

90. U.S. Department of Agriculture. *Dietary Guidelines for Americans, 2020–2025.* 9th ed. https://www.dietaryguidelines.gov/sites/default/files/2021-03/Dietary_Guidelines_for_Americans-2020-2025.pdf. Published December 2020. Accessed October 12, 2021.

91. Ribeiro MM, Andrade A, Nunes I. Physical exercise in pregnancy: benefits, risks and prescription. *J Perinat Med.* 2021 Sep 6;50(1):4-17. doi:10.1515/jpm-2021-0315. PMID: 34478617.

92. U.S. Department of Health and Human Services. *Physical Activity Guidelines for Americans.* 2nd ed. https://health.gov/our-work/nutrition-physical-activity/physical-activity-guidelines/current-guidelines. Published 2018. Accessed December 10, 2022.

93. Patnode CD, Evans CV, Senger CA, et al. Behavioral counseling to promote a healthful diet and physical activity for cardiovascular disease prevention in adults without known cardiovascular disease risk factors: updated evidence report and systematic review for the US Preventive Services Task Force. *J Am Med Assoc.* 2017;318(2):175-193. doi:10.1001/jama.2017.3303.

94. *Facing Addiction in America: The Surgeon General's Report on Alcohol, Drugs, and Health.* Washington, DC: U.S. Department of Health and Human Services, Office of the Surgeon General; 2016.

95. National Institute on Alcohol Abuse and Alcoholism. Alcohol facts and statistics: alcohol use in the United States. https://www.niaaa.nih.gov/publications/brochures-and-fact-sheets/alcohol-facts-and-statistics. Published 2021. Accessed December 10, 2022.

96. Lipari RN, Van Horn SL. Children living with parents who have a substance use disorder. Substance Abuse and Mental Health Services Administration. https://www.samhsa.gov/data/sites/default/files/report_3223/ShortReport-3223.html. Published 2017. Accessed December 10, 2022.

97. National Institute on Alcohol Abuse and Alcoholism. Underage drinking. https://www.niaaa.nih.gov/sites/default/files/publications/NIAAA_Underage_Drinking_1.pdf. Published 2021. Accessed December 10, 2022.

98. White AM, Slater ME, Ng G, et al. Trends in alcohol-related emergency department visits in the United States: results from the nationwide emergency department sample, 2006 to 2014. *Alcohol Clin Exp Res.* 2018;42(2):352-359. doi:10.1111/acer.13559.

99. Taylor B, Irving HM, Kanteres F, et al. The more you drink, the harder you fall: a systematic review and meta-analysis of how acute alcohol consumption and injury or collision risk increase together. *Drug Alcohol Depend.* 2010;110(1-2):108-116. doi:10.1016/j.drugalcdep.2010.02.011.

100. Bagnardi V, Rota M, Botteri E, et al. Light alcohol drinking and cancer: a meta-analysis. *Ann Oncol.* 2013;24(2):301-308. doi:10.1093/annonc/mds337.

101. White AM, Castle I-JP, Hingson RW, Powell PA. Using death certificates to explore changes in alcohol-related mortality in the United States, 1999 to 2017. *Alcohol Clin Exp Res.* 2020;44(1):178-187. doi:10.1111/acer.14239.

102. Fuller-Rowell T, Curtis DS, El-Sheikh M, et al. Racial discrimination mediates race differences in sleep problems: a longitudinal analysis. *Cultur Divers Ethnic Minor Psychol.* 2017;23(2):165-173. doi:10.1037/cdp0000104.

103. Gomes T, Tadrous M, Mamdani MM, et al. The burden of opioid-related mortality in the United States. *JAMA Netw Open.* 2018;1(2):e180217. doi:10.1001/jamanetworkopen.2018.0217.

104. Mattson CL, Tanz LJ, Quinn K, et al. Trends and geographic patterns in drug and synthetic opioid overdose deaths—United States, 2013–2019. *Morb Mortal Wkly Rep.* 2021;70(6):202-207. doi:10.15585/mmwr.mm7006a4.

105. Curry SJ, Krist AH, Owens DK, et al. Screening and behavioral counseling interventions to reduce unhealthy alcohol use in adolescents and adults: US Preventive Services Task Force recommendation statement. *J Am Med Assoc.* 2018;320(18):1899-1909. doi:10.1001/jama.2018.16789.

106. Samet JH, O'Connor PG. Alcohol abusers in primary care: readiness to change behavior. *Am J Med.* 1998;105(4):302-306. doi:10.1016/s0002-9343(98)00258-7.

107. Smith PC, Schmidt SM, Allensworth-Davies D, Saitz R. Primary care validation of a single-question alcohol screening test. *J Gen Intern Med.* 2009;24(7):783-788. doi:10.1007/s11606-009-0928-6.

108. Bush K, Kivlahan DR, McDonell MB, et al. The AUDIT Alcohol Consumption Questions (AUDIT-C): an effective brief screening test for problem drinking. Ambulatory Care Quality Improvement Project (ACQUIP). Alcohol Use Disorders Identification Test. *Arch Intern Med.* 1998;158(16):1789-1795. doi:10.1001/archinte.158.16.1789.

109. Krist AH, Davidson KW, Mangione CM, et al. Primary care-based interventions to prevent illicit drug use in children, adolescents, and young adults: US Preventive Services Task Force recommendation statement. *J Am Med Assoc.* 2020;323(20):2060-2066. doi:10.1001/jama.2020.6774.

110. Substance Abuse and Mental Health Services Administration. NIDA drug screening tool. https://archives.drugabuse.gov/nmassist/. Accessed December 10, 2022.

111. McNeely J, Strauss SM, Wright S, et al. Test-retest reliability of a self-administered Alcohol, Smoking and Substance Involvement Screening Test (ASSIST) in primary care patients. *J Subst Abuse Treat.* 2014;47(1):93-101. doi:10.1016/j.jsat.2014.01.007.

112. Yudko E, Lozhkina O, Fouts A. A comprehensive review of the psychometric properties of the drug abuse screening test. *J Subst Abuse Treat.* 2007;32(2):189-198. doi:10.1016/j.jsat.2006.08.002.

113. Johnson K, Posner SF, Biermann J, et al. Recommendations to improve preconception health and health care—United States: a report of the CDC/ATSDR Preconception Care Work Group and the Select Panel on Preconception Care. *MMWR Recomm Rep.* 2006;55(RR-6):1-23. https://www.cdc.gov/mmwr/preview/mmwrhtml/rr5506a1.htm. Accessed December 10, 2022.

114. Callegari LS, Ma EW, Schwarz EB. Preconception care and reproductive planning in primary care. *Med Clin North Am.* 2015;99(3):663-682. doi:10.1016/j.mcna.2015.01.014.

115. Liu F, Parmerter J, Straughn M. Reproductive life planning: a concept analysis. *Nurs Forum.* 2016;51(1):55-61. doi:10.1111/nuf.12122.

116. Sanders LB. Reproductive life plans: initiating the dialogue with women. *MCN Am J Matern Child Nurs.* 2009;34(6):342-347. doi:10.1097/01.NMC.0000363681.97443.c4.

117. Malnory ME, Johnson TS. The reproductive life plan as a strategy to decrease poor birth outcomes. *J Obstet Gynecol Neonatal Nurs.* 2011;40(1):109-119. doi:10.1111/j.1552-6909.2010.01203.x.

118. Files JA, Frey KA, David PS, et al. Developing a reproductive life plan. *J Midwifery Womens Health.* 2011;56(5):468-474. doi:10.1111/j.1542-2011.2011.00048.x.

119. Callegari LS, Aiken ARA, Dehlendorf C, et al. Addressing potential pitfalls of reproductive life planning with patient-centered counseling. *Am J Obstet Gynecol.* 2017;216(2):129-134. doi:10.1016/j.ajog.2016.10.004.

120. Gordon PR, Senf J, Campos-Outcalt D. Is the annual complete physical examination necessary? *Arch Intern Med.* 1999;159(9):909-910. doi:10.1001/archinte.159.9.909.

121. Krogsbøll LT, Jørgensen KJ, Gøtzsche PC, Krogsbøll LT. General health checks in adults for reducing morbidity and mortality from disease. *Cochrane Database Syst Rev.* 2019;1(1):CD009009. doi:10.1002/14651858.CD009009.pub3.

122. Himmelstein DU, Phillips RS. Should we abandon routine visits? There is little evidence for or against. *Ann Intern Med.* 2016;164(7):498-499. doi:10.7326/M15-2097.

123. ACOG Committee Opinion No. 755: well-woman visit. *Obstet Gynecol.* 2018;132(4):e181-e186. doi:10.1097/AOG.0000000000002897.

124. American College of Obstetricians and Gynecologists' Committee on Adolescent Health Care. The initial reproductive health visit: ACOG Committee Opinion, Number 811. *Obstet Gynecol*. 2020;136(4):e70-e80. doi:10.1097/AOG.0000000000004094.

125. Laine C. The annual physical examination: needless ritual or necessary routine? *Ann Intern Med*. 2002;136(9):701-703. doi:10.7326/0003-4819-136-9-200205070-00013.

126. World Health Organization. Social determinants of health. https://www.who.int/health-topics/social-determinants-of-health#tab=tab_1. Accessed December 10, 2022.

127. Committee on Educating Health Professionals to Address the Social Determinatns of Health, Board on Global Health, National Academies of Sciences, Engineering, and Medicine. *A Framework for Educating Health Professionals to Address the Social Determinants of Health*. Washington, DC: National Academies Press; 2016. doi:10.17226/21923.

128. Krist MD, Davidson KW, Ngo-Metzger Q. What evidence do we need before recommending routine screening for social determinants of health? *Am Fam Physician*. 2019;99(10):602-605.

129. Davidson KW, Kemper AR, Doubeni CA, et al. Developing primary care-based recommendations for social determinants of health: methods of the U.S. Preventive Services Task Force. *Ann Intern Med*. 2020;173(6):461-467. doi:10.7326/M20-0730.

130. Feltner C, Wallace I, Berkman N, et al. Screening for intimate partner violence, elder abuse, and abuse of vulnerable adults: evidence report and systematic review for the US Preventive Services Task Force. *J Am Med Assoc*. 2018;320(16):1688-1701. doi:10.1001/jama.2018.13212.

131. Shakoor S, Theobald D, Farrington DP. Intergenerational continuity of intimate partner violence perpetration: an investigation of possible mechanisms. *J Interpers Violence*. 2022;37(7-8):NP5208-NP5227. doi:10.1177/0886260520959629.

132. World Health Organization. Health equity. https://www.who.int/health-topics/health-equity#tab=tab_1. Accessed December 10, 2022.

133. Smedley BD, Stith AY, Nelson AR, Committee on Understanding Racial and Ethnic Disparities in Health Care, Board on Health Sciences Policy. *Unequal Treatment: Confronting Racial and Ethnic Disparities in Healthcare*. Washington, DC: National Academies Press; 2003. http://www.nationalacademies.org/hmd/Reports/2002/Unequal-Treatment-Confronting-Racial-and-Ethnic-Disparities-in-Health-Care.aspx. Accessed December 10, 2022.

134. Davidson KW, Mangione CM, Barry MJ, et al. Actions to transform US Preventive Services Task Force methods to mitigate systemic racism in clinical preventive services. *J Am Med Assoc* 2021;326(12):2405-2411. doi:10.1001/jama.2021.17594.

135. American College of Nurse-Midwives. Code of ethics. http://www.midwife.org/ACNM/files/ACNMLibraryData/UPLOADFILENAME/000000000048/Code-of-Ethics.pdf. Published 2005. Accessed December 10, 2022.

136. Midwives Association of North America. MANA statement of values and ethics. https://mana.org/sites/default/files/pdfs/MANAStatementValuesEthicsColor.pdf. Published 2010. Accessed December 10, 2022.

137. American Nurses Association. *Code of Ethics for Nurses: With Interpretive Statements*. Silver Spring, MD: American Nurses Association; 2015.

138. American Nurses Association. *Nursing's Social Policy Statement: The Essence of the Profession*. Silver Spring, MD: American Nurses Association; 2010.

139. Hirschhorn LR, Magge H, Kiflie A. Aiming beyond equality to reach equity: the promise and challenge of quality improvement. *BMJ*. 2021;374:n939. doi:10.1136/bmj.n939.

140. National Quality Forum. https://www.qualityforum.org/Home_New/Working_with_NQF.aspx. Accessed December 10, 2022.

141. Congress.gov. H.R.1318: Preventing Maternal Deaths Act of 2018: summary. https://www.congress.gov/bill/115th-congress/house-bill/1318. Accessed December 10, 2022.

APPENDIX

# 4A

# Skillful Communication to Mitigate Clinician Bias

HEATHER BRADFORD, SIGNEY OLSON, ELIZABETH MUÑOZ, AND ELLEN SOLIS

## Introduction

When engaging in client conversations and promoting person-centered care, a hallmark of midwifery care is use of therapeutic communication, guidance, and counseling.[1,2] Therapeutic communication is defined as an exchange between the clinician and the client using verbal and nonverbal methods, and incorporates many widely accepted techniques. The midwifery philosophy of care affirms a professional obligation to recognize the unconditional value and human dignity of each person, regardless of their health status, and to respect their diverse history, background, and identity.[1] Person-centered language and communication are at the heart of clinical care. Effective and empathic communication can increase client knowledge, empower the client, build trust, enhance shared decision making, alleviate anxiety of both clinicians and clients, and improve health outcomes and client satisfaction.[3,4] Use of effective communication has also been associated with lower rates of clinician burnout due to increased self-efficacy and comfort in skillful communication to handle emotionally charged situations.[5]

Despite the role of therapeutic communication as a foundational component of midwifery care and its well-documented benefits, communication with clients surrounding their health and health behaviors can be challenging to negotiate, especially when discussing topics potentially associated with bias or shame. Bias occurs when a judgment is made (either consciously as explicit bias or unconsciously as implicit bias) about a group of people or a person and a prejudice is formed.[6] Because of the unconscious nature of implicit bias, it may be harder to identify

and mitigate; it is more prevalent under high work demands and cognitive "busyness" with time pressures.[7] Biases can be either "good" (positive bias) or "bad" (negative bias). A person's culture and life experiences influence the development of biases.[8]

Some clinicians may believe there is a "correct" set of behaviors and feel judgment toward clients who do not conform to their expectations, leading to various types of bias seen in the clinical setting (Table 4A-1).[9-12] An extensive literature describes the stigmatizing language used by clinicians and the association of clinician bias, poor quality care, and adverse health outcomes.[6,13-16] When clinician bias interferes with communication and the client relationship, clients are more likely to be inadequately assessed and to receive inappropriate diagnoses and treatment decisions, and less likely to be allotted sufficient time for clinical care.[17] They are also less likely to seek care, including preventive care and screening,[18,19] and are less likely to follow treatment recommendations.[20] This leads to poorer health outcomes and perpetuates a cycle of health disparities and mistrust in the healthcare system.[6]

Bias toward clients and/or their health behaviors presents in several communication methods, including verbal and nonverbal communication with the client, verbal communication about the client with colleagues, and health records.[16] This appendix focuses on opportunities for improvement in clinician–client communication, aiming to disrupt harmful narratives that perpetuate health disparities and contribute to adverse health outcomes in sexual and reproductive health care. It also reviews clinical scenarios that focus on conversations regarding weight, substance use, and sexual behaviors.

| Table 4A-1 | Types of Bias Among Clinicians | |
|---|---|---|
| **Type of Bias** | **Description** | **Clinical Example** |
| Affinity bias and homophily | Attraction to individuals most like ourselves in interest, experiences, and backgrounds<br>Homophily: People are drawn to people who were culturally similar to themselves in terms of leisure pursuits, experiences, and self-presentation styles | Spending more time during a clinical encounter with a client because they attended the same school |
| Appearance bias | Beauty: View that attractiveness equates to success in role<br>Height: Perception that taller individuals are more successful | Engaging in shorter clinical dialogue with a client perceived as unattractive |
| Attribution bias | Positive or negative evaluation of an individual based on prior interaction or healthcare condition | Making decisions on lab tests and a plan of care without consent because of current or history of substance use<br>Believing that development of a chronic condition such as type 2 diabetes or hypertension is a direct result of a person's health behaviors |
| Racial bias | Prejudgment about an individual based on race | Ignoring or dismissing concerns or symptoms from a client of color who is racially discordant from your own race |
| Bias based on sexual orientation and gender expression/identity | Preference for certain types of sexual orientations, gender expression/identities over another | Not recommending routine cervical cancer screening in a cisgender lesbian client |
| Weight bias | Preference for individuals with smaller-sized or lower-weight bodies | Recommending weight loss for lower back strain instead of a comprehensive assessment, consideration of diagnostic imaging, and pain management |

Data from Banaji MR. *Blindspot: Hidden Biases of Good People*. New York, NY: Bantam; 2016; Dilmaghani M. Beauty perks: physical appearance, earnings, and fringe benefits. *Econ Hum Biol*. 2020;38:100889. doi:10.1016/j.ehb.2020.100889; Lawrence BJ, Kerr D, Pollard CM, et al. Weight bias among health care professionals: a systematic review and meta-analysis. *Obesity (Silver Spring)*. 2021;29(11):1802-1812. doi:10.1002/oby.23266; Marcelin JR, Siraj DS, Victor R, et al. The impact of unconscious bias in healthcare: how to recognize and mitigate it. *J Infect Dis*. 2019;220(220 suppl 2):S62-S73. doi:10.1093/infdis/jiz214.

## Self-Reflection

While bias cannot be eliminated, clinicians can become more aware of their bias and attempt to mitigate it. Acknowledging this is an important component in providing evidence-based care and striving toward empathic and professional discourse with clients.[21] Self-reflection is a necessary clinician skill and should occur before having any clinical conversation where clinician bias may be a concern, particularly around health behaviors. While identification of personal and societal bias can be valuable in a person's initial reflection process, it is not always enough to result in changes in behaviors, thoughts, or actions. Furthermore, intersectionality of multiple types of bias can add to the challenges of unlearning the biased behaviors.

After reflecting on their personal biases, clinicians should assess their clinical environment, personal social spheres, and community resources. Evaluating their own exposure and/or distance to a wide variety of health-related decisions can support clinicians in further reflecting on that exposure and building empathy from experience. Additionally, direct experiences with diverse populations that involve active listening and centering of oppressed voices may improve clinical care. By increasing their interactions with individuals of varying backgrounds, clinicians' bias can be mitigated. However, clinicians must also take steps to avoid tokenization, which increases the emotional labor of marginalized and historically oppressed populations.

"Healthism" is a form of bias in which people view individuals as being solely in control of their own health, and believe that achieving optimal health is a large part of societal worth. In reality, "good health," as traditionally defined, is not possible for many individuals in a variety of circumstances to achieve. This may include those persons with chronic health concerns and/or certain disabilities, limited socioeconomic opportunities, limited healthcare access, genetic predispositions, and generational trauma contributing to high allostatic load. Additionally, by focusing on individual responsibility, healthism does not acknowledge the significant role that systemic and institutional oppression play in health care. Examples include the lack of grocery stores or safe spaces for physical activity in a community, as well as concerns regarding access to health care.

Weight bias is another form of bias that stigmatizes individuals whose weight exceeds a certain standard. Midwives should explore their historical relationship to their own bodies, food, and physical movement. Although research on the effectiveness of strategies to reduce weight bias is limited, engaging in reflection about personal relationships with specific health behaviors such as eating and exercise can help clinicians reduce bias in their own interactions.[22] This reflection may trigger harmful memories of experiences with others in school, the workplace, and/or a healthcare setting because of one's body shape or size. Discussions of and work toward eliminating bias may also trigger prior memories of not providing the best care or causing harm in clinical conversations. Seeking healing from one's own past and critically evaluating the evidence regarding contributors to health is an important step to providing and advancing person-centered care.

Table 4A-2 and Table 4A-3 provide a stepwise approach to examining personal and department/institutional bias in health care.

## Basics of Therapeutic Communication

Therapeutic communication is a method used by clinicians to connect with clients during healthcare visits. This style of communication encompasses various techniques (Table 4A-4) that aid in conveying a clear message to the client and prompting them to offer more information or detail to the clinician.[23,24] Therapeutic communication techniques include open-ended questioning by avoiding yes/no questions, reflection or restatement of the client's thoughts or ideas, and silence to promote the client to continue speaking, among others.

| Table 4A-2 | Self-Reflective Questions to Identify and Mitigate Bias Among Clinicians |
|---|---|

1. What is your personal lens/framework when discussing health concepts and behaviors, including others' potential initial assumptions about your choices?
2. What does "healthy" mean to you, and in what ways have you incorporated this understanding into your life?
3. Do you have any pride or shame related to the choices you have made surrounding your health?
4. What are ways in which you believe certain health behaviors are linked with health outcomes (this may be research-based, anecdotal, or both)?
5. How do your beliefs about client behaviors challenge you if a client does not meet your definition of healthy or does not take the steps you would take toward health?
6. Which health behaviors, topics, choices, or populations bring out your bias most?
7. Do you know of available resources to identify and address your own bias?

| Table 4A-3 | Questions for Department or Institutional Leadership |
|---|---|

1. How can this organization most effectively request and receive client and community feedback regarding opportunities for improving care?
2. What are common health-related behaviors and needs in our client population that may elicit clinician and staff bias?
3. What evidence-based research is available regarding care delivery for clients presenting with these health-related behaviors and needs?
4. What client resources and materials are available that are culturally humble, incorporate individuals' needs and preferences, and use affirming terminology?
5. What resources are available to support evidence-based care among our clinicians and staff?
6. How do individuals from this community or with a particular diagnosis want to receive health care or be treated for their condition? What language and word choices are preferred? What approaches to care are most valued by the community?
7. How would the intersection of a client's culture, multiple identities, diagnoses, and personal desires affect their needs and communication preferences?

| Table 4A-4 | Techniques for Navigating Conversations About Health |
|---|---|
| **Technique** | **Description** |
| Create a safe space for the conversation. | Assure privacy and comfort for the client, and evaluate power dynamics between you and the client. |
| Center yourself, quickly review your plan to optimize the visit. | Assess your body language and tone of voice. Present yourself in a genuine fashion, sitting at eye level or with the client in a higher sitting position. |
| Introduce yourself using your first and last names and gender pronouns, and ask the client's gender pronouns and what name they would like to use in conversation and the chart. | This demonstrates respect for the client, their dignity, and their autonomy. |
| Open by asking the individual their needs for the visit, open with curiosity, and focus on the expressed selected health needs. | Provide space for the client's own narrative surrounding the health concern. Ask permission prior to asking questions regarding potentially sensitive topics and convey a willingness to listen with curiosity rather than ego. Use person-centered language and terminology preferred by individual(s) with this concern or condition. For example, instead of using the term "obese woman," consider "person in a larger body." |
| Find common ground and shared goals surrounding the health topic. | Prioritize reframing your discussion as a partnership. |
| Check in with yourself. | Take a momentary pause to acknowledge that it may be uncomfortable for you to shift how you talk about health if you are used to another approach. |
| Actively listen. | Ask open-ended questions when possible and explore the client's narrative and needs. Use nonverbal cues and verbal cues to continue the conversation, demonstrating to the client that they are being heard. Use eye contact and facial expressions that demonstrate interest. |
| Stay focused. | Use "I" statements to own your words. Repeat back what the client said to demonstrate engagement. Ask questions when needed to obtain additional information. |
| Identify the goal for the conversation. | Establish goals by exploring questions together. What is the problem we are trying to solve? What is the bigger picture? |
| Continue genuine exploration of health topic. | What questions do you need to ask? What information or modifications do you need? |
| Work collaboratively to develop potential plans of action in light of evidence-based care for the client's health needs, personal preferences, and constraining factors. | Allow the client to generate potential steps toward their goal, and provide evidence-based and locally available assistance as needed. Confirm understanding of the plan from the client. Document the encounter in the chart using respectful person-centered language, conveying the client's needs and values. |
| After the visit, self-reflect on your performance. | Evaluate the success of the interaction. |

Data from from Sharma N, Gupta V. Therapeutic communication. In: *StatPearls*. Boca Raton, FL: StatPearls Publishing; 2022. Copyright © 2022, StatPearls Publishing LLC; Brown B. *Dare to Lead: Brave Work, Tough Conversations, Whole Hearts*. New York, NY: Random House; 2018.

## Examples of Clinical Conversations

When engaging in conversations that involve clients' behaviors, it is helpful for clinicians to consider specific examples of scenarios in which bias may occur. This section's approach will bridge from more abstract concepts to real-life applications that can improve a client's health and satisfaction with care. Table 4A-5, Table 4A-6, and Table 4A-7 provide examples of common conversations where clinician bias may occur (weight, substance use, and sexual health practices, respectively).[24,25] The basic techniques of therapeutic communication are utilized throughout. Examples of possible clinician responses are written in italics.

| Table 4A-5 | Guidance for Navigating Conversations About Health and Weight | | | |
|---|---|---|---|---|
| **Techniques for Therapeutic Communication** | **Four Examples Regarding Conversations About Weight** | | | |
| | **Scenario 1:** A person presents for an annual exam and requests guidance on weight loss to improve their health. They have no chronic health conditions. (This applies to individuals of BMI of 18.5 kg/m² or higher. For those with BMI < 18.5 who state they want to lose weight, an eating disorder diagnosis is highly likely and appropriate referrals should be offered.) | **Scenario 2:** A person presents for an annual exam and does not bring up weight directly. They have no chronic health conditions. (This applies to individuals of most to all BMI categories.) | **Scenario 3:** A pregnant person with a BMI > 30.0 kg/m² at their first prenatal visit asks about their weight gain limit of a maximum of 20 pounds for the pregnancy. | **Scenario 4:** A pregnant person with a BMI < 18.0 kg/m² at their first prenatal visit asks about what their weight gain limit should be. |

Prior to seeing the clinician, many clients are routinely weighed. While this may not be evidence-based practice, if it occurs, consent should always be obtained before a client is asked to step on the scale.
*"Part of our clinic's routine is to weigh clients prior to their visit. However, you always have the right to decline that altogether or face away from the scale. I can also collect it and not record it in the chart, if you prefer."*

**Center yourself, quickly review your plan to optimize the visit, assess your body language, and tone of voice.**

| | | | |
|---|---|---|---|
| **Open with curiosity by asking the individual their needs for the visit and focus accordingly.**<br><br>**Provide space for the person's own narrative surrounding the health concern.**<br><br>**Ask permission prior to asking questions regarding potentially sensitive topics and convey a willingness to listen with curiosity rather than ego.**<br><br>**Use the language and terminology preferred by the individual with this concern or condition.** | *"How can I help today?"* | *"I'm so glad you came in! One of the goals I have for today's visit is to check in about whether you have any health-related questions or priorities. Tell me how I can help!"*<br><br>While discussion of healthy eating and exercise is an essential component of the annual exam, it is unlikely that weight is a necessary component of this visit.<br><br>Examples of when weight is most relevant: *Clients who are severely underweight, during dosing of medications/anesthesia, and when analyzing pediatric growth chart measurements* | *"This is a question I get often and I'm happy to discuss this today if you like. Would you tell me what your thoughts are about weight gain in pregnancy and anything about your relationship with your body? I'd love to hear more about where you're coming from."*<br><br>Prior to discussing weight gain/loss with clients, clinicians should consider how they would treat the client if they were in a smaller body or a larger body. |

| Techniques for Therapeutic Communication | Four Examples Regarding Conversations About Weight | | |
| --- | --- | --- | --- |
| **Find common ground and shared goals surrounding the health topic. Prioritize reframing your discussion as a partnership. Stay focused. Use "I" statements to own your parts.** | *"Thank you so much for sharing that with me, I appreciate it. One of the goals of today's visit for me is to check in about whether you have any health-related questions or priorities. That's such a great question and one a lot of people bring up."* | | *"I'm so glad you feel able to talk to me about this. I get the sense that you really want to do what is best for the baby and yourself. That's what my goal is as well!*<br><br>*I understand that being weighed can be triggering. It is always your right to decline being weighed or ask not to know the number on the scale. We will routinely monitor your baby's growth at each visit by measuring your uterus."* |
| **Check in with yourself and take a momentary breath to acknowledge that it may be uncomfortable for you to talk about weight and health.** | | | |
| **Listen, ask open-ended questions when possible, and explore the person's narrative and needs.** | | | |
| **Identify the goal for the conversation. Get on the same page by exploring questions together. Is there a concern that needs to be addressed? What is the bigger picture?** | *"Bodies go through a lot of changes in our lives, most of which are entirely normal. The culture we live in tends to be pretty focused on weight as a primary indication of our health, but there are multiple components to health. Tell me what is important to you."* | *"I am happy to work with you on those concerns you mentioned. Let's talk about a few of the strategies we have to address that. Please feel free to ask any and all questions I can help with."* | *"How are you feeling chatting with me? Is this a topic you would like to keep discussing?"*<br><br>*"Bodies go through a lot of changes during pregnancy, most of which are entirely normal. It can definitely bring up a lot of feelings related to body image and health. Bodies will typically gain the amount of weight that they're intended to gain, and that amount might look different for different people."* |
| **Continue genuine exploration of the topic or health concern. Are there questions you need to ask? Any information or modifications that need to be addressed?** | *"Would you be open to telling me more about your relationship with your body and food? Do you have any history of disordered eating or chronic dieting?"*<br><br>If the client responds yes to having a history of disordered eating, the clinician should pause the conversation regarding weight and nutrition and ask:<br><br>*"Would you be open to sharing a little bit more about that with me and ways that might impact your daily life more recently?"* | *"Would you be open to telling me more about your relationship with your body and food? Do you have any history of disordered eating or chronic dieting?"*<br><br>If the client responds yes to having a history of disordered eating, the clinician should pause the conversation regarding weight and nutrition and ask:<br><br>*"Would you be open to sharing a little bit more about that with me and ways that might impact your daily life more recently?"* | *"Can you tell me more about your relationship with your body and food prior to pregnancy? Do you have any history of disordered eating or chronic dieting?"*<br><br>If the client responds yes to having a history of disordered eating, the clinician should pause the conversation regarding weight/nutrition and ask"<br><br>*"Would you be open to sharing a little bit more about that with me and ways that might impact your daily life more recently?"*<br><br>For clinicians who do not have knowledge regarding treatment of disordered eating, any recommendations regarding weight and nutrition should be deferred and the client should be offered a referral to a registered dietitian and/or therapist. |

*(continues)*

| Table 4A-5 | Guidance for Navigating Conversations About Health and Weight (*continued*) | | | |
|---|---|---|---|---|
| **Techniques for Therapeutic Communication** | **Four Examples Regarding Conversations About Weight** | | | |
| **Work collaboratively with the individual to develop potential plans of action in light of evidence-based care for their health needs, personal preferences, and constraining factors. Allow the person to generate potential steps toward their goal, and provide evidence-based and locally available assistance as needed.**<br><br>**Confirm understanding of the plan from the client.** | *"Interestingly, many factors influence health, like not smoking, moderate alcohol intake, and including fresh foods in our meals. Know that I will support you in meeting your health goals, and it is normal for you to need some time to learn more about this. I have lots of excellent resources on the topic of weight. There are also dietitians and therapists in my network who practice specifically from a health-focused perspective.*<br><br>*Reframing exercise to be joyful or intentional movement to improve health without the intention of weight loss can be a good place to start. When making nutrition choices, I recommend getting curious about which foods your body intuitively wants and not engaging in calorie-counting or app-based tracking. Are those referrals something you would be interested in today?"*<br><br>*If financial constraints, clinicians can consider referring to cost-free resources either locally or virtually.* | *"Many people are used to having their weight taken at annual exams as part of their care. I don't do this routinely for my clients unless we identify a potential concern. There are many ways to assess someone's health.*<br><br>*I'm here to support your health needs moving forward. Please feel free to schedule an in-person or virtual appointment with me anytime you'd like to talk more."* | *"There are recommendations that exist regarding weight gain in pregnancy that have been around for a long time. What we know from current research is that there may be some additional risks in pregnancy for those with a higher BMI—these are things like diabetes, high blood pressure, and growing large-for-gestational-age babies. While this is the most accepted information we have, I also recognize that it cannot be free of bias (much like other guidelines). There are many ways that we can measure health and many ways a person can keep themselves healthy and we don't need to focus on weight."* | *"There are a few recommendations that exist regarding recommended weight gain in pregnancy that have been around for a long time. What we know from current research is that there may be some additional risks in pregnancy for those with a lower BMI—these are things like fetal growth restriction, premature labor and birth, and small-for-gestational-age babies. While this is the most accepted information we have, I also recognize that it cannot be free of bias (much like other guidelines) and for some people talking about weight can cause anxiety.*<br><br>*There are many ways that we can measure health and many ways a person can keep themselves healthy and we don't need to focus on weight."* |
| **After the visit, self-reflect on your performance and evaluate the success of the interaction as permissible.** | | | | |

Abbreviation: BMI, body mass index.

Data from Albury C, Strain WD, Brocq SL, et al. The importance of language in engagement between health-care professionals and people living with obesity: a joint consensus statement. *Lancet Diabetes Endocrinol.* 2020;8(5):447-455. doi:10.1016/s2213-8587(20)30102-9; Brown B. *Dare to Lead: Brave Work, Tough Conversations, Whole Hearts.* New York, NY: Random House; 2018.

| Table 4A-6 | Guidance for Navigating Conversations About Health and Substance Use |||||
|---|---|---|---|---|
| **Techniques for Therapeutic Communication** | **Four Examples Regarding Conversations About Substance Use** ||||
| Center yourself, quickly review your plan to optimize the visit, and assess your body language and tone of voice. |||||
| | **Scenario 1:** A person presents for an annual exam and reports using medications that are not prescribed to them to address their chronic back pain. | **Scenario 2:** A person presents for an annual exam and asks about the health risks of having five alcoholic beverages most evenings. | **Scenario 3:** A pregnant person presents for their first prenatal visit and reports using cannabis daily. | **Scenario 4:** A pregnant person reports opioid use in pregnancy and states they are ready to begin medication to treat opioid use disorder at their prenatal visit. |
| **Open by asking the individual their needs for the visit, open with curiosity, and focus on the expressed selected health needs. Provide space for the person's own narrative surrounding the health concern.** **Ask permission prior to asking questions regarding potentially sensitive topics and convey a willingness to listen with curiosity rather than ego.** **Use the language and terminology preferred by individual(s) with this concern or condition.** | *"I'm so glad you brought this up today. I am wondering if you want to chat about the specific medications you're taking and how you feel when you've taken them."* | *"Thanks for asking that question. If you're open to it, I'd like to talk a bit about when and how you drink alcohol and what you typically drink. Would that be okay with you?"* | *"Thanks so much for sharing that with me. If it's okay with you, I'd like to chat more about using cannabis during pregnancy, if that's something you're open to?"* | *"Thanks so much for sharing this with me. I can absolutely talk with you about the process of getting started on medications for opioid use disorder. Would it be okay with you if we talked a bit more about your experience using opioids? When was the last time you used opioids and how much did you use?"* |
| **Find common ground and shared goals surrounding the health topic. Prioritize reframing your discussion as a partnership.** | *"I understand that your lower back pain has been an issue this year. I want to help you find a way to treat this pain effectively and safely."* | *"You mentioned drinking wine after stressful work days, and were concerned about the health effects. It might be helpful to look at other ways that have worked in the past to decrease your stress level. Do you have any specific health-related goals?"* | *"I want you to feel as good as possible during pregnancy, and I know nausea can be a challenge in these early weeks. Would it be okay to talk about some other options available for treating nausea in the first trimester?"* | *"I know this can be scary, and I want you to know I'm here for you during your treatment. You can share honestly with me, and I will do the same."* |

*(continues)*

| Table 4A-6 | Guidance for Navigating Conversations About Health and Substance Use (*continued*) | | | |
|---|---|---|---|---|
| **Techniques for Therapeutic Communication** | **Four Examples Regarding Conversations About Substance Use** | | | |
| **Check in with yourself and the client. Take a momentary breath to acknowledge that it may be uncomfortable for you to shift how you talk about substance use if you are used to another approach.** | How are you feeling about the client's use of multiple medications that were not prescribed to them? What feelings come up for you in this interaction? | How are you feeling about the client's alcohol consumption? Does this client elicit negative feelings you have related to alcohol? What can you examine about your own or your family history of alcohol use? | What feelings does this interaction bring up? Are your feelings more negative or positive because the client is pregnant? Are you able to educate the client of the risks of cannabis use in a bias-informed manner? | How do you feel knowing the fetus has been exposed to opioids in pregnancy? Are you able to show the compassion this client needs at this time? Do you need to collaborate with or refer to a clinician who specializes in providing this care? |
| **Listen, ask open-ended questions when possible, and explore the person's narrative and needs.** | | | | |
| **Stay focused. Use "I" statements to own your parts.** | *"I am concerned about your health and safety and want to have a conversation about the use of medication that was not prescribed to you. Would it be okay to talk about this today?"* | *"I understand what you're saying about stress and I hear where you're coming from."* | *"I have several options to recommend that can help with the nausea and vomiting symptoms. Would it be okay if I run through them now?"* | *"I am so happy you've talked with me. I am here to help you along the way. I want you to know that I will always be honest with you, and I hope you'll do the same with me. It is so important that we trust each other as we work together."* |
| **Identify the goal for the conversation. Get on the same page by exploring questions together. Is there a concern that needs to be addressed? What is the bigger picture?** | *"What is your goal for pain control and medication use?"* | *"Do you have concerns or goals about your alcohol consumption or your stress level?"* | *"It sounds like you're looking for a way to treat the nausea and vomiting of early pregnancy in a more natural way than through the use of prescription medications. I can recommend vitamin $B_6$ as a nonprescription supplement that has been shown to help."* | *"Now that we've discussed your options for treatment, I'd like to talk about follow-up. The goal in pregnancy is to treat your cravings and prevent withdrawal from opioids. Know that I will support you no matter how your treatment for opioid use turns out. I would like to see you weekly to prescribe your medication and make sure your needs are being met with the dosage. It may take a bit of adjusting, but you'll get there."* |

| Techniques for Therapeutic Communication | Four Examples Regarding Conversations About Substance Use | | | |
|---|---|---|---|---|
| **Continue genuine exploration of the topic or health concern. Are there questions you need to ask? Any information or modifications that need to be addressed?** | *"What has/has not worked before? In the past few days, how often have you used medication that was not prescribed for you to help with pain? Would you be willing to see the chronic pain clinic for your medications instead of using a friend's prescription when your symptoms flare?"* | *"Have you experienced a time of increased drinking before? If so, was it because of a stressor? How did you manage that experience? I have some recommendations regarding decreasing alcohol intake. Would it be okay to review those today? Could you reduce your drinking to the 'moderate' amount I mentioned, or would that be a struggle?"* | *"Can you tell me a bit more about the timing of the nausea and vomiting you're experiencing? Is it mostly in the morning before you've eaten, or is it on and off all day long?"* | *"There may come a time in the pregnancy that we need to involve specialists due to the risks of opioid use in pregnancy. Would you be willing to meet with a clinician who has experience working with substance use and can assist in making a plan of care with you?"* |
| **Work collaboratively with the individual to develop potential plans of action in light of evidence-based care for their medical needs, personal preferences, and constraining factors. Allow the person to generate potential steps toward their goal, and provide evidence-based and locally available assistance as needed. Confirm understanding of the plan from the client.** | *"I will submit a referral today and have my team follow up with you to get scheduled with the chronic pain clinic and physical therapy for an assessment within the next 1 to 2 weeks. Does that sound like an okay plan?"* | *"After your visit, I will send you the resources we discussed today through the electronic health record portal. I would like you to check in with me via message within the next 2 weeks to let me know how you're doing. Does that sound like an okay plan?"* | *"I'll plan to check in with you over the next 3 days to see how the vitamins are working for you. We can reevaluate the plan if you're not having the relief you want. I'm here if you need me in the meantime."* | *"You're scheduled to see my colleagues in the specialist clinic in 1 week, and we'll meet again that day as well. Now before you go today, I'll get you started with medications for opioid use disorder now. Do you have any questions about the plan of care?"* |

**Self-reflect on your performance and evaluate the success of the interaction as permissible.**

| Table 4A-7 | Guidance for Navigating Conversations About Health and Sexual Practices |
|---|---|

| Techniques for Therapeutic Communication | Four Examples Regarding Conversations About Sexual Health Practices | | | |
|---|---|---|---|---|
| | **Scenario 1:** A client comes to you for an annual exam and their intake form notes multiple sexual partners in the last 6 months. They told the medical assistant they do not want STI screening today. | **Scenario 2:** A person presents for an annual exam and during the discussion regarding sexual health and safety, they explain they engage in consensual rope bondage. | **Scenario 3:** A pregnant person presents for a 28-week visit, and you note that your clinic nurse called the client with positive chlamydia results several days ago. You also note they tested positive for chlamydia at 12 weeks' gestation. The chart indicates they are not in a relationship but have multiple sexual partners. | **Scenario 4:** A pregnant person presents for their initial prenatal visit and makes a request to the medical assistant that both of their romantic partners be present for the visit since they are a polyamorous family and are all planning to co-parent. |
| **Open by asking the individual their needs for the visit, open with curiosity, and focus on the expressed selected health needs. Provide space for the person's own narrative surrounding the health concern.**<br><br>**Ask permission prior to asking questions regarding potentially sensitive topics and convey a willingness to listen with curiosity rather than ego.**<br><br>**Use the language and terminology preferred by individual(s) with this concern or condition.** | *"Thanks for sharing this information with me. Normally, for all my clients, I include a discussion regarding sexual health as part of the visit. Would it be okay if I ask a few more questions about your sexual health practices?"* | *"Thanks so much for sharing that with me. Part of my job is to support individuals in their sexual health goals, whatever that looks like for them. Is there anything else about your sexual health that you would like to share with me?"* | *"Thanks so much for sharing how you're feeling with me. I know the third trimester of pregnancy can bring about a lot of changes.*<br><br>*I noticed that one of our nurses called you a few days ago to give you some STI results. Would it be okay if we reviewed the recommended next steps to complete a test of cure to assure the infection has resolved?"* | *"Hi there, I'm XX, the midwife you're scheduled with today. The medical assistant let me know that the three of you are all co-parents and excited to participate in today's visit. You're absolutely welcome here."* |
| **Find common ground and shared goals surrounding the health topic. Prioritize reframing your discussion as a partnership.** | *"I'm here to talk through any questions you might have and talk about the pros and cons of any testing that would be recommended. Are there any specific goals you have related to your sexual health?"* | *"Sexual expression exists in so many forms, and I'm glad you've had space to explore what that looks like for you."* | *"Some people can feel embarrassed to talk about positive STI testing results. I want to let you know that I hold absolutely no judgment about these things. STIs are incredibly common, and I'm so glad you requested testing when you were concerned."* | *"This kid is going to be so lucky to have three parents! Thanks so much for sharing that with me. What questions do each of you have about the pregnancy and parenting?"* |

| Techniques for Therapeutic Communication | Four Examples Regarding Conversations About Sexual Health Practices | | | |
|---|---|---|---|---|
| **Check in with yourself and take a momentary breath to acknowledge that it may be uncomfortable for you to shift how you talk about sex or sexual behaviors due to your own beliefs about the topic.**<br><br>**Sexual health bias can appear in the clinical environment as unintentionally using language that shames or blames the client. Take a moment to think about how your bias may or may not affect the advice you give in this scenario.** | What feelings does this interaction bring up? Are you experiencing any judgment toward the person for not wanting STI testing? What might be some reasons a person feels that way? Are you able to educate the client respectfully regarding the risks of undiagnosed STIs in a bias-informed manner? | What feelings does this interaction bring up? Do you feel comfortable or uncomfortable talking about kink-related sexual activity? Does this topic feel like a knowledge gap for you? Are you able to understand the difference between consensual kink-related activity and abusive behavior? | What feelings does this interaction bring up? Are your feelings more negative or positive because the client is pregnant? Are you able to educate the client about the risks of STIs in a bias-informed manner? | What feelings does this interaction bring up? Are your feelings more negative or positive because the client is pregnant? How do you feel answering questions and discussing the plan of care with all three co-parents? |
| **Listen, ask open-ended questions when possible, and explore the person's narrative and needs.** | | | | |
| **Stay focused. Use "I" statements to own your parts.** | *"I will always defer to what tests you want to have run because I trust that people know how to make the best decisions for themselves."* | *"Rope bondage isn't a topic I know a lot about, but I'm open to learning anything that you would like to share that's connected to your health."* | *"I recognize that it can be challenging to navigate pregnancy, test results, and the overall life demands."* | *"I've cared for a few families who are in polyamorous relationships, but every family is unique."* |
| **Identify the goal for the conversation. Get on the same page by exploring questions together. Is there a concern that needs to be addressed? What is the bigger picture?** | *"You've shared with me that having a safe sex life is very important to you. It might be helpful to talk through what that means to you."* | *"You've shared with me that having a safe sex life is very important to you. It might be helpful to talk through what that means to you."* | *"You've shared with me that having a safe sex life is very important to you. It might be helpful to talk through what that means to you."* | *"My goal for you in this pregnancy is to have your questions answered and feel supported in your decision making along the way."* |
| **Continue genuine exploration of the topic or health concern. Are there questions you need to ask? Any information or modifications that need to be addressed?** | *"Would you be open to discussing the current recommendations for how often to do STI screening? Would you be open to tests that you can collect yourself or use urine and do not involve a pelvic examination or a blood draw?"* | *"Are there any concerns you have about the types of activities you engage in and what effect they may have on your health?"* | *"It's common for people to experience a reinfection of this STI. Would it be okay to discuss ways to help prevent a similar infection in the future and other recommendations for STI testing?"* | *"I'd love to know if there are any specific concerns or worries you have about your pregnancy or ways that we can better support your family?"* |

*(continues)*

| Table 4A-7 | Guidance for Navigating Conversations About Health and Sexual Practices (*continued*) |
|---|---|
| **Techniques for Therapeutic Communication** | **Four Examples Regarding Conversations About Sexual Health Practices** |

<table>
<tr>
<td>Work collaboratively with the individual to develop potential plans of action in light of evidence-based care for their medical needs, personal preferences, and constraining factors. Allow the person to generate potential steps toward their goal, and provide evidence-based and locally available assistance as needed. Confirm understanding of the plan from the client.</td>
<td>"I so appreciate you sharing those thoughts and questions with me today. It sounds like for the time being, you'd like to hold off on any STI testing, which is okay. In the future, if at any point you want to review recommendations or have me order testing, know that you can easily make that request through our portal and you can get testing quickly. Does that sound like an okay plan?"</td>
<td>"I so appreciate you sharing those thoughts and questions with me today. It sounds like you're doing a great job advocating for yourself and taking care of your body. In the future, if at any point you have additional questions or want to talk with me about anything related to your health, know that you can easily contact me through our portal for brief questions or come in for an in-person or telehealth visit. Does that sound like an okay plan?"</td>
<td>"I so appreciate you sharing those thoughts with me today, I'm so glad you felt comfortable talking about the best ways to keep you safe and healthy. It sounds like there's a few strategies you're going to try to reduce the chance of a similar infection down the line. But just like you did this time, if you have any concerns, don't hesitate to come in any time for additional testing. If at any point you want to review recommendations or have me order testing, know that you can easily make that request through our portal and get in within a few days. Does that sound like an okay plan?"</td>
<td>"I so appreciate you sharing those thoughts and questions with me today. It sounds like everything is going really well in your pregnancy so far, and it was great to meet you and your partners. As your pregnancy continues, please don't hesitate to let me know if there are any specific things you need help navigating. If you have brief questions, know that you can easily send me a message through our portal or schedule an in-person or telehealth visit. Does that sound like an okay plan?"</td>
</tr>
<tr>
<td colspan="5">After the visit, self-reflect on your performance, and evaluate the success of the interaction as permissible.</td>
</tr>
</table>

Abbreviation: STI, sexually transmitted infection.

## Conclusion

Connection and communication are central to the midwifery model of care, and effective, empathic, and skillful communication is essential. Communicating well can increase the client's knowledge, build trust, enhance shared decision making, and positively affect healthcare outcomes and satisfaction. Through self-awareness, intentional language, and a respectful, stepwise, common-ground approach, midwives can improve their communication with clients and minimize harmful narratives that perpetuate health disparities and contribute to adverse health outcomes in health care.

## Resources

| Organization and Resource | Description |
| --- | --- |
| Health at Every Size Framework from the Association for Size Diversity in Health | Website provides resources for people and clinicians consistent with the Health at Every Size Framework. |
| HIV Risk Reduction Tool from the Centers for Disease Control and Prevention | Interactive website provides strategies for reducing human immunodeficiency virus (HIV) acquisition or transmission; includes suggestions for less risky sexual behaviors while supporting overall sexual health. |
| National Harm Reduction Coalition | This organization provides harm-reduction strategies for people who use drugs. |
| Project Implicit | Website provides easy-to-use tests for implicit bias on a range of topics as well as information on mitigation strategies to decrease effects of bias. |

## References

1. American College of Nurse-Midwives. Our philosophy of care. https://www.midwife.org/Our-Philosophy-of-Care#:~:text=Equitable%2C%20ethical%2C%20accessible%20quality%20health,participation%20in%20health%20care%20decisions. Accessed July 27, 2022.

2. American College of Nurse-Midwives. *ACNM Core Competencies for Basic Midwifery Practice.* Silver Spring, MD: American College of Nurse-Midwives; 2020.

3. Littell RD, Kumar A, Einstein MH, et al. Advanced communication: a critical component of high quality gynecologic cancer care: a Society of Gynecologic Oncology evidence based review and guide. *Gynecol Oncol.* 2019;155(1):161-169. doi:10.1016/j.ygyno.2019.07.026.

4. Boissy A, Windover AK, Bokar D, et al. Communication skills training for physicians improves patient satisfaction. *J Gen Intern Med.* 2016;31(7):7557-61. doi:10.1007/s11606-016-3597-2.

5. Hlubocky FJ, Rose M, Epstein RM. Mastering resilience in oncology: learn to thrive in the face of burnout. *Am Soc Clin Oncol Educ Book.* 2017;37:771-781. doi:10.1200/edbk_173874.

6. FitzGerald C, Hurst S. Implicit bias in healthcare professionals: a systematic review. *BMC Med Ethics.* 2017;18(1):19. doi:10.1186/s12910-017-0179-8.

7. Staats C. *State of the Science: Implicit Bias Review.* https://search.issuelab.org/resource/state-of-the-science-implicit-bias-review-2013.html. Published 2013.

8. Dovidio JF, Penner LA, Albrecht TL, et al. Disparities and distrust: the implications of psychological processes for understanding racial disparities in health and health care. *Soc Sci Med.* 2008;67(3):478-86. doi:10.1016/j.socscimed.2008.03.019.

9. Banaji MR. *Blindspot: Hidden Biases of Good People.* New York, NY: Bantam; 2016.

10. Dilmaghani M. Beauty perks: physical appearance, earnings, and fringe benefits. *Econ Hum Biol.* 2020;38:100889. doi:10.1016/j.ehb.2020.100889.

11. Lawrence BJ, Kerr D, Pollard CM, et al. Weight bias among health care professionals: a systematic review and meta-analysis. *Obesity (Silver Spring).* 2021;29(11):1802-1812. doi:10.1002/oby.23266.

12. Marcelin JR, Siraj DS, Victor R, et al. The impact of unconscious bias in healthcare: how to recognize and mitigate it. *J Infect Dis.* 2019;220(220 suppl 2):S62-S73. doi:10.1093/infdis/jiz214.

13. Dehon E, Weiss N, Jones J, et al. A systematic review of the impact of physician implicit racial bias on clinical decision making. *Acad Emerg Med.* 2017;24(8):895-904. doi:10.1111/acem.13214.

14. Puhl RM. What words should we use to talk about weight? A systematic review of quantitative and qualitative studies examining preferences for weight-related terminology. *Obesity Rev.* 2020;21(6):e13008. doi:10.1111/obr.13008.

15. Ashford RD, Brown AM, McDaniel J, Curtis B. Biased labels: an experimental study of language and stigma among individuals in recovery and health professionals. *Substance Use Misuse.* 2019;54(8):1376-1384. doi:10.1080/10826084.2019.1581221.

16. Healy M, Richard A, Kidia K. How to reduce stigma and bias in clinical communication: a narrative review. *J Gen Intern Med.* 2022;37(10):2533-2540. doi:10.1007/s11606-022-07609-y.

17. Narayan MC. Addressing implicit bias in nursing: a review. *Am J Nurs.* 2019;119(7):36-43. doi:10.1097/01.NAJ.0000569340.27659.5a.

18. Alberga AS, Edache IY, Forhan M, Russell-Mayhew S. Weight bias and health care utilization: a scoping review. *Prim Health Care Res Dev.* 2019;20:e116. doi:10.1017/s1463423619000227.

19. Phelan SM, Burgess DJ, Yeazel MW, et al. Impact of weight bias and stigma on quality of care and outcomes for patients with obesity. *Obesity Rev.* 2015;16(4):319-26. doi:10.1111/obr.12266.

20. Hall WJ, Chapman MV, Lee KM, et al. Implicit racial/ethnic bias among health care professionals and its influence on health care outcomes: a systematic review. *Am J Public Health*. 2015;105(12):e60-e76. doi:10.2105/ajph.2015.302903.

21. Edgoose JY, Regner CJ, Zakletskaia LI. BREATHE OUT: a randomized controlled trial of a structured intervention to improve clinician satisfaction with "difficult" visits. *J Am Board Fam Med*. 2015;28(1):13-20. doi:10.3122/jabfm.2015.01.130323.

22. Popeski N, Kuzio C, Fowler M, et al. Incorporating obesity and weight bias training improved attitudes of hospital staff towards people with obesity in Alberta. *Can J Diabetes*. 2021;45(7):S12. doi:https://doi.org/10.1016/j.jcjd.2021.09.039.

23. Sharma N, Gupta V. Therapeutic communication. In: *StatPearls*. Boca Raton, FL: StatPearls Publishing; 2022. https://www.ncbi.nlm.nih.gov/books/NBK567775/.

24. Brown B. *Dare to Lead: Brave Work, Tough Conversations, Whole Hearts*. New York, NY: Random House; 2018.

25. Albury C, Strain WD, Brocq SL, et al. The importance of language in engagement between health-care professionals and people living with obesity: a joint consensus statement. *Lancet Diabetes Endocrinol*. 2020;8(5):447-455. doi:10.1016/s2213-8587(20)30102-9.

APPENDIX

# 4B

# Preconception Care

AMY ALSPAUGH

*The editors acknowledge Mary C. Brucker and Mary Ann Faucher, who
were authors of this appendix in the previous edition.*

## Introduction

What we now call preconception health came out of
a movement that looked to improve perinatal outcomes by looking beyond the small window of prenatal care and childbirth, rationalizing that healthy
individuals tend to have healthy pregnancies and
healthy children. Thus, both public health and clinical interventions began to target this preconception
period in an effort to improve perinatal outcomes.
While the period prior to pregnancy is important for
the identification and modification of some specific
risks, this effort should not come at the expense of,
but rather augment, discussions of person-centered
health care.

Since the concept of preconception health arose,
much of our understanding about reproductive and
sexual health needs has evolved. We better understand many key concepts, from the limitations of
reproductive life planning[1,2] to the nuances of pregnancy ambivalence,[3–5] and we frame these topics
within a lens of health equity.[6]

## Origins, Uses, and Limitations of Preconception Health and Reproductive Life Planning

The concept that health prior to pregnancy should
be optimized to improve pregnancy-related outcomes began to take hold in the last quarter of the
twentieth century.[7] Preconception health was born
from this movement, and relies upon the notion
of reproductive life planning to identify when preconception health care is needed. Reproductive life
planning is a counseling method to help individuals proactively identify their reproductive goals and

from these goals, create a reproductive life plan.
The reproductive life planning movement is a direct attempt to address the high rates of unintended
pregnancy in the United States and assumes that unintended pregnancies are both problematic for individuals and society and a cause of adverse perinatal
outcomes. It is essential to remember that pregnancy intention is an imperfect measure, meaning
that individuals are capable of ambiguous, complicated, and even contradictory feelings toward both
pregnancy and pregnancy prevention.[3,8] The very
notion of unintended pregnancy does not resonate
with the broad public, so clinical use of this term
is greatly limited. Further, adverse health events related to unintended pregnancy are likely related to
the structural inequities experienced by those who
are more likely to have an unintended pregnancy,
and using unintended pregnancy as a marker of success or failure places the burden of change on the individual instead of on the systems that created and
uphold these inequities.[8]

Some approaches to preconception care advocate for treating all individuals with the capacity
for pregnancy as being in need of preconception
counseling and advice.[9] This approach is problematic for many reasons, one of which is the assumption that all individuals with the capacity for
pregnancy will desire a pregnancy at some point.
Additionally, the focus on preconception health
in individuals not planning a pregnancy can take
away time from addressing the person's health concerns or can make them feel unheard if a discussion about pregnancy ensues after they expressly
say it is not desired.

Preconception care must exist within an overarching framework that, first and foremost, values individuals and their health as having intrinsic

value. Using the lens of patient-centered health and health equity, health provision must view the individual as an autonomous being with broad health needs that are not centered solely on their value as a person who may reproduce.[6] This foundation is necessary to provide preconception care in a way that is just and respectful.

## Preconception Care

Preconception health is, without question, valuable for many individuals who do report a desire for pregnancy now or in the near future. Using one of many screening methods (Table 4B-1), reproductive life planning can help the clinician to identify those persons who may need preconception health care. Each of these approaches has unique strengths and weaknesses, but the importance of framing these inquiries as open-ended questions with no right or wrong answers is critical. One Key Question[10] is the shortest approach but may not create open dialogue for those persons who have more nuanced or complicated feelings about pregnancy and raising children. The PATH questions[11] offer a person an opening to talk about the degree of uncertainty regarding their goals, while the last question provides context on the relative importance of contraceptive efficacy.

| Table 4B-1 | Different Approaches to Reproductive Planning and Counseling |
|---|---|
| **Approach** | **Questions** |
| One Key Question[10] | Would you like to become pregnant in the next year? |
| Reproductive life plan[9] | 1. Do you have any children now? 2. Do you want to have (more) children? 3. How many (more) children would you like to have and when? |
| PATH questions[11] 1. Pregnancy Attitudes 2. Timing 3. How important is prevention | Do you think you might like to have (more) children at some point? If person is considering future parenthood: What do you think that might be? How important is it to you to prevent pregnancy (until then)? |

## General Health Promotion and Preconception Care

All individuals can benefit from health promotion, as discussed in the *Health Promotion Across the Lifespan* chapter. However, individuals who are planning a pregnancy within the near future merit a review of some topics that can impact both fertility and the course of pregnancy.

### Oral Health

Several myths exist regarding oral health in pregnancy. Some individuals may have heard that loss of teeth is inherently associated with pregnancy and, therefore, may not seek dental care while pregnant. Other individuals may avoid such care due to fear of risk of X rays. In any case, research has demonstrated an increased risk of preterm birth, low birth weight, and preeclampsia when individuals have significant periodontal disease during pregnancy.[12] This increase in the incidence of preterm birth in conjunction with periodontal disease is likely linked to the inflammatory process. Ideally, dental work necessary to correct periodontal disease or dental caries should be completed prior to pregnancy.[13]

### Substance Use

Counseling that is particularly important during a preconception visit includes recommendations regarding substance use. Individuals who use alcohol during pregnancy run the risk that their child will develop a fetal alcohol spectrum disorder, including fetal alcohol syndrome, the most severe form.[14] Smoking or other tobacco use, including e-cigarettes, remains the leading preventable cause of premature death for individuals in the United States.[15,16] Tobacco is fetotoxic, and its use in pregnancy is associated with an increased incidence of low birth weight. Particular attention also should be paid to the increasing number of individuals dealing with opioid use. Opioid use is harmful to the pregnant person and associated with neonatal opioid withdrawal syndrome.

The preconception period represents an opportunity for individuals to seek help in adjusting their patterns of use—and if applicable, misuse—of these substances, particularly since it usually takes time and sometimes several attempts to quit successfully. Additionally, nicotine and cannabis are modifiable causes of subfertility for both those with the capacity for pregnancy and those who produce sperm, and should be explored in individuals who are considering a pregnancy or having difficulty achieving pregnancy.[17,18,19]

## Immunizations

The preconception period is an important time to assess for and provide immunizations for those persons who do not have immunity. All individuals of reproductive age should have their immunization status for tetanus–diphtheria–acellular pertussis toxoid (Tdap); measles, mumps, and rubella (MMR); hepatitis B; and varicella reviewed annually. If immunity is lacking, these immunizations should be offered. Current recommendations are to give one dose of Tdap to every pregnant person during every pregnancy (27–36 weeks) regardless of the duration of time since the last Tdap vaccination. This is true for all pregnant individuals, including those vaccinated preconceptionally. Individuals at risk for acquiring hepatitis B or who have not received the vaccine should be offered the immunization series prior to pregnancy. Vaccines containing live attenuated virus are contraindicated during pregnancy, such as MMR, varicella, and the live attenuated version of the flu vaccine, so ensuring these vaccines are up-to-date prior to pregnancy is important.[20] Additionally, all Food and Drug Administration (FDA)–approved COVID-19 vaccines appear to be safe during pregnancy and are recommended for individuals prior to or during pregnancy, although long-term studies are lacking.[21]

Rubella is a known teratogen, causing congenital rubella syndrome when nonimmune women are infected during the first 16 weeks of pregnancy. Individuals who receive the rubella immunization should be counseled to avoid pregnancy for 1 month, based on a theoretical risk of passing rubella to a developing embryo. However, there are no reports of teratogenicity secondary to receiving rubella vaccine in early pregnancy; thus, pregnancy termination is not recommended for individuals who are inadvertently vaccinated for rubella within 4 weeks of becoming pregnant or when they are pregnant.[22]

## Nutrition: Counseling and Folic Acid Supplementation

All individuals should be counseled to avoid vitamins or multivitamin preparations that exceed the current recommended daily allowances because of the potential adverse effects associated with higher doses. For example, vitamin A in the form of retinol is associated with fetal malformations if very high doses of supplements are consumed in the first trimester.[23] Generally speaking, a diet high in intake of fruit, with minimal intake of fast food and sugar-sweetened beverages, and lower in glycemic load has been suggested to decrease time-to-pregnancy.[24] Thus, nutritional counseling should be part of a preconception health visit.

The most important nutritional counseling that should be done during preconception is education on folic acid supplementation. Most individuals in the United States do not consume the recommended amounts of folate from diet alone. All professional organizations recommend that individuals planning a pregnancy take a daily supplement that contains 400 to 1000 micrograms of folic acid to reduce the risk of having a fetus with a neural tube defect.[25] Most over-the-counter multivitamins contain 400 micrograms (0.4 milligram) of folic acid, and generic preparations are appropriate.

Vitamin D deficiency is widespread, yet data are still emerging with regard to the value of vitamin D supplementation.[26] At present, regular screening of pregnant persons for vitamin D deficiency and targeted supplementation of vitamin D during pregnancy are not recommended. However, clinicians may consider screening individuals at increased risk of vitamin D deficiency, such as vegetarians, those who live in cold climates and along northern latitudes, those who wear sunscreen regularly, and those who belong to a racial/ethnic group with dark skin.[27] When a deficiency is identified, ingestion of 1000 to 4000 IU/day is considered to be reasonable and safe by most experts.[27]

## Decreasing Environmental Risks

The most common environmental toxins in the United States and their known health effects are listed in **Table 4B-2.** No person can totally avoid exposure to toxins, though it is critical to note that many marginalized groups, such as communities of color and those who are economically marginalized, are exposed to a disproportionate amount of environmental toxins.[28] These same communities are also more likely be employed in jobs that incur an increased risk of exposure, such as work in a factory, on a farm, or with harsh cleaning solvents.[29]

The most prevalent environmental toxins are manufactured chemicals, including pesticides, polychlorinated biphenyls, and perfluorochemicals. Most of these chemicals degrade slowly and are absorbed by individuals through ingestion of contaminated food and water or inhalation of particles. Environmental toxins have broad deleterious effects on reproductive health, including decreased sperm quality, congenital anomalies, spontaneous miscarriage, stillbirth, low birth weight, and preterm labor. Many environmental toxins also cross the placenta and have been found in cord blood and fetal tissue as well as breast/chest milk.[30]

| Table 4B-2 | Environmental Toxins | |
|---|---|---|
| **Type of Environmental Exposure** | **Toxin and Reported Association** | **Counseling to Minimize Exposure** |
| **Home Environment** | | |
| Older homes with lead paint and water pipes | Lead: Neurologic delays and lowered intelligence,[31] attention deficits and behavioral problems[32,33] | Use a wet cloth or mop to clean floors and surfaces. Because lead can be present in dust, sweeping and dusting may spread the lead instead of removing it. Check homes built before 1978 for lead paint, which may also be present in the soil and dust. Test home drinking water for lead, use cold water for cooking, run water before drinking, and use lead-removing filters.[34] Call the National Lead Information Center for more information (1-800-424-LEAD). |
| Smoking in the home | Inhaled cigarette smoke: Increased risk of a low-birth-weight infant[35,36] | Avoid secondhand exposure; promote tobacco cessation and relapse prevention. Increase ventilation when smoking is present by opening windows or remaining outside. |
| Flame retardants in foam furniture | Polybrominated diphenyl ether (PBDE) flame retardants: Decreased executive function, poorer attention, behavioral problems in children[37,38] | Select foam products that are labeled as "flame retardant free." |
| Air pollution | Polycyclic aromatic hydrocarbons (PAHs): Preterm birth,[39] low birth weight,[40] asthma,[41] neurodevelopmental problems such as autism[42] | Use a wet mop/cloth to clean surfaces. Wash hands frequently, especially before eating. Antibacterial gel alone does not remove toxins. Follow local recommendations related to air and water quality, including avoiding outdoor exercise in times of peak air pollution. |
| Cleaning products | Liquid solvents: Infertility, miscarriage, and low birth weight[43–45] | Use nontoxic products, or cheaply and easily make your own effective, nontoxic cleaners using common household ingredients. Avoid dry cleaning clothes to avoid exposure to solvents. |
| Home and garden pesticides | Pesticides: Childhood cancer,[46,47] autism spectrum disorders,[48,49] problems with intelligence and working memory[50,51] | Avoid or minimize pesticides at home, including sprays, bug bombs, chemical tick-and-flea collars, flea baths, and flea drips. Minimize the risk of insects and rodents in your house by storing food in tightly closed containers, sealing cracks, repairing drips, and using baits and traps as needed. Use nontoxic or natural pesticides in the garden. Purchase organic fruits and vegetables. |
| Personal care products | Phthalates: Neurodevelopment disorders,[47] pregnancy complications,[52] infertility[47,53] | Use "fragrance-free" products instead of products with a fragrance; use phthalate-free products when available. |
| **Diet and Nutrition** | | |
| Seafood consumption | Mercury: Decreased cognitive functions and memory impairments[54,55] | Avoid fish with high levels of mercury, such as shark, swordfish, king mackerel, and tilefish. If fishing locally, use trusted sites to find local fish advisories. Don't eat fish you catch before checking local warnings to ensure the fish is safe to eat. |

| Type of Environmental Exposure | Toxin and Reported Association | Counseling to Minimize Exposure |
|---|---|---|
| Produce | *Listeria monocytogenes*: Infection can result in fetal loss, preterm labor, neonatal sepsis, meningitis, and death[56,57] | Thoroughly wash raw produce, and keep raw meat, poultry, eggs, seafood, and their juices separate from other food. Avoid specific foods with a high risk of contamination with *Listeria*, such as unpasteurized milk and foods with unpasteurized milk, luncheon meats and hot dogs unless heated until steaming hot just before serving, refrigerated meat spreads, and smoked seafood. |
| Food storage containers | Bisphenol A: Infertility,[58] miscarriage,[52] and neurodevelopmental disorders[33,59] | Select glass, ceramic, or stainless-steel containers for food and drink instead of plastic. Avoid microwaving foods in plastic or covered with plastic wrap. |
| **Workplace or Occupational Exposure** | | |
| Agriculture, custodial services, manufacturing, beauty salon, and health care | Pesticides, organic solvents, heavy metals, biologics, and radiation: See above | Ensure patients are aware that they have a right not to be exposed to workplace hazards that may harm their health. Pregnant individuals have a right to a safe and healthy workspace. |

Based on McCue K, DeNicola N. Environmental exposures in reproductive health. *Obstet Gynecol Clin North Am.* 2019;46(3): 455-468. doi:10.1016/j.ogc.2019.04.005.

An important first step in decreasing exposure to environmental toxins is risk identification through the collection of a thorough history of occupational, recreational, residential, or dietary exposures. Counseling should include sources of environmental toxins and approaches used to limit exposure. To conduct this kind of counseling, clinicians need a working knowledge of local and regional environmental pollutants, including soil contaminated by past and present industry and agricultural pesticides. Clinicians can also provide guidance to reduce exposure to toxins for all individuals, including recommendations to rinse fruits and vegetables to remove pesticide residue and to avoid consuming contaminated foods.

## Special Considerations

A complete history may reveal reproductive problems including extremes of age, genetic conditions of the person or family, and chronic illnesses and treatments. In these situations, preconception care can be invaluable. It is also important to note that preconception health and pregnancy planning can be a source of stress and fear especially for those individuals who fall within the following categories, so every effort should be made to engage in supportive counseling and coordination of care among healthcare providers, when needed.[60,61]

### Risk for Genetic Disorders

Knowledge about genetic inheritance, screening, and counseling has increased greatly during the past decades. Collection of a three-generation history is needed to identify genetic conditions. If a specific risk factor is identified or if the future parents have concerns, referral to a genetic specialist is required. Population genetics suggest that some screening can be focused based on the individual's ethnic or racial background. For example, Ashkenazi Jews have a higher risk of Tay–Sachs disease than other groups. Sickle cell disease is more common among African Americans, while cystic fibrosis has a higher incidence among Northern Europeans.[62] Because many individuals' ancestry can be complex or unknown, screening for genetic conditions can be offered to all patients.

When a person with a capacity for pregnancy has been identified as a carrier for a condition, the reproductive partner should also be offered screening. If applicable, the reproductive partner should be evaluated for a history of personal or family health conditions, with necessary follow-up for an evaluation of their health and potentially genetic counseling.[63] In the event that a referral for genetic counseling is necessary, clinicians must remain sensitive to the costs and insurance coverage of genetic counseling services and provide individuals with affordable options. A detailed discussion of this subject is found in the *Assessment for Genetic and Fetal Abnormalities* chapter.

## Reproductive History

Previous adverse pregnancy outcomes suggest the need for additional attention in the preconception period. For example, individuals who have had a previous pregnancy complicated by conditions such as preterm birth or fetal growth restriction are at risk for similar outcomes in a subsequent pregnancy.[64,65] If the etiology of a previous adverse perinatal outcome is known, further assessment and therapies may be instituted preconceptionally to mitigate the risk of recurrence. Health education about birth spacing, nutrition, and healthy habits may be useful in improving outcomes, but systemic and structural causes often remain unchanged.

## Effect of Age on Reproductive Outcomes

Declines in fertility and adverse reproductive outcomes are more likely as pregnancy-capable individuals become older—this decline starts around age 32 and accelerates more rapidly around age 37.[66,67] In addition, as individuals age, their risks for diabetes, hypertension, and other chronic diseases increase. These chronic conditions independently increase the risk for poor perinatal outcomes.[68-70] Thus, it is often difficult to distinguish the risks that are secondary to age from those that are secondary to a combination of age and a chronic condition.

The effects of age on reproductive outcomes form a continuum. Although 35 years is often used as a cut-off for identifying individuals at increased risk, most of these risks increase incrementally over time. Based on a person's desires regarding future pregnancies, discussion about a variety of options related to fertility and pregnancy, including egg banking and other aspects of reproductive artificial technology, may be warranted.[71] These topics are beyond the scope of this appendix.[72]

## Medical Conditions

Individuals who have medical conditions that can adversely affect pregnancy (e.g., diabetes, hypertension, epilepsy, autoimmune disorders) should be referred for care by a specialist prior to attempting pregnancy. Table 4B-3 lists selected chronic health conditions that can adversely affect the course of pregnancy, though it is not all-inclusive. Several of these conditions have risks associated with the disease; others require treatments that may be teratogenic or fetotoxic.

# Medications

Medications used by the person, including herbal preparations, botanicals, and over-the-counter agents, should be evaluated for potential teratogenic effects, and the continuing need for the medication should be assessed. Individuals should not be automatically counseled to discontinue medications because they are considering pregnancy, as this may negatively affect their medical or mental health. Ideally, a plan should be in place for use of any specific medication in the preconception period and during the early stages of organogenesis. When a person reports taking a medication that has identified risks during pregnancy, the clinician should discuss the implications with the person and recommend safer alternative medications as available. Easy-to-use smartphone apps (e.g., Epocrates and InfantRisk) are helpful for identifying medications that are safe to use during pregnancy and those for which an alternative should be identified.

# Preparing for Pregnancy

The decision to seek pregnancy is unique to each person. A preconception visit enables the individual to optimize their health—although ideally all healthcare encounters should share this goal. Health is more than the mere absence of disease, and exploration of the person's level of stress, socioeconomic stability, family dynamics, support networks, and other social determinants of health can also be considered during this time. Short interpregnancy spacing, as defined as 6 months or less, has been found to be an independent risk factor for adverse perinatal outcomes, and that information may influence a person's timing of pregnancy.[89]

The preconception period is also an ideal time for individuals to consider their access to and availability of health care. An essential question to consider at a preconception visit is whether the birthing person wishes to see a midwife, obstetrician-gynecologist, family practice physician, or maternal–fetal medicine specialist when pregnant. Place of birth and provider options may be controlled by the person's insurance coverage and subject to certain limitations. If individuals investigate these options early, they may be able to make the arrangements for the birth provider and the environment they need and prefer.

Counseling for those persons who may desire pregnancy soon should also involve a discussion about how and when to stop using contraception, if applicable. Generally speaking, return to fertility is relatively quick after cessation of many hormonal contraceptives,[90] and occurs immediately after cessation of a nonhormonal method. Injectable

| Table 4B-3 | Preconception Care Interventions for Chronic Medical Conditions | |
|---|---|---|
| **Medical Condition** | **Preconception Considerations** | **Management** |
| Asthma | Asthma increases the risk for adverse outcomes in both the birthing person and the neonate, although active management of symptoms mitigates risk. Most asthma medications are safe for use during pregnancy, and the risks posed by uncontrolled asthma symptoms are greater than those posed by any medication.[73] | Prior to pregnancy, a complete assessment of asthma control should be initiated. Preferred medications include albuterol for short-acting treatment and inhaled corticosteroids, and specifically budesonide, for long-acting control, with intranasal corticosteroids being used to treat concomitant allergic rhinitis, if needed.[74] |
| Autoimmune conditions (e.g., rheumatoid arthritis, systemic lupus erythematosus) | Preconception care should focus on identification of serious organ damage that might affect the ability to safely carry a pregnancy, evaluation of disease activity, serologic evaluation for the identification of autoantibodies associated with adverse outcome, and review of current medications and their safety in pregnancy.[75] Ideally, the disease should be stable with a pregnancy-safe medication for 4 to 6 months prior to conception. | The following medications require a washout period prior to conception: mycophenolate mofetil, leflunomide, and methotrexate.[76]<br>The following immunosuppressive medications are compatible with pregnancy: prednisone, azathioprine, cyclosporine, and tacrolimus.<br>Refer individuals considering pregnancy to their specialist for evaluation and management. |
| Cardiovascular disease | Preconception care should include a discussion of genetic counseling.<br>Perinatal outcomes are closely associated with the severity of the heart disease (e.g., mitral valve prolapse is associated with minimal risks; pulmonary hypertension is potentially life threatening). | ACE inhibitors should be discontinued prior to pregnancy. The use of warfarin (Coumadin) in pregnancy is especially toxic to the fetus during the first trimester when given at doses greater than 5 mg/day.[77] |
| Diabetes | Preconception visits should include baseline labs (HbA1c, creatinine, TSH, urine albumin–creatinine ratio). Folic acid of up to 5 mg/day should be prescribed and continued until 12 weeks' gestation. Higher levels of folic acid may be prescribed to mitigate the increased risk of neural tube defects that has been associated with preexisting diabetes.[77] | Good glycemic control (i.e., HbA1c < 6.0%) at the time of conception lowers the risk of miscarriage and congenital anomalies that are associated with hyperglycemia, although any improvement in HbA1c prior to pregnancy improves outcomes.<br>Discontinue ACEs, ARBs, statins, and hypoglycemic agents other than metformin and insulin, with the addition of glucagon if the person is on insulin.[78] |
| Hypertension | During preconception care, consider evaluation for secondary causes of hypertension. Have persons with long-standing hypertension be evaluated by a specialist for silent ventricular hypertrophy, retinopathy, and renal disease prior to pregnancy.[79] | Use of ACE inhibitors and ARBs should be discontinued prior to pregnancy, as their use is associated with increased risks of fetal malformation, oligohydramnios, fetal growth restriction, and fetal death. Preferred drugs include methyldopa and labetalol. Education should include maintaining a diet low in sodium.[79] |
| Intimate partner violence (IPV) | IPV has been associated with preterm birth, low birth weight, postpartum depression, and maternal mortality. Interventions before pregnancy can focus on identifying a safe environment for the person and any existing children. | IPV has often been left out of preconception care but is a critical factor to address to improve health outcomes for both the birthing person and the neonate.[80] |

(continues)

| Table 4B-3 | Preconception Care Interventions for Chronic Medical Conditions (*continued*) | |
|---|---|---|
| **Medical Condition** | **Preconception Considerations** | **Management** |
| Mental health conditions | Although debate continues regarding the potential teratogenic effects of some psychotropic agents, there is a general consensus that the benefits associated with treatment generally outweigh the risks, because mental health disorders in pregnancy are associated with poor perinatal outcomes, higher risk of postpartum psychiatric illnesses, increased rates of substance use, lower participation in prenatal care, and adverse infant outcomes.[81] | Valproate should be discontinued prior to pregnancy.[82] |
| Obesity | Persons with obesity may take longer to conceive, with time-to-pregnancy increasing with the degree of obesity.[83]<br>Considered the most common of the chronic diseases, obesity increases risks of hypertensive disorders of pregnancy and gestational diabetes as well as preterm birth, birth defects, and perinatal death. Education and counseling during the preconception period can assist a person in losing weight in a healthy manner before attempting pregnancy. | Weight-loss drugs should be avoided, as they may be associated with increased risk of congenital anomalies when used in pregnancy.<br>For those persons who have undergone bariatric surgery, it is suggested that they wait 12 to 24 months before trying to conceive.[84] |
| Renal disease | For individuals with renal disease who get pregnant, there is an increased risk of complications including preeclampsia, preterm birth, fetal growth restriction, and neonatal intensive care admission.[85] | Because individuals who have severe renal disease are likely to experience a worsening of the condition during pregnancy, including severe associated conditions such as hypertension, they should be carefully counseled by a specialist and their medications evaluated prior to becoming pregnant.[85] |
| Seizure disorders | Persons with epilepsy may have a mild reduction in fertility.[86]<br>Those with well-controlled epilepsy (seizure free for 2–5 years) may be eligible to stop or reduce their medication prior to pregnancy, and individuals taking more than one antiepileptic drug may consider a trial of monotherapy. | Valproic acid, a high-risk teratogenic drug, can be replaced with levetiracetam to treat epilepsy.[87]<br>High-dose (5 mg) folic acid is recommended at least 1 month prior to conception and throughout the first trimester.[86] |
| Thyroid disorders | Overt hypothyroidism during the first trimester of pregnancy is associated with dwarfism and intellectual impairment. Other pregnancy complications associated with hypothyroidism include miscarriage, preterm birth, preeclampsia, placental abnormalities, and low birth weight.<br>Ideally, persons with thyroid disorders should have achieved a euthyroid state prior to conception. | Medications for hypothyroidism are safe to use during pregnancy. The general recommendation is to avoid pregnancy for 6 months after receiving radioactive treatment.<br>Individuals with Graves' disease will need to seek care from a specialist before and during pregnancy due to the complexity of disease management.[88] |

Abbreviations: ACE, angiotensin-converting enzyme; ARB, angiotensin II receptor blocker; HbA1c, hemoglobin A1c; IPV, intimate partner violence.

contraception is a notable exception, with a median time to conception of 10 months after the last injection that is unrelated to duration of use.[91] Discussion of return to fertility with the person planning a pregnancy should center on their desire for when to stop a method. Additionally, monitoring fertility indicators (e.g., basal body temperature, cervical fluid, menstrual charting) that allow for better identification of the fertile window has been shown to increase fecundability.[92]

When couples engage in regular, unprotected penile–vaginal intercourse, pregnancy is typically achieved in 3 to 6 months, and 90% of individuals becoming pregnant within the first year. If pregnancy does not ensue after 12 months, an infertility evaluation should be offered. Alternatively, individuals age 35 years and older may wish to seek infertility care after only 6 months of trying to become pregnant because fertility wanes with increasing age.[71]

## Conclusion

Preconception planning is an important topic for clinicians and individuals alike, but should be centered within the desires and priorities of the person with capacity for pregnancy. A healthy person is more likely to have a healthy pregnancy and a healthy newborn. Health care during the preconception period is especially important for some groups—namely, those with a chronic health condition—but is also an excellent opportunity to provide health education, offer counseling, and encourage habits that are congruent with health and wellness.

## Resources

| Organization | Description |
|---|---|
| Centers for Disease Control and Prevention (CDC) | U.S. government site with specific information regarding preconception care. Includes download of the free consumer-oriented app *Show Your Love* to help women maintain healthy habits, chart ovulation, and plan for pregnancy. |
| National Preconception Health and Health Care Initiative | Partnership among more than 70 public and private organizations to promote preconception health care. Source of extensive materials and information. |
| Office of Women's Health Website | Patient-centered information on enhancing preconception health, information for reproductive partners, and an explanation of genetic counseling options. |

## References

1. Callegari LS, Aiken ARA, Dehlendorf C, et al. Addressing potential pitfalls of reproductive life planning with patient-centered counseling. *Am J Obstet Gynecol.* 2017;216(2):129-134. doi:10.1016/j.ajog.2016.10.004.

2. Morse JE, Moos M-K. Reproductive life planning: raising the questions. *Matern Child Health J.* 2018;22(4):439-444. doi:10.1007/s10995-018-2516-z.

3. Askelson NM, Losch ME, Thomas LJ, Reynolds JC. "Baby? Baby not?": exploring women's narratives about ambivalence towards an unintended pregnancy. *Women Health.* 2015;55(7):842-858. doi:10.1080/03630242.2015.1050543.

4. Gómez AM, Arteaga S, Villaseñor E, et al. The misclassification of ambivalence in pregnancy intentions: a mixed-methods analysis. *Perspect Sex Reprod Health.* 2019;51(1):7-15. doi:10.1363/psrh.12088.

5. Higgins JA, Popkin RA, Santelli JS. Pregnancy ambivalence and contraceptive use among young adults in the United States. *Perspect Sex Reprod Health.* 2012;44(4):236-243. doi:10.1363/4423612.

6. Dehlendorf C, Akers AY, Borrero S, et al. Evolving the preconception health framework: a call for reproductive and sexual health equity. *Obstet Gynecol.* 2021;137(2):234-239. doi:10.1097/AOG.0000000000004255.

7. Freda MC, Moos M-K, Curtis M. The history of preconception care: evolving guidelines and standards. *Matern Child Health J.* 2006;10(5 suppl):S43-S52. doi:10.1007/s10995-006-0087-x.

8. Potter JE, Stevenson AJ, Coleman-Minahan K, et al. Challenging unintended pregnancy as an indicator of reproductive autonomy. *Contraception.* 2019;100(1):1-4. doi:10.1016/j.contraception.2019.02.005.

9. Tydén T, Verbiest S, Van Achterberg T, et al. Using the reproductive life plan in contraceptive counselling. *Ups J Med Sci.* 2016;121(4):299-303. doi:10.1080/03009734.2016.1210267.

10. Bellanca HK, Hunter MS. One Key Question®: preventive reproductive health is part of high quality primary care. *Contraception.* 2013;88(1):3-6. doi:10.1016/j.contraception.2013.05.003.

11. Geist C, Aiken AR, Sanders JN, et al. Beyond intent: exploring the association of contraceptive choice with questions about Pregnancy Attitudes, Timing and How important is pregnancy prevention (PATH) questions. *Contraception.* 2019;99(1):22-26. doi:10.1016/j.contraception.2018.08.014.

12. Daalderop LA, Wieland BV, Tomsin K, et al. Periodontal disease and pregnancy outcomes: overview of systematic reviews. *JDR Clin Transl Res.* 2018;3(1):10-27. doi:10.1177/2380084417731097.

13. Bobetsis YA, Graziani F, Gürsoy M, Madianos PN. Periodontal disease and adverse pregnancy outcomes. *Periodontol 2000.* 2020;83(1):154-174. doi:10.1111/prd.12294.

14. Dejong K, Olyaei A, Lo JO. Alcohol use in pregnancy. *Clin Obstet Gynecol.* 2019;62(1):142-155. doi:10.1097/GRF.0000000000000414.

15. Centers for Disease Control and Prevention. Fast facts and fact sheets: smoking and cigarettes. https://www.cdc.gov/tobacco/data_statistics/fact_sheets/fast_facts/index.htm. Published June 2, 2021. Accessed December 10, 2022.

16. Rollins LG, Sokol NA, McCallum M, et al. Electronic cigarette use during preconception and/or pregnancy: prevalence, characteristics, and concurrent mental health conditions. *J Womens Health 2002.* 2020;29(6):780-788. doi:10.1089/jwh.2019.8089.

17. Fonseca BM, Rebelo I. Cannabis and cannabinoids in reproduction and fertility: where we stand. *Reprod Sci (Thousand Oaks, A).* Published online May 10, 2021. doi:10.1007/s43032-021-00588-1.

18. Marom-Haham L, Shulman A. Cigarette smoking and hormones. *Curr Opin Obstet Gynecol.* 2016;28(4):230-235. doi:10.1097/GCO.0000000000000283.

19. Payne KS, Mazur DJ, Hotaling JM, Pastuszak AW. Cannabis and male fertility: a systematic review. *J Urol.* 2019;202(4):674-681. doi:10.1097/JU.0000000000000248.

20. Psarris A, Sindos M, Daskalakis G, et al. Immunizations during pregnancy: how, when and why. *Eur J Obstet Gynecol Reprod Biol.* 2019;240:29-35. doi:10.1016/j.ejogrb.2019.06.019.

21. American College of Obstetricians and Gynecologists. ACOG and SMFM recommend COVID-19 vaccination for pregnant individuals. https://www.acog.org/en/news/news-releases/2021/07/acog-smfm-recommend-covid-19-vaccination-for-pregnant-individuals. Published July 30, 2021. Accessed December 10, 2022.

22. Dontigny L, Arsenault M-Y, Martel M-J. No. 203: rubella in pregnancy. *J Obstet Gynaecol Can.* 2018;40(8):e615-e621. doi:10.1016/j.jogc.2018.05.009.

23. Clagett-Dame M, Knutson D. Vitamin A in reproduction and development. *Nutrients.* 2011;3(4):385-428. doi:10.3390/nu3040385.

24. Grieger JA. Preconception diet, fertility, and later health in pregnancy. *Curr Opin Obstet Gynecol.* 2020;32(3):227-232. doi:10.1097/GCO.0000000000000629.

25. Chitayat D, Matsui D, Amitai Y, et al. Folic acid supplementation for pregnant women and those planning pregnancy: 2015 update. *J Clin Pharmacol.* 2016;56(2):170-175. doi:10.1002/jcph.616.

26. Pilz S, Zittermann A, Obeid R, et al. The role of vitamin D in fertility and during pregnancy and lactation: a review of clinical data. *Int J Environ Res Public Health.* 2018;15(10). doi:10.3390/ijerph15102241.

27. ACOG Committee Opinion No. 495: vitamin D: screening and supplementation during pregnancy. *Obstet Gynecol.* 2011;118(1):197-198. doi:10.1097/AOG.0b013e318227f06b.

28. Mikati I, Benson AF, Luben TJ, et al. Disparities in distribution of particulate matter emission sources by race and poverty status. *Am J Public Health.* 2018;108(4):480-485. doi:10.2105/AJPH.2017.304297.

29. Morelli V, Ziegler C, Fawibe O. Environmental justice and underserved communities. *Prim Care.* 2017;44(1):155-170. doi:10.1016/j.pop.2016.09.016.

30. ACOG Committee Opinion, Number 832: reducing prenatal exposure to toxic environmental agents. *Obstet Gynecol.* 2021;138(1):e40-e54. doi:10.1097/AOG.0000000000004449.

31. Marshall AT, Betts S, Kan EC, et al. Association of lead-exposure risk and family income with childhood brain outcomes. *Nat Med.* 2020;26(1):91-97. doi:10.1038/s41591-019-0713-y.

32. Caito S, Aschner M. Developmental neurotoxicity of lead. *Adv Neurobiol.* 2017;18:3-12. doi:10.1007/978-3-319-60189-2_1.

33. Arbuckle TE, Davis K, Boylan K, et al. Bisphenol A, phthalates and lead and learning and behavioral problems in Canadian children 6–11 years of age: CHMS 2007–2009. *Neurotoxicology.* 2016;54:89-98. doi:10.1016/j.neuro.2016.03.014.

34. Environmental Protection Agency. Basic information about lead in drinking water. https://www.epa.gov/ground-water-and-drinking-water/basic-information-about-lead-drinking-water#getinto. Updated November 15, 2022. Accessed December 10, 2022.

35. Kalayasiri R, Supcharoen W, Ouiyanukoon P. Association between secondhand smoke exposure and quality of life in pregnant women and postpartum women and the consequences on the newborns. *Qual Life Res Int J Qual Life Asp Treat Care Rehabil.* 2018;27(4):905-912. doi:10.1007/s11136-018-1783-x.

36. Zhou S, Rosenthal DG, Sherman S, et al. Physical, behavioral, and cognitive effects of prenatal tobacco and postnatal secondhand smoke exposure. *Curr Probl Pediatr Adolesc Health Care.* 2014;44(8):219-241. doi:10.1016/j.cppeds.2014.03.007.

37. Sagiv SK, Kogut K, Gaspar FW, et al. Prenatal and childhood polybrominated diphenyl ether (PBDE) exposure and attention and executive function at 9–12 years of age. *Neurotoxicol Teratol.* 2015;52(pt B):151-161. doi:10.1016/j.ntt.2015.08.001.

38. Vuong AM, Yolton K, Poston KL, et al. Prenatal and postnatal polybrominated diphenyl ether (PBDE) exposure and measures of inattention and impulsivity in children. *Neurotoxicol Teratol.* 2017;64:20-28. doi:10.1016/j.ntt.2017.09.001.

39. Liu C, Sun J, Liu Y, et al. Different exposure levels of fine particulate matter and preterm birth: a meta-analysis based on cohort studies. *Environ Sci Pollut Res Int.* 2017;24(22):17976-17984. doi:10.1007/s11356-017-9363-0.

40. Jedrychowski WA, Majewska R, Spengler JD, et al. Prenatal exposure to fine particles and polycyclic aromatic hydrocarbons and birth outcomes: a two-pollutant approach. *Int Arch Occup Environ Health.* 2017;90(3):255-264. doi:10.1007/s00420-016-1192-9.

41. Hehua Z, Qing C, Shanyan G, et al. The impact of prenatal exposure to air pollution on childhood wheezing and asthma: a systematic review.

*Environ Res.* 2017;159:519-530. doi:10.1016/j .envres.2017.08.038.

42. Liu X-Y, Wang B-L, Yi M-J, Zhang F-H. [Association of exposure to polycyclic aromatic hydrocarbons during pregnancy with autism spectrum disorder–related behaviors in toddlers: a birth cohort study]. *Zhongguo Dang Dai Er Ke Za Zhi [Chin J Contemp Pediatr].* 2019;21(4):332-336. doi:10.7499/j .issn.1008-8830.2019.04.006.

43. Doyle P, Roman E, Beral V, Brookes M. Spontaneous abortion in dry cleaning workers potentially exposed to perchloroethylene. *Occup Environ Med.* 1997;54(12):848-853. doi:10.1136/oem.54.12.848.

44. Olsen J, Hemminki K, Ahlborg G, et al. Low birthweight, congenital malformations, and spontaneous abortions among dry-cleaning workers in Scandinavia. *Scand J Work Environ Health.* 1990;16(3):163-168. doi:10.5271/sjweh.1800.

45. Hruska KS, Furth PA, Seifer DB, et al. Environmental factors in infertility. *Clin Obstet Gynecol.* 2000;43(4): 821-829. doi:10.1097/00003081-200012000-00014.

46. Patel DM, Jones RR, Booth BJ, et al. Parental occupational exposure to pesticides, animals and organic dust and risk of childhood leukemia and central nervous system tumors: findings from the International Childhood Cancer Cohort Consortium (I4C). *Int J Cancer.* 2020;146(4):943-952. doi:10.1002/ijc.32388.

47. Kahn LG, Philippat C, Nakayama SF, et al. Endocrine-disrupting chemicals: implications for human health. *Lancet Diabetes Endocrinol.* 2020;8(8):703-718. doi:10.1016/S2213-8587(20)30129-7.

48. von Ehrenstein OS, Ling C, Cui X, et al. Prenatal and infant exposure to ambient pesticides and autism spectrum disorder in children: population based case-control study. *BMJ.* 2019;364:l962. doi:10.1136/bmj.l962.

49. Biosca-Brull J, Pérez-Fernández C, Mora S, et al. Relationship between autism spectrum disorder and pesticides: a systematic review of human and preclinical models. *Int J Environ Res Public Health.* 2021;18(10). doi:10.3390/ijerph18105190.

50. Cimino AM, Boyles AL, Thayer KA, Perry MJ. Effects of neonicotinoid pesticide exposure on human health: a systematic review. *Environ Health Perspect.* 2017;125(2):155-162. doi:10.1289/EHP515.

51. Furlong MA, Barr DB, Wolff MS, Engel SM. Prenatal exposure to pyrethroid pesticides and childhood behavior and executive functioning. *Neurotoxicology.* 2017;62:231-238. doi:10.1016/j .neuro.2017.08.005.

52. Filardi T, Panimolle F, Lenzi A, Morano S. Bisphenol A and phthalates in diet: an emerging link with pregnancy complications. *Nutrients.* 2020;12(2). doi:10.3390/nu12020525.

53. Bonde JP, Flachs EM, Rimborg S, et al. The epidemiologic evidence linking prenatal and postnatal exposure to endocrine disrupting chemicals with male reproductive disorders: a systematic review and meta-analysis. *Hum Reprod Update.* 2016;23(1): 104-125. doi:10.1093/humupd/dmw036.

54. Bellinger DC, O'Leary K, Rainis H, Gibb HJ. Country-specific estimates of the incidence of intellectual disability associated with prenatal exposure to methylmercury. *Environ Res.* 2016;147:159-163. doi:10.1016/j.envres.2015.10.006.

55. Bennett D, Bellinger DC, Birnbaum LS, et al. Project TENDR: Targeting Environmental Neuro-Developmental Risks. The TENDR consensus statement. *Environ Health Perspect.* 2016;124(7): A118-A122. doi:10.1289/EHP358.

56. Madjunkov M, Chaudhry S, Ito S. Listeriosis during pregnancy. *Arch Gynecol Obstet.* 2017;296(2): 143-152. doi:10.1007/s00404-017-4401-1.

57. Wadhwa Desai R, Smith MA. Pregnancy-related listeriosis. *Birth Defects Res.* 2017;109(5):324-335. doi:10.1002/bdr2.1012.

58. Pivonello C, Muscogiuri G, Nardone A, et al. Bisphenol A: an emerging threat to female fertility. *Reprod Biol Endocrinol RBE.* 2020;18(1):22. doi:10.1186 /s12958-019-0558-8.

59. Jiang Y, Li J, Xu S, et al. Prenatal exposure to bisphenol A and its alternatives and child neurodevelopment at 2 years. *J Hazard Mater.* 2020;388:121774. doi:10.1016/j.jhazmat.2019.121774.

60. Steel A, Lucke J, Adams J. The prevalence and nature of the use of preconception services by women with chronic health conditions: an integrative review. *BMC Womens Health.* 2015;15:14. doi:10.1186 /s12905-015-0165-6.

61. McCorry NK, Hughes C, Spence D, et al. Pregnancy planning and diabetes: a qualitative exploration of women's attitudes toward preconception care. *J Midwifery Womens Health.* 2012;57(4):396-402. doi:10.1111/j.1542-2011.2011.00143.x.

62. Delatycki MB, Laing NG, Moore SJ, et al. Preconception and antenatal carrier screening for genetic conditions: the critical role of general practitioners. *Aust J Gen Pract.* 2019;48(3):106-110. doi:10.31128/AJGP-10-18-4725.

63. Rose NC, Wick M. Carrier screening for single gene disorders. *Semin Fetal Neonatal Med.* 2018;23(2):78-84. doi:10.1016/j.siny.2017.06.001.

64. Phillips C, Velji Z, Hanly C, Metcalfe A. Risk of recurrent spontaneous preterm birth: a systematic review and meta-analysis. *BMJ Open.* 2017;7(6):e015402. doi:10.1136/bmjopen-2016-015402.

65. Kinzler WL, Kaminsky L. Fetal growth restriction and subsequent pregnancy risks. *Semin Perinatol.* 2007;31(3):126-134. doi:10.1053/j. semperi.2007.03.004.

66. Wesselink AK, Rothman KJ, Hatch EE, et al. Age and fecundability in a North American preconception

cohort study. *Am J Obstet Gynecol.* 2017;217(6):667. e1-667.e8. doi:10.1016/j.ajog.2017.09.002.

67. ACOG Committee Opinion No. 589: female age-related fertility decline. *Fertil Steril.* 2014;101(3):633-634. doi:10.1016/j.fertnstert.2013.12.032.

68. Casteleiro A, Paz-Zulueta M, Parás-Bravo P, et al. Association between advanced maternal age and maternal and neonatal morbidity: a cross-sectional study on a Spanish population. *PLoS One.* 2019;14(11):e0225074. doi:10.1371/journal.pone.0225074.

69. Kortekaas JC, Kazemier BM, Keulen JKJ, et al. Risk of adverse pregnancy outcomes of late- and post-term pregnancies in advanced maternal age: a national cohort study. *Acta Obstet Gynecol Scand.* 2020;99(8):1022-1030. doi:10.1111/aogs.13828.

70. Kahveci B, Melekoglu R, Evruke IC, Cetin C. The effect of advanced maternal age on perinatal outcomes in nulliparous singleton pregnancies. *BMC Pregnancy Childbirth.* 2018;18(1):343. doi:10.1186/s12884-018-1984-x.

71. Dillon CM, Ennen CS, Bailey KJ, Thagard AS. A Comprehensive approach to care of women of advanced maternal age. *Nurs Womens Health.* 2019;23(2):124-134. https://doi.org/10.1016/j.nwh.2019.02.002.

72. Chronopoulou E, Raperport C, Serhal P, et al. Pre-conception tests at advanced maternal age. *Best Pract Res Clin Obstet Gynaecol.* Published online 2020. https://doi.org/10.1016/j.bpobgyn.2020.11.003.

73. Popa M, Peltecu G, Gica N, et al. Asthma in pregnancy: review of current literature and recommendations. *Maedica.* 2021;16(1):80-87. doi:10.26574/maedica.2020.16.1.80.

74. Vatti RR, Teuber SS. Asthma and pregnancy. *Clin Rev Allergy Immunol.* 2012;43(1-2):45-56. doi:10.1007/s12016-011-8277-8.

75. Sammaritano LR. Contraception and preconception counseling in women with autoimmune disease. *Best Pract Res Clin Obstet Gynaecol.* 2020;64:11-23. doi:10.1016/j.bpobgyn.2019.09.003.

76. Somers EC. Pregnancy and autoimmune diseases. *Best Pract Res Clin Obstet Gynaecol.* 2020;64:3-10. doi:10.1016/j.bpobgyn.2019.11.004.

77. Hebson C, Saraf A, Book WM. Risk assessment and management of the mother with cardiovascular disease. *Clin Perinatol.* 2016;43(1):1-22. doi:10.1016/j.clp.2015.11.001.

78. Egan AM, Dow ML, Vella A. A review of the pathophysiology and management of diabetes in pregnancy. *Mayo Clin Proc.* 2020;95(12):2734-2746. doi:10.1016/j.mayocp.2020.02.019.

79. Lu Y, Chen R, Cai J, Huang Z, Yuan H. The management of hypertension in women planning for pregnancy. *Br Med Bull.* 2018;128(1):75-84. doi:10.1093/bmb/ldy035.

80. Morgan IA, Robbins CL, Basile KC. Addressing intimate partner violence to improve women's preconception health. *J Womens Health 2002.* 2018;27(10):1189-1194. doi:10.1089/jwh.2018.7366.

81. Howard LM, Khalifeh H. Perinatal mental health: a review of progress and challenges. *World Psychiatry.* 2020;19(3):313-327. doi:10.1002/wps.20769.

82. Sharma V, Sharma P, Sharma S. Managing bipolar disorder during pregnancy and the postpartum period: a critical review of current practice. *Expert Rev Neurother.* 2020;20(4):373-383. doi:10.1080/14737175.2020.1743684.

83. Poston L, Caleyachetty R, Cnattingius S, et al. Preconceptional and maternal obesity: epidemiology and health consequences. *Lancet Diabetes Endocrinol.* 2016;4(12):1025-1036. doi:10.1016/S2213-8587(16)30217-0.

84. Dutton H, Borengasser SJ, Gaudet LM, et al. Obesity in pregnancy: optimizing outcomes for mom and baby. *Med Clin North Am.* 2018;102(1):87-106. doi:10.1016/j.mcna.2017.08.008.

85. Wiles K, Chappell L, Clark K, et al. Clinical practice guideline on pregnancy and renal disease. *BMC Nephrol.* 2019;20(1):401. doi:10.1186/s12882-019-1560-2.

86. Walker SP, Permezel M, Berkovic SF. The management of epilepsy in pregnancy. *BJOG Int J Obstet Gynaecol.* 2009;116(6):758-767. doi:10.1111/j.1471-0528.2009.02141.x.

87. Kuo C-Y, Liu Y-H, Chou I-J, et al. Shifting valproic acid to levetiracetam in women of childbearing age with epilepsy: a retrospective investigation and review of the literature. *Front Neurol.* 2020;11:330. doi:10.3389/fneur.2020.00330.

88. Alexander EK, Pearce EN, Brent GA, et al. 2017 Guidelines of the American Thyroid Association for the diagnosis and management of thyroid disease during pregnancy and the postpartum. *Thyroid.* 2017;27(3):315-389. doi:10.1089/thy.2016.0457.

89. Brunner Huber LR, Smith K, Sha W, Vick T. Interbirth interval and pregnancy complications and outcomes: findings from the pregnancy risk assessment monitoring system. *J Midwifery Womens Health.* 2018;63(4):436-445. doi:10.1111/jmwh.12745.

90. Girum T, Wasie A. Return of fertility after discontinuation of contraception: a systematic review and meta-analysis. *Contracept Reprod Med.* 2018;3:9. doi:10.1186/s40834-018-0064-y.

91. Food and Drug Administration. Depo-Provera prescribing information. https://www.accessdata.fda.gov/drugsatfda_docs/label/2010/020246s036lbl.pdf. Accessed December 10, 2022/.

92. Stanford JB, Willis SK, Hatch EE, et al. Fecundability in relation to use of fertility awareness indicators in a North American preconception cohort study. *Fertil Steril.* 2019;112(5):892-899. doi:10.1016/j.fertnstert.2019.06.036.

CHAPTER

# 5

# Common Conditions in Primary Care

JAN M. KRIEBS AND BUNNY POUNDS

## Introduction

To some, the primary care provider role for midwives in the United States might appear to be a new phenomenon, but its roots harken back decades, if not centuries. This nation's first midwives were esteemed healers in their communities, and the first nurse-midwives were public health nurses, all providing elements of primary care as we know it today. Their scope of practice included general health and well-being for the whole family.[1] By the 1990s, competencies in primary care had been added to midwifery education and practice standards, and they were made even clearer in subsequent core competency revisions.[2,3] Despite state-by-state variations in legislative and regulatory support for this aspect of the midwife's role, as well as irregularities in reimbursement for primary care services, midwives have embraced their role as primary care providers and the responsibilities that come with it.[4]

By the end of the twentieth century, it had become clear that midwives can increase access to primary care services when they are integral members of the primary care workforce.[5] Diversification of the workforce to better represent the clients served,[6] in addition to midwifery education that incorporates concepts such as cultural humility, positionality, and intersectionality, are supports that make midwifery primary care not only physically accessible but also safe for all clients.[7]

Midwifery care focuses on normalcy, and the chapters focusing on primary care in *Varney's Midwifery* present the knowledge needed to help people of all ages maintain and promote healthy lifestyles. Yet people who receive primary care from midwives experience a range of inequities that can influence their health and well-being and result in health disparities.

Midwives care for racially and ethnically diverse populations, and midwives will be more effective when the workforce has similar diversity. The disparate effects of social determinants of health and systemic racism can be found in many communities. Some populations who receive care from midwives have documented increased risks of inequalities in access and health disparities, such as people of color or people of young or old age, low education and low literacy, low income, religious affiliation, disability status, gender and sexual minority status, use of substances, and place of residence (especially remote, rural, or urban areas). The intersectionality of these population characteristics can further magnify health problems, as in the case of racial/ethnic disparities among rural residents.[8-10]

With these imperatives in mind, this chapter presents an overview of the common health conditions encountered in primary care. It covers care of individuals who are not pregnant, but who have disorders or conditions that can be characterized as belonging to the realm of primary care rather than sexual or reproductive health care. This chapter begins with a definition of primary care, and then addresses some of the more common primary care conditions managed by midwives. Readers are additionally directed to the *Health Promotion Across the Lifespan* chapter, which summarizes current recommendations for primary and secondary prevention.

## Defining Primary Care

No universally accepted definition of *primary care* exists. Variations exist among insurers, providers, professional organizations, and consumers. Perhaps the most widely accepted definition is the one introduced in 1996 by the Institute of Medicine, which characterized primary care as:

*The provision of integrated, accessible health care services by clinicians who are accountable for addressing a large majority of personal health care needs, developing a sustained partnership with patients, and practicing in the context of family and community.*[11]

For some individuals, the "large majority" has been defined as provision of 80% of the care needed by a person annually. However, this definition of primary care fails to highlight the importance of health maintenance, age-appropriate screening, and health education—all activities that are discussed in depth in the *Health Promotion Across the Lifespan* chapter.

## Social Determinants of Health and Primary Care

It is increasingly appreciated that social determinants of health can dramatically affect the health of individuals and their families and should be part of the primary care assessment. Organizations such as the Centers for Disease Control and Prevention (CDC), the National Institutes of Health (NIH), and the Health Resources and Services Administration (HRSA) have called for integration of population health into primary care with the goal of creating a more unified approach to care.[12] Use of programs such as the National Vital Signs to monitor effectiveness of care and geocoding to better recognize potential socioeconomic factors impacting health can provide for better evaluation of care quality.[13-15]

Examples of social determinants of health include safe neighborhoods and the ability to access transportation; safe spaces for physical activity, including both sports and safe streets; opportunities for education leading to literacy and numeracy; job opportunities that provide a living wage; clean air and water; and access to food. Two examples of social determinants are discussed briefly here, as illustrations of how these concerns play into the primary care assessment.

Screening for food insecurity is essential to assist in the provision of resources for a patient and to determine the parameters for discussing diet. Food insecurity is associated with a host of chronic diseases, including obesity, and with frailty in the elderly population. Before engaging in a discussion of nutritional diets or dietary changes, it is important to find out if the patient has enough of any kind of food to eat. Many professional societies and electronic medical record systems use the two-question Hunger Vital

| Table 5-1 | Food Insecurity Screen |
|---|---|

A person is considered food insecure if they respond "often true" or "sometimes true" to at least one of these questions:

1. "We worried whether our food would run out before we got money to buy more." Was that often true, sometimes true, or never true for your household in the last 12 months?
2. "The food we bought just didn't last, and we didn't have money to get more." Was that often true, sometimes true, or never true for your household in the last 12 months?

Signs Screener for this purpose (Table 5-1).[16] This tool, which is easily administered, opens the door to offering food assistance through programs such as the Special Supplemental Nutrition Program for Women, Infants, and Children (WIC), the Summer Food Service Program, the Supplemental Nutrition Assistance Program (SNAP), and others.[17]

A study of patients' preferences about food insecurity screening indicated they preferred these questions be asked by the person doing the initial patient screen, such as a nurse or nursing assistant. The receipt of a list of food bank locations, local community organizations, and financial assistance programs was deemed the most helpful by at least 75% of study participants.[18]

As is true for food insecurity, housing insecurity may not always be readily apparent. Homelessness is only one aspect of housing insecurity, albeit the most severe. From difficulty in paying housing costs, to frequent moves or sleeping in the homes of relatives or friends, to overcrowding, to substandard housing—every aspect of housing insecurity impacts individuals' health and stress levels.[19,20]

As with food insecurity, questions about housing may feel insensitive or disrespectful, implying that the individual is not able to care for their own family. The use of a standard tool, which can be offered as part of "the questions we ask all our clients," can help reduce discomfort whether administered by a clinician or a member of the office staff.

Numerous tools are available (Table 5-2). One of the simplest is the Homelessness Screening Clinical Reminder adopted by the Veterans Health Administration in 2012.[21] Several other tools are summarized by the Social Interventions Research & Interventions Network at the University of California, San Fransisco.[22] The Accountable Health Communities tool included in this summary directly addresses the issue of homelessness as well as

| Table 5-2 | Housing Insecurity Screening Tools |
|---|---|

**Homelessness Screening Clinical Reminder**

1. In the past 2 months, have you been living in stable housing that you own, rent, or stay in as part of a household? (A negative response indicates housing instability.)

2. Are you worried or concerned that in the next 2 months you may not have stable housing that you own, rent, or stay in as part of a household? (A positive response indicates risk.)

**Accountable Health Communities Tool**

What is your living situation today?

- I have a steady place to live.
- I have a place to live today, but am worried about losing it in the future.
- I do not have a steady place to live. I am temporarily staying with others; in a hotel; in a shelter; living outside on the street, on a beach, in a car, in an abandoned building, in a bus or train station, or in a park.

Based on Chhabra M, Sorrentino AE, Cusack M, et al. Screening for housing instability: providers' reflections on addressing a social determinant of health. *J Gen Intern Med.* 2019;34(7):1213-1219. doi:10.1007/s11606-019-04895-x; Social Interventions Research & Evaluation Network. Housing insecurity/instability/homelessness questions. https://sirenetwork.ucsf.edu/housing-insecurity-instability-homelessness-questions. Accessed June 20, 2022.

| Table 5-3 | Signs and Symptoms of Severe Anemia | |
|---|---|---|
| **Signs** | **Symptoms** | |
| Pallor | Fatigue, drowsiness | |
| Jaundice | Weakness | |
| Orthostatic hypotension | Dizziness | |
| Peripheral edema | Headaches | |
| Pale mucous membranes and nail beds | Malaise | |
| | Pica | |
| Smooth, sore tongue | Poor appetite, changes in food preferences | |
| Splenomegaly | | |
| Tachypnea, dyspnea on exertion | Changes in sleep habits | |
| | Changes in mood | |
| Tachycardia or flow murmur | | |

instability. It asks only two questions; each question indicates risk.

One issue for practices to consider before they start screening is how to address a response indicating risk. Time constraints are universal. Having materials, local resources, and referrals ready to share can provide a partial solution.

The remainder of this chapter covers common primary care conditions encountered by midwives. The material is organized by system, beginning with hematologic conditions and proceeding through the major body systems. Mental health is presented in the *Mental Health Conditions* chapter, and other primary care content is covered throughout the text.

## Hematologic Conditions

### Anemia

Anemia is defined as a decrease in red blood cell (RBC) mass or a decrease in hemoglobin. Hemoglobin is the protein within RBCs that carries oxygen away from the lungs to supply the cells, and returns carbon dioxide to the lungs for exhalation. Hematocrit, the blood count value usually reported with (or instead of) hemoglobin, is the ratio of RBC volume to the total blood volume. It typically is about three times as large a number as the hemoglobin concentration, so long as the RBCs are both normocytic and normochromic.

Most often, anemia remains a silent condition unless it is acute or severe. Signs and symptoms of anemia are listed in Table 5-3.[23] Anemia can be caused by decreased RBC production, increased RBC destruction, or blood loss, and is diagnosed in nonpregnant people when the hemoglobin level is less than 12.0 g/dL in women and less than 13.0 g/dL in men.[24] No well-defined standard has been established for diagnosing anemia in transgender individuals. These limits were established by the World Health Organization for use in international nutrition studies and do not apply to all populations. The hemoglobin level that indicates anemia can vary based on the individual's personal health profile. Individuals who smoke (because of competition for oxygen-binding sites on RBCs) and those living at high altitudes (because of lower oxygen concentration in the atmosphere) have higher hemoglobin and hematocrit levels; their bodies adapt to maintain adequate oxygenation and their hemoglobin levels increase as the altitude or the number of cigarettes smoked per day increases.[24] The threshold for anemia should be higher in these individuals. The U.S. Preventive Services Task Force does not address whether screening for anemia should be a routine part of health care for nonpregnant people.

### Differential Diagnosis of Anemia

Anemia can be acquired through iron deficiency or result from hemorrhage, or it can be inherited in persons with hemoglobinopathies, such as thalassemia or sickle cell disease. The clinical evaluation and diagnosis of anemia are based on the mean corpuscular volume (MCV), which is how this chapter reviews this condition.

Anemia can be subclassified as normocytic, microcytic, or macrocytic depending on the amount and type of hemoglobin present in RBCs, as reflected in the MCV. *Microcytic anemias* include iron deficiency, the thalassemias, and anemia of chronic diseases, often related to inflammation. *Macrocytic anemias* include folate and vitamin $B_{12}$ deficiency, as well as anemia associated with liver disease, increased reticulocyte production, and some medication effects. *Normocytic anemias* commonly reflect acute blood loss or conditions such as autoimmune diseases, sickle cell disease, hemoglobin C disease, or glucose-6-phosphate dehydrogenase (G6PD) deficiency. Aplastic anemia, while normocytic, is characterized by pancytopenia, meaning a reduction in the number of RBCs, white blood cells (WBCs), and platelets. Table 5-4 lists the laboratory values associated with some common causes of anemia.

A complete blood count (CBC) provides the first level of assessment and helps differentiate many of the underlying causes of anemia. Among adults who have menses, the history and review of systems should include obtaining a history of how heavy the menstrual flow is, even though the accuracy of an individual's estimation of their flow has been demonstrated to vary. Any information about prior anemia diagnoses can contribute to the differential diagnosis. For individuals who menstruate and have a hemoglobin value of less than 12.0 g/dL, a laboratory panel including serum folate, iron and ferritin measurements, total iron-binding capacity, and reticulocyte count should be ordered, and a hemoglobin electrophoresis performed. The ferritin level is the most sensitive and specific predictor of iron stores and, therefore, true iron deficiency. Specific minor causes of anemia may require further evaluation, but should not be part of the initial evaluation.

### Iron-Deficiency Anemia

Normal daily iron loss through excretion, sweat, and cellular shedding amounts to 1 mg; menses causes an additional monthly loss of iron. The Recommended Daily Intake (RDI) of iron is 15 mg for girls from 14 to 18 years old and 18 mg for women from 19 to 50 years old. For all other adults older

| Table 5-4 | Laboratory Values Associated with Common Anemias | | | | |
|---|---|---|---|---|---|
| Laboratory Test | Iron Deficiency | Vitamin $B_{12}$ Deficiency | Folate Deficiency | Thalassemia | Chronic Disease |
| Red blood cells (RBCs) | Low | Low | Low | Normal | Low |
| Hemoglobin (Hgb) | Low | Low | Low | Low | Low |
| Mean corpuscular volume (MCV) | Low | High | High | Low | Normal-low |
| Mean corpuscular hemoglobin (MCH) | Low | High | High | Low | Low |
| Reticulocytes | Low | Low | Low | High | Low |
| Ferritin | Low | High | High | Normal–high | Normal–high |
| Iron | Low | High | High | Normal–decreased | Low |
| Total iron-binding capacity (TIBC) | High | Normal | Normal | Variable | Low |
| Other | | Low vitamin $B_{12}$ | Low folate | Teardrop red cells | |
| | | Elevated methylmalonate | Normal methylmalonate | Target cells | |
| | | Elevated homocysteine | Elevated homocysteine | Abnormal hemoglobin electrophoresis | |

than age 18, the RDI drops to 8 mg.[25] Dietary iron intake is often lower than the recommended level. During pregnancy, the RDI is 27 mg.

The most common anemia in the United States is due to iron deficiency, which usually is mild and easily reversible. Occult blood loss, excessive menstrual loss, and inadequate nutritional intake are the most common causes of iron deficiency in adults. If nutritional deficiency is ruled out and there is no identifiable source of bleeding such as heavy menses, an inquiry about use of aspirin and nonsteroidal anti-inflammatory drugs (NSAIDs) as well as assessment for gastrointestinal bleeding is warranted. Nutritional deficiencies causing significant iron depletion include restrictive vegetarian diets as well as pica; therefore, a careful diet history is part of the work-up.

A ferritin level less than 100 to 150 ng/mL confirms the diagnosis of iron-deficiency anemia and renders serum iron and total iron-binding capacity measurements unnecessary. Based on the severity of the anemia and its cause, consultation or referral may be indicated; when the hemoglobin indicates severe anemia (less than 9.0 g/dL), consultation is appropriate, even when the anemia is clearly caused by iron deficiency.

First-line treatment for iron-deficiency anemia is to increase dietary intake of iron-rich foods to enhance the body's absorption of iron. Nutritional counseling should stress the importance of including non-heme iron-rich foods in the diet—such as green leafy vegetables, collard greens, egg yolks, raisins, prunes, liver, oysters, and some fortified cereals— particularly for individuals who eat little or no animal protein. Assessment and counseling about the elimination of picas (e.g., eating ice or laundry starches) is also important. A detailed discussion of dietary sources of iron can be found in the *Nutrition* chapter.

Iron supplementation, either through the diet or with oral medications, should be recommended for nonpregnant adults when the hemoglobin is less than 12.0 g/dL[25] When uncomplicated iron deficiency is the cause of the anemia, oral medications are used empirically, including ferrous sulfate, ferrous fumarate, and ferrous gluconate. Each of these preparations is readily available and marketed under several brand names. Multiple daily doses of iron have been a standard recommendation. However, taking the equivalent of 325 mg of ferrous sulfate daily or every other day should be sufficient; every-other-day dosing will decrease side effects and has been shown to be equally effective as daily dosing.[26-28] Taking iron preparations with meals will usually decrease absorption of this nutrient, but will also improve gastrointestinal side effects such as nausea and reflux. Certain drugs, such as antacids, decrease the absorption of iron supplements and should not be taken at the same time. After the hemoglobin level has returned to normal, continued supplementation for 3 months should adequately replenish iron stores in the body.

While no clear standard for follow-up exists, the CBC and reticulocyte (immature RBCs) count are generally repeated 1 to 3 months following treatment initiation, depending on the severity of the original deficiency and the person's age. Response to iron supplementation is often rapid in cases of uncomplicated iron-deficiency anemia, as evidenced by rebounding hemoglobin and hematocrit levels and elevated reticulocyte counts. Menstruating individuals who are unresponsive to iron therapy and anyone who has ceased menstruating or is older than age 50 with iron-deficiency anemia should be referred for a consultation with a specialist. People may also require referral to a hematologist for further evaluation and possible treatment with intravenous iron therapy if they are unable to tolerate or absorb oral iron therapy. In extreme cases, an urgent referral to the emergency room for immediate evaluation or blood transfusion is warranted if the anemia is severe or symptomatic.

## Hemoglobin Abnormalities

As noted earlier, the hemoglobin in RBCs functions to carry oxygen from the lungs to cells. Normal adult hemoglobin is genetically composed of four polypeptide subunits (two alpha-globin chains and two beta-globin chains) plus a heme molecule containing iron (HbA). Adult hemoglobin also includes 2% to 3% hemoglobin $A_2$ (HbA$_2$), a normal variation in which delta chains substitute for beta chains. An additional 1% to 2% may be fetal hemoglobin (HbF), in which the molecule contains gamma chains rather than beta chains. Small traces of other hemoglobin subtypes, such as HbA$_1$, may be seen as well.[23]

Hemoglobinopathies are structural abnormalities that occur when one or two of the subunits are replaced by a variant type of globin chain. The resulting hemoglobin molecule is designated by a letter. The main hemoglobinopathies are sickle cell (HbS), HbC, and HbE. Alpha- or beta-thalassemia occurs when deficient amounts of either alpha- or beta-globin chains are made. Common hemoglobinopathies and thalassemias are listed in Table 5-5.

| Table 5-5 | Disorders of Abnormal Hemoglobin | |
|---|---|---|
| **Name** | **Description** | **Clinical Significance** |
| **Hemoglobinopathies** | | |
| Sickle cell disease | HbSS | Severe illness with sickle cell crisis |
| Sickle cell trait | HbSA | Mild anemia; increased risk for urinary tract infections; sickle cell crisis may occur at high altitudes, if dehydrated, or during extreme physical activity |
| Sickle cell hemoglobin C disease | HbSC | Mild to moderate anemia; sickle cell crises may occur, but less frequently than in persons with HbSS; increased risk for infection; risk for retinopathy and blindness in adulthood |
| Hemoglobin C disease | HbCC | Usually asymptomatic; may have symptoms associated with splenomegaly. No therapy needed; normal life expectancy. |
| Hemoglobin C trait | HbCA | Usually asymptomatic |
| Hemoglobin E disease | HbEE | Microcytic, hypochromic anemia. Hemolysis associated with infection or medications. |
| Hemoglobin E trait | HbEA | Variable mild anemia similar to $\beta$ thalassemia minor |
| **Thalassemias: Alpha-Thalassemias** | | |
| Alpha-thalassemia silent carrier | 1 of 4 alpha genes deleted | Asymptomatic and difficult to detect |
| Alpha-thalassemia trait | 2 of 4 alpha genes deleted; heterozygous form (i.e., aa/– –) or homozygous form (i.e., a–/a–) | Mild microcytic anemia; individual is asymptomatic |
| Hemoglobin H disease | 3 of 4 alpha genes deleted (i.e., a–/– –), or 2 of 4 alpha genes deleted and the third mutated to the constant spring (cs) form (i.e., – –/aacs) | Enlarged spleen; bone abnormalities; severe illness |
| Hemoglobin Bart's hydrops fetalis | 4 of 4 alpha genes deleted (i.e., – –/– –) | Incompatible with life; causes hydrops fetalis |
| **Thalassemias: Beta-Thalassemias** | | |
| Beta-thalassemia (Cooley's anemia) | Beta-thalassemia major, homozygous Beta0/Beta0 or heterozygous Beta0/Beta+[a], leading to absence of beta-chain formation | Severe anemia; jaundice; splenomegaly; requires frequent blood transfusions; often experience iron overload. Classic facial features. |
| Thalassemia intermedia | Beta+/Beta+, resulting in decreased beta-chain formation | Significant anemia but does not need blood transfusions |
| Thalassemia minor | Normal beta-chain/Beta+ or Beta0 | Mild microcytic anemia; individual is asymptomatic |

Abbreviations: Beta0, absence of beta-globin formation; Beta+, reduced beta-globin formation.

[a] Depending on the authority, Beta0/Beta+ has been classified as either beta-thalassemia major or intermedia. It is generally less severe than the Beta0/Beta0 presentation because some beta-chain production is possible with Beta+ mutations.

## Thalassemias

Most thalassemias are autosomal recessive inherited disorders of the globin chains that form normal adult hemoglobin (hemoglobin A). Worldwide, approximately 1.7% of the population is heterozygous for either alpha-thalassemia ($\alpha$-thalassemia) or beta-thalassemia ($\beta$-thalassemia), and approximately 0.04% of the global population is affected by homozygous or multiple heterozygous mutations.[29] However, due to increased immigration from parts of the world where the thalassemias are more prevalent (Southeast Asia, the Mediterranean, Africa, Middle East, and the Indian subcontinent), the prevalence of these conditions has increased by 7.5% in the United States over the last 50 years.[30]

Alpha-thalassemia is most common among individuals of Chinese and Southeast Asian descent. Two genes on chromosome 16 control for alpha-globin chain production. As alpha-globin production decreases, the percentage accounted for by the beta-globin subunit, which is less efficient at carrying and distributing oxygen to cells, increases. A single deletion will create an asymptomatic carrier state; two deletions will cause a smaller MCV without anemia; and the three-deletion state leads to the microcytic hypochromic state known as hemoglobin H disease, of which hemoglobin Constant Spring is the most common variety. Effects include shortened red cell lifespan, splenomegaly, and severe hemolytic anemia. The absence of the alpha chains found in hemoglobin A and the resultant increase in the hemoglobin B subunit (HbBarts) population produces non-immune fetal hydrops, which results in fetal demise.[31]

Beta-thalassemia is most common among people of Mediterranean origin and, to a lesser degree, among those with Chinese, Asian, and African ancestry, with a global incidence of 1.5% for carriers. Estimates of its frequency in the most affected populations range from 3% to 10%.[32] More than 200 different point mutations can be involved in the beta-globin changes associated with thalassemia, leading to a wide spectrum of disease. Asymptomatic individuals with a mutation affecting a single beta-globin gene may remain in a silent carrier state or may present with only mild anemia (beta-thalassemia minor). For these individuals, the diagnosis in most likely made based on routine screening or incidental findings. Those with more severe disease—that is, beta-thalassemia intermediate and beta-thalassemia major—have mutations affecting multiple genes. The two conditions are differentiated by the age at diagnosis and the degree of anemia, and both require lifelong therapy.[31–33]

The diagnosis of thalassemia is often made in childhood in persons in whom more genes are affected. However, milder presentations may not be identified until later in life, and the diagnosis is often made for the first time in pregnancy when screening for hemoglobinopathies is commonly performed. Identification of thalassemia in pregnancy is important because a child could be born with a severe hemoglobinopathy if the partner or sperm donor also is a carrier of a gene for abnormal hemoglobin.

Several laboratory findings can suggest the presence of a thalassemia. Among persons with alpha-thalassemias, decreased HbA production causes abnormal proportions of hemoglobins A, $A_2$, and F. The beta-thalassemias are associated with elevated levels of hemoglobin F and hemoglobin $A_2$ (greater than 3.5%). In both cases, the trait will appear as a microcytic anemia in which the MCV is markedly low relative to the hemoglobin level, usually less than 75 femtoliters (fL). The Metzer index is a calculation derived by dividing the MCV by the number of RBCs. When the Metzer index is less than 13, a thalassemia is strongly suspected. Values greater than 13 suggest iron-deficiency anemia. Even with values less than 13, a complete anemia panel is justified to rule out a combination of iron deficiency and hemoglobinopathy.

When the diagnosis of thalassemia is established, folic acid supplementation may be employed, but iron therapy is inappropriate. The anemia associated with the thalassemias is due to a combination of low hemoglobin production and mild hemolysis, since the associated abnormal RBCs are more vulnerable to destruction and have a shorter lifespan. Consequently, people with thalassemia may not be iron deficient. Simple iron supplementation will not correct the anemia and can be dangerous if it contributes to iron overload.[31]

### Sickle Cell Disease

Sickle cell disease (homozygous SS disease) is an autosomal recessive inherited disorder in which hemoglobin S is produced instead of hemoglobin A. Sickle cell trait (Hb AS) is found most commonly among persons of African descent compared to individuals of other racial and/or ethnic backgrounds. The incidence of sickle cell trait in the United States has been estimated to be 73.1 per 1000 Black births, 6.9 per 1000 Hispanic births, 3.0 per 1000 white births, and 2.2 per 1000 Asian/Native Hawaiian/other Pacific Islander births.[34] The most recent data show that the rate of sickle cell disease is 1 in 135 for individuals identifying as Black or African American, and 1 in 13 Black infants will have sickle trait.[35] Sickle cell trait is rarely associated with hematuria, bacteriuria, or splenic infarct. Although the trait itself is often asymptomatic and does not commonly cause severe health complications, identifying individuals carrying the sickle trait enables appropriate genetic counseling and testing prior to pregnancy. The primary complication, other than the risk of genetic inheritance, is an increase in the development of urinary tract infections. Interestingly, sickle cell trait may lessen the accuracy of hemoglobin $A_{1c}$

testing, making screening for diabetes in individuals with sickle trait more difficult.

In sickle cell disease, the HbS changes shape (polymerizes) when deoxygenated, which causes the RBCs to form a permanent crescent moon or "sickle" shape, rendering these cells less able to bend their shape as they traverse through smaller vessels. The sickle-shape RBCs are also more adhesive and clump together to block the microvasculature. Sickle cell crises involve acute episodes of severe pain from ischemia and infarction of tissue and organs downstream from the area of vascular blockage. The disease has a multi-organ effect and is associated with a shortened lifespan as a consequence of renal damage, cardiac damage, infection, acute chest syndrome, and increased risk for infection. Effective interventions, including universal newborn screening, interventions to reduce the chance of infections, and prophylactic transfusions to decrease strokes, have all contributed to extending lifespans. Hydroxyurea remains the only treatment that reduces both acute and chronic complications. The average lifespan for individuals living with sickle cell disease is now about 40 years, with estimates that it may rise over time to 54 years as childhood interventions shift the risk from early stroke or infection to more chronic effects of the disease.[36]

Hemoglobin S may also be present in heterozygous form as HbSC disease or sickle thalassemia (HbS-B thalassemia), conditions that are associated with somewhat milder forms of sickle crisis. Regardless of the hemoglobinopathy or its presentation, genetic counseling for couples planning a child is recommended.

### Glucose-6-Phosphate Dehydrogenase Deficiency

Glucose-6-phosphate dehydrogenase (G6PD) deficiency is an X-linked genetic disease found most frequently among individuals of Mediterranean or African descent. Lack of the G6PD enzyme leads to increased breakdown of RBCs. Because it is an X-linked condition, G6PD deficiency is rarely symptomatic among those assigned female at birth. Even among individuals who have the condition, the clinical presentation ranges from being asymptomatic to presenting with severe acute or chronic hemolytic anemia. Hemolysis occurs when the individual has an infection or receives oxidative drugs. Among the contraindicated medications for persons with this disorder are sulfa drugs and sulfa derivatives, nitrofurantoin (Macrobid), NSAIDs, toluidine blue, and methylene blue. Consumption of fava beans and some other legumes should be avoided as well, because these foods can produce hemolysis among individuals with the Mediterranean variant. Infections can prompt acute hemolysis. Because surgery can also precipitate an episode of hemolysis, referrals should include documentation of the diagnosis.[37]

### Von Willebrand's Disease

Von Willebrand's disease is an autosomal dominant mutation that causes defects in a protein necessary for platelet adhesion and affects clotting factor VIII.[38] This condition is associated with development of heavy menses; indeed, it accounts for approximately 20% of cases of diagnosed heavy menstrual bleeding, particularly among adolescents.[39] Von Willebrand's disease or another bleeding disorder should be suspected if the individual reports heavy menstrual bleeding in association with prolonged bleeding after surgery or a family history of bleeding problems.[40] The initial assessment for von Willebrand's disease includes obtaining a platelet count, ferritin level, and bleeding time and coagulation studies. When platelets are normal, the ferritin level is low, and the bleeding time is prolonged, von Willebrand's disease is a strong possibility. Although the midwife may continue to provide general care for the patient, referral to a hematologist for evaluation is warranted. Individuals with this condition should avoid aspirin or other agents with anticoagulant properties.

### Thrombocytopenia

Thrombocytopenia is any condition defined by a low platelet count. Since platelets have a 10-day lifespan, normal platelet counts are dependent on the continual production of healthy platelets. Symptoms of thrombocytopenia can include easy bruising (purpura), superficial bleeding that appears as pinpoint red spots (petechiae), long bleeding time from cuts or injuries, bleeding from the gums or nose, blood in the urine or stool, fatigue, and heavy menses. Mild thrombocytopenia can initially be diagnosed on routine blood counts; a peripheral blood smear can then refine the basic diagnosis. On examination, an enlarged spleen may be noted. Categories of thrombocytopenia include increased platelet destruction, decreased platelet production, and retention of platelets within the spleen. Although any decrease in the platelet count below approximately 150,000 cells per microliter is considered a thrombocytopenia and should be noted, serious injury in nonpregnant individuals is unlikely if the platelet count remains greater than 10,000 to 20,000 cells per microliter.[41]

| Table 5-6 | Causes of Thrombocytopenia |
|---|---|
| **Cause** | **Comments** |
| Medication use | Nonsteroidal anti-inflammatory drugs, valproic acid, statins, penicillin, sulfonamides, chemotherapy |
| Environmental exposures | Chemical exposure including benzene, pesticides, arsenic |
| Excessive alcohol intake | More common in persons with vitamin $B_{12}$ or folate deficiency |
| Autoimmune diseases | Immune thrombocytopenia, rheumatoid arthritis, lupus |
| Cancers | Leukemia, lymphoma |
| Splenic retention | Infection<br>Hemolytic anemias<br>Sarcoidosis<br>Metastatic tumors<br>Blood cancers |

When thrombocytopenia is diagnosed and a transient cause (such as mild late pregnancy decreases in platelet count) cannot be identified, referral to a competent professional is necessary (Table 5-6).[42] able

While von Willebrand's disease is the most commonly encountered clotting disorder identified in midwifery practice, there are a number of other inherited coagulopathies, of which the hemophilias are the most common. Some other, less common disorders can lead to abnormal bleeding; most are rare and will not present in an office practice as an undiagnosed condition.

Some patients may also have acquired coagulopathies. Vitamin K deficiency, intentional anticoagulation therapy, liver disease, and disseminated intravascular coagulation are the most common.

## Cardiovascular Conditions

Assessment of cardiovascular health begins with a history and review of systems that assess for hypertension, cardiac events, and vascular changes in the patient and their immediate family. Assessment of heart sounds and of the pulses during the physical examination is essential, as is an accurate measurement of blood pressure.

Cardiovascular diseases include cerebrovascular disease or stroke, dyslipidemia, heart disease, and hypertension. Heart disease is the number one cause of death in the United States, and stroke is the fifth leading cause of death.[43] Risk factors for cardiovascular disease include age, family history, high-fat diet, lack of exercise, smoking, excess alcohol, obesity, diabetes, hypertension, and dyslipidemia. The incidence of cardiovascular risk factors is increasing; nearly 11% of adults older than the age of 20 have high total cholesterol levels and 47% have hypertension.[44,45] Socioeconomic disparities play a major role in risk as well; recognized risk factors include housing or food instability, lack of available transportation, interpersonal safety or violence, and need for assistance with utilities as a measure of financial need.[46]

### Hypertension

Hypertension—an arterial disease characterized by persistent high blood pressure—is the most frequent specific diagnosis associated with primary care visits in the United States.[47] Hypertension is a major risk factor for a number of conditions, such as coronary artery disease, stroke, heart failure, and renal failure. It is more common among African Americans and among the elderly.[48] Hypertension can be categorized as primary or secondary. Primary hypertension—the more common form—is thought to be related to factors such as genetics, age, and obesity. Secondary hypertension occurs as the result of another disorder, such as a renal or heart condition. A third variation of hypertension is white coat hypertension, which refers to the observation that a person's blood pressure is higher in the presence of a healthcare provider. The prevalence of white coat hypertension ranges from 13% to 35%; thus, this condition must be included in the differential diagnosis when a high blood pressure is noted.[49] A fourth variation called masked hypertension refers to individuals who have normal blood pressure during an office visit but demonstrate hypertension at home. It is estimated to occur in 1 in 7 persons. Definitions for blood pressure levels are listed in Table 5-7.[50]

### Diagnosis of Hypertension

Several professional organizations in the United States have published guidelines for care of persons with hypertension. The most widely accepted guidelines for the diagnosis and treatment of hypertension were originally established by the Joint National Committee (JNC).[51,52] In 2014, the Seventh Joint National Committee (JNC 7) guidelines were vigorously reviewed by the panel members of the Eighth Joint National Committee (JNC 8); however, the JNC 8 panel was discontinued by the National Heart, Lung, and Blood Institute. The

| Table 5-7 | Classification of Blood Pressure Levels for Adults | | | |
|---|---|---|---|---|
| **Blood Pressure Classification** | **Systolic (mm Hg)** | | **Diastolic (mm Hg)** | **Corresponding Values** |
| Normal | < 120 | and | < 80 | Office reading of 120/80 equals: Home: 120/80 Nighttime ABPM: 100/65 |
| Elevated | 120–129 | and | < 80 | Not defined |
| Stage 1 hypertension | 130–139 | or | 80–89 | Office reading of 130/80 equals: Home: 130/80 Nighttime ABPM: 110/65 |
| Stage 2 hypertension | ≥ 140 | or | ≥ 90 | Office reading of 140/90 equals: Home: 140/90 Nighttime ABPM: 140/85 Office reading of 160/100 equals: Home: 140/95 Nighttime ABPM: 140/90 |

Abbreviation: ABPM, ambulatory blood pressure monitoring.

Based on Whelton PK, Carey RM, Aronow WS, et al. 2017 ACC/AHA/AAPA/ABC/ACPM/AGS/APhA/ASH/ASPC/NMA/PCNA guideline for the prevention, detection, evaluation, and management of high blood pressure in adults: a report of the American College of Cardiology /American Heart Association Task Force on Clinical Practice Guidelines. *Hypertension*. 2017. [Epub ahead of print]. doi:10.1016/j .jacc.2017.11.006.

panel members published their recommendations, which focus on pharmacologic management of persons with hypertension.[51] To resolve confusion, in 2017, the American Heart Association, in conjunction with multiple other professional organizations, updated the JNC 7 and published new guidelines for detection, evaluation, and management of high blood pressure in adults; these guidelines are presented in Table 5-8.[50]

The initial steps in screening and diagnosis of hypertension are (1) accurate assessment of blood pressure, (2) identification of signs that suggest primary versus secondary hypertension, (3) screening for other cardiovascular risk factors, and (4) assessment for possible white coat hypertension or masked hypertension.

***Accurate Measurement of Blood Pressure*** Many clinicians take action based on blood pressure results that are inaccurate because the technique of assessment is incorrect. Blood pressures should always be taken with a properly sized cuff placed at the level of the heart. The patient should have had 10 minutes to sit quietly and should not have ingested tobacco or caffeine for at least 30 minutes prior to measuring the blood pressure. They should be seated with their back against a chair, legs uncrossed, and forearm resting comfortably on a table. The diagnosis should be made on an average of two

or more readings taken on two or more occasions. Out-of-office or home blood pressure readings are recommended for the confirmation of this diagnosis. If hypertension is diagnosed, many midwives refer the patient to a physician to establish a plan for care and monitoring.

***Signs That Suggest Primary Versus Secondary Hypertension*** Signs that suggest primary hypertension include family history, slowly increasing blood pressure over time, and lifestyle factors such as obesity, smoking, low level of physical activity, and excessive use of alcohol. Signs that suggest secondary hypertension include labile blood pressure and other systemic symptoms such as dizziness, snoring, muscle cramps or weakness, weight loss, edema, fatigue, or weakness. Disorders that are associated with secondary hypertension include hyperthyroidism, kidney disease, Cushing's syndrome, use of medications such as amphetamines and NSAIDs, and use of illicit drugs including cocaine.[50]

***Atherosclerotic Cardiovascular Disease Risk*** Screening for cardiovascular risks is a critical component of this evaluation because the benefit of pharmacologic management of hypertension is directly related to the risk for atherosclerotic cardiovascular disease (ASCVD). Pharmacologic treatment is recommended for persons with a systolic blood pressure of 130 mm Hg or higher or an average diastolic blood pressure of 80 mm Hg or higher.[50] Cardiovascular risk calculators are listed in the Resources section at the end of this chapter.

***White Coat Hypertension and Masked Hypertension*** The 2017 guidelines include recommendations for screening individuals for white coat hypertension.[51] As noted earlier, white coat hypertension is the diagnosis for persons who have hypertension in an office setting but no hypertension at home. There are no data about the benefits or risks associated with treating persons with white coat hypertension.

Masked hypertension is not common but should be included in the differential diagnosis if the person reports a history of occasional hypertension but is normotensive during a primary care visit. Home blood pressure monitoring or ambulatory blood pressure monitoring can be helpful in establishing this diagnosis.

***Laboratory Evaluation*** If hypertension is detected, laboratory evaluation includes tests that will assess for complications of hypertension and the presence of comorbidities. Recommended laboratory evaluations include fasting blood glucose, thyroid indices, serum creatinine, lipid profile, serum sodium, potassium, and calcium, all of which may be part of a metabolic panel. An electrocardiogram should also be performed.

### Treatment of Primary Hypertension

Table 5-8 outlines the general management of persons with hypertension after the initial evaluation. Many cases of primary hypertension are related to lifestyle, rather than underlying disease. These causes are directly modifiable through lifestyle changes such as weight loss, nutritional counseling for a low-sodium diet, exercise, smoking cessation, and moderation in alcohol consumption.[52–54] A weight loss of as little as 10 pounds can have a salutary effect on blood pressure. Table 5-9 demonstrates the effect of lifestyle modification on blood pressure as reported by the JNC 7 and supported by the 2017 guidelines.[50,52] Achieving more than one modification has an independent effect on blood pressure, so a combination of modifications can achieve better results.[53]

In addition to lifestyle modifications, several categories of drugs can be prescribed to treat hypertension. Low-dose thiazide diuretics are an effective first-line choice; they have been demonstrated to

| Table 5-8 | Overview of Treatment and Recommended Follow-Up Following Initial Diagnosis of Hypertension |
|---|---|
| **Diagnosis** | **Treatment and Recommended Follow-Up** |
| Normotensive | Promote optimal lifestyle and repeat blood pressure evaluation annually |
| Elevated blood pressure | Nonpharmacologic lifestyle modifications and repeat evaluation in 3–6 months |
| Stage 1 hypertension with 10-year estimated ASCVD risk < 10% | Nonpharmacologic lifestyle modifications and repeat evaluation in 3–6 months |
| Stage 1 hypertension with 10-year estimated ASCVD risk > 10% | Nonpharmacologic lifestyle modifications and antihypertensive medication Repeat evaluation in 1 month |
| White coat hypertension | If blood pressure is ≥ 130 mm Hg but < 160 mm Hg systolic or > 80 mm Hg but < 100 mm Hg diastolic, HBPM or ABPM can be used to establish the diagnosis; if white coat hypertension is present, lifestyle modification and annual monitoring with HBPM or ABPM to detect sustained hypertension |
| Masked hypertension | If office blood pressure is 120–129/80 mm Hg but the individual has a history of hypertension, HBPM or ABPM can be used to establish the diagnosis; if daytime HBPM or ABPM are ≥ 130/80 mm Hg, institute lifestyle modification and start antihypertensive medication |

Abbreviations: ABPM, ambulatory blood pressure monitoring; ASCVD, atherosclerotic cardiovascular disease; HBPM, home blood pressure monitoring.

Based on Whelton PK, Carey RM, Aronow WS, et al. 2017 ACC/AHA/AAPA/ABC/ACPM/AGS/APhA/ASH/ASPC/NMA/PCNA guideline for the prevention, detection, evaluation, and management of high blood pressure in adults: a report of the American College of Cardiology/American Heart Association Task Force on Clinical Practice Guidelines. *Hypertension*. 2017. [Epub ahead of print]. doi:10.1016/j.jacc.2017.11.006.

reduce all-cause mortality, stroke, and cardiovascular disease.[55] Angiotensin-converting enzyme (ACE) inhibitors, calcium-channel blockers (CCBs), beta blockers, angiotensin II receptor blockers (ARB),

| Table 5-9 | Lifestyle Modifications to Prevent and Manage Hypertension[a] | |
|---|---|---|
| Modification | Recommendation | Approximate SBP Reduction (Range)[b] |
| Weight reduction | Maintain normal body weight (BMI: 18.5–24.9 kg/m$^2$) | 5–20 mm Hg/10 kg |
| Adopt DASH eating plan | Consume a diet rich in fruits, vegetables, and low-fat dairy products with reduced saturated and total fat, and reduce dietary sodium to ≤ 100 mmol/day (2.4 g of sodium) | 8–14 mm Hg |
| Physical activity | Engage in regular aerobic physical activity such as brisk walking (at least 30 minutes per day, most days of the week) | 4–9 mm Hg |
| Moderation of alcohol[c] | Men: No more than 1 oz of ethanol per day (2 drinks) Women: No more than 0.5 oz of ethanol per day (1 drink) | 2–4 mm Hg |

Abbreviations: BMI, body mass index; DASH, Dietary Approaches to Stop Hypertension; SBP, systolic blood pressure.

[a] For overall cardiovascular risk reduction, stop smoking.

[b] The effects of implementing these modifications are dose and time dependent, and could be greater for a specific individual.

[c] Ethanol in a standard drink: 1 oz of ethanol = 12 oz beer, 5 oz wine, or 1.5 oz distilled spirits.

Based on Whelton PK, Carey RM, Aronow WS, et al. 2017 ACC/AHA/AAPA/ABC/ACPM/AGS/APhA/ASH/ASPC/NMA/PCNA guideline for the prevention, detection, evaluation, and management of high blood pressure in adults: a report of the American College of Cardiology /American Heart Association Task Force on Clinical Practice Guidelines. Hypertension. 2017. [Epub ahead of print]. doi:10.1016/j .jacc.2017.11.006; National High Blood Pressure Education Program. *The Seventh Report of the Joint National Committee on Prevention, Detection, Evaluation, and Treatment of High Blood Pressure: Complete Report.* Bethesda, MD: National Heart, Lung, and Blood Institute; August 2004.

and other drug categories are used either alone or in combination; ACE inhibitors have shown evidence of similar efficacy to thiazide diuretics, but are not superior and are more costly.[55] A meta-analysis of trials of antihypertensive drugs concluded that all classes of these medications had similar effectiveness in preventing coronary heart disease.[56] The choice of agent recommended for use may vary depending on the presence or absence of other risk factors or comorbidities. An algorithm for managing hypertension can be found in the JNC 7 and JNC 8 guidelines.[51,52] Among adults on antihypertensive therapy, only 44% achieve effective control, with lower rates associated with non-Hispanic Black race, age greater than 60, diabetes, kidney disease, and high overall cardiovascular risk. Both lack of awareness of a hypertension diagnosis and failure to be treated effectively have been associated with lack of access to care and lack of health insurance.[57]

Those persons who need pharmacologic therapies are often referred to a physician to initiate treatment. However, many midwives will provide care for people being treated or at risk for hypertension. Based on the practice setting, a midwife may consult with a specialist, refer the individual at the time of diagnosis to a specialist, or initiate an initial antihypertensive agent. If the initial pharmacologic agent proves inadequate, as evidenced by not achieving the goal blood pressure in the algorithm, consultation and/or referral is warranted.

## Dyslipidemia

Dyslipidemia—that is, elevated fat or cholesterol in the blood—is another major risk factor associated with cardiac disease, and often is preventable or modifiable. Low-density lipoprotein (LDL) is the major component of cholesterol, accounting for approximately 65% to 70% of total cholesterol. LDL has been used as a surrogate biomarker to assess for risk for cardiac disease. An elevation in LDL level is directly associated with the development of atherosclerotic plaques.

Specific risk factors for dyslipidemia include obesity, hypertension, diabetes, smoking, preexisting coronary heart disease, and a family history of early cardiovascular disease. Risk increases with age: For menstruating people, the clinically relevant increased risk is related to menopause, and age 55 years and older often is used as the point at which risk begins to spike upward. Conditions that increase the risk of dyslipidemia include diabetes; thyroid disease; kidney diseases including chronic renal failure and nephrotic syndrome; obstructive liver disease such as gallstones, hepatitis, and cirrhosis; and use of medications such as protease inhibitors, progestins, corticosteroids, and anabolic steroids.[58] Modifiable risks include physical inactivity, a diet high in fats or sugars, smoking, and obesity.[59] Data suggest that among women age 20 to 45 years, the majority have coronary heart disease, related conditions such as diabetes, or one or more coronary heart disease risk factors, although most do not receive screening for this condition.[57]

Screening for dyslipidemia is not standardized in the same manner as screening for hypertension. The CDC recommends that adults at low risk for this condition should have cholesterol testing every 5 years, with testing occurring more frequently based on cardiovascular risk factors.[59]

Screening for dyslipidemia includes first conducting a global risk assessment of risk factors. For example, people with type 2 diabetes, type 1 diabetes for more than 15 years, two risk factors for cardiovascular disease, or metabolic syndrome should be considered to have a high or very high risk for ASCVD. The second step in screening is to obtain a complete lipid panel after an overnight fast. The panel will include blood values of LDL cholesterol (LDL-C), total cholesterol, and high-density lipoprotein (HDL) cholesterol. The third step is to calculate the 10-year risk for having a coronary event. Clinicians are advised to use an online calculator to predict 10-year risk for a first ASCVD event.[60] This calculation incorporates medical history risks and the results of the lipid panel, then predicts 10-year risk of ASCVD and compares the individual's 10-year and lifetime risks to a hypothetical individual with optimal characteristics. Online calculators are included in the Resources section at the end of this chapter.

When an individual is identified as having a high cholesterol level, counseling includes making diet changes to decrease total and dietary fat to between 25% and 35% of total calories, adding dietary fiber, stopping smoking, and increasing exercise levels. Medication therapy can be deferred while a trial of healthy lifestyle changes is undertaken, as long as there is no family history suggestive of genetic predisposition to coronary artery disease and the LDL-C level is less than 160 mg/dL for those persons without other cardiac risk factors. Determining who needs intervention and how their progress should be followed may be an indication for consultation or referral to a specialist. Pharmacologic therapy is instituted based on LDL level and risk profile.

The most widely accepted guidelines for the management of dyslipidemia are those established by the American College of Cardiology and the American Heart Association.[45,46] The most recent guidelines, which were released in 2018, focus on 10 take-home messages designed to simplify the guidelines to reduce risk of ASCVD by managing cholesterol levels, along with algorithms for appropriate statin use for primary and secondary ASCVD prevention.[45] The first take-home message emphasizes that a heart-healthy lifestyle should be encouraged for all individuals regardless of age, LDL-C level, presence of existing ASCVD, or risk profile. The sixth take-home message encourages shared decision making in the form of a clinician–patient discussion of risks before starting statin therapy. The remaining take-home messages provide the recommended course of action for various patient management groups based on risk, LDL-C level, ASCVD severity, and comorbidities. Liberal initiation of statins is recommended as the primary mode of treatment for individuals with clinical indications of atherosclerotic cardiovascular disease, including LDL-C cholesterol levels of 190 mg/dL or higher or conditions such as diabetes. The guidelines recommend the use of other products as adjunctive therapy in rare cases such as statin resistance cases or in individuals unable to tolerate statins.[56] According to the American College of Cardiology and the American Heart Association, the strongest evidence supports the use of statins for the following indications:[58,61]

- Primary prevention of atherosclerotic cardiovascular disease in individuals with LDL-C levels of 190 mg/dL or higher by using maximally tolerated statins

- Primary prevention of atherosclerotic cardiovascular disease in individuals with diabetes age 40 to 75 years with LDL-C levels of 70 to 189 mg/dL by using a moderate-intensity statin

- Primary prevention of atherosclerotic cardiovascular disease in individuals without diabetes with an estimated 10-year ASCVD risk of 7.5% or greater, with LDL-C levels of 70 to 189 mg/dL, and age 40 to 75 years

- Secondary prevention of additional morbidity and mortality in individuals with clinical ASCVD

Statins are categorized by how well they lower LDL-C on average. Table 5-10 categorizes the common statins as either high, moderate, or low intensity, which is consistent with the terminology used in the current guidelines.[61]

| Table 5-10 | High-, Moderate-, and Low-Intensity Statin Therapies[a] | | |
|---|---|---|
| **High Intensity (Daily Dosage Lowers LDL-C by Average of ≥ 50%)** | **Moderate Intensity (Daily Dosage Lowers LDL-C by Average of 30–50%)** | **Low Intensity (Daily Dosage Lowers LDL-C by Average of < 30%)** |
| **Statins and Doses Approved by the FDA and Tested in RCTs** | | |
| Atorvastatin (Lipitor), 40 mg[b] to 80 mg | Atorvastatin (Lipitor), 10 (20) mg | Lovastatin (Mevacor), 20 mg |
| Rosuvastatin (Crestor), 20 (40) mg | Rosuvastatin (Crestor), (5) 10 mg | Pravastatin (Pravachol), 10–20 mg |
| | Simvastatin (Zocor), 20–40 mg[c] | |
| | Pravastatin (Pravachol), 40 (80) mg | |
| | Lovastatin (Mevacor), 40 mg | |
| | Fluvastatin (Lescol), 40 mg 2 times daily | |
| **Statins and Doses Approved by the FDA but Not Tested in RCTs** | | |
| | Fluvastatin XL (Lescol XL), 80 mg | Simvastatin (Zocor), 10 mg |
| | Pitavastatin (Livalo), 2–4 mg | Fluvastatin (Lescol), 20–40 mg |
| | | Pitavastatin (Livalo), 1 mg |

Abbreviations: FDA, U.S. Food and Drug Administration; LDL-C, low-density lipoprotein cholesterol; RCT, randomized controlled trial.

[a] Individual responses to statin therapy varied in the RCTs and should be expected to vary in clinical practice. There might be a biologic basis for less than average response.

[b] Evidence from one RCT only. Down-titration was initiated if the participant was unable to tolerate atorvastatin 80 mg in the IDEAL (Incremental Decrease Through Aggressive Lipid Lowering) study.

[c] Although simvastatin 80 mg was evaluated in RCTs, initiation of simvastatin 80 mg or titration to 80 mg is not recommended by the FDA because of the increased risk of myopathy, including rhabdomyolysis.

Data from Grundy SM, Stone NJ, Bailey AL, et al. 2018 AHA/ACC/AACVPR/AAPA/ABC/ACPM/ADA/AGS/APhA/ASPC/NLA/PCNA guideline on the management of blood cholesterol: a report of the American College of Cardiology/American Heart Association Task Force on Clinical Practice Guidelines. *J Am Coll Cardiol.* 2019;73(24):e285-e350. doi:10.1016/j.jacc.2018.11.003.

Some midwives may consult or refer a person with dyslipidemia to a specialist upon discovery of the condition, whereas others may initiate statin therapy but will consult or refer if the response is inadequate as measured by serum cholesterol levels.

## Respiratory Conditions

### Upper Respiratory Infections

Upper respiratory infections (URIs) include the common cold, rhinosinusitis, influenza, and pharyngitis. Commonly viral in nature, nonspecific URIs and influenza are a frequent reason for calls to healthcare providers, with individuals often asking for antibiotics that will not cure the problem. Although rates of inappropriate prescribing have decreased slightly, rates of overtreatment remain high.[62] Both overtreatment and inappropriate treatment have led to a 30% or greater rate of antibiotic resistance in *Streptococcus pneumoniae* infections, despite the availability of a vaccine.[63]

Many URIs can be avoided through the use of simple hygiene techniques, most particularly the practice of hand washing. The use of antibacterial soaps and environmental sprays usually is not necessary in the home, but has not been linked to adverse ecological effects. Hand sanitizers have become useful items in public areas, especially when respiratory infections are prevalent.

The diagnosis of nonspecific URI is made based on the presence of nasal congestion and a clear, white, or yellow/green discharge, as well as sore throat, muscle aches, headache, and cough. The symptoms of colds and influenza overlap, although high fever, profound malaise, and dry cough are more typical of influenza than of a cold. Symptomatic management can reduce the severity of symptoms, although many interventions commonly implemented lack evidence of effectiveness. Treatments include rest, increased fluids, saline gargle or spray, and a variety of medications. Pharmacologic remedies are best targeted to specific symptoms, such as dextromethorphan (Delsym) for coughs; therefore, combination drugs are not advised. Antibiotics are not indicated for treatment of individuals with nonspecific URI or influenza.[64]

Ipratropium bromide (Atrovent), an anticholinergic nasal spray, can be used if needed to relieve rhinorrhea, sneezing, and congestion. Initial use consists of two sprays in each nostril, three to four times daily.[65] Antihistamines can provide limited relief in the first few days after the onset of a URI.[66] Intranasal corticosteroids have not shown any benefit for URIs, but are not harmful and may be continued if being used for another condition.[67] Regardless of pharmacologic treatments, resolution of symptoms should be complete within a week.

A bacterial cause for URI should be suspected when the symptoms persist or worsen after 8 to 10 days; when maxillofacial pain is present (especially if only one side of the face is affected); when the symptoms over the first 3 to 4 days are severe; when symptoms are associated with a fever higher than 39°C (102.2°F); when purulent discharge is present; or when symptoms worsen after a viral infection had appeared to be resolving. If antibiotic therapy is needed, the narrowest-spectrum drug effective against *S. pneumoniae* and *Haemophilus influenzae* should be used.

### Common Cold

The common cold is a self-limited syndrome that can be caused by many different viruses. This type of mild URI is the most frequent illness experienced by adults and children in industrialized nations. Symptoms include varying patterns of nasal discharge, headache, sore throat, sore muscles, cough, or sneezing. The common cold is usually spread via droplets and hard-surface contamination. The incubation period is 24 to 72 hours, and the period of infectivity starts approximately on the second day of illness and peaks on the third day of illness. Nevertheless, viruses that cause the common cold can be infective for several days. The initial differential diagnosis is allergic or bacterial rhinitis, bacterial pharyngitis, pertussis, and influenza. Complications associated with the common cold include rhinosinusitis, lower respiratory tract infections, exacerbation of asthma, and bronchitis.

### Rhinosinusitis

When an acute URI has spread into the sinus cavities, the term *rhinosinusitis* usually is preferred to the older term *sinusitis*. A green or yellow nasal discharge commonly is noted, in addition to pain and pressure over the affected sinus. Other symptoms can include a toothache near the affected sinus, fever, and a cough that worsens when lying down. More than 95% of these infections are viral.[68] Acute rhinosinusitis lasts less than 4 weeks, and most such infections resolve spontaneously.[68] Although fewer cases of rhinosinusitis are bacterial in origin, overuse of antibiotics is common with these conditions. One study found these medications were prescribed in more than 80% of rhinosinusitis episodes.[68] Clinical scenarios that suggest a bacterial infection include persistent symptoms for more than 10 days without improvement; severe onset with a high fever of at least 39°C (102.2°F) and purulent nasal discharge for 3 or more days beginning with the onset of symptoms; and unilateral predominance of sinus pain "double-sickening," in which viral symptoms begin to improve but then suddenly worsen near the end of the first week.[65] The combination of unilateral pain and purulent drainage is a reliable indicator of bacterial infection in 85% of cases.[69]

Therapy for rhinosinusitis includes supportive management with over-the-counter (OTC) decongestants, analgesics, and antipyretics. As with the common cold, antihistamines should not be used unless the congestion includes an allergic component. When symptoms of a bacterial infection or super-infection are present, then antibiotics should be initiated. Amoxicillin or ampicillin/clavulanate are first-line therapies; doxycycline would be recommended for individuals with a type 1 penicillin allergy or as a second-line therapy. Clindamycin plus cefixime or cefpodoxime can be used in those persons with a non-type 1 penicillin allergy or as a second-line therapy. The fluoroquinolones offer no greater therapeutic benefit and have significant adverse effects.[65] When symptoms persist for more than 12 weeks, referral to a specialist is warranted for evaluation of possible chronic rhinosinusitis or another underlying condition.

### Influenza

The onset of viral influenza is abrupt, marked by fever, rhinitis, cough, sore throat, headache, muscle pain, and general malaise. Most symptoms will resolve in a week or less, although malaise and tiredness can persist. Approximately 3% to 11% of the U.S. population has symptomatic influenza during a normal season, and it should be suspected as the cause of URI during the flu season, which typically begins in October and lasts through April.[70] Herd immunity achieved by widespread vaccination is the best protection against influenza outbreaks.

Vaccines for the seasonal flu types anticipated by the CDC become available in early fall and are recommended for all persons. Recommendations for different vaccine formulations, such as inactivated, recombinant, and live attenuated, vary by age and the person's medical history, and may change yearly.[71] It is important to refer to the latest CDC annual guidance. Table 5-11 indicates which individuals are at greater risk of severe complications of influenza.

The CDC recommends the use of the inhaled neuraminidase inhibitors oseltamivir or zanamivir, oral baloxavir, or intravenous peramivir to treat influenza. In particular, individuals with increased complication risks and those with severe or progressive disease should be treated.[72] Treatment of infections suspected of being influenza within 48 hours of the onset of symptoms can shorten the duration of infection by approximately 1 day. Without pharmacologic treatment, in healthy adults, influenza is a self-limiting disease and may be best treated with rest and supportive therapy.

### Pharyngitis

Approximately 5% to 15% of cases of sore throat are caused by group A beta-hemolytic *Streptococcus* (GAS); the remainder are primarily viral in origin and require only supportive care while symptoms resolve. Testing for GAS is not necessary when symptoms—cough, runny nose, oral sores, and hoarseness—clearly indicate a viral infection. In contrast, tonsillar exudate, tender anterior cervical lymph nodes, fever, and lack of a cough suggest a bacterial infection. Either a rapid antigen detection test or culture can be performed if symptoms do not exclude GAS. Follow-up culture after a negative rapid antigen detection test is no longer recommended in adults. Penicillin and amoxicillin regimens lasting 10 days are the most appropriate first-line treatments for GAS. The first-generation cephalosporins—clindamycin (Cleocin), clarithromycin (Biaxin), or azithromycin (Zithromax)—are all acceptable alternatives when penicillin allergy exists. An analgesic or antipyretic can be used for supportive therapy; corticosteroids are not recommended. It is not necessary to treat household contacts.[73]

### Bronchitis

Infections of the lower respiratory tract limited to the trachea and bronchi are termed *bronchitis*; they can appear as an inflammatory response to an otherwise uncomplicated URI. In healthy people of reproductive age, acute bronchitis is typically a viral syndrome of low-grade fever, malaise, fatigue, sore throat, chest pain, and cough. The cough can be productive or nonproductive. The cough of bronchitis can be differentiated from the cough of the common cold when it persists more than 5 days. Smoking, exposure to irritating fumes in the environment, and gastric reflux that irritates the bronchi can also precipitate acute bronchitis. Long-term exposure to smoking or environmental pollutants can lead to chronic bronchitis. On auscultation, areas of the lung other than over the bronchi should have normal findings; a chest X ray, if performed, should not show infiltrates. Worsening chest pain with shortness of breath or pain on inspiration suggests pneumonia.

In most cases, the infection and the cough will resolve within 1 to 2 weeks with supportive therapy.

| Table 5-11 | Individuals at Increased Risk of Complications of Influenza |
|---|---|

Persons with the following conditions:

- Asthma
- Neurologic and neurodevelopment conditions
- Blood disorders such as sickle cell disease
- Respiratory diseases including asthma, cystic fibrosis, and chronic obstructive pulmonary disease
- Endocrine disorders
- Heart disease including congenital heart disease, congestive heart failure, and coronary artery disease
- Kidney diseases
- Liver disorders
- Metabolic disorders
- Body mass index > 40 kg/m$^2$
- Stroke survivors
- Weakened immune system due to disease or medications
- Age 65 or older
- Pregnancy through 2 weeks after the end of pregnancy
- Living in nursing homes and other long-term care facilities
- People from certain racial and ethnic groups are at increased risk for hospitalization with flu, including non-Hispanic Black persons, Hispanic or Latino persons, and American Indian or Alaska Native persons

Adapted from Centers for Disease Control and Prevention. Influenza. https://www.cdc.gov/flu/highrisk/index.htm. Last reviewed September 6, 2022. Accessed December 27, 2022.

If cough is persistent after the primary infection has resolved and wheezing is noted, the use of an albuterol inhaler can provide relief. If an inhaler is prescribed, the directions should be for two puffs every 4 to 6 hours as needed to relieve symptoms.[74] Asthma should be considered as an alternative diagnosis.

Antibiotics are not useful in the case of viral bronchitis, but under certain circumstances suspected bacterial infections of the bronchi can require antibiotic therapy. Antibiotics should be avoided in healthy adults with moderate symptoms; their potential benefit is outweighed in most cases by the potential for increased resistance and the expense of therapy.[74]

If the diagnosis is unclear, or if symptoms persist and worsen, both pneumonia and pertussis should be ruled out. Signs and symptoms that indicate the diagnosis is pneumonia include temperature greater than or equal to 38°C (100.4°F), tachycardia at more than 100 beats per minute, crackles, decreased breath sounds, and the absence of a prior asthma diagnosis. If four of these five signs are present, the likelihood of pneumonia increases.[75] Symptoms suggestive of pneumonia warrant referral of the patient to a specialist for evaluation.

### Community-Acquired Pneumonia

Together, influenza and pneumonia are the ninth most frequent cause of death in the United States.[43] Current CDC recommendations are for all persons age 65 and older to receive the pneumococcal vaccine, and for persons younger to receive this vaccine if they have certain health conditions. Predisposing factors for pneumonia include damage to the cilia of the respiratory tract from chronic cough, viral infections, or smoking. The common infecting organisms are *Streptococcus pneumoniae*, *Haemophilus influenzae*, *Mycoplasma pneumoniae*, *Chlamydia pneumoniae*, *Staphylococcus aureus*, and a variety of viruses, most commonly influenza. Because bacterial causes of community-acquired pneumonia predominate, antibiotic therapy should be instituted promptly when a diagnosis is made. Risk factors for community-acquired pneumonia include age older than 65 years, underweight or body mass index (BMI) less than 19 kg/m$^2$, smoking, excessive alcohol intake, decreased ciliary activity, prior episodes of pneumonia or chronic bronchitis, chronic obstructive pulmonary disease, use of antihistamines, immunosuppression, and chronic illnesses.[76,77]

The onset of symptoms with community-acquired pneumonia is usually abrupt, with fatigue, cough, difficulty breathing, chills/sweats, anorexia, headache,

and chest pain being the most common. Fever of 38°C (100.4°F) or higher, tachycardia, tachypnea, rales, and lung consolidation can be found on examination. When the cause is bacterial, high fever and a productive cough are more likely, whereas viral causes produce a more generalized malaise. Chest X ray is indicated to confirm the diagnosis and to identify underlying complications. Testing to confirm the pathogen is not routinely recommended before empiric therapy is initiated in the outpatient setting, except for influenza testing when the virus is circulating in the community.[77] Nevertheless, at least one expert has argued that this practice runs counter to the need for better targeting of antibiotic therapy to reduce risk of resistance in common pathogens.[62]

Outpatient versus inpatient treatment of patients with community-acquired pneumonia is a decision with significant consequences in terms of treatment modalities, testing schemes, and costs. While uncomplicated pneumonia should be treated promptly with antibiotics and can safely be managed on an outpatient basis in healthy adults, consultation with or referral to a specialist is necessary for any person with suspected pneumonia.

### Pertussis

*Bordetella pertussis* is an increasingly important respiratory pathogen; prior to the availability of a vaccine for this bacterium, the average number of cases was 150 per 100,000 population. The incidence of pertussis (also called whooping cough) began to rise again in the 1980s, with epidemic peaks occurring after 2000. In 2017, nearly 19,000 cases of this infection were diagnosed in the United States, though the CDC suggests that many cases go unreported.[78]

Pertussis affects the ability to clear the respiratory tract by paralyzing the cilia lining the respiratory tract and causing inflammation, as well as by directly invading the alveoli.[78] The incubation period is approximately 7 to 10 days, but symptoms can first occur as distant in time as 6 weeks following exposure. Clinically, the first symptoms resemble a mild URI, with little temperature elevation. Although pertussis is milder in adults than in infants or young children, it can persist with an increasingly violent cough over several weeks. Table 5-12 describes the stages of the disease.[79]

Common complications of untreated pertussis in adults include rib fracture, pneumothorax, superimposed bacterial pneumonia, and urinary incontinence. Other, less common risks include dehydration, epistaxis, hernia, and—rarely—encephalopathy, pneumothorax, rectal prolapse, subdural hematoma, and seizure.[80]

In addition to vaccinating infants and children, vaccination against pertussis with the tetanus/ diphtheria/acellular pertussis (Tdap) combination vaccine among adults is an effective measure to control the spread of this disease. The action of vaccinating others around the child is called *cocooning*, and is accomplished by administering the Tdap vaccine to all adults who have close interaction with newborns. Pregnant individuals are vaccinated during the third trimester to promote passive immunity for the newborn.

Therapy for pertussis includes a macrolide antibiotic; the original recommendation for erythromycin was expanded to include azithromycin (Zithromax) and clarithromycin (Biaxin), as these macrolides are better tolerated. Post-exposure prophylaxis with the same drugs is recommended for all close contacts of a pertussis case, for individuals at high risk of severe disease (i.e., newborns, pregnant people in the third trimester, and individuals with preexisting conditions such as moderate to severe asthma or immunosuppression that could be exacerbated by infection), and for persons who have close contact with those at risk of severe disease.

It is not known whether post-exposure vaccination has any benefit.[80]

## Asthma

Asthma is a chronic inflammation of the airways associated with intermittent worsening of symptoms; reversible obstruction from bronchospasm, edema, and mucus production; and hyper-responsiveness to stimuli. An individual's personal genetics play a role in developing asthma, as well as social determinants of health and where someone lives. Approximately 8% of all Americans have current asthma diagnoses; almost half of those adults will report an asthma attack within the last 12 months.[81]

Signs and symptoms suggestive of asthma are listed in Table 5-13. On examination, wheezing when breathing normally, prolonged expiratory phase, use of accessory muscles, increased nasal swelling, secretions or polyps, and evidence of atopy all increase the likelihood of an asthma diagnosis. Pulmonary function testing is required for diagnosis.[82] The differential diagnosis in adults includes chronic obstructive

| Table 5-12 | Stages of Pertussis (Whooping Cough) | |
|---|---|---|
| **Stage** | **Duration** | **Symptoms** |
| Catarrhal | 1–2 weeks | Cough, runny nose, low-grade fever, sneezing |
| Paroxysmal | 1–6 weeks | Episodes of rapid coughing 15 or more times per day, ending with a long inspiratory gasp and high-pitched "whooping" sound, occurring more often at night, accompanied by possible vomiting, exhaustion |
| Recovery | Weeks to months | Slowly resolving symptoms: cough disappears within 2–3 weeks, may return with subsequent respiratory illnesses |

Based on Centers for Disease Control and Prevention. *Epidemiology and Prevention of Vaccine-Preventable Diseases.* Hall E, Wodi AP, Hamborsky J, et al., eds. 14th ed. Washington, DC: Public Health Foundation; 2021.

| Table 5-13 | Characteristic Signs and Symptoms of Asthma |
|---|---|

Wheezing (not required for diagnosis)
History of:
- Persistent cough (particularly at night)
- Recurrent wheezing
- Recurrent difficulty in breathing
- Nighttime symptoms that wake one from sleep

Symptoms occur or are worsened by:
- Exercise
- Comorbid conditions (rhinitis, reflux)
- Exposure to airborne pollutants (smoking, chemicals, perfume)
- Allergies, either seasonal (such as pollen) or perennial (usually an indoor allergen such as dander, mold, or dust)
- Temperature extremes
- Strong emotional expression (laughing or crying hard)
- Stress
- Menstrual cycles

Based on National Asthma Education and Prevention Program. *Expert Panel Report: Guidelines for the Diagnosis and Management of Asthma (EPR-3).* Bethesda, MD: National Heart, Lung, and Blood Institute; 2007; Wu TD, Brigham EP, McCormack MC. Asthma in the primary care setting. *Med Clin North Am.* 2019;103(3):435-452. doi:10.1016/j.mcna.2018.12.

pulmonary disease, vocal cord dysfunction, congestive heart failure, medication-related cough, pulmonary embolism, and gastroesophageal reflux disease, among other possibilities.[83] Four classes of asthma are distinguished based on severity of disease, as shown in Table 5-14.[84] Midwives practicing in areas characterized by high asthma rates may want to keep flow meters in their offices either to assist in the presumptive diagnosis of asthma or to assess lung function when someone with asthma presents for care or is symptomatic.

Important components of the management of asthma include patient education, management of environmental factors and comorbidities that worsen symptoms, and use of medication. The key to control of asthma and prevention of its worsening is involving the patient in decisions about care, awareness of environmental triggers and the need to minimize exposure when possible, and knowledge of the role that other health problems play in asthma management.[82,83] Medication management is based on a stepwise approach.[82,84] Intermittent symptoms of asthma (occurring fewer than 2 days per week, disturbing nighttime rest fewer than 2 days per month, not interfering with activities of daily living, and with one or fewer exacerbations per year) can be managed with short-acting beta-agonists such as albuterol sulfate (Proventil) on an as-needed basis. When a rescue inhaler is needed on more than 2 days per week, a diagnosis of persistent asthma should be considered.

Anyone with persistent asthmatic symptoms needs to be on daily medication. Inadequate treatment limits physical activity, decreases pulmonary function, and increases the risk of recurrent attacks. The choice of medications is based on both the severity and the persistence of symptoms. The main classes of asthma drugs for long-term maintenance include inhaled corticosteroids, immunomodulators, leukotriene receptor antagonists, long-acting beta-agonists, 5-lipoxygenase inhibitors, mast cell mediators, methylxanthines, and combination drugs. The preferred agents for all patients with asthma, regardless of stage, are inhaled corticosteroids because they reduce inflammation and are theorized to minimize the risk of airway remodeling.

Individuals with newly diagnosed asthma should be evaluated in consultation with or by referral to a specialist experienced in respiratory care. Individuals with known mild intermittent, persistent mild, or persistent moderate asthma can be cared for by a midwife for primary care and monitoring. However, consultation with an asthma specialist is warranted if a person requires more than medium-dose inhaled corticosteroids to achieve control (Stage 3 or higher) or has unstable asthma.[82,84,85]

| **Table 5-14** | **Classification of Asthma** | | | | | |
|---|---|---|---|---|---|---|
| **Disease Severity** | **Daytime Symptoms** | **Nighttime Symptoms** | **PEF or FEV** | **Interference with Normal Activity** | **Use of Short-Acting Medication** | **Asthma Exacerbation Frequency**[a] |
| Mild intermittent | ≤ 2 days/week | ≤ 2 nights/month | > 80% | None | ≤ 2 days/week | 0–1/year |
| Persistent mild | > 2 days/week but not daily | > 2 nights/month | > 80% | Minor | > 2 days/week but not daily and not more than 1 time/day | ≥ 2/year |
| Persistent moderate | Daily | > 1 night/week but not nightly | > 60 and < 80% | Some | Daily | ≥ 2/year |
| Persistent severe | Continual | Frequent | ≤ 60% | Extremely limited | Several times/day | ≥ 2/year |

Abbreviations: FEV, forced expiratory volume; PEF, peak expiratory flow.

[a] Data are insufficient to link frequency of exacerbations to different levels of severity. Generally, more frequent and intense exacerbations are an indication of increasing severity. Persons with two or more exacerbations per year may be considered to have persistent asthma even in the absence of impairment levels consistent with persistent asthma.

Modified from National Heart, Lung, and Blood Institute. Asthma care quick reference. https://www.nhlbi.nih.gov/files/docs/guidelines/asthma_qrg.pdf. Published 2012. Accessed April 24, 2022.

# Gastrointestinal Disorders and Abdominal Pain

Stomach aches and pains, diarrhea and constipation, and bloating are all common symptoms. As part of the history for any person of capable of childbearing, last menstrual period and potential pregnancy risk are routinely assessed. Ruling out pregnancy is an essential first step whenever abdominal symptoms are present because diagnosis and management can be influenced by this condition. This section focuses on general gastrointestinal health concerns common to all. Complications that occur during pregnancy and produce abdominal symptoms are addressed in the *Pregnancy-Related Conditions* and *Medical Complications in Pregnancy* chapters. Similarly, gynecologic concerns are addressed in the *Menstrual Cycle Abnormalities* and *Malignant and Chronic Gynecologic Disorders* chapters.

## Gastroesophageal Reflux Disease

Gastroesophageal reflux disease (GERD) is the more severe and persistent form of gastroesophageal reflux, caused by involuntary relaxation of the sphincter muscle separating the esophagus and the stomach. In 2014, GERD was the indication for more than 5.6 million office visits.[86] When gastric reflux occurs more than twice a week, GERD is diagnosed. GERD produces symptoms of heartburn that worsen with meals, bending over, and lying down. Other, less easily recognizable symptoms include an asthma-like wheeze, cough, laryngitis, and chest pain. Persistent severe disease can produce complications such as injury to the epithelium of the esophagus (Barrett's esophagus), stricture formation, and adenocarcinoma. Hiatal hernia—separation of the diaphragm that allows the sphincter and upper portion of the stomach to penetrate into the chest cavity—is common in healthy older adults and can contribute to the symptoms of GERD. Obesity and smoking influence the development of GERD, as can pregnancy. *Helicobacter pylori* infection, the dominant cause of gastroduodenal ulcers, does not appear to have an effect on the emergence of GERD.[87]

Therapy for GERD includes weight reduction, consumption of a low-fat diet, and avoidance of triggers such as caffeine, tobacco, and spicy or acidic foods. Eating small meals and remaining upright after meals can help prevent or ameliorate symptoms. If reflux occurs primarily at night, elevating the head while in bed will also help avoid discomfort. Certain medications, including beta-adrenergic agonists, tranquilizers, sedatives, progesterone, and calcium-channel blockers, can worsen symptoms.

The use of antacids is likely to provide short-term relief of intermittent symptoms but can interfere with absorption of other medications. Step-up therapy for more severe symptoms begins with an 8-week course of a proton pump inhibitor, such as omeprazole (Prilosec), esomeprazole (Nexium), or lansoprazole (Prevacid). No specific proton pump inhibitor appears to be more effective than another. A proton pump inhibitor should be taken in the morning, before the first meal of the day. A second dose in the evening may be needed for nighttime symptoms. If only partial relief is achieved, adding a second dose or changing to a different proton pump inhibitor may be effective.[87] If symptoms are unresolved following an 8-week trial of a proton pump inhibitor, referral for consultation with a specialist is indicated.

## Ulcers

Peptic ulcers are open lesions of the stomach or duodenum, penetrating through the mucosa into smooth muscle. An estimated 15 million people—that is, 5.9% of adults in the United States—have these lesions.[88] Common etiologies include *Helicobacter pylori* infection, a condition responsible for 70% of gastric ulcers and 95% of duodenal ulcers, and excessive use of NSAIDs, such as ibuprofen or aspirin.[89] Smoking, advancing age, and chronic medical conditions are associated with increased risk of disease.[90]

Testing for *H. pylori* is indicated in adults with a peptic ulcer, history of peptic ulcers, or undiagnosed dyspepsia. Noninvasive testing methods include antibody screens, urea breath testing, and fecal antigen testing.[90] Endoscopy is warranted in individuals older than 50 years and those with alarming symptoms such as bleeding, unexplained weight loss, change in bowel habits, or recurrent vomiting. Endoscopic testing has excellent sensitivity and specificity, but is invasive and expensive.[87] Thus, for midwives, the decision to consult or refer a patient for management of suspected *H. pylori* ulceration is made early in the evaluation process.

In addition to medication, counseling about avoiding use of aspirin and NSAIDs, stress reduction, and smoking cessation are all useful interventions for management of persons with ulcers. By themselves, these lifestyle interventions are not curative; instead, antibiotic therapy is necessary to eliminate *H. pylori* from the gastrointestinal tract and is essential for healing. Recommended initial therapies include a proton pump inhibitor and clarithromycin (Biaxin) plus either amoxicillin (Amoxil) or metronidazole (Flagyl) for 14 days. Common side effects of these regimens include headache, altered taste, diarrhea, and stomach upset; patients should be made aware that they will have gastrointestinal symptoms during therapy as a means to decrease nonadherence.[87] The use of probiotics may offer some relief for side effects and assist in maintaining normal gastric flora.[91] Sucralfate (Carafate) is also often used to promote healing and reduce inflammation. Gastric ulcers that remain unresolved need to be evaluated to exclude cancerous lesions of the stomach.

## Abdominal Pain

Abdominal pain has many causes, both gynecologic and non-gynecologic. Table 5-15 lists some of these etiologies. The diversity of differential diagnoses for abdominal pain reinforces the idea that midwives confronted with a patient having acute abdominal pain should not hesitate to seek consultation when the diagnosis is unclear.

| Table 5-15 | Abdominal Pain Differential Diagnosis | |
|---|---|---|
| **Right Upper Quadrant** | **Periumbilical** | **Left Upper Quadrant** |
| Cholecystitis | Acute pancreatitis | Gastric ulcer |
| Duodenal ulcer | Aortic aneurysm/ dissection | Pneumonia |
| Hepatitis | | Pancreatitis |
| Hepatomegaly | Diarrhea | Perforated colon |
| Pneumonia | Diverticulitis | Ruptured spleen |
| **Right Lower Quadrant** | Early appendicitis | **Left Lower Quadrant** |
| Appendicitis | Intestinal obstruction | Constipation |
| Meckel's diverticulitis | Hernia | Diarrhea |
| Ectopic pregnancy | Ulcer | Sigmoid diverticulitis |
| Endometriosis | | Ectopic pregnancy |
| Hernia | | Endometriosis |
| Mittelschmerz | | Hernia |
| Ovarian torsion | | Mittelschmerz |
| Ovarian cyst | | Ovarian torsion |
| Pelvic inflammatory disease | | Ovarian cyst |
| Perforated cecum | | Pelvic inflammatory disease |
| Regional ileitis | | Regional ileitis |
| Renal/ureteral stone | | Renal/ureteral stone |
| Salpingitis | | Salpingitis |
| | | Ulcerative colitis |

Note: This list is not comprehensive.

When a person presents with abdominal pain, assessment begins with a comprehensive history. The onset, description, duration, associated symptoms, and precipitating or relieving factors are determined, and the patient is asked whether the pain is localized and, if so, to which quadrant.

### Acute Abdomen

Acute abdomen, defined as sudden severe abdominal pain, is a medical emergency. Characteristics that distinguish the acute abdomen include abdominal rigidity or distension, guarding, rebound pain, tachycardia, and decreased or absent bowel sounds. Fever can be present but is not essential to the diagnosis. Vomiting as well as urinary, bowel, or vaginal symptoms can be present. Immediate referral for prompt surgical evaluation is needed.

### Gallbladder Disease

Gallbladder disease occurs in 15% to 20% of the population, but only 20% of affected individuals will have symptomatic cholecystitis that eventually requires evaluation or treatment.[92] Cholecystitis is an inflammation of the gallbladder—the organ that collects, concentrates, and dispenses into the digestive tract the bile produced by the liver. When excess cholesterol triggers a crystallization process, gallstones form. If the gallstones become symptomatic, they usually cause only mild biliary colic or a sharp pain after a fatty or large meal; this pain may last a few hours and then resolve. Choledocholithiasis is blockage of the common bile duct by gallstones.[93]

Risk factors for developing gallbladder disease include female sex, obesity followed by rapid weight loss, hypertriglyceridemia, pregnancy, older age, diabetes, and genetic predisposition. When cholecystitis develops, the sharp epigastric pain can last for several hours or days and is often associated with nausea and vomiting. People with acute attacks present with severe, persistent right upper quadrant pain, often radiating to the right shoulder blade or the central back opposite the epigastrium. Murphy's sign (Figure 5-1) is considered to be positive if the person stops inspiration with deep palpation of the right upper quadrant of the abdomen. Leukocytosis, elevated liver function tests, and elevated bilirubin are common laboratory findings. Ultrasound is the most effective diagnostic tool for identifying gallbladder disease.

In individuals with only mild pain and intermittent symptoms, dietary and lifestyle changes can be a first-line intervention. These include reducing fat intake; increasing intake of high-fiber foods, vegetables, and fruits; and increasing exercise.

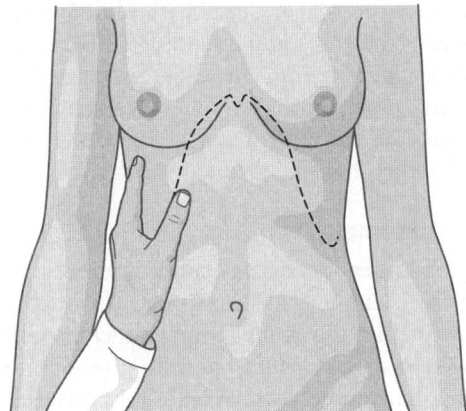

**Figure 5-1** Murphy's sign.

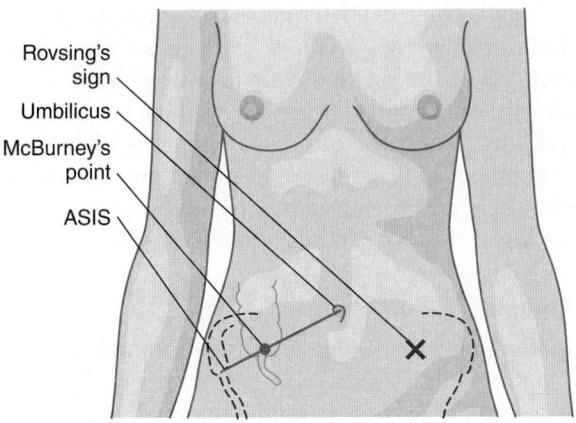

**Figure 5-2** McBurney's point and Rovsing's sign. McBurney's point is on the abdominal wall on a line between the umbilicus and the anterior superior iliac spine (ASIS), and is usually two-thirds the distance from the umbilicus toward the ASIS. The most common placement is at the base of the appendix.

Nonsteroidal pain medications can be used for pain relief. If symptoms are improved, then referral for medical management is indicated. The use of urso-deoxycholic acid, a bile stone solvent, accompanied by the use of antibiotics can delay or prevent the need for surgery.[93] Prompt surgical removal of the gallbladder is the usual treatment for severe, symptomatic disease.

### Appendicitis

When the appendix becomes obstructed, enlarged, and unable to drain, the subsequent bacterial response leads to appendicitis. Appendicitis is the most common abdominal surgical emergency.[94] The relative increase in appendicitis incidence is often attributed to improved diagnostic accuracy, particularly the accuracy of computed tomography, which decreases the risk of misidentifying the symptoms as other, usually gynecologic, pelvic symptoms.[95]

The classic symptoms of appendicitis are anorexia and generalized abdominal pain, resolving into acute right lower quadrant abdominal pain, vomiting, and fever. A CBC will show leukocytosis with an increased neutrophil ratio. Deep tenderness over McBurney's point in the lower right abdomen is an early sign of acute appendicitis. Rebound pain with release of pressure from the left lower abdomen is known as Rovsing's sign. **Figure 5-2** illustrates the locations of McBurney's point and Rovsing's sign.

Although appendectomy has been considered the standard management of appendicitis, patients with uncomplicated cases can be offered antibiotic management, with the understanding that this approach may fail. If this occurs, usually within 1 to 2 days, surgery is required. Additionally, as many as 20% of individuals choosing this route may have a recurrence and require surgical intervention.[96]

### Gastroenteritis and Acute Diarrhea

Some people report diarrhea when they have any change in bowel habits that produces soft, frequent, or less-formed stools. True diarrhea is characterized by increased water content and can include mucus or bloody discharge. Individuals who report having diarrhea are asked about associated symptoms such as cramping, nausea or vomiting, and fever. Careful examination of the abdomen, including auscultation of bowel sounds, palpation, and percussion, is necessary.

Acute diarrhea is predominantly infectious; chronic diarrhea, lasting for more than 2 consecutive weeks, can result from a variety of infections, medication use, chronic illness, malabsorption syndromes, stress, and irritable bowel syndrome. Recent travelers, the elderly, members of a community with an identified outbreak, and individuals recently prescribed antibiotics require closer attention to a specific diagnosis. Anyone with chronic watery diarrhea should be referred to a gastroenterologist for further testing.

Viral gastroenteritis is a generally self-limiting disease, in which oral exposure to a pathogenic virus such as norovirus or rotavirus leads to explosive onset of nausea, vomiting, and/or diarrhea, fever, and malaise within 1 to 3 days of exposure. The abdomen is tender; no guarding is present. Bowel sounds are increased. Norovirus alone accounts for 58% of acute foodborne illnesses.[97] Other causes of diarrhea-linked infections include *Escherichia coli* species, *Salmonella*, and a host of other bacteria, most of which are foodborne pathogens.

The majority of cases of diarrhea in healthy adults will spontaneously resolve within 1 to 4 days. Rest and oral fluids are the basic components of care. Medications such as diphenoxylate (Lomotil) or loperamide (Imodium) may be offered to decrease the frequency of stools. Intravenous rehydration with electrolytes is indicated for severe dehydration and for individuals at increased risk, such as the elderly and immunocompromised persons.

Investigation of acute diarrhea includes a stool sample to check for white blood cells or frank bleeding. Laboratory evaluation of electrolytes should be reserved for more severe or persistent cases when dehydration is suspected. If symptoms do not resolve or the patient becomes dehydrated, stool samples for culture and for ova and parasites (depending on the suspected pathogen) as well as a toxin assay for *Clostridium difficile* (if the patient has recent antimicrobial use) would be indicated.

Traveler's diarrhea (TD), as distinguished from norovirus infections acquired in large travel group settings such as cruises, will be bacterial in 80% of cases—specifically, the pathogenic agent will likely be *E. coli* or another enterococcus. Prevention through hand washing and food selection can help reduce the risk of contracting TD, though it can never be completely eliminated in high-risk regions. When infection occurs, early rehydration is essential, and antimotility agents, such as loperamide, can provide symptom relief. When antibiotic treatment does not resolve symptoms, parasitic pathogens should be considered based on the location of travel.[98]

## Constipation

Straining to produce hard stools, infrequent bowel movements (fewer than once in 3 days), and painful defecation are characteristic of constipation. Estimates of the prevalence of constipation average 15%.[99] Constipation is classified as primary or secondary (i.e., resulting from another disorder). Initial questioning regarding these symptoms should include an assessment of the person's usual bowel function. Inadequate dietary fiber, decreased fluid intake, and iron therapy for anemia, whether prescribed or self-initiated, are common causes of constipation. Other medications, such as tricyclic antidepressants (e.g., amitriptyline [Elavil]), anticholinergics (e.g., ipratropium bromide [Atrovent]), and calcium-channel blockers (e.g., diltiazem [Cardizem] and verapamil [Calan]), can slow peristalsis and increase stool transit time, leading to constipation. Misuse of laxatives leading to decreased natural stimulation of the bowel is also common,

particularly among the elderly. Stress, anxiety, and depression can lead to changes in bowel habits, as can a history of sexual abuse. Pelvic floor dysfunction can also contribute to constipation. Other serious causes include hypothyroidism, cancer, strictures, and opioid use. A careful history is necessary to rule out serious underlying disease that would require a referral. A careful history for prior abuse is essential in evaluating prolonged constipation, particularly if it relates to functional difficulty. A stool diary kept for 2 weeks and descriptions of stool appearance can aid diagnosis.[99] The physical examination includes both abdominal assessment and digital rectal exam, which can identify physical problems such as anal fissures or hemorrhoids as well as impaction.[99] Assessment for rectocele is also useful.

Management of chronic constipation includes counseling about diet and exercise, as well as increased fluid intake. Avoidance of straining and recognizing the physical cues that indicate the need to defecate are included in teaching. Patients should also be counseled to stop the overuse of laxatives, cathartics, and enemas. If any medication is necessary during early treatment, a bulk-forming OTC drug such as Metamucil should be used; however, adding fiber to the diet is a better strategy because a pattern of healthy eating will help maintain normal function. If symptom relief is not obtained with the preceding measures, a trial of laxatives such as docusate sodium (Colace) is in order before referring the patient to a physician.

## Irritable Bowel Syndrome Versus Inflammatory Bowel Diseases

Irritable bowel syndrome (IBS) is a functional bowel disorder that consists of lower gastrointestinal tract symptoms of increased bloating, diarrhea, or constipation in the absence of any structural or biochemical cause. This condition is chronic in nature, tends to wax and wane, and is one of the most common presentations in primary care practice. The current definition (Rome IV) includes recurrent abdominal pain at least 1 day per week for 3 months and two or more of the following criteria: an association of the pain with defecation, change in frequency of bowel movements, or change in appearance of the stool. Symptoms must have been present for at least 6 months.[100] Increased or decreased stool frequency, abnormal stool formation (either hard or watery), bloating, difficulty in the passage of stool (straining, urgency, or failure to completely empty the bowel), and mucus in the stool are further confirmation of the diagnosis. Because the symptoms are unstable, the terms "IBS with diarrhea" and "IBS with constipation" are commonly used.

The onset of IBS usually occurs during the young adult years. Because organic causes of bowel changes are more frequent with increasing age, a new diagnosis should be made with care in adults older than 40 years. Assessment includes evaluation for bowel obstruction, including malignancies, and for gastrointestinal bleeding. Irritable bowel syndrome should not be confused with inflammatory bowel diseases such as Crohn's disease and ulcerative colitis, which are chronic, recurrent inflammations of the bowel. Symptom relief after having a bowel movement is strongly suggestive of IBS.

Education about IBS should include reassurance about the course and management possibilities, and information on dietary modifications such as increasing fiber (although increasing bran can provoke symptoms) and possibly decreasing gluten. Probiotics may relieve bloating and flatulence for some individuals. Medication use should be based on the predominant symptoms.[100]

Because of the strong likelihood of underlying psychological distress among persons with IBS, a careful assessment for anxiety disorders and depression is warranted. Considerations in managing this aspect of the disease include the use of antidepressants, psychotherapy, and supportive behavioral therapy.

In contrast to IBS, inflammatory bowel diseases are autoimmune disorders that affect the small and large intestines. Examples include Crohn's disease and ulcerative colitis. Inflammatory bowel diseases often have a genetic component. The symptoms of these diseases overlap with those of irritable bowel disorder, but also have some dissimilarities. For example, both disorders are associated with intestinal symptoms, but IBS is more likely to be triggered by dietary factors whereas inflammatory bowel disease is more unpredictable. Persons with inflammatory bowel diseases need physician care and often require medications that can be complex to manage.

## Hepatitis

*Hepatitis* is the generic term used to describe inflammation of the liver, regardless of etiology. The most common causes of hepatitis include the infections caused by pathogenic viruses identified by the letters A through E and linked to liver disease by the acute and chronic nature of the conditions. While hepatitis A and E are spread by the fecal–oral route, hepatitis B, C, and D are spread by contact with blood and body fluids and can be contracted sexually. Hepatitis A and B are the most common forms of hepatitis in the United States. Although there are fewer new cases of hepatitis C than cases of hepatitis

A and B on an annual basis, infection with the C variant becomes chronic in approximately 75% to 85% of persons who are infected with it.[101] Together, hepatitis B and C are responsible for 65% of all liver cancers in the United States, with hepatitis C responsible for half. Collectively, the A, B, and C strains are responsible for most new viral hepatitis diagnoses in the United States.

Hepatitis D occurs as a coinfection with hepatitis B or as a secondary infection, and requires the presence of hepatitis B for its transmission. Hepatitis D is uncommon in the general population of North America, although it can occur in individuals who use intravenous drugs and persons with frequent exposure to blood products (e.g., persons with hemophilia) as well as their sexual contacts.[102]

Hepatitis E is an enterically transmitted virus, often associated with contaminated water sources; it is most commonly found in Asia, the Middle East, South America, and Latin America. Hepatitis E has been diagnosed in the United States primarily in individuals traveling from low-resource countries, although it can be associated with foodborne transmission. This disease often manifests with only mild symptoms, and does not result in a carrier state.[102]

Hepatitis can also result from generalized infection by other viruses, including cytomegalovirus, Epstein-Barr virus, herpes simplex virus, and measles virus. Nonviral causes of liver inflammation include autoimmune disease, bacterial sepsis, and syphilis. Hepatitis can also be chemically induced by chronic alcohol ingestion or by use of medications such as acetylsalicylic acid (aspirin), acetaminophen (Tylenol), phenytoin (Dilantin), isoniazid (Niazid), and rifampin (Rifadin).

Symptoms common to all types of hepatitis include jaundice, dark-colored urine, abdominal pain, clay-colored stools, fatigue, loss of appetite, and nausea or vomiting. Laboratory abnormalities include elevated liver function tests. Testing for antibodies to the various viral causes of hepatitis, followed by consultation or referral for management, is appropriate.

### Hepatitis A

Hepatitis A virus (HAV) is an RNA virus transmitted through the fecal–oral route. Most cases of hepatitis A arise during community-wide outbreaks. In the United States, vaccination has been successful in limiting the rate of infection, although outbreaks still occur occasionally. In adults, most cases are symptomatic.[102] Contaminated water and food (especially shellfish) are typical sources of infection, with most cases being associated with close personal contact with an infected person, although blood-borne transmission has been documented in both infants and adults.[102]

Hepatitis A has an incubation period of 28 days (range: 15–50 days), with the virus being shed through the feces approximately 2 weeks prior to the emergence of clinical symptoms. The infection has a short acute phase of 10 to 15 days, with symptoms resolving within 2 months. However, as many as 15% of symptomatic persons have prolonged or relapsing disease lasting up to 6 months.[102] This self-limited disease does not result in chronic infection and is managed with symptomatic treatment and monitoring for worsening liver disease.

Serologic testing with a finding of immunoglobulin M (IgM) antibody is required to confirm infection. IgM anti-HAV usually becomes detectable 5 to 10 days before the onset of symptoms and can persist for up to 6 months after infection. Immunoglobulin G (IgG) anti-HAV appears early in the course of the disease and indicates lifelong protection against the disease.[102]

Since 1995, two licensed inactivated hepatitis A vaccines have been available in the United States. The CDC does not currently recommend routine vaccinations for all adults, but does make this recommendation for persons working in high-risk settings such as healthcare or group homes, traveling to countries where hepatitis A is endemic, or with certain health conditions.

### Hepatitis C

Hepatitis C virus (HCV) infection is rarely identified at the time of exposure. The CDC estimated that more than 57,000 cases occurred in the United States in 2019, but only 2194 cases were reported.[101] Approximately 2.4 million people in the United States have chronic hepatitis C, which, if left untreated, can lead to liver cancer. The majority were probably exposed during the 1970s and 1980s, when rates of this infection reached their highest point. Risk factors for HCV infection include birth between 1945 and 1965, ever use of injectable or intranasal drugs, long-term hemodialysis, known exposure (healthcare worker, organ or blood recipient from a positive donor), human immunodeficiency virus (HIV) infection, and abnormal liver enzyme test results. As of 2020, the CDC recommended testing all adults for hepatitis C once, testing every pregnant individual during pregnancy, and regular testing for people with risk factors.[102]

Transfusion with unscreened blood is an uncommon risk today for contracting hepatitis C. In contrast, unsterile tattoos from unlicensed providers, whether in social settings or during incarceration, have been linked to an increased risk of hepatitis C.[103] All-cause mortality is increased by infection with hepatitis C; racial disparities in rates of infection and mortality from hepatitis C are apparent in the higher rates among Mexican Americans, Hispanic Americans, and Black individuals compared to white individuals.[104]

The period of incubation for hepatitis C ranges from 2 weeks to 6 months. Approximately 30% of individuals newly infected with HCV are symptomatic.[101,102] Chronic disease develops slowly, and both excessive alcohol use and obesity have been associated with its progression.

Diagnosis of hepatitis C infection is made by serum enzyme immunoassay (EIA) or chemiluminescent immunoassay (CLIA) detection of antibody to the virus. Hepatitis C antibody testing is accurate 4 weeks to 6 months after exposure. If the test for antibody to hepatitis C is positive, qualitative and quantitative HCV-RNA polymerase chain reaction (PCR) testing should be performed. Because of the high incidence of chronic disease, serum alanine aminotransferase (ALT) and quantification of HCV-RNA (viral load) should be performed.[101,102]

Currently, no vaccine is available that can prevent infection with hepatitis C, although identification of treatments—including curative therapies—is rapidly evolving.[102] At the system level, screening blood supplies, providing opioid use disorder treatment programs and needle exchange programs, and quality improvement programs for facilities that aim to reduce the risk of iatrogenic exposure of staff are all significant ways to reduce incidence of HCV infection. Counseling, including use of barriers with sexual activity and avoiding sharing intravenous drug paraphernalia, is essential to decrease transmission between individuals.[105] The primary goal of treatment is undetectable HCV RNA after completion of treatment (clinical cure). Treatment for acute and chronic hepatitis C should be managed by a specialist familiar with the currently available therapeutic regimens.

## Conditions of the Genitourinary System

The close proximity of the urinary tract to the reproductive organs means that individuals with female genitalia frequently call a midwife for management of urinary tract symptoms. Outpatient evaluation and management of uncomplicated cystitis is an essential skill for midwives, as are prompt recognition and triage of more serious conditions. Definitions

| Table 5-16 | Definitions and Diagnosis of Urinary Tract Infections |
|---|---|
| **Type of Infection** | **Definition and Diagnostic Method** |
| Asymptomatic bacteriuria | In a patient without a urinary catheter, a voided urine culture with no more than two organisms, one of which has $> 10^5$ colonies of no more than two organisms without signs or symptoms of UTI |
| Cystitis | Infection limited to the lower urinary tract, typically with symptoms of dysuria, frequency, and urgency |
| Pyelonephritis | Infection ascending to the kidneys system, accompanied by fever, flank pain with or without lower urinary tract symptoms but with bacteriuria |
| Uncomplicated UTI | Cystitis or pyelonephritis occurring in a person with an anatomically and functionally normal genitourinary tract and no predisposing factors for infection |
| Complicated UTI | Cystitis or pyelonephritis occurring in a person with anatomic of functional abnormalities of the urinary tract, immunocompromised status, drug-resistant bacteria, or other comorbidities increasing susceptibility to worsening infections. |
| Recurrent UTI | Two separate episodes of acute bacterial cystitis proven by culture within 6 months or three separate episodes within 12 months. |
| Relapse | Reoccurrence of acute cystitis with the same organism within 2 weeks of treatment completion, related to persistence of the organism within the urinary tract. |
| Reinfection | New infection with the same or different organism greater than 2 weeks after original treatment completion or after negative urine culture between infections. |
| Diagnostic criteria for acute UTI | In a person with a normal urinary tract and no other recognized cause for signs and symptoms, and no urinary catheter in place within the previous 48 hours, the diagnosis of UTI is confirmed by the presence of urgency, frequency, dysuria, suprapubic tenderness, costovertebral angle pain or tenderness, or fever ($> 38°C$) if $\leq 65$ years of age. In the absence of complicating factors, urinalysis or urine culture is not necessary for diagnosis. |
| Laboratory confirmation | Urinalysis positive for leukocyte esterase and/or nitrites positive urine culture of $\geq 10^3$ CFU/mL with no more than two species of microorganisms |

Abbreviations: CFU, colony-forming units; UTI, urinary tract infection; WBC, white blood cell.

Based on Nicolle LE, Gupta K, Bradley SF, et al. Clinical practice guideline for the management of asymptomatic bacteriuria: 2019 update by the Infectious Diseases Society of America. *Clin Infect Dis.* 2019;68(10):e83-e110. doi:10.1093/cid/ciy1121. Anger J, Lee U, Ackerman AL, et al. Recurrent uncomplicated urinary tract infections in women: AUA/CUA/SUFU guideline. *J Urol.* 2019 Aug;202(2): 282-289. doi:10.1097/JU.0000000000000296. Epub 2019 Jul 8. Update in: *J Urol.* 2022 Oct;208(4):754-756. PMID: 31042112. Gupta K, Grigoryan L, Trautner B. Urinary Tract Infection. *Ann Intern Med.* 2017 Oct 3;167(7):ITC49-ITC64. doi:10.7326/AITC201710030. PMID: 28973215.

and diagnostic criteria for urinary tract infections are listed in **Table 5-16**.[106]

## Acute Cystitis

Uncomplicated acute cystitis is defined variously as the presence of 1000 or more colony-forming units (CFU) per milliliter of urine in a culture from a catheter specimen for symptomatic individuals or, more traditionally, as 100,000 or more CFU per milliliter whether or not symptoms of a lower urinary tract infection (UTI) are present. However, lower CFU counts can be associated with infection.

In particular, in a person with symptoms, a finding of less than 100,000 CFU per milliliter should be interpreted with caution.

The predominant organism implicated in uncomplicated lower urinary tract infection is *E. coli*, with *Staphylococcus saprophyticus, Klebsiella pneumoniae, Proteus mirabilis,* and *Enterobacter* and *Enterococcus* species making up the majority of the other pathogens that are associated with UTI.[106,107]

*Asymptomatic bacteriuria* is the term applied when symptoms are absent and 100,000 CFU per milliliter or more of a single organism grow in a urine culture. The current recommendation is not to screen community-dwelling individuals without symptoms.[107] However, routine urine culture in pregnant patients to identify asymptomatic bacteriuria is recommended due to the pregnancy-related physiologic changes in the urinary tract, which facilitate the migration of bacteria to the upper urinary tract.

Lower UTIs are among the most common infections that people experience. Individuals with female genitalia have a greater risk of UTI, particularly after intercourse, in large part due to the shorter passage through the urethra. Individuals who have such an infection are at risk for recurrence, often within a few months. Risk factors for UTI include sexual activity, use of a barrier contraceptive and/or spermicide, vaginal infections, trauma to the vagina, increasing age, and genetic susceptibility.[107,108] Symptoms of a lower UTI include pain on urination, increased voiding frequency, and persistent suprapubic or low back pain. Because the symptoms of UTI overlap with those of sexually transmitted infections (STIs) such as chlamydia, sexually active young people should be screened for STIs.

Lower UTI is frequently diagnosed based on symptoms including dysuria, frequency, and urgency in the absence of vaginal pain or discharge. Urinalysis showing nitrates or WBCs may potentially indicate the presence of a lower UTI, but may also identify cases of asymptomatic bacteriuria not requiring treatment; urinalysis should not be used to diagnose a UTI independent of symptoms. The presence of vaginal discharge decreases the likelihood that a UTI is present.[109] When cystitis is suspected, a culture and sensitivity should be obtained during the symptomatic phase to confirm that a UTI is the cause of symptoms and to ensure that an antibiotic is prescribed to which the pathogen is sensitive. Between 30% and 50% of women with one UTI will have a recurrence within 1 year.[109]

Recurrent lower UTI is diagnosed after more than two infections proven by culture within a year. Identifying characteristics of uncomplicated recurrences include frequent sexual activity, a prior history of pyelonephritis, and rapid symptom resolution after treatment. Nocturia, hematuria, dyspareunia, and persistent symptoms after antibiotic therapy are indicative of another source of irritation, such as interstitial cystitis. Among postmenopausal individuals, recurrent lower UTI is associated with urinary incontinence, cystocele, and prolapse. The use of vaginal estrogen creams or rings can help prevent recurrent lower UTI in this population by restoring integrity to the vaginal and urethral tissues affected by lower estrogen levels.[110]

Prior to obtaining culture and sensitivity results, treatment with an appropriate antibiotic can be started based on reported symptoms and urinalysis. Patients should be cautioned that if the culture is negative, or if the sensitivities suggest a preferred course, they may be called and advised to stop or to change to a different medication. Recommendations for treatment of lower UTI have become more complicated as resistance to various antibiotics has emerged.[109] Nitrofurantoin (Macrodantin) or the combination of nitrofurantoin monohydrate with macrocrystals (Macrobid) is preferred if there is no suspicion of pyelonephritis, or trimethoprim–sulfamethoxazole (TMP-SMX; Bactrim) if the local resistance rate is less than 20%. Amoxicillin or ampicillin should never be used as a sole agent; fluoroquinolones, amoxicillin–clavulanate (Augmentin), and beta-lactams should be reserved for more serious infections or if the recommended drugs are contraindicated.[108,109]

Phenazopyridine HCl (Pyridium) can be offered as a dose of 200 mg orally three times daily after meals for temporary relief of pain associated with a UTI. It should never be used for this purpose for more than 48 hours, nor should it be recommended for use without a plan to evaluate the individual for the cause of pain. When it is prescribed, the orangish urinary discoloration caused by the drug should be mentioned.

The use of cranberry either as juice or in other formulations as an adjuvant to prescriptive therapy has been debated. Recent meta-analyses suggest that the use of cranberry products may reduce risk of recurrent infection.[111–113]

## Interstitial Cystitis

Interstitial cystitis is a persistent inflammatory bladder condition that is associated with suprapubic or retropubic pain, dysuria, frequency and urgency, dyspareunia, and nocturia. A single symptom, such as frequency or pain, may appear first. Over time, the bladder wall can become irritated or scarred, leading to the development of submucosal bleeding. Diagnosis is often delayed because the symptoms are mistaken for lower UTI. No evidence can be found for a microbial pathogen; however, some people report an acute UTI prior to the onset of symptoms. Numerous potential contributors to causation have been proposed, and links to other chronic pain syndromes are recognized.[114,115] A conservative estimate puts the number of adult women with pain and urinary symptoms of interstitial cystitis/painful bladder syndrome in the United States at greater than 3 million.[116]

The history includes questions regarding flow, volume, and pain. Measurement of a post-void residual and urinalysis are needed. Midwives can offer patients with interstitial cystitis/painful bladder syndrome counseling on restricting alcohol and possible food triggers such as spicy or high-acid foods, caffeine, and chocolate; tobacco cessation; self-care; stress management techniques; and bladder training. If these steps do not resolve the issue, referral for further evaluation, including a possible biopsy to rule out bladder cancer, and medication is warranted.[114,115]

## Pyelonephritis

Patients with abdominal pain should be evaluated for acute pyelonephritis, an inflammation of the kidneys. The characteristic presentation of pyelonephritis is severe flank pain and fever with associated chills, nausea or vomiting, and painful urination. Assessment of costovertebral angle tenderness (CVAT) by striking beneath the 12th rib in the acute angle formed with the spine can help to assess the location of the pain (Figure 5-3). The risk factors and pathogens associated with pyelonephritis are the same as those for lower UTI. The diagnosis should be confirmed by a urinalysis, which will be positive for WBCs or the presence of pyuria, and by urine culture with sensitivities. Additional laboratory tests include blood urea, creatinine, and CBC; an elevated leukocyte count is an indicator of severity.[117]

Indications for physician consultation or referral in urinary tract disorders include evidence of severe upper urinary tract infection, frequent recurrence of a UTI, infection with resistant organisms or in people with multiple antibiotic allergies, comorbidities that can affect immune status, comorbidities that can affect the structure or function of the urinary tract, hematuria that persists after treatment, and observed anatomic abnormality.[109] Physician consultation is required when pyelonephritis is suspected; a pending urine culture should not delay consultation. Treatment varies depending on whether it is delivered on an inpatient basis or at an outpatient site. Commonly prescribed drugs for uncomplicated infections include various combinations of fluoroquinolones; TMP-SMP is a common first-line therapy. Before prescribing any pharmacologic therapy, local resistance patterns as well as medication allergies should be reviewed. If the local resistance rate is greater than 10%, a single dose of an intravenous medication should be added while waiting for sensitivity data.[109,117,118]

## Kidney Stones

The prevalence of nephrolithiasis (kidney stones) is estimated to be 8.8% nationally.[119] Conditions that can precipitate new onset of kidney stones include heat or dehydration associated with climate or working conditions, obesity, and weight gain. A substantial number of individuals in whom stones form are asymptomatic. The usual symptoms of nephrolithiasis include severe pain in the flank or upper abdomen (renal colic) caused by the stone passing into the ureter. As the stone enters the bladder, it triggers nausea and symptoms resembling those of a UTI. Hematuria is a common finding, but is not required for diagnosis.[119]

When kidney stones are suspected, referral to a specialist for management is needed. While arranging referral, NSAIDs can be initiated for pain management and are as effective as opioids for this purpose. Small stones, less than 0.8 centimeter in diameter, can be allowed to pass without surgery. Surgical management of kidney stones that are large, obstructive, or associated with infection now relies on extracorporeal shock-wave lithotripsy, ureteroscopy, and percutaneous nephrolithotomy as means to avoid open procedures.[119]

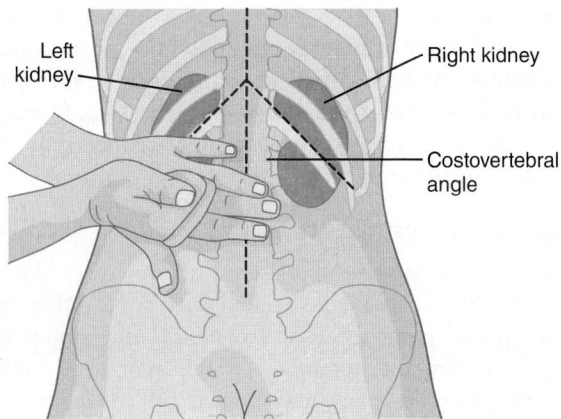

Left kidney — Right kidney — Costovertebral angle

**Figure 5-3** Assessing for costovertebral angle tenderness.
Note: Choose the technique that is most comfortable for both examiner and patient.

1. With the patient seated on the examination table, place the palm of one hand over their costovertebral angle on one side of their back. Make a fist out of your other hand. Use the ulnar surface of your fist for striking. Strike the back of the hand that is over the costovertebral angle with the fist of your other hand.

OR

2. Put your hands around the person's waist and locate by the palpation the costovertebral angles with the flat part of your index and middle fingers on each hand. Alternately strike each costovertebral angle with your fingers by a sudden, upward motion of your hand.

# Endocrine Conditions

## Metabolic Syndrome

Obesity, especially central obesity, is associated with an increased risk of insulin resistance and elevated blood cholesterol. The National Cholesterol Education Program has defined metabolic syndrome as atherogenic dyslipidemia, elevated blood pressure, dysglycemia, a prothrombotic state, and a pro-inflammatory state.[119] Table 5-17 provides one commonly accepted definition of metabolic syndrome.[120]

Individuals with one or more of these characteristics should be assessed with blood pressure measurement, waist circumference measurement, fasting glucose, and a full cholesterol panel. Counseling about lifestyle changes, including weight loss, increased exercise, and dietary changes, is essential. Patients should be referred as appropriate for evaluation and pharmacologic treatment and/or management of hyperlipidemia, hypertension, or diabetes.

## Diabetes Mellitus

The definition of diabetes mellitus is based on the underlying cause of hyperglycemia. Table 5-18 distinguishes between four types of diabetes.[121] In addition to the four classifications listed in Table 5-18, a fifth term, prediabetes, is used to identify persons with abnormal plasma glucose values that do not meet the criteria for diabetes. These individuals are at increased risk for developing diabetes and should be monitored closely.

*Type 1 diabetes* is almost universally mediated by the immune system, which causes destruction of pancreatic B cells. It is most commonly diagnosed in children or young adults (hence the older name of "juvenile" diabetes) and accounts for approximately 5% to 10% of all cases of diabetes.[122] *Type 2 diabetes*, which is the most common form of diabetes, is the result of resistance to insulin and the inability of the pancreas to increase insulin production to compensate for this resistance.

Together, diabetes types 1 and 2 affect more than 37 million persons in the United States, of whom approximately 8.5 million (23.0% of adults with diabetes) remain undiagnosed.[122] Increasingly, addressing issues of food and housing insecurity, access to care, and communication barriers, including health literacy and numeracy, are seen as key to improving community-level care for diabetes.[121]

Rates of diabetes increase as persons age, and in persons with obesity. A first-degree family member with diabetes, lack of physical activity, and smoking are other factors that increase risk. A diet high in red meat, high-fat dairy, and processed carbohydrates and sweets increases the risk for developing diabetes regardless of other risk factors. Ethnic groups with an increased prevalence of diabetes include non-Hispanic Black individuals, Mexican Americans and Puerto Ricans, Southwest American Indians, and Asian Americans. Although having a large-for-gestational-age infant is no longer considered a risk

| Table 5-17 | National Cholesterol Education Program Diagnostic Criteria for Metabolic Syndrome |
|---|---|

Positive diagnosis with any three of the following:

- Waist circumference ≥ 88 cm in women or > 101 cm in men
- Serum triglycerides ≥ 150 mg/dL or treatment to reduce triglyceride levels
- Serum HDL-C < 50 mg/dL for women or < 40 mg/dL for men or treatment for reduced HDL-C
- Blood pressure ≥ 130/85 mm Hg or treatment for hypertension
- Fasting plasma glucose ≥ 110 mg/dL or treatment for hyperglycemia

Abbreviation: HDL-C, high-density lipoprotein cholesterol.

Based on National Cholesterol Education Program (NCEP) Expert Panel on Detection, Evaluation, and Treatment of High Blood Cholesterol in Adults (Adult Treatment Panel III). Third report of the National Cholesterol Education Program (NCEP) Expert Panel on Detection, Evaluation, and Treatment of High Blood Cholesterol in Adults (Adult Treatment Panel III): final report. *Circulation.* 2002;106(25):3143-3421.

| Table 5-18 | Classification of Diabetes |
|---|---|
| **Classification** | **Description** |
| Gestational diabetes | Diabetes diagnosed in the second or third trimester of pregnancy that is not clearly overt or preexisting to the pregnancy (type 1 or type 2) diabetes |
| Type 1 diabetes | Diabetes resulting from beta-cell destruction, usually leading to absolute insulin deficiency |
| Type 2 diabetes | Diabetes resulting from progressive loss of pancreatic beta-cell insulin secretion in the face of increased insulin resistance |
| Other types of diabetes | Diabetes due to other causes such as cystic fibrosis, pancreatic disease, drug-induced, or chemically induced |

Based on American Diabetes Association. Standards of medical care in diabetes—2022. *Diab Care.* 2021;45(suppl 1):S1-S264.

factor for diabetes, pregnant people with a history of gestational diabetes and/or polycystic ovary syndrome have demonstrated increased risk.[121–123]

Screening for diabetes mellitus should be performed for everyone older than 35 years, and for anyone with a BMI of 25 kg/m$^2$ or greater (BMI ≥ 23 kg/m$^2$ among Asian Americans) and one or more risk factors for cardiac disease.[121] Screening tests include glycosylated hemoglobin A1c (HbA1c), fasting blood glucose, and the 2-hour glucose tolerance test. HbA1c measures the average plasma glucose level over the last month; its results are expressed as the percentage of total hemoglobin. This test can be used to assess either the degree of elevated blood glucose over time in persons with a new diagnosis of diabetes or the degree of glycemic control in persons who are being treated for diabetes. Type 2 diabetes is diagnosed if the HbA1c result is equal to or greater than 6.5%.

Table 5-19 summarizes the criteria for the diagnosis of diabetes.[121] Any one of the three tests can be used to assess for this condition, but the diagnosis is not made until the same test is repeated twice. The repeat test requires a new blood sample and can be performed right away. The person newly diagnosed with diabetes should be referred to a healthcare provider skilled in treating diabetes.

Midwives can play an important role in some components of care for persons with diabetes, including diet education, promotion of moderate exercise, counseling for weight loss, and smoking cessation. If individuals have female genitalia, they may have an increased risk for developing vaginal infections with candidiasis when glucose control is not optimal. Anyone with diabetes who desires a pregnancy should be encouraged to achieve glucose control prior to becoming pregnant. Hyperglycemia in early pregnancy is associated with miscarriage and congenital anomalies. Preconception counseling and care can have an important positive effect on pregnancy outcomes. Counseling guidelines for those persons with diabetes who are planning a pregnancy can be found in the *Preconception Care* appendix.

The American Diabetes Association recommends beginning lifestyle changes with the addition of the pharmacologic agent metformin (Glucophage) as soon as prediabetes or type 2 diabetes is diagnosed.[121] Tight glucose control can reduce the incidence of microvascular complications, and glycemic targets are based on long-term clinical studies that have identified plasma glucose levels associated with minimal progression of disease. However, diabetes is a progressive disease, and frequently second or third medications are added over time to help maintain euglycemia. Multiple new therapies have been developed in the last several years so that treatment can be individualized to minimize side effects and maximize glucose control. Most medications for diabetes work by improving insulin secretion or insulin sensitivity. Others suppress appetite or promote weight loss. Insulin therapy may also be recommended.

If a midwife is participating in primary care services for a person using medication to control diabetes, additional knowledge about the medications and their effects is needed because these medications have wide-ranging physiologic effects.

## Thyroid Disease

An estimated 12% of the U.S. population will develop thyroid disease at some point in their lifetime,

| Table 5-19 | Diagnosis of Diabetes Mellitus | |
|---|---|---|
| Test | Description | Glycemic Goals Following Treatment |
| *Any one of the following three tests will confer the diagnosis of diabetes if repeated twice:* | | |
| Hemoglobin A$_{1c}$[a] ≥ 6.5% | Fasting not required. | < 7.0% |
| Fasting plasma glucose ≥ 126 mg/dL | Fasting is defined as no caloric intake for at least 8 hours. | 80–130 mg/dL |
| 2-hour plasma glucose ≥ 200 mg/dL after a 75-g glucose load | This test will diagnose more individuals with diabetes than will hemoglobin A1c or a fasting plasma glucose level. | < 180 mg/dL 2-hour post-meal |

Abbreviation: RBC, red blood cell.

[a] Hemoglobin A1c measures the percentage of glycosylated hemoglobin present; glycosylated hemoglobin is hemoglobin that is coated in glucose. As plasma glucose levels rise, the amount of glycosylated hemoglobin increases. Glucose stays attached to an RBC for the life of the RBC and, therefore, is a measure of average plasma glucose levels for the prior 3 months.

Based on American Diabetes Association, Professional Practice Committee. Standards of medical care in diabetes—2022. *Diab Care.* 2022;45(suppl 1):S1-S264.

| Table 5-20 | Thyroid Hormone Values in Thyroid Disorders | | |
|---|---|---|---|
| **Condition** | **Thyroid-Stimulating Hormone** | **Free $T_4$** | **Serum $T_3$** |
| Graves' disease (hyperthyroid) | Absent | Elevated | Elevated |
| Subclinical hyperthyroid | < 0.1 mU/L | Normal | Normal |
| Hypothyroid | High with primary hypothyroidism<br>Low with secondary hypothyroidism | Low | Low/normal |
| Subclinical hypothyroid | Mildly elevated (< 10.0 mU/L) | Low/normal | Normal |

with this disease impacting approximately 20 million Americans; as many as 60% are unaware of their condition.[124] Thyroid disease can be as much as 5 to 8 times more likely in women than in men. If not diagnosed and treated appropriately, thyroid disease in pregnancy can result in increased risk of miscarriage, preterm delivery, and severe developmental issues with the child. To date, the U.S. Preventive Services Task Force reports insufficient evidence to recommend for or against screening asymptomatic, nonpregnant adults for thyroid conditions.[125] Other experts recommend screening in adults, with the age of first testing ranging from 35 to 60 years.[126]

Thyroid-releasing hormone from the hypothalamus stimulates pituitary release of thyroid-stimulating hormone (TSH). In turn, TSH stimulates the production and release of triiodothyronine ($T_3$) and thyroxine ($T_4$) from the thyroid gland. Although $T_3$ is the more active form of the thyroid hormones, little is produced in the thyroid itself. Instead, most $T_3$ is produced from circulating $T_4$ by enzymatic conversion.

When screening for or diagnosing thyroid disease, the first tests performed usually are measurements of TSH and free $T_4$. Among the various antibody tests, confirmation of thyroid peroxidase antibodies is associated with chronic autoimmune thyroiditis (Hashimoto's thyroiditis), the predominant cause of overt hypothyroidism. Table 5-20 identifies the changes in screening laboratory values associated with common thyroid disorders. Table 5-21 lists the common signs and symptoms of thyroid disease.

### Hypothyroidism

Hypothyroid conditions result primarily from failure of the thyroid gland to produce adequate hormone and are more common than hyperthyroidism. The most common cause of hypothyroidism in the United States is the autoimmune disorder known as Hashimoto's thyroiditis. Other causes include

| Table 5-21 | Common Clinical Features of Thyroid Disease | |
|---|---|---|
| **Hypothyroidism** | **Hyperthyroidism** |
| Bradycardia | Anxiety, nervousness |
| Cold intolerance | Diarrhea |
| Constipation | Fatigue |
| Delay in deep tendon reflex relaxation | Goiter |
| | Increased sweating |
| Depression | Heat intolerance |
| Decreased sweating | Hyperreflexia |
| Dry skin, brittle nails, thinning hair | Irregular menses |
| Edema (nonpitting) | Increased appetite with weight loss |
| Fatigue, sleepiness | Lid lag, stare |
| Goiter | Ophthalmopathy |
| Headaches | Palpitations with angina |
| Hoarseness | Tremor |
| Lethargy | Warm, moist skin |
| Loss of appetite | Weakness |
| Muscle weakness | |
| Muscle cramping or pain | |
| Heavy menstrual bleeding | |
| In advanced disease, amenorrhea | |
| Pallor | |
| Slowed speech and body movements | |
| Weight gain (occasionally loss) | |

treatment for Graves' disease, thyroidectomy, and medications. Secondary hypothyroidism, caused by pituitary or hypothalamic disorders, is uncommon. In primary hypothyroid states, the TSH level will be elevated; the pituitary gland secretes excess TSH in response to low levels of $T_3$ and $T_4$.

Uncomplicated primary hypothyroidism usually is treated with thyroid hormone supplementation.

Management of hypothyroidism is complex; medication dosage is based on laboratory values and symptom relief. The midwife plays an important role in screening patients who present with symptoms of hypothyroidism. When thyroid disease is suspected or confirmed with laboratory values, midwives can initiate treatment and refer patients to a healthcare provider competent in the treatment of thyroid disease. Midwives can prescribe thyroid supplementation based on the patient's weight, 1.6 mcg/kg per day, or begin with a low dose such as 50 mcg/day and titrate the dose every 4 to 6 weeks until a euthyroid state is achieved. The first approach is quicker but patients can initially have hyperthyroid symptoms such as tachycardia.[127]

### Hyperthyroidism

The single most common cause of a hyperthyroid state (also referred to as thyrotoxicosis) is Graves' disease, an autoimmune disease that has a higher incidence among women than men, and that is the cause of more than 10% of all cases of thyrotoxicosis in young adults. The thyroid is typically enlarged and tender in hyperthyroidism. Many patients will notice irritation of the conjunctiva, diplopia, or blurred vision, or present with proptosis (bulging of the eye or displacement forward of the eye in its orbit) and periorbital edema.

Other causes of hyperthyroidism include toxic multinodular goiter, toxic adenomas, early stages of Hashimoto's thyroiditis, and postpartum thyroiditis. This disease has also been associated with very high levels of circulating human chorionic gonadotropin (hCG), such as those found in persons who have a hydatidiform mole. Subclinical hyperthyroidism is most commonly associated with suppressive thyroid therapy, although mild Graves' disease is a possible cause.

The midwife should refer for consultation any patient in whom hyperthyroidism is diagnosed or suspected. Patients who are being treated for thyroid disease will need frequent laboratory assessment of their circulating thyroid hormone levels.

## Neurologic Conditions

### Headaches

Headaches have many causes and differing degrees of risk, and often are divided into two types: primary and secondary. Primary headaches include tension headaches, migraine, and cluster headaches, whereas secondary headaches are rarer and are related to underlying disease such as a neoplasm. A complete health history should be collected for individuals with headaches, including a clear description of symptoms associated with onset and duration of headaches, frequency of severe headache, frequency of mild headache, level of interference with normal activities, and frequency of medication use to relieve symptoms. Additional questions can be asked about nausea, light sensitivity, and noise sensitivity, all of which suggest a migraine headache. A headache diary can be valuable in diagnosis and treatment.[128]

Conditions that can provoke headache as a symptom, such as sinus infection or concussion, are not discussed here, nor are vascular emergencies such as aneurysm and arteriovenous (AV) malformation. Warning signs identified during the history taking and physical examination that require emergency attention are summarized in Table 5-22.

### Tension Headache

According to the International Headache Society (IHS), tension headaches are characterized by bilateral pain, with a pressing or tightening quality and mild to moderate intensity.[129] Such headaches are relatively common, with prevalence rates ranging from 30% to 78%. Sensitivity to light or sound can be present. While the duration of tension headaches can vary from minutes to multiple days, normal physical activity does not affect the sensation. Other than in the most severe cases, nausea does not occur.[129]

Tension-type headaches are classified based on their frequency: infrequent episodic (less than

| Table 5-22 | Warning Signs of Headache Emergencies |
|---|---|

Rapid onset of severe symptoms ("thunder clap") or worst headache experienced

Alteration in consciousness or mental status

High fever

Severe vomiting, especially without nausea

Neck stiffness

Neurologic symptoms:
- Weakness
- Loss of balance
- Numbness
- Paralysis

Vision changes

Pattern of worsening headache

Increasing medication use to control headache

Direct association with exercise or position change

1 day/month), frequent episodic (1–14 days/month), and chronic.[129] Most individuals with infrequent or moderate-frequency tension headaches do not seek treatment. Among persons with chronic tension headaches, it has been reported that most are able to continue working and managing daily activities, but they are more likely to have mood or anxiety disorders, decreased ability to function, disturbed sleep, and decreased emotional well-being.[130]

Caring for people with episodic tension headaches includes respecting their report of symptoms, assessing for the presence of anxiety or depression, and promoting lifestyle changes that include relaxation and stress reduction. NSAIDs or acetaminophen can be used as initial therapy to relieve symptoms, especially with episodic tension headaches. Combination medications that include caffeine with aspirin (e.g., Excedrin), ibuprofen (Advil), or acetaminophen (Tylenol) are useful when a single medication is not adequate.[131] Both acupuncture[132] and cognitive-behavioral therapy[133] have shown promise in treating tension-type headaches. Prophylactic treatment is not effective or useful in managing episodic headache.[134]

Chronic tension headache is a more severe condition that often requires prophylactic medication. The tricyclic antidepressants—most commonly, amitriptyline—can be used for this purpose; biofeedback, stress reduction, and other nonpharmacologic interventions to interrupt the cycle of headaches can be used as additional modalities.[135,136] When people report chronic headache over several months while using pain relievers, a medication overuse headache should be suspected, and a plan to stop or taper the drugs in question should be implemented. Individuals with chronic headache should be referred to a neurologist for management.

### Migraine Headache

Migraine headache is both common and frequently underdiagnosed in primary care settings, with an estimated 25% of cases being missed. This tendency suggests that a person with episodic headaches should be assumed to have migraines unless otherwise diagnosed.[137] The prevalence of migraine among women is estimated to be more than 20%.[138] Among people of all races, women are more likely than men to be diagnosed with migraine. Individuals who are poor, unemployed, or disabled show a higher burden of disease. The incidence increases between the ages of 18 and 44.[138] Migraine is relatively rare after menopause, and new-onset headaches in this age group should be evaluated carefully for other causes.

Both genetic predisposition and environmental triggers appear to be involved in the development of migraine headache. The underlying cause is an abnormally increased sensitization to neuronal stimuli, beginning in the cerebral cortex and affecting the trigeminovascular system.

The diagnosis of migraine is subdivided based on the presence or absence of an aura, complications, and associated conditions. The IHS defines *migraine without aura* as a "recurrent headache disorder manifesting in attacks lasting 4–72 hours."[129] Typical characteristics of such headaches are unilateral location, pulsating quality, moderate or severe intensity, aggravation by routine physical activity, and association with nausea and/or photophobia and phonophobia.[129] Migraine without aura in individuals of childbearing age is often related to the menstrual cycle. *Migraine with aura* is characterized by "recurrent attacks, lasting minutes, of unilateral fully reversible visual, sensory or other central nervous system symptoms that usually develop gradually and are usually followed by headache and associated migraine symptoms."[129] The visual, sensory, and speech symptoms associated with aura are reversible.

Migraine is an intermittently recurring event, which proceeds through well-defined stages: (1) the premonitory stage, (2) aura (if present), (3) headache, and (4) postdrome.[129] The premonitory stage is noted in approximately 30% of those individuals with the condition and occurs up to 48 hours before onset of the actual headache; tiredness, fatigue, malaise, mood changes, and stomach upset are the most common symptoms.[129] Following the headache, variable symptoms can persist for hours or days. Over time, migraine can progress from an episodic to a persistent condition with almost daily symptoms. Chronic migraine (defined as migraine headaches occurring on 15 or more days per month) is accompanied in some individuals by both physiologic changes in pain perception and anatomic alterations within the brain.[129] The International Headache Society defines migraines by the criteria shown in **Table 5-23**.[129]

A number of lifestyle changes can improve the frequency of migraine. These modifications include the avoidance of substances that the individual can identify as headache triggers (e.g., cheese, alcohol, chocolate), stress reduction, and stable patterns of eating and rest.

Pharmacologic therapy is used to treat acute attacks (abortive therapy) or reduce the severity and frequency of subsequent episodic attacks (preventive therapy).[139] Abortive treatments for individuals with mild, infrequent cases of migraine include NSAIDs taken in maximal doses, or acetaminophen (Tylenol) 1000 mg. Either type of medication may also be combined with caffeine in OTC preparations.

| Table 5-23 | **Migraine Types** |
|---|---|
| **Migraine Without Aura** | **Migraine with Aura** |
| A. At least five attacks fulfilling criteria B–D | A. At least two attacks fulfilling criteria B and C |
| B. Headache attacks lasting 4–72 hours (untreated or unsuccessfully treated) | B. One or more of the following fully reversible aura symptoms:<br>1. Visual<br>2. Sensory<br>3. Speech and/or language<br>4. Motor<br>5. Brainstem<br>6. Retinal |
| C. Headache has at least two of the following characteristics:<br>1. Unilateral location<br>2. Pulsating quality<br>3. Moderate or severe pain intensity<br>4. Aggravation by or causing avoidance of routine physical activity | C. At least three of the following characteristics:<br>1. At least one aura symptom spreads gradually over ≥ 5 minutes<br>2. Two or more symptoms occur in succession<br>3. Each individual aura symptom lasts 5–60 minutes<br>4. At least one aura symptom is unilateral<br>5. At least one aura symptom is positive (adding something to the vision)<br>6. The aura is accompanied, or followed within 60 minutes, by headache |
| D. During headache at least one of the following:<br>1. Nausea and/or vomiting<br>2. Photophobia and phonophobia | |

Data from Headache Classification Committee of the International Headache Society. The international classification of headache disorders, 3rd edition. *Cephalalgia*. 2018;38(1):1-211.

Historically, the most common abortive therapies were ergotamine preparations such as ergotamine tartrate/caffeine (Cafergot). Ergotamine is teratogenic, so individuals of childbearing age must use an effective and reliable contraceptive method when using this medication, and people planning a pregnancy require a change in therapeutic management. Ergotamines are less frequently used today, as more effective medications have been introduced. The triptans, such as sumatriptan (Imitrex) and naratriptan (Amerge), are serotonin receptor agonists and are quite effective as abortive therapy. Triptans are available as oral, intranasal, oral disintegrating tablets, or subcutaneous formulations. The U.S. Food and Drug Administration (FDA) has issued a caution with regard to use of triptans and selective serotonin reuptake inhibitors (SSRIs) because both drug classes increase serotonin levels, which can place the individual at risk for serotonin syndrome. If the triptan is used infrequently, the risk of serotonin syndrome is very small.

Preventive therapy for migraine includes agents from a number of drug classes, such as the tricyclic antidepressants, antiepileptics, beta blockers, calcium-channel blockers, ACE inhibitors, and angiotensin receptor blockers. Individuals requiring long-term migraine management should receive care from a neurologist or another practitioner skilled in the management of headache.

Menstrual-related migraines may benefit from long-cycle combined hormonal therapy or progesterone-only contraception, particularly the levonorgestrel intrauterine system (IUS). Decreasing the frequency of estrogen withdrawal minimizes the headache response. When estrogen is included in treatment, the patient should be monitored for possible increases in the frequency of headache, which would mandate the use of progesterone-only methods. Combined hormonal contraception is contraindicated in those persons who have migraine with aura, due to increased risk of stroke (Medical Eligibility Criteria for Contraceptive Use [MEC] category 4); among women who experience migraine without aura, the CDC considers the use of combined hormonal contraception acceptable but not optimal (MEC category 2).[140] Additional discussion can be found in the *Hormonal Contraception* chapter. Short-term use of a triptan in the days prior to menses may also interrupt the headache cycle.

Midwives can care for patients with migraines. To do so, however, additional education regarding different presentations, danger signs, drug effects, and prescribing considerations is needed.[139]

### Epilepsy

Epileptic seizures are transient bursts of excessive aberrant or synchronous neuron activity that causes physical signs or symptoms.[141] Diagnosis requires two unprovoked or reflex seizures more than 24 hours apart; or one such seizure and a likelihood greater than 60% that further seizures will occur within 10 years; or diagnosis of a syndrome that includes epilepsy as one of its features.[141]

The classification of seizure disorders is based on whether the seizures are generalized or partial, with these categories being further subdivided by specific patterns of associated symptoms. Generalized seizures are caused by significant activity in both lobes of the brain, and almost always involve changes in consciousness. Tonic–clonic seizures (grand mal), absence (petit mal) seizures, and brief myoclonic seizures are all examples of generalized seizure activity. Partial seizures may or may not involve alteration in consciousness; if this symptom is present, they are referred to as complex partial seizures.

Seizure activity during the childbearing years can peak around the times of ovulation and menstruation, or less commonly with an inadequate luteal phase—a condition known as catamenial epilepsy.[142] The midwife's role in caring for individuals diagnosed with a seizure disorder primarily focuses on the effect of epilepsy medications on reproductive health, the management of contraception, and assessment of risks associated with epilepsy or medications used to treat epilepsy. Menstrual disorders, polycystic ovary syndrome, decreased libido, and infertility are all associated with epilepsy and with some antiepileptic medications.[142] Decreased bone mineral density has also been linked to the use of antiepileptic drugs, although seizure-associated falls' contribution to overall fracture rates is not clear.[143] Some anticonvulsants are associated with an increased risk for teratogenic effects, and pregnant individuals taking these medications should be referred to a genetic specialist for counseling. The *Preconception Care* appendix addresses some of these issues.

Contraceptive management when the patient has epilepsy is complicated by the interaction of estrogen-containing hormonal products with antiepileptic medications that affect the cytochrome P450 metabolic pathway—for example, barbiturates, carbamazepine (Tegretol), lamotrigine (Lamictal), phenytoin (Dilantin), and topiramate (Topamax; in larger doses).[144] These medications can interfere with the effectiveness of hormonal contraceptives and increase the risk of unintended pregnancy. All forms of contraception are considered Category 1 in the CDC's Medical Eligibility Criteria, which caution that specific drug interactions should be reviewed before prescribing such medications.[145] Use of a barrier method as a secondary method of contraception can be recommended. More information about contraception, including evidence-based criteria for eligibility, can be found in the *Fertility, Family Building, and Contraception* chapter. All people with epilepsy should receive counseling regarding risks associated with pregnancy, and referral to a maternal–fetal medicine specialist should be considered.

Another important concern with epilepsy is the increased risk of depression and suicide. Both the psychological and physical stresses of living with the disease and the side effects of medication factor into these risks.[146] Screening for mood changes and suicidal ideation during sexual and reproductive health visits is particularly appropriate.

## Carpal Tunnel Syndrome

The carpal tunnel carries the median nerve through the wrist, where compression from edema, inflammation of the tissue, or anatomic distortion can produce the classic symptoms of carpal tunnel syndrome (CTS)—tingling, numbness, or altered sensation across the palmar surface of part of the thumb, the first two fingers, and part of the ring finger in the affected hand. Over time, CTS almost always becomes bilateral. A person may report that pain and numbness are worse at night. Figure 5-4 illustrates the area affected by carpal tunnel syndrome.

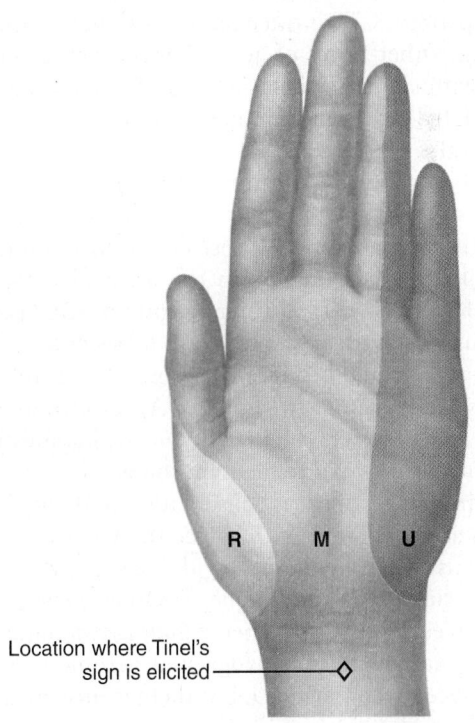

**Figure 5-4** Distribution of sensation by the radial (R), median (M), and ulnar (U) nerves.

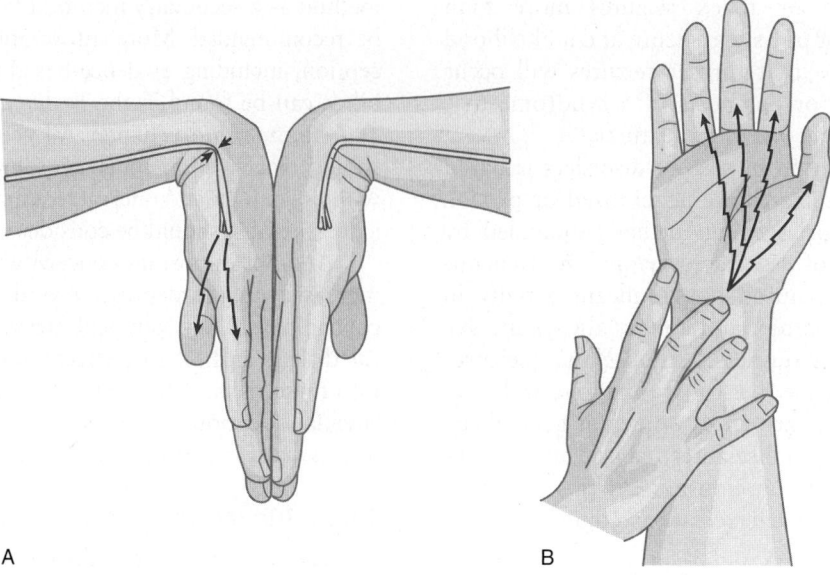

A                                    B

**Figure 5-5  A.** Phalen test. **B.** Tinel's sign.

Female sex, pregnancy, increasing age, obesity, history of wrist injury or arthritis, diabetes, and hypothyroidism have all been associated with increased risk of developing CTS.[147] Research indicates that work-related activities also play a significant role in the development of this condition.[148] When persons engaged in a repetitive motion of the wrists report numbness or loss of sensation in this pattern, CTS is often assumed to be a causative factor. Other forms of nerve damage can also present with similar symptoms. If additional symptoms unrelated to the median nerve are present, prompt referral is warranted.

Two simple tests can help to confirm that a patient's report is consistent with CTS (**Figure 5-5**). First, tapping over the wrist crease in the midline should produce tingling in the affected area; this is referred to as Tinel's sign (**Figure 5-5B**). Second, holding the wrist flexed for 45 to 60 seconds and releasing it should produce symptoms; this is referred to as the Phalen test (**Figure 5-5A**). Electromyography and nerve conduction studies will confirm the diagnosis of carpal tunnel syndrome.

Initial treatment is conservative, and may begin with splinting at night to place the wrist in a neutral position. Only limited evidence supports the effectiveness of this technique.[149] Other conservative therapies, ranging from nerve gliding techniques, to wrist manipulation, to yoga and aerobic exercise, have been recommended, but there is little evidence of their effectiveness.[150] If symptoms are severe, persist, or worsen with conservative management, the individual should be referred to an orthopedic surgeon or neurologist for further evaluation. Treatment can then include injections of steroids or surgical release of the nerve. If left untreated, the condition will worsen over time and eventually lead to permanent decrease in sensation.

## Musculoskeletal Disorders

### Low Back Pain

Pain in the lower back, with or without sciatic nerve pain, is divided into acute pain lasting less than 7 weeks and chronic pain. In 2018, the rates of low back pain within the past 3 months were reported as 28% in men and 31.6% in women.[151] Approximately 25% of all individuals who experience an episode of acute, nonspecific low back pain will have a recurrence within 1 year.[152] Risk factors include female sex, increasing age, obesity, smoking, psychological factors, and physically intensive work.[153] The differential diagnoses range from sprain/strain to spinal conditions that include herniated discs, compression fractures, spinal stenosis; systemic diseases including cancer and connective tissue disease; and referred pain from pelvic or abdominal disease.[154]

Assessment of the patient presenting with symptoms consistent with acute lower back pain includes history and related symptoms, subjective evaluation of the pain, associated psychological factors, ability to function normally, environmental or work-related risks, prior episodes, and questioning regarding red-flag symptoms of more serious disorders. Red-flag signs and symptoms include history of trauma, parenteral drug use, unexplained weight loss, cancer history, long-term use of steroids, fever, incontinence, neurologic deficits, and intense localized pain on physical examination. Referral to a specialist is necessary if any red flags are identified, even if measures to relieve discomfort (as described later in this section) are offered as well.

Clinical assessment does not require imaging for acute, episodic low back pain.[155] Instead, magnetic resonance imaging (MRI) is required only for those individuals with progressive neurologic deficit. The assessment should allow for differentiation of pain into nonspecific causes, possible radiculopathy or stenosis, and other risks including progressive neurologic disease.[155]

Initial management of acute low back pain includes health education about exercise, encouragement to remain physically active, nonpharmacologic measures, and pharmacologic management. Heat may offer relief from strains. Bed rest or prolonged immobilization is of no benefit for persons with acute low back pain.[153–155]

Pharmacologic therapy for acute low back pain begins with NSAIDs or acetaminophen (Tylenol). Short-term use (fewer than 4 days) of a muscle relaxant can assist when acute pain is severe. No strong evidence exists to recommend one agent over another, although cyclobenzaprine (Flexeril) is commonly prescribed for this indication.[154,155] Management of back pain requiring longer or more complex treatment should be referred to a specialist. While opioid medications can be effective pain relievers, their benefit in treating low back pain is often outweighed by their potential for misuse. Prolonged use of opioids occurs frequently and is associated with higher rates of adverse outcomes, including slower recovery, addiction, overdose, and accidental death.[156] Among women with chronic low back pain, tricyclic antidepressants have been shown to offer some benefit.

Nonpharmacologic therapies have also shown some benefit in the treatment of individuals with chronic low back pain. Cognitive-behavioral therapy, spinal manipulation, acupuncture, massage, and yoga, as well as interdisciplinary approaches, have all demonstrated moderate to significant benefits.[152,154]

## Dermatologic Conditions

When assessing a skin lesion or rash, a history specific to the current concern, including the pattern of recurrence, timing and progression, and potential environmental exposures, will facilitate identification of the dermatologic condition. The physical examination includes assessment of the appearance, shape, and texture of the lesion; the pattern of multiple lesions; and the distribution of lesions across the body. Knowing the terminology for common skin changes (Table 5-24) allows for standardized descriptions and facilitates identification. Several of the more common or significant conditions found during the delivery of primary care by midwives are described in this section.

### Psoriasis

Psoriasis is a chronic skin disorder caused by an underlying immune defect that produces thick pruritic, scaly plaques on the skin. Commonly the head and neck, elbow and knee joints, and lower back are affected. Although lesions can occur anywhere on the body, the extremities are more often affected than the trunk. The prevalence of psoriasis in the United States is reported to be approximately 3% of the population, with the incidence of new cases peaking among young adults.[157] The condition is markedly more prevalent among white individuals.[157] Among the various expressions of psoriasis, plaque psoriasis accounts for almost 90% of all cases.[158] In this form, well-defined areas of thickened, erythematous skin with silvery, scaly patches are seen, usually with a symmetric distribution.

Anyone in whom psoriasis is suspected should be referred to a dermatologist for evaluation and creation of a plan of care. If plaques cover less than 5% of the body surface, topical therapy may be sufficient, although this treatment rarely is associated with complete remission. Initial topical treatments include corticosteroids, salicylic acid (to soften keratinized skin), and moisturizers. Ultraviolet light therapy, retinoids, methotrexate (Trexall), cyclosporine-A (Neoral, Sandimmune), and biologic agents are used both for more severe cases and for more complete healing.[158]

Psoriasis is a complex condition that can remit, but rarely resolves. It has been associated with a number of comorbidities, including metabolic syndrome, cardiovascular disease, and autoimmune disorders. Associated psychological conditions include depression and suicidal ideation Ongoing assessment of depression status and stressors is an important part of providing care for individuals who have psoriasis. Counseling can include use of stress reduction techniques and comfort measures such as oatmeal baths.

| Table 5-24 | Terms and Definitions for Common Skin Manifestations |
|---|---|
| **Term** | **Definition** |
| Acne | A dermatologic condition primarily of the sebaceous skin glands, characterized by papules, pustules, or comedones. This condition is more properly termed acne vulgaris to differentiate it from other, less common types of acne. |
| Actinic keratosis (AK) | A premalignant skin condition that manifests with multiple crusty patches. Also termed solar keratosis. |
| Calcineurin inhibitors | Immunosuppressant agents that are theorized to act by selectively inhibiting inflammation through action on T-cell activation. |
| Carbuncle | A skin infection composed of a cluster of boils (furuncles). This infection is most frequently caused by *Staphylococcus aureus*. |
| Cellulitis | An acute spreading dermatologic bacterial infection characterized by significant edema, erythema, and pain. |
| Cosmeceutical | A word coined from the terms "cosmetic" and "pharmaceutical," which is used to describe agents that both have therapeutic effects and promote attractiveness. |
| Dermatophytes | Parasites that may infect the skin. An example is the fungus that causes athlete's foot. |
| Eczema | Inflammatory dermatologic process that is characterized by pruritus, erythema, and lesions that can be encrusted and scaly. |
| Furuncle | Skin infection commonly involving a hair follicle. Also called a boil. |
| Humectant | Agent that absorbs water and promotes maintenance of moisture on the skin. |
| Intertrigo | Rash or inflammation of the body folds or intertriginous areas of the skin. |
| Keratinocyte | Epidermal cell that synthesizes keratin. |
| Langerhans cell | Dendritic skin cell that transports antigens to lymph nodes. |
| Melanin | Skin pigment produced by special cells (melanocytes). |
| Melanocyte | Cell located in the bottom layer (stratum basale) of the skin's epidermis that produces melanin. |
| Merkel cell | Cell found in the middle layers of the skin around hair follicles. Cancer originating among these cells—Merkel cell carcinoma—tends to be highly aggressive. |
| Onychomycosis | Fungal infection of the nails on either the fingers or the toes. |
| Psoriasis | Skin condition caused by overgrowth of keratinocytes, resulting in patchy thickened skin. |
| Pyoderma | Skin condition characterized by purulent-filled lesions. |
| Retinoids | Natural or synthetic derivative of vitamin A that is widely used in pharmacotherapeutics in dermatology. |
| Seborrheic keratoses | Wart-like, benign skin lesions. |
| Solar lentigo | Flat pigmented lesions on sun-exposed skin, more common in individuals older than age 40. |
| Sun protection factor (SPF) | A measure of the degree to which a sunscreen provides protection from the sun's ultraviolet rays. A sunscreen with an SPF factor of 15 or greater is recommended by the American Academy of Dermatology. |
| Telangiectasia | Thread-like red lines on the skin, often seen in clusters and referred to as "spider veins." Thought to be caused primarily by exposure to the sun and extreme temperatures. |
| Xerosis | Dry skin. |

## Skin Cancers

Unprotected exposure to ultraviolet radiation is directly related to development of malignant melanomas and other skin cancers, as well as precursor lesions such as actinic keratosis, squamous cell carcinoma, and basal cell carcinoma. Exposure can occur via natural sun or a tanning facility. All of the skin cancers share the risk factors of fair skin with a tendency to freckle or burn, blond/red hair, blue or green eyes, history of severe sunburns, immunosuppression, and family history. Each year, more than 3 million persons in the United States are estimated to be diagnosed with a non-melanotic skin cancer, and rates continue to rise.[159]

Several types of skin cancer are discussed here to provide midwives with an understanding of abnormal findings on examination of the skin. The diagnosis and management of skin cancers are beyond the scope of practice for midwives. All individuals with suspicious skin lesions should be referred to a dermatologist for further evaluation and treatment.

### Actinic Keratosis

Actinic keratoses are small, dry, rough textured papules or plaques caused by excess exposure to ultraviolet (UV) radiation. In the United States, as much as 25% of the population may develop actinic keratoses over a lifetime, with persons older than 40 years being at increased risk. Early actinic keratosis lesions are usually smaller than 2 cm; they may remain the color of the underlying skin, or be gray or pink. Over time, actinic keratoses can progress to a harder, warty texture. There is disagreement about whether actinic keratosis is itself a precancerous lesion or a squamous carcinoma in situ.[160]

### Basal Cell Carcinoma/Squamous Cell Carcinoma

Together, basal and squamous carcinomas are referred to as keratinocyte carcinomas. The rates of their diagnosis are increasing. Basal cell carcinomas have a waxy or translucent appearance with a raised edge and central erosion, and can bleed. Like actinic keratoses, squamous cell carcinomas are scaly, but the lesions will be thickened, poorly defined, occasionally hard (horn-like), on an erythematous base. Risk factors for keratinocyte carcinoma include advancing age, white race, sun exposure, radiation exposure, and immune suppression. Sun-exposed fair skin is the most common location for lesions, but individuals with darker skin tones can also develop skin cancer, and not all lesions occur on exposed tissue.[161]

### Melanoma

The incidence of melanoma has been steadily increasing in the United States; the lifetime risk is approximately 2.6% among white individuals, with much lower rates among Hispanic and Black individuals.[162] Unlike the other skin cancers, which are relatively easy to treat and have excellent prognoses, melanoma has the highest mutation risk of any cancer. It is virulent, complex, and heterogenous in nature—characteristics that cause difficulties in its treatment. Disease-free survival depends on early diagnosis and prompt surgical excision. Five-year survival rates for individuals diagnosed with a localized tumor are near 99%; individuals with distant metastases have a survival rate of approximately 30%.[162]

Melanoma is more common among individuals with large numbers of moles, and among women with dysplastic nevi. Dysplastic nevi are larger than common moles, with a rough texture, often irregular in outline, and of different colors. Among women, melanomas are more common on the legs and trunk. Lesions also can appear on the genital area, and they should be carefully noted for follow-up. The midwife should initiate a referral to a dermatologist for any patient with a suspicious lesion.

## Common Skin Infections

### Herpes Zoster

Herpes zoster, also called shingles or zoster, is a reactivation of the varicella virus (chickenpox) as immunity to the virus wanes. This virus lies dormant along one or more dermatomes, in the dorsal root of sensory nerve ganglia. Approximately 4 per 1000 Americans and 1% of adults older than age 60 will have an outbreak annually. The incidence rises with age and in persons with impaired cellular immunity.[163] Although generally recognizable, the zoster-associated lesions can be confused with herpes simplex or, in the initial stages, with impetigo, folliculitis, and other skin lesions. Physical trauma at the affected dermatome and psychological stress can also play a role in the reactivation of the varicella virus.

Clinically, zoster often presents with a prodrome of burning pain along the affected dermatome, accompanied by headache, fatigue, and malaise. The typical painful rash of papules on an erythematous base that progresses to vesicles, ruptures, and crusts over may take 7 days to develop. The entire cycle from initial rash to complete healing takes 2 to 3 weeks.

Management of acute herpes zoster includes antiviral drugs such as acyclovir (Zovirax) or valacyclovir (Valtrex), with the addition of analgesics to treat the pain. Initially, acetaminophen (Tylenol) or an NSAID should be given, with opioids being reserved for severe or intractable pain. When postherpetic neuralgia develops, severe pain can persist for months. Treatment of individuals with postherpetic neuralgia is complicated and requires referral to a pain specialist.

Transmission of the varicella virus by direct contact with lesions is possible, but such contact will produce chickenpox, not herpes zoster. Only those persons who have not been vaccinated or who have not experienced prior varicella infection are at risk for chickenpox. Unlike with chickenpox, droplet transmission does not occur with zoster. Vaccination against herpes zoster is now recommended for adults age 50 years or older.[164]

### Tinea Versicolor (Pityriasis)

Tinea versicolor is a chronic infection, in which normal skin fungi that are present on the outer layer of the epidermis, in hair follicles and sebaceous glands, overgrow and become pathogenic. Factors that increase the risk for outbreaks include heat and humidity; oily skin; other conditions including steroid therapy, immune suppression, malnutrition, burns, adrenalectomy, and Cushing's disease; and oral contraceptive use.

The associated rash consists of flat macules of discolored skin on the neck, upper back, or chest. Light-skinned individuals will notice hyperpigmented lesions, while those with darker skin can notice either hypopigmented or hyperpigmented lesions. The macules spread to form large patches, and pruritus may be associated with outbreaks.

To treat tinea versicolor, topical antifungals, including clotrimazole (Lotrimin, Mycelex) and ketoconazole (Nizoral), can be applied daily for 2 to 4 weeks. Ketoconazole shampoo (Nizoral) can also be used daily for 3 days as a body wash from the scalp to the hips. When the spread of the rash is extensive or treatment with topical medications proves ineffective, a course of oral antifungals can be prescribed. The affected individual should be advised that the presence of tinea versicolor is not secondary to poor hygiene, and that they need to continue the prescribed treatment even if the lesions resolve during the course of therapy. Areas of hypopigmentation that arise with sun exposure or tanning may persist until the melanocytes destroyed by the fungus have become reestablished.

## Bacterial Skin Infections

Bacterial skin infections are a common reason for healthcare visits. Knowledge of the presentation of the most common bacterial skin infections informs proper management of these conditions. Among the normal skin flora, *Staphylococcus epidermis* and *Staphylococcus aureus* are the most common bacteria, along with the corynebacteria and mycobacteria; *Streptococcus pyogenes* is less common. The most significant pathogens within this group are *S. aureus* and *S. pyogenes* (group A beta-hemolytic *Streptococcus*). Risk factors for the development of cellulitis and other soft-tissue infections include trauma, bite injuries, prior cellulitis, diabetes, comorbidities that damage the venous or lymphatic systems, chronic renal disease, cirrhosis, and intravenous drug use.[165]

### Erysipelas

The most likely source of erysipelas is infection with *S. pyogenes*. This infection most often presents as a superficial infection of the skin producing a painful erythematous plaque with well-defined edges. It is treated similarly to cellulitis.[165]

### Cellulitis

Penetration of fluid into subcutaneous tissue, causing erythema, warmth, edema, pain, and possibly lymphadenopathy, is the hallmark of cellulitis. An elevated WBC count and fever can be present. When ulcers or other open lesions are present, *S. aureus* infection is the likely culprit. By comparison, diffuse infection is more likely to occur when the pathogen present is *S. pyogenes*.

Both erysipelas and cellulitis usually are treated orally with a penicillinase-resistant semi-synthetic penicillin (e.g., dicloxacillin [Dynapen]), cephalosporin (e.g., cephalexin [Keflex]), or clindamycin (Cleocin). When systemic symptoms are present, infections require parenteral therapy.[165] When purulent cellulitis is present, treatment should include an antibiotic that is effective against methicillin-resistant *S. aureus* (MRSA). When cellulitis or erysipelas do not resolve with antibiotic treatment, the individual should be referred to a specialist for further assessment.

### Purulent Soft-Tissue Infections

Conditions such as furuncles and carbuncles are most commonly found in areas of the body where restrictive clothing is worn or chafing occurs. A small, firm, red papule will enlarge and become painful as pus increases inside, then may either resolve or open and drain spontaneously. When several furuncles coalesce into a carbuncle, the affected individual can experience systemic symptoms of fever or chills in addition to the local pain. Carbuncles will become fluctuant, thinning the skin above the site and drain, possibly from several openings.

Treatment of people with sporadic lesions can be accomplished with warm soaks to help open and drain the site. More severe lesions may require incision and drainage. Treatment should be based on the presence of a systemic response with alterations in temperature (greater than 38°C or less than 36°C), tachypnea, tachycardia, or WBC counts outside the normal range. An antibiotic effective against *S. aureus* should be used; in recurrent infection, a culture should be taken. Treatment for MRSA should be considered in areas where the incidence of this infection is high, and in those individuals with an impaired immune system.[165]

### Necrotizing Soft-Tissue Infection

Necrotizing fasciitis is a soft-tissue infection caused by secondary or polymicrobial extension of a surface infection, often involving mixed anaerobes or group A *Streptococcus*. The infection encompasses the subcutaneous tissue and extends to the muscle layer. In 80% of cases, there is a direct relationship to a skin lesion.[165] To distinguish cellulitis from a necrotizing infection, the following signs and symptoms can be identified in necrotizing infections: severe pain, development of bullae, skin bruising, rapid progression to systemic symptoms, edema, surface anesthesia, and a wooden or rigid texture of the underlying tissue.[165] If a deep-tissue infection associated with a skin lesion is suspected, the patient should be immediately referred to a physician, urgent care, or an emergency department so that the patient can be promptly evaluated for antibiotic therapy and possibly surgical treatment.

### Methicillin-Resistant Staphylococcus aureus

*S. aureus* is one of a group of common bacteria—including *Enterococcus*, *E. coli*, and *Neisseria gonorrhoeae*—that have developed increasing resistance to the traditional antibiotic therapies. In office settings, MRSA is most commonly seen as boils or carbuncles. These lesions begin with a "spider bite" appearance before enlarging and becoming painful.

The Infectious Disease Society of America's guidelines continue to recommend incision and drainage of boils as the most appropriate treatment. This organization's recommendation is to defer antibiotics unless the individual has cellulitis or severe disease with multiple locations. If MRSA is suspected, antibiotics that offer adequate coverage, including TMP-SMX (Bactrim), clindamycin (Cleocin), a tetracycline, or linezolid (Zyvox), should be prescribed for 5 to 10 days, and a culture taken prior to treatment.[166] Regardless of the midwife's choice to use supportive measures, incise the lesion for drainage, or prescribe antibiotics, patients should be advised that signs of worsening infection or failure to begin healing are indications to seek further care.

## Weight Management Counseling and Dietary Patterns

Numerous health conditions are associated with increasing BMI, including cardiovascular disease, osteoarthritis, and metabolic disorders such as diabetes and polycystic ovary syndrome. Midwives assist many individuals with weight management concerns. Consistent weight management is a very challenging task for many people, and the best evidence shows that the kind of low- to moderate-intensity counseling that a busy clinician can provide is not the most effective approach.[167] In addition, community resources such as those that provide a high-intensity comprehensive lifestyle intervention, entailing a minimum of 14 sessions over 6 months, may be unavailable. When a midwife has limited time, direct referral of the patient to a dietician or a specific weight management program may be most helpful. The midwife should seek interventions that are short, precisely targeted, easily administered, understandable, and validated.

### Assessment of Weight-Related Health Risk

Assessment customarily begins with a calculation of the person's BMI. Web-based BMI calculators can readily be found on the Internet (sources are listed in the Resources section at the end of this chapter), but the calculation involves only simple arithmetic and can be done by hand using the following formula:

$$BMI = [(\text{weight in pounds}) \div (\text{height in inches})^2] \times 703 \text{ } or$$

$$BMI = (\text{weight in kg}) \div (\text{height in m})^2$$

For most individuals, including adolescents, a BMI in the "normal" range (18.5–24.9 kg/m²) is associated with improved health outcomes.

BMI is not a holistic measure of health, only a ratio of weight to height. This assessment technique is also clearly inaccurate for body builders or elite athletes, who have much less body fat than the average person and, therefore, might have a "high" BMI but actually be at normal or even reduced risk. In addition, BMI is not as accurate after menopause. The typical loss of muscle mass that can happen after menopause can result in a deceptively "normal" BMI but higher than normal risk for obesity-related morbidities.

Waist circumference has been found to be an additional indicator of increased disease risk. Data reveal that an even better measure for identifying persons at risk for cardiovascular disease and diabetes is a waist circumference-to-height ratio of more than 0.5.[168] For example, a waist measurement of 37 inches and a height measurement of 65 inches would translate into a ratio of 0.57. The waist-to-height ratio identifies abdominal adiposity in the many different populations in which it has been tested, and the cut-off ratio of 0.5 is applicable to all persons. The ease, usefulness, and relative accuracy of the waist-to-height ratio argue strongly for making waist circumference measures a regular part of every health assessment examination.

### Counseling About Weight and Health

The weight management and treatment algorithm developed by the National Heart, Lung, and Blood Institute (NHLBI) uses BMI as the primary decision indicator and is available on the Internet.[169] Within this algorithm, weight management counseling is not advised if a person is overweight (BMI of 25–29.9 kg/m$^2$) in the absence of risk factors for diabetes or cardiovascular disease. However, assessment of readiness for lifestyle changes is recommended for anyone with a BMI of 30 or greater, or for individuals with a BMI in the range of 25 to 29.9 with any additional risk factors (e.g., prediabetes, diabetes, hypertension, dyslipidemia, elevated waist circumference, or other obesity-related condition). If they are ready to make a behavior change, then referral to a comprehensive lifestyle program is recommended, although the counseling may also be undertaken by the provider.[169]

If weight management will be helpful, or if the patient is expressing concern about their weight, the next step should be a brief assessment of readiness to change. It can be helpful to conceive of the process of weight management as providing *cues* rather than providing *cures*. If and when a person is receptive, they will receive and welcome a supportive and factual weight management conversation and be able to consider strategies proposed by the midwife as cues to their own behavior and incorporate them into their lives. If a person is not ready to change, attempts to intervene from a healthcare professional will seem irrelevant, irritating, or even threatening as an advertisement for a product or behavior in which they have no interest.

Accordingly, a midwife seeing a person who meets the NHLBI criteria for weight-loss management might use a few brief questions to obtain a general concept of where the person is in their journey using the "stages of change" model: precontemplation (motivation), contemplation (acknowledgment), preparation (commitment to a change), action, maintenance.[170] **Table 5-25** presents a sample question sequence that is supportive, brief, and factual for the stages of change model.

Although it would be ideal to have people complete a 24-hour or 3-day food diary prior to their healthcare visit, and then have the time to analyze these data for macronutrient and micronutrient content together, the reality is that busy midwives do not usually have the time to do this kind of counseling. Another option is to ask all individuals being seen for an initial or annual visit to complete a "Starting the Conversation About Healthy Eating" questionnaire, which incorporates questions to assess readiness to change, along with seven questions to assess dietary patterns.[171] The questionnaire includes practical suggestions for each question on how this aspect of eating can be improved, as well as a section for making goals for each stage of change.

A more comprehensive and validated instrument is the easy-to-use "Rapid Eating and Activity Assessment for Patients" (REAP), which contains 31 questions.[172] The accompanying "REAP Physician Key for Diet Assessment and Counseling" provides

| Table 5-25 | Sample Question Sequence for the Stages of Change Model Related to Weight Loss Intent |
|---|---|

"There's no right or wrong answer to this question, but for me to better understand where you are right now, have you been thinking about losing weight?"

[In response to either yes or no] "That's fine." (That is, briefly give support.)

[If yes] "Have you been thinking about a plan?"

[If yes] "Is this something you intend to do soon, like within the month, or is this more of a long-term goal?"

"Would you like me to be involved in this process with you, and be a support for you, no matter what happens?"

clear directions for further assessment, treatment, and counseling based on responses to each of the questions. All behavioral changes must be made, freely accepted, and committed to by the individual. Principles of healthy eating patterns are discussed in the *Nutrition* chapter.

Weight is a delicate subject for many people, and repeatedly offering warm support rather than remedies will build trust. When specific plans and strategies seem relevant to discuss, offering cues to become more active in weight management rather than imposing cures should be the goal. Cures are imposed; cues are freely accepted or freely put on hold. Finally, if the individual will be seeing the same healthcare provider again, this provider can offer continuing support. It is important for the midwife to take into account and be supportive of weight management failures as well as successes, as both may occur. Repeated, honest, and realistic offers of support "no matter what happens" can help build the needed trust. More information on how to conduct counseling can be found in the *Health Promotion Across the Lifespan* chapter and the *Skillful Communication to Mitigate Clinician Bias* appendix.

While a weight-loss intervention can be part of the nutritional choices made by someone (in consultation with their healthcare provider), the more fundamental issue remains adopting a healthier dietary pattern. The healthiest and safest weight-loss diets usually involve following the same healthier dietary patterns that would be recommended for anyone, with the modification of eating smaller portions, so as to create a daily calorie deficit in the range of 500 to 750 kcal/day. A minimum weight-loss goal to improve an individual's health has been shown to be 5% of total body weight. Anyone attempting weight

loss should be offered a follow-up assessment with the midwife or another clinician after 6 months. At the 6-month visit, the midwife can evaluate weight loss, review attempted changes in behaviors, and reinforce these efforts. It is important to initiate plans with the individual to maintain weight loss, since weight loss usually plateaus at this time. A midwife can remind everyone that learning and adopting a healthier dietary pattern will be valuable throughout life, whatever the weight, and whatever the health and life goals.

Persons who are unable to meet a healthy weight goal with diet and exercise, especially after attempting intensive comprehensive lifestyle programs, may be candidates for pharmacologic therapy or referral for possible bariatric surgery. Weight-loss drugs work by suppressing appetite, increasing satiety by altering neurotransmitters that regulate appetite and food intake in the central nervous system, or limiting fat absorption. More recently, drugs used for type 2 diabetes, which stimulate the pancreas, have been shown to assist in weight loss by limiting serum glucose. The most common side effects are gastrointestinal symptoms. Currently, there are five FDA-approved drugs for long-term weight loss.[173] They are listed in **Table 5-26** in the order of their relative weight-loss results, from largest to smallest mean amount of weight lost.

Individuals with BMIs greater than 40 kg/m$^2$ or BMIs between 35 and 40 kg/m$^2$, who have a comorbidity such as hypertension, hyperlipidemia, diabetes, or obstructive sleep apnea, should be offered a referral to a bariatric surgeon in addition to a comprehensive lifestyle program. Bariatric surgery has been shown to be the most successful strategy for weight loss for this population.[174] Weight reduction can decrease the effect of comorbidities such

| Table 5-26 | **FDA-Approved Prescription Weight-Loss Medications for Adults** | | |
|---|---|---|---|
| **Drug** | **Average Weight Loss (% body weight lost)** | **Notes** | **Warnings** |
| Semaglutide (Wegovy) | 15 kg (15%) | Once weekly self-injection | Risk of pancreatitis |
| Phentermine and topiramate combination therapy (Qsymia) | Highest dose (11%) Lower doses (7%) | Schedule IV drug | Teratogenic potential; contraindicated in pregnancy and breastfeeding |
| Naltrexone/bupropion (Contrave) | 5–8 kg (5–10%) | Combination of addiction drug and antidepressant | May increase suicidal thoughts |
| Liraglutide (Saxenda) | 4–6 kg (5–10%) | Daily injection | Risk of pancreatitis |
| Orlistat (Xenical) | 2.5–4 kg (3%) | Reduces fat absorption | May need supplements of fat-soluble vitamins |

as diabetes.[175] Additionally, recent evidence demonstrates that patients who are obese and experiencing infertility (undergoing assisted reproductive technologies) increase their ability to conceive and have a live birth by one-third following bariatric surgery compared to attempts prior to surgery.[176]

## Surgical Weight Loss

Several approaches for surgical weight loss are or have been in use (**Figure 5-6** and **Table 5-27**). Even though surgical weight loss is the most efficient strategy for weight loss and has multiple other health benefits, it is not without risk. Weight-loss surgery works by two mechanisms: restriction and malabsorption of food intake. Malabsorption works to speed weight loss, but it predisposes patients to nutritional deficiencies. Lifelong follow-up, including supplementation for prevention of such deficiencies and routine screening, is mandatory. For clinicians, understanding the physical and hormonal changes within the body is paramount when caring for individuals who have undergone bariatric surgery.

Only one surgery works by restriction alone—the adjustable gastric band. With this technique, an inflatable band is placed around the upper portion of the stomach, creating a small pouch above it. The result is a sense of satiety after the individual eats a smaller portion of food. The size of the stomach opening can be adjusted by injecting sterile saline into the band or by removing it to enlarge the opening.

The gastric sleeve, also called sleeve gastrectomy, uses both restriction and malabsorption to induce weight loss. Approximately 80% of the stomach is removed, leaving behind a tube. The smaller stomach reduces the amount of food the person can eat. More importantly, the removal of a large portion of the stomach impacts the gut hormones and results in decreased hunger, faster satiety, and better blood sugar control. The sleeve gastrectomy is the most commonly performed bariatric procedure globally. In a 15-year follow-up study, 32% of patients maintained their weight loss after the original sleeve gastrectomy, but nearly 50% needed surgical conversion to the classic Roux-en-Y gastric bypass for gastroesophageal reflux or regained weight.[162]

The Roux-en-Y gastric bypass has been the gold standard to which the other surgeries are compared for some time. It induces weight loss through both restriction and malabsorption. The procedure has two parts. First, a small pouch is created by removing the top part of the stomach. Then, the first part of the small intestine (mostly duodenum) is cut: The bottom portion is connected to the new pouch, and the top portion (which is still attached to the remainder of the stomach) is attached farther down on the small intestine so that stomach acids and enzymes can drain. The new stomach pouch restricts the amount of food that can be eaten, thereby reducing calorie consumption. Less absorption of calories also occurs because less digestion of food takes place in the stomach, and the food does not go through the portion of

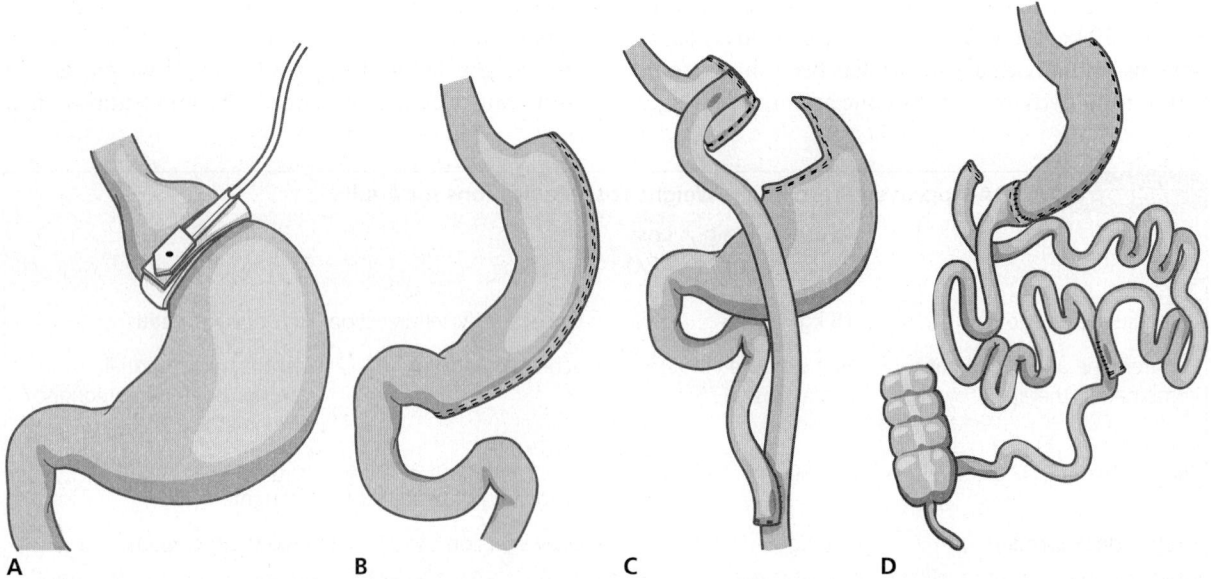

A     B     C     D

**Figure 5-6** Methods of bariatric surgery. **A.** Adjustable gastric band. **B.** Gastric sleeve or sleeve gastrectomy. **C.** Roux-en-Y gastric bypass. **D.** Biliopancreatic diversion with duodenal switch.

| Table 5-27 | Characteristics of Types of Bariatric Surgery | | | |
|---|---|---|---|---|
| | **Adjustable Gastric Band** | **Gastric Sleeve or Sleeve Gastrectomy** | **Roux-en-Y Gastric Bypass** | **Biliopancreatic Diversion with Duodenal Switch** |
| Mechanism of action | Restriction | Restriction and minimal malabsorption | Restriction and malabsorption | Restriction and malabsorption |
| Initial loss of excess weight | 40–50% in 3–5 years | > 50% in 3–5 years | 60–80% in 1 year | 60–70% in 1 year |
| Maintenance | < 50% | > 50% | > 50% | 60–70% |
| Potential for deficiencies | Possible | Likely | Definite | Definite |
| Advantages | No cutting or rerouting<br>Shorter hospital stays<br>Reversible and adjustable<br>Lowest risk for vitamin/mineral deficiency | No rerouting<br>Approximately 2-day hospital stay<br>Hunger suppression, appetite reduction, and increased satiety | May increase energy expenditure<br>Reduces appetite, enhances satiety<br>Better initial and long-term weight loss than with gastric band | Greater maintainable weight loss overall<br>Reduces appetite, improves satiety<br>Most effective for patients with diabetes mellitus |
| Disadvantages | Slower weight loss<br>Greater percentage of failure to lose at least 50% of body weight<br>Requires foreign device in body<br>Mechanical problems, slippage, erosion<br>Highest rate of reoperation | Nonreversible<br>Potential for vitamin/mineral deficiencies<br>Highest risk of reflux<br>Slightly higher complication rate than for gastric band | Long-term vitamin/mineral deficiency risk<br>2- to 3-day hospital stay if laparoscopic<br>Lifelong adherence to diet, vitamin/mineral supplements, and follow-up<br>Higher complication rate than for gastric band or sleeve | Highest complication rate and risk of mortality<br>Longest hospital stays<br>Greatest potential for protein deficiencies<br>Long-term vitamin/mineral deficiencies common<br>Strict adherence to diet, supplements, and follow-up |

the intestine that would normally absorb some of the calories. The rerouting of the food stream produces changes in those gut hormones that promote satiety, suppress hunger, and improve blood sugar control.

It is less common to see patients who have had biliopancreatic diversion with duodenal switch (BPD/DS), but it is still an approved procedure for a subset of patients. This procedure also has two parts. First, the stomach is reduced to a tube (as in the sleeve surgery). Then, a large portion (about three-fourths) of the small intestine is bypassed—namely, the duodenum and jejunum. This procedure has the same effects of restriction and impact on the gut hormones as the sleeve and gastric bypass, but because the bypassed section of the small intestine carries the bile and pancreatic enzymes necessary for breaking down protein and fat, this approach significantly reduces the amount of calorie and fat-soluble nutrient absorption.

Considering how surgical weight-loss procedures change the anatomy, it is clear why nutrient deficiencies can be a problem post-surgery—which is why lifelong follow-up, supplementation for prevention of these deficiencies, and monitoring are required. The number of people opting for surgical weight loss has grown consistently in recent years.[177] Follow-up rates reported in the literature vary, but patients lost to follow-up is the primary issue noted in monitoring long-term results of weight-loss surgery.[178] Many patients are not receiving the recommended monitoring for nutritional imbalances after weight-loss surgery, and many stop taking their supplements as well, putting them at increased risk for deficiencies in several micronutrients and macronutrients. Additionally, many are unaware of the effects of nutritional deficiencies when pregnant.

Midwives can make a considerable impact on the overall health of patients who have undergone weight-loss surgery by assessing for routine supplementation intake, screening for common nutritional deficiencies at least annually, including nutritional imbalance in the differential diagnosis for a variety of complaints, and ensuring prompt treatment once deficiency has been discovered. Since it is common for patients to have multiple deficiencies and for the signs and symptoms of nutritional deficiencies to be vague and mimic other illnesses, screening for these conditions early in a work-up may avoid further costly diagnostic testing. Specific guidelines for recommended screening can be found in the Clinical Practice Guideline for the Perioperative Nutrition, Metabolic, and Nonsurgical Support of Patients Undergoing Bariatric Procedures—2019 Update.[179] Table 5-28 summarizes potential common nutritional deficiencies following different types of bariatric surgery.[180–183]

## Eating Disorders

The lifetime prevalence of eating disorders in Western countries is estimated to be 1.89%, but the paucity of studies using standardized criteria and the fact that eating disorders often go undetected suggest this number may be significantly higher.[184] Primary care providers may not automatically recognize eating disorders. Due to the difficulties of detection and the complex etiology of eating disorders, successful detection, diagnosis, and treatment require a multidisciplinary effort by a team of health professionals, preferably with special education in the field. Although midwives in busy practices may lack the education needed to provide in-depth counseling and treatment of women with eating disorders, they should be able to rule out some instances of eating disorders through use of a brief screening and provide follow-up referrals when necessary.

The SCOFF is a brief five-question instrument with a high negative predictive value in the general population. That is, when used among a normal clinical population, the SCOFF questionnaire is not reliable in detecting eating disorder, but it is reliable in ruling it out.[185] Originally designed as a mnemonic, the initials reflect its origin in British English. While SCOFF does not work as a mnemonic in American usage, the five questions are universal. They assess whether individuals are making themselves vomit to relieve a feeling of fullness; whether they are concerned that they have lost control over what or how much they eat; whether they have recently lost a significant amount of weight (15 pounds or more); whether they feel that they are "fat" even when others comment that they are thin; and whether they feel that thoughts and feelings about food are

dominating their life. An answer of "yes" to two or more questions is indicative of an eating disorder. Two questions from the SCOFF instrument that can be particularly associated with pica (another eating order) are the two "F" questions related to feeling fat and thinking a lot about food.[186] Individuals with some symptoms of disordered eating should be assessed in more detail by professionals in the area.

## Conclusion

Modern midwifery has often been viewed as possessing a limited, albeit well-recognized, scope of practice—that is, midwives take care of healthy pregnant women and help them give birth. Historically, however, midwives have never limited their care exclusively to healthy pregnant women, if for no other reason than that many of the women traditionally served by midwives were at risk because of age, socioeconomic status, or lack of access to other healthcare resources. In addition, midwives have often provided first-line care for families and sometimes larger populations. As has always been true, the needs of the community and the skills of the midwives who serve that community help define midwifery scope of practice. Today midwifery is practiced in a healthcare system in which the only provider whom many people see is their "women's health" provider. While midwives still care for pregnant individuals, they are also obliged to correctly identify common conditions, minor and major, and facilitate treatment of people with these conditions by themselves or through other strategies such as collaborative management and referral.

Midwives must be able to describe abnormal or unusual symptoms or signs accurately, even when they cannot make a diagnosis with any certainty. These professionals must be prepared to assess and triage anyone with these conditions, and to determine which can be managed autonomously by the midwife and which cannot. All midwives need to know to whom they will refer cases beyond their personal or professional scopes of practice. Referral can be to nurse practitioners or physician assistants, as well as to physicians, dieticians, social workers, physical therapists, and others. Creation of a large network of healthcare contacts serves both midwives and their patients well.

The astute reader may have noticed the frequency with which reference has been made to lifestyle changes that can help prevent or treat diseases. One of the assets that midwives bring to primary care for is an understanding of the importance of health maintenance as well as disease prevention. Every midwife has the ability and responsibility to provide this aspect of primary care.

| Table 5-28 | Vitamin/Mineral Role, Site of Absorption, and Signs and Symptoms of Deficiency | | |
|---|---|---|---|
| **Vitamin/Mineral** | **Role** | **Absorption** | **Signs and Symptoms** |
| Calcium | Formation of bone and teeth, muscle contraction, nerve function, blood clotting, heart rhythm | Duodenum Upper jejunum | Muscle cramps<br>Numbness and tingling<br>Fatigue<br>Abnormal heart rhythm<br>Dry skin<br>Confusion and memory loss<br>Osteopenia and osteoporosis |
| Vitamin D | Bone health, calcium–phosphate metabolism | Duodenum Jejunum | Brittle bones<br>Fractures<br>Muscle weakness<br>Fatigue<br>Mood changes |
| Vitamin E | Protects from oxidative damage, healthy immune system, RBC production, prevention of platelet aggregation | Duodenum Jejunum | Ataxia<br>Muscle weakness<br>Hemolytic anemia<br>Retinopathy<br>Impaired immune response |
| Iron | Hemoglobin and myoglobin synthesis | Duodenum Proximal jejunum | Anemia<br>Fatigue<br>Pale skin |
| Selenium | Liver, kidney, heart, skeletal muscle, eye lens metabolism | Duodenum | Cardiomyopathy<br>Myopathy<br>Osteoarthropathy<br>Keshan disease |
| Copper | Neurotransmitter synthesis, respiratory oxidation, iron absorption | Duodenum Proximal jejunum | Neuropathy<br>Anemia<br>Neutropenia<br>Optic neuropathy<br>Fatigue<br>Myelopathy |
| Zinc | Cellular metabolism, DNA synthesis, protein synthesis, immune function, wound healing | Duodenum Proximal jejunum | Hair loss<br>Diarrhea<br>Glossitis<br>Hypogonadism<br>Taste alteration<br>Delayed wound healing |
| Vitamin A | Healthy teeth, bones, muscles, skin, vision, and immune system | Duodenum Jejunum | Night blindness<br>Xerophthalmia<br>Dry, scaling skin<br>Infections |

*(continues)*

| Table 5-28 | Vitamin/Mineral Role, Site of Absorption, and Signs and Symptoms of Deficiency (*continued*) | | |
|---|---|---|---|
| **Vitamin/Mineral** | **Role** | **Absorption** | **Signs and Symptoms** |
| Vitamin $B_1$ (thiamine) | Enzymatic cofactor, nerve function and structure, brain metabolism | Upper jejunum | Lactic acidosis<br>Delayed gastric emptying<br>Peripheral neuropathy<br>Ataxia<br>Ocular changes<br>Beriberi<br>Wernicke encephalopathy |
| Vitamin $B_6$ (pyridoxine) | Cellular metabolism<br>Cofactor | Proximal jejunum | Muscle weakness<br>Paresthesia<br>Abnormal gait |
| Vitamin $B_9$ (folate) | DNA/RNA biosynthesis, cell division and repair, RBC formation | Jejunum | Neural tube defects<br>Macrocytic anemia<br>Weakness<br>Fatigue<br>Shortness of breath<br>Heart palpitations<br>Red, swollen tongue |
| Vitamin $B_{12}$ | Neurologic function, RBC formation, fatty acid and amino acid metabolism | Terminal ileum | Peripheral neuropathy<br>Megaloblastic anemia |
| Vitamin C (ascorbic acid) | Cell growth, tissue repair, collagen synthesis, absorption of nonheme iron, immune function | Intestine | Scurvy<br>Bleeding gums<br>Fatigue<br>Impaired wound healing |

Abbreviation: RBC, red blood cell.

Based on Chu AS, Matalga MA, Krueger L, Barr PA. Nutrient deficiency-related dermatoses after bariatric surgery. *Adv Skin Wound Care.* 2019;32(10):443-455; Patel JJ, Mundi MS, Hurt RT, et al. Micronutrient deficiencies after bariatric surgery: an emphasis on vitamins and trace minerals. *Nutr Clin Pract.* 2017;32(4):471-480; Parretti HM, Subramanian A, Adderley NJ, et al. Post-bariatric surgery nutritional follow-up in primary care: a population-based cohort. *Br J Gen Pract.* 2021. [Epub ahead of print]. http://doi.org/10.3399/bjgp20X714161; Lupoli R, Lemo E, Saldalamacchia G, et al. Bariatric surgery and long-term nutritional issues. *World J Diabetes.* 2017;8(11):464-474. https://doi.org/10.4239/wjd.v8.i11.464.

Finally, the importance of combining an evidence-based approach with a holistic awareness of the various factors playing into the person's life is increasingly recognized as positively influencing an individual's ability to adhere to treatment recommendations, whether these recommendations focus on lifestyle changes, medication, or other therapeutic interventions. The provision of effective health care requires an awareness and assessment of how poverty, insurance coverage, literacy, mental health, and other factors affect the ability to achieve the goals set with the midwife from whom an individual obtains care.

## Resources

| Organization | Description |
|---|---|
| American College of Cardiology (ACC) | 10-year calculator for atherosclerotic cardiovascular disease. This risk calculator can also be downloaded from iTunes as an app. |
| Framingham Risk Assessment Tool | Based on the Framingham Heart Study. |
| Multi-Ethnic Study of Atherosclerosis (MESA) | Coronary artery calcification calculator. |

| Organization | Description |
|---|---|
| Reynolds Risk Score | This calculator is particularly sensitive for women in assessing risk for coronary event. |
| American Association of Clinical Endocrinologists and American College of Endocrinology (AACE/ACE) | Diabetes treatment algorithms. |
| American College of Cardiology (ACC) | *High Blood Pressure in Adults: Guideline for the Prevention, Detection, Evaluation and Management.* 2017 American Heart Association and American College of Cardiology Hypertension guidelines. |
| | This site has multiple links to the executive summary, slides, patient handouts, and key points for clinicians. |
| National Heart, Lung, and Blood Institute (NHLBI) | JNC 7 reference card and link to complete guideline. |
| American Headache Society | Migraine resources and guidelines. |

## References

1. Phillippi JC, Barger MK. Midwives as primary care providers for women. *J Midwifery Womens Health.* 2015;60:250-257.

2. Varney H, Thompson JB. *A History of Midwifery in the United States: The Midwife Said Fear Not.* New York, NY: Springer; 2016.

3. American College of Nurse-Midwives. *Core Competencies for Basic Midwifery Practice.* Silver Spring, MD: American College of Nurse-Midwives; 2012.

4. Phillippi JC, Avery M. The 2012 American College of Nurse-Midwives core competencies for basic midwifery practice: history and revision. *J Midwifery Womens Health.* 2014;59:82-90.

5. American College of Nurse-Midwives. Position statement: midwives are primary care providers and leaders of maternity care homes. http://www.midwife.org/ACNM/files/ACNMLibraryData/UPLOADFILENAME/000000000273/Primary%20Care%20Position%20Statement%20June%202012.pdf. Published 2012; revised 2018. Accessed March 21, 2022.

6. Dau KQ. Organizational change in the pursuit of equity. *J Midwifery Womens Health.* 2016;61:685-687.

7. Tervalon M, Murray-Garcia J. Cultural humility versus cultural competence: a critical distinction in defining physician training outcomes in multicultural education. *J Health Care Poor Underserved.* 1998;9(2):117-125.

8. Goodman D. Improving access to maternity care for women with opioid use disorders: colocation of midwifery services at an addiction treatment program. *J Midwifery Womens Health.* 2015;60:706-712.

9. Womack JA, Brandt CA, Justice AC. Primary care of women aging with HIV. *J Midwifery Womens Health.* 2015;60:146-157.

10. James CV, Moonesinghe R, Wilson-Frederick SM, et al. Racial/ethnicity health disparities among rural adults—United States, 2012–2015. *MMWR Surveill Summ.* 2017;66(SS-23):1-9. http://dx.doi.org/10.15585/mmwr.ss6623a1.

11. Donaldson MS, Yordy KD, Lohr KN, Vanselow NA, eds. *Primary Care: America's Health in a New Era.* Washington, DC: National Academy Press; 1996.

12. Linde-Feucht S, Coulouris N. Integrating primary care and public health: a strategic priority. *Am J Public Health* 2012;102(S3):S310-S311.

13. Dzau VJ, McClellan MB, McGinnis JM, et al. Vital directions for health and health care: priorities from a National Academy of Medicine initiative. *JAMA.* 2017;317(14):1461–1470. doi:10.1001/jama.2017.1964.

14. Fiscella K, Sanders MR, Carroll JK. Transforming health care to address value and equity: national vital signs to guide vital reforms. *JAMA.* 2021;326(2):131-132. doi:10.1001/jama.2021.9938.

15. Bazemore AW, Cottrell EK, Gold R, et al. "Community vital signs": incorporating geocoded social determinants into electronic records to promote patient and population health. *J Am Med Inform Assoc.* 2016;23(2):407-412. doi:10.1093/jamia/ocv088.

16. Hager ER, Quigg AM, Black MM, et al. Development and validity of a 2-item screen to identify families at risk for food insecurity. *Pediatrics.* 2010;126(1):e26-e32.

17. Cutts D, Cook J. Screening for food insecurity: short-term alleviation and long-term prevention. *Am J Public Health.* 2017;107(11):1699-1700. doi:10.2105/AJPH.2017.304082.

18. Kopparapu A, Sketas G, Swindle T. Food insecurity in primary care: patient perception and preferences. *Fam Med.* 2020;52(3):202-205. https://doi.org/10.22454/FamMed.2020.964431.

19. Stahre M, VanEenwyk J, Siegel P, Njai R. Housing insecurity and the association with health outcomes

and unhealthy behaviors, Washington State, 2011. *Prev Chronic Dis.* 2015;12:140511. http://dx.doi.org/10.5888/pcd12.140511.

20. Housing and health: an overview of the literature. *Health Aff Health Policy Brief.* June 7, 2018. doi:10.1377/hpb20180313.396577.

21. Chhabra M, Sorrentino AE, Cusack M, et al. Screening for housing instability: providers' reflections on addressing a social determinant of health. *J Gen Intern Med.* 2019;34(7):1213-1219. doi:10.1007/s11606-019-04895-x.

22. Social Interventions Research & Evaluation Network. Housing insecurity/instability/homelessness questions. https://sirenetwork.ucsf.edu/housing-insecurity-instability-homelessness-questions. Accessed June 20, 2022.

23. Bunn HF. Chapter 3: Overview of the anemias. In: Aster JC, Bunn HF, eds. *Pathophysiology of Blood Disorders.* 2nd ed. New York, NY: McGraw-Hill Education; 2017:32-46.

24. Centers for Disease Control and Prevention. Recommendations to prevent and control iron deficiency in the United States. *MMWR Recomm Rep.* 1998;47(RR-3):1-36.

25. National Institutes of Health. Iron: dietary supplement fact sheet. https://ods.od.nih.gov/factsheets/Iron-HealthProfessional. Published 2022. Accessed April 23, 2022.

26. Moretti D, Goede JS, Zeder C, et al. Oral iron supplements increase hepcidin and decrease iron absorption from daily or twice-daily doses in iron-depleted young women. *Blood.* 2015;126:1981.

27. Stoffel NU, Cercamondi CI, Brittenham G, et al. Iron absorption from oral iron supplements given on consecutive versus alternate days and as single morning doses versus twice-daily split dosing in iron-depleted women: two open-label, randomised controlled trials. *Lancet Haematol.* 2017;4:e524.

28. Stoffel NU, Zeder C, Brittenham GM, et al. Iron absorption from supplements is greater with alternate day than with consecutive day dosing in iron-deficient anemic women. *Haematologica.* 2020;105:1232.

29. Rund D, Rachmielewitz E. β-Thalassemia. *N Engl J Med.* 2005;353:1135-1146.

30. Sayani FA, Kwiatkowski JL. Increasing prevalence of thalassemia in America: implications for primary care. *Ann Med.* 2015;47(7):592-604.

31. Muncie H, Campbell J. Alpha and beta thalassemia. *Am Fam Physician.* 2009;80(4):339-344.

32. Olivieri NF. The β-thalassemias. *N Engl J Med.* 1999;341:99-109.

33. Kattamis A, Forni GL, Aydinok Y, Viprakasit V. Changing patterns in the epidemiology of β-thalassemia. *Euro J Haematol.* 2020;105(6):692-703. doi:10.1111/ejh.13512.

34. Centers for Disease Control and Prevention. Incidence of sickle cell trait—United States, 2010. *MMWR.* 2014;63(49):1155-1158.

35. Centers for Disease Control and Prevention. Sickle cell disease: data and statistics on sickle cell disease. https://www.cdc.gov/ncbddd/sicklecell/data.html. Last reviewed March 30, 2022. Accessed April 22, 2022.

36. Payne AB, Mehal JM, Chapman C, et al. Trends in sickle cell disease-related mortality in the United States, 1979 to 2017. *Ann Emerg Med.* 2020;76(3S):S28-S36. doi:10.1016/j.annemergmed.2020.08.009.

37. Frank JE. Diagnosis and management of G6PD deficiency. *Am Fam Physician.* 2005;72(7):1277-1282.

38. Leebeek FW, Eikenboom JC. Von Willebrand's disease. *N Engl J Med.* 2016;375(21):2067-2080. doi:10.1056/NEJMra1601561.

39. Dilley A, Drews C, Miller C, et al. Von Willebrand disease and other inherited bleeding disorders in women with diagnosed menorrhagia. *Obstet Gynecol.* 2001;97:630-636.

40. National Heart, Lung, and Blood Institute. *The Diagnosis, Evaluation and Management of von Willebrand Disease.* NIH Publication No. 08-5832. Bethesda, MD: U.S. Department of Health and Human Services, National Institutes of Health, National Heart, Lung, and Blood Institute; 2007.

41. National Heart, Lung, and Blood Institute. Platelet disorders. https://www.nhlbi.nih.gov/health/platelet-disorders. Accessed April 27, 2022.

42. Bunn HF, Furie B. Chapter 14: platelet disorders. In: Aster JC, Bunn HF, eds. *Pathophysiology of Blood Disorders.* 2nd ed. New York, NY: McGraw-Hill Education; 2017:171-184.

43. Murphy SL, Kochanek KD, Xu JQ, Arias E. *Mortality in the United States, 2020.* NCHS Data Brief, no 427. Hyattsville, MD: National Center for Health Statistics. 2021. https://dx.doi.org/10.15620/cdc:112079.

44. Virani SS, Alonso A, Aparicio HJ, et al. Heart disease and stroke statistics—2021 update: a report from the American Heart Association. *Circulation.* 2021;143(8):e254-e743. doi:10.1161/CIR.0000000000000950.

45. Grundy SM, Stone NJ, Bailey AL, et al. 2018 AHA/ACC/AACVPR/AAPA/ABC/ACPM/ADA/AGS/APhA/ASPC/NLA/PCNA guideline on the management of blood cholesterol: a report of the American College of Cardiology/American Heart Association Task Force on Clinical Practice Guidelines. *J Am Coll Cardiol.* 2019;73(24):e285-e350. doi:10.1016/j.jacc.2018.11.003.

46. Centers for Disease Control and Prevention. *Hypertension Cascade: Hypertension Prevalence, Treatment and Control Estimates Among U.S. Adults Aged 18 Years and Older Applying the Criteria from the American College of Cardiology and American*

*Heart Association's 2017 Hypertension Guideline—NHANES 2015–2018.* Atlanta, GA: U.S. Department of Health and Human Services; 2021.

47. Santo L, Okeyode T. National Ambulatory Medical Care Survey: 2018 national summary tables. https://www.cdc.gov/nchs/data/ahcd/namcs_summary/2018-namcs-web-tables-508.pdf. Accessed April 23, 2022.

48. Arnett DK, Blumenthal RS, Albert MA, et al. 2019 ACC/AHA guideline on the primary prevention of cardiovascular disease: a report of the American College of Cardiology/American Heart Association Task Force on Clinical Practice Guidelines *Circulation.* 2019;140(11):e596-e646. doi:10.1161/CIR.0000000000000678. [Published correction appears in *Circulation.* 2019;140(11):e649-e650.] [Published correction appears in *Circulation.* 2020; 141(4):e60.] [Published correction appears in *Circulation.* 2020;141(16):e774.]

49. Ostchega Y, Fryar CD, Nwankwo T, Nguyen DT. *Hypertension Prevalence Among Adults Aged 18 and Over: United States, 2017–2018.* NCHS Data Brief, no 364. Hyattsville, MD: National Center for Health Statistics; 2020.

50. Whelton PK, Carey RM, Aronow WS, et al. 2017 ACC/AHA/AAPA/ABC/ACPM/AGS/APhA/ASH/ASPC/NMA/PCNA guideline for the prevention, detection, evaluation, and management of high blood pressure in adults: a report of the American College of Cardiology/American Heart Association Task Force on Clinical Practice Guidelines. *Hypertension.* 2017. [Epub ahead of print]. doi:10.1016/j.jacc.2017.11.006.

51. James PA, Oparil S, Carter BL, et al. Evidence-based guideline for the management of high blood pressure in adults: report from the panel members appointed to the Eighth Joint National Committee (JNC 8). *JAMA.* 2014;311(5):507-520.

52. National High Blood Pressure Education Program. *The Seventh Report of the Joint National Committee on Prevention, Detection, Evaluation, and Treatment of High Blood Pressure: Complete Report.* Bethesda, MD: National Heart, Lung, and Blood Institute; August 2004.

53. Weber MA, Schiffrin EL, White WB, et al. Clinical practice guidelines for the management of hypertension in the community: a statement by the American Society of Hypertension and the International Society of Hypertension. *J Clin Hypertens.* 2014;16(1):14-26.

54. Appel L, Champagne C, Harsha D, et al. Effects of comprehensive lifestyle modification on blood pressure control: main results of the PREMIER clinical trial. Writing Group of the PREMIER Collaborative Research Group. *JAMA.* 2003;289:2083-2093.

55. Wright JM, Musini VM, Gill R. First-line drugs for hypertension. *Cochrane Database Syst Rev.* 2018;4(4):CD001841. doi:10.1002/14651858.CD001841.pub3.

56. Law M, Morris J, Wald N. Use of blood pressure lowering drugs in the prevention of cardiovascular disease: meta-analysis of 147 randomised trials in the context of expectations from prospective epidemiological studies. *BMJ.* 2009;338:b1665.

57. Dorans KS, Mills KT, Liu Y, He J. Trends in prevalence and control of hypertension according to the 2017 American College of Cardiology/American Heart Association (ACC/AHA) guideline. *J Am Heart Assoc.* 2018;7(11). doi:10.1161/JAHA.118.008888.

58. Jellinger PS, Handelsman Y, Rosenblit PD, et al. American Association of Clinical Endocrinologists and American College of Endocrinology guidelines for management of dyslipidemia and prevention of cardiovascular disease. *Endocr Pract.* 2017;23(suppl 2): 1-87.

59. Centers for Disease Control and Prevention. Cholesterol. https://www.cdc.gov/cholesterol/cholesterol_screening.htm?CDC_AA_refVal=https%3A%2F%2Fwww.cdc.gov%2Fcholesterol%2Fchecked.htm. Accessed December 27, 2022.

60. American College of Cardiology, American Heart Association. ASCVD risk calculator. http://tools.acc.org/ASCVD-Risk-Estimator-Plus/#!/calculate/estimate/. Accessed April 23, 2022.

61. Hoover LE. Cholesterol management: ACC/AHA updates guideline. *Am Fam Physician.* 2019;99(9): 589-591.

62. Hersh AL, King LM, Shapiro DJ, et al. Unnecessary antibiotic prescribing in US ambulatory care settings, 2010–2015. *Clin Infect Dis.* 2021;72(1):133-137. doi:10.1093/cid/ciaa667.

63. Centers for Disease Control and Prevention. Antibiotic resistance threats in the United States, 2019. https://www.cdc.gov/drugresistance/pdf/threats-report/2019-ar-threats-report-508.pdf. Revised December 2019. Accessed December 27, 2022.

64. Chow A, Benninger M, Brook I, et al. IDSA clinical practice guideline for acute bacterial rhinosinusitis in children and adults. *Clin Infect Dis.* 2012; 54(8):1041-1045.

65. Graves BW. Respiratory conditions and cardiovascular conditions. In: Brucker MC, King TL, eds. *Pharmacology for Women's Health.* 2nd ed. Burlington, MA: Jones & Bartlett Learning; 2017:549-586.

66. De Sutter A, Saraswat A, van Driel M. Antihistamines for the common cold. *Cochrane Database Syst Rev.* 2015;11:CD009345. doi:10.1002/14651858.CD009345.pub2.

67. Hayward G, Thompson MJ, Perera R, et al. Corticosteroids for the common cold. *Cochrane Database Syst Rev.* 2015;10:CD008116. doi:10.1002/14651858.CD008116.pub3.

68. Meltzer EO, Hamilos DL. Rhinosinusitis diagnosis and management for the clinician: a synopsis of recent consensus guidelines. *Mayo Clin Proc*. 2011;86(5):427-443.

69. Aring AM, Chan MM. Current concepts in adult acute rhinosinusitis. *Am Fam Physician*. 2016;94(2):97-105.

70. Centers for Disease Control and Prevention. Influenza. https://www.cdc.gov/flu/about/index.html. Last reviewed September 20, 2022. Accessed December 27, 2022.

71. Grohskopf LA, Alyanak E, Ferdinands JM, et al. Prevention and control of seasonal influenza with vaccines: recommendations of the Advisory Committee on Immunization Practices, United States, 2021–22 influenza season. *MMWR Recomm Rep*. 2021;70(RR-5):1-28. http://dx.doi.org/10.15585/mmwr.rr7005a1.

72. Centers for Disease Control and Prevention. Influenza antiviral medications: summary for clinicians. https://www.cdc.gov/flu/professionals/antivirals/summary-clinicians.htm#overview. Last reviewed September 9, 2022. Accessed December 27, 2022.

73. Shulman S, Bisno A, Clegg H, et al. Clinical practice guideline for the diagnosis and management of group A streptococcal pharyngitis: 2012 update by the Infectious Disease Society of America. *Clin Infect Dis*. 2012;55(10):e86-e102.

74. Kinkade S, Long NA. Acute bronchitis. *Am Fam Physician*. 2016;94(7):560-565.

75. Hunton R. Updated concepts in the diagnosis and management of community-acquired pneumonia. *J Am Acad Physician Assist*. 2019;32(10):18-23. doi:10.1097/01.JAA.0000580528.33851.0c.

76. Metlay JP, Waterer GW, Long AC, et al. Diagnosis and treatment of adults with community-acquired pneumonia: an official clinical practice guideline of the American Thoracic Society and Infectious Diseases Society of America. *Am J Respir Crit Care Med*. 2019;200(7):e45-e67. doi:10.1164/rccm.201908-1581.

77. Musher DM, Thorner AR. Community-acquired pneumonia. *N Engl J Med*. 2014;371(17):1619-1628.

78. Blaine A, Skoff T, Cassiday P, et al. Chapter 10: pertussis. In: *Manual for the Surveillance of Vaccine Preventable Diseases*. Centers for Disease Control and Prevention. https://www.cdc.gov/vaccines/pubs/surv-manual/index.html. Last reviewed May 11, 2020. Accessed April 24, 2022.

79. Centers for Disease Control and Prevention. *Epidemiology and Prevention of Vaccine-Preventable Diseases*. Hall E, Wodi AP, Hamborsky J, et al., eds. 14th ed. Washington, DC: Public Health Foundation: 2021.

80. Havers F, Moro PL, Hariri S, Skoff T. Pertussis. In: *Epidemiology and Prevention of Vaccine-Preventable Diseases*. Hall E, Wodi AP, Hamborsky J, et al., eds. 14th ed. Washington, DC: Public Health Foundation; 2021.

81. Pate CA, Zahran HS, Qin X, et al. Asthma surveillance—United States, 2006–2018. *MMWR Surveill Summ*. 2021;70(SS-5):1-32. http://dx.doi.org/10.15585/mmwr.ss7005a1external icon.

82. National Asthma Education and Prevention Program. *Expert Panel Report: Guidelines for the Diagnosis and Management of Asthma (EPR-3)*. Bethesda, MD: National Heart, Lung, and Blood Institute; 2007.

83. Wu TD, Brigham EP, McCormack MC. Asthma in the primary care setting. *Med Clin North Am*. 2019;103(3):435-452. doi:10.1016/j.mcna.2018.12.

84. National Heart, Lung, and Blood Institute. Asthma care quick reference. http://www.nhlbi.nih.gov/files/docs/guidelines/asthma_qrg.pdf. Published 2012. Accessed April 24, 2022.

85. Cloutier MM, Baptist AP, Blake KV, et al. 2020 focused updates to the asthma management guidelines: a report from the National Asthma Education and Prevention Program Coordinating Committee Expert Panel Working Group. *J Allergy Clin Immunol*. 2020;146(6):1217-1270. doi:10.1016/j.jaci.2020.10.003.

86. Peery AF, Crockett SD, Murphy CC, et al. Burden and cost of gastrointestinal, liver, and pancreatic diseases in the United States: update 2018. *Gastroenterology*. 2019;156(1):254-272. doi:10.1053/j.gastro.2018.08.063. [Published correction appears in *Gastroenterology*. 2019;156(6):1936.]

87. Chey WD, Leontiadis GI, Howden CW, Moss SF. ACG clinical guideline: treatment of *Helicobacter pylori* infection. *Am J Gastroenterol*. 2017;112:212-238.

88. National Center for Health Statistics. Summary health statistics tables for U.S. adults: National Health Interview Survey, 2018, Table A-4b, A-4c. https://ftp.cdc.gov/pub/Health_Statistics/NCHS/NHIS/SHS/2018_SHS_Table_A-4.pdf. Accessed April 27, 2022.

89. Fashner J, Gitu J. Diagnosis and treatment of peptic ulcer disease and H. pylori infection. *Am Fam Physician*. 2015;91(4):236-242.

90. Kavitt RT, Lipowska AM, Anyane-Yeboa A, Gralnek IM. Diagnosis and treatment of peptic ulcer disease. *Am J Med*. 2019;132(4):447-456. doi:10.1016/j.amjmed.2018.12.009.

91. Wilhelm S, Johnson J, Kale-Pradhan P. Treating bugs with bugs: the role of probiotics as adjunctive therapy for *Helicobacter pylori*. *Ann Pharmacother*. 2011;45(7-8):960-966.

92. Littlefield A, Lenahan C. Cholelithiasis: presentation and management. *J Midwifery Womens Health*. 2019;64(3):289-297. doi:10.1111/jmwh.12959.

93. Schmidt M, Dumot JA, Søreide O, Søndenaa K. Diagnosis and management of gallbladder calculus disease. *Scand J Gastroenterol.* 2012;47(11):1257-1265.

94. D'Souza N, Nugent K. Appendicitis. *Am Fam Physician.* 2016;93(2):142-143.

95. Buckius M, McGrath B, Monk J, et al. Changing epidemiology of acute appendicitis in the United States: study period 1993–2008. *J Surg Res.* 2012;175(2):185-190.

96. Podda M, Gerardi C, Cillara N, et al. Antibiotic treatment and appendectomy for uncomplicated acute appendicitis in adults and children. *Ann Surg.* 2019;270(6):1028-1040. doi:10.1097/SLA.0000000000003225.

97. Scallan E, Hoekstra R, Angulo F, et al. Foodborne illness acquired in the United States—major pathogens. *Emerg Infect Dis.* 2011;17(1):7-16.

98. Connor BA. Travelers' diarrhea. In: *CDC Health Information for International Travel.* https://wwwnc.cdc.gov/travel/yellowbook/2020/preparing-international-travelers/travelers-diarrhea. Published 2020. Accessed April 27, 2022.

99. Bharucha AE, Lacy BE. Mechanisms, evaluation, and management of chronic constipation. *Gastroenterology.* 2020;158(5):1232-1249.e3. doi:10.1053/j.gastro.2019.12.034.

100. Mearin F, Lacy BE, Chang L, et al. Bowel disorders. *Gastroenterology.* 2016;150(6):1393-1407. doi:10.1053/j.gastro.2016.02.031.

101. Centers for Disease Control and Prevention. Surveillance for viral hepatitis—United States, 2019. https://www.cdc.gov/hepatitis/statistics/2019surveillance/pdfs/2019HepSurveillanceRpt.pdf. Published May 2021. Accessed April 27, 2022.

102. Centers for Disease Control and Prevention. Viral hepatitis. https://www.cdc.gov/hepatitis/index.htm. Last reviewed September 27, 2021. Accessed April 27, 2022.

103. Tohme R, Holmberg SD. Transmission of hepatitis C virus infection through tattooing and piercing: a critical review. *Clin Infect Dis.* 2012;54(8):1167-1178.

104. Emmanuel B, Shardell MD, Tracy L, et al. Racial disparity in all-cause mortality among hepatitis C virus–infected individuals in a general US population, NHANES III. *J Viral Hepat.* 2016:24(5):380-388.

105. Spearman CW, Dusheiko GM, Hellard M, Sonderup M. Hepatitis C. *Lancet.* 2019;394(10207):1451-1466. doi:10.1016/S0140-6736(19)32320-7.

106. O'Dell KK. Pharmacologic management of asymptomatic bacteriuria and urinary tract infections in women. *J Midwifery Womens Health.* 2011;56:248-265.

107. Nicolle LE, Gupta K, Bradley SF, et al. Clinical practice guideline for the management of asymptomatic bacteriuria: 2019 update by the Infectious Diseases Society of America. *Clin Infect Dis.* 2019;68(20):e83-e110. https://doi.org/10.1093/cid/ciy1121.

108. Chu CM, Lowder JL. Diagnosis and treatment of urinary tract infections across age groups. *Am J Obstet Gynecol.* 2018;219(1):40-51. doi:10.1016/j.ajog.2017.12.231.

109. Foxman B. Urinary tract infection syndromes: occurrence, recurrence, bacteriology, risk factors, and disease burden. *Infect Dis Clin North Am.* 2014;28(1):1-13.

110. Rahn DD, Carberry C, Sanses TV, et al. Vaginal estrogen for genitourinary syndrome of menopause: a systematic review. *Obstet Gynecol.* 2014;124(6):1147-1156.

111. Centers for Disease Control and Prevention. Antibiotic prescribing and use. https://www.cdc.gov/antibiotic-use/clinicians/adult-treatment-rec.html. Last reviewed October 3, 2017. Accessed April 28, 2022.

112. Barbosa-Cesnik C, Brown MB, Buxton M, et al. Cranberry juice fails to prevent recurrent urinary tract infection: results from a randomized placebo-controlled trial. *Clin Infect Dis.* 2011;52(1):23-30.

113. Fu Z, Liska D, Talan D, Chung M. Cranberry reduces the risk of urinary tract infection recurrence in otherwise healthy women: a systematic review and meta-analysis. *J Nutr.* 2017;147(12):2282-2288. doi:10.3945/jn.117.254961.

114. Xia JY, Yang C, Xu DF, et al. Consumption of cranberry as adjuvant therapy for urinary tract infections in susceptible populations: a systematic review and meta-analysis with trial sequential analysis. *PLoS One.* 2021;16(9):e0256992.

115. McLennan MT. Interstitial cystitis: epidemiology, pathophysiology, and clinical presentation. *Obstet Gynecol Clin North Am,* 2014;41(3):385-395.

116. Hanno PM, Erickson D, Moldwin R, Faraday MM. Diagnosis and treatment of interstitial cystitis/bladder pain syndrome: AUA guideline amendment. *J Urol.* 2015;193(5):1572-1580. doi:10.1016/j.juro.2015.01.086.

117. Berry SH, Elliott MN, Suttorp M, et al. Prevalence of symptoms of bladder pain syndrome/interstitial cystitis among adult females in the United States. *J Urol.* 2011;186:540-544.

118. Herness J, Buttolph A, Hammer NC. Acute pyelonephritis in adults: rapid evidence review. *Am Fam Physician.* 2020;102(3):173-180.

119. Bishop K, Momah T, Ricks J. Nephrolithiasis. *Primary Care.* 2020;47(4):661-671. doi:10.1016/j.pop.2020.08.005.

120. National Cholesterol Education Program (NCEP) Expert Panel on Detection, Evaluation, and Treatment of High Blood Cholesterol in Adults (Adult Treatment Panel III). Third report of the

National Cholesterol Education Program (NCEP) Expert Panel on Detection, Evaluation, and Treatment of High Blood Cholesterol in Adults (Adult Treatment Panel III): final report. *Circulation*. 2002;106(25):3143-3421.

121. American Diabetes Association, Professional Practice Committee. Standards of medical care in diabetes—2022. *Diabetes Care*. 2022;45(suppl 1):S1-S264.

122. Centers for Disease Control and Prevention. National diabetes statistics report. https://www.cdc.gov/diabetes/data/statistics-report/index.html. Last reviewed June 29, 2022. Accessed April 28, 2022.

123. Reis JP, Loria CM, Sorlie PD, et al. Lifestyle factors and risk for new-onset diabetes in a large population-based prospective cohort study. *Ann Intern Med*. 2011;155(5):292-299.

124. American Thyroid Association. General information: prevalence and impact of thyroid disease. https://www.thyroid.org/media-main/press-room/#:~:text=Prevalence%20and%20Impact%20of%20Thyroid,are%20unaware%20of%20their%20condition. Accessed April 28, 2022.

125. U.S. Preventive Services Task Force. Final recommendation statement: thyroid dysfunction: screening. https://www.uspreventiveservicestaskforce.org/uspstf/recommendation/thyroid-dysfunction-screening. Published March 24, 2015. Accessed April 28, 2022.

126. Garber JR, Cobin RH, Gharib H, et al. Clinical practice guidelines for hypothyroidism in adults: cosponsored by the American Association of Clinical Endocrinologists and the American Thyroid Association. *Endocr Pract*. 2012;18(6):989-1028.

127. Davis MG, Phillippi JC. Hypothyroidism: diagnosis and evidence-based treatment. *J Midwifery Womens Health*. 2022;67:394-397. https://doi.org/10.1111/jmwh.13358.

128. Maizels M, Houle T. Results of screening with the brief headache screen compared with a modified ID-Migraine. *Headache*. 2008;48:385-394.

129. Headache Classification Committee of the International Headache Society. The International Classification of Headache Disorders, 3rd edition. *Cephalalgia*. 2018;38(1):1-211. doi:10.1177/0333102417738202.

130. Holroyd KA, Stensland M, Lipchik GL, et al. Psychosocial correlates and impact of chronic tension-type headaches. *Headache*. 2000;40:3-16.

131. Diener H-C, Gold M, Hagen M. Use of a fixed combination of acetylsalicylic acid, acetaminophen and caffeine compared with acetaminophen alone in episodic tension-type headache: meta-analysis of four randomized, double-blind, placebo-controlled, crossover studies. *J Headache Pain*. 2014;15(1):76.

132. Linde K, Allais G, Brinkhaus B, et al. Acupuncture for the prevention of tension-type headache. *Cochrane Database Syst Rev*. 2016;4:CD007587. doi:10.1002/14651858.CD007587.pub2.

133. Christiansen S, Jürgens T, Klinger R. Outpatient combined group and individual cognitive-behavioral treatment for patients with migraine and tension-type headache in a routine clinical setting. *Headache*. 2015;55(8):1072-1091.

134. Verhagena AP, Damena L, Bergera MY, et al. Lack of benefit for prophylactic drugs of tension-type headache in adults: a systematic review. *Fam Pract*. 2010;27(2):151-165.

135. Jackson JL, Shimeall W, Sessums L, et al. Tricyclic antidepressants and headaches: systematic review and meta-analysis. *BMJ*. 2010;341:c5222. doi:10.1136/bmj.c5222.

136. Yancey JR, Sheridan R, Koren KG. Chronic daily headache: diagnosis and management. *Am Fam Physician*. 2014;89(8):642-648.

137. Tepper SJ, Dahlöf CGH, Dowson A, et al. Prevalence and diagnosis of migraine in patients consulting their physician with a complaint of headache: data from the landmark study. *Headache*. 2004;44:856-864.

138. Burch R, Rizzoli P, Loder E. The prevalence and impact of migraine and severe headache in the United States: figures and trends from government health studies. *Headache*. 2018;58(4):496-505. doi:10.1111/head.13281.

139. Deneris A, Allen PR, Hayes EH, Latendresse G. Migraines in women: current evidence for management of episodic and chronic migraines. *J Midwifery Womens Health*. 2017;62(3):270-285.

140. Curtis KM, Tepper NK, Jatlaoui TC, et al. U.S. medical eligibility criteria for contraceptive use, 2016. *MMWR Recomm Rep*. 2016;65(RR-3):1-104.

141. Fisher R, Acevedo C, Wiebe S, et al. ILAE official report: a practical clinical definition of epilepsy. *Epilepsia*. 2014;55(4):475-482.

142. Samba Reddy D. Neuroendocrine aspects of catamenial epilepsy. *Horm Behav*. 2013;63(2):254-266.

143. Pack AM, Olarte LS, Morrell MJ, et al. Bone mineral density in an outpatient population receiving enzyme-inducing antiepileptic drugs. *Epilepsy Behav*. 2003;4(2):169.

144. Gaffield ME, Culwell KR, Lee CR. The use of hormonal contraception among women taking anticonvulsant therapy. *Contraception*. 2011;83(1):16-29.

145. Curtis KM, Tepper NK, Jatlaoui TC, et al. U.S. medical eligibility criteria for contraceptive use, 2016. *MMWR Recomm Rep*. 2016;65(RR-3):1-104. http://dx.doi.org/10.15585/mmwr.rr6503a1external icon.

146. Yuen AW, Thompson PJ, Flugel D, et al. Mortality and morbidity rates are increased in people with epilepsy: is stress part of the equation? *Epilepsy Behav*. 2007;10(1):1-7.

147. Becker J, Norab DB, Gomesa I, et al. An evaluation of gender, obesity, age and diabetes mellitus as risk factors for carpal tunnel syndrome. *Clin Neurophysiol*. 2002;113:1429-1434.

148. Kozak A, Schedlbauer G, Wirth T, et al. Association between work-related biomechanical risk factors and the occurrence of carpal tunnel syndrome: an overview of systematic reviews and a meta-analysis of current research. *BMC Musculoskelet Disord*. 2015;16:231. doi:10.1186 /s12891-015-0685-0.

149. Page MJ, Massy-Westropp N, O'Connor D, Pitt V. Splinting for carpal tunnel syndrome. *Cochrane Database Syst Rev*. 2012;7:CD010003.

150. Page MJ, O'Connor D, Pitt V, Massy-Westropp N. Exercise and mobilisation interventions for carpal tunnel syndrome. *Cochrane Database Syst Rev*. 2012;6:CD009899.

151. QuickStats: percentage of adults aged ≥18 years who had lower back pain in the past 3 months, by sex and age group—National Health Interview Survey, United States, 2018. *MMWR*. 2020;68:1196. http://dx.doi.org/10.15585/mmwr.mm685152a5external icon.

152. Golob AL, Wipf JE. Low back pain. *Med Clin North Am*. 2014;98(3):405-428.

153. Casazza BA. Diagnosis and treatment of acute low back pain. *Am Fam Physician*. 2012;85(4): 343-350.

154. Goertz M, Thorson D, Bonsell J, et al. *Adult Acute and Subacute Low Back Pain*. Bloomington, MN: Institute for Clinical Systems Improvement; 2012.

155. Qaseem A, Wilt TJ, McLean RM, Forciea MA, for the Clinical Guidelines Committee of the American College of Physicians. Noninvasive treatments for acute, subacute, and chronic low back pain: a clinical practice guideline from the American College of Physicians. *Ann Intern Med*. February 14, 2017. [Epub ahead of print]. doi:10.7326/M16-2367.

156. Cifuentes M, Webster B, Genevay S, Pransky G. The course of opioid prescribing for a new episode of disabling low back pain: opioid features and dose escalation. *Pain*. 2010;151(1):22-29.

157. Menter A, Gottlieb A, Feldman SR, et al. Guidelines for the management of psoriasis and psoriatic arthritis. Section 1. Overview of psoriasis and guidelines of care for the treatment of psoriasis with biologics. *J Am Acad Dermatol*. 2008;5:826-850.

158. Menter A, Korman NJ, Elmets CA, et al. American Academy of Dermatology guidelines of care for the management of psoriasis and psoriatic arthritis. Section 3. Guidelines of care for the management and treatment of psoriasis with topical therapies. *J Am Acad Dermatol*. 2009;60:643-659.

159. American Academy of Dermatology. Skin cancer. https://www.aad.org/media/stats-skin-cancer#:~: text=Skin%20cancer%20is%20the%20most%20 common%20cancer%20in%20the%20United %20States.&text=Current%20estimates%20 are%20that%20one,skin%20cancer%20in%20their %20lifetime.&text=It%20is%20estimated%20 that%20approximately,with%20skin%20cancer %20every%20day9. Last updated April 22, 2022. Accessed December 27, 2022.

160. Rosen T, Lebwohl MG. Prevalence and awareness of actinic keratosis: barriers and opportunities. *J Am Acad Dermatol*. 2013;68:S2-S9.

161. Fahradyan A, Howell AC, Wolfswinkel EM, et al. Updates on the management of non-melanoma skin cancer (NMSC). *Healthcare*. 2017;5(4):82. doi:10.3390/healthcare5040082.

162. American Cancer Society. Melanoma skin cancer. https://www.cancer.org/cancer/melanoma-skin -cancer.html. Accessed May 19, 2022.

163. Thomas SL, Hall AJ. What does epidemiology tell us about risk factors for herpes zoster? *Lancet Infect Dis*. 2004;4(1):26-33.

164. Dooling KL, Guo A, Patel M, et al. Recommendations of the Advisory Committee on Immunization Practices for use of herpes zoster vaccines. *MMWR*. 2018;67:103-108. http://dx.doi.org/10.15585/mmwr .mm6703a5external icon.

165. Stevens DL, Bisno AL, Chambers HF, et al. Practice guidelines for the diagnosis and management of skin and soft tissue infections: 2014 update by the Infectious Diseases Society of America. *Clin Infect Dis*. 2014;59(2):e10-e52. doi:10.1093/cid/ciu444.

166. Liu C, Bayer A, Cosgrove SE, et al. Management of patients with infections caused by methicillin-resistant *Staphylococcus aureus*: clinical practice guidelines by the Infectious Diseases Society of America (IDSA). *Clin Infect Dis*. 2011;e18-e55. doi:10.1093 /cid/ciq146.

167. Jensen MD, Ryan DH, Apovian CM, et al. 2013 AHA/ACC/TOS guideline for the management of overweight and obesity in adults: a report of the American College of Cardiology/American Heart Association Task Force on Practice Guidelines and the Obesity Society. *Circulation*. 2014;129(25 suppl 2): S102-S138.

168. Browning LM, Hsieh SD, Ashwell M. A systematic review of waist-to-height ratio as a screening tool for the prediction of cardiovascular disease and diabetes: 0.5 could be a suitable global boundary value. *Nutr Res Rev*. 2010;23(2):247-269.

169. NHLBI Obesity Education Initiative Expert Panel on the Identification, Evaluation, and Treatment of Obesity in Adults (US). *The Practical Guide: Identification, Evaluation, and Treatment of Overweight and Obesity in Adults*. Bethesda, MD: National Heart, Lung, and Blood Institute; 2002.

170. Raihan N, Cogburn M. Stages of change theory. In: *StatPearls [Internet]*. https://www.ncbi.nlm.nih.gov

/books/NBK556005/. Treasure Island, FL: Stat-Pearls Publishing; March 9, 2022.

171. Widen E, Siega-Riz AM. Prenatal nutrition: a practical guide for assessment and counseling. *J Midwifery Womens Health*. 2010;55(6):540-549. doi:10.1016/j.jmwh.2010.06.017.

172. Gans KM, Risica PM, Wylie-Rosett J, et al. Development and evaluation of the nutrition component of the Rapid Eating and Activity Assessment for Patients (REAP): a new tool for primary care providers. *J Nutr Ed Behav*. 2006;38(5):286-292.

173. National Institute of Diabetes and Digestive and Kidney Diseases. Prescription medications to treat overweight & obesity. https://tinyurl.com/2p9xn2kn. Last reviewed June 2021. Accessed December 27, 2022.

174. Colquitt JL, Pickett K, Loveman E, Frampton GK. Surgery for weight loss in adults. *Cochrane Database Syst Rev*. 2014;8:CD003641.doi:10.1002/14651858. CD003641.pub4.

175. Felsenreich DM, Artemiou E, Steinlechner K, et al. Fifteen years after sleeve gastrectomy: weight loss, remission of associated medical problems, quality of life, and conversions to Roux-en-Y gastric bypass: long-term follow-up in a multicenter study. *Obes Surg*. 2021;31(8):3453-3461. doi:10.1007/s11695-021-05475-x.

176. Milone M, Sosa Fernandez LM, Sosa Fernandez LV, et al. Does bariatric surgery improve assisted reproductive technology outcomes in obese infertile women? *Obesity Surg*. 2017;27(8):2106-2112.

177. American Society for Metabolic and Bariatric Surgery. Estimate of bariatric surgery numbers, 2011–2019. https://asmbs.org/resources/estimate-of-bariatric-surgery-numbers. Accessed May 20, 2022.

178. Parretti HM, Hughes CA, Jones LL. "The rollercoaster of follow-up care" after bariatric surgery: a rapid review and qualitative synthesis. *Obes Rev*. 2019;20(1):88-107. doi:10.1111/obr.12764.

179. Mechanick JI, Apovian C, Brethauer S, et al. Clinical practice guidelines for the perioperative nutrition, metabolic, and nonsurgical support of patients undergoing bariatric procedures—2019 update: cosponsored by American Association of Clinical Endocrinologists/American College of Endocrinology, the Obesity Society, American Society for Metabolic and Bariatric Surgery, Obesity Medicine Association, and American Society of Anesthesiologists. *Obesity*. 2020;28(4):O1-O58. doi:10.1002/oby.22719.

180. Chu AS, Matalga MA, Krueger L, Barr PA. Nutrient deficiency-related dermatoses after bariatric surgery. *Adv Skin Wound Care*. 2019;32(10):443-455.

181. Patel JJ, Mundi MS, Hurt RT, et al. Micronutrient deficiencies after bariatric surgery: an emphasis on vitamins and trace minerals. *Nutr Clin Pract*. 2017;32(4):471-480.

182. Parretti HM, Subramanian A, Adderley NJ, et al. Post-bariatric surgery nutritional follow-up in primary care: a population-based cohort. *Br J Gen Pract*. 2021. [Epub ahead of print]. http://doi.org/10.3399/bjgp20X714161.

183. Lupoli R, Lemo E, Saldalamacchia G, et al. Bariatric surgery and long-term nutritional issues. *World J Diabetes*. 2017;8(11):464-474. https://doi.org/10.4239/wjd.v8.i11.464.

184. Qian J, Wu Y, Liu F, et al. An update on the prevalence of eating disorders in the general population: a systematic review and meta-analysis. *Eating and Weight Disorders: Studies on Anorexia, Bulimia and Obesity*. 2022;27(2):415-428. doi: 10.1007/s40519-021-01162-z. Epub 2021 Apr 8. PMID: 33834377; PMCID: PMC8933366.

185. Solmi F, Hatch SL, Hotopf M, et al. Validation of the SCOFF questionnaire for eating disorders in a multiethnic general population sample. *Int J Eating Disord*. 2015;48(3):312-316.

186. Santos AM, Benute GR, Nomura RM, et al. Pica and eating attitudes: a study of high-risk pregnancies. *Matern Child Health J*. 2016;20(3):577-582.

CHAPTER

# 6

# Nutrition

MARY K. BARGER

## Nutrition and Health

Health and nutrition are intimately interrelated. Proper nutrition is essential to human growth, development, and well-being. Increasing attention to the role of the body's microbiome, especially in the gastrointestinal tract, in metabolic, cellular, and neurologic functioning has, in turn, increased our knowledge about the direct connection between what we eat and our health.[1] Our dietary patterns and food preferences begin in utero from the pregnant person's diet flavoring the amniotic fluid,[2] and they continue after birth based on family tradition and culture, geographic residence, financial resources, and educational levels.

Since the average individual in the United States can expect to live for at least 75 years, they should be aware of the growing body of evidence that suggests a healthy diet can prevent several detrimental conditions, such as cardiovascular disease (including myocardial infarction and stroke), cancer, adult-onset diabetes, osteoporosis, and age-related vision loss. Measures to reduce this disease burden are relatively simple and well researched: maintaining a healthy weight; eating a well-balanced, nutrient-dense diet; not smoking; and exercising regularly. Although Americans have increased their physical activity in the last 10 years[3] and decreased their alcohol[4] and tobacco consumption, not much progress has been made on improving the quality of their diet. Indeed, their Healthy Eating Index (HEI) scores remain low, averaging 59 points out of 100 over the last 10 years.[5] Additionally, the rate of obesity in the United States continues to increase, with 11.5% of women and 6.9% of men in the United States experiencing severe obesity, defined as a body mass index (BMI) of 40 or greater.[6]

The role of social determinants of health in determining nutritional consumption, dietary patterns, and their consequences cannot be overlooked by the midwife. A person's experience of the food environment is determined by the combination of food availability, perceived affordability, and acceptability.[7] It is not surprising that fruit and vegetable consumption varies by income level and that often-cited barriers to higher consumption include cost, accessibility, and availability.[8] Food availability depends on transportation systems and refrigeration to move a variety of foods, particularly perishable fruits and vegetables, to grocery stores. Food availability also depends on the geographic location of grocery stores and farmers markets, and the ability to access these food sources via public transit systems or other means. Many locations in the United States are considered "food deserts." (See the U.S. Department of Agriculture [USDA] maps in the Resources list at the end of this chapter.) Perceived affordability of food depends on a combination of absolute and relative judgments. Absolute judgments include not only the actual cost but the potential waste due to package size, limited longevity of fresh foods, and satiability of the food.[9] Relative judgments include price compared to another food—often a less healthy alternative—or to prepared fast food.[9] Food acceptability is shaped by taste, texture, smell, convenience, and familiarity. Some of these food environment–related factors can be lessened with education and nutritional counseling or innovative clinical practice such as produce prescriptions,[10] but many require policy strategies at the local and national levels to overcome the barriers to healthy eating.

If midwives are to promote healthy eating habits to their patients, they need to understand some basic principles of nutrition, appreciate the physiologic response of the body to ingested food, and be familiar with current recommendations and the numerous ways these guidelines are measured and communicated to the public. Healthy nutritional intake is essential in all phases of life, including preconception and during pregnancy, and the key principles remain the same for everyone whether they want to lose weight, gain weight, or maintain their current weight. Although understanding individual components of the diet is important for health professionals, counseling people about diet should be positively focused on types of preferred foods and the need to eat a variety of nutrient-dense foods, rather than emphasizing individual macronutrients and micronutrients. Increasingly, midwives are caring for transgender and nonbinary individuals, and more research is needed to develop evidence-based guidelines to support the unique nutritional needs of this population.[11,12]

## Principles of Nutrition and Nutrient Recommendations

Nutrients are the chemical components of food. Humans require more than 40 different nutrients for good health. These nutrients are classified as either macronutrients (fats, carbohydrates, and protein) or micronutrients (vitamins and minerals). Water is also a necessary nutrient, but it does not fit into either category. Water, vitamins, and minerals provide no calories but are necessary, although not totally sufficient, for the body to be able to utilize the energy provided by fat, carbohydrates, and protein.

Vitamin and mineral supplements have become increasingly popular in recent years, and some people incorrectly think these agents can supply all needed nutrients. Ideally, people should obtain both macronutrients and micronutrients from a diet composed of a variety of nutrient-dense foods rather than from nutritional supplements. This diet must be balanced in a way that prevents nutritional deficiencies and excesses. Variety is essential both to guarantee proper intake of all necessary nutrients and to benefit from the protective effects of certain dietary components against diseases such as cancer and heart disease. Today's research suggests that decreased health risks associated with a healthy diet are due to combinations of substances in foods and food groups rather than to the effect of any single substance or nutrient.[13]

## Nomenclature for Nutritional Standards

The *U.S. Dietary Guidelines for Americans* are updated regularly, with the ninth edition (the most recent version) being published in 2020.[4] The *Dietary Guidelines* emphasize healthy *dietary patterns* that people should follow, rather than concentrating on the *individual nutrient levels* they should consume. Nevertheless, labeling on packaged foods regarding the overall nutritive value of a product can still be useful. Therefore, it is important to be familiar with the nomenclature used by various U.S. governmental organizations for nutritional standards setting.

U.S. nutritional standards have two origins: the Food and Nutrition Board, which is part of the Health and Medicine Division (HMD) of the National Academy of Medicine (formerly the Institute of Medicine [IOM]), and the Food and Drug Administration (FDA). The Food and Nutrition Board standards were originally developed during World War II as part of an effort to ensure adequate nutrition for members of the armed services. Since then, these standards have been used to set government policy related to food programs such as the School Lunch Program and food relief efforts globally. The FDA guidelines are more recent and are intended to assist consumers in obtaining recommended nutrients in their diets.

**Table 6-1** compares the terms used by the HMD's Food and Nutrition Board and by the FDA.[14,15] An important characteristic of the Daily Reference Intakes (DRIs) is that they not only aim to determine minimum nutrient intake levels necessary to prevent nutritional deficiencies, but also strive to set standards to decrease the incidence of chronic diseases such as osteoporosis and cancer.

Most food labels are based on a "typical" diet of 2000 calories per day. However, the number of calories actually needed in a day depends on the individual's daily expenditure of calories. Several formulas are available to calculate how many calories an individual needs daily, but clinicians may not have the time to make those calculations. Another option is to use a website that calculates the number of calories needed to maintain or lose weight when provided with the individual's specific sex, age, height, weight, and daily activity levels (see the Resources section at the end of this chapter). In general, women of average stature and weight will need between 1600 to 2000 calories per day to maintain their current weight depending on their activity level. Those with obesity or who are very active will

| Table 6-1 | U.S. Nutritional Standards |
|---|---|

### Food and Nutrition Board, Health and Medicine Division, National Academy of Medicine

**Dietary Reference Intakes (DRIs)**

- DRIs aim to determine the minimum nutrient intake levels necessary to prevent nutritional deficiencies, and set standards to decrease chronic diseases such as osteoporosis and cancer. This term has more or less supplanted Recommended Daily Allowance (RDA).
- DRIs are a combination of the RDA and Adequate Intake (AI).
- DRIs also specify the Tolerable Upper Limit (UL), RDAs, estimated average requirement (EAR), and AIs.

**Tolerable UL**

- The maximum level of daily nutrient intake that is unlikely to pose risks of adverse health effects to almost all of the individuals in the group for whom it is designed.

**RDAs**

- Developed and updated periodically.
- Set the recommended average intake over a 3- to 7-day period for each nutrient specified.
- Fewer than half of the more than 40 necessary nutrients have an established RDA.
- RDAs are set quite high to meet the needs of almost all (97–98%) individuals in a group, so they may be too high for individual needs.

**EAR**

- The intake value that is estimated to meet the requirement defined by a specified indicator of adequacy in 50% of an age- and gender-specific group. At this level of intake, the remaining 50% of the specified group would not have their needs met.

**AIs**

- Used to develop a recommended intake when a scientific basis for establishing the EAR is lacking.

### Food and Drug Administration

**Daily Value (DV)**

- DVs appear on FDA-regulated products.
- DVs are not meant to set levels of nutrients to be consumed every day, but rather to help determine how particular foods fit into an overall healthy diet.
- DVs are calculated based on a diet of 2000 calories per day (unless otherwise stated).
- DVs are calculated from two sources—DRVs and RDI.

**Daily Reference Value (DRV)**

- Recommended proportions of protein, carbohydrate, and fat in the diet.
- Recommended grams per 1000 calories of dietary fiber intake.
- Recommended daily maximums for sodium and potassium.

**Reference Daily Intake (RDI)**

- Refers to vitamins and minerals as well as protein for younger children and pregnant and lactating persons per day. To ensure that the nutritional needs of all age groups are met, the RDI is calculated from the highest DRI for each nutrient.

Abbreviations: AIs, adequate intakes, DRI, dietary reference intake; DRV, Daily Reference Value; DVs, Daily Values; EAR, estimated average requirement; FDA, U.S. Food and Drug Administration; RDAs, Recommended Dietary Allowances; RDI, Reference Daily Intake; UL, upper intake level.

Based on Food and Nutrition Board. *Dietary Reference Intakes (DRIs): Recommended Intakes for Individuals*. Washington, DC: National Academy of Sciences; 2004, updated 2011; Food and Drug Administration. Food Labeling: Revision of the Nutrition and Supplement Facts Labels. *Federal Register* 81(103):33742-33999.

need more calories to maintain their current weight, whereas those who are older, or who are trying to lose weight, will require fewer calories. However, all food is not the same, so calories are simply one consideration within the full scope of an individual's diet. The sections that follow review macronutrients, micronutrients, and the physiologic response to ingested food.

## Macronutrients

Macronutrients contain calories and are the energy-providing nutrients for the human body. The three basic macronutrients are fat, carbohydrates, and proteins. Macronutrients are needed in large quantities and meet the bulk of the human body's energy needs. One of the primary components of a healthy diet is consuming fat, carbohydrate, and protein in balanced proportions.

### Fats

Fats are an important source of energy, providing more calories per gram than either protein or carbohydrates. Fat provides energy at a rate of 9 kcal/g, compared to 4 kcal/g for protein and carbohydrates. Fats are composed of fatty acids and have various roles in the human body, including transport and digestion of the fat-soluble vitamins and components of cell structure. Stored body fat facilitates temperature regulation by serving as insulation, and it helps to protect vital organs by providing a cushioning effect. In addition, dietary fat intake increases the pleasure of eating and helps signal satiety during a meal.

Although in the last half of the twentieth century the American Heart Association (AHA) led a campaign to decrease intake of fats, particularly saturated fats, due to their purported association with heart disease, evidence to date has not substantially supported a causal link between chronic disease and the consumption of most fats. The AHA campaign succeeded in decreasing Americans' fat intake from 45% of total calories to 33%.[16] However, the percentage of calories consumed from fats is *not* linked to chronic diseases; instead, what matters is the *type and source* of fats consumed. Therefore, the focus of nutrition recommendations has shifted to dietary patterns and instead of individual macronutrients.

### Body Fats

Body fats need to be distinguished from dietary fat. For example, the cholesterol (a fatlike substance present in all animal tissues) consumed as part of the diet is different than the cholesterol in blood that is measured as part of a lipid panel. Dietary cholesterol is found in foods of animal origin such as meat and eggs, while blood cholesterol is a waxy, fatlike substance manufactured by the body and stored in the liver.

Fifty years of evidence has shown that although there is a slight association between dietary cholesterol and serum cholesterol, dietary cholesterol has a minimal effect on risk for cardiovascular disease due to the complexities of the metabolic effects of ingested food. However, dietary cholesterol may affect the liver.[17] For example, eggs—a common source of cholesterol—are rich in other nutrients that may counterbalance the cholesterol's detrimental effects on the cardiovascular system. In addition, more harmful physiologic effects can occur when an individual substitutes an egg for breakfast with a high-glycemic food, such as a large muffin, as discussed later in this chapter.

The body uses blood cholesterol to make steroid hormones such as estrogen and progesterone, as described in the *Anatomy and Physiology of the Reproductive System* chapter. Blood cholesterol is also required for production of vitamin D and bile, as well as being an important component of cell membranes.

Several subtypes of cholesterol are found in the body, with the two primary forms being low-density lipoprotein (LDL) and high-density lipoprotein (HDL). LDL transports cholesterol out of the liver to other parts of the body. Cells attach to these particles and then extract either LDL or cholesterol. Excess amounts of LDL promote the production of fatty plaques on arterial walls, causing them to lose elasticity and narrow, resulting in arteriosclerosis. If a plaque breaks free, it may cause a cardiac event such as a heart attack or stroke. LDL is often characterized as "bad" or "lousy" cholesterol. Conversely, HDL carries excess cholesterol away from the arteries and back to the liver; thus, it is known as "good" or "healthy" cholesterol. A high level of HDL appears to have a protective effect against coronary heart disease and heart attacks. Exercise is strongly associated with higher levels of HDL in the body and, therefore, with lower risk of cardiovascular disease.

Another way in which fats are transported through the blood to cells is in the form of triglycerides. Serum triglycerides are either derived from consumed fat, especially trans fats, or synthesized de novo by body fat or the liver. The amount of triglycerides synthesized de novo is positively correlated with the individual's consumption of refined carbohydrates. Triglycerides store excess calories in adipose cells and are released when a source of energy is needed, especially by the brain. Whether a high triglyceride level is an independent cause of heart disease remains controversial, because many individuals with high triglyceride levels also have high LDL and low HDL cholesterol levels, which are known risk factors for heart disease. Data collected for the National Health and Nutrition Examination Survey (NHANES) reveal that serum levels of total cholesterol, LDL, and triglycerides declined from the 1990s through 2014 in all population subgroups of women, regardless of lipid-lowering medication use.[18]

### Dietary Fats

Dietary fats are characterized by the chemical structure of their fatty acids. They are classified into four types: trans fats, saturated fats, polyunsaturated fats, and monounsaturated fats.

**Trans Fats.** Trans fats are produced when vegetable oils are heated in the presence of hydrogen gas and a catalyst, resulting in a partially hydrogenated oil. Such oils become a solid when they cool, making them easier to transport; they are more stable and unlikely to spoil, providing a longer shelf life; and they can be reheated without breaking down, so they are ideal for making fried foods. Although trans fats are found in small amounts in beef and dairy fat, they are largely consumed in the form of commercially made products. Trans fats are harmful because they elevate LDL cholesterol levels and lower HDL cholesterol levels; they also stimulate production of prostaglandins and other eicosanoids that increase inflammation, platelet aggregation, and vasoconstriction. The combination of these effects results in an increased risk for cardiovascular disease, diabetes, gallstones, weight gain, and ovulatory infertility.[19] In 2015, the FDA declared trans fats "unfit for human consumption" and banned them from processed foods in 2018, with a final deadline of 2020 for their removal from these products.[20]

**Saturated Fats.** Saturated fats are derived from both animal and plant sources. These fats often are solid at room temperature and are found in highest amounts in meat fat, butter, whole-milk products, coconut oil, palm oil, and palm kernel oil. Consumption of these fats worsens individuals' serum lipoprotein profiles.

**Unsaturated Fats.** In contrast to saturated fats, unsaturated fats have several beneficial roles in the body, including improving serum cholesterol levels, reducing inflammation, and stabilizing heart rhythms. These fats are found primarily in vegetable oils, nuts, and seeds, and are liquid at room temperature.

Unsaturated fats are of two types: *monounsaturated* and *polyunsaturated*. Monounsaturated fats are found in high concentrations in olives, peanuts, oils such as canola oil, avocados, nuts such as almonds and pecans, and seeds such as pumpkin and sunflower seeds. Polyunsaturated fats are grouped into two types, distinguished by their chemical bonds: omega-6 (n-6) and omega-3 (n-3) fatty acids. There are several kinds of n-3s but the most studied are alpha-linolenic acid (ALA), eicosapentaenoic acid (EPA), and docosahexaenoic acid (DHA). Both n-6 and n-3 are considered "essential fatty acids" due to the body's limited ability to produce them, which means they must be obtained from dietary sources. Omega-6 fatty (linoleic) acids are found in safflower, sunflower, corn, soybean, and flaxseed oils, as well as canola oils. The omega-3 fatty acids DHA and EPA are found in oily fish such as salmon, mackerel, anchovies, and sardines, as well as algae. Plant sources of omega-3 fatty acids, such as chia and flax seeds, walnuts, soybean, and canola oil, are rich in ALA.

The amount of n-3 fats in the U.S. diet has decreased significantly since the 1950s, in part due to changes in the food chain. Today most meat comes from grain-fed animals; relatively speaking, grain-fed animals have less n-3 fats in their meat than do grass-fed animals. The consumption of oily fish has also decreased over the same period of time, perhaps due to warnings about heavy metals in fish. Observational studies have shown an association between n-3s and a range of health outcomes, including heart disease mortality, mood disorders, cancer prevention, rheumatoid arthritis improvement, and infant development.[21] Results from clinical trials that used n-3 fats supplements to prevent myocardial infarction and stroke have been somewhat mixed, with some evidence suggesting higher supplements in the range of 4 g/day are required to realize a benefit.[22]

In summary, the total number of calories obtained from fat is unimportant for cardiovascular and general health; rather, it is the type of fats consumed that is important for health outcomes. Trans fats should be eliminated from the diet as much as possible. Replacing saturated fats with monounsaturated and polyunsaturated fats will provide modest improvements in protection against heart disease. Consumers should be cautious about the foods they choose to substitute for trans fats and saturated fats, as some seemingly healthy alternatives are not necessarily healthier substitutes. Nevertheless, a good recommendation is to reduce consumption of red meat and whole-milk dairy products, increase intake of fish to at least two 6-ounce servings per week, and increase consumption of soy products, nonhydrogenated vegetable oils, and nuts. Table 6-2 provides the distribution of daily recommended values of macronutrients for women age 19 to 30 years,[14,15] and **Table 6-3** shows the recommended DRIs for women.[15,23]

| Table 6-2 | Recommended Daily Values for Macronutrients for Women 19–30 Years | |
|---|---|---|
| | **Percent Daily Calories (Actual Daily Amount)** | |
| | **Food and Drug Administration** | **Health and Medicine Division** |
| **Fat** | 30% | 20–35% |
| Saturated fat | < 10% | As little as possible |
| Cholesterol | (< 300 mg) | As little as possible |
| Trans fat | 0 | 0 |
| **Carbohydrates** | 60% | 45–65% |
| Dietary fiber | (25 g) | (28 g) |
| **Protein** | 10% | 10–35% |

Based on Food and Nutrition Board. *Dietary Reference Intakes (DRIs): Recommended Intakes for Individuals.* Washington, DC: National Academy of Sciences; 2004, updated 2011; Food and Drug Administration. Food Labeling: Revision of the Nutrition and Supplement Facts Labels. *Federal Register* 81(103):33742-33999.

## Carbohydrates

Carbohydrates, which can be found in grains, vegetables, fruits, and sugars, are the major dietary source of glucose, the body's essential energy for cellular metabolism. All carbohydrates except insoluble fibers are broken down by the body into the basic sugars and absorbed in the bloodstream. Glucose, galactose, and fructose can be used immediately by the body or can be stored in the liver or muscle tissue in the form of glycogen, which is then converted to glucose whenever this reserve energy is needed.

In the past, carbohydrates have been described as simple or complex, with people being encouraged to eat more complex carbohydrates. However, this recommendation does not distinguish between the different physiologic consequences that occur after eating different types of complex carbohydrates. Because the amount of insulin production that is stimulated in response to carbohydrate intake is a key factor in the body's physiologic response, researchers have developed two measures to assess this response: the glycemic index and the glycemic load.[24] In general, ingestion of high-glycemic foods results in a worsened lipoprotein profile, more thrombotic activity, abnormal glucose metabolism, increased inflammation, and more cellular proliferation.

### Glycemic Index

The glycemic index is a measure of the blood glucose response during the 2 hours after ingesting 50 grams of a carbohydrate contained in a food, compared to a standard 50 grams of glucose. This index is influenced by the amount of fiber and fat in the consumed food, both of which slow the absorption of the carbohydrate. Highly processed grains such as those found in white bread, white

| Table 6-3 | Daily Reference Intakes of Macronutrients for Women | | | | |
|---|---|---|---|---|---|
| | **Nonpregnant** | | **Pregnant** | | |
| | **14–18 Years** | **Adults** | **Singleton** | **Multiple** | **Lactation** |
| Carbohydrate (g) | 130 | 130 | 175 | 330 | 210 |
| Fiber (g) | 26 | 21–25 | 28 | 28 | 29 |
| Fat (g) | ND | ND | ND | 156 | ND |
| Protein (g) | 46 | 46 | 71 | 175 | 71 |
| Water (L) | 2.3 | 2.7 | 3.0 | 3.0 | 3.0 |

Abbreviation: ND, not determined.

Data from Food and Nutrition Board. *Dietary Reference Intakes (DRIs): Recommended Intakes for Individuals.* Washington, DC: National Academy of Sciences; 2004, updated 2011; Goodnight W, Newman R. Optimal nutrition for improved twin pregnancy outcome. *Obstet Gynecol.* 2009;114(5):1121-1134.

rice, and semolina-flour pasta have a high index. For example, white rice's glycemic index is 89, whereas that for brown rice is 45. Vegetables have a low glycemic index due to their fiber content and low natural sugar content; indeed, in some cases, it is hard to even measure their glycemic index. For example, obtaining 50 grams of carbohydrate from broccoli requires ingesting 16 cups. Fruits, although naturally sweet, if consumed as the whole fruit, have a low glycemic index due to the fruit's fiber; for example, an apple has a glycemic index of about 10. Riper fruits have a higher glycemic index. In general, low-glycemic foods have a glycemic index of 55 or less, whereas those with a glycemic index of 70 or greater are considered high-glycemic foods.[24]

### Glycemic Load

Compared to the glycemic index, the glycemic load is a better measure of the amount of insulin production stimulated by consumption of specific foods. The glycemic load is calculated by multiplying the glycemic index of the food by the amount of carbohydrate consumed, expressed in grams, and then dividing by 100. A low glycemic load is less than 10 grams per serving and a high glycemic load is greater than 20 grams per serving, with values in between considered intermediate.[24] For example, the glycemic index for one cup of brown rice is 45, but the glycemic load is 20. The same amount of white rice would have a glycemic index of 89 and a glycemic load of 40. This is a typical example, in which unprocessed grain products stimulate the production of less insulin than do processed foods such as white rice. The same is true for whole fruits as compared to consuming only the juice of the fruit. A person would need to consume three or four oranges to ingest the same glycemic load as contained in 8 ounces of orange juice.

### Fiber

Fiber is a type of complex carbohydrate composed of nonstarch polysaccharides that cannot be digested by enzymes in the small intestine. Fiber is characterized as either soluble or insoluble based on its solubility in water. Soluble fiber types include pectin found in fruits, beta-glucans found in oats and barley, and gums found in beans and cereals. Insoluble fiber types include cellulose found in leaves, root vegetables (e.g., beets and carrots), bran, and whole wheat; hemicellulose found in bran and whole grains; and lignin found in plant stems and leaves.

The typical U.S. diet is relatively low in dietary fiber. Fiber intake among adults in the United States averages approximately 16 grams, or only 60% of the recommended amounts.[25] Research has revealed that dietary fiber is associated with a decreased risk of heart disease, most likely through lowering total cholesterol and LDL cholesterol levels, and with decreased risk of type 2 diabetes, diverticulitis, and constipation.

The Health and Medicine Division of the National Academies of Science, Engineering, and Medicine and USDA recommend that carbohydrates make up 45% to 65% of daily caloric intake. People should attempt to maximize their intake of low-glycemic foods rich in fiber, such as whole grains, vegetables, and fruits, and to minimize their intake of high-glycemic foods, such as sweetened and energy drinks; refined grains such as white bread, white rice, and russet potatoes; and high-sugar snacks. A desirable intake of fiber for women is 20 to 28 grams per day.

### Protein

Protein is a basic component of cells and is needed for cellular growth, replacement, and repair. Enzymes—the substances responsible for controlling the processes that keep the human body functioning smoothly—are composed of protein. Hormones, hemoglobin, and antibodies also are composed partly or entirely of protein. Protein, in turn, is composed of organic compounds known as amino acids. The different arrangements of amino acids into proteins determine the particular properties of each protein.

Approximately 20 amino acids exist that are necessary for human growth and metabolism. The body produces the majority of these necessary amino acids. Approximately nine amino acids, however, must be obtained through foods; thus, they are called *essential amino acids*. Foods of animal origin, such as meat, poultry, fish, eggs, and dairy products, provide all of these essential amino acids and are known as complete proteins. Proteins derived from plants, such as legumes, nuts, and grains, lack certain essential amino acids and are termed incomplete proteins. Even so, a vegetarian diet can supply all of the essential amino acids as long as a variety of plant-based proteins are eaten throughout the day.[26]

Proteins cannot be stored in the body, so each day they must be consumed to avoid the body breaking down nonessential tissue, such as muscle, to supply proteins vital for survival. Recommended protein intake is 0.8 to 1.0 g/kg, or 10% to 35% of total calories. While protein intake deficiencies are common in the developing world, most persons in the United States consume adequate amounts of protein. The average intake of women in the United States is approximately 70 g/day or 15% to 16% of kilocalories consumed, with adolescents and older women having less than average intakes.[27]

The body does not distinguish between animal and plant sources of amino acids. However, protein food sources usually contain other nutrients, such as saturated fat. Evidence from the Nurses' Health Study suggests that substituting plant-based protein for high-glycemic carbohydrates can decrease the risk for heart disease and type 2 diabetes among women.[28]

## Physiologic Response to Food Intake

The quality of human nutrition encompasses not only the type of food that is consumed, but also the physiologic and chemical responses to it. Food is a hormonal stimulant whose effects are more powerful than those of most drugs. Understanding this reality may be the impetus providers need to spend time with patients assessing their diets and helping them to choose better foods. The body's response to food intake depends on the composition of both the macronutrients and the micronutrients ingested. With regard to prevention of inflammation and other processes that promote disease, especially chronic disease, the most important physiologic response to food intake is how much insulin production is stimulated.

Distinguishing high-glycemic meals from low-glycemic meals is important in understanding the body's physiologic response to carbohydrates.[29] A high-glycemic meal creates a rapidly rising and high blood glucose response, which results in a similar insulin production response. Subsequently, the blood glucose level falls more rapidly than the insulin level decreases, which results in high insulin levels, low glucose levels, and suppression of glucagon production. Faced with these conditions, the body responds as if adequate glucose is present—that is, it suppresses the secretion of free fatty acids, thereby blocking the body's access to stored fat for energy. Low glucose levels also cause poor brain function, which stimulates the appetite, especially for a high-glycemic meal. After several more hours, to maintain a euglycemic state, skeletal muscles become insulin resistant, decreasing their glucose uptake. In turn, free fatty acids and cortisol are secreted to allow access to stored glucose from the liver. In addition, other inflammatory hormones

are released, causing oxidative stress and potentially damage from the production of excessive free radicals. Over time, this cycle of increased levels of glucose, insulin, and free fatty acids damages pancreatic beta cells, potentially resulting in type 2 diabetes, as well as affecting other processes associated with a variety of conditions, including cardiovascular disease, cancer, neural tube defects in the fetus (if the individual is pregnant), and gallbladder disease.

Eating a diet rich in carbohydrates from whole grains, beans, fruits, and vegetables results in a much more modulated glucose response, in which insulin levels follow but never exceed glucose levels. Therefore, insulin levels are maintained within a narrower range. As glucose levels slowly decline and do not overshoot insulin levels, there is also appropriate glucagon stimulation, which permits access to stored fat as an alternative energy source until the next meal.

## Micronutrients: Vitamins and Minerals

Micronutrients are dietary elements that the body needs in trace amounts. Metabolism and use of macronutrients by the body require a host of enzymatic and hormonal processes that are also influenced by the necessary presence of micronutrients—specifically, vitamins and minerals, which for the most part cannot be synthesized by the body. Micronutrient deficiencies can have profound adverse health effects. Such deficiencies are a common health problem in developing nations and in some geographic areas in developed nations.

Vitamins are organic substances used by the body as catalysts for intracellular metabolic reactions, whereas minerals are inorganic substances. Both vitamins and minerals are essential for physiologic function, but must be obtained via the diet. Vitamins are classified as fat-soluble or water-soluble: Water-soluble vitamins are excreted from the body and are not stored, whereas fat-soluble vitamins are stored in body fat.

A few of these micronutrients are highlighted here because they play a special role in women's health, pregnancy, or lactation, or because women in the United States are likely to be deficient in them. The roles of vitamins and minerals in pregnancy are discussed later in this chapter. **Table 6-3** lists the recommended intakes for selected vitamins and minerals in women ages 14 to 70 years, the requirements in pregnancy and lactation, and common food sources of these nutrients.[15,30,31]

## Fat-Soluble Vitamins

Large doses of fat-soluble vitamins are stored in the body and can reach toxic levels that have dangerous effects. For example, accumulation of vitamin A, which occurs when this nutrient is ingested as retinol, can result in liver toxicity, visual problems, and increased risk for hip fractures. Vitamin A is important for vision (especially night vision), a healthy immune system, and cell growth. Vitamin A deficiency is rare in the U.S. population, but it may be an important nutrient to attend to in low-resource countries. Table 6-4 presents the current recommended daily reference intake of vitamins and micronutrients in women in the United States.[32]

Vitamin D promotes absorption of calcium and phosphate and helps deposit these minerals in teeth

| Table 6-4 | Recommended Daily Reference Intakes[a] of Vitamins and Micronutrients in Women | | | | | |
|---|---|---|---|---|---|---|
| | **Nonpregnant Women** | | | | | |
| **Vitamin/Mineral** | **14–18 Years** | **19–50 Years** | **51–70 Years** | **Pregnancy** | **Lactation** | **Dietary Source** |
| Vitamin A (mcg) | 700 | 700 | 700 | 770 | 1200 | DGLV, yellow/orange vegetables and fruits |
| Vitamin C (mg) | 65 | 75 | 75 | 85 | 120 | Citrus fruits |
| Vitamin D (IU) | 600 | 600 | 600 | 600–4000[b] | 600–4000[b] | Fortified dairy and nondairy milks |
| Vitamin E (mg) | 15 | 15 | 15 | 15 | 19 | Nuts, vegetable oils |
| Thiamin (mg) | 1.1 | 1.1 | 1.1 | 1.4 | 1.4 | Pork, enriched grain |
| Riboflavin (mg) | 1.1 | 1.1 | 1.1 | 1.4 | 1.4 | Meat, enriched grain |
| Niacin (mg) | 14 | 14 | 14 | 18 | 17 | Meat, nuts, legumes |
| Vitamin $B_6$ (mg) | 1.2 | 1.3 | 1.5 | 1.9 | 2.0 | Chicken, fish, enriched grains |
| Folate (mcg) | 400 | 400 | 400 | 600 | 500 | DGLV, liver, fortified cereal, quinoa |
| Vitamin $B_{12}$ (mcg) | 2.4 | 2.4 | 2.4 | 2.6 | 2.8 | Animal-based food, fortified nondairy milk |
| Calcium (mg) | 1300 | 1000 | 1200 | 1300 | 1300 | Dairy, canned fish with bones, bivalves |
| Choline (mg) | 400 | 425 | 425 | 450 | 550 | Egg yolks, organ meats |
| Iodine (mcg) | 150 | 150 | 150 | 220 | 290 | Seaweed, seafood, iodized salt, dairy, eggs |
| Iron (mg) | 15 | 18 | 8 | 27 | 9 | Organ meats, dried small fish, meat, DGLV |
| Magnesium (mg) | 360 | 320 | 320 | 350–360 | 310–320 | Seafood, legumes, grains |
| Phosphorus (mg) | 1250 | 700 | 700 | 700 | 700 | Meat, seafood, dairy, legumes, nuts |
| Potassium[a] (mg/dL) | 2300 | 2600 | 2600 | 2900 | 2800 | Apricots, figs, nuts, soy, wheat germ |
| Sodium[a] (mg/dL) | 1500 | 1500 | 1500 | 1500 | 1500 | Salted and canned foods |
| Zinc (mg) | 9 | 8 | 8 | 11 | 12 | Egg yolk, organ meats, bivalves |

Abbreviation: DGLV, dark green leafy vegetables.

[a] Some nutrients do not have Dietary Reference Intake (DRI) but an Adequate Intake (AI) has been established.

[b] Lower values: Food and Nutrition Board; higher values: Hollis and Wagner.[31]

Data from Food and Nutrition Board. *Dietary Reference Intakes (DRIs): Recommended Intakes for Individuals*. Washington, DC: National Academy of Sciences; 2004, updated 2011; Hollis BW, Wagner CL. Substantial vitamin D supplementation is required during the prenatal period to improve birth outcomes. *Nutrients*. 2022;14(4).

and bones, but it also plays a role in health beyond bone formation. Most body tissues have vitamin D receptors; thus, this vitamin is involved with regulation of many systems, such as blood pressure, glucose and insulin regulation, and modulation of the immune system. Vitamin D is a not a true vitamin, as humans synthesize $D_3$ when their skin is exposed to ultraviolet sunlight. Vitamin $D_3$ synthesis from sunlight is affected by the intensity of sunlight, especially related to latitude and season; the presence of air pollution; and factors that limit the skin's absorptive ability, such as the amount of pigmentation, presence of sunscreen, and increasing age. Oily fish and fish liver oils are other sources of vitamin $D_3$, although absorption is decreased in people with intestinal malabsorptive conditions. Vitamin $D_2$—another form of vitamin D—is derived from plant sterols, such as those found in mushrooms. Vitamin D is also consumed through fortified products, such as dairy and nondairy milks. Both $D_3$ and $D_2$ are inactive forms that require metabolism in the liver to convert the vitamin D to 25(OH)D, the form most commonly used to assess a person's vitamin D levels, followed by metabolism in the kidney to convert it to $1,25(OH)_2D$, the physiologic active form.

Vitamin D deficiency has historically been defined as a serum 25(OH)D concentration less than 10 ng/mL (25 nmol/L), which is the level at which rickets or myopathy develops. Currently, there is some controversy about what constitutes vitamin D deficiency in adults based on whether the goal is bone health only or whether other general health conditions are also considered. HMD's Food and Nutrition Board, using bone health as the goal, has defined a vitamin D level of less than 50 nmol/L (20 ng/mL) as inadequate, with the recommended range for this vitamin being 50 to 100 nmol/L (20 to 40 ng/mL).[33] This agency recommends supplement intakes of 600 to 800 IU in the absence of adequate sunlight, with an upper tolerable limit of 4000 IU. However, the U.S. Endocrine Society, the American Geriatrics Society, and Central Europe guidelines recommend a minimum of 75 nmol/L (30 ng/mL) as the vitamin D level, with a level in the range of 75 to 155 nmol/L (40 to 60 ng/mL) considered ideal.[34] These organizations acknowledge that individuals may need to consume 1500 to 2000 IU daily to achieve these levels, with an upper tolerable level of 10,000 to 40,000 IU. Adults who have obesity; who take anticonvulsants, glucocorticoids, some antifungals, or antiretroviral drugs; or who have inflammatory bowel disease or gastric bypass surgery may require two to three times this dose to achieve healthy levels.[34]

Despite the current controversy about precisely which serum values represent vitamin D deficiency—vitamin D 25(OH)D levels of less than 20 ng/mL (50 nmol) versus less than 30 ng/mL (75 nmol)—there is no question that vitamin D deficiency is prevalent in all ethnic groups of women in the United States (**Table 6-5**). More than 50% of American women have serum vitamin D levels less than 50 nmol/L (20 ng/mL), and non-Hispanic Black and Mexican women have particularly low average levels.[32]

## Water-Soluble Vitamins

### Folic Acid

Among the water-soluble B vitamins, folic acid (vitamin $B_9$) has a great import for childbearing people due its role in preventing neural tube defects. Folate is essential for RNA and DNA synthesis. Observational studies have shown that high folate levels are associated with lower rates of cancer (especially intestinal cancer), cardiovascular disease, dementia, and depression. Supplementation with folate and other B vitamins has proved effective in lowering homocysteine levels, which are associated with cardiovascular disease. However, randomized trials involving fairly large populations have not found that vitamin B supplements decrease the incidence of any of these conditions. Nevertheless, folate deficiency is clearly associated with megaloblastic anemia. People at risk for megaloblastic anemia include those with poor diets, those with alcohol use disorder, and those who have malabsorptive disorders or take pharmacologic agents that act as folic acid antagonists (e.g., anticonvulsants, sulfasalazine [Azulfidine]).

Folate is found in liver and leafy greens such as spinach, but the primary dietary sources of this micronutrient in the United States are fortified cereals and flours as well as multivitamin supplements. Folate status can be assessed by either serum folate or red blood cell (RBC) folate tests, with the latter being a better indicator of tissue levels or long-term status.

In general, the U.S. population is not folate deficient. Since food fortification began in the mid-1990s, the percentage of the population that is folate deficient, defined as being at risk for hypersegmented RBCs, in all age and ethnic groups has been 1% or less.[35] However, approximately 20% of U.S. reproductive-age women have folate levels considered inadequate for protection from neural tube defects.[35] Although there is little risk of toxicity from high folic acid intake, concern has arisen that consumption of excess amounts could

| Table 6-5 | Recommended and Actual Status of Selected Micronutrients in U.S. Women 20–39 Years of Age by Race/Ethnicity According to National Nutrition and Health Examination Survey, 2003–2006 |

| | | Actual Status for Women 20–39 Years of Age, Median Values | | | |
|---|---|---|---|---|---|
| Micronutrient (Measurement) | Adequate Levels in Women | All Women | Mexican | Non-Hispanic Black | Non-Hispanic White |
| Vitamin A (mcg/dL) | > 20 | 49.3 | 43.2 | 42.4 | 53.1 |
| Folate as RBC folate (ng/mL) | > 95[a]<br>> 330[b] | **248** | **250** | **210** | **263** |
| Vitamin B$_{12}$ (pg/mL) | > 400 | 431 | 476 | 487 | 405 |
| Vitamin D 25(OH)D (nmol/L) | ≥ 50 or 75 | **57.6** | **44.9** | **32.4** | **66.6** |
| Vitamin E (mcg/dL) | > 500 | 997 | 1000 | 892 | 1020 |
| Iron as serum ferritin (ng/mL) | > 15 | 40.5 | 37.1 | 31.1 | 42.3 |
| Iodine: urinary excretion (mcg/L) | >100<br>>150 (pregnancy) | **119** | 187 | **123** | **115** |

Abbreviation: RBC, red blood cell.

[a] Amount to prevent hypersegmented RBCs.

[b] Amount to prevent neural tube defects.

**Bolded text:** Deficient levels using the highest standard (e.g., for pregnancy if applicable).

Data from National Center for Environmental Health. *Second National Report on Biochemical Indicators of Diet and Nutrition in the U.S. Population*. Atlanta, GA: Centers for Disease Control and Prevention; 2012.

exacerbate the anemia and cognitive symptoms associated with vitamin B$_{12}$ deficiency. Therefore, folic acid supplements of 1 mg or more require a provider prescription.

### Vitamin B$_{12}$

Vitamin B$_{12}$ deficiency can lead to anemia, as well as neurologic and cognitive dysfunction including depression. Everyone needs vitamin B$_{12}$ in their diet; human beings do not make this vitamin on their own, and the vitamin B$_{12}$ that may be produced by bacteria in the colon is mostly not bioavailable. Subgroups at risk for vitamin B$_{12}$ deficiency are those with small bowel or inflammatory bowel disease, those with a history of gastric bypass surgery, vegans, and elderly persons. If a pregnant person is vitamin B$_{12}$ deficient, they should be quickly treated, since this condition may affect the developing fetus.

Beef liver, beef, fatty fish (e.g., salmon), and dairy products are good dietary sources of vitamin B$_{12}$. For vegans, this nutrient may be obtained from soy and other products such as nutritional yeast, which is fortified with vitamin B$_{12}$.

Recommended routine supplementation of vitamin B$_{12}$ and eating vitamin B$_{12}$–fortified foods is recommended by the Food and Nutrition Board for all adults older than age 50 due to the prevalence of atrophic gastritis in older adults, which inhibits absorption of vitamin B$_{12}$.[15] There is no evidence that supplementation in those without neurologic disease or vitamin B$_{12}$ deficiency improves cognition, depression, or fatigue.[36]

Vitamin B$_{12}$ supplements may be provided as injections, orally, or intranasally. Oral supplements are relatively inexpensive and widely available. Methylcobalamin, adenosylcobalamin, and hydroxycobalamin are natural bioidentical forms of vitamin B$_{12}$ found in commercial supplements. However, the most common form in supplements and the best studied is the synthetic compound cyanocobalamin. However, smokers should be aware that cyanocobalamin supplements may not be effective for them due to their higher excretion rates of this compound and should consider a different bioidentical form of the supplement.[37] Polymorphisms may affect the bioavailability of different forms, so individuals may need to try different formulations to improve their serum levels.[38] A typical oral vitamin B$_{12}$ supplementation regimen might be 250 to 500 mcg/day, which would probably compensate for poor absorption of the supplements. Few data are available on differences in bioavailability between sublingual and oral doses, but it appears that sublingual doses are equivalent to injections for elderly persons.[39] Intake of relatively high doses of vitamin $B_{12}$ does not appear to be associated with any detrimental health problems, so no upper tolerable limit has been established.

In summary, most women in the United States have adequate intakes of vitamins, except for vitamin D and, in some subpopulations, folate or vitamin $B_{12}$ (e.g., in the elderly subpopulation). Nutrition scientists have been learning more about the roles that vitamins play in health beyond the basic understanding achieved in the twentieth century. Randomized trials on the use of vitamin supplements to prevent chronic disease have yielded disappointing results, but it may be that, without addressing the content of the entire diet, vitamin supplementation is not powerful enough to overcome the physiologic effects of types and amounts of macronutrients in the diet.

## Minerals

Minerals are chemical compounds found in the earth and absorbed by plants or animals, or dissolved in water. The five major minerals found in the human body are calcium, magnesium, phosphorus, potassium, and sodium. The other minerals needed in minute quantities, called "trace minerals," have specific functions within the body; they include cobalt, copper, iodine, iron, manganese, molybdenum, and selenium. The minerals reviewed in this chapter are those commonly associated with deficiencies and their resulting adverse health conditions.

### Calcium

Calcium is essential not only for healthy bone and teeth formation, but also for nerve conduction, muscle contraction, and blood clotting; given the last function, it plays a role in cardiovascular health. Additionally, it is an important treatment for hypoparathyroidism. Because approximately 20% of women in the United States older than 50 years are at risk for bone fracture due to osteoporosis,[40] maximizing peak bone mass through adolescence and early adulthood is essential. Unfortunately, adolescent girls have the lowest total intakes of calcium, 918 mg ± 30 mg per day, with only 13% to 15% meeting the daily requirement of 1300 mg from both diet and supplements.[41] In addition to calcium's role in building bone mass during adolescence and early

adulthood, it is important that women obtain adequate amounts of calcium throughout the lifespan to maintain bone mass. Among women using supplements who are older than age 40, more than 40% of their calcium intake comes from daily supplements or calcium carbonate antacids. Recent studies have highlighted the potential adverse effects of taking calcium supplement doses of 1000 mg or more per day, such as an increase in myocardial infarction events and increased incidence of hip fractures and kidney stones.[42] Some evidence suggests that these adverse effects occur with excessive amounts in the form of supplements, but not dietary sources.[42]

### Iodine

Iodine is essential for normal thyroid function, and deficiency of this mineral can lead to an enlargement of the thyroid gland known as goiter; it can also have devasting effects on fetal and infant neurobehavioral development. Iodine deficiency has been associated with decreased ability to conceive.[43] The leading sources of dietary iodine in the United States are dairy foods, eggs, seafood, and seaweed.[44] From the late 1970s through 2010, iodine levels in the U.S. population declined by 50%, though these levels have since stabilized.[41] This decline is probably due to a combination of decreased intake of salt, especially iodized salt, fish, and possibly dairy products, or a decrease in the amount of iodine in cow feed,[40] which collectively account for 60% of iodine intake. The recommended daily intake of iodine is 150 mcg in nonpregnant women and 220 mcg in pregnancy, which would result in the World Health Organization's (WHO's) recommended sufficient urinary iodine levels of 100 mcg/L and 150 mcg/L, respectively. The most recent data show that, in general, the U.S. population obtains sufficient iodine, but 40% of childbearing-age women have deficient urinary iodine levels (<100 mcg/L) and all population groups are below the pregnancy recommendation, but especially non-Hispanic Asian women (see Table 6-5).[44] However, since 2005, when the American Thyroid Association made the recommendation that prenatal vitamins be formulated to contain 150 mcg of iodine, the NHANES data suggest that mean urinary iodine levels in pregnant people have increased to 144 mcg/L; they may be higher now, given that the latest data are from 2014.[45]

### Iron

The most common nutritional deficiency globally is iron deficiency, which disproportionally affects women. Iron is essential to the production of hemoglobin and, therefore, for the transport of oxygen. RBCs contain 80% of the body's iron, where it can be measured as hemoglobin. Iron not in RBCs is stored as ferritin; transferrin is a protein needed for this stored iron to be transported in the circulation. Women who are not pregnant are at risk of anemia because of iron loss during menstruation, coupled with inadequate iron intake or decreased iron stores associated with close spacing of pregnancies. Special populations of people at higher risk for iron-deficiency anemia include pregnant people and those with malabsorption conditions, such as individuals with inflammatory bowel disease and those who have undergone bariatric surgery. Slightly less than 1 mg of iron is lost from the intestines daily; this daily iron loss is more than 1 mg among people with *Helicobacter pylori* infection, malaria, or infection with intestinal parasites.

Two forms of iron are found in food: heme and non-heme. Heme iron found in animal products is absorbed more efficiently than non-heme iron. For example, 20% to 30% of heme iron is absorbed, compared to 2% to 10% of non-heme iron. Iron uptake also varies according to the specific needs of a person's body. If a person has adequate iron stores, only approximately 10% of ingested iron is absorbed. In the presence of iron deficiency, however, as much as 40% of ingested iron can be absorbed.

Some foods or supplements can enhance or inhibit iron absorption, and these items should be discussed when counseling patients. Iron uptake enhancers include animal muscle from meat, chicken, or seafood; fermented vegetables and sauces (e.g., sauerkraut, kimchee, and soy sauce); and, in populations deficient in vitamin A, vitamin A. The current evidence does not support a role of vitamin C in enhancing non-heme iron absorption or absorption of iron supplements.[46] Iron uptake inhibitors include foods containing phytates (e.g., whole grains, oats, bran, nuts, spinach), phenols (e.g., tea, especially green tea; coffee; cocoa; and red wine), calcium, and soy proteins. Iron absorption also is decreased in the presence of antacids.

*Pica*—a condition characterized by persistent and compulsive eating of non-nutritive substances, including excessive consumption of ice—can be either a symptom of iron-deficiency anemia or a contributing cause. Frequently, correcting the anemia will eliminate the pica.

The loss of iron stores is followed by anemia. Adequacy of iron stores can be measured in several ways. The most commonly available tests assess characteristics of the RBCs, such as hemoglobin level, and a peripheral smear to characterize the morphology of the RBCs. However, biochemical tests of serum ferritin and transferrin saturation measure earlier stages of iron depletion prior to actual iron deficiency as evidenced by a low hemoglobin level. The primary laboratory and clinical findings with differing states of anemia are discussed in the *Common Conditions in Primary Care* and *Pregnancy-Related Conditions* chapters. Although iron-deficiency anemia typically is associated with pale (hypochromic) and small (microcytic) RBCs, changes in RBC morphology occur relatively late in the process.

In a large study of a multi-ethnic sample of non-pregnant women age 25 to 44 years in the United States and Canada, the prevalence of iron-deficiency anemia (strictly defined as a ferritin level less than 15 ng/dL and transferrin saturation less than 10%) ranged from nearly 3% for non-Hispanic white women to more than 6% for Native American, Hispanic, and non-Hispanic Black women.[47] The rates of deficiency were significantly higher in pregnancy compared to nonpregnancy in white women (4.4% versus 2.8%) and Native American women (25% versus 6.3%), while non-Hispanic Black women had a lower prevalence of anemia in pregnancy (3.5% versus 6.1%).[47] These rates are considerably lower than those reported for low-income pregnant populations in the United States using Special Supplemental Nutrition Program for Women, Infants, and Children (WIC) services, which used hemoglobin to define anemia. In 2018, the overall prevalence of anemia among WIC participants was 11.4%, with non-Hispanic Black women having the highest prevalence.[48]

People diagnosed with iron-deficiency anemia who increase their dietary consumption of iron-rich foods and avoid taking antacids 2 hours before or 4 hours after meals may correct the problem nutritionally. The other option for remedying this deficiency is iron supplementation. After the addition of 30 to 100 mg of elemental iron taken daily, an increase in the reticulocyte count should be noted within 2 weeks and an increase in the hemoglobin noted within 3 to 4 weeks.

Ferrous salts are the first-line choice for oral iron supplementation for the treatment of iron-deficiency anemia. Other types of iron supplements are not more effective, do not appear to have a more benign side-effect profile, and cost approximately four times as much as ferrous salts. Because only a maximum amount of absorption is possible at one time, divided doses are preferable. Also, separating administration of iron from ingestion of a multivitamin can maximize absorption. A key safety issue is that iron supplements—particularly those

| Table 6-6 | Iron Supplements | |
|---|---|---|
| **Iron (Fe) Group** | **Generic Name (Brand)** | **Total Dose (Dose of Elemental Iron), mg** |
| **Iron Salts** | | |
| Tablets | Iron sulfate (FeoSol) | 325 (65) |
| | Iron fumarate (Feostat, Hemocyte) | 200 (66) |
| | Iron gluconate (Fergon) | 240 (27) |
| Liquid | Iron sulfate elixir (FeoSol Elixir) | 220 (44) per 5 mL 300 (60) per 5 mL |
| | Iron gluconate + herbs (Floradix or Floravital—gluten free) | (10) per 10 mL— higher absorption rate |
| **Polysaccharide Iron/Carbonyl Iron** | | |
| Tablets | Carbonyl iron (FeoSol caplets) | 50 (45) |
| | Polysaccharide iron (Ferrex-150) | 150 (150) |
| Liquid | Polysaccharide iron elixir (Niferex Elixir) | 100 (100) per 5 mL |

prescribed prenatally—are a source of childhood poisoning.[49]

Side effects of iron therapy, such as nausea, bloating, abdominal cramping, and constipation, are proportional to the dose. In many cases, people discontinue the therapy due to these side effects. Patients should be counseled about the potential side effects and measures they can take to lessen them. An alternative to daily iron supplementation is taking 120 mg of elemental iron once or twice weekly. It is not recommended that people double their multivitamin supplement in an effort to obtain added iron, as this approach could result in excessive levels of fat-soluble vitamins.

Table 6-6 lists types of iron supplements and the amounts of elemental iron in each dose. Enteric-coated and slow-release iron formulations are not recommended because iron is absorbed in the small intestine and these products provide iron that is excreted unabsorbed.

## Role of Vitamin and Mineral Supplementation

Ideally, micronutrients should be obtained through intake of a variety of fruits and vegetables each day—at a minimum, five servings per day—and exposure to adequate sunlight. Unfortunately, fruit and vegetable intake among Americans remains very low, with the median daily intakes being 1 and 1.6 servings per day, respectively; fewer than one in eight individuals meets the daily fruit recommendation and only 10% meet the recommendation for vegetables.[8]

Use of supplements is not a substitute for a healthy diet. Currently half of U.S. adults take a daily supplement, 33% of whom take a multivitamin/mineral version.[50] For some micronutrients, U.S. adult intake from supplements is much higher than from food (e.g., B-vitamin intake is 5 times higher from supplements than from food).[46] In some cases, supplements make up for intake shortfalls (e.g., for vitamin D); in other cases, their ingestion may result in excess intake (e.g., of calcium and folic acid).[51] Too much of these micronutrients can be harmful to cardiovascular health. The U.S. Preventive Services Task Force (USPSTF) states there is insufficient evidence to recommend routine multivitamin/mineral supplementation for the general population.[52] However, this recommendation does not apply to populations at risk for deficiencies, including persons who have undergone gastric bypass and those who have malabsorptive conditions or take medications that can result in lower absorption. As discussed in the section "Dietary Patterns," limited supplementation should be at least considered by those consuming a vegetarian or vegan diet.

There is no conclusive evidence to support the use of supplements in generally healthy populations to prevent chronic diseases, such as cardiovascular disease, cancer, and diabetes. A randomized controlled trial among 21,000 older adults followed for 3.6 years showed no effect of multivitamin supplements on cardiovascular outcomes or total cancers.[53] Of note, the USPTF has assigned a "D" rating (moderate certainty of harm) to intake of beta-carotene and found no effect for vitamin E supplements in the prevention of cardiovascular disease and cancer.[52] Surprisingly, studies have shown supplements of vitamin D and calcium in older adults do not prevent fractures.[54] There are problems with supplement studies, such as a lack of uniformity of definition, identification of the micronutrients in the multi-supplements, reliance on self-reports for dose data, and length of studies. Additionally, as pointed out in the physiologic section, micronutrients are important for certain enzymatic processes but the quality and type of macronutrients initiate important physiologic responses that probably have a larger effect on long-term health. Rarely do studies examine the macronutrient effect in combination with the supplement. At the very least, multivitamin/mineral supplements do not seem to cause any harm. Therefore, in general, taking a multivitamin/mineral supplement "just in case" seems to do no harm, although it may not be money well spent.

## Dietary Patterns

In research studies, the quality of the totality of what participants eat and drink are typically measured one of three ways: the Healthy Eating Index (HEI), the Alternative Healthy Eating Index (AHEI), or the Dietary Approaches to Stop Hypertension (DASH) score. The HEI measures how a set of foods aligns with the latest recommendations; the maximum score is 100. Revised HEI scoring for the latest 2020 USDA recommendations is in progress. The AHEI assigns scores to foods based on their predictive value in preventing chronic disease. DASH scores measure adherence with the DASH diet out of 70 points. All three indexes demonstrate that populations with high diet scores have lower rates of all-cause mortality, cancer, diabetes, and cardiovascular and neuro-generative disease.[55] Emphasizing the importance of the totality of what we eat is important.

When discussing nutrition, a healthcare provider will probably be of most value to patients by emphasizing healthier dietary patterns that are relevant at any weight and applicable throughout the life course. The word "diet" is often interpreted by many laypersons too narrowly—that is, as meaning "a weight-loss diet." It may be helpful, therefore, to use a less-familiar term such as "dietary pattern" with patients when counseling them on nutrition. The *USDA Dietary Guidelines for Americans 2020–2025* highlight three food patterns that are recommended as healthy dietary patterns: (1) the Healthy U.S. style pattern; (2) the Mediterranean-style eating pattern; and (3) the Healthy Vegetarian eating pattern. A 2020 systematic review identified moderate support for these patterns in the prevention of chronic disease. When making dietary suggestions, it is key to consider the individual's preferences, culture, and budget.

The same graphic, MyPlate, can be applied to all three dietary patterns (see the *Health Promotion Across the Lifespan* chapter). Essentially half of a food plate should be occupied by whole vegetables and fruits (minimum of five servings per day), one-quarter with whole grains, and one-quarter with protein, with low-fat dairy pictured as the drink. Not part of the MyPlate graphic but part of the more detailed description is limitation

| Table 6-7 | Key Principles in a Healthy Eating Pattern |
|---|---|

1. Choose healthy fats instead of unhealthy fats.
   - Avoid trans fats; choose monounsaturated and polyunsaturated fats.
2. Choose slowly digested carbohydrates over highly refined ones.
   - Emphasize whole fruits, vegetables, beans, and nuts.
   - Choose whole grains, such as brown rice, bulgur, barley, quinoa, and wheat berries.
3. Choose proteins that are plant based at least half of the time, and choose fish, eggs, and poultry the rest of the time, eating little red meat.
4. Eat large amounts of fruits and vegetables—a minimum of five servings per day.
5. Choose low-calorie hydration—water is best.
   - Drink coffee and tea in moderation.
   - If milk is part of the diet, choose low-fat types.
   - Limit juice to one small glass per day.
   - Avoid high-sugar drinks.
   - Limit alcohol intake to one glass per day.
6. Meet daily recommendations for vitamins and minerals.
7. Get daily exercise—30 minutes of brisk walking daily.
   - Calories expended are important to maintain a healthy weight.

Data from Skerrett PJ, Willett WC. Essentials of healthy eating: a guide. *J Midwifery Womens Health*. 2010;55(6):492-501.

of added sugar, especially in the form of sweetened drinks (which are the leading source of sugar for Americans);[4] saturated fats; and sodium. The AHEI promotes the Healthy Eating Plate, which differs slightly from MyPlate in that the drink illustration replaces dairy with water, fruit is a smaller portion than vegetables, and healthy oil is visually depicted. If a clinician uses the MyPlate graphic in counseling, it is important to discuss what a person drinks during the day because fruit juices and sweetened beverages have a high glycemic index, are high in calories, and not nutritionally dense. General principles for following a Healthy U.S. style or Mediterranean-style eating pattern are summarized in Table 6-7.[56]

### Variety of Plant-Based Diet Patterns

The number of Americans stating they consume a vegetarian or vegan diet has increased rapidly in recent years, with 10% reporting that they follow one of these diet patterns.[26] Reasons cited for a change to a plant-based diet, besides religious or cultural issues, are concerns for animal welfare, personal health, and the environment. In general, a vegetarian diet does not include meat, poultry, or fish. A vegetarian diet is subclassified as either *lacto-ovo-vegetarian*, which includes dairy products and eggs, or *vegan*, which does not contain any animal products. Both types of vegetarian diets can be nutritionally sound throughout the lifespan, including during pregnancy and lactation. Because vegetarian diets are generally lower in saturated fat and higher in fruits, vegetables, and whole grains, this dietary pattern can reduce the risk of some chronic diseases. Population studies of vegetarians have found a lower incidence of obesity, hypertension, type 2 diabetes, and ischemic heart disease, and lower LDL cholesterol levels, compared to nonvegetarian populations.[26] People adhering to a vegetarian-type diet pattern also have lower body fat and a more favorable body fat distribution.[57]

When consuming a vegetarian diet, attention must be paid to some nutrients that are not found in large quantities in vegetarian food sources, such as vitamin $B_{12}$, vitamin D, calcium, and n-3 fatty acids. Essential amino acid needs can be met by eating a wide variety of plant foods during the day.

Vitamin $B_{12}$ deficiency is the most common nutrient deficiency in persons who eat a vegetarian diet. Unfortunately, the foods in a typical vegan dietary pattern cannot guarantee uptake of sufficient dietary vitamin $B_{12}$ for normal functioning. Thus, vegans should assiduously supplement their vitamin $B_{12}$ intake with vitamin $B_{12}$–fortified foods and supplements. Such fortified foods can include vitamin $B_{12}$–fortified nutritional yeasts, vitamin $B_{12}$–fortified breakfast cereals, and vitamin $B_{12}$–fortified meat and milk alternatives.

No food available to a vegan contains adequate vitamin D and calcium. Vegans appear to have a 40% increased risk of bone fracture risk and more than twice the risk of hip fracture compared to omnivores,[58] so they need to consciously choose fruit and plant sources of vitamin D and calcium. Sunshine on human skin is a significant "source" of vitamin D, but it may not be available to everyone depending on the geographic location and time of year. Fortunately, the FDA increased the amount of vitamin D supplementation in non-dairy milks in 2016, so they are now a good source of this nutrient, as are fortified cereals. Vegans should consider vitamin D supplementation with vitamin $D_3$, the best source of this nutrient. Calcium supplements should also be considered.

Cardiovascular disease appears to be less prevalent among vegetarians, even though vegetarians' n-3 fatty acid concentration is often lower than that of omnivores.[59] People consuming a vegan diet must rely on endogenous ALA conversion to EPA and DHA to achieve adequate n-3 levels. However, most vegans' intake is high in linoleic acid (LA), which inhibits this conversion. It is recommended that to increase their n-3 fatty acid intake, people consuming vegan and vegetarian diets consider algae supplements; decreasing their intake of high-LA-content food sources, such as nuts, meat analogs, and high-LA oils (e.g., soybean and safflower); and increase their intake of ALA-rich foods such as flaxseed, canola oil, and walnuts and walnut oil.

### Gluten-Free Diet

The number of people choosing a gluten-free diet has increased rapidly in the United States in the last few years, with the latest estimates suggesting that approximately 1.7% of people living in the United States adhere to a gluten-free diet, including 1.8 million people with celiac disease and 2.7 million people without celiac disease.[60] For persons with celiac disease, adherence to a gluten-free diet decreases inflammation and symptoms of the disease. Although celiac disease and wheat allergy sensitivity are clearly defined disorders related to gluten intake, the health benefits of gluten avoidance in individuals without these issues is questionable. The evidence does not support that a gluten-free diet decreases weight loss[61] or inflammatory bowel conditions, and a gluten-free diet may increase the risk for cardiovascular disease.[62]

The midwife should be aware of potential dietary concerns related to a gluten-free diet. People consuming gluten-free products are at risk for excessive intake of high-glycemic carbohydrates and saturated fat, and deficiencies of fiber, vitamin C, vitamin $B_{12}$, folic acid, and vitamin D as well as calcium, zinc, and magnesium.[61] However, it should be noted that gluten-free pseudo-cereals, such as quinoa and amaranth, have twice the mineral content (including calcium and iron) of traditional cereals. Therefore, the principle of opting for whole-grain forms of food, instead of processed foods, is an important message to communicate.

Persons with celiac disease are at increased risk for poor pregnancy outcomes and osteoporosis. The pregnancy-related risks include prematurity, fetal growth restriction, small-for-gestational-age newborns, and stillbirth; these risks are lower if the disease is well controlled.[63] Therefore, preconception counseling about a gluten-free diet in these persons has the potential to improve their pregnancy outcomes. Additionally, persons with celiac disease are at risk for low bone density that may or may not normalize with a gluten-free diet.[63]

## Nutrition Across the Lifespan

Nutritional needs change significantly over the course of a person's lifetime. The latest *Dietary Guidelines for Americans*[4] highlight nutritional needs from infancy through older age. This section highlights some key issues for reproductive-age individuals, including those related to pregnancy and lactation; nutrition issues for persons of older ages are discussed in the *Menopause* chapter.

### Nutrition During Adolescence

Adolescence is a period of rapid physical growth and, therefore, high nutritional need. During adolescence, girls gain 40% of their skeletal mass and 50% of their body weight. Inadequate nutrition, especially calcium intake, can compromise their peak bone mass. Unfortunately, the diet pattern of adolescents tends to be poor, with 65% of adolescents having poor food quality scores.[64] Besides poor intake of fruits, vegetables, and whole grains, adolescents consume more than 30% of their calories from calorie-dense, nutrient-poor drinks.[65] Of perhaps greatest concern is the increased rate of obesity among U.S. children and adolescents. However, a prospective study of a multiethnic sample of youth from grades 10 through 1 year post high school found no association between quality of food intake and baseline weight.[65,66]

In recent decades, the age of onset of puberty has decreased. Earlier onset of puberty can pose significant self-image and psychosocial problems for young children, who may be seen as more socially and emotionally mature than they really are. The reasons for this trend may include increased exposure to environmental pollutants and chemicals, as well as stress; being born small for gestational age, experiencing fetal growth restriction, and not being fed human milk are also risk factors.[61] Likewise, increased body fat in childhood is a strong risk factor for earlier onset of puberty. For every one-point increase in BMI, menstruation occurs 1 month earlier.[67] Stage 2 or greater breast development is no longer uncommon at ages 7 and 8 years; the median age for this stage among U.S. girls varies by race/ethnicity from 8.8 for African Americans to 9.7 for Asian Americans. Beyond body fat and environmental factors, type of food consumed plays a role in the development of puberty. Data from national surveys show that the onset of puberty is delayed approximately 7 months in children who consume large amounts of plant protein, whereas those with a high intake of animal protein enter puberty approximately 7 months earlier.[67] Also, greater intake of isoflavone—a nutrient found in soy products, chickpeas, and lentils—delays breast development by 7 months.

### Nutrition, the Menstrual Cycle, and Fertility

Nutrition also affects, and is affected by, the menstrual cycle. Studies suggest that caloric intake varies during the menstrual cycle, peaking once in the follicular phase and once in the luteal phase, and reaching a nadir during menses.[68] These changes are theorized to coincide with cyclical fluxes in a woman's basal metabolic rate that are affected by hormones. Women also appear to increase their intake of carbohydrates and fat during the luteal phase, and their intake of protein and fat in the follicular phase, as compared to the menstrual phase. Persons with premenstrual syndrome have similar intakes as those without this condition, but increase their intakes of non-milk sugars and alcohol in the luteal phase.[63] Women with very low body fat levels become anovulatory. There is an association between vitamin deficiency, particularly deficiencies of calcium and vitamin D, and increased physical symptoms of premenstrual disorder.[69]

According to the Centers for Disease Control and Prevention, in the United States, 2.8 million married women are infertile, and another 9.5 million have impaired fecundity.[70] Risk of ovulatory disorders and an inability to conceive is about 60% lower in those adhering to a Mediterranean-type diet pattern or the Fertility Diet compared to a typical Western-style diet, which is low in fruits and vegetables and high in fat and sugar.[71] The Fertility Diet was derived from the Nurses' Health Study.[72] Similar to the Mediterranean-style diet pattern, the Fertility Diet eliminates trans fats; favors consumption of low-glycemic carbohydrates, including choosing more plant-based proteins; and temporarily trades nonfat or low-fat dairy products for the full-fat versions. These diet patterns also increase the ability to achieve and maintain a pregnancy among those persons using assisted reproductive technologies.[71] It appears that in high levels, glucose is not only a teratogen for the growing fetus but also severely affects a developing oocyte; thus, individuals who follow a diet pattern that features a lower glycemic load and who maintain their insulin levels within a narrow range are more fertile.

Women at the extremes in body weight are more likely to have reduced fertility. Therefore, aiming for a healthy body weight is important for improving fertility. Data from the Nurses' Health Study indicate that for people with high BMIs, losing 5% to 10% of body weight may improve ovulation, especially if regular exercise is incorporated into the regimen.[67] Lean women who exercise strenuously should reduce this activity to a moderate level to improve their fertility.

## Prenatal Nutrition and Gestational Weight Gain

Individuals who have a healthy diet before becoming pregnant need only subtle changes in their eating pattern to optimize nutrition in pregnancy. Energy requirements increase by approximately 200, 300, and 400 calories per day in the first, second, and third trimesters, respectively[73]—an increase that is equivalent to the addition of one healthy snack per day.

Diet quality both preconception and during pregnancy has lasting effects not only on the fetus but also on the child as they grow into adulthood.[74] Increasing evidence supports the effects of diet during pregnancy on the epigenetics of the fetus, which genes become activated through DNA methylation, and placental functioning.[75,76] These epigenetic changes can have short-term effects on closure of the neural tube and oral cleft anomalies as well as long-term effects on cardiometabolic health and cancer.[75] Adverse epigenetic effects occur in the presence of both over- and under-nutrition, the high glucose levels seen with diabetes in pregnancy, oxidative stress, and the lack of key substrates such as fatty acids (e.g., DHA).[76] Male fetuses appear more vulnerable to epigenetic changes than female fetuses.[76] Therefore, specific and accurate nutrition counseling during pregnancy is more important now than ever.

### Weight Gain

Gestational weight gain (GWG) is just one aspect of a pregnant person's nutritional status. Indeed, routine weight measurements during pregnancy are not the standard of care in all developed nations.[73] The United States is one of the few developed nations in which weight gain is routinely tracked over the course of pregnancy.

A relationship exists between both insufficient and excess gestational weight gain and adverse outcomes for both the pregnant person and the fetus. Pregestational weight and subsequent GWG affects the offspring's weight gain and adiposity. In turn, birth adiposity affects adult weight and long-term health.[74] Inadequate weight gain is associated with low birth weight, small-for-gestational-age infants, preterm birth, increased perinatal mortality, and long-term increased risk for obesity and diabetes.[74] Conversely, infants of pregnant persons who gain excessive weight or enter pregnancy with obesity are at increased risk of being large for gestational age, hypoglycemia, and birth trauma associated with difficult birth.[74] For pregnant people, excessive GWG is associated with cesarean birth, postpartum weight retention, and decreased lactation success.[77] Long-term outcomes associated with excessive GWG may can include metabolic syndrome, type 2 diabetes, and cardiovascular disorders.

Guidelines for GWG have changed over the years. In 1990, the Institute of Medicine (IOM) issued pregnancy weight gain guidelines aimed at ensuring adequate weight gain to prevent low birth weight. At the time, the weight gain recommended by IOM was higher than the 12-pound weight gain typically recommended in clinical practice. Since then, obesity and excessive weight gain in pregnancy have become public health concerns in the United States. In 2009, IOM revisited its recommendations by considering the evidence accumulated since the early 1990s, with a particular focus on the role of retention of GWG in the development of long-term obesity in women, and issued new GWG guidelines (**Table 6-8**).[78]

The recommended GWG differs based on the individual's pregestational BMI. The IOM recommendations are for the general population in the United States; subpopulations—such as adolescents, people who smoke, and those with chronic illness—may require individualized weight gain targets.

Persons are provided with information about their BMI category and target prenatal weight gain using the IOM recommendations at the first prenatal visit. Weight gain is then assessed and nutrition counseling reviewed at subsequent prenatal visits. Charting weight gain on a graph gives both the pregnant person and the prenatal care provider a pictorial representation for easy visualization of the GWG. Although a composite weight gain graph is often available in prenatal charts, weight gain graphs that show the mean and range specific for each BMI category are available. (See the Resources section at the end of this chapter for weight chart sources.) It is essential that pregnant individuals are provided with useful information to help manage their GWG. Besides ascertaining food insecurity, conversation starters can include the questions in **Table 6-9**.

| Table 6-8 | Recommended Gestational Weight Gain for Pregnant People with a Singleton Pregnancy[a] | |
|---|---|---|
| Prepregnancy | | Gestational Weight Gain Recommendations |
| Category | BMI, kg/m² | Total Weight Gain at Term, pounds |
| Underweight | <18.5 | 28–40 |
| Normal weight | 18.5–24.9 | 25–35 |
| Overweight | 25.0–29.9 | 15–25 |
| Obesity | ≥30 | 11–20 |

Abbreviation: BMI, body mass index.

[a] Calculations assume a mean first trimester weight gain of 2 kg (range: 1–3 kg) for people who are underweight, normal weight, and overweight. The assumed first trimester weight gain for people who are obese is 1.5 kg (range: 0.5–2 kg).

Based on Institute of Medicine. *Weight Gain During Pregnancy: Reexamining the Guidelines*. Washington, DC: Institute of Medicine; 2009.

| Table 6-9 | Nutrition Conversation Starters |
|---|---|

**Food Insecurity Questions ("Yes" to either one indicates some level of insecurity.)**

- Within the past 12 months, we were worried whether our food would run out before we got money to buy more.
- Within the past 12 months, the food we bought just did not last and we did not have money to get more.

**Starter Questions**

- Tell me about the food you usually eat.
- Are there foods you tend to avoid?
- Do you prepare your own food?
- How many times a week do you eat food that you do not prepare yourself?
- When asked about GWG, respond with "How do you feel about your food intake?" Strategize about ways to improve nutrition for maternal and fetal health and appropriate GWG.

Abbreviation: GWG, gestational weight gain.

Modified with permission from Marshall NE, Abrams B, Barbour LA, et al. The importance of nutrition in pregnancy and lactation: lifelong consequences. *Am J Obstet Gynecol*. 2022;226(5):607-632. doi:10.1016/j.ajog.2021.12.035.

## Dietary Advice

The recommended Daily Reference Intakes for macronutrients and micronutrients for women during pregnancy are summarized in Tables 6-3 and 6-4. Diet can play a powerful role in maintaining a healthy pregnancy, and prenatal care is an ideal time to start the conversation about a healthy dietary pattern. This is a life event when people are willing to make lifestyle changes for the health of the fetus.

Frequency of meals also plays a role during pregnancy. A substantial body of research supports the recommendation that pregnant people eat three meals a day and at least two snacks. Some people will want to observe their religion's periods of fasting, even though Catholicism, Judaism, and Islam all customarily exempt a pregnant woman from any obligation to fast. As part of prenatal care, the midwife elicits this information and provides teaching as required.

Table 6-10 summarizes dietary recommendations during pregnancy, which are designed to meet the unique nutritional needs of pregnancy while reducing the risk of exposure to infections and teratogens.[79,80] These recommendations are consistent with the healthy, nutrient-dense dietary patterns discussed previously. However, some popular diet patterns are not recommended in pregnancy, including the Atkins Diet, the Paleo diet, and the Ketogenic diet.[74] These diet patterns substantially restrict some macronutrients, which can be harmful during pregnancy due to the resulting micronutrient deficiencies or induced ketosis. The basic message to pregnant people is "Eat better, not more."[74]

### Vitamin and Mineral Supplementation.
Prenatal vitamins are multivitamin supplements formulated to provide the vitamins and minerals needed most by pregnant women. Although prenatal vitamins are one of the hallmarks of prenatal care, the actual value of vitamin and micronutrient supplements for pregnant women is more nuanced and complex. First, a balanced diet generally provides all the nutrients needed for health during pregnancy. Unfortunately, most pregnant people in the United States do not consume a diet that provides all the vitamins and micronutrients needed during pregnancy. The specific vitamins and micronutrients that have documented adverse effects on fetal development if present in insufficient amounts in the diet are folic acid, vitamin D, iron, iodine, and choline.[76]

**Folic Acid.** Supplemental folic acid is recommended for all pregnant persons. This supplementation needs to be started in the preconception period

| Table 6-10 | Summary of Dietary Advice for All Pregnant People |
|---|---|

**Supplements**

Take folic acid in a multivitamin at least 1 month prior to conception and for the first 3 months after conception to prevent neural tube defects.

**Diet**

Gain the recommended weight for BMI by eating the following:
- Three meals a day and two snacks to avoid prolonged periods of fasting
- Five servings of fruits and vegetables, at minimum, per day
- Whole-grain carbohydrates; limit food with high sugar content like desserts, juices, and sodas
- Adequate amounts of protein, choosing more plant-based sources such as nuts and beans
- At least two 4-oz servings of best-choices fish weekly or one serving of good-choices fish:
  - Examples of best choices: anchovy, catfish, clam, crab, flounder, pollock, salmon, sardines, shrimp, sole, tilapia, trout, whitefish
  - Examples of good choices: bluefish, carp, Chilean sea bass, halibut, snapper, tuna (albacore, white tuna, canned and fresh or frozen, yellowfin)
- Limit canned tuna to twice a week

Drink 8–10 glasses of water per day.
- Limit caffeine to 200 mg/day (2 cups of coffee or 4 cups of black tea)
- Avoid all alcoholic drinks
- Limit sweetened drinks

Ensure adequate intake of these micronutrients:
- Vitamin A as beta-carotene; limit food sources with preformed vitamin A such as liver ($<$ 4 oz/week) or cod liver oil
- Vitamin D from exposure to sunlight (amount will vary by geography, BMI, and skin pigmentation); if not feasible, consider supplementation with vitamin $D_3$ (1000–4000 IU depending on intake of vitamin D–fortified dairy products and vitamin D serum levels)
- Folic acid through a multivitamin supplement
- Individuals adhering to strict vegan diets: Take vitamin $B_{12}$ supplements or consume vitamin $B_{12}$–fortified products
- Iodine through diet (dairy and fish) or a multivitamin with iodide (preferably as potassium iodide)
- Iron through diet, multivitamin, or additional low-dose supplement if anemic
- Calcium through diet, with supplementation suggested for individuals at risk for preeclampsia
- Choline-rich food sources such as meat, poultry, and eggs, since this nutrient is not typically included in prenatal vitamins

**Foods to Avoid**

Soft cheeses unless they clearly state they are made from pasteurized milk, including Brie, feta, Camembert, blue-veined cheeses, and Mexican-style cheeses such as queso blanco, queso fresco, and queso panela

Uncooked meats or refrigerated pâtés or meat spreads

Raw eggs, cookie dough

Raw fish

Mercury-concentrating fish: king mackerel, marlin, orange roughy, shark, swordfish, tilefish (Gulf of Mexico), tuna (bigeye)

Deli meat salads or smoked seafood

Raw sprouts

Raw unpasteurized fruit juice, raw milk, or unpasteurized dairy products

Refrigerated perishable foods that have not been consumed in 2–3 days

| Food Handling |
|---|
| Wash cutting boards and equipment used to cut raw meat with hot soap and water |
| Wash and peel raw fruits and vegetables before eating |
| Wash hands after handling hot dogs, luncheon meats, or deli meats |
| **Food Processing** |
| Cook all deli meats, hot dogs, smoked meats, pâtés, and luncheon meats to steaming hot before eating |
| Cook meat and eggs to 71.1°C (160°F) |
| Cook seafood to 62.8°C (145°F) |

Abbreviation: BMI, body mass index.

Based on U.S. Food and Drug Administration. Food safety for pregnant women, their unborn babies, and children under five. https://www.fda.gov/media/83740/download. Published January 2022. Accessed June 20, 2022; Barger MK. Maternal nutrition and perinatal outcomes. *J Midwifery Womens Health*. 2010;55(6):502-511.

since closure of the neural tube occurs by 6 weeks after the last menstrual period. Folic acid supplementation begun preconception and taken through the first trimester lowers the risk of neural tube defects (NTDs) by approximately 30% to 70%, with the amount of decrease depending on the study conducted and the amount of folic acid used by study participants.[81] The recommended dose is 400 micrograms per day for persons who do not have an a priori risk for NTDs. Those who had a previous pregnancy complicated by an NTD, have diabetes, have a BMI greater than 30, or are taking antiepileptic medication are advised to take 4 mg of folic acid per day starting 1 month prior to conception and through the first 4 months of pregnancy.[82]

**Iron.** Iron is the single most difficult nutrient to obtain via the diet during pregnancy. Iron intake needs are approximately doubled during pregnancy, but iron absorption is also increased with increasing gestational age.[83,84] However, unlike folic acid supplementation, routine iron supplementation is controversial. Currently, the USPSTF does not find sufficient evidence to recommend routine iron supplementation in pregnancy, and its updated evidence report from 2020 does not provide any more convincing evidence.[85] Iron supplementation increases plasma hemoglobin levels but does not affect overall maternal and neonatal outcomes unless iron is used specifically to treat anemia during pregnancy.[84] Moreover, iron supplements frequently cause gastrointestinal distress.

There is clear evidence that the change in diet patterns away from consumption of red meat has led to decreased iron consumption in the United States.[86] Although the rate of iron deficiency increases during pregnancy from 7% in the first trimester to nearly 40% in the third trimester, the rate of actual anemia is low.[76] Some pregnant populations are especially at risk for anemia in pregnancy, including individuals with multiple gestation, adolescents, non-Hispanic Black people, and vegetarians.[76] Additionally, pregnant individuals with pica may have iron deficiency.

The absorption of iron in prenatal vitamins can depend on the amount of calcium in the vitamin. For example, more iron may be absorbed from a vitamin with a lower iron content and no calcium than from a vitamin containing both calcium and iron. The absorption of iron in supplements depends on the amount of elemental iron in the formulation, whether it is a quick-release or extended-release formulation, and whether the iron is in the ferric, ferrous, or iron polymaltose complex form.[82] Since iron is absorbed in the small intestine, extended-release formulations make little physiologic sense. Table 6-6 identifies the equivalent amounts of elemental iron for different iron preparations.

Because iron absorption increases in pregnancy, some authors have proposed that intermittent iron supplementation may be preferable to daily iron supplementation. Exposure of the intestinal mucosal cells to iron supplements on an intermittent basis may improve iron absorption because these cells might absorb iron better if not exposed to it continuously. Randomized controlled trials of intermittent iron supplementation rather than daily iron supplementation demonstrated equally positive pregnancy outcomes when iron supplements were taken one to three times per week rather than daily.[87]

**Iodine.** Iodine deficiency in pregnancy is the leading cause of intellectual impairment worldwide, with data showing that even a mild deficiency is associated with attention-deficit disorders.[76,88] Due to the increased production of thyroid hormone in pregnancy and the 30% to 50% increased urinary excretion of iodine in pregnant individuals, the demand for iodine increases both in pregnancy and during lactation. Most U.S. women are mildly iodine deficient, with only one subpopulation meeting the iodine requirements for pregnancy (see Table 6-5). The decreased food intake of iodine in recent years has led the American Thyroid Association to recommend routine iodine supplementation during pregnancy.[88] A review by this chapter author of the 18 most recommended prenatal multivitamins from three different "best" lists on the Internet showed that all included iodine, although the source of iodine may not have been the most reliable form.

**Choline.** Newer research has focused on the importance of choline in pregnancy due to its role in central nervous system development, cell division, and cellular methylation, and its synergistic effect with DHA in delivering nutrients to the fetus. Choline demand is very high in pregnancy, with newborns having serum concentrations 3 to 5 times greater than of the birthing person; human milk has 15 times that of maternal serum. Only 8% of pregnant people in the United States have adequate intake of choline according to the current standard, with those following a vegan diet pattern being most at risk for deficiencies.[76,89] The previously mentioned review of 18 recommended prenatal vitamin formulations showed that only 44% contained choline.

**Vitamin D.** Vitamin D not only plays a role in assuring bone homeostasis in the pregnant person and fetus, but also is essential for placental functioning and neural development in the fetus.[90] The vitamin D levels in the pregnant person determine the vitamin D levels in the fetus. Certain populations of U.S. women are generally vitamin D deficient (see Table 6-5), which has implications for their pregnancy outcomes. Studies of vitamin D supplementation during pregnancy show that pregnant individuals who receive this therapy have lower incidence of preeclampsia and gestational diabetes, and may be at lower risk of a low-birth-weight infant and postpartum hemorrhage.[91,92] In contrast, the evidence for decreased risk of preterm birth with vitamin D supplementation is conflicting.[91] Vitamin D deficiency has also been associated with infant asthma, slowed infant growth, and infant cognitive issues.[91,92]

There are no current recommendations for routine screening of all pregnant people for vitamin D deficiency, but providers who care for those at risk, such as people who expose little skin to the sun or people with darker-colored skin living in northern climates, might selectively do so. Studies have supplemented pregnant participants with 2000 to 4000 IU daily.[91]

**Prenatal Multivitamins.** Prenatal multivitamins generally contain enough of the vitamins and minerals needed by a pregnant person and, therefore, are a convenient vehicle for delivering those micronutrients. Prenatal multivitamins are specifically recommended for people who are in one of the following categories: nutritionally inadequate diet, multiple gestation, cigarette smoking, substance use or alcohol use disorder, adolescent, vegetarian diet, history of bariatric surgery, eating disorder, or lactase deficiency.

The amounts of specific vitamins and minerals in commercially marketed prenatal vitamins vary greatly. Also, the lack of uniform labeling makes it difficult to compare different products. Prenatal vitamins should contain iodine and choline, since levels of these nutrients are low in the general population. With the addition of extra calcium and the omega-3 long-chain polyunsaturated fats (DHA and EPA), however, many prenatal vitamins become difficult to swallow. Some manufacturers provide chewable or liquid formulations, whereas others recommend twice-daily dosing. If calcium, iron, and omega-3 supplementation are needed, midwives might consider recommending separate tablets for each nutrient needed.

Prenatal multivitamins can cause increased gastrointestinal distress and constipation in some people. These symptoms presumably arise secondary to the iron content in the vitamin. For individuals who experience nausea and vomiting, discontinuing iron-containing pills does appear to improve nausea symptoms.[93] When a prenatal vitamin is discontinued, even if temporarily, it should be replaced with a folic acid supplement.

Vitamins are not always beneficial. For example, vitamin A in the form of retinol, when taken in large doses, can be a teratogen. Studies have shown that cranial neural crest anomalies may occur when a pregnant person takes as little as 10,000 IU of retinol daily.[94] Routine supplementation of vitamin A is unnecessary in the United States, and, if supplementation is used, it should not exceed 5000 IU of retinol daily. Typical prenatal multivitamins contain at least 800 IU of vitamin A, usually as beta-carotene, which is not a concern as a teratogen. Pregnant individuals should be cautioned not to double or triple their intake of multivitamins to get additional folic acid or calcium.

## Special Nutritional Needs
### Plant-Based Diets in Pregnancy

With the increased popularity of plant-based diets, more studies have examined the effects of these diets on pregnancy outcomes. A meta-analysis of 22 studies of various degrees of plant-based dietary patterns showed no differences in infant outcomes,[95] with a subsequent systematic review identifying two studies showing an increase in hypospadias.[96] A cohort study conducted after this meta-analysis indicated that pregnant individuals who were vegans or lacto-ovo vegetarians had 2.5 the odds of a small-for-gestational-age infant but no difference in infant morbidities.[97] Greater adherence to a healthy plant-based diet is also associated with a lower risk of gestational diabetes and decreased excessive GWG and possibly preeclampsia.[96]

Individuals who eat plant-based diet can meet all their nutritional needs in pregnancy, although some modifications in their eating pattern may be needed. Those who follow a vegetarian diet during pregnancy may not obtain the recommended daily amounts of protein, vitamins $B_{12}$ and D, or iron, calcium, iodine, choline, zinc, and omega-3s. The increased protein demands of pregnancy can be met by increasing consumption of legumes, nuts, and soy protein. Vitamin $B_{12}$ intake can be adequate among those vegetarians who consume eggs, dairy products, and fortified foods; if their diet lacks a regular source of vitamin $B_{12}$, however, persons consuming a vegan diet need to be certain that they are receiving vitamin $B_{12}$ from either fortified soy and rice beverages, fortified foods, or nutritional yeast supplements. Fermented soy products are not a source of vitamin $B_{12}$. It may be appropriate to screen persons on a vegan diet for vitamin $B_{12}$ deficiency.[96]

Iron from plant sources is non-heme iron; thus, it is less easily absorbed and more foods can inhibit its absorption than is the case with heme iron. Nevertheless, iron can be obtained in a vegetarian diet.

Nonanimal sources of zinc include nuts and beans. Just as happens with iron, phytates can bind zinc, thereby preventing absorption of this micronutrient. Another source of zinc is fortified cereals.

If they do not consume any dairy products, pregnant persons may not have adequate vitamin D levels and, in the absence of sufficient sunlight exposure, may need vitamin D supplements. The same is true for choline, which mostly comes from eggs and animal proteins. Intake of iodine, which comes from fish, sea vegetables, and dairy products, will be low if these foods or iodized salt are not part of the diet.

Studies have shown that vegetarian diets, and especially vegan diets, are lower in the omega-3 long-chain polyunsaturated fats, DHA, and EPA, compared to an omnivorous diet. These fatty acids are essential for development of the fetus's retina and central nervous system. It is generally assumed that they must be obtained from the diet, although the exact amounts needed per day and the adverse effects of deficiencies have not been determined. Persons who eat eggs can increase their DHA by consuming DHA-fortified eggs from hens fed microalgae; otherwise, consumption of microalgae-derived DHA supplements is an alternative method for obtaining enough of these fatty acids.

### Pregnant with Medical Conditions

Medical conditions that adversely impact nutrition during pregnancy include eating disorders,[98,99] a history of bariatric surgery,[100] conditions associated with malabsorption, and a need for medications that affect folic acid metabolism. These conditions result in nutritional deficiencies from diminished ability to absorb or metabolize both macronutrients and micronutrients. People with these conditions are at risk for pregnancy outcomes related to decreased supply of nutrients to the fetus—specifically, small for gestational age, low birth weight, preterm birth, and, in the case of a person who has a recent history of hospitalization for anorexia nervosa, stillbirth.[99] Midwives caring for these persons will want to consult with a nutritionist to individualize their care.

Midwives are increasingly providing care for persons after bariatric surgery. Two types of bariatric surgery procedures are commonly performed: (1) restrictive (laparoscopic gastric banding or Lap-Band) and (2) restrictive/malabsorptive (gastric bypass). Lap-Band slippage and movement can occur during pregnancy and result in severe vomiting. Some sources advocate for deflating the band prior to pregnancy to allow for adequate nutrition, though no national guidelines have been established. Current recommendations advise persons to wait 12 to 18 months after bariatric surgery before starting a pregnancy, so that weight loss is stabilized.[101] However, a meta-analysis showed no differences for those conceiving less than 12 months post surgery except for less GWG.[102] Knowing the type of bariatric procedure done and when it was performed allows the midwife to provide appropriate nutritional advice and risk screening.

Notably, people tend to become less adherent in taking their multivitamin supplements with increasing time since their bariatric surgery.[103] GWG recommendations are based on pregravid BMI even after bariatric surgery. Any type of malabsorptive surgery will reduce food, micronutrient, and medication absorption. Therefore, baseline vitamin and mineral status of the pregnant person post bariatric surgery is evaluated at the first prenatal visit, with supplements recommended as needed. A complete blood count and measurement of vitamin $B_{12}$ and D, ferritin, and calcium levels every trimester should also be considered,[101] along with early glucose screening. The midwife providing prenatal care for someone following bariatric surgery must effectively coordinate care among a network of clinicians, including maternal–fetal medicine physicians, nutritionists, and ultrasonographers. Such team-based care optimizes the pregnant person's chance for a safe and satisfying birth.

Pregnant people who are taking anticonvulsant medications (e.g., valproate [Depakote, Depakene], carbamazepine [Tegretol]) should take 4 mg of folic acid per day starting 1 month prior to conception and continue that regimen throughout the pregnancy, as these medications have an antifolate effect.

### Multifetal Gestation

There are no national guidelines on the increased nutritional requirements for persons with multiple gestations, but extrapolations have been made from singleton to twin pregnancies. There is a consensus for the need for more calories per day, in the range of 40 to 45 kcal/kg daily for someone with a BMI between 18.5 and 24.9 or about 2400 calories per day.[23] Additionally, 1 mg of folic acid per day is recommended. Although individuals with multifetal gestation have lower vitamin D levels, as do their infants, there is no national consensus on how much vitamin D requirements increase in such cases.[104] It is generally recommended that women with

multiple fetuses take two prenatal vitamin supplements beginning in the second trimester to obtain the additional iron, folate, calcium, magnesium, and zinc that are needed.[23] This recommendation is safe as long as the vitamin A in the supplements is not retinol; if it is retinol, then the dose needs to remain less than 10,000 IU.

### Pica

*Pica* is the term applied to the unusual condition in which an individual purposefully ingests nonfood items. Pica is more common in pregnant people than in those who are not pregnant. The prevalence of pica varies by geographic region and culture, but has been noted to affect as many as 50% of pregnant people in some settings.[105] The most common substances eaten are earth, clay, or dirt; raw starches such as cornstarch; and ice and freezer frost. The etiology of pica is unknown, although several theories exist. There is a clear association between pica and iron-deficiency anemia.[106,107] Pica can cause lead poisoning and may be associated with other micronutrient deficiencies. Management consists of diagnosis and treatment of nutritional deficiencies, assessment of hunger or eating disorders, and health education. Motivational interviewing may assist in behavior change and replacing the nonfood substance with a healthy food.

### People with Limited Resources

People with low incomes are at increased risk for dietary deficiencies. As mentioned earlier, assessment for food insecurity is essential before any nutritional education. The Special Supplemental Nutrition Program for Women, Infants, and Children (WIC)—an income-based, supplemental food program provided by the USDA—provides food resources and cultural-based nutrition education for pregnant and lactating people, infants, and children younger than the age of 5. Current WIC policy is aimed at promoting consumption of healthier foods and access to farmers markets, and has expanded access to fresh fruits and vegetables and improved dietary intakes among this program's participants.[108] The program is also able to connect participants with other important community resources to help improve their pregnancy outcomes. WIC is not an entitlement program, but rather a grant program that requires reallocation of funding annually. Therefore, changes may occur at any time based on federal and state funding.

## Conclusion

Research increasingly confirms that good nutrition is essential during all phases of life, and the basic principles of good nutrition remain remarkably consistent throughout the life course. Albeit with some caveats, good nutrition is good nutrition—for those who are pregnant, or who want to lose weight, gain weight, or maintain their weight. The midwife should understand the basics of nutrition and how dietary patterns affect normal physiology. Nutrition counseling should be gently incorporated into a midwife's regular practice so that each person can understand some basic principles of nutrition, the physiologic response of the body to ingested food, and current evidence-based dietary guidelines. Although understanding individual components of the diet is important for health professionals, counseling a person about diet should remain positively focused on the types of preferable foods to eat and the need to eat a variety of nutrient-dense foods, rather than emphasizing individual macronutrients and micronutrients. Of course, a midwife should also be prepared with nutrition information specific to pregnancy, be alert to the possibility of eating disorders and refer clients appropriately in such cases, and be ready with encouragement, information, and possible referral to a registered dietician if a person indicates a desire to achieve a healthier weight.

## Resources

| Organization | Description |
|---|---|
| **Guidelines and Tools** | |
| National Institutes of Health (NIH) | Body mass calculator (English and Spanish) |
| Centers for Disease Control and Prevention (CDC) | Nutrition topics |
| U.S. Department of Agriculture (USDA) | Data & Research section: mapping food resources |
| | *Dietary Guidelines for Americans*: "Current Guidelines" |
| | MyPlate: "Lifestages" for guidance for different age groups and pregnancy and lactation |
| | Food Data Central: interactive database of nutrient content of food and prepared meals |
| Brown University School of Public Health | Nutrition tools: Rate My Plate (English, Spanish) |
| | Rapid Eating Assessment for Patients (REAP) tool |
| | WAVE Assessment: a one-page tool to assess weight, activity, and variety of foods eaten |
| University of Sydney | Glycemic index for foods |
| Harvard University School of Public Health | The Nutrition Source |
| **Free Smartphone Apps** | |
| MyPlate Calorie Counter | Tracks nutrient and exercise with meal plans and recipes |
| MyFitness Pal | Site to track weight, food intake, and exercise over time with a large database of foods or can be customized to personal intake of food |
| Yumly Recipes and Cooking Tools | Provides healthy cooking recipes |
| Calorie Counter by Fat Secret | Easy to use, with large database for easy tracking |
| **Handouts About Nutrition** | |
| Share with Women handouts from the *Journal of Midwifery and Women's Health* | Currently nine handouts on nutrition and health such as *Staying Healthy on a Vegetarian Diet in Pregnancy*, *Vitamin D*, and *Eating Safely in Pregnancy*. Available in English with two also in Spanish. |

## References

1. Hills RD Jr, Pontefract BA, Mishcon HR, et al. Gut microbiome: profound implications for diet and disease. *Nutrients.* 2019;11(7):1613.

2. De Cosmi V, Scaglioni S, Agostoni C. Early taste experiences and later food choices. *Nutrients.* 2017;9(2):107.

3. Whitfield GP, Hyde ET, Carlson SA. Participation in leisure-time aerobic physical activity among adults, National Health Interview Survey, 1998–2018. *J Phys Act Health.* 2021;18(S1):S25-S36.

4. Brenan M. U.S. alcohol consumption on low end of recent readings. *Gallup.* https://news.gallup.com/poll/353858/alcohol-consumption-low-end-recent-readings.aspx. Published August 19, 2021. Accessed June 30, 2022.

5. U.S. Department of Agriculture, U.S. Department of Health and Human Services. *Dietary Guidelines for Americans, 2020–2025.* 9th ed. Washington, DC: U.S. Government Printing Office; 2020.

6. Hales CM, Carroll MD, Fryar CD, Ogden CL. Prevalence of obesity and severe obesity among adults: United States, 2017–2018. *NCHS Data Brief.* No. 20. Hyattsville, MD: National Center for Health Statistics; 2020.

7. Sawyer ADM, van Lenthe F, Kamphuis CBM, et al. Dynamics of the complex food environment underlying dietary intake in low-income groups: a systems map of associations extracted from a systematic umbrella literature review. *Int J Behav Nutr Phys Act.* 2021;18(1):96.

8. Lee SH, Moore LV, Park S, et al. Adults meeting fruit and vegetable intake recommendations—United States, 2019. *Morb Mortal Wkly Rep.* 2022;71(1):1-9.

9. Daniel C. Is healthy eating too expensive? How low-income parents evaluate the cost of food. *Soc Sci Med.* 2020;248:112823.

10. Rodriguez ME, Drew C, Bellin R, et al. *Produce Prescription Programs. US Field Scan Report: 2010–2020.* DAISA Enterprises. https://drive.google.com/file/d/1KllO_7e4-WmBEdXiNa1Hzvbrnf-rWPqC/view. Published 2021. Accessed May 26, 2022.

11. Gomes SM, Jacob MC, Rocha C, et al. Expanding the limits of sex: a systematic review concerning food and nutrition in transgender populations. *Public Health Nutr.* 2021;24(18):6436-6449.

12. Rozga M, Linsenmeyer W, Cantwell Wood J, et al. Hormone therapy, health outcomes and the role of nutrition in transgender individuals: a scoping review. *Clin Nutr.* 2020;40:42-56.

13. Tapsell LC, Neale EP, Satija A, Hu FB. Foods, nutrients, and dietary patterns: interconnections and implications for dietary guidelines. *Adv Nutr.* 2016;7(3):445-454.

14. U.S. Food and Drug Administration. Food labeling: revision of the nutrition and supplement facts labels. *Federal Register.* 2016;81:33742-33999.

15. Institute of Medicine. *Dietary Reference Intakes: The Essential Guide to Nutrient Requirements.* Washington, DC: National Academies Press; 2006.

16. Wright JD, Wang C-Y. Trends in intake of energy and mcaronutrients in adults from 1999–2000 through 2007–2008. Hyattsville, MD: National Center for Health Statistics; 2010.

17. Püschel GP, Henkel J. Dietary cholesterol does not break your heart but kills your liver. *Porto Biomed J.* 2018;3(1):e12.

18. Rosinger A, Carroll MD, Lacher D, Ogden C. Trends in total cholesterol, triglycerides, and low-density lipoprotein in US adults, 1999–2014. *JAMA Cardiol.* 2017;2(3):339-341.

19. Chavarro JE, Rich-Edwards JW, Rosner BA, Willett WC. Dietary fatty acid intakes and the risk of ovulatory infertility. *Am J Clin Nutr.* 2007;85(1):231-237.

20. U.S. Food and Drug Adminsitration. Trans fat. https://www.fda.gov/food/food-additives-petitions/trans-fat. Published 2018. Updated May 18, 2020. Accessed May 20, 2022.

21. Office of Dietary Supplements. Omega-3 fatty acids. National Institutes of Health website. https://ods.od.nih.gov/factsheets/Omega3FattyAcids-HealthProfessional/. Published August 4, 2021. Accessed May 25, 2022.

22. Bhatt DL, Steg PG, Miller M, et al. Cardiovascular risk reduction with icosapent ethyl for hypertriglyceridemia. *N Engl J Med.* 2019;380(1):11-22.

23. Goodnight W, Newman R. Optimal nutrition for improved twin pregnancy outcome. *Obstet Gynecol.* 2009;114(5):1121-1134.

24. Barclay AW, Augustin LSA, Brighenti F, et al. Dietary glycaemic index labelling: a global perspective. *Nutrients.* 2021;13(9):3244.

25. Hoy MK, Goldman JD. Fiber intake of the U.S. population: What We Eat in America, NHANES 2009–2010. *Food Survey Research Group Dietary Data Brief.* 2014;12.

26. Melina V, Craig W, Levin S. Position of the Academy of Nutrition and Dietetics: vegetarian diets. *J Acad Nutr Diet.* 2016;116(12):1970-1980.

27. Energy intakes: percentages of energy from protein, carbohydrate, fat, and alcohol, by gender and age. In: *What We Eat in America, NHANES 2017–2018.* Washington, DC: U.S. Department of Agriculture; 2020.

28. Chen M, Li Y, Sun Q, et al. Dairy fat and risk of cardiovascular disease in 3 cohorts of US adults. *Am J Clin Nutr.* 2016;104(5):1209-1217.

29. Ludwig DS. The glycemic index: physiological mechanisms relating to obesity, diabetes, and cardiovascular disease. *J Am Med Assoc.* 2002;287(18):2414-2423.

30. Beal T, Ortenzi F. Priority micronutrient density in foods. *Front Nutr.* 2022;9:806566.

31. Hollis BW, Wagner CL. Substantial vitamin D supplementation is required during the prenatal period to improve birth outcomes. *Nutrients.* 2022;14(4):899.

32. National Center for Environmental Health. *Second National Report on Biochemical Indicators of Diet and Nutrition in the U.S. Population.* Atlanta, GA: Centers for Disease Control and Prevention; 2012.

33. Institute of Medicine. *Dietary Reference Intakes for Calcium and Vitamin D.* Washington, DC: National Academies Press; 2011.

34. Holick MF, Binkley NC, Bischoff-Ferrari HA, et al. Evaluation, treatment, and prevention of vitamin D deficiency: an Endocrine Society clinical practice guideline. *J Clin Endocrinol Metab.* 2011;96(7):1911-1930.

35. Pfeiffer CM, Sternberg MR, Zhang M, et al. Folate status in the US population 20 y after the introduction of folic acid fortification. *Am J Clin Nutr.* 2019;110(5):1088-1097.

36. Markun S, Gravestock I, Jäger L, et al. Effects of vitamin $B_{12}$ supplementation on cognitive function, depressive symptoms, and fatigue: a systematic review, meta-analysis, and meta-regression. *Nutrients.* 2021;13(3).

37. Forsyth JC, Mueller PD, Becker CE, et al. Hydroxocobalamin as a cyanide antidote: safety, efficacy and pharmacokinetics in heavily smoking normal volunteers. *J Toxicol Clin Toxicol.* 1993;31(2):277-294.

38. Paul C, Brady DM. Comparative bioavailability and utilization of particular forms of $B_{12}$ supplements with potential to mitigate $B_{12}$-related genetic polymorphisms. *Integr Med.* 2017;16(1):42-49.

39. Bensky MJ, Ayalon-Dangur I, Ayalon-Dangur R, et al. Comparison of sublingual vs. intramuscular administration of vitamin $B_{12}$ for the treatment of patients with vitamin $B_{12}$ deficiency. *Drug Deliv Transl Res.* 2019;9(3):625-630.

40. Sarafrazi N, Wambogo EA, Shepherd JA. Osteoporosis or low bone mass in older adults: United States, 2017–2018. *NCHS Data Brief.* 2021;405:1-8.

41. Hoy M, Goldman J. Calcium intake of the U.S.population: *What We Eat in America, NHANES 2009–2010.* In: *Food Surveys Research Group Dietary Data Brief No. 13.* Washington, DC: U.S. Department of Agriculture; 2014.

42. Li K, Wang X-F, Li D-Y, et al. The good, the bad, and the ugly of calcium supplementation: a review of calcium intake on human health. *Clin Interv Aging.* 2018;13:2443-2452.

43. Mills JL, Buck Louis GM, Kannan K, et al. Delayed conception in women with low-urinary iodine concentrations: a population-based prospective cohort study. *Hum Reprod.* 2018;33(3):426-433.

44. Panth P, Guerin G, DiMarco NM. A review of iodine status of women of reproductive age in the USA. *Biol Trace Elem Res.* 2019;188(1):208-220.

45. Perrine CG, Herrick KA, Gupta PM, Caldwell KL. Iodine status of pregnant women and women of reproductive age in the United States. *Thyroid.* 2019;29(1):153-154.

46. Cook JD, Reddy MB. Effect of ascorbic acid intake on nonheme-iron absorption from a complete diet. *Am J Clin Nutr.* 2001;73(1):93-98.

47. Barton JC, Wiener HH, Acton RT, et al. Prevalence of iron deficiency in 62,685 women of seven race/ethnicity groups: the HEIRS Study. *PLoS One.* 2020;15(4):e0232125.

48. Kanu FA, Hamner HC, Scanlon KS, Sharma AJ. Anemia among pregnant women participating in the Special Supplemental Nutrition Program for Women, Infants, and Children—United States, 2008–2018. *Morb Mortal Wkly Rep.* 2022;71:813-819.

49. Chang TP, Rangan C. Iron poisoning: a literature-based review of epidemiology, diagnosis, and management. *Pediatr Emerg Care.* 2011;27(10):978-985.

50. Cowan AE, Jun S, Gahche JJ, et al. Dietary supplement use differs by socioeconomic and health-related characteristics among U.S. adults, NHANES 2011–2014. *Nutrients.* 2018;10(8):1114.

51. Chen F, Du M, Blumberg JB, et al. Association among dietary supplement use, nutrient intake, and mortality among U.S. adults: a cohort study. *Ann Intern Med.* 2019;170(9):604-613.

52. U.S. Preventive Services Task Force. Vitamin, mineral, and multivitamin supplementation to prevent cardiovascular disease and cancer. *JAMA.* 2022;327(23):2326-2333. doi: 10.1001/jama.2022.8970.

53. Sesso HD, Rist PM, Aragaki AK, et al. Multivitamins in the prevention of cancer and cardiovascular disease: the COcoa Supplement and Multivitamin Outcomes Study (COSMOS) randomized clinical trial. *Am J Clin Nutr.* 2022;115(6):1501-1510.

54. Yao P, Bennett D, Mafham M, et al. Vitamin D and calcium for the prevention of fracture: a systematic review and meta-analysis. *JAMA Netw Open.* 2019;2(12):e1917789.

55. Morze J, Danielewicz A, Hoffmann G, Schwingshackl L. Diet quality as assessed by the Healthy Eating Index, Alternate Healthy Eating Index, Dietary Approaches to Stop Hypertension Score, and health outcomes: a second update of a systematic review and meta-analysis of cohort studies. *J Acad Nutr Diet.* 2020;120(12):1998-2031.

56. Skerrett PJ, Willett WC. Essentials of healthy eating: a guide. *J Midwifery Womens Health*. 2010;55(6):492-501.

57. Fontes T, Rodrigues LM, Ferreira-Pêgo C. Comparison between different groups of vegetarianism and its associations with body composition: a literature review from 2015 to 2021. *Nutrients*. 2022;14(9):1853.

58. Tong TYN, Appleby PN, Armstrong MEG, et al. Vegetarian and vegan diets and risks of total and site-specific fractures: results from the prospective EPIC-Oxford study. *BMC Med*. 2020;18(1):353.

59. Segovia-Siapco G, Sabaté J. Health and sustainability outcomes of vegetarian dietary patterns: a revisit of the EPIC-Oxford and the Adventist Health Study-2 cohorts. *Eur J Clin Nutr*. 2019;72(suppl 1):60-70.

60. Kim HS, Patel KG, Orosz E, et al. Time trends in the prevalence of celiac disease and gluten-free diet in the US population: results from the National Health and Nutrition Examination Surveys 2009–2014. *JAMA Intern Med*. 2016;176(11):1716-1717.

61. Sabença C, Ribeiro M, Sousa TD, et al. Wheat/gluten-related disorders and gluten-free diet misconceptions: a review. *Foods*. 2021;10(8):1765.

62. Lebwohl B, Cao Y, Zong G, et al. Long term gluten consumption in adults without celiac disease and risk of coronary heart disease: prospective cohort study. *BMJ*. 2017;357:j1892.

63. Saccone G, Berghella V, Sarno L, et al. Celiac disease and obstetric complications: a systematic review and metaanalysis. *Am J Obstet Gynecol*. 2016;214(2):225-234.

64. Liu J, Rehm CD, Onopa J, Mozaffarian D. Trends in diet quality among youth in the United States, 1999–2016. *J Am Med Assoc*. 2020;323(12):1161-1174.

65. Lipsky LM, Nansel TR, Haynie DL, et al. Diet quality of US adolescents during the transition to adulthood: changes and predictors. *Am J Clin Nutr*. 2017;105(6):1424-1432.

66. Calcaterra V, Cena H, Regalbuto C, et al. The role of fetal, infant, and childhood nutrition in the timing of sexual maturation. *Nutrients*. 2021;13(2):419.

67. Cheng G, Buyken AE, Shi L, et al. Beyond overweight: nutrition as an important lifestyle factor influencing timing of puberty. *Nutr Rev*. 2012;70(3):133-152.

68. Davidsen L, Vistisen B, Astrup A. Impact of the menstrual cycle on determinants of energy balance: a putative role in weight loss attempts. *Int J Obes*. 2007;31(12):1777-1785.

69. Abdi F, Ozgoli G, Rahnemaie FS. A systematic review of the role of vitamin D and calcium in premenstrual syndrome. *Obstet Gynecol Sci*. 2019;62(2):73-86.

70. Centers for Disease Control and Prevention. FastStats: infertility. https://www.cdc.gov/nchs/fastats/infertility .htm. Published 2017. Accessed May 20, 2022.

71. Montagnoli C, Santoro CB, Buzzi T, Bortolus R. Maternal periconceptional nutrition matters: a scoping review of the current literature. *J Matern Fetal Neonat Med*. 2021:1-18.

72. Chavarro JE, Rich-Edwards JW, Rosner BA, Willett WC. Diet and lifestyle in the prevention of ovulatory disorder infertility. *Obstet Gynecol*. 2007;110(5):1050-1058.

73. Kominiarek MA, Peaceman AM. Gestational weight gain. *Am J Obstet Gynecol*. 2017;217(6):642-651.

74. Marshall NE, Abrams B, Barbour LA, et al. The importance of nutrition in pregnancy and lactation: lifelong consequences. *Am J Obstet Gynecol*. 2022;226(5):607-632.

75. Barua S, Junaid MA. Lifestyle, pregnancy and epigenetic effects. *Epigenomics*. 2015;7(1):85-102.

76. National Academies of Sciences Engineering and Medicine, Health and Medicine Division, Food and Nutrition Board. *Nutrition During Pregnancy and Lactation: Exploring New Evidence: Proceedings of a Workshop*. National Academies Press; July 31, 2020. https://www.ncbi.nlm.nih.gov/books /NBK560007/. Accessed May 20, 2022.

77. Nomura K, Minamizono S, Nagashima K, et al. Maternal body mass index and breastfeeding non-initiation and cessation: a quantitative review of the literature. *Nutrients*. 2020;12(9):2684.

78. Institute of Medicine, National Research Council, Committee to Reexamine IOM Pregnancy Weight Guidelines. *Weight Gain During Pregnancy: Reexamining the Guidelines*. Washington, DC: National Academies Press; 2009.

79. U.S. Food and Drug Administration. Food safety for pregnant women, their unborn babies, and children under five. https://www.fda.gov/media/83740 /download. Published 2022. Accessed June 20, 2022.

80. Barger MK. Maternal nutrition and perinatal outcomes. *J Midwifery Womens Health*. 2010;55(6):502-511.

81. Wilson RD, O'Connor DL. Maternal folic acid and multivitamin supplementation: international clinical evidence with considerations for the prevention of folate-sensitive birth defects. *Prevent Med Rep*. 2021;24:101617.

82. Dwyer ER, Filion KB, MacFarlane AJ, et al. Who should consume high-dose folic acid supplements before and during early pregnancy for the prevention of neural tube defects? *BMJ*. 2022;377:e067728.

83. Graves BW, Barger MK. A "conservative" approach to iron supplementation during pregnancy. *J Midwifery Womens Health*. 2001;46(3):159-166.

84. Peña-Rosas JP, De-Regil LM, Garcia-Casal MN, Dowswell T. Daily oral iron supplementation during pregnancy. *Cochrane Database Syst Rev*. 2015;7:Cd004736.

85. U.S. Preventive Services Task Force. *Literature Surveillance Report: Screening ror Iron Deficiency Anemia and Iron Supplementation in Pregnant Women to Improve Maternal Health and Birth Outcomes.* https://www.uspreventiveservicestaskforce.org/uspstf/document/literature-surveillance-report-/iron-deficiency-anemia-in-pregnant-women-screening-and-supplementation. Published 2020. Accessed June 20, 2022.

86. Sun H, Weaver CM. Decreased iron intake parallels rising iron deficiency anemia and related mortality rates in the US population. *J Nutr.* 2021;151(7):1947-1955.

87. Peña-Rosas JP, De-Regil LM, Gomez Malave H, et al. Intermittent oral iron supplementation during pregnancy. *Cochrane Database Syst Rev.* 2015;10:Cd009997.

88. Alexander EK, Pearce EN, Brent GA, et al. 2017 guidelines of the American Thyroid Association for the diagnosis and management of thyroid disease during pregnancy and the postpartum. *Thyroid.* 2017;27(3):315-389.

89. Wallace TC, Fulgoni VL 3rd. Assessment of total choline intakes in the United States. *J Am Coll Nutr.* 2016;35(2):108-112.

90. Larqué E, Morales E, Leis R, Blanco-Carnero JE. Maternal and foetal health implications of vitamin D status during pregnancy. *Ann Nutr Metabol.* 2018;72(3):179-192.

91. Bi WG, Nuyt AM, Weiler H, et al. Association between vitamin D supplementation during pregnancy and offspring growth, morbidity, and mortality: a systematic review and meta-analysis. *JAMA Pediatr.* 2018;172(7):635-645.

92. Palacios C, Kostiuk LK, Peña-Rosas JP. Vitamin D supplementation for women during pregnancy. *Cochrane Database Syst Rev.* 2019;7:Cd008873.

93. Gill SK, Maltepe C, Koren G. The effectiveness of discontinuing iron-containing prenatal multivitamins on reducing the severity of nausea and vomiting of pregnancy. *J Obstet Gynaecol.* 2009;29(1):13-16.

94. Rothman KJ, Moore LL, Singer MR, et al. Teratogenicity of high vitamin A intake. *N Engl J Med.* 1995;333(21):1369-1373.

95. Piccoli GB, Clari R, Vigotti FN, et al. Vegan–vegetarian diets in pregnancy: danger or panacea? A systematic narrative review. *BJOG.* 2015;122(5):623-633.

96. Sebastiani G, Herranz Barbero A, Borrás-Novell C, et al. The effects of vegetarian and vegan diet during pregnancy on the health of mothers and offspring. *Nutrients.* 2019;11(3):557.

97. Yisahak SF, Hinkle SN, Mumford SL, et al. Vegetarian diets during pregnancy, and maternal and neonatal outcomes. *Int J Epidemiol.* 2021;50(1):165-178.

98. Sebastiani G, Andreu-Fernández V, Herranz Barbero A, et al. Eating disorders during gestation: implications for mother's health, fetal outcomes, and epigenetic changes. *Front Pediatr.* 2020;8:587.

99. Ante Z, Luu TM, Healy-Profitós J, et al. Pregnancy outcomes in women with anorexia nervosa. *Int J Eat Disord.* 2020;53(5):403-412.

100. Akhter Z, Rankin J, Ceulemans D, et al. Pregnancy after bariatric surgery and adverse perinatal outcomes: a systematic review and meta-analysis. *PLoS Med.* 2019;16(8):e1002866.

101. ACOG Practice Bulletin No. 105: bariatric surgery and pregnancy. *Obstet Gynecol.* 2009;113(6):1405-1413.

102. Chen W, Liang Y, Chen G, et al. Early pregnancy (≤ 12 months) after bariatric surgery: does it really influence maternal and perinatal outcomes? *Obes Surg.* 2022;32(4):979-990.

103. Smelt HJM, Pouwels S, Smulders JF, Hazebroek EJ. Patient adherence to multivitamin supplementation after bariatric surgery: a narrative review. *J Nutr Sci.* 2020;9:e46.

104. Wierzejska RE. Review of dietary recommendations for twin pregnancy: does nutrition science keep up with the growing incidence of multiple gestations? *Nutrients.* 2022;14(6):1143.

105. Fawcett EJ, Fawcett JM, Mazmanian D. A meta-analysis of the worldwide prevalence of pica during pregnancy and the postpartum period. *Int J Gynaecol Obstet.* 2016;133(3):277-283.

106. Lumish RA, Young SL, Lee S, et al. Gestational iron deficiency is associated with pica behaviors in adolescents. *J Nutr.* 2014;144(10):1533-1539.

107. Miao D, Young SL, Golden CD. A meta-analysis of pica and micronutrient status. *Am J Hum Biol.* 2015;27(1):84-93.

108. Hamad R, Batra A, Karasek D, et al. The impact of the revised WIC food package on maternal nutrition during pregnancy and postpartum. *Am J Epidemiol.* 2019;188(8):1493-1502.

C H A P T E R

# 7

# Mental Health Conditions

JAIN LATTES AND JULIA S. SENG

## Introduction

Mental health disorders affect millions of individuals in the United States. Primary care providers, including midwives, care for many of these individuals, who may experience either a single disorder or disorders that are comorbid with other illnesses. This chapter presents an overview of mental health conditions that commonly affect patients, a framework for identifying the most common disorders, and screening strategies for determining if there is a need for urgent referral to a mental health expert.

Controversy exists regarding use of the terms "mental health" and "behavioral health." As no clear consensus is available, this chapter uses the term "mental health."

The diagnostic standard for psychiatric disorders is the American Psychiatric Association's (APA's) *Diagnostic and Statistical Manual of Mental Disorders (DSM-5-TR)*, which has evolved as knowledge about mental health has increased.[1] The *DSM-5* delineates specific diagnostic criteria for each distinct psychiatric diagnosis and is the reference for the tables that appear throughout this chapter. It is important to be mindful that even if the patient does not meet the full criteria for a specific diagnosis according to the *DSM-5*, their level of distress or impairment may still be significant and warrant treatment or referral.

Mental health conditions are the most common and costly cause of disability in the United States.[2] Common mental health conditions include depression, anxiety, and post-traumatic stress. Almost one-third of persons who reside in the United States will suffer from an anxiety disorder in their lifetime, and between 15% and 20% will experience a major depressive episode. The lifetime rate of post-traumatic stress in the United States is approximately 6% to 7% overall[3,4] but closer to 10%

for women.[4] Data from 2019 indicate that approximately 20% of all adults in the United States had at least one mental, behavioral, or emotional disorder during that year.[5] Unfortunately, many individuals with mental health disorders do not seek treatment, and of those who do, many are not able to access care due to widespread shortages of mental health providers and/or lack of financial resources. Members of uninsured, underinsured, low-income, and other marginalized populations are among those who are least likely to receive treatment.[4]

Midwives working as primary care providers can assess, initiate, and sometimes continue treatment for patients with unipolar depression (including perinatal and postpartum depression), as well as some of the more common anxiety disorders. Although most primary care providers do not have the training needed to provide counseling or therapy, they can recommend lifestyle changes to improve symptoms while also prescribing psychopharmacologic medications for treatment. This chapter provides an overview of how to screen, evaluate, and treat the most common mental health disorders.

The management of patients with complex major mental health disorders, such as schizophrenia, bipolar disorder (BPD), obsessive–compulsive disorder (OCD), and eating disorders, is beyond the scope of care for most primary care practitioners. The role of the midwife in caring for individuals with one of these disorders is restricted to screening and referral for treatment.

This chapter also discusses substance use disorder (SUD) and its treatments, which are available for all individuals, including perinatal patients. As SUD has become more prevalent and as the emphasis of care for SUD has shifted to the primary care provider, some midwives will have the opportunity to manage treatment of patients with these disorders.

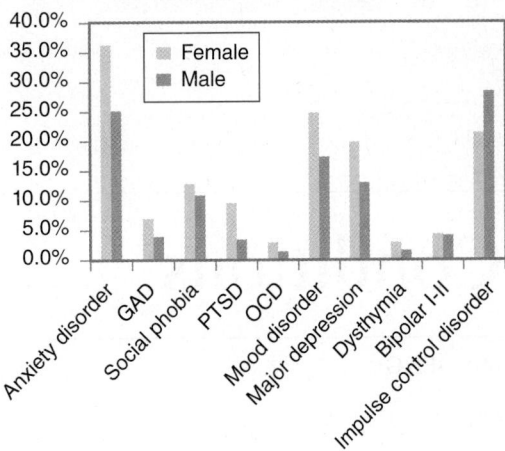

**Figure 7-1** Lifetime prevalence of selected disorders identified in the *Diagnostic and Statistical Manual of Mental Disorders, Fourth Edition* (*DSM-IV*) from the World Mental Health Survey version of the Composite International Diagnostic Interview.
Abbreviations: GAD, generalized anxiety disorder; OCD, obsessive–compulsive disorder; PTSD, post-traumatic stress disorder.
Data from Kessler RC, Berglund P, Demler O, et al. Lifetime prevalence and age-of-onset distributions of *DSM-IV* disorders in the National Comorbidity Survey Replication. *Arch Gen Psychiatry*. 2005;62(6):593-602.

Figure 7-1 presents the lifetime prevalence of selected mental health disorders in men and women.[4] A cross-national survey of 72,933 individuals in Africa, Asia, Europe, the Middle East, and the Americas found that among all cohorts in all countries, women had an odds ratio (OR) of 1.9 (95% confidence interval [CI], 1.8–2.0) for experiencing depression and an OR of 1.7 (95% CI, 1.6–1.8) for experiencing an anxiety disorder when compared to men. No significant sex difference was found among those with a bipolar disorder, and the sex difference for social phobia (OR, 1.3; 95% CI, 1.2–1.4) was less than that for other anxiety disorders.[6]

## Etiology of Mental Health Disorders

Two main pathophysiology theories have been proposed to explain the development of anxiety, unipolar mood disorders, and post-traumatic stress disorder (PTSD). The first is the monoamine theory, which assumes that dysregulation or deficiency in the monoamine neurotransmitters in the brain contributes to depression or anxiety symptoms. Monoamine neurotransmitters include serotonin, norepinephrine, and dopamine. The second biologic theory for the development of mood disorders is called the hypothalamic–pituitary–adrenal (HPA) axis theory; it suggests that chronic activation of the stress response cycle leads to chronic brain changes such as a smaller hippocampus and fluctuations in stress hormones such as cortisol, corticotropin-releasing hormone (CRH), and adrenocorticotropic hormone (ACTH). An imbalance of these stress hormones is thought to increase neurotransmitter reuptake (making less available for use by the brain), which leads to the development of mood symptoms.

Mental health disorders have a complex etiology, with genetic factors, environmental factors, and gene-by-environment interactions all contributing to an individual's risk for developing symptoms.[7] The two most frequently encountered mental health disorders in primary care, and the ones on which this chapter primarily focuses, are unipolar depression and anxiety, both of which are multifactorial in origin. Studies of twins have found that genetic factors are a significant contributor to the development of both major depression and anxiety disorders, although perhaps more for depression than for anxiety. Epidemiologic studies have shown that the heritability of major depression is between 31% and 42%.[8] Awareness of PTSD is increasing, and this disorder is beginning to be addressed in primary care with the use of a trauma-informed approach first promoted by the Substance Abuse and Mental Health Services Administration (SAMHSA) for addiction and mental health services.[9]

Environmental factors can lead to chemical changes at the cellular level without altering specific DNA sequences. How an individual interacts with their environment can modify gene expression either positively or negatively. Current research indicates that adverse psychosocial experiences, such as witnessing or experiencing trauma, are associated with numerous mental health disorders, including anxiety, depression, addiction, schizophrenia, and PTSD.

Environmental influences on mental health can include cultural and religious practices and beliefs, as well as systemic discrimination in the forms of racism, sexism, and classism. The correlation of minority status with fewer resources and barriers to access also decreases options for treatment. These factors can shape how an individual perceives their symptoms as well as how they present to providers (somatic versus emotional complaints) and even how they seek treatment (psychiatric provider, social worker, primary care provider, or clergy). While considering the etiology of mental illness, it is important to acknowledge that as a result of the United States' long history of medical racism and discrimination, marginalized people in this country are less likely to seek out, and more likely to delay, treatment for mental illness.

## Evaluating the Patient

Mental health cannot be completely separated from physical health. In consequence, a comprehensive evaluation is indicated when screening for mental health disorders. This requires obtaining both subjective and objective information, provided directly by the patient and, when possible, from their health record. Screening should begin with an evaluation of the patient's current health status, a review of systems and a review of the patient's known medical, psychiatric, family, and trauma history. Information gathering can be targeted to elicit data specific to the mental health assessment. A complete review of symptoms may clarify what is affecting the patient at the time of evaluation, even if the patient does not recognize connections between their symptoms and possible psychiatric illness. Chronic pain, headache, gastrointestinal complaints, and sleep changes are among the most common somatic complaints of patients with mental health disorders when seen in the primary care setting.

Evaluations should also be based on a physical examination of the patient, a mental status assessment, and laboratory tests, as indicated. The physical exam can target specific areas of concern identified during the review of systems and is helpful in identifying signs of self-injurious behaviors or trauma. Vital signs may show signs of malnutrition or excessive weight changes. Information for the mental status exam is gathered throughout the entire patient interview. The provider assesses and makes note of the patient's appearance, orientation, motor activity, speech, mood, affect, thought process and content, insight, judgment, and impulse control. Laboratory tests are performed, when necessary, to rule out other conditions that might mimic or exacerbate mental health conditions. For example, thyroid disorders can present with symptoms like those seen with major depression and with anxiety. Anemia, menopause, and both hyperglycemia and hypoglycemia can also cause symptoms similar to those seen with the most common mental health disorders and should be screened for accordingly.

## Mood Disorders

Mood disorders are separated into two major categories: unipolar and bipolar. Unipolar mood disorders with *DSM-5* diagnoses include forms of depression known as major depressive disorder (MDD), persistent depressive disorder (dysthymia), and premenstrual dysphoric disorder. "Major depressive disorder with peripartum onset," a diagnosis that has replaced the formerly used term "postpartum depression," is discussed later in the chapter. The *DSM-5* uses this term for any MDD episode that first occurs during pregnancy and up until 4 weeks following birth. Bipolar mood disorders are further subdivided into bipolar I and bipolar II, or less commonly, described as cyclothymia. These disorders are discussed later in the chapter.

MDD is the most common mood disorder among adults in the United States, and is four times more prevalent than either persistent depressive disorder or bipolar I/II. It is important to note that each of these disorders is associated with significant suffering and financial costs to individuals, families, and society.

### Unipolar Mood Disorders
#### Major Depressive Disorder

Depression affects millions of persons in the United States. Approximately 21% of the U.S. population experiences major depressive disorder during their lifetime.[10] Women are at increased risk compared to men, as are individuals who are members of ethnic minority groups, living in poverty, or lacking adequate access to health care. Additional risk factors are listed in Table 7-1.

Major depressive disorder is the mental health disorder most frequently diagnosed by primary care providers. Even so, it is common for depression to go undiagnosed or be treated suboptimally, depending on the demands of the practice and the provider's attitude. Overall rates of depression screening are less than 5% in primary care settings, with even lower rates seen among patients of color and the elderly population,[11] although more recent data show that electronic medical records are facilitating better screening. According to the 2019 National Survey on Drug Use and Health, approximately 65% of adults with a diagnosed major depressive episode receive treatment.[12]

Depression has a major impact on quality of life and is the third leading cause of "years lived with disability."[13] Depressive disorders often are associated with other comorbid medical conditions, such as chronic disease, and may lead to decreased quality of life for those persons whose health conditions are aggravated by depression. In addition, individuals with depression may have other psychiatric

| Table 7-1 | Risk Factors for Major Depression |
|---|---|

Stressful life events such as divorce, job change, financial problems, or pregnancy

Recent death of a loved one or friend

Family members with depression

History of abuse or trauma

Exposure to traumatic event (e.g., car accident, hurricane)

Intimate-partner violence

Racism, discrimination, micro-aggressions

A serious or chronic medical condition

Alcohol or drug abuse

Prior episodes of depression

Many medications can contribute to depression or cause symptoms of depression

| Table 7-2 | Symptoms of Major Depressive Disorder (SIGECAPS) |
|---|---|

Symptoms must include either depressed mood or anhedonia (lack of interest) PLUS any of the following symptoms (to total five symptoms), which occur nearly every day for at least 2 weeks, and are severe enough to impede function:

1. **S**leep disorder (insomnia or hypersomnia)
2. **I**nterest deficit or a lack of feeling pleasure
3. **G**uilt (worthlessness, hopelessness, regret)
4. **E**nergy deficit (fatigue or loss of energy nearly every day)
5. **C**oncentration deficit
6. **A**ppetite disorder (increased or decreased), unplanned weight loss or gain
7. **P**sychomotor retardation or agitation
8. **S**uicidality (recurrent thoughts of death)

There has never been a manic or hypomanic episode.

Symptoms are not attributable to a medical condition or substance use.

Must be qualified as a single episode or recurrent.

Based on American Psychiatric Association. *Diagnostic and Statistical Manual of Mental Disorders. 5th ed. Text revision (DSM-5-TR)*. VA: American Psychiatric Association; 2022.

disorders, including personality disorders, anxiety disorders, eating disorders, and substance use disorders.[14] Individuals with combined diagnoses, including those exhibiting any psychotic features such as delusions or hallucinations, require more specialized care. They should be referred appropriately by the midwife for evaluation and treatment by psychiatric providers.[15]

The diagnostic criteria for major depression are described in Table 7-2. The number and severity of symptoms, including how much they interfere with normal daily activities, will determine the severity of the person's depression. Individuals with severe major depression often report significant impacts on their daily life.[16]

Persistent depressive disorder, also known as dysthymia, is a unique diagnosis in that the level of depression is usually not severe enough to meet the criteria for MDD. Individuals with this condition must experience a depressed mood most days plus two or more symptoms for at least 2 years, with no longer than 2 months without symptoms.

### Differential Diagnoses for Major Depressive Disorder

As discussed earlier in this chapter, additional assessment for depression should include an evaluation for conditions or diseases that can either mimic depression or worsen depression. Thyroid function tests are usually indicated in these instances. Hypothyroidism can cause fatigue, weight change, and symptoms of depression, whereas hyperthyroidism can present as anxiety, irritability, and restlessness. Anemia, menopause, chronic fatigue, and substance use also can cause individuals to present with symptoms that mimic or worsen MDD, so these conditions should be ruled out during the initial assessment.

Individuals with bipolar disorders (defined later in this chapter) also may present with depression symptoms, although this depression is distinct from unipolar depression. All patients should be screened for mania/hypomania because treating bipolar depression with typical antidepressants can worsen the disease process and prognosis. Anyone with symptoms of mania/hypomania should be referred to a psychiatric provider for treatment.

Figure 7-2 presents a simplified algorithm that can aid the differential diagnosis of mood disorders. This algorithm is based on a thorough process that is outlined in the *DSM-5*.[1,17]

### Screening Tools for Unipolar Mood Disorders

The U.S. Preventive Services Task Force and other professional organizations including the American

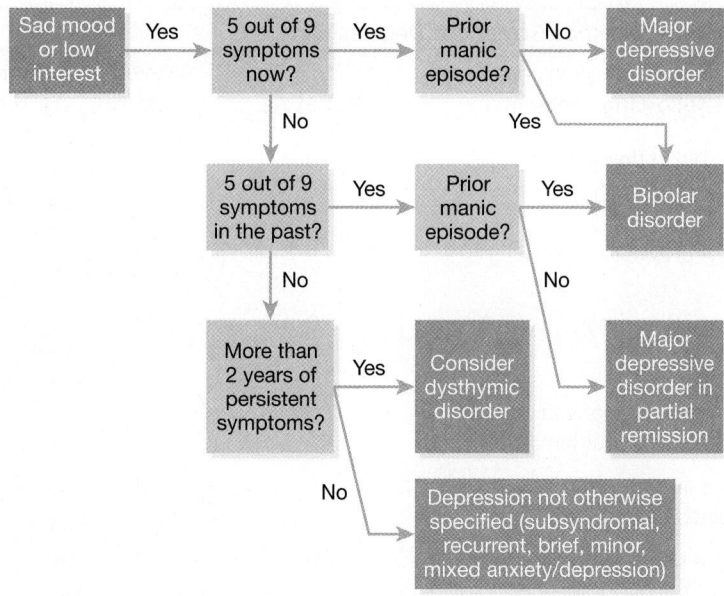

**Figure 7-2** Differential diagnosis of mood disorders.
Reproduced from U.S. Department of Health and Human Services. *Depression in Primary Care: Volume 1. Detection and Diagnosis.* AHCPR Publication No. 93-0550. Rockville, MD: Agency for Health Care Policy and Research; 1993:20.

College of Nurse-Midwives (ACNM), American Academy of Pediatrics (AAP), and American College of Obstetricians and Gynecologists (ACOG) recommend universal depression screening for all adolescents and adults, including pregnant and postpartum individuals. Screening must exist within a system that can provide appropriate referrals when indicated.[17] Validated screening tools, by definition, are proven to provide reliable, reproducible, and highly sensitive measurement of what they are designed to measure. Several screening tools for major depressive disorder are available for use in clinical practice, and those most used in the midwifery setting are presented in this chapter.

The two depression screening tools most widely used in primary care practices and midwifery practices are the Patient Health Questionnaire-9 (PHQ-9)[18] and the Edinburgh Postnatal Depression Scale (EPDS).[19] Both of these tools are free to access by providers, are easily administered (consisting of only 9 or 10 questions), and have been validated for use in other languages and cultures. They are equally sensitive screening tools for depression.

The PHQ-9 (Table 7-3) is available in the public domain, has nine items, and is commonly used for monitoring response to treatment as well as screening for depression.[18] Depression screening can be conducted quickly, using a two-step

screening process. The patient is asked the two questions of the PHQ-2 (the first two questions of the PHQ-9), which are then followed up with the PHQ-9 as needed. This two-step screen provides a balance of sensitivity and specificity.[20] The midwife can then provide primary care or refer the patient to a mental health specialist, depending on available resources.

Originally developed in the United Kingdom by Cox et al.,[19] the EPDS has been validated for use both in pregnancy and postpartum in diverse populations and in 18 languages (Table 7-4).[21] It consists of a self-report series of 10 questions that takes approximately 5 minutes to complete. This tool is freely available to any who want to use it. It also has a higher level of accuracy for individuals in low-resource settings compared to other tools. Evidence indicates that the EPDS is a reliable and valid measure for use in geographically diverse and non-English-speaking populations (and is now valid with men and those identifying as men). The EPDS, which also assesses for anxiety, can be used to monitor the effect of treatment in patients over the course of pregnancy and into the postpartum period (Figure 7-3).[22,23]

The Center for Epidemiologic Studies—Depression Scale (CES-D) and the Beck Depression Inventory (BDI) are two other screening tools for

| Table 7-3 | PHQ-9: Nine-Question Screen for Depression | | | | |
|---|---|---|---|---|---|
| **Over the last 2 weeks, how often have you been bothered by any of the following problems?** | | **Not at All** | **Several Days** | **More Than Half the Days** | **Nearly Every Day** |
| 1. Little interest or pleasure in doing things | | 0 | 1 | 2 | 3 |
| 2. Feeling down, depressed, or hopeless | | 0 | 1 | 2 | 3 |
| 3. Trouble falling or staying asleep, or sleeping too much | | 0 | 1 | 2 | 3 |
| 4. Feeling tired or having little energy | | 0 | 1 | 2 | 3 |
| 5. Poor appetite or overeating | | 0 | 1 | 2 | 3 |
| 6. Feeling bad about yourself or that you are a failure or have let yourself or your family down | | 0 | 1 | 2 | 3 |
| 7. Trouble concentrating on things, such as reading the newspaper or watching television | | 0 | 1 | 2 | 3 |
| 8. Moving or speaking so slowly that other people could have noticed; or the opposite—being so fidgety or restless that you have been moving around a lot more than usual | | 0 | 1 | 2 | 3 |
| 9. Thoughts that you would be better off dead, or of hurting yourself in some way | | 0 | 1 | 2 | 3 |
| | Column Totals | ____ | ____ | ____ | |
| | TOTAL SCORE | ____ | | | |

10. If you indicated any problems, how difficult have those problems made it for you to do your work, take care of things at home, or get along with other people?

☐ Not difficult at all   ☐ Somewhat difficult   ☐ Very difficult   ☐ Extremely difficult

| *Total Score* | *Depression Severity* |
|---|---|
| 1–4 | Minimal depression |
| 5–9 | Mild depression |
| 10–14 | Moderate depression |
| 15–19 | Moderately severe depression |
| 20–27 | Severe depression |

- Consider a depressive disorder if there are at least four responses in the shaded section (including Questions 1 and 2). Add up the score to determine severity.
- Consider a major depressive disorder if there are at least five responses in the shaded section (one of which corresponds to Question 1 or 2).
- Consider another depressive disorder if there are two to four responses in the shaded section (one of which corresponds to Question 1 or 2).

Abbreviation: PHQ-9, Patient Health Questionnaire-9.

Question 10 Note: All responses should be verified by the clinician. Diagnoses of major depressive disorder or other depressive disorder also require impairment of social, occupational, or other important areas of functioning (Question 10) and ruling out normal bereavement, a history of a manic episode (bipolar disorder), and a physical disorder, medication, or other drug as the biologic cause of the depressive symptoms.

Developed by Drs. Robert L. Spitzer, Janet B. W. Williams, Kurt Kroenke, and colleagues, with an educational grant from Pfizer Inc. http://www.phqscreeners.com.

| Table 7-4 | Edinburgh Postnatal Depression Scale |
|---|---|

1. I have been able to laugh and see the funny side of things.

**0** As much as I always could
**1** Not quite so much now
**2** Definitely not so much now
**3** Not at all

2. I have looked forward with enjoyment to things.

**0** As much as I ever did
**1** Rather less than I used to
**2** Definitely less than I used to
**3** Hardly at all

3. I have blamed myself unnecessarily when things went wrong.

**3** Yes, most of the time
**2** Yes, some of the time
**1** Not very often
**0** No, never

4. I have been anxious or worried for no good reason.

**0** No, not at all
**1** Hardly ever
**2** Yes, sometimes
**3** Yes, very often

5. I have felt scared or panicky for no good reason.

**3** Yes, quite a lot
**2** Yes, sometimes
**1** No, not much
**0** No, not at all

6. Things have been getting on top of me.

**3** Yes, most of the time I haven't been able to cope at all
**2** Yes, sometimes I haven't been coping as well as usual
**1** No, most of the time I have coped quite well
**0** No, I have been coping as well as ever

7. I have been so unhappy that I have had difficulty sleeping.

**3** Yes, most of the time
**2** Yes, quite often
**1** Not very often
**0** No, not at all

8. I have felt sad or miserable.

**3** Yes, most of the time
**2** Yes, quite often
**1** Not very often
**0** No, not at all

9. I have been so unhappy that I have been crying.

**3** Yes, most of the time
**2** Yes, quite often
**1** Only occasionally
**0** No, never

10. The thought of harming myself has occurred to me.

**3** Yes, quite often
**2** Sometimes
**1** Hardly ever
**0** Never

The scores for each item are totaled. Scores greater than 12 require evaluation and possible referral to a mental health specialist. Scores between 10 and 12 indicate the presence of symptoms of distress. The test should be repeated in 1 to 2 weeks and referral considered. Scores between 0 and 9 indicate that any symptoms of distress may be short-lived and are not likely to interfere with day-to-day function. If they persist more than 1 to 2 weeks, further evaluation is recommended.

Reproduced with permission from Cox JL, Holden JM, Sagovsky R, Detection of postnatal depression: development of the 10-item Edinburgh Postnatal Depression Scale. *Br J Psychiatry.* 1987;150:782-786.

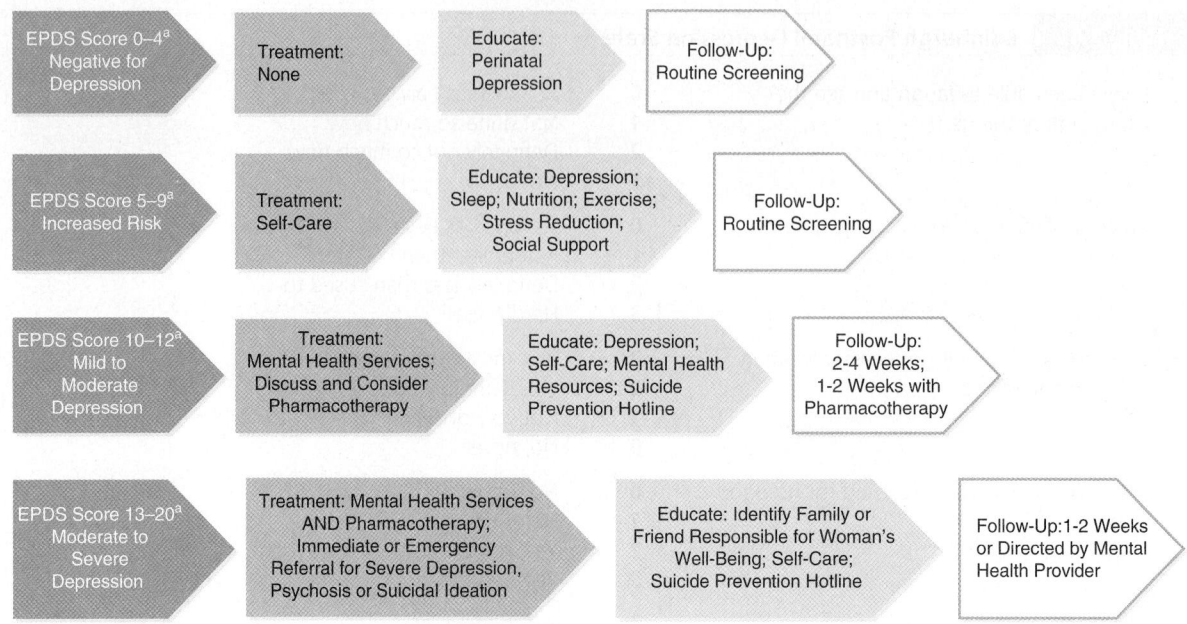

**Figure 7-3** Screening and treatment algorithm for perinatal depression.
Abbreviation: EPDS, Edinburgh Postnatal Depression Scale.
[a] Regardless of EPDS score, a response indicating thoughts of harming self or others should be addressed directly.
Reproduced with permission from Latendresse G, Deneris A. Selective serotonin reuptake inhibitors as first line antidepressant therapy for perinatal depression. *J Midwifery Womens Health.* 2017;62(3):317-328. © 2017, with permission from Wiley.

unipolar depression, and have similar sensitivities to the PHQ-9 and the EPDS. However, they have some drawbacks that can be prohibitive to using these tools in clinical practice. The CES-D is the longest of the commonly used screening instruments for depression, consisting of 20 questions, and the BDI is proprietary and requires a fee for each use.

All of the instruments mentioned in this chapter are written at the sixth-grade level and are easy to complete, and several can be completed and scored online. The accuracy of all these questionnaires is comparable for identifying individuals at risk for depression.[24]

Three points must be kept in mind when using one of these screening tools:

- The screening tools detect an increased risk for depression, but do not *diagnose* depression. The diagnosis is made via a more in-depth assessment by a mental health professional.

- Any answer that indicates the patient is severely depressed or may have suicidal ideation must be explored further and may be a medical emergency requiring immediate evaluation. Thus, screening should be done within a system that provides access to mental health providers.

- It is extremely important to distinguish unipolar depressive illness from bipolar depression, as the treatment and prognosis for these disorders are quite different, and because use of an antidepressant medication may exacerbate bipolar illness.[23]

## Suicidal Ideation and Intent

The midwife should always assess for suicidal ideation in patients who have screened positive for depression and in anyone who expresses a sense of hopelessness. Individuals with PTSD are at risk for suicide as well, with the greatest risk being found among women who have comorbid MDD.[25] Common statements that are red flags for suicidal ideation include "Life is not worth living," "My family would be better off without me," "I won't be around to deal with that," and "There is nothing I can do to make this better." Individuals at highest risk for suicide include those who have a specific plan or have access to the means to commit suicide, such as guns, cutting, or prescription or street drugs. Other risk factors for suicide include previous hospitalizations or suicide attempts; family history of suicide; a sense of hopelessness; experiencing family, romantic, or legal conflicts; social isolation; and insomnia.[26]

| Table 7-5 | Questions to Assess for Suicidal Ideation and Intent |
|---|---|
| **Question** | **Clinical Notes** |
| 1. Are you currently thinking about or have you recently thought about death or harming yourself? | If answer is yes, consider additional questions that assess frequency, intensity, and duration of suicidal ideation. |
| 2. Have you thought about how you would harm yourself? | If answer is yes, consider additional questions that assess frequency of suicidal thoughts about a possible method of suicide. |
| 3. Do you have access to a method such as gun and bullets or pills? | If answer is yes, consider additional questions that assess location of methods. |
| 4. Do you have any intention of following through with thoughts of self-harm? | If answer is yes, consider additional questions that assess:<br>• Preparatory acts (e.g., collected pills, wrote a suicide note, obtained a gun)<br>• Rehearsals for suicide (e.g., loading gun) versus non-suicidal self-injurious acts |

Screening instruments are used to identify individuals at risk for suicide. Although no single instrument is considered the best, or even the most frequently used, they all address the questions listed in Table 7-5. Midwives are mandatory reporters and must act to safeguard any patient deemed at risk for self-harm by transferring care when needed to emergency mental health services.

## Bipolar Disorders

Bipolar disorders are characterized by sustained extreme mood swings. Depression was defined earlier in the chapter. At the opposite end of the spectrum from depression exist mania and hypomania, which are characterized as a sustained abnormal increase in energy and activity. The criteria for diagnosis of mania include persistent elevated mood for at least a week, with symptoms such as inflated self-esteem, decreased need for sleep, flight of ideas, pressure to keep talking, and distractibility. The mood disturbance needs to interfere with social functioning and work or include psychotic features.[1] Even though bipolar disorders have a strong genetic component behind their etiology, the predominant theory behind the disorder is that multiple environmental, genetic, and neural processes play a role in lowering the threshold at which mood changes occur. Both phases of the disorder have adverse effects on thoughts, behaviors, judgment, and relationships. The onset of bipolar disorder symptoms occurs in late adolescence, and the disease process often occurs concomitantly with substance use disorder and other mental health diagnoses such as anxiety, personality disorders, and attention-deficit/hyperactivity disorder (ADHD).

Management of bipolar disorders is outside the scope of care for most primary care providers and midwives. Nevertheless, all providers must be able to screen for these conditions because improper treatment can exacerbate symptoms or worsen long-term prognosis. Bipolar disorders also share overlapping features with PTSD. Consequently, individuals are sometimes misdiagnosed and mistreated, and potential comorbidities can be overlooked, again highlighting the importance of utilizing the appropriate assessment tools by properly trained clinicians.

An individual with bipolar I disorder must meet the criteria for a manic episode. They may or may not experience major depressive episodes (as defined earlier in the chapter). Bipolar II disorder differs from bipolar I disorder in that the individual must meet the criteria for hypomania *and* must have met the criteria for a current or past major depressive episode.

Cyclothymic disorder (cyclothymia) is a separate condition from bipolar disorders that is characterized by multiple periods of hypomanic and depressive symptoms for at least 2 years, with periods of stable mood within that time that last less than 2 months. The symptoms cause significant distress or impairment in functioning but do not meet the full criteria for hypomania or MDD. This disorder is less prevalent than bipolar disorders are but its treatment is similar.

Some specific components of a patient's history should alert a primary care provider to the possibility of a bipolar disorder. These include onset of depression prior to age 18, history of suicide attempt, irritability or anger management issues, previous episodes of decreased need for sleep or food,

| Table 7-6 | Symptoms of Bipolar Disorder (DIGFAST) |
|---|---|

1. **D**istractibility, poorly focused, multitasking
2. **I**ndiscretion, risky behaviors
3. **G**randiosity, increased self-esteem
4. **F**light of ideas, racing thoughts
5. **A**ctivity, increase in goal directed activity
6. **S**leep, decreased need for sleep
7. **T**alkative

and a history of adverse response to antidepressant therapy. Further exploration of the patient's current mental status and family history will provide more information that can be used to determine the correct course of management going forward. As with the mnemonic for depression screening (SIGE-CAPS), a mnemonic is available to help the provider assess for signs and symptoms of bipolar disorder (DIGFAST) (Table 7-6).

### Screening Tool for Bipolar Disorder

The Mood Disorder Questionnaire is a 15-item validated self-report questionnaire that can be completed in less than 5 minutes and is designed to help providers identify patients with bipolar disorder.[27] It focuses on the symptoms of mania and hypomania. Most midwives and primary care providers will not provide psychiatric care for individuals with a bipolar diagnosis and likely will not use the questionnaire in their clinical practice, but they should be aware of its availability. The Mood Disorder Questionnaire should not be used for diagnostic purposes and has been shown to have a lower sensitivity rate for detection of illness than the screening tools used for MDD. Any positive screen should be followed up with a diagnostic evaluation by a trained provider.

## Anxiety Disorders

Anxiety disorders, a group of disorders characterized by anxiety and/or fear, include generalized anxiety disorder (GAD), panic disorder, and phobias (e.g., social anxiety disorder, specific phobias). Phobias are the most prevalent subcategory of anxiety disorders. As a group, anxiety disorders are more prevalent than mood disorders in the United States, yet they are less often screened for or detected in primary care practices.[28] Women are

almost twice as likely as men to experience both anxiety and mood disorders.[6] The diagnostic criteria for anxiety disorders includes significant stress; impairment of social, family, or occupational functioning; and fears that are out of proportion to any actual threat.

The reported lifetime prevalence of anxiety and its related disorders varies considerably from 14% to 33%, perhaps secondary to different survey techniques and populations used as samples in the various studies.[29,30] The overall prevalence of reported anxiety symptoms in the United States decreases with age, and women are more likely to experience any severity of symptoms than men. There is a dearth of data regarding racial and ethnic disparities in the documented prevalence of anxiety disorders in the United States, although the Centers for Disease Control and Prevention (CDC) does report that non-Hispanic white adults experience more generalized anxiety symptoms than other populations and non-Hispanic Asians report the least amount of anxiety symptoms.[30] Most of the research on anxiety has been conducted on European-white individuals, yet persons from underrepresented groups are less likely to have access to mental health services, are more likely to have comorbid conditions, and are differentially exposed to many of the risks for anxiety.[31] These factors need to be taken into consideration by clinicians, as they have significant repercussions for affected individuals.

All anxiety disorders, including obsessive–compulsive disorder (OCD), are frequently compounded by other anxiety or mood disorders—more so than other psychiatric disorders.[28] It is common to have a three-way interaction that involves anxiety disorders, depression, and somatic conditions, including respiratory disease, irritable bowel syndrome, chronic pain or malaise, fatigue, atopic disorders, and even cardiac disease. Anxiety disorders are highly internalizing conditions that contribute to associated somatic complaints such as palpitations, chest pain, shortness of breath, and dizziness.[32] These experiences mimic symptoms of other diseases or conditions, which leads to increased healthcare utilization and reduced quality of life for the individual.[28]

Phobias and OCD typically develop during childhood, adolescence, or early adulthood. Panic disorders and GAD have significant variations in age of onset.[30] Neuroimaging data suggest a significant neurobiologic contribution to the development of anxiety disorders.[32]

Until the *DSM-5* was published in 2013, PTSD was classified as an anxiety disorder. Elements of PTSD are shared with anxiety disorders and mood disorders.[33] However, distinct symptom and neuro-imaging patterns[34,35] and the external trauma etiologic factor led to creation of a new "Trauma-Related Disorders" classification. Symptoms that appear to be anxiety or depressed mood warrant assessment that extends into PTSD hallmarks to ensure the PTSD diagnosis is not missed.

While much public effort has been made to identify individuals with major depression, less attention has been directed at screening for individuals with anxiety disorders. An approach for evaluation of a suspected anxiety disorder that is recommended by the British Association for Psychopharmacology is presented in Figure 7-4.[36] The *DSM-5* includes a more complex algorithm that captures all possible differential diagnoses,[1] but the approach shown in the figure can be helpful for initial screening performed by a midwife.

## Phobias

A phobia is described as extreme or irrational fear or anxiety about a specific object or situation. This fear or anxiety is persistent, lasting more than 6 months.[1] Social anxiety disorder, also referred to as social phobia, is a specific phobia related to social situations in which the individual is exposed to potential scrutiny by others.[1] Studies suggest that phobias can be caused by a traumatic experience or may be learned behavior within a family environment. Parental stress, overprotection, hypercriticism, abuse, and neglect may all contribute to the development of social phobia.

## Generalized Anxiety Disorder

Generalized anxiety disorder is characterized by excessive worry or anxiety concerning family, health, finances, work, or school. As with all anxiety disorders, women are at greater risk for GAD compared to men.[30] GAD is associated with numerous somatic symptoms, leading to frequent primary care, specialist, and emergency department visits, and absences from work.

Generalized anxiety is characterized by the following signs:

- Excessive anxiety and worry (apprehensive expectation) about two (or more) domains of activities or events (e.g., family, health, finances, and school/work difficulties) occurs on more days than not, for 3 months or more.

- Anxiety and worry are difficult to control.

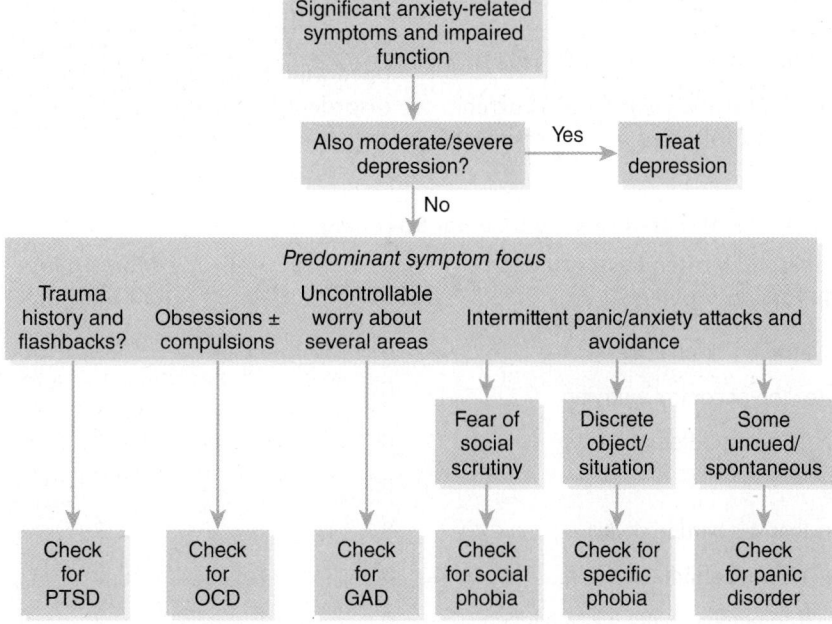

**Figure 7-4** One scheme for exploration of a suspected anxiety disorder.
Abbreviations: GAD, generalized anxiety disorder; OCD, obsessive–compulsive disorder; PTSD, post-traumatic stress disorder.
Reproduced with permission from Baldwin DS, Anderson IM, Nutt DJ, et al. Evidence-based pharmacological treatment of anxiety disorders, post-traumatic stress disorder and obsessive–compulsive disorder: a revision of the 2005 guidelines from the British Association for Psychopharmacology. *J Psychopharm.* 2014;28(5):403-439.

- Anxiety and worry are associated with restlessness and/or muscle tension.
- Anxiety and worry are associated with marked avoidance of activities or events with possible negative outcomes, excessive time and effort preparing for activities or events with possible negative outcomes, marked procrastination in behavior or decision making due to worries, and repeatedly seeking reassurance due to worries.[1]

## Panic Attacks

Panic attacks are periods of intense anxiety or fear that have a sudden onset. Although these attacks can be predicted to occur in the presence of a particular trigger, they can also occur unexpectedly. The symptoms of a panic attack are dramatic and usually frightening to the person who is experiencing the event. The attack usually peaks at approximately 10 minutes, but full recovery can take days. Symptoms can include sweating, trembling, or shaking, sensation of shortness of breath or smothering, nausea, chest pain or discomfort, dizziness, lightheadedness, unsteadiness or fainting, fear of losing control or going crazy, fear of dying, paresthesia, and chills or hot flashes. Individual attacks may occur in conjunction with any of the anxiety disorders, although the presence of recurrent attacks is characterized as panic disorder.[1]

## Panic Disorder

The primary symptom of panic disorder is recurrent unexpected panic attacks, followed by (1) persistent concern or worry about additional panic attacks or their consequences (e.g., losing control, having a heart attack, "going crazy") or (2) significant maladaptive change in behavior related to the attacks (e.g., behaviors designed to avoid having panic attacks, such as avoidance of exercise or unfamiliar situations).[1]

Individuals who experience frequent anxiety or have a history of being fearful are more likely to have panic disorder. Additional risk factors include childhood physical or sexual abuse, as well as parents with a history of depression, anxiety, or bipolar disorder. There may be a genetic component to panic disorder as well.

## Differential Diagnoses for Anxiety Disorders

As with MDD, anxiety disorders can present with symptoms that mimic or be compounded by some other common conditions such as MDD, substance abuse, hyperthyroidism, cardiac arrhythmias, and hyperglycemia or hypoglycemia. Careful screening and referral are crucial for proper diagnosis and treatment.

## Screening for Anxiety Disorders

In general, anxiety disorders are under-detected and, therefore, undertreated. Like the PHQ-2 and the PHQ-9 screening instruments, the GAD-2 and GAD-7 questionnaires (Table 7-7) have been developed and validated as means to screen for anxiety disorders. While the GAD-7 was initially developed specifically to screen for GAD, it has since been

| Table 7-7 | GAD-7: Generalized Anxiety Disorder Screening Tool | | | |
|---|---|---|---|---|
| Over the last 2 weeks, how often have you been bothered by the following problems? | Not at All | Several Days | More Than Half the Days | Nearly Every Day |
| 1. Feeling nervous, anxious, or on edge | 0 | 1 | 2 | 3 |
| 2. Not being able to stop or control worrying | 0 | 1 | 2 | 3 |
| 3. Worrying too much about different things | 0 | 1 | 2 | 3 |
| 4. Trouble relaxing | 0 | 1 | 2 | 3 |
| 5. Being so restless that it is hard to sit still | 0 | 1 | 2 | 3 |
| 6. Becoming easily annoyed or irritable | 0 | 1 | 2 | 3 |
| 7. Feeling afraid as if something awful might happen | 0 | 1 | 2 | 3 |
| **Column Scores** | _____ | _____ | _____ | _____ |
| Total Score (add column scores) _____ | | | | |
| Scores of 5, 10, and 15 are cut-off points for mild, moderate, and severe anxiety, respectively. Further evaluation is recommended for a score ≥ 10. | | | | |

Developed by Drs. Robert L. Spitzer, Janet B. W. Williams, Kurt Kroenke, and colleagues, with an educational grant from Pfizer Inc. http://www.phqscreeners.com.

validated as a screen for panic and social anxiety too.[37] This instrument was also found to be equally effective at screening among four racial/ethnic groups of undergraduate students: African American, white, Hispanic/Latinx, and Asian.[38] The GAD-2 questionnaire consists of the first two questions of the GAD-7, with a score 3 or higher suggesting the presence of an anxiety disorder.

## Substance Use Disorders

Although midwives will not likely be the provider who initially diagnoses a patient with a SUD, they will certainly care for these individuals in practice. It is crucial to understand the etiology of SUD, recognize it occurs alongside other mental health disorders, and be aware of how primary care providers and midwives can facilitate treatment and support for patients experiencing addiction issues. The prevalence of SUD co-occurring with other mental illness is very high. Roughly half of all individuals diagnosed with significant mental illness will also experience a SUD in their lifetime, and vice versa.[39] The existence of one mental health disorder with a comorbid substance use disorder is called a *dual diagnosis*. When a patient has a dual diagnosis, their symptoms are often more persistent and severe, and more treatment resistant, than in a person with either diagnosis alone.

The *Health Promotion Across the Lifespan* chapter addresses screening and counseling related to substance use, and the *Prenatal Care* chapter addresses substance use screening during pregnancy. The *DSM-5* classifies substance-related disorders according to the type of substance being used (e.g., alcohol, opioids, stimulants, tobacco). These disorders are further categorized on a continuum from mild to severe based on symptoms.

In general, use is described as "disordered" when the following criteria[1] are met:

- Cravings and/or tolerance exist.
- Use leads to clinically significant impairment and distress.
- A significant amount of time is spent obtaining and recovering from the substance.
- The substance is used in situations that are physically hazardous.
- Use persists despite social or interpersonal problems caused by or worsened by the substance.
- There is a persistent desire or effort to cut down or control use.

Substance use disorder is classified as a mental health disorder due to the fundamental changes that occur in the brain with addiction. These changes impact decision making, memory, and behavior. Individuals with SUD can demonstrate compulsive and impulsive behaviors in an effort to obtain and use substances, thereby exhibiting common hallmark features of other mental health disorders. While the effects of certain substances can mimic the symptoms of other mental health disorders, such as psychosis, delirium, and panic symptoms, the permanent change in brain function also predisposes an individual to developing other significant mental illness.

The etiology of SUD is similar to that of other mental health disorders. Genetic vulnerability may predispose someone to dependency and can also alter how individuals cope with stress. In addition, evidence suggests that racial and socioeconomic inequities in individuals' environment may give rise to substance use.[40] Increased access and exposure to drugs, poverty, and trauma all increase the propensity for developing SUD. Chronic stress is thought to activate the HPA axis, changing dopamine signals, which reinforces the properties of certain drugs.[39] In 2021, the American Society of Addiction Medicine released a public policy statement addressing racial justice in addiction medicine. Among other things, they call for training and practice that acknowledges a patient's experience of racism, training for trauma-informed care, recognition of social determinants of health that are linked to racism, and policies that ensure equitable access to prevention and treatment programs.[41] Chronic stress has also been shown to induce changes in gene expression and impact behavior, further increasing the individual's vulnerability to developing SUD. This is a result of long-term genetic adaptation, influencing gene expression. Fortunately, evidence exists that these changes can be reversed with environmental interventions.

While SUD can alter brain function, predisposing someone to developing other mental health disorders, it is important to note that having significant mental illness, such as schizophrenia, anxiety, depression, or PTSD, can contribute to substance use and the development of SUD. Often, individuals self-medicate to temporarily minimize the symptoms of mental illness. Mental illness causes changes in brain activity (as does substance use) and subsequently enhances the "reward" effect of substances while decreasing awareness of the adverse effects associated with the same substance.

The vast majority of overdose-related deaths in the United States involve opioid use, with nearly 76,000 people dying from this cause in 2020 alone.[42] The CDC has declared this issue to be an epidemic because of the alarming rates of hospitalization and deaths caused by misuse and overuse of opioids and synthetic opioids. Current treatment standards for opioid use disorder include opioid agonist therapy along with counseling and behavioral therapies to assist with treatment and sustain recovery.

Three medications are approved for treatment of opioid dependence: methadone, naltrexone, and buprenorphine. Methadone is a synthetic opioid agonist that works to eliminate withdrawal symptoms and cravings. Unfortunately, it can be dispensed only by specialized treatment centers, which usually do not provide primary care or perinatal care. These regulations can become prohibitive, especially for individuals in rural communities who need treatment.

Naltrexone works to block the euphoric and sedative effects of opioids and may reduce cravings. It is approved for use in treatment of opioid use disorders, but only in an intramuscular extended-release form, which requires a risk evaluation and mitigation strategy (REMS) to ensure proper and safe use of the medication. Again, this restriction creates barriers to accessing treatment.

Buprenorphine is a partial opioid agonist, binding to the same opioid receptors as methadone albeit less strongly. Like methadone, it works to reduce cravings and withdrawal symptoms, but has fewer side effects. Most often, buprenorphine is administered orally in combination with naloxone, which is an opioid antagonist. When injected, the naloxone component has increased bioavailability and produces uncomfortable withdrawal symptoms—a phenomenon that helps to prevent diversion or misuse of buprenorphine. Buprenorphine is more readily accessible than either of the other opioid agonist treatment options.

In 2016, the Comprehensive Addiction and Recovery Act was authorized. It increased allocation of funds toward fighting the opioid epidemic and expanded access to buprenorphine by expanding the number of patients on opioid agonist therapy a prescriber can have as well as the list of providers who can prescribe the medication. Midwives were inadvertently left out of the initial legislation, though this omission was amended in 2018. Acknowledging continued barriers to prescribing buprenorphine, in 2021 the U.S. government removed the requirement for providers to complete specific certification requirements to prescribe buprenorphine if they maintain a limited number of qualifying patients in their practice. This greatly improves access to opioid agonist therapy in the primary care setting and acknowledges that midwives care for populations disproportionately affected by the country's opioid epidemic.

## Trauma- and Stressor-Related Disorders

Trauma is now understood to be an etiology of significant mental health morbidity, both in the immediate 1-month period after the traumatic event (i.e., acute stress disorder) and over the long term (e.g., PTSD). In the World Mental Health Survey of 68,894 people in 24 countries, 70% of adults reported that they had experienced a significant trauma exposure.[43] In the United States, 7.8% of adults have had PTSD in their lifetime.[4] Through its guidelines, SAMHSA has led the social care sector toward providing "trauma-informed care" as a standard approach because the vast majority of people using mental health, substance use, or other social services have been exposed to a traumatic event. Trauma that is unresolved can lead to distress and impairment in social, family, and school or work functioning as well as to mental health problems. SAMHSA defines trauma as follows:

> *Individual trauma results from an event, series of events, or set of circumstances that is experienced by an individual as physically or emotionally harmful or life threatening and that has lasting adverse effects on the individual's functioning and mental, physical, social, emotional, or spiritual well-being.*[9p7]

The pattern over time, or "natural history," of PTSD begins with trauma exposure, followed by acute stress disorder; the acute distress order usually resolves but can persist beyond the 1-month period and evolve into PTSD, which becomes chronic (persisting or recurring) in more than half of cases.[4] When PTSD persists, depression comorbidity often accrues as a secondary disorder,[44] and affected individuals may turn to substance use and misuse in an effort to manage the noxious symptoms of PTSD and low mood.[45] PTSD also is associated with suicide.[46] Among people whose PTSD stems from relational trauma in early life, such as childhood abuse or neglect, some develop a complex form of PTSD that includes dissociation. This dissociative subtype affects 14% of people with PTSD.[47] It is characterized by reacting to stress or an overwhelming environment with altered consciousness—that is, an out-of-body experience or a sense that what is happening is not real.

Developing PTSD after trauma exposure is not inevitable. Though individuals' specific outcomes depend on the extent of life threat or intrusion upon body integrity during the trauma, most people will be resilient or will recover. Although resilience comes to some extent from personal attributes (e.g., engaged coping style), it is increasingly understood that resilience to trauma depends strongly on a person's context (e.g., social support, safety, resources).[48] It is also useful to know that PTSD symptoms can remit but recur when something "triggers" a reminder of the trauma. PTSD can also occur with delayed onset; that is, the person can become symptomatic long after the exposure if a life event (e.g., death of an abuser, birth of a child) triggers PTSD reactions for the first time.

Risks of developing PTSD are not equal across a population. Risk for PTSD varies by sex and gender in ways not yet fully understood. The research to date, which has been largely conducted in binary groups, consistently shows that women develop PTSD at twice the rate of men (10.4% versus 5.0%).[4] Trauma exposure, and therefore risk for PTSD, is also higher among marginalized groups such as LGBTQ people and Black, Indigenous, and People of Color (BIPOC), incarcerated people, and asylum seekers and refugees, all of whom experience human rights violations, discrimination, micro-aggressions, and hate crimes. Post-traumatic stress is transmissible across generations in the forms of historical trauma (e.g., slavery, forced migration, genocide) and intrafamilial violence and abuse.[49] Causal factors include family context, the trauma exposure itself, female sex, ancestry, and gene-by-environment interaction.[34]

PTSD is the only diagnosis in the field of psychiatry that includes an exogenous factor (trauma) in its etiology. The *DSM-5* diagnostic criterion "A" defines qualifying trauma as "exposure to actual or threatened death, serious injury, or sexual violence" by direct experiencing, witnessing, learning that it occurred to a close family member or friend, or experiencing it repeatedly due to one's work role (e.g., first responder).[1] It is worth noting that APA's definition excludes forms of childhood abuse and neglect, making the diagnosis restrictive, and leading many professionals to seek work-arounds for getting people with maltreatment-related PTSD access to services that depend on a diagnosis.

## Acute Stress Disorder

Acute stress disorder is defined as "the development of specific fear behaviors that last from three days to one month after a traumatic event."[1] Rates of this disorder vary from 19% of people exposed to any kind of trauma to 59% of those exposed to rape.[1] Making this diagnosis is useful because with a diagnosis it becomes possible to gain access to therapy.[50] In the immediate aftermath of a trauma exposure,

mental health treatment and support usually are directed at preventing PTSD or other long-term sequelae of the traumatic event. The symptoms of acute stress disorder are similar to those of PTSD, except that dissociation symptoms are also on the list (e.g., feeling numb, feeling detached from others, not recalling parts of the trauma). The main distinction is that acute stress disorder is considered to end at 1 month; at that point, it is appropriate to assess for PTSD if symptoms linger.

## Post-Traumatic Stress Disorder

As with other disorders, diagnosis of PTSD is best made by a mental health professional. PTSD is a syndrome with eight criteria that must be met to make the diagnosis. Examples of criteria associated with the traumatic events include avoidance of stimuli, intrusive symptoms, negative alterations of mood, and alterations in reactivity.[1] Although a minimum of six symptoms across the four clusters is required to meet the diagnostic threshold, partial PTSD is associated with impairment and care-seeking at levels similar to full diagnosis.[51] The syndrome includes several elements that must occur in relation to the original trauma exposure.

PTSD is a complex syndrome that is among the common mental health disorders, yet it remains an oft-missed diagnosis.[52] Thus, screening and making a referral that states the patient's trauma history and the provider's suspicion of PTSD strongly enhances the likelihood of accurate evaluation and evidence-based treatment.

Even without having a firm diagnosis of PTSD, providers who suspect PTSD are well positioned to provide trauma-informed care and offer adaptations to decrease the likelihood that individuals with past trauma and some post-traumatic stress reactions will be triggered by the care they receive. PTSD is strongly associated with early morbidity in multiple body systems (e.g., immune, cardiorespiratory, metabolic, neuroendocrine), so the ability to seek healthcare services depends on receiving trauma-informed care. In primary care, the focus of trauma-informed care means the impact of PTSD on the individual's life and healthcare experience is being understood and addressed knowledgeably.

### Screening for Trauma History and PTSD

Screening for trauma history and PTSD can involve choosing and pairing two tools—a trauma history questionnaire and a PTSD symptom screener. Clinically, a main reason for inquiring about past trauma is to start a conversation with the patient about potential triggers to avoid. In healthcare settings, screening for adverse childhood experiences (ACEs) is nearly always salient. Other trauma exposures can be asked about depending on whether they are likely to be related to the care being provided. Examples of other trauma exposures that may affect care offered in primary care and reproductive healthcare settings include adult sexual assault, intimate-partner violence, prior perinatal loss, prior traumatic birth, prior medical trauma (e.g., life threatening, disrespectful, uncontrolled pain or fear), and discrimination in health care. Including an item that asks "Other?" and allows space to explain on the questionnaire is also often useful.

The ACEs Questionnaire, developed by the California Surgeon General's Office and designed for ease of use in healthcare settings, is freely available.[53] Screening for PTSD symptoms should follow a positive trauma history disclosure. The National Center for PTSD also has freely available, reliable, valid PTSD screeners. The Primary Care PTSD Screen for *DSM-5* (PC-PTSD-5) is available from this source and is widely used.[54] Although the PC-PTSD-5 validation studies set a cut-off of four "yes" answers, researchers found that three or even two "yes" answers is a more accurate cut-off for women.[54,55]

A positive screen should lead to referral to a mental health professional for a diagnostic interview and treatment with an evidence-based therapy for PTSD. However, PTSD is a "disorder of avoidance"; indeed, avoiding reminders of the trauma is one of the diagnostic criteria for this condition. It is not surprising that many people avoid treatment for PTSD because it is likely to involve talking about and reexperiencing the sensations and emotions of the past trauma. Demonstrating empathy in case of a declined referral leaves the door open to further discussions about PTSD-related needs in the reproductive health and primary care settings.

## Menstruation-Related Mood Changes

Mental health disturbances related to the menstrual cycle are divided into "core" and "variant" groups (Table 7-8).[1,56] The core premenstrual disorders include premenstrual syndrome (PMS) and premenstrual dysphoric disorder (PMDD). Approximately 20% to 30% of menstruating people have PMS, and 3% to 9% meet the criteria for PMDD.[57] Variant premenstrual disorders include those not associated with a regular ovulatory cycle.

## Premenstrual Syndrome and Premenstrual Dysphoric Disorder

The core premenstrual disorders are defined by the timing of somatic and/or psychological symptoms that occur during all or part of the 2-week premenstrual phase and resolve during or after menses starts in individuals with ovulatory cycles. Patients with any one of these disorders have a symptom-free interval between menses and ovulation.

The etiology of premenstrual disorders is poorly understood, but cyclic changes in progesterone and estrogen levels appear to trigger the symptoms. Premenstrual disorders share features associated with anxiety and depression, which have been linked to serotonergic dysregulation. It is thought that changes in estrogen and progesterone levels affect serotonin and dopamine levels, although other neurotransmitters may also be involved.[57] Recent research suggests PMDD may be the result of extreme neurologic sensitivity to normal hormone variations.[58] Genetic vulnerability is thought to also play a role in determining which people experience PMDD.[59]

Diagnosis of PMS or PMDD is based on the amount, severity, cyclicity, and chronicity of symptoms.[56,60,61] The Daily Record of Severity of Problems, an instrument validated by Endicott et al., is the most widely used daily symptom scale because it measures all 11 of the *DSM-5* symptoms of PMDD.[62] This record can be printed and used by patients to record their symptoms over a few months. Smartphone users also now have access to many different applications to help them track symptoms over time, which can be helpful when discussing their cycles with a provider. Diagnostic and laboratory testing should be done to rule out other conditions that can cause symptoms similar to PMS and PMDD, such as anemia, hypothyroidism, migraine, and endometriosis.

PMDD is a the most severe, yet least common, of the menstrual disorders. The most frequent and disabling symptoms of PMDD are extreme irritability and mood lability. Disordered sleep (either insomnia or hypersomnia) and extreme changes in tension or energy have also been reported. Confusion and alterations in mental status are prominent features of PMDD, which can result in affected individuals being unable to work. Patients experiencing PMDD may have difficulty with relationships on the days that they are symptomatic. They may also experience comorbidity of their PMDD with other mood or anxiety disorders such as MDD, bipolar disorder, or OCD.[63]

| Table 7-8 | Classification of Premenstrual Disorders: Consensus Criteria of the International Society for Premenstrual Disorders |
|---|---|
| **Definition** | **Characteristics** |
| **Core Premenstrual Disorders** | |
| Premenstrual syndrome (PMS) | Multiple symptoms appear only during the luteal phase of an ovulatory cycle and are relieved within 4 days of the onset of menses without recurrence until the approximate time of ovulation. ACOG requires at least one affective symptom and one somatic symptom for diagnosis.[a] |
| | Must not be an exacerbation of another condition. Symptoms are not severe enough to interfere with daily function and cause significant distress. Affective symptoms include angry outbursts, anxiety, depression, irritability, confusion, and social withdrawal. Somatic symptoms include abdominal bloating, breast tenderness, headache, joint or muscle pain, extremity swelling, and weight gain. |
| Premenstrual dysphoric disorder (PMDD) | Classified separately from PMS based on severe psychological symptoms that occur during the luteal phase and remit entirely during the rest of the menstrual cycle.[b] |
| | • At least five symptoms are present in the final week before menses. They improve within a few days of the onset of menses, and become minimal or absent in the week after menses. |
| | • One or more of the following symptoms must be present: marked affective lability, marked irritability, marked depressed mood, and marked anxiety or tension. |
| | • One or more of the following must be present to reach the total of five symptoms: decreased interest in usual activities, difficulty concentrating, lethargy, change in appetite, hypersomnia or insomnia, sense of being overwhelmed, and physical symptoms such as breast tenderness or abdominal bloating. |
| | • Symptoms are associated with significant distress and are not an exacerbation of another disorder or attributable to the effects of a substance or medication. |
| **Variant Premenstrual Disorders** | |
| Premenstrual exacerbation | Luteal-phase exacerbation of another condition such as depression, diabetes, migraine, epilepsy, or asthma |
| Nonovulatory premenstrual disorders | Symptoms result from ovarian activity other than ovulation. |
| Progesterone-induced premenstrual disorders | Women receiving exogenous progestogens may develop PMS symptoms. |
| Premenstrual disorders without menstruation | Symptoms arise from continuous ovarian activity, although menstruation is suppressed. |

Abbreviation: ACOG, American College of Obstetricians and Gynecologists.

[a] Diagnosis is based on structured interview, self-report, and prospective recording of at least two menstrual cycles.

[b] See *DSM-5* for a full description of the diagnostic criteria for PMDD.

Based on American Psychiatric Association. *Diagnostic and Statistical Manual of Mental Disorders.* 5th ed. Arlington, VA: American Psychiatric Association; 2013; Ismaili E, Walsh S, O'Brien PMS, et al. Fourth consensus of the International Society for Premenstrual Disorders (ISPMD): auditable standard for diagnosis and management of premenstrual disorder. *Arch Womens Mental Health.* 2016;19:953-958.

## Premenstrual Exacerbation of Psychiatric Conditions

Mood disorders can worsen in the premenstrual period and can mimic PMDD symptoms. Many patients who present with a concern about PMDD actually have an underlying mood disorder. Reviewing the patient's daily symptom diary can be the key in distinguishing between PMDD and another psychiatric diagnosis.

## Borderline Personality Disorder

Personality disorders in general are characterized as rigid and unhealthy patterns of thinking, functioning, and behavior. Often the individuals exhibiting these behaviors see nothing wrong or out of the ordinary with how they react to others and blame everyone but themselves for challenges they face in life. This causes significant issues with maintaining both relationships and employment and can lead to social isolation and substance use issues. Like other mental health disorders, personality disorders are thought to stem from both genetic and environmental influences, specifically trauma and neglect in childhood.

Borderline personality disorder is one of the 10 personality disorders classified by the *DSM-5*. It presents as a long-standing pattern of instability with interpersonal relationships and self-image, along with extreme impulsivity. Individuals with this disorder have an intense fear of abandonment (real or imagined), chronic feelings of emptiness, marked mood reactivity, recurrent suicidal or self-harming behavior or threats, and inappropriate anger. They often experience paranoia or dissociative symptoms and see the world in extremes, such as all good or all bad characteristics. Because of common comorbidities such as substance abuse, anxiety, and bipolar disorder, borderline personality disorder can be missed or misdiagnosed.

In the healthcare setting, individuals with this disorder have historically been labeled as "difficult patients" rather than as someone with a diagnosable mental health condition. It is important to remember that patients with borderline personality disorder have difficulties with boundaries in all types of relationships, including with their providers. Providers should take care to set clear boundaries with all patients, avoid responding to difficult or provocative behaviors, and encourage continuity of care between as few providers as possible when interacting with patients with borderline personality disorder.

## Attention-Deficit/Hyperactivity Disorder

Attention-deficit/hyperactivity disorder (ADHD) is a diagnosis usually made in childhood or adolescence due to its effect on academic performance. Hallmark inattention symptoms include impulsivity, difficulty organizing tasks, being easily distracted, inability to pay attention to details or sustain attention in professional or academic settings, and failure to follow through on instructions. Hyperactivity symptoms include difficulty sitting still, excessive talking, interrupting others, and chronic feelings of restlessness. There is a strong genetic component to the risk for ADHD. Prevalence estimates suggest that between 2.5% and 5% of U.S. adults have ADHD, with a marked increase in the rate of diagnosis occurring over the past 20 years.[64] With or without a formal diagnosis, this disorder presents in adulthood along with psychosocial dysfunction, substance abuse, nicotine use, and increased suicide rates. The results of the World Mental Health Survey indicate that 18% of adults with ADHD meet criteria for three or more other mental health conditions.[64]

If a patient presents for care with concern for ADHD or symptoms consistent with this disorder, they should be referred for further evaluation by a psychiatric provider. Diagnosis is made by a comprehensive clinical assessment, a clinical interview, and occasionally a physical exam. If the individual already has a historical diagnosis of ADHD, the midwife can suggest psychosocial interventions to limit the disorder's impact, and should refer the patient for proper medication management. The standard treatment for adult ADHD is stimulant medications—controlled substances that are often subject to diversion or misuse. For this reason, it is unlikely that a midwife will manage ADHD treatment, especially on a long-term basis.

## Treatment of Mental Health Disorders

The two primary therapeutic modalities for most mental health disorders are psychotherapy and pharmacotherapy. Several different forms of psychotherapy exist, and several different classes of drugs have effects on the neurotransmitters relevant to mental health disorders. For some conditions, such as depression, a combination of pharmacotherapy and psychotherapy is most effective as treatment; for others, such as anxiety disorders, psychotherapy is considered to be more effective.

In brief, psychotherapy helps individuals understand emotions, behaviors, and ideas that contribute to their mental health, and identifies ways to help modify emotions, behaviors, and/or ideas. Therapy can be conducted individually, in groups, or for the family unit. Table 7-9 summarizes the primary forms of psychotherapy used to treat the most common mental health conditions that a midwife may identify in clinical practice.

Cognitive-behavioral therapy (CBT)—a time-limited therapy that aims to change maladaptive patterns of thinking and behaviors—has been the

| Table 7-9 | Common Types of Psychotherapy | |
|---|---|---|
| **Therapy** | **Description** | **Conditions for Which Effectiveness Is Established** |
| Cognitive-behavioral therapy (CBT) | Well-established, effective short-term therapy. Focus is on identifying and changing thinking and behavior patterns. Benefits are usually seen in 12–16 weeks. Therapy may involve reading and keeping records between therapy sessions. | Depression[a] <br> Anxiety disorders <br> Eating disorders <br> Phobias |
| Exposure therapy | A form of CBT. Exposure therapy is used to reduce anxiety and fear responses via gradual or simulated exposure to the anxiety-provoking stimulus. | Phobias <br> Obsessive–compulsive disorder <br> Post-traumatic stress disorder |
| Dialectical behavioral therapy | A blend of CBT and Eastern meditation that focuses on combining acceptance and change. May include individual and group therapy. Originally developed for persons with suicidal thoughts. Useful for anyone with high emotional reactivity. | Depression[a] <br> Panic disorder <br> Post-traumatic stress disorder <br> Eating disorders <br> Obsessive–compulsive disorder |
| Interpersonal therapy | Limited structured therapy usually delivered over a 16-week period. Focuses on how interpersonal difficulties affect mental health and, in particular, depression. | Depression[a] |
| Eye-movement desensitization and reprocessing (EMDR) | Eye movement training and focus on external stimuli can reduce the intensity of disturbing thoughts. EMDR may be similar to what happens during rapid eye movement (REM) sleep. | Post-traumatic stress disorder <br> Panic attacks <br> Phobias |

[a] Includes perinatal depression.

subject of the most research and is effective for treating individuals with major depressive disorders and anxiety disorders. Topics, or "lessons," for sessions often include psychoeducation, behavioral activation, cognitive restructuring, problem solving, graded exposure, relapse prevention, and assertiveness skills. While CBT has traditionally been delivered by mental health specialists, the scarcity of such providers has limited its impact. More recently, CBT has been delivered or supported by primary care providers, specially trained nurses, and social workers. In this approach, therapy may be delivered face-to-face, virtually, or as a computer-based program.

Because the first-line medication treatment for most anxiety disorders (GAD, panic disorder, social anxiety disorder) and unipolar mood disorders (MDD, dysthymia, PMDD) is the same, this chapter will sometimes refer to these medications as "antidepressants," regardless of their intended use.

Antidepressant medications are formulated to target the neurotransmitters that play a role in mood regulation—namely, serotonin, norepinephrine, and dopamine. The psychotropic medications most commonly used to treat unipolar mood and anxiety disorders are selective serotonin reuptake inhibitors (SSRIs). Other prescription antidepressant medications target norepinephrine and dopamine, either in combination with serotonin or alone. Figure 7-5 depicts the effects and interactions of these neurotransmitters.[65]

Although neurotransmitters have many complex functions, they exert those functions only when released into the synaptic space between neurons. SSRIs, which block reuptake and subsequent degradation of the neurotransmitter into the presynaptic neuron, ensure increased availability of serotonin. A downstream effect of increased serotonin availability is believed to be responsible for the reduction in symptoms linked to SSRIs. This chapter presents a broad overview of these therapies for midwives who may collaborate with a mental healthcare professional in the care of patients with the more common mental health disorders.

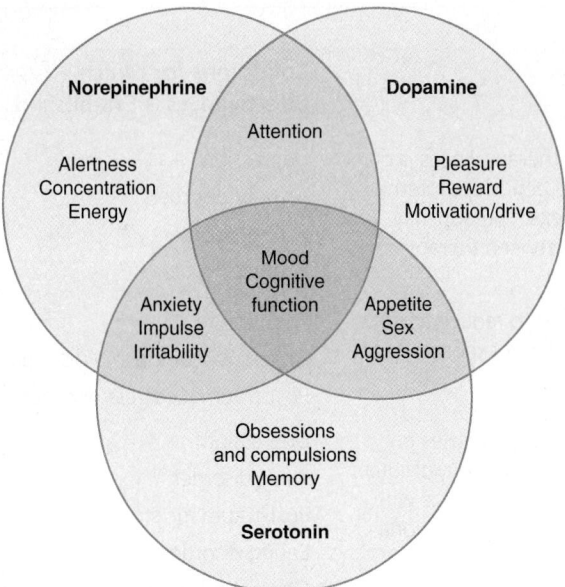

**Figure 7-5** Role of dopamine, norepinephrine, and serotonin. Reproduced with permission from Early NK. Mental health. In: Brucker MC, King TL, eds. *Pharmacology for Women's Health*. 2nd ed. Burlington, MA: Jones & Bartlett Learning; 2017:727-764.

## Treatment of Unipolar Mood and Anxiety Disorders

Many treatment modalities exist for patients with depression and anxiety, including CBT, counseling, faith-based therapy, group work, complementary therapies, and psychotropic medications. Education and recommendations for sleep hygiene, participation in pleasurable activities, and exercise are beneficial adjuncts to other interventions.[66,67] Regardless of the treatment modality selected, the goal is not just a reduction of symptoms, but full remission of those symptoms.

The decision to initiate treatment with psychotherapy or medication is based on many factors, such as the affected individual's preferences, severity of depression, access to and acceptability of counseling, insurance coverage, and the individual's ability to commit to the time involved in therapy. Medication and psychotherapy are associated with similar rates of initial improvement for individuals with an MDD diagnosis, but the combination of the two improves quality of life and acceptability among patients.[68,69] Current guidelines published in the United States recommend psychotherapy and pharmacotherapy in combination for treatment of MDD when possible.[67] This improves the likelihood of remission and decreases the risk of relapse. The effectiveness of pharmacotherapy compared to psychotherapy is similar for individuals with anxiety

disorders as well, and combined therapy has been shown to have the highest success rate in treating them.[70] Pharmacotherapy should be the initial therapy for anyone with severe major depression or any debilitating anxiety that affects daily functioning.[67]

More patients with persistent depressive disorder (PDD) have symptoms considered resistant to treatment. However, this may be due to a combination of inadequate dose or duration or poor adherence to taking medication.[71] A combination of psychotherapy and psychopharmacology is preferred by patients and improves life functioning and cost-effectiveness.[71]

### Psychotherapy

Several types of psychotherapy are available for treating persons with MDD and anxiety disorders. To date, CBT has the most evidence for its effectiveness in treatment of MDD.[72] CBT, mindfulness-based cognitive therapy, exposure-based therapy, and therapist-supported Internet-based and video-conferencing CBT have all been found to be effective for treatment of women with anxiety.[73–75]

Most midwifery practices are not structured to provide ongoing psychotherapy. Nevertheless, the midwife's responsibility for follow-up continues even after referral to a mental health specialist to ensure continuity of care and follow-through with further treatment. The midwife may also be uniquely situated to provide targeted time-limited counseling from having developed an ongoing therapeutic relationship with the patient. This relationship provides an opportunity to discuss behaviors that may improve depression symptoms, such as adequate sleep, exercise,[66,76] and engaging in pleasurable activities, also known as behavioral activation.

### Pharmacologic Therapies

Due to the challenges of entering into and following through with psychotherapy, many individuals with depression and anxiety will opt to initiate pharmacotherapy rather than counseling when seeking treatment. Prior to beginning pharmacotherapy for depression or anxiety, it is critical that the clinician has ruled out bipolar disorder, as treatment with an antidepressant may trigger mania,[77] suicidal ideation, or psychosis in persons with this condition.[65]

Second-generation antidepressants, which include SSRIs, norepinephrine–dopamine reuptake inhibitors (NDRIs), and serotonin–norepinephrine reuptake inhibitors (SNRIs), are the first-line medications for treating depression.[78] SSRIs and SNRIs are the first-line treatments for anxiety. The dosages for the treatment of anxiety disorders are similar to those for depression. These agents have been well studied, are safe and effective, and are well tolerated overall.

Research has failed to demonstrate significant differences in effectiveness among the various SSRIs, SNRIs, and NDRIs.[78] The choice of medication to initiate therapy is based on several factors, including the patient's preferences, past history of antidepressant use and effects noted, concurrent medications and their potential risk of interactions, family members' response to specific medications, and plans for pregnancy or breastfeeding in the near future. An additional consideration when choosing a specific therapy is the patient's ability to consistently take medication as prescribed, because abrupt discontinuation of antidepressants with a shorter half-life can lead to serotonin withdrawal (or discontinuation) syndrome—an uncomfortable constellation of symptoms including dizziness, ataxia, agitation, headache, tremor, and confusion.[15]

It may take up to 4 weeks for an individual to show a noticeable or measurable response to antidepressant therapy. If no clinical response occurs by 6 weeks of treatment at a therapeutic dose, there is a low likelihood of eventual response and switching to another medication in the same class may be indicated.[78] Further treatment of patients who fail to respond to initial therapy or after two trials of antidepressants is best managed with referral to, or in consultation with, a psychiatric provider.

Another choice for depression treatment is bupropion (Wellbutrin, Zyban), an NDRI that has fewer sexual side effects compared to SSRIs. This medication is an appropriate for treatment of depression in adults 18 years or older, but has no therapeutic effect on anxiety and may actually aggravate those symptoms.[78] Bupropion lowers the threshold for seizures, so it should not be used with other medications that also lower the seizure threshold or for individuals with risk factors for seizures.

Benzodiazepines, usually clonazepam (Klonopin) or lorazepam (Ativan), may be beneficial for short-term use by patients with significant impairment from anxiety while waiting for the therapeutic effect of an SSRI to begin.[79] These medications can also be useful for the episodic treatment of individuals with panic disorder. Benzodiazepines can lead to dependency, cause drowsiness, may aggravate depression, and should be used with caution with older adults. These risks must be balanced against the benefits that benzodiazepines can offer with short-term or intermittent use.

Older-generation antidepressant medications include monoamine oxidase inhibitors and tricyclic antidepressants. These psychotropic medications have a narrow therapeutic range, a potential for high toxicity, and serious interactions with many foods and other medications. Because of these limitations, they are rarely prescribed by primary care providers.

### Antidepressant Medications: Common Side Effects

All of the SSRIs and SNRIs may cause gastrointestinal upset, jitteriness, and headache after their initiation as the body adapts to higher levels of neurotransmitters. Within approximately 2 weeks, the receptors are desensitized and downregulated, leading to the disappearance or significant decrease in these symptoms.[65] Psychotropic medications should always be started at a low dose for the first 1 to 2 weeks to minimize the initiation side effects. The lower dose, when accompanied by anticipatory guidance, will improve the likelihood of patients continuing the medication as directed. Table 7-10 lists other drug-specific side effects related to the most commonly used antidepressant medications. Weight gain and sleep disturbances are commonly reported side effects of long-term antidepressant use. Management strategies for bothersome side effects include waiting for spontaneous resolution, reducing or dividing the dose, or ultimately switching to another antidepressant.

Sexual side effects are also commonly reported with SSRI and SNRI use, affecting as many as 65% of adult women treated with these medications.[80] These side effects include decreased libido, anorgasmia, and erectile dysfunction. Anticipatory counseling is essential prior to initiating therapy with antidepressants so that patients are aware of this possible effect. Sometimes the initial sexual dysfunction resolves spontaneously with time, but management strategies also include lowering the dose of medication, switching to a different antidepressant, and augmenting the antidepressant with bupropion. This last option may fall outside the scope of midwifery care in many practices, but primary care providers should be aware of management options and know when to refer patients for further treatment or adjustment of medications.

### Antidepressant Medications: Adverse Effects and Drug–Drug Interactions

Serotonin syndrome is a potentially life-threatening reaction that results from excess serotonergic

| Table 7-10 | Antidepressant Medications Prescribed by Primary Care Providers | | | |
|---|---|---|---|---|
| **Generic Agent (Brand Name)** | **Starting Dose** | **Dosage Range and Maximum Dose** | **Side-Effect Profile** | **Pharmacokinetic Half-Life** |
| **Selective Serotonin Reuptake Inhibitors** | | | | |
| Citalopram (Celexa) | 10–20 mg/day for 7 days, then may increase to 40 mg/day. Maintain initial dose for 4 weeks before increasing it. | 20–40 mg/day | Minimal drug interactions. Weight gain is common, and more likely after 6 months of use. Good choice for those with anxiety and who are pregnant. May cause QT prolongation.<br><br>Lowest risk for liver toxicity; higher risk for sexual dysfunction. | Half-life of 35 hours; few metabolites |
| Escitalopram (Lexapro) | 5–10 mg to start. Increase to 20 mg if partial response after 4 weeks. | 10–20 mg/day | Minimal drug interactions. Weight is gain common, and more likely after 6 months of use. Good choice for patients with anxiety in pregnancy. May cause QT prolongation. | Half-life of 27–32 hours |
| Fluoxetine (Prozac) | 10–20 mg/day; may increase to 20 mg/day after 7 days. Maintain at 20 mg/day for 4–6 weeks; then 30 mg for 2–4 weeks before additional increases. | 20–80 mg/day | May worsen anxiety. Higher risk for switching to the mania phase if the individual has bipolar disorder. Lowest risk for sexual dysfunction. Weight gain is common, and more likely after 6 months of use. More activating than other SSRIs. | Longer half-life of 3–4 days; long elimination of active metabolites. Withdrawal symptoms are less likely than with all other SSRIs. |
| Paroxetine (Paxil) | 10–20 mg/day for 7 days; may increase dose by 10 mg/week | Maximum dose: 50 mg/day | Not recommended during pregnancy. Weight gain is more likely than with other SSRIs; may be sedating. Higher risk for sexual dysfunction. Anticholinergic. Recommended during breastfeeding/chestfeeding. | Short half-life; no active metabolites. Users are more likely to experience serotonin withdrawal symptoms. |
| Sertraline (Zoloft) | 25–50 mg for 7 days, then may increase in 25-mg increments | Maximum dose: 200 mg/day | Weight gain is common, and more likely after 6 months of use. Limited CPY450 interactions.<br><br>Mildly stimulating. Recommended for patients who breastfeed/chestfeed. | Half-life of 2–4 days; some minimally active metabolites. Withdrawal symptoms are less likely. |
| **Selective Norepinephrine Reuptake Inhibitors** | | | | |
| Duloxetine (Cymbalta) | 20–60 mg as one or two doses/day; 30 mg/day for 7 days, then may increase to 60 mg/day | Maximum dose: 60 mg/day | Weight-neutral in the short term; uncertain if weight gain occurs in the long term. Fewer sexual side effects than some SSRIs in the short term; no long-term difference. No impact on blood pressure. | Half-life of 12 hours. Withdrawal symptoms have been reported, but their frequency is unknown. |

| Generic Agent (Brand Name) | Starting Dose | Dosage Range and Maximum Dose | Side-Effect Profile | Pharmacokinetic Half-Life |
|---|---|---|---|---|
| Venlafaxine (Effexor) | 37.5 mg | 75–300 mg/day in 2–3 divided doses | Weight-neutral. Fewer sexual side effects than SSRIs. May reduce vasomotor symptoms related to perimenopause. Increases blood pressure in a dose-dependent fashion. More agitation and gastrointestinal side effects than SSRIs. | Withdrawal symptoms have been reported. Frequency of withdrawal symptoms is unknown. |
| Venlafaxine IR | 37.5 mg | 37.5–300 mg/day | | |
| **Norepinephrine–Dopamine Reuptake Inhibitors** | | | | |
| Bupropion (Wellbutrin, Zyban) | 200 mg in divided doses, twice daily | 450 mg in four divided doses. Single dose should not exceed 150 mg. | May be stimulating. No sexual side effects. Weight-neutral or minor weight loss. Lowers seizure threshold | Half-life is 29 hours for sustained release. Withdrawal symptoms have not been reported. |
| Bupropion XR | 150 mg daily in morning | Maximum dose: 450 mg daily | | |

Abbreviations: IR, immediate release; NDRI, norepinephrine–dopamine reuptake inhibitor; SNRI, serotonin–norepinephrine reuptake inhibitor; SR, sustained release; SSRI, selective serotonin reuptake inhibitor.
Based on Hackley B, Sharma C, Kedzior A, Sreenivasan S. Managing mental health conditions in primary care settings. *J Midwifery Womens Health.* 2010;55(1):9-19; U.S. Department of Veterans Affairs. The management of major depressive disorder: clinical guideline summary. https://www.healthquality.va.gov/guidelines/MH/mdd/. Updated 2022. Accessed January 14, 2023.

activity. Although it remains rare, its incidence is suspected to be rising due to more frequent prescribing of serotonergic medications, and a possible toxic reaction when therapeutic doses of an SSRI or SNRI are potentiated by an interaction with a number of other agents. Combination treatment with more than one SSRI or SNRI, monoamine oxidase inhibitors, lithium, or concurrent use of St. John's wort may precipitate serotonin syndrome and should be avoided. Some other classes of drugs—such as triptans, anticonvulsants, and some opioids—also have serotonergic activity. Many recreational drugs, including amphetamines, cocaine, and MDMA (Ecstasy), can trigger serotonin syndrome as well.

Signs and symptoms of serotonin syndrome include autonomic instability such as hypertension or hypotension, hyperthermia, tachycardia and tachypnea, and diaphoresis; changes in mental status, including agitation, confusion, or hypomania; and neuromuscular changes such as myoclonus, hyperreflexia, tremor, ataxia, and rigidity.[81] The clinical manifestations can be highly variable, and patients who are suspected of experiencing serotonin syndrome should be referred for emergency evaluation for supportive care and treatment with a serotonin antagonist.[81]

The risk of suicidal ideation and behavior increases during the first 1 to 2 months after beginning treatment with antidepressant medication, especially among adolescents and young adults.[82] Depression is also associated with suicide attempts at any age. In 2004 (and updated in 2007), the U.S. Food and Drug Administration (FDA) placed a black box warning on these agents' labels, alerting prescribers of a possible increase in suicidality at time of initiation or dosage change in patients younger than 25 years of age. Because antidepressants can take several weeks to become effective, close monitoring is indicated for the first few months after therapy is initiated. The black box warning explanation should always be included in documentation of counseling with patients under the age of 25.

SSRIs and duloxetine are metabolized through the CPY450 enzyme system. As such, they interact with a wide variety of other medications that are metabolized by the same system. Some of the medications that are known to interact with these second-generation antidepressants include older antidepressants such as tricyclic antidepressants, digoxin (Lanoxin), warfarin (Coumadin), anticonvulsants, beta blockers, and theophylline (Theo-Dur).[65]

Prior to prescribing any psychotropic medication, the clinician is responsible for reviewing all the medications the patient is taking to avoid potentially serious interactions.

### Follow-Up and Monitoring

Frequent ongoing monitoring of psychotropic medications is recommended until remission of symptoms is achieved, at which point reducing the frequency of visits is appropriate. The initial follow-up visit within 2 to 4 weeks is an important time to discuss whether the individual has filled the prescription and is taking it as prescribed, and if not, to identify the barriers or reasons. It also allows for assessment of side effects or worsening suicidal thoughts or behaviors. Most individuals will benefit from a dose adjustment from the initial dose, with slow titration being important to minimize adverse effects and subsequent abrupt discontinuation of therapy. A partial response to treatment is usually an indication that an increased dose is indicated. Some patients may experience an improvement in their depression or anxiety symptoms within 1 to 2 weeks, although many will not appreciate a response until as late as 6 weeks after beginning medication.

Repeated use of the same screening instrument employed during the initial diagnosis allows the provider and the patient to determine whether they have achieved an objective, quantifiable response to the therapy. There is no absolute rule for how often the measurement-based screening tools should be repeated or which criteria should be used to determine adequate treatment. A decrease in score should indicate some treatment response and guides the clinician toward decisions regarding dose adjustments. Repeated screening also reduces the rate of relapse and allows for the patient and provider to recognize improvement and the presence of any residual symptoms.

### Relapse/Recurrence

Relapse is common in persons who suffer from depression, with 50% to 85% of affected individuals experiencing at least one lifetime recurrence.[83] The risk of recurrence is lower when antidepressant therapy is continued for 4 to 9 months after remission has been achieved, for a total duration of 6 to 12 months.[84] Individuals who have had or are at high risk for relapses will benefit from more long-term maintenance therapy. Characteristics of patients for whom maintenance therapy should be considered are listed in Table 7-11. These patients

| Table 7-11 | Indications for Possible Maintenance Antidepressant Therapy |
|---|---|

Residual symptoms after adequate treatment

Persistent sleep disturbance

Family history of mood disorders

Ongoing psychosocial stressors

Three or more previous episodes of major depression

Two or more closely spaced episodes

Dysthymia

Dysthymia with an episode of major depression (double depression)

are encouraged to continue therapy for at least 2 years, during which time follow-up should occur every 3 to 12 months as long as the patient's mental health status remains stable.[78,83]

### Discontinuing Antidepressant Medications

When a decision is made to discontinue psychotropic medications, the dose should be tapered over several weeks to months to avoid serotonin withdrawal syndrome.[67] In general, the longer the duration the patient has taken the medication, the longer the taper should take to avoid discontinuation effects. Medications with a longer half-life, such as fluoxetine, can be discontinued in a shorter amount of time than others.

Discontinuation symptoms may include dizziness, fatigue, nausea, agitation, irritability, and headache. It is best to provide patients with information regarding discontinuation symptoms when initiating therapy to reduce the occurrence of skipping doses or abrupt discontinuation. This caution should also be reinforced at each follow-up encounter. Counseling should also include reassurance that these symptoms do not indicate a dependency or addiction to the medication. Because of their effect on the metabolism of other medications, discontinuation of antidepressants may necessitate a dose adjustment of other medications. Patients should be counseled to notify their other providers if needed to discuss medication adjustment at that time.

### Complementary and Alternative Treatments for Depression and Anxiety

More and more people are using complementary and alternative medicine (CAM) for treatment of

| Table 7-12 | Complementary and Alternative Treatments for Depression and Anxiety | | |
|---|---|---|---|
| **Category** | **Recommendation** | **Cautions/Side Effects** | **Dose and Education** |
| Light therapy | First line: Seasonal MDD<br>Second line/adjunctive:<br>Mild to moderate MDD | Eyestrain, headache | 10,000 lux 30 min/day for 6 weeks[85,86] |
| Exercise | First line: Mild to moderate MDD<br>Second line/adjunctive: Moderate to severe MDD | | 30 min 3 times per week for minimum 9 weeks[66,85,86] |
| Yoga | Second line/adjunctive: Mild to moderate MDD | Results for perinatal depression mixed[87] | 60–90 min once weekly[85–87]<br>↑ effect with ↑ frequency |
| Acupuncture | Third line/adjunctive | Evidence is limited | Frequency varies widely in studies[85,86,88] |
| **Herbs** | | | |
| St. John's wort | First line: Mild to moderate MDD<br>Second line/adjunctive: Moderate to severe MDD | Drug interactions with many medications. GI symptoms; headache. | 500–1800 mg/day for 4–12 weeks. Wear sunscreen; avoid alcohol.[85,86,88] |
| Omega-3s | Second line/monotherapy: Mild to moderate MDD<br>Second line/adjunctive: Moderate to severe MDD | Close monitoring if taking antiplatelet or anticoagulant medications | 3–9 g/day omega-3 OR 1–2 g EPA + 1–2 g DHA for 4–16 weeks[85,86,88,89] |
| SAMe | Second line/adjunctive: Mild to severe MDD | GI symptoms, insomnia, headache | 800–1600 mg in divided doses with meals for 4–12 weeks[85,86,88] |
| Crocus sativa (saffron) | Third line/monotherapy or adjunctive: Mild to moderate MDD | Nausea, headache, insomnia | 20–30 mg/day for 6–8 weeks[85,86] |

Abbreviations: DHA, docosahexaenoic acid; EPA, eicosapentaenoic acid; GI, gastrointestinal; MDD, major depressive disorder; RCT, randomized controlled trial; SAMe, S-adenosyl L-methionine.

*Recommendations:*

First line = Evidence from meta-analysis and/or one or more RCTs with adequate sample size plus clinical support.

Second line = Includes first-line evidence plus small RCTs or observational studies plus clinical support.

Third line = First- and second-line evidence and expert opinion plus clinical support.

Based on Ravindran AV, Balneaves LG, Faulkner G, et al. Canadian Network for Mood and Anxiety Treatments (CANMAT) 2016 clinical guidelines for the management of adults with major depressive disorder: Section 5. Complementary and alternative medicine treatments. *Can J Psychiatry*. 2016;61(9):576-587.

mental illness. Although data are somewhat lacking, existing studies suggest that approximately 50% of people with anxiety and/or depression use CAM. Unfortunately, this use is often unsupervised and may occur in combination with other more conventional medications, which can lead to significant drug interactions.[85,86] Table 7-12 outlines these potential treatments and current evidence to support them. Midwives and primary care providers should be aware of the available evidence supporting the use of the most common methods and be prepared to provide education regarding possible side effects, drug interactions, and contraindications to use.

### Treatment of Bipolar Disorder

Treatment for bipolar disorders involves the use of medications that are not normally prescribed by midwives or primary care providers. As discussed previously, giving a serotonergic agent to an individual with bipolar disorder can precipitate a manic or hypomanic episode and make long-term treatment more difficult. Therefore, careful screening and proper referral for bipolar disorder are essential prior to initiating antidepressants.

Medications for treating bipolar disorder include lithium, anticonvulsants, and atypical antipsychotic medications, all of which have significant side effects, potential for adverse or drug–drug interactions (including oral contraceptives), and require frequent follow-up including blood tests at regular intervals. Weight gain, sexual dysfunction, sedation, movement disorders, and dermatologic issues are just some of the adverse effects associated with use of these medications. In addition, some of these medications are teratogenic (e.g., valproic acid, carbamazepine, lithium), so extreme caution should be used when prescribing them to patients with childbearing capacity.

### Treatment of PTSD

In 2020, the two major professional organizations specialized in trauma and PTSD published treatment guidelines for PTSD that substantially agree.[90,91] First-line treatment for PTSD is psychotherapy. The strongest recommendations of evidence-based psychotherapies that result in remission of PTSD all focus on processing the traumatic experience using theory-based and empirically supported techniques to reduce PTSD symptoms. Table 7-13 summarizes the evidence-based PTSD psychotherapies in order of the strength of the evidence of their benefit.

| Table 7-13 | Evidence-Based Psychotherapies for Treating Individual Adults with PTSD |
|---|---|
| **Strong** recommendation | Cognitive processing therapy, cognitive therapy, eye-movement desensitization and reprocessing (EMDR), CBT with a trauma focus, prolonged exposure |
| **Standard** recommendation | CBT without a trauma focus, narrative exposure therapy (NET), present-centered therapy |
| **Emerging evidence** for recommendation | Reconsolidation of traumatic memories, single-session CBT, virtual reality therapy, written exposure therapy (WET) |
| **Insufficient evidence** to recommend | Other approaches have been tested and found not to result in significant improvement or have not been sufficiently tested to inform recommendation. |

Abbreviation: CBT, cognitive-behavioral therapy.

Based on Forbes D, Bisson JI, Monson CM, Berliner L, eds. *Effective Treatments for PTSD: Practice Guidelines from the International Society for Traumatic Stress Studies*. 3rd ed. New York, NY: Guilford; 2020:170, Table 11.1.

Because most therapies for PTSD that have a solid evidence base involve processing the trauma, and because avoidance of reminders is a diagnostic criterion for PTSD, it can be a difficult decision to engage in therapy. An important implication is that only the patient can judge when they have the capacity to seek treatment. If referral is declined, it can be very helpful to simply move on to mutual collaboration about how best to identify and avoid triggers so the client can continue to engage in needed health care.

Psychoeducation—learning about PTSD and how to manage it—can also be beneficial and does not require confronting trauma memories. Psychoeducation is defined by three components: information about the condition, skills building to manage the symptoms, and emotional support while learning. Although not likely to achieve remission of PTSD when used alone, psychoeducation can provide self-efficacy to manage PTSD. Examples of stand-alone psychoeducation programs include Skills Training for Affect and Interpersonal Regulation, Dialectical Behavior Therapy, and Survivor Moms' Companion.[92–94]

Psychopharmacology for PTSD helps with symptom severity, but it does not cure the disorder. Nevertheless, it can bring some relief, which the International Society for Traumatic Stress Studies treatment guidelines characterize as low effect.[90] Medication is considered a useful adjunct to support engagement in psychotherapy. First-line medications for PTSD are the SSRIs, with sertraline (Zoloft), paroxetine (Paxil), fluoxetine (Prozac), and the SNRI venlafaxine (Effexor) having the most evidence for efficacy, although only sertraline and paroxetine have FDA approval for this indication.[90]

Given the chronic and complex nature of PTSD for some people, evidence supports some other strategies that help with well-being and functioning as useful adjuncts to treatment. These modalities include acupuncture, neurofeedback, saikokeishikankyoto (traditional herbal formula), somatic experiencing, transcranial magnetic stimulation, and yoga.[90]

It is also becoming common to think of PTSD treatment as "modular," in the sense that the client and the provider work together to make a tailored plan aligned with the client's priorities, preferences, and values.[95] This may include developing a plan for the order in which to begin and continue different treatment modalities to gain better health and functioning and potentially self-understanding or even post-traumatic growth.

Finally, it is vital to keep in mind that PTSD is rarely a stand-alone condition. Treatments effective for depression, anxiety, substance use, and self-harm all may also be useful and act synergistically for severely affected individuals.

### Treatments for PMS and PMDD

Treatments for PMS and PMDD include (1) nonpharmacologic approaches such as diet, supplements, exercise, and psychotherapy; (2) SSRIs; and (3) hormonal agonists and antagonists.

Nonpharmacologic approaches to premenstrual-related mood changes may help stabilize mood and relieve physical symptoms, but there is little evidence to support these approaches as monotherapy specifically for PMDD. Vitex agnus castus (chasteberry) has been shown to be effective and well tolerated in reducing minor PMS symptoms.[96] A diet that includes complex carbohydrates, consumed during the luteal phase, may be helpful because this type of diet boosts the amount of serotonin present in neural synapses.[97] CBT has also been shown to help women manage their symptoms. There is no consistent evidence that primrose oil, B vitamins, or vitamin E are any more effective in reducing symptoms than a placebo.

The strongest evidence for effective treatment of individuals with PMDD involves boosting neurotransmitter presence or suppressing ovulation. SSRIs are the most-studied antidepressants used as pharmacotherapy for women with PMDD. All of the SSRIs appear to be equally effective, and both continuous and intermittent dosing regimens are used. A low to moderate dose may be effective and well tolerated.[98] The action of SSRIs for PMDD differs from their action for other psychiatric conditions in two basic ways:

- Relief of symptoms occurs in the first cycle of use. Ordinarily, SSRIs require up to 2 months before reaching full effectiveness.
- The SSRI is effective when taken only at intervals, rather than every day. Withdrawal symptoms do not appear when the SSRI is discontinued after several days or a week of use.

The third strategy to treat premenstrual-related mood changes aims to create a steady hormonal state, without the cyclic fluctuations that appear to trigger the neurologic cascade resulting in PMDD. Hormonal contraceptives can suppress ovulation and are widely acceptable for individuals who do not want to become pregnant. Oral contraceptives containing drospirenone (e.g., Yaz, Yasmin) have been the most specifically studied for their effectiveness in treating PMDD and PMS.[99] Patients who

use drospirenone-containing contraceptives have an increased risk for deep vein thrombosis; this risk should be taken into consideration before prescribing these medications. Fluctuation of hormone levels can be further minimized by using shorter pill-free intervals or continuous-dosing regimens.[100] Hormonal contraceptives have also been used as an adjunct treatment for underlying depression that worsens prior to menses,[101] and the midwife who is familiar with the range of products and dosing regimens can fine-tune treatment for an individual patient's needs in consultation with their psychiatric provider. Long-term suppression of ovulation with a gonadotropin-releasing hormone (GnRH) agonist plus low-dose estrogen–progesterone is reserved for those individuals who have not responded to trials of an SSRI or combined oral contraceptive to reduce the severe symptoms associated with PMDD.[97]

## Mental Health Disorders During Perinatal and Postpartum Period

### Depression and Anxiety in Pregnancy

Most, if not all, of the governing bodies for obstetric and midwifery care worldwide recommend routine screening for mental health issues during pregnancy. Many U.S. states also mandate that providers screen for depression during pregnancy. As discussed earlier in the chapter, the most widely used screening tool for this purpose is the Edinburgh Postnatal Depression Scale. Unfortunately, there is no consensus on how often pregnant individuals should be screened—although at the very minimum, they should be screened at least once and anyone who has risks for or symptoms of depression should be rescreened to monitor depression or anxiety severity or treatment response. Even more unfortunate is the lack of resources available to pregnant persons who do screen positive. There is an increasingly more urgent call for integrating mental health care into the perinatal care setting, as a step toward reducing gendered and racial health disparities. Evidence shows that nurses and midwives can effectively deliver behavioral interventions that decrease symptoms and improve depression.[102] Working with insurance companies and medical billers for better reimbursement will be the key to creating a system that allows providers to offer these services all in one place.

The prevalence of various psychiatric conditions during pregnancy mirrors their prevalence in the general population. Mood and anxiety disorders are the most diagnosed psychiatric conditions during pregnancy. Individuals of childbearing potential are more likely to be diagnosed with a psychiatric disorder during their fertile years than at any other time in their lives. These same individuals are most vulnerable to psychiatric illness while they are pregnant or during the postpartum period. An estimated 10% to 20% of individuals will experience minor or major depression during pregnancy,[103] though these numbers likely underrepresent the true incidence of depression in pregnancy. The prevalence of at least one anxiety disorder diagnosis in pregnancy is also about 20%.[104] Mental health problems are frequently associated with comorbid psychiatric conditions; thus, when one disorder is identified in a pregnant patient, the possibility that more than one psychiatric condition might be present should always be considered.

Some symptoms of depression and anxiety are like the transient normal discomforts and changes associated with pregnancy. Changes in sleep, energy, appetite, weight, and libido are appropriate concerns of prenatal patients, but providers should be alerted to the possibility of mental health issues when those symptoms are accompanied with a constellation of other symptoms such as anxiety, irritability, or emotional detachment to pregnancy. Formal screening is crucial to help differentiate between the two situations.

Ample evidence of the adverse outcomes associated with untreated mental health disorders in pregnancy has been documented. For example, 11% of the pregnancy-related deaths in the United States between 2008 and 2017 were attributed to mental health conditions;[105] all of these deaths were determined to be preventable by review committees. Untreated depression during pregnancy is associated with substance use, smoking, and other behaviors that can independently affect pregnancy outcomes. Pregnant individuals with untreated depression also have increased risks for preterm birth and fetal growth restriction, and are at increased risk for postpartum depression and anxiety and the risks associated with those conditions.[106] These same patients have a higher rate of substance use in pregnancy as well.

Perinatal anxiety is associated with the same adverse pregnancy outcomes as depression.[107] Perinatal anxiety is a very strong predictor of postpartum depression. In terms of its effects on affected individuals' children, it is associated with almost twice the risk for ADHD in boys[108] and for hyperactivity.[109] Infants whose mothers had perinatal depression and anxiety have higher cortisol levels than infants whose mothers did not, and these elevations continue through adolescence. Treatment of patients with depression during pregnancy appears to normalize this elevation.[110]

Someone with a previous history of psychiatric illness should be counseled about the significant risk of relapse in pregnancy, especially if they discontinue their psychotropic medications. Patients should be cautioned that pregnancy is not protective with respect to mental illness and that the majority of people who discontinue medications for mood disorders and anxiety disorders will experience a relapse in pregnancy or the postpartum period. A comprehensive discussion of the risks associated with exposure to psychotropic medication as well as the risks associated with untreated mental illness is essential when counseling a pregnant patient or someone considering pregnancy in the near future. Both the patient and the provider need to be able to make informed decisions regarding care.

## Postpartum Blues

Postpartum blues, also known as baby blues, is the most common mood change that occurs after childbirth, occurring in 14% to 76% of new mothers worldwide.[111] The symptoms of crying, anxiety, emotional lability, irritability, and fatigue peak within 2 to 5 days of their onset, but usually do not interfere with functioning. Although postpartum blues is usually benign and self-limiting, it can be frightening for a new parent who is experiencing such drastic mood changes. If a patient in the early postpartum period calls with concerns about their mood, utilizing the first two questions of the PHQ-9 can be helpful in assessing their risk for developing MDD or postpartum anxiety. If the individual reports anhedonia—the inability to feel pleasure—a more thorough screen for postpartum depression is warranted.

Once postpartum blues is determined to be the likely cause of symptoms, anticipatory guidance that these mood swings are commonly experienced and usually resolve spontaneously within 10 to 14 days can reassure new parents. These patients should also be counseled to contact their provider if the symptoms do not resolve within 2 weeks following birth because as many as one in five people with postpartum blues will develop MDD.

## Postpartum Depression and Anxiety

Changes in mood are experienced by a majority of individuals after childbirth. Estrogen levels, which have a significant influence on neurotransmitter systems, rapidly decrease during the postpartum period. In addition, lower serotonergic activity following birth has been noted. Likewise, downregulation of the HPA axis following birth may contribute to increased vulnerability to depression.[112] Disturbances in sleep patterns and circadian rhythms are also universal in new parents. Melatonin release is suppressed by exposure to light when a person would normally be sleeping (e.g., when a new parent wakes frequently throughout the night to feed and change their infant). Postpartum insomnia may both contribute to and be aggravated by MDD.[113] While these physiologic changes do not lead to depression in all individuals who have given birth, when they are coupled with prior history of depression or bipolar disorder, a genetic predisposition, inadequate social support, and multiple stressors, it is not surprising that childbirth can present a challenge to one's mental health and well-being. This adjustment to childbirth and parenting should be normalized to destigmatize the perception of postpartum mood changes.

As noted earlier in this chapter, the U.S. Preventive Services Task Force, ACNM, and ACOG recommend regularly screening for depression, including screening in the postpartum period. Although several instruments are available to screen for postpartum depression, the EPDS is the most widely used tool.[19] It has been validated for use both during pregnancy and postpartum for men and women, screens for anxiety, and is accessible without cost. Recognizing the impact of postpartum depression (including paternal depression) on the whole family, and acknowledging that new parents often have limited access to other providers after the first 6 weeks postpartum, the AAP now recommends frequent screening of all parents at well-child visits within the first year after birth.[114] This guidance highlights how pediatric providers are on the frontlines for recognition, referral, and support for new parents. It also recognizes the importance of caring for the

parent–baby dyad as a unit and seeks to destigmatize postpartum mental health care.

As in pregnancy and primary care, a positive screen should be followed up with a diagnostic evaluation by a qualified clinician to establish an accurate diagnosis. The screening questionnaires reviewed earlier in this chapter do not differentiate between unipolar or bipolar depression; patients identified as being depressed should be evaluated for a history or symptoms of mania or hypomania. A positive response to the questions that assess suicidality (question 9 on the PHQ-9 and question 10 on the EPDS) requires immediate attention by the clinician and possible referral for emergency mental health services.

The peak onset for postpartum depression is in the second month after childbirth, and the risk for this disorder remains elevated up to a year following childbirth. As many as 19% of individuals will have a major depressive episode at some time during the first 3 months postpartum.[115] New data suggest that individuals with persistent depression symptoms in the first year postpartum are more likely to continue to experience significant depression symptoms up to 11 years after childbirth, highlighting the importance of proper and timely treatment for this population.[115] Risk factors for postpartum depression are listed in Table 7-14.

Research suggests that postpartum depression increases the risk of adverse outcomes in children. Moreover, untreated depression has been associated with impaired child development. New parents who are depressed may be less responsive to their infants and less likely to engage in face-to-face interactions that would contribute to infant communication skills, such as vocalizing, smiling, imitation, and game-playing, compared to those who are not depressed. They also display less synchrony in

| Table 7-14 | Risk Factors for Postpartum Depression and Anxiety | |
|---|---|
| **Strong Risk Factors** | **Additional Risk Factors** |
| Anxiety during pregnancy | Biologic vulnerability |
| Depression during pregnancy | Family history of depression, anxiety, or postpartum depression |
| Stressful life events during pregnancy | |
| Low level of social support: single marital status | Unplanned pregnancy |
| History of depression, anxiety, post-traumatic stress disorder | Young age at time of birth |
| Postpartum depression after a prior pregnancy | Lower socioeconomic status, financial insecurity |
| Identifying as a person of color (lived experience of racism and bias) | History of interpersonal violence |
| | Thyroid dysfunction |
| | Negative perceived birth experience |

their parent–baby interactions. Children of a parent with postpartum depression are more likely to have delayed language development, poor cognitive functioning, disruptive behaviors, and emotional maladjustment.[116] There is also increasing evidence of an association between postpartum depression rates and rates of depression in children in late adolescence. As mentioned throughout this chapter in reference to any unipolar mood disorder, when assessing a patient for postpartum depression, it is critical to rule out postpartum bipolar disorder, which can be severe and possibly lead to postpartum psychosis.

For several reasons, the prevalence of postpartum anxiety is less clear but is thought to be higher than that for postpartum depression. Research on postpartum anxiety is lacking. While the EPDS was originally developed to screen for MDD, three of the questions target anxiety symptoms. Unfortunately, many providers do not consider anxiety disorders when interpreting the results from this tool. Postpartum anxiety shares overlapping symptoms with postpartum depression, but is even more challenging to identify because some anxiety and emotional lability in the postpartum period are expected as a parent transitions into a new role, copes with lack of sleep, and gets accustomed to changes in the dynamics and expectations in their relationships with others.

Individuals with postpartum anxiety present with signs and symptoms that can often be overlooked or dismissed as "normal" postpartum behavior. They may be preoccupied with a fear of anything that could possibly go wrong. They may be more irritable toward others. Often, these individuals exhibit symptoms of obsessive–compulsive disorder in the postpartum period. Repetitive and intrusive thoughts can coincide with compulsive behaviors that are meant to control the anxiety but interfere with normal functioning. Compulsive behaviors seen in the postpartum period can include repeatedly checking on the baby, constant cleaning, or counting or reorganizing. Affected individuals may refuse to let others care for the baby—even trusted and responsible family members. They may report that they stay up even when the baby is sleeping, watching and monitoring to make sure the infant is breathing, rather than taking advantage of the time to sleep and recover. Panic attacks and intrusive thoughts are common in these cases. In severe cases, patients may exhibit paranoia and psychosis. Postpartum anxiety is consistently linked to postpartum depression, worsening insomnia, reduced rates of breastfeeding/chestfeeding, impaired

parent–child bonding, and altered socioemotional development.[117] It can be debilitating for a new parent and impair their ability to safely care for their children, which can have profound effects on the family unit.

While postpartum depression is an MDD, the *DSM-5* does not identify depression in pregnancy or postpartum as a specific diagnosis. Instead, it qualifies depression that is diagnosed either in pregnancy or within 4 weeks postpartum as "major depressive disorder with peripartum onset."[1] There is no specific diagnosis for anxiety disorders in the peripartum period identified within the *DSM-5*. As a clinician, it is important to remember that the postpartum period extends beyond the first 4 weeks after birth and to recognize that clinically significant symptoms often do not appear within that first month following parturition. Providers should also be cognizant that meeting the diagnostic criteria for a specific diagnosis is not the only measure of impairment for an individual patient.

Identifying a vulnerability to postpartum depression may allow the midwife an opportunity to recommend interventions that may decrease the patient's risk for this disorder. Interventions that may help prevent postpartum depression include interpersonal psychotherapy, regular physical activity, improving or developing a social support system, and arranging to obtain sufficient sleep postpartum.[118] Many of these behaviors can be fostered prior to or during pregnancy. For example, counseling regarding exercise (especially outdoors), healthy eating, and good sleep habits can be reinforced at each prenatal visit—not just to ensure physical well-being during pregnancy, but also to promote the pregnant person's emotional well-being. Joining postpartum support groups may also help new parents develop coping skills and destigmatize the notion that postpartum mood changes are a sign of weakness. Psychotherapy can help the parent learn to identify and access sources of support from family and friends, thereby avoiding the development of postpartum depression. Those who are at risk for postpartum depression but have a desire to avoid medication may be especially receptive to this advice.

## Pharmacotherapy for Perinatal and Postpartum Depression and Anxiety

Management of mental health disorders that appear or recur during pregnancy and postpartum requires collaborative decision making between patient and provider. Each patient needs to make individual informed choices based on their diagnosis, the likely progression of their illness, and the results of shared decision making. Information provided as part of shared decision making includes possible adverse effects over the course of the pregnancy, including the risks associated with no treatment (reviewed earlier in the chapter), fetal effects, newborn effects, and neurobehavioral effects on the child. The decision to treat the condition with medication should also consider the severity of the illness, with pharmacotherapy being more strongly considered in persons with a history of severe and incapacitating mental illness or recurrent episodes. Patients who perceive that a plan of care has been imposed on them are less likely to follow through with the treatment as prescribed.

The combination of psychotherapy with psychotropic medication has been shown to have higher remission and lower relapse rates than either type of treatment alone. Midwives who are knowledgeable about common mental health disorders and the pharmacology of the medications used to treat them may feel comfortable prescribing for these patients but should do so only if they have the ability to provide follow-up care and have access to other mental health resources including emergency services if needed. They should not manage medications in situations involving complicated dual diagnoses, bipolar disorder, or active suicidal ideation.

The choice to use medication during pregnancy can be complicated. Randomized controlled trials (RCTs) are impossible to conduct with pregnant individuals as participants, leaving clinicians to consider the conflicting findings of many observational, anecdotal, retrospective, and open trials of the various antidepressant medications. To date, no absolute rules for prescribing antidepressants during pregnancy have emerged, although some general guidelines related to psychopharmacology management in pregnancy and breastfeeding/chestfeeding have been issued (Table 7-15).

Very few high-quality studies have examined the effectiveness of complementary treatments in pregnancy and breastfeeding. Some women who opt not to participate in therapy or take psychotropic medications may consider complementary therapies to help manage their perinatal depression. General recommendations for the most used alternative therapies for depression and anxiety in pregnancy were provided earlier in this chapter.

Identifying individuals who are at risk is only half the battle. Helping these patients access appropriate treatment is also necessary to have the desired impact on the overall health of new parents

| Table 7-15 | Guidelines for Psychopharmacology Management in Pregnancy and Lactation |
|---|---|

- Rule out bipolar disorder first.
- Use what has worked in the past (after considering safety information) and minimize switching medications in pregnancy if possible.
- Patients should always use the lowest effective dose.
- Patients should avoid polypharmacy when possible. Fewer data are available on the safety of combined pharmacology on pregnancy and breastfeeding.
- Patients will likely need dose adjustments as pregnancy progresses. Blood volume expansion begins early in pregnancy, and normal hemodilution usually necessitates a dose increase as pregnancy progresses to maintain a therapeutic response.
- The questionnaire that was used to initially screen for depression or anxiety—whether the Patient Health Questionnaire-9 or the Edinburgh Postnatal Depression Scale—should also be used to monitor response to treatment.

and the family unit. The primary care provider or midwife is in the best position to maintain ongoing contact with the parent to reinforce ongoing treatment. Such follow-up will decrease the chance that individuals fall through the cracks or discontinue treatment before achieving a satisfactory response.

## Potential Risks Associated with SSRI Use During Pregnancy and Lactation

Antidepressants are one of the most commonly prescribed drug classes in the United States. Approximately 8% of individuals in the United States use an antidepressant during their pregnancy, and this usage rate is much higher than anywhere else in the world.[119] As use of SSRIs—the most commonly prescribed pharmacotherapy for treating perinatal depression—increases, information about both their positive and adverse effects is changing rapidly.

Studies that have found associations between antidepressants and perinatal outcomes have encountered many methodologic challenges, including small sample sizes, recall bias, self-reported data, and outcome measures that are too rare to detect. Thus, large epidemiologic population-based observational studies are the current best resource for detecting an association between medication taken during pregnancy and an adverse outcome. These studies are not able to conclusively prove an etiologic relationship. Notably, most studies do not account for the effects of systemic and institutional racism, underlying mental illness, or other social determinants of health that negatively impact pregnancy outcomes. Table 7-16 summarizes the known risks associated with SSRI/NSRI use during pregnancy and lactation.[23,119–123]

Reputable evidence-based online resources are available to clinicians and their clients to help guide decisions about medication use during pregnancy and breastfeeding/chestfeeding. Although the transfer rates for the different drugs vary, in all cases the infant is exposed to a lower concentration of SSRI during breastfeeding/chestfeeding than during pregnancy.[123] The relative infant dose (RID) is the estimated infant dose in human milk (in mg/kg) divided by the maternal dose (in mg/kg) times 100.[124] In general, the accepted value for safety in breastfeeding/chestfeeding is 10% or less.

All SSRIs are considered first-line treatment for depression and anxiety with breastfeeding/chestfeeding. When initiating pharmacotherapy for the first time ever in the postpartum period, sertraline or paroxetine should be considered before other medications in the same class. This is based on the RID (0.5% and 1.5%, respectively) and reports

| Table 7-16 | Risk Summary for SSRIs/SNRIs Used During Pregnancy and Breastfeeding/Chestfeeding |
|---|---|
| **Risk** | **Description** |
| Pregnancy loss (miscarriage and stillbirth) | No increase in risk. |
| Congenital birth defects | No increase in risk. |
| Congenital cardiac defects | Exposure to paroxetine, but not other SSRIs/SNRIs, is associated with cardiovascular abnormalities in some but not all case-control studies. The absolute increased risk is up to 2 per 1000 exposed pregnancies in the first trimester. |
| Preterm birth | Depression and SSRI exposure are both associated with an increased risk for preterm birth; studies have been unable to disentangle the effects of depression and treatments on risk of preterm birth. |
| Low birth weight | Most, but not all, well-controlled studies indicate no increase in risk. |
| Postpartum hemorrhage | A meta-analysis of studies shows increased risk for SSRIs (RR, 1.20; 95% CI 1.04–1.38) and SNRIs (RR, 1.62; 95% CI, 1.41–1.85). |
| Persistent pulmonary hypertension of the newborn | The absolute increased risk is approximately 1 per 1000 pregnancies exposed after 20 weeks' gestation. |
| Neonatal adaptation syndrome | Up to 30% of in-utero exposed newborns demonstrate a poorly defined syndrome with mild symptoms such as transient tachypnea, jitteriness, weak cry, poor muscular tone. The syndrome is more common with fluoxetine, paroxetine, and venlafaxine. Symptoms begin by 48 hours after birth and resolve within a few days to 2 weeks. |
| Autism spectrum disorder | Most studies show no increased risk after adjusting for parental psychiatric diagnoses. |
| Effects on breastfeeding/chestfeeding infant | Very little evidence of adverse effects on breastfeeding infants. Relative exposure during lactation is much less than in utero. |

Abbreviations: CI, confidence interval; RR, relative risk; SNRI, serotonin–norepinephrine reuptake inhibitor; SSRI, selective serotonin reuptake inhibitor.

Based on Latendresse G, Deneris A. Selective serotonin reuptake inhibitors as first line antidepressant therapy for perinatal depression. *J Midwifery Womens Health*. 2017;62(3):317-328; Betcher HK, Wisner KL. Psychotropic treatment during pregnancy: research synthesis and clinical care principles. *J Womens Health (Larchmt)*. 2020 Mar;29(3):310-318. doi:10.1089/jwh.2019.7781. Epub 2019 Dec 3; Lusskin SI, Khan SJ, Ernst C, Habib S, Fersh ME, Albertini ES. Pharmacotherapy for perinatal depression. *Clin Obstet Gynecol*. 2018 Sep 1;61(3):544-561. doi:10.1097/GRF.0000000000000365; ACOG Practice Bulletin No. 92: use of psychiatric medications during pregnancy and lactation. *Obstet Gynecol*. 2008 Apr;111(4):1001-1020. doi:10.1097/AOG.0b013e31816fd910; Jiang HY, Xu LL, Li YC, Deng M, Peng CT, Ruan B. Antidepressant use during pregnancy and risk of postpartum hemorrhage: a systematic review and meta-analysis. *J Psychiatr Res*. 2016 Dec;83:160-167. doi:10.1016/j.jpsychires.2016.09.001. Epub 2016 Sep 4.

of side effects in infants. Fluoxetine (Prozac) has a higher rate of transfer to human milk, although still less than 10%, and is more often associated with infant behavioral side effects.[124] However, if the parent was already taking fluoxetine during pregnancy, it is not recommended to change antidepressants during breastfeeding/chestfeeding.[123] Switching in the postpartum period would expose the neonate to unnecessary polypharmacy during the transition period due to this medication's longer half-life, and the patient risks having a poor or adverse response to the new medication, which could worsen the course of their mental illness.

Venlafaxine and duloxetine are the SNRIs for which the most information is available regarding lactation; both show RID values within the acceptable range. Fewer published data are available regarding bupropion's effects on human milk–fed infants. The active metabolites of bupropion also have acceptable RID values, but this agent should be used with caution in breastfeeding/chestfeeding individuals due to its dose-related seizure potential.[123]

## Substance Use Disorders in the Perinatal Period

There has been slow progress in reducing the stigma related to SUD in pregnancy and parenthood. Although access to proper treatment has expanded, recent data show that fewer than 1 in 10 women in need of SUD treatment actually receive it.[125] Unfortunately, barriers do still exist for those who seek treatment. A lot of work remains to be done to educate and properly guide healthcare providers and their staff about SUD and proper treatment guidelines. Shame and fear of legal consequences prevent some pregnant individuals from accessing treatment or even from receiving prenatal care. Drug-related events are becoming the leading preventable cause of death during pregnancy and up to 12 months postpartum,[126] and the gender gap is closing for SUD. More women and transgender individuals are experiencing addiction issues, and healthcare providers are not meeting their needs at this time.

Untreated SUD, like other mental health conditions, can negatively impact pregnancy and neonatal outcomes. Miscarriage, preterm birth, fetal growth restriction, sudden infant death syndrome, placental abruption, neonatal withdrawal symptoms, and neurobehavioral developmental delays are the most common adverse effects of substance use in pregnancy. Many of these outcomes are similar to the risks associated with untreated metal health disorders. Further complicating a provider's assessment of risk are the confounding factors of polysubstance abuse and comorbid psychiatric diagnoses that are so common with addiction.

Neonatal abstinence syndrome (NAS) constitutes a constellation of physiologic and neurobehavioral signs of withdrawal in a newborn who was exposed in utero to alcohol, tobacco, and/or illicitly used substances. More recently, NAS has been used to describe withdrawal symptoms specific to opioid use exposure in pregnancy. Withdrawal caused by in utero exposure to opioids is also called *neonatal opioid withdrawal syndrome* (NOWS), and the two terms are used interchangeably in much of the literature. Approximately 50% to 80% of opioid-exposed newborns develop NAS.[126] The number of affected infants has risen dramatically over the past 20 years, with higher rates being seen in rural areas of the United States.

Primary care providers and advanced practitioners now can provide office-based opioid agonist therapy for their clients with opioid use disorders. This creates opportunities for improved access for pregnant patients to receive proper treatment and support in recovery through the perinatal period, especially in rural areas where opioid use rates are at their highest and access to treatment was limited until recently. As midwives, we are uniquely situated to provide intensive, comprehensive, and long-term continuity of care for our patients.

In pregnancy, patients should be maintained on an opioid agonist medication such as methadone or buprenorphine because opioid withdrawal can have significant effects on pregnancy outcomes. Sudden discontinuation of opioids can cause preterm labor, miscarriage, and fetal distress. Usually, buprenorphine is used alone because there is limited information on the safety of naltrexone in pregnancy, although emerging research supports the safety of naltrexone in pregnancy.[127] In response to the physiologic changes that occur in pregnancy, the patient will likely need periodic dose adjustments to opioid agonist therapy to avoid withdrawal symptoms.

NAS can be an expected condition after birth when birthing persons have SUD, and communication is needed with pediatric providers to assure proper monitoring and treatment. However, there is no evidence that the dose of opioid agonist has any correlation to the degree of NAS. In addition, breastfeeding/chestfeeding has been shown to reduce the severity of NAS in opioid-exposed newborns.[126] These are two key points to emphasize when counseling and reassuring patients regarding their treatment plans. Rooming-in with the parent after birth, soothing techniques such as swaddling, rocking the baby, and keeping the lights and noise levels low are all interventions meant to improve symptoms of NAS. These interventions also work to involve the newly postpartum parent in the newborn's care, and support them through their transitions, which in return supports long-term recovery. Sometimes the neonate experiences more severe withdrawal signs and may need medical interventions in addition to supportive care.

In the postpartum period, patients should continue with their opioid agonist therapy, while recognizing that dose adjustments may be needed. Breastfeeding/chestfeeding parents should be counseled to continue opioid agonists until the baby stops taking human milk and is sleeping through the night.[126] Ensuring that proper social supports for the patient and their family are in place is vital before considering stopping opioid agonist therapy, and patients should be counseled that many people safely continue opioid agonist therapy for years.

## PTSD During the Perinatal Period

PTSD affects individuals in their childbearing years in numerous ways that warrant using a trauma-informed approach in perinatal services. Effects occur across the biologic, psychological, social, and spiritual realms. In the psychological and parenting domains, the idea of "ghosts in the nursery" from unresolved parental trauma has been understood since the 1970s.[128] Biologic effects of PTSD on pregnancy are now being studied, including mechanisms of illness such as hyperemesis and adverse outcomes including prenatal complications, shorter gestation, lower birth weight, and less breastfeeding despite intention and initiation (whether the PTSD stems from prepregnancy or birth trauma).[129,130]

Among those persons expecting their first infant, salient past trauma exposures include childhood maltreatment, sexual trauma, medical trauma, and previous reproductive loss. In subsequent pregnancies, prior birth trauma, stillbirth, and sickness or death of the infant are additional sources of PTSD.[131]

Rates of PTSD in pregnancy vary from the rate seen in the nonpregnant female population (approximately 4% to 5%) to much higher rates (14% to 30%) among vulnerable populations.[132,133] Research suggests that pregnancy itself, invasive contact, dependence on a caregiver in prenatal care, dynamics of labor, and numerous aspects of early

parenting may be triggers for PTSD reactions. Marginalized populations may have higher incidence rates because they are often younger at first pregnancy and have had less time to recover from childhood maltreatment and fewer resources for effective treatment of prepregnancy PTSD. They also may be living in less-safe environments and have more recent or ongoing trauma exposures.[133] This individual focus should be augmented by the understanding, from a human rights perspective, that BIPOC and other marginalized group members can experience cultural and historical trauma[49] that can make using prenatal care in the dominant culture's healthcare system triggering and stressful.

Birth can be a trauma exposure that leads to recurrence of preexisting PTSD or to new onset PTSD.[132] Birth trauma can occur due to perinatal emergency. However, it also can occur during births that seem normal to the providers but were interpersonally traumatic to the patient because of perceptions of incompetent or uncaring staff.[134]

PTSD adversely affects health, so it may also affect gestational health status and risk behaviors. The chronic wear and tear on the body from PTSD-generated "fight or flight" arousal and sleep disturbance leads to allostatic overload, which takes a toll on the metabolic, cardiorespiratory, immune, and neuroendocrine systems, including in pregnancy.[135] This allostatic overload or "weathering" can be a way of understanding the greater rates of pregnancy complications among marginalized (i.e., highly traumatized, unrecovered) populations.[136] Hormone levels can be altered in ways that have not yet been well studied. Evidence also suggests rates of substance use in pregnancy are higher among those persons with PTSD.[136] In survey research, individuals who were not able to stop smoking in pregnancy may have been self-medicating for noxious symptoms of PTSD. They were more likely to use nicotine to cope with difficult emotions and had levels of PTSD arousal higher than in smokers who were able to quit.[137] PTSD has also been associated with having less social support.[138] Thus, taking a holistic view of the impacts of PTSD suggests that avoiding retraumatization at the very least, enhancing social support, and encouraging treatment for recovery, if possible, are all likely worthwhile as ways to achieve good outcomes.

Pharmacotherapy for PTSD could be helpful during pregnancy. The risk–benefit discussion of this course of action can take the risks of potential self-medication with substances into account. Medications with evidence supporting their recommendation in general include sertraline (Zoloft), which has the best safety profile for pregnancy and breast-feeding/chestfeeding, and which has expert opinion support as a treatment for PTSD across the child-bearing years.[139] It may be helpful for clinicians to recall the dynamics of past trauma and PTSD when considering individuals' specific risk. Patients with PTSD may have negative attention bias or a strong sense that "if something bad can happen, it will" based on their life experience of danger and harm and the hypervigilance of PTSD. This hypervigilance may include very strong efforts to protect the fetus, making the risks of pharmacologic treatment unacceptable to some.

Therapies such as CBT and eye movement desensitization and reprocessing are first-line treatments for PTSD, and the perinatal period is a time when most clients would have access to insurance coverage and integrated behavioral health services. Pregnancy is also a time of high emotional and practical demands, making it hard to engage in trauma-focused therapy, even when it is accessible. The evidence base for trauma treatment during pregnancy is growing, but as of this writing it remains low-level evidence. Qualitative and anecdotal evidence indicates that when their PTSD is frequently and severely triggered during pregnancy, individuals who have sought therapy have made very satisfying progress in processing trauma and achieving their desired outcomes.[140,141]

Positive experiences with providers across the childbearing years—especially during labor—have also been recognized as healing opportunities.[141] Providers can become informed about common concerns and learn how to ask about triggers. A qualitative meta-synthesis of eight qualitative studies conducted with women survivors of sexual abuse found six themes: control, remembering (i.e., reexperiencing), vulnerability, dissociation, concerns about disclosure, and healing.[142] This background information can be applied to inform individual midwives' approach to providing trauma-specific practices within a system of trauma-informed care.

A system of trauma-informed care follows the public health framework of "tiers."[143] The bottom and broadest tier is *universal* trauma-informed care; this requires changing habits of mind to align with knowledge that a significant proportion of clients have experienced trauma and are still affected by it. The middle tier is *targeted* trauma-specific practices and programs; these respond to people who can self-identify as a trauma survivor with some unmet needs. Programs are frontline evidence-based interventions that can be offered by perinatal team members. Practices are responses that individual

providers offer to meet those needs and that may be uniquely tailored or co-created with the client (e.g., a trigger-avoiding birth plan, recommending a doula who is experienced in working with sexual assault survivors in labor). The top tier is *trauma-focused* treatment provided by a mental health specialist; this is the most restrictive tier since often there are not enough resources and not all therapists have training in evidence-based therapies for PTSD.

Some brief specialist help that stops short of trauma-processing therapy may sometimes be needed. Members of the perinatal care team may be able to provide this care. Problems that may require team member expertise could include fear of childbirth, difficulty with breastfeeding/chestfeeding, or dissociation in labor. Midwives, lactation consultants, and nurses or doulas who have strategies that are grounded in their clinical experience and understanding of trauma and PTSD may be well equipped to address these issues.

During the postpartum year, preexisting PTSD and birth-related new-onset PTSD are likely to persist and may be comorbid with depression.[144] It may comfort new parents to know that birth-related PTSD alone has not been associated with bonding problems. The birthing parents most at risk for delayed or impaired bonding are those who had both preexisting PTSD and major depression prenatally and postnatally.[145]

It is possible to screen for trauma history and PTSD at the same time that screening for depression takes place—in pregnancy and postpartum. Case-finding for PTSD and depression prenatally provides an opportunity for mutual collaboration to avoid triggering and retraumatizing and to provide a positive, healing birth experience, strengthening the trauma survivor to get off to a great start at parenting.[146]

## Bipolar Disorder in the Perinatal Period

Pregnancy has not been shown to be protective against mood disorders. As many medications used to treat bipolar disorder are known to be teratogenic, patients with this disorder often discontinue their medications abruptly at first awareness of pregnancy. This greatly increases their risk for an early relapse. Consequences of relapse include poor self-care, poor weight gain in pregnancy, reduced overall prenatal care, increased substance use, increased rates of self-harm, and increased rates of postpartum psychosis. Although the general prevalence of bipolar disorder is low,[4] there is a significant risk of relapse following birth. In addition, patients who experience their first episode of depression in the postpartum period are more likely to have bipolar disorder, with rates varying between 15% and 50%, depending on the diagnostic criteria used.[147]

Perinatal and postpartum patients with a known or suspected diagnosis of bipolar disorder should be co-managed with a multidisciplinary team including the primary care provider, perinatal provider, and psychiatric prescriber.

## Postpartum Psychosis

Postpartum psychosis is a rare and life-threatening emergency that requires immediate psychiatric evaluation. Postpartum psychosis occurs in 1 to 2 women per 1000 live births,[148] and may occur anytime in the first year postpartum. Its peak incidence is during the first 4 weeks postpartum, and it can often be recognized within the first few days postpartum.[148]

Little is known about postpartum psychosis, but it is thought to represent an episode of bipolar illness.[148] Genetics, rapidly changing hormones, and environmental factors all appear to play a role in this condition. In addition, autoimmune thyroid disease may contribute to the development of postpartum psychosis. Patients diagnosed with postpartum psychosis have a 4% to 5% risk of either suicide or infanticide. Treatment of postpartum psychosis often involves hospitalization, mood stabilizers, and benzodiazepines or other medications to improve sleep.

The primary differences among postpartum blues, postpartum depression, and postpartum psychosis relate to the duration and severity of the symptoms. Table 7-17 lists characteristics that can help the clinician distinguish between these conditions when assessing a birthing person who reports disordered mood during the postpartum period.[149]

| Table 7-17 | Diagnostic Criteria for Postpartum Depressive Disorders |
|---|---|

**Postpartum Blues (Baby Blues)**

Affects 80% of new mothers

Onset: first 7–10 days after birth

Peak prevalence: postpartum days 3–5

No specific diagnostic criteria

Most common symptom: weepiness

Other symptoms: mood lability, feeling overwhelmed, sadness and frustration, fatigue/exhaustion

**Postpartum Depression**

Affects 10–20% of new mothers

Onset: first 2–3 months postpartum

Peak prevalence: 2–6 months postpartum

Must include depressed mood or anhedonia and any of the following symptoms, which occur nearly every day for at least 2 weeks and are severe enough to impede function:

1. Sleep disorder (insomnia or hypersomnia)
   a. Must be evaluated in the context of the expected sleep pattern with a newborn
   b. Can the new parent sleep when their infant is asleep?
2. Interest deficit or a lack of feeling pleasure
   a. Inability to appreciate infant, not bonding
   b. Persistent sadness
3. Guilt (worthlessness, hopelessness, regret)
   a. More common than feeling sad
   b. Feeling inadequate as a mother (parent)
4. Fatigue or loss of energy nearly every day
   a. Feeling of being overwhelmed, unable to cope

5. Concentration deficit
   a. Persistent difficulty with normal daily tasks
   b. Difficulty remembering things
6. Appetite disorder (increased or decreased)
   a. Is the woman drinking enough and urinating regularly based on normal postpartum physiology?
7. Psychomotor retardation or agitation
   a. Unable to get out of bed or go to sleep
   b. Loss of interest in caring for oneself
   c. Obsessive thoughts of harm to the infant
8. Suicidality (recurrent thoughts of death)
   a. Thoughts of harming oneself
   b. Do you wish you could go to sleep and not wake up? (passive suicidal ideation)
   c. Do you think about ways to kill yourself? (active suicidal ideation)

**Postpartum Psychosis**

Affects 1–2 women per 1000 live births

Onset: usually starts within 2–4 weeks of birth, but can start as early as 2–3 days after birth and often progresses rapidly

Emergency psychiatric condition characterized by symptoms of:
• Confusion, restlessness, disorganized behavior
• Delusional beliefs, hallucinations, and disordered thinking
• "Everything is black or dark"
• Feeling of hopelessness
• Delusions about the infant
• Auditory hallucinations, which can be instructions to harm the infant
• Visual hallucinations

Modified with permission from NIHCM Foundation. *Identifying and Treating Maternal Depression: Strategies and Considerations for Health Plans*. Issue Brief. Rockville, MD: U.S. Public Health Service, Health Resources and Services Administration, Maternal and Child Health Bureau; 2010. https://nihcm.org/publications/identifying-treating-maternal-depression-strategies-considerations-for-health-plans. Accessed January 16, 2023.

## Conclusion

Millions of individuals develop mental health disorders in the United States, and these conditions are likely to affect the well-being of both the individual and their family. For some people, the midwife may be the first or only healthcare provider available to address their needs. As primary care providers, midwives are, at a minimum, responsible for appropriate screening and referral for those clients at risk for mental health conditions. A system of universal screening can help identify the individuals at risk for mental illness, and determine who can be treated safely within a primary care setting and who should be referred for more specialized treatment. With psychiatric consultation and collaboration, midwives can provide first-line treatment for many patients.

Psychopharmacology is an important component of treatment of mental health disorders. With careful screening, counseling, follow-up, and potential referral, this approach to treatment can be within the scope of midwifery practice. As when prescribing any medication regimen, it is essential that the midwife be familiar with psychotropic medications.

An individual's susceptibility to mental health is influenced by their life stage and hormonal status, among other factors. Pregnancy and the puerperium are times characterized by dramatic hormonal shifts, which when compounded with the stresses of becoming a parent can place someone at increased risk for mood and anxiety disorders. For those persons who have trauma from childhood maltreatment, sexual violence, or previous medical or perinatal traumatic experiences, PTSD can be activated by pregnancy, parenting an infant, or prenatal and labor care. Early identification and treatment can decrease long-term morbidity, but the potential effects of medications on the fetus and nursing newborn must also be considered.

## Resources

| Organization | Resource |
| --- | --- |
| MGH Center Women's Mental Health | Perinatal Information Resource Center (PIRC) website provides a listing of women's mental health resources for providers and patients, updates from the literature, and continuing education. |
| 988 Suicide and Crisis Lifeline | The 988 dialing code across the United States offers 24/7 call, text, and chat access to trained crisis counselors for help with mental health crises including suicidal thoughts, substance use, and emotional distress. People can also call if they are worried about a loved one who may need crisis support. |

## References

1. American Psychiatric Association. *Diagnostic and Statistical Manual of Mental Disorders. 5th ed. Text revision (DSM-5-TR)*. Arlington, VA: American Psychiatric Association; 2022.

2. Roehrig C. Mental disorders top the list of the most costly conditions in the United States: $201 billion. *Health Aff.* 2016;35(6):1130-1135. doi:10.1377/hlthaff.2015.1659Mayor E.

3. Goldstein RB, Smith SM, Chou SP, et al. The epidemiology of DSM-5 posttraumatic stress disorder in the United States: results from the National Epidemiologic Survey on Alcohol and Related Conditions-III. *Soc Psychiatry Psychiatr Epidemiol.* 2016;51(8):1137-1148. doi:10.1007/s00127-016-1208-5.

4. Kessler RC, Berglund P, Demler O, et al. Lifetime prevalence and age-of-onset distributions of *DSM-IV* disorders in the National Comorbidity Survey Replication. *Arch Gen Psychiatry.* 2005;62(6):593-602. doi:10.1001/archpsyc.62.6.593.

5. National Institute for Mental Health. Prevalence of any mental illness. https://www.nimh.nih.gov/health/statistics/mental-illness. Updated January 2, 2022. Accessed February 3, 2022.

6. Seedat S, Scott KM, Angermeyer MC, et al. Cross-national associations between gender and mental disorders in the World Health Organization World Mental Health Surveys. *Arch Gen Psychiatry.* 2009;66(7):785-795. doi:10.1001/archgenpsychiatry.2009.36.

7. Kumsta R. The role of epigenetics for understanding mental health difficulties and its implications for psychotherapy research. *Psychol Psychother.* 2019;92(2):190-207. doi:10.1111/papt.12227.

8. Kendall K, Van Assche E, Andlauer T, et al. The genetic basis of major depression. *Psychol Med.* 2021;51(13):2217-2230. doi:10.1017/S0033291721000441.

9. Substance Abuse and Mental Health Services Administration. *SAMHSA's Concept of Trauma and Guidance for a Trauma-Informed Approach*. HHS Publication No. (SMA) 14-4884. Rockville, MD: Substance Abuse and Mental Health Services Administration; 2014.

10. Hasin DS, Sarvet AL, Meyers JL, et al. Epidemiology of adult DSM-5 major depressive disorder and its specifiers in the United States. *JAMA Psychiatry.* 2018;75(4):336-346. doi:10.1001/jamapsychiatry.2017.4602.

11. Akincigil A, Matthews EB. National rates and patterns of depression screening in primary care: results from 2012 and 2013. *Psychiatr Serv.* 2017;68(7):660-666. doi:10.1176/appi.ps.201600096.

12. National Institute of Mental Health. Prevalence of any mental illness. https://www.nimh.nih.gov/health/statistics/major-depression. Updated January 2022. Accessed February 3, 2022.

13. GBD 2017 Disease and Injury Incidence and Prevalence Collaborators. Global, regional, and national incidence, prevalence, and years lived with disability for 354 diseases and injuries for 195 countries and territories, 1990–2017: a systematic analysis for the Global Burden of Disease Study 2017. *Lancet.* 2018;392(10159):1789-1858. doi:10.1016/S0140-6736(18)32279-7. [Published correction appears in *Lancet.* 2019;393(10190):e44.]

14. Merikangas KR, Ames M, Cui L, et al. The impact of comorbidity of mental and physical conditions on role disability in the US adult household population. *Arch Gen Psychiatry.* 2007;64(10):1180-1188. doi:10.1001/archpsyc.64.10.1180.

15. Hackley B, Sharma C, Kedzior A, Sreenivasan S. Managing mental health conditions in primary care settings. *J Midwifery Womens Health.* 2010;55(1):9-19. doi:10.1016/j.jmwh.2009.06.004.

16. Roest AM, de Vries YA, Al-Hamzawi A, et al. Previous disorders and depression outcomes in individuals with 12-month major depressive disorder in the World Mental Health surveys. *Epidemiol Psychiatr Sci.* 2021;30:e70. doi:10.1017/S2045796021000573.

17. U.S. Department of Health and Human Services. *Depression in Primary Care: Volume 1. Detection and Diagnosis*. AHCPR Publication No. 93-0550. Rockville, MD: Agency for Health Care Policy and Research; 1993:20.

18. Pfizer, Inc. The Patient Health Questionnaire-9. http://www.phqscreeners.com. Accessed February 3, 2022.

19. Cox JL, Holden JM, Sagovsky R. Detection of post-natal depression: development of the 10-item Edinburgh Postnatal Depression Scale. *Br J Psychiatry.* 1987;150:782-786. doi:10.1192/bjp.150.6.782.

20. Levis B, Sun Y, He C, et al. Accuracy of the PHQ-2 alone and in combination with the PHQ-9 for screening to detect major depression: systematic review and meta-analysis. *JAMA.* 2020;323(22):2290-2300. doi:10.1001/jama.2020.6504.

21. Levis B, Negeri Z, Sun Y, et al. Accuracy of the Edinburgh Postnatal Depression Scale (EPDS) for screening to detect major depression among pregnant and postpartum women: systematic review and meta-analysis of individual participant data. *BMJ.* 2020;371:m4022. doi:10.1136/bmj.m4022.

22. Smith-Nielsen J, Egmose I, Wendelboe KI, et al. Can the Edinburgh Postnatal Depression Scale-3A be used to screen for anxiety? *BMC Psychol.* 2021;9:118. doi.org/10.1186/s40359-021-00623-5.

23. Latendresse G, Elmore C, Deneris A. Selective serotonin reuptake inhibitors as first-line antidepressant therapy for perinatal depression. *J Midwifery Womens Health.* 2017;62(3):317-328. doi:10.1111/jmwh.12607.

24. Maurer DM. Screening for depression. *Am Fam Physician.* 2012;85(2):139-144.

25. Cougle JR, Resnick H, Kilpatrick DG. PTSD, depression, and their comorbidity in relation to suicidality: cross-sectional and prospective analyses of a national probability sample of women. *Depress Anxiety.* 2009;26(12):1151-1157. doi:10.1001/archpsyc.1995.03950240066012.

26. Claassen CA, Trivedi MH, Rush AJ, et al. Clinical differences among depressed patients with and without a history of suicide attempts: findings from the STAR*D trial. *J Affect Disord.* 2007;97(1-3):77-84. doi:10.1016/j.jad.2006.05.026.

27. Hirschfeld RM, Williams JB, Spitzer RL, et al. Development and validation of a screening instrument for bipolar spectrum disorder: the Mood Disorder Questionnaire. *Am J Psychiatry.* 2000;157(11):1873-1875. doi:10.1176/appi.ajp.157.11.1873.

28. Bandelow B, Michaelis S. Epidemiology of anxiety disorders in the 21st century. *Dialog Clin Neurosci.* 2015;17(3):327-335. doi:10.31887/DCNS.2015.17.3/bbandelow.

29. Terlizzi E, Villarroel M. Symptoms of generalized anxiety disorder among adults: United States, 2019. *NCHS Data Brief.* 2020;(378):1-8. https://www.cdc.gov/nchs/products/databriefs/db378.htm. Accessed January 14, 2023.

30. Kessler RC, Petukhova M, Sampson NA, et al. Twelve-month and lifetime prevalence and lifetime morbid risk of anxiety and mood disorders in the United States. *Int J Methods Psychiatr Res.* 2012;21(3):169-184. doi:10.1002/mpr.1359.

31. Zolensky MJ, Garey L, Bakshaie J. Disparities in anxiety and its disorders. *J Anxiety Disord.* 2017;48:1-5. doi:10.1016/j.janxdis.2017.05.004.

32. Patriquin MA, Mathew SJ. The neurobiological mechanisms of generalized anxiety disorder and chronic stress. *Chronic Stress (Thousand Oaks).* 2017 Jan-Dec;1:2470547017703993. doi:10.1177/2470547017703993. Epub 2017 Jun 8.

33. Barbano AC, van der Mei WF, deRoon-Cassini TA, et al. Differentiating PTSD from anxiety and depression: lessons from the ICD-11 PTSD diagnostic criteria. *Depress Anxiety.* 2019;36(6):490-498. doi:10.1002/da.22881.

34. Nievergelt CM, Maihofer AX, Klengel T, et al. International meta-analysis of PTSD genome-wide association studies identifies sex- and ancestry-specific genetic risk loci. *Nat Commun.* 2019;10(1):4558. doi:10.1038/s41467-019-12576-w.

35. Neria Y. Functional neuroimaging in PTSD: from discovery of underlying mechanisms to addressing diagnostic heterogeneity. *Am J Psychiatry.* 2021;178(2):128-135. doi:10.1176/appi.ajp.2020.20121727/.

36. Baldwin DS, Anderson IM, Nutt DJ, et al. Evidence-based pharmacological treatment of anxiety disorders, post-traumatic stress disorder and obsessive–compulsive disorder: a revision of the 2005 guidelines from the British Association for Psychopharmacology. *J Psychopharm.* 2014;28(5):403-439. doi:10.1177/0269881114525674.

37. Spitzer RL, Kroenke K, Williams JB, Löwe B. A brief measure for assessing generalized anxiety disorder: the GAD-7. *Arch Intern Med.* 2006;166(10):1092-1097. doi:10.1001/archinte.166.10.1092.

38. Robinson CM, Klenck SC, Norton PJ. Psychometric properties of the Generalized Anxiety Disorder Questionnaire for *DSM-IV* among four racial groups. *Cognitive Behav Ther.* 2010;39(4):251-261. doi:10.1080/16506073.2010.486841.

39. National Institutes of Health, National Institute on Drug Abuse. Common comorbidities with substance use disorders research report. https://www.drugabuse.gov/publications/research-reports/common-comorbidities-substance-use-disorders/introduction. Updated April 2020. Accessed February 9, 2023.

40. Mennis J, Stahler GJ, Mason MJ. Risky substance use environments and addiction: a new frontier for environmental justice research. *Int J Environ Res Public Health.* 2016;13(6):607. doi:10.3390/ijerph13060607.

41. American Society of Addiction Medicine. Public policy statement on advancing racial justice in addiction medicine. https://www.asam.org/advocacy/public-policy-statements/details/public-policy-statements/2021/02/25/public-policy-statement-on-advancing-racial-justice-in-addiction-medicine. Published February 25, 2021. Accessed February 2, 2022.

42. Centers for Disease Control and Prevention. Drug overdose deaths in the U.S. top 100,000. https://www.cdc.gov/nchs/pressroom/nchs_press_releases/2021/20211117.htm. Published November 17, 2021. Accessed February 3, 2022.

43. Kessler RC, Aguilar-Gaxiola S, Alonso J, et al. Trauma and PTSD in the WHO World Mental Health Surveys. *Eur J Psychotraumatol.* 2017;8(sup5):1353383. doi:10.1080/20008198.2017.1353383.

44. Breslau N, Davis GC, Peterson EL, Schultz LR. A second look at comorbidity in victims of trauma: the posttraumatic stress disorder–major depression connection. *Biol Psychiatry.* 2000;48(9):902-909. doi:10.1016/s0006-3223(00)00933-1.

45. Khantzian EJ. The self-medication hypothesis of substance use disorders: a reconsideration and recent applications. *Harv Rev Psychiatry.* 1997;4(5):231-244. doi:10.3109/10673229709030550.

46. Fox V, Dalman C, Dal H, et al. Suicide risk in people with post-traumatic stress disorder: a cohort study of 3.1 million people in Sweden. *J Affect Disord.* 2021;279:609-616. doi:10.1016/j.jad.2020.10.009.

47. Stein DJ, Koenen KC, Friedman MJ, et al. Dissociation in posttraumatic stress disorder: evidence from the World Mental Health Surveys. *Biol Psychiatry.* 2013;73(4):302-312. doi:10.1016/j.biopsych.2012.08.022.

48. Herrenkohl TI. Person–environment interactions and the shaping of resilience. *Trauma Violence Abuse.* 2013;14(3):191-194. doi:10.1177/1524838013491035.

49. Butler LD, Carello J, Critelli F, eds. *Trauma and Human Rights: Integrating Approaches to Address Human Suffering.* London, UK: Palgrave Macmillan; 2019. doi.org/10.1007/978-3-030-16395-2.

50. U.S. Department of Veteran Affairs, National Center for PTSD. Acute stress disorder. https://www.ptsd.va.gov/professional/treat/essentials/acute_stress_disorder.asp. Updated October 2019. Accessed January 14, 2023.

51. Breslau N, Lucia VC, Davis GC. Partial PTSD versus full PTSD: an empirical examination of associated impairment. *Psychol Med.* 2004;34(7):1205-1214. doi:10.1017/s0033291704002594.

52. Kostaras P, Bergiannaki JD, Psarros C, et al. Posttraumatic stress disorder in outpatients with depression: still a missed diagnosis. *J Trauma Dissociation.* 2017;18(2):233-247. doi:10.1080/15299732.2016.1237402.

53. California Surgeon General's Clinical Advisory Committee. Adverse childhood experiences revised questionnaire. Aces Aware, State of California Department of Health Care Services. https://www.acesaware.org/wp-content/uploads/2019/11/ACEs-Screener-Identified-English.pdf. Accessed January 14, 2023.

54. U.S. Department of Veteran Affairs, National Center for PTSD. Primary care PTSD screen for *DSM-5* (PC-PTSD-5). https://www.ptsd.va.gov/professional/assessment/screens/pc-ptsd.asp. Updated August 12, 2021. Accessed January 14, 2023.

55. Prins A, Bovin MJ, Kimerling R, et al. The primary care PTSD screen for DSM-5 (PC-PTSD-5). *J Gen Intern Med.* 2016;(31):1206-1211. https://doi.org/10.1007/s11606-016-3703-5. Accessed January 14, 2023.

56. Ismaili E, Walsh S, O'Brien PMS, et al. Fourth consensus of the International Society for Premenstrual Disorders (ISPMD): auditable standard for diagnosis and management of premenstrual disorder. *Arch Womens Mental Health.* 2016;19:953-958. doi:10.1007/s00737-016-0631-7.

57. Robinson LL, Ismail KM. Clinical epidemiology of premenstrual disorder: informing optimized patient outcomes. *Int J Womens Health.* 2015;7:811-818. doi:10.2147/IJWH.S48426.

58. Rubinow DR, Schmidt PJ. Is there a role for reproductive steroids in the etiology and treatment of affective disorders? *Dialogues Clin Neurosci.* 2018;20(3):187-196. doi:10.31887/DCNS.2018.20.3/drubinow.

59. Li HJ, Goff A, Rudzinskas SA, et al. Altered estradiol-dependent cellular $Ca^{2+}$ homeostasis and endoplasmic reticulum stress response in premenstrual dysphoric disorder. *Mol Psychiatry.* 2021;26(11):6963-6974. doi:10.1038/s41380-021-01144-8.

60. Eisenlohr-Moul TA, Girdler SS, Schmalenberger KM, et al. Toward the reliable diagnosis of *DSM-5* premenstrual dysphoric disorder: the Carolina Premenstrual Assessment Scoring System (C-PASS). *Am J Psychiatry.* 2017;174:51-59. doi:10.1176/appi.ajp.2016.15121510.

61. Epperson CN, Hantsoo LV. Making strides to simplify diagnosis of premenstrual dysphoric disorder. *Am J Psychiatry.* 2017;174(1):6-7. doi:10.1176/appi.ajp.2016.16101144.

62. Endicott J, Nee J, Harrison W. Daily Record of Severity of Problems (DRSP): reliability and validity. *Arch Womens Mental Health.* 2006;9:41-49. doi:10.1007/s00737-005-0103-y.

63. Direkvand-Moghadam A, Sayehmiri K, Delpisheh A, Sattar K. Epidemiology of premenstrual syndrome (PMS): a systematic review and meta-analysis study. *J Clin Diagn Res.* 2014;8(2):106-109. doi:10.7860/JCDR/2014/8024.4021. [Published correction appears in *J Clin Diagn Res.* 2015;9(7):ZZ05.]

64. Chung W, Jiang SF, Paksarian D, et al. Trends in the prevalence and incidence of attention-deficit/hyperactivity disorder among adults and children of different racial and ethnic groups. *JAMA Netw Open.* 2019;2(11):e1914344. doi:10.1001/jamanetworkopen.2019.14344.

65. Early NK. Mental health. In: Brucker MC, King TL, eds. *Pharmacology for Women's Health.* 2nd ed. Burlington, MA: Jones & Bartlett Learning; 2017:727-764.

66. Cooney GM, Dwan K, Greig CA, et al. Exercise for depression. *Cochrane Database Syst Rev.* 2013;9:CD004366. doi:10.1002/14651858.CD004366.pub6.

67. Trangle M, Gursky J, Haight R, et al. Adult depression in primary care. Institute for Clinical Systems Improvement. https://www.icsi.org/wp-content/uploads/2021/11/Depr.pdf. Updated March 2016. Accessed February 8, 2022.

68. Kamenov K, Twomey C, Cabello M, et al. The efficacy of psychotherapy, pharmacotherapy and their combination on functioning and quality of life in depression: a meta-analysis. *Psychol Med.* 2017;47(3):414-425. doi:10.1017/S0033291716002774.

69. Cuijpers P, Noma H, Karyotaki E, et al. A network meta-analysis of the effects of psychotherapies, pharmacotherapies and their combination in the treatment of adult depression. *World Psychiatry.* 2020;19(1):92-107. doi:10.1002/wps.20701.

70. Bandelow B, Michaelis S, Wedekind D. Treatment of anxiety disorders. *Dialogues Clin Neurosci.* 2017;19(2):93-107. doi:10.31887/DCNS.2017.19.2/bbandelow.

71. Schramm E, Klein DN, Elsaesser M, et al. Review of dysthymia and persistent depressive disorder: history, correlates, and clinical implications. *Lancet Psychiatry.* 2020;7(9):801-812. doi:10.1016/S2215-0366(20)30099-7.

72. Zhang A, Franklin C, Jing S, et al. The effectiveness of four empirically supported psychotherapies for primary care depression and anxiety: a systematic review and meta-analysis. *J Affect Disord.* 2019;245:1168-1186. doi:10.1016/j.jad.2018.12.008.

73. Hofmann SG, Asnaani A, Vonk IJ, et al. The efficacy of cognitive behavioral therapy: a review of meta-analyses. *Cognit Ther Res.* 2012;36(5):427-440. doi:10.1007/s10608-012-9476-1.

74. Olthuis JV, Watt MC, Bailey K, et al. Therapist-supported Internet cognitive behavioural therapy for anxiety disorders in adults. *Cochrane Database Syst Rev.* 2016;3:CD011565. doi:10.1002/14651858.CD011565.pub2.

75. Matsumoto K, Hamatani S, Shimizu E. Effectiveness of videoconference-delivered cognitive behavioral therapy for adults with psychiatric disorders: systematic and meta-analytic review. *J Med Internet Res.* 2021;23(12):e31293. doi:10.2196/31293.

76. Schuch FB, Vancampfort D, Rosenbaum S, et al. Exercise improves physical and psychological quality of life in people with depression: a meta-analysis including the evaluation of control group response. *Psychiatry Res.* 2016;241:47-54. doi:10.1016/j.psychres.2016.04.054.

77. Daveney J, Panagioti M, Waheed W, Esmail A. Unrecognized bipolar disorder in patients with depression managed in primary care: a systematic review and meta-analysis. *Gen Hosp Psychiatry.* 2019;58:71-76. doi:10.1016/j.genhosppsych.2019.03.006.

78. U.S. Department of Veterans Affairs. The management of major depressive disorder: clinical guideline summary. https://www.healthquality.va.gov/guidelines/MH/mdd/. Updated 2022. Accessed January 14, 2023.

79. Garakani A, Murrough JW, Freire RC, et al. Pharmacotherapy of anxiety disorders: current and emerging treatment options. *Front Psychiatry.* 2020;11:595584. doi:10.3389/fpsyt.2020.595584.

80. Montejo AL, Montejo L, Baldwin DS. The impact of severe mental disorders and psychotropic medications on sexual health and its implications for clinical management. *World Psychiatry.* 2018;17(1):3-11. doi:10.1002/wps.20509.

81. Wang RZ, Vashistha V, Kaur S, Houchens NW. Serotonin syndrome: preventing, recognizing, and treating it. *Cleve Clin J Med.* 2016;83(11):810-817.

82. Boaden K, Tomlinson A, Cortese S, Cipriani A. Antidepressants in children and adolescents: meta-review of efficacy, tolerability and suicidality in acute treatment. *Front Psychiatry.* 2020;11:717. doi:10.3389/fpsyt.2020.00717.

83. Severe J, Greden JF, Reddy P. Consequences of recurrence of major depressive disorder: is stopping effective antidepressant medications ever safe? *Focus (Am Psychiatr Publ).* 2020;18(2):120-128. doi:10.1176/appi.focus.20200008.

84. Pence BW, O'Donnell JK, Gaynes BN. The depression treatment cascade in primary care: a public health perspective. *Curr Psychiatry Rep.* 2012;14(4):328-335. doi:10.1007/s11920-012-0274-y.

85. Ng JY, Nazir Z, Nault H. Complementary and alternative medicine recommendations for depression: a systematic review and assessment of clinical practice guidelines. *BMC Complement Med Ther.* 2020;20(1):299. doi:10.1186/s12906-020-03085-1.

86. Ravindran AV, Balneaves LG, Faulkner G, et al. Canadian Network for Mood and Anxiety Treatments (CANMAT) 2016 clinical guidelines for the management of adults with major depressive disorder: Section 5. Complementary and alternative medicine treatments. *Can J Psychiatry.* 2016;61(9):576-587. doi:10.1177/0706743716660290.

87. Gong H, Ni C, Shen X, et al. Yoga for prenatal depression: a systematic review and meta-analysis. *BMC Psychiatry.* 2015;15:14.

88. National Institutes of Health, National Center for Complementary and Integrative Health. Depression and complementary health approaches: what the science says. *NCCIH Clin Dig.* October 2019. https://www.nccih.nih.gov/health/providers/digest/depression-and-complementary-health-approaches. Accessed February 3, 2022.

89. Deane KHO, Jimoh OF, Biswas P, et al. Omega-3 and polyunsaturated fat for prevention of depression and anxiety symptoms: systematic review and meta-analysis of randomised trials. *Br J Psychiatry.* 2021;218(3):135-142. doi:10.1192/bjp.2019.234.

90. Forbes D, Bisson JI, Monson CM, Berliner L, eds. *Effective Treatments for PTSD: Practice Guidelines from the International Society for Traumatic Stress Studies.* 3rd ed. New York, NY: Guilford; 2020.

91. Ford JD, Courtois C, eds. *Treating Complex Traumatic Stress Disorders in Adults: Scientific Foundations and Therapeutic Models,* 2nd ed. New York, NY: Guildford Press; 2020.

92. Cloitre M, Koenen KC, Cohen LR, Han H. Skills training in affective and interpersonal regulation followed by exposure: a phase-based treatment for PTSD related to childhood abuse. *J Consult Clin Psychol.* 2002;70(5):1067-1074. doi:10.1037//0022 -006x.70.5.1067.

93. Lynch TR, Chapman AL, Rosenthal MZ, et al. Mechanisms of change in dialectical behavior therapy: theoretical and empirical observations. *J Clin Psychol.* 2006;62(4):459-480. doi:10.1002/jclp.20243.

94. Sperlich M, Seng JS, Rowe H, et al. The Survivor Moms' Companion: feasibility, safety, and acceptability of a posttraumatic stress specific psychoeducation program for pregnant survivors of childhood maltreatment and sexual trauma. *Int J Childbirth.* 2011;1(2):122-135.doi:10.1891/2156-5287.1.2.122.

95. Karatzias T, Cloitre M. Treating adults with complex posttraumatic stress disorder using a modular approach to treatment: rationale, evidence, and directions for future research. *J Trauma Stress.* 2019;32(6):870-876. doi:10.1002/jts.22457.

96. Csupor D, Lantos T, Hegyi P, et al. Vitex agnus-castus in premenstrual syndrome: a meta-analysis of double-blind randomised controlled trials. *Complement Ther Med.*2019;47:102190.doi:10.1016/j.ctim .2019.08.024.

97. Lanze di Scalea T, Pearlstein T. Premenstrual dysphoric disorder. *Psychiatr Clin North Am.* 2017;40: 201-216. doi:10.1016/j.mcna.2019.02.007.

98. Marjoribanks J, Brown J, O'Brien PM, Wyatt K. Selective serotonin reuptake inhibitors for premenstrual syndrome. *Cochrane Database Syst Rev.* 2013;6:CD001396.doi:10.1002/14651858.CD00 1396.pub3.

99. Lopez LM, Kaptein AA, Helmerhorst FM. Oral contraceptives containing drospirenone for premenstrual syndrome. *Cochrane Database Syst Rev.* 2012;2:CD006586. doi:10.1002/14651858.CD006 586.pub4.

100. Naheed B, Kuiper JH, Uthman OA, et al. Non-contraceptive oestrogen-containing preparations for controlling symptoms of premenstrual syndrome. *Cochrane Database Syst Rev.* 2017;3(3): CD010503.

101. Peters W, Freeman MP, Kim S, et al. Treatment of premenstrual breakthrough of depression with adjunctive oral contraceptive pills compared with placebo. *J Clin Psychopharmacol.* 2017;37(5):609-614. doi: 10.1097/JCP.0000000000000761.

102. Wang TH, Pai LW, Tzeng YL, et al. Effectiveness of nurses and midwives-led psychological interventions on reducing depression symptoms in the perinatal period: a systematic review and meta-analysis. *Nurs Open.* 2021;8(5):2117-2130. doi:10.1002 /nop2.764.

103. Woody CA, Ferrari AJ, Siskind DJ, et al. A systematic review and meta-regression of the prevalence and incidence of perinatal depression. *J Affect Disord.* 2017;219:86-92. doi:10.1016/j.jad.2017.05.003.

104. Fawcett EJ, Fairbrother N, Cox ML, et al. The prevalence of anxiety disorders during pregnancy and the postpartum period: a multivariate Bayesian meta-analysis. *J Clin Psychiatry.* 2019;80(4): 18r12527. doi:10.4088/JCP.18r12527.

105. Trost S. Preventing pregnancy-related mental health deaths: insights from 14 US maternal mortality review committees, 2008–17. *Health Aff.* 2021;40(10):1551-1559. doi:10.1377/hlthaff.2021 .00615.

106. Simonovich SD, Nidey NL, Gavin AR, et al. Meta-analysis of antenatal depression and adverse birth outcomes in US populations, 2010–20. *Health Aff.* 2021;40(10):1560-1565. doi:10.1377 /hlthaff.2021.00801.

107. Grigoriadis S, Graves L, Peer M, et al. Maternal anxiety during pregnancy and the association with adverse perinatal outcomes: systematic review and meta-analysis. *J Clin Psychiatry.* 2018;79(5):17r 12011. doi:10.4088/JCP.17r12011.

108. Shao S, Wang J, Huang K, et al. Prenatal pregnancy-related anxiety predicts boys' ADHD symptoms via placental C-reactive protein. *Psychoneuroendocrinology.* 2020;120:104797. doi:10 .1016/j.psyneuen.2020.104797.

109. Bolea-Alamañac B, Davies SJC, Evans J, et al. Does maternal somatic anxiety in pregnancy predispose children to hyperactivity? *Eur Child Adolesc Psychiatry.* 2019;28(11):1475-1486. doi:10.1007/s007 87-019-01289-6.

110. Chisolm MS, Payne JL. Management of psychotropic drugs during pregnancy. *BMJ.* 2016;532:h5918. doi:10.1136/bmj.h5918.

111. Rezaie-Keikhaie K, Arbabshastan ME, Rafiemanesh H, et al. Systematic review and meta-analysis of the prevalence of the maternity blues in the postpartum period. *J Obstet Gynecol Neonatal Nurs.* 2020;49(2): 127-136. doi:10.1016/j.jogn.2020.01.001.

112. Stewart DE, Vigod SN. Postpartum depression: pathophysiology, treatment, and emerging therapeutics. *Annu Rev Med*. 2019;70:183-196. doi:10.1146/annurev-med-041217-011106.

113. Sharma V, Palagini L, Riemann D. Should we target insomnia to treat and prevent postpartum depression? *J Matern Fetal Neonatal Med*. 2021;1-3. doi:10.1080/14767058.2021.2005021.

114. Rafferty J, Mattson G, Earls MF, Yogman MW; Committee on Psychosocial Aspects of Child and Family Health. Incorporating recognition and management of perinatal depression into pediatric practice. *Pediatrics*. 2019;143(1):e20183260. doi:10.1542/peds.2018-3260.

115. Gavin NI, Gaynes BN, Lohr KN, et al. Perinatal depression: a systematic review of prevalence and incidence. *Obstet Gynecol*. 2005;106(5 pt 1):1071-1083. doi:10.1097/01.AOG.0000183597.31630.db.

116. Netsi E, Pearson RM, Murray L, et al. Association of persistent and severe postnatal depression with child outcomes. *JAMA Psychiatry*. 2018;75(3):247-253. doi:10.1001/jamapsychiatry.2017.4363.

117. Polte C, Junge C, von Soest T, et al. Impact of maternal perinatal anxiety on social-emotional development of 2-year-olds, a prospective study of Norwegian mothers and their offspring: the impact of perinatal anxiety on child development. *Matern Child Health J*. 2019;23(3):386-396. doi:10.1007/s10995-018-2684-x.

118. Werner E, Miller M, Osborne LM, Kuzava S, Monk C. Preventing postpartum depression: review and recommendations. *Arch Womens Ment Health*. 2015 Feb;18(1):41-60. doi:10.1007/s00737-014-0475-y.

119. Betcher HK, Wisner KL. Psychotropic treatment during pregnancy: research synthesis and clinical care principles. *J Womens Health*. 2020;29(3):310-318. doi:10.1089/jwh.2019.7781.

120. Munk-Olsen T, Bergink V, Rommel AS, et al. Association of persistent pulmonary hypertension in infants with the timing and type of antidepressants in utero. *JAMA Netw Open*. 2021;4(12):e2136639. doi:10.1001/jamanetworkopen.2021.36639.

121. Huybrechts KF, Bateman BT, Palmsten K, et al. Antidepressant use late in pregnancy and risk of persistent pulmonary hypertension of the newborn. *JAMA*. 2015;313(21):2142-2151. doi:10.1001/jama.2015.5605.

122. Leshem R, Bar-Oz B, Diav-Citrin O, et al. Selective serotonin reuptake inhibitors (SSRIs) and serotonin norepinephrine reuptake inhibitors (SNRIs) during pregnancy and the risk for autism spectrum disorder (ASD) and attention deficit hyperactivity disorder (ADHD) in the offspring: a true effect or a bias? A systematic review and meta-analysis. *Curr Neuropharmacol*. 2021;19(6):896-906. doi:10.2174/1570159X19666210303121059.

123. Sriraman NK, Melvin K, Meltzer-Brody S. ABM Clinical Protocol #18: use of antidepressants in breastfeeding mothers. *Breastfeed Med*. 2015;10:290-299. doi:10.1089/bfm.2015.29002.

124. Anderson PO. Antidepressants and breastfeeding. *Breastfeed Med*. 2021;16(1):5-7. doi:10.1089/bfm.2020.0350.

125. Martin CE, Scialli A, Terplan M. Addiction and depression: unmet treatment needs among reproductive age women. *Matern Child Health J*. 2020;24(5):660-667. doi:10.1007/s10995-020-02904-8.

126. Substance Abuse and Mental Health Services Administration. *Clinical Guidance for Treating Pregnant and Parenting Women with Opioid Use Disorder and Their Infants*. HHS Publication No. (SMA) 18-5054. Rockville, MD: Substance Abuse and Mental Health Services Administration; 2018.

127. Towers CV, Katz E, Weitz B, Visconti K. Use of naltrexone in treating opioid use disorder in pregnancy. *Am J Obstet Gynecol*. 2020;222(1):83.e1-83.e8. doi:10.1016/j.ajog.2019.07.037.

128. Fraiberg S, Adelson E, Shapiro V. Ghosts in the nursery: a psychoanalytic approach to the problems of impaired infant–mother relationships. In: Raphael-Leff J, ed. *Parent–Infant Psychodynamics: Wild Things, Mirrors, and Ghosts*. London, UK: Routledge; 2018: 87-117.

129. Seng J, Miller J, Sperlich M, et al. Exploring dissociation and oxytocin as pathways between trauma exposure and trauma-related hyperemesis gravidarum: a test-of-concept pilot. *J Trauma Dissociation*. 2013;14(1):40-55. doi:10.1080/15299732.2012.694594.

130. Cook N, Ayers S, Horsch A. Maternal posttraumatic stress disorder during the perinatal period and child outcomes: a systematic review. *J Affect Disord*. 2018;225:18-31. doi:10.1016/j.jad.2017.07.045.

131. Turton P, Hughes P, Evans CD, Fainman D. Incidence, correlates and predictors of post-traumatic stress disorder in the pregnancy after stillbirth. *Br J Psychiatry*. 2001;178:556-560. doi:10.1192/bjp.178.6.556.

132. Yildiz PD, Ayers S, Phillips L. The prevalence of posttraumatic stress disorder in pregnancy and after birth: a systematic review and meta-analysis. *J Affect Disord*. 2017;208:634-645. doi:10.1016/j.jad.2016.10.009.

133. Seng JS, Low LK, Sperlich M, et al. Prevalence, trauma history, and risk for posttraumatic stress disorder among nulliparous women in maternity care. *Obstet Gynecol*. 2009;114(4):839-847. doi:10.1097/AOG.0b013e3181b8f8a2.

134. Beck CT. Birth trauma and its sequelae. *J Trauma Dissociation*. 2009;10(2):189-203. doi:10.1080/15299730802624528. PMID: 19333848.

135. Li Y, Rosenberg MS, Seng JS. Allostatic load: a theoretical model for understanding the relationship between maternal posttraumatic stress disorder and adverse birth outcomes. *Midwifery*. 2018;62:205-213. doi:10.1016/j.midw.2018.04.002.

136. Morland L, Goebert D, Onoye J, et al. Posttraumatic stress disorder and pregnancy health: preliminary update and implications. *Psychosomatics*. 2007;48(4):304-308. doi:10.1176/appi.psy.48.4.304.

137. Lopez WD, Konrath SH, Seng JS. Abuse-related post-traumatic stress, coping, and tobacco use in pregnancy. *J Obstet Gynecol Neonatal Nurs*. 2011;40(4):422-431. doi:10.1111/j.1552-6909.2011.01261.x.

138. Zalta AK, Tirone V, Orlowska D, et al. Examining moderators of the relationship between social support and self-reported PTSD symptoms: a meta-analysis. *Psychol Bull*. 2021;147(1):33-54. doi:10.1037/bul0000316.

139. Thomson M, Sharma V. Pharmacotherapeutic considerations for the treatment of posttraumatic stress disorder during and after pregnancy. *Expert Opin Pharmacother*. 2021;22(6):705-714. doi:10.1080/14656566.2020.1854727.

140. Seng JS, Sparbel KJ, Low LK, Killion C. Abuse-related posttraumatic stress and desired maternity care practices: women's perspectives. *J Midwifery Womens Health*. 2002;47(5):360-370. doi:10.1016/s1526-9523(02)00284-2.

141. Sperlich M, Seng JS. *Survivor Moms: Women's Stories of Birthing, Mothering and Healing After Sexual Abuse*. Eugene, OR: Motherbaby Press; 2008.

142. Montgomery E. Feeling safe: a metasynthesis of the maternity care needs of women who were sexually abused in childhood. *Birth*. 2013;40(2):88-95. doi:10.1111/birt.12043.

143. World Health Organization. The World Health Report 2001: mental health: new understanding, new hope. https://apps.who.int/iris/handle/10665/42390. Published 2001. Accessed January 14, 2023.

144. Dekel S, Ein-Dor T, Dishy GA, Mayopoulos PA. Beyond postpartum depression: posttraumatic stress-depressive response following childbirth. *Arch Womens Mental Health*. 2020;23(4):557-564. doi:10.1007/s00737-019-01006-x.

145. Seng JS, Sperlich M, Low LK, et al. Childhood abuse history, posttraumatic stress disorder, postpartum mental health, and bonding: a prospective cohort study. *J Midwifery Womens Health*. 2013;58(1):57-68. doi:10.1111/j.1542-2011.2012.00237.x.

146. Sperlich M, Seng J, Rowe H, et al. A cycles-breaking framework to disrupt intergenerational patterns of maltreatment and vulnerability during the childbearing year. *J Obstet Gynecol Neonatal Nurs*. 2017;46(3):378-389. doi:10.1016/j.jogn.2016.11.017.

147. Sharma V, Doobay M, Baczynski C. Bipolar postpartum depression: an update and recommendations. *J Affect Disord*. 2017;219:105-111. doi:10.1016/j.jad.2017.05.014.

148. Perry A, Gordon-Smith K, Jones L, Jones I. Phenomenology, epidemiology and aetiology of postpartum psychosis: a review. *Brain Sci*. 2021;11(1):47. doi:10.3390/brainsci11010047.

149. NIHCM Foundation. *Identifying and Treating Maternal Depression: Strategies and Considerations for Health Plans*. Issue Brief. Rockville, MD: U.S. Public Health Service, Health Resources and Services Administration, Maternal and Child Health Bureau; 2010. https://fhop.ucsf.edu/sites/fhop.ucsf.edu/files/wysiwyg/NIHCM_IssueBrief_MaternalDepression_June2010.pdf. Accessed March 28, 2023.

# Sexual, Gynecologic, and Reproductive Health Care

Section Editors

TEKOA L. KING—Chapter 8

MELISSA D. AVERY—Chapters 9-18

CHAPTER

# 8

# Anatomy and Physiology of the Reproductive System

VANESSA R. GARCIA

*The editors acknowledge Mary C. Brucker and Tekoa L. King, who were authors of this chapter in the previous edition.*

## Introduction

Midwifery practice begins with an understanding of reproductive anatomy and physiology. Five chapters in this text specifically focus on the anatomy and physiology underpinning clinical practice. This chapter provides a general overview of the anatomy of the reproductive systems of those persons assigned female and male at birth. It focuses on individuals assigned female at birth and includes content on the breast, bony pelvis, and menstrual physiology as well as a brief overview of sexual response. The anatomy of individuals with disorders of sexual differentiation, also known as intersex conditions, and the anatomy of those persons who have undergone hormonal or surgical therapies that result in physical/anatomic changes are beyond the scope of the chapter.

Throughout this edition of *Varney's Midwifery*, a deliberate effort to utilize gender-neutral language has been applied. When such language could negatively impact clarity, the term "female" may be used to describe the anatomy and physiology of those persons assigned female at birth. Additionally, there is updated terminology related to several aspects of the pelvis and its attendant musculature. This may seem odd, since anatomy is presumed to be static and unchanging. While it is true that anatomic structures have not changed for millennia, our understanding of anatomy is evolving, as are the words we use to describe anatomic structures. While the anatomic terms in common usage primarily derive from Latin, anatomists have used different terminology and nomenclature throughout history. The majority of anatomic terminology arose from

knowledge based on dissections completed before the 1800s. These terms are based in Latin or Greek and often have many meanings, some of which appear demeaning to women. One meaning of the word "pudendum," for example, is "shame."

Additionally, technologies like magnetic resonance imaging are now being used to identify anatomic structures and have demonstrated that some prior knowledge about anatomic structures is incorrect, particularly regarding the female pelvis. In addition, there is a growing recognition that anatomic terms related to the reproductive system of the female body need revision both to correct misunderstandings and to address those terms whose meanings are no longer appropriate.[1-4]

To provide standardization for anatomic terms, the International Federation of Associations of Anatomists first published the *Terminologia Anatomica* in 1998, with an update in 2019.[5] In recent years, anatomic terms originally based on individuals' names or on historical belief systems about race and ethnicity have begun to be phased out. However, since some of these terms are still used in clinical practice, this text will include the common clinical term in parentheses after the first usage of the currently recommended anatomic term. Thus, this text offers the reader the opportunity to update terminology that has, historically, reflected prevalent biases.[1]

## The Breast

The breast undergoes dramatic changes in size, shape, and function during an individual's lifetime.

Growth, differentiation, and lactogenesis are the result of complex hormonal stimuli. Breast development starts during embryonic life, although full development of breast tissue does not occur until pregnancy and lactation.

## Breast Anatomy

After pubertal exposure to estrogen and maturation, the adult breast extends vertically from approximately the second rib to the sixth rib, and horizontally from the edge of the sternum to the mid-axillary line, with an extension of tissue into the axilla known as the axillary tail (tail of Spence) (Figure 8-1).[6] The breast is composed of skin, subcutaneous tissue, and breast tissue. The shape of the breast is maintained primarily by suspensory ligaments (Cooper's ligaments) that connect the dermis of the breast to the deep pectoral fascia, which overlays the pectoralis major and serratus anterior muscles of the chest.

The nipple, which is located slightly below the center of each breast, is surrounded by a circular area of pigmented skin known as the areola. The skin of the breast includes both the nipple and the areola. The nipple's elastic tissue contains smooth muscle fibers and is innervated by both sensory and autonomic nerve endings. The nipple becomes smaller and firmer in response to cold, touch, and sexual stimulation under the influence of oxytocin. The darker, circular areola surrounding the nipple is somewhat elastic and varies in diameter.

The nipple has approximately five to nine mammary ductal orifices and is abundantly innervated with sensory nerve endings. The nipple/areola complex also has many sebaceous and apocrine sweat glands. For example, the openings of the sebaceous glands (Montgomery tubercles) under the areola form round elevations just under the skin that become enlarged in pregnancy; they produce secretions that keep the nipple/areola complex lubricated and may assist in the initiation of lactation by providing olfactory cues to the newborn.

The breast tissue is composed of epithelial (glandular or secretory) tissue, between which is interspersed stromal (adipose and connective) tissue. These two types of tissue are present in approximately equal amounts in the breasts of those persons who are not pregnant or lactating.[7] During pregnancy and lactation, however, the glandular tissue proliferates under the influence of progesterone and becomes the predominant breast tissue.[8] Postmenopausally, the glandular tissue tends to shrink

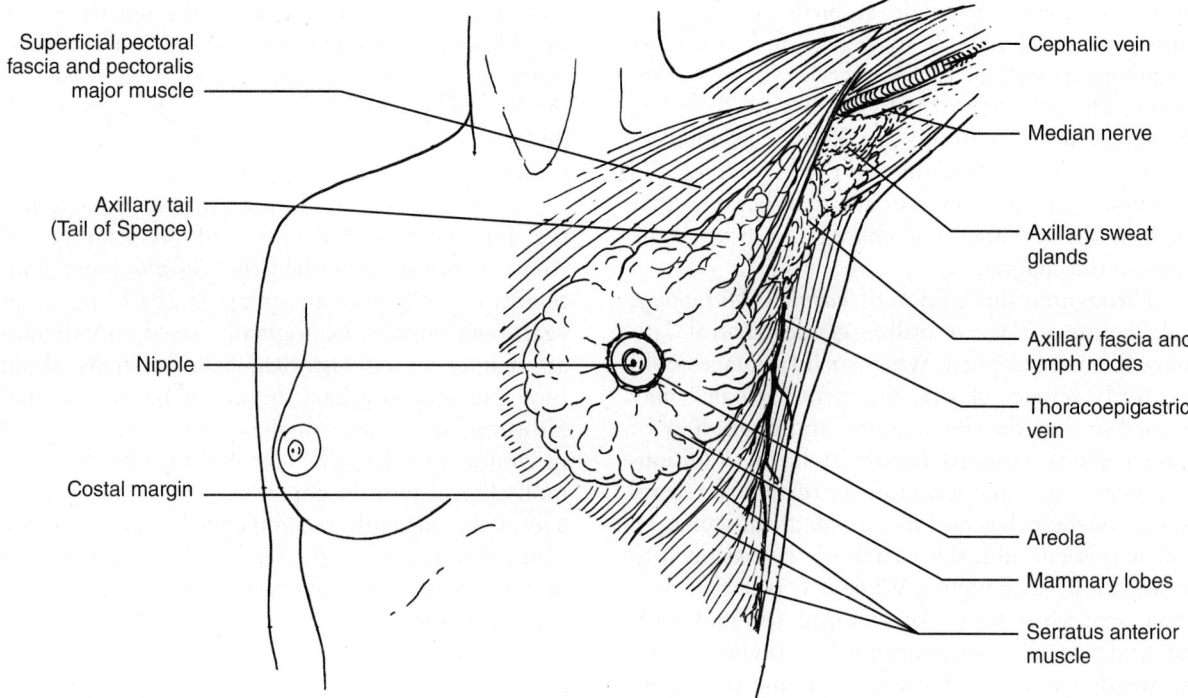

**Figure 8-1** Anterior pectoral dissection.
Modified with permission from Clemente CD. *Anatomy: A Regional Atlas of the Human Body* . 6th ed. Philadelphia, PA: Lippincott Williams & Wilkins; 2011. Reprinted by permission of the author.

and is generally replaced by fat, resulting in changes in breast shape and size.

The glandular tissue in each breast of a reproductive-age person is organized into several lobes that are made up of clusters of 10 to 100 alveoli, referred to as lobules (Figure 8-2). Traditionally, the lobes have been depicted as separate, distinct entities that terminate in a lactiferous sinus just under the nipple.[7] More recently, some controversy has arisen regarding the structure of the breast ductal system. First, the lactiferous sinus may not be an anatomic structure per se, but rather a transient dilation of the terminal duct that occurs during lactation.[7] A few studies have found anastomoses between lobes, while others have not found connections; the majority, however, have shown that each ductal system is independent.[9] Because breast cancer forms in ductal systems, a thorough understanding of this anatomy has important clinical implications.

The alveoli that comprise the lobules are sac-like structures composed of two layers of cells. The inner luminal cells are responsible for synthesis and secretion of milk. They are surrounded by myoepithelial cells that eject milk during lactation. During pregnancy, the alveoli gain the capacity to produce and excrete milk. These differentiated alveoli are referred to as acini when they become milk-secreting sacs. The secretory cells in these acinar units are stimulated by prolactin to secrete milk into the lumen of the acini. During lactation, the myoepithelial cells are stimulated by oxytocin to contract, which compresses the alveolar sacs so that milk is ejected into the milk ductules. The ductules are connected to larger lactiferous ducts, which merge to form a smaller number of ducts leading to openings at the nipple, through which milk exits the breast. The exact number of these openings is not known, but the most recent evidence suggests there are, on average, five to nine patent ducts in each nipple of a lactating individual.[8]

Blood is supplied to the breast primarily by the mammary artery and by the lateral thoracic arteries. Venous flow from the breast drains into the internal thoracic, axillary, and cephalic veins. While these veins are not typically visible, they may become so as they dilate during pregnancy and/or lactation. The lymphatic vessels of the breast serve an important function during lactation by draining milk molecules that are too large to move into blood vessels.

Lymphatic flow to and from the breast is also significant because it determines the location of metastasis of cancer cells from the breast to other parts of the body. Most breast lymph flows to the axillary lymph nodes and is, therefore, the main route of cancer metastasis from the breast. Thus, it is important to include palpation of the axillary tail during clinical breast exams to account for this route of metastasis (Figure 8-1). The intermammary lymph nodes are the other main group of lymph nodes that drain the breast but, compared with the axillary tail, they receive only a small fraction of the lymph flow from the breast.

The breast is innervated by the lateral and anterior cutaneous branches of the second to the sixth intercostal nerves and by the supraclavicular nerves. The nipple and areola are innervated primarily by the cutaneous branch of the fourth intercostal nerve.

## Breast Development

Human breast development begins during the embryologic period with the appearance of the bilateral primitive milk streaks that extend from the axilla to the groin. This ridge then regresses everywhere except in the region destined to become the mammary gland. On occasion, areas of this ridge do not regress, but instead develop into supernumerary nipples and, sometimes, into glandular mammary tissue capable of milk production and excretion. These accessory nipples may be noted on a physical examination in a parallel line down the chest under the breast. They do not, however, have any clinical significance.

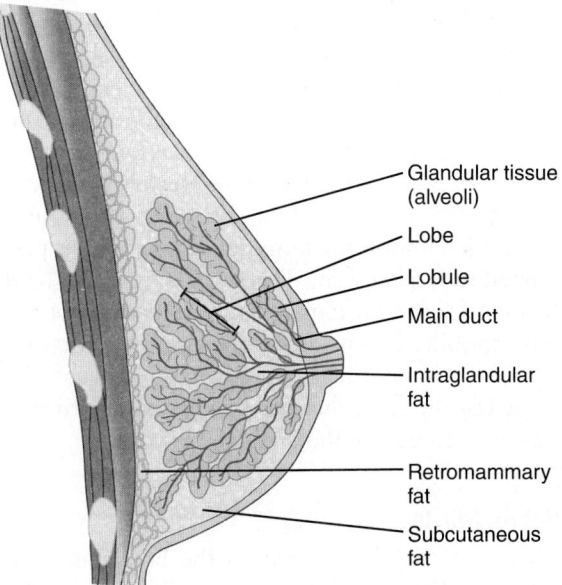

Glandular tissue (alveoli)
Lobe
Lobule
Main duct
Intraglandular fat
Retromammary fat
Subcutaneous fat

**Figure 8-2** Schematic diagram of the ductal anatomy of the breast based on the findings of Ramsay et al.[8] Milk ducts are small and branch a short distance from the base of the nipple. The ductal system is nonlinear and glandular tissue is situated directly beneath the nipple.

At birth, newborns have an opening of a primitive ductal system to the surface, a protruding nipple, and a circular area of skin that has proliferated into the areola. The structures present at birth can range from simple blunt-ended tubular structures to well-developed branching ductal systems with lobular–alveolar structures.[10] Under the influence of maternal and neonatal pro-lactation hormones, these structures are capable of producing milk shortly after birth. In some cases, this milk is excreted and exits via the neonate's nipple (this secretion is sometimes referred to as "witch's milk"). Once the maternal hormones of pregnancy are no longer affecting the newborn, the infant breast tissue undergoes a period of involution. By the time the child reaches 2 years of age, only a small ductal system remains. Some growth in this tissue is noted during childhood, but no development occurs until puberty, when the breast undergoes a period of extensive development with exposure to estrogen.

With the onset of puberty, a process of elongation and branching of the ductal system begins, along with formation of lobules through development of some of the ductal endings into clusters of ductules and alveolar buds. This gradual process of branching and lobule formation occurs primarily under the influence of estrogen and other hormones, including growth hormone. While this process continues through sexual maturity, full glandular differentiation and formation of the secretory acini capable of producing and secreting milk does not occur until pregnancy. The changes in breast structure that take place in pregnancy and lactation are referred to as mammogenesis and lactogenesis. Both processes are detailed in the *Anatomy and Physiology of Pregnancy* and *Anatomy and Physiology of Postpartum* chapters, respectively. Following lactation, the breast glandular tissue undergoes regression and atrophy with tissue remodeling. The breast tissue atrophies further after menopause, with the number of lobes decreasing and fibrous connective tissue and adipose tissue accumulating during this phase of the life span.

## The Bony Pelvis

The bony pelvis has multiple functions. First, it provides an attachment site for the muscles and connective tissue of the pelvis, thereby providing support and stability to the pelvic organs. Second, it provides the site of attachment and articulation for the lower limbs. Third, it supports the weight of the upper trunk and distributes it to the lower extremities.

Finally, at the conclusion of pregnancy, the fetus passes through the bony pelvis during birth.

### Pelvic Bones

While the pelvis appears to be a single large structure, it is actually three bones separated by ligaments, all of which are important when assessing the pregnant or laboring individual. The bones of the pelvis are the innominate bones (comprising the two lateral sides of the pelvis), the sacrum, and the coccyx (Figure 8-3).

The innominate bones are the large bones commonly referred to as "pelvic bones." Each has three parts: the ilium, the ischium, and the pubis. The ilium is the upper and posterior portion; the two ilia connect to the sacrum. The ischium is the lower and medial portion of the innominate bone. The ischium has important bony landmarks that are assessed during labor as the fetus passes through the pelvis—namely, the ischial spine, the ischial tuberosity, and the pelvic sidewall. The pubis is the anterior portion of the innominate bone. The pubic bones join at the pubic symphysis, where they are attached to an avascular fibrocartilage disc. The inferior margin of the pubic symphysis and the descending rami create the pubic arch, another important bony landmark of the pelvis for the fetus to negotiate during birth and one that can impact fetal descent. More details on the bony pelvis can be found in the chapter *Anatomy and Physiology of Pregnancy*. A review of how the fetus passes through the pelvis during labor can be found in the *First Stage of Labor* chapter.

The sacrum and the coccyx make up the posterior portion of the pelvis. The sacrum is formed by the fusion of the five sacral vertebrae. The superior part of the sacrum, the sacral promontory, is another important bony landmark of the pelvis related to fetal descent. The coccyx is formed by the fusion of several rudimentary vertebrae and is modestly mobile. Extension of the coccyx occurs during relaxation of the levator ani and rectal sphincter muscles—an event that occurs normally during defecation and during the birthing process.

### Pelvic Joints

There are three joints within the bony pelvis: the pubic symphysis and the two sacroiliac joints. These joints are made of a network of cartilage and/or ligaments that join the bones of the pelvis. During pregnancy, the joints of the pelvis soften under the influence of the hormones of pregnancy, including relaxin. This softening allows for movement and

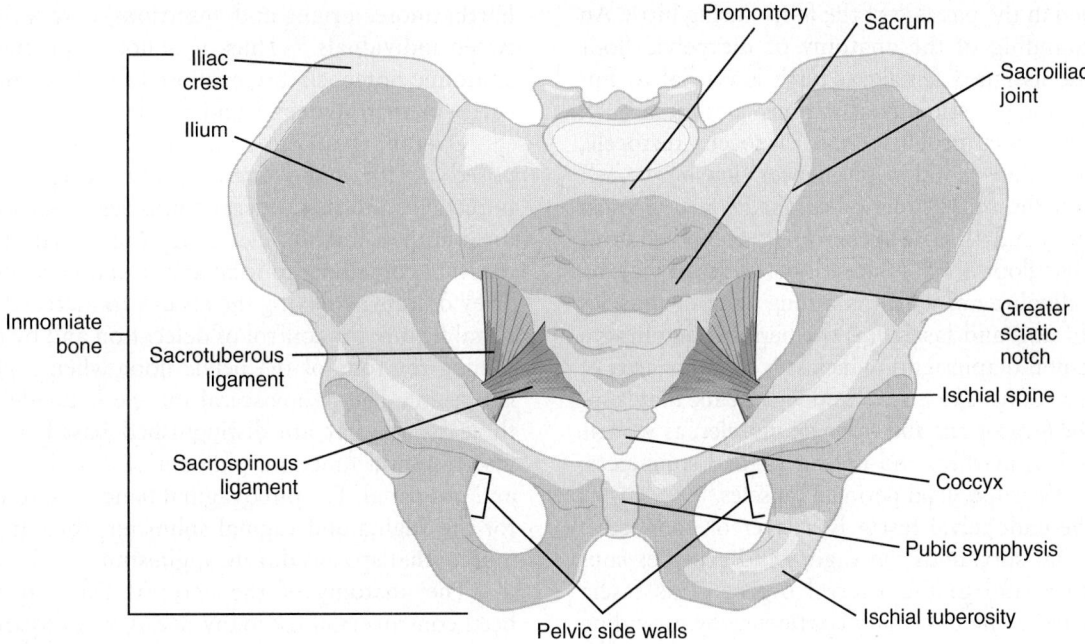

**Figure 8-3** Front view of the bony pelvis with ligaments.

widening of the pelvis in both the longitudinal and horizontal planes, which increases the area within the pelvic bones to facilitate birth.

The pubic symphysis is composed of fibrocartilaginous tissue. During pregnancy, it widens marginally and becomes slightly more mobile. Although this widening usually does not exceed 10 millimeters, it may cause tenderness, particularly with motion.[11,12] In clinical practice, managing the pain caused by this common pregnancy discomfort is one with which every midwife becomes familiar. Rarely, the pubic symphysis may separate spontaneously (or surgically) during labor.

The sacroiliac joints are primarily weight-bearing joints that take the weight of the upper body and distribute it to the lower limbs. They are synovial joints, meaning that the surfaces of the articulating bones are covered by a thin membrane of cartilage and are separated by a joint cavity lined by a synovial membrane that produces a lubricating fluid. The resulting hinge-type movement gives the sacrum the ability to rotate slightly as the individual assumes different postures, enlarging the measurements of two of the three pelvic planes through which the fetus passes during birth.

### Pelvic Ligaments

In this section, the pelvic ligaments of those persons assigned female at birth are discussed; the anatomy of individuals assigned male at birth differ. The term "ligament" is generally used to describe connective tissue that joins two bones. In the pelvis, in addition to indicating a connection between bones, the term "ligament" is used to describe a variety of tissues that connect pelvic organs to bones. Nevertheless, the sacrospinous and sacrotuberous ligaments of the sacrum are "true" ligaments in the bony pelvis that help provide stability to the pelvis in part by supporting the sacrum and restricting its ability to tilt.

The sacrospinous ligaments are triangular, with a broad base that attaches to the lateral margins of the sacrum and coccyx and inserts at the apex of the ischial spine. The coccygeus muscle lies along the pelvic aspect of this ligament. The pudendal nerve, which innervates the skin and muscles of the perineum, lies just posterior to the sacrospinous ligaments where it attaches to the ischial spine. The sacrotuberous ligaments attach to the sacrum at the level of the S3 through S5 vertebrae and extend to the inferior spine of the ilium, where it becomes the ischial tuberosity, extending inferior and lateral to the sacrospinous ligaments.

### The Pelvic Floor

The pelvic floor is composed of major muscle groups as well as ligaments and fascia that together support the abdominal and pelvic organs and maintain urinary and anal continence. The pelvic floor differs between individuals assigned male and female at birth. In pregnant individuals, these tissues are also involved in the passage of the fetus during birth. An understanding of the anatomy of the pelvic floor of those assigned female at birth is crucial to understanding the etiology of various conditions such as pelvic organ prolapse (e.g., cystocele, rectocele, uterine prolapse) and incontinence. Viewing the pelvis from the most superior (cephalic) to the most inferior (caudal) region, the major components of the pelvic floor are (1) the endopelvic fascia; (2) the pelvic diaphragm, which is a long sling of muscles (levator ani) and fascia; (3) the perineal diaphragm (urogenital diaphragm), which is a complex area of muscle, connective tissue and ligaments that support the levator ani and perineal muscles, as well as the vagina, urethra, and urethrovaginal sphincters; and (4) the superficial perineal muscles.

The endopelvic fascia is a layer of connective tissue that surrounds the vagina and provides support to it and to the visceral organs. This fascia also plays a role in urinary continence by providing support to the urethra and neck of the bladder.[13,14]

The pelvic diaphragm separates the pelvic cavity from the perineal space and can be envisioned as a diamond-shaped hammock that supports the viscera, abdominal organs, and pelvic organs. The pelvic diaphragm consists of the levator ani and coccygeus muscles and their associated fascia (Figure 8-4). Nomenclature for the muscles of the pelvic floor is classically based on their attachment points (origin and insertion). However, this area is dense with fascia, muscular subdivisions, and insertions that intermingle with each other, as this muscle group supports the urethra, vagina, and anus.

Furthermore, origin and insertions may vary between individuals.[15] Thus, it is not surprising that anatomic nomenclature proposed for these muscles varies in anatomic texts and articles.

Overall, the levator ani muscle group is composed of the pubovisceral (pubococcygeus), puborectalis, and iliococcygeus muscles. Insertions of the pubovisceral muscle create functional sphincters that contribute to fecal and urinary continence. They do this by flexing the coccyx to increase anal–rectal flexure for control of defecation and by maintaining the tone of the pelvic floor when a person is upright. The pubovisceral muscle is divided into three bands that are distinguished based on their insertion and function: puboperineal, pubovaginal, and puboanal. The pubovaginal band acts as a sling for the vagina and vaginal sphincter; thus, it is the muscle that spasms during vaginismus.

The anatomy of the perineal diaphragm has been controversial for many decades. Although this area generally separates the internal levator muscles from the superficial perineal muscles, the exact structures in the perineal diaphragm are not clearly delineated in all anatomic dissection studies.[16]

When the muscles of the pelvic floor become damaged, as can occur during childbirth, support of the urethra and other pelvic structures becomes increasingly dependent upon the ligaments and fascia. Under the strain of continuous or prolonged stretching, these ligaments and fascia can weaken and become incapable of preventing organ prolapse and/or stress incontinence. The muscles of the pelvic floor are described further in Table 8-1.

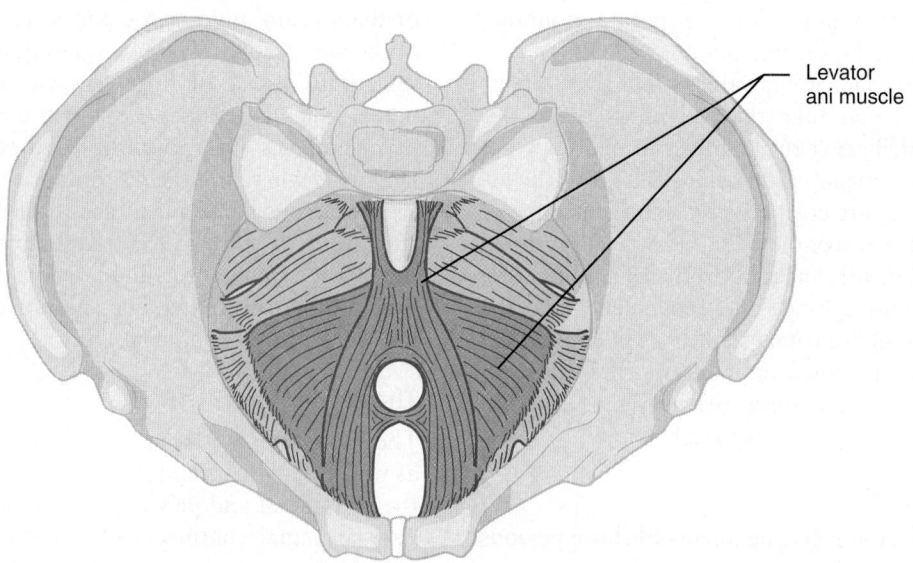

Levator
ani muscle

**Figure 8-4** View of the structures of the pelvic floor muscles from above.

| Table 8-1 | Muscles of the Pelvic Floor |
|---|---|
| Levator ani | This muscle group originates at the posterior border of the pubic symphysis and sweeps back to insert on the lateral margins of the coccyx (i.e., pelvic sidewalls).<br><br>**Pubovisceral** (formerly pubococcygeus): Fibers originate at the pubis to form a Y, passing backward around the urethra, vagina, and rectum. Some authors separate the pubovisceral muscle into three subdivisions based on the three different insertions of this muscle. The *puboperineal* portion pulls the perineal body ventrally toward the pubis. The *pubovaginal* aspect has an origin at the posterior aspect of the pubis and inserts on the fascia of the vagina and perineal body, thereby elevating the vagina to the mid-urethra. This muscle forms a U-shape around the vagina. The *puboanal* inserts between the internal and external anal sphincters.<br><br>**Puborectalis**: These intermediate fibers form a U-loop around the anal–rectal junction and insert into the posterior wall of the rectum, blending with the anal sphincter.<br><br>**Iliococcygeus**: This muscle starts lateral to the pubovisceral muscle and has two sides. Both arise from a fascial line on the obturator internus muscle along the pelvic wall of the obturator foramen and extend to fuse at the insertion on the lateral margins of the coccyx and anococcygeal body. |
| Coccygeus | Triangular muscle between the ischial spine and the coccyx. |

## Perineal Membrane and Muscles of the Perineum

The perineal membrane is a single layer of muscle and fascial tissue that forms a fibrous sheet spanning the area just inferior to the pelvic diaphragm. The perineal membrane was previously thought to be an equilateral triangle defined by the pubic symphysis and ischial tuberosities and was called the urogenital diaphragm. In the past, it was thought this area had both a superficial region and a deeper region. The deeper region was thought to hold the urethral sphincter muscles and contain a deep transverse perineal muscle, and the superficial region to contain the superficial genital muscles, erectile tissue of the clitoris, and vestibular glands. Recent studies suggest this area does not have distinct deep and superficial compartments; indeed, many now believe that the deep transverse perineal muscle does not exist in the female body. Furthermore, the term *perineal membrane* has replaced urogenital diaphragm.[17] The urethra and the vagina pass through this membrane. In the female body, the muscles within this membrane are involved in urethral support and sphincter mechanics. An overview of the perineal membrane and the muscles of the perineum is provided in Table 8-2.

Superficial to the perineal membrane are the three external genital muscles: (1) the bulbocavernosus, (2) ischiocavernosus, and (3) superficial transverse perineal muscles (Figure 8-5).[18] The two bulbocavernosus muscles are also known as the sphincter vaginae. Contraction of these muscles reduces the size of the vaginal orifice, whereas contraction of the anterior muscle fibers contributes to clitoral erection. Similarly, the ischiocavernosus muscles help maintain clitoral erection. The perineal body, which crosses the midline of the perineum between the vaginal and anal openings, is the point of convergence of the superficial transverse perineal, bulbocavernosus, and levator ani muscles, as well as the urogenital and external anal sphincters. This perineal body is also the point of attachment of the two sides of the perineal membrane, provides support to the posterior vaginal wall, and helps prevent rectal prolapse. Damage to the perineal body, in addition to stretching of the levator ani muscles that may occur during the second stage of labor, can result in rectal prolapse. One of the goals of proper repair of the perineum following birth is to provide additional support to the perineal body during healing.

## Urogenital Anatomy

### Bladder and Urethra

Knowledge of how pelvic floor anatomy promotes urinary and fecal continence is necessary for understanding how changes related to pregnancy, childbirth, and aging result in some individuals developing pelvic floor dysfunction, including urinary stress incontinence.

Two sphincter structures are involved in urinary continence: the inner sphincter at the neck of the bladder and the external urethral rhabdosphincter/urethrovaginal sphincter complex. The inner sphincter is an extension of the detrusor smooth

| Table 8-2 | Muscles of the Perineum |
|---|---|
| **Muscle** | **Description** |
| Perineal membrane | A musculofascial layer that arises from the inferior ramus of the ischium, spans the anterior pelvic outlet, and is attached to the lateral vaginal walls. The urethra-related sphincter muscles pass through this membrane. |
| Bulbocavernosus | This one muscle has two parts functioning as a muscular tube. Posteriorly, the bulbocavernosus muscle attaches to the perineal body; anteriorly, it inserts into the corpus cavernosus of the clitoris; laterally, the two parts of the muscle surround the orifice of the vagina, covering the vestibular bulbs and greater vestibular glands (Bartholin's glands) on either side. |
| Ischiocavernosus | The perineum has two ischiocavernosus muscles, one on either lateral boundary of the perineum. Posteriorly, they arise from the inner surface of the ischial tuberosities; anteriorly, they cover and insert into the sides and posterior surface of the crus clitoris; laterally, they extend from the clitoris to the ischial tuberosities along the ischial ramus, from which they derive some of their fibers. |
| Superficial transverse perineal (transversus perinei superficialis) | Two superficial transverse perineal muscles arise from the inner and anterior surfaces of the ischial tuberosity of the superior ramus of the ischium by a small tendon; they span the posterior edge of the perineal membrane and insert into the perineal body. |
| Perineal body (central tendinous point of the perineum) | A fat and fibromuscular structure that is located midline between the vagina and the anus, and at the base of the perineal diaphragm. The tissue is fibrous because it is the point of fusion for both the superior and inferior fascia of the perineal diaphragm and the external perineal and membranous layer of perineal subcutaneous tissue (Colles' fascia); it has muscular fibers because it is a common point of attachment for a number of muscles. |

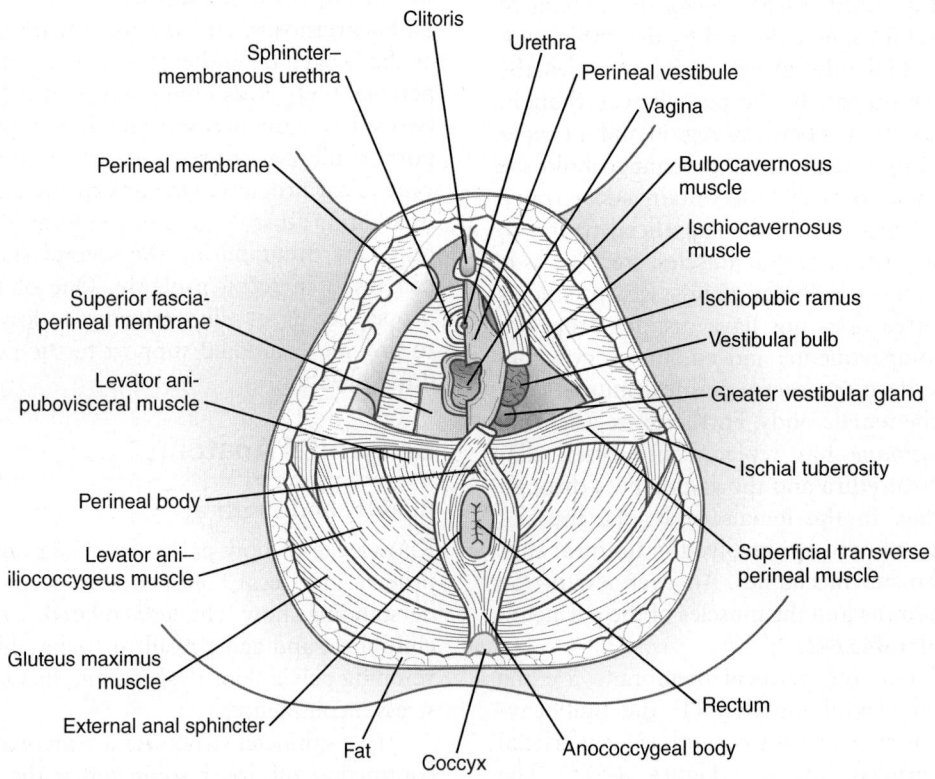

**Figure 8-5** Muscles and structures of the perineum.
Modified from Clark NR. Gynecologic anatomy and physiology. In: Schuiling KD, Likis FE, eds. *Gynecologic Health Care*. 4th ed. Burlington, MA: Jones & Bartlett Learning; 2022.

muscle of the bladder that is under autonomic control, whereas the urethral rhabdosphincter/urethrovaginal sphincter complex is composed of skeletal muscle and is under voluntary control. Support by the pelvic floor musculature is also critical to maintaining urinary continence. The major components of this supportive structure are the vaginal wall, the endopelvic fascia, the arcus tendineus fasciae pelvis, and the levator ani muscles. The endopelvic fascia surrounds the vagina and attaches to the arcus tendineus fascia, which serves to suspend and support the urethra.

The urethra is approximately 4 centimeters long and runs posteriorly along the pubic symphysis from the external opening (urethral meatus) to the bladder. The urethra is composed of an inner layer of epithelium surrounded by a layer of vascular tissue and a layer of muscular tissue, which together help maintain the urethra in a constricted position. The urethra is stabilized by the pubourethral ligaments, which attach the anterior portion of the urethra to the pubic symphysis.

To maintain urinary continence, urethral constricting pressure must be greater than bladder pressure. This pressure balance is achieved in part by the constriction provided by the urethral muscles and sphincters and in part by the support/compression provided by the pelvic floor muscles and their associated structures. The urethra exits the pelvis via the urogenital hiatus of the levator ani, through which the vagina also passes. The baseline muscle tone of the levator ani, therefore, is critical in maintaining urinary continence by keeping the urethra compressed.

### Anorectal Anatomy

The rectum is the terminal portion of the colon, just as the anal canal is the terminal portion of the rectum; the anus is the opening where stool exits the body. The anal canal is approximately 2.5 to 5 centimeters in length, compared to the 10 to 12 centimeters of the rectum. The internal and external anal sphincters are rings of muscle at the opening of the anus, which surround the anal canal with the anal mucosal lining. The internal anal sphincter comprises a layer of muscle that is a continuation of the muscular layer of the rectum, ending approximately 1 centimeter from the anus.[19] Similar to the internal sphincter, the external anal sphincter is a cylindrical muscular structure; it is partially interwoven with the levator ani muscle and extends to the anus. The external anal sphincter is composed of striated muscle under voluntary control. The ability

to identify the striated muscle of the sphincter and the tissue of the sphincter itself is important in differentiating between second-, third-, and fourth-degree perineal lacerations.

### Pelvic Nerves and Vasculature

The perineum is perfused by the internal pudendal artery and branches of the pudendal artery, including the inferior rectal artery. These vessels are branches of the anterior division of the internal iliac (hypogastric) artery. Perineal innervation occurs via the pudendal nerve and its branches, which originate from S2, S3, and S4 vertebrae. The pudendal nerve also innervates the levator ani, rectal sphincter, skin of the vulva and lower portion of the vagina, and muscles of the urogenital diaphragm. Anesthetic can be injected near the ischial spines to numb this nerve for repair and to reduce sensation in the perineum during the second stage of labor, as described in the *Pudendal Nerve Block* appendix.

## External Genitalia

The external genitalia, also referred to as the vulva, are those structures located between the pubis and the perineum (Figure 8-6). They include the mons pubis, labia minora, labia majora, clitoris, urethra,

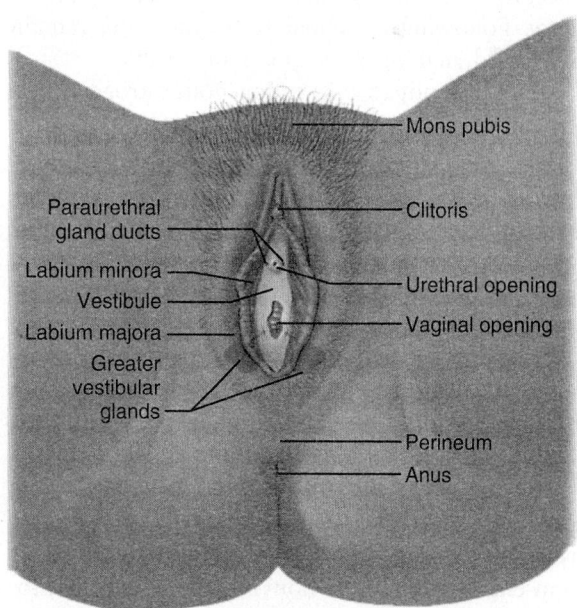

**Figure 8-6** External genitalia of the female body.
Modified from Clark NR. Gynecologic anatomy and physiology. In: Schuiling KD, Likis FE, eds. *Gynecologic Health Care.* 4th ed. Burlington, MA: Jones & Bartlett Learning; 2022.

vestibule, and vaginal opening. Although not externally visible, the paraurethral (Skene's glands) and greater vestibular glands and ducts, the vestibular bulbs, and the hymen/hymenal ring are also considered part of the external genitalia.

### Vulva

The mons pubis is the layer of fatty tissue that overlays the pubic bone. After puberty, the skin of the mons is covered with coarse, curly hair. In addition to providing cushioning during sexual activity, the mons pubis contains sebaceous glands that emit pheromones.[20]

The labia majora are folds of connective and adipose tissue that extend inferiorly from the mons and merge posteriorly into the perineal body to form the posterior commissure. Medial to the labia majora are the labia minora, which are two thin folds of connective tissue. During sexual arousal, both the labia majora and labia minora become engorged with blood and may appear edematous.[20] The area between the labia minora that extends from the clitoris to the fourchette is referred to as the vestibule and is the area into which the urethra, the ducts of the paraurethral glands, the greater vestibular glands, and the vagina all open. The labia minora merge superiorly to form the prepuce/hood of the clitoris and inferiorly to form the fourchette. Prior to an individual's first vaginal birth, the labia meet to cover the vaginal opening, obscuring it from view. Following a vaginal birth, the labia remain separated, making the vagina more visible.

After menopause, as endogenous estrogen levels fall, pubic hair tends to thin and gray. The vulva also may thin and flatten, losing some of its fullness.

### Clitoris

The clitoris is a highly innervated, erectile sex organ considered to be the center for orgasmic response. It resides in the superior portion of the vestibule where the labia minora fuse. The glans is the only visible portion of the clitoris and comprises a small fraction of the total structure, the majority of which is under the tissue of the vulva. The glans is covered by the prepuce/hood and is estimated to contain approximately 8000 nerve endings.[20] While the glans is approximately 1.5 to 2 centimeters long in its non-engorged state, the nonvisible body of the clitoris may be up to 4 centimeters in length.

The body of the clitoris splits proximally into two crura to create an inverted V structure attached to the pubic arch by the suspensory ligament and extending along the ischiopubic rami (Figure 8-7A).[21]

These crura can reach 9 centimeters in length and are composed of erectile tissue called the corpus cavernosa.[20] Adjacent to the crura and surrounding the lateral aspect of the urethra and vaginal orifice are the vestibular bulbs. These are composed of corpus spongiosum tissue, the same vascular, erectile tissue found in the penis. The vestibular bulbs become engorged with blood during sexual arousal and contract during orgasm. Some have argued that these structures should be renamed the bulbs of the clitoris due to their direct relationship with other components of the clitoris and urethra.[22] Additionally, when the entirety of the clitoris is viewed next to the penis, it is evident that they are homologues of each other (Figure 8-7B). Indeed, during embryologic development, the penis arises from same tissue as the clitoris, explaining their structural similarities and tissue types.

The clitoris is attached to the pubic symphysis by the suspensory ligaments. This organ is innervated by the dorsal nerve of the clitoris, branches of the pudendal nerve, and cavernous nerves that supply the erectile tissue arteries.

### Paraurethral and Vestibular Glands

The greater vestibular glands are located beneath the fascia of the vestibule on either side of the vaginal opening at about the 4 o'clock and 8 o'clock positions. Each gland has a duct that opens into the inferior aspect of the vestibule between the labia minora and the hymenal ring. These glands secrete mucus that functions as a lubricant during sexual arousal and as a general moisturizer for the vulva.[20]

The paraurethral glands, also known as the lesser vestibular glands, usually open into the vestibule on either side of the urethra, but sometimes open at the posterior wall of the urethra. These glands also secrete mucus during sexual arousal and are the source of ejaculate in individuals with paraurethral glands.[23] This ejaculate contains prostate-specific antigen and may have antimicrobial properties that serve to protect the urethra. Interestingly, the paraurethral glands may be absent in some individuals. Both the paraurethral and greater vestibular glands can become infected, causing swelling and/or painful abscesses.

## Internal Genitalia

A midsagittal view of the internal organs and associated structures that make up the reproductive system in the female body is shown in Figure 8-8.[18] These organs and structures include the vagina, uterus, cervix, ovaries, and oviducts (fallopian

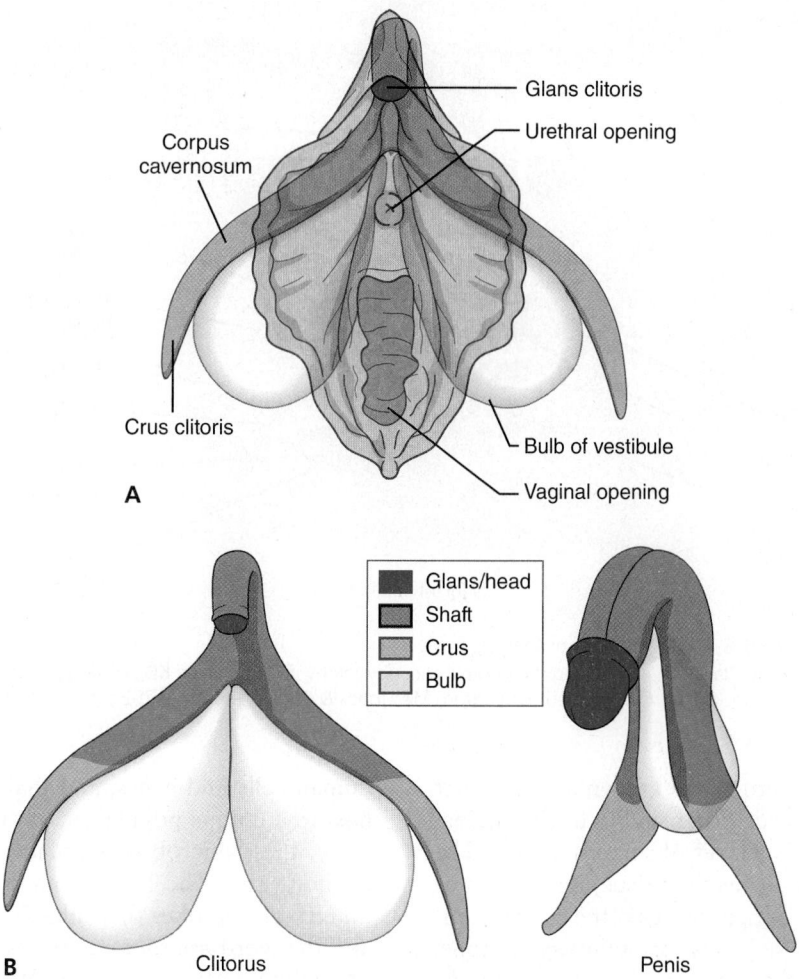

**Figure 8-7  A.** Internal and external view of the clitoris and adjacent anatomy.
**B.** Commonalities between the clitoris and the penis.

tubes, also referred to as uterine tubes or salpinges). A detailed description of each component follows.

## Vagina

The vagina is a muscular, tubular structure extending from the vulva inward to the cervix. An understanding of vaginal anatomy is crucial for assessing myriad clinical conditions, as well as for repair following birth.

Anteriorly, the vagina is separated from the bladder by connective tissue known as the vesicovaginal septum. Posteriorly, the vagina is separated from the rectum by the rectovaginal septum (in the lower segment) and by the rectouterine pouch (also referred to as the cul-de-sac or pouch of Douglas). The rectouterine pouch is an extension of the peritoneal cavity that lies between the vagina and rectum. When a person develops a hematoma during birth, this is a large potential space that can rapidly fill with a significant quantity of blood. The pressure

from a hematoma in this site will often be reported as rectal pain and pressure.

The walls of the vagina, which are referred to as the anterior, posterior, and lateral vaginal walls, run from the vaginal opening at the vestibule to the cervix posteriorly, where they create a pouch. The spaces created between the cervix and the ends of the vaginal walls are called the vaginal fornices. There are four fornices: the anterior fornix, the posterior fornix, and two lateral fornices. The ability to recognize these fornices is important for accurate vaginal exams, determining cervical length, correct application of a speculum and performance of Papanicolaou (Pap) tests, lateral examination of the ovaries during bimanual exam, and assessment of vaginal lacerations into the fornices.

The vagina has three layers: mucosa, muscularis, and adventitia. The vaginal mucosa is lined with a layer of stratified squamous epithelium; in a person who is past puberty but premenopausal,

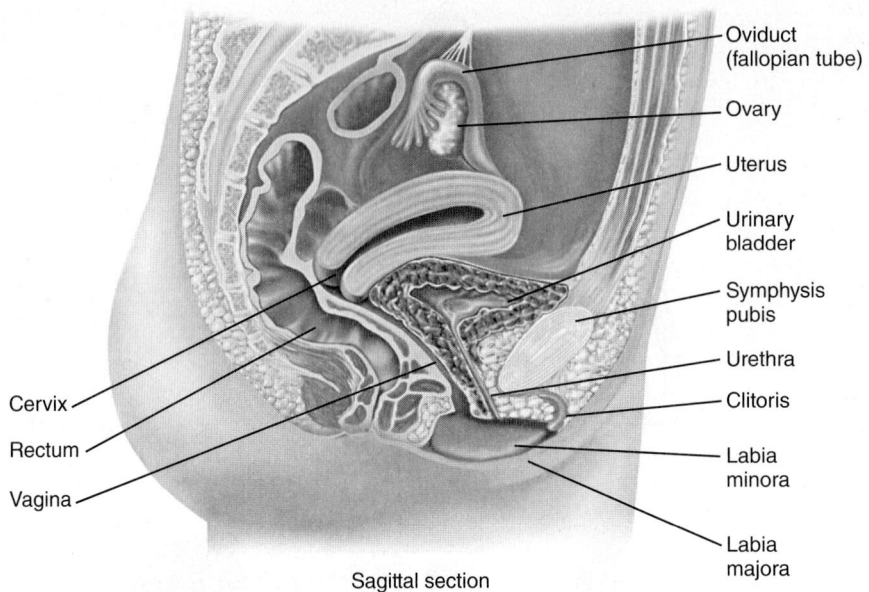

Sagittal section

**Figure 8-8** Midsagittal view of a female pelvis.
Modified Clark NR. Gynecologic anatomy and physiology. In: Schuiling KD, Likis FE, eds. *Gynecologic Health Care.* 4th ed. Burlington, MA: Jones & Bartlett Learning; 2022.

this tissue is folded into ridges known as rugae that can stretch and provide distensibility to the vagina. Beneath this lining is a layer of smooth muscle. The outermost layer of connective tissue, referred to as the adventitia, is contiguous with the visceral endopelvic fascia. These layers maintain vaginal tone. Postmenopausally, the vaginal walls become thinner, the rugae become less apparent, and elasticity and moisture lessen with the decrease in estrogen levels.

The blood supply to the vagina emerges from the vaginal artery, which branches from the uterine artery, or directly from the internal iliac artery, the inferior vesical arteries, and the middle rectal and internal pudendal arteries. Blood is drained from the vaginal area by a venous plexus that follows the arteries, and lymph is drained primarily via the inguinal lymph nodes.

The upper portion of the vagina is innervated primarily by the uterovaginal plexus, which arises from the inferior hypogastric or pelvic plexus. This uterovaginal plexus contains sympathetic efferent fibers from the second, third, and fourth sacral nerves. In addition, the vagina is innervated by a few filaments from the first two sacral ganglia that are sensitive to pain. The lower portion of the vagina is primarily innervated by the pudendal nerve.

### The Vaginal Microbiome

Many scientists believe that human bodies are composed of more cells and genes from microbes than human cells and genes, and that each individual is host to a unique population of microbes.[24] Furthermore, these microbial populations vary depending on body site. The microbiota comprises the community of microbes that inhabit a part of the body and the word *microbiome* refers to the genomes of that community of microbes. While invisible to the naked eye, the vaginal microbiome is crucial to vaginal health.

The vaginal microbiome evolves over the life span and is influenced by a variety of factors, such as diet, smoking, socioeconomic status, and sexual practices. In reproductive-age people, the vagina is typically dominated by *Lactobacillus* species (spp.), which produce lactic acid, hydrogen peroxide, and antimicrobial compounds to maintain vaginal homeostasis.[25,26] These bacteria maintain a low enough pH to deter overgrowth of bacteria and to defend against pathogenic bacteria. When the microbiome is disrupted, a state called dysbiosis may ensue. Dysbiosis can occur without definitive etiology and is more likely to occur with douching, antibiotic use, and use of noncotton underwear.[27] In the vagina, low levels of *Lactobacillus* spp. may contribute to development of bacterial vaginosis (BV), a dysbiotic state characterized by a more diverse microbiome consisting of *Gardnerella vaginalis*, *Atopobium vaginae*, and *Megasphaera*. Vaginal yeast infections, which are caused by an overgrowth of *Candida* fungi, are another form of dysbiosis.

Currently, researchers are investigating the use of *Lactobacillus* isolates that secrete anti-*Candida* factors as a means to prevent vaginal candidiasis, further emphasizing the role of *Lactobacillus* spp. in vaginal health.[25]

In pregnancy, the vaginal microbiome is typically very stable and is dominated by *Lactobacillus* spp. It has been theorized that the dominance of *Lactobacillus* spp. during pregnancy demonstrates their importance in sustaining a healthy vaginal microbiome for the pregnant person.[28,29]

During menopause, the decreasing levels of circulating estrogen change the vaginal microbiome structure as well as contribute to vulvovaginal atrophy and vaginal dryness. It has been found that hormone replacement therapy directly impacts the dominance of *Lactobacillus* spp. in the vaginal microbiome of menopausal individuals and that this effect contributes to the resolution of vaginal symptoms of menopause, such as vulvovaginal atrophy and vaginal dryness.[26] Furthermore, research into the role of oral and vaginal probiotics for individuals during menopause holds promise

for informing care, though its results are not yet conclusive enough to change clinical practice. This interplay of hormones and vaginal microbiome ecology is further illustrative of the complexity of the microbiome.

## Uterus

The uterus is a pear-shaped, muscular organ that, in the nonpregnant state, is situated in the pelvic cavity superior to the bladder. The uterus is anchored in place by the uterine ligaments (Figure 8-9).

The long axis of the uterine body can be *anteverted*, meaning that it is tilted toward the person's abdomen at a right angle to the long axis of the vagina. In some people, the angle is *retroverted* and the uterus is tipped toward the back. When the uterine fundus is tilted more severely forward, it is said to be *anteflexed*; when tilted severely backward, it is said to be *retroflexed* (Figure 8-10).

The adult nulliparous uterus measures approximately 6 to 8 centimeters in length, 5 centimeters across, and 4 centimeters in thickness; it weighs approximately 50 grams. The functions of the uterus

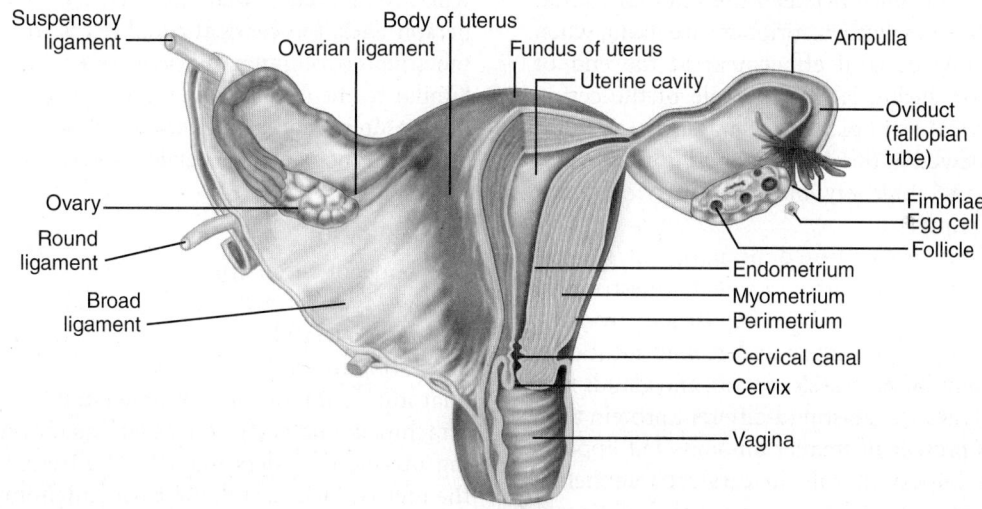

**Figure 8-9** Anterior view of internal reproductive anatomy including ligaments and uterine layers.

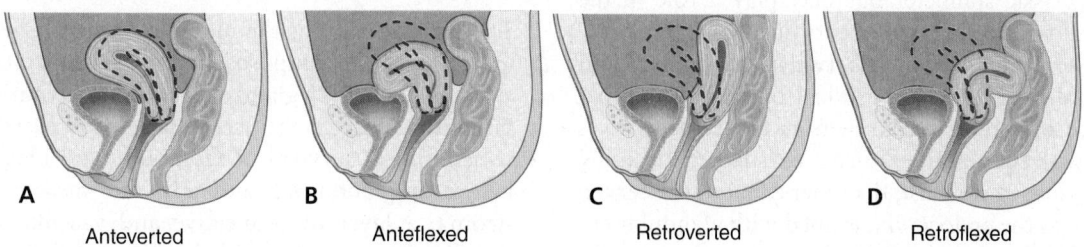

**Figure 8-10** Positions of the long axis of the uterus. **A.** Anteverted. **B.** Anteflexed. **C.** Retroverted. **D.** Retroflexed. Midline positioning is shown in dotted blue.

include sexual response, receiving a fertilized ovum, providing the environment for the embryo and the fetus, and contracting to aid in the expulsion of the fetus and placenta.

The uterus has two main parts: the cervix and the corpus or body. During pregnancy, the body of the uterus differentiates into an upper segment called the fundus and a lower segment called the isthmus.

### Cervix

The cervix is the entrance to the uterus from the vagina. As such, assessment and manipulation of the cervix are integral to midwifery practice. The cervix is the cylindrical, fibromuscular lower portion of the uterus that is sometimes referred to as the neck of the uterus. It has two areas of constriction at each end: the internal os, which is found at the junction of the cervix and the uterine body, and the external os, which opens into the vagina. The external os of the cervix can be palpated toward the back of the vagina, though its position may be more anterior or posterior depending upon the flexion of the uterus. Assessing the distance between the internal os and the external os is what practitioners are doing when they determine cervical effacement at the end of pregnancy or during labor. The role of the cervix and the cervical os in pregnancy and birth are additionally reviewed in the *Anatomy and Physiology of Pregnancy* and *Anatomy and Physiology of Labor and Birth* chapters.

The cervix is composed primarily of subepithelial stroma, along with a smaller proportion of smooth muscle fibers.[30] The subepithelial stroma is approximately 80% collagen and ground substance, which contains blood vessels, nerves, and glands that secrete thick mucus. Elastin (a different protein than collagen) is present in smaller amounts but appears to play an important role in cervical remodeling during pregnancy, in labor, and after birth.[30] Recent studies have found that smooth muscle lies in a circular pattern around the internal os.[31] This tissue is not a classic sphincter but may play a role in the cervical remodeling that occurs during early labor.

The tunnel-like area between the internal and external os is called the cervical canal. The external surface of the cervix, known as the ectocervix, is lined with squamous epithelial cells like those lining the vagina. In contrast, the inner canal of the cervix, known as the endocervix, is lined with glandular epithelial cells, also termed columnar epithelial cells. The area where the endocervix and the exocervix meet is the squamocolumnar junction.

Although the term "squamocolumnar junction" is often used interchangeably with the term "transformation zone," these are two separate entities. The transformation zone is the location of carcinogenesis mediated by oncogenic subtypes of human papillomavirus (HPV). It is a dynamic area of metaplasia over an individual's lifetime and, histologically, is the area where glandular epithelium has been replaced by squamous epithelium. As a result, the squamocolumnar junction is part of the transformation zone, but the transformation zone encompasses an area greater than simply that of the squamocolumnar junction. Nonetheless, collection of cells from the squamocolumnar junction during Pap testing is crucial, since some research demonstrates that cervical cancers originate from a small population of cells at this junction.[32] Depending on several factors, including age, pregnancy status, and hormonal contraceptive use, the squamocolumnar junction may or may not be visible. When the columnar cells are visible, this benign condition usually is known as ectopy or eversion. A prepubescent individual has a pink, smooth cervix without eversion. Those using estrogen-containing hormonal contraception or who are pregnant often have marked eversion. As a person ages, the cervical canal tends to recede and the squamocolumnar junction often is not visible. Similar to the upper vagina, the cervix is innervated by the uterovaginal plexus, which arises from the inferior hypogastric or pelvic plexus.

### Uterine Body

The body of the uterus is made up of an external serosal layer formed by the peritoneum, a muscular (myometrial) layer, and a mucosal (endometrial) layer (Figure 8-9). An understanding of uterine anatomy is important for understanding placental attachment and perfusion, as well as for understanding uterine disorders that affect different layers of the uterus, such as endometriosis, adenomyosis, and leiomyomas, among others.

### Endometrium

The endometrium is the mucosal lining of the uterine cavity. It is composed of (1) ciliated columnar epithelial cells; (2) glands that secrete a thin, alkaline mucus rich in proteins, sugars, and secretions, which allows survival of the zygote and blastocyst before implantation; and (3) the mesenchymal stroma, a layer of connective and vascular tissue that lies between the epithelial layer and the myometrium. This stroma can be subdivided into two layers: (1) the stratum basalis, which is closest to the myometrium and is not shed during menstruation, and (2) the stratum functionalis, the layer of the endometrium that proliferates and degenerates cyclically in menstruating individuals.

The endometrium receives blood from two different sets of arteries: a "straight" set of arteries that supply the stratum basalis and a set of "coiled" spiral arterioles that supply the stratum functionalis (Figure 8-11).[33] During the menstrual cycle, these vessels and the rest of the endometrium undergo marked changes. As part of the proliferative phase of the menstrual cycle, under the effects of rising levels of estrogen and progesterone, the endometrium becomes increasingly vascularized and the glands of the endometrium become longer and increasingly convoluted, filling with secretions. As a result, there is a 10-fold increase in thickness of the myometrium during the proliferative phase, from 0.5 to 5 millimeters.

If fertilization and implantation do not occur, the subsequent decline in estrogen and progesterone levels leads to atrophy of the functional layer of the endometrium, which in turn leads to increased coiling of the spiral arterioles and a regression of the glandular development. The excessive coiling of the spiral arterioles diminishes the blood flow to the endometrial layer, which then produces tissue ischemia, necrosis, and endometrial bleeding. Menstrual flow is the result of this bleeding and shedding of necrotic endometrial tissue. A more detailed description of the menstrual cycle appears later in this chapter.

Once a person reaches menopause, the endometrium becomes atrophic. The epithelium flattens, the glands gradually disappear, and the endometrial stroma becomes increasingly fibrous. In some cases, however, the endometrium retains a weak proliferative capacity, which may contribute to the development of endometrial hyperplasia and perhaps, ultimately, endometrial cancer.[34]

### Myometrium

The bulk of the uterus is made up of the myometrium, which is composed of bundles of smooth muscle fibers separated by connective tissue that consists primarily of collagen and elastin. The muscle fibers of the myometrium are arranged in three distinct patterns that contribute to this tissue's ability to contract effectively. In the inner layer of the myometrium, the fibers run in a circular pattern that spirals in a perpendicular orientation to the long axis of the uterus. In the middle layer, the muscle fibers are interlaced and form figure-eight patterns running diagonally along the long axis of the uterus.[35] In the outermost layer of the myometrium, fibers are arranged in both longitudinal and spiral patterns.

The arrangement of muscle fibers in these three patterns maximizes the contractility of the uterus during labor and birth. It is also an important anatomic factor following birth. As these muscles constrict after the fetus and placenta are expelled, the muscles form a ligature around the uterine blood vessels that supplied the placenta, thereby controlling bleeding and initiating uterine involution during the postpartum period. Additionally, these layers

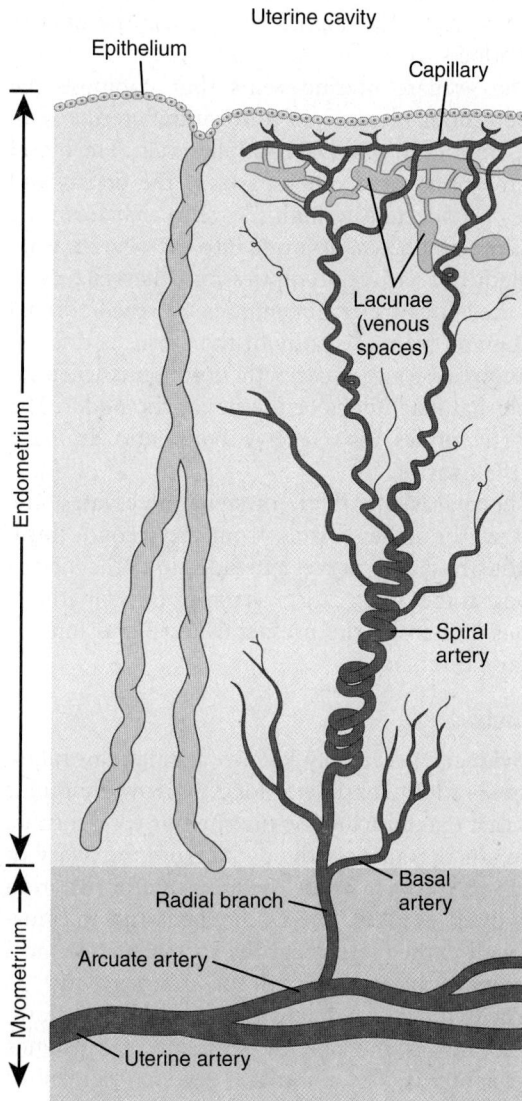

**Figure 8-11** Anatomy and circulation of the endometrium. Reproduced with permission from Moore KL, Persaud TVN, Torchia MG. *The Developing Human: Clinically Oriented Embryology.* 10th ed. Philadelphia, PA: Elsevier; 2016. Copyright Elsevier 2016. Reprinted with permission from Elsevier.

become more differentiated in pregnancy with the hypertrophy of the myometrial cells that occurs in pregnancy. Changes in the uterus during pregnancy are discussed in the *Anatomy and Physiology of Pregnancy* chapter, and the *Anatomy and Physiology of Labor and Birth* chapter contains a detailed description of the physiology of uterine contractions.

A gradient in the amount of muscle tissue found throughout the uterus is apparent, such that at the fundus, the myometrium contains primarily muscle fibers, whereas only 10% to 15% of the tissue mass in the cervix is composed of muscle fibers. The proportion of muscle fibers present determines the contractile strength of the uterine muscle. Thus, the distribution of muscle within the uterus creates a contraction strength gradient along its length.

### Uterine Ligaments, Blood Supply, and Innervation

The broad ligaments of the uterus are composed of folds in the peritoneum. These two wing-like structures extend from the sides of the uterus to the pelvic sidewalls. The superior part of the broad ligaments forms the suspensory ligament of the ovary and the mesosalpinx (the part of the broad ligament that encloses the oviducts). The round ligaments attach on either side of the uterus just below and in front of the insertion of the oviducts; they then cross the broad ligament in a fold of peritoneum, pass through the inguinal canal, and insert in the anterior (upper) portion of the labia majora on either side of the perineum. The ligaments are composed largely of smooth muscle that is continuous with the smooth muscle of the uterus. The round ligaments hypertrophy during pregnancy and stretch as the uterus enlarges, contributing to the common discomfort of "round ligament pain" experienced during the second and third trimesters. The peritoneal ligaments (uterosacral, cardinal, and pubocervical) extend from the cervix to different parts of the pelvis and help to stabilize the uterus. They are also the source of the discomfort that pregnant individuals describe as pelvic or vaginal pain toward the end of pregnancy.

The vessels that supply the uterus are derived primarily from the uterine and ovarian arteries. The uterine artery is a branch of the anterior branch of the internal iliac arteries (also referred to as the hypogastric arteries). The uterine artery enters the side of the uterus through the broad ligament and divides into several branches supplying the lower cervix and upper vagina, the upper portion of the cervix, and the body of the uterus. One large branch of the uterine artery travels along the margin of the uterus toward the fundus. At approximately the height of the round ligament, this branch of the uterine artery furcates into three vessels: One vessel joins the terminal branch of the ovarian artery, one supplies part of the salpinx, and one supplies the uterine fundus. These vessels that supply and drain blood from the uterus are collectively referred to as the arcuate vessels of the uterus.

The ovarian artery is a direct branch of the aorta that enters the broad ligament. The main stem of the ovarian artery travels near the mesosalpinx all the way to the upper, lateral portion of the uterus to join with the ovarian branch of the uterine artery. Branches from this main stem perfuse the ovaries and oviducts.

The arcuate uterine veins that compose the uterine venous plexus join to form the uterine vein, which empties into the internal iliac vein. The blood from the upper and outer parts of the uterus and ovaries is collected by multiple veins that form the pampiniform plexus, draining into the ovarian vein. The right ovarian vein empties into the vena cava, while the left ovarian vein empties into the left renal vein. Lymph from the body of the uterus is drained by lymph vessels that carry their contents to either the internal iliac nodes or the periaortic nodes. The periaortic nodes also receive lymphatic drainage from the ovaries.

The parasympathetic system innervates the uterus via branches arising from the second, third, and fourth sacral nerves. In addition, the uterus receives some innervation from the sympathetic nervous system by the presacral nerve and lumbar sympathetic chain.

### Oviducts

The oviducts, previously known as fallopian tubes, are the 8- to 14-centimeter-long, narrow, muscular tubes that extend from the uterine horns or cornua. The oviducts transport the ovum from the ovary to the uterus. It is also in the oviducts that fertilization normally takes place. These tubes penetrate the muscular wall of the uterus near the cornua and connect the cavity of the salpinx with the uterine cavity.

The oviducts can be divided into three sections. The isthmus is the narrow segment that extends from the uterus. The ampulla is a wider segment of the oviduct, where fertilization of the ovum most commonly occurs. The infundibulum is the fimbriated, open distal end of the salpinx, often referred to as the fimbriae. The fimbriae are fine, fingerlike mucosal projections at the end of the salpinx that sweep near the ovaries but are not connected to the ovaries.

Consequently, the oviducts open directly into the abdominal cavity. The oviducts vary in diameter at the different segments, with the isthmus measuring approximately 2 to 3 millimeters in thickness and the ampulla reaching a diameter of 5 to 8 millimeters.

The structure of the oviducts promotes movement of the ovum from the ovary into the salpinx and down toward the uterine cavity. The cilia of the mucosa move in waves to assist with transport of the ovum, and the fibers of the muscularis layer are arranged so that the oviducts can move and contract in a way that promotes transport of the ovum. Notably, recent research suggests that as many as 70% of cases of the most common form of ovarian cancer may originate in the oviducts, not the ovaries.[36] These cancerous cells may exit the oviducts and attach to the ovary or even distant organs. As a result, many "tubal ligations" are now salpingectomies, in which the oviducts are entirely removed to reduce lifetime risk of ovarian cancer.

## Ovaries

The ovaries are the organs of gamete production in the female body. Gamete production begins in fetal development by the third month of gestation. By the fourth month of gestation, each ovary contains approximately 10 million primary oocytes. The oocytes remain in a state of arrested meiosis until puberty. By puberty, only about 200,000 oocytes are present.[37] Ovulation is discussed in more detail in the next section on the menstrual cycle.

The two almond-shaped ovaries vary in size from each other, from person to person, and in the same person at different stages of life. During the reproductive years, the size of the ovaries ranges from approximately 2.5 to 5 cm long to 1.5 to 3 cm wide; to use an analogy, they range in size from an almond to a lime. These organs are located in the upper part of the pelvic cavity. Each ovary attaches in three ways: (1) to the broad ligament by the mesovarium; (2) to the uterus by the utero-ovarian ligaments, which extend from below the insertion points of the oviducts in the posterior part of the uterus; and (3) to the pelvic wall by the suspensory ligament of the ovary (also referred to as the infundibulopelvic ligament). The suspensory ligament of the uterus is a fold of the peritoneum that extends from the ovary to the pelvic wall. This fold also contains blood vessels and nerves that supply the ovary. If an ovary completely or partially rotates on its ligamentous supports, the condition is known as ovarian torsion. This twisting obstructs blood flow to the ovary, causing pain; if not corrected, it can result in ischemia and loss of ovarian function.

Each ovary is made up of two main parts: the cortex and the medulla. The cortex—the outer layer of the ovary—is composed of connective tissue and contains follicles at different stages of development. It is lined with germinal epithelium, and its dull, whitish outer layer is referred to as the tunica albuginea. The medulla of the ovary also consists of connective tissue and contains arteries, veins, and smooth muscle fibers.

In addition to producing ova, the ovaries manufacture the steroid hormones estrogen and progesterone and, therefore, are also part of the endocrine system. Within the ovarian follicles, two types of glandular cells are primarily involved in the synthesis of steroids—thecal cells and granulosa (or luteal) cells, both of which are important during the menstrual cycle and, therefore, to fertility. Theca cells differentiate from the interfollicular stroma of ripening follicles in response to proteins secreted by growing follicles.[38] These cells produce the androgen substrate required for ovarian estrogen biosynthesis, another key component of the menstrual cycle.

## Congenital Uterine Anomalies

Congenital uterine anomalies, also referred to as Müllerian anomalies, are present in as many as 10% of individuals assigned female at birth, although the majority of these anomalies are minor.[39-41] These conditions often go undiagnosed until an individual presents for evaluation due to infertility, recurrent miscarriages, pelvic pain, difficulty with vaginal penetrative sexual activity, or ectopic pregnancy.[42] The diagnosis may be made by pelvic examination, by ultrasound, or during a surgical procedure.

During development of the embryo, the two Müllerian ducts differentiate to form the uterus, cervix, superior portion of the vagina, and oviducts. Abnormal development results in a wide range of anatomic malformations. Classification of congenital uterine anomalies has been proposed by the American Society for Reproductive Medicine (ASRM). Although attempts have been made to update this classification system with more detailed categorizations, the ASRM system remains the standard for describing uterine anomalies and is presented in Table 8-3.[42]

Normal fertilization may not be possible for individuals with some Müllerian anomalies, such as agenesis of the oviducts. Other anomalies such as a communicating unicornuate uterus have been found to be associated with endometriosis and dysmenorrhea. However, an arcuate uterus may have no negative impact on conception and pregnancy.

| Table 8-3 | Classification of Congenital Uterine Anomalies |
|---|---|
| **Classification** | **Description** |
| **Class I Hypoplasia or Agenesis** | |
| I A | Vagina (with or without uterine abnormality) |
| I B | Cervix |
| I C | Fundus of uterus |
| I D | Oviducts |
| I E | Combination of above |
| **Class II Unicornuate Uterus (One Single Horn of Uterus)** | |
| II A | Rudimentary horn with endometrial cavity and communicating with single horn of uterus |
| II B | Rudimentary horn with endometrial cavity but noncommunicating with single horn of uterus |
| II C | Rudimentary horn without endometrial cavity |
| II D | No rudimentary horn |
| **Class III Uterus Didelphys** | |
| III | Two separate cavities with two separate cervices |
| **Class IV Bicornuate Uterus** | |
| IV A | Complete: Two separate uterine cavities separated by myometrial tissue and one cervix |
| IV B | Partial: Septum confined to fundus |
| **Class V Septate Uterus** | |
| V A | Complete: The septum extends into the internal cervical os with two cavities separated by avascular tissue and one cervix |
| V B | Partial: The septum does not reach the internal os |
| **Class VI Arcuate Uterus** | |
| VI | Concave fundus instead of convex or straight |
| **Class VII Diethylstilbestrol-Related Anomalies** | |
| VII A | T-shaped uterus |
| VII B | T-shaped uterus with dilated horns |
| VII C | Uterine hypoplasia |

Based on American Fertility Society. The American Fertility Society classifications of adnexal adhesions, distal tubal occlusion, tubal occlusion secondary to tubal ligation, tubal pregnancies, Müllerian anomalies and intrauterine adhesions. *Fertil Steril.* 1988;49:944-955.[42]

The most recent classification of congenital anomalies by ASRM relates to changes due to the use of diethylstilbestrol (DES), a nonsteroidal estrogen that was widely prescribed from 1948 to 1971 in an effort to prevent a number of pregnancy-related complications. Approximately 5 to 10 million pregnant women received DES during this time frame, after which DES was discovered to be not only ineffective but actually harmful to the fetus.[39,43] A number of structural and functional abnormalities have been identified as the direct effects of in utero exposure to DES, including changes to the uterus, vagina, and cervix. Reproductive health risks in DES daughters (i.e., individuals assigned female at birth and exposed to DES in utero) include infertility, ectopic pregnancy, spontaneous abortion, and premature birth. In addition, DES daughters are at greater risk for cervical and uterine carcinomas at age 30 years or younger, and at greater risk for breast cancer at age 40 years and older.[39,43]

To date, the limited data on the outcomes of DES-exposed grandchildren have not demonstrated uterine abnormalities in these individuals. In contrast, animal studies have shown a significant increase in uterine cancers, ovarian tumors, and lymphomas in third-generation offspring of DES-exposed subjects.[39,43] Thus, when obtaining an individual's health history, it is recommended that the midwife inquire whether they know if their gestational parent was exposed to DES, especially if they had a history of infertility, difficult pregnancies, or reproductive organ cancers.[44]

## The Menstrual Cycle: An Introduction

*Menstrual cycle* is the general term used to describe ovulation, menstruation, and the complex interplay of hormones regulating this cycle. While the menstrual cycle is often presented as being 28 days in length, the normal menstrual cycle can, in fact, range from 24 to 35 days in duration and is typically more variable in the first 5 to 7 years after menarche and in the last 10 years before menopause. The overall menstrual cycle encompasses two cycles within it: the ovarian cycle and the endometrial/uterine cycle. Each of these cycles has two phases that correspond with each other and occur simultaneously. Specifically, the ovarian cycle includes follicular and luteal phases, which correspond to the proliferative and secretory phases of the endometrial cycle, respectively.

This chapter divides the physiology of the menstrual cycle into several sections, beginning with hormonal production and regulation through steroidogenesis and the hypothalamic–pituitary–ovarian axis, respectively. This is followed by a discussion of the anatomy of the ovarian cycle, along with its associated physiology and anatomic developments. We conclude with a description of the endometrial cycle.

The physiology of the menstrual cycle is a sophisticated process. Over the last few decades, scientific discoveries have revealed more information about the interplay between functions of the reproductive organs, hormones, and the immune system. Evidence suggests that the body responds to infection, illness, and chronic disease differently at different points in the menstrual cycle, with these variations being partly due to fluctuations in sex hormones.[45,46] Some researchers have found that athletes are more likely to sustain injuries when their estrogen levels are high just prior to ovulation and theorize that this propensity is related to collagen metabolism, a process influenced by estrogen.[31] Furthermore, the menstrual cycle may affect immune cell numbers in a cyclic fashion, and disturbances in these cell numbers and functions have been noted in persons with conditions such as endometriosis and heavy menstrual bleeding.[45,47] Additionally, in an ovulating person, androgen levels begin to increase prior to ovulation, perhaps to stimulate the libido.[48] Non-ovulatory cycles, induced by ovulation-suppressing contraceptives, may also be associated with lower libido. As additional discoveries have been made about this exquisitely complex process, our understanding of the menstrual cycle has become more nuanced and new avenues of inquiry have opened.[49]

## Steroidogenesis

Many hormones exist in the human body, which are generally one of three different types: those made from amino acids, those made from peptides, and steroid hormones, which are derived from cholesterol. One type of steroid hormone is the gonadocorticoid group, also referred to as the sex hormones; it includes androgens, estrogen, and progestogens. All gonadocorticoids are synthesized from cholesterol through a series of chemical reactions known as steroidogenesis. This process of steroidogenesis proceeds through a few efficient chemical steps that reduce the number of carbon atoms in cholesterol from 27 to 18.

The major site of biosynthesis for all sex steroid hormones in a healthy ovulating person is the ovary. Other peripheral sites in the body, including adipose tissue and skeletal muscle, produce small amounts of these hormones. The role of these tissues in gonadocorticoid production explains why an individual with a very high or low level of adipose tissue or skeletal muscle can experience disruptions within the ovulatory and/or menstrual cycle. Additionally, for steroidogenesis to occur, there must be interaction between gonadotropins, follicle-stimulating hormone (FSH), luteinizing hormone (LH), and the ovaries. Production of FSH and LH is part of the hypothalamic–pituitary–ovarian axis, as illustrated in Figure 8-12.

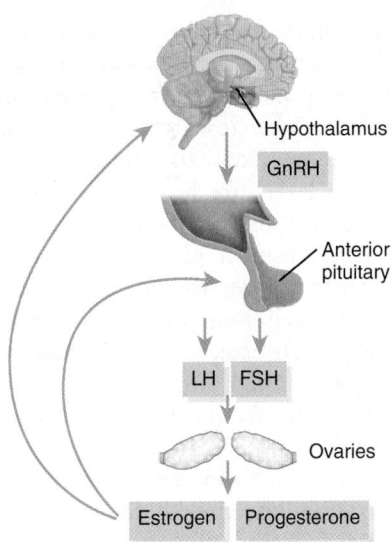

**Figure 8-12** The hypothalamic–pituitary–ovarian axis. Abbreviations: FSH, follicle-stimulating hormone; GnRH, gonadotropin-releasing hormone; LH, luteinizing hormone.

## The Hypothalamic–Pituitary–Ovarian Axis

*Hypothalamic–pituitary–ovarian axis* (H-P-O axis) is a term used to refer to the effects created by these individual endocrine organs when they work in concert as a system. These organs respond to positive and negative feedback loops to regulate steroid hormone production in a complex and coordinated manner. An understanding of the H-P-O axis is critical when assisting those individuals with amenorrhea, polycystic ovarian syndrome, abnormal uterine bleeding, dysmenorrhea, and infertility. Additionally, understanding the H-P-O axis is crucial to understanding the mechanism of action for hormonal contraceptives, which aids the practitioner in providing accurate contraceptive counseling.

The hypothalamus controls anterior pituitary function by secreting releasing and inhibiting factors that affect the pituitary. The hypothalamus also controls the production of steroid and peptide hormones, which act as chemical messengers that regulate the entire gynecologic system. The four key hormones in this system are FSH, LH, estrogen, and progesterone. These hormones stimulate the reproductive organs and are collectively referred to as gonadotropins. The hypothalamus releases gonadotropin-releasing hormone (GnRH) in a pulsatile fashion. The frequency of the pulses varies over the course of the ovarian cycle; GnRH is secreted at the highest frequency during the follicular phase, with secretion decreasing during the luteal phase. When FSH and

LH travel from the pituitary via the circulatory system to the ovaries, they stimulate the ovarian cells to secrete estrogen (as estradiol) and progesterone, which are the final members of the hormonal group that regulates the menstrual cycle.

While this description may appear one directional, the H-P-O axis functions through both negative and positive feedback loops in response to estrogen and progesterone levels, which in turn affect FSH and LH secretion. This system includes two negative feedback loops. First, when estrogen and progesterone levels rise above a set point, the hypothalamus decreases secretion of GnRH, which leads to a decrease in the secretion of FSH and LH. Conversely, when estrogen and progesterone levels fall below a set point, the hypothalamus increases secretion of GnRH, which then causes an increase in the secretion of FSH and LH. An interesting positive feedback loop occurs when estrogen levels reach a peak just before ovulation, which triggers the hypothalamus to increase secretion of GnRH, causing a surge of FSH and, primarily, LH and the release of a mature ovum from the ovary.

Among the factors that influence feedback are three specific peptides—inhibin, activin, and follistatin—that are synthesized by ovarian granulosa cells and secreted into the ovarian follicular fluid. As the names imply, activin simulates FSH secretion, while inhibin and follistatin inhibit FSH secretion by binding to activin.

Other factors are also known to have important actions on ovarian function. Because hormones are receptor specific, the cells within the ovary contain receptor sites that are essential for normal ovarian function and a normal menstrual cycle. As the various changes occur in the ovary during the monthly cycle, hormonal receptors on ovarian cells upregulate and can interact with the feedback system. For example, the ovary is a primary site of production for insulin-like growth factor, which stimulates steroidogenesis by increasing the size and number of receptors for both FSH and LH. This growth factor also amplifies androgen production and FSH action within the ovaries at specific sites.

## The Ovarian Cycle

The ovarian cycle is defined by changes that occur in the ovary during the menstrual cycle. This cycle has two phases, the follicular phase and the luteal phase, with ovulation occurring between the two. The follicular phase starts with the onset of menses and ends on the day before the LH surge occurs.

Ovulation is defined by release of the ovum from the ovary. The luteal phase begins on the day of the LH surge and ends at the onset of menses. Although ovulation is a distinct event, it usually occurs 10 to 12 hours after the LH peak, which is why some texts divide the ovarian cycle into the follicular and luteal phases only, while others define ovulation as a distinct middle phase.

## Follicular Phase

During each ovarian cycle, oocytes undergo monthly meiosis as a part of ovum maturation. During this process, each oocyte splits into secondary oocytes that contain 23 chromosomes. Then, through a series of steps, each oocyte becomes surrounded by cells, thereby forming an oocyte-containing follicle that has hormone receptor sites.

The length of the follicular phase varies, but averages 10 to 14 days. This phase of the ovarian cycle produces an ovum for fertilization and begins on the first day of menses. At the beginning of the follicular phase, estrogen and progesterone levels are low following the end of the previous cycle. These low levels cause the hypothalamus to release GnRH, which stimulates the anterior pituitary gland to release FSH and LH. FSH and LH stimulate the maturation of a cohort of follicles in the ovaries that then produce estrogen. Specifically, the follicles develop receptors for FSH and LH on their granulosa and theca cells, respectively. As the follicles grow, these cells produce androgens that are converted to estrogen, thereby increasing estrogen levels.

As estrogen levels increase, FSH production by the pituitary decreases. The follicle with the most FSH receptors, and thus the most estrogen receptor sites, becomes dominant. As the dominant follicle uses the available FSH, the other follicles atrophy. As the level of estrogen peaks owing to production by the dominant follicle, the hypothalamus increases its secretion of GnRH, priming the cycle for a surge in LH, which triggers ovulation, or release of an ovum (Figure 8-13).

## Ovulation

Ovulation usually occurs 10 to 12 hours after the LH surge and 24 to 36 hours after the estrogen peak. The LH surge is the most reliable single indicator of ovulation.[38] During this time, prostaglandins and proteolytic enzymes break down the wall of the dominant follicle, causing it to rupture and release the oocyte. The oocyte is then swept up by the fimbria and caught within the salpinx, where it can be fertilized for approximately 12 to 24 hours after release.

At the time of follicular rupture, some people experience abdominal discomfort, known as mittelschmerz. Other physiologic events also occur around ovulation. For example, under the influence of estrogen in the mid- to late follicular phase, the cervix softens, the external cervical os opens slightly, and cervical mucus becomes clear, thin, and more profuse. These changes in the cervical mucus facilitate sperm transport to aid in fertilization. After ovulation, higher progesterone levels lead to the production of thick cervical mucus, which inhibits the entry of sperm into the uterus. Interestingly, this cervical mucus also inhibits entry of microbes, which explains why intrauterine infections are less likely during the luteal phase and in those individuals using progesterone-based contraceptives.

## Luteal Phase

The luteal phase begins after ovulation occurs. Whereas the length of the follicular phase of the ovarian cycle may vary, the duration of the luteal phase is generally constant at 14 days. Following ovulation, the dominant follicle is transformed into a structure called the corpus luteum (yellow body). The consistent length of the luteal phase is directly related to the longevity of the corpus luteum, assuming no interference by fertilization and implantation. If fertilization and implantation do occur, cells that will become the placenta produce human chorionic gonadotropin hormone to maintain the corpus luteum. This structure becomes the initial source of progesterone to sustain the pregnancy until the placenta starts producing progesterone around week 12 of gestation.

If implantation does not occur, the corpus luteum produces high levels of progesterone that peak at 7 to 8 days after ovulation. These high levels of progesterone trigger a negative feedback loop of the H-P-O axis: The hypothalamus decreases its secretion of GnRH, which leads to a decrease in the secretion of FSH and LH, thereby suppressing new follicular growth.

Because progesterone is associated with an elevation in basal body temperature (BBT), daily measurement of BBT will demonstrate a rise *after* ovulation has occurred, which is when the corpus luteum is producing progesterone. This makes BBT assessment useful as a post hoc measure and as the basis of some natural family planning methods. A variety of other factors, including oxytocin, are likely to be involved in this phase of the menstrual cycle.

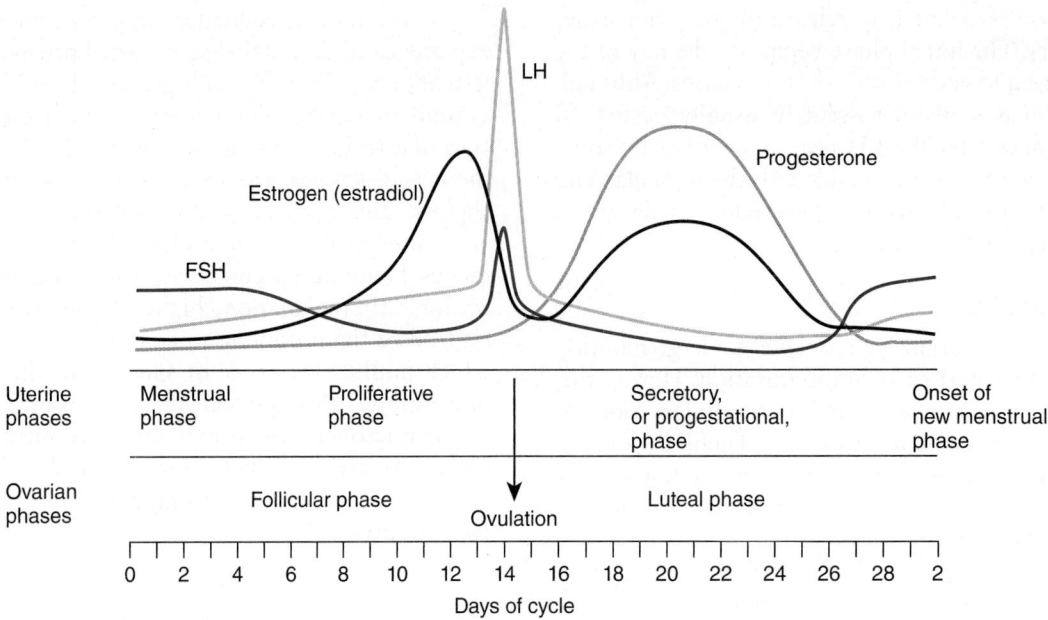

**Figure 8-13** Hormonal changes throughout the menstrual cycle.
Abbreviations: FSH, follicle-stimulating hormone; LH, luteinizing hormone.

If no pregnancy occurs, the corpus luteum regresses and estrogen, progesterone, and inhibin levels eventually decrease such that there is transitional time between one cycle and the next. As production of inhibin drops, FSH levels begin to increase. Conversely, because estrogen and progesterone levels are low, GnRH pulses increase, which in turn facilitates production and release of FSH and LH from the hypothalamus and pituitary. FSH helps rescue a group of follicles from atresia, and the cycle begins anew.

Table 8-4 presents an overview of the hormones of the ovarian cycle, their location of production, their primary functions, and conditions occurring with altered levels of these hormones.

## The Endometrial/Uterine Cycle

The endometrial or uterine cycle is defined by the changes that occur in the endometrium during the menstrual cycle. It is divided into two phases: the proliferative phase and the secretory phase. The proliferative phase corresponds to the follicular phase of the ovarian cycle and is under the influence of estrogen. The secretory phase corresponds to the luteal phase of the ovarian cycle and is under the influence of progesterone.

### Proliferative Phase

During the proliferative phase, the endometrial tissue develops under the increasing influence of estrogen. Endometrial glands change from being narrow and tubular to being enlarged to the extent that they link to one another, forming a continuous lining.

In situations when the uterine lining is exposed to estrogen but not progesterone, such as during chronic anovulation or when an individual receives exogenous estrogen without progesterone, a proliferative endometrium becomes persistent. When this occurs, there is a higher risk of endometrial hyperplasia; this state is associated with endometrial cancer. These conditions are discussed in more detail in the *Menstrual Cycle Abnormalities* chapter.

### Secretory Phase

The rising progesterone levels that occur following ovulation have a major influence on the endometrium, turning a proliferative endometrium into a secretory one. The thickness of the endometrium does not regress, but the appearance of the tissue does change. Notably, the coiling of the spiral vessels and the tortuosity of the glands increase. The stroma become edematous such that at the time of implantation (approximately 21 to 27 days into the cycle), three distinct zones have appeared: the stratum spongiosum (the most superficial layer), the stratum compactum (midportion), and the stratum basale (the innermost layer). Once an endometrium becomes secretory, the risks associated with

| Table 8-4 | | Hormones That Regulate the Ovarian Cycle and Clinical Implications of Altered Physiology | |
|---|---|---|---|
| Hormone | Origin | Physiologic Action | Clinical Implications When Hormone Levels Are Increased or Decreased |
| Estrogen: steroid hormone (Estradiol is the most potent form during the reproductive years) | Ovaries: produced in response to FSH and LH | Regulation of menstrual cycle; Maturation of reproductive organs and development of secondary sex characteristics; Closure of long bones following puberty; Physiologic changes in pregnancy; Metabolic effects on other organs | **Increased:** Hyperthyroidism, irregular menstrual cycle, estrogen-producing or adrenal tumor **Decreased:** Ovarian failure, dyspareunia, postmenopause, osteoporosis, Turner syndrome, anorexia nervosa |
| Progesterone: steroid hormone | Ovaries: produced in response to FSH and LH | Regulation of menstrual cycle; Mammary gland development; Physiologic changes in pregnancy | **Increased:** Pregnancy, ovulation, ovarian cysts, hydatidiform mole, progesterone-secreting tumor/cyst **Decreased:** Threatened miscarriage, fetal demise, preeclampsia, spotting between periods, migraines, short luteal phase syndrome |
| Follicle-stimulating hormone (FSH): gonadotropin | Anterior pituitary: released in response to GnRH | Stimulates growth and development of the primary follicles; Stimulates production of estrogen and progesterone in the ovaries | **Increased:** Postmenopause, ovarian failure, infertility, Turner syndrome, gonadotropin-secreting pituitary tumor **Decreased:** Pregnancy, PCOS, infertility, pituitary or hypothalamic dysfunction (may cause amenorrhea), hyperprolactinemia, anorexia nervosa |
| Luteinizing hormone (LH): gonadotropin | Anterior pituitary: released in response to GnRH | Ovulation; Corpus luteum formation; Stimulates production of estrogen and progesterone in the ovaries | **Increased:** PCOS, ovarian failure, postmenopause **Decreased:** Pituitary or hypothalamic dysfunction (may cause amenorrhea), infertility, anorexia nervosa |

Abbreviations: GnRH, gonadotropin-releasing hormone; PCOS, polycystic ovarian syndrome.

persistent proliferative endometrium are diminished. Since the discovery that exogenous progesterone facilitates development of a secretory endometrium, it has become standard practice to include progesterone as an adjunctive treatment with estrogen in menopausal hormone therapy, if the individual has a uterus.

If no implantation occurs, the decreasing levels of estrogen and progesterone from the corpus luteum result in disorganization of the endometrium by approximately day 25 of the cycle. The tissue shrinks, venous drainage diminishes, and blood flow within the spiral arteries is compromised, resulting in rhythmic constriction and relaxation. The cells of the uterine lining go through a physiologic death,

known as apoptosis, and the uterus is ready for the next step—menses.

## Menstruation

As the lining of the uterus weakens, blood and uterine tissue (stroma) escape into the endometrial cavity. The appearance of blood marks the first day of the menstrual period. The onset of bleeding, which occurs after the large drop in plasma levels of estrogen and progesterone, is indicative of a normal menstrual cycle with functional organs and endocrine system. Investigation of amenorrhea often involves a challenge test (called a progesterone withdrawal test) in which oral progesterone is ingested over a period of days. When the dose is complete, it causes a sudden drop in progesterone levels. If vaginal bleeding occurs after the progesterone dose is complete, the assumption is made that the individual has adequate endogenous estrogen and that there is no end-organ disorder. More information about this testing is found in the *Menstrual Cycle Abnormalities* chapter.

Figure 8-14 presents an overview of the fascinating and complex menstrual cycle, including the ovarian, hormonal, and uterine cycles.[50]

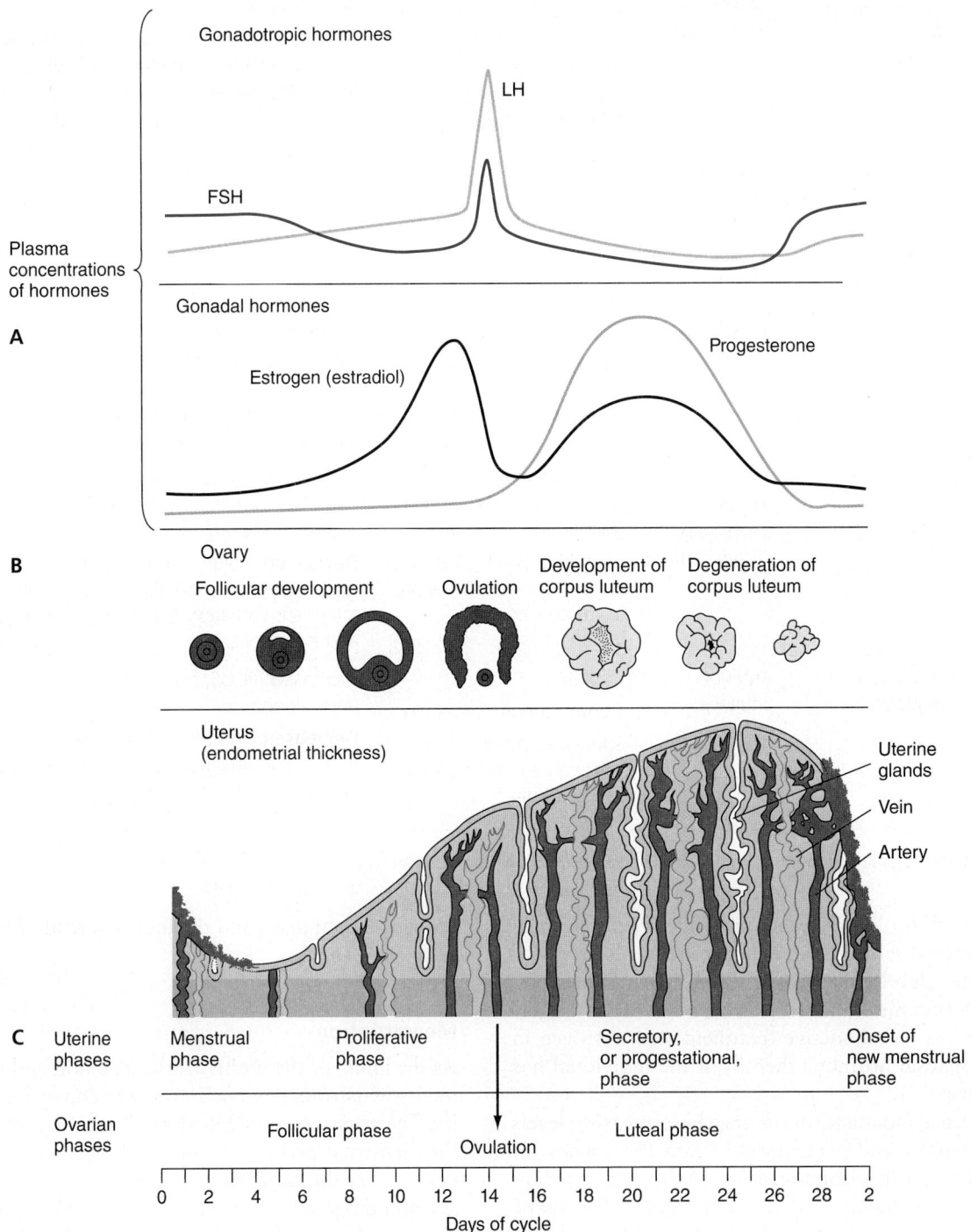

**Figure 8-14** The menstrual cycle. **A.** Hormonal cycles. **B.** The ovarian cycle. **C.** The uterine (endometrial) cycle.
Abbreviations: FSH, follicle-stimulating hormone; LH, luteinizing hormone.
Reproduced from Chiras DD. *Human Biology.* 9th ed. Burlington, MA: Jones & Bartlett Learning; 2019.

# Reproductive Anatomy in Individuals Assigned Male at Birth

In this section, the reproductive anatomy of individuals assigned male at birth, and who have not had any surgery on their genitalia, is discussed. This reproductive system consists of both internal and external structures. The many glands and ducts of these structures are well vascularized to promote the formation, storage, and ejaculation of sperm for fertilization and to produce important androgens for development of secondary sex characteristics. The primary androgen is testosterone, whose function is to maintain reproductive function and produce gametes, or sperm. The regulation of hormones that contribute to gamete production, sexual development, and sexual function is performed by the hypothalamic–pituitary–gonadal axis. In this system, FSH and LH are released from the anterior pituitary and are regulated by GnRH produced in the hypothalamus.

The reproductive anatomy consists of both external and internal structures. The external structures include the penis and scrotum, while the internal structures consist of the testes, epididymis, vas deferens, seminal vesicles, prostate, and bulbourethral glands (**Figure 8-15**).[51] A brief description of each structure follows.

## Penis

The penis is the organ used for urination, sexual response, and reproduction via the transport of sperm out of the body. It consists of three parts: the root, the body, and the glans. The root of the penis attaches the penis to the lower abdomen and contains erectile tissue. The body of the penis, which is the main portion of the penis, is shaped like a tube or cylinder. It has three chambers containing the corpora cavernosa and corpus spongiosum tissue, which can fill with blood during sexual arousal to create an erection. The glans is the most distal portion of the penis and is shaped like an asymmetrical cone. It is covered with a loose layer of skin called the foreskin, which retracts during erection. The foreskin is the skin that is removed or altered during male circumcision. The external opening of the urethra is located at the tip of the glans; the urethra is the tube through which urine and sperm exit the body.

## Scrotum

The scrotum is a thin external sac located under the penis. It is composed of skin and smooth muscle and is divided into two compartments by the scrotal septum. The purposes of the scrotum are twofold: to protect the testes and to provide thermoregulation. The scrotum keeps the testes several degrees below body temperature, which is crucial for sperm production and health.

## Testes

The testes are small oval organs suspended within the scrotum. They produce both testosterone and immature sperm. The immature sperm cells are produced through the process of spermatogenesis in the seminiferous tubules, which are coiled masses of tubes within the testes. Most male bodies have two testes, one on either side of the scrotal septum.

## Epididymis

The epididymis is a long, coiled tube that rests at the posterior portion of each testicle. Sperm are stored in the epididymis while they mature. The epididymis connects the testes to the vas deferens. During sexual arousal, contractions force sperm into the vas deferens.

## Vas Deferens

The vas deferens is a long, muscular tube that connects the epididymis of each testicle to the pelvic cavity just behind the bladder. Mature sperm are propelled through the vas deferens to the urethra in preparation for ejaculation.

## Seminal Vesicles

The seminal vesicles are two pouches attached to the vas deferens at the base of the bladder. These vesicles produce a fructose-rich fluid that constitutes the majority of ejaculate or semen. The purposes of this fluid are to provide sperm with an energy source and to aid in motility.

## Prostate Gland

Located below the bladder and anterior to the rectum is the prostate. This gland provides additional fluid to ejaculate that also nourishes the sperm and aids in their motility. The urethra passes through the center of the prostate. The prostate normally enlarges with aging.

## Bulbourethral Gland (Cowper's gland)

There are two bulbourethral glands, one located on either side of the urethra just below the prostate. These glands produce a clear, slippery fluid that empties directly into the urethra and lubricates it. In

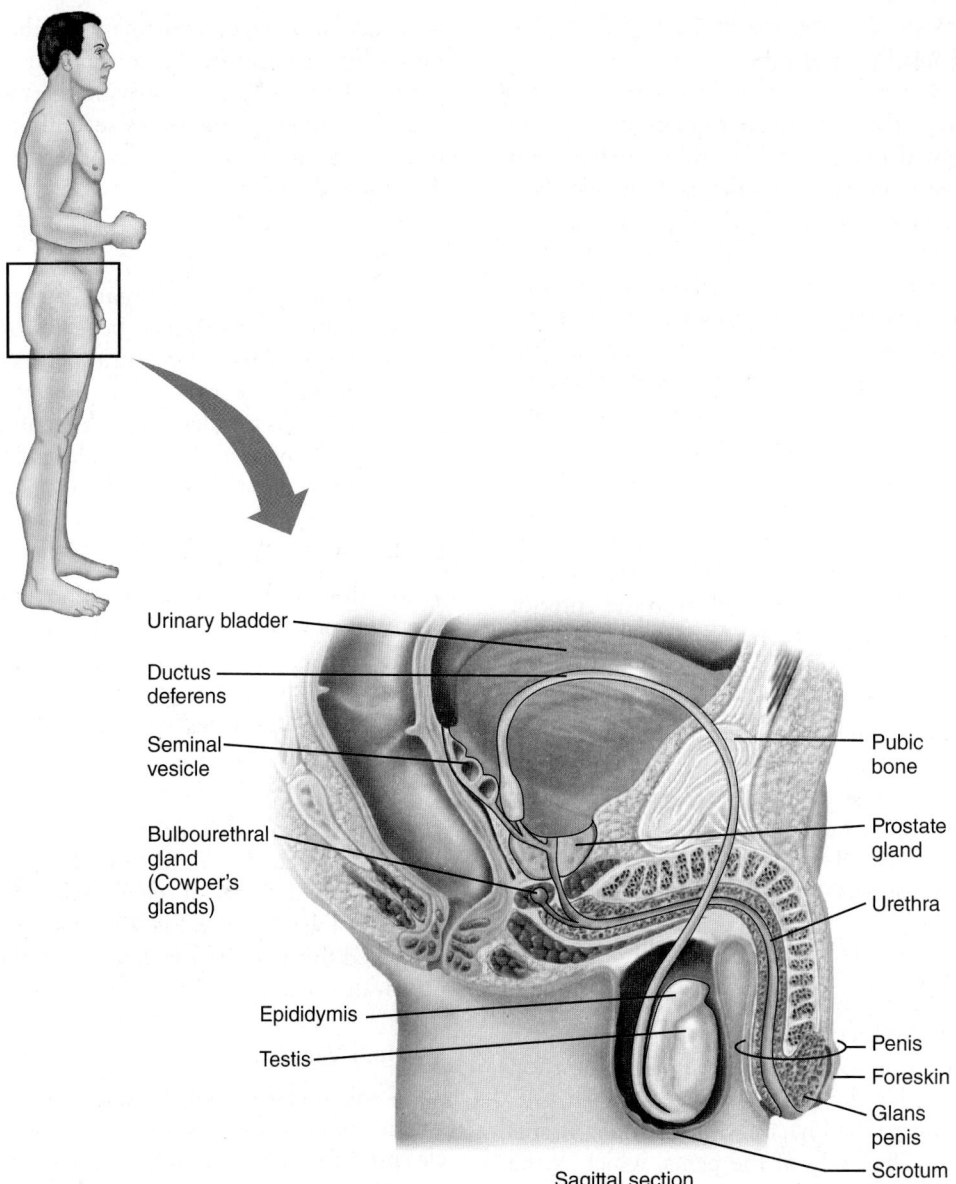

**Figure 8-15** Midsagittal view of the reproductive system of those assigned male at birth.
Modified from Harbison HS. Male sexual and reproductive health. In: Schuiling KD, Likis FE, eds. *Gynecologic Health Care*. 4th ed. Burlington, MA: Jones & Bartlett Learning; 2022.

addition to assisting with sperm motility, this fluid neutralizes acid from any residual drops of urine in the urethra, which supports sperm viability.

## Sexual Response in the Female Body

Sexual response, especially for individuals assigned female at birth, is a complex interaction between mental processes and physical stimulation that has an infinite number of individual variations. Sexual activity can include many different expressions.

Additionally, sexual response has many influences and is not merely physiologic in nature. An individual's mental perspective, history, and circumstances all affect sexual response. Furthermore, recent research confirms that culture may influence sexual response.[52] Although this section describes the physiologic response, it is important to recognize that individual sexuality and sexual responses cannot be adequately described by knowing the basic physiology of sexual response. More information is found in the *Sexuality* chapter.

Descriptions of sexual response have for years been based on the model developed by Masters and Johnson in the 1960s. Indeed, this linear model has been applied to all individuals regardless of sex. Masters and Johnson's model depicted sexual response as comprising four phases: excitement (sexual stimulation leads to vasoconstriction), plateau (increased vasoconstriction and pelvic floor muscle tension), orgasm (generalized genitopelvic muscle contraction), and resolution (return to a nonstimulated state).[53] A weakness of this model is that it focuses exclusively on physiologic responses to stimuli.

A newer model first developed by Basson in 2000 focused on sexual response in the female body and incorporates emotional, cognitive, and psychological factors. This model, which was developed based on information from cis-gendered women, suggests that for this group, sexual response may arise more from need for intimacy rather than from a desire for sexual arousal. It may be that emotional intimacy and physical satisfaction are the goal, not simply orgasm. Furthermore, the sense of sexual arousal may be only minimally linked to awareness of physiologic changes such as genital congestion. Lastly, this model does not identify orgasm as the goal of all sexual response. It recognizes that sexual motivation is complex and not simply an innate physiologic occurrence. A model that provides an expanded understanding of "female" sexual response and offers a more detailed template for elucidating this complex phenomenon is presented in Figure 8-16.[54,55]

While orgasm may not always be the goal of sexual response, it is an aspect of it. Orgasm may be stimulated by vaginal penetration or clitoral stimulation in people with this anatomy, although it may also occur without these actions. In general, for those assigned female at birth, clitoral stimulation is the most common source of physical stimulation for initiation of orgasm. One interesting controversy about the anatomy of sexual response in the female body is the "G-spot," which was proposed to be an anatomic collection of nerves in the anterior vagina that is the source of vaginally stimulated orgasm. Subsequent anatomic and physiologic studies have not confirmed that this spot exists.[56,57]

Orgasm is regulated by both sensory and autonomic nerves. It starts when the pudendal nerve transmits information from the clitoris and external genitalia; this is followed by increased blood flow to the area. A reflex wave of smooth and skeletal muscle contractions then occurs in the vagina, urethra, anus, and uterus.

Estrogen—in particular, estradiol—is the primary hormone that mediates sexual response in the female body, but the roles of the hormones of import are not fully understood. However, the lower levels of estradiol that occur following menopause are the etiology of vaginal atrophy, as well as difficulty with vasoconstriction and vaginal lubrication. These changes associated with aging can lead to diminished sexual interest, arousal, and orgasm.[58]

## Conclusion

This chapter has presented a brief overview of reproductive anatomy and physiology, focusing on individuals assigned female at birth. Midwives caring for those individuals with specific disorders such as pelvic floor dysfunction, sexual dysfunction, or menstrual disorders will need additional detailed knowledge about how the anatomy and physiology of these organs affect a person's health. Some resources for reviewing these topics are included in the Resources section.

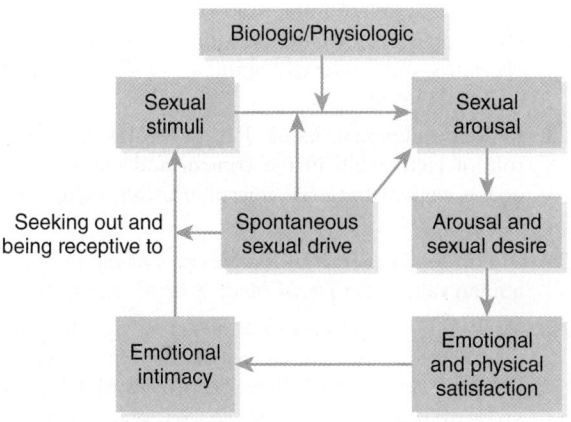

**Figure 8-16** Intimacy-based model of sexual response in the female body.
Sources: Based on Basson R. Human sexual response. *Handbook Clin Neurol.* 2015;130:11-18; Bachmann G, Stern L, Ramos J. Female sexual function. *Glob Libr Womens Med.* https://www.glowm.com/section-view/heading/female-sexual-function/item/428#.YZLBWy-cZUc.

## Resources

| Organization | Description |
|---|---|
| Bartleby.com | *Gray's Anatomy of the Human Body* online; free access to the book and illustrations |
| Association of Reproductive Health Professionals (ARHP) | Female sexual response |

## References

1. Draper A. The history of the term pudendum: opening the discussion on anatomical sex inequality. *Clin Anat*. 2021;34(2):315-319.

2. Hill AJ, Balgobin S, Mishra K, et al. for Society of Gynecologic Surgeons Pelvic Anatomy Group. Recommended standardized anatomic terminology of the posterior female pelvis and vulva based on a structured medical literature review. *Am J Obstet Gynecol*. 2021;225(2):169.e1-169.e16.

3. Balgobin S, Jeppson PC, Wheeler T, et al. for Society of Gynecologic Surgeons Pelvic Anatomy Group. Standardized terminology of apical structures in the female pelvis based on a structured medical literature review. *Am J Obstet Gynecol*. 2020;222(3):204-218.

4. Jeppson PC, Balgobin S, Washington BB, et al. for Society of Gynecologic Surgeons Pelvic Anatomy Group. Recommended standardized terminology of the anterior female pelvis based on a structured medical literature review. *Am J Obstet Gynecol*. 2018;219(1):26-39.

5. Chimielwski, PP. New *Terminologia Anatomica* highlights the importance of clinical anatomy. *Folia Morphol (Warsz)*. 2020;79(1):15-20.

6. Clemente CD. *Anatomy: A Regional Atlas of the Human Body*. 6th ed. Philadelphia, PA: Lippincott Williams & Wilkins; 2011.

7. Geddes DT. Inside the lactating breast: the latest anatomy research. *J Midwifery Womens Health*. 2007;52:556-563.

8. Ramsay DT, Kent JC, Hartmann RA, Hartman PE. Anatomy of the human breast redefined with ultrasound imaging. *J Anat*. 2005;206:525-534.

9. Love RM, Barsky SH. Anatomy of the nipple and breast ducts revisited. *Cancer*. 2004;101:1947-1957.

10. Howard BA, Gusterson BA. Human breast development. *J Mammary Gland Biol Neoplasia*. 2000;5(2):120-137.

11. Huseynov A, Zollikofer CP, Coudyzer W, et al. Developmental evidence for obstetric adaptation of the human female pelvis. *Proc Natl Acad Sci USA*. 2016;113(19):5227-5232.

12. Ritchie JR. Orthopedic considerations during pregnancy. *Clin Obstet Gynecol*. 2003;46(2):456-466.

13. Chermansky CJ, Moalli PA. Role of pelvic floor in lower urinary tract function. *Auton Neurosci*. 2016;200:43-48.

14. Ashton-Miller JA, DeLancey JOL. Functional anatomy of the female pelvic floor. *Ann NY Acad Sci*. 2007;1101:266-296.

15. Kearney R, Sawhney R, DeLancey JO. Levator ani muscle anatomy evaluated by origin-insertion pairs. *Obstet Gynecol*. 2004;104(1):168-173.

16. Stein TA, DeLancey JO. Structure of the perineal membrane in females: gross and microscopic anatomy. *Obstet Gynecol*. 2008;111(3):686-693.

17. Stoker J. Anorectal and pelvic floor anatomy. *Best Pract Res Clin Gastroenterol*. 2009;23(4):463-475.

18. Clark NR. Gynecologic anatomy and physiology. In: Schuiling KD, Likis FE, eds. *Gynecologic Health Care*. 4th ed. Burlington, MA: Jones & Bartlett Learning; 2022: 87-98.

19. Barleben A, Mills S. Anorectal anatomy and physiology. *Surg Clin North Am*. 2010;90:1-15.

20. Nguyen J, Duong H. Anatomy, abdomen and pelvis, female external genitalia. In: *StatPearls*. Treasure Island, FL: StatPearls Publishing; 2021. https://www.ncbi.nlm.nih.gov/books/NBK547703/. Accessed August 8, 2022.

21. Pauls RN. Anatomy of the clitoris and the female sexual response. *Clin Anat*. 2015;28:376-384.

22. O'Connell HE, Hutson JM, Anderson CR, Plenter RJ. Anatomical relationship between urethra and clitoris. *J Urol*. 1998;159(6):1892-1897.

23. Rodriguez FD, Camacho A, Bordes SJ, et al. Female ejaculation: an update on anatomy, history, and controversies. *Clin Anat*. 2021;34(1):103-107.

24. Integrative Human Microbiome Project. The Integrative Human Microbiome Project. *Nature*. 2019;569(7758):641-648.

25. Jang SJ, Lee K, Kwon B, et al. Vaginal lactobacilli inhibit growth and hyphae formation of *Candida albicans*. *Sci Rep*. 2019;9(1):1-9.

26. Muhleisen AL, Herbst-Kralovetz MM. Menopause and the vaginal microbiome. *Maturitas*. 2016;91: 42-50.

27. Ahrens P, Andersen, LOB, Lilje B, et al. Changes in the vaginal microbiota following antibiotic treatment for *Mycoplasma genitalium*, *Chlamydia trachomatis* and bacterial vaginosis. *PloS One*. 2020; 15(7):e0236036.

28. Redondo-Lopez V, Cook RL, Sobel JD. Emerging role of lactobacilli in the control and maintenance of the vaginal bacterial microflora. *Rev Infect Dis*. 1990;12(5):856-872.

29. Witkin SS, Ledger WJ. Complexities of the uniquely human vagina. *Sci Transl Med*. 2012;4(132):132fs11.

30. Vink JY, Qin S, Brock CO, et al. A new paradigm for the role of smooth muscle cells in the human cervix. *Am J Obstet Gynecol*. 2016;215(4):478.e1-478.e11.

31. Nott JP, Bonney EA, Pickering JD, Simpson NAB. The structure and function of the cervix during pregnancy. *Translat Res Anatom*. 2016;2:1-7.

32. Herfs M, Yamamoto Y, Laury, A, et al. A discrete population of squamocolumnar junction cells implicated in the pathogenesis of cervical cancer. *Proc Natl Acad Sci*. 2012;109(26):10516-10521.

33. Moore KL, Persaud TVN, Torchia MG. *The Developing Human: Clinically Oriented Embryology*. 10th ed. Philadelphia, PA: Elsevier; 2016.

34. Sivridis E, Giatromanolaki A. Proliferative activity in the postmenopausal endometrium: the lurking potential for giving rise to an endometrial carcinoma. *J Clin Pathol*. 2004;57(8):840-844.

35. Deveduex D, Marque C, Masour S, et al. Uterine electromyography: a critical review. *Am J Obstet Gynecol*. 1993;169(6):1636-1653.

36. Labidi-Galy S, Papp E, Hallberg D, et al. High grade serous ovarian carcinomas originate in the fallopian tube. *Nat Comm*. 2017;8(1):1-11.

37. Gilbert SF. The saga of the germ line. In: *Developmental Biology*. 6th ed. Sunderland, MA: Sinaur Associates; 2000. http://www.ncbi.nlm.nih.gov/books/NBK10008. Accessed October 1, 2012.

38. Rimon-Dahari N, Yerushalmi-Heinemann L, Alyagor L, Dekel N. Ovarian folliculogenesis. *Results Probl Cell Differ*. 2016;58:167-190.

39. Goodman A, Schorge J, Greene M. The long-term effects of in utero exposures: the DES story. *N Engl J Med*. 2011;364:2083-2084.

40. Venetis C, Papadopoulos S, Campo R, Gordts S, Tarlatzis B, Grimbizis G. Clinical implications of congenital uterine anomalies: a meta-analysis of comparative studies. *Reprod Biomed Online*. 2014;29:665-683.

41. Dreisler E, Stampe Sørensen S. Müllerian duct anomalies diagnosed by saline contrast sonohysterography: prevalence in a general population. *Fertil Steril*. 2014;102:525-529.

42. American Fertility Society. The American Fertility Society classifications of adnexal adhesions, distal tubal occlusion, tubal occlusion secondary to tubal ligation, tubal pregnancies, Müllerian anomalies and intrauterine adhesions. *Fertil Steril*. 1988;49:944-955.

43. Reed C, Fenton S. Exposure to diethylstilbestrol during sensitive life stages: a legacy of heritable health effects. *Birth Defects Res C: Embryo Today*. 2013;99:134-146.

44. Centers for Disease Control and Prevention. Information to identify and manage DES patients. February 2017. https://www.cdc.gov/DES/hcp/information/daughters/risks_daughters.html#cca. Accessed May 20, 2017.

45. Oertelt-Prigione S. Immunology and the menstrual cycle. *Autoimmun Rev*. 2012;11(6-7):A486-A492.

46. Alvergne A, Tabor VH. Is female health cyclical? Evolutionary perspectives on menstruation. *Trends Ecol Evol*. 2018;33(6):399-414.

47. Berbic M, Fraser IS. Immunology of normal and abnormal menstruation. *Womens Health*. 2013;9(4): 387-395.

48. Bullivant SB, Sellergren SA, Stern K, et al. Women's sexual experience during the menstrual cycle: identification of the sexual phase by noninvasive measurement of luteinizing hormone. *J Sex Res*. 2004;41(1):82-93.

49. Sherman JJ, LeResche L. Does experimental pain response vary across the menstrual cycle? A methodological review. *Am J Physiol Regul Integr Comp Physiol*. 2006;291(2):R245-R256.

50. Chiras DD. *Human Biology*. 9th ed. Burlington, MA: Jones & Bartlett Learning; 2019.

51. Harbison HS. Male sexual and reproductive health. In: Schuiling KD, Likis FE, eds. *Gynecologic Health Care*. 4th ed. Burlington, MA: Jones & Bartlett Learning; 2022:133-147.

52. Abdolmanafi A, Nobre P, Winter S, et al. Culture and sexuality: cognitive–emotional determinants of sexual dissatisfaction among Iranian and New Zealand women. *J Sex Med*. 2018;15(5):687-697.

53. Masters WH, Johnson VE. *Human Sexual Response*. New York, NY: Bantam; 1966.

54. Basson R. Human sexual response. *Handbook Clin Neurol*. 2015;130:11-18.

55. Bachmann G, Stern L, Ramos J. Female sexual function. *Glob Libr Womens Med*. https://www.glowm.com/section-view/heading/female-sexual-. Accessed August 9, 2022.

56. Mazloomdoost D, Pauls RN. A comprehensive review of the clitoris and its role in female sexual function. *Sex Med Rev*. 2015;3(4):245-263.

57. Puppo V, Puppo G. Anatomy of sex: revision of the new anatomical terms used for the clitoris and the female orgasm by sexologists. *Clin Anat*. 2015; 28(3):293-304.

58. Clayton AH, Harsh V. Sexual function across aging. *Curr Psychiatry Rep*. 2016;18(3):28.

C H A P T E R

# 9

# Sexuality

MELODY J. CASTILLO AND ALICE R. SATTLER

## Introduction

Sexuality is defined by the World Health Organization (WHO) as "a central aspect of being human throughout life that encompasses sex, gender identities and roles, sexual orientation, eroticism, pleasure, intimacy and reproduction."[1,2] Most simply, sexual health is the ability to embrace and enjoy sexuality throughout the lifespan[3] and is widely recognized as an inextricable component of overall health.[4] Sexual health is a state of well-being in relation to sexuality, not just the absence of disease, dysfunction, or infirmity. Sexual health requires a positive and respectful approach to sexuality and sexual relationships, as well as the possibility of having pleasurable and safe sexual experiences, free of coercion, discrimination, and violence.[1] The American Sexual Health Association (ASHA) adds that the experiences of sexually transmitted infections (STIs) or unplanned pregnancy do not prevent individuals from experiencing or attaining sexual health.[3]

Sexual health is dependent on the recognition and respect for sexual rights,[1] widely recognized as inherent human rights[2,5] and defined by a variety of professional, nongovernmental, and governmental organizations.[6] The Sexual Rights Initiative defines sexual rights as including the individual right to freely decide and control matters of sexuality, to be free from violence or coercion, to be able to access sexual and reproductive healthcare information and services, and to be free of discrimination based on sexual identification or practices.[6]

The midwifery model of care, informed by a philosophy of respect for human dignity, individuality, and diversity that honors normal life experiences, is well suited to support healthy experiences and expressions of sexuality beyond reproduction.[7] Additionally, assessing safety in interpersonal relationships and sexual function, as well as providing counseling and care that support healthy sexual behaviors throughout the lifespan, are core components of midwifery identified by the American College of Nurse-Midwives (ACNM).[8]

Midwives provide care to a diverse populace, including women (both cis and transgender), individuals of all genders with female-assigned reproductive and sexual systems (FARSS), and individuals with a range of anatomic presentations, gender identities, sexual orientations, partners, and practices. Midwifery care encompasses some of the most personal and stigmatized components of life as well as pivotal transitions, such as pregnancy and menopause. Developing an understanding of sexual function and dysfunction in individuals of all sexes and genders, and knowing how to best approach sexuality and sexual function from existing frameworks are essential to the provision of inclusive sexual midwifery care. This chapter provides a framework for approaching sexuality, sexual health, and alterations in sexual function in all sexes and genders across the lifespan.

## Sexual Response Models

Sexual function is characterized in models that conceptualize human sexual response as the compilation of psychological and physiologic occurrences that define a sexual event. Influenced by physiologic, psychological, interpersonal, social, and cultural factors, sexual response is variable both within and between individuals.[9] As a result, defining what constitutes a typical sexual response remains a challenge. Since the first sexual response model was proposed by Masters and Johnson in 1966,[10] numerous models have been introduced to better characterize the complexity of factors involved. No single model

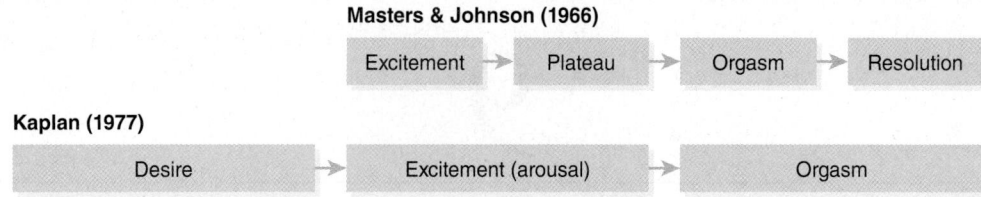

**Figure 9-1** Linear models of sexual response.

has emerged as universally representative. Understanding the strengths and limitations of the various models of sexual response facilitates the development of a clinical framework to describe sexual function, identify alterations, and develop a clinical approach to the assessment and management of sexual concerns.

## Limitations

Sexual response models are limited by their origins in cisnormative and heteronormative paradigms based on phallo-centric and coitus-centric bias, where sex is defined as insertive penovaginal sexual activity.[11] Evolution of the understanding of sex, gender, and sexuality is ongoing, and contemporary research methods are changing to better represent the diversity of lived experiences. Nevertheless, disparities in representation in the evolution of sexual response models must be considered in the greater discussion of sexuality. Early investigations of sexual response in animal studies centered on male ejaculation as an endpoint of sexual motivation and rarely discussed sexual motivation or function in populations with FARSS.[12] Later models sought to better characterize and incorporate sexual responses in women. While pivotal in addressing sexual health disparities in cisgender women, those models implicitly affirmed sexual dichotomy, gender binary, and cisnormativity at the risk of excluding intersex and gender-expansive individuals.[13,14] The extent to which experiences of intersex or transgender individuals are reflected in these models is still largely unknown.[15] Additionally, models generally reflect the experiences of heterosexual and coupled individuals, overlooking experiences of individuals in LGBTQIA+ populations, in solo and multipartnered sexual experiences, and outside the context of a coupled relationship structure.[11,16]

No model explicitly incorporates consent into the characterization of sexual response. Affirmative consent (e.g., free, explicit, and verbal consent, not simply the absence of "no") is recognized as an essential component of healthy sexual activity.[17] Although some models discuss a willingness or openness to sexual stimuli and activity, openness is not equivalent to consent or sexual agency, and the latter components' omission cannot be overlooked. Additionally, sexual response can occur outside the context of consensual sexual stimulation as a function of autonomic response and does not imply a desire for, openness to, or consent to sexual activity.

## Linear Models

Early models of sexual response as a linear process continue to impact current research and understanding (Figure 9-1). Masters and Johnson's first formal model characterized sexual response as a buildup of tension culminating in orgasmic release.[10] Based on clinical observations of roughly 700 individuals, identified as women and men, this model centered on physiologic processes, primarily the genitals, and conceptualized sexual response in a linear model of four successive phases: excitement, plateau, orgasm, and resolution.[10] Recognizing the role of psychological components in sexual response, Kaplan later introduced a triphasic model that included three phases: desire, excitement, and orgasm; this model incorporated desire as an explicit precursor to the essentially unchanged components of the Masters and Johnson model.[13]

Early linear models portrayed desire as exclusively spontaneous and precursory in the initiation of sexual response. However, they failed to characterize the complexity of psychological and physiologic components of sexual response, depict nonlinear trajectories through components of sexual response, and accommodate individual variations in motivations and responses. Although characterizations of sexual response continue to evolve, the dual control model[18] and the composite circular incentives model[14] have been pivotal in shaping contemporary understandings of sexual function, dysfunction, and approaches to their clinical management.

## Nonlinear Models

The dual control model (DCM) differentiates between psychological and physiologic sexual excitement, or arousal,[18,19] and creates a framework

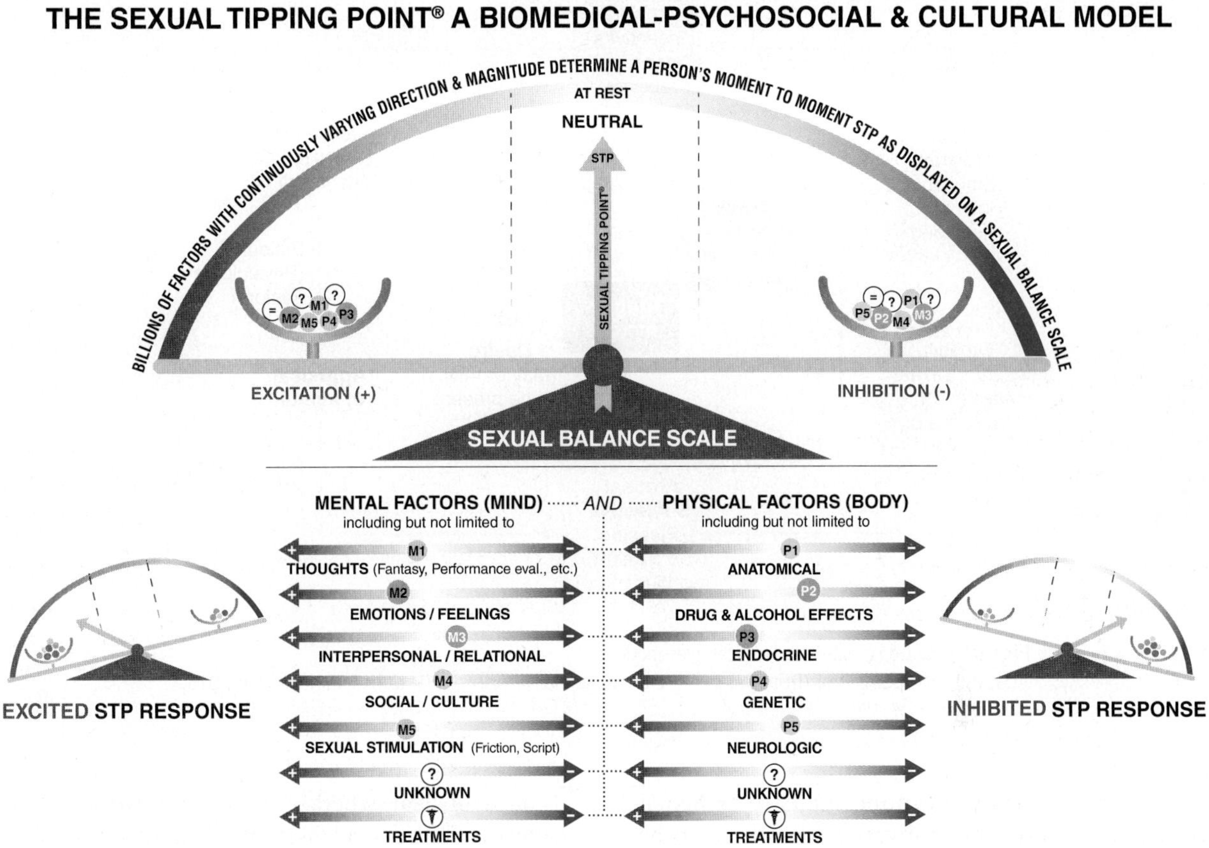

## THE SEXUAL TIPPING POINT® A BIOMEDICAL-PSYCHOSOCIAL & CULTURAL MODEL

**Figure 9-2** Sexual Tipping Point Model.
Adapted with permission from Michael A. Perelman, Ph.D, based on the Sexual Tipping Point Model, owned by and used with the permission of the MAP Education & Research Foundation (mapedfund.org).

that better accounts for understanding individual variations in sexual response[20,21] and approaches to sexual dysfunction management. Unlike previous models that centered on genitalia, this model focuses on the role of cognitive processing in sexual response, which varies among individuals and is influenced by numerous biopsychosocial factors. Sexual response, mediated by the context of a sexual encounter, is dependent on the co-occurring appraisal of both sexually exciting or arousing stimuli and sexually inhibiting stimuli. The DCM proposes that a functional sexual response requires both the presence of sexual stimuli and the absence of a stimulus blockade. In other words, sexual response is dependent on the presence of sexual stimuli potent enough to overcome a threshold of hindering factors, which vary from person to person and from encounter to encounter.[22] The DCM evolved into the Sexual Tipping Point Model, which explains that the variety of psychosocial and physical factors that can excite and inhibit the sexual response are variable control rather than on-off switches

(Figure 9-2).[23] Popularizations of this model have contextualized sexual stimuli as stepping on the "gas" and stimulus blockades as stepping on the "brakes" of sexual response.[24]

Basson's composite circular incentives model (CCIM) of sexual response incorporates relevant components from earlier models into a more comprehensive, integrated framework and is currently regarded as the preeminent, evidence-based model of sexual response.[25] The CCIM accounts for desire as either spontaneous or a response to stimuli, sexual or nonsexual; variation in the trajectory of phases of sexual response; and experiences of overlapping phases of sexual response (Figure 9-3).[25]

In the CCIM, sexual response may be initiated by spontaneous sexual desire or activated from a state of neutrality by a willingness to respond to arousing stimuli.[26,27] Sexual desire is characterized as either spontaneous (i.e., the intrinsic urge for sexual satisfaction) or responsive (i.e., a reaction to antecedent or co-occurring cognitive or physical arousal), and is not an essential component of sexual response.

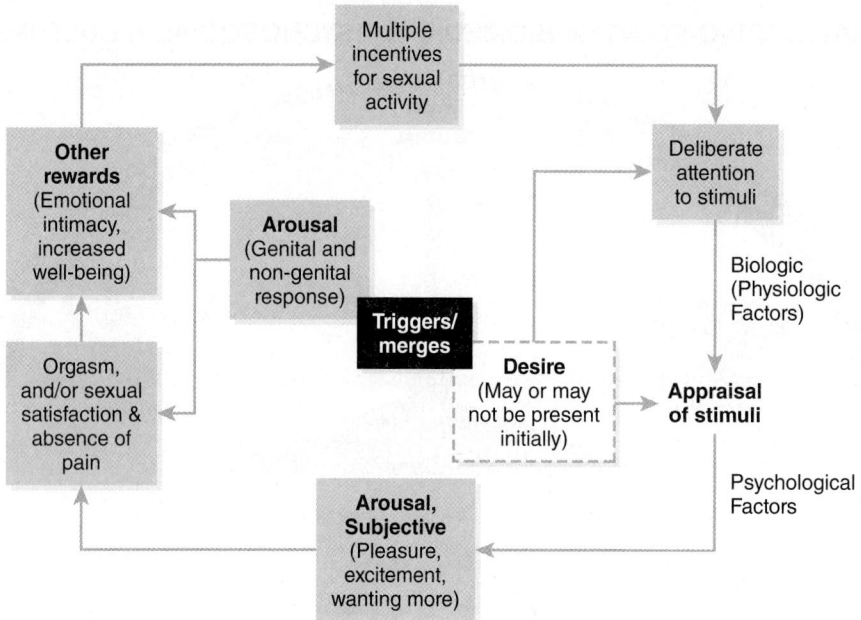

**Figure 9-3** Composite circular incentives model.
Adapted with permission from Basson R. Human sexual response. *Handbook Clin Neurol.* 2015; 130:11-18.

When an incentivizing opportunity to be sexual presents, whatever the motivation, a choice can be made to seek or respond to stimulation to kindle sexual arousal and desire. Motivation for sexual activity may stem from emotional or interpersonal incentives that enhance intimacy, rather than a desire for sexual stimulation or orgasm. Factors such as a desire for intimacy, to feel wanted, or to feel loved may, by themselves, provide sufficient motivation for initiating sexual response.[26] Arousal, referred to as excitement in linear models, is conceptualized as having distinct psychological (subjective) and physiologic components (characterized as genital vasocongestion), which may or may not be congruent and which are dependent on the context of the sexual event as well as physical sexual stimulation.[26] With access to arousal and desire, sensitivity to stimuli increases, reinforcing the motivation for sexual response. Movement through the phases of sexual response involves overlapping and merging of the phases. Each phase is reinforced by the previous phase and supports the subsequent phase. Additionally, progression through the phases of sexual response may occur via a variety of pathways, modulated by the context of the sexual experience. Examples of biopsychosocial contextual factors are presented in Table 9-1.[28] Satisfaction with the sexual experience, with or without orgasm, provides motivation for future sexual encounters.

It is unclear whether desire and arousal, particularly subjective arousal, are distinct psychological constructs.[29] Some research has demonstrated that individuals, especially with FARSS, can have difficulty distinguishing their experiences of desire versus arousal,[30–34] while other research supports desire and arousal as distinct constructs.[35,36] Genital arousal may occur in the absence of desire in unwanted sexual contact and assault as a result of autonomic nervous system function.[37,38] The CCIM accommodates experiences of desire and arousal as both distinct and overlapping experiences, as illustrated in Figure 9-3.

The peak of the sexual event or sexual climax is not inherently linked to orgasm in the CCIM. Satisfaction may be tied to the initial motivations for sexual activity, such as communication, affection, intimacy, or pleasure, with or without orgasm.[26]

The composite model does not reject early linear models. Instead, it centers the emotional and interpersonal aspects of motivation in partnered sexual activity and accommodates experiences of innate sexual desire, self-stimulation, and sexual responses that follow a linear trajectory. From a practical standpoint, linear models may be more helpful in orienting individuals and clinicians to the physical components of sexual response, while the composite model may better support the conceptualization of the complexity and interaction of the

| Table 9-1 | Biopsychosocial Factors That Contribute to Sexual Dysfunction | | |
|-----------|-----------|-----------|-----------|
| **Biologic** | **Psychological** | **Social/Cultural** |
| Aging | Boredom | Believing sex to be shameful |
| Cardiovascular/pulmonary disease | Distraction | Cultural beliefs about sexuality and gender roles |
| Endocrinopathies: | Negative body image | Duration of relationship(s) |
|   Diabetes | Poor self-worth | Dissatisfaction with relationship(s) |
|   Hypothyroidism | Pressure to "perform" | Family teachings |
|   Hyperprolactinemia/prolactinoma | Psychiatric disorders: | Interpersonal difficulty |
| Genitourinary conditions: |   Anxeity | Lack of knowledge/experience |
|   Urinary incontinence |   ADD/ADHD | Life stressors |
| Gynecologic disorders: |   Depression | Poor communication skills |
|   Endometriosis |   PTSD | Poverty, unemployment, financial stress |
|   Fibroids | Self-observation during sexual activity | Working conditions |
|   Pelvic floor dysfunction | Sexual dysfunction in partner(s) | |
|   Pelvic organ prolapse | Sexual trauma or abuse | |
|   Vulvar dermatoses | | |
|   Vulvovaginaldynia | | |
| Neurologic/neuromuscular conditions: | | |
|   Epilepsy | | |
|   CNS lesions | | |
|   Multiple sclerosis | | |
|   Nerve injury, especially pudendal or hypogastric | | |
|   Spinal cord injury | | |
|   Parkinson's disease | | |
| Malignancy/treatment: | | |
|   Mastectomy | | |
|   Gynecologic/colorectal surgery | | |
|   Pelvic radiation | | |
| Medications | | |
| Pain, chronic | | |
| Poor health | | |
| Sleep dysfunction | | |
| Vascular disorders: | | |
|   Atherosclerosis | | |
|   Endothelial dysfunction | | |

Abbreviations: ADD, attention-deficit disorder; ADHD, attention-deficit/hyperactivity disorder; CNS, central nervous system; PTSD, post-traumatic stress disorder.

biopsychosocial aspects of sexual response.[28] Similarly, the DCM and Sexual Tipping Point Model are helpful to conceptualize facilitators and barriers to sexual response, making them very useful for assessing sexual dysfunction and guiding management strategies. The integration of these models provides a practical framework for approaching sexual response and alterations in sexual function for individuals of all genders, in all stages of life. As efforts to validate established sexual response models and develop more inclusive models continue, midwives can support the experiences and concerns of individuals accessing care by integrating current characterizations of sexual response with an understanding of their limitations and an awareness of the wide individual variations in patterns of response.

## Anatomy and Physiology of Sexual Response

Sexual response is a neurobiologic process regulated by the central and peripheral nervous systems, particularly the autonomic nervous system, and involving all major body systems. The reproductive and sexual tract includes the internal and external genitalia, as well as blood vessels, nerves, pelvic muscles, and support structures. Extragenital peripheral anatomic structures involved in sexual response include cutaneous blood vessels, salivary and sweat glands, the nipples, and the anus.[39] Sensitivity to sexual stimulation is not limited to these structures, and anatomy relevant to sexual response varies within and between individuals.

The phenotypic presentation of the natal reproductive and sexual tract is primarily influenced by biologic sex, and this presentation varies both within the constructs of female-assigned and male-assigned natal genitalia and across the spectrum of sexual presentations. Individual variations in genital appearance are influenced by genetics, epigenetics, hormonal exposure (endogenous and exogenous), and surgical intervention. Because natal reproductive and sexual tracts assigned-female and assigned-male generally arise from the same embryologic tissues, anatomic function and physiology are generally shared, particularly in the genitals. Prominent homologous genital structures include the clitoris and glans penis, the labia minora and shaft of the penis, and the labia majora and scrotum (see Figure 8-7A).

To facilitate an inclusive approach to understanding sexual response, this section approaches the anatomy and physiology of sexual response by emphasizing how sexually differentiated systems work similarly. The anatomy and physiology of the reproductive system are covered more generally in the *Anatomy and Physiology of the Reproductive System* chapter. Note that there are many variations of external phenotypes of reproductive anatomy, and anatomy references may use varied terminology to describe similar structures.

### Natal Female-Assigned Reproductive and Sexual Tract

#### Vulva

The external genitalia include the clitoris, labia majora, and labia minora and comprise a combination of keratinized hair-bearing skin and mucosal surfaces.

The pudendal nerve, including both deep and superficial branches, provides somatic innervation.

#### Clitoris

The tissue structure of the clitoris is formed externally by a glans covered by a prepuce and internally by two crura of erectile corpora cavernosa that run laterally to the vaginal canal, as well as two bulbs of erectile corpus spongiosum (vestibular/vaginal/clitoral bulbs) that run medially between the crura (see Figure 8-7A). The corpora cavernosa and corpus spongiosum become vasocongested during sexual response. The clitoris is somatically innervated via the pudendal nerve and autonomically innervated via the cavernous nerve. The clitoris is a key site for sexual stimulation and pleasure.

#### Vagina

The vagina is a canal formed by autonomically innervated smooth muscle lined with mucosa that connects the uterus to the external genitalia. It is lubricated by secretions from the mucous membranes and vaginal glands, which increase during genital arousal and orgasm as part of the sexual response. The mucosal epithelia are influenced by hormones, particularly estrogen. Somatic sensation is primarily a function of the lower one-third of the vagina, which is innervated by the pudendal nerve. The upper two-thirds of the vaginal canal is primarily innervated by the uterovaginal plexus. The concept of a universal "G-spot" in the anterior vaginal canal continues to be debated in research.[40] However, clitoral structures along the anterior vaginal wall can be a source of pleasure when stimulated. Periurethral glands, colloquially referred to as "the female prostate," can excrete fluid into the urethra at the time of orgasm in some individuals. The definition and composition of female ejaculation are debated, but this phenomenon is colloquially referred to as "female ejaculation."[41]

#### Cervix

Although the cervix is typically considered an insensitive structure, stimulation of the cervix and associated uterine movement can be a source of pleasure in some individuals and a trigger for pain in others. The cervix is innervated by the hypogastric nerve. Sensitivity to sexual stimulation in this area is colloquially referred to as the "A-spot."

#### Pelvic Muscles

Skeletal muscles surround the vagina, provide support to the pelvic organs, and contract during sexual arousal and orgasm. Examples include the bulbo-spongious, ischiocavernosus, and levator ani muscles.

### Anus

The anus is a potential site of sexual stimulation. It is innervated by the pudendal nerve.[42]

### Natal Male-Assigned Reproductive and Sexual Tract

#### Penis

The penis is an erectile structure, homologous to the clitoris, that is formed by two cylinders of corpora cavernosa and a single cylinder of corpus spongiosum. It consists of the glans penis, covered by a prepuce, and a shaft. The penis is a key site for sexual stimulation and pleasure, as well as the output tract for urine and ejaculate. The penis is innervated autonomically by both parasympathetic and sympathetic pathways via the cavernous nerve and somatically by the pudendal nerve.

#### Testes and Scrotum

The scrotum is the hair-bearing keratinized skin covering the gonads (testes). The scrotum is homologous to the labia majora and can be a source of sexual pleasure. The cremaster muscle lines the scrotum and contracts during arousal and orgasm.

#### Prostate

The prostate gland is involved in secretion of seminal fluid and may also be a site of sexual stimulation.[43] Colloquially it may be referred to as the "P-spot" when stimulated as part of sexual activity.

### Gender-Affirming Surgically Reconstructed Sexual Systems

#### Neovagina or Neophallus

The anatomy and architecture of the neovagina and neophallus vary depending on the surgical approach used to create these structures, but are typically composed of reconstructed natal tissue of varying origin with the goal of preserving sensation and sexual function. The neophallus may not contain erectile tissue. If desired, erection can often be accomplished with surgical implantation of a prosthesis. More information on anatomic variation is included in the *Gender-Affirming Care* chapter.

### Physiology of Sexual Response

#### Desire

Physiologically, sexual desire is conceptualized as a neurobiologic process that reflects a balance between inhibitory and excitatory processes.[18] Many mediating components, including neurotransmitters, hormones, and psychological factors, have both excitatory and inhibitory effects. Excitatory neurotransmitters include dopamine, norepinephrine, and melanocortins. Inhibitory neurotransmitters include serotonin, endocannabinoids, and opioids. Sex hormones typically have an excitatory impact on desire. Acting on neurotransmitters, they amplify sensitivity and response to sexual stimuli.[44,45] Psychosocial factors that affect excitatory or inhibitory mechanisms include mood, relationship satisfaction, cultural narratives on gender roles, and level of sexual education.

#### Arousal

Arousal is characterized by sexual response models as both psychological and physiologic. Physiologically, it is defined as a state resulting from sexual contact or erotic stimulation (e.g., dreams, fantasies, objects, or sensations) that stimulates the central nervous system (CNS) to the sacral spinal cord.[46] Vascular engorgement and vasodilation of genital erectile tissues occur with physiologic arousal, particularly in the corpora cavernosa and the corpus spongiosum, resulting in increased temperature and sensitivity to touch. In individuals with FARSS, increased blood flow is associated with clitoral erection, congestion in the vaginal walls, increased length and plasticity of the vaginal canal, and onset of lubrication. In individuals with male-assigned reproductive and sexual systems (MARSS), increased blood flow is associated with penile erection, testicular congestion, and production of prostatic secretions. Outside the genitals, vascular dilation is associated with increased sensitivity of the skin, flushing of the face, and nipple erection.

Other physical changes include increased tension in the pelvic floor muscles, the smooth muscles of the pelvis, and the peripheral skeletal muscles, especially in the face and limbs. Arousal is associated with CNS symptoms of increased focus, wakefulness, and concentration. Sympathetic nervous system activation results in increased heart rate, respiratory rate, and blood pressure.

Cognitive sexual arousal or mental sexual arousal is defined as an awareness of or mental engagement in response to sexual stimulation, or to the physical symptoms of arousal.[47–49] Physical and psychological arousal can occur either at the same time or separately in a healthy sexual response.[48,50,51] For example, some individuals will experience an increase in subjective sexual arousal when they become aware of their genital arousal, and some individuals may experience subjective sexual arousal prior to genital arousal, or not be subjectively aware of physical changes of sexual arousal at that time.[48]

### Orgasm

Defining the experience of orgasm is notoriously difficult. Orgasm is generally defined as a distinct cortical state, involving an altered state of consciousness and experience of peak sexual pleasure, accompanied by involuntary contractions of the pelvic musculature. Physiologically, orgasm is the result of a complex interplay of endocrine and neurologic activity, mediated by pelvic, hypogastric, pudendal, sacral, and vagal nerve pathways, and triggered by central (e.g., audiovisual input, mental imagery, or fantasy) and peripheral (e.g., clitoris, vagina, cervix, uterus, penis, prostate, or anus) stimuli. Oxytocin, released at the time of orgasm, is associated with uterine contraction in individuals with an intact FARSS.[52,53] In individuals with an intact MARSS, orgasm is associated with ejaculation. Relaxation of myotonia—that is, voluntary or involuntary muscle contractions—results in resolution of genital and peripheral vasocongestion. In conjunction, the individual typically experiences an overall sense of relief, well-being, and contentment.[52–57]

Although orgasm and ejaculation typically occur concurrently in individuals with MARSS, they are distinct physiologic processes.[58] Nevertheless, the terms *orgasm* and *ejaculation* are often used interchangeably, colloquially and in research. Where data are unavailable, this chapter uses *ejaculation* as a surrogate for *orgasm*.

The experience of orgasm is highly variable due to physiologic factors including the hormonal environment, neurologic processes, and the strength of the pelvic floor muscles. Endogenous and exogenous hormones can cause intrapersonal and interpersonal variations in the subjective experience. Variations in the pudendal, hypogastric, sacral, and vagal neuropathways and cortical activation have similar impacts and can explain reported differences in the subjective experience of orgasm depending on the primary site of sexual stimulation (e.g., penile versus prostatic orgasm, clitoral versus vaginal orgasm).[56] Type, intensity, and duration of stimulation preceding orgasm contribute to variations as well. Differences in the ease of triggering orgasm during solitary and partnered sexual activity are common, particularly for women, both cisgender and transgender, and other individuals with FARSS.[57]

While typically considered a positive component of sexual activity, orgasm can be a physiologic reflex to any sexual stimulation, independent of desire, subjective arousal, or consent. Reflexive orgasm

in nonconsensual situations can be profoundly distressing to individuals who experience it, resulting in self-blame, shame, and confusion. It is estimated that approximately 5% of individuals subjected to sexual abuse and assault have experienced orgasm during abuse or assault.[37]

After orgasm, a resolution period occurs in which the physiologic changes related to arousal return to baseline. In individuals with intact natal MARSS, a refractory period also occurs that is associated with a physiologic inability to respond to sexual stimuli. The duration of this period varies from a few minutes to a few days, and tends to increase with age. Individuals with FARSS may or may not experience a refractory period, as multiple and successive orgasms can occur.[59]

## Alterations (Dysfunctions) in Sexual Response

The prevalence of sexual dysfunctions is difficult to characterize due to the variety of definitions and research methods used, and their sociocultural contexts.[60] Additionally, individuals often endorse overlapping sexual concerns, making differentiation of dysfunctions difficult and the determination of their prevalence even more challenging.[61] One of the most comprehensive studies on the prevalence of sexual concerns surveyed 31,581 presumed women in the United States. Overall, 38.7% reported low sexual desire, 26.1% reported low sexual arousal, and 20.5% reported problems with orgasm.[62] Lifetime estimates of sexual pain disturbances also vary widely, ranging from approximately 8% to 30%.[63] Sexual dysfunction (disturbance with distress) is also fairly common, with prevalence of desire, arousal, and orgasm dysfunctions ranging from 5% to 10%.[60,62] Data are limited, but the prevalence of sexual dysfunctions in intersex, gender-nonconforming, and transgender populations appears to be similar.[64]

### Biopsychosocial Risk Factors and Protective Factors for Sexual Dysfunction

Research has demonstrated very few truly universal risk factors and protective factors for sexual dysfunction across all populations. Instead, culturally and socially specific differences in risk and protective factors exist in a global context. Furthermore, apparently modifiable risk factors such as exercise or sex education can be constrained by the sociocultural context.[65]

A disturbance in any phase or component of the sexual response cycle can result in an associated dysfunction. Any condition affecting the excitatory and/or inhibitory processes of sexual response can be a risk factor for sexual dysfunction (Table 9-1). Protective factors that promote sexual function and reduce the risk of sexual dysfunction may be biologic, psychological, or social in nature. Some common, though not universal, protective factors include regular exercise, a higher subjective sense of health and well-being, a positive body image, access to sex education, older age at the time of partnering, daily affection, and intimate communication.[65]

Studies on the sexual functioning of intersex, gender-nonconforming, gender-nonbinary, and transgender individuals are scarce, but the extant research suggests that risk and protective factors are similar to those for cisgender individuals.[66] Limited research suggests that gender-affirming interventions such as hormone therapy or gender-affirming surgery reduce the risk of sexual dysfunction.[64]

## Diagnostic Criteria for Sexual Dysfunction
### General Principles

Diagnostic criteria for sexual dysfunction vary by professional organization, as does the language used to discuss alterations in sexual function. This chapter uses the term *dysfunction* rather than *disorder* to emphasize the role of individually defined function in sexual health and to avoid the stigma associated with the latter term.

Initially characterized as psychiatric in origin, the introduction of sexual dysfunctions as diagnoses is closely tied to the development of the *Diagnostic and Statistical Manual of Mental Disorders* (DSM), published by the American Psychiatric Association.[67–69] Better understanding of the biologic and sociocultural components of sexual response and dysfunction have led to the development of diagnostic systems for sexual dysfunction that incorporate both biologic and psychological factors into the diagnostic criteria.[68] Sexual dysfunctions are defined diagnostically by four major systems: *DSM-IV, DSM-5*, International Consultation in Sexual Medicine (ICSM), and International Society for the Study of Women's Sexual Health (ISSWSH) Nomenclature Committee (Table 9-2).[70,71] Advantages and disadvantages exist for each system, and all are used concurrently. Understanding the similarities across the various diagnostic systems facilitates a simple, but comprehensive approach to diagnosing sexual dysfunctions. Key similarities in diagnostic criteria include duration of symptoms, context of symptoms, associated distress, and an assumption of adequate sexual stimulation.

### Duration of Symptoms.
Diagnosis requires that symptoms affect the majority of an individual's sexual experiences, typically defined as 75% to 100% of experiences, for a duration of 3 (ICSM) to 6 (ISSWSH, *DSM*) months.[63,68] Such criteria are established to avoid pathologizing normal and transient fluctuations in sexual function due to episodic factors such as major life events, relationship changes, or health changes.[72]

### Context of Symptoms.
Diagnoses are based on the contexts of their onset—that is, lifelong (primary) versus acquired (secondary). Differentiating these contexts clarifies the nature of the dysfunction, and helps to identify management strategies.

### Distress.
Understanding distress and how it is described by individuals accessing care facilitates diagnosis and management of sexual dysfunction. In research, frustration is a common term used to express distress,[73] but distress may also be described as guilt, incompetence, loss, sadness, sorrow, or worry.[74] The antithesis of distress is sexual satisfaction. Sexual distress and the diagnosis of sexual dysfunction are characterized in relationship to sexual satisfaction. For example, anorgasmia may be reported, but if it is not associated with distress and there is sexual satisfaction, there is not sexual dysfunction.

Distress alone does not confer dysfunction. For example, an individual who can easily experience orgasm with self-stimulation but has difficulty experiencing orgasm during partnered sexual activity may experience distress, but does not have a dysfunction.[75] Distress is essential to making a sexual dysfunction diagnosis, but dysfunction is not required to intervene.

### Adequate Sexual Stimulation.
The diagnosis of any sexual dysfunction can be made only in the context of adequate sexual stimulation. However, there is no universal definition for what constitutes adequate stimulation. Many forms of sexual stimulation are possible, and response to sexual stimulation varies within and between individuals. Distinguishing between adequate and inadequate sexual stimulation relies heavily on clinical judgment and requires a thorough clinical history.

Sociocultural messages about adequate sexual stimulation can affect sexual practices and shape expectations about anticipated sexual responses. Particularly for individuals with FARSS, a commonly held misconception is that the individual should be able to experience orgasm from insertive penile and receptive vaginal sexual activity alone. However, research suggests that sexual stimulation from insertive penile and receptive vaginal sexual activity

| Table 9-2 | **Major Classification Systems of Sexual Dysfunctions** | | | |
|---|---|---|---|---|
| | **Fourth International Consultation in Sexual Medicine (ICSM)[70]** | **ISSWSH Nomenclature Committee[33,63,68]** | **DSM-IV (*Diagnostic and Statistical Manual of Mental Disorders*, fourth edition)[71]** | **DSM-5 (*Diagnostic and Statistical Manual of Mental Disorders*, fifth edition, text revision)[67]** |
| **Year of Publication** | 2015 | 2019 | 1994 | 2022 |
| **Publishing Organization** | International Society for Sexual Medicine (ISSM)<br><br>Founded in 1978 to study male erectile dysfunction; scope later expanded to all human sexuality. | International Society for the Study of Women's Sexual Health (ISSWSH)<br><br>Founded as a nonprofit multidisciplinary academic and scientific organization that supports the standards of ethics and professionalism in the research, education, and clinical practice of women's sexual health.[63] | American Psychiatric Association (APA)<br><br>Founded in 1892; largest psychology professional organization in the United States.<br><br>*DSM* is revised using expert working groups of researchers and clinicians. | |
| **Key Similarities and Differences** | Diagnoses are differentiated by male and female categories, but criteria are parallel.<br><br>Applicable to biopsychosocial contexts. | Diagnostic criteria are specifically for women.<br><br>Applicable to biopsychosocial contexts. | Diagnostic criteria are nonspecific to sex; where differentiated by sex, diagnoses are parallel.<br><br>Lack of duration criteria for diagnoses.<br><br>Applicable to psychiatric contexts only. | Diagnoses are differentiated by male and female categories, but criteria are parallel.<br><br>Applicable to psychiatric contexts only.<br><br>Controversially merged desire/arousal dysfunctions and merged pain dysfunctions under a single diagnosis. |

alone is insufficient for triggering the experience of orgasm in at least half, if not a majority, of individuals with FARSS. Additional stimulation during partnered sexual activity is often needed to experience orgasm. In cases of inadequate sexual stimulation, desire, arousal, or orgasm-related distress may present, but dysfunction cannot be diagnosed.[54,76,77]

### Diagnostic Criteria

Sexual dysfunctions are organized into four main categories: desire, arousal, orgasm, and pain dysfunctions. The diagnostic criteria presented in Tables 9-3, 9-4, and 9-5 integrate the various diagnostic systems to facilitate a simplified diagnostic approach to desire-, arousal-, and orgasm-related

dysfunctions in clinical contexts. Pain dysfunctions are discussed separately.

***Sexual Desire Dysfunction.*** Sexual desire dysfunction is the most common sexual dysfunction reported in population-based surveys across genders and sexualities.[60] Approximately 8% to 20% of respondents endorse low sexual desire with distress.[62,64,66,78] The etiology of desire dysfunction is attributed to an imbalance of excitatory and inhibitory processes centrally and peripherally.[62] This is supported by neuroimaging studies, which demonstrate excessive neurobiologic inhibitory mechanisms and inadequate excitatory and disinhibiting mechanisms in individuals with desire dysfunctions.[44] The primary

| Table 9-3 | Sexual Desire Dysfunction |
|-----------|---------------------------|
| **Diagnosis** | **Definition/Criteria** |
| Hypoactive sexual desire dysfunction (ICSM)[70] | Persistent or recurrent deficiency or absence of sexual or erotic thoughts or fantasies and desire for sexual activity. Symptoms are:<br>1. Present for least 3 months<br>2. Occur in 75% to 100% of sexual experiences<br>3. Associated with distress. |

Abbreviation: ICSM, International Consultation on Sexual Medicine.

Based on McCabe MP, Sharlip ID, Atalla E, et al. Definitions of sexual dysfunctions in women and men: a consensus statement from the Fourth International Consultation on Sexual Medicine 2015. *J Sex Med.* 2016;13(2):135-143.

diagnosis associated with desire dysfunction is hypoactive sexual desire dysfunction (Table 9-3).

Biologic risk factors for desire dysfunctions include endocrine disruptions such as hyperprolactinemia (suppresses dopamine, inhibits excitatory response) and hypogonadism (e.g., natural or surgical menopause),[79] as well as iatrogenic factors such as administration of selective serotonin reuptake inhibitors (SSRIs; increase serotonin, inhibit sexual response) and antipsychotics (suppress dopamine, inhibit excitatory response).[62] Psychological risk factors include an impaired body image or sense of self-worth, a decreased feeling of connection to the partner(s), a history of unwanted sexual experience(s), caregiving relationship with a partner(s),[11] over-familiarity associated with long-term relationship status, boredom, situational stress, and distraction.[80] Social risk factors include internalization of sex-negative cultural attitudes and beliefs about sexuality and gender roles, homophobia or transphobia, and family teachings, as well as inadequate sexual education.[65]

### Sexual Arousal Dysfunction.

Sexual arousal dysfunctions include hypoactive and hyperactive sexual arousal responses. Due to differences in the function of natal female-assigned and male-assigned genitals during sexual activities, differentiating dysfunction by female and male categories can be clinically useful to clarify involved natal anatomy and physiology, but does not describe the gender of affected individuals. Hypoactive sexual arousal dysfunctions include female hypoactive cognitive arousal disorder, female hypoactive genital arousal disorder, and [penile] erectile dysfunction (ED). Hyperactive sexual arousal dysfunction is defined by the diagnosis of persistent genital arousal disorder or genital dysesthesia disorder (PGAD). The nomenclature and definitions of arousal dysfunctions are the most controversial, due to ongoing debate regarding the differentiation of physiologic versus subjective arousal. Diagnostic criteria are presented in Table 9-4.

The prevalence of arousal disorders varies by diagnosis. The incidence of female hypoactive arousal dysfunctions is reportedly as low as 10% and as high as 49% depending on the population in question.[60,64,81] The prevalence of erectile dysfunction increases with age, affecting approximately 1% to 10% of individuals with MARSS 21 years of age and 50% to 100% of those 70 years of age and older.[60] Although PGAD can affect any individual, current research is almost exclusively limited to cisgender women; in this population, reported prevalence ranges from 0.6% to 3%.[82,83]

Biologically, any disruption in the excitatory and inhibitory mechanisms of the neurovascular and endocrine systems can result in genital sexual arousal dysfunction. As a result, the biopsychosocial risk factors for arousal disorders closely mirror those for desire dysfunctions, explaining why desire and arousal disorders often coexist. PGAD, specifically, is associated with abnormal pudendal nerve innervation. The exact etiology is not known, but the onset of symptoms has been associated with the discontinuation of SSRIs.[82,83]

### Orgasm Dysfunction.

As many as 8% to 29% of individuals in the general population experience orgasm dysfunction.[56,64] Orgasm dysfunctions are characterized by alterations in the frequency, intensity, and timing of orgasm, as well as by a diminished experience or absence of pleasure.[63,68] Despite the ISSWSH orgasm dysfunction diagnostic criteria arising from a gendered diagnostic taxonomy, these criteria are inclusive of orgasm dysfunctions across all genders and sexes and are presented in Table 9-5. The etiology is attributed to dysfunction in the afferent pathways of the pudendal, hypogastric, sacral, and vagal nerves; excessive neurobiologic inhibitory mechanisms; and hyposensitivity and/or inattention to sexual cues and stimuli.[84,86] Acquired orgasm dysfunctions are often iatrogenic in nature (e.g., SSRI use or prostatectomy).[55]

Psychosocial factors associated with orgasm dysfunction include the belief that orgasm is the goal of sexual activity, and can be affected by social and cultural narratives regarding who "gets" to experience orgasm—in particular, who "gives" and "receives" orgasm. Other factors include inadequate or inaccurate sexual education, performance anxiety, poor body image, excessive self-observation, life stressors, and interpersonal conflict.[86]

| Table 9-4 | Sexual Arousal Dysfunction | | |
|---|---|---|---|
| **Diagnosis** | **Definition** | **Criteria** | **Comments** |
| | **Hypoactive Sexual Arousal Dysfunctions** | | |
| Female cognitive arousal dysfunction | Difficulty or inability to attain or maintain adequate mental excitement associated with sexual activity as manifested by problems with feeling turned on, engaged, and/or mentally sexually aroused. | Symptoms are:<br>1. Present for least 6 months<br>2. Associated with distress | |
| Female genital arousal dysfunction | The distressing difficulty or inability to attain or maintain adequate genital response, including (1) vulvovaginal lubrication, (2) engorgement of the genitalia, and (3) sensitivity of the genitalia associated with sexual activity. Symptoms are related to (1) vascular injury or dysfunction and (2) neurologic injury or dysfunction. | | Exclude vaginitis, vulvovaginal atrophy, vestibulodynia, and/or clitorodynia. |
| [Penile] erectile dysfunction (ED) | Consistent or recurrent inability to attain and/or maintain penile erection sufficient for sexual satisfaction[70] | Symptoms are:<br>1. Present for least 3 months<br>2. Occur in 75% to 100% of sexual experiences<br>3. Associated with distress<br>4. Distinguished as lifelong or acquired (primary or secondary) | Most common sexual dysfunction in individuals with natal MARSS |
| | **Hyperactive Sexual Arousal Dysfunction** | | |
| Persistent genital arousal disorder/genital dysesthesia (PGAD) | Persistent or recurrent, unwanted or intrusive, distressing sensations of genital arousal. Symptoms are most commonly experienced in the clitoris, but can also occur in other genito-pelvic regions (e.g., mons pubis, vulva, vestibule, vagina, urethra, perineal region, bladder, and/or rectum); may include a sensation of being on the verge of orgasm, experiencing uncontrollable orgasms, and/or having an excessive number of orgasms; may include other types of genito-pelvic dysesthesia (e.g., buzzing, tingling, burning, twitching, itch, pain). | Symptoms are not associated with concomitant sexual interest, thoughts, or fantasies AND may be associated with:<br>1. Limited resolution, no resolution, or aggravation of symptoms by sexual activity with or without aversive or compromised orgasm<br>2. Aggravation of genital symptoms by certain circumstances<br>3. Despair, emotional lability, catastrophization, or suicidality | In one survey, 46% of individuals with PGAD had approached more than five healthcare providers about their symptoms before being diagnosed.[83]<br><br>Associated with significant impairments to ADLs and quality of life, and increased suicidality. |

Abbreviations: ADLs, activities of daily living; MARSS, male-assigned reproductive and sexual systems.

Based on McCabe MP, Sharlip ID, Atalla E, et al. Definitions of sexual dysfunctions in women and men: a consensus statement from the Fourth International Consultation on Sexual Medicine 2015. *J Sex Med.* 2016;13(2):135-143; Parish SJ, Cottler-Casanova S, Clayton AH, et al. The evolution of the female sexual disorder/dysfunction definitions, nomenclature, and classifications: a review of *DSM*, ICSM, ISSWSH, and ICD. *Sex Med Rev.* 2021;9(1):36–56; and Goldstein I, Komisaruk BR, Pukall CF, et al. International Society for the Study of Women's Sexual Health (ISSWSH) review of epidemiology and pathophysiology, and a consensus nomenclature and process of care for the management of persistent genital arousal disorder/genito-pelvic dysesthesia (PGAD/GPD). *J Sex Med.* 2021;18(4):665-697.

| Table 9-5 | Orgasm Dysfunction |
|---|---|

| **Domain Definition** |
|---|

A persistent or recurrent distressing compromise of orgasm frequency, timing, intensity and/or pleasure associated with sexual activity. Symptoms are:

1. Present for at least 3 months (ICSM) to 6 months (ISSWSH)
2. Occur in 75% to 100% of sexual experiences
3. Associated with distress
4. May be lifelong or acquired

| Context of Dysfunction | | Specific Dysfunctions | | Comments |
|---|---|---|---|---|
| *Frequency* | *Absent* | Anorgasmia | The inability to experience orgasm despite adequate sexual arousal and adequate and prolonged sexual stimulation | The ability to experience orgasm by masturbation, even if unable to during partnered sexual activity, excludes the diagnosis of anorgasmia. |
| | *Decreased* | Diminished frequency of orgasm | Orgasm occurs with decreased frequency despite adequate sexual arousal and adequate and prolonged sexual stimulation | |
| *Timing* Average time from arousal to orgasm (latency) during partnered penovaginal sexual activity: FARSS: 10–15 minutes[54,85] MARSS: 5–7 minutes[85] | *Too Soon* | Premature orgasm | Orgasm occurs earlier than desired by the individual | Associated with negative personal consequences, such as distress, bother, frustration, and/or the avoidance of sexual intimacy. |
| | | Premature ejaculation (MARSS) | Ejaculation that always or nearly always occurs before or within approximately 1 minute of penetrative sexual activity from the first sexual experience (lifelong) or a clinically significant and bothersome decrease in latency time, to approximately 3 minutes or less (acquired premature ejaculation) (ICSM)[70] | |
| | *Late* | Delayed orgasm | Orgasm occurs later than desired by the individual. | Ejaculation occurring by nonpartnered sexual activity, including masturbation, does NOT exclude diagnosis. Associated with voluntary cessation of partnered sexual activity to avoid frustration, physical exhaustion, or genital irritation of self and/or partner(s). |
| | | Delayed ejaculation (MARSS) | Inability to ejaculate in all or almost all occasions of partnered sexual activity, which causes distress (ICSM)[70] | |
| *Intensity* | *Diminished* | Muted orgasm | Orgasm occurs with decreased intensity | |

*(continues)*

| Table 9-5 | Orgasm Dysfunction (*continued*) | | |
|---|---|---|---|
| | | **Domain Definition** | |
| Pleasure | Absent — Anhedonic orgasm | Absent sexual pleasure with orgasm | |
| | Decreased — Hypohedonic orgasm | Orgasm occurs with decreased pleasure | |

Dysorgasmia (painful orgasm) is discussed in the "Sexual Pain Dysfunction" section.

Abbreviations: FARSS, female-assigned reproductive and sexual systems; ISSM, International Society for Sexual Medicine; ISSWSH, International Society for the Study of Women's Sexual Health; MARSS, male-assigned reproductive and sexual systems.

Based on Parish SJ, Goldstein AT, Goldstein SW, et al. Toward a more evidence-based nosology and nomenclature for female sexual dysfunctions: Part II. *J Sex Med.* 2016;13(12):1888-1906; Parish SJ, Cottler-Casanova S, Clayton AH, et al. The evolution of the female sexual disorder/dysfunction definitions, nomenclature, and classifications: a review of *DSM*, ICSM, ISSWSH, and ICD. *Sex Med Rev.* 2021;9(1):36-56; and McCabe MP, Sharlip ID, Atalla E, et al. Definitions of sexual dysfunctions in women and men: a consensus statement from the Fourth International Consultation on Sexual Medicine 2015. *J Sex Med.* 2016;13(2):135-143.

## Sexual Pain Dysfunction

Burning, stinging, rawness, irritation, cutting, tearing, and cramping are examples of how painful sexual activity is described. Pain associated with sexual activity is a common concern. Studies show that most pain experienced with sexual activity is intermittent, occasional, and transient (lasting 5 minutes or less).[87] Pain that is experienced with the majority of sexual experiences, and associated with distress, is identified as dysfunction. The prevalence of painful vaginal or neovaginal sex in cisgender and transgender women ranges from approximately 10% to 30%,[63,88] with most estimates around 25% to 30%. Postcoital pain is less studied. The ENIGI Follow-Up Study found that 16% of transgender women and 7% of transgender men reported pain after intercourse. The prevalence of anodyspareunia (pain with anal penetration) has been reported as occurring in 10% of cisgender men who have sex with men, and in as many as 72% of cisgender women.[89] There is very little research on the prevalence of painful sexual activity for cisgender men who have sex with women. In one study of cisgender men engaging in penetrative sex, 7% reported pain with penovaginal activity and 15% reported pain with insertive penile–anal activity.[89]

Sexual pain dysfunctions can quickly disrupt other domains of sexual function and overall health, inhibiting sexual response. Once sexual activity is associated with pain, the threshold for sexual response shifts and over time, pain becomes an inhibitory mechanism and typically affects other domains of sexual response.

It is important to note that for some individuals who practice *kink* (such as bondage, discipline, dominance, submission, sadism, and masochism [BDSM]), the experience of pain during sexual activity may play a part in heightening the desire, arousal, and orgasm response. The experience of consensual pain that does not cause clinically significant distress does not represent a sexual dysfunction.

### Pain Pathophysiology

The experience of pain is not itself a threat or insult to the body. Instead, it represents the body's adaptation and response. Pain is a cortically mediated subjective experience that occurs when input from sensory nerves is integrated into the peripheral and central nervous system.[90]

Two physiologic types of pain are distinguished: *nociceptive* and *inflammatory*. Nociceptive pain arises from dedicated sensory neurons in the body (*nociceptors*) that detect potential threats to tissue by detecting changes to—among other things—pressure, temperature, and mechanical forces. Inflammatory pain is an adaptive response to inflammation that discourages movement and contact until healing has occurred.[91]

Pathologic pain can arise directly from a disease or injury of the nervous system (neuropathic pain), or it can be dysfunctional pain that occurs without the presence of any noxious stimuli (no nociceptive input) or any (or only minimal) inflammatory processes.[91] An initial insult or inflammation can lead to dysfunctional pain and chronic pain syndromes through processes of *sensitization*.[90,92]

Sensitization is either *peripheral* or *central*, depending on whether the sensory nerves in the periphery of the body are being affected. Peripheral sensitization leads to sensory neuron changes such as a lowered threshold of detecting potentially noxious stimuli. Central sensitization occurs where increased excitability of nerves and altered synaptic connections alter the perception or inhibition of pain in the central nervous system. This sensitization lowers the threshold of detection to ultimately result in *allodynia* (i.e., nonpainful input that becomes perceived as painful) and *hyperalgesia* (i.e., painful input that becomes perceived as more painful). Sensitization is the perception of pain continuing despite the original insult (such as recurrent vaginal candidiasis) resolving, or in the absence of any original outside stimulus.[90]

Another concept central to understanding sexual pain dysfunction, particularly deep dyspareunia, is the system of visceral and somatic nociceptors that are responsible for referred pain. The human body has sensory neurons that act to receive information from the external and internal surroundings; these neurons can broadly be divided into *somatic* (nociceptors primarily in skin, muscle, and bone; sensitive to specific qualities of input such as sharp or dull) and *visceral* (nociceptors in internal organs; sensitive to distension and traction, such as bladder filling).[93] These receptors converge as they reach the spinal cord, and their close proximity can allow signals from visceral and somatic sensory nerves to interact. Visceral pain may affect somatic sensory nerves, and vice versa (or different viscera). This phenomenon, known as "cross-talk," is the origin of referred pain. Low back pain during menses is an example of referred pain, as the visceral pain from uterine nerve activity influences nearby somatic nerves from muscle, skin, and bone of the lower back. Because the vulva is extensively innervated with both visceral and somatic nociceptors, and the pelvis has extensive somatic innervation of the musculoskeletal system as well as the visceral innervation from pelvic organs, "cross-talk" can create complex patterns and presentations of pelvic pain.

### Risk Factors

Biologic risk factors may include any comorbid pain condition or physical condition affecting the neurovascular or tissue integrity of the genitalia.

Conditions that commonly co-occur with sexual pain dysfunction include painful bladder syndrome and fibromyalgia. Psychological risk factors include low self-efficacy (the belief that one can control or affect their experience of pain), dysfunctional thought patterns (e.g., catastrophizing), mood disorders (e.g., anxiety, depression), and post-traumatic stress disorder (PTSD). Social risk factors are affected by varying cultural norms and taboos related to sex and what should or should not be painful. Risk factors include poor communication about sex and having an unsupportive partner, especially one who responds negatively to attempts to communicate about the experience of pain. Other risk factors include internalized homophobia and transphobia.[94]

### Diagnostic Criteria

Historically, the study of sexual pain dysfunctions focused entirely on psychiatric explanations for pain inhibiting penovaginal sex. However, as sexual pain dysfunctions have become better understood, they have been reframed as chronic pain conditions that can affect any aspect of genital sexual function. In the past, sexual pain dysfunctions were typically divided into categories of *dyspareunia* (broad definition for pain associated with intercourse), *vaginismus* (inability to experience vaginal penetration due to spasm of circumvaginal musculature), and *vestibulodynia/vulvodynia* (pain of the vaginal vestibule/vulva). However, vaginal and pelvic muscle spasms are not typically observed in individuals diagnosed with vaginismus.[95] Individuals may experience a defensive musculature contraction in response to superficial pain, making it difficult to distinguish vaginismus from superficial dyspareunia and provoked vestibulodynia. Therefore, new nomenclature to describe sexual pain dysfunctions has been introduced by professional medical and psychological organizations.[67,68,71,96] Both *DSM-5* and ICSM criteria are especially useful for discussing sexual pain dysfunctions.

### *Genital–Pelvic Pain Dysfunction*

Current diagnostic criteria for sexual pain dysfunctions reflect a consolidation of previous definitions into larger, more inclusive diagnoses as standardized by the ICSM and the *DSM-5*. These criteria are presented in Table 9-6.

Although formal diagnostic systems have moved away from the term *dyspareunia*, it remains useful as an inclusive description of "pain experienced during penetrative sexual activities."[90] Some individuals may not meet the formal criteria for GPPPD, yet do

| Table 9-6 | Pain Dysfunction Terminology | | |
|---|---|---|---|
| | **Diagnosis** | **Definition** | **Criteria** |
| **Sexual Activity and Penetration Associated Pain Dysfunctions** | Genito-pelvic pain/ penetration disorder (GPPPD) | Persistent or recurrent difficulties with at least one of the following:<br>• Vaginal penetration during sex<br>• Marked vulvovaginal or pelvic pain during genital contact<br>• Marked fear or anxiety about vulvovaginal or pelvic pain in anticipation of, during, or as a result of genital contact<br>• Marked hypertonicity or over-activity of pelvic floor muscles with or without genital contact | 1. Symptoms must be present for at least 1 month<br>2. Occur in 75% to 100% of sexual experiences<br>3. Lead to distress |
| | Painful orgasm (dysorgasmia) or ejaculation | The occurrence of genital and/or pelvic pain during or shortly after orgasm or ejaculation. | 1. Symptoms must be present for at least 3 months<br>2. Occur in 75% to 100% of sexual experiences<br>3. Lead to distress |

Based on American Psychiatric Association. *Diagnostic and Statistical Manual of Mental Disorders.* 5th ed. Text revision (DSM-5-TR). Arlington, VA: American Psychiatric Association; 2022; McCabe MP, Sharlip ID, Atalla E, et al. Definitions of sexual dysfunctions in women and men: a consensus statement from the Fourth International Consultation on Sexual Medicine 2015. *J Sex Med.* 2016;13(2):135-143; and Parish SJ, Cottler-Casanova S, Clayton AH, et al. The evolution of the female sexual disorder/dysfunction definitions, nomenclature, and classifications: a review of DSM, ICSM, ISSWSH, and ICD. *Sex Med Rev.* 2021;9(1):36-56.

experience dyspareunia. Dyspareunia has many potential etiologies (Table 9-7).[92,97,98] Attention to comorbid conditions and the anatomy and physiology of the human pelvis is useful when attempting to identify the underlying cause.[92,97]

Genital–pelvic pain associated with anal receptive sexual activities and in individuals with MARSS is not represented in formal definitions of sexual dysfunction. However, these phenomena occur, can lead to distress, and similarly can necessitate intervention. Anodyspareunia (pain with anal intercourse) is not well researched. The anal sphincter has a higher resting tone than the circumvaginal musculature, and penetration of the anus requires a greater degree of relaxation for comfortable sexual activity.[94] Lesions of the anus and rectum are also common in the general population (e.g., hemorrhoids) and can potentially cause anodyspareunia.[99]

The prevalence of penodynia (pain of the penis) is uncertain, but appears to be rare. Similarly to the vulva, the penis is innervated by the pudendal nerve, and it shares many of the same anatomic and physiologic considerations.

### Dysorgasmia or Painful Ejaculation

The prevalence of dysorgasmia and painful ejaculation are unclear. In individuals with FARSS, dysorgasmia is likely due to pain associated with contractions of the pelvic musculature and uterus that occur with orgasm. Hypertonic or dysfunctional pelvic floor musculature, as well as venous reflux associated with pelvic congestion syndrome, can also contribute to this condition. Certain conditions, such as reproductive tract atrophy, endometriosis, and pelvic adhesions, appear to be associated with dysorgasmia. Some medications, such as SSRIs and tricyclic antidepressants (TCAs), can potentially include dysorgasmia as a side effect.[100] Intrauterine device (IUD) use has also been associated with dysorgasmia in some individuals, possibly related to the presence of a foreign body in the uterus.

Dysorgasmia in individuals with MARSS is generally studied under the rubric of painful ejaculation, which can be due to urethritis (infectious or noninfectious), prostatitis (infectious or noninfectious), pelvic surgery, adverse effects of some medications, and, most commonly, prostatectomy for treatment of prostate cancer.[55,101]

### Vulvar Pain and Vulvodynia

The International Society for the Study of Women's Sexual Health (ISSWSH), the International Society for the Study of Vulvovaginal Disease (ISSVD), and the International Pelvic Pain Society (IPPS) issue specific consensus diagnostic nomenclature for vulvar

| Table 9-7 | Conditions Associated with Dyspareunia |
|---|---|
| **System/Domain** | **Examples** |
| **Gastrointestinal** | Irritable bowel syndrome (IBS), inflammatory bowel disease (IBD) (e.g., Crohn's disease, ulcerative colitis), constipation |
| **Hormonal** | Genitourinary syndrome of menopause (GSM), vulvovaginal atrophy, lactational amenorrhea |
| **Iatrogenic** | Radiation therapy, hysterectomy, laparotomy or laparoscopy |
| **Infectious/ inflammatory** | Vulvovaginal candidiasis, herpes, pelvic inflammatory disease (PID), recurrent urinary tract infection (UTI) |
| **Musculoskeletal** | Hypertonic pelvic floor, physiologic defensive contraction of musculature as pain response, myofascial pain syndrome, symphysis pubis misalignment, previous fracture |
| **Neoplastic** | Ovarian cancer, Paget's disease |
| **Neurologic** | Nerve compression, postherpetic neuralgia, referred sensation from other organs |
| **Reproductive** | Endometriosis, uterine leiomyoma, ovarian cyst |
| **Trauma** | Intrapartum injury, female genital mutilation |
| **Urinary** | Interstitial cystitis, painful bladder syndrome |

Based on Yong PJ, Williams C, Yosef A, et al. Anatomic sites and associated clinical factors for deep dyspareunia. *Sex Med.* 2017;5(3):e184-e195; Caruso S, Monaco C. Dyspareunia in women: updates in mechanisms and current/novel therapies. *Curr Sex Health Rep.* 2019;11(1):9-20; and Orr N, Wahl K, Joannou A, et al. Deep dyspareunia: review of pathophysiology and proposed future research priorities. *Sex Med Rev.* 2020;8(1): 3-17. doi:10.1016/j.sxmr.2018.12.007.

| Table 9-8 | 2015 ISSVD Classification of Persistent Vulvar Pain | |
|---|---|---|
| **Diagnosis** | **Etiology** | **Examples** |
| Vulvar pain | Infectious | Herpes, candidiasis |
| | Inflammatory | Lichen sclerosis, lichen planus |
| | Neoplastic | Paget's disease, squamous cell carcinoma |
| | Neurologic | Postherpetic neuralgia, nerve injury or compression |
| | Trauma | Genital mutilation, intrapartum injury |
| | Hormonal deficiencies | Genitourinary syndrome of menopause, vulvovaginal atrophy |

Abbreviation: ISSVD, International Society for the Study of Vulvovaginal Disease.

Based on Bornstein J, Goldstein AT, Stockdale CK, et al. 2015 ISSVD, ISSWSH and IPPS consensus terminology and classification of persistent vulvar pain and vulvodynia. *Obstet Gynecol.* 2016;127(4):745-751. doi:10.1097/aog.0000000000001359.

| Table 9-9 | 2015 ISSVD Classification of Persistent Vulvar Pain |
|---|---|
| **Diagnosis** | **Potential Associated Factors** |
| Vulvodynia | Comorbidities and other pain syndromes (e.g., painful bladder syndrome, fibromyalgia, irritable bowel syndrome, temporomandibular disorder) |
| | Genetics |
| | Hormonal factors (e.g., pharmacologically induced) |
| | Inflammation |
| | Musculoskeletal (e.g., pelvic muscle overactivity, myofascial, biomechanical) |
| | Neurologic mechanisms: Central (spine, brain) Peripheral (neuroproliferation) |
| | Structural defects (e.g., perineal descent) |
| | Psychosocial factors (e.g., mood, interpersonal, coping, role, sexual function) |

Abbreviation: ISSVD, International Society for the Study of Vulvovaginal Disease.

Based on Bornstein J, Goldstein AT, Stockdale CK, et al. 2015 ISSVD, ISSWSH and IPPS consensus terminology and classification of persistent vulvar pain and vulvodynia. *Obstet Gynecol.* 2016;127(4):745-751. doi:10.1097/aog.0000000000001359.

pain disorders. Vulvar pain describes pain caused by a specific and identifiable etiology, such as infection, inflammation, neoplasm, trauma, or neurologic processes or hormonal deficiencies (Table 9-8). Vulvodynia describes pain of at least 3 months duration, without a clearly identifiable cause, but may have potential associated factors (Table 9-9). Vulvodynia is further defined by location (localized, generalized, or mixed), onset (spontaneous, provoked, or mixed; primary or secondary), temporality (immediate, delayed) and duration (intermittent, persistent, constant).[96] Evaluating vulvodynia using standard approaches for symptom analysis (OLDCARTS) facilitates a specific diagnosis and approach to management.

Vulvar pain and vulvodynia are the most prevalent sexual pain dysfunctions in reproductive-age individuals with FARSS, with estimates between 5% and 15%. The prevalence of vulvodynia, specifically, is estimated to be between 3% and 16%.[93,102,103] Vulvar pain has numerous etiologies (Table 9-9), including but not limited to inflammation, neurologic dysfunction (in either the central or peripheral nervous system), referred pain from another structure, loss of tissue integrity, and neuroproliferative changes (over-proliferation of nociceptors at the vestibule, either congenital or acquired).[96]

Neurologically, the pudendal nerve plays a significant role in vulvar pain. It has deep branches to the clitoris, and superficial branches to the vulva and vestibule that can become compressed, entrapped, or damaged through stretching, such as during birth. Due to the phenomenon of "cross-talk" and the complex viscero-somatic nociceptors of the vulva, referred pain can also occur, from visceral organs (e.g., the bladder) or musculoskeletal structures (e.g., the bulbocavernosus muscle).

A relapsing–remitting pattern of vulvar pain and vulvodynia is believed to be the most common form, rather than a stable and persistent chronic pain pattern.[93] In one study approximately 10% of individuals with vulvodynia reported persistent pain over 36 months, with half experiencing remission and 40% experiencing relapse after a period of remission.[102]

## Approach to Sexual Wellness and Dysfunction

The frameworks of structural competency, trauma-informed care, and sex-positivity provide structure for an integrated and inclusive midwifery approach to sexual health care. This section describes an approach to sexuality and sexual health in midwifery practice, as well as a practical approach to supporting sexual function, screening for violence and dysfunction, and addressing sexual health concerns using the midwifery model of care.

### Framework for Approach to Sexual Care

#### Structural Competency

Many factors influence sexual health. The framework of structural competency provides a mechanism to

begin to address complex systemic and organizational structures. Structural competency is the learned ability to distinguish and appreciate how issues that are defined clinically as symptoms, attitudes, or diseases also represent the consequences and results of systemic factors such as health care and food delivery systems, urban and rural infrastructure, medicalization, and the ways in which systems define illness and health.[104]

The structural competency framework asks clinicians to consider the ways health disparities reflect systems of privilege and oppression, such as racism, ableism, fat-phobia, sexism, ageism, cisnormativity, and heteronormativity, and how they shape the healthcare encounter and relationship. Limitations in an individual healthcare provider's ability to buffer the impact of systemic forces are acknowledged, and structural competency challenges clinicians to integrate awareness of local, national, and global structures into their approach. Incorporating humility, clinicians are encouraged to consider the limits of their personal ability to develop insights into the unique intersection of structural forces shaping individual experiences of health and health care.

The structural competency framework is a particularly useful clinical approach to sexuality, centered at the intersection of characteristics such as sex, gender, and sexual orientation, which are fraught with stigma. The sexuality of individuals belonging to marginalized groups is stigmatized disproportionately, creating additional barriers to care and health disparities.[105–107] Midwives can use the structural competency framework to approach sexual health from an informed, but humble perspective by considering how structural forces shape the messages that individuals receive about their sexuality and ultimately their experience of sexual health. Midwives can integrate structural competency into their care by developing an awareness of systems of oppression, listening to individuals and communities about how to best address them in healthcare settings, and facilitating access to resources that might buffer disparities related to social determinants of health.

Resources to support a structurally competent approach are provided in the Resources section at the end of the chapter. Within the clinical system, peer advocates, cultural brokers, community health workers, social workers, and case managers may provide additional support.

#### Trauma-Informed Care

Sexual health care occurs within a setting characterized by greater historical, sociocultural, political, and personal contexts. The adverse health effects associated with trauma are well established.[108] In recognition of this relationship, a trauma-informed approach to care is quickly becoming the standard for all care.[109] The inherent intimacy of sexual health care and patients' vulnerability to healthcare-associated trauma warrant explicit discussion of trauma-informed care in sexual healthcare contexts.

Trauma-informed care is a strengths-based service delivery approach rooted in an understanding of the ubiquity of trauma and its impact. It emphasizes safety for survivors and providers and avoidance of institutional processes and individual practices that might potentially retraumatize individuals, and underscores the importance of survivor participation in the development and evaluation of healthcare services.[110] When they implement a trauma-informed approach to care, clinicians are cognizant of the power asymmetry inherent in the patient–provider relationship and are intentional about centering patient autonomy to engage in health care. Clinicians also recognize that trauma shapes general and health behaviors, the way that care is accessed and interpreted, and the ability to feel safe in a new environment.[111] Trauma-informed care is introduced in the *Introduction to Sexual, Reproductive, and Primary Care* chapter.

### Contexts of Historical and Contemporary Sexual Trauma in Health Care.

Healthcare systems, being influenced by and influencing social norms, have a history of legitimizing the marginalization of LGBTQI+ persons by equating some sexual orientations and genders with mental illness.[112] In the United States, nonconsensual physical examinations and experiments were performed on enslaved Black women to develop gynecologic instruments and procedures,[113] people suspected of having STIs were forced to undergo pelvic examinations,[114] and Black, Indigenous, and People of Color (BIPOC) have undergone forced sterilization.[115] The United States also saw decades of intentional mismanagement of syphilis in Black men as part of the Tuskegee Study,[116] as well as the nonconsensual collection and commercialization of a biospecimen, now called HeLa cells, from Henrietta Lacks, a Black woman.[117] These examples, and many others that have gone unwritten, characterize the historical contexts of trauma in the sexual and reproductive health care provided by midwives, particularly for BIPOC.[117] Current professional cultures and practices with respect to consent and physical examination underline ongoing patient vulnerability to healthcare-associated

trauma,[109,118–121] as do reports of intentional professional misconduct, which limited data suggest is prevalent.[121,122]

The prevalence of sexual violence in the United States is staggering. It is estimated that 81% of cis-women and 43% of cismen have experienced some form of sexual harassment and/or assault in their lifetime.[123] The 2015 National Intimate Partner and Sexual Violence Survey (NISVS) reported that more than 1 in 3 women and 1 in 4 men experienced some type of intimate-partner violence (IPV), defined as rape, physical violence, or stalking by an intimate partner.[124] Cisgender women, nonbinary persons, and transgender individuals are disproportionately affected by such incidents. The 2015 NISVS found that 1 in 5 cisgender women, compared to 1 in 33 cisgender men, reported experiencing attempted or completed rape.[124] In the 2015 U.S. Transgender Survey, almost half (47%) of transgender respondents reported sexual assault at some point during their lifetime. Transgender people of color and sex workers reported even higher rates of sexual assault.[125] The 2016 NISVS revealed that 44% of lesbian women and 61% of bisexual women reported a history of rape, physical violence, and/or stalking compared to 35% of heterosexual women.[124] In the same survey, 37% of bisexual men reported that they had experienced rape, physical violence, or stalking, compared to 26% of heterosexual men and 29% of gay men.[124]

The provision of trauma-informed care includes organizational, clinic, provider, and personnel considerations. Establishing organizational components such as antidiscrimination policies and policies for reporting and responding to IPV, sexual violence, and professional sexual misconduct is crucial.[126] Clinic components include the physical environment, workflows, educational materials, and electronic health records. Welcoming visual cues, such as pride flags; the provision of diverse and inclusive educational materials in appropriate languages; and gender-inclusive and private bathrooms in patient care spaces all help to establish safety and trust.[127] Supports for adapting exemplar organizational and clinical models are described in the Resources section at the end of the chapter.

Provider and personnel components include beliefs, values, awareness, communication, and practices. In general, employing "universal trauma precautions"—including operating under the assumption that everyone has experienced trauma—can guide provider and personnel behavior that facilitates trust and safety.[128] Trainings are available to assess implicit and explicit provider beliefs and values and improve awareness of factors that impact health and the healthcare experience.[129]

### Sex-Positivity

Sex-positivity arises from feminist and queer theories advocating for the liberation of female and queer sexuality through transgressive sexual acts and can be understood as a framework that promotes being open-minded, being nonjudgmental, and respecting personal sexual autonomy.[130] A sex-positive approach to sexuality and sexual health views consensual sexual activity as a healthy and enjoyable part of life and celebrates the diversity of sexual expressions and behaviors. The Sexual Exploration in America Study (2015), part of the largest nationally representative survey focused on understanding sexual behaviors and practices,[131] gathered data regarding the incidence of more than 50 lifetime sexual activities; its findings, which are summarized in Table 9-10, demonstrate a wide variety of typical sexual behaviors.[132]

A sex-positive framework also incorporates the concepts of body-positivity, relationship-positivity, and kink-positivity.[133] A body-positive approach acknowledges that the stigmatization of obesity (fat-phobia) and disability is rooted in racist, sexist, and ableist ideals, and that sexuality cannot be separated from body image, dysphoria, or disability.[133] A relationship-positive approach to care acknowledges the validity of relationships and relationship structures outside of hetero-patriarchal monogamy, such as the many forms of consensual non-monogamy and polyamory,[133] and avoids judgment of nonconsensual non-monogamy to facilitate open communication and risk-reduction strategies. A kink-positive approach to sexuality avoids pathologizing sexual identities and consensual behaviors that eroticize power or pain, such as BDSM and other sexual fetishism. It embraces the many forms of pleasure associated with consent, respect, and communication.[134] Access to a provider who is sex-positive is particularly important for kink-oriented individuals who, depending on the nature of sexual practices, face unique health risks associated with sexual activity.

### Midwifery Management Process Applied to Sexual Health

Concerns regarding sexuality and sexual health may be identified as the primary reason for a healthcare visit, may be introduced to the midwife during a visit for other concerns, or may be disclosed in response to screening. The midwifery management process can be used to maximize sexual health and address sexual concerns no matter how the concern is raised. This section describes the application of the midwifery management process to sexuality and sexual health.

### Investigate, Identify, and Anticipate

The first steps of the midwifery management process involve comprehensively collecting data pertinent to the situation, identifying any problems, and anticipating other health issues related to the identified problem. The approach to and depth of data collection related to sexual health depend on the context of the concern and visit type. Reviewing past health histories and medications can help identify factors associated with sexual dysfunction, allowing the midwife to inquire about associated dysfunctions specifically, or it may identify potential etiologies of dysfunctions introduced by the individual. Some of these health conditions and medications are detailed in Table 9-1 and Table 9-11.[135] Currently, no validated, comprehensive sexual health screening tool is available. To support their clients' sexual health, midwives must adopt an approach to care that integrates screenings for safety, a comprehensive sexual history, assessment of sexual function, and screening for sexual dysfunction.[136]

**Sexual History.** A sexual history may be completed as a part of general health history at the time of a wellness visit, during the investigation of a sexual concern, or when otherwise prompted. Establishing rapport and obtaining consent to discuss sexuality is an essential first step. It is also important to establish the legal boundaries of confidentiality when abuse or violence is disclosed. Legal requirements for mandatory reporting vary from state to state.

Disclosing why questions are being asked, explaining how the information informs the plan of care, and giving permission and respecting the decision to decline to answer any question all help to create a safe environment and build trust. If consent is not given, affirming the decision communicates respect for the patient's autonomy and avoids nudging or coercive behavior. When consent is given, it is important that the midwife indicates that the individual may withdraw consent at any time.

As jargon for sexual organs and behaviors can be stigmatizing or socially charged, asking which terms the patient prefers to use when describing anatomy and then using that language

| Table 9-10 | Diversity of Sexual Activity in the United States | | |
|---|---|---|---|
| | **Percentage of Population (%)** | | |
| **Lifetime Behavior** | **Total** | **Women** | **Men** |
| **Solo and Partnered Sexual Behaviors** | | | |
| Vaginal intercourse | 89 | 91 | 86 |
| Masturbation | 85 | 78 | 92 |
| Received oral sex | 85 | 85 | 85 |
| Gave oral sex | 83 | 83 | 83 |
| Masturbation with someone else | 55 | 53 | 58 |
| Worn sexy underwear or lingerie for a partner | 52 | 75 | 26 |
| Partnered sex in a public place | 44 | 43 | 45 |
| Masturbation in front of partner | 42 | 39 | 44 |
| Spanked or been spanked as part of sex | 31 | 34 | 30 |
| Receptive anal sex | 24 | 37 | 9 |
| Role played with partner | 23 | 22 | 26 |
| Insertive anal sex | — | — | 43 |
| Partner or self tied-up as part of sex | 21 | 21 | 22 |
| Sucked/licked partner's feet/toes | 18 | 11 | 26 |
| Playfully whipped or been whipped as part of sex | 15 | 14 | 16 |
| **Sexual Behaviors Involving Enhancement Products** | | | |
| Watched sexually explicit videos or DVDs (pornography) | 71 | 60 | 82 |
| Looked through sexually explicit magazine | 66 | 55 | 79 |
| Read erotic stories | 57 | 57 | 57 |
| Used a vibrator/dildo | 42 | 50 | 33 |
| Flirted with someone over texting/chat | 38 | 36 | 40 |
| Received nude or semi-nude photo of someone | 34 | 27 | 41 |
| Read guidebook or self-help book | 33 | 34 | 32 |
| Sent nude or semi-nude photo of self to someone | 26 | 27 | 24 |
| Used anal sex toys | 17 | 16 | 18 |
| Used over-the-counter sexual enhancement pill or supplement | 14 | 8 | 21 |
| Had sex with someone over Facetime/Skype | 12 | 11 | 14 |
| Used a phone app related to sex | 9 | 6 | 12 |
| **Social Sexual Experiences** | | | |
| Gone to strip club | 44 | 30 | 59 |
| Has a threesome | 14 | 10 | 18 |
| Had group sex | 9 | 6 | 12 |
| Gone to sex or swingers party | 6 | 5 | 6 |
| Taken class/workshop to learn about sex | 4 | 4 | 4 |
| Gone to BDSM party or dungeon | 3 | 3 | 4 |

Abbreviation: BDSM, bondage, discipline, dominance, submission, sadism, and masochism.

Data from Herbenick D, Bowling J, Fu TC, et al. Sexual diversity in the United States: results from a nationally representative probability sample of adult women and men. *PLoS One*. 2017;12(7). doi: 10.1371/journal.pone.0181198.

| Table 9-11 | Medications That Contribute to Sexual Dysfunction |
|---|---|
| **Medications** | |

| | |
|---|---|
| Anticholinergics | Hormonal agents: |
| Antiemetics | Antiandrogens (finasteride, spironolactone, etc.) |
| Antispasmodics | |
| Anticonvulsants: | Gonadotropin-releasing hormone (GnRH) agonists |
| Carbamazepine | Combined hormonal contraceptives |
| Phenytoin | |
| Primidone | Selective estrogen receptor modulators (SERMs; e.g., Tamoxifen) |
| Cardiovascular medications: | |
| Amiodarone | Aromatase inhibitors |
| Beta blockers | Pain medications: |
| Calcium-channel blockers | Nonsteroidal anti-inflammatory drugs (NSAIDs) |
| Clonidine | Opioids |
| Digoxin | Psychotropic medications: |
| Hydrochlorothiazide | Antidepressants; selective serotonin reuptake inhibitors (SSRIs), serotonin–norepinephrine reuptake inhibitors (SNRIs), tricyclic antidepressants (TCAs) |
| Methyldopa | |
| Statins | |
| | Antipsychotics |
| | Benzodiazepines |
| | Lithium |

Based on Parish SJ, Hahn SR, Goldstein SW, et al. The International Society for the Study of Women's Sexual Health process of care for the identification of sexual concerns and problems in women. *Mayo Clin Proc.* 2019;84:842-856.

builds rapport.[137] When colloquial terms need to be clarified or may make the individual accessing care or the midwife uncomfortable if repeated, using diagrams or asking to use a different term may be helpful. If handled sensitively, these moments can be an opportunity to facilitate present and future patient–provider communication. If not, they can be harmful and even create a barrier to future care.

Sensitively asking about sex, sexual presentation, gender, sexual orientation and identity, and relationship structures and status, when pertinent, avoids the perpetuation of implicit assumptions, destigmatizes discussing these topics, and opens the door to important health discussions. For example, asking "Do you have sex with men, women, or both?" implies a cisnormative relationship between

sex assigned at birth, sexual presentation, and gender, and the response provides little information that is relevant to risks for STIs or unintended pregnancy. If intending to ask about sexual identity or orientation, ask, "Do you identify with any particular sexual orientation or identity? How do you identify?" If intending to evaluate risk for unintended pregnancy, questions can include "Do you have sex with a partner? Tell me about your partner(s)?" or "Do you have sex with anyone that could result in pregnancy, such as someone with a penis?" If gathering information about a partner's sexual presentation or gender identity is pertinent, ask specifically about those characteristics. Taking a sexual history is also covered in the *Collecting a Health History* appendix.

***5 P's Model.*** The Centers for Disease Control and Prevention's (CDC) 5 P's Model provides a practical framework for sexual history taking.[138] This model organizes the components of a sexual history into five categories: partners, practices, protection from STIs, past history of STIs, and pregnancy intention. Though convenient, its utility is limited to assessing risk for and identifying opportunities to prevent STIs and unintended pregnancy. It does not cover sex, sexual presentation, gender identity, sexual orientation or identity, relationship structures or status, or screening for sexual violence or dysfunction.

Some components may be addressed by collecting demographic data through routine intake forms and processes, or the relevant data may be collected prior to beginning the 5 P's questions. If data are collected with intake forms, an option to respond to any question with "decline to state" gives the individual accessing care explicit control over which information is shared. A two-step method of sex and gender data collection—asking first about sex assigned at birth, then about gender identity—is preferred.[139] For example, the question "What sex were you assigned at birth?" may be followed by "What gender do you identify with?" As disclosure of sex assigned at birth and gender identity does not specify current sexual presentation, a thorough history also includes an anatomic inventory, facilitating a risk assessment for unintended pregnancy and appropriate anatomic-based health screenings, such as cervical cancer screening.

***Screening for Intimate-Partner and Sexual Violence.*** Rapport established during sexual history taking can be used to seamlessly screen for intimate-partner and sexual violence. If not completed as part of the sexual history, screening can be completed with other periodic assessments and when otherwise indicated (suggestive injury, chronic pelvic pain, unexplained pelvic or bladder pain, dyspareunia).[140] Screening for sexual and intimate-partner violence creates opportunities to coordinate resources and intervene as determined by the victim, and as required by state law.[141] Although most tools have only been validated in women, examples of screening tools are presented in Table 9-12.

*Screening for Sexual Dysfunction.* Assessing sexual function and screening for sexual dysfunction can be done periodically at wellness visits and when risk factors for sexual dysfunction are present. Numerous models and screening tools are available to guide the assessment,[142] with their implementation

| Table 9-12 | Screening Tools for Sexual and Intimate-Partner Violence | |
|---|---|---|
| **Tool** | **Types of Violence[a]** | **Number of Questions** |
| Abuse Assessment Screen (AAS) | Physical, sexual, emotional, fear | 5 |
| Extended Hurt, Insult, Threaten, Scream (E-HITS) | Physical, sexual, emotional, verbal | 5 |
| Humiliation, Afraid, Rape, Kick (HARK) | Physical, sexual, emotional, fear | 4 |
| Partner Violence Screening (PVS) | Physical, current safety | 3 |

[a] Most questions ask about the previous 12 months.

Based on Soeken KL, McFarlane J, Parker B, et al. The Abuse Assessment Screen: a clinical instrument to measure frequency, severity, and perpetrator of abuse against women. In: Campbell JC, ed. *Empowering Survivors of Abuse: Health Care for Battered Women and Their Children.* Sage Publications; 1998:195-203; Chan CC, Chan YC, Au A, Cheung GOC. Reliability and validity of the 'Extended-Hurt, Insult, Threaten, Scream' (E-HITS) screening tool in detecting intimate partner violence in hospital emergency departments in Hong Kong. *Hong Kong J Emerg Med.* 2010;17(2):109; Sohal H, Eldridge S, Feder G. The sensitivity and specificity of four questions (HARK) to identify intimate partner violence: a diagnostic accuracy study in general practice. *BMC Fam Pract.* 2007 Aug 29;8:49. doi:10.1186/1471-2296-8-49. PMID: 17727730; PMCID: PMC2034562; and Feldhaus KM, Koziol-McLain J, Amsbury HL, Norton LM, Lowenstein SR, Abbott JT. Accuracy of 3 brief screening questions for detecting partner violence in the emergency department. *JAMA.* 1997;277(17):1357-1361. doi:10.1001/jama.1997.03540410035027.

depending on the clinical scenario. If completing a comprehensive sexual history using the 5 P's Model, assessment of sexual function can be incorporated by adding a sixth domain or "P," pleasure.[136] Table 9-13 outlines the process of taking a sexual history using this adaptation.

Independent of a comprehensive sexual history, a targeted history to assess sexual function can be performed. Assessing by domain of sexual function, desire, arousal, and orgasm or satisfaction, and for pain facilitates a thorough assessment (Table 9-14). Screening tools in the form of questionnaires are available for this purpose—though not all are validated—and their utility ranges from screening for dysfunctions across all domains of sexual response to screening for individual sexual dysfunctions.[143]

When risk for sexual dysfunction is evident, the Ex-PLISSIT model[144] provides a simple framework for clinicians to draw connections between those factors and sexual function (Table 9-15). Use of this model explicitly creates space to discuss sexuality and sexual concerns, encouraging the patient to discuss sexual concerns they may otherwise be hesitant to ask about, and establishes the midwife as a partner to address their specific needs.

When a sexual concern or dysfunction is recognized, a targeted but comprehensive history that evaluates biopsychosocial factors that may be contributing to it is essential to identifying potential etiologies and approaches to intervention (Table 9-16).

In summary, history taking should be tailored to the individual and situation. The goal is assessment and optimization of sexual health. Not all questions need to be asked or answered.[138] In many cases, a sexual history is not required to provide sexual health care. If an individual accessing care does not consent to completing a sexual history, a brief overview of sexual healthcare options available to the individual can be provided as an alternative. Creating a safe clinical space by respecting individual autonomy is always appropriate.[109]

## Physical, Laboratory, and Diagnostic Imaging Assessments

The comprehensive evaluation of sexual concerns does not always require physical or pelvic examination. When indicated, physical examination is performed as appropriate to the situation to identify or exclude etiologies of dysfunction. Midwives already possess the assessment skills required for basic physical evaluation of sexual dysfunctions. In addition to general physical assessment skills, midwives are experts in genitourinary, speculum, bimanual, and rectovaginal examinations. When sexual dysfunction is associated with extragenital symptoms, a more comprehensive physical examination is warranted. For example, in an individual assigned female at birth with new-onset orgasm dysfunction associated with bowel or bladder dysfunction, musculoskeletal and neurologic evaluation are an important component of assessment to exclude central and peripheral nervous system disease. Other times, a more targeted physical examination is indicated.

For example, in an individual with MARSS reporting pain with ejaculation associated with frequent urination, genitourinary and prostate examination are appropriate to assess for prostatitis. When assessments outside the scope of the midwifery expertise are indicated, referring the patient to an appropriate healthcare provider facilitates comprehensive evaluation.

In general, physical assessment for the evaluation of sexual dysfunctions follows established practices for physical and pelvic examination. However,

| Table 9-13 | Sexual History Taking: The Five P's | | |
|---|---|---|---|
| | **Goals** | **Dialogue** | **Practices** |
| **Opening** | Provide context, orient the individual accessing care to the role of sexual health in overall health.<br><br>Establish boundaries of confidentiality.<br><br>Obtain consent to discuss sexuality and sexual health.<br><br>Explicitly give permission to withdraw consent and discuss individual questions or concerns. | Sexuality and sexual health are an important part of your overall health. I ask all my patients about their gender and sexuality to address any questions or concerns and identify opportunities to prevent infections, help them avoid unplanned pregnancy, and improve sexual health. Like the rest of your care, all of this information is kept completely confidential, unless you or someone else is in danger. We do not have to discuss this topic any further if you do not want to. Declining this conversation now does not mean that we cannot have it in the future. Is it okay for me to ask a few questions about your sexual history and health?<br><br>• What sex were you assigned at birth?<br>• What is your gender? How do you identify?<br>• Have you had any hormonal, surgical, or cosmetic interventions that have affected or enhanced your reproductive/sexual organs or genitals?<br>• How do you identify in terms of sexual orientation or identity?<br>• Do you have any questions or concerns about your sexual health? | |
| **Partners** | Assess risk for and opportunities for prevention of STIs and pregnancy. | • Are you currently having sex with anyone?<br>• If no, have you ever had sex of any kind with anyone?<br>• If no, is it because you were unsafe or experiencing any problems that you would like to discuss?<br>• In the last 12 months, how many partners have you had?<br>• How do your partners identify in terms of sex and gender?<br>• Do you or your partner(s) currently have any other sexual partners? | Avoid cisnormative and heteronormative assumptions about relationship structures and the sex, gender identity, or sexual orientation of partner(s).<br><br>If not currently sexually active, but has been in the past, taking a sexual history is still important. |

| | Goals | Dialogue | Practices |
|---|---|---|---|
| **Practices** | Assess risk for and opportunities for prevention of STIs and pregnancy. Establish where specimens should be collected for appropriate screening. | I need to ask some more specific questions about the kinds of sex you have had over the last 12 months to better understand your risk for STIs and what screening tests to offer. Different tests are used for the different body parts people use to have sex. Is it okay for me to continue?<br>• What parts of your body are involved when you have sex?<br>   ◆ Mouth?<br>   ◆ Genitals?<br>   ◆ Anus?<br>   ◆ Other?<br>• How are you using those parts of your body? Follow-up questions will be dependent on which anatomy is present and what was disclosed in the previous question (i.e., Are you using your penis for oral, vaginal, or anal sex?).<br>• Do you meet your partners online or through apps?<br>• Have you or any of your partners used drugs?<br>• Have you exchanged sex for your needs (money, housing, drugs, etc.)? | Ask open-ended questions that are focused on the information you need to know based on what you have already learned. |
| **Past History/Protection from STIs** | Assess risk for and opportunities for prevention of STIs. | • Have you ever been tested for STIs and HIV? Would you like to be tested?<br>• Have you been diagnosed with an STI or HIV in the past? When? Were you treated?<br>• What about your partner(s)?<br>• Do you have any symptoms that you are concerned about?<br>• Do you and your partner(s) discuss STI prevention?<br>• If you use prevention tools, what methods do you use (e.g., external or internal condoms, dental dams)?<br>• How often do you use this/these method(s)?<br>• If "sometimes," in which situations, or with whom, do you use each method?<br>• Have you received HPV, hepatitis A, and/or hepatitis B vaccines?<br>• Are you aware of PrEP, a medicine that can prevent HIV? Have you ever used it or considered using it? | Focusing on sexual health goal setting for healthy and safer sexual experiences can be paired with risk-reduction strategies.<br>For those persons at risk for STIs, be certain to encourage testing and give positive feedback about prevention methods that the patient is willing or able to use.<br>STI/HIV prevention strategies can include:<br>• Not having sex<br>• Mutual monogamy, or both partners having sex with only each other<br>• Using PrEP<br>• Using condoms appropriately with every sexual event |

*(continues)*

| Table 9-13 | Sexual History Taking: The Five P's (*continued*) | | |
|---|---|---|---|
| | **Goals** | **Dialogue** | **Practices** |
| **Pregnancy Intention** | Determine pregnancy intention, identify opportunities for family planning, preconception, or contraceptive counseling. | • Do you think you would like to have (more) children at some point?<br>• When do you think that might be?<br>• How important is it to you to prevent pregnancy (until then)?<br>• Are you or your partner using contraception or practicing any form of birth control? Would you like to talk about ways to prevent pregnancy? Do you need any information on birth control? | Information gathered in earlier questions should establish the possibility of pregnancy in the individual or a partner. |
| **Pleasure** | Establish and normalize the role of pleasure in sexual health.<br>Identify opportunities to improve sexual pleasure and create space to discuss concerns related to sexual function. | • Do you use any products or devices to enhance your sexual experience?<br>• Are there any you are considering using that you have questions about?<br>• How satisfied are you with your and/or your partner(s)' sexual functioning?<br>• Do you have any concerns regarding your or your partner(s)' sexual desire or frequency of sexual activity?<br>• Do you have any concerns about arousal or the way that your mind or your body responds to sexual stimulation?<br>• Do you have difficulty obtaining or maintaining an erection?<br>• Do you have any concerns about ejaculation?<br>• Do you ever experience pain during or after sex?<br>• Is there anything about your (or your partner's) sexual activity (as individuals or as a couple) that you would like to change? | If using sexual devices or aids, assess risk for spreading infection, such as sharing with others or use with multiple partners, condom use, cleaning, and sterilization practices. |
| **Safety/Closing** | Screen for intimate-partner violence and sexual assault.<br>Create an opportunity for further or future discussion. | • Has anyone ever threatened your mental or physical safety, made you do something sexual that you did not want to, or sabotaged your birth control plan?<br>• What other things about your sexual health and sexual practices should we discuss to help ensure your good health?<br>• What other concerns or questions regarding your sexual health or sexual practices would you like to discuss? | Allow time for questions or concerns that the individual may not have been ready to discuss earlier. |

Abbreviations: HIV, human immunodeficiency virus; HPV, human papillomavirus; STI, sexually transmitted infection.

Adapted from Reno H, Park I, Workowski K, et al. A guide to taking a sexual history. Centers for Disease Control and Prevention. https://www.cdc.gov/std/treatment/sexualhistory.pdf. Accessed January 29, 2023; and Savoy M, O'Gurek DT, Brown-James A. Sexual health history: techniques and tips. *Am Fam Physician*. 2020;101(5):286-293.

| Table 9-14 | General Assessment of Sexual Function |
|---|---|
| **Domain** | **General Questions** |
| Desire | Frequency of interest in any type of sexual activity? |
| | Level of desire affecting self and/or relationship(s)? |
| | Spontaneous desire experienced? |
| | Responsive desire experienced? |
| Arousal | Difficulties with lubrication, engorgement, and sensation? |
| | Difficulty attaining or sustaining erection? |
| | Difficulties general or specific to sex partner(s), practice(s), or situation(s)? |
| | Sufficient sexual stimulation? |
| Orgasm/ satisfaction | Is orgasm an important component of sexual satisfaction? |
| | What is? |
| | Frequency of orgasm? |
| | Ease of orgasm? |
| | Methods of achieving orgasm? |
| | Intensity and satisfaction with orgasm? |
| | Sufficient sexual stimulation? |
| Pain | Pain? |
| | Constant or provoked? |
| | During genital contact or penetrative activities? |
| | Superficial or deep? |
| | Relationship between pain and arousal? |

Based on Parish SJ, Hahn SR, Goldstein SW, et al. The International Society for the Study of Women's sexual health process of care for the identification of sexual concerns and problems in women. *Mayo Clin Proc.* 2019;94:842-856.

heightened attention is paid to factors that may be contributing to the identified sexual dysfunction to facilitate a plan of care. Physical assessment always begins with obtaining explicit consent and establishing how the patient can signify to the midwife that they want to pause or discontinue the examination; it then proceeds with inspection and hands-on assessments. Particularly when sexual pain dysfunctions are present, it may take multiple visits to build rapport and obtain consent for pelvic assessment, which will almost certainly be a painful experience. Examination approaches and interpretation are dependent on the anatomy present. In any individual with a history of pelvic surgery, a thorough history is key to interpreting physical examination findings. In individuals with a history of gender-affirming genital surgery, a detailed surgical history facilitates identification of anatomy and tissues present and analogous tissue types, and assists in the interpretation of assessment findings. Use of mirrors can facilitate teaching about anatomy and function, and can support a neutral or positive self-image—both of which are factors associated with sexual health.

In individuals with FARSS, anogenital inspection facilitates identification of alterations in anatomy, such as female genital mutilation, adhesions, scarring, dermatoses, injuries, and active infections like human papillomavirus (HPV), herpes, or vulvovaginal candidiasis. Depending on the patient's anatomy, gentle traction on the genital architecture may be indicated to visualize or identify changes in function. When an alteration in the integument is identified, skin biopsy may provide additional diagnostic information. A cotton swab can be used to map pain on the vulva (Q-tip test) when pain dysfunction is present. Vaginal speculum examination facilitates assessment of the architecture of the vaginal vault to rule out pelvic organ prolapse, Müllerian anomaly, stricture, and stenosis, and allows assessment of the vaginal mucosa. It also facilitates assessment of the cervix and collection of genital specimens to identify infectious causes of sexual dysfunction. Bimanual examination can be used to identify signs of infection or anatomic dysfunction, such as urethral or bladder tenderness, cervical motion tenderness, pelvic mass, or uterine immobility. Point tenderness can indicate pelvic floor dysfunction, endometriosis, or a symptomatic fibroid. Localized pain and increased pelvic tone can suggest pelvic floor dysfunction.[145] Rectovaginal examination allows assessment of the anus, rectum, and posterior vaginal wall for integrity, tenderness, and masses.

In individuals with vaginas, any factor associated with decreased estrogen levels can precipitate vaginal atrophy, including masculinizing hormone therapy, lactation, and perimenopausal or postmenopausal hormonal changes. When any of these factors is a barrier to the indicated vaginal assessment and there are no contraindications, a short course of topical vaginal estrogen can facilitate examination.

When the patient's genitals have been altered by gender-affirming surgery, interpretation of the assessment findings depends on the tissue type present. Typically, a neovulva is constructed from scrotal tissue, which is analogous to the labia majora and

| Table 9-15 | Ex-PLISSIT Model | |
|---|---|---|
| **Stage** | **Description** | **Examples** |
| Explicit-permission giving (Ex-P) | Establishes that it is appropriate to discuss sexuality with the midwife and creates the opportunity to discuss potential concerns. | • People with [risk factor] often experience sexual difficulties, such as loss of desire or problems with enjoyment. Have you been affected? Do you want to talk about it?<br>• Many people are concerned about how this [condition and/or intervention] might affect their sexuality. Would you like to discuss your experience?<br>• How has [risk factor] affected you as a couple? Has it affected your sexual relationship? Would you like to discuss this? |
| Limited information (LI) | Establishes the midwife as a source of information, by clarifying misinformation, and providing health education and resources limited to the situation. | • You are right that some symptoms of menopause can be associated with changes in sexual function. But, you can still enjoy a rewarding sex life. If you are experiencing bothersome symptoms, we can explore medications and/or therapies that can help.<br>• It is not uncommon for new parents to be apprehensive about resuming sex after the birth of a baby. It's okay to explore and take things slow. |
| Specific suggestions (SS) | Problem-solving approach to address specific concerns. | • If you want to have sex more often, but don't because the mood never strikes, consider scheduling time for sex. You can create an event on your phone and send your partner an invite to make it fun.<br>• If pelvic congestion causes pain during sex, try positions that elevate your hips during and after sexual activity. |
| Intensive therapy (IT) | Referral to services outside the midwifery scope. | • It sounds like communication issues are a barrier to your sexual health. Psychotherapists specialize in these kinds of problems. Would you like me to refer you?<br>• Urologists specialize in erectile disorders. A urologic evaluation might be helpful. Would you like a referral? |

Adapted from Taylor B. Using the extended PLISSIT model to address sexual healthcare needs. *Nurs Standard*. 2006;21(11):35-40. doi:10.7748 /ns2006.11.21.11.35.c6382. PMID: 17165482.

can be assessed similarly. There is more variation in tissues used to construct neovaginas, but general assessment principles still apply. For example, penile inversion vaginoplasty results in keratinized epithelium lining the vaginal canal; thus, individuals who have undergone this surgery can experience dermatoses like eczema, psoriasis, or lichen sclerosis in the vaginal vault.[137] Postoperatively, granulation tissue is a common cause of bleeding, discharge, and pain. The neovagina, unlike the natal vagina, does not self-clean. Regular douching and dilation are often necessary. If there are concerns about vaginal constriction or stricture, referral to an experienced surgeon for further evaluation and management is necessary.[137]

In individuals with MARSS, genitourinary examination facilitates inspection of the external genitals; evaluation for inguinal hernia; palpation of the inguinal lymph nodes, penis, and testes for tenderness and masses; and collection of urethral specimens. Examination can facilitate diagnosis or exclusion of conditions such as phimosis, paraphimosis, balanitis, epididymitis, varicocele, and STI. Prostate examination is indicated whenever the patient has symptoms of prostatitis, including hematospermia, painful ejaculation, alterations in urination, dysuria, or unexplained pelvic pain.[146]

In individuals born with MARSS who have had gender-affirming vaginoplasty, the prostate typically remains intact postoperatively and indications for prostate examination are the same. However, prostate examination is performed endovaginally, as postoperatively the prostate is located along the urethra, above the anterior wall of the vaginal canal.[137]

| Table 9-16 | Comprehensive Targeted Biopsychosocial History for Sexual Concerns | | |
|---|---|---|---|
| | **Biologic** | **Psychosocial** | **Sexual** |
| Symptoms | Establish current health status.<br><br>Any current conditions associated with sexual dysfunction? | Establish current mood and mental health status.<br><br>Consider mood screening like the Patient Health Questionaire-9 (PHQ-9) instrument for depression or the General Anxiety Disorder-7 (GAD-7) tool for anxiety. | Establish the problem.<br><br>What is the sexual concern in the patient's own words? |
| Present context | Evaluate medications list, substance use. | Nature and duration of current sexual relationship(s)?<br><br>Values/beliefs about sex or the current problem? | Context in which the concern occurs. For example, solo or partnered, all partners, feelings toward partner(s) at the time, type of sexual stimulation, environment, safety, and privacy of the situation? |
| Past context | Review past health history. | Consider screening for adverse childhood events or traumas. | Past sexual experiences, solo and partnered, rewarding? Coercive? Abusive?<br><br>Consider screening for sexual abuse. |
| Onset | Do any physical or mental health events align with onset of concern? | Relationship/social circumstances at the time of onset of concern? | Was there a time that this problem was not present? When? What were the circumstances then? |
| Full clinical picture | If the general health context is relevant, get details on how it is impacting sexual function (e.g., malignancy). | Any major psychosocial stressors outside of the sexual context, such as at home or work?<br><br>Any nonsexual personal or relationship issues, such as ability to express emotions or communication? | Evaluate the rest of the sexual response cycle (desire/arousal/satisfaction) and for pain. |
| Role of partner(s) | Any health problems? | Mood? Mental health? Reaction to sexual problems? | Any disturbance in sexual response? |
| Distress | Level of distress regarding health or health issues? | Level of distress regarding psychosocial/relationship issues? | Level of distress caused by sexual concern? |

Based on Basson R, Althof S, Davis S, et al. Summary of the recommendations on sexual dysfunctions in women. *J Sex Med*. 2004; 1(1):24-34.

In any individual, anorectal examination is indicated when there is a history of receptive anal sexual activity and a report of anorectal bleeding, lesions, pain, or discharge. This examination may include inspection, palpation, and collection of anorectal specimens.

Diagnostic imaging and laboratory evaluation in persons with sexual health concerns are dictated by the individual presentation. Pelvic ultrasound, magnetic resonance imaging (MRI), and computed tomography (CT) enhance and deepen assessment of pelvic anatomy. Imaging can also identify vasocongestive disorders that may not be evident on gross physical examination.

Aside from microscopy and other evaluations of pelvic specimens, such as pH, cultures, or nucleic acid amplification tests (NAAT), laboratory investigation of sexual dysfunction can include screening for conditions associated with sexual dysfunction (e.g., anemia, prolactinoma, thyroid disorders, diabetes) and hormonal changes (e.g., hypogonadism).

Midwives may not perform assessments such as the genitourinary examination of individuals with MARSS often enough to be confident and competent to safely complete them. When a physical assessment is indicated that is outside the midwife's assessment skills, safely evaluating for immediate referral to urgent or emergency services, considering empiric treatment based on history, and coordinating referral to an appropriate provider promotes inclusive care. Referral to a specialist or physician may also be necessary when the initial findings are indeterminate, when first-line therapies fail, or when specialized or surgical assessment and management is indicated, such as vulvoscopy, cystoscopy, hysteroscopy, anoscopy, colonoscopy, venous Doppler sonography, nerve conduction studies, or exploratory laparoscopy.

### Immediate Intervention

Although most sexual health care occurs in ambulatory settings, emergent midwifery, medical, or legal intervention may be necessary, altering the anticipated plan of care. Examples of conditions necessitating such care include emergency contraception, IPV, and sexual assault.

The midwife's response to a client's report of IPV or sexual assault varies depending on the situation and factors such as when the abuse happened, the age of the survivor or victim, clinical protocols, local resources, and state laws. Clinical management is guided by practice guidelines or protocols that integrate local and clinical resources, as well as state legal requirements, into the general plan of care. Familiarity with reporting requirements facilitates an upfront disclosure of legal limits on confidentiality.

How midwives respond to the disclosure of sexual violence matters. Negative reactions or redirecting attention to one's own feelings, rather than the victim's/survivor's response, has been associated with increased risks to the victim/survivor for depression, severity of PTSD symptoms, and substance use. Alternatively, reactions that validate the victim's/survivor's experience, reassure the victim/survivor that the violence was not their fault, and provide resources are associated with fewer symptoms of PTSD.[147]

Midwives do not typically complete forensic examinations as part of their response to sexual violence. If such an exam is required, the International Association of Forensic Nurses (IAFN) publishes protocols for sexual assault medical forensic examinations of adults, adolescents, and children and provides technical assistance to providers.[148] Midwives interested in adding this skill to their practice can complete the training requirements established by the IAFN and the ACNM's Position Statement Expansion of Midwifery Practice and Skills Beyond Basic Core Competencies.[149]

### Comprehensive Plan of Care: General Principles

Facilitation of sexual health and management of sexual dysfunction is guided by the principle of shared decision making and is dependent on individual needs, working diagnoses, and available resources. Aside from facilitating the identification of sexual concerns, the Ex-PLISSIT model provides a practical framework for care management (Table 9-15). Often, a comprehensive plan of care involves no more than midwifery presence, reassurance, and basic behavioral or pharmacologic intervention that can be managed by the midwife. However, because any disturbance in biopsychosocial functioning can impact sexual function, interdisciplinary collaboration is frequently indicated. Whenever evaluation or management of a sexual dysfunction requires skills or resources beyond the midwife's scope of practice, referral to the appropriate professional is indicated. Understanding the role of other health professionals in the management of sexual dysfunction facilitates appropriate use of resources and avoids delays in care.

### Follow-Up Evaluation

Midwifery management of sexuality and sexual health concerns can occur in the context of a single visit or over multiple encounters and involve ongoing reevaluation of function and efficacy of intervention. Continuity of care is an important component of safety, quality, and satisfaction, and can ensure future access to care.[150,151] Intentional coordination of follow-up care and anticipatory guidance regarding indications for reevaluation and a preview of next steps facilitates a comprehensive midwifery approach to sexuality from start to finish.

## Midwifery Management of Alterations in Sexual Function

Addressing sexual concerns often involves an interdisciplinary approach, including management of health problems that do not initially appear related to sexual function. Examples include optimizing blood pressure control or blood glucose levels to minimize effects of microvascular disease or neuropathies, and general health promotion. As members of an interdisciplinary team, midwives can support sexual health by educating individuals on the connections between their health conditions and sexual health, and by encouraging optimal management of those conditions where possible. Sexuality and sexual health can be a source of joy, pleasure, or resilience for individuals. Identifying sexuality as a healthy component of the human experience and as a potential health resource employs a sex-positive and strengths-based approach to support overall health.

## Promotion of General Health and Well-Being

Good health, a subjective sense of well-being, and comprehensive sex education are protective factors against sexual dysfunction. Basic information and health education that draws connections between daily behaviors and sexual health are well within the midwifery scope of practice.

### Exercise

Exercise, in the form of both short-term and long-term exercise habits, has positive effects on sexual function. Positive effects are related to mediation of hormonal activity, engagement of the sympathetic nervous system, and improvements to autonomic nervous system tone. Acutely, cardiovascular exercise improves physiologic sexual arousal for 15 to 30 minutes after exercise.[152] Chronic (habitual) exercise habits improve cardiovascular health, vascular tone, mood, and body image—all factors associated with improved sexual health and well-being.[153–155] However, excessive physical activity is associated with negative impacts on sexual health.[152]

### Sleep

Sleep disturbances and deprivation, especially in association with conditions such as obstructive sleep apnea (OSA), have been linked to disturbances in sexual function.[156] Interventions for sleep disorders can range from reviewing basic sleep hygiene to specialty referral for management of insomnia or sleep-disturbing conditions.[157] Any suspicion of OSA should prompt referral for a sleep study.

## Sexual Aids and Devices

In addition to general health promotion, the promotion of sexual well-being often includes discussing the use of sexual aids and devices. Sexual aids and devices are commonly used in solitary and partnered sexual activity to increase comfort (i.e., reduce friction, reduce depth of penetration) or to increase sexual stimulation and arousal (e.g., vibrators, penis rings to reduce venous outflow). Most sexual devices are widely available without prescription, can be easily and privately purchased online, and require minimal instructions and guidance for use.

### Lubricants

Lubricants are used to decrease friction and enhance comfort and sensation during sexual activity. They are important to prevent condom breakage and can be useful for treatment of health conditions and sexual dysfunctions such as genitourinary syndrome of menopause or dyspareunia. Lubricants can be used by anyone for any sexual activity. The choice of lubricant depends on the sexual activity and personal preference.

Lubricants come in a variety of forms, commonly water-, silicone-, or oil-based. Water-based lubricants are compatible with all types of condoms and sexual devices, but can be perceived as being sticky or drying too quickly. Inclusion of preservatives and glycerin is associated with mucosal irritation and an increased risk for vaginal yeast infections in some individuals. Silicone- and oil-based lubricants have increased longevity and require less application, but are not compatible with all sexual device and condom materials, and are more difficult to clean. Device and barrier materials and lubricant compatibilities are listed in Table 9-17.[158] Most importantly, silicone lubricants cannot be used with silicone sexual devices, and oil-based lubricants cannot be used with latex barriers or condoms. Petroleum products such as baby oil and petroleum jelly should never be used as lubricants, as they are difficult to remove and are associated with irritation and infection.

Some lubricants have properties designed to enhance sexual function, such as cooling, warming, or numbing effects to increase arousal, delay ejaculation, or facilitate penetration. To avoid irritation, lubricants that are free of preservatives, glycerin, fragrances, dyes, and heating, cooling, or numbing properties are recommended. Additionally, lubricants with spermicides (nonoxynol-9) have irritant effects and are not recommended. If using such a lubricant is strongly desired, harm-reduction patch testing of the lubricant on the skin and mucosa is recommended.

| Table 9-17 | Device, Lubricant, and Barrier Compatibilities | | | | | | |
|---|---|---|---|---|---|---|---|
| | | **Device Material** | | | **Barrier Material** | | |
| | | **Silicone** | **Glass, Metal, Ceramic, Plastic** | **Jelly Rubber, Silicone Blend, Vinyl, or Cyberskin** | **Latex** | **Nitrile/ Lambskin** | **Polyisoprene** | **Polyurethane** |
| **Lubricant** | Water-Based | X | X | X | X | X | X | X |
| | Silicone | | X | X | X | X | X | |
| | Oil | X | X | | | X | | X |

Data from Rubin ES, Deshpande NA, Vasquez PJ, Kellogg Spadt S. A clinical reference guide on sexual devices for obstetrician-gynecologists. *Obstet Gynecol.* 2019;133(6):1259-1268.

## Sexual Devices

Sexual aids and devices are designed to aid or enhance sexual activity.[158] They include stimulatory, engorgement-enhancing, insertable, penetration-limiting, positioning, and mobility aids and devices (Table 9-18).[158,159] Although research is lacking, sexual devices are widely used, facilitate sexual function in the presence of some chronic illnesses or disabilities, and are important tools in managing arousal, orgasm, and pain dysfunctions.[159] They are generally considered safe, although emergency room visits associated with sexual device use have been reported[160] and sharing of devices or use with a partner(s) poses risk for transmission of pathogens. Familiarity with safe use of sexual aids and devices is an essential component of inclusive and comprehensive sexual health care.

In general, most devices should be cleaned with soap and warm water and be stored in individual containers (e.g., bags or boxes) after every use. Sanitizing procedures are dependent on device materials, waterproofing, and the inclusion of batteries or electronics. The CDC provides guidelines for disinfection.[161] Devices should be sanitized whenever they may have come into contact with body fluids or parts that are harboring active infection, the device is used in the anus, or there is an odor to the device. Due to limited research regarding the efficacy of sanitization strategies and the wide variety of devices on the market, any device made of porous materials (any material other than borosilicate glass, medical-grade silicone, or metal) or that will be used by multiple users should be used with a barrier, such as a condom. When used by multiple individuals or if inserted into multiple body parts (i.e., vagina and anus), both sanitizing and condom use can be used to minimize the risk for transmission of pathogens.[158]

## Psychological and Pharmacologic Management of Sexual Dysfunctions

### Psychological Management of Sexual Dysfunctions

Psychological intervention is a key component of a comprehensive biopsychosocial approach to managing sexual dysfunctions. Psychological interventions include psychoeducation, self-help educational materials (bibliotherapy), cognitive-behavioral sex therapy, mindfulness-based therapy, sex therapy, and counseling.[75,162,163] When referral to a specialist is indicated, it is important to consider accessibility. Psychotherapists that specialize in sexual dysfunction are not available in all geographic regions, and patients seeking their services may incur a significant out-of-pocket expense. Furthermore, these treatment modalities are only beneficial when the individual is engaged in the therapeutic regimen and completes prescribed activities as directed. If full engagement in therapeutic modalities is not feasible, an alternative plan of care can be explored.

### Psychoeducation

Psychoeducation is the provision of accurate and accessible information on sexual response and sexual health and is the foundation for all interventions for sexual dysfunction. Comprehensive sexual education is protective against sexual dysfunction,[65] and psychoeducation is a core component of the management of sexual disturbances and dysfunctions.[163] Psychoeducation for the individual or couple improves understanding of how cognitive and physical sexual stimulation are involved in their own sexual response. Well within the midwife's scope of practice and an effective intervention, psychoeducation can be incorporated into any plan of care.[65,164]

| Table 9-18 | Sexual Devices and Aids | |
|---|---|---|
| **Type** | | **Description** |
| Vibrators/stimulatory devices | Vibrator | Available in a variety of styles, shapes, and sizes. Designed to provide vibratory stimulation to internal and external genitalia, as well as the anus. |
| | Air pulsation device | Air pulsations produce clitoral stimulation, distinct from vibratory or manual stimulation. |
| | | Device shapes and sizes vary. Selection is guided by individual anatomy and intention for solo or partnered activity. |
| Engorgement/ erectile-enhancing devices | Pump/vacuum constriction | Available for vulvas and phalluses; can be used alone, or with medications to improve engorgement of the external genitals. |
| | | Use with caution if taking anticoagulants, or when blood disorders or risks for blood clotting are present. |
| | Ring | Tourniquet-like device used to maximize phallic engorgement and duration of erection. Can be used alone or with a genital pump. Available in a variety of materials, with varying rigidity, and/or with vibratory stimulation for self and partner(s). |
| | | Limit use to 30 minutes at a time to avoid adverse effects. |
| Insertable devices | Dilator | Rod- or cylinder-shaped device with a rounded end. Inserted into the vagina in programs to serially increase the width/depth tolerated to facilitate penetrative vaginal sexual activity by improving vaginal tissue flexibility and control of pelvic floor muscles. |
| | Dildo | Provides penetrative stimulation of the vagina or anus. Available in a variety of sizes and shapes, some with features like heat or vibration. Can be used with hip, thigh, or hand harnesses to facilitate partnered sexual activity. |
| | Anal | Come in a variety of materials, shapes, and sizes to provide anal and/or prostate stimulation. Nonporous materials and a flared base to prevent the device from being drawn fully into the rectum are essential safety features of any device intended for anal stimulation. |
| Penetration-limiting devices | | Also known as a "bumper." Soft, ring-shaped device designed to limit penetration during insertive sexual activities. Helpful for management of deep dyspareunia with partnered sexual activity. |
| Positioning/mobility aids | | Any device designed to overcome positional or mobility barriers to sexual function. Include specially designed pillows, cushions, and furniture, as well as bouncers and swings. |

Based on Rubin ES, Deshpande NA, Vasquez PJ, Kellogg Spadt S. A clinical reference guide on sexual devices for obstetrician-gynecologists. *Obstet Gynecol*. 2019;133(6):1259-1268; and Dewitte M, Reisman Y. Clinical use and implications of sexual devices and sexually explicit media. *Nat Rev Urol*. 2021;18(6):359-377.

### Self-Help Educational Materials

Bibliotherapy—the use of printed materials as part of therapeutic intervention for a condition—has been shown to have positive effects on sexual dysfunctions across all domains.[165] Educational materials are available as handouts, books, websites, and applications. Best practice is to be familiar with any material being recommended, if possible.

This approach is particularly helpful for individuals who are unable to access specialized therapy or medications.

### Sex Therapy

Sex therapy is a specific, highly specialized form of psychotherapy intended to help individuals and couples with sexual dysfunctions. Sex therapy usually includes 8 to 12 weekly sessions with home assignments for individuals and their partner(s). In the United States, qualified sex therapists can be found most easily using the American Association of Sexuality Educators, Counselors, and Therapists (AASECT) online database.[166] Two core components of sex therapy are *sensate focus,* and *directed masturbation.*[163]

*Sensate Focus.* A progressive series of sensual touching and feeling exercises for couples, sensate focus therapy is used to decrease anxiety and avoidance of touching or sexual activity, improve communication between individuals, and improve intimacy by reintroducing sexual activity in a progressive way. Mindfulness techniques are incorporated to facilitate redirection of goal-oriented, orgasm-focused thought processes into the conscious experience of present sensations.[75]

*Directed Masturbation.* Directed masturbation, also known as *masturbation training,* is a progressive series of self-awareness and exploration exercises intended to help patients become more familiar with their own genitals and erotic areas of the body. An individual becomes more aware of sexually arousing stimuli, and eventually masturbates to orgasm.[75]

### Cognitive-Behavioral Therapy

Cognitive-behavioral therapy (CBT) focuses on identifying and altering cognitions (patterns of thought, such as unrealistic expectations or catastrophizing) and behaviors (such as avoidance of sexual activity) that can contribute to sexual dysfunction, particularly sexual desire dysfunction. CBT can be incorporated into a sex therapy program, or it can be utilized as a stand-alone therapy. CBT is usually limited to approximately 10 to 12 weekly sessions, and may occur in individual, couple, or group settings. Sessions usually occur on a weekly basis and include homework, to help reinforce changes in patterns of cognitions and behaviors.

### Mindfulness-Based Therapy

A concept that originates in Buddhist meditation, mindfulness is defined as "the awareness that emerges through paying attention on purpose, in the present moment, and non-judgmentally to things as they are."[167] Mindfulness-based therapies teach individuals how to remain present in the moment, to acknowledge distracting thoughts as a passing phenomenon, and not to dwell on or judge these distractions. Mindfulness-based therapy is often

incorporated into sex therapy and CBT modalities.[75] However, mindfulness can be learned and practiced in a variety of settings, including phone-based apps, physical fitness activities, and meditation practices. Mindfulness can be particularly helpful in addressing distraction, as distraction from sexual stimuli during sexual activity plays a role in diminished responsive desire, as well as arousal and orgasm dysfunction.[86] Mindfulness can also be helpful for individuals who experience significant self-criticism, poor self-image, or depression and anxiety, as it improves self-compassion and self-acceptance.[75,167,168]

### Counseling

When comorbid mood disorders or other psychiatric conditions present with sexual dysfunction, individual counseling may be indicated. Trauma-focused therapy is particularly helpful for individuals with a history of trauma, including sexual abuse. Couples counseling is helpful in the management of sexual dysfunctions that involve maladaptive relationship behaviors. Couples counseling focuses on avoiding blame for interpersonal problems and aims to find solutions to resolve identified problems.

### Pharmacologic Management of Sexual Dysfunctions

Due to the complexity and entanglement of the excitatory and inhibitory processes that regulate sexual response and functioning, there is significant overlap in pharmacologic management between all sexual dysfunction domains.

First-line medication management of sexual dysfunction focuses on the treatment of any modifiable neuroendocrine or vascular factors that may be negatively affecting an individual's sexual function. Examples include the treatment of hyperprolactinemia or thyroid disease, chronic hypertension, or hyperglycemia. Evaluation of an individual's current medical treatment for any comorbid condition is also necessary, especially if individuals experiencing sexual dysfunction are using medications known to be associated with high rates of sexual disturbances, such as SSRIs.[36]

Pharmacologic treatment of sexual dysfunction involves shared decision making. Few medications have official Food and Drug Administration (FDA)–approved indications related to sexual dysfunction in the United States, so most pharmacologic management occurs on an off-label basis. A verbal informed consent should be obtained from the patient that acknowledges this reality, and should be documented appropriately. Prior to prescribing any medication, it is important to check medication interactions in an evidence-based prescribing reference. Some medications used to treat sexual dysfunction, such as flibanserin, have many potential interactions. Indications and prescribing information for commonly used FDA-approved and off-label medications are presented in Table 9-19, Table 9-20, and Table 9-21.

### Domain-Specific Approaches to Management

Midwifery management of sexual disorders should be tailored to the specific condition, based on the best available evidence, and utilize a shared decision-making process. This section reviews recommended psychological and pharmaceutic approaches, as well as the use of sexual aids and devices, for each condition.

#### Desire Dysfunctions

**Hypoactive Sexual Desire Dysfunction.** The most well-established evidence-based interventions for sexual desire dysfunctions are psychological. Additionally, these interventions have benefits for multiple domains of sexual function, in addition to desire—which is advantageous because most individuals present with sexual dysfunction in more than one domain.

Flibanserin and bremelanotide are both FDA-approved medications for use in premenopausal cisgender women in the United States, and a variety of medications are used on an off-label basis (Table 9-20). Evidence supports off-label use of low-dose systemic testosterone therapy in cisgender and transgender women who are postmenopausal or otherwise hypogonadal.[15,189,190]

#### Arousal Dysfunctions

**Hypoactive Sexual Arousal.** Treatment approaches can vary depending on individual presentation and comorbid health conditions, which should be addressed with a first-line treatment. Such comorbid conditions include pelvic health conditions—for example, genitourinary syndrome of menopause and atrophic vaginitis. When hyposensitivity of the genitalia is the primary concern, determining whether the concern is related to inattention to genital changes can help the provider decide if specialty referral is indicated to exclude neurologic dysfunction.

When neurovascular disruptions are not apparent, interventions to address subjective sexual arousal are a good place to start. This includes mindfulness-based interventions to increase awareness of sexual cues and improve cue engagement. Sensate focus and directed masturbation therapies are well-supported interventions for hypoactive sexual arousal.

Sexual aids and devices are also helpful in the management of arousal dysfunctions to enhance sexual stimulation. Types of sexual devices with various functions are presented in Table 9-18.

A urology referral is recommended for arousal dysfunction in transgender individuals with MARSS who are using testosterone suppression therapy and have a history of (erectile) dysfunction prior to testosterone suppression.

Flibanserin and bremelanotide have been used off-label for the treatment of hypoactive sexual arousal. Most studies demonstrating their efficacy involved individuals who experienced both desire dysfunction and arousal dysfunction.[61,169]

#### Persistent Genital Arousal Syndrome/ Genito-Pelvic Dysesthesia

Concerns about excessive arousal or unprovoked orgasm are often misunderstood, trivialized, or dismissed. Given the high rates of co-occurring anxiety, depression, and suicidality, persistent genital arousal must be taken seriously. Timely recognition of this dysfunction and referral to specialty care (e.g., neurology, psychotherapy) is critical. ISSWSH publishes guidelines for the assessment and management for persistent genital arousal syndrome that midwives can use as a reference.[82]

#### Orgasm Dysfunction

The language used to discuss orgasm dysfunction can be therapeutic. By intentionally using the phrase "experience orgasm" rather than "achieve orgasm" or "successfully having an orgasm," midwives can create space to reframe beliefs about orgasm and the goals of sexual activity.

Sensate and directed masturbation, psychotherapy, and the use of sexual aids to enhance or introduce novel sexual stimulation can be effective in treating orgasm dysfunction.[191] When individuals can experience orgasm through masturbation, they are more likely to experience orgasm during partnered sexual activity.[192] It is reasonable to counsel patients about this relationship, and to encourage paralleling solo and partnered sexual activities where possible and desired.

There are no FDA-approved medications for orgasmic dysfunction. Off-label medications used for orgasmic dysfunction include amphetamine/ dextroamphetamine salts, bupropion, dopamine agonists, and oxytocin, as well as off-label use of flibanserin and bremelanotide (see Table 9-19 and Table 9-20).

| Table 9-19 | FDA-Approved Medications for Sexual Dysfunctions | | | | | |
|---|---|---|---|---|---|---|
| **Medication** | **Drug Class/ Mechanism of Action** | **Potential Adverse Effects** | **Comments*** | **Sexual Dysfunction** | | |
| | | | | **Desire** | **Arousal** | **Orgasm** |
| **Bremelanotide** 1.75 mg subcutaneous autoinjector once as needed 45 minutes prior to sexual activity Repeat every 24 hours as needed, but no more than 8 times in 1 month | Melanocortin 3 and 4 receptor agonist; MOA is uncertain, but melanocortins interact both centrally and peripherally to promote desire and arousal[169] | Nausea, facial flushing, headache[163] | Improvements can be seen as soon as 4 weeks after initiating treatment. Transient increase in blood pressure after use. Not recommended for use in individuals with uncontrolled hypertension or cardiovascular disease.[163,169] | Female: FDA approved Male: off-label | Off-label | Off-label |
| **Flibanserin** 100 mg once daily at bedtime | 5-HT$_{1A}$ agonist, 5-HT$_{2A}$ antagonist; Decreases inhibitory processes by serotonin blockade; increases dopamine and norepinephrine;[170] increases brain's response to sexual cues and reduces inhibition to sexual cues | Dizziness, somnolence (12%), nausea, headache, insomnia (4.9%)[171] Interacts with moderate/strong CYP3A4 inhibitors (e.g., fluconazole, grapefruit juice)[172] | Therapeutic effect may take up to 8 weeks to be seen. Discontinue after 8 weeks if no improvement. Avoid drinking alcohol within 2 hours of administration due to risk of severe hypotension.[44,163] | Female: FDA approved Male: off-label | Off-label | Off-label |
| **Sildenafil** 25–100 mg taken as needed, 1 hour prior to sexual activity | PDE$_5$ inhibitor, promotes vasodilation, facilitating vasocongestion of erectile tissue[173] | Headache, flushing, nausea, rhinitis, transient visual disturbances | Requires intact erectile and vascular tissue as well as sexual stimulation to function. Highly effective for genital arousal dysfunction for male-assigned individuals; mixed evidence for female-assigned individuals, with the exception of specific subgroups (DM1, SCI, SSRI-induced arousal dysfunction, MS). | | **Male: FDA approved** Female: off-label | |

*Unless otherwise indicated, MOA is not dependent on biologic sex.

Abbreviations: DM1, type 1 diabetes mellitus; FDA, Food and Drug Administration; MOA, mechanism of action; MS, multiple sclerosis; SCI, spinal cord injury; SSRI, selective serotonin reuptake inhibitor.

**Table 9-20  Off-Label Medications for Sexual Dysfunctions**

| Medication | Drug Class/ Mechanism of Action | Potential Adverse Effects | Comments* | Desire | Arousal | Orgasm |
|---|---|---|---|---|---|---|
| | | | **Modulation of Excitatory Processes** | | | |
| **Amphetamine or dextroamphetamine mixed salts** 2.5–10 mg taken 30 minutes prior to sexual activity[63,174] | Modulates norepinephrine and dopamine release;[174] stimulant—increases sensitivity and attention to sexual cues | Hypertension, palpitations, tachycardia, headache, insomnia, weight loss, constipation, xerostomia[175] | Controlled substance; use with caution due to potential for dependency or abuse. Dose escalation may be needed to maintain effect.[174,176] Can interfere with sleep if taken too late in the day. | | Off-label | Off-label |
| **Bupropion** 150 mg SR twice daily or 300 mg XL once daily | Inhibition of dopamine and norepinephrine reuptake; antagonist at nicotinic acetylcholine receptors | Anxiety, irritability, headache, seizures, dry mouth, nausea, gastrointestinal disturbances, sweating[179] | Particularly helpful with SSRI-induced sexual dysfunction. | Off-label | Off-label | Off-label |
| **Cabergoline** 0.25 mg twice weekly (e.g., every Monday and Thursday), up to a maximum of 1 mg twice weekly[178] | Dopamine (D$_2$) agonist; pro-excitatory neurotransmitter | Nausea, headache, gastrointestinal disturbances[177] | Administration with food reduces gastrointestinal disturbances. Must be titrated slowly (minimum of 4 weeks between dose changes). Contraindicated with uncontrolled hypertension. | | Off-label | Off-label |
| **Oxytocin lozenges** 250 units sublingually 1 hour prior to sexual activity[63] 24 IU nasal spray as needed during intercourse[179] | Numerous roles in sex, orgasm, pair bonding, pelvic muscle contractions during orgasm | Unpleasant taste (lozenges, nasal spray), flushing, headaches[177] | Short half-life (1 to 6 minutes); can be impractical for use. | | Off-label | Off-label |

*(continues)*

**Table 9-20** Off-Label Medications for Sexual Dysfunctions (*continued*)

| Medication | Drug Class/ Mechanism of Action | Potential Adverse Effects | Comments* | Sexual Domains Addressed | | |
|---|---|---|---|---|---|---|
| | | | | Desire | Arousal | Orgasm |
| **Testosterone** 300 mcg/day transdermal patch[180] or a product formulated for cisgender men, at 1/10 the typical dose[181] | Mediates numerous mechanisms of sexual response both centrally and peripherally, acts to increase sensitivity to sexual cues[182] Supports genital erectile tissue integrity[183] | Acne, hirsutism, weight gain, possible long-term negative cardiovascular effects, requires ongoing monitoring[184] | Therapeutic effect may not be seen for 6 to 8 weeks; discontinue after 6 months if ineffective.[184] Groups most likely to benefit are individuals assigned female at birth with hypogonadism (such as individuals in menopause), and transgender women who have had gender-affirming genital surgery.[15,62,181] | Off-label | Off-label | |
| **Modulation of Inhibitory Processes** | | | | | | |
| **Buspirone** 10 mg – 60 mg twice daily in two divided doses | Partial agonist of the 5-HT$_{1A}$ receptor; reduces serotonergic tone; reduces inhibitory response to sexual cues | Flushing, headache, light-headedness, nausea | Use caution when taking other serotonergic medications. | Off-label | Off-label | |
| **Trazodone** 50–100 mg once daily at bedtime | 5-H$_{T1}$ agonist, 5-HT$_{2A}$ receptor antagonist; heterocyclic antidepressant; reduces inhibitory response to sexual cues | Somnolence, dizziness, headaches | Use caution when taking other serotonergic medications. Best evidence for use in cisgender women with hypogonadism experiencing sleep and sexual dysfunctions.[75] | Off-label | Off-label | |

*Unless otherwise indicated, MOA is not dependent on biologic sex.

Abbreviations: MOA, mechanism of action; SR, sustained release; SSRI, selective serotonin reuptake inhibitor; XL, extended release.

| Table 9-21 | Medications for Vulvovaginal Conditions Associated with Sexual Dysfunction | | | | | | |
|---|---|---|---|---|---|---|---|
| Medication | Drug Class/ Mechanism of Action | Potential Adverse Effects | Comments* | Sexual Domains Addressed | | | |
| | | | | Desire | Arousal | Orgasm | Pain |
| **Alprostadil** | Synthetic prostaglandin $E_1$; topical vasodilator; smooth muscle relaxant; enhances sensory nerve activity[173,185] | Topical irritation or burning[186] | Must be compounded in nonoffensive base.[90]<br>Topical efficacy shown only for use on vaginal/vulvar tissue.[173] | | Off-label | | |
| **DHEA (prasterone)** 6.5 mg intravaginal suppository once nightly | "Pre-hormone"; converted to estrogen and testosterone within the vaginal tissue[187] | Vaginal discharge, abnormal cervical cytology results | Does not increase serum estrogen or testosterone levels.[183]<br>Indicated for individuals assigned female at birth experiencing sexual dysfunction secondary to vulvovaginal atrophy.[183,188] | | Off-label | Off-label | Off-label |
| **Estrogen, topical vaginal** Available as a topical cream, intravaginal tablet, or low-dose intravaginal ring. | Improves tissue integrity, elasticity; modulates nociceptors; improves tissue lubrication[188] | Topical use may cause burning or irritation, especially with initial use on atrophied tissue | Systemic exposure is negligible with most vaginal preparations, but caution is advised when any contraindication to exogenous estrogen is present.<br>Most effective for genital arousal in individuals assigned female at birth who are experiencing vulvovaginal atrophy.[66,188] | | Off-label | Off-label | Off-label |
| **Ospemifene** 60 mg once daily | Selective estrogen receptor modulator; functions as an estrogen agonist in genital tissues[188] | Hot flash, headache, vaginal discharge<br>Increases risk of venous thromboembolism | FDA recommends use of an opposing progestin due to potential endometrial effects, but no data are available to support this recommendation at this time.[163]<br>Indicated for individuals assigned female at birth experiencing vulvovaginal atrophy.[183] | | Off-label | | Off-label |

*Unless otherwise indicated, MOA is not dependent on biologic sex.

Abbreviations: DHEA, dehydroepiandrosterone; FDA, Food and Drug Administration; MOA, mechanism of action.

## Approach to Sexual Pain Dysfunction Management

Addressing intermittent or occasional sexual pain facilitates wellness and prevents future inhibitory effects on sexual response, even when formal criteria are not met for a sexual pain dysfunction. Typical approaches include encouraging communication with partner(s), changing sexual positions, adding a lubricant or sex aid (e.g., a penetration-limiting device), changing sexual activities (e.g., reduce penetrative sexual activity and increase oral sexual activity), and taking a break from sexual activity.[87] Assessing whether pain is present during self-stimulating sexual activities can also help to guide management. Often, individuals have already discovered ways to experience desire, arousal, and orgasm without pain, but struggle with partnered sexual activity.

Individuals experiencing sexual pain dysfunction are often seen by numerous providers and have their concerns dismissed. In one study, 60% of participants were seen by at least three providers before being diagnosed with a sexual pain dysfunction.[47]

Because pain dysfunctions are inherently multifactorial, are complex, and involve multiple organ systems, multiple treatment modalities are frequently indicated.[98] A comprehensive plan of care typically includes psychological intervention, pharmacologic intervention, and pelvic floor physical therapy. When more conservative therapies are ineffective or there is another indication (e.g., resection of endometrial implants, myomectomy for bulky fibroids), referral for surgical consultation is indicated. Vestibulectomy (removal of the vaginal vestibule) is highly effective for treating provoked vestibulodynia.[193] Specialist referral can also provide patients with access to other interventions, such as nerve blocks, botulinum toxin A injections into the pelvic musculature, laser therapy of atrophic vaginal tissue, or combinations of these treatments.[194]

### Pharmacologic Management

If medication administration is contributing to sexual pain dysfunction (e.g., anticholinergic-associated vaginal dryness), working with the care team to discontinue the offending medication is ideal, but may not always be feasible. This situation can arise with the use of combined hormonal contraceptives, which are a known risk factor for vestibulodynia due to associated hypoestrogenic effects in the vestibule. Especially when used for the management of other conditions associated with pelvic and sexual pain (e.g., endometriosis), discontinuation of these agents may not be practical. In such cases, a topically applied estrogen/testosterone mixed compound is a reasonable approach.[183] Similarly, transmasculine individuals using masculinizing hormone therapy can experience dysorgasmia in relation to testosterone use, but discontinuing testosterone is not appropriate. When this is the case, titrating the testosterone dose to lower physiologic levels, as tolerated, or exploring other options is more appropriate.

Table 9-22 summarizes the pharmacologic agents used for sexual pain dysfunctions. Shared decision making is the cornerstone of pharmacologic management, as there are no FDA-approved medications for sexual pain dysfunctions. Patients should be aware that treatment recommendations are based on limited research, expert consensus (where there is often disagreement), and clinical experience.[195] With the exception of topical treatments, pharmacologic management of sexual pain dysfunction mirrors that for other chronic non-malignancy-related pain conditions. Opioids are not recommended, as their common side effects are associated with an increased risk for sexual pain dysfunction (e.g., opioid-induced constipation) and they confer a high risk for dependence.

### Psychosocial and Behavioral Management

Because pain is a cortically mediated experience, much chronic pain management relies on "retraining" the brain and body's responses. Psychotherapy and behavioral techniques can be employed to alter the experience of pain, desensitize, cognitively reframe, or improve self-efficacy related to pain.[198]

**Psychoeducation.** Education is a key component of the management of sexual pain dysfunctions. Midwives can help set expectations regarding sexual activity and the body's capabilities, and dispel misunderstandings regarding how a body should respond to any given sexual stimulus. An explanation of the physiology of chronic pain can be a validating experience to individuals experiencing pain. Research demonstrates that education about the physiology of pain reduces sexual and psychological distress, pain, disability, and anxiety.[91] It can also increase engagement in care by increasing self-efficacy—that is, the belief that the individual can influence their experience of pain.

**Yoga and Meditation.** Yoga is an exercise that involves stretching, relaxation, physical awareness, and the practice of mindfulness. It may be helpful for some individuals with sexual pain dysfunction. When hypertonic pelvic musculature is contributing to sexual

**Table 9-22  Pharmacologic Management of Sexual Pain Dysfunctions**

| Medication | Drug Class and Mechanism of Action | Potential Adverse Effects | Comments |
|---|---|---|---|
| **Systemic** | | | |
| **Amitriptyline** 12.5–50 mg at bedtime; starting dose 12.5 mg | Tricyclic antidepressant; serotonin–norepinephrine reuptake inhibitor  Reduces peripheral nerve sensitization | Sedation, dry eyes, dry mouth, constipation[196] | Must be titrated up for initiation and tapered down for discontinuation  Can take several weeks to see beneficial effects  Possibly more effective for generalized vulvodynia  Small risk for desire/arousal/orgasm disturbances (however, also used for dysorgasmia) |
| **Duloxetine** 60 mg once daily; starting dose 30 mg once daily | Serotonin–norepinephrine reuptake inhibitor | Nausea, dizziness, sweating | Must be titrated up for initiation and tapered down for discontinuation  Can take several weeks to see beneficial effects  Small risk for desire/arousal/orgasm disturbances (<5%)[197] |
| **Gabapentin** 300 mg three times daily; starting dose 300 mg at bedtime; maximum daily dose 2400 mg | Inhibits glutamate release; modulates neuron calcium channels[103] | Sedation, dizziness | Must be titrated up for initiation and tapered down for discontinuation  Can take up to 3 weeks at a therapeutic dose to achieve beneficial effects[196]  Three-times-daily dosing may not be feasible for all individuals |
| **Lamotrigine** 25–200 mg once daily; starting dose 25 mg once daily | Inhibits glutamate release, the main neurotransmitter of nociceptors | Risk of Stevens-Johnson syndrome (SJS) | Must be titrated slowly (dose packs are available) and discontinued immediately if any signs of rash to avoid rare risk of SJS  Must be tapered down for discontinuation  Can take several weeks to see beneficial effects  Numerous medication interactions (including estrogen) |
| **Topical** | | | |
| As part of a gradual desensitization and self-familiarization process, the process of applying topical medications can be therapeutic in and of itself. | | | |
| **Lidocaine 5% ointment** Applied 1–2 times daily to the vestibule and 30 minutes prior to any sexual activity (or use of capsaicin). | Topical anesthetic | May experience topical irritation or burning | Can cause numbness to partner(s) |
| **Capsaicin 0.025%** 30 minutes after application of lidocaine, apply at thin layer to the affected area for 20 minutes, then rinse off at bedtime, for 12 weeks | Produces long-lasting desensitization of nociceptors at the vaginal vestibule after chronic use[193] | Topical irritation, burning, risk for chemical burn at excessively high dose or prolonged contact | Used in conjunction with lidocaine (for premedication) due to severe burning sensation  Indicated for vestibulodynia—namely, neuroproliferative vulvodynia[90] |

*(continues)*

| Table 9-22 | Pharmacologic Management of Sexual Pain Dysfunctions (*continued*) | | |
|---|---|---|---|
| **Medication** | **Drug Class and Mechanism of Action** | **Potential Adverse Effects** | **Comments** |
| **Baclofen, topical**<br>Vaginal suppository; dosage recommendations vary | Skeletal muscle relaxant | Topical use may limit some systemic side effects, but absorption through mucous membranes may result in sedation or nausea | Must be compounded<br>Can be indicated for overactive pelvic floor |
| **Diazepam, topical**<br>Vaginal suppository; dosage recommendations vary | Benzodiazepine; acts on GABA receptors; antianxiolytic, antispasmodic | Sedation, medication interactions, respiratory depression, or dependence[93] | Must be compounded<br>Readily absorbed through mucous membranes; risk of systemic absorption, systemic effects, dependency and abuse<br>Helpful with dysfunctions associated with an overactive pelvic floor |
| **Estrogen (topical):**<br>Topical cream, intravaginal tablet, or low-dose intravaginal ring | Improve tissue integrity, elasticity; modulate nociceptors; improve tissue lubrication[188] | Local irritation | Risk of systemic absorption negligible for most formulations and applications; use with caution when contraindications to systemic estrogens are present<br>Helpful with provoked vulvodynia and pain secondary to VVA from any condition decreasing endogenous sex hormones (hyperprolactinemia, menopause, lactation, CHC use) |
| **Estradiol 0.01%/ testosterone 0.1%**<br>Apply to affected area at bedtime | Acts on local estrogen and androgen receptors; promotes tissue integrity | Small, but potential risk for androgenizing effects; monitor serum total testosterone levels as needed | Must be compounded (preferably in a methylcellulose gel base)<br>Risk of systemic absorption negligible for most formulations and applications; use with caution when contraindications to systemic estrogens are present<br>Helpful with provoked vulvodynia and pain secondary to VVA from any condition decreasing endogenous sex hormones (hyperprolactinemia, menopause, lactation, CHC use) |
| **Prasterone (DHEA)**<br>Insert 6.5-mg suppository into the vagina once nightly at bedtime | DHEA is converted to both estrogen and testosterone locally in the genital tissues where it is applied | Vaginal discharge, abnormal Pap test results | Does not increase serum estrogen or testosterone levels<br>Indicated for dyspareunia and vulvodynia secondary to VVA, for female-assigned individuals with hypogonadism |

Abbreviations: CHC, combined hormonal contraceptive; DHEA, dehydroepiandrosterone; VVA, vulvovaginal atrophy.

pain dysfunction, caution is advised against practices that involve excessive core or pelvic muscle exercise.

***Mindfulness-Based Therapy.*** See the "Psychological Management of Sexual Dysfunctions" section.

***Sex Therapy.*** Sensate focus and directed masturbation components of sex therapy can be used to facilitate the exploration of one's own body and ultimately improve familiarity with responses to varying sexual stimuli and physical boundaries.

*Individual and Partnered Psychotherapy.* Individual or partnered therapy can be beneficial to improve sexual communication skills in general, but also to help partners learn to communicate with each other about sexual pain.[199] Individual psychotherapy can assist individuals in addressing associated psychosocial factors that can complicate treatment, such as poor sense of self-worth or self-efficacy, a history of trauma, ongoing depression or anxiety, or internalized gender norms and roles.

Partnered therapy or couples counseling can be helpful for individuals who are struggling with navigating sexual pain dysfunction in their relationship.[199] An estimated 40% to 60% of individuals do not share their experience of pain during sexual activity with their sexual partner(s).[87] Individuals who communicate with their partner(s) about the experience of sexual pain have less pain and higher sexual satisfaction. The way in which a partner responds to the disclosure of pain with sexual activity affects the individual's pain experience.[89]

### Pelvic Floor Physical Therapy

Pelvic floor physical therapy is helpful for individuals with FARSS and MARSS who are experiencing sexual pain dysfunction. Pelvic floor physical therapists provide very detailed neuromusculoskeletal evaluations and tailor treatment plans to the individual. Treatment modalities include desensitization exercises, pelvic floor relaxation exercises, transcutaneous electrical nerve stimulation (TENS) units, and biofeedback.[200] Treatments are often provided in weekly sessions, with regular home activities for patients between appointments, over the course of 10 to 16 sessions. As with any other physical therapy program, the home practice of these skills and activities is critical for success.[199]

*Desensitization.* Desensitization refers to the overall process in which an individual is slowly and gradually presented with intensifying stimulation known to cause pain to increase the pain threshold. By removing the pressures of the sexual context, processing painful sensations in a controlled and supportive clinical setting can help reduce anxiety and fear. Concurrent CBT can help amplify this effect.[201]

*Biofeedback.* Biofeedback allows an individual, through the use of electromyography (EMG), to monitor their own muscle activity with visual and/or auditory feedback, so as to improve their own kinesthetic awareness of the pelvic floor muscles and how they can control their function.[200]

*Pelvic Floor Relaxation Exercises.* Individuals experiencing sexual dysfunction due to pain with sexual activity are more likely to have over-active pelvic floor muscles. Many will benefit from exercises that target awareness of the pelvic floor musculature and their relaxation.

*Vaginal Dilators.* Designed for vaginal insertion, vaginal dilators are made of nonporous materials, such as silicone or borosilicate, and typically come as a set of graduated diameters of increasing size. Under the guidance of a pelvic floor therapist, sex therapist, or clinician, they can be used for desensitization. Individuals who listen to soothing music or practice mindfulness meditation during dilation can experience more benefits from vaginal dilation.[202]

*Genital TENS Units.* TENS units use low-voltage electrical current to stimulate multiple nerve receptors at the area of pain. The competing signals block or modulate the experience of pain and release natural endorphins. TENS units designed for genital use are particularly helpful for individuals experiencing dyspareunia and vulvodynia.[93]

*Myofascial Release and Manual Techniques.* Internal manual therapy is used to release trigger points, mobilize scar tissue, and relieve pelvic adhesions that restrict the movement of muscles and organs within the pelvis to improve pelvic pain.[200,203]

*Bladder and Bowel Training.* Urinary and bowel dysfunction are common comorbidities with pelvic pain dysfunction, particularly when related to a hypertonic pelvic floor. Pelvic floor physical therapists work with patients to develop more functional bladder and bowel evacuation habits as part of a comprehensive plan of care.

### Dysfunction-Specific Management
#### Genital–Pelvic Pain Dysfunction and Dyspareunia

The core component of managing genital–pelvic pain dysfunction is addressing any underlying or co-occurring pelvic pathologies that may have causal or contributory roles in the disorder. Due to the sensitization that occurs with chronic pain, sexual pain can persist despite treatment of the original pathology, and additional management follows the principles outlined earlier.

In individuals with genital–pelvic pain dysfunction associated with endometriosis, nonpenetrative sexual activities are associated with significantly higher sexual satisfaction.[204] Recommending modification of sexual activities accordingly is reasonable. Penetration-limiting sex devices (such as the Ohnut) can prevent pain associated with deeper penetrative sexual activities. Positional variation can also help.

### Dysorgasmia and Painful Ejaculation

Few resources are available to guide the management of dysorgasmia. Of all pharmacologic interventions, amitriptyline has the most support for use in individuals with FARSS.

Once infectious causes are ruled out, individuals with MARSS experiencing painful ejaculation are best served by referral to urology for further evaluation and management.

### Vulvar Pain and Vulvodynia

Management of any modifiable associated factors, including general advice for vulvar care and avoidance of irritants, and prompt treatment of infectious vaginitis are important preventive components of a comprehensive plan of care. Optimizing tissue integrity is pivotal in the management of vulvar pain dysfunction. This is often more obvious at mid-life and menopause, but is pertinent anytime an individual has risk factors for local hypoestrogenism or hypoandrogenism (e.g., combined hormonal contraceptive or spironolactone use). In these cases, a trial of topical estrogen or of compounded topical estrogen and testosterone is a reasonable intervention.

## Lifespan Considerations

Sexuality is an important component of health throughout the lifespan. However, major life transitions, including pregnancy, parenting, and menopause, can create stressors that present challenges to sexual wellness. Additionally, mischaracterization of older adults as asexual beings creates a barrier to sexual health in later stages of life. Supporting individuals throughout the perinatal period, in the menopausal transition, and into older adulthood are essential components of midwifery care. Understanding challenges to sexual health during these periods of life is essential for holistic and sex-positive midwifery care.

### Pregnancy

The perinatal period is associated with numerous biopsychosocial factors that affect sexuality, including a rapidly changing body that may be accompanied by dysphoria, changes in body image,

neuroendocrine changes, discomforts of pregnancy, lactation, mood disturbances, fatigue, stress, and shifting priorities.[205] These factors are particularly impactful for individuals, couples, and families that are also experiencing a transition to parenthood, where new aspects of their identities and relationships as co-parents are emerging.[206] Sexual satisfaction is a component of relationship function and impacts the wellness of both gestational and nongestational parents, as well as offspring.[206] As many as 73% of pregnant individuals report difficulties with sexual functioning during pregnancy, and more than half report decreased sexual satisfaction. In the postpartum period, 21% to 64% of parents report sexual and/or relationship problems,[207] with evidence of a steep increase in incidence compared to the prepregnancy period.[208]

Perinatal sex education[209] and research to guide recommendations for perinatal sexual practices are limited. Misconceptions about the safety of sexual activity during pregnancy are common and affect experiences of sexuality and sexual satisfaction.[207] Yet, sexual activity with and without vaginal penetration, and with and without orgasm, is generally safe in uncomplicated pregnancies. Table 9-23 outlines general principles for providing advice on sexual activity during pregnancy.[210–212]

Multiple components of sexual activity can trigger uterine contractions, primarily due to endogenous oxytocin production, and to a lesser extent exogenous prostaglandin exposure (i.e., sexual activity where semen is introduced into the vagina). These activities include nipple stimulation, sexual activities that elicit the Ferguson reflex (i.e., any vaginal or anal insertive sexual activity that applies force to the cervix or lower uterine segment), and orgasm. Not all individuals will experience uterine contractions in response to sexual activity. In uncomplicated pregnancies, contractions that are not painful and that are limited to 1 to 2 hours after sexual activity are generally not concerning. When complications of pregnancy arise, particularly those that would be exacerbated by uterine activity or mechanical force, recommendations for sexual practices are individualized. Due to limited research in this area, advice relies heavily on the precautionary principle (i.e., in the absence of validated scientific data, an abundance of caution is warranted where potential complications can be catastrophic) and harm reduction (i.e., reducing the potentially negative consequences of an activity when the activity is ongoing).

Avoiding sexual stimulation that triggers uterine contractions is prudent when contractions associated with sexual activity last longer than 1 to 2 hours or

| Table 9-23 | General Considerations for Sexual Activity in Pregnancy |
| --- | --- |

- In uncomplicated pregnancies, sexual activity is generally considered safe. The cervix and lower uterine segment tolerate the impact of mechanical force from penetrative sexual activity. The fetus is protected from force by the cervix, uterus, and amniotic fluid. Contractions that are not painful and that are limited to 1–2 hours after sexual activity are generally not concerning

- Individualize advice whenever possible. Recommendations are based on pregnancy history, comorbidities, individual sexual practices, and the patient's and partner(s)' fears and emotional needs.

- Individual responses to sexual stimuli vary (i.e., impact on uterine activity, bleeding) and help guide recommendations.

- It is common to experience changes in sexuality during pregnancy.

- When discomforts of pregnancy are present, desire or the experience of sexual activity can be impacted.

- Increased blood flow and tissue sensitivity in the breasts/chest and genitals can be associated with positive experiences like pleasure, or more negative experiences like swelling and discomfort.

- Communication with partner(s), trying different positions, and using a lubricant can be helpful to accommodate physical changes associated with pregnancy.

- In high-risk pregnancies, research is very limited, and more is needed to make validated recommendations. Utilize the precautionary principle and harm reduction strategies when necessary.

Based on MacPhedran SE. Sexual activity recommendations in high-risk pregnancies: what is the evidence? *Sex Med Rev.* 2018;6(3): 343-357; Sex during pregnancy. *J Midwifery Womens Health.* 2017;62(5). doi:10.1111/jmwh.12677; and Jones C, Chan C, Farine D. Sex in pregnancy. *CMAJ.* 2011;183(7):815-818.

are painful, and in any pregnancy in which a problematic condition would be exacerbated by contractions or is a contraindication to a contraction stress test (CST). This includes situations in which there is an indication for or presence of cervical cerclage, or when there is a history of preterm labor or birth, shortened cervix, placental abruption, placental insufficiency, placenta previa, or vasa previa. Approaches such as wearing a supportive bra during sexual activity, avoiding or modifying insertive sexual activities with penetration-limiting devices or positioning, using withdrawal or condoms, and avoiding sexual stimulation that leads to contractions can be considered. Similar strategies can be employed in pregnancies where mechanical forces (e.g., rhythmic movement, thrusting) during sexual activity could have adverse impacts (e.g., cervical cerclage, placental abruption, placenta previa, or vasa previa).

## Postpartum

In the postpartum period, when to resume sexual activity is the most common sexuality concern. At 6 weeks postpartum, fewer than half of gestational parents have resumed sexual activity. At 8 and 12 weeks postpartum, 51% to 65% and 78% have resumed sexual activity, respectively.[208] Deciding when to resume sexual activity is highly individualized and is influenced by factors such as mode of delivery, birth-associated trauma or injury, the presence of postpartum complications, lactation, cultural practices, individual/partner preferences, body image, sleep, and support. There is no particular time at which resuming sexual activity is appropriate, with the exception of waiting for lacerations or surgical wounds to heal and for the birthing individual to be ready. Additional recommendations include using a vaginal lubricant, particularly if the individual is lactating; trying alternative positions for comfort during penetrative vaginal intercourse; and engaging in other sexual and nonsexual forms of intimacy. Scheduling additional postpartum visits after the resumption of sexual activity or after 12 to 16 weeks postpartum can facilitate the identification and management of postpartum sexual concerns.

In the absence of pain or distress, waiting to resume sexual activity does not imply dysfunction. However, if dysfunction is inhibiting a return to sexual activity, it should be addressed. Trauma to the pelvic floor and pelvic floor dysfunction can take longer to heal and resolve than the typically conceptualized recovery period of 6 to 8 weeks and may require an intervention such as pelvic floor physical therapy. Once resumed, the frequency of coupled sexual activity tends to decrease, but does return to prepregnancy rates at about 12 months postpartum.[208]

## Menopause, Middle, and Later Life

The onset of menopause and increasing incidence of erectile dysfunction (ED) during midlife are associated with a mischaracterization of midlife as an inflection point for sexual function. Sexual satisfaction has a positive association with well-being, quality of life, and relationship quality in mid and later life.[213-215] Data from the U.S. National Social, Life, Health and Aging Project (2007) indicate that more than half of adults aged 57 to 85 and about one-third of adults aged 75 to 85 years are sexually active.[216] Except for ED and orgasmic dysfunction in individuals with MARSS, increasing biologic age and the menopausal transition are not inevitably or directly associated with sexual problems in the general population.[217,218] Challenges to sexual wellness in mid and later life are better characterized as responses to biopsychosocial factors affecting individuals during that particular stage of life, rather than as being related to age itself.[217] Decline in health is associated with diminished sexual activity and satisfaction.[213] Increased incidence of chronic health conditions, illness, and malignancy with advancing age can pose barriers to sexual health. Health conditions can have both direct (e.g., disruption in genital response owing to disease, surgery, chemotherapy, or pain) and indirect (e.g., diminished self-image, energy level, or mobility) effects on sexual function.[219] Psychosocial and cultural factors at midlife can also contribute to risks for sexual dysfunction, such as the stress of family and work obligations, caregiving responsibilities, and changes in body and body image. Having a partner, and gaining a new partner, are positively associated with sexual function in women.[220] Conversely, relationship factors such as partner health conditions or sexual dysfunction, relationship discord, or loss of a partner (divorce, death) can contribute to dysfunction.[221] Subjective age or feeling older and attitudes about aging are factors that can impact sexuality in mid and later life as well.[222]

Menopause has a unique impact on sexuality. Individuals report both negative and positive changes in sexuality with this life transition.[223]

Biologic factors associated with menopause and the decrease in ovarian steroidogenesis (e.g., genitourinary syndrome of menopause [GSM]) as well as genitourinary and reproductive system conditions (e.g., pelvic organ prolapse) can contribute to sexual dysfunctions such as diminished desire or arousal, vaginal dryness, or pain dysfunctions.[221] Treating or facilitating access to care for conditions associated with sexual dysfunction, such as management of GSM for new-onset dyspareunia, typically improve sexual function.

Many individuals develop adaptations that facilitate a fulfilling sex life as challenges to sexual health arise; these changes are then associated with positive experiences. Such adaptations include changes in behavior (e.g., trying new sexual activities or positions, or using sexual aids and devices) and prioritizing different aspects of sex (e.g., valuing orgasm less and emotional connections more).[221] Changes associated with experience gained in mid and later life, including improved self-knowledge, self-acceptance, and self-confidence, also positively impact sexuality. Some individuals, particularly women, report less inhibition and feeling freer to enjoy sexual activity as their concerns about unplanned pregnancy or caring for younger children diminish.[224]

Normalizing physical changes that occur with age, especially weight gain and breast changes, can help support a positive body image and sexual health.[225] Addressing sexual concerns during mid and later life draws on the same principles as the general midwifery approach to sexual health. Considerations include biopsychosocial changes associated with menopause, midlife, and later life, and may require specific anticipatory guidance or more frequent screening for sexual dysfunction. Management goals may vary to accommodate physiologic and psychosocial changes associated with aging, the impact of chronic conditions and their long-term sequelae, and polypharmacy.

## Resources
### Approach to Care Resources

| Organization/Project | Description |
| --- | --- |
| American Academy of Family Physicians (AAFP) Everyone Project Toolkit | Online resource to assist the healthcare team to address social determinants of health. |
| Substance Abuse and Mental Health Services Administration (SAMHSA) | SAMHSA's Concept of Trauma and Guidance for a Trauma-Informed Approach. |
| Trauma-Informed Care Implementation Resource Center | Resources from trauma-informed care leaders across the United States. |
| Supporting Organizational Sustainability to Address Violence Against Women Institute (SOS Institute) | Online toolkit of resources for creating a trauma-informed organizational culture and environment. |

| Organization/Project | Description |
|---|---|
| The Alternative Sexualities Health Research Alliance (TASHRA) | Nonprofit organization dedicated to championing kink competent health care. |
| | Publications: |
| | *Elemental Kink Readiness to Advanced Kink Proficiencies for Medical and Mental Health Providers* |
| | *Clinical Practice Guidelines for Working with People with Kink Interests* |
| National Coalition for Sexual Freedom's (NCLR) Kink and Poly Aware Professionals (KAP) Directory | Directory of psychotherapeutic, medical, legal and other professionals who self-identify as knowledgeable about and sensitive to diverse expressions of sexuality. |

*Mandatory Reporting Resources*

| Report Type | Resources |
|---|---|
| Sexual assault | Rape, Abuse, & Incest National Network (RAINN) |
| Child abuse | Rape, Abuse, & Incest National Network (RAINN) Mandatory Reporting by State Database, Children |
| | Futures Without Violence Compendium of State and U.S. Territory Statutes and Policies on Domestic Violence and Health Care |
| Elderly/disabled adult abuse | Rape, Abuse, & Incest National Network (RAINN) Mandatory Reporting by State Database, Disabled/Elderly Adults |
| | Futures Without Violence Compendium of State and U.S. Territory Statutes and Policies on Domestic Violence and Health Care |
| | National Center on Elder Abuse (NCEA) |

*National Hotlines/Helplines*

| Hotline/Helpline | Contact Information |
|---|---|
| National Domestic Violence Hotline | 1-800-799-7233 |
| | 1-800-787-3224 (TTY) |
| National Dating Abuse Helpline | 1-866-331-9474 |
| | 1-866-331-8453 (TTY) |
| | Text "Loveis" to 22522 |
| National Sexual Assault Hotline | 1-800-656-HOPE (4673) |
| National Victims of Crime Hotline | 1-855-4-VICTIM (1-855-484-2846) |
| National Child Abuse Hotline | 1-800-4-A-CHILD (1-800-422-4453) |
| U.S. Administration of Aging Eldercare Locator | 1-800-677-1116 |
| StrongHearts Native Helpline | 1-844-7NATIVE (1-844-762-8483) |
| The Network/La Red Hotline | 1-800-832-1901 |
| 24-hour support for LGBTQI+ and kink/polyamorous individuals who are or have been abused by a partner(s) | |
| National Human Trafficking Hotline | 1-888-373-7888 |

*Sexual Violence Resources*

| Organization | Resources |
|---|---|
| National Coalition Against Domestic Violence (NCADV) | Personalized safety plan<br>Tips for accessing resources after sexual assault (getting help from law enforcement, seeking legal advice) |
| Futures Without Violence; National Health Resource Center on Domestic Violence Family Violence Prevention Fund (FVPF) | Coding and documentation for domestic violence<br>Healthcare guide for survivors of domestic and sexual violence |
| Justice Department Office on Violence Against Women (OVW) | List of local resources and coalitions by state, quick identification of resources for victims |
| National Sexual Violence Resource Center | Directory of organizations |
| Rape, Abuse, & Incest National Network (RAINN) | Rape and sexual assault crime definitions by state<br>Consent laws by state |
| National Center on Elder Abuse (NCEA) | Directory listing of state reporting numbers, government agencies, state laws, state-specific data and statistics, and other resources |

*Professional Roles and Resources for Interdisciplinary Collaboration*

| Profession | Title | Role | Professional Organization |
|---|---|---|---|
| Health Education | Sexuality educator | Develop curriculum, train, and teach in one-on-one sessions, lectures, workshops, or courses on a range of sexuality topics including sexual health, pregnancy prevention, sexually transmitted infection prevention, sexual orientation, gender identity, and sexual function and dysfunction across the lifespan. | American Association of Sexuality Educators, Counselors and Therapists (AASECT) |
| Behavioral Health | Sexuality counselor | Represent a variety of professions, including healthcare professionals and clergy. Assist individuals with concerns through education, problem-solving techniques of communication, and suggestion of exercises and techniques in sexual expression. Sexuality counseling is generally short term, focusing on an immediate concern. | |
| Behavioral Health | Sex therapist | Licensed mental health professionals trained to assess, diagnose, and provide in-depth psychotherapy to individuals with sexual issues and concerns. May provide comprehensive and intensive psychotherapy over an extended period of time in more complex cases. | |
| Nursing | Sexual Assault Nurse Examiner (SANE) | Registered nurses who have completed specialized training in the medical forensic care of individuals who have experienced sexual assault or abuse. SANEs are certified in accordance with the population that they serve: Sexual Assault Nurse Examiner-Adult/Adolescent (SANE-A) and the Sexual Assault Nurse Examiner-Pediatric (SANE-P). | International Association of Forensic Nurses (IAFN) |

| Profession | Title | Role | Professional Organization |
|---|---|---|---|
| Medical/Surgical | Gynecologist | Physician/surgeon who specializes in the care of individuals with female-assigned reproductive and sexual systems (breasts, vulva, vagina, uterus, ovaries). | American College of Obstetricians and Gynecologists (ACOG) |
| | Urologist | Physician/surgeon who specializes in health issues of the urinary tract (urethra, bladder, ureters, kidneys) and the male-assigned reproductive and sexual systems (penis, testes, scrotum, prostate). | American Board of Urology (ABU) American Urological Association |
| | Urogynecologist/ female pelvic medicine and reconstructive surgery | Physician/surgeon who specializes in the care of individuals with female-assigned reproductive and sexual systems (vulva, vagina, uterus, ovaries) and pelvic floor disorders. | American Urogynecologic Society (AUGS) |
| Physical Therapy | Pelvic health physical therapists | Licensed physical therapists (PTs) who complete additional training in pelvic health and treat pelvic pain, pelvic floor dysfunction, sexual dysfunction, urinary and bowl dysfunction, and pregnancy and postpartum musculoskeletal dysfunction, as well as other conditions. Use education, exercise, manual therapy, biofeedback, and therapeutic tools to restore strength, mobility, and function in the affected area/system. | American Physical Therapy Association (APTA) Academy of Pelvic Health Physical Therapy (APTA Pelvic Health) |
| Interdisciplinary Professional Organizations | Sexuality specialist/ sexologist | Content specialists within the role and scope of a corresponding profession (e.g. nursing, midwifery, medicine, psychology, behavioral health, social work). Available for consultation, collaboration, co-management, and referral. | America College of Sexologists (ACS) International Society of Sexual Medicine (ISSM) International Society of Women's Sexual Health (ISSWSH) |
| | Gender specialist | | World Professional Association for Transgender Health (WPATH) |

## Bibliotherapy Resources

| Title | Description |
|---|---|
| **Internet** | |
| Sex Positive Families | Provides education and resources that help families discuss and navigate sexuality with children. |
| ScarleTeen | Inclusive, comprehensive, supportive sexuality and relationships information for teens and emerging adults. |
| Native Youth Sexual Health Network (NYSHN) | Works with Indigenous peoples across Canada and the United States to advocate for and build strong, comprehensive, and culturally safe sexuality and reproductive health, rights, and justice initiatives in their own communities. |

*(continues)*

| Title | Description |
|---|---|
| **Internet** | |
| OMGYes! | Web-based paid sex education resource center for cis-women and sexual pleasure; develops large-scale studies in partnership with Indiana University and the Kinsey Institute on women ages 18–95. Focuses on sexual stimulation techniques. |
| Kinsey Institute FAQs & Sex Information | Answers, statistics, and resources that address frequently asked questions about sexuality. |
| American Psychological Association's (APA) Aging & Human Sexuality Resource Guide | Compilation of resources for providers and patients including journal articles, books, book chapters, handouts, and organizations. |
| **Books** | |
| *Our Bodies, Our Selves* | A historically influential health education book that has been translated in more than 33 different languages; it is no longer being updated, but is still in wide circulation. First published in 1970 and most recently published in 2011; provides evidence-based information on girls' and women's health. In 2018, in partnership with Suffolk University's Center for Women's Health and Human Rights, began to develop a new online platform for girls, women, nonbinary, and transmasculine individuals called Our Bodies Ourselves Today. |
| *Come as You Are: The Surprising New Science That Will Transform Your Sex Life* by Emily Nagoski | Accessible presentation of relevant research regarding desire, pleasure, and mindfulness. A complementary workbook for use in conjunction while reading the book is also available (*The Come as You Are Workbook*). |
| *Trans Bodies, Trans Selves: A Resource for the Transgender Community* | Resource guide for transgender, gender-expansive, and nonbinary populations, covering health, legal issues, cultural and social questions, history, theory, and more. |
| *The Ultimate Guide to Sex and Disability: For All of Us Who Live with Disabilities, Chronic Pain, and Illness* by Miriam Kaufman | Written by a physician and sex educator for the general public, regardless of sex, gender, or sexual orientation. |
| *Naked at Our Age: Talking Out Loud About Senior Sex* by Joan Price | Informative guide to sex for seniors, including single and coupled, heterosexual and gay. |
| *Mating in Captivity: Unlocking Erotic Intelligence* by Esther Perel | Written by an experienced couples therapist, this book explores the complexities of maintaining desire in long-term relationships and provides practical suggestions for improving erotic connection. |
| *The State of Affairs: Rethinking Infidelity* by Esther Perel | Examines love and relationship structures from multiple angles, inviting readers into an honest and entertaining exploration of modern marriage in its many variations. |
| *Heal Pelvic Pain: A Proven Stretching, Strengthening, and Nutrition Program for Relieving Pain, Incontinence, IBS, and Other Symptoms Without Surgery* by Amy Stein | Written by a physical therapist for the general population, but is also useful for clinicians. Provides practical strategies and techniques for addressing pelvic pain associated with pelvic floor dysfunction. |

*Professional Resources*

| National | Global |
|---|---|
| American Association of Sexuality Educators, Counselors, and Therapists (ASSECT) | International Society of Sexual Medicine (ISSM) (Publishes the *Journal of Sexual Medicine*) |
| America College of Sexologists (ACS) | International Society of Women's Sexual Health (ISSWSH) |
| American Sexual Health Association (ASHA) | World Association for Sexual Health (WAS) |
| Association of Black Sexologists and Clinicians (ABSC) | World Health Organization (WHO) |
| GLMA: Health Professionals Advancing LGBTQ Equality (GLMA) | Sexual Medicine Society of North America (SMSNA) |
| International Society for the Study of Vulvovaginal Disease (ISSVD) | Society for the Scientific Study of Sexuality (SSSS) |
| National Vulvodynia Association (NVA) | |
| Society for Sex Therapy & Research (STARR) (Publishes the *Journal of Sex and Marital Therapy*) | |
| Women of Color Sexual Health Network (WoCSHN) | |
| SIECUS: Sex Ed for Social Change (Formerly the Sexuality Information and Education Council of the United States) | |

## References

1. Sexual health. World Health Organization. https://www.who.int/health-topics/sexual-health#tab=tab_2. Accessed January 29, 2023.

2. Declaration of sexual rights. World Association for Sexual Health. 2014. https://worldsexualhealth.net/wp-content/uploads/2013/08/Declaration-of-Sexual-Rights-2014-plain-text.pdf. 2014. Accessed February 14, 2023.

3. Understanding sexual health. American Sexual Health Association. https://www.ashasexualhealth.org/sexual-health/. Last updated December 9, 2022. Accessed January 29, 2023.

4. Sexual health and its linkages to reproductive health: an operational approach. World Health Organization. Published 2017. https://apps.who.int/iris/handle/10665/258738. License: CC BY-NC-SA 3.0 IGO. Accessed February 14, 2023.

5. Sexual rights: an IPPF declaration. International Planned Parenthood Federation. Published 2008. https://www.ippf.org/resource/sexual-rights-ippf-declaration. Accessed February 14, 2023.

6. Sexual rights. Sexual Rights Initiative. https://www.sexualrightsinitiative.org/sexual-rights.

7. Our philosophy of care. American College of Nurse Midwives. https://www.midwife.org/our-philosophy-of-care. Accessed January 29, 2023.

8. Core competencies for basic midwifery practice. American College of Nurse-Midwives. https://www.midwife.org/acnm/files/acnmlibrarydata/uploadfilename/000000000050/ACNMCoreCompetenciesMar2020_final.pdf. Published 2020. Accessed January 29, 2023.

9. Basson R. Women's sexual function and dysfunction: current uncertainties, future directions. *Int J Impot Res*. 2008;20(5):466-478.

10. Masters WH, Johnson VE. *Human Sexual Response*. New York, NY: Ishi Press International; 1966.

11. van Anders SM, Herbenick D, Brotto LA, et al. The heteronormativity theory of low sexual desire in women partnered with men. *Arch Sex Behav*. 2021:1-25. doi: 10.1007/s10508-021-02100-x. Epub 2021 Aug 23. PMID: 34426898; PMCID: PMC8382213.

12. Singer B, Toates FM. Sexual motivation. *J Sex Res*. 1987;23(4):481-501.

13. Kaplan HS. Hypoactive sexual desire. *J Sex Marital Ther*. 1977;3(1):3-9.

14. Basson R. Human sex-response cycles. *J Sex Marital Ther*. 2001;27(1):33-43.

15. Holmberg M, Arver S, Dhejne C. Supporting sexuality and improving sexual function in transgender persons. *Nat Rev Urol*. 2019;16(2):121-139.

16. Baber KM, Murray CI. A postmodern feminist approach to teaching human sexuality. *Fam Relat*. 2001;50(1):23-33.

17. Willis M, Hunt M, Wodika A, et al. Explicit verbal sexual consent communication: effects of gender, relationship status, and type of sexual behavior. *Int J Sex Health*. 2019;31(1):60-70.

18. Bancroft J. Central inhibition of sexual response in the male: a theoretical perspective. *Neurosci Biobehav Rev*. 1999;23(6):763-784.

19. Janssen E, Bancroft J. The dual control model: the role of sexual inhibition and excitation in sexual arousal and behavior. *Psychophysiol Sex*. 2007;15:197-222.

20. Bancroft J, Graham CA, Janssen E, Sanders SA. The dual control model: current status and future directions. *J Sex Res.* 2009;46(2-3):121-142.

21. Kurpisz J, Mak M, Lew-Starowicz M, et al. The dual control model of sexual response by J. Bancroft and E. Janssen: theoretical basis, research and practical issues. *Postępy Psychiatrii i Neurologii.* 2015;24(3):156-164.

22. Jabs F, Brotto LA. Identifying the disruptions in the sexual response cycles of women with sexual interest/arousal disorder. *Can J Hum Sex.* 2018;27(2):123-132.

23. Perelman MA. The Sexual Tipping Point: a mind/body model for sexual medicine. *J Sex Med.* 2009;6(3):629-632.

24. Nagoski E. *Come as You Are: The Surprising New Science That Will Transform Your Sex Life.* New York, NY: Simon and Schuster; 2015.

25. Driscoll M, Basson R, Brotto L, et al. Empirically supported incentive model of sexual response ignored. *J Sex Med.* 2017;14(5):758-759.

26. Basson R. The female sexual response: a different model. *J Sex Marital Ther.* 2000;26(1):51-65.

27. Basson R. Using a different model for female sexual response to address women's problematic low sexual desire. *J Sex Marital Ther.* 2001;27(5):395-403.

28. Thomas HN, Thurston RC. A biopsychosocial approach to women's sexual function and dysfunction at midlife: a narrative review. *Maturitas.* 2016;87:49-60.

29. Althof SE, Meston CM, Perelman MA, et al. Opinion paper: on the diagnosis/classification of sexual arousal concerns in women. *J Sex Med.* 2017;14(11):1365-1371. doi:10.1016/j.jsxm.2017.08.013.

30. Balon R, Clayton AH. Female sexual interest/arousal disorder: a diagnosis out of thin air. *Arch Sex Behav.* 2014;43(7):1227-1229. doi:10.1007/s10508-013-0247-1.

31. Sarin S, Amsel R, Binik YM. A streetcar named "Derousal"? A psychophysiological examination of the desire–arousal distinction in sexually functional and dysfunctional women. *J Sex Res.* 2016;53(6):711-729. doi:10.1080/00224499.2015.1052360.

32. Spurgas AK. Interest, arousal, and shifting diagnoses of female sexual dysfunction, or: how women learn about desire. *Stud Gend Sex.* 2013;14(3):187-205. doi:10.1080/15240657.2013.818854.

33. Derogatis LR, Sand M, Balon R, et al. Toward a more evidence-based nosology and nomenclature for female sexual dysfunctions: Part I. *J Sex Med.* 2016;13(12):1881-1887. doi:10.1016/j.jsxm.2016.09.014.

34. O'Loughlin JI, Basson R, Brotto LA. Women with hypoactive sexual desire disorder versus sexual interest/ arousal disorder: an empirical test of raising the bar. *J Sex Res.* 2018;55(6):734-746. doi:10.1080/00224499.2017.1386764.

35. Parish SJ, Meston CM, Althof SE, et al. Toward a more evidence-based nosology and nomenclature for female sexual dysfunctions: Part III. *J Sex Med.* 2019;16(3):452-462. doi:10.1016/j.jsxm.2019.01.010.

36. Parish SJ, Hahn SR, Goldstein SW, et al. The International Society for the Study of Women's sexual health process of care for the identification of sexual concerns and problems in women. *Mayo Clin Proc.* 2019;94(5):842-856. doi:10.1016/j.mayocp.2019.01.009.

37. Levin RJ, van Berlo W. Sexual arousal and orgasm in subjects who experience forced or non-consensual sexual stimulation: a review. *J Clin Forensic Med.* 2004;11(2):82-88. doi:10.1016/j.jcfm.2003.10.008.

38. Lalumière ML, Sawatsky ML, Dawson SJ, Suschinsky KD. The empirical status of the preparation hypothesis: explicating women's genital responses to sexual stimuli in the laboratory. *Arch Sex Behav.* 2020. doi:10.1007/s10508-019-01599-5.

39. Goldstein I. The central mechanisms of sexual function. Boston University School of Medicine. https://www.bumc.bu.edu/sexualmedicine/publications/the-central-mechanisms-of-sexual-function/. Published February 3, 2003. Accessed January 29, 2023.

40. Vieira-Baptista P, Lima-Silva J, Preti M, et al. G-spot: fact or fiction? A systematic review. *Sex Med.* 2021;9(5). doi:10.1016/j.esxm.2021.100435.

41. Pastor Z. Female ejaculation orgasm vs. coital incontinence: a systematic review. *J Sex Med.* 2013;10(7):1682-1691. doi:10.1111/jsm.12166.

42. Female genital anatomy. Boston University School of Medicine. https://www.bumc.bu.edu/sexualmedicine/physicianinformation/female-genital-anatomy/. Published November 26, 2002. Accessed January 29, 2023.

43. Levin RJ. Prostate-induced orgasms: a concise review illustrated with a highly relevant case study. *Clin Anat.* 2018;31(1):81-85. doi:10.1002/ca.23006.

44. Croft HA. Understanding the role of serotonin in female hypoactive sexual desire disorder and treatment options. *J Sex Med.* 2017;14(12):1575-1584. doi:10.1016/j.jsxm.2017.10.068.

45. Kingsberg SA, Clayton AH, Pfaus JG. The female sexual response: current models, neurobiological underpinnings and agents currently approved or under investigation for the treatment of hypoactive sexual desire disorder. *CNS Drugs.* 2015;29(11):915-933. doi:10.1007/s40263-015-0288-1.

46. Sexual arousal. *American Psychological Association Dictionary of Psychology.* https://dictionary.apa.org/sexual-arousal. Accessed January 29, 2023.

47. Ishak WW, ed. *The Textbook of Clinical Sexual Medicine.* Cham, Switzerland: Springer; 2017. doi:10.1007/978-3-319-52539-6.

48. Meston CM, Stanton AM. Understanding sexual arousal and subjective–genital arousal desynchrony in women. *Nat Rev Urol.* 2019;16(2):107-120. doi:10.1038/s41585-018-0142-6.

49. Velten J, Milani S, Margraf J, Brotto LA. Visual attention and sexual arousal in women with and without sexual dysfunction. *Behav Res Ther.* 2021;144. doi:10.1016/j.brat.2021.103915.

50. Meston CM, Stanton AM. Desynchrony between subjective and genital sexual arousal in women: theoretically interesting but clinically irrelevant. *Curr Sex Health Rep.* 2018;10(3):73-75. doi:10.1007/s11930-018-0155-4.

51. Bouchard KN, Chivers ML, Pukall CF. Effects of genital response measurement device and stimulus characteristics on sexual concordance in women. *J Sex Res.* 2017;54(9):1197-1208. doi:10.1080/00224499.2016.1265641.

52. Levin RJ. The pharmacology of the human female orgasm: its biological and physiological backgrounds. *Pharmacol Biochem Behav.* 2014;121:62-70.

53. Alwaal A, Breyer BN, Lue TF. Normal male sexual function: emphasis on orgasm and ejaculation. *Fertil Steril.* 2015;104(5):1051-1060.

54. Bhat GS, Shastry A. Time to orgasm in women in a monogamous stable heterosexual relationship. *J Sex Med.* 2020;17(4):749-760. doi:10.1016/j.jsxm.2020.01.005.

55. Clavell-Hernández J, Martin C, Wang R. Orgasmic dysfunction following radical prostatectomy: review of current literature. *Sex Med Rev.* 2018;6(1):124-134. doi:10.1016/j.sxmr.2017.09.003.

56. Shaeer O, Skakke D, Giraldi A, et al. Female orgasm and overall sexual function and habits: a descriptive study of a cohort of U.S. women. *J Sex Med.* 2020;17(6):1133-1143. doi:10.1016/j.jsxm.2020.01.029.

57. Garcia JR, Lloyd EA, Wallen K, Fisher HE. Variation in orgasm occurrence by sexual orientation in a sample of U.S. singles. *J Sex Med.* 2014;11(11):2645-2652. doi:10.1111/jsm.12669.

58. Alwaal A, Breyer BN, Lue TF. Normal male sexual function: emphasis on orgasm and ejaculation. *Fertil Steril.* 2015;104(5):1051-1060. doi:10.1016/j.fertnstert.2015.08.033.

59. What is the refractory period? International Society for Sexual Medicine. https://www.issm.info/sexual-health-qa/what-is-the-refractory-period/#:~:text=It%20may%20take%20a%20half,can%20last%20a%20few%20days. Accessed January 29, 2023.

60. McCabe MP, Sharlip ID, Lewis R, et al. Incidence and prevalence of sexual dysfunction in women and men: a consensus statement from the Fourth International Consultation on Sexual Medicine 2015. *J Sex Med.* 2016;13(2):144-152. doi:10.1016/j.jsxm.2015.12.034.

61. Pyke RE, Clayton AH. Lumping, splitting, and treating: therapies are needed for women with overlapping sexual dysfunctions. *Sex Med Rev.* 2019;7(4):551-558. doi:10.1016/j.sxmr.2019.04.002.

62. Kingsberg SA, Simon JA. Female hypoactive sexual desire disorder: a practical guide to causes, clinical diagnosis, and treatment. *J Womens Health.* 2020;29(8):1101-1112. doi:10.1089/jwh.2019.7865.

63. Goldstein I, Clayton AH, Goldstein AT, et al., eds. *Textbook of Female Sexual Function and Dysfunction: Diagnosis and Treatment.* Hoboken, NJ: Wiley Blackwell; 2018.

64. Kerckhof ME, Kreukels BPC, Nieder TO, et al. Prevalence of sexual dysfunctions in transgender persons: results from the ENIGI follow-up study. *J Sex Med.* 2019;16(12):2018-2029. doi:10.1016/j.jsxm.2019.09.003.

65. McCool-Myers M, Theurich M, Zuelke A, et al. Predictors of female sexual dysfunction: a systematic review and qualitative analysis through gender inequality paradigms. *BMC Womens Health.* 2018;18(1). doi:10.1186/s12905-018-0602-4.

66. Holmberg M, Arver S, Dhejne C. Supporting sexuality and improving sexual function in transgender persons. *Nat Rev Urol.* 2019;16(2):121-139. doi:10.1038/s41585-018-0108-8.

67. Based on American Psychiatric Association. *Diagnostic and Statistical Manual of Mental Disorders.* 5th ed. Text revision *(DSM-5-TR).* Arlington, VA: American Psychiatric Association; 2022.

68. Parish SJ, Cottler-Casanova S, Clayton AH, et al. The evolution of the female sexual disorder/dysfunction definitions, nomenclature, and classifications: a review of DSM, ICSM, ISSWSH, and ICD. *Sex Med Rev.* 2021;9(1):36-56. doi:10.1016/j.sxmr.2020.05.001.

69. Spurgas AK. Interest, arousal, and shifting diagnoses of female sexual dysfunction, or: how women learn about desire. *Stud Gend Sex.* 2013;14(3):187-205.

70. McCabe MP, Sharlip ID, Atalla E, et al. Definitions of sexual dysfunctions in women and men: a consensus statement from the Fourth International Consultation on Sexual Medicine 2015. *J Sex Med.* 2016;13(2):135-143. doi:10.1016/j.jsxm.2015.12.019.

71. American Psychiatric Association. *Diagnostic and Statistical Manual of Mental Disorders.* 4th ed. Washington, DC: American Psychiatric Association; 1994.

72. Moor A, Haimov Y, Shreiber S. When desire fades: women talk about their subjective experience of declining sexual desire in loving long-term relationships. *J Sex Res.* 2021;58(2):160-169. doi:10.1080/00224499.2020.1743225.

73. Kingsberg SA, Tkachenko N, Lucas J, et al. Characterization of orgasmic difficulties by women: focus group evaluation. *J Sex Med.* 2013;10(9):2242-2250. doi:10.1111/jsm.12224.

74. Parish SJ, Goldstein AT, Goldstein SW, et al. Toward a more evidence-based nosology and nomenclature for female sexual dysfunctions: Part II. *J Sex Med.* 2016;13(12):1888-1906. doi:10.1016/j.jsxm.2016.09.020.

75. Kingsberg SA, Althof S, Simon JA, et al. Female sexual dysfunction: medical and psychological treatments, Committee 14. *J Sex Med.* 2017;14(12):1463-1491. doi:10.1016/j.jsxm.2017.05.018.

76. Herbenick D, Fu TC, Arter J, et al. Women's experiences with genital touching, sexual pleasure, and orgasm: results from a U.S. probability sample of women ages 18 to 94. *J Sex Marital Ther.* 2018;44(2):201-212. doi:10.1080/0092623X.2017.1346530.

77. Frederick DA, John HKS, Garcia JR, Lloyd EA. Differences in orgasm frequency among gay, lesbian, bisexual, and heterosexual men and women in a U.S. national sample. *Arch Sex Behav.* 2018;47(1):273-288. doi:10.1007/s10508-017-0939-z.

78. Laumann EO, Paik A, Raymond Rosen MC. Sexual dysfunction in the United States: prevalence and predictors. *JAMA.* 1999;281(6):537-544. doi:10.1001/jama.281.6.537.

79. Nimbi FM, Tripodi F, Rossi R, et al. Male sexual desire: an overview of biological, psychological, sexual, relational, and cultural factors influencing desire. *Sex Med Rev.* 2020;8(1):59-91. doi:10.1016/j.sxmr.2018.12.002.

80. Nimbi FM, Tripodi F, Rossi R, Simonelli C. Expanding the analysis of psychosocial factors of sexual desire in men. *J Sex Med.* 2018;15(2):230-244. doi:10.1016/j.jsxm.2017.11.227.

81. Shifren JL, Monz BU, Russo PA, et al. Sexual problems and distress in United States women. *Obstet Gynecol.* 2008;112(5):970-978.

82. Goldstein I, Komisaruk BR, Pukall CF, et al. International Society for the Study of Women's Sexual Health (ISSWSH) review of epidemiology and pathophysiology, and a consensus nomenclature and process of care for the management of persistent genital arousal disorder/genito-pelvic dysesthesia (PGAD/GPD). *J Sex Med.* 2021;18(4):665-697. doi:10.1016/j.jsxm.2021.01.172.

83. Jackowich RA, Boyer SC, Bienias S, et al. Healthcare experiences of individuals with persistent genital arousal disorder/genito-pelvic dysesthesia. *Sex Med.* 2021;9(3). doi:10.1016/j.esxm.2021.100335.

84. Tavares IM, Laan ETM, Nobre PJ. Sexual inhibition is a vulnerability factor for orgasm problems in women. *J Sex Med.* 2018;15(3):361-372. doi:10.1016/j.jsxm.2017.12.015.

85. Rowland DL, Kolba TN. Understanding orgasmic difficulty in women. *J Sex Med.* 2016;13(8):1246-1254. doi:10.1016/j.jsxm.2016.05.014.

86. Moura CV, Tavares IM, Nobre PJ. Cognitive-affective factors and female orgasm: a comparative study on women with and without orgasm difficulties. *J Sex Med.* 2020. doi:10.1016/j.jsxm.2020.08.005.

87. Herbenick D, Schick V, Sanders SA, et al. Pain experienced during vaginal and anal intercourse with other-sex partners: findings from a nationally representative probability study in the United States. *J Sex Med.* 2015;12(4):1040-1051. doi:10.1111/jsm.12841.

88. Kerckhof ME, Kreukels BPC, Nieder TO, et al. Prevalence of sexual dysfunctions in transgender persons: results from the ENIGI follow-up study. *J Sex Med.* 2019;16(12):2018-2029.

89. Carter A, Ford JV, Luetke M, et al. "Fulfilling his needs, not mine": reasons for not talking about painful sex and associations with lack of pleasure in a nationally representative sample of women in the United States. *J Sex Med.* 2019;16(12):1953-1965. doi:10.1016/j.jsxm.2019.08.016.

90. Goldstein AT, Pukall CF, Goldstein I, eds. *Female Sexual Pain Disorders: Evaluation and Management.* 2nd ed. Hoboken, NJ: Wiley Blackwell.

91. Henzell H, Berzins K, Langford JP. Provoked vestibulodynia: current perspectives. *Int J Womens Health.* 2017;9:631-642. doi:10.2147/IJWH.S113416.

92. Orr N, Wahl K, Joannou A, et al. Deep dyspareunia: review of pathophysiology and proposed future research priorities. *Sex Med Rev.* 2020;8(1):3-17. doi:10.1016/j.sxmr.2018.12.007.

93. di Biase M, Iacovelli V, Kocjancic E. Vulvodynia: current etiology, diagnosis, and treatment. *Curr Bladder Dysfunct Rep.* 2016;11(3):248-257. doi:10.1007/s11884-016-0381-4.

94. Grabski B, Kasparek K. Sexual anal pain in gay and bisexual men: in search of explanatory factors. *J Sex Med.* 2020;17(4):716-730. doi:10.1016/j.jsxm.2020.01.020.

95. Lahaie MA, Amsel R, Khalifé S, et al. Can fear, pain, and muscle tension discriminate vaginismus from dyspareunia/provoked vestibulodynia? Implications for the new DSM-5 diagnosis of genito-pelvic pain/penetration disorder. *Arch Sex Behav.* 2015;44(6):1537-1550. doi:10.1007/s10508-014-0430-z.

96. Bornstein J, Goldstein AT, Stockdale CK, et al. 2015 ISSVD, ISSWSH, and IPPS Consensus Terminology and Classification of Persistent Vulvar Pain and Vulvodynia. *Obstet Gynecol.* 2016 Apr;127(4):745-751. doi:10.1097/AOG.0000000000001359. PMID: 27008217.

97. Yong PJ, Williams C, Yosef A, et al. Anatomic sites and associated clinical factors for deep dyspareunia. *Sex Med.* 2017;5(3):e184-e195. doi:10.1016/j.esxm.2017.07.001.

98. Caruso S, Monaco C. Dyspareunia in women: updates in mechanisms and current/novel therapies. *Curr Sex Health Rep.* 2019;11(1):9-20. doi:10.1007/s11930-019-00188-w.

99. Štulhofer A, Ajduković D. Should we take anodyspareunia seriously? A descriptive analysis of pain during receptive anal intercourse in young heterosexual women. *J Sex Marital Ther.* 2011;37(5):346-358. doi:10.1080/0092623X.2011.607039.

100. Sundström-Poromaa I, Bixo M, Björn I, Nordh O. Compliance to antidepressant drug therapy for treatment of premenstrual syndrome. *J Psychosom Obstet Gynaecol.* 2000;(4):205-11. doi: 10.3109/01674820009085589.

101. Chiles KA. Musings on male dysorgasmia. *J Sex Med.* 2017;14(4):489-490.doi:10.1016/j.jsxm.2017.01.019.

102. Reed BD, Harlow SD, Plegue MA, Sen A. Remission, relapse, and persistence of vulvodynia: a longitudinal population-based study. *J Womens Health.* 2016;25(3):276-283. doi:10.1089/jwh.2015.5397.

103. Bachmann GA, Brown CS, Phillips NA, et al. Effect of gabapentin on sexual function in vulvodynia: a randomized, placebo-controlled trial. *Am J Obstet Gynecol.* 2019;220(1):89.e1-89.e8. doi:10.1016/j.ajog.2018.10.021.

104. Metzl JM, Hansen H. Structural competency: theorizing a new medical engagement with stigma and inequality. *Soc Sci Med.* 2014;103:126-133.

105. Courtwright AM. Justice, stigma, and the new epidemiology of health disparities. *Bioethics.* 2009;23(2):90-96.

106. Herek GM. A nuanced view of stigma for understanding and addressing sexual and gender minority health disparities. *LGBT Health.* 2016;3(6):397-399.

107. Williams SL, Mann AK. Sexual and gender minority health disparities as a social issue: how stigma and intergroup relations can explain and reduce health disparities. *J Soc Issues.* 2017;73(3):450-461.

108. Gerber MR, Gerber EB. An introduction to trauma and health. In: *Trauma-Informed Healthcare Approaches.* Cham, Switzerland: Springer; 2019:3-23.

109. Tillman S. Consent in pelvic care. *J Midwifery Womens Health.* 2020;65(6):749-758.

110. SAMHSA's concept of trauma and guidance for a trauma-informed approach. Substance Abuse and Mental Health Services Administration. https://ncsacw.acf.hhs.gov/userfiles/files/SAMHSA_Trauma.pdf. 2014.

111. Tips for creating a welcoming environment. National Center on Domestic Violence, Trauma & Mental Health. http://nationalcenterdvtraumamh.org/wp-content/uploads/2012/01/Tipsheet_Welcoming-Environment_NCDVTMH_Aug2011.pdf. Published 2011.

112. Spurlin WJ. Queer theory and biomedical practice: the biomedicalization of sexuality/the cultural politics of biomedicine. *J Med Humanities.* 2019;40(1):7-20.

113. Owens DC. *Medical Bondage: Race, Gender, and the Origins of American Gynecology.* Athens, GA: University of Georgia Press; 2017.

114. Stern SW. The venereal doctrine: compulsory examinations, sexually transmitted infections, and the rape/prostitution divide. *Berkeley J Gender L Just.* 2019;34:149.

115. Pegoraro L. Second-rate victims: the forced sterilization of Indigenous peoples in the USA and Canada. *Settler Colonial Stud.* 2015;5(2):161-173.

116. Hammond BA, James C. Creating an intergroup dialogue curriculum on race for psychiatry residents. *Acad Psychiatry.* 2020;44(4):498-499.

117. Beskow LM. Lessons from HeLa cells: the ethics and policy of biospecimens. *Annu Rev Genomics Hum Genet.* 2016;17:395-417.

118. Friesen P. Educational pelvic exams on anesthetized women: why consent matters. *Bioethics.* 2018;32(5):298-307.

119. Hammoud MM, Spector-Bagdady K, O'Reilly M, et al. Consent for the pelvic examination under anesthesia by medical students: recommendations by the Association of Professors of Gynecology and Obstetrics. *Obstet Gynecol.* 2019;134(6):1303.

120. Salwi S, Erath A, Patel PD, et al. Aligning patient and physician views on educational pelvic examinations under anaesthesia: the medical student perspective. *J Med Ethics.* 2021;47(6):430-433.

121. Shalowitz DI, Anderson TL. Safeguarding against sexual misconduct. *Obstet Gynecol.* 2020;135(1):6-8.

122. Teegardin C, Norder L. Abusive doctors: how the Atlanta newspaper exposed a system that tolerates sexual misconduct by physicians. *Am J Bioethics.* 2019;19(1):1-3.

123. Kearl H. The facts behind the #metoo movement: a national study on sexual harassment and assault (executive summary). https://www.nsvrc.org/resource/facts-behind-metoo-movement-national-study-sexual-harassment-and-assault. Published 2018. Accessed February 14, 2023.

124. Smith SG, Zhang X, Basile KC, et al. The National Intimate Partner and Sexual Violence Survey: 2015 data brief—updated release. National Center for Injury Prevention and Control, Centers for Disease Control and Prevention. https://www.cdc.gov/violenceprevention/pdf/2015data-brief508.pdf. Published 2018.

125. James SE, Herman JL, Rankin S, et al. The Report of the 2015 U.S. Transgender Survey. Washington, DC: National Center for Transgender Equality. Published 2016. https://transequality.org/sites/default/files/docs/usts/USTS-Full-Report-Dec17.pdf.

126. Clemens V, Brähler E, Fegert JM. #patientstoo: professional sexual misconduct by healthcare

professionals towards patients: a representative study. *Epidemiol Psychiatr Sci.* 2021;30. doi:10.1017/S2045796021000378. PMID: 34402421; PMCID: PMC8220485.

127. DeMeester RH, Lopez FY, Moore JE, et al. A model of organizational context and shared decision making: application to LGBT racial and ethnic minority patients. *J Gen Intern Med.* 2016;31(6):651-662.

128. Palmieri J, Valentine JL. Using trauma-informed care to address sexual assault and intimate partner violence in primary care. *J Nurs Pract.* 2021;17(1):44-48.

129. The EveryONE Project Toolkit. American Academy of Family Physicians. https://www.aafp.org/family-physician/patient-care/the-everyone-project/toolkit.html. Accessed January 29, 2023.

130. Ivanski C, Kohut T. Exploring definitions of sex positivity through thematic analysis. *Can J Hum Sex.* 2017;26(3):216-225.

131. National Survey of Sexual Health and Behavior. Indiana University Bloomington. https://nationalsexstudy.indiana.edu/. Accessed January 29, 2023.

132. Herbenick D, Bowling J, Fu TC, et al. Sexual diversity in the United States: results from a nationally representative probability sample of adult women and men. *PLoS One.* 2017;12(7):e0181198-e0181198.

133. Mosher CM. Historical perspectives of sex positivity: contributing to a new paradigm within counseling psychology. *Couns Psychol.* 2017;45(4):487-503.

134. Burnes TR, Singh AA, Witherspoon RG. Sex positivity and counseling psychology: an introduction to the major contribution. *Couns Psychol.* 2017;45(4):470-486.

135. Parish SJ, Hahn SR, Goldstein SW, et al. The International Society for the Study of Women's sexual health process of care for the identification of sexual concerns and problems in women. *Mayo Clin Proc.* 2019;94:842-856.

136. Savoy M, O'Gurek DT, Brown-James A. Sexual health history: techniques and tips. *Am Fam Physician.* 2020;101(5):286-293.

137. Grimstad F, McLaren H, Gray M. The gynecologic examination of the transfeminine person after penile inversion vaginoplasty. *Am J Obstet Gynecol.* 2021;224(3):266-273.

138. Reno H, Park I, Workowski K, et al. A guide to taking a sexual history. Centers for Disease Control and Prevention. https://www.cdc.gov/std/treatment/sexualhistory.pdf. Accessed January 29, 2023.

139. Herman JL. Best practices for asking questions to identify transgender and other gender minority respondents on population-based surveys. Gender Identity in US Surveillance (GenIUSS). https://williamsinstitute.law.ucla.edu/publications/geniuss-trans-pop-based-survey. Published 2014.

140. Ammerman B, Jones H. Him too: a case report on male sexual violence and screening in primary care. *Urol Nurs.* 2020;40(1):36-39.

141. El-Serag R, Thurston RC. Matters of the heart and mind: interpersonal violence and cardiovascular disease in women. *J Am Heart Assoc.* 2020;9(4):e015479-e015479.

142. Punjani NS. Application of the extended-PLISSIT model to improve sexual health in the adolescent population: a theory. *J Comm Pub Health Nursing.* 2019;5:4. https://www.omicsonline.org/open-access/application-of-the-extendedplissit-model-to-improve-sexual-health-in-the-adolescent-population-a-theory-analysis.pdf.

143. Grover S, Shouan A. Assessment scales for sexual disorders: a review. *J Psychosex Health.* 2020;2(2):121-138.

144. Taylor B. Using the extended PLISSIT model to address sexual healthcare needs. *Nurs Standard.* 2006;21(11). doi: 10.7748/ns2006.11.21.11.35.c6382. PMID: 17165482.

145. Kingsberg SA, Janata JW. Female sexual disorders: assessment, diagnosis, and treatment. *Urol Clin North Am.* 2007;34(4):497-506.

146. Marcell AV. *Preventive Male Sexual and Reproductive Health Care: Recommendations for Clinical Practice.* Philadelphia, PA: Male Training Center for Family Planning and Reproductive Health/Rockville, MD: Office of Population Affairs; 2014.

147. Sherman MD, Hooker S, Doering A, Walther L. Communication tips for caring for survivors of sexual assault. *Fam Pract Manag.* 2019;26(4):19-23.

148. Sexual Assault Forensic Examiners. https://www.safeta.org/. Accessed January 29, 2023.

149. Expansion of midwifery practice and skills beyond basic core competencies. American College of Nurse-Midwives. http://www.midwife.org/acnm/files/ACNMLibraryData/UPLOADFILENAME/000000000066/Expansion-of-Midwifery-Practice-June-2015.pdf. Published 2015.

150. Gray DJP, Sidaway-Lee K, White E, et al. Continuity of care with doctors: a matter of life and death? A systematic review of continuity of care and mortality. *BMJ Open.* 2018;8(6):e021161-e021161.

151. Levy-Carrick NC, Lewis-O'Connor A, Rittenberg E, et al. Promoting health equity through trauma-informed care: critical role for physicians in policy and program development. *Fam Community Health.* 2019;42(2):104-108.

152. Maseroli E, Rastrelli G, di Stasi V, et al. Physical activity and female sexual dysfunction: a lot helps, but not too much. *J Sex Med.* 2021;18(7):1217-1229. doi:10.1016/j.jsxm.2021.04.004.

153. Stanton AM, Handy AB, Meston CM. The effects of exercise on sexual function in women. *Sex*

*Med Rev.* 2018;6(4):548-557. doi:10.1016/j.sxmr .2018.02.004.

154. Kumagai H, Myoenzono K, Yoshikawa T, et al. Regular aerobic exercise improves sexual function assessed by the Aging Males' Symptoms questionnaire in adult men. *Aging Male.* 2021;23(5): 1194-1201. doi:10.1080/13685538.2020.1724940.

155. Lopes IP, Ribeiro VB, Reis RM, et al. Comparison of the effect of intermittent and continuous aerobic physical training on sexual function of women with polycystic ovary syndrome: randomized controlled trial. *J Sex Med.* 2018;15(11):1609-1619. doi:10.1016/j.jsxm.2018.09.002.

156. Seehuus M, Pigeon W. The sleep and sex survey: relationships between sexual function and sleep. *J Psychosom Res.* 2018;112:59-65. doi:10.1016/j .jpsychores.2018.07.005.

157. Maness DL, Khan M. Nonpharmacologic management of chronic insomnia. *Am Fam Physician.* 2015 Dec 15;92(12):1058-1064. PMID: 26760592.

158. Rubin ES, Deshpande NA, Vasquez PJ, Kellogg Spadt S. A clinical reference guide on sexual devices for obstetrician-gynecologists. *Obstet Gynecol.* 2019;133(6):1259-1268. doi:10.1097/AOG.00000 00000003262.

159. Dewitte M, Reisman Y. Clinical use and implications of sexual devices and sexually explicit media. *Nat Rev Urol.* 2021;18(6):359-377. doi:10.1038 /s41585-021-00456-2.

160. Forrester MB. Vibrator and dildo injuries treated at emergency departments. *J Sex Marital Ther.* 2021;47(7):687-695. doi: 10.1080/0092623X.2021. 1938319. Epub 2021 Jun 18. PMID:34142642.

161. Rutala WA, Weber DJ. *Guideline for Disinfection and Sterilization in Healthcare Facilities, 2008.* 2008.

162. Weinberger JM, Houman J, Caron AT, et al. Female sexual dysfunction and the placebo effect: a meta-analysis. *Obstet Gynecol.* 2018;132(2): 453-458. doi:10.1097/AOG.0000000000002733.

163. Wheeler LJ, Guntupalli SR. Female sexual dysfunction: pharmacologic and therapeutic interventions. *Obstet Gynecol.* 2020;136(1):174-186. doi:10.1097/AOG.0000000000003941.

164. Kilmann PR, Mills KH, Bella B, et al. The effects of sex education on women with secondary orgasmic dysfunction. *J Sex Marital Ther.* 1983;9(1):79-87. doi:10.1080/00926238308405835.

165. van Lankveld JJDM, van de Wetering FT, Wylie K, Scholten RJPM. Bibliotherapy for sexual dysfunctions: a systematic review and meta-analysis. *J Sex Med.*2021;18(3):582-614.doi:10.1016/j.jsxm.2020 .12.009.

166. American Association of Sexuality Educators, Counselors and Therapists. Home page. https:// www.aasect.org/. Accessed February 10, 2022.

167. Arora N, Brotto LA. How does paying attention improve sexual functioning in women? A review of mechanisms. *Sex Med Rev.* 2017;5(3):266-274. doi:10.1016/j.sxmr.2017.01.005.

168. Jaderek I, Lew-Starowicz M. A systematic review on mindfulness meditation–based interventions for sexual dysfunctions. *J Sex Med.* 2019;16(10): 1581-1596. doi:10.1016/j.jsxm.2019.07.019.

169. Clayton AH, Althof SE, Kingsberg S, et al. Bremelanotide for female sexual dysfunctions in premenopausal women: a randomized, placebo-controlled dose-finding trial. *Womens Health.* 2016; 12(3):325-337. doi:10.2217/whe-2016-0018.

170. Gao Z, Yang D, Yu L, Cui Y. Efficacy and safety of flibanserin in women with hypoactive sexual desire disorder: a systematic review and meta-analysis. *J Sex Med.* 2015;12(11):2095-2104. doi:10.1111 /jsm.13037.

171. Gelman F, Atrio J. Flibanserin for hypoactive sexual desire disorder: place in therapy. *Ther Adv Chronic Dis.* 2017;8(1):16-25. doi:10.1177 /2040622316679933.

172. Lexi-Comp. Flibanserin: drug information. *UpToDate.* https://www.uptodate.com/contents/flibanserin -drug-information. Accessed December 28, 2021.

173. Miller MK, Smith JR, Norman JJ, Clayton AH. Expert opinion on existing and developing drugs to treat female sexual dysfunction. *Expert Opin Emerg Drugs.* 2018;23(3):223-230. doi:10.1080 /14728214.2018.1527901.

174. Levine LA, Betcher HK, Ziegelmann MJ, Bajic P. Amphetamine/dextroamphetamine salts for delayed orgasm and anorgasmia in men: a pilot study. *Urology.* 2020;142:141-145. doi:10.1016/j .urology.2020.04.081.

175. Lexi-Comp. Dextroamphetamine and amphetamine: drug information. *UpToDate.* https://www .uptodate.com/contents/dextroamphetamine-and -amphetamine-drug-information. Accessed December 28, 2021.

176. Moll JL, Brown CS. The use of monoamine pharmacological agents in the treatment of sexual dysfunction: evidence in the literature. *J Sex Med.* 2011;8(4):956-970. doi:10.1111/j.1743-6109.2010 .02190.x.

177. Martin-Tuite P, Shindel AW. Management options for premature ejaculation and delayed ejaculation in men. *Sex Med Rev.* 2020;8(3):473-485. doi:10.1016/j.sxmr.2019.09.002.

178. Hollander AB, Pastuszak AW, Hsieh TC, et al. Cabergoline in the treatment of male orgasmic disorder: a retrospective pilot analysis. *Sex Med.* 2016;4(1): e28-e33. doi:10.1016/j.esxm.2015.09.001.

179. Althof SE, McMahon CG. Contemporary management of disorders of male orgasm and

ejaculation. *Urology.* 2016;93:9-21. doi:10.1016/j.urology.2016.02.018.

180. ACOG Practice Bulletin: clinical management guidelines for obstetrician-gynecologists female sexual dysfunction. doi:10.1097/AOG.0000000000003324. PMID: 31241598. 2019.

181. Parish SJ, Simon JA, Davis SR, et al. International Society for the Study of Women's Sexual Health clinical practice guideline for the use of systemic testosterone for hypoactive sexual desire disorder in women. *J Womens Health.* 2021;30(4):474-491. doi:10.1089/jwh.2021.29037.

182. Bloemers J, van Rooij K, Poels S, et al. Toward personalized sexual medicine (part 1): integrating the "dual control model" into differential drug treatments for hypoactive sexual desire disorder and female sexual arousal disorder. *J Sex Med.* 2013;10(3):791-809. doi:10.1111/j.1743-6109.2012.02984.x.

183. Simon JA, Goldstein I, Kim NN, et al. The role of androgens in the treatment of genitourinary syndrome of menopause (GSM): International Society for the Study of Women's Sexual Health (ISSWSH) expert consensus panel review. *Menopause.* 2018;25(7):837-847. doi:10.1097/GME.0000000000001138.

184. Davis SR, Baber R, Panay N, et al. Global consensus position statement on the use of testosterone therapy for women. *J Clin Endocrinol Metab.* 2019;104(10):4660-4666. doi:10.1210/jc.2019-01603.

185. Goldstein SW, Gonzalez JR, Gagnon C, Goldstein I. Peripheral female genital arousal as assessed by thermography following topical genital application of alprostadil vs placebo arousal gel: a proof-of-principle study without visual sexual stimulation. *Sex Med.* 2016;4(3):e166-e175. doi:10.1016/j.esxm.2016.03.026.

186. Liao Q, Zhang M, Geng L, et al. Efficacy and safety of alprostadil cream for the treatment of female sexual arousal disorder: a double-blind, placebo-controlled study in Chinese population. *J Sex Med.* 2008;5(8):1923-1931. doi:10.1111/j.1743-6109.2008.00876.x.

187. Wang J, Wang L. The therapeutic effect of dehydroepiandrosterone (DHEA) on vulvovaginal atrophy. *Pharmacol Res.* 2021;166. doi:10.1016/j.phrs.2021.105509.

188. Faubion SS, Sood R, Kapoor E. Genitourinary syndrome of menopause: management strategies for the clinician. *Mayo Clin Proc.* 2017;92(12):1842-1849. doi:10.1016/j.mayocp.2017.08.019.

189. Parish SJ, Simon JA, Davis SR, et al. International Society for the Study of Women's Sexual Health clinical practice guideline for the use of systemic testosterone for hypoactive sexual desire disorder in women. *J Sex Med.* 2021;18(5):849-867. doi:10.1016/j.jsxm.2020.10.009.

190. Cocchetti C, Ristori J, Mazzoli F, et al. Management of hypoactive sexual desire disorder in transgender women: a guide for clinicians. *Int J Impot Res.* 2020;33(7):703-709. doi:10.1038/s41443-021-00409-8.

191. Jenkins LC, Mulhall JP. Delayed orgasm and anorgasmia. *Fertil Steril.* 2015;104(5):1082-1088. doi:10.1016/j.fertnstert.2015.09.029.

192. Rowland DL, Hevesi K, Conway GR, Kolba TN. Relationship between masturbation and partnered sex in women: does the former facilitate, inhibit, or not affect the latter? *J Sex Med.* 2020;17(1):37-47. doi:10.1016/j.jsxm.2019.10.012.

193. Goldstein AT, Pukall CF, Brown C, et al. Vulvodynia: assessment and treatment. *J Sex Med.* 2016;13(4):572-590. doi:10.1016/j.jsxm.2016.01.020.

194. Pacik PT, Geletta S. Vaginismus treatment: clinical trials follow up 241 patients. *Sex Med.* 2017;5:e114-e123. doi:10.1016/j.esxm.2017.02.002.

195. Lamvu G, Alappattu M, Witzeman K, et al. Patterns in vulvodynia treatments and 6-month outcomes for women enrolled in the national vulvodynia registry: an exploratory prospective study. *J Sex Med.* 2018;15(5):705-715. doi:10.1016/j.jsxm.2018.03.003.

196. Committee Opinion No 673: Persistent vulvar pain. *Obstet Gynecol.* 2016 Sep;128(3):e78-e84. doi:10.1097/AOG.0000000000001645.

197. Montejo AL, Prieto N, de Alarcón R, et al. Management strategies for antidepressant-related sexual dysfunction: a clinical approach. *J Clin Med.* 2019;8(10). doi:10.3390/jcm8101640.

198. Flanagan E, Herron KA, O'Driscoll C, de Williams ACC. Psychological treatment for vaginal pain: Does etiology matter? A systematic review and meta-analysis. *J Sex Med.* 2015;12(1):3-16. doi:10.1111/jsm.12717.

199. Padoa A, McLean L, Morin M, Vandyken C. The overactive pelvic floor (OPF) and sexual dysfunction. Part 2: evaluation and treatment of sexual dysfunction in OPF patients. *Sex Med Rev.* 2021;9(1):76-92. doi:10.1016/j.sxmr.2020.04.002.

200. Stein A, Sauder SK, Reale J. The role of physical therapy in sexual health in men and women: evaluation and treatment. *Sex Med Rev.* 2019;7(1):46-56. doi:10.1016/j.sxmr.2018.09.003.

201. Lindström S, Kvist LJ. Treatment of provoked vulvodynia in a Swedish cohort using desensitization exercises and cognitive behavioral therapy. *BMC Womens Health.* 2015;15(1). doi:10.1186/s12905-015-0265-3.

202. Liu M, Juravic M, Mazza G, Krychman ML. Vaginal dilators: issues and answers. *Sex Med Rev.* 2021;9(2):212-220. doi:10.1016/j.sxmr.2019.11.005.

203. Ross V, Detterman C, Hallisey A. Myofascial pelvic pain: an overlooked and treatable cause of

chronic pelvic pain. *J Midwifery Womens Health.* 2021;66(2):148-160. doi:10.1111/jmwh.13224.

204. Hämmerli S, Kohl-Schwartz A, Imesch P, et al. Sexual satisfaction and frequency of orgasm in women with chronic pelvic pain due to endometriosis. *J Sex Med.* 2020;17(12):2417-2426. doi:10.1016/j.jsxm.2020.09.001.

205. Lévesque S, Bisson V, Fernet M, Charton L. A study of the transition to parenthood: new parents' perspectives on their sexual intimacy during the perinatal period. *Sex Relationship Ther.* 2021;36(2-3):238-255.

206. Rosen NO, Dawson SJ, Leonhardt ND, et al. Trajectories of sexual well-being among couples in the transition to parenthood. *J Fam Psychol.* 2021;35(4):523.

207. Beveridge JK, Vannier SA, Rosen NO. Fear-based reasons for not engaging in sexual activity during pregnancy: associations with sexual and relationship well-being. *J Psychosomatic Obstet Gynecol.* 2018;39(2):138-145.

208. O'Malley D, Higgins A, Smith V. Exploring the complexities of postpartum sexual health. *Curr Sex Health Rep 13.* 2021:1-8. doi.org/10.1007/s11930-021-00315-6.

209. Foux R. Sex education in pregnancy: does it exist? A literature review. *Sex Relationship Ther.* 2008;23(3):271-277.

210. MacPhedran SE. Sexual activity recommendations in high-risk pregnancies: what is the evidence? *Sex Med Rev.* 2018;6(3):343-357.

211. Sex during pregnancy. *J Midwifery Womens Health.* 2017;62(5). doi:10.1111/jmwh.12677.

212. Jones C, Chan C, Farine D. Sex in pregnancy. *CMAJ.* 2011;183(7):815-818.

213. Paine EA, Umberson D, Reczek C. Sex in midlife: women's sexual experiences in lesbian and straight marriages. *J Marriage Fam.* 2019;81(1):7-23.

214. Sinkovic´ M, Towler L. Sexual aging: a systematic review of qualitative research on the sexuality and sexual health of older adults. *Qual Health Res.* 2019;29(9):1239-1254.

215. Smith L, Yang L, Veronese N, et al. Sexual activity is associated with greater enjoyment of life in older adults. *Sex Med.* 2019;7(1):11-18.

216. Lindau ST, Schumm LP, Laumann EO, et al. A study of sexuality and health among older adults in the United States. *N Engl J Med.* 2007;357(8):762-774.

217. Laumann EO, Waite LJ. Sexual dysfunction among older adults: prevalence and risk factors from a nationally representative US probability sample of men and women 57–85 years of age. *J Sex Med.* 2008;5(10):2300-2311.

218. Avis NE, Zhao X, Johannes CB, et al. Correlates of sexual function among multi-ethnic middle-aged women: results from the Study of Women's Health Across the Nation (SWAN). *Menopause.* 2005;12(4):385-398.

219. Basson R, Rees P, Wang R, et al. Sexual function in chronic illness. *J Sex Med.* 2010;7(1):374-388.

220. Thomas HN, Hess R, Thurston RC. Correlates of sexual activity and satisfaction in midlife and older women. *Ann Fam Med.* 2015;13(4):336-342.

221. Thomas HN, Neal-Perry GS, Hess R. Female sexual function at midlife and beyond. *Obstet Gynecol Clin.* 2018;45(4):709-722.

222. Estill A, Mock SE, Schryer E, Eibach RP. The effects of subjective age and aging attitudes on mid-to late-life sexuality. *J Sex Res.* 2018;55(2):146-151.

223. Shifren JL. Midlife sexuality in women's words. *Menopause.* 2019;26(10):1088-1089.

224. Thomas HN, Hamm M, Hess R, et al. Patient-centered outcomes and treatment preferences regarding sexual problems: a qualitative study among midlife women. *J Sex Med.* 2017;14(8):1011-1017.

225. Thomas HN, Hamm M, Borrero S, et al. Body image, attractiveness, and sexual satisfaction among midlife women: a qualitative study. *J Womens Health.* 2019;28(1):100-106.

CHAPTER

# 10

# Fertility, Family Building, and Contraception

MELICIA ESCOBAR AND SIGNEY OLSON

## Introduction

Rooted in the midwifery hallmarks of patient-centered care, informed choice, shared decision making, and the right to self-determination, fertility care is a core component of midwifery care.[1] In this chapter, fertility care is conceptualized as a spectrum that includes working with individuals toward achieving and preventing pregnancy in accordance with their goals, and through a spectrum of ambivalence and certainty regarding parenthood and family building.

The definition of family is not universal, but rather relies on individual beliefs regarding personal identity and roles, as well as the potential identity and roles of any other family members. The concept of family may vary in different social and cultural contexts, including ways in which individual members view and define themselves. Outdated connotations of family may imply this structure can exist only in the context of marriage and offspring, but these definitions are no longer recognized in many areas.[2] There is no specific number of members who must be involved to qualify as family, and this grouping does not need to involve a parent–child dynamic. Many individuals, particularly in the lesbian, gay, bisexual, transgender, and queer (LGBTQ+) communities, may consider nonbiologic *chosen family* to be an essential structure, often linked to safety and survival. In other contexts, communities may use familial terms to refer to those with certain roles or significance but who are not biologically related. At its core, family represents sources of committed support, regardless of geographic location and biologic connection.[2] Many intentional single parents planning for pregnancy may have differing definitions of family, and clinicians should take care to avoid making assumptions about a patient's desired family structure.

Given the numerous structures and definitions of family, people generally enter into midwifery care already part of a family constellation that may shape their goals for fertility care and how they wish to expand family building, whether through their own fertility or other options. Preconceived notions stemming from childhood and social upbringing influence an individual's goals, acceptance, and definitions of family. People may be further shaped by their intersecting identities and oppressions. The reality of family building is fluid and impacted by various factors (e.g., personal, social, cultural, political, economic, religious) across one's lifespan. Midwives must be aware of, and responsive to, these dynamics if they are to provide holistic care.

Family and parenthood may not always be synonymous with an individual's role and identity. Additionally, parenthood can be independent from current familial circumstances.[2] Many individuals who have experienced miscarriage or pregnancy loss still maintain an identity of parenthood, as do individuals who have experienced the death of a child.[3] Noncustodial parents and parents who place their children for adoption often continue to hold an identity of parenthood and do not become any less of a parent without legal rights or in case of a different geographic location from those children.[4] Other individuals may play a less defined, parent-like role in the raising of children, whether incidentally or intentionally. Communal child raising is a natural structure that has existed throughout time, often out of necessity, and generally offers significant benefits to children, parents, and caregivers alike.[5-7]

This chapter builds on other chapters and appendices in this text, including the *Anatomy and Physiology of the Reproductive System* and *Anatomy and Physiology of Pregnancy* chapters, the *Preconception Care* appendix, and the *Context of Individuals Seeking Midwifery Care* chapter. Multiple ways to conceive and build family (e.g., ovulation induction methods, adoption, fertility awareness–based methods, assisted reproductive technologies) are reviewed. This chapter also serves as an introduction to pregnancy prevention through behavioral, hormonal, and nonhormonal methods of contraception. More specific details on pregnancy prevention strategies can be found in the *Nonhormonal Contraception* and *Hormonal Contraception* chapters. The *Early Pregnancy Loss and Abortion* chapter explores options counseling.

## Reproductive Goals Counseling and Reproductive Justice

Centering a patient's reproductive goals or plan can be achieved through reproductive goals counseling (RGC). RGC is a widely endorsed method in the United States for proactively exploring fertility preferences and priorities[8,9] and can be used as a component of general preventive health care. Individuals can use questions posed during RGC as a process, ideally separate from the clinical encounter, to explore their fertility preferences and priorities to ensure that their choices support their goals. Midwives can also use RGC in their health counseling to support those preferences and priorities by providing patient-centered, relevant, and tailored health information (see Tables 10-2, 10-3, and 10-4 later in the chapter for examples of how to integrate RGC into clinical practice). However, midwives should exercise caution when engaging in RGC and seek to mitigate personal bias, a harmful dichotomy of *intended* and *unintended* pregnancy, and assumptions that *planning* and *choice* are meaningful or relevant for everyone.[10,11]

Approaching RGC using the Reproductive Justice (RJ) framework can help midwives avoid harmful assumptions and maintain a patient-centered position throughout the process wherein the person's wishes and context, including the intersecting ways in which they may be oppressed, are fully acknowledged. This is especially crucial for members of the most marginalized groups—Black, Indigenous, other people of color, and transgender people—who are often de-centered in their health care and for whom access to holistic and comprehensive services are often limited or restricted. The RJ framework has three core values that apply to all

people and can guide the RGC process: (1) the right to *not* have a child; (2) the right *to* have a child; and (3) the right to parent children in safe and healthy environments (Table 10-1).[12] While centering

| Table 10-1 | Reproductive Justice |
| --- | --- |

Utilized as a framework to guide conversations regarding reproductive decisions, Reproductive Justice (RJ) distinctly clarifies that reproductive health—specifically that of marginalized individuals—cannot be separated from systems of oppression that have direct influence over individual bodily autonomy. External influences regarding ability for reproductive choice may include political, economic, geographic, community and familial factors.

This term was coined in 1994 by Loretta Ross, co-founder of SisterSong Women of Color Reproductive Justice Collective.

Examples of instances where RJ may be applied:[13]

- Reproductive coercion of individuals based on race or ethnicity
- Lack of Medicaid coverage for fertility treatment
- Anti-Crisis Pregnancy Center advocacy
- Pressure by clinicians for certain populations to utilize long-acting reversible contraception (LARC) methods
- Lack of ethnic and racially diverse sperm and egg donors[14]
- National and global impact of climate changes on reproductive health
- Ethical debates regarding non-medically necessary egg freezing
- Mass incarceration of Black, Indigenous, and other people of color[15]
- Right for legally disabled individuals to marry and conceive
- Parental leave policies for all parents involved in raising a child
- Sterilization requirement of transgender individuals to change documentation
- Pregnancy and birthing experiences of incarcerated individuals
- Rural reproductive health disparities
- Police violence, unsafe neighborhoods, and racial profiling
- Access to safe and respectful childcare
- Medical and birth trauma

The American College of Nurse-Midwives' position statement on racism and racial bias is supported by the RJ framework, and antiracism efforts within midwifery must acknowledge the inherent intersection of both racism and body-based oppression regarding reproductive health.[16]

| Table 10-2 | Reproductive Life Plan |
|---|---|
| **Do you hope to have any (more) children?** | |
| **Yes** | **No** |
| How many (more) children do you hope to have? | What are you planning to do to prevent becoming pregnant (again)? |
| How long would you like to wait until you become pregnant (again)? | What can your healthcare clinician do to help you achieve your plan? |
| [Do you have a partner with whom you would like to parent?] Is your partner on board with the plan? | [Do you have a partner with whom you would like to parent?] Is your partner on board with the plan? |
| What do you plan to do to prevent getting pregnant until then? | What can your healthcare clinician do to help you achieve your plan? |
| What can your healthcare clinician do to help you achieve your plan? | |

Based on Morse JE, Moos M. Reproductive life planning: raising the questions. *Matern Child Health J.* 2018;22(4):439-444. doi:10.1007/s10995-018-2516-z.

patients on an individual level, the RJ approach to RGC also creates a structural-level opportunity for midwives to analyze relevant systems of power that impact people's self-determination in family building so that harmful structures can be understood and eliminated.

## Counseling Approaches

Recommendations for best practice when implementing RGC include investing in high-quality interpersonal relationships with patients characterized by openness, trust, and caring; using shared decision making; employing patient-centered communication through the use of open-ended questions; and using the person's feedback to guide the health encounter.[10] There is no prescribed formula for asking questions when implementing RGC.

The Reproductive Life Planning[17] (Table 10-2) and One Key Question[18] (Table 10-3) approaches have been used in recent years to provide a structured way for a patient and clinician to begin to discuss plans for pregnancy, and to guide the approach to reproductive health education during a visit. While not inherently lesser options, the line of questioning posed in these approaches runs the risk of causing harm or being too reductive without a patient-centered approach.[17] Another approach designed to be inclusive of gender identity and sexual orientation, the PATH (Pregnancy/Parenthood Attitudes, Timing, How important) framework, aligns well with these recommendations for best practice and with the RJ framework.[10,19–21] Table 10-4 provides an overview of the PATH framework and how it can be used in clinical practice.[21] This approach

| Table 10-3 | One Key Question |
|---|---|

Would you like to become pregnant in the next year?
- Yes
- No
- Unsure
- OK either way

Power to Decide. One Key Question. https://powertodecide.org/one-key-question. Updated 2022. Accessed January 28, 2022.

| Table 10-4 | Questions Utilized in the PATH Framework |
|---|---|
| PA: Pregnancy/ Parenthood Attitudes | Do you think you might like to have (another; more) children at some point? *If **NO**, skip to H: How important. If **YES**, continue to T: Timing.* |
| T: Timing | When do you think that might be? *Regardless of time frame, continue to H: How important.* |
| H: How important | How important is it to you to prevent pregnancy (until then)? *Or* How important is it to you not to cause a pregnancy (until then)? |

Based on Hatcher RL, Nelson A, Trussell J, et al. *Contraceptive Technology,* 21st ed. Atlanta, GA: Managing Contraception; 2018.

also allows space for a more expansive discussion around family building that moves beyond pregnancy and contraception and may include goals such as being child-free by choice, adoption, use of a gestational carrier, guardianship, co-parenting with or without romantic partners, or use of assisted reproductive technologies.

## Unassisted and Assisted Reproductive Care

Throughout discussions regarding reproductive and fertility care in this chapter, terms such as *male infertility* and *female infertility* are avoided, as these are nonspecific and do not accurately represent the spectrum of genders who may desire parenthood with or without pregnancy. While minimization of an individual to their reproductive organs should be generally avoided, in the context of a healthcare conversation, specification of reproductive organ function is valuable from a clinical lens. Use of the word *donor* when applicable is important, as it conveys the use of third-party genetic material and may have necessary legal implications.

Additionally, the term *partner* should be used with caution. Framing the process of conception as always involving two biologically and/or sexually involved romantic partners excludes many individuals, such as those pursuing intentional single parenthood. Polyamorous or genetically blended families also deserve representation and are often excluded from family building conversations due to assumptions about intended parenthood.

### Fertility and Infertility

From a medical perspective, fertility is the capacity for pregnancy and infertility is the lack of conception after 1 year or more of regular, unprotected, penile–vaginal intercourse.[22] This narrowed definition through a heteronormative lens thus excludes many individuals who may desire evaluation and discussion of fertility. Many queer individuals do not have prior knowledge of fertility issues before they arrive at a clinician's office, as they may not fit the preceding definition.[23] Categorizing infertility leads to one of two diagnoses: *primary infertility* for individuals who have not been pregnant previously, and *secondary infertility* for individuals who have been pregnant at least once in the past.[24] Any person with a uterus and ovaries 35 years or older who has been trying to conceive should seek care after 6 months of attempting to become pregnant instead of waiting 1 year. While age may be a potential physiologic factor that increases length of time

to conception for some individuals, the purpose of this recommendation is to discuss available testing options earlier and offer the opportunity to initiate treatment if desired so as to maximize the reproductive window. The reproductive window will vary by individual and includes the period of time when that person can become pregnant.

Infertility may exist for individuals of all genders. In the context of two people with reproductive capabilities, it affects approximately 15% of couples in the United States.[25] Most individuals assigned-male-at-birth will be born with two testes and the ability to produce sperm post puberty. However, as described in the *Gender-Affirming Care* chapter, approximately 1.7% of the population is born intersex (the defined parameters of this term are not fully agreed upon in the medical community) and, therefore, may have variation in the reproductive organs or gametes present.[26] Such variation is often not visible at birth and may be discovered initially during a fertility work-up in adulthood. Most individuals assigned-female-at-birth will be born with a typically shaped uterus, two uterine tubes, and two ovaries containing approximately 1 to 2 million oocytes (Table 10-5).[27] It is generally believed that those persons with ovaries are born with all of the eggs they will have in their lifetime and that by the time of puberty, only 300,000 to 400,000 oocytes are left in the ovaries.[28]

### Likelihood of Conception

Monthly fecundity refers to the likelihood of pregnancy occurring on a per-month basis. In the context of two individuals younger than age 30, with all necessary appropriate gametes for conception and who have no established fertility concerns, each cycle has an approximate 20% to 25% chance of conception.[29] Thus, it is estimated that 80% of couples will conceive within the first 6 months of trying to conceive, with the first 3 months having the highest probability. After 12 months of trying to conceive,

| Table 10-5 | Egg Quantity Through the Various Life Stages |
|---|---|
| In utero: 5–7 million eggs | |
| At birth: 1–2 million eggs | |
| Puberty: 300,000–500,000 eggs | |
| 30 years: 120,000 eggs | |
| 37 Years: 25,000 eggs | |
| 51 years/menopause: 1000 eggs | |

average fecundity decreases to less than 5% per cycle. On average, fertility peaks for individuals with a uterus and ovaries sometime in their late 20s or early 30s. By age 40, the chances of conceiving per month are likely near 5%. Many narratives surrounding age-related changes in fertility may conjure up feelings of shame or guilt for patients, and clinicians must take care to structure conversations regarding age in an emotionally sensitive manner. While testing results and statistical probability may be a helpful component of fertility counseling, human conception can be a humbling process and outcomes are not always predictable. It is important for clinicians and patients to note that the experience of medically defined infertility does not necessarily equal sterility. Outside of menopause and/or absent reproductive organs, individuals continue to possess reproductive capabilities. Likelihood of conception is also influenced by the establishment of an existing concern, such as meeting the definition of infertility. If the medical criteria for infertility are not met, such as with same-sex individuals using donor sperm, it is more difficult to predict the probability of conception.[30]

### Age-Related Fertility Discussions

One important aspect of reproductive care with which midwives should be familiar is the prevention of infertility at the outset. Although many causes of infertility involve chromosomal, anatomic, or physiologic factors that are beyond an individual's control, early discussion of desired reproductive life goals can assist individuals in family building.[31] For example, asking individuals at their routine preventive health visits if they happen to know the age at which their mother entered menopause can help to easily identify individuals at risk for premature ovarian insufficiency. However, clinicians should be sensitive to the reality that individuals may not have access to that information for a variety of reasons.

Age is considered the most influential factor related to fertility for both egg- and sperm-producing individuals, although the correlation is much stronger for those with eggs. Sperm-producing individuals older than the age of 40 may experience lower rates of pregnancy and fertilization.[32] Many client-facing resources discuss age 35 as the age at which fertility begins to decline for individuals with ovaries.[27] However, significant deceleration of overall pregnancy rates typically occurs closer to age 37 and again at age 40, although this can vary. While overall pregnancy rates decline with increasing age, risk of fertility-related complications increases. This trend results in lower fertilization rates, higher

miscarriage rates, higher rates of chromosomal conditions, and, ultimately, lower pregnancy rates. These increased risks are believed to most commonly represent decreased egg quality secondary to altered oogenesis (egg maturation). Most eggs that experience chromosomal changes will not become fertilized or will undergo arrested development in the early embryonic stages. While some chromosomal anomalies may not be compatible with ongoing fetal development, some variations in chromosomes are more likely to result in pregnancy and live birth, such as Down syndrome and trisomy 23.

Because age is a nonmodifiable factor that may be tied to feelings of guilt and regret, clinicians should take caution in discussing this potentially sensitive aspect of conception and avoid shaming older parents or prospective parents.[33,34] When employing RGC techniques for patients on the younger side of the reproductive age spectrum, discussions surrounding future fertility should remain objective and factual. Care should be taken to avoid making fear-based assumptions that view fertility as being universally subject to an inevitable, steep decline after age 35. Doing so may suggest or imply to patients an urgency to conceive that conflicts with their goals. Conversely, discussing future fertility frequently and beginning at a young age may help patients to understand the biologic limitations of the reproductive system. While taking care to avoid placing additional pressure on patients, RGC can also help clinicians identify patients who may benefit from additional education about age-related fertility decline. This can be important to prevent scenarios in which individuals remain uninformed about the potential for age-related fertility changes until fewer options are open to them. With counseling, patient outcomes may or may not be altered, but the decision making lies with the patient, a powerful difference.[35] Studies show that various demographic groups hold differing beliefs regarding the ideal age for pregnancy, peak of fertility, and approximate age of age-related fertility decline.[36] Additionally, with increased screening of patients, appropriate candidates for cryopreservation (egg freezing) are more easily identified, although many barriers exist regarding access to cryopreservation.

Ultimately, the goal of age-related fertility discussions should focus on empowering patients with the knowledge they need to move forward with an approach that is in alignment with their goals. Counseling on health-promoting habits such as safer sex practices, adequate nourishment, regular intentional body movement or exercise, and avoidance of smoking, heavy alcohol use, and potentially harmful environmental toxins may help facilitate desired fertility.[37] For example, cigarette smoking may be linked to development of menopause at an earlier age in some individuals.[38] However, many of these topics have the potential to invoke shame and personal responsibility for fertility, and clinicians should take care to counsel their clients through a lens of harm reduction, using objective, judgment-free language.

### Potential Causes of Infertility

For sperm-producing individuals, causes of infertility are usually secondary to sperm abnormalities related to sperm size or shape, count, and/or quality, in addition to transport issues. Table 10-6 lists the most common sperm-related causes of infertility.[39] Azoospermia refers to a complete lack of sperm, and oligospermia refers to a low sperm count.[40]

In individuals with a uterus and/or ovaries, infertility may be caused by, or correlated with, numerous gynecologic or endocrine conditions. These can often be divided into three general categories: structural, hormonal, and multifactorial. Table 10-7 highlights factors contributing to these three categories.[42,43]

In many pronatalist cultures, long-standing patriarchal narratives ascribe the concern of infertility exclusively to women and perpetuate inaccurate beliefs regarding the amount of control a person has over their own fertility. This perspective may focus on perceived egg or menstrual abnormalities.[44,45] In some cases, these harmful perceptions can lead to social isolation and violence.[46] Such stereotypes may also be perpetuated in a healthcare setting, with frequent emphasis on the diagnostic work-up for the gestational parent and limited conversation involving the sperm-producing partners, many of whom find it difficult to believe they may be contributing to infertility concerns.[47]

In reality, one-third of infertility is believed to result from conditions affecting individuals with a uterus and/or ovaries, one-third from conditions affecting the sperm-producing individual, and one-third from conditions affecting a combination of both individuals.[48] Thus, when discussing infertility with a patient, it is important to consider all individuals involved in conception and discuss options for testing for all parties. Approximately 22% to 30% of the time, the cause is unknown, resulting in unexplained infertility, a diagnosis of exclusion.[49] This diagnosis is often noted as one of the most frustrating diagnoses for patients, as it can feel disappointing to be without a lead theory on the cause of infertility and, in turn, without a clear

| Table 10-6 | Common Causes of Sperm-Related Infertility |
|---|---|

**Structural or physiologic changes**

- Retrograde ejaculation: Sperm move backward into the bladder
- Testicular injury or trauma
- Obstruction in epididymis, vas deferens, or ejaculatory duct
- Congenital absence of the vas deferens, which is common in carriers of cystic fibrosis
- Erectile dysfunction
- Cryptorchidism: One or both testicles are not descended
- Varicocele: Enlarged vein(s) in the testicle(s), altering blood flow and temperature, which decreases sperm production
- Viral infections leading to testicular swelling or scar tissue (most commonly mumps, gonorrhea, or chlamydia)
- Diabetes
- Prior vasectomy, disclosed or undisclosed

**Increasing age**

**Testicular cancer**

**Hormone imbalance**

- Hyperprolactinemia
- Androgen insensitivity
- Thyroid disorder

**Chromosomal variance**

- Most commonly Klinefelter syndrome

**Medications[41]**

- Antiandrogenic agents, anabolic steroids
- Immunosuppressive agents, corticosteroids
- Opiates
- Antidepressants
- Antihypertensive agents
- Statins
- Antiepileptic agents
- Antiviral agents
- Antifungal agents
- Sildenafil (Viagra)

Data from Punab M, Poolamets O, Paju P, et al. Causes of male infertility: a 9-year prospective monocentre study on 1737 patients with reduced total sperm counts. *Hum Reprod.* 2016;32(1):18-31. doi:10.1093/humrep/dew284.

| Table 10-7 | Causes of Infertility for Individuals with Uterus and/or Ovaries | |
|---|---|---|
| **Structural Causes** | | |
| Endometriosis adhesions | | |
| Adenomyosis | | |
| Diethylstilbestrol (DES) exposure (exact mechanism unknown)[43] | Discontinued in the United States in 1971; used in other countries until more recently | |
| Uterine fibroid(s) | | |
| Uterine polyp(s) | | |
| Uterine tubal blockage, unilateral or bilateral | May be idiopathic, or caused by endometriosis, a history of pelvic inflammatory disease, or sexually transmitted infection | |
| Uterine anomalies such as bicornuate or unicornuate uteri, septate uterus | | |
| Uterine scar tissue secondary to prior surgery | | |
| **Hormonal/Endocrinologic Causes** | | |
| Absent ovulation (anovulation) or irregular ovulation; may be caused by a variety of conditions | Polycystic ovarian syndrome (PCOS)<br>Hyperprolactinemia<br>Hypothalamic hypogonadism<br>Thyroid dysfunction<br>Malnourishment, either unintentional or as seen with restrictive eating disorders and chronic dieting; frequently resulting in menstrual disturbances | |
| Luteal-phase insufficiency of progesterone | | |
| Autoimmune conditions | | |
| **Multifactorial Causes** | | |
| Inflammatory endometriosis or adenomyosis | | |
| Pelvic masses such as endometriomas or malignancies | | |
| Recurrent miscarriage or pregnancy loss | Timing of loss may give insight into underlying cause | |
| Genetic or chromosomal variance | | |
| Geographic infertility, partners living apart, unable to attempt conception | | |
| Social infertility, lack of necessary gametes | | |
| Age | | |
| Immune dysregulation or autoimmune conditions | | |
| Premature ovarian insufficiency (POI) | Early-onset low ovarian reserve with irregular menses; cannot be diagnosed by low anti-Müllerian hormone (AMH) levels with regular menses | |
| Tubal ligation, known or unknown | | |
| Prior cancer, particularly types requiring radiation | | |

Based on Practice Committee of the American Society for Reproductive Medicine. Diagnostic evaluation of the infertile male: a committee opinion. *Fertil Steril*. 2021;116:18. https://www.ncbi.nlm.nih.gov/pubmed/25597249. doi:10.1016/j.fertnstert.2015.03.019.

sense of the optimal approach to remedy this condition.[50] Treatment (discussed later in this chapter) often involves a broad, high-intervention approach intended to address the maximum number of potential concerns preventing pregnancy, even if those concerns cannot be pinpointed.[51]

Occasionally, unexplained infertility may have a diagnosable cause if a thorough history is taken. During the COVID-19 pandemic, one study found that some couples previously diagnosed with long-standing unexplained infertility actually conceived during this time, leading researchers to believe that the frequency of sexual intercourse may have been the actual underlying cause.[49]

### Focused History

The initial evaluation for an individual who has not yet experienced a pregnancy despite trying to conceive should begin with a detailed history to ascertain whether they meet the medical definition of infertility. Once it has been determined that an individual's history meets this criterion, clinicians should use respectful discussion and system-specific questions to explore potential factors related to conception (Table 10-8).[52–57]

### Physical Examination

In addition to assessing vital signs, particular attention should be given to any signs of potential genetic or hormonal variances indicating possible excess androgen. For example, short stature could indicate Turner syndrome (also called 45,X or monosomy X); acne, alopecia, or hirsutism may indicate elevated androgen levels; and galactorrhea can be a sign of hyperprolactinemia.[58] A pelvic examination may be offered in the context of shared decision making to assess for conditions related to anatomy (e.g., fibroids, bicornuate uterus), infections (e.g., sexually transmitted infections [STIs]), and hormonal states (e.g., hypoestrogenic signs, such as a lack of vaginal moisture and a cervix deficient in mucus) that could contribute to infertility. However, many of these evaluations may be accomplished by other diagnostic methods such as ultrasound.

The sperm-contributing individual may also be offered examination, by either a midwife experienced with conducting andrology-related exams, a reproductive specialist, or a urologist. During assessment, the clinician looks for signs of anatomic conditions (e.g., enlarged testicular veins causing a varicocele or absent vas deferens), infectious conditions (e.g., prostatitis), and hormonal conditions (e.g., gynecomastia, which could be an indication of hyperthyroidism,

or Klinefelter syndrome [47,XXY]), which can cause infertility.[40] If indicated, the clinician should refer the sperm-producing individual to a reproductive endocrinologist who specializes in andrology and fertility.

Prior to offering or initiating diagnostic testing, the midwife should review basic concepts of fertility and strategies that optimize the possibility of conception. These concepts, which are listed in Table 10-9, should be presented in the appropriate context of the patient's social scenario and can apply equally to those conceiving with a sperm-producing partner at home and to those planning insemination.[29,59–62] Education may include discussion on daily basal body temperature (BBT), self-evaluation of cervical mucus, ovulation over-the-counter tests, and smartphone apps. Details about using these methods can be found in the *Nonhormonal Contraception* chapter.

### Diagnostic Testing

Diagnostic evaluation is warranted for anyone meeting the medical criteria for infertility and any person with a gynecologic or endocrine disorder known to have an association with infertility. Additionally, due to the high cost of donor-assisted conception, many individuals planning on using donor gametes may opt for a more in-depth evaluation to proactively identify possible barriers to fertility. To avoid overmedicalizing or pathologizing donor-assisted conception, these tests should always be presented as optional after a discussion of their potential benefits. Some of these tests may be performed at the same time, such as a sperm analysis and hormonal bloodwork. It is recommended to begin with the least invasive testing options prior to discussing more in-depth testing.

### Basic Semen Analysis

Because comprehensive testing of a patient with a uterus and/or ovaries can be intensive and costly, an assessment of the sperm-contributing individual's fertility status is recommended to be conducted early in the process of evaluation for infertility.[40] A basic semen analysis (BSA) allows evaluation of sperm count number, concentration, motility, morphology, progression, and structure of sperm per ejaculate. Ideally, one sperm sample contains 20 to 100 million/mL sperm, though only 1000 per ejaculation ever get as far as the uterus. Sperm production takes approximately 72 days from immature to mature development. Thus, if an individual plans to discontinue a potentially impactful medication, it is advisable to wait this duration of time before testing

| Table 10-8 | Factors Associated with Infertility | |
|---|---|---|
| **History for Both Individuals** | **Additional Medical History for Individual with a Uterus/Ovary** | **Additional Medical History for Sperm-Producing Individual** |
| **Current Pattern of Intercourse (if applicable)** | | |
| Frequency of intercourse or sperm contact | | |
| Duration of infertility | | |
| Prior pregnancy attempts | | |
| Periods of intercourse or sperm contact without pregnancy occurring, with current or past partners | | |
| **Medical History** | | |
| History of any prior pregnancies | Prior contraception use | History of varicocele |
| History of sexually transmitted infections | Dyspareunia or other pain with insertion | History of mumps |
| History of genitourinary infection | Abnormal Pap smears or treatment | History of testicular torsion |
| Symptoms or known diagnosis of endocrine disorders | Pelvic or abdominal surgeries | Prior pelvic or testicular trauma or injury |
| Prior chemotherapy or treatments for cancer | Menstrual history[a] | History of cystic fibrosis |
| Current prescribed or over-the-counter medications | | |
| History of sexual dysfunction | | |
| History of sleep apnea[55] | | |
| **Social History** | | |
| Substance use (i.e., alcohol, tobacco, or other unprescribed medications) | Increased adverse childhood events/experiences (ACE) scores and sexual trauma have been linked to higher rates of difficulty conceiving[56] | History or current use of anabolic steroids[57] |
| | | Frequent use of hot tubs |
| **Occupational History** | | |
| Regular exposure to toxic environmental or chemical substances such as dry-cleaning solvents, pesticides | | Regular exposure to high levels of heat (e.g., factory workers), laptop use |
| **Family History** | | |
| Family history of infertility | Family history of early menopause Family history of painful and/or heavy menses | Family history of testicular cancer |
| Family history of congenital anomalies, genetic disorders | Family history of hirsutism and/or irregular menses | |

[a] Menstrual history includes age of menarche, interval, regular or irregular, amount of flow, history of oligomenorrhea or amenorrhea, and dysmenorrhea.

Data from Koroma L, Stewart L. Infertility: evaluation and initial management. *J Midwifery Womens Health*. 2012;57(6):614-621. https://www.ncbi.nlm.nih.gov/pubmed/23078197. doi:10.1111/j.1542-2011.2012.00241.x; Moore M. Infertility. In: Schuiling KD, Likis FE, eds. *Gynecologic Health Care*. 4th ed. Burlington, MA: Jones & Bartlett Learning; 2022:383-398; Lindsay TJ, Vitrikas KR. Evaluation and treatment of infertility. *Am Fam Physician*. 2015;91(5):308-314. https://www.ncbi.nlm.nih.gov/pubmed/25822387.

| Table 10-9 | Techniques for Optimizing Fertility |
|---|---|
| **Topic** | **Content** |
| Fertile window | The fertile window varies considerably even in individuals with regular cycles, but is usually considered to last 6 days. Conception is most likely when sperm contact occurs within the 3 days before ovulation, though it is important to note that ovulation is a process that can take 12–30 hours. |
| | Three ways of determining the fertile window are available: |
| | • BBT recorded at rest at the same time each day before rising. Fertility is highest 2 days after BBT increases by at least 0.4°F. |
| | • Teaching individuals to self-monitor their cervical mucus. Fertility is highest when the mucus is slippery and clear and sperm contact occurs on the day when cervical mucus is most profuse. |
| | • Ovulation detection kits are based on the surge of LH that is associated with ovulation. These kits may not fully display an accurate window, as ovulation can occur up to 2 days after the LH surge. When educating patients, it is helpful to emphasize that LH is a marker for impending ovulation, not an indication that ovulation is necessarily occurring at that time. Because sperm can live in the vagina, cervix, and/or uterus for several days, the overlap between an LH surge and sperm contact may not always need to be precise. |
| Timing of vaginal–penile intercourse or sperm contact via insemination | Intercourse every 1–2 days during the fertile window results in the highest pregnancy rates, though patients should be encouraged to time intercourse without putting too much emotional pressure on themselves or partner. Several sequential days of daily intercourse are unlikely to be beneficial. Conversely, while age is likely to impact the optimal period of abstinence, most individuals should limit abstinence to 2–4 days when trying to conceive. Abstinence may be detrimental to sperm count and progression (i.e., how fast and forward-moving sperm are on a scale of 0–4). Thus, it is recommended for a sperm-producing partner to ejaculate (via sexual intercourse or masturbation) within several days prior to timing of intercourse or sperm contact with ovulation. |
| | Given the cost of intrauterine insemination and/or donor sperm obtained via a cryobank, it may be feasible to time sperm contact to occur near ovulation. Those using readily available fresh donor sperm to conceive may wish to plan for vaginal insemination multiple times near ovulation. |
| Sexual practices | There is no evidence that any specific position improves the chance of pregnancy. Sperm with strong forward progression have been documented in the uterine tubes within 2 minutes after ejaculation. |
| | Some vaginal lubricants may decrease sperm motility and progression, though many sperm-friendly products now exist. Lubrication may also increase comfort during sex. |
| Lifestyle considerations | Tobacco use and excessive caffeine consumption (more than 5 cups of coffee per day) are associated with decreased chance of pregnancy. The effects of heavy alcohol use or marijuana use have not been fully studied. |
| | Sauna use does not decrease fertility. |
| Stress | While high levels of stress are well documented in people experiencing infertility, there is minimal evidence of causation. Stress management strategies may improve the experience of dealing with infertility or undergoing fertility treatment, but it is unclear whether they can directly improve the chances of pregnancy. |
| | Assessment for worsening mental health is often warranted, as studies show persons experiencing infertility and undergoing treatment are at significantly higher risk for depression, anxiety, marital stress, lower quality of life, suicide, and reproductive trauma. |

Abbreviations: BBT, basal body temperature; LH, luteinizing hormone.

Data from Practice Committee of the American Society for Reproductive Medicine, Practice Committee of the Society for Reproductive Endocrinology and Infertility. Optimizing natural fertility: a committee opinion. *Fertil Steril*. 2022;117(1):53-63; Zarek SM, Hill MJ, Richter KS, et al. Single-donor and double-donor sperm intrauterine insemination cycles: does double intrauterine insemination increase clinical pregnancy rates? *Fertil Steril*. 2014;102(3):739-743. https://www.ncbi.nlm.nih.gov/pubmed/24934490. doi:10.1016/j.fertnstert.2014.05.018; Suarez SS, Pacey AA. Sperm transport in the female reproductive tract. *Hum Reprod Update*. 2006;12(1):23-37. https://www.ncbi.nlm.nih.gov/pubmed/16272225. doi:10.1093/humupd/dmi047; Sandhu RS, Wong TH, Kling CA, Chohan KR. In vitro effects of coital lubricants and synthetic and natural oils on sperm motility. *Fertil Steril*. 2014;101(4):941-944. https://www.ncbi.nlm.nih.gov/pubmed/24462060. doi:10.1016/j.fertnstert.2013.12.024; Rooney KL, Domar AD. The relationship between stress and infertility. *Dialog Clin Neurosci*. 2018;20(1):41-47. https://www.ncbi.nlm.nih.gov/pubmed/29946210.

again. If intended parents plan to use a known sperm donor, a BSA is recommended prior to finalizing plans to freeze sperm samples.

### Blood Work

Evaluating internal endocrine biomarkers may provide clinicians with a possible source of infertility or potential fertility concern, sometimes incidentally.[58] Note, however, that no reliable tests are currently available to determine the quality of oocytes in the preconception period. Even with more extensive fertility testing or treatment, clinicians are unable to guarantee or definitively predict who will have desired fertility outcomes. When discussing laboratory results with patients, clinicians must understand the associated hormonal nuances and potential testing limitations. Table 10-10 outlines relevant lab work, considerations, and results interpretations.[58,63–67]

| Table 10-10 | Infertility Laboratory Studies | |
|---|---|---|
| **Lab Study** | **Consideration** | **Results Interpretation** |
| **Reproductive Hormones**[a] | | |
| Estradiol | This level gradually increases over the follicular phase, as the oocyte in the follicle produces increased amounts of estrogen as it matures. | Baseline levels should be < 60 pg/mL ideally. Each mature follicle produces an average of 200 pg/mL. |
| Follicle-stimulating hormone (FSH) | Produced in pulsatile fashion by pituitary gland. FSH holds an inverse relationship to estradiol, so an accurate FSH reading must be accompanied by a baseline estradiol reading. | Results < 10 mIU/mL demonstrate good ovarian function; higher results are common in perimenopause. Normal variation seen cycle to cycle. |
| Progesterone | Produced only by the corpus luteum created by the follicular remnants post ovulation. Luteal-phase progesterone should be drawn 1 week post ovulation; calculation consideration should be given in regard to the patient's menstrual cycle length and adjusted accordingly. | Results < 1.0 ng/mL show appropriate baseline levels after resolution from the prior month's corpus luteum. Results > 2 or 3 ng/mL demonstrate ovulation has very recently occurred, likely within a day. Results > 10.0 ng/mL show appropriate mid-luteal levels high enough to support a pregnancy if desired. |
| Luteinizing hormone (LH) | Produced in pulsatile fashion by pituitary gland. The LH:FSH ratio may be helpful in evaluating for PCOS. | Normal levels vary, but typically range between 4 and 10 mIU/mL prior to ovulation, except in some cases of PCOS. LH surges may reach peaks as high as 50–100 mIU/mL, though these results are rarely seen in serum findings, as the window of elevation is brief. |
| Anti-Müllerian hormone (AMH) | A test of ovarian reserve that can be checked any day of the cycle; used as an indicator of egg quantity. This test cannot predict the likelihood of pregnancy or egg quality, only the approximate quantity of eggs remaining in the ovary. Its primary use is determining medication dosage and expected egg yield in IVF cycles. AMH levels are similar in those persons experiencing infertility and those with no history of infertility. Should not be drawn if a patient is currently taking a combined hormonal contraceptive method, as this may decrease the result by up to 50%. This test will be elevated in persons with PCOS. | Levels of 1.0 ng/mL and greater are considered to have a favorable response to IVF stimulation medications. Levels correlate directly with age and decline with increasing age. Levels > 8 ng/mL are strongly correlated with PCOS. Levels are typically checked no more than annually if patients desire monitoring to assist in decision-making for family building, though a significant drop in levels should be repeated using the same lab. |

*(continues)*

| Table 10-10 | Infertility Laboratory Studies (*continued*) | |
|---|---|---|
| **Other Blood Work** | | |
| Thyroid-stimulating hormone (TSH) with free thyroxine (T$_4$) | Hypothyroidism and subclinical hypothyroidism. | Titration may vary slightly, but TSH levels are commonly recommended to be kept between 0.5 and 2.5 uIU/mL, a narrower range than in those not trying to conceive. |
| Thyroid peroxidase antibodies (TPO) | Presence of antibodies helps determine a diagnosis of Hashimoto's thyroiditis. | Negative antibodies are typically reported as 0–34 IU/mL. |
| Vitamin D | Deficiency may lower fertility rates. | Guidelines vary but the generally accepted range is 35–100 ng/mL. Many clinicians aim for mid-range goals. |
| Complete blood count | Evaluation for anemia, which is associated with lower rates of fertility. | Evaluate as usual. |
| Hemoglobin A1c | Insulin resistance or poorly controlled diabetes may decrease rates of fertility. | Evaluate as usual. |
| Genetic carrier screening | Allows individuals to learn of genetic changes in their own DNA prior to conception. If two individuals screen positive for the same variance, IVF with genetic testing may be offered. Many donor sperm cryobanks screen many or all of their donors. Similar to genetic testing in pregnancy, these tests are never mandatory and may be accompanied by ethical considerations. | Given the number of genetic variances included in screening, it is common for individuals to screen positive for one or more mutations, many of which may be inconsequential. |
| Genetic karyotype | Some variation in karyotype may be linked to fertility concerns. | Variation in karyotype is normal, and human genetics exists on a spectrum. |

Abbreviations: CD, cycle day; DNA, deoxyribonucleic acid; IVF, in vitro fertilization; PCOS, polycystic ovarian syndrome.

[a] Reproductive hormones are menstrual cycle day dependent and, therefore, contextual. Baseline labs should be drawn on CD 2, 3, 4 or 5, counting the first day of full flow as CD 1.

Data from Penzias A, Azziz R, Bendikson K, et al. Fertility evaluation of infertile women: a committee opinion. *Fertil Steril*. 2021;116(5):1255-1265. https://www.ncbi.nlm.nih.gov/pubmed/34607703. doi:10.1016/j.fertnstert.2021.08.038; González-Foruria I, Martínez F, Rodríguez-Purata J, et al. Can anti-Müllerian hormone predict success outcomes in donor sperm inseminations? *Gynecol Endocrinol*. 2019;35(1):40-43. https://www.ncbi.nlm.nih.gov/pubmed/30324829. doi:10.1080/09513590.2018.1499089; Hvidman HW, Bentzen JG, Thuesen LL, et al. Infertile women below the age of 40 have similar anti-Müllerian hormone levels and antral follicle count compared with women of the same age with no history of infertility. *Hum Reprod*. 2016;31(5):1034-1045. https://www.ncbi.nlm.nih.gov/pubmed/26965431. doi:10.1093/humrep/dew032; Orouji Jokar T, Fourman LT, Lee H, et al. Higher TSH levels within the normal range are associated with unexplained infertility. *J Clin Endocrinol Metab*. 2018;103(2):632-639. https://www.ncbi.nlm.nih.gov/pubmed/29272395. doi:10.1210/jc.2017-02120; Turan OD. Vitamin D level and infertility. *Adnan Menderes Üniversitesi Tıp Fakültesi/J Adnan Menderes University Medical Faculty*. 2015. https://doi.org/10.5152/adutfd.2015.2399; Poornima S, Daram S, Devaki RK, Qurratulain H. Chromosomal abnormalities in couples with primary and secondary infertility: genetic counseling for assisted reproductive techniques (ART). *J Reprod Infertil*. 2020;21(4):269-274. https://www.ncbi.nlm.nih.gov/pubmed/33209743. doi:10.18502/jri.v21i4.4331.

Sperm-contributing individuals may also be assessed for thyroid conditions, testosterone levels and genetic variances.

### Baseline Sonogram

A vaginal sonogram is recommended to be performed at the same time as the baseline hormonal blood work. Performing a vaginal sonogram during the initial cycle days helps to ensure minimal ovarian activity and an appropriately thin endometrium.[58] If findings differ from expected, the blood testing results can help to determine the potential cause. While image quality may be altered, for individuals who experience pain with vaginal insertion or with a disclosed history of sexual trauma, an abdominal ultrasound should always be offered to minimize retraumatization. Ultrasound does have some limitations, as it does not allow the clinician to visualize the microscopic oocyte, cannot evaluate tubal patency, and does not allow for the full internal endometrial wall to be appreciated.

### Hysterosalpingogram

A hysterosalpingogram (HSG) is a radiologic test that utilizes a small catheter placed into the uterus, followed by introduction of fluid containing dye and X-ray evaluation of tubal spillage to determine uterine tube patency or blockage. If bilateral spillage is visualized, the uterine tubes are documented as patent. Unilateral spillage suggests a tubal blockage, spasm, or hydrosalpinx. This procedure can cause minimal discomfort for some individuals and significant pain for others. The clinician should instruct the patient to take ibuprofen prior to the procedure to increase comfort and assess for the need of an antianxiety medication if desired by the patient. Spontaneous pregnancy rates have been shown to increase post HSG, likely owing to the removal of small tubal blockages during this procedure.

### Saline Ultrasound

This procedure may be recommended if the clinician suspects possible uterine polyps.[68] Easily performed in the midwife's office, this test involves placement of a small catheter into the uterus, followed by introduction of normal saline and sonographic evaluation of the endometrial contour, highlighting any areas of possible polypoid or fibroid tissue encroaching into the uterine cavity and preventing pregnancy.

Once these basic assessments have been completed, a series of more intensive procedures may be recommended, including magnetic resonance imaging (MRI) of the pelvis and/or pituitary, hysteroscopy, and laparoscopy. For individuals with secondary infertility who have had a previous cesarean, specialists may recommend a hysteroscopic or laparoscopic post-cesarean scar evaluation to assess for a niche—that is, a small myometrial indentation.[69]

### Treatment of the Individual with Infertility

The role of midwives within the context of a fertility or reproductive endocrinology clinic may vary, though the emphasis on patient education makes these clinicians a valuable contribution to this field. Many midwives specialize in and offer nonsurgical fertility treatment, including counseling, patient education, medication management, and intrauterine insemination (see the *Intrauterine Insemination* appendix). Additionally, they may collaborate with physician colleagues to care for individuals undergoing more intensive or surgical treatments, such as in vitro fertilization (IVF; discussed later in this chapter).[70] Given the increased utilization of fertility treatment, midwives should be familiar with the general options for diagnosis and treatment and have a clear understanding of optimal timing for referral to increase access to care.

Clinicians should approach this care through an RJ lens, framing fertility as a matter of ethical right to parenthood. *Body-based oppression* refers to the ways in which society poorly treats certain people based on the way their body appears externally.[71,72] This mistreatment is often more prevalent among persons with marginalized identities and those with certain health conditions. Withholding and delaying treatment or referrals creates additional barriers and upholds harmful cultural narratives regarding whether certain individuals are worthy of parenthood. These marginalized groups may include individuals who are LGBTQ+; older; Black, Indigenous, people of color (BIPOC); imprisoned; disabled; or human immunodeficiency virus (HIV)–positive.[73] In many cases, the barriers imposed by one clinic or provider may lead patients to believe they will receive similar negative treatment at other facilities so that—quite understandably—they do not pursue second opinions. Provision of expanded fertility treatment access is essential in continuing to support reproductive bodily autonomy.

The least invasive fertility treatment includes patient education on menstrual cycle and ovulation tracking, which helps an individual to learn their body's cues and optimize monthly fecundity. Fertility awareness methods (FAM) may be used for both pregnancy prevention and planned conception, often focusing on monitoring cervical mucus, basal body temperature, breast tenderness, mood, and other symptoms. While these methods may not be effective for all individuals, especially those with irregular menses, a conversation regarding ovulation timing is often a helpful place for the clinician to start. This first step is appropriate for persons planning to conceive with either donor sperm or sperm from their partner. FAM differs from other forms of *natural family planning* slightly in that it utilizes current data as opposed to estimating ovulation based on prior data and does not assume that all menstrual cycles have a frequency of 28 days. See the *Fertility Awareness Methods* appendix for a detailed description of how to counsel clients in the use of FAM.

Complementary approaches that have been assessed to increase conception chances include the use of acupuncture, chiropractic, prayer, antioxidant supplements (e.g., selenium intake to improve the properties of sperm), and psychotherapy, although evidence for the success rates of these approaches is conflicting.[74]

### Emotional Considerations

Experiencing infertility has been shown to have effects similar to those experienced by individuals who have survived significant trauma, with resulting symptoms that may resemble post-traumatic stress disorder (PTSD). Feelings of failure, worthlessness, and anxiety regarding lack of control are common themes when debriefing individuals on the reality of experiencing infertility.[75] Patients experiencing infertility report levels of depression similar to those noted in patients who have been diagnosed with cancer.[76] Some studies also demonstrate increased rates of divorce and destabilization of family structure.[77] In addition, individuals who conceive through fertility treatment have a higher risk of postpartum depression.[78] Clinicians should assess patients' mental health throughout the infertility work-up and treatment process, and provide appropriate mental health referrals as needed.[79] Some patients may experience less distress or regret after unsuccessful infertility treatment cycles if they receive a higher level of perceived emotional support.[80]

The invasive nature of frequent internal monitoring may be triggering for patients who have experienced sexual trauma and necessitate abdominal ultrasound.[81] Because many patients are not able to disclose previous traumas, fertility specialists must use a trauma-sensitive approach with all patients.[82] Additionally, patients may report that their sexuality feels altered in this process, and higher rates of sexual dysfunction are found with those undergoing fertility treatment.[83,84] Sexual desire is often strongly connected to personal body image and self-esteem, both of which can be negatively impacted by infertility.[84,85] These important discussions regarding sexuality throughout infertility are a frequent missed opportunity for clinicians and should be included in care.

### Ovulation Induction

For individuals with irregular menses or anovulation, such as is seen commonly with polycystic ovarian syndrome (PCOS), the use of oral ovulation induction medications is often appropriate. The two

| Table 10-11 | Comparison of Clomiphene Citrate and Letrozole | |
|---|---|
| **Clomiphene Citrate (Clomid)** | **Letrozole (Femara)** |
| Consider as first-line option for ovulation induction (FDA approval) | Not FDA-approved for ovulation induction<br>May use as a first-line option for patients with PCOS |
| 50-mg tablets available | 50 mg tablets available |
| Side effects include hot flashes, night sweats, mood irritability, headache | Side effects include joint or muscle pain, headaches and hot flashes |
| May cause temporary endometrial thinning | Possible improved endometrial response |
| Risk of multiple-gestation pregnancy approximately 7–8% due to higher likelihood of polyfollicular response | Fewer multiple-gestation pregnancies due to higher likelihood of monofollicular response |
| Higher chance of side effects | Significantly fewer bothersome side effects reported as compared to Clomid |

Abbreviations: FDA, Food and Drug Administration; PCOS, polycystic ovarian syndrome.

agents most commonly used for this purpose are clomiphene citrate (Clomid) and letrozole (Femara). Table 10-11 compares these two drugs.[86] Both are typically used in conjunction with a one-time injection of choriogonadotropin alfa (Ovidrel; 250 mcg of recombinant human chorionic gonadotropin [hCG]), commonly referred to as the *trigger shot*. Molecularly similar to LH, this medication causes the body to react in the same way it would to endogenous LH and to initiate the beginning of ovulation. Letrozole is gradually becoming the first-line medication recommended for persons with PCOS, as multiple studies have demonstrated slightly improved rates of pregnancy and lower rates of multiple pregnancy with this agent.[87,88] Additionally, it may have advantages for patients with higher body mass indexes (BMIs).[89] Table 10-12 provides an overview of ovulation induction protocols for the two medications.

These medications vary in their mechanism of action but seek to accomplish the same goal—namely, stimulating the ovaries to produce one or

| Table 10-12 | Ovulation Induction Protocol |
|---|---|
| **Clomiphene Citrate (Clomid)** | **Letrozole (Femara)** |
| Begin at 50 mg or 100 mg, may increase to 150 mg; dosage taken daily for 5 consecutive days | Begin at 2.5 mg or 5 mg, may increase to 7.5 mg; dosage taken daily for 5 consecutive days |
| Evaluate baseline blood work on cycle day 2, 3 or 4. This includes estradiol, progesterone, LH, FSH, and hCG. | |
| Begin medication on cycle days 3, 4 or 5 and take × 5 days. | |
| Reevaluate with bloodwork/sonogram to determine ovarian response. | |
| Titration upward may occur if no dominant follicle (roughly defined as > 14 mm) is seen on sonogram 5 days after the last pill is taken. A mature follicle ready to ovulate will measure approximately 18–25 mm, and both oral medications may cause more than one follicle to mature. Mature follicles may be accompanied by immature follicles; follicles smaller than 16 mm at the time of ovulation are unlikely to contain a mature egg capable of fertilization and therefore are less likely to result in pregnancy. | |

Abbreviations: FSH, follicle-stimulating hormone; hCG, human chorionic gonadotropin; LH, luteinizing hormone.

more mature follicles. Once one or more follicles reach maturity (typically measuring 18 mm in diameter or greater on sonogram), choriogonadotropin alfa is administered subcutaneously to trigger the process of ovulation, essentially ensuring that ovulation occurs at the optimal time.

It is within the scope of reproductive health clinicians to discuss and prescribe these medications to be taken at home. Nevertheless, some organizations recommend routine pelvic sonographic monitoring and serum hormone testing with available same-day results to assess ovarian response to the medications.[90,91] This testing is often logistically possible only within a fertility clinic set up to manage the frequency of these visits. The rationale cited for this approach is often two-fold: (1) Both medications may result in multiple mature follicles that go on to ovulate and thus increase the chance of multiple gestation, and (2) for those persons with irregular menses, it may take several rounds of medication administration to discover the optimal dose needed to achieve a mature follicle or follicles.

Without sonographic monitoring of the number of mature follicles, patients cannot be fully informed as to their risk of multiple gestation. While this risk is relatively low (7% to 8% for clomiphene citrate versus 3% to 5% for letrozole versus 1% with spontaneous pregnancy), discussion about risk and informed consent may alter a patient's comfort in moving forward with timed conception.[87] In cases where the patient determines the multiple gestation risk to be unacceptable, if applicable, the clinician should advise the patient to use barrier methods or to abstain from sexual activity.[87,92]

Additionally, without monitoring, clinicians are unable to determine a patient's ovarian response, which means that patients may spend several months taking a medication that is not producing the desired effect. However, in the context of rural reproductive health, it is appropriate and encouraged for clinicians to learn how to prescribe these medications.

When caring for historically oppressed or marginalized populations desiring conception, access to appropriate and respectful fertility care is a matter of RJ. Providing this care, even without monitoring, conveys the message to patients that their bodies are worthy of reproduction, family building, and specialized care.

### Treatment of Luteal-Phase Insufficiency

While the increasing level of estrogen during the follicular phase initially thickens the endometrial lining, progesterone secreted from the corpus luteum during the luteal phase after ovulation occurs has a supportive effect on maintaining the endometrial lining and receptivity.[93,94] The typical length of the luteal phase is 14 days, with minimal variability except in the case of luteal-phase insufficiency: That condition can result in a shortened time frame from ovulation to the next menses, usually less than 10 days. The clinician should take care to discuss the timing of a progesterone level if one will be drawn, as the peak progesterone will occur 1 week post ovulation and it can be challenging to pinpoint timing in patients with irregular menses. Additionally, luteal-phase insufficiency is often accompanied by an increase in the number of days of light bleeding or spotting leading up to the first day of menses.

Many clinicians choose to measure luteal-phase progesterone levels in patients wishing to conceive. However, an individual measurement of progesterone cannot diagnose luteal-phase insufficiency because of the pulsatile nature of hormonal release.

Thus, this diagnosis should be made primarily through a documented shorter number of days between ovulation and menses.

Because luteal-phase insufficiency has been shown to be present in both individuals able to conceive and those experiencing infertility, controversy exists regarding the role that luteal-phase progesterone levels play in sustaining pregnancy. Traditionally, luteal-phase insufficiency has been treated with oral or vaginal micronized progesterone.[95] While this approach is unlikely to be harmful and remains the most commonly utilized intervention, research suggests it provides only minimal to no improvement in pregnancy rates for most individuals not undergoing other fertility treatments. This suggests that low luteal-phase progesterone levels are not necessarily the underlying cause of infertility and should not necessarily be treated by simply supplementing the individual with more progesterone. The likely explanation is that low luteal-phase progesterone and corpus luteum secretion may be more directly related to an alteration or deviation in follicular development and maturation, which is not a phenomenon easily measured in the clinical setting. Clinicians may also consider use of oral clomiphene citrate or injectable hCG to increase progesterone levels after completing patient counseling regarding the multiple gestation risk with clomiphene citrate.[93]

## Intrauterine Insemination

Intrauterine insemination (IUI) is a clinical procedure in which a washed sperm sample is placed directly into an individual's uterus near the time of ovulation using a soft, thin, flexible catheter with the intention to increase the chance of conception.[96] This process bypasses the cervix, which may act as a potential barrier to sperm motility, and expedites the transportation of the sperm to the fundus. When timed appropriately, the chance of contact between the oocyte and the sperm, and thus pregnancy, is higher. The sperm used in IUI may come from a partner or donor and may consist of either fresh or frozen sperm, though there are both medical and legal aspects to consider, depending on the clinical setting and context. IUI is within the scope of practice of a midwife or advanced practice registered nurse (APRN) and uses a similar skill set to other gynecologic procedures such as intrauterine device (IUD) insertion and endometrial biopsy.[97] Though most commonly performed in the setting of a fertility clinic, IUI with a trained clinician can be safely performed in a client's home as well.

Prior to recommending IUI, patient fertility goals and potential fertility concerns are taken into account to aid in the process of shared decision making. If a physiologic cause of infertility exists, this should align with an indication for the IUI procedure.[97] Though IUI is commonly viewed as the first-line treatment for infertility or for those without infertility wanting to conceive with the use of donor sperm, other higher-level intervention options, such as in vitro fertilization (IVF), should also be objectively reviewed as options because the physical, emotional, and financial effort involved with fertility treatment is significant. Additionally, the benefits of IVF may ultimately align most closely with the patient's desired family-building goals, particularly for those persons desiring additional pregnancies in the future.[97] With shared decision making, a discussion comparing the financial and emotional costs of multiple IUI cycles to one IVF cycle is appropriate and proactive.

Intrauterine insemination (IUI) has several benefits for those individuals desiring conception—some medical, some social, and some functional. Contrary to common belief, IUI is often not recommended as the best primary approach to all cases of infertility. Specifically, IUI has minimal utility in scenarios in which an individual is using partner sperm to conceive and the partner has a normal sperm count. Scenarios where IUI is more likely to be recommended include the following:[98]

- Individuals who are conceiving with donor sperm.
- Individuals who are conceiving with a partner who has a lowered sperm count or altered sperm parameters.
- Individuals who are conceiving with a partner who experiences ejaculatory anxiety with sex.
- Individuals with scant or absent cervical mucus.
- Individuals with dyspareunia.
- Individuals with cervical stenosis or abnormalities.
- Individuals who are HIV-serodiscordant from their sperm-producing partner, including scenarios in which the sperm-producing partner is HIV-positive and scenarios in which the sperm-producing partner is negative.[99] Sperm washing and fertility procedures have been shown to reduce seroconversion, although use of antiretroviral agents and pre-exposure prophylaxis (PrEP) are also excellent approaches to reduce transmission.
- Individuals with unexplained infertility. While there may be only modest benefit if one

of the preceding reasons is not present, many individuals may be offered IUI in conjunction with oral induction medications.

- Individuals who report any other reason in which vaginal–penile sex is not the preferred method of conception.

While IUI in the absence of a physiologic indication may provide only modest benefits, some individuals choose to undergo this procedure as a lower-cost, minimally interventive option or when higher-level intervention options such as IVF are not accessible. Prior to an IUI procedure, the patient may have utilized oral ovulation induction medication (e.g., clomiphene citrate, letrozole) or injectable gonadotropins containing FSH or FSH plus LH (e.g., follitropin beta [Follistim], follitropin alpha [Gonal-F], menotropins [Menopur]), all of which may be recommended as a means to mature multiple follicles. These medications are administered for an average of 12 to 14 days prior to the injection of hCG and the process of IUI.[98]

This procedure is well within the scope of a midwife. In IUI, a 3-mL syringe containing 0.5 to 2 mL of washed sperm is placed into the uterus via a small catheter guided through the cervix.[96] Unlike other procedures involving the cervix, a tenaculum is not traditionally used, although its use may be considered for stabilization when needed. Mild to moderate cramping is common, similar to the cramping that patients may experience during IUD sounding. The *Intrauterine Insemination* appendix offers a step-by-step approach to this procedure.

The term *intracervical insemination* (ICI) appears in some fertility-related literature and by definition refers to the placement of a sperm sample within the cervical canal, stopping short of entering the uterus. However, ICI is not a commonly performed procedure when IUI is an option. Occasionally ICI is used colloquially to refer to *vaginal insemination*, a procedure in which an individual inserts sperm into their vaginal canal, near the cervix, using a needle-free syringe; ICI does not require the use of washed sperm.[97]

Patients and clinicians may inquire about the use of planning for a single IUI attempt versus two IUI procedures within the fertile window.[100] There is unlikely to be a clinical advantage to more than one IUI, though more research is needed when frozen donor sperm is used.[59] Existing IUI research primarily focuses on cisgender, heterosexual couples who have intercourse in addition to the IUI, thus creating a scenario in which resultant pregnancies may have occurred from intercourse.[97]

## Contraindications for Intrauterine Insemination

When counseling a patient on recommendations regarding IUI, the clinician's initial step is to ensure no contraindications for this procedure exist. Although absolute contraindications are uncommon, an active uterine infection such as pelvic inflammatory disease (PID) or other known infections should be treated prior to performing an IUI. Other contraindications include bilateral uterine tubal blockage or previously removed uterine tubes, as this prevents contact between oocyte and sperm, regardless of the use of IUI.[96] While unilateral uterine tubal blockage or removal is not considered a contraindication, patients with these histories should be counseled on the lower rates of pregnancy with IUI compared to other fertility treatments such as IVF, which bypasses tubal concerns altogether.[98]

Unwashed sperm samples represent another contraindication to IUI. Due to elevated levels of prostaglandins present in seminal fluid, the IUI procedure must be performed with the use of washed sperm to reduce the level of prostaglandins present in the sample. Forgoing the step of washing sperm will likely result in painful uterine cramping and inflammation, creating an disadvantageous environment for implantation.[97] Sperm washing involves centrifuging the sperm and extracting only the sperm cells while removing the components that make up semen, such as proteins, sugars, and prostaglandins. This procedure is within the scope of midwives and APRNs, but is commonly the responsibility of laboratory personnel in the clinic setting. Donor sperm purchased through a cryobank is typically available in both washed and unwashed vials.[97] Vaginal insemination does not require washed sperm, as the seminal fluid containing prostaglandins remains outside the cervical os and only sperm cells travel upward to the uterine cavity and tubes.

While IUI can be recommended in the case of oligospermia (low sperm count), it should not be used in cases of very low sperm count, as pregnancy is unlikely. Each vial of sperm should contain a minimum of 10 million sperm. Individuals with oligospermia may choose to freeze multiple sperm samples and combine them so as to reach the threshold sperm count needed to perform IUI with a good chance of achieving pregnancy. However, it may be laborious for patients to go through the sample freezing process to reach this threshold.[97]

## Benefits Associated with Intrauterine Insemination

IUI allows the transport of sperm beyond the cervix, directly into the uterus, increasing the chance of conception by optimizing both the timing and the location of sperm contact. Additionally, it allows an increased chance of pregnancy when utilizing anonymous frozen donor sperm purchased through a cryobank. Most anonymous donor vials of sperm contain sperm that may live for a shorter duration of time and have a lower sperm count compared to fresh sperm. The standard for frozen donor sperm count is 10 million per vial, and patients may be able to contact the cryobank for a replacement if a vial is found to be below that threshold.

## Risks Associated with Intrauterine Insemination

### Infection and Uterine Perforation

Although rare, all intrauterine procedures carry a theoretical risk of both infection and uterine perforation. However, due to the low likelihood of uterine perforation with a IUI catheter, the use of a tenaculum is not standard during this procedure, although some clinicians may choose to use this device occasionally when needed to access the internal os of the cervix.[98]

### Multiple-Gestation Pregnancy

While IUI alone does not increase the incidence of multiple-gestation pregnancy, the chance is increased with the concurrent use of oral ovulation induction medications such as clomiphene citrate and letrozole.[98]

### Procedure Not Resulting in Pregnancy

Success rates for IUI depend heavily on the individual's reproductive and gynecologic history, including age, previous pregnancies, and presence or absence of physiologic infertility. The diagnostic parameters of the sperm, including count, motility, progression, and morphology, are also predictive. On average, the success rate of IUI is typically 10% to 20% per cycle, similar to the chance of pregnancy for individuals without infertility who conceive through vaginal–penile intercourse. Although there is not a specific number of IUI procedures that are recommended prior to consideration of other treatment options, patients commonly opt for 3 to 6 cycles of IUI to account for cycle-to-cycle variation.[97]

When IUI is utilized without prior discussion of a thorough reproductive and gynecologic history of the patient, unknown barriers to fertility may exist, such as bilateral tubal blockage. Given the high cost of both IUI and prepared sperm, whether fresh or frozen, it is recommended to review the potential for existing, yet unknown fertility concerns that may prevent pregnancy from occurring via IUI.[97]

## Assisted Reproductive Technologies

### In Vitro Fertilization

The term *assisted reproductive technologies* (ART) primarily refers to the utilization of IVF. Table 10-13 reviews the steps involved in the IVF process.

### Intracytoplasmic Sperm Injection

In addition to basic IVF, patients are presented with the option of additional laboratory procedures that

| Table 10-13 | Steps for In Vitro Fertilization |
|---|---|

1. Injectable gonadotropins containing FSH or FSH plus LH, such as follitropin beta (Follistim), follitropin alpha (Gonal-F), and menotropins (Menopur) are used to stimulate multiple eggs to maturation.

   a. On average, these medications are taken for 10–12 days, with frequent blood work and ultrasound monitoring occurring throughout this time.

2. A *trigger shot* or injection of hCG is given to initiate the process of ovulation.

3. Immediately prior to release of the eggs from the ovary, an ultrasound-guided transvaginal egg retrieval is performed under anesthesia to aspirate mature oocytes.

4. These oocytes are combined with sperm utilizing either conventional methods or intracytoplasmic sperm injection.

5. At 24 hours post egg retrieval, it can be determined how many eggs were fertilized successfully and progressed to the embryo stage of development.

6. Over the course of 3–5 days, embryologists closely monitor this development, most frequently monitoring until day 5.

   a. If genetic testing is desired, a biopsy is performed on day 5 or 6 and embryos are frozen while the results are processed.

7. Embryo(s) transfer to the uterus is performed under ultrasound guidance in the clinician's office. Similar to IUI, no anesthesia is required. Guidelines from the American Society for Reproductive Medicine recommend a single embryo transfer for most patients, although transferring more than one embryo may be reasonable in certain circumstances.

*Note*: Oocyte cryopreservation (also called egg freezing) is discussed later in this chapter and utilizes all of the steps in the IVF process until Step 4.

Abbreviations: FSH, follicle-stimulating hormone; hCG, human chorionic gonadotropin; IUI, intrauterine insemination; IVF, in vitro fertilization; LH, luteinizing hormone.

may benefit their chance of pregnancy. Intracytoplasmic sperm injection (ICSI) involves embryologist selection of one healthy-appearing sperm, followed by the manual injection of that sperm into the oocyte via a pipette under microscopic supervision.[101] This procedure is frequently recommended for issues of low sperm count and can be completed with a single sperm cell per egg in rare cases.[102] If oocytes are suspected to have an altered external zona pellucida that may be preventing sperm from undergoing the typical acrosomal reaction and subsequent fertilization, ICSI may also be an appropriate choice to increase fertilization rates.[101] For individuals who have previously undergone a vasectomy or do not have sperm present in their seminal fluid, a percutaneous epididymal sperm aspiration (PESA), which entails fine-needle extraction of the sperm from the epididymis, or testicular sperm aspiration (TESA), which involves fine-needle extraction of the sperm from the testes and seminiferous tubules, may be done prior to ICSI to bypass the typical route of sperm transport.

## Preimplantation Genetic Testing

Preimplantation genetic testing for aneuploidy (PGT-A) is another optional procedure involving a microscopic biopsy of the trophectoderm of the embryo (the cells that ultimately create the placenta), which provides the clinician and patient with information about the chromosomal makeup of each individual embryo. Embryos with the expected number of chromosomes are then typically utilized first during the embryo transfer procedure. The proposed benefits of genetic testing are highly debated, with some studies showing significant advantages and others showing minimal advantages only in certain scenarios.[103] Some data suggest that when using untested embryos, overall IVF pregnancy rates range from approximately 30% to 50%, highly dependent on age; by comparison, those rates may be as high as 50% to 70% with the use of PGT-A tested embryos shown to have the typical number of chromosomes.[104,105] Other studies argue that the live birth rate is more important and that PGT-A may simply reduce the number of embryo transfers needed and/or prevent a patient from undergoing miscarriage prior to successful pregnancy. Preimplantation genetic testing for monogenic disorders (PGT-M) is a similar optional procedure done for individuals with positive known genetic mutations and is performed to identify single-gene disorders.

Similar to discussions about genetic testing in pregnancy, the use of this technology in the prepregnancy time frame can bring up important ethical

discussions. The motivation for using preimplantation genetic testing can vary, and may include screening out specific inherited genetic conditions, screening out chromosomal conditions, decreasing miscarriage risk, and sex selection of the embryo for either social reasons or avoidance of sex-specific genetic conditions. It is important to explain to patients during counseling that PGT-A and PGT-M cannot change existing DNA, but rather assist in the identification of embryos with typical DNA patterns shown to correlate closely with increased pregnancy rates.[105] For example, PGT-A is often offered in the case of recurrent pregnancy loss thought to be caused by chromosomal conditions. Patients must understand that PGT-A is just a valuable tool in miscarriage prevention. While it can help in prioritizing transfer of embryos screened to be genetically typical, it cannot alter DNA. Thus, some causes of recurrent pregnancy loss may be modifiable, while others are not.[22]

## Reciprocal In Vitro Fertilization

Reciprocal IVF (sometimes called co-IVF) typically involves two individuals with a uterus, usually partners, who utilize one set of DNA; that is, one acts as the egg-contributing partner and the other partner becomes the gestational parent. Polyamorous families may also plan for reciprocal IVF in a variety of ways.[106,107] For example, a family of three individuals may consist of a partner who undergoes egg retrieval, a second partner who contributes sperm to create an embryo, and a third partner who carries a pregnancy created by combining the egg and sperm of their partners. While many factors increase risk for preeclampsia, it is theorized that pregnancy resulting from use of oocytes other than the gestational parent may increase this risk.[108]

## Gestational Carriers

The term *gestational carrier* typically refers to an individual who is not an intended parent and has no genetic connection to a pregnancy, but carries the pregnancy with the acknowledgment and agreement that they will give the resulting child to the intended parent(s).[109] The egg and sperm used to create the embryo can originate from one or both of the intended parent(s) and/or a third party (or parties). A traditional gestational carrier is an individual who both donates their eggs to be used and is the gestational carrier for a pregnancy resulting from an ART procedure or insemination. Many clinicians may be familiar with the term *surrogate*, which has now been largely replaced by the previously mentioned terms.

When considering the legality of these two types of gestational carriers, it is helpful to consider the three primary components needed for pregnancy: egg, sperm, and a uterus. When a gestational carrier maintains two out of these three components, there are greater legal challenges regarding parental custody after the birth of the child. Because of these potential challenges, many states do not permit traditional gestational carriers, and there is wide variation in state-specific and international laws.

### Risks Associated with In Vitro Fertilization

Short-term risks of IVF include ovarian hyperstimulation syndrome, ovarian torsion, electrolyte and fluid shifts, and temporary abdominal discomfort such as cramping, tenderness, and bloating. Long-term risks related to IVF may not be fully understood or recognized given the difficulty of proving causation. The risk of multiple pregnancies in IVF using single embryo transfer is statistically lower than in non-IVF medicated cycles using ovulation induction methods, often contrary to the common perception of IVF procedures resulting in multiple gestation.[88,102] This difference arises because oocytes are obtained through surgical retrieval in the former case, which enables patients and clinicians to determine the number of embryos transferred back to the body through shared decision making. However, if the parties plan to purposefully transfer back more than one embryo, the risk of multiple gestation does exist. Placental anomalies and increased postpartum hemorrhage are also frequently noted during the labor and birth of those conceiving through IVF, although there is not a clearly defined underlying etiology.

While some research suggests an increase in fetal anomalies with IVF, a direct mechanism has not been identified. When IVF procedures are utilized for individuals experiencing unexplained infertility, it is possible these procedures might be assisting fetal DNA with higher risks of anomalies to bypass the typical conception barriers. Therefore, it may not be the technological procedures themselves that cause complications, but rather the underlying, unidentified cause of infertility. For individuals who opt for preimplantation genetic testing and have a resulting pregnancy, other recommended prenatal genetic testing should be offered, because all screening procedures have the potential for false-negative results.

The rate of subchorionic hemorrhage (SCH) is approximately doubled for those pregnant persons who have undergone IVF.[103,104] This finding is often incidental and not associated with a decreased chance of live birth or preterm birth after IVF. Given the anxiety that pregnant individuals may experience, clinicians should take care to provide anticipatory guidance regarding early first trimester bleeding and cramping and to explain that SCH does not necessarily indicate a threat to ongoing pregnancy.

### Egg Cryopreservation

Oocyte cryopreservation can be pursued for any person desiring a delay in conception. Reasons for making this decision vary widely, but may include family history of early menopause, unknown readiness for parenthood, and planning for potential impact of fertility-altering medications or treatments with known reproductive toxicity, such as chemotherapy.[110] Long-term risks are minimal. In essence, the egg cryopreservation procedure is nearly identical to the IVF process but stops short of fertilization.

Many patients are concerned they may deplete their ovarian reserve faster by freezing eggs, so it is helpful for the clinician to explain this is not the case. Although the ovary typically matures and ovulates only one mature egg per cycle, a cohort of eggs is recruited every cycle; the remaining immature eggs in this cohort undergo atrophy and do not continue to be stored in the body. Thus, the injectable gonadotropin medication used in the egg freezing process aims to stimulate multiple eggs to the point of maturity, allowing for collection during the egg retrieval versus being lost to atrophy.

Advantages of egg freezing include maintaining the genetic age and health of the eggs at the time they were frozen, thereby providing for a lower risk of genetic anomalies and miscarriage if used in the future. With current technology, there is no known expiration date for cryopreserved oocytes, and many years may pass between freezing and use for conception. Egg freezing can feel liberating for many individuals as a way to control their biologic clock, although it is important to explain that without knowledge of how eggs will interact with sperm, it is difficult to predict the potential for pregnancy in the future.[111] On average, an estimated 20 frozen eggs are needed to result in one live birth, although this number likely varies with the individual's age.

For those persons who would like to pursue egg freezing but feel confident they will not be paired with a sperm-producing partner in the future, embryo freezing using donor sperm may be an excellent option instead of egg freezing. In such a case, the individual has more information upfront regarding the statistical chance of pregnancy by removing the unknown sperm variable in the case of egg freezing.

## Donor-Assisted Conception and Reproduction

For those persons who do not have access to all necessary gametes for conception, use of donor biologic material may be considered. This may include donor sperm, donor eggs, or donor embryos. While the majority of individuals who utilize donor-assisted conception are members of the LGBTQ+ community, individuals in other social scenarios may pursue these options as well. Examples include a heterosexual couple in which the cisgender male partner does not produce sperm, a heterosexual cisgender woman planning for intentional single parenthood, a cisgender woman with early menopause seeking an egg donor, and a couple whose IVF treatment results in recurrent genetic anomalies incompatible with pregnancy. Initial discussions with patients may include who will be involved in the conception and if the situation involves a partnership, whose biologic material will be used. If more than one intended parent would like to use their own eggs to conceive, the clinician should offer testing and discuss age as an important prognostic factor for planning purposes.

For individuals using any donor biologic material (eggs, sperm, embryos), the American Society for Reproductive Medicine (ASRM) recommends that intended parents meet with a mental health provider who specializes in third-party reproduction prior to initiation of fertility treatment. Ideally, the goal of this recommendation is not to pathologize queer family building or create unnecessary barriers, but rather to address unique considerations of using donor material that is not obtained from an intended parent.[112] Donor sperm is available in two broad categories: (1) donor sperm purchased through a cryobank and (2) sperm donated by a known acquaintance, friend, or relative of the patient's partner (and thus without biological connection to the patient but with the ability to incorporate both familial genetics).

Cryobanks typically divide their donors into two subcategories, *open ID* and *nondisclosure ID*, indicating whether the donor is open to contact from children conceived through the use of their donor sperm. Those who are open to future contact may grant permission for the child to contact the cryobank after the child turns 18 years of age. Given the accessibility of information on the Internet and research indicating the psychological benefits of the option to contact their donor, many experts believe fully anonymous donor sperm may not exist within the same limits in the future.[113]

Known donors, also called directed donors, are individuals known to the intended parent(s) prior to conception. The Food and Drug Administration (FDA) requires similar testing for known donors as the comprehensive testing that is completed in cryobanks.[114] For some people, this process may be more expensive upfront but more cost-effective over the long term because known donors have an FDA-mandated 7-day window to produce multiple vials of sperm, all of which will legally belong to the intended parent(s). This 7-day window is to assure that STI testing is current and most accurate.

Donor sperm commercially available through cryobanks is usually offered in three preparation types: ICI, IUI, and IVF. Vials of ICI-prepared sperm should be used only with vaginal insemination, such as in at-home insemination without a medical provider. The term ICI technically refers to the placement of sperm within the cervix as opposed to the uterus or vaginal canal. Although this is an outdated procedure, the terminology persists. Vials of IUI-prepared sperm typically contain washed sperm and can be used for either an IUI or IVF procedure because IUI vials contain a higher sperm count than IVF vials. Vials of IVF-prepared sperm are recommended only for use in IVF cycles, as the sperm count is not considered high enough to result in pregnancy if used in conjunction with IUI or intravaginal insemination.

Given all the costs associated with the donor sperm process, many individuals may prefer to proceed directly to IVF instead of undergoing many cycles of less intensive treatment with a lower chance of conception. While IVF may be utilized without known medical reasons (i.e., medically defined infertility), it may prevent emotional burnout and, in some cases, may actually be more cost-efficient when compared to many cycles of other treatment coupled with the cost of donor sperm. When the patient is utilizing insurance benefits, most private insurance plans will require a minimum of three to six IUIs prior to the patient accessing any available IVF coverage.

Transgender or nonbinary individuals with a uterus and ovaries who have previously taken testosterone are likely to return to their baseline fertility 1 to 6 months after stopping testosterone therapy. Although earlier research suggested that transmasculine individuals may be more likely to have PCOS, more recent research has yielded conflicting results, possibly related to variance in the PCOS criteria.[115–117] It is important to note that the administration of testosterone does change ovarian appearance but does not induce or cause PCOS.[118] If an individual stops testosterone and does not resume menses, the clinician should offer a work-up to evaluate for PCOS. Individuals may become pregnant while on testosterone, even in the absence of menstruation, despite a desire to prevent pregnancy. Transgender or nonbinary individuals assigned-male-at-birth (AMAB) who take estrogen may still produce sperm, although standard doses are likely to decrease the sperm count for most patients. A small body of research also suggests that AMAB individuals may have overall lower sperm counts prior to use of gender-affirming hormones, suggesting perhaps there is an underlying hormonal correlation. Refer to the *Gender-Affirming Care* chapter for more information on transgender and nonbinary fertility options.

## Ethical Considerations and Disparities in Fertility Treatment

Numerous ethical considerations arise with various aspects of fertility treatment, including financial, racial, weight, and identity-related disparities.[119] Patients of all backgrounds may experience difficulty in accessing fertility care, whether for geographic or insurance-related reasons. Private insurance coverage has wide variations, and patients should be thoroughly counseled on the anticipated fertility treatment costs prior to initiation of treatment. Clinicians should not withhold or refuse treatment because of their personal beliefs about family. Such actions effectively prevent a significant portion of the population from being able to pursue parenthood, even when treatment may involve low-cost, low-level intervention. Infertility is considered a disability under the American with Disabilities Act, and many believe infertility treatment should not be considered elective care, given that most causes of infertility are not within the control of an individual.[120,121] Between the disparities in accessing care and the ethical considerations of genetic technology, the field of fertility has frequently been associated with unsavory aspects of the modern eugenics movement, including discrimination, racism, sexism, and ableism.[73]

While some U.S. states may provide Medicaid coverage for initial fertility testing when such testing is coded as a gynecologic concern, no U.S. state Medicaid program currently provides coverage for fertility treatment procedures.[120] In the case of certain conditions such as tubal blockage or very low sperm count, IVF may be the only chance an individual or couple has for conception. The lack of insurance coverage effectively prevents parenthood entirely for some patients. Table 10-14 lists many of the potential benefits of fertility treatment

| Table 10-14 | Benefits of Broadening Access to Infertility Treatments |
| --- | --- |

- Lower all-cause mortality
- Lower cancer-related mortality
- Lower healthcare costs related to chronic health problems
- Strengthen relationships between individuals and families
- Couples less likely to divorce when states adopt infertility insurance mandates
- Fewer mental health concerns
- Avoid undue financial burden on Medicaid recipients who choose to pursue fertility treatment and improved relationship between Medicaid recipients and government
- Decrease existing discriminatory health disparities regarding family building

Data from Cintina I, Wu B. How do state infertility insurance mandates affect divorce? *Contemp Econ Policy.* 2019;37(3): 560-570. https://doi.org/10.1111/coep.12416; Kissin DM, Boulet SL, Jamieson DJ. Fertility treatments in the United States: improving access and outcomes. *Obstet Gynecol.* 2016;128(2):387-390; Ethics Committee of the American Society for Reproductive Medicine. Disparities in access to effective treatment for infertility in the United States: an Ethics Committee opinion. *Fertil Steril.* 2021;116(1):54-63. https://doi.org/10.1016/j.fertnstert.2021.02.019; Stentz NC, Koelper N, Barnhart KT, Sammel MD, Senapati S. Infertility and mortality. *Obstet Gynecol.* 2020;222(3):251.e1. doi:10.1016/j.ajog.2019.09.007.

expansion.[77,120,122,123] Individuals with fewer socioeconomic resources report feeling discouraged from accessing fertility treatment due to costs and a perception of specialized care being out of reach.[47] Due to the historical economic effects of structural racism, a large racial wealth gap continues to persist, creating conditions in which Black, Indigenous, and other people of color have more limited access to fertility treatment options. Additionally, many gynecologic conditions that directly influence fertility, such as fibroids, pelvic pain, and endometriosis, are linked to minority stress, increased allostatic load, adverse childhood experiences (ACE) scores, and weathering.[124] Organizations in support of expanded reproductive rights and coverage include the World Health Organization (WHO), ASRM, RESOLVE: National Infertility Association, and the United Nations.[122,125–129]

Some LGBTQ+ patients may find it challenging to identify safe, inclusive providers who understand the process of donor-assisted conception without over-medicalization or over-pathologizing queer conception. Given that many individuals in the LGBTQ+ community may not have access to the gametes needed to create a pregnancy, the available guidelines and research may not readily apply, making it more difficult to understand options regarding treatment.[129] For example, much of the research conducted on IUI has been done with participants who also engage in vaginal–penile intercourse, which makes it is difficult to determine which route of sperm transport resulted in pregnancy. Donor-assisted conception is also associated with significant increased cost. The average vial of frozen donor sperm may cost approximately $800 to $1500,[130–132] with one vial necessary per conception attempt. Differences in how insurance plans and clinicians define infertility may also act as a barrier to accessing necessary services.

Individuals in higher-weight bodies have long experienced discrimination within the fertility field, with both clinicians and insurance companies often citing higher risk as a medically acceptable reason to withhold treatment. Research is conflicting regarding the impact that body weight may have on pregnancy rates or live birth, although proper access to fertility treatment is likely to improve rates.[133–135] Additionally, research examining risks and poor outcomes in individuals with higher body weights cannot be separated from the significant weight bias that exists within health care and society at large.[135,136] Disparaging narratives around risk of pregnancy for those with high BMIs can feel defeating to patients, endorsing the dialogue that they are putting their future child at risk.[133] Given that robust evidence suggests BMI is not an accurate representation of health, at best these policies are not protective; at worst, they perpetuate deeply harmful weight stigma and induce feelings of worthlessness for patients denied treatment.[137–140] Additionally, when the right to parenthood is withheld based on perceived health, the healthcare system minimizes an individual's bodily autonomy and right to determine acceptable risk. Because higher BMIs are correlated with PCOS, one of the most common fertility concerns, this disparity is incredibly common, often veiled in concern for the future neonate. Many fertility clinics both in the United States and internationally enforce strict BMI limits for patients desiring treatment initiation.[141–143] Stigmatization often causes an increase in anxiety, depression, and hopelessness, anecdotally leading many individuals to stop seeking treatment for mental health preservation or a fear of being turned away.[144] Those who are on the cusp of the BMI limit, which is frequently set at 40, may engage in physically and psychologically unhealthy behaviors such as restriction, starvation, laxative use, and overexercise in an effort to reach the BMI threshold. Given the harms associated with weight cycling, coupled with the risk for rebound insulin resistance, these policies have the potential to create long-lasting harm.[139] Strategies to communicate with patients without bias are covered in the *Skillful Communication to Mitigate Clinician Bias* appendix.

Political and public discourse on the ethics and morals of individual reproductive choices and bodily autonomy—ranging from abortion to assisted reproductive technology—is common in the United States. Legislation resulting from that ongoing discourse impacts a clinician's ability to provide, and a patient's ability to receive, patient-centered reproductive care. Specific to assisted reproductive technologies, embryo personhood laws that define life as beginning at conception effectively limit or ban the creation, testing, management, and disposal of embryos.[145] Such laws have been proposed in some states and may be potentially intertwined with laws aimed at prohibiting abortion. With the *Dobbs v. Jackson Women's Health Organization* decision on June 24, 2022, which overturned 50 years of protection of the right to obtain an abortion afforded by *Roe v. Wade*, state-specific trigger laws and forthcoming legislation will adversely impact clinical aspects of infertility care and present legal risk to patients and clinicians alike.[145,146]

For example, a 1986 Louisiana law, the only one of its kind in the United States at the time of this writing, granted all created embryos juridical personhood.[147] By requiring an embryo to have a reasonable chance at life, this law prevents all patients with currently frozen embryos from discarding extra embryos, regardless of the reason. These frozen embryos also have associated storage fees and patients must decide between indefinite storage, thawing for a planned embryo transfer, or embryo adoption to another individual or couple. Two other 2022 laws in Indiana have legally defined life as "when a human ovum is fertilized by a human sperm and [assert] a compelling state interest in protecting human physical life from the moment that human physical life begins."[148,149] As a result, it is likely the destruction of embryos will become illegal when abortion becomes illegal in Indiana. Arizona also has a 2021 law that prohibits all abortions in the presence or presumption of a fetal anomaly, which has the potential to impact the use of embryo genetic testing within in vitro fertilization.[150] Other such legislation is emerging in states nationally in the wake of the *Dobbs* decision.

| Table 10-15 | Critical Elements to Include in a Referral Note for an Individual with Infertility |
|---|---|

Social history of individual and partner(s) if appropriate

Length of time attempting pregnancy and whether the definition of infertility is met (>1 year if the individual with uterus and ovaries is < 35 years; > 6 months if they are ≥ 35 years)

Risk factors, if any, that are identified

Menstrual history

Current medications

Past health history potentially affecting fertility

Care provided: procedures and results for individual; laboratory results or if pending

Summary of rationale for transfer

Request for information about the treatment plan for follow-up

## Summary

Overall, it is very difficult to predict the success rates of completed pregnancies and live births resulting from treatment for infertility.[96] Many factors contribute to the cause of infertility as well as to the subsequent availability, access, and success of treatment. Midwives caring for individuals with infertility who are undergoing treatment can provide both clinical and emotional support in recognition of the physical, emotional, and social pressures that these patients may face. Additionally, clinicians providing prenatal care should be able to honor and appreciate the journey that individuals have experienced. Normalization of the infertility experience by the clinician and society as a whole can offer a coping mechanism for individuals with infertility diagnoses.[45] Table 10-15 provides a list of critical elements included in a transfer note after a midwife has performed initial evaluation and determines that more specialized care is needed by patients with infertility.

## Pregnancy Prevention

Another aspect of providing fertility care is supporting patients in achieving their goal to prevent pregnancy. In the PATH framework, understanding a person's attitudes or feelings about timing and importance of pregnancy prevention can help facilitate shared decision making around options for pregnancy prevention. This section explores key concepts when pregnancy prevention is identified as a reproductive goal and prefaces the more comprehensive overview of contraceptive options presented in the *Nonhormonal Contraception* and *Hormonal Contraception* chapters.

### Key Definitions and Concepts

Although the terms *birth control*, *contraception*, and *family planning* are often used interchangeably when discussing pregnancy prevention, they are not analogous in meaning, nor are they always used accurately. Additionally, when reviewing contraceptive options, concepts such as *efficacy* and *effectiveness* may be conflated. These terms are defined in Table 10-16.[151,152]

### Unintended Pregnancy

The Pregnancy Risk Assessment Monitoring System (PRAMS), which is implemented by the Centers for Disease Control and Prevention (CDC) in collaboration with state health departments, has historically informed estimates of the rate of *unintended* pregnancies. In 2012, the PRAMS survey included an additional response option to measure pregnancy intention that captured recollections of uncertainty about the desire for pregnancy prior to becoming pregnant. The data collected from respondents are more reflective of uncertainty and varying preferences or plans for timing of their pregnancies.[153] Table 10-17 outlines the current question and responses that inform how pregnancy intention has been understood and interpreted.[154]

Rather than perpetuate a binary characterization of pregnancy intention (intended or unintended), reporting data in terms of desire may be more accurate. The rate of unintended pregnancy in 2011 was reported to be approximately 45%.[155] More recently, the national proportion of pregnancies wanted later or not wanted ranged from 26% to 46% (95% confidence interval). The proportion of pregnancies characterized by uncertainty (I wasn't sure what I wanted) ranged from 8% to 20% (95% confidence interval).[156] Among those persons who wanted to be pregnant later or not at all, pregnancy rates are highest among the poor, the young, and people of color.[155] Contributing factors to this disparity are complex, and such outcomes cannot be attributed to contraceptive misuse alone. Salient factors include social and economic injustices that lead to poverty; historical injustices with regard to reproductive autonomy and health, including forced sterilization, that adversely impact attitudes and norms; reproductive coercion; limited access to contraception, emergency contraception, and abortion care services; racial discrimination and bias;

| Table 10-16 | Definitions of Terms Used in Discussing Pregnancy Prevention |
|---|---|
| **Term** | **Definition** |
| Birth control | Limitation of the number of children who are conceived, or ways to control reproduction via use of methods that improve or diminish fertility. |
| Contraception | Use of specific methods to prevent conception; does not include methods that act after conception, such as interference with or after implantation. Note that medications with contraceptive effects can be used for other purposes aside from preventing pregnancy. |
| Effectiveness | The success of a method in preventing pregnancy when used typically, including pregnancies that occur because of incorrect or inconsistent use of a given contraceptive method; poor effectiveness for a contraceptive method usually is attributed to user failure. |
| Efficacy | The chance that conception will occur despite consistent and correct (perfect) use of a specific method; poor efficacy for a contraceptive method often is termed *true method failure*. |
| Family planning | A broad term generally considered to include methods to assist an individual to plan if or when a pregnancy is desired. Most often this involves the use of various contraceptive or birth control methods, but not exclusively. |
| Pregnancy | Physiologic state following the implantation of a blastocyst(s). |

Data from American College of Obstetricians and Gynecologists. Gynecology data definitions. https://www.acog.org/practice-management/health-it-and-clinical-informatics/revitalize-gynecology-data-definitions. Accessed February 15, 2022; Brucker MC, King TL. *Pharmacology for Women's Health.* 2nd ed. Burlington, MA: Jones & Bartlett Learning; 2017.

| Table 10-17 | Pregnancy Intentions Question from PRAMS Questionnaire |
|---|---|

Thinking back to just before you got pregnant with your new baby, how did you feel about becoming pregnant? Check ONE answer.

| Current Responses | Traditional Responses |
|---|---|
| I wanted to be pregnant later. | Mistimed/unintended |
| I didn't want to be pregnant then or at any time in the future. | Unwanted/unintended |
| I wanted to be pregnant sooner. | Intended |
| I wanted to be pregnant then. | Intended |
| I wasn't sure what I wanted. | Not applicable |

Abbreviation: PRAMS, Pregnancy Risk Assessment Monitoring System.

Data from Centers for Disease Control and Prevention. Pregnancy Risk Assessment Monitoring System (PRAMS): phase 8 core questionnaire. https://www.cdc.gov/prams/pdf/questionnaire/Phase-8-Core-Questions-508.pdf. Updated 2016. Accessed December 15, 2021.

misinformation among both healthcare providers and patients; and restrictive policies and regulations that limit opportunities for providers to engage in complete, evidence-based family planning.[157]

## Childfree by Choice

The childfree movement consists of individuals intentionally opting out of parenthood for a variety of reasons (e.g., political, economic, climate-related, shifting gender norms, and decreasing stigmatization). It is distinct from desiring pregnancy and being unable to become pregnant. As the birth rate in the United States continues to decline, increasingly more adults and young people who are not parents report that they are not likely to have children.[158,159] In the context of providing RGC that is unbiased, patient-centered, and within a reproductive justice framework, these trends are important for clinicians to acknowledge when in engaging in shared decision making with the goal of pregnancy prevention. Parenthood in the United States is often viewed as a moral imperative. In turn, people who choose a childfree life may face moral outrage, stigma, and biased care.[160] This personal clinician bias, reinforced by and combined with pronatalist policies and cultural norms, can impact the way counseling is provided, such that individuals seeking sterilization to achieve their reproductive goal may encounter restricted care.[160,161] Shared decision making should be utilized when discussing a patient's reproductive goal of sterilization, including a referral to a physician. Nonjudgmental and objective language should be used in these conversations, indicating to the patient that their bodily autonomy is a high priority when choosing a method of pregnancy prevention that is aligned with this goal.

## Efficacy and Effectiveness Considerations

The terms *efficacy* and *effectiveness* are both used to describe how well a form of contraception works, but are distinctly different concepts. Efficacy is the chance that conception will occur despite consistent and correct (perfect) use of a given method. Effectiveness describes the success of a method in preventing pregnancy when used typically, including pregnancies that occur because of incorrect or inconsistent use of a given contraceptive method. To clarify these concepts, efficacy can be viewed as true method failure, while effectiveness is associated with instances where factors related to individual use (e.g., forgetting a pill dose) or systems issues (e.g., insurance coverage termination after the postpartum period).[162] Certain methods are known to be efficacious, such as oral contraceptives when used perfectly. However, because of real-life factors such as missed pills and drug–drug interactions, their effectiveness may be less than that of other methods.

### Calculation of Effectiveness of Contraceptive Methods

The Pearl index, also called the Pearl rate, has been used for more than seven decades in clinical trials to report the effectiveness of a contraceptive method. This index is calculated by dividing the number of unintended pregnancies by the number of years of exposure to the risk of unintended pregnancy among all the participants in the study[163,164] A lower Pearl index indicates a lower risk of unintended pregnancy.

Some studies report two Pearl indices, one of which is labeled as typical or actual use for a contraceptive method (effectiveness). The data from which this effectiveness index is calculated include all pregnancies, regardless of whether they involved user error or method failure. Other reports cite the second, perfect-use Pearl index, which is calculated based on data limited to cycles in which there is assurance that the method was correctly and consistently used (efficacy).[163]

Major problems have been found when using the Pearl index to assess a contraceptive method. For example, average amounts of exposure may differ from study to study, thus making the indices noncomparable. Over longer periods of time, individuals who become pregnant may leave the study, leaving behind only those participants who are less likely to become pregnant. Furthermore, for some methods such as the diaphragm, the longer the method is used, the more likely users are to become experienced with correct use. Conversely, the effectiveness of other contraceptive methods can expire, such as implants. These methods are associated with more pregnancies if they are used for periods beyond the recommended duration of use.

In addition, the Pearl index does not recognize other confounding factors. Reasons for self-discontinuation (e.g., side effects), dissatisfaction or change in desire to attempt pregnancy, and loss to follow-up of individuals who may continue to use the method correctly and successfully avoid pregnancy are not incorporated in index calculations.

To compensate for problems with the Pearl index, some researchers use life tables for statistical calculations of unintended pregnancy rates.[165] These tables present separate effectiveness rates for each month of study among a group of individuals using a specific contraceptive method over a set period of time (e.g., 12 months). When the results are subdivided by months, the assumption that contraceptive failure rates remain static is corrected. Other statistical analyses using life tables may differentiate between net effectiveness, which allows for comparison of reasons for dropping out of a study, and gross effectiveness, which enables comparison of one study to another. Studies today tend to use both the Pearl index and life table analysis, although many do not clearly designate which approach was used.

In addition to these statistical problems, studies reporting data often are part of clinical trials undertaken in pursuit of FDA approval of a method. Trials involving contraceptives differ from the more traditional drug trials. Phase 2 and 3 clinical trials are typically randomized, are often double-masked, and compare an agent to a placebo. In Phase 3 trials, the participants are individuals with a health condition that the new drug is likely to treat. Obvious ethical and methodologic problems prohibit the use of this approach for investigation of new contraceptive methods. Therefore, most clinical trials include typical participants who are healthy and seeking a method to use for contraception. The concept of the "typical" participant in clinical trials is also problematic because people younger than the age of 18 years are minors who are subject to pediatric research policies and, therefore, are not included in contraceptive trials. In addition to eliminating most adolescents, clinical trials of contraceptives tend to enroll participants of average weight and BMI, excluding people with higher body weights. Exempting people from both of these subpopulations limits the generalizability of the findings from clinical trials to all people using contraceptives in the United States. Furthermore, a lack of research on the care of gender-diverse individuals, who may also be taking gender-affirming hormones, contributes to the problem of limited generalizability.[166]

The manner in which contraceptive methods are compared to one another can be problematic. The effectiveness of one method can usually be compared to the effectiveness of another method only by using results from previously conducted research, rather than by conducting a direct comparison study. For example, assume a new oral contraceptive was found to be associated with a 20% rate of amenorrhea in users. Previously published research about an older contraceptive will most likely be used as the basis for comparison with this new contraceptive. Therefore, the assumption is made that both of the studies in question, old and new, used similar methodologic approaches and populations. In reality, reasonable comparisons cannot be guaranteed. Most studies provide relatively similar results regarding effectiveness and efficacy, and the rates included in this chapter are generally agreed upon by several references.[163]

Efficacy and effectiveness are not the only considerations when presenting contraceptive options. In a patient-centered approach, a variety of considerations, including potential medical risks and side effects, are equally important to consider when engaging in shared decision making.[11] By reflecting on personally held biases and preferences, clinicians can help their patients identify other priorities that may impact their selection. See the "Choice of a Specific Contraceptive Method" section later in this chapter for further discussion of additional considerations that may be important for patients. Bertotti et al. found that the commonly used tiered-effectiveness approach, in which clinicians use method efficacy to inform discussions of pregnancy risk that drive contraceptive decision making, may downplay the risks of contraceptive methods, which can threaten patients' autonomy and runs the risk of becoming coercive.[167] Notably, this approach can lead to an imbalanced presentation of risks and impair decision making when methods other than those with the highest efficacy may be more desirable and most appropriate for a given patient.

## Permanent Versus Reversible Contraceptive Methods

The first categorization of contraceptive methods is permanent versus reversible. Sterilization, through tubal ligation and vasectomy, remains the most efficacious and effective of all contraceptive methods and is the method used by approximately 20.6% of women between ages 15 and 44 years.[168] Different types of sterilization are discussed in the *Nonhormonal Contraception* chapter. However, millions of individuals of childbearing age desire a reversible contraceptive method.

Reversible contraceptive methods can be categorized as either long acting (LARCs) or short acting (SARCs), and as either hormonal or nonhormonal. LARCs, when placed in the uterus or subdermally, offer contraception for extended periods of time. They may be hormonal or nonhormonal methods, and possess different mechanisms of action. LARCs include IUDs (levonorgestrel [LNG] and copper) and implants. These methods require a visit to a healthcare provider for placement and removal. SARCs, when taken, placed, or injected weekly or monthly, offer a shorter period of contraception and utilize hormones. They include oral contraceptive pills, rings, patches, and injectables. These methods require a prescription from a healthcare provider in the United States, and with the exception of the injectable option, can be initiated and stopped by the user on their own at any time. Hormonal contraceptives are among the most commonly used forms of birth control in the United States. Nonhormonal methods include behavior strategies, spermicidal agents, barriers, and the copper IUD.

In addition to considering hormonal content and autonomy in starting or stopping a chosen method, individuals seeking contraception may consider how quickly it becomes effective, its ability to provide protection from STIs, its ability to be used discreetly, and cost. Table 10-18 provides an overview of available contraceptive methods and these factors for comparison.

The CDC has identified increasing access to LARCs as one of the top public health priorities for reducing adolescent pregnancy and unintended pregnancy in the United States.[169] LARCs have been identified as the most effective form of contraception, regardless of age or parity, for people with a uterus. Guidelines published by the American College of Obstetricians and Gynecologists (ACOG) state that LARCs should be considered as a highly effective option for most people seeking contraception, including adolescents.[170,171] The American Academy of Pediatrics similarly recommended LARCs as an appropriate highly effective option for adolescents, and subsequent studies have found that they tend to continue to use the methods for several years.[172,173]

Initially, LARCs are the most expensive reversible methods because of the healthcare costs incurred for both the device and the visit for its insertion. However, once implanted or inserted, the annualized

| Table 10-18 | Comparing Reversible Contraceptive Methods | | | | | |
|---|---|---|---|---|---|---|
| Method | Contains Hormone | High Autonomy | Immediately Effective | STI Protection | Discreet Use | High Initial Cost[a] |
| **Long-Acting Reversible Contraception (LARC)** | | | | | | |
| Intrauterine device | | | | | | |
| • LNG | X | | X | | X | X |
| • Copper | | | X | | X | X |
| Implant | X | | | | X | X |
| **Short-Acting Reversible Contraception (SARC)** | | | | | | |
| Oral contraceptive pills | X | X | | | | |
| Patch | X | X | | | | |
| Ring | X | X | | | | |
| Injectable | X | | | | X | |
| **Other Methods** | | | | | | |
| Condoms | | X | X | X | | |
| Diaphragm, sponge, cervical cap | | X | X | | | |
| Spermicide | | X | X | | | |
| Fertility awareness | | X | X | | | |
| Withdrawal | | X[b] | | | | |
| Abstinence | | X[b] | | | | |
| Lactation amenorrhea | | X | X | | | |

Abbreviations: LNG, levonorgestrel; STI, sexually transmitted infection.

[a] Cost may vary depending on insurance coverage. Likewise, the cost of LARC over a year may be relatively less compared to monthly SARC cost for 12 months. Reflected here are upfront cost considerations in case of no or inadequate insurance coverage, which can pose a barrier.
[b] Not true in every instance.

cost is the same or less than that for less effective methods. Several studies have found that state funding of free or low-cost LARCs decreases the costs associated with unplanned births and abortions and, therefore, that these methods are cost-effective.[174]

Like any contraceptive method, LARCs are not perfect, nor are they the best choice for everyone. Access to this highly effective method has increased since the implementation of the Affordable Care Act in 2010. Availability of LARC, and other moderately effective methods, has become recognized as an indicator of high-quality reproductive care.[175] In striving to provide high-quality reproductive care, however, the contraception paradox emerges:

Contraception can be empowering as a means of controlling one's fertility but, at the same time, can become an oppressive force, especially among historically marginalized communities.[176] Both the American College of Nurse-Midwives (ACNM) and ACOG recognize the need for comprehensive, evidence-based, and unbiased shared decision making using am RJ framework.[177,178]

In addition, some relatively rare conditions exist that preclude the use of some contraceptive methods. To further inform these discussions, national medical eligibility criteria for different contraceptive methods provide insights into the advisability of specific contraceptive methods.

## Medical Eligibility Criteria for Contraceptive Use

In 1996, the first edition of WHO's *Medical Eligibility Criteria for Contraceptive Use* (WHO MEC) was published. This document is regularly updated based on new evidence.[179] The WHO MEC is currently in its fifth edition and is especially useful for midwives working internationally. WHO has encouraged countries to modify the MEC as needed. In recognition that practice in the United States may differ in some respects from international care, the CDC has published nationally focused guidelines known as the *U.S. Medical Eligibility Criteria for Contraceptive Use, 2016* (U.S. MEC). Both the WHO MEC and the U.S. MEC offer specific recommendations for the use of specific contraceptive methods by people with certain medical conditions or characteristics. These publications are available as free apps and are listed in the Resources section of this chapter.

Modifications of the WHO MEC for contraceptive users in the United States include exclusion of methods not available in the United States and inclusion of several additional health conditions of note in this country. In particular, modifications that address breastfeeding/chestfeeding, IUD use, valvular heart disease, ovarian cancer, uterine fibroids, and venous thromboembolism were made to the WHO MEC to better reflect the U.S. population and practice.[179,180]

A companion to the U.S. MEC is a document focusing on selected practices that, although common, can be complicated. Titled *U.S. Selected Practice Recommendations for Contraceptive Use, 2016* (U.S. SPR), this publication is available as a free app and is listed in the Resources section of this chapter. The U.S. SPR focuses on frequently occurring conditions associated with controversial or complex interventions for people seeking contraception in the United States. The most recent changes to the U.S. SPR include guidelines on when to start a method after emergency contraception as well as use of medications to ease insertion of IUDs.[181]

The U.S. MEC primarily focuses on the safety of use of various contraceptives, especially for both initiation and continuation. The clinician and the patient can quickly verify recommendations for use of a specific method by referring to multiple tables in the publication. Note that the U.S. MEC is a set of guidelines—compliance with its recommendations is not mandatory. Thus, deviations from its recommendations may occur after considering an individual's specific situation. Nevertheless, variations in practice are becoming rarer and the U.S.

MEC guidelines are used widely throughout the United States, augmented with information from the U.S. SPR.

In summary, many factors are considered when providing care for a person who desires to prevent pregnancy. Although the effectiveness and eligibility of specific methods are important considerations, counseling is a prerequisite to facilitating an informed choice. The best contraception for anyone is the method that they personally desire, that is accessible, and that can be well adapted into their lives.

## Contraceptive Counseling and Clinical Practice

The hallmarks of midwifery care include concepts such as promoting family-centered care, facilitating empowerment of patients as partners in health care, promoting public health, and advocating for shared decision making and the right to self-determination.[1] Responsibilities of midwives in this area include identification of individual needs, health education, assisting in decision making, and provision of contraceptive methods. To appropriately provide comprehensive sexual and reproductive health care, midwives must be aware of their own biases and attitudes about sexuality, gender roles, contraception, religious beliefs, and other beliefs that could affect contraceptive counseling.

Obtaining a comprehensive health history, including screening for intimate-partner violence (IPV) and reproductive coercion (see the *Health Promotion Across the Lifespan* chapter for recommended screening), is the initial step in contraceptive counseling. In combination, IPV and reproductive coercion have synergistic effects on unintended pregnancy.[182] This information will allow midwives to assess for the risk factors outlined in the U.S. MEC and tailor counseling to the individual. Certain medical conditions may affect a person's eligibility for some contraceptive methods. For example, combined hormonal contraceptives are not safe for a person with severe hypertension.[180]

## Choice of a Specific Contraceptive Method

Engaging in sexual activity does not automatically place someone at risk for pregnancy. Yet, more than 60% of women between ages 15 and 44 years use a contraceptive method.[168] To effectively provide any counseling, midwives must be able to personally detach from the decision that the patient may make, acknowledging that their decision may not be the one a midwife would make or recommend. In fact, the patient's decision may even conflict with the midwife's personal beliefs.

A person's preference is the major foundation for choice of a specific method.[11] Incorporation of a partner into the process of choosing a contraceptive method is also their choice. In some cases, midwives may provide education to couples; in other situations, the patient alone consults with the professional. Throughout this chapter, content regarding education and care may be extrapolated to include significant others when their inclusion is preferred.

Some patients may prefer not to share information about a chosen contraceptive method with their partners because of personal privacy concerns, fear of contraceptive sabotage, or pregnancy pressure. The latter two instances are types of reproductive coercion that occur when a partner or other interferes with autonomous reproductive health decisions and may not be perceived or identified as such by the patient.[172] Evidence suggests that individuals experiencing IPV may seek contraceptive methods that are undetectable (e.g., a LARC method), which may contribute to clinician bias toward LARC in cases of reproductive coercion.[182] To avoid further limitations of a patient's contraceptive choice, it is important for midwives to avoid making assumptions about contraceptive preferences and to center the patient's desires in their counseling, which may include other methods (i.e., spermicides, SARCs, and access to emergency contraception and abortion care).[183]

Some individuals may seek contraceptives because they are anticipating exposure to pregnancy, voluntarily or not. For example, a deployment in the military may place the individual in a setting where they are vulnerable to sexual violence, or where contraceptive-associated amenorrhea may be preferable because of deployment to areas with lack of hygienic conditions.[184,185] People who have physical or intellectual disabilities also have unique needs in the area of contraception and menstruation.[186] These needs may be related to or separate from voluntary sexual activity.

An individual's preference for a specific contraceptive method also can be influenced by a variety of individual factors that may emerge from reproductive goals counseling and should be acknowledged by the midwife. Desired family size and choices about contraceptive methods are strongly influenced by culture, attitudes, and religion. Although pregnancy is defined by implantation, some people may view pregnancy as starting at conception, and this belief may affect adoption of certain contraceptive methods that do not impede conception based on their mechanism of action. Some may believe exogenous hormones are unnatural and opt for only nonhormonal methods. The contraceptive experiences and usage of a particular method among friends and family may also influence how someone approaches their options. Cost and insurance availability can cause a person to discount certain methods. These are only a few examples, but in general, understanding a person's intersecting identities, circumstances, and the way they experience oppression will inform this discussion. Table 10-19 outlines other factors often involved in a patient's selection of a contraceptive method.

| Table 10-19 | Common Factors Involved in a Patient's Selection of Contraceptive Methods |
|---|---|
| **Factor** | **Example** |
| Acceptance of critical aspects of the method | View that a daily method or one that is coital dependent is inconvenient |
| Acceptance of unintended pregnancy | Failure of method is inconvenient but not troublesome to the individual and/or their family |
| Access to the method and ability to use it successfully | Unable to manipulate diaphragm for insertion and removal<br>Expense of methods and no insurance to cover cost |
| Beliefs | Desire not to have device reside in the individual's body<br>Wariness about using any exogenous hormones |
| Eligibility based on risk factors | Age and concomitant health conditions identified as Level 3 or 4 in the *U.S. Medical Eligibility Criteria* |
| Health benefits | Personal risk factors that can be ameliorated by specific methods |
| Need for a discreet method and privacy | Desire not to let the partner or others know of sexual activity or contraception |

| Factor | Example |
|---|---|
| Need for protection from STIs | Most methods provide contraception but not STI protection unless condoms are added |
| Opinions of partner or significant others | Family members' opinions about the benefits or complications of use of a specific method |
| Past history | Desire to restart or not restart a method |
| Pattern of sexual activity | Sexual activity is infrequent |
| Side effects and tolerance | Interpretation/tolerance of intermenstrual bleeding; amenorrhea; other common side effects |
| Support and counseling from healthcare provider | Healthcare provider with a negative opinion about a specific method or about adolescents engaging in sexual intercourse |
| Time to return to fertility after discontinuation | Desires a pregnancy within a short period, which may preclude certain methods including LARCs |

Abbreviations: LARC, long-acting reversible contraception; STI, sexually transmitted infection.

Practice varies as to how the informed consent or shared decision-making processes are acknowledged and documented. Some healthcare institutions require that the patient sign consent forms. In any case, decision making that engages and empowers the patient is essential.[187] Written consent must always be obtained prior to initiation of any invasive method, such as an implant or IUD.

## Conclusion

This chapter reviewed various ways that clinicians can support their patients in managing their fertility through family building and pregnancy prevention.

Reproductive goals counseling in the context of any patient encounter is an opportunity to promote the hallmarks of midwifery care—namely, patient-centered care, informed choice, shared decision making, and the right to self-determination. Discussions regarding future family building can and should start in the younger reproductive years. Approaching fertility care with a reproductive justice lens is also essential for reducing harm and promotion of health and wellness. Clinicians should understand their individual scope of practice and know when to utilize appropriate referrals, while recognizing that many aspects of fertility care are within the scope of the midwife or advanced practice nurse.

## Resources

| Organization | Description |
|---|---|
| American Society for Reproductive Medicine (ASRM) | U.S. professional organization for reproductive medicine specialists. Continuing education courses for healthcare professionals available. |
| Centers for Disease Control and Prevention (CDC) | *U.S. Medical Eligibility Criteria for Contraceptive Use* (U.S. MEC). *U.S. Selected Practice Recommendations for Contraceptive Use* (U.S. SPR). Both resources are available as apps for download for iOS and Android operating systems. |
| Guttmacher Institute | Research and policy organization committed to advancing sexual and reproductive health and rights in the United States and globally. |
| The PATH Framework | A patient-centered framework with a shared decision-making model at its core for use with any population. |
| Power to Decide: Bedsider Providers | Articles, digital tools, and educational materials to support quality sexual and reproductive health care. |

| Organization | Description |
|---|---|
| SisterSong | Women of Color reproductive justice (RJ) collective providing RJ training and leadership development. |
| World Health Organization (WHO) | Downloadable wheel (to be printed and assembled). |
| RESOLVE: National Infertility Association | Free support groups in more than 200 communities, patient advocacy, information for anyone challenged in their infertility. |
| Fat Positive Fertility | Online platform offering workshops, support groups, and resources for both patients and healthcare professionals. Run by fertility coach Nicola Salmon, author of *Fat and Fertile*. |
| Fertility for Colored Girls | Organization that provides education, awareness, support, and encouragement to African American women/couples and other women of color experiencing infertility. |
| Broken Brown Egg | Organization that provides resources and support for three major targets: Reproductive Justice and Health Equity, the Reproductive Health Careers Pipeline, and Empowerment and Community. |
| Cade Foundation | Organization that provides information, support, and financial assistance to help needy infertile families overcome infertility. |

## References

1. American College of Nurse-Midwives. ACNM core competencies for basic midwifery practice. https://www.midwife.org/acnm/files/acnmlibrarydata/uploadfilename/000000000050/ACNMCore CompetenciesMar2020_final.pdf. Updated 2020. Accessed September 21, 2020.

2. Baltor MRR, Rodrigues JSM, Ferreira N, Dupas G. The text in its context: what is family for you? *Revista de Pesquisa Cuidado é Fundamental Online*. 2014;6(1):293-304. https://doi.org/10.9789/2175-5361.2014.v6i1.293-304.

3. Diamond DJ, Diamond MO. Parenthood after reproductive loss: how psychotherapy can help with postpartum adjustment and parent–infant attachment. *Psychotherapy*. 2017;54(4):373-379. https://www.ncbi.nlm.nih.gov/pubmed/28967766. doi:10.1037/pst0000127.

4. Weitz YS, Karlsson M. Professional or authentic motherhood? Negotiations on the identity of the birth mother in the context of foster care. *Qual Soc Work*. 2021;20(3):703-717. doi:10.1177/1473325020912815.

5. Mulaudzi FM, Peu MD. Communal child-rearing: the role of nurses in school health. *Curationis*. 2014;37(1):1158. doi:10.4102/curationis.v37i1.1158.

6. Cirulli F, Berry A, Bonsignore LT, et al. Early life influences on emotional reactivity: evidence that social enrichment has greater effects than handling on anxiety-like behaviors, neuroendocrine responses to stress and central BDNF levels. *Neurosci Biobehav Rev*. 2010;34(6):808. doi:10.1016/j.neubiorev.2010.02.008.

7. Bradshaw D, Jay S, McNamara N, et al. Perceived discrimination amongst young people in socio-economically disadvantaged communities: parental support and community identity buffer (some) negative impacts of stigma. *Br J Develop Psychol*. 2016;34(2):153-168. https://www.ncbi.nlm.nih.gov/pubmed/26490256. doi:10.1111/bjdp.12120.

8. Gavin L, Pazol K, Ahrens K. Providing quality family planning services: recommendations of CDC and the U.S. office of population affairs, 2017. *MMWR Recomm Rep*. 2017;66(1):1383-1385.

9. ACOG Committee Opinion No. 755: well-woman visit. *Obstet Gynecol*. 2018;132(4):e181-e186. doi:10.1097/AOG.0000000000002897.

10. Callegari LS, Aiken ARA, Dehlendorf C, et al. Addressing potential pitfalls of reproductive life planning with patient-centered counseling. *Obstet Gynecol*. 2017;216(2):129-134. doi:10.1016/j.ajog.2016.10.004.

11. Brandi K, Fuentes L. The history of tiered-effectiveness contraceptive counseling and the importance of patient-centered family planning care. *Obstet Gynecol*. 2020;222(4):S873-S877. doi:10.1016/j.ajog.2019.11.1271.

12. Ross LJ, Solinger R. *Reproductive Justice*. Berkeley, CA: University of California Press; 2017.

13. Eaton AA, Stephens DP. Reproductive justice special issue introduction: "reproductive justice: moving the margins to the center in social issues research." *J Soc Iss*. 2020;76(2):208-218. doi:10.1111/josi.12384.

14. Karpman HE, Ruppel EH, Torres M. "It wasn't feasible for us": queer women of color navigating family formation: queer women of color family formation.

*Fam Relations.* 2018;67(1):118-131. doi:10.1111/fare.12303.

15. Oleson JC. The new eugenics: Black hyper-incarceration and human abatement. *Soc Sci.* 2016;5(4):66. doi:10.3390/socsci5040066.

16. American College of Nurse-Midwives. Position statement: racism and racial bias. https://www.midwife.org/acnm/files/ACNMLibraryData/UPLOADFILENAME/000000000315/PS-Racism-and-Racial-Bias-26-Apr-18.pdf. Updated 2018. Accessed September 20, 2020.

17. Morse JE, Moos M. Reproductive life planning: raising the questions. *Matern Child Health J.* 2018;22(4):439-444. doi:10.1007/s10995-018-2516-z.

18. Power to Decide. One Key Question. https://powertodecide.org/one-key-question. Updated 2022. Accessed January 28, 2022.

19. Geist C, Aiken ARA, Sanders JN, et al. Beyond intent: exploring the association of contraceptive choice with questions about pregnancy attitudes, timing and how important is pregnancy prevention (PATH) questions. *Contraception.* 2019;99(1):22-26. doi:10.1016/j.contraception.2018.08.014.

20. Bonnington A, Dianat S, Kerns J, et al. Society of Family Planning clinical recommendations: contraceptive counseling for transgender and gender diverse people who were female sex assigned at birth. *Contraception.* 2020;102(2):70-82. doi:10.1016/j.contraception.2020.04.001.

21. Hatcher RL, Nelson A, Trussell J, et al. *Contraceptive Technology.* 21st ed. Atlanta, GA: Managing Contraception; 2018.

22. Practice Committee of the American Society for Reproductive Medicine. Definitions of infertility and recurrent pregnancy loss: a committee opinion. *Fertil Steril.* 2020;113(3):533-535. doi:10.1016/j.fertnstert.2019.11.025.

23. Epstein R. Space invaders: queer and trans bodies in fertility clinics. *Sexualities.* 2018;21(7):1039-1058. doi:10.1177/1363460717720365.

24. Kolanska K, Uddin J, Dabi Y, et al. Secondary infertility with a history of vaginal childbirth: ready to have another one? *J Gynecol Obstet Hum Reprod.* 2022;51(1):102271. doi:10.1016/j.jogoh.2021.102271.

25. Infertility workup for the women's health specialist: ACOG Committee Opinion, Number 781. *Obstet Gynecol.* 2019;133(6):e377-e384. https://www.ncbi.nlm.nih.gov/pubmed/31135764. doi:10.1097/AOG.0000000000003271.

26. United Nations for LGBT Equality. Fact sheet: intersex. https://www.unfe.org/wp-content/uploads/2017/05/UNFE-Intersex.pdf. Updated 2017. Accessed July 2, 2022.

27. American College of Obstetricians and Gynecologists Committee on Gynecologic Practice, Practice Committee. Female age-related fertility decline: Committee Opinion No. 589. *Fertil Steril.* 2022;101(3):633-634. https://www.ncbi.nlm.nih.gov/pubmed/24559617. doi:10.1016/j.fertnstert.2013.12.032.

28. Silber S. Unifying theory of adult resting follicle recruitment and fetal oocyte arrest. *Reprod BioMed Online.* 2015;31(4):472-475. https://www.sciencedirect.com/science/article/pii/S1472648315003582. https://doi.org/10.1016/j.rbmo.2015.06.022.

29. Practice Committee of the American Society for Reproductive Medicine, Practice Committee of the Society for Reproductive Endocrinology and Infertility. Optimizing natural fertility: a committee opinion. *Fertil Steril.* 2022;117(1):53-63. https://www.ncbi.nlm.nih.gov/pubmed/34815068. doi:10.1016/j.fertnstert.2021.10.007.

30. Gerkowicz SA, Crawford SB, Hipp HS, et al. Assisted reproductive technology with donor sperm: national trends and perinatal outcomes. *Obstet Gynecol.* 2018;218(4):421.e1-421.e10. https://www.ncbi.nlm.nih.gov/pubmed/29291411. doi:10.1016/j.ajog.2017.12.224.

31. Wyndham N, Marin Figueira PG, Patrizio P. A persistent misperception: assisted reproductive technology can reverse the "aged biological clock." *Fertil Steril.* 2012;97(5):1044-1047. https://www.ncbi.nlm.nih.gov/pubmed/22386844. doi:10.1016/j.fertnstert.2012.02.015.

32. de La Rochebrochard E, Thonneau P. Paternal age >or=40 years: an important risk factor for infertility. *Obstet Gynecol.* 2003;189(4):901-905. https://www.ncbi.nlm.nih.gov/pubmed/14586322. doi:10.1067/s0002-9378(03)00753-1.

33. Kearney AL, White KM. Examining the psychosocial determinants of women's decisions to delay childbearing. *Hum Reprod.* 2016;31(8):1776-1787. https://www.ncbi.nlm.nih.gov/pubmed/27240695. doi:10.1093/humrep/dew124.

34. Adachi T, Endo M, Ohashi K. Regret over the delay in childbearing decision negatively associates with life satisfaction among Japanese women and men seeking fertility treatment: a cross-sectional study. *BMC Public Health.* 2020;20(1):886. https://www.ncbi.nlm.nih.gov/pubmed/32513145. doi:10.1186/s12889-020-09025-5.

35. Adachi T, Endo M, Ohashi K. Uninformed decision-making and regret about delaying childbearing decisions: a cross-sectional study. *Nurs Open.* 2020;7(5):1489-1496. https://www.ncbi.nlm.nih.gov/pubmed/32802369. doi:10.1002/nop2.523.

36. Jensen RE, Martins N, Parks MM. Public perception of female fertility: initial fertility, peak fertility, and age-related infertility among U.S. adults. *Arch Sex Behav.* 2018;47(5):1507-1516. https://www.ncbi.nlm.nih.gov/pubmed/29582267. doi:10.1007/s10508-018-1197-4.

37. Segal TR, Giudice LC. Before the beginning: environmental exposures and reproductive and obstetrical outcomes. *Fertil Steril.* 2019;112(4):613-621. https://www.ncbi.nlm.nih.gov/pubmed/31561863. doi:10.1016/j.fertnstert.2019.08.001.

38. Hyland A, Piazza K, Hovey KM, et al. Associations between lifetime tobacco exposure with infertility and age at natural menopause: the Women's Health Initiative Observational Study. *Tob Control.* 2016; 25(6):706-714. https://www.ncbi.nlm.nih.gov/pubmed/26666428. doi:10.1136/tobaccocontrol-2015-052510.

39. Punab M, Poolamets O, Paju P, et al. Causes of male infertility: a 9-year prospective monocentre study on 1737 patients with reduced total sperm counts. *Hum Reprod.* 2016;32(1):18. doi:10.1093/humrep/dew284.

40. Schlegel PN, Sigman M, Collura B, et al. Diagnosis and treatment of infertility in men: AUA/ASRM guideline part I. *Fertil Steril.* 2021;115(1):54-61. https://www.ncbi.nlm.nih.gov/pubmed/33309062. doi:10.1016/j.fertnstert.2020.11.015.

41. Semet M, Paci M, Saïas-Magnan J, et al. The impact of drugs on male fertility: a review. *Andrology.* 2017; 5(4):640-663. https://www.ncbi.nlm.nih.gov/pubmed/28622464. doi:10.1111/andr.12366.

42. Practice Committee of the American Society for Reproductive Medicine. Diagnostic evaluation of the infertile male: a committee opinion. *Fertil Steril.* 2021;116:18. https://www.ncbi.nlm.nih.gov/pubmed/25597249. doi:10.1016/j.fertnstert.2015.03.019.

43. National Cancer Institute, National Institutes of Health. Diethylstilbestrol (DES) exposure and cancer. https://www.cancer.gov/about-cancer/causes-prevention/risk/hormones/des-fact-sheet. Updated 2021. Accessed February 5, 2021.

44. Davis G, Loughran T. *The Palgrave Handbook of Infertility in History.* London, UK: Palgrave Macmillan; 2017.

45. Benyamini Y, Gozlan M, Weissman A. Normalization as a strategy for maintaining quality of life while coping with infertility in a pronatalist culture. *Int J Behav Med.* 2017;24(6):871-879.

46. Akpinar F, Yilmaz S, Karahanoglu E, et al. Intimate partner violence in Turkey among women with female infertility. *Sex Relationship Ther.* 2019;34(1):3-9. https://doi.org/10.1080/14681994.2017.1327711.

47. Bell AV. "I don't consider a cup performance; I consider it a test": masculinity and the medicalisation of infertility. *Sociol Health Illn.* 2016;38(5):706-720. https://www.ncbi.nlm.nih.gov/pubmed/26683445. doi:10.1111/1467-9566.12395.

48. Practice Committee of the American Society for Reproductive Medicine. Diagnostic evaluation of the infertile female: a committee opinion. *Fertil Steril.* 2015; 103(6):e44-e50.

49. Pacchiarotti A, Frati G, Saccucci P. A surprising link with unexplained infertility: a possible COVID-19

paradox? *J Assist Reprod Genet.* 2020;37(11):2661-2662. https://www.ncbi.nlm.nih.gov/pubmed/32845433. doi:10.1007/s10815-020-01911-6.

50. Aisenberg Romano G, Ravid H, Zaig I, et al. The psychological profile and affective response of women diagnosed with unexplained infertility undergoing in vitro fertilization. *Arch Womens Mental Health.* 2012;15(6):403-411. https://www.ncbi.nlm.nih.gov/pubmed/22847827. doi:10.1007/s00737-012-0299-6.

51. Pandian Z, Gibreel A, Bhattacharya S. In vitro fertilisation for unexplained subfertility. *Cochrane Database Syst Rev.* 2015;11. doi:10.1002/14651858.CD003357.pub4.

52. Koroma L, Stewart L. Infertility: evaluation and initial management. *J Midwifery Womens Health.* 2012;57(6):614-621. https://www.ncbi.nlm.nih.gov/pubmed/23078197. doi:10.1111/j.1542-2011.2012.00241.x.

53. Moore M. Infertility. In: Schuiling KD, Likis FE, eds. *Gynecologic Health Care.* 4th ed. Burlington, MA: Jones & Bartlett Learning; 2022:383-398.

54. Lindsay TJ, Vitrikas KR. Evaluation and treatment of infertility. *Am Fam Physician.* 2015;91(5):308-314. https://www.ncbi.nlm.nih.gov/pubmed/25822387.

55. Lim ZW, Wang I, Wang P, et al. Obstructive sleep apnea increases risk of female infertility: a 14-year nationwide population-based study. *PloS One.* 2021;16(12):e0260842. https://www.ncbi.nlm.nih.gov/pubmed/34910749. doi:10.1371/journal.pone.0260842.

56. Jacobs MB, Boynton-Jarrett R, Harville EW. Adverse childhood event experiences, fertility difficulties and menstrual cycle characteristics. *J Psychosom Obstet Gynaecol.* 2015;36(2):46-57. https://www.ncbi.nlm.nih.gov/pubmed/25826282. doi:10.3109/0167482X.2015.1026892.

57. Durairajanayagam D. Lifestyle causes of male infertility. *Arab J Urol.* 2018;16(1):10-20. https://www.ncbi.nlm.nih.gov/pubmed/29713532. doi:10.1016/j.aju.2017.12.004.

58. Penzias A, Azziz R, Bendikson K, et al. Fertility evaluation of infertile women: a committee opinion. *Fertil Steril.* 2021;116(5):1255-1265. https://www.ncbi.nlm.nih.gov/pubmed/34607703. doi:10.1016/j.fertnstert.2021.08.038.

59. Zarek SM, Hill MJ, Richter KS, et al. Single-donor and double-donor sperm intrauterine insemination cycles: does double intrauterine insemination increase clinical pregnancy rates? *Fertil Steril.* 2014;102(3):739-743. https://www.ncbi.nlm.nih.gov/pubmed/24934490. doi:10.1016/j.fertnstert.2014.05.018.

60. Suarez SS, Pacey AA. Sperm transport in the female reproductive tract. *Hum Reprod Update.* 2006;12(1):23-37. https://www.ncbi.nlm.nih.gov/pubmed/16272225. doi:10.1093/humupd/dmi047.

61. Sandhu RS, Wong TH, Kling CA, Chohan KR. In vitro effects of coital lubricants and synthetic and natural oils on sperm motility. *Fertil Steril*. 2014; 101(4):941-944. https://www.ncbi.nlm.nih.gov/pubmed /24462060. doi:10.1016/j.fertnstert.2013.12.024.

62. Rooney KL, Domar AD. The relationship between stress and infertility. *Dialog Clin Neurosci*. 2018; 20(1):41-47. https://www.ncbi.nlm.nih.gov/pubmed /29946210.

63. González-Foruria I, Martínez F, Rodríguez-Purata J, et al. Can anti-Müllerian hormone predict success outcomes in donor sperm inseminations? *Gynecol Endocrinol*. 2019;35(1):40-43. https://www.ncbi.nlm .nih.gov/pubmed/30324829. doi:10.1080/09513590 .2018.1499089.

64. Hvidman HW, Bentzen JG, Thuesen LL, et al. Infertile women below the age of 40 have similar anti-Müllerian hormone levels and antral follicle count compared with women of the same age with no history of infertility. *Hum Reprod*. 2016;31(5):1034-1045. https://www.ncbi.nlm.nih.gov/pubmed/26965431. doi:10.1093/humrep/dew032.

65. Orouji Jokar T, Fourman LT, Lee H, et al. Higher TSH levels within the normal range are associated with unexplained infertility. *J Clin Endocrinol Metab*. 2018;103(2):632-639. https://www.ncbi.nlm.nih. gov/pubmed/29272395. doi:10.1210/jc.2017-02120.

66. Turan OD. Vitamin D level and infertility. *Adnan Menderes Üniversitesi Tıp Fakültesi/J Adnan Menderes University Medical Faculty*. 2015. https://doi. org/10.5152/adutfd.2015.2399.

67. Poornima S, Daram S, Devaki RK, Qurratulain H. Chromosomal abnormalities in couples with primary and secondary infertility: genetic counseling for assisted reproductive techniques (ART). *J Reprod Infertil*. 2020;21(4):269-274. https://www .ncbi.nlm.nih.gov/pubmed/33209743. doi:10.18502/ jri.v21i4.4331.

68. Singh V, Mishra B, Sinha S, et al. Role of saline infusion sonohysterography in infertility evaluation. *J Hum Reprod Sci*. 2018;11(3):236-241. https://www.ncbi.nlm.nih.gov/pubmed/30568352. doi:10.4103/jhrs.JHRS_47_18.

69. Vissers J, Hehenkamp W, Lambalk CB, Huirne JA. Post-caesarean section niche-related impaired fertility: hypothetical mechanisms. *Hum Reprod*. 2020; 35(7):1484-1494. https://www.ncbi.nlm.nih.gov/ pubmed/32613231. doi:10.1093/humrep/deaa094.

70. Barber D. Research into the role of fertility nurses for the development of guidelines for clinical practice. *J Br Fertil Soc*. 1997;2(2):195-197.

71. Gordon A. Having a better body image won't end body-based oppression. https://www.self.com/story /body-neutrality. Updated 2020. Accessed July 2, 2022.

72. O'Hara L, Ahmed H, Elashie S. Evaluating the impact of a brief Health at Every Size®–informed health promotion activity on body positivity and internalized weight-based oppression. *Body Image*. 2021; 37:225-237. https://www.ncbi.nlm.nih.gov/pubmed /33744684. doi:10.1016/j.bodyim.2021.02.006.

73. Barnes L, Fledderjohann J. Reproductive justice for the invisible infertile: a critical examination of reproductive surveillance and stratification. *Sociol Compass*. 2020;14(2). https://doi.org/10.1111/soc4.12745.

74. Smith JF, Eisenberg ML, Millstein SG, et al. The use of complementary and alternative fertility treatment in couples seeking fertility care: data from a prospective cohort in the United States. *Fertil Steril*. 2010;93(7): 2169-2174. https://www.ncbi.nlm.nih.gov/pubmed /20338559. doi:10.1016/j.fertnstert.2010.02.054.

75. Roozitalab S, Rahimzadeh M, Mirmajidi SR, et al. The relationship between infertility, stress, and quality of life with posttraumatic stress disorder in infertile women. *J Reprod Infertil*. 2021;22(4):282-288. https://www.ncbi.nlm.nih.gov/pubmed/34987990. doi:10.18502/jri.v22i4.7654.

76. Domar AD, Zuttermeister PC, Friedman R. The psychological impact of infertility: a comparison with patients with other medical conditions. *J Psychosom Obstet Gynaecol*. 1993;14(suppl):45-52. https://www .ncbi.nlm.nih.gov/pubmed/8142988.

77. Cintina I, Wu B. How do state infertility insurance mandates affect divorce? *Contemp Econ Policy*. 2019; 37(3):560-570. https://doi.org/10.1111/coep.12416.

78. Lee SH, Liu LC, Kuo PC, Lee MS. Postpartum depression and correlated factors in women who received in vitro fertilization treatment. *J Midwifery Womens Health*. 2011;56(4):347-352. https://www .ncbi.nlm.nih.gov/pubmed/21733105. doi:10.1111/j .1542-2011.2011.00033.x.

79. RESOLVE: National Infertility Association. Coping with infertility tips. https://resolve.org/get-help /helpful-resources-and-advice/managing-infertility -stress/. Accessed February 10, 2022.

80. Huang D, Ransohoff A, Boscardin J, et al. Patients' perceived level of counseling and emotional support, not number of cycles, strongly impacts decision regret after failed autologous IVF in women age 42 and over. *Fertil Steril*. 2021;116(1):e8. https://doi .org/10.1016/j.fertnstert.2021.05.013.

81. Harrington R. Childless. *Psychoanal Dialog*. 2019; 29(1):35-50. https://doi.org/10.1080/10481885.2018 .1560868.

82. Ventegodt S, Morad M, Merrick J. Clinical holistic medicine: holistic pelvic examination and holistic treatment of infertility. *Sci World J*. 2004;4:148-158. https://www.ncbi.nlm.nih.gov/pubmed/15010569. doi:10.1100/tsw.2004.14.

83. Uriart BN, Guerr MP, Penad AM. P-499 infertility impact on perceived quality of life and sexual

satisfaction in Spanish women with primary and secondary infertility. *Hum Reprod.* 2021;36. https://doi.org/10.1093/humrep/deab130.498.

84. Okobi OE. A systemic review on the association between infertility and sexual dysfunction among women utilizing female sexual function index as a measuring tool. *Cureus.* 2021;13(6):e16006. https://www.ncbi.nlm.nih.gov/pubmed/34336497. doi:10.7759/cureus.16006.

85. Sater AC, Miyague AH, Schuffner A, et al. Impact of assisted reproduction treatment on sexual function of patients diagnosed with infertility. *Arch Gynecol Obstet.* 2022:1. https://www.ncbi.nlm.nih.gov/pubmed/35066622. doi:10.1007/s00404-021-06367-2.

86. Bergh CM, Moore M, Gundell C. Evidence-based management of infertility in women with polycystic ovary syndrome. *J Obstet Gynecol Neonatal Nurs.* 2016;45(1):111-122. https://www.ncbi.nlm.nih.gov/pubmed/26815805. doi:10.1016/j.jogn.2015.10.001.

87. Legro RS, Brzyski RG, Diamond MP, et al. Letrozole versus clomiphene for infertility in the polycystic ovary syndrome. *Obstet Gynecol Surv.* 2014;69(10):599-601. https://doi.org/10.1097/01.ogx.0000456355.64379.77.

88. Wang R, Li W, Bordewijk EM, et al. First-line ovulation induction for polycystic ovary syndrome: an individual participant data meta-analysis. *Hum Reprod Update.* 2019;25(6):717-732. https://www.ncbi.nlm.nih.gov/pubmed/31647106. doi:10.1093/humupd/dmz029.

89. McKnight KK, Nodler JL, Cooper JJ Jr, et al. Body mass index–associated differences in response to ovulation induction with letrozole. *Fertil Steril.* 2011;96(5):1206-1208.

90. Vause TD, Cheung AP, Sierra S, et al. Ovulation induction in polycystic ovary syndrome: No. 242, May 2010. *Int J Gynaecol Obstet.* 2010;111(1):95-100. https://www.ncbi.nlm.nih.gov/pubmed/20848729. doi:10.1016/j.ijgo.2010.07.001.

91. Kousta EW. Modern use of clomiphene citrate in induction of ovulation. *Hum Reprod Update.* 1997;3(4):359. doi:10.1093/humupd/3.4.359.

92. Practice Committee of the Society for Reproductive Endocrinology and Infertility, Quality Assurance Committee of the Society for Assisted Reproductive Technologies, Practice Committee of the American Society for Reproductive Medicine. Multiple gestation associated with infertility therapy: a committee opinion. *Fertil Steril.* 2022. https://www.ncbi.nlm.nih.gov/pubmed/35115166. doi:10.1016/j.fertnstert.2021.12.016.

93. Practice Committees of the American Society for Reproductive Medicine and the Society for Reproductive Endocrinology and Infertility. Diagnosis and treatment of luteal phase deficiency: a committee opinion. *Fertil Steril.* 2021;115(6):1416-1423. https://www.ncbi.nlm.nih.gov/pubmed/33827766. doi:10.1016/j.fertnstert.2021.02.010.

94. Mesen TB, Young SL. Progesterone and the luteal phase: a requisite to reproduction. *Obstet Gynecol Clin North Am.* 2015;42(1):135-151. https://www.ncbi.nlm.nih.gov/pubmed/25681845. doi:10.1016/j.ogc.2014.10.003.

95. Sallam HN, Rahman AF, Abou-Ali A, et al. Oral micronized progesterone versus human menopausal gonadotropins for the treatment of repeated early pregnancy loss due to luteal phase insufficiency. *Fertil Steril.* 2002;78:S277. https://doi.org/10.1016/S0015-0282(02)03923-7.

96. Allahbadia GN. Intrauterine insemination: fundamentals revisited. *J Obstet Gynaecol India.* 2017;67(6):385-392. https://www.ncbi.nlm.nih.gov/pubmed/29162950. doi:10.1007/s13224-017-1060-x.

97. Olson S. Intrauterine insemination: clinical training. 2022. Unpublished training offered by the author.

98. American Society for Reproductive Medicine, Reproductive Facts. Intrauterine insemination (IUI). https://www.reproductivefacts.org/news-and-publications/patient-fact-sheets-and-booklets/documents/fact-sheets-and-info-booklets/intrauterine-insemination-iui/. Updated 2016. Accessed February 15, 2022.

99. Ethics Committee of the American Society for Reproductive Medicine. Human immunodeficiency virus and infertility treatment: an Ethics Committee opinion. *Fertil Steril.* 2021;115(4):860-869. https://www.ncbi.nlm.nih.gov/pubmed/33832741. doi:10.1016/j.fertnstert.2021.01.024.

100. Rakic L, Kostova E, Cohlen BJ, Cantineau AE. Double versus single intrauterine insemination (IUI) in stimulated cycles for subfertile couples. *Cochrane Database Syst Rev.* 2021(7). doi:10.1002/14651858.CD003854.pub2.

101. Practice Committees of the American Society for Reproductive Medicine and the Society for Assisted Reproductive Technology. Intracytoplasmic sperm injection (ICSI) for non-male factor indications: a committee opinion. *Fertil Steril.* 2020;114(2):239-245. https://www.ncbi.nlm.nih.gov/pubmed/32654822. doi:10.1016/j.fertnstert.2020.05.032.

102. Ding CC, Thong KJ. "One sperm, one embryo, one baby"? *Asian J Androl.* 2010;12(2):284-286. https://www.ncbi.nlm.nih.gov/pubmed/19935674. doi:10.1038/aja.2009.72.

103. Sanders KD, Silvestri G, Gordon T, Griffin DK. Analysis of IVF live birth outcomes with and without preimplantation genetic testing for aneuploidy (PGT-A): UK Human Fertilisation and Embryology Authority data collection 2016–2018. *J Assist Reprod Genet.* 2021;38(12):3277-3285. https://www.ncbi.nlm.nih.gov/pubmed/34766235. doi:10.1007/s10815-021-02349-0.

104. Greco E, Litwicka K, Minasi MG, et al. Preimplantation genetic testing: where we are today. *Int J Mol Sci*. 2020;21(12):4381. https://www.ncbi.nlm.nih.gov/pubmed/32575575. doi:10.3390/ijms21124381.

105. Awadalla MS, Bendikson KA, Ho JR, et al. A validated model for predicting live birth after embryo transfer. *Sci Rep*. 2021;11(1):10800. https://www.ncbi.nlm.nih.gov/pubmed/34031492. doi:10.1038/s41598-021-90254-y.

106. Aharon D, Sekhon L, Lee JA, et al. Perinatal outcomes in reciprocal vs. anonymous donor oocyte IVF cycles. *Fertil Steril*. 2020;114(3):e271. https://doi.org/10.1016/j.fertnstert.2020.08.752.

107. Roth A. (Queer) family values and "reciprocal IVF": what difference does sexual identity make? *Kennedy Inst Ethics J*. 2017;27(3):443-473. https://www.ncbi.nlm.nih.gov/pubmed/28989168. doi:10.1353/ken.2017.0034.

108. Mascarenhas S, Suff N, Shennan A. Concurrent reciprocal IVF and risk of pre-eclampsia. *J Obstet Gynaecol*. 2021:1-2. https://www.ncbi.nlm.nih.gov/pubmed/34907816. doi:10.1080/01443615.2021.1971177.

109. Pfeifer S, Butts S, Fossum G, et al. Recommendations for practices utilizing gestational carriers: a committee opinion. *Fertil Steril*. 2017;107(2):e3. doi:10.1016/j.fertnstert.2016.11.007.

110. Baldwin K, Culley L, Hudson N, Mitchell H. Running out of time: exploring women's motivations for social egg freezing. *J Psychosom Obstet Gynaecol*. 2019;40(2):166-173. https://www.ncbi.nlm.nih.gov/pubmed/29648960. doi:10.1080/0167482X.2018.1460352.

111. Greenwood EA, Pasch LA, Hastie J, Jordan, et al. To freeze or not to freeze: decision regret and satisfaction following elective oocyte cryopreservation. *Fertil Steril*. 2018;109(6):1097. doi:10.1016/j.fertnstert.2018.02.127.

112. Practice Committee and Mental Health Professional Group of the American Society for Reproductive Medicine. Guidance on qualifications for fertility counselors: a committee opinion. *Fertil Steril*. 2021;115(6):1411. doi:10.1016/j.fertnstert.2021.02.016.

113. Ravelingien A, Provoost V, Pennings G. Open-identity sperm donation: how does offering donor-identifying information relate to donor-conceived offspring's wishes and needs? *J Bioeth Inq*. 2015;12(3):503-509. https://www.ncbi.nlm.nih.gov/pubmed/24996630. doi:10.1007/s11673-014-9550-3.

114. Penzias A, Azziz R, Bendikson K, et al. Recommendations for reducing the risk of viral transmission during fertility treatment with the use of autologous gametes: a committee opinion. *Fertil Steril*. 2020;114(6):1158-1164. https://www.ncbi.nlm.nih.gov/pubmed/33280723. doi:10.1016/j.fertnstert.2020.09.133.

115. Baba T, Endo T, Honnma H, et al. Association between polycystic ovary syndrome and female-to-male transsexuality. *Hum Reprod*. 2007;22(4):1011-1016. https://www.ncbi.nlm.nih.gov/pubmed/17166864. doi:10.1093/humrep/del474.

116. Bosinski HA, Peter M, Bonatz G, et al. A higher rate of hyperandrogenic disorders in female-to-male transsexuals. *Psychoneuroendocrinology*. 1997;22(5):361-380.

117. Liu M, Murthi S, Poretsky L. Polycystic ovary syndrome and gender identity. *Yale J Biol Med*. 2020;93(4):529-537. https://www.ncbi.nlm.nih.gov/pubmed/33005117.

118. Ikeda K, Baba T, Noguchi H, et al. Excessive androgen exposure in female-to-male transsexual persons of reproductive age induces hyperplasia of the ovarian cortex and stroma but not polycystic ovary morphology. *Hum Reprod*. 2013;28(2):453-461.

119. Komorowski AS, Jain T. A review of disparities in access to infertility care and treatment outcomes among Hispanic women. *Reprod Biol Endocrinol*. 2022;20(1):1. https://www.ncbi.nlm.nih.gov/pubmed/34980166. doi:10.1186/s12958-021-00875-1.

120. Kissin DM, Boulet SL, Jamieson DJ. Fertility treatments in the United States: improving access and outcomes. *Obstet Gynecol*. 2016;128(2):387-390. https://www.ncbi.nlm.nih.gov/pubmed/27399992. doi:10.1097/AOG.0000000000001419.

121. Khetarpal A, Singh S. Infertility: inability or disability? *Australasian Med J*. 2012;05(06):334. https://doi.org/10.21767/AMJ.2012.1290.

122. Ethics Committee of the American Society for Reproductive Medicine. Disparities in access to effective treatment for infertility in the United States: an Ethics Committee opinion. *Fertil Steril*. 2021;116(1):54-63. https://doi.org/10.1016/j.fertnstert.2021.02.019.

123. Stentz NC, Koelper N, Barnhart KT, Sammel MD, Senapati S. Infertility and mortality. *Obstet Gynecol*. 2020;222(3):251.e1. doi:10.1016/j.ajog.2019.09.007.

124. Harris HR, Wieser F, Vitonis AF, et al. Early life abuse and risk of endometriosis. *Hum Reprod*. 2018;33(9):1657-1668. https://www.ncbi.nlm.nih.gov/pubmed/30016439. doi:10.1093/humrep/dey248.

125. United Nations. *Universal Declaration of Human Rights*. United Nations; 1948.

126. United Nations. The crucial role of families. https://www.un.org/ecosoc/sites/www.un.org.ecosoc/files/files/en/integration/2017/IFFD.pdf. Updated 2017.

127. RESOLVE: National Infertility Association. Learn about RESOLVE's mission and the history of this organization. https://resolve.org/about-us/mission/.

128. Askew I. Message from the director SRH/HRP. https://www.who.int/news/item/28-01-2021-message-from-director-srh-hrp. Updated January 28, 2021.

129. Tam MW. Queering reproductive access: reproductive justice in assisted reproductive technologies. *Reprod Health.* 2021;18(1):164. https://www.ncbi.nlm.nih.gov/pubmed/34340704. doi:10.1186/s12978-021-01214-8.

130. Fairfax Cryobank. Fees. https://fairfaxcryobank.com/fees. Accessed February 14, 2022.

131. California Cryobank. Sperm bank pricing: donor semen cost. https://www.cryobank.com/services/pricing/. Accessed February 14, 2022.

132. Seattle Sperm Bank. Our prices. https://www.seattlespermbank.com/services/prices/. Accessed February 14, 2022.

133. Ward P, McPhail D. Fat shame and blame in reproductive care: implications for ethical health care interactions. *Womens Reprod Health.* 2019;6(4):225-241. https://doi.org/10.1080/23293691.2019.1653581.

134. Cook KM, Lamarre A, Rice C, Friedman M. "This isn't a high-risk body": reframing risk and reducing weight stigma in midwifery practice. *Can J Midwifery Res Pract.* 2019;18(1):26-34. https://www.cjmrp.com/files/v18n1-weight-stigma-and-pregnancy.pdf.

135. Pandey S, Maheshwari A, Bhattacharya S. Should access to fertility treatment be determined by female body mass index? *Hum Reprod.* 2010;25(4):815-820. https://www.ncbi.nlm.nih.gov/pubmed/20129994. doi:10.1093/humrep/deq013.

136. Pearl RL, Puhl RM. Weight bias internalization and health: a systematic review. *Obes Rev.* 2018;19(8):1141-1163. https://www.ncbi.nlm.nih.gov/pubmed/29788533. doi:10.1111/obr.12701.

137. Tomiyama AJ, Carr D, Granberg EM, et al. How and why weight stigma drives the obesity "epidemic" and harms health. *BMC Med.* 2018;16(1):123. https://www.ncbi.nlm.nih.gov/pubmed/30107800. doi:10.1186/s12916-018-1116-5.

138. Matheson EM, King DE, Everett CJ. Healthy lifestyle habits and mortality in overweight and obese individuals. *J Am Board Fam Med.* 2012;25(1):9. doi:10.3122/jabfm.2012.01.110164.

139. Dulloo AG, Montani J-P. Pathways from dieting to weight regain, to obesity and to the metabolic syndrome: an overview. *Obes Rev.* 2015;16(suppl 1):1-6. https://www.ncbi.nlm.nih.gov/pubmed/25614198. doi:10.1111/obr.12250.

140. Bacon L. *Health at Every Size: The Surprising Truth About Your Weight.* Dallas, TX: Benbella Books; 2010.

141. Kelley AS, Badon SE, Lanham MSM, et al. Body mass index restrictions in fertility treatment: a national survey of OB/GYN subspecialists. *J Assist Reprod Genet.* 2019;36(6):1117-1125. https://www.ncbi.nlm.nih.gov/pubmed/30963351. doi:10.1007/s10815-019-01448-3.

142. Kaye L, Sueldo C, Engmann L, et al. Survey assessing obesity policies for assisted reproductive technology in the United States. *Fertil Steril.* 2016;105(3):703-706. https://doi.org/10.1016/j.fertnstert.2015.11.035.

143. Dayan N, Spitzer K, Laskin CA. A focus on maternal health before assisted reproduction: results from a pilot survey of Canadian IVF medical directors. *J Obstet Gynaecol Can.* 2015;37(7):648-655. https://www.ncbi.nlm.nih.gov/pubmed/26366823. doi:10.1016/S1701-2163(15)30204-8.

144. Gameiro S, Boivin J, Peronace L, Verhaak CM. Why do patients discontinue fertility treatment? A systematic review of reasons and predictors of discontinuation in fertility treatment. *Hum Reprod Update.* 2012;18(6):652-669. https://www.ncbi.nlm.nih.gov/pubmed/22869759. doi:10.1093/humupd/dms031.

145. Cohen IG, Daar J, Adashi EY. What overturning *Roe v Wade* may mean for assisted reproductive technologies in the US. *JAMA.* 2022 Jul 5;328(1):15-16. doi:10.1001/jama.2022.10163.

146. ASRM Center for Policy and Leadership. State abortion trigger laws: potential implications for reproductive medicine. *Am Soc Reprod Med.* 2022. https://www.asrm.org/globalassets/asrm/asrm-content/news-and-publications/dobbs/cpl-report_impact-of-state-trigger-laws-on-reproductive-medicine_final.pdf.

147. Catchings HC. A "modern family" issue: recategorizing embryos in the 21st century. *La Law Rev.* 2019;80:1521.

148. King J. HB 1217 coerced abortion. 2022(2022). https://iga.in.gov/legislative/2022/bills/house/1217.

149. Nisly C. Protection of life. 2022(2022). https://iga.in.gov/legislative/2022/bills/house/1282.

150. Barto N. Abortion; unborn child; genetic abnormality. 2021(55th). Senate Bill 1457, State of Arizona. https://www.azleg.gov/legtext/55leg/1R/bills/sb1457c.pdf.

151. American College of Obstetricians and Gynecologists. Gynecology data definitions. https://www.acog.org/practice-management/health-it-and-clinical-informatics/revitalize-gynecology-data-definitions. Accessed February 15, 2022.

152. Brucker MC, King TL. *Pharmacology for Women's Health.* 2nd ed. Burlington, MA: Jones & Bartlett Learning; 2017.

153. Maddow-Zimet I, Kost K. Effect of changes in response options on reported pregnancy intentions: a natural experiment in the United States. *Public Health Rep.* 2020;135(3):354-363.

154. Centers for Disease Control and Prevention. Pregnancy Risk Assessment Monitoring System (PRAMS): phase 8 core questionnaire. https://www.cdc.gov/prams/pdf/questionnaire/Phase-8-Core-Questions-508.pdf. Updated 2016. Accessed December 15, 2021.

155. Finer LB, Zolna MR. Declines in unintended pregnancy in the United States, 2008–2011. *N Engl J Med.* 2016;374(9):843-852.

156. Kost K, Maddown-Zimet I, Little AC. Pregnancies and pregnancy desires at the state level: estimates for 2017 and trends since 2012. 2021. https://www.guttmacher.org/report/pregnancy-desires-and-pregnancies-state-level-estimates-2017.

157. Troutman M, Rafique S, Plowden TC. Are higher unintended pregnancy rates among minorities a result of disparate access to contraception? *Contracept Reprod Med.* 2020;5(1):1-6.

158. Martin JA, Hamilton BE, Osterman MJ. Births in the United States, 2013. NCHS data brief, no 175. Hyattsville, MD: National Center for Health Statistics. 2014. https://www.cdc.gov/nchs/products/databriefs/db175.htm#:~:text=There%20were%203.93%20million%20births,all%2Dtime%20low%20in%202013.

159. Brown A. Growing share of childless adults in the US don't expect to ever have children. Pew Research Center; 2021. https://www.pewresearch.org/fact-tank/2021/11/19/growing-share-of-childless-adults-in-u-s-dont-expect-to-ever-have-children/.

160. Ashburn-Nardo L. Parenthood as a moral imperative? Moral outrage and the stigmatization of voluntarily childfree women and men. *Sex Roles.* 2017; 76(5):393-401.

161. Hintz EA, Brown CL. Childfree by choice: stigma in medical consultations for voluntary sterilization. *Womens Reprod Health.* 2019;6(1):62-75.

162. Murphy PA, Elmore CE. Contraception. In: Brucker MC, King TL, eds. *Pharmacology for Women's Health.* Burlington, MA: Jones & Bartlett Learning; 2017.

163. Trussell J. Understanding contraceptive failure. *Best Pract Res Clin Obstet Gynaecol.* 2009;23(2): 199-209.

164. Pearl R. Factors in human fertility and their statistical evaluation. *Lancet.* 1933;222(5741):607-611.

165. Kuo T, Suchindran CM, Koo HP. The multistate life table method: an application to contraceptive switching behavior. *Demography.* 2008;45(1):157-171.

166. Boudreau D, Mukerjee R. Contraception care for transmasculine individuals on testosterone therapy. *J Midwifery Womens Health.* 2019;64(4):395-402.

167. Bertotti AM, Mann ES, Miner SA. Efficacy as safety: dominant cultural assumptions and the assessment of contraceptive risk. *Soc Sci Med.* 2021;270:113547.

168. Daniels K, Daugherty JD, Jones J, Mosher WD. Current contraceptive use and variation by selected characteristics among women aged 15–44: United States, 2011–2013. 2015 Nov 10;(86):1-14.

169. Division of Reproductive Health. Strategic plan: improving women's reproductive health, pregnancy health, and infant health. Centers for Disease Control and Prevention; 2019. https://www.cdc.gov/reproductivehealth/drh/about-us/DRH-strategic-plan.htm.

170. Committee on Gynecologic Practice, Long-Acting Reversible Contraception Working Group. Committee Opinion No. 642: increasing access to contraceptive implants and intrauterine devices to reduce unintended pregnancy. *Obstet Gynecol.* 2015;126(4): e44-e48.

171. ACOG Committee Opinion No. 735: adolescents and long-acting reversible contraception: implants and intrauterine devices. *Obstet Gynecol.* 2018; 131(5):e130-e139. https://www.ncbi.nlm.nih.gov/pubmed/29683910. doi:10.1097/AOG.0000000000002632.

172. Menon S; Committee on Adolescence. Long-acting reversible contraception: specific issues for adolescents. *Pediatrics.* 2020;146(2):e2020007252. https://www.ncbi.nlm.nih.gov/pubmed/32690806. doi:10.1542/peds.2020-007252.

173. Diedrich JT, Klein DA, Peipert JF. Long-acting reversible contraception in adolescents: a systematic review and meta-analysis. *Obstet Gynecol.* 2017; 216(4):364.e1-364.e12. https://www.ncbi.nlm.nih.gov/pubmed/28038902. doi:10.1016/j.ajog.2016.12.024.

174. Trussell J, Hassan F, Lowin J, et al. Achieving cost-neutrality with long-acting reversible contraceptive methods. *Contraception.* 2015;91(1):49-56. https://www.ncbi.nlm.nih.gov/pubmed/25282161. doi:10.1016/j.contraception.2014.08.011.

175. National Quality Forum. Perinatal and reproductive health 2015–2016 final report. https://www.qualityforum.org/Publications/2016/12/Perinatal_and_Reproductive_Health_2015-2016_Final_Report.aspx. Updated 2016. Accessed January 4, 2022.

176. Gomez AM, Mann ES, Torres V. "It would have control over me instead of me having control": intrauterine devices and the meaning of reproductive freedom. *Crit Public Health.* 2018;28(2):190-200.

177. American College of Nurse-Midwives. Position statement: access to comprehensive sexual and reproductive health care. https://www.midwife.org/acnm/files/ACNMLibraryData/UPLOADFILENAME/000000000087/Access-to-Comprehensive-Sexual-and-Reproductive-Health-Care-Services-FINAL-04-12-17.pdf. Updated 2016. Accessed January 4, 2022.

178. Postpartum Contraceptive Access Initiative. Support patient autonomy. https://pcainitiative.acog.org /contraceptive-counseling/supporting-patient-autonomy/. Updated 2017. Accessed January 6, 2022.

179. World Health Organization. *Medical Eligibility Criteria for Contraceptive Use.* Geneva, Switzerland: World Health Organization; 2015.

180. Curtis KM, Tepper NK, Jatlaoui TC, et al. US medical eligibility criteria for contraceptive use, 2016. *MMWR Recomm Rep.* 2016;65(3):1-103.

181. Curtis KM, Jatlaoui TC, Tepper NK, et al. US selected practice recommendations for contraceptive use, 2016. *MMWR Recomm Rep.* 2016;65(4):1-66.

182. Grace KT, Anderson JC. Reproductive coercion: a systematic review. *Trauma Violence Abuse.* 2018;19(4):371-390.

183. Fay KE, Corry S, Simmons RG, Baayd J. Coerced choice: resigned contraceptive usership among individuals affected by reproductive coercion. *J Midwifery Womens Health.* 2022. Sep;67(5):593-597. doi:10 .1111/jmwh.13396. Epub 2022. Jul 21. PMID: 35861284; PMCID: PMC9561046.

184. Doherty ME, Scannell-Desch E. Women's health and hygiene experiences during deployment to the Iraq and Afghanistan wars, 2003 through 2010. *J Midwifery Womens Health.* 2012;57(2):172-177.

185. Borrero S, Callegari LS, Zhao X, et al. Unintended pregnancy and contraceptive use among women veterans: the ECUUN study. *J Gen Intern Med.* 2017;32(8):900-908.

186. Mosher W, Hughes RB, Bloom T, et al. Contraceptive use by disability status: new national estimates from the National Survey of Family Growth. *Contraception.* 2018;97(6):552-558.

187. Childress JF, Childress MD. What does the evolution from informed consent to shared decision making teach us about authority in health care? *AMA J Ethics.* 2020;22(5):423-429.

APPENDIX

# 10A

# Fertility Awareness Methods

MELISSA A. SAFTNER

*The editors acknowledge Mary C. Brucker, who was the author of this appendix in the previous edition.*

## Introduction

Although fewer than 1% of individuals who use contraception in the United States employ fertility awareness methods, in some areas of the world these methods are the predominant form of birth control.[1,2] Some reasons for the limited use of these strategies in the United States include the complexity of the methods, lack of available education about fertility awareness methods, and personal beliefs of consumers and providers that these methods are not effective.[3] It is important to note that high-quality studies on fertility awareness method effectiveness are limited.[4]

Formal education programs exist for both clinicians, patients, and partners. Many midwives complete certification courses for a particular type of fertility awareness method, whereas others prefer to refer interested individuals to a specialist in the area. This appendix provides general information about fertility awareness methods and discusses the most commonly used fertility awareness methods. This appendix uses the term *intercourse* to mean penile-vaginal sex with ejaculation.

## Assumptions

Fertility awareness methods are based on regularly occurring biologic events during the menstrual cycle that should be understood by the clinician and the patient:

1. Ovulation occurs once, approximately 14 days before menses begins, not 14 days after the last menstrual period started.

2. The maximum lifespan of the ovum is 12 to 24 hours.

3. Sperm are viable after ejaculation for approximately 3 to 5 days.

4. The most likely time for conception to occur is during the fertile window, which spans from approximately 5 days prior to ovulation until the day after ovulation, for a total of 6 days each month.[5]

## Considerations for Use

Table 10A-1 lists the main criteria that a patient and their partner should consider before adopting a fertility awareness method for contraception. Although no devices are required with these methods, it is necessary for the couple to be dedicated to consistent and correct use of the chosen fertility awareness method.

| Table 10A-1 | Considerations for Use of Fertility Awareness Methods |
|---|---|
| Commitment by both sexual partners to consistently use the method month after month | |
| Comfort in observing for signs of fertility, including touching the vulva | |
| Commitment to recognize and document even subtle signs of fertility | |
| Ability to practice abstinence for at least one month, during which time baseline signs of fertility are observed and documented before initiating the method | |

## Contraindications

Relative contraindications to fertility awareness methods include conditions that result in irregular menstrual cycles, including recent childbirth, onset of menarche, perimenopause, breastfeeding, frequent anovulatory cycles, and recent discontinuation of hormonal contraceptives. Patients with the following conditions also may have difficulty using some fertility awareness methods: persistent vaginitis or other infections that may disrupt signs of cervical changes; not being comfortable examining cervical mucus; intermenstrual bleeding; and inability to correctly interpret the signs of fertility.[6]

## Types of Fertility Awareness Methods

Currently, several fertility awareness methods are in common use. Table 10A-2 summarizes the majority of these methods based on the available data.[5,6] Fertility awareness methods can be generally categorized as either calendar methods or symptom-based methods.[6] Both are discussed in this section. For methods that are considered proprietary, their

developers usually charge and/or restrict use of their educational materials, including provider and consumer charts, to maintain integrity and accuracy. Many of the proprietary organizations also have educational programs for accreditation or certification.

## Calendar Methods

The "rhythm" method, also known as the calendar method, is the oldest fertility awareness–based method; it was developed in the 1930s. The Standard Days Method (SDM) is a more recent adaptation of the calendar method.

### Standard Days Method

SDM is based entirely on tracking the days of the menstrual cycle for individuals with regular cycles.[7] The user notes the first day of menstruation and abstains from intercourse or uses another birth control method between days 8 and 19 after the first day that menses starts during each menstrual cycle.[7] Individuals with irregular menstrual cycles, breastfeeding individuals who have not had at least three

| Table 10A-2 | Description, Observations, Fertile Day, and Estimated Effectiveness of Selected Fertility Awareness–Based Methods | | | | |
|---|---|---|---|---|---|
| **Method** | **Signs or Symptoms Used by Method** | **Observations** | **Days to Avoid Unprotected Intercourse** | **Efficacy, First Year of Typical Use** | **Unintended Pregnancies, First Year of Use with Perfect Use[a]** |
| Standard Days Method (calendar) | Day of cycle | Track cycle days beginning with first day of menses<br>Note days 8–19 of cycle | Days 8–19 of cycle<br>Total: 12 days per cycle | 88% | 5 |
| Ovulation method (symptoms-based) | Cervical secretions | Monitor cervical secretions daily<br>Assess quality and quantity of secretions<br>Record data | Menses<br>Preovulatory days following days with intercourse<br>All days with fertile-type secretions<br>Until 4 days past "peak" day<br>Total: Approximately 14–16 days each cycle | 77% | 3 |
| TwoDay Method (symptoms-based) | Cervical secretions | Note presence or absence of cervical secretions<br>Record data | All days with secretions<br>One day following days with secretions<br>Total: Approximately 10–14 days each cycle | 86% | 4 |

| Method | Signs or Symptoms Used by Method | Observations | Days to Avoid Unprotected Intercourse | Efficacy, First Year of Typical Use | Unintended Pregnancies, First Year of Use with Perfect Use[a] |
|---|---|---|---|---|---|
| Symptothermal method (symptoms-based) | Cervical secretions Vaginal mucus BBT | Monitor cervical secretions daily Assess quantity and quality of secretions Take BBT daily Record observations on chart | Menses Preovulatory days following days with intercourse All days with fertile-type secretions Until 3 days of higher temperatures, or 4 days past peak Total: Approximately 14–16 days each cycle | 98% | 2 |

Abbreviation: BBT, basal body temperature.

[a] Number of pregnancies per 100 individuals per year of use with perfect use.

Based on Arevalo M, Sinai I, Jennings V. A fixed formula to define the fertile window of the menstrual cycle as the basis of a simple method of natural family planning. *Contraception*. 1999;60(6):357-360; Jennings, VH, Polis, CB. Fertility awareness-based methods. In: Hatcher RA, Nelson AL, Trussell J, et al, eds. *Contraceptive Technology*. 21st ed. New York, NY: Ayer Company Publishers; 2018:395-416; World Health Organization. *Family Planning: A Global Handbook for Providers*. WHO Press; 2018. https://www.who.int/publications/i/item/9780999203705. Accessed September 16, 2022.

normal menstrual cycles, or those with a recent birth, miscarriage, or abortion are not good candidates for SDM.[6]

SDM has been promoted globally, although some questions exist regarding standardization and effectiveness of the educational programs. These educational programs often advocate use of a bead-like device called CycleBeads, whose colors an individual uses to determine whether they should be considered fertile or infertile on a particular day.[7] CycleBeads and SDM programs are proprietary, with the former device being marketed by a for-profit company. A number of apps using SDM are available.

## Symptoms-Based Methods

The three common symptoms-based methods focus on using physical signs that indicate ovulation to identify the days of fertility and infertility for a specific cycle. These signs include changes in amount and characteristics of cervical mucus, basal body temperature (BBT), and the position and consistency of the cervix (Figure 10A-1).[8] Although cervical mucus is to be assessed, it is most commonly determined by wetness of the vulva. Ovulation methods that use BBT require use of an appropriate thermometer—one of the few devices associated with fertility awareness methods.

### Billings Ovulation Method

The Billings Ovulation Method focuses on changes in cervical mucus. During the infertile period in both the preovulatory phase and the postovulatory phase of the cycle, cervical mucus is absent or results in no sensation of wetness at the vulva. Fertile days are signaled by vulvar wetness or slippery cervical mucus. The individual observes the sensation of wetness at the vulva and the presence of mucus throughout the day and records their observations at the end of each day. During the entire first cycle of charting, abstinence is necessary for the individual to become familiar with their pattern of cervical mucus and sensations of vulvar wetness. The Billings Ovulation Method uses two patterns to describe monitoring cervical mucus (Table 10A-3).[8]

Use of spermicides, lubricants, vaginal treatments, or barriers with spermicides may interfere with use of this method. Individuals are also advised to refrain from intercourse on days with heavy menstrual bleeding because it masks the signs of mucus associated with ovulation.

### Creighton Model Fertility Care System

This fertility awareness method is a modification of the Billings Ovulation Method, yet is considered a separate method. The Creighton Model Fertility Care System has a standardized teaching

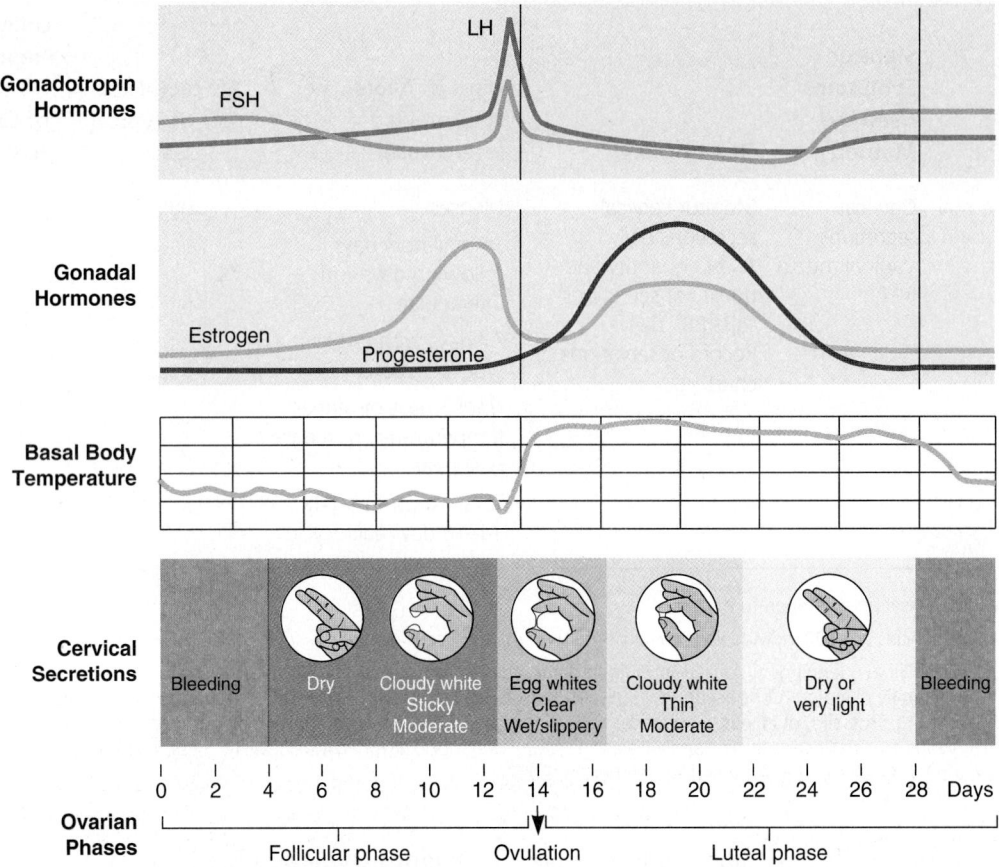

**Figure 10A-1** Hormonal, temperature, secretions, and ovarian phases during the menstrual cycle.

| Table 10A-3 | Billings Ovulation Method | |
|---|---|---|
| **Cervical Mucus Pattern** | **Characteristics** | **Timing of Intercourse** |
| Basic infertile pattern (BIP) | Days immediately after menstruation Consistent dryness at the vulva | Intercourse every other day to avoid confusing seminal fluid with mucus |
| Peak pattern | Change in vulvar sensation from wet to slippery | Avoid intercourse during peak and for 3 days after peak day |
| | Under the influence of estrogen, the mucus increases in volume and becomes clear and stretchy, with an egg-white consistency (spinnbarkeit) | |
| | Last day of peak is also called "peak day" | |

plan, is trademarked, and relies on a code system for charting.[9,10]

## TwoDay Method

The TwoDay Method simplifies observation of cervical mucus.[11,12] This particular method does not require distinguishing the quality of the mucus. Instead, an individual using this method asks two specific questions (Table 10A-4). Individuals with

| Table 10A-4 | TwoDay Method |
|---|---|
| **Question** | **Fertility** |
| 1. Did I note secretions today?<br>2. Did I note secretions yesterday? | Both questions must be answered. If the answer is "yes" to either one, it should be assumed the individual is fertile. |

| Table 10A-5 | Patterns of Ovulatory Temperature Rises | |
|---|---|---|
| **Physical Signs of Ovulation** | **Description** | **Comments** |
| Rise in basal body temperature (BBT) | BBT rise of at least at least 0.4°F above the previous six daily BBT measurements | Rise is characterized as a sustained elevation or a plateau of the temperature for 3 days, or when there have been 5 days of progressive increase |
| Abrupt rise pattern | Rise over 1–2 days | |
| Saw-tooth pattern | Rise and fall over several days, with overall increase | For example, an increase of 0.4°F, decrease of 0.2°F, increase of 0.4°F, and so on |
| Slow rise or staircase pattern | Gradual rise over several days | |
| Sharp dip and rise pattern | Sharp dip in temperature followed by a rise | Occasionally occurs with ovulation but is not required |
| Changes in cervical mucus | Increase in volume and change to clear and elastic consistency | Same as peak pattern in Billings Ovulation Method |
| Cervical changes | From firm to soft and moves higher into vaginal canal | |

irregular cycles can use this method because it relies entirely on observing one physical sign of fertility.

Similar to the Standard Days Method, the Two-Day Method is proprietary. The app associated with this method is available as a free download.

## Symptothermal Method

The symptothermal method combines observation of three physical signs of ovulation: BBT, cervical mucus, and changes in the cervix itself.[4,8] Table 10A-5 lists physical signs of ovulation that suggest fertile days on the basis of ovulation.

The rise in BBT occurs as more progesterone is released by the corpus luteum, signaling that ovulation has occurred.[8] The pattern of the rise in temperature varies for each individual and can be altered by inconsistent schedules or illness. Observing cervical mucus changes augments the BBT pattern to help identify fertile and infertile days. As with the Billings Ovulation Method, fertile days are characterized by elastic, thin, clear mucus.

In addition to BBT and cervical mucus observation, the third component of this method is changes in the cervix itself, which can be felt by palpating the cervix. As ovulation approaches, the cervix softens, the os dilates slightly, and the cervix is positioned higher in the vaginal canal. After ovulation, the cervix returns to being firm, closed, and lower in the vaginal canal.[13] Detection of the cervical position is an optional sign. An individual using this method documents observation of the three parts of the method—BBT, cervical mucus, and cervical characteristics.

## References

1. Sundaram A, Vaughan B, Kost K, et al. Contraceptive failure in the United States: estimates from the 2006–2010 National Survey of Family Growth. *Perspect Sex Reprod Health*. 2017;49(1):7-16.
2. United Nations, Department of Economic and Social Affairs. Contraceptive use by method 2019. https://digitallibrary.un.org/record/3849735?ln=en. Accessed September 8, 2021.
3. Han L, Taub R, Jensen JT. Cervical mucus and contraception: what we know and what we don't. *Contraception*. 2017;96(5):310-321.
4. Urrutia RP, Polis CB, Jensen ET, et al. Effectiveness of fertility awareness-based methods for pregnancy prevention. *Obstet Gynecol*. 2018:132(3):591-604.
5. Arevalo M, Sinai I, Jennings V. A fixed formula to define the fertile window of the menstrual cycle as the basis of a simple method of natural family planning. *Contraception*. 1999;60(6):357-360.
6. Jennings, VH, Polis, CB. Fertility awareness-based methods. In: Hatcher RA, Nelson AL, Trussell J, et al, eds. *Contraceptive Technology*. 21st ed. New York, NY: Ayer Company Publishers; 2018:395-416.
7. World Health Organization. *Family Planning: A Global Handbook for Providers*. Geneva, Switzerland: WHO Press; 2018. https://www.who.int/publications/i/item/9780999203705. Accessed October 5, 2021.
8. Simmons RG, Jennings V. Fertility awareness-based methods of family planning. *Best Pract Res Clin Obstet Gynaecol*. 2020:66;68-82.
9. Stanford JB, Porucznik CA. Enrollment, childbearing motivations, and intentions of couples in the

Creighton Model Effectiveness, Intentions, and Behaviors Assessment (CEIBA) study. *Front Med (Lausanne)*. 2017;4:147. doi:10.3389/fmed.2017.00147. Accessed October 6, 2021.

10. Saint Paul VI Institute for the Study of Human Reproduction. *Creighton Model*. https://creightonmodel.com/. Published 2020. Accessed October 6, 2021.

11. Dunson D, Sinai I, Colombo B. The relationship between cervical secretions and the daily probabilities of pregnancy: effectiveness of the TwoDay algorithm. *Hum Reprod*. 2001;16:2278-2282.

12. Institute for Reproductive Health. *TwoDay method*. https://www.irh.org/twoday-method/. Published 2021. Accessed October 6, 2021.

13. Weschler T. *Taking Charge of Your Fertility, 20th Anniversary Edition: The Definitive Guide to Natural Birth Control, Pregnancy Achievement, and Reproductive Health*. New York, NY: William Morrow Paperbacks; 2015:Table 10A-2.

APPENDIX

# 10B

# Intrauterine Insemination

SIGNEY OLSON

## Intrauterine Insemination Counseling

Prior to performing intrauterine insemination (IUI), an informed consent process should be completed, explaining the procedural steps and providing permission for the clinician to perform the IUI. A consent form signed by the patient should be placed in the patient's health record. Additionally, the sperm sample identification must be carefully verified with the patient prior to beginning the procedure.[1] Typically, at the time of the procedure, at least two separate members of the healthcare team provide close monitoring to ensure the correct sperm sample is utilized. During the process of sperm washing in a laboratory setting, typically another two or three personnel are involved in confirming the identity of the sperm-producing partner or donor and ensuring that proper protocol is followed in handling the sperm processing.[1]

## Choosing an Intrauterine Insemination Catheter

Two main styles of IUI catheters are currently available in the United States, the firm catheter and the soft-tip catheter. Within each style, brands have slight differences in design, and variations in rigidity, tip shape, and length. All catheters are designed as single-use devices. The soft catheters utilize a firm outer sheath with an internal flexible channel (Figure 10B-1), whereas the firm catheters utilize a wire-like malleable stylet (Figure 10B-2).[2] The choice of catheter may depend on cervical characteristics such as os size and curvature of the cervical canal. No difference in pregnancy or live birth rates has been demonstrated with use of a specific style of catheter.[2]

## Timing of the Intrauterine Insemination(s)

Determining the appropriate timing to perform IUI depends on whether ovulation induction medication is used. If so, a second medication, injectable human chorionic gonadotropin (hCG), is typically administered at a precise time to trigger ovulation.[3] Typically, the IUI is scheduled at approximately 36 hours after the hCG injection. This allows adequate time for the oocyte to release from the mature follicle and begin to move through the uterine tube.[3]

When ovulation induction medication is not used, another method of pinpointing ovulation must be used, typically in the form of ovulation prediction test strips, which measure the concentration of luteinizing hormone (LH) in the urine.[1] The IUI is typically scheduled between 12 and 24 hours after a positive LH surge has been detected. This range is often broader than the timing of IUI with the use of hCG, as LH test strips offer slightly less specific timing and instructions may vary on the optimal time to test.[1]

## Intrauterine Insemination Procedure

Few clinical instruction resources for IUI exist. The following key points and steps for insertion are general guidelines and are best used along with hands-on experience.

### Premedication

During an IUI, patients are likely to briefly experience mild to moderate uterine cramping as the catheter is inserted through the cervical canal and the specimen is released at the fundus. Patients may premedicate with over-the-counter analgesics such as

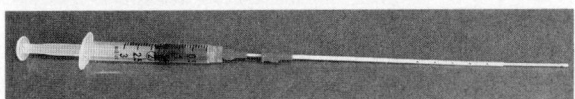

**Figure 10B-1** Soft-tip IUI catheter with outer sheath.

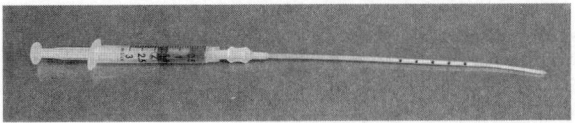

**Figure 10B-2** Firm IUI catheter with malleable stylet.

aspirin, acetaminophen, or ibuprofen, all of which are considered safe within the context of IUI.[1]

### Equipment for Intrauterine Insemination

- Clean gloves of appropriate size
- Sterile speculum
- Adequate lighting for visualization
- IUI catheter
- 3-mL syringe containing 0.5–2 mL of thawed sperm sample[1,3]

### Steps for Performing Intrauterine Insemination[1,3]

1. Using shared decision making, ensure that ovulation has been properly timed and counsel the patient regarding possible risks and side effects of the IUI.
2. Encourage the patient to retain a partially filled urinary bladder.
3. Ensure the washed sperm sample has been processed and/or thawed appropriately and placed into a syringe.
4. Put on clean gloves.
5. Adhere the IUI catheter securely onto the 3-mL syringe holding 0.5–2 mL fluid media containing the sperm sample.
6. Heightened attention to detail should be employed when verifying and confirming sperm identification numbers to prevent incorrect sample use.
7. Introduce the speculum into the vaginal canal and obtain visualization of the cervix.
8. Introduce the IUI catheter through the cervix, into the uterus.
   a. If using a soft-tipped IUI catheter with an outer sheath, ensure the outer sheath is advanced through the internal os before advancing the soft inner channel through to the fundus.
      i. If resistance is encountered, consider switching to a firm catheter and/or utilizing cervical dilation.
   b. If using a firm IUI catheter, take care not to push the catheter into the fundus to avoid endometrial injury.
      i. If resistance is encountered, bend the wire within the catheter to align it with the cervical shape.
9. Slowly release the sperm sample into the uterine cavity by exerting pressure on the syringe plunger.
10. Slowly withdraw the IUI catheter from the uterus and cervix.
11. Slowly withdraw the speculum from the vaginal canal.
12. Review the next steps with the patient, including 5 to 10 minutes of bed rest if desired.

### Follow-Up Care

After completion of the IUI procedure, several points of anticipatory guidance are appropriate to review. Some individuals may experience spotting and/or ongoing mild to moderate cramping for 1 to 2 days after the procedure. Patients are instructed to contact their clinician if symptoms worsen and can plan to return to their normal activities immediately following the IUI.[1] For those who engage in vaginal–penile intercourse, there is no need to abstain after an IUI, and there may be a modest benefit toward pregnancy. A pregnancy test is recommended approximately 2 weeks after the IUI procedure and may entail a urine hCG test or serum hCG test.[1]

### References

1. Olson SM. *Signey Olson Health: Intrauterine Insemination: Clinical Training.* 2022.
2. Abou-Setta AM, Mansour RT, Al-Inany HG, et al. Intrauterine insemination catheters for assisted reproduction: a systematic review and meta-analysis. *Hum Reprod.* 2006;21(8):1961-1967. https://doi.org/10.1093/humrep/del139.
3. Allahbadia GN. Intrauterine insemination: fundamentals revisited. *J Obstet Gynaecol India.* 2017;67(6):385-392. doi:10.1007/s13224-017-1060-x.

CHAPTER

# 11

# Nonhormonal Contraception

MELISSA A. SAFTNER

*The editors acknowledge Mary C. Brucker, who was the author of this chapter in the previous edition.*

## Introduction

Contemporary forms of contraception include an array of both hormonal and nonhormonal methods. Many individuals choose a nonhormonal option. Some choose a nonhormonal method because they have general concerns about the use of exogenous hormones or want to avoid exposure to additional hormones. Others have preexisting health conditions, such as thromboembolic disorders that preclude the use of some hormonal types of contraception.[1] Still other individuals use nonhormonal methods as a secondary contraceptive method while initiating or transferring between hormonal methods or as one of multiple contraceptive methods used simultaneously.

This chapter reviews the contraceptive methods that do not contain hormones as their mechanism of action. Nonhormonal reversible methods can be categorized as behavioral, spermicidal, pH altering, barrier methods, or copper intrauterine devices (IUDs). Contraceptives within the behavioral, spermicidal, pH altering, and barrier categories are controlled by the user, are relatively inexpensive, and have few or minor side effects. Many nonhormonal methods do not require a prescription (e.g., foam, condoms), and most are used only when coitus is anticipated or during coitus. Behavioral methods use no device at all, relying instead on biologic processes such as breastfeeding/chestfeeding or observing changes during the menstrual cycle for contraceptive effectiveness. The newest nonhormonal contraceptive, Phexxi, alters vaginal pH and is available by prescription. Both the copper and levonorgestrel-containing IUDs are highly effective, long-acting reversible contraceptives (LARC) with multiple commonalities. Because the copper

type of IUD does not contain any hormone, it is discussed in depth in this chapter, whereas those IUDs containing levonorgestrel are reviewed in the *Hormonal Contraception* chapter. Finally, sterilization (e.g., tubal ligation or vasectomy) is a permanent nonhormonal method of contraception.

Most nonhormonal contraceptive methods are safe, and with few exceptions, these forms of contraception have no absolute contraindications. Thus, they are listed as Category 1 in the Centers for Disease Control and Prevention's (CDC's) guideline, "U.S. Medical Eligibility Criteria (MEC) for Contraceptive Use."[1] Health risks associated with these products are detailed in the section specific to each method in this chapter.

## Effectiveness of Nonhormonal Methods in Preventing Pregnancy

Each individual has personal reasons to choose one contraceptive method instead of another. For the majority of individuals, effectiveness is a major consideration in the choice of a contraceptive method, albeit not necessarily the *most* important. The best method for an individual is the one that they desire and will use consistently and correctly.

If individuals use no contraceptive method, approximately 85 of every 100 will conceive a pregnancy in the first year of no contraceptive use.[2] Effectiveness rates for typical use of the nonhormonal reversible methods vary widely, ranging from fewer than 1 unintended pregnancy per 100 individuals who use the copper IUD to 28 unintended pregnancies per 100 individuals who use spermicide only.[2,3] The lactational amenorrhea method is highly effective, but the duration of its effectiveness is approximately 6 months; this method also depends on meeting specific requirements, which can be socially difficult to fulfill for the average person in the United States.[3] Fertility awareness methods have quite variable rates of effectiveness and are highly dependent upon health education and the user's clear understanding and commitment to following them.[4] Some individuals may consider effectiveness to be less important than other factors and view a pregnancy that occurs a bit earlier than planned as acceptable. For other individuals, effectiveness is a primary consideration. Ultimately, the decision about the type of contraception (if any) to use belongs to the individual and their partner, and providers should be aware of their own beliefs to avoid injecting personal bias when counseling individuals about these issues.[5]

## Behavioral Methods

Behavioral contraceptive methods focus on identifying the likely fertile time for an individual.[6] These methods are highly dependent upon the person's and their partner's motivation, understanding of fertility, and having normal menstrual cycles, and they are particularly attractive to individuals who do not want to use artificial interventions. Behavioral methods can be used for pregnancy prevention, attainment of pregnancy, or pregnancy spacing. Globally, behavioral methods are among the oldest and more popular methods, with more than 8% of people worldwide using coitus interruptus or fertility awareness.[7]

### Abstinence

When undertaken for the purpose of avoiding pregnancy, abstinence is defined as refraining from penile–vaginal intercourse. However, if abstinence is defined to include prevention of sexually transmitted infections (STIs), then abstinence includes not engaging in sexual contact that has a risk of STI transmission. For example, anal intercourse with an infected partner confers a higher risk of transmission of human immunodeficiency virus (HIV) than vaginal penetration. By comparison, oral intercourse confers a higher risk of transmission of human papillomavirus (HPV) and herpes simplex virus (HSV).[8,9]

Abstinence is cost free, controlled by the individual, does not require a healthcare provider, is free of side effects, and is available at any time. Complete abstinence is 100% effective and prevents exposure to STIs as well as pregnancy. Planned abstinence can be unrealistic for some people, however, and is difficult for individuals to achieve in coercive situations.

### Coitus Interruptus/Withdrawal Method

With the coitus interruptus (withdrawal) method, the penis is completely removed from the vagina and away from the labia and external genitalia before ejaculation. The number of individuals using withdrawal as their contraceptive method of choice was reported to have increased from 1994 to 2019.[7] Approximately 5% (47 million) of reproductive-age women worldwide use withdrawal. In addition, some individuals and their partners use this method interchangeably or in combination with other methods, such as fertility awareness or condoms.[10] Coitus interruptus is cost free, requires no contact with healthcare services, has no side effects, and is a contraceptive method that is always available. With typical use, 12 of 100 people with a uterus will experience an unintended pregnancy within the first year of use.[3]

Using coitus interruptus relies to a great extent on the partner with a penis having both awareness of the sensation of imminent ejaculation and the ability to withdraw consistently and completely from the vagina in time to avoid semen coming in contact with the vagina. Of note, pre-ejaculate fluid may contain sperm, and could potentially result in pregnancy.[11] Interrupting the sexual response cycle also may diminish pleasure for either or both partners. Moreover, individuals with a uterus may not be comfortable with the idea of relinquishing control of contraception.

Coitus interruptus, including correct use and estimated effectiveness, should be included in a discussion of contraceptive methods, especially as use rates have been reported to be high among adolescents in the United States.[12] However, coitus interruptus does not protect against STIs, nor does it have any noncontraceptive benefits.

### Lactational Amenorrhea Method

The lactational amenorrhea method (LAM) relies on physiologic changes associated with breastfeeding/chestfeeding for contraception. Breastfeeding confers a natural method of contraception in the initial postpartum period because the high levels of prolactin that occur during breastfeeding/chestfeeding inhibit secretion of gonadotropin-releasing hormone from the hypothalamus, thereby preventing ovulation. Pumping or manual expression of milk may reduce the effectiveness of LAM.[10,11] To be successful

| Table 11-1 | Criteria for the Lactational Amenorrhea Method |
|---|---|

1. The nursing infant is aged 6 months or younger.
2. The nursing infant receives all nutrition from suckling, with no more than 5% from food or formula supplementation, and is nursing on demand, with no more than 4 hours between feeds in the daytime and no more than 6 hours between feeds in the night.
3. Menstruation has not resumed since the infant's birth.

Based on King J. Contraception and lactation. *J Midwifery Womens Health*. 2007;52(6):614-620; Van der Wijden C, Manion C. Lactational amenorrhea method for family planning. *Cochrane Database Syst Rev*. 2015;10:CD001329. doi:10.1002/14651858. CD001329.pub2.

as a means of contraception, LAM requires that three essential conditions be present, as outlined in Table 11-1.[13,14]

Globally, LAM is widely used as a birth spacing method. The major advantages of LAM include that it is immediately available, requires no healthcare visit, and is free, with effectiveness rates as high as 98% to 99.5% during the first 6 months postpartum when the three essential conditions are operational.[14] Unfortunately, this method has a limited lifespan because of the short period of effectiveness. In the United States, it can be difficult to meet the three essential conditions for LAM, especially for individuals who return to work and are separated from their infant for several hours each day.

### Fertility Awareness Methods

Fertility awareness methods (FAM) of contraception are based on identifying the fertile days in the menstrual cycle when an ovum can be fertilized. The use of FAM varies globally; in the United States, approximately 3% of individuals report using FAM.[15] There is often underreporting of this method because FAM has been characterized as a "traditional" method when compared to "modern" methods, perhaps causing individuals and providers to discount their use.[16] The most common concern about FAM is poor effectiveness for pregnancy prevention. Reliable data for many of the FAM strategies are generally lacking because of the rarity of randomized controlled trials and overall low quality of research studies.[17]

FAM encompasses a number of low-cost, user-controlled contraceptive methods that are available at any time. A multi-country survey of more than 2000 couples using FAM reported that

the majority were not only satisfied with the method, but also believed that the methods improved their sex lives.[18] Like many contraceptive methods, FAM does not protect against transmission of STIs. The *Fertility Awareness Methods* appendix provides an overview of the various FAM options.

All of the fertility awareness–based methods are highly dependent on the couple's motivation and desires; consequently, it is difficult to recommend one method over the others. Technology may be used in combination with these methods, thereby potentially increasing their effectiveness. More than 100 apps are available with varying accuracy. Proper training in FAM along with accurate use of the app is critical to prevent pregnancy.[19]

### Spermicidal Agents

Spermicides are chemical agents that kill sperm. They may be formulated as gels, creams, aerosol foam, suppositories, vaginal film, or sponges. The active agent in all spermicidal preparations available in the United States is nonoxynol-9, a surfactant that destroys the sperm cell membrane. This agent is combined with an inert base that creates the specific formulation, such as a cream or gel. The inert base material serves as a mechanical barrier to the cervical os and facilitates vaginal distribution and formation of a surface film that withstands coital activity. The effectiveness of any contraceptive method using the spermicide is directly related to the nonoxynol-9 dose. Products with at least 100 mg of nonoxynol-9 are more effective than preparations with lower doses.[20]

Table 11-2 provides detailed information on spermicidal products. Spermicidal preparations are relatively easy to use, are controlled by the individual, and are effective within 15 minutes. These agents are available widely in stores and online without a prescription. Figure 11-1 depicts the Today sponge, which is impregnated with nonxynol-9.

For this contraceptive method to be effective, the individual must use the spermicide consistently with each act of vaginal intercourse. Also, for some preparations, as noted in Table 11-2, timing of insertion is critical for effectiveness. For example, the contraceptive film and suppositories require 15 minutes in the vagina to become effective prior to being exposed to sperm. Patients who object to inserting a finger into their vagina may find film and suppositories problematic, as both need to be placed deep into the vagina to cover the cervix. Some postcoital leakage is common with all of the spermicidal preparations except film, which some patients

| Table 11-2 | Spermicidal Preparations | | | |
|---|---|---|---|---|
| **Preparation** | **Nonoxynol-9 (mg/dose)** | **Timing of Application[a]** | **Duration of Action** | **Comments** |
| Creams | 52.5–150 | Up to 1 hour before coitus | 1 hour[b] | Use alone or with a diaphragm |
| Film | 72–100 | Insert 15 minutes before coitus | 3 hours[b] | Becomes a gel as it dissolves under body temperature<br><br>Use dry fingers to place the film deep into the vagina |
| Foam | 100–125 | Insert immediately before coitus | 1 hour[b] | Aerosol, under pressure in a container; apply with an applicator that is inserted into the vagina in a similar manner to a tampon applicator |
| Gels | 52.5–150 | Insert immediately before coitus | 1 hour[b] | Use alone or with a diaphragm |
| Suppository or insert | 100–125 | Insert 15 minutes before coitus | 1 hour[b] | Activated when melted; spermicide is embedded in cocoa butter or glycerin<br><br>Remove the covering and insert the suppository deep into the vagina |
| Sponge | 1000 | Anytime up to 24 hours before coitus | Leave in place for 6 hours after coitus, but no longer than 30 hours total to avoid the rare risk of toxic shock syndrome | Polyurethane "pillow"; moistening with tap water until suds appear prior to use activates nonoxynol-9<br><br>Fold the sponge by using the dimple; place it deeply within the vagina, with the string loop on the bottom for easy removal |

[a] Insert another application of nonoxynol 9 for additional acts of intercourse.

[b] Do not douche for this method for a minimum of 6 hours post coitus.

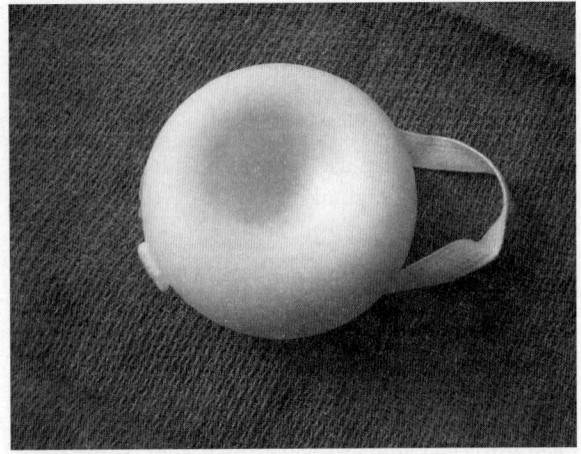

**Figure 11-1** Today sponge.
Photograph courtesy of Tekoa L. King, CNM, MPH.

consider esthetically unpleasing. The film melts at body temperature and does not result in any additional vaginal discharge.

Spermicidal preparations have a low effectiveness rate for typical use. Among typical users during the first year of use, approximately 18% to 28% will have an unintended pregnancy—a rate similar to that for the withdrawal method.[3,21] The one exception is the sponge, for which effectiveness rates differ according to a person's parity. The rates of unintended pregnancy in the first year of use are 12% and 27% for nulliparous and multiparous individuals, respectively.[3] Even with this limited effectiveness, using any form of this contraceptive method is more effective than using no method.

Side effects and adverse effects of nonoxynol-9 include a contact dermatitis/local irritation of the vulva, vagina, or penis, which is often mischaracterized as an allergic reaction. Nonoxynol-9 is a surfactant with the potential to damage the vaginal epithelium, increasing risks of infections, including STIs. Spermicides are absolutely contraindicated for individuals at high risk for exposure to HIV per the U.S. MEC for Contraceptive Use.[1] The risk of microabrasions to the vaginal epithelium increases with use more than twice a day, which in turn increases the risk of HIV infection.[22] In addition, individuals who are HIV positive or who have acquired immunodeficiency syndrome (AIDS) likely should not use spermicides because of the increased risk for genital lesions and HIV transmission associated with this contraceptive method.[23]

A rare but serious side effect of sponge use is toxic shock syndrome—an immunologic-mediated, potentially fatal, septic reaction to bacterial toxins of the species *Staphylococcus aureus* and/or *Streptococcus pyogenes*. This condition was discovered in the 1980s and associated with use of the contraceptive sponge as well as super-absorbent tampons that were composed of carboxymethylcellulose and polyester instead of cotton.[24] Such factors as recent childbirth, use for more than 24 hours, difficult removal, or fragmentation of the aforementioned items appear to increase the risk of toxic shock syndrome.[25] However, the absolute risk of toxic shock syndrome is extremely low.[24] This infection usually presents as 2 to 3 days of mild symptoms, such as low-grade fever, muscle aches, chills, and malaise. The symptoms worsen rapidly, and include fever higher than 38°C (101.4°F), with diffuse macular erythema and hypotension. Individuals using diaphragms or the sponge should be educated about the symptoms of toxic shock syndrome, and can decrease their risk of this rare disorder by removing the device within 24 hours of its insertion.

## pH Altering

Phexxi is a prescription, pH-altering vaginal gel containing 1.8% lactic acid, 1% citric acid, and 0.4% potassium bitartrate. It works by maintaining the vagina's acidic pH level between 3.5 and 4.5, which in turn decreases sperm motility. Patients insert one dose of Phexxi into the vagina within 1 hour before intercourse. The vaginal gel provides protection for one act of vaginal intercourse; an additional dose is needed with each subsequent episode of intercourse.[26] With perfect use, Phexxi has a 93% efficacy rate; with typical use, the efficacy rate is 86%. A study of more than 1100 individuals found 49 pregnancies occurred following more than 26,000 acts of intercourse with Phexxi in place.[27]

Phexxi is not absorbed and has no systemic side effects. The most commonly reported adverse reactions include a vulvovaginal burning sensation (18%) and pruritus (14.5%).[26] Local discomfort was reported by 9.8% of partners. Phexxi is not recommended for individuals with a history of recurrent urinary tract infections or urinary tract abnormalities. Because the gel is water-based, it does not interact with other vaginal medications and can safely be used with other methods of hormonal and nonhormonal contraception (e.g., condoms, diaphragms). However, it cannot be combined with the vaginal ring.[26] Phexxi can be used postpartum with the resumption of intercourse.

## Barrier Methods

Diaphragms, cervical caps, and condoms are among the oldest contraceptive methods. These methods are usually described as barrier methods because of their mechanism of action. To achieve the maximum effectiveness, spermicides must be used with these barriers so that sperm can be killed before conception occurs. The "barrier" refers to the combination of the physical product that traps ejaculate in the vagina and the chemical barrier supplied by the spermicide. Effectiveness of barrier methods ranges from approximately 88% for diaphragms to an estimated 80% for condoms.[3]

### Diaphragm

The diaphragm is a dome-shaped silicone cup with a flexible rim that permits compression of the device to facilitate insertion into the vagina, but then allows it to regain its shape so that it fits snugly against the vaginal walls. When properly positioned, the diaphragm rim rests against the anterior vaginal wall (posterior to the symphysis pubis) and lateral vaginal walls and extends posteriorly to completely cover the cervix. A diaphragm is used with a spermicidal gel or cream that is applied inside the dome of the diaphragm and lightly around the rim, thereby providing both physical and chemical barriers to sperm.[28]

Diaphragms come in four types. The Caya is a one-size-fits-most diaphragm, and the other three types are classified based on the presence or absence of a spring in the rim. The latter three types are available in several sizes. All diaphragms require a prescription. The diaphragm is a private, patient-controlled, and not necessarily coital-dependent contraceptive

| Table 11-3 | Types of Diaphragms | |
| --- | --- | --- |
| **Type** | **Description** | **Indications** |
| Wide-seal rim | Has a flexible 1½-cm-wide "skirt" extending from the inner edge of the rim | Latex-free diaphragm composed of silicone. The small skirt is designed to hold gel in place and improve the seal. May have one of two types of springs. |
| | Arcing spring | Strongest type of rim. May be used by individuals who have cystocele, rectocele, uterine prolapse, retroverted uterus, or an anteverted or retroverted cervix. |
| | Omniflex | Has a distortion-free spring that provides an arc, no matter where the rim is compressed. This type of rim is proposed to provide increased suction for added protection. The wide-seal rim omniflex replaced the "all-flex" diaphragm, which was once the most popular diaphragm but was discontinued by the manufacturer in approximately 2014. However, it folds on only two axes. |
| Silicone single size | Purple diaphragm with rim dimples for gripping during insertion and a finger dome for ease of removal | Marketed with the Caya brand name, this silicone diaphragm is designed to fit most people. It is a single size, and no measuring is required. Like all diaphragms, Caya is available by prescription only. Some providers suggest that proper placement should be verified by a clinician because the diaphragm is not marketed as fitting all people with a cervix. |

method. All of today's diaphragms are made with silicone. Table 11-3 provides detailed information on types of diaphragms. A silicone wide-seal diaphragm is illustrated in Figure 11-2 and a one-size diaphragm is depicted in Figure 11-3.

Approximately 12% of typical diaphragm users will have an unintended pregnancy in the first year of use, making the diaphragm more effective than external condoms and all other vaginal barrier methods.[3] External condoms can be used simultaneously with diaphragms, enhancing contraceptive effectiveness and adding protection against STI transmission.

Except for Caya, the size of the diaphragm must be determined individually for each person, because the distance from the posterior vaginal fornix to the posterior aspect of the symphysis pubis varies among individuals. Sizing is not specifically associated with parity, although nulliparous individuals are generally fit with size 65, 70, or 75 and multiparous individuals fit with size 75, 80, or 85.

To fit a diaphragm, ask the patient to empty their bladder prior to the fitting. Insert a gloved index and middle finger into the vagina until the middle finger reaches the posterior wall of the vagina, to determine the distance between the posterior symphysis and the posterior vagina behind the cervix. Mark the point at which the index finger touches the

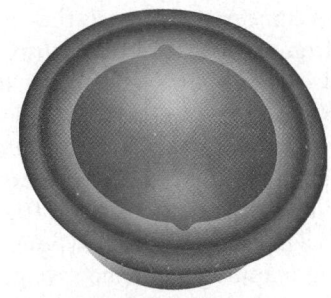

**Figure 11-2** Wide-seal diaphragm.

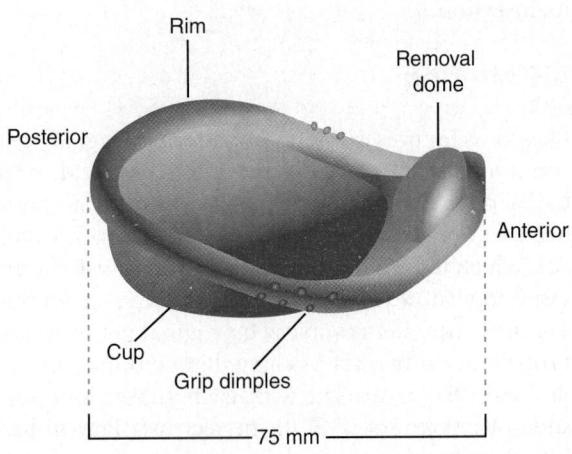

**Figure 11-3** Single-size contoured diaphragm.

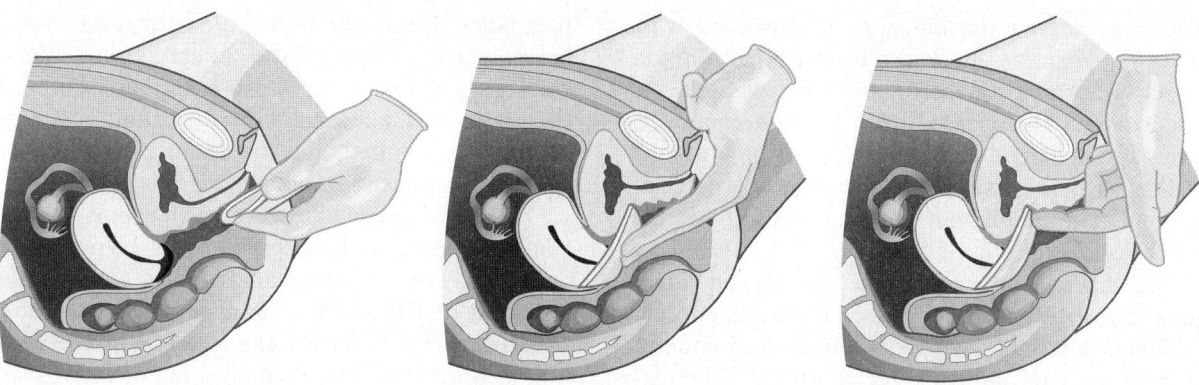

**Figure 11-4** Diaphragm fitting.

inferior pubic arch. Remove the fingers and place a diaphragm rim on the tip of the middle finger. The opposite rim of the correct size of diaphragm should lie approximately in front of the mark. Lubricate or moisten the diaphragm or fitting ring, compress the sides together with the fingers and thumb of one hand, and introduce it into the vagina (Figure 11-4). Be certain to direct the diaphragm or fitting ring downward and inward, thereby applying pressure against the posterior vaginal wall and avoiding the more sensitive anterior structures.

Once the diaphragm is inserted, check its placement with a gloved finger. It is the correct size if (1) the rim is behind the cervix in the posterior fornix, (2) the circumference is against the lateral vaginal walls, (3) a fingertip can be inserted between the diaphragm rim and the posterior surface of the pubis, and (4) the cervix is covered. The diaphragm is too small if (1) there is more than enough space for the flat portion of a fingertip to be inserted between the rim of the diaphragm and the posterior surface of the pubis, (2) it moves about freely in the vagina, or (3) it dislodges when the patient coughs or bears down. The diaphragm is too large if (1) it fits tightly against the symphysis pubis, (2) the rim buckles forward against the lateral vaginal walls, (3) it dislodges or protrudes out the vagina when the patient performs the Valsalva maneuver, or (4) the patient feels discomfort when the diaphragm is in place. Many midwives will verify the appropriate size by inserting diaphragms of successive size until the correct size is ascertained and then inserting one size larger for confirmation, although this is not required. It is important that the midwife asks the patient to demonstrate insertion and removal of the diaphragm after verifying the correct fit. After patient insertion, the midwife should then confirm the placement via a digital exam.[21,28]

Little evidence regarding timing of insertion and removal of diaphragms is available, but the usual instructions state that the diaphragm should be coated with approximately 1 teaspoon of a spermicide inside the dome and rim, inserted less than 3 hours before coitus, and left in place for at least 6 hours after intercourse (so that the spermicide remains effective), but no more than 24 hours.[21] If another act of intercourse occurs, the diaphragm should not be removed, but another application of spermicide is then applied intravaginally.

Side effects of diaphragm use include an increased risk for urinary tract infections as compared to other contraceptive methods, perhaps due to pressure on the urethra exerted by the diaphragm's rim, causing incomplete bladder emptying, or from the spermicide altering the vaginal flora, which may increase the risk of *Escherichia coli* bacteriuria.[21] If the patient experiences recurrent urinary tract infections, the diaphragm may be too large or the rim too rigid, and refitting is indicated.[28] If refitting does not resolve the problem, the patient can be counseled to select another contraceptive method.

Local irritation from the nonoxynol-9 spermicidal agent may occur. If the diaphragm has been improperly fitted or is left in place longer than 24 hours after having intercourse, vaginal wall abrasions can occur. When recurrent vaginal or vulvar irritation occurs without evidence of an infection, these symptoms may indicate allergy to the diaphragm itself, especially if it is an older latex diaphragm. In addition, the risk of toxic shock syndrome may increase—though it remains low—if the diaphragm is left in place for more than 24 hours.[1,21]

Contraindications to use of a diaphragm are the same as those for a spermicide and are related to the spermicide component of this contraceptive method. Diaphragms are classified as U.S. MEC for Contraceptive Use Category 3 for patients with a history of toxic shock syndrome, because toxic shock syndrome has been associated with use of these devices.[1] Occasionally, a diaphragm cannot be fitted for an individual who has an anatomic abnormality such as pelvic organ prolapse or a vaginal septum. The diaphragm does not protect against STI transmission.

A general consensus exists that an individual should be examined for a refit of a fitted diaphragm following a weight change of more than 15 pounds, a birth, or a second-trimester abortion.[21] The diaphragm should not be used after giving birth until uterine involution is complete and the vagina has regained its tone. All patients using a diaphragm should be instructed about the symptoms of toxic shock syndrome.

## Cervical Cap

The cervical cap is a dome-shaped silicone cap (Figure 11-5). The concave dome fits snugly over the cervix and is held in place by the muscular walls of the vagina. The brim is slightly wider on the side that fits into the posterior fornix. The cap has a strap that stretches over the diameter of the dome, which facilitates removal. Spermicide is applied inside the dome, around the brim, and in the groove between the dome and the brim prior to insertion of the device.[21,29]

The only cervical cap currently available in the United States is marketed with the brand name Fem-Cap.[21,30] Originally approved by the U.S. Food and Drug Administration (FDA) in 2003, it is available in three sizes, with size determined by a patient's

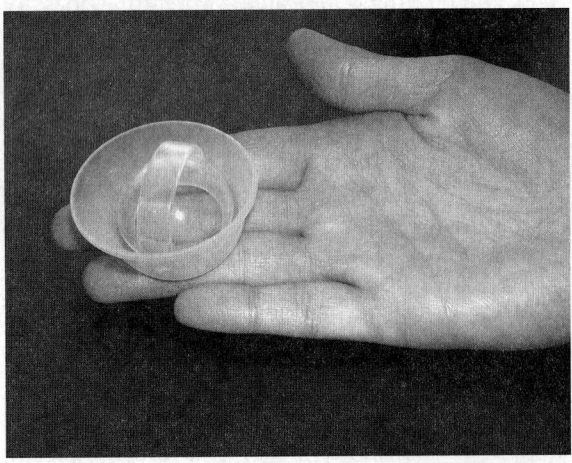

**Figure 11-5** Cervical cap (FemCap).
Reproduced with permission from The Cervical Barrier Advancement Society and Ibis Reproductive Health.

pregnancy history: 22 mm if the patient has never been pregnant; 26 mm if the patient has had a miscarriage, abortion, or cesarean birth; and 30 mm if the patient has had a full-term vaginal birth. A prescription is required, and the device is available at selected pharmacies or online.

The advantage of the cervical cap is that it can be inserted as long as 42 hours before intercourse, thereby avoiding interruption of foreplay; it should be left in place for at least 6 hours after intercourse.[21,31] When the cap is inserted more than 1 hour prior to coitus, an application of spermicide should be added intravaginally without removing the cap. If another act of intercourse occurs, the cervical cap should not be removed and an additional application of spermicide should be applied intravaginally.

In the original clinical trial reported to the FDA prior to approval of the originally designed cap, the 6-month effectiveness rate for FemCap was 77% overall, but 86% for nulliparous individuals.[29,31] The current FDA-approved FemCap is a different design; only limited data on its effectiveness are available, and it is unclear whether it is as effective or even more effective than the diaphragm.[31]

Contraindications to using the cervical cap are the same as the contraindications to using spermicides and diaphragms, with a few additions. Individuals who have cervical cancer, cervical intraepithelial neoplasia, or a marked abnormally shaped cervix should be advised to use another form of contraception.[21,29] Using the cervical cap during menstruation may increase the risk of toxic shock syndrome and, therefore, should be avoided.[31] The cap does not protect against STI transmission, so using an external condom in combination with the cap adds this protection.

While a pelvic examination is not needed to select the correct size of cervical cap, a clinician should insert and remove the device to illustrate proper technique for the patient, and then have the patient perform a return demonstration. Figure 11-6 illustrates how a patient can insert a cervical cap in a manner similar to inserting a diaphragm. The mild suction exerted by the device allows it to fit snugly next to the cervix; it is properly placed when it does not move easily away from the cervix. The cap is most easily inserted before sexual arousal because sexual arousal can cause the cervix to become slightly soft. Removal is accomplished in a manner similar to removing a diaphragm. The patient inserts a clean finger into the vagina, firmly moves the cap off the cervix, and removes it by slipping it down the vagina and forward.

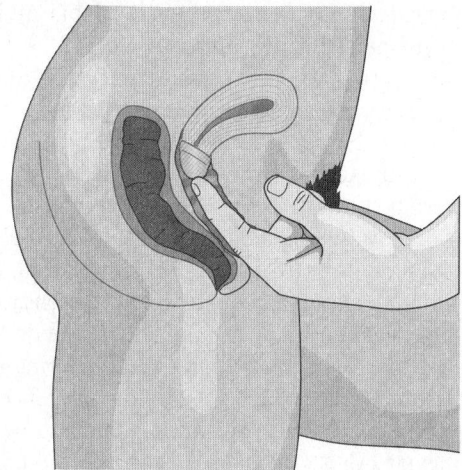

**Figure 11-6** Proper insertion of a cervical cap by a patient.

Urinary tract infections occur less frequently in patients using the cap compared to the diaphragm, and vaginitis occurs at similar rates as in diaphragm users.[29] The cap should be replaced after each year of use.[21,29] The size should not need to be changed unless the person's history changes—for example, if the patient had never been pregnant when originally fitted and now has experienced a miscarriage, abortion, or given birth.

### External Condom

Contraceptives for individuals with a penis have long been a subject of research.[32,33] Even so, only two reversible methods are currently available: the external condom and coitus interruptus. External condoms usually are sold over the counter and packaged inside a foil or plastic wrapper.

Many external condoms are available in the United States, including those made of natural rubber latex. Condoms composed of polyurethane, a synthetic material, provide an option for individuals who are allergic to latex. Compared to latex condoms, the polyurethane condoms are odorless and colorless, fit more loosely, have a longer shelf life, and can be used with any lubricant.[34] Latex condoms are effective in preventing transmission of HIV and STIs; however, the effectiveness of nonlatex condoms in protecting against HIV and STIs has not been well established.[34]

Condoms come in a variety of colors, textures, transparencies, sizes, and shapes, with the polyurethane condoms being more expensive than the latex ones. Both types can be used either dry or with lubricants. Oil-based lubricants such as petroleum jelly or massage oils should not be used, as they can cause breakage of the latex. Condoms used in conjunction with spermicides have enhanced effectiveness compared to those used either dry or with nonspermicidal lubricants. However, the spermicide should be used judiciously, as applying too much of the agent can cause slippage of the condom.

External condoms remain the most widely available and commonly used barrier method in the United States. Approximately 21% of individuals using a contraceptive have reported that their partners with a penis use condoms, making it a popular method for preventing pregnancy.[7] When used correctly and consistently with each coitus, during the first year of use among typical users, approximately 18% of individuals would be expected to have an unintended pregnancy.[35] Most condom failures result from breakage or slippage during intercourse or while removing the condom. In a meta-analysis of 11 randomized trials that compared latex and synthetic condoms, failure rates were comparable for all latex and synthetic condoms, although most synthetic condoms had higher reported rates of breakage and slippage.[34]

Condoms can cause vaginal irritation or discomfort; synthetic condoms are reported to cause less vaginal irritation and discomfort than the latex versions.[35] Disadvantages include perceived reduced sensitivity and lack of spontaneity during sexual activity, especially during foreplay when the condom should be worn, as well as latex allergy of either partner. Some individuals have difficulty maintaining an erection while the condom is on, and some individuals may be embarrassed to use a condom or to ask that the partner use one. Lastly, external condoms are controlled by the partner who wears it on their penis. The individual with a vagina who cannot negotiate condom use by their partner may be exposed to risks of unwanted pregnancy and STIs.

Condoms can be used as an adjunct to other contraceptives. For example, if a patient using combined oral contraceptives misses one or more pills, using condoms for the duration of the pill cycle provides protection from pregnancy. Dual use of condoms with another contraceptive should also be advocated for individuals with multiple or new partners to reduce risk of STIs, and for those seeking added protection against unintended pregnancy.[36,37]

Reviewing correct use is best done by demonstration, using a penile model or a simple substitute such as a banana. Basic instructions include the description that the external condom is a strong, thin, elastic sheath that is applied to the tip of an erect penis and unrolled to catch the seminal fluid during ejaculation and prevent it from being deposited in the vagina. Some space should be left in the tip of the condom to have a repository for semen; otherwise, the fluid can be forced outside the base. In the event of condom breakage or slippage, emergency contraception is available as an option, as described in the *Hormonal Contraception* chapter.

### Internal Condom

The internal condom is a soft, loosely fitting, thin sheath (Figure 11-7).[38] It has two flexible rings—one on the closed end of the sheath that is inserted into the vagina, and a larger ring on the open end that remains outside the vagina and covers the introitus. The internal condom is available in only one size and does not need to be fitted by a healthcare professional.[39] Although the product may be prelubricated with a silicone-based, nonspermicidal agent, additional lubricants or spermicidal preparations may be used in combination with the condom. Each condom is intended for one-time use. Current internal condoms are made of nitrile, latex, or silicone to diminish the issue of a crinkling sound with the previous generation of polyurethane-based internal condoms.

The effectiveness of the internal condom is generally considered slightly less than that of external condoms, with approximately 79% of users in the first year of typical use avoiding unintended pregnancy.[3] The discrepancy in failure rates between perfect use (95%) and typical use may reflect problems mastering insertion as well as inconsistent use.[40] The internal condom protects as effectively as external condoms against STIs and HIV transmission when used correctly, in part because the internal condom

also provides a barrier between the labia and the base of the penis during intercourse.[3,41]

The internal condom can be inserted as long as 8 hours before sexual intercourse, but must be in place before the penis enters vagina. Some couples prefer the freedom of movement and looseness of the internal condom compared to the external condom. Some individuals have reported that the edge of the outer ring provides clitoral stimulation. Both partners may experience uncomfortable sensations, including feeling the inner ring, having the condom adhere to the penis, and feeling the outer ring press against the vulva during intercourse. Checking for correct placement and adding more lubricant can alleviate these problems. Learning the correct steps for insertion may be challenging, but can be achieved with detailed instruction. Table 11-4 reviews the steps involved in correct use of the internal condom. Most individuals need to practice two to three times to successfully place the condom.[21]

The internal condom usually moves from side to side in the vagina during vaginal intercourse. However, if the penis slips between the condom and the walls of the vagina, or if the outer ring is pushed into the vagina, there is risk of pregnancy. As long as ejaculation has not occurred, the condom can be removed or repositioned, and additional spermicide

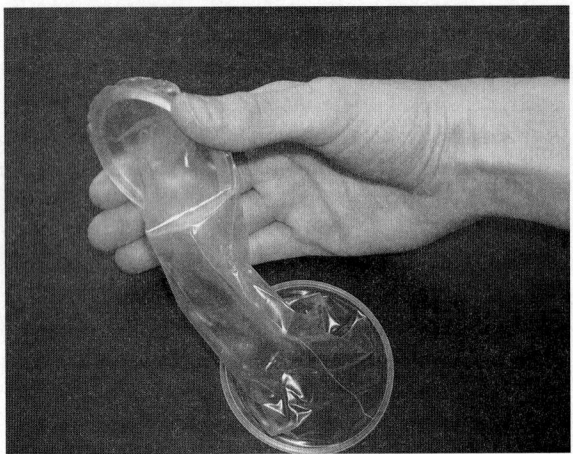

**Figure 11-7** Internal condom.
Reproduced with permission from The Cervical Barrier Advancement Society and Ibis Reproductive Health.

| Table 11-4 | General Instructions for Use of Internal Condom |
|---|---|
| **Insertion** | |
| Lubricate the outside of the closed end with spermicide. | |
| Relax in a comfortable position (e.g., lie down, squat, stand with one foot on a chair). | |
| Squeeze the sides of the inner ring at the closed end together. | |
| Insert the condom deep in the vagina, in similar fashion as inserting a tampon. | |
| Slip the inner ring into the vagina as far as possible (until it reaches the cervix). | |
| Allow the outer ring to hang approximately 1 inch (2.5 cm) outside the vagina. | |
| **Removal** | |
| Squeeze and twist the outer ring to keep semen inside the pouch. | |
| Gently remove the condom directly out of the vagina. | |
| Discard the condom, but do not flush it down the toilet. | |

added. The internal condom is used by some individuals for anal intercourse; this use is not FDA approved. In the event of condom breakage or slippage, emergency contraception is available as an option, as described in the *Hormonal Contraception* chapter. The internal condom does protect against STIs.

## Intrauterine Devices

Several synonyms are used to describe IUDs, including intrauterine contraceptives (IUCs), intrauterine contraceptive devices (IUCDs), and intrauterine systems (IUSs). For consistency, the term IUD is used throughout this chapter. IUDs and contraceptive implants are the two types of long-acting reversible contraceptive (LARC) devices available in the United States. IUDs are the most commonly used reversible contraceptive globally, although in the United States among individuals with a uterus using a birth control method, more people choose oral contraceptives.[42]

Rates of IUD use were increasing in the United States during the 1970s, but decreased significantly following the highly publicized association between pelvic inflammatory disease (PID) and the Dalkon Shield before this device's eventual removal from the market in 1974.[43] The problems associated with the Dalkon Shield changed the perception of IUD safety; a generation of reproductive-age people chose non-IUD options given these safety concerns. Multiple factors have contributed to the lower prevalence of IUD use in the United States, including a lack of widespread marketing, especially compared to oral contraceptives; common misconceptions about the IUDs' mechanism of action; misinformation about associated risks; and a history of negative publicity. Recent surveys of contraceptive preference, however, indicate that IUDs are increasing in favor among individuals, perhaps indicating a resurgence of this method's acceptability in the United States.[43]

IUDs have been found to be among the most effective reversible forms of contraception. In addition to their effectiveness, an emerging body of research suggests that these methods may provide protection against cervical cancer.[44] Additional research needs to be conducted to confirm this benefit.

### Types of Intrauterine Devices

IUDs are classified as either hormonal or nonhormonal. Two types of T-shaped IUDs are available in the United States: one that incorporates copper (Copper T 380A [ParaGard]), and another that releases levonorgestrel (LNG; levonorgestrel-releasing intrauterine system [LNG-IUS or LNG-IUD]). These two types of IUDs have much in common. This chapter focuses on the Copper T 380A, nonhormonal IUD, although some information about the LNG-IUD is also provided.

The copper IUD (ParaGard) is a nonhormonal contraceptive that has been available for decades in the United States. This IUD is associated with irregular bleeding, dysmenorrhea, and heavier menses, which on rare occasions may lead to anemia.[45,46] Individuals who are aware of these menstrual changes and accept them prior to insertion may be able to tolerate the device better than those in whom these effects occur unexpectedly. Although the copper IUD is currently approved by the FDA for 10 years of use, emerging research supports its effectiveness beyond 10 years.[45,46]

Four LNG-IUDs (Mirena, Liletta, Skyla, and Kyleena) exist; they are described in more detail in the *Hormonal Contraception* chapter. While all of these devices contain the same hormone (LNG), they differ in size, duration of effectiveness, and dose of hormone. Additionally, Mirena and Liletta each have unique FDA approvals: Mirena is approved for the treatment of individuals with heavy menstrual bleeding who also desire an IUD, whereas Liletta is approved specifically for use in nulliparous individuals.[47] When considering the side effects and the therapeutic benefit of amenorrhea conferred by the presence of LNG in these devices, it may be helpful to consider the patient's baseline menstrual flow. Patients who report light to moderate bleeding may be more likely to experience amenorrhea within the first year of use.[47]

### Copper T 380A (ParaGard)

ParaGard, the only nonhormonal IUD currently available in the United States, is composed of polyethylene and an inert plastic material that is flexible, is non-inflammatory, and resumes its original shape easily after being flexed for insertion (Figure 11-8). The vertical stem of the polyethylene body is wrapped with 176 mg of copper wire, while each of its horizontal arms has a 68.7-mg copper collar attached.[45,46] The copper components of ParaGard release ions into the endometrial cavity that affect tubal and endometrial fluids, and subsequently incapacitate sperm. The ParaGard IUD has a length of plastic thread attached to the lower segment that facilitates its removal and enables both the midwife and the patient to confirm the presence of the device. Embedded within this IUD's polyethylene body

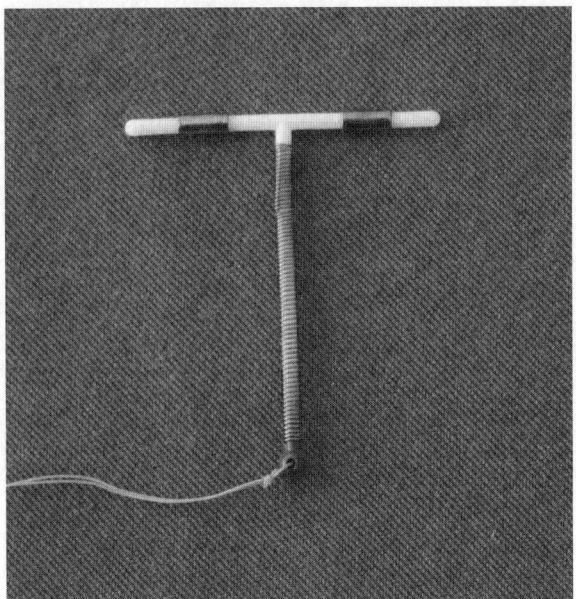

**Figure 11-8** Paragard IUD.
© Jones & Bartlett Learning. Photographed by Kimberly Potvin.

is a small amount of barium sulfate, which provides for localization of the device with standard X-ray imaging. ParaGard provides contraception for as long as 12 years after insertion. Other types of non-hormonal IUDs are available in countries outside the United States.

The effectiveness rate for ParaGard is high, with fewer than 1 patient in 100 experiencing an unintended pregnancy in the first year of use.[3] The copper in the IUD alters sperm tubal transport, has toxic effects on the ovum, and impairs normal sperm activity by slowing motility, reducing sperm capacitation, and increasing sperm destruction. In addition, the copper creates a localized reaction in the endometrial tissue that renders the uterine endometrium unfavorable for implantation.[47–49]

The copper IUD is associated with menstrual changes such as 1 to 3 more days of bleeding per cycle, increased severity of dysmenorrhea, and a potential increase in blood loss, which can exacerbate iron-deficiency anemia.[49] Consequently, ParaGard is not a good choice of contraception for patients with heavy menstrual bleeding.

Use of a copper IUD is not coitus dependent, does not require additional cost after the initial insertion, and is effective for 10 years or longer.[49] Some patients do not like the IUD-associated side effects such as increased bleeding, and others do not like the idea of having a foreign object inside their body. When patients do not have these concerns and they do not desire hormones for contraception, the copper-containing IUD may be a good choice.

## Contraindications to Use of Intrauterine Devices

Contraindications to the copper IUD and LNG-IUD are listed in Table 11-5.[1] The copper IUD is also contraindicated for people with Wilson's disease and those with systemic lupus erythematosus with severe thrombocytopenia. Additional contraindications for the LNG-IUD include current breast cancer, history of breast cancer, current heart disease, history of heart disease, systemic lupus erythematosus (SLE), and liver disease (e.g., cirrhosis).[1] The LNG-IUD is not recommended for use as an emergency contraceptive (EC), perhaps because of ethical issues in conducting a rigorous study and lack of compelling need because the copper IUD has well-recognized spermicidal effects, and has been on the market for approximately four decades with a body of research demonstrating its effectiveness as an EC. Any abnormal uterine bleeding should be evaluated for pathologic causes prior to IUD insertion. An IUD should not be used if the patient has a known hypersensitivity to any device component.

The procedures for inserting and removing an IUD are described in the *Intrauterine Device Insertion and Removal* appendix. This appendix includes discussion of timing and pre-insertion medication and side effects associated with insertion for both types of IUDs. Information on vasovagal responses and uterine perforation, which can occur during insertion, are also included in the appendix.

## Adverse Effects Associated with Intrauterine Devices

Patients should be counseled that the copper IUD may be associated with changes in menstrual bleeding patterns. It often increases the amount of menstrual bleeding and the number of days of bleeding. The IUD also has inherent risks related to its insertion and removal. Bleeding, infection, perforation of the uterus, and pain may occur, although serious complications are rare. Table 11-6 lists conditions that should be considered for follow-up visits, which can be remembered by using the mnemonic "PAINS."

### Intrauterine Device Expulsion

Expulsion rates for the various types of IUDs are relatively similar. These rates are generally low (2.3%) following insertion of the copper IUD in a nonpregnant person and are highest in the first

| Table 11-5 | Contraindications for the Use of Copper-Containing and Levonorgestrel-Releasing Intrauterine Devices: U.S. Medical Eligibility Criteria for Contraceptive Use Categories 3 or 4[a] |
|---|---|
| **Contraindications** | **Medical Eligibility Criteria for Contraceptive Use Category** |
| Cervical cancer awaiting treatment | 4 for initiation; 2 for continuation |
| Distorted uterine cavity | 4 |
| Endometrial cancer | 4 for initiation; 2 for continuation |
| Gestational trophoblastic disease with persistently elevated ß-hCG levels or malignant disease, with evidence or suspicion of intrauterine disease | 4 for initiation; 2 for continuation |
| Immediately post septic abortion | 4 |
| Pelvic inflammatory disease (current) | 4 for initiation; 2 for continuation |
| Pelvic tuberculosis | 4 for initiation; 3 for continuation |
| Pregnancy | 4 |
| Postpartum sepsis | 4 |
| Current purulent cervicitis or chlamydial infection or gonococcal infection | 4 for initiation; 2 for continuation |
| Solid organ transplant | 3 for initiation; 2 for continuation |
| Unexplained vaginal bleeding that is suspicious for a serious condition | 4 for initiation; 2 for continuation |

Abbreviation: hCG, human chorionic gonadotropin.

[a] U.S. Medical Eligibility Criteria for Contraceptive Use Categories: Category 1: a condition for which there is no restriction; Category 2: a condition for which the advantages of using the method generally outweigh the theoretical or proven risks; Category 3: a condition for which the theoretical or proven risks usually outweigh the advantages of using the method; Category 4: a condition that represents an unacceptable health risk if the contraceptive method is used.

Modified from Curtis KM, Tepper NK, Jatlaoui TC, et al. U.S. Medical Eligibility Criteria for Contraceptive Use, 2016. *MMWR.* 2016;65(3):1-106.

| Table 11-6 | PAINS Mnemonic for Adverse Effects of Intrauterine Devices |
|---|---|
| **P**eriod | Amenorrhea, especially sudden onset; with the copper IUD, may be associated with pregnancy. Light bleeding and amenorrhea are side effects of LNG-IUDs. |
| **A**bdominal pain | General abdominal pain can suggest an ectopic pregnancy, sexually transmitted infection, or intolerance of copper. |
| **I**nfection | Vaginal discharge, pelvic pain, history of exposure, or any suspicion of sexually transmitted infections. |
| **N**ot feeling well | Malaise, fever, nausea, and vomiting suggesting infection or sepsis. |
| **S**trings | Strings or threads of the IUD changing in length or missing entirely. |

Abbreviations: IUD, intrauterine device; LNG-IUD, levonorgestrel-releasing intrauterine device.

year after insertion.[50] Adolescents are more likely to experience expulsion regardless of parity.[51] The rate of expulsion in the immediate postpartum period is typically higher than at other times, but patients who receive immediate insertion of an IUD following childbirth are more likely to demonstrate continued use as compared to those who defer IUD insertion until a postpartum office visit.[50,52] Insertion after the 14th postpartum day is associated with an expulsion rate equal to that of insertion at 6 weeks or later.[53]

Encouraging regular string or thread checks can help detect expulsion. Education should include signs and symptoms of expulsion, including detection of the device at the cervical os, pain and cramping, abnormal uterine bleeding, discharge, or fever.

### Missing Intrauterine Device Strings

A clinician's inability to find IUD strings during an examination may indicate a complication and warrants further investigation. Sometimes the strings have simply receded into the cervix or uterine cavity, the strings were cut too short, or the threads have curled behind the cervix and become difficult to palpate. Gentle cervical exploration with a cytobrush or cotton swab may be able to guide and straighten the strings—a technique colloquially termed "fishing" for the strings. Care should be taken not to pull on the threads and dislodge the device. If the strings are not apparent to the clinician during a clinical examination, it is possible that the device was spontaneously expelled and the patient is unaware of its loss. Pregnancy should be considered whenever strings are not visible[54,55] because the IUD can rise in the uterus as it enlarges.

An ultrasound can identify whether the IUD is in situ; if the IUD is not visible by ultrasound, then other imaging modalities should be employed to determine whether the IUD is in the abdomen after uterine perforation. If imaging reveals that the IUD either is dislodged and no longer in the expected location (e.g., in a uterine tube or the cervical canal) or has perforated the uterus and entered the abdomen, immediate referral is indicated.

In the unusual event that the IUD is appropriately positioned in the fundus but the threads are not palpable, the patient needs to make an informed decision regarding IUD removal and replacement or to continue with the IUD in place. Contraceptive effectiveness is not dependent upon the threads extending from the uterus into the vagina.

### Pregnancy with an Intrauterine Device in Situ

A patient who becomes pregnant with an IUD in place should be informed of the risks involved if the pregnancy is continued—namely, chorioamnionitis, miscarriage with or without sepsis, and preterm birth.[55] Although the risk of pregnancy is small with an IUD in place, patients who become pregnant with an IUD in place should also be evaluated for ectopic pregnancy, as the risk of an ectopic pregnancy is higher with an IUD in situ.

If pregnancy is confirmed, an ultrasound reveals the placement of the IUD, and the IUD strings are visible, the IUD should be removed to decrease the risk of miscarriage. The incidence of miscarriage is slightly higher if the IUD remains in place than if the device is removed.[55] This benefit is most apparent when the IUD is removed during the first 12 weeks' gestation. Removing the IUD for a patient who wishes to terminate the pregnancy reduces their risk of uterine infection.[55] The IUD is removed as described in the *Intrauterine Device Insertion and Removal* appendix.

When pregnancy is confirmed and the strings of the IUD are not visible, ultrasound may reveal that the device has been covertly expelled, such as with a heavy menses; the patient may not have been aware of its loss. If the ultrasound reveals the IUD is placed abnormally (e.g., within a uterine tube) or is in the uterus but without strings visible or accessible, the patient should be referred to a specialist.

### Ectopic Pregnancy and Intrauterine Devices

A smaller number of ectopic pregnancies occur in patients who use an IUD than in patients who do not use any contraceptive method because of the overall contraceptive effectiveness of the device. However, IUDs are more effective in preventing intrauterine pregnancies than ectopic pregnancies. Therefore, if a pregnancy does occur when an IUD is in place, careful evaluation for the presence of an ectopic pregnancy is required.[49]

## Permanent Contraception: Sterilization

Sterilization is the surgical interruption or closure of pathways for sperm or ova to unite, which prevents fertilization. Sterilization is considered a safe, highly effective, and permanent form of contraception.[56]

The term "tying tubes" is a common phrase for tubal sterilization or ligation, but this wording should be avoided as it may incorrectly connote that the uterine tubes could later be easily untied. Reversal of a tubal ligation is actually a complicated and costly procedure. Tubal sterilization procedures can be performed soon after a vaginal birth (postpartum sterilization), in conjunction with a cesarean birth, immediately following an uncomplicated first trimester abortion, or independent of pregnancy (interval sterilization).

Vasectomy, or ligation of the vas deferens, is also a safe and simple procedure. A vasectomy is approximately half the cost of tubal sterilization, although tubal sterilization is more common in the United States.[57] In fact, in the United States, sterilization is one of the most frequently performed surgeries for a person with a uterus. Overall, both tubal sterilization and vasectomy are more than 99% effective in preventing pregnancy.[3]

### Tubal Sterilization

Tubal sterilization is accomplished by one of two procedures: laparoscopy and minilaparotomy.[57] Minilaparotomy is typically reserved for the immediately postpartum period.[57] Laparoscopic procedures provide tubal occlusion via electrocoagulation, mechanical devices such as clips or rings, and tubal excision. Early studies conducted when tubal occlusion techniques were relatively new found that electrosurgery and micro-clips were associated with higher pregnancy rates compared to tubal ligation. However, recent studies have found that all techniques for occluding or cutting the uterine tube have similar effectiveness. Thus, the technique chosen is based on the surgeon's preference and skill.

Sterilization is a surgical procedure that requires the services of a skilled surgeon. It has been reported that some surgeons have personal requirements of age or parity prior to offering sterilization to individuals. Such requirements based on age or parity are not justified.[57] Only 0.5% of patients experience an unintended pregnancy within the first year following surgical sterilization, which translates into a 99.5% effectiveness rate.[3] This number includes patients with an unsuspected pregnancy at the time the procedure is performed. Failure can also happen many years after the procedure is performed. Because spontaneous pregnancy after tubal ligation is rare, the overall risk of ectopic pregnancy is lower in patients who undergo surgical sterilization than in the general population. If pregnancy does occur after tubal sterilization, however, there is a high risk that it will be an ectopic pregnancy.[57]

Counseling prior to obtaining informed consent includes a review of alternatives, risks associated with the procedure and use of anesthesia, the permanency of contraception, and the risk of ectopic pregnancy should a pregnancy occur after the procedure. Individuals also should be informed that sterilization does not prevent transmission of STIs or HIV. Sterilization is not coital dependent, nor does it require any partner agreement or purchase of supplies. Some studies show a positive effect on sexuality, which is likely related to reduced worry about unintended pregnancy.[57] The long-term effects of tubal sterilization on menstrual pattern (post-tubal ligation syndrome) appear to be negligible. Most recent studies have not found any difference in menstrual patterns between individuals before and after sterilization.[57] Complications are those associated with any surgery.

Regret that a sterilization procedure was performed has been reported.[58] Various studies indicate that the percentage of people who regret their decision to undergo tubal sterilization ranges from 1% to slightly less than 30%.[58,59] Higher rates of regret are found in individuals who are younger than age 30 at the time of sterilization, report an unstable relationship, change partners after the surgical procedure, have experienced the death of a child, or have a low parity.[58–60] Historically, persons of color have been sterilized without consent, and even today a disproportionate number of persons of color undergo tubal sterilization. Among these patients, more persons of color appear to believe that the procedure can be reversed compared to their white counterparts, perhaps indicating the need for improved communication or education as part of shared decision making.[59]

The midwife must be aware of applicable federal and state regulations about sterilization. Because of past abuses related to forced sterilization, strict criteria should be met to verify informed consent, including the requirement that the consenting individual is an adult. Consent must be obtained within a specified time period (usually 30 days) before giving birth, and the time interval may differ by state, facility, and payer.[57] As with any shared decision-making discussion, the patient should receive information that is at the appropriate health literacy level, and in the individual's native language. The patient should understand that the procedure can be declined at any time, even after the consent form has been signed.

Reversal of sterilization is expensive, requiring either costly assisted reproductive technology or highly technical microsurgery, and results cannot be guaranteed. The rate of pregnancy following sterilization reversal varies with the type of tubal occlusive method used and with the age of the patient. Rates of successful reanastomosis following reversal procedures are in the range of approximately 50% to 80%.[61]

### Hysteroscopic Sterilization (Transcervical Sterilization)

The transcervical sterilization method involves gaining access to the uterine tubes via hysteroscopy that is introduced through the cervix. This method is not currently available in the United States, but was previously marketed as Essure. The Essure system consists of stainless steel coils that are soft and flexible because they are wrapped in polyethylene terephthalate covered with a nickel–titanium alloy. The small metal springs are placed into the proximal end of each uterine tube. Upon release, they expand and anchor to the tube, creating scar tissue.[62] Thus, the mechanism of action involves irritation and growth of new tissue that results in permanent occlusion of the uterine tubes as the tubes respond to the polyester fibers within the micro-inserts. Tubal occlusion occurs approximately 3 months after the procedure is performed. The tissue response has been found to be localized to the insert.[62]

Essure was removed from the market in 2018. Bayer, the company that manufactured the device, noted that there was less demand for the product; however, multiple reports also cited adverse events including chronic pelvic pain, migration of the device, perforation of the uterus and or uterine tubes, autoimmune-like reactions, and hypersensitivity to the device.[63] Long-term data on safety, effectiveness, and pregnancy rates for Essure continue to be collected although the device is no longer available.[64–66] U.S. and worldwide literature indicates that this sterilization technique has a greater than 98% effectiveness.[67]

### Vasectomy

Vasectomy is one of the few contraceptive options currently available for individuals with a penis. Sterilization is achieved by cutting or occluding the vas deferens so that sperm can no longer pass out of the body in the ejaculate. This procedure can be done in an outpatient setting under local anesthesia by a trained provider. Advantages of this method include the short procedure time and the reduced risk of hematoma, infection, and postoperative discomfort when compared to uterine tubal ligation.[68]

Vasectomy is a highly effective and relatively low-cost permanent method of sterilization with a low morbidity rate and an extremely low mortality rate. The incidence of pregnancy 5 years after the procedure is less than 1%.[3] Vasectomy is not immediately effective; it may take 12 weeks or more, or between 12 and 20 ejaculations, before the ejaculate is sperm free. Alternative contraception needs to be used until azoospermia is confirmed in the laboratory.[57]

Individuals should be informed that recanalization does occur, albeit infrequently. Regret about undergoing a vasectomy has been reported among approximately 3% to 5% of men who have the procedure done.[69] The majority of men who report regret had the procedure when they were younger than age 30 years, were in an unstable marriage, had no or very young children, or made the decision to have a vasectomy during a time of financial crisis or for reasons related to a pregnancy.[70]

### Conclusion

This chapter reviewed currently available nonhormonal methods of contraception for both partners in the United States. Options for contraception change frequently, as do aspects of individuals' lives; therefore, it is imperative for midwives to remain informed of the latest options so that they can engage in meaningful shared decision making with their patients. Each patient has individual needs, which makes each decision-making process unique. For many patients, nonhormonal methods can provide the primary or secondary contraceptive method that they desire.

### Resources

| Organization | Description |
| --- | --- |
| U.S. Medical Eligibility Criteria (MEC) for Contraceptive Use and U.S. Selected Practice Recommendations for Contraceptive Use (SPR) app | Includes recommendations for the use of specific nonhormonal contraceptive methods and addresses how to initiate and use them. Charts, apps, and lists are available from the website. |
| Bedsider | An online birth control support network for women age 18–29 operated by the National Campaign to Prevent Teen and Unplanned Pregnancy, a private nonprofit organization. |
| Guttmacher Institute | A leading research and policy organization committed to advancing sexual and reproductive health and rights worldwide. |

### References

1. Curtis KM, Tepper NK, Jatlaoui TC, et al. U.S. Medical Eligibility Criteria for Contraceptive Use 2016. *MMWR*. 2016;65(3):1-106.

2. Trussell J, Aiken ARA, Micks E, Guthrie KA. Contraceptive efficacy. In: Hatcher RA, Nelson AL, Trussell J, et al., eds. *Contraceptive Technology*. 21st ed. New York, NY: Ayer; 2018:829-928.

3. Sundaram A, Vaughan B, Kost K, et al. Contraceptive failure in the United States: estimates from the 2006–2010 National Survey of Family Growth. *Perspect Sex Reprod Health*. 2017;49(1):7-16.

4. Jennings VH, Polis CB. Fertility awareness-based methods. In: Hatcher RA, Nelson AL, Trussell J, et al., eds. *Contraceptive Technology*. 21st ed. New York, NY: Ayer; 2018:395-416.

5. Trussell J, Aiken ARA, Micks E, Guthrie KA. Efficacy, safety, and personal considerations. In: Hatcher RA, Nelson AL, Trussell J, et al., eds. *Contraceptive Technology*. 21st ed. New York, NY: Ayer; 2018:95-128.

6. Altshuler AL, Blumenthal PD. Behavioral methods of contraception. In: Shoupe D, Mishell D Jr, eds. *The Handbook of Contraception: Current Clinical Practice*. Cham, Switzerland: Humana Press Springer; 2016:247-262.

7. United Nations, Department of Economic and Social Affairs. Contraceptive use by method 2019: data booklet. https://digitallibrary.un.org/record/3849735?ln=en. Published 2019. Accessed September 8, 2021.

8. U.S. Department of Health and Human Services. How can you prevent getting or transmitting HIV through sex? https://www.hiv.gov/hiv-basics/hiv-prevention/reducing-sexual-risk/preventing-sexual-transmission-of-hiv. Updated June 14, 2022. Accessed December 29, 2022.

9. Centers for Disease Control and Prevention. STD risk and oral sex: CDC fact sheet. https://www.cdc.gov/std/healthcomm/stdfact-stdriskandoralsex.htm. Last reviewed December 31, 2021. Accessed December 29, 2022.

10. Arteaga S, Gomez AM. "Is that a method of birth control?": a qualitative exploration of young women's use of withdrawal. *J Sex Res.* 2016;53(4-5):626-632.

11. Killick S, Leary C, Trussell J, Guthrie K. Sperm content of pre-ejaculatory fluid. *Hum Fertil.* 2011;14(1):48-52.

12. Jones RK. Coitus interruptus (withdrawal, pulling out). In: Hatcher RA, Nelson AL, Trussell J, et al., eds. *Contraceptive Technology.* 21st ed. New York, NY: Ayer; 2018:451-458.

13. Labbok MH. Postpartum sexuality and the lactational amenorrhea method for contraception. *Clin Obstet Gynecol.* 2015;58(4):915-927.

14. Van der Wijden C, Manion C. Lactational amenorrhea method for family planning. *Cochrane Database Syst Rev.* 2015;10:CD001329. doi:10.1002/14651858.CD001329.pub2.

15. Polis CB, Jones RK. Multiple contraceptive method use and prevalence of fertility awareness based methods in the United States, 2013–2015. *Contraception.* 2018;98:188-192.

16. Malarcher S, Spieler J, Fabic MS, et al. Fertility awareness methods: distinctive modern contraceptives. *Glob Health Sci Pract.* 2016;25;4(1):13-15.

17. Urrutia RP, Polis CB, Jensen ET, et al. Effectiveness of fertility awareness-based methods for pregnancy prevention: a systematic review. *Obstet Gynecol.* 2018;132(3):591-604.

18. Unseld M, Rötzer E, Weigl R, et al. Use of natural family planning (NFP) and its effect on couple relationships and sexual satisfaction: a multi-country survey of NFP users from US and Europe. *Front Public Health.* 2017;13(5):42.

19. Al-Rshoud F, Qudsi A, Naffa FW, et al. The use and efficacy of mobile fertility-tracking applications as a method of contraception: a survey. *Curr Obstet Gynecol Rep.* 2021;10(2):25-29. doi: 10.1007/s13669-021-00305-4.

20. Raymond EG, Chen PL, Luoto J. Contraceptive effectiveness and safety of five nonoxynol-9 spermicides: a randomized trial. *Obstet Gynecol.* 2004;103:430-439.

21. Nelson A, Harwood B. Vaginal barriers and spermicides. In: Hatcher RA, Nelson AL, Trussell J, et al., eds. *Contraceptive Technology.* 21st ed. New York, NY: Ayer; 2018:367-394.

22. Van Damme L, Ramjee G, Alary M, et al. Effectiveness of COL-1492, a nonyxynol-9 vaginal gel, on HIV-1 transmission in female sex workers: a randomized controlled trial. *Lancet.* 2002;360:971-977.

23. Tepper NK, Curtis KM, Cox S, Whiteman MK. Update to CDC's U.S. Medical Eligibility Criteria for Contraceptive Use, 2016: updated recommendations for the use of contraception among women at high risk for HIV infection. *MMWR.* 2020;69(14):405-410.

24. Faich G, Pearson K, Fleming D, et al. Toxic shock syndrome and the vaginal contraceptive sponge. *JAMA.* 1986;255(2):216-218.

25. Schwartz B, Brome C. Nonmenstrual toxic shock syndrome associated with barrier contraceptives: report of a case-control study. *Rev Infect Dis.* 1989;1(suppl S43-S48):S48-S49.

26. Phexxi® [Prescribing information]. San Diego, CA: Evofem Biosciences; May 2020.

27. Chappell BT, Culwell K, Dart C, Howard B. Perfect-use pregnancy rates with the vaginal pH regulator: efficacy results from AMPOWER [30I]. *Obstet Gynecol.* 2020;135:99S.

28. Allen RE. Diaphragm fitting. *Am Fam Physician.* 2004;69(1):97-100.

29. Koeniger-Donohue R. The FemCap: a non-hormonal contraceptive. *Womens Health Care.* 2006;5(4):79-91.

30. Cervical Barrier Advancement Society, Ibis Reproductive Health. Cervical cap (FemCap). https://cervicalbarriers.org/cervical-caps/. Accessed September 9, 2021.

31. Gallo MF, Grimes DA, Schulz KF, Lopez LM. Cervical cap versus diaphragm for contraception. *Cochrane Database Syst Rev.* 2002;4:CD003551.

32. Kogan P, Wald M. Male contraception: history and development. *Urol Clin North Am.* 2014;41(1):145-161.

33. Thirumalai A, Page ST. Male hormonal contraception. *Annu Rev Med.* 2020;71:17-31. doi:10.1146/annurev-med-042418-010947.

34. Gallo MF, Grimes DA, Lopez LM, Schulz KF. Nonlatex versus latex male condoms for contraception. *Cochrane Database Syst Rev.* 2006;1:CD003550. doi:10.1002/14651858.CD003550.pub2.

35. Warner L, Steiner MJ. Male condoms. In: Hatcher RA, Nelson AL, Trussell J, et al., eds.

*Contraceptive Technology.* 21st ed. New York, NY: Ayer; 2018:431-450.

36. Higgins J, Cooper A. Dual use of condoms and contraceptives in the US. *Sex Health.* 2012;9(1): 73-80.

37. Lemoine J, Teal SB, Peters M, Guiahi M. Motivating factors for dual-method contraceptive use among adolescents and young women: a qualitative investigation. *Contraception.* 2017;96(5):352-356. doi:10.1016/j.contraception.2017.06.011.

38. Cervical Barrier Advancement Society. Internal/female condoms. https://cervicalbarriers.org/internal-condoms/. Accessed September 15, 2021.

39. Witte SS, MacPhee C, Ginsburg N, Deshmukh N. Medicaid reimbursement for the female condom. *Am J Public Health.* 2017;107(10):1633-1635.

40. Beksinska M, Smit J, Joanis C, Hart C. Practice makes perfect: reduction in female condom failures and user problems with short-term experience in a randomized trial. *Contraception.* 2012;86(2):127-131.

41. Wiyeh AB, Mome RKB, Mahasha PW, et al. Effectiveness of the female condom in preventing HIV and sexually transmitted infections: a systematic review and meta-analysis. *BMC Public Health.* 2020;20(1):319. doi:10.1186/s12889-020-8384-7.

42. Nelson AL, Cohen S, Galitsky A, et al. Women's perceptions and treatment patterns related to contraception: results of a survey of US women. *Contraception.* 2018;97(3):256-273. doi:10.1016/j.contraception.2017.09.010.

43. Bougie O, Singh SS. Dalkon Shield: forgotten but not yet gone. *J Obstet Gynaecol Can.* 2016;38(8):695.

44. Cortessis VK, Barrett M, Brown Wade N, et al. Intrauterine device use and cervical cancer risk: a systematic review and meta-analysis. *Obstet Gynecol.* 2017;130(6):1226-1236. doi:10.1097/AOG.0000000000002307.

45. Food and Drug Administration. Intrauterine copper contraceptive. https://www.accessdata.fda.gov/drugsatfda_docs/label/2005/018680s060lbl.pdf. Published September 2005. Accessed September 15, 2021.

46. Cooper Surgical. Mechanism of action. https://hcp.paragard.com/about-paragard/moa/. Published October 2022. Accessed December 29, 2022.

47. Horvath S, Schreiber CA, Sonalkar S. Contraception. In: Feingold KR, Anawalt B, Boyce A, et al., eds. *Endotext [Internet].* South Dartmouth, MA: MDText.com; 2018. https://www-ncbi-nlm-nih-gov.ezp2.lib.umn.edu/books/NBK279148/. Accessed December 29, 2022.

48. Gemzell-Danielsson K, Berger C, Lalitkumar PGL. Emergency contraception: mechanisms of action. *Contraception.* 2013;87(3):300-308.

49. Dean G, Bimla Schwarz E. Intrauterine devices (IUDs). In: Hatcher RA, Nelson AL, Trussell J, et al., eds. *Contraceptive Technology.* 21st ed. New York, NY: Ayer; 2018:157-194.

50. Cooper Surgical. Prescribing information. https://hcp.paragard.com/wp-content/uploads/2018/09/ParaGard-PI.pdf. Revised February 2020. Accessed September 20, 2021.

51. Deans EI, Grimes DA. Intrauterine devices for adolescents: a systematic review. *Contraception.* 2009;79:418-423.

52. Escobar M, Shearin S. Immediate postpartum contraception: intrauterine device insertion. *J Midwifery Womens Health.* 2019;64(4):481-487.

53. Zerden ML, Stuart GS, Charm S, et al. Two-week postpartum intrauterine contraception insertion: a study of feasibility, patient acceptability and short-term outcomes. *Contraception.* 2017;95(1):65-70.

54. Ramesh SS, Charm S, Kalinowski A, et al. Management of intrauterine contraception in early pregnancy. *South Med J.* 2017;110(8):550-553.

55. Brahmi D, Steenland M, Renner R-M, et al. Pregnancy outcomes with an IUD in situ: a systematic review. *Contraception.* 2012;85(2):131-139.

56. Stuart GS, Ramesh SS. Interval female sterilization. *Obstet Gynecol.* 2018;131(1):117-124.

57. American College of Obstetricians and Gynecologists. Benefits and risks of sterilization: Practice Bulletin No. 208. *Obstet Gynecol.* 2019;133(3):e194-e207.

58. Shreffler KM, Greil AL, McQuillan J, Gallus KL. Reasons for tubal sterilization, regret and depressive symptoms. *J Reprod Infant Psychol.* 2016;34(3): 304-313.

59. Shreffler KM, McQuillan J, Greil AL, Johnson DR. Surgical sterilization, regret, and race: contemporary patterns. *Soc Sci Res.* 2015;50:31-45.

60. Eeckhaut MCW, Sweeney MM. Understanding sterilization regret in the United States: the role of relationship context. *J Marriage Fam.* 2018;80(5):1259-1270.

61. Karayalcin R, Ozcan S, Tokmak A, et al. Pregnancy outcome of laparoscopic tubal reanastomosis: retrospective results from a single clinical centre. *J Int Med Res.* 2017;45(3):1245-1252. doi:10.1177/0300060517709815. Epub 2017 May 23. PMID: 28534697; PMCID: PMC5536424.

62. Bayer. Essure permanent birth control. https://labeling.bayerhealthcare.com/html/products/pi/essure_ifu.pdf?r=1. Published 2002. Accessed September 20, 2021.

63. U.S. Food and Drug Administration. Essure benefits and risks. https://www.fda.gov/medical-devices/essure-permanent-birth-control/essure-benefits-and-risks. Current as of March 14, 2022. Accessed December 29, 2022.

64. U.S. Food and Drug Administration. FDA activities related to Essure. https://www.fda.gov/medical-devices/essure-permanent-birth-control/fda-activities-related-essure. Current as of October 6, 2022. Accessed December 29, 2022.

65. Câmara S, de Castro Coelho F, Freitas C, Remesso L Essure present controversies and 5 years' learned lessons: a retrospective study with short- and long-term follow-up. *Gynecol Surg.* 2017;14(1):20.

66. Fantasia HC. Update on the Essure system for permanent birth control. *Nurs Womens Health.* 2017; 21(5):401-405.

67. Hurskainen R, Hovi S-L, Gissler M, et al. Hysteroscopic tubal sterilization: a systematic review of the Essure system. *Fertil Steril.* 2010;94(1):16-19.

68. Zeitler M, Rayala B. Outpatient vasectomy. *Primary Care Clin Office Pract.* 2021;48(4):613-625.

69. Amory JK. Male contraception. *Fertil Steril.* 2016;106(6):1303-1309.

70. Potts J, Pasqualotto F, Nelson D, et al. Patient characteristics associated with vasectomy reversal. *J Urol.* 1999;161:1835-1839.

CHAPTER

# 12

# Hormonal Contraception

AMY ALSPAUGH

*The editors acknowledges Mary C. Brucker, who was the author of this chapter in the previous edition.*

## Introduction

Hormonal methods of contraception include combined oral contraceptives (COCs) and progestin-only pills (POPs), as well as non-oral hormonal formulations, including vaginal rings, transdermal patches, intrauterine devices (IUDs), and subdermal implants. The copper IUD and other nonhormonal methods of contraception are reviewed in the *Non-hormonal Contraception* chapter. Hormonal contraceptives can be further subclassified as either short-acting reversible contraceptives (SARCs) or long-acting reversible contraceptive (LARCs).

The manufacturers of the hormonal intrauterine agents—which have the brand names Liletta, Mirena, Skyla, and Kyleena—use the terms *intrauterine system* (IUS) and *intrauterine device* (IUD) interchangeably in their descriptions. Other sources use the term *intrauterine contraceptive device* (IUCD). For consistency, IUD is the abbreviation used throughout this chapter for intrauterine devices.

## Evolution of Hormonal Contraceptive Methods

For the last several decades, modifications of the types of hormones and doses in contraceptives have been made in attempts to decrease the adverse effects associated with these agents while maintaining their effectiveness at preventing pregnancy. Notably, the original contraceptive pill had approximately three times the amounts of both progestin and estrogen as are present in modern formulations. Thus, the lower doses of the newer formulations have greatly decreased the severity and prevalence of side effects.[1] Because daily dosing of contraceptive pills is burdensome and results in decreased efficacy if the medication is not used as directed, much of the innovation in the contraceptive field has been focused on non-oral, longer-term methods.[2] Contraceptive options other than the oral formulations offer individuals a wider variety of choices for the hormone delivery method and duration of action with lower maintenance that may be appealing for some individuals.

Several hormonal methods combine estrogen and a progestin, whereas others contain only progestin (Table 12-1). Understanding which hormones are present in a particular contraceptive method can assist the provider in presenting anticipatory guidance to the patient related to both the common side effects and the rare adverse effects associated with that method.

## Mechanism of Action of Hormonal Contraceptives

Hormonal contraceptives prevent pregnancy in a variety of ways. The primary mechanisms of action of contraception are (1) inhibition of ovulation and (2) changes to cervical mucus so that sperm transport is impaired.[3] Hormonal contraceptives also alter uterine tube motility, which inhibits sperm motility, and cause the endometrium to become atrophic. Hormonal methods of contraception contain synthetic steroidal hormones that act centrally, altering the functions of the pituitary gland and hypothalamus.[3] Although it may seem counterintuitive that supplementing natural progesterone and estrogen with synthetic analogues of the same hormones can prevent ovulation and impede sperm transport,

| Table 12-1 | Contraceptive Methods and Types of Hormones | |
|---|---|---|
| Hormonal Method | Estrogen and Progestin | Progestin Only |
| Combined oral contraceptives (COCs) | X | |
| Progestin-only contraceptives (POPs) | | X |
| Transdermal contraceptive patch | X | |
| Intravaginal contraceptive ring | X | |
| Depot medroxyprogesterone acetate injections (DMPA) | | X |
| Subdermal implants | | X |
| Levonorgestrel-releasing intrauterine device (LNG-IUD) | | X |
| Emergency contraception | | X |

the steadiness of the dosing, as opposed to the natural fluctuations, causes these effects.

## Mechanism of Action of Estrogen

A major action of estrogen in hormonal contraception is to stabilize the endometrium, thereby providing cycle control and minimizing breakthrough bleeding.[4] Estrogen also suppresses gonadotropin-releasing hormone (GnRH) and pituitary release of both GnRH and follicle-stimulating hormone (FSH). These actions inhibit development of a dominant follicle and subsequent ovulation. Several pharmacologic formulations of estrogen exist. The major estrogen used in hormonal contraception is ethinyl estradiol. Mestranol, the form of estrogen used in the first birth control pill, is now rarely used[4] while a new formulation, estradiol valerate, has been shown to be helpful in individuals with especially heavy menstrual bleeding.[5]

Estrogen is a lipophilic intracellular hormone that has many physiologic effects. For example, estrogen increases the plasma concentrations of clotting factors, which explains why it is associated with an increased risk for venous thromboembolism (VTE).[6] Estrogen also increases insulin resistance and the concentrations of very low-density lipids and high-density lipids, and it may cause a slight rise

in blood pressure.[4] Although these estrogen effects could be potentially dangerous for individuals who have an a priori risk for VTE or cardiovascular disease, today's COCs contain forms of estrogen and low doses that are associated with markedly lowered to negligible risks.[7]

Ethinyl estradiol is metabolized by the cytochrome P-450 (CYP450) enzymes, which are highly polymorphic. Many drugs can inhibit or accelerate the function of CYP450 enzymes. More than 150 drugs have been suggested as agents that have drug interactions with ethinyl estradiol. These drug interactions potentiate or inhibit the effects of either estrogen or the interacting drug. Concomitant use of ethinyl estradiol and any other pharmacologic agent should be individually evaluated. Clinically relevant drug interactions are discussed later in this chapter.

## Mechanism of Action of Progestins

Unlike the case for estrogen, for which a single type (ethinyl estradiol) is used almost exclusively for contraception, several progestins are prescribed for this indication. Progestins include both synthetic and natural progesterone. Progestins are typically described by the "generation" in which they reached the market, which range from the first generation to the fourth generation[8] (Figure 12-1). All synthetic progestins bind to the progesterone receptor and have varying affinities for androgen, glucocorticoid, mineralocorticoid, and estrogen receptors. The side effects of different progestins are largely related to their individual affinity for these other receptors.

In contraceptive methods, progestins prevent pregnancy through a combination of actions. One such mechanism is inhibition of the release of luteinizing hormone (LH), thereby preventing the LH surge necessary for ovulation. Another mechanism is alteration of cervical mucus, which results in cervical mucus that is more similar to mucus of the postovulatory phase. This mucus, though smaller in volume, has more viscosity and cellular content, and an altered molecular structure that makes it hostile to sperm entrance into the uterus.[3] Progestin-only agents lack the endometrial stabilization from estrogen, which results in increased irregular vaginal bleeding.

## General Considerations for Hormonal Contraceptives

When providing individuals with the information they need to make a choice about hormonal

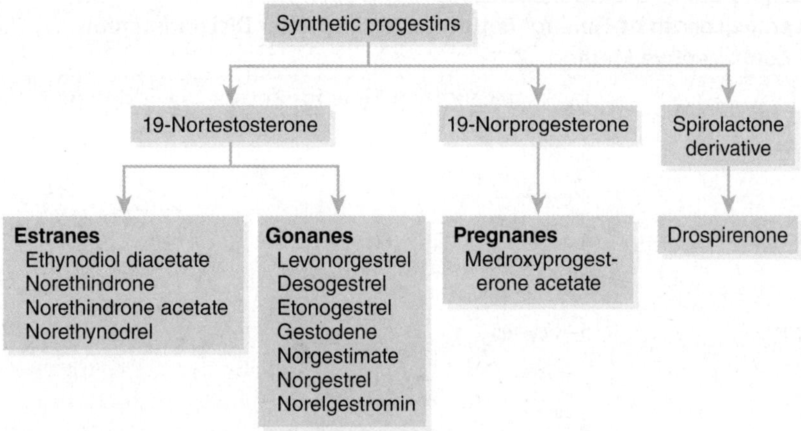


**Figure 12-1** Progestins used for contraception.

**Table 12-2 Effectiveness of Hormonal Contraceptive Methods**

| Contraceptive Method | Type of Method | Pregnancies per 100 Individuals per Year with Consistent and Correct Use[a] | Pregnancies per 100 Individuals per Year as Commonly Used |
|---|---|---|---|
| Oral method (pills containing either combined estrogen/progestin or progestin only) | SARC | 0.3 | 7 |
| Transdermal patch | SARC | 0.3 | 7 |
| Contraceptive ring | SARC | 0.3 | 7 |
| Contraceptive injections | SARC | 0.2 | 4 |
| Emergency contraception | SARC/LARC | <1–2 | |
| Levonorgestrel IUD | LARC | 0.5 | 0.7 |
| Subdermal implants | LARC | 0.1 | 0.1 |

Abbreviations: IUD, intrauterine device; LARC, long-acting reversible contraceptive; SARC, short-acting reversible contraceptive.

Data from World Health Organization, Johns Hopkins Bloomberg School of Public Health. *Family Planning: A Global Handbook for Providers.* https://apps.who.int/iris/bitstream/handle/10665/260156/9780999203705-eng.pdf?sequence=1. Published 2018. Accessed March 13, 2023.

contraception, midwives should review several topics. These include each option's effectiveness, how long it takes for fertility to return when the agent is discontinued, noncontraceptive benefits and side effects, possible drug interactions, and contraindications.

### Effectiveness

Hormonal contraceptives are the most effective method of all reversible contraception products. Table 12-2 summarizes the effectiveness of the hormonal methods, with the least effective options listed first.[9] Because of their lack of dependency upon user actions, LARCs—unsurprisingly—are more effective than SARCs.

### Return to Fertility

For most hormonal methods, including LARCs, return to fertility after discontinuing use is relatively rapid, rarely taking more than a few months.[9] The exception is depot medroxyprogesterone acetate (DMPA), for which a median of 7 months usually passes after the last injection before pregnancy is achieved.[10] Table 12-3 lists the length of time for the average person capable of pregnancy to attain fertility after discontinuation of specific hormonal methods.[11]

### Noncontraceptive Benefits

Discussion of hormonal contraceptives often focuses on the side effects and adverse effects associated with their use, rather than on their benefits.

| Table 12-3 | Average Length of Time for Return to Fertility After Discontinuation of Contraceptive Method | |
|---|---|---|
| **Contraceptive Method** | **Average Length of Time for Return to Fertility (in Menstrual Cycles)** | |
| Combined oral contraceptives | 3 cycles | |
| Progestin-only pills | 3 cycles | |
| Transdermal patch | 4 cycles | |
| Contraceptive ring | 3 cycles | |
| Contraceptive injections | 5–8 cycles | |
| Levonorgestrel IUD | 2 cycles | |
| Subdermal implants | 2 cycles | |
| Emergency contraception | 1 cycle | |

Based on Yland JJ, Bresnick KA, Hatch EE, et al. Pregravid contraceptive use and fecundability: prospective cohort study. *BMJ.* 2020;371:m3966. doi:10.1136/bmj.m3966.

Although adverse effects are always reviewed, most of the side effects are minor, and serious adverse effects are rare. However, a number of noncontraceptive benefits are also associated with these agents, as described in Table 12-4. Counseling about the noncontraceptive benefits of these products should be balanced with discussion of their untoward effects.[12] Is it essential to remember that individuals may desire hormonal contraception for many different reasons. For example, in addition to or unrelated to pregnancy prevention, individuals may desire hormonal contraception for cycle control, to induce amenorrhea, for the treatment of polycystic ovarian syndrome (PCOS) or endometriosis, or to manage perimenopausal symptoms.[13,14] Centering the desires of the individual helps the provider identify the various reasons for seeking contraception to ensure that an individualized plan of care may be offered.

## Contraindications to Use of Hormonal Contraceptives

Although most individuals can use hormonal contraceptives, there are some situations in which these agents are not recommended or are even contraindicated. Contraindications to hormonal contraceptive use are primarily contraindications to estrogen, progestins, or both, and include—most notably—breast cancer and pregnancy. There are more contraindications to estrogen than to progestins. For example, individuals with a history of cardiovascular disease or coagulopathy should not use estrogen-containing products. Contraindications defined as Category 3 or 4 in the *U.S. Medical Eligibility Criteria for Contraceptive Use* are found in Table 12-5.[15]

Individuals seeking to use hormonal contraceptives should always be screened for the presence of any contraindications first; if any are present, alternative contraceptive methods should be discussed and recommended. The *U.S. Medical Eligibility Criteria* (U.S. MEC) recommendations, which are summarized in the *Fertility, Family Building, and Contraception* chapter, include specific contraceptive eligibility guidelines for individuals who have a variety of disorders and health conditions.[15] The U.S. MEC are also available as an app for smartphones, and on the Centers for Disease Control and Prevention (CDC) website.

## Side Effects and Adverse Effects of Hormonal Contraceptives

The U.S. MEC,[15] as described in the *Fertility, Family Building, and Contraception* chapter, provides guidelines for use of the different hormonal methods based on clinical trials as well as national and international studies. In 2016, the CDC published a set of recommendations on some common issues related to use of contraceptives as a companion to the U.S. MEC, as discussed in the *Fertility, Family Building, and Contraception* chapter.[15]

### Side Effects of Estrogen and Progestins in Contraceptives

Both estrogens and progestins have multiple biologic effects. Given the different forms, doses, and routes of administration available, it can be difficult to determine which side effect is related to estrogen and which is related to progestin in a particular product. In general, the most common side effects

| Table 12-4 | Noncontraceptive Benefits of Hormonal Contraceptives | | | | |
|---|---|---|---|---|---|
| **Noncontraceptive Benefit** | **Combined Oral, Transdermal, and Vaginal Contraception** | **Progestin-Only Oral Contraception** | **DMPA** | **LNG-IUD** | **Implant** |
| **Reduction of Menstrual-Associated Conditions** | | | | | |
| Dysmenorrhea | X | X | X | X | X |
| Heavy menstrual flow | X | X | X | X | X |
| Irregularity | X | X | X | X | X |
| Menstrual migraines | X | X | X | X | X |
| Perimenopausal symptoms (e.g., hot flashes) | X | | | | |
| Premenstrual syndrome | X | | | | |
| **Therapeutic Use—Management of the Following Conditions** | | | | | |
| Uterine fibroids | X | X | X | X | X |
| Endometriosis | X | X | X | X | X |
| Heavy menstrual bleeding | X | | | X | |
| Acne | X | | | | |
| Polycystic ovarian syndrome | X | | | | |
| Hirsutism | X | | | | |
| **Decreased Risk of the Following Conditions** | | | | | |
| Anemia | X | X | X | X | X |
| Endometrial cancer | X | | | X | |
| Ovarian cancer | X | | | X | |

Based on Schrager S, Larson M, Carlson J, et al. Beyond birth control: noncontraceptive benefits of hormonal methods and their key role in the general medical care of women. *J Womens Health (Larchmt).* 2020;29(7):937-943. doi:10.1089/jwh.2019.7731.

of estrogen are headaches and nausea. Bloating, leukorrhea, chloasma, and increased cholesterol in bile (which increases the risk of gallstones) have also been reported.[16]

All progestin-only methods are safer than the combined products, but progestins are associated with bleeding irregularities including amenorrhea. Common side effects of progestins include acne, decreased libido, pruritus, mood changes, premenstrual-type symptoms such as edema, and transient, but usually mild, depression.[16] DMPA is associated with a decrease in bone mass or bone mineral density that is thought to be reversible in individuals who are not in the perimenopausal period.[17] Studies that have evaluated the effects of progestin on mood changes and depression have reported conflicting findings, and depression is not a contraindication for use of progestin-containing contraceptives. That

said, when an individual reports mood changes associated with progestin (or any other contraceptive method), an alternative form of contraception should be considered.[18]

Both estrogen and progestin methods may have similar or overlapping side effects, especially during the first few months of use. Headaches and nausea may be more common with estrogen-containing pills, but nausea is often encountered with any oral method. Other problems that individuals may report with hormonal contraceptives include breast tenderness, acne, and premenstrual symptoms.[2] The latter two are most likely to occur when using progestin-only methods.

## Adverse Effects of Hormonal Contraceptives

Estrogen use increases the risk for some rare, but severe, adverse effects. Notably, estrogen is associated

| Table 12-5 | Contraindications for Hormonal Contraceptives Based on Category 3 or Category 4 Status in *U.S. Medical Eligibility Criteria for Contraceptive Use* |
|---|---|

| Absolute Contraindications: MEC Category 4 | Not Recommended: MEC Category 3 |
|---|---|
| **Combined Oral Contraceptives (COCs)** | |
| Breastfeeding and < 21 days postpartum | Anticonvulsant therapy |
| Current breast cancer | Antiviral therapy with ritonavir-boosted protease inhibitor |
| Cirrhosis (severe) | Breast cancer history and no evidence of current disease for 5 years |
| DVT history and not on an anticoagulant, or acute DVT or PE or DVT/PE and established anticoagulation for at least 3 months but still high risk | Breastfeeding and 21–42 days postpartum |
| Diabetes mellitus: nephropathy, retinopathy, neuropathy, or other vascular disease, or diabetes of > 20 years' duration | DVT history and low risk for recurrent DVT/PE |
| History of stroke | Fosamprenavir use |
| Hypertension with systolic blood pressure ≥ 160 mm Hg or diastolic blood pressure ≥ 100 mm Hg or vascular disease | Gallbladder disease (current or medically treated) |
| Ischemic heart disease (current or history) | Headaches (migraine) without aura < 35 years[b] |
| Known thrombogenic mutations | History of bariatric surgery with malabsorptive procedures (oral contraception only) |
| Liver tumors: hepatocellular or malignant | Hypertension adequately controlled or systolic blood pressure 140–159 mm Hg or diastolic blood pressure 90–99 mm Hg |
| Major surgery with prolonged immobilization | Inflammatory bowel disease and at increased risk for VTE |
| Migraine with aura | Postpartum cardiomyopathy ≥ 6 months |
| Multiple risk factors for atherosclerotic cardiovascular disease | Postpartum < 40 days and breastfeeding with additional risk factors for venous thromboembolism |
| Peripartum cardiomyopathy (< 6 months) or moderate impaired cardiac function | Prior history of COC-related cholestasis |
| Postpartum < 21 days | Rifampin or rifabutin therapy |
| Smoking ≥ 15 cigarettes a day | Smoking < 15 cigarettes |
| Solid-organ transplant, complicated | Superficial venous thrombosis (acute or history) |
| Stroke: history of cerebrovascular accident | |
| Systemic lupus erythematosus positive or unknown antiphospholipid antibodies | |
| Valvular disease, complicated | |
| Viral hepatitis (acute or flare) | |
| **Contraceptive Implant** | |
| Current breast cancer | Breast cancer history and no evidence of current disease for 5 years |
| | Cirrhosis (severe) |
| | History of bariatric surgery with malabsorptive procedures |
| | Ischemic heart disease (current or history, continuation only) |
| | Liver tumors: hepatocellular or malignant |
| | Solid organ transplant, complicated |
| | Stroke: history of cerebrovascular accident (continuation only) |
| | Systemic lupus erythematosus with positive or unknown antiphospholipid antibodies |
| | Unexplained vaginal bleeding suspicious for serious condition before evaluation |

| Absolute Contraindications: MEC Category 4 | Not Recommended: MEC Category 3 |
|---|---|
| **Depot Medroxyprogesterone Acetate (DMPA)** | |
| Current breast cancer | Breast cancer history and no evidence of current disease for 5 years |
| | Cirrhosis (severe) |
| | Diabetes mellitus: nephropathy, retinopathy, neuropathy, or other vascular disease, or diabetes of > 20 years' duration |
| | Hypertension with systolic blood pressure ≥ 160 mm Hg or diastolic blood pressure ≥ 100 mm Hg or vascular disease |
| | Ischemic heart disease (current or history) |
| | Liver tumors: hepatocellular or malignant |
| | Long-term use of corticosteroid therapy in individuals with a history or risk of nontraumatic fractures |
| | Multiple risk factors for atherosclerotic cardiovascular disease |
| | Rheumatoid arthritis on long-term corticosteroid therapy |
| | Stroke: history of cerebrovascular accident |
| | Systemic lupus erythematosus positive or unknown antibodies or severe thrombocytopenia |
| | Unexplained vaginal bleeding suspicious for serious condition before evaluation |
| **Levonorgestrel-Releasing Intrauterine Device** | |
| Current breast cancer | Breast cancer history and no evidence of current disease for 5 years |
| Cervical cancer awaiting treatment (initiation only) | Cirrhosis (severe) |
| Distorted uterine cavity | Ischemic heart disease (current or history, continuation only) |
| Endometrial cancer (initiation only) | |
| Gestational trophoblastic disease with persistency elevated beta-hCG levels or malignant disease, with evidence of or suspicion of intrauterine disease | Liver tumors: hepatocellular or malignant |
| | Pelvic tuberculosis (continuation only) |
| Pelvic inflammatory disease, current (initiation only) | Solid-organ transplantation, complicated (initiation only) |
| Pelvic tuberculosis (initiation only) | Stroke: history of cerebrovascular accident |
| Pregnancy | Systemic lupus erythematosus with positive or unknown antiphospholipid antibodies |
| Sexually transmitted infection with current purulent cervicitis or chlamydial infection or gonococcal infection (initiation only) | |
| Immediate postseptic abortion or postpartum sepsis | |
| Pelvic tuberculosis | |
| Unexplained vaginal bleeding (initiation only) | |

*(continues)*

| Table 12-5 | Contraindications for Hormonal Contraceptives Based on Category 3 or Category 4 Status in *U.S. Medical Eligibility Criteria for Contraceptive Use* (continued) | |
|---|---|---|
| **Absolute Contraindications: MEC Category 4** | | **Not Recommended: MEC Category 3** |
| **Progestin-Only Pills (POPs)** | | |
| Current breast cancer | | Anticonvulsant therapy |
| | | Breast cancer history and no evidence of current disease for 5 years |
| | | History of bariatric surgery with malabsorptive procedures |
| | | Ischemic heart disease (current or history, continuation only) |
| | | Liver tumors: hepatocellular or malignant |
| | | Rifampin or rifabutin therapy |
| | | Stroke: history of cerebrovascular accident (continuation only) |
| | | Systemic lupus erythematosus with positive or unknown antiphospholipid antibodies |

Abbreviations: DVT, deep vein thrombosis; hCG, human chorionic gonadotropin; PE, pulmonary embolus; VTE, venous thromboembolism.

Based on Curtis KM, Tepper NK, Jatlaoui TC, et al. U.S. Medical eligibility criteria for contraceptive use, 2016. *MMWR Recomm Rep.* 2016;65(3):1-103. https://www.cdc.gov/reproductivehealth/contraception/mmwr/mec/summary.html. Accessed March 13, 2023.

with an increased risk for cardiovascular events such as stroke and myocardial infarction, and thromboembolic events such as deep vein thrombosis (DVT).[19] Individuals who smoke, who are older than age 35 years, and who use estrogen are at a higher risk for myocardial infarction. In addition, estrogen use slightly increases the risk of developing breast cancer.[20,21] Although the risk of breast cancer is low among reproductive-age individuals, evidence indicates that the risk from combined contraception increases with longer duration of use; thus, use of these agents should be carefully considered for individuals with a familial history of breast cancer. An increased risk of VTE may be associated with use of certain progestins. For example, the risk of venous thrombosis associated with COCs containing the progestins gestodene, desogestrel, and drospirenone plus 30–35 micrograms of ethinyl estradiol is approximately 50% to 80% greater than the risk associated with the same estrogen combined with levonorgestrel.[22] Relationships between progestins and cardiovascular risk and bone health continue to be studied.

### Counseling About Side Effects and Adverse Effects of Hormonal Contraceptives

Midwives can assist individuals in reviewing their individualized risks and benefits. It is important to remember that hormonal contraceptives do not protect a person from acquiring a sexually transmitted infection (STI)—condoms are the only contraceptive method that serve the dual purpose of pregnancy prevention and STI protection. For example, an individual may decide that the benefits in terms of the reliability and effectiveness of a hormonal method for preventing pregnancy outweigh a relatively minor increase in their risk for a specific condition. Consideration of risk of a condition also should be viewed in light of the risk of pregnancy with a less reliable method. For example, the risk of DVT is known to increase with use of estrogen-containing contraceptives. However, for an individual who does not have a history of coagulopathy or a medical disorder that increases their a priori risk for coagulopathy, the risk of DVT associated with estrogen-containing contraceptives is less than the risk of developing DVT during pregnancy. Thus, shared decision making and a careful cost–benefit assessment are essential steps prior to prescribing any hormonal contraception unless an absolute contraindication exists.

### Drug–Drug Interactions

All hormonal contraceptive methods are considered to have potential drug interactions, including implants and IUDs. The effect of one or both of the agents can be potentiated; one or both can be inhibited; one can be inhibited and the other potentiated; or nothing clinically relevant can occur. Most of these effects occur because the same liver enzymes in the CYP450 family metabolize the two drugs, and one or the other drug alters the function of the enzymes, thereby affecting metabolism of the other agent.

Many drug interactions occur secondary to use of pharmacologic agents that are CYP450 enzyme inducers (i.e., they potentiate the effect of the enzyme, which leads to rapid metabolism of the other drug). Fortunately, healthy individuals do not commonly use most of the drugs that decrease contraceptive effectiveness. The majority of known drug interactions occur with oral (rather than non-oral hormonal) contraceptives. Nevertheless, healthcare providers should be particularly alert for potential interactions if an individual is taking medications to treat tuberculosis, a seizure disorder, a clotting disorder, human immunodeficiency virus (HIV) infection, or mild depression. Importantly, despite widespread assumptions about interactions between antibiotics and hormonal contraception, broad-spectrum antibiotics, antifungals, and antiparasitic agents have no effect on contraceptive efficacy.[15]

Among the drugs that have been suggested to decrease the effectiveness of COCs are anti-infectives (specifically rifampin [Rifadin]), anticonvulsants (e.g., carbamazepine [Tegretol], phenytoin [Dilantin], phenobarbital [Luminal]), antifungals (specifically griseofulvin [Fulvicin]), protease inhibitors (e.g., saquinavir [Invirase], ritonavir [Norvir]), and non-nucleoside reverse transcriptase inhibitors (e.g., efavirenz [Sustiva], nevirapine [Viramune]).[15] St. John's wort—a nutritional supplement marketed as a treatment for mild depression—also appears to decrease the effectiveness of COCs.[23,24]

Several of these agents have been suggested to impact the effectiveness of POPs as well—specifically, rifampin, anticonvulsants, and potentially St. John's wort.[15] Thus, a secondary contraceptive method is recommended for individuals using any of these agents.

Pharmacogenomics may play a role in drug interactions with contraceptives, although more information is needed to verify these relationships. A history of problems with a particular contraceptive method in the past can direct the choice of a new method. As always, it is good practice to obtain an individual's complete history regarding medications (both prescribed and over-the-counter [OTC] agents), botanicals, and nutritional supplements and to verify whether any potential drug interaction exists, as information about such interactions is constantly evolving.

## Clinical Evaluation When Initiating or Changing a Hormonal Contraceptive Method

This section reviews clinical considerations that apply to all hormonal contraceptives. Table 12-6 summarizes the components of management for any individual initiating or changing a contraceptive method.

## Special Considerations for Hormonal Contraception

### Adolescents and Young People

In most locales, individuals younger than 18 years are considered minors and cannot give consent for care. However, legal provisions typically exist that allow adolescents to obtain contraception if desired. All methods of hormonal contraception can be appropriate for adolescents. The Food and Drug Administration [FDA] requires a black box warning on DMPA that states adolescents should not use DMPA longer than 2 years given the effects on bone density at a time when bone mineralization is maximal.[10] This recommendation is not supported by all professional associations, but should be considered when discussing this option with an adolescent who is considering use of DMPA.[25]

Some noncontraceptive benefits associated with several options—such as decrease in acne, menstrual bleeding, and dysmenorrhea—can be of particular value to adolescents.[12,26] The sections of this chapter that review the different methods contain information that is generally appropriate to persons in this age group. Counseling provided to adolescents should be accurate, be age-appropriate, and include sexual health education, contraception, and STI prevention. A lack of high-quality sexual health education may mean that adolescent patients need more time and information to ensure that they are able to make the best decision for their needs and comfort. No contraceptive options should be denied due to age alone, and it is essential to ensure that contraceptive decisions are made without coercion or pressure from the healthcare provider, partner, or family of the adolescent.[27]

### Lesbian, Gay, Bisexual, Queer, Gender-Nonbinary, Gender-Expansive, and Transgender Men Clients

Seeking reproductive health care as a queer individual can be an uncomfortable and harmful experience for a variety of reasons.[28] As the healthcare provider, it is essential to signal an openness and competence to discussing contraception and reproductive health for queer individuals.[29] Sexual identity, gender identity, and sexual behavior are all distinct concepts, and the provider should inquire about each without making assumptions. When offering contraceptive services for a person who identifies as lesbian,

| Table 12-6 | Care of an Individual Initiating or Changing a Hormonal Contraceptive Method |
|---|---|

Assure that no contraindications exist for the chosen method.

If the method is Category 3 according to the U.S. Medical Eligibility Criteria, discuss both risks and benefits with the individual so they can make an informed choice.

Obtain reasonable assurance that the individual is not pregnant, which includes having no signs or symptoms of pregnancy and meeting one of the following criteria:[7]

- ≤ 7 days after the start of normal menses
- Has not had sexual intercourse since the start of last normal menses
- Has been correctly and consistently using a reliable method of contraception
- ≤ 7 days after miscarriage or induced abortion
- Within 4 weeks postpartum
- Fully or nearly fully breastfeeding/chestfeeding (exclusively breastfeeding/chestfeeding or the vast majority [≥85%] of feeds are from human milk), amenorrheic, and < 6 months postpartum

Verify that the method to be initiated is one that the individual desires and is likely to use correctly. Because hormonal methods influence menstrual flow, it is important to explore the individual's feelings and concerns about decreased flow, irregular bleeding, and amenorrhea.

Verify the individual is not taking any drugs likely to interact with hormonal contraceptives.

For all individuals using hormonal contraceptives, review the following points:

- Signs or symptoms indicating serious complications (danger or warning signs)
- Common side effects
- Effect on menstrual flow
- Noncontraceptive benefits
- Average time for return to fertility
- Lack of protection from sexually transmitted infections
- Date and time for follow-up appointment
- Health promotion or screening activities as appropriate, separate from contraceptive needs

For all individuals using a short-acting reversible contraceptive (e.g., daily pills, weekly patch) that is user dependent, review the following points:

- When and how to initiate the method
- Back-up or secondary protection when indicated (and additional supplies for occasional use if needed)
- How to use the method correctly and continuously
- Common mistakes to avoid
- What to do if they fail to use the method correctly (e.g., missed pills)
- Safe disposal of used contraceptives and packages
- Specific information regarding prescriptions, including when to be renewed and general cost
- Consider providing a prescription for emergency contraception for the individual to have on hand in case the method is forgotten

Provide opportunities for the individual to ask questions and ensure they know how to contact the clinic with questions.

gay, bisexual, or queer (LGBQ), or as transgender or gender-nonconforming (TGNC), care should be individualized to the person's priorities and needs.[29] The National LGBTQ Task Force is a source of more in-depth information about sexual and reproductive health for such individuals.

A transgender man often retains the ability to conceive and should be offered contraception and other preventive care as indicated.[30] Although gender-affirming hormone therapy (testosterone) limits fertility, pregnancy can still occur in individuals engaged in sexual activity with reproductive potential (see the *Gender-Affirming Care* chapter). Therefore, transgender men who have not undergone gender-affirming surgery such as hysterectomy and who are sexually active may desire or need contraception. No method is contraindicated based on the use of testosterone alone.[30] Contraceptive methods such as IUDs and implants that tend to promote amenorrhea may be appealing; IUD use should involve a thorough discussion of the placement procedure.[30]

### Postpartum, Postabortion, and/or Lactation

Hormonal contraception is not contraindicated for a healthy postpartum individual, although the timing at which such contraception is initiated or resumed is controversial for postpartum individuals who are lactating. Additional discussion of this subject can be found in the *Postpartum Care* chapter. There are minimal contraindications to all hormonal contraception methods following a miscarriage or abortion.[15]

In general, individuals who recently have given birth, regardless of whether they are breastfeeding/chestfeeding, should delay use of contraceptive methods containing estrogen until at least 21 days after the birth because of the increased risk for venous thrombosis resulting from the hypercoagulable state during pregnancy and the early postpartum period.[15] Progestin-only methods, including implants, injections, and pills, may be initiated earlier than estrogen-containing methods because progestin-only methods are not associated with thrombotic activity. There is some concern about immediate postpartum DMPA initiation due to reports of difficulty with lactation, though this has not been demonstrated in existing data.[31,32] Misinformation regarding postpartum DMPA is common, however.[33]

The American College of Obstetricians and Gynecologists suggests that either an implant or an IUD can be inserted within 10 minutes after birth.[34] Although some evidence shows a higher rate of expulsion of the latter option, this risk may be outweighed by the benefit of having a method that does not require follow-up care or for those who may lose health insurance postpartum.[35] The insertion procedure immediately postpartum is the same as that used outside of pregnancy, although the midwife should use caution because the uterine isthmus is much softer and more prone to perforation at this time. IUDs also may be placed following spontaneous or elective abortion, either immediately or at 4 to 8 weeks post abortion/miscarriage.[36,37] The only contraindication to immediate insertion of an IUD is for individuals with postpartum sepsis following a birth or abortion, who should wait until the infection has resolved before placement can safely occur.[15]

### Body Mass Index and Contraceptive Effectiveness

For the majority of hormonal contraceptive methods, there is little evidence to suggest that high or low weight or body mass index (BMI) impacts efficacy.[38,39] For two specific methods, however, some considerations must be kept in mind. The hormonal patch is marketed as less effective in individuals who weigh more than 90 kg (198 pounds) and is not recommended for individuals who have a BMI greater than 30 kg/m$^2$.[40] This recommendation is based on two studies that reported a high risk of pregnancy among individuals with obesity compared to individuals without obesity; importantly, though, the patch provided better protection against pregnancy than barrier methods in both studies.[41,42] Data regarding the efficacy of emergency contraception in individuals with obesity tends to be of lower quality and findings are inconsistent. While some data suggest that hormonal emergency contraception, using either levonorgestrel or ulipristal acetate, is less efficacious in individuals with obesity,[43] the majority of studies indicate no difference in efficacy based on body weight or BMI.[44-46] Currently, data are generally lacking for the highest categories of BMI, and recommendations will continue to evolve over time as more is understood about the pharmacokinetic interaction of hormonal contraception and body weight.[39]

### HIV or Risk Factors for HIV

No method of contraception is contraindicated for individuals living with human immunodeficiency virus/acquired immunodeficiency syndrome (HIV/AIDS), regardless of viral load or use of antiviral agents. All hormonal contraceptive methods are considered Category 1 by the World Health Association.[47] Additionally, no hormonal contraceptive methods are contraindicated for individuals at higher risk of acquiring HIV.[47] There was once concern that injectable hormonal contraception increased an individual's risk for acquiring HIV, but findings from a recent, large, randomized controlled trial (RCT) indicate no increased risk for HIV acquisition among individuals using DMPA, hormonal IUDs, or nonhormonal IUDs.[48] An important component of patient education is sharing the information that hormonal contraceptive methods do not currently offer any protection against HIV or other STIs.

### Individuals with Disabilities

Disabilities often have no impact on fertility, and individuals with disabilities are just as likely to be sexually active as those without disabilities.[49] Unfortunately, individuals with disabilities have long been subject to eugenic and ableist programs that have sought to control their fertility through compulsory contraception or sterilization, and this trend continues to this day.[50] Thus, it is imperative to center the desires and needs of the individual with disabilities in contraceptive counseling while acknowledging their autonomy, promoting their comfort, and advocating for their needs.[51]

No contraceptive methods are contraindicated based on any specific disability, although use of certain anticonvulsants—as noted in the "Drug–Drug Interactions" section—may limit the available options. Thus, all methods are safe for the majority of individuals with disabilities, and should be offered to an individual without provider bias. Short- and long-acting methods, as well as sterilization, should be provided based on the desires of the individual, rather than the preferences of the family, other healthcare providers, or a care facility. While individuals with disabilities are more likely to experience sexual assault than those without a disability,[52] the impetus should be on assault prevention, not coercive contraceptive practices to prevent pregnancy.[53]

Some changes may need to be made in facilities to accommodate provision of care to individuals with disabilities, who often delay or avoid care because of lack of appropriate accommodations or provider knowledge.[54] Examples included exam tables that can be elevated or lowered and avoiding the use of stirrups during pelvic exams.[54] Menstrual suppression may be desired by individuals with special cognitive or physical disabilities, but selection of a method that achieves that goal should be made in concert with the wishes of the individual.[55]

### Individuals in the Military

Contraception should be available to active-duty members of the military and based on Department of Defense policies. Some active-duty individuals are deployed in areas where the working environment presents unique circumstances related to contraception. For example, personnel working in combat areas or at geographically isolated bases may not have full access to every method.[56] Scheduling challenges may make both healthcare visits and pharmacy pickups difficult and can create challenges with daily dosing of a method like pills.[56] Methods that decrease menstrual bleeding may be appealing for individuals in the military, especially those about to be deployed.[57]

### Individuals Who Are Incarcerated

Incarceration rates for individuals with the capacity for pregnancy are increasing, with disproportionately high rates of incarceration noted among communities of color.[58] Individuals who enter the carceral system are disproportionately from marginalized backgrounds, such as communities of color and socioeconomically marginalized groups, and often lack access to reproductive health care before, during, and after incarceration.[59] Individuals who are incarcerated may want to initiate or remain on hormonal contraception for a variety of reasons, including both contraceptive and noncontraceptive reasons. Facilitating access to high-quality health care, including contraceptive care, is imperative to treating all people with respect and dignity.[60]

Every method should be made available to the incarcerated individual. There is a long history of incarcerated individuals being targeted for reproductive coercion, including forced sterilization, so providing patient-centered, respectful care is critically important.[61,62] Because a majority of the people with the capacity for pregnancy who are incarcerated have a history of sexual assault, health care must be trauma-informed in a carceral setting.[59]

### Perimenopausal Period

Age is not a contraindication for use of hormonal contraceptive methods. The exception is use of estrogen-containing contraception for an individual who smokes more than 15 cigarettes per day and is 35 years or older.[15] The combination of these factors places an individual at higher risk of myocardial infarction from exogenous estrogen, but also places them at greater risk of stroke during pregnancy. In contrast, COCs can safely be used by nonsmokers who are perimenopausal.

Individuals in their 40s continue to be sexually active and fertile, even if their degree of fertility is less than when they were younger. Fertility declines gradually and varies individually, making it clinically challenging to identify an exact point in time at which contraception can be stopped. Additionally, many individuals continue to desire pregnancy at an older age, so the provider should avoid making assumptions about a desire to avoid or achieve pregnancy based on an individual's age.[63] Specific concerns related to aging can influence risk perception and priorities as well, so considering contraception from a holistic view is helpful.[64]

Some perimenopausal individuals opt for permanent sterilization, but some forms of hormonal contraception provide additional noncontraceptive benefits that may be especially appealing during midlife. COCs can provide relief from many peri-menopausal discomforts such as irregular bleeding, hot flashes, and dyspareunia.[65] The hormonal IUD has an FDA indication as a therapy for individuals experiencing heavy menses. Likewise, other contraceptive methods associated with the side effect of amenorrhea may be of value for perimenopausal individuals.[65]

For the individual in the perimenopausal period, hormonal contraceptive methods both mask the progression toward natural menopause (because of the changes in bleeding patterns) and render hormonal levels inaccurate for predicting the onset of menopause.[13] No evidence exists to guide the provider in deciding when it is best to discontinue a hormonal method; however, many providers discontinue the hormone contraceptive method when an individual is 55 years old. At that time, almost all individuals are postmenopausal.

### Menstrual-Related Conditions

Hormonal contraception was originally developed for pregnancy prevention, but the mechanisms of action also mean that hormonal contraception can be used to treat a variety of menstrual-related conditions. Such contraception, especially methods containing estrogen, can be used to treat dysmenorrhea, metrorrhagia, menorrhagia, acne, and hirsutism.[66–68] For individuals with endometriosis, both combined hormonal contraception and progestin-only contraception have been shown to decrease dysmenorrhea, pelvic pain, and dyspareunia, and to improve quality of life.[69] For individuals with PCOS, hormonal contraception can reduce hyperandrogenic symptoms such as acne, hirsutism, and metrorrhagia; thus, it is considered first-line treatment for long-term management of PCOS in individuals not desiring a pregnancy in the near future.[14,70] It is important to remember that individuals who may not want or need pregnancy prevention from hormonal contraception may benefit from these additional effects in treating menstrual-related conditions.

## Initiation of Hormonal Contraceptives

For decades, healthcare providers delayed initiation of a hormonal contraceptive method until after a woman's next menstrual period to reassure both the provider and the individual that the individual was not pregnant. Timing initiation in tandem with a menstrual period also represented an attempt to minimize breakthrough bleeding, although this

connection has not been proven. Some providers advocated starting a method on the first day of menses, others within 5 days of a menses, and yet others within a week of menses. For years, many providers advised individuals to start oral contraceptives on the Sunday after a menses started to avoid having menses start over the weekend. Although all these approaches to initiation were based on opinion and not evidence, they continue to be used in some practices today.

### Quick Start or Same-Day Start

In 2002, a study was published advocating a new initiation method called *Quick Start*.[71] Quick Start is the term used to describe an initiation method in which the individual begins using oral, dermal, or vaginal contraceptives as soon as they get them, regardless of where they are in their menstrual cycle. Quick Start was developed in response to consumer desires. As many as 25% of individuals provided with a prescription for contraceptive pills never had it filled, often using another, less reliable method or no method of contraception at all.[72] Individuals reported being more satisfied when they were able to obtain the contraceptive method they desired in a timely manner. In addition, waiting for a menses is a questionable practice often deemed unnecessary because of the improved reliability of pregnancy tests. Even in the rare event that an individual is pregnant and is inadvertently exposed to contraceptive hormones, there is no evidence of an increase in the risk of miscarriage or any teratogenic effects from hormonal contraceptives.[73] Quick Start was also initially promoted as a way to ensure longer continuation rates as compared to traditional approaches, although only limited evidence supports this effect.[74,75]

The Quick Start practice has since expanded from its initial use with oral contraceptives. Studies suggest it can be used for initiation of patches, rings, and injections as well as pills.[38,17] Figure 12-2 provides an algorithm for Quick Start and various other hormonal methods.[39]

In general, regardless of when an individual begins a hormonal method, there should be some reasonable assurance that they are not pregnant. This assurance can take the form of a normal menses within the last 5 days, a negative pregnancy test, or history indicating that they have not had sexual intercourse that could result in a pregnancy since their last menses. In instances where sexual intercourse that could result in pregnancy has recently occurred, providing emergency contraception in combination with the Quick Start method reduces

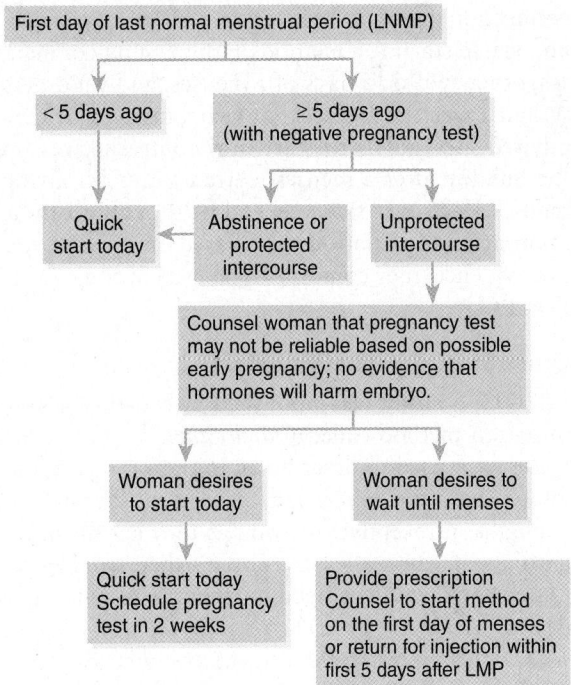

**Figure 12-2** Quick Start for pills, patches, rings, and injections.
Modified with permission from Center for Reproductive Health Education in Family Medicine. Quick Start Algorithm. 2017. www.rhedi.org. Used by permission of RHEDI/Center for Reproductive Health Education in Family Medicine, Montefiore Medical Center, New York City, 2007.

the risk of pregnancy, and can be used with combined contraception and progestin-only pills, implant, and injection.[76,77]

### Use of Back-Up Methods

Evidence regarding the optimal duration of use of back-up contraception is lacking, and most guidelines are empirical at best. Years ago, it was not uncommon to recommend back-up use for a full month after initiation of COCs. Today, the CDC recommends that a back-up method is used for 7 days when not starting contraception within 5 to 7 days of the start of menses and engaging in sexual intercourse with the potential for pregnancy.[7] Progestin-only pills are the exception: They need only 2 days of use of a back-up method.[7] Additionally, a back-up method should be used when contraception has been missed. (Method-specific information is provided later in this chapter.) The exact type of back-up method recommended will vary based on the individual's desire and level of comfort, but generally any short-term nonhormonal method, such as condoms or a diaphragm, can serve as a back-up method.

### Changing from One Hormonal Method to Another

Individuals may change from one method to another or even discontinue use of contraception for a variety of personal reasons. When an individual desires to switch from one hormonal method to another, their rationale may be based on cost, convenience, desire for increased effectiveness, or a number of other reasons. In this situation, a strategy of briefly overlapping methods can be implemented to manage the small window of time in which the new method is not yet preventing pregnancy. If overlap cannot be arranged, a back-up method can provide temporary contraception if the individual will be engaging in sexual intercourse with the potential for pregnancy.

Table 12-7 provides information on how to switch from one hormonal method to another while maintaining maximum protection from pregnancy.[40,41] Individuals switching from oral contraceptives should follow the guidance in this table and not necessarily finish a package of pills.

## Managing Common Side Effects Associated with Hormonal Contraceptive Methods

Assisting an individual who is experiencing the side effects of any contraceptive is a key aspect of midwifery practice to help individuals optimally use the method. Studies regarding contraceptive use reveal that side effects are the primary reason that the majority of individuals discontinue their hormonal contraceptive.[78,79] In addition to counseling individuals about potential side effects, it is important to include in health education the caveats that not all individuals will experience these side effects, and that not all discomforts or health concerns experienced while using hormonal contraception will be related to the contraceptive method being used. With those points in mind, it is essential to take an individual's report of a side effect seriously regardless of the possible source, as minimizing side effects hinders patient trust and reduces bodily autonomy.[80–82]

### Vaginal Bleeding Irregularities

Changes in menstrual bleeding occur with all hormonal contraceptive methods and may be viewed as either an advantage or a disadvantage. Lighter menses generally are well received by most individuals; however, while some may be comfortable with amenorrhea, others are not.[83] The majority of individuals find unpredictable or breakthrough

| Table 12-7 | When to Start a New Hormonal Method When Switching from Another Method to Minimize Risk of Pregnancy | | | | | | | |
|---|---|---|---|---|---|---|---|---|
| | **New Method** | | | | | | | |
| **Current Method** | **COC or POP** | **Transdermal Patch** | **Vaginal Ring** | **Progestin Injection** | **Implant** | **LNG-IUD (Kyleena, Skyla)** | **LNG-IUD (Liletta, Mirena)** | **Copper IUD** |
| **COC or POP** | No gap: take first pill of new pack the day after taking any pill in old pack | 1 day before stopping pill | No gap: insert ring the day after taking any pill | 7 days before stopping pill | 4 days before stopping pill | 7 days before stopping pill | Insert up to 5 days after stopping pill | Insert up to 5 days after stopping pills |
| **Transdermal patch** | 1 day before stopping patch | | No gap: insert ring same day as stopping patch | 7 days before stopping patch | 4 days before stopping patch | 7 days before stopping patch | Insert up to 5 days after stopping patch | Insert up to 5 days after stopping patch |
| **Vaginal ring** | 1 day before stopping ring | 2 days before stopping ring | | 7 days before stopping ring | 4 days before stopping ring | 7 days before stopping ring | Insert up to 5 days after stopping ring | Insert up to 5 days after stopping ring |
| **Progestin injection** | Any day up to 15 weeks after injection | Any day up to 15 weeks after injection | Any day up to 15 weeks after injection | | Any day up to 15 weeks after injection | Any day up to 15 weeks after injection | Insert up to 15 weeks after injection | Insert up to 16 weeks after last injection |
| **Implant** | 7 days before implant is removed | 7 days before implant is removed | 7 days before implant is removed | 7 days before implant is removed | | Insert 7 days before implant is removed | Insert up to 5 days after implant is removed | Insert up to 5 days after implant is removed |
| **LNG-IUD** | 7 days before LNG-IUD is removed | 7 days before LNG-IUD is removed | 7 days before LNG-IUD is removed | 7 days before LNG-IUD is removed | 4 days before LNG-IUD is removed | | | No gap: insert immediately after LNG-IUD is removed |
| **Copper IUD** | 7 days before IUD is removed | 7 days before IUD is removed | 7 days before IUD is removed | 7 days before IUD is removed | 4 days before IUD is removed | No gap: insert immediately after copper IUD is removed and use back-up method for 7 days | Insert immediately after copper IUD is removed; no back-up needed | |

Abbreviations: COC, combined oral contraception; IUD; intrauterine device; LNG-IUD, levonorgestrel-releasing intrauterine device; POP, progestin-only pill.

Modified with permission from Reproductive Health Access Project. How to switch birth control methods. https://www.reproductiveaccess.org/wp-content/uploads/2014/12/switching_bc.pdf. Published June 2021. Accessed February 24, 2022.

bleeding to be at least a nuisance. An individual's attitude toward different bleeding patterns is shaped by both individual and social influences and should be considered when exploring contraceptive options to ensure greater satisfaction with the method.[83]

Progestin-only methods are more likely than combined hormonal contraception to be associated with irregular bleeding, including amenorrhea, because progestin-only methods lack estrogen's endometrial-stabilizing properties. Strong evidence has not yet emerged regarding how to manage hormone-associated bleeding, although extended and combined regimens have been suggested to suppress menstrual bleeding.[43,44] Many providers base their practice in this area on observation or expert opinions. Figure 12-3 provides a sample algorithm for basic management of problematic irregular bleeding.[43-45] The pharmacologic treatments included in the algorithm are based on common clinical practices and should not be accepted as evidence based. Most medications provide temporary relief at best.

### Headaches

Many individuals have mild occasional headaches, usually associated with tension or allergies. However, for some, headaches can be disabling and may even herald a severe adverse effect such as a cerebral vascular accident (CVA). Some contraceptive methods are associated with increased incidence of headaches, such that the healthcare provider is faced with the perplexing problem of identifying whether the headache is minor or signals a significant healthcare problem. If an individual presents with neurovascular symptoms such as flashing lights, loss of vision, muscle weakness, slurred speech, dizziness, or abnormal cranial nerve changes as well as a headache, these symptoms are an emergency, and the individual requires immediate care to rule out a CVA. They also should discontinue the hormonal contraceptive method as quickly as possible and be counseled to use a nonhormonal method until the neurologic condition is resolved. For those who have headaches but no neurologic symptoms, and for whom no abnormalities are found upon examination, the healthcare provider may consider alternative hormonal therapies. For example, individuals using COCs can have headaches during the withdrawal period (menstrual headaches) and may benefit from an extended-cycle method.[84]

### Nausea

Nausea is a common side effect reported by individuals using any drug, but it is more likely with oral and transdermal contraceptives. There is no simple remedy. No single type of COC or POP is superior to another in terms of mitigating nausea. Ultimately, if the nausea and vomiting prove onerous for an individual, they should consider another contraceptive method, especially a contraceptive ring, implant, or IUD.[85]

If the nausea is mild but problematic, several suggestions for its management may be made, although evidence is lacking regarding the effectiveness of these interventions. Among the most frequently used empirical management strategies for individuals experiencing nausea with oral contraceptives are taking the pill before sleep or taking it with a meal to avoid ingestion on an empty stomach. Ginger often is suggested as a food with antinausea effects.

## Short-Acting Reversible Contraceptives

Short-acting reversible hormonal contraceptives (SARCs) include pills, injectable agents, transdermal patches, and intravaginal rings that contain either the combination of estrogen and a progestin or only a progestin. Once initiated, the duration of action of these methods can range from a single day to as long as 13 weeks. Advantages of these methods include high rates of effectiveness, relative ease of use, high levels of user control, and reduction in dysmenorrhea. Disadvantages of SARCs include the need to remember to use the method on a daily or routine basis, the potential for recurring costs, and lack of protection against transmission of STIs.

## Combined Oral Contraceptives

COCs produce a pharmacologic—rather than a physiologic—cycle. When the placebo pills are taken, the exogenous estrogen and progestin are withdrawn and endometrial wall shedding takes place. This bleeding is sometimes called a pseudomenstruation, also the more commonly used term is withdrawal bleeding. However, most individuals will characterize it as a normal menses or a period. Typically, this bleeding is scant and of shorter duration as compared to an individual's menses when not using hormonal contraception because the endometrial lining has not built up as it would in a physiologic cycle.

The main variations among the formulations of the combined pill relate to the hormonal dose, the relative proportions of estrogen and progestin, and the particular progestin component used. As a result, a wide variety of pills are available, each with

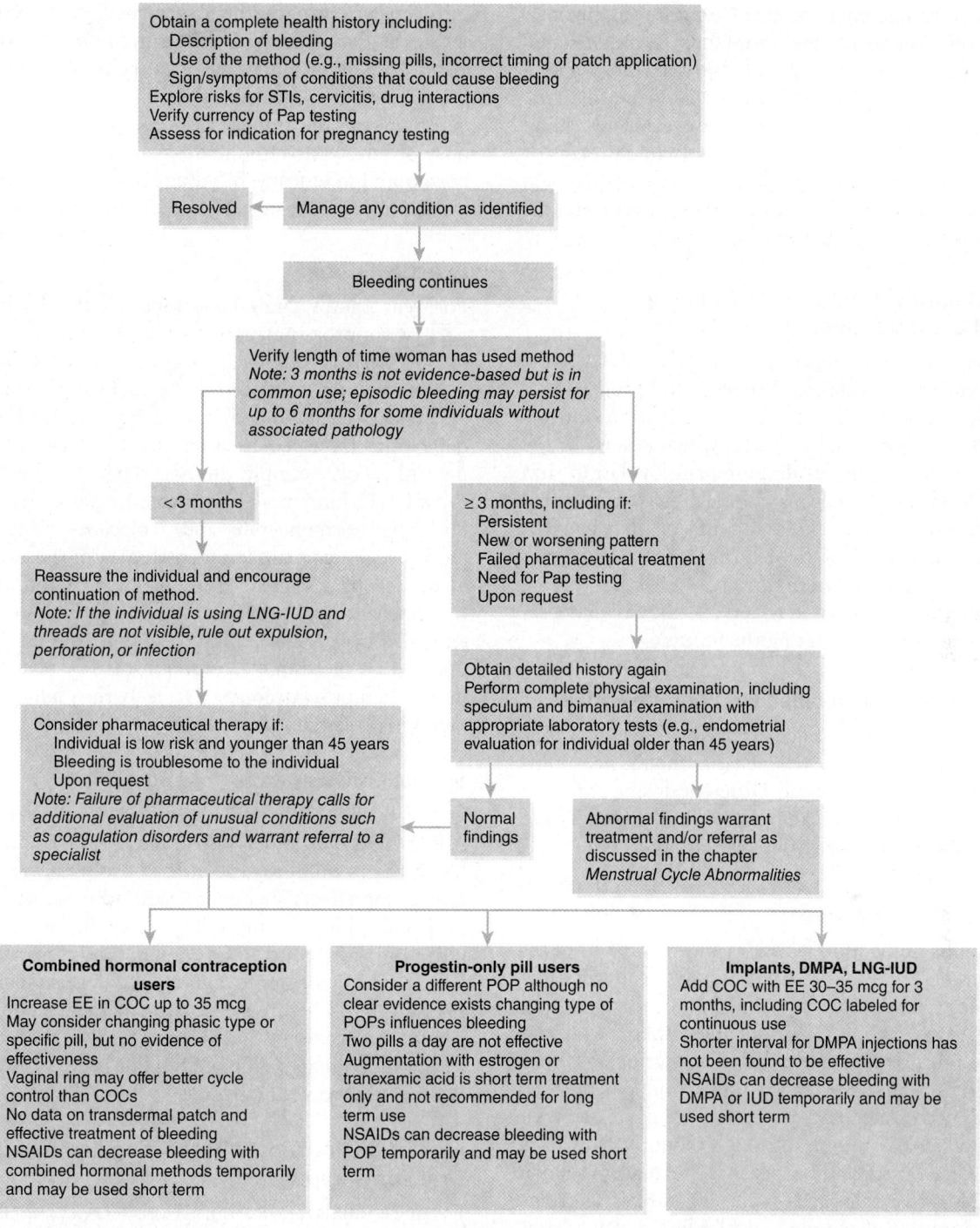

**Figure 12-3** Sample algorithm for management of individuals using a hormonal contraceptive method and experiencing associated troublesome bleeding.

Abbreviations: COCs, combined oral contraceptives; DMPA, depot medroxyprogesterone acetate; EE, ethinyl estradiol; IUD, intrauterine device; LNG-IUD, levonorgestrel-releasing intrauterine device; NSAIDs, nonsteroidal anti-inflammatory drugs; POP, progestin-only pill; STIs, sexually transmitted infections.

[a] Medical therapy is primarily based on expert opinion and common practice. Little strong evidence exists in this area.

Based on Edelman A, Micks E, Gallo MF, et al. Continuous or extended cycle vs. cyclic use of combined hormonal contraceptives for contraception. *Cochrane Database Syst Rev.* 2014;7:CD004695. doi:10.1002/14651858.CD004695.pub3; Faculty of Sexual and Reproductive Healthcare Clinical Effectiveness Unit Clinical guidance: problematic bleeding with hormonal contraception (July 2015). https://www.fsrh.org/standards-and-guidance/documents/ceuguidanceproblematicbleedinghormonalcontraception/. Accessed March 13, 2023; Grossman Barr N. Managing adverse effects of hormonal contraceptives. *Am Fam Physician.* 2010;82(12):1499-1506.

a different side-effect profile. Complicating this discussion is the reality that more than 75 brand-name COCs are currently available. In years past, it had been suggested that individuals could be matched to specific pills. Other practices advocated switching certain COCs to others via a complicated process of estimating strength of progestin or dose of estrogen. For most individuals, however, there is little clinical difference among the formulations.

## Mechanism of Action for Combined Oral Contraceptives

The primary mechanism of action for COCs is the prevention of ovulation. Estrogen and progestin, in combination, inhibit pituitary production and secretion of both FSH and LH, which results in the inhibition of follicular development, ovulation, and development of a corpus luteum.[3] Estrogen or progestin could inhibit FSH and LH on its own, but the combination of these drugs greatly enhances the ovulation-inhibition effects.[3] COCs also create scanty, thick, and viscous cervical mucus that prevents sperm from entering the uterus.[3]

## Regimens for Combined Oral Contraceptives

COCs often are identified according to whether they involve one of three regimens: monophasic, multiphasic, or extended cycle. Different dosing regimens can have various advantages or disadvantages, and individuals may prefer one over another.

### Monophasic Regimen

The pills in the monophasic regimen come in packs of either 21 or 24 pills that are identical every day in terms of the amount and type of estrogen and progestin. The packs also include either 7 or 4 placebo pills, respectively. Some formulations have replaced the placebo with a folate supplement. One pill is taken each day for a total of 28 days, and then a new pack is begun. Although monophasic COCs have been marketed for decades, the newer regimen of 24 active pills and 4 placebo tablets shortens the duration of withdrawal bleeding and increases effectiveness.

### Multiphasic Regimen

The hormone-containing pills in the multiphasic pack vary in the amount of estrogen and/or progestin provided during particular weeks of the cycle of pills and also include either 4 or 7 days of placebo pills. Multiphasic regimens often are referred to as biphasic when two different combinations of

estrogen and progestin are provided, or triphasic when the pack has three different combinations or doses. Most multiphasic COCs vary the dose of the progestin, but a few are estrophasic—that is, they maintain a stable amount of progestin and vary the dose of ethinyl estradiol. Minimal differences have been noted in efficacy, bleeding changes, or adverse events in monophasic versus multiphasic COCs.[86]

### Extended Cycle

For years, individuals have taken COCs back to back without stopping for a placebo week. Based on this desire for convenience, new regimens were introduced. An extended cycle includes hormone and placebo pills, but the hormone pills are taken daily for three consecutive months instead of monthly. For example, in one type of extended-cycle COC, known as Seasonale, the pack includes 84 active hormone pills and 7 placebos. This extended regimen results in menstrual suppression, as evidenced by a decreased frequency of withdrawal bleeding and potential amenorrhea.[87] Some of the extended-cycle regimens use pills that contain a reduced dose of ethinyl estradiol instead of placebos, in an attempt to decrease dysmenorrhea and other menstrual-related symptoms.[88]

## Special Considerations for Use of Combined Oral Contraceptives

Adolescents can safely use COCs but are more likely than adults to discontinue use if they experience side effects such as nausea; adolescents may also find taking a daily pill more challenging than older individuals do.[89] Counseling about common side effects, strategies to enhance regular use such as taking the pill before sleep, and emergency contraception are generally included in health education for all individuals taking COCs but may be of particular value to young people.

## Care of the Individual Requesting Combined Oral Contraceptives

For individuals requesting to use COCs, the steps in initiating these contraceptives are summarized in Table 12-6. Physical examination should include blood pressure and weight, but a pelvic examination is not required. When selecting the specific COC, the lowest dose of estrogen possible should be chosen to minimize risks and side effects. Prescribing up to 13 packs of COCs—the equivalent of a year's supply—has been shown to support contraceptive continuation and avoid an increased risk for undesired pregnancy.[7]

Of all the SARCs, COCs have the largest number of contraindications or Category 3 or 4 considerations in the U.S. MEC.[15] Most of these conditions are significant disorders, especially those associated with cardiovascular events such as hypertension, stroke, headaches with aura, and myocardial infarction. Thrombotic diseases, severe liver disease, breast cancer, lupus, diabetes with neuropathies, and vascular disease also are commonly included in the Category 3 or 4 considerations. The U.S. MEC should be reviewed for any individuals who want to consider COCs as the most efficient way to identify potential contraindications.[7]

Figure 12-4 provides a guide that can be used to counsel individuals about missed pills. Most individuals, even when using an extended-cycle regimen, will resume normal ovulatory function within 90 days or 3 months of taking the last pill.[9] For years, individuals have been advised to postpone pregnancy until 3 months after COCs are discontinued to ensure credible dating of a pregnancy. However, there is no evidence that earlier conception is associated with untoward perinatal outcomes.

Table 12-8 lists content that should be specifically emphasized when counseling individuals using COCs, in addition to the health education reviewed for any hormonal contraception (Table 12-6).

## Progestin-Only Pills

Progestin-only pills (POPs) contain a low dose of a single progestin and, therefore, can be used by individuals who want to use contraceptive pills but for whom estrogen is contraindicated. Originally FDA approved in the early 1970s, these agents tend to occupy a niche market for individuals who are breastfeeding/chestfeeding, but can safely be used by most individuals.[90] Although some call these agents mini-pills, use of that term can be confusing because of the number of low-dose COCs available. Therefore, progestin-only pills or POPs is the preferred term. Currently, several POPs are available. Most POP formulations have no hormone-free days, thereby providing a constant low-level dose of the progestin norethindrone. A newer POP containing drospirenone has a longer half-life and 4 hormone-free days, meaning that this formulation is less sensitive to dosing windows and may provide a withdrawal bleed similar to COCs.[91]

### Mechanism of Action of Progestin-Only Pills

The dose of progesterone contained in POPs is much less than the amount found in COCs. In consequence, POPs do not prevent ovulation consistently, and as many as 40% of individuals will continue

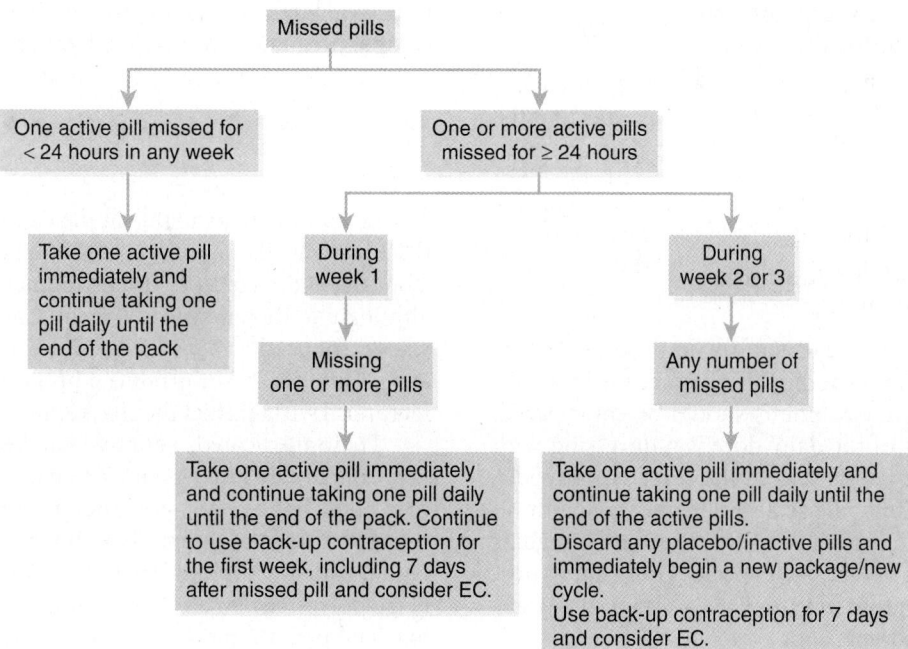

**Figure 12-4** Algorithm for counseling individuals who have missed pills (combined oral contraceptives or progestin-only pills).
Abbreviation: EC, emergency contraception.

| Table 12-8 | Educational Content to Be Emphasized When Counseling Individuals Using Combined Oral Contraceptives[a] |
|---|---|

Pills should be taken daily, preferably at approximately the same time.

Conditions that should be reported are identified by the mnemonic ACHES:

**A**bdominal pain

**C**hest pain

**H**eadache (severe)

**E**ye problems or loss of vision

**S**evere leg pain or swelling in a calf or thigh

[a] In addition to the information in Table 12-6.

| Table 12-9 | Educational Content to Be Emphasized When Counseling Individuals Using Progestin-Only Contraceptive Pills[a] |
|---|---|

The pill should be taken within 3 hours of the designated time every day.

Conditions that should be reported are identified by the mnemonic ACHES:

**A**bdominal pain

**C**hest pain

**H**eadache (severe)

**E**ye problems or loss of vision

**S**evere leg pain or swelling in a calf or thigh

[a] In addition to the information in Table 12-6.

to ovulate while using these contraceptives.[3] Progesterone also creates cervical mucus that is hostile to sperm, resulting in little to no sperm penetration into the uterus.[3] To minimize risk of pregnancy, the daily dose of POPs with norethindrone must be taken at the same time each day to maintain a steady-state plasma level of the progestin. If more than 24 hours elapses between doses, the plasma level falls and escape ovulation can occur, meaning that pregnancy is possible during this time.

## Special Considerations for Use of Progestin-Only Pills

Although individuals who are lactating often use POPs, there is conflicting information regarding the amount of progestin transmitted to human milk. POPs have not been associated with an increased risk of VTE.[92]

## Care of Individuals Requesting Progestin-Only Pills

While the management plan for individuals choosing to initiate POPs is the same as that for individuals using COCs, two points should be emphasized. The regularity of the daily dose is unforgiving with norethindrone-containing POPs; that is, individuals must take the pills at 24-hour intervals with no more than 3 hours of variation. Second, irregular spotting and bleeding are expected, not simply possible, because progestin alone does a poor job of stabilizing the endometrium.

Table 12-9 lists topics to be emphasized for the individual regarding POP use in addition to the health education required for individuals using any type of hormonal contraception (Table 12-6).

Prescribing 13 packs will help improve continuation rates.[7] Similar to the case for individuals using COCs, the majority of individuals using POPs resume ovulatory function within 90 days or 3 months after discontinuing this contraceptive method.[9]

While it is not unusual for individuals using POPs to have irregular bleeding and amenorrhea, if an individual misses two periods, even they have taken all of their pills on time, a pregnancy test is warranted.[2] Anytime an individual uses POPs and experiences severe abdominal pain, they will need to be evaluated emergently for possible ovarian cyst, ectopic pregnancy, or pelvic inflammatory disease.

## Transdermal Contraception (Patch)

Currently, two transdermal delivery systems for contraception are available in the United States. Ortho Evra was FDA approved in 2002 but withdrawn from the U.S. market by the manufacturer in 2015, although it remains available in Canada. Xulane was introduced as a replacement for Ortho Evra; it is the same patch but produced by a different manufacturer. Twirla joined the market in 2020.[93]

These medicated, adhesive patches have a surface contact area of 14 cm². The patch is composed of a thin, lightweight polyester material and constructed in three layers. The outer surface of the patch, called a backing layer, consists of a flexible, beige polyester film and serves as a protective covering. The patch's middle layer contains both the adhesive component and the active drug compounds. A third layer of clear polyethylene film protects the adhesive layer during storage and is removed prior to use. The contraceptive patch is a combined hormonal method containing both a synthetic estrogen and a progestin, with each brand having a unique type and dose of exogenous hormones.

## Mechanism of Action of the Contraceptive Patch

The primary mechanism of action for the contraceptive patch is similar to that for COCs. The transdermal absorption of exogenous estrogen and progestin inhibits ovulation by suppressing release of gonadotropins within the hypothalamic–pituitary–ovarian axis. Alterations in cervical mucus and endometrial lining are secondary mechanisms of contraceptive action. The active drug is absorbed through the skin, thereby avoiding a first-pass effect through the liver. Therefore, this route can decrease the total dose of exogenous hormones delivered when compared to oral contraceptive methods.

The contraceptive patch is self-applied by the individual. Each patch is infused with hormones that are adequate for approximately 1 week. To mimic the normal 28-day menstrual cycle, a single contraceptive patch is applied for 7 days and then immediately replaced with a new patch. Three patches are used in a month, resulting in 21 consecutive days of hormone exposure. The fourth week is a patch-free week, and a withdrawal bleed is expected following that interval. The contraceptive cycle is then restarted with the application of a new patch immediately following the 7-day patch-free week. Situations in which the transdermal delivery of the active drugs is disrupted (e.g., partial detachment) can result in decreased effectiveness. However, the adhesive component of the contraceptive patch is not generally affected by heat, humidity, or exercise. Additionally, the patch can be safely used as extended/continuous contraception—for example, using a new patch every week for 3 months before removing the patch for a 7-day hormone-free period.[94]

Four application sites have been approved for use with the patch and have been studied for their therapeutic effectiveness: the buttocks, the upper outer arm, the abdomen, and the upper torso. The area around the breasts should not be used for patch application—not because of known problems, but because of general concerns about breast tissue being exposed to hormones. To avoid problems with adherence/effectiveness, patches should be applied to clean, dry skin and individuals should be counseled to avoid areas that have been recently exposed to perfumes, gels, lotions, shampoos, and other topical products unless they clean and dry the skin first.

## Special Considerations for Use of the Contraceptive Patch

Contraindications to the use of the contraceptive patch are the same as contraindications for any combined hormonal contraceptive. Side effects include headaches and breast discomfort. There have also been reports of application-site reactions, a non-hormonal-related side effect.[95]

Unlike oral contraceptives, the patch does not require daily maintenance. When dispensed from a pharmacy as a single-month supply, the contraceptive patch is packaged as a set of three individual patches. Even though the patch is marketed for 7 days of use, studies have found that after the second week of method use, a single patch will continue to deliver a sufficient amount of hormones for an additional 2 days, providing some forgiveness at that time should the individual be delayed in making the patch change after week 2 or 3.[14]

The contraceptive patch has received a significant amount of media attention regarding its association with VTE. A Cochrane review estimated that the risk of VTE with patch use is 53 cases per 100,000 individuals.[85] The general consensus is that the risk of VTE with the patch is higher than the risk associated with levonorgestrel-containing COCs, but still less than the risk of VTE during pregnancy.[95]

## Care of Individuals Requesting Contraceptive Patches

When transdermal patches are requested as the contraceptive method, the provider should screen the individual for previous skin allergies such as reactions to bandages or other medicated patches. The individual's current weight should also be considered. If their weight exceeds 90 kg (198 pounds), the individual should be advised of the potentially decreased effectiveness of the patch: The package label carries a precaution related to this weight threshold.[40,93]

Prescribing 13 packs can improve continuation rates.[7] The follow-up visit should include assessment of the individual's satisfaction with this contraceptive method and experience of any side effects or problems with method use. Table 12-10 discusses health education specifically related to use of a transdermal contraceptive patch.

Providers may furnish two prescriptions: one for the ongoing monthly supply and a second for a single replacement patch in case one becomes prematurely detached. If the individual forgets to apply a second or third patch of the cycle and no more than 1 to 2 days has elapsed since the day they would normally apply the patch (9 days from the application of their current patch), they should apply a new patch

| Table 12-10 | Educational Content to Be Emphasized When Counseling Individuals Using the Contraceptive Patch[a] |
|---|---|

When removing the patch from packaging, the individual should not touch the medicated side. Instead, remove only half of the release liner, apply that half to the skin, and then remove the liner for the remaining half, applying with gentle pressure to ensure adhesion.

Only one patch at a time should be used. Use of multiple patches is more likely to increase side/adverse effects than to improve effectiveness.

Verify attachment daily. If it appears that the patch may be detaching, gently press on the patch for approximately 10 seconds. If that effort is unsuccessful, remove the patch and replace it with a new one.

Patches should not be reused or relocated to another site.

Patches should not be secured by other tape or wrapping.

If the patch becomes nonadherent for less than 1 day, remove it and apply a new patch. Do not attempt to reapply a patch that has adhered to clothing, as this may decrease effectiveness.

If the patch is off for more than 1 day during the 3 weeks, apply another patch and start a new 4-week cycle, and use a back-up method for the first week.

Used patches can be discarded in the trash, away from pets and children as they may contain residual hormones. They should never be flushed down a toilet.

[a] In addition to the information in Table 12-6.

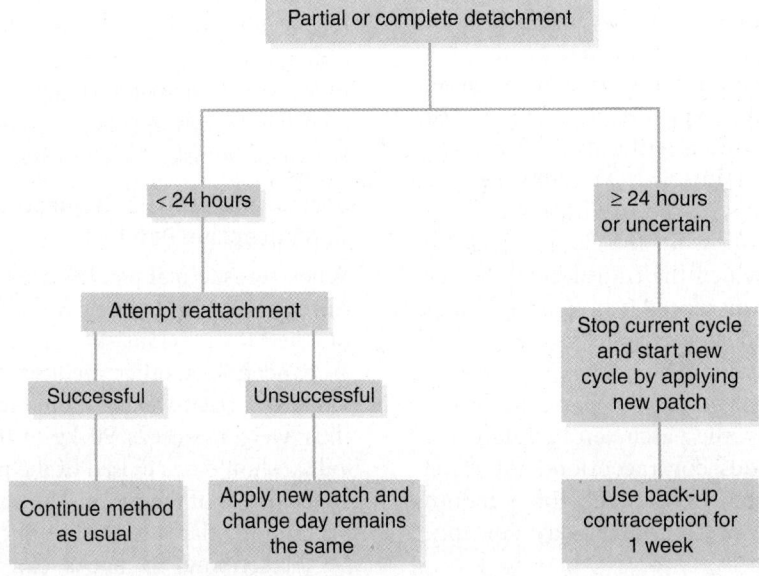

**Figure 12-5** Algorithm for management of individuals with a partial or completely detached transdermal contraceptive patch.

as soon as possible (Figure 12-5). The original patch change schedule remains unaltered. If more than 9 days has elapsed since the application of the current patch, the individual should understand that they are not protected from pregnancy and should start a new 21-day cycle by applying a new patch and using a back-up contraceptive method for the first week.[40]

If the individual forgets to take off the patch at the beginning of the patch-free week, they should remove it as soon as they remember. If more than 9 days has elapsed since placement of the third patch, they should replace the patch according to the original schedule. Depending on how far into the patch-free week they remove the third patch, they may or may not experience a withdrawal bleed, although contraceptive protection is maintained.

If the individual forgets to restart a new patch following the patch-free week, they need to understand that they are not protected from pregnancy. In such a case, they should put on a new patch and use a secondary method for pregnancy prevention for the first week of this new cycle.

## Intravaginal Contraceptive Ring

Currently, two intravaginal delivery systems for contraception are available in the United States. NuvaRing, manufactured by Merck Pharmaceuticals, was introduced in the U.S. market in 2001. It is a flexible, vinyl ring measuring approximately 4 mm thick and 54 mm in diameter. The ring is composed of ethylene vinyl acetate, which encases the active components and controls the daily release of the drugs. This combined hormonal method of contraception contains both estrogen and progestin components: 11.7 mg etonorgestrel and 2.7 mg ethinyl estradiol.[96]

Annovera, made by TherapeuticsMD and the Population Council, was introduced in 2019. Unlike NuvaRing, the Annovera ring is intended to be used for 1 year. It is made of silicone and contains 103 mg segesterone acetate (SA) and 17.4 mg ethinyl estradiol (EE), which releases, on average, 0.15 mg/day of segesterone acetate and 0.013 mg/day of ethinyl estradiol.[97]

### Mechanism of Action of Intravaginal Contraceptive Ring

The primary mechanism of action for the contraceptive ring is similar to that of COCs. The vaginal mucosa absorbs the exogenous estrogen and progestin compounds, inhibiting ovulation via suppression of gonadotropins within the hypothalamic–pituitary–ovarian axis.[3] Alterations in cervical mucus and the endometrial lining are secondary mechanisms of contraceptive action. Because the hormones are released directly into the vagina, a lower daily dose of hormones is required in comparison to COCs.[2]

The contraceptive ring is self-administered by the individual, who inserts a ring once per month. To mimic the normal 28-day menstrual cycle, a single contraceptive ring is inserted and left in place for 21 days. It is then removed for 7 days, thereby inducing a withdrawal bleed. The contraceptive cycle restarts with the insertion of a new NuvaRing or the same Annovera ring immediately following the 7-day ring-free week. As with the patch and combined pill, extended or continuous use of the rings is possible, without the need for a withdrawal bleed.[94]

The vaginal ring comes in only one size, does not require fitting, and is not position dependent. That is, as long as the ring remains in contact with the vaginal mucosa, the hormones will be absorbed. The contraceptive ring can be used concurrently with tampons and left in place during sexual intercourse. It can also be removed for up to 3 hours without compromising its effectiveness.[2]

### Special Considerations for Use of the Intravaginal Contraceptive Ring

The most prevalent side effects with the vaginal ring include headache, dysmenorrhea, and breast discomfort. Additionally, a method-specific, nonhormonal side effect is vaginal irritation and discharge, although individuals with vaginal dryness may find this an added benefit.[98] When dispensed from a pharmacy, the contraceptive ring comes individually packaged in a resealable foil pouch (NuvaRing) or a storage container (Annovera). Prior to dispensing, NuvaRing is stored refrigerated, but it can be stored for up to 4 months at room temperature afterward. Temperature extremes should be avoided when storing the contraceptive ring, as there is potential for decreased effectiveness in those situations.

The contraceptive ring is convenient for many individuals because it does not require daily or weekly maintenance, and its insertion and removal are not difficult. The ring usually is not perceived by the individual user and only occasionally felt by a partner during penetrative vaginal intercourse. The NuvaRing ring should be rinsed only with cool water, while the Annovera can be cleaned in between uses with soap and water.

Contraceptive rings may be of value for adolescents. Not only does this method offer more privacy than oral contraceptives or patches, but it also provides the same benefits as other combined hormonal methods—namely, lighter menses, less dysmenorrhea, no weight gain, and no effect on bone mineral density.[26]

### Care of Individuals Requesting an Intravaginal Contraceptive Ring

The management plan for individuals using the contraceptive ring is similar to that for other combined hormonal contraceptive methods. Providers should screen for contraindications to combined hormonal contraception.[15] A prescription for emergency contraception should be considered, and individuals should be encouraged to have spermicide and condoms available in the event that the ring is expelled or an error occurs in removing or starting a new ring on schedule. Like the other hormonal methods, neither ring will protect against STIs or HIV.

Prescribing 13 packs helps maintain continuation rates.[7] The follow-up visit is the same as that for any combined hormonal contraceptive, and should include assessment of the individual's satisfaction with the method and their experience of any side effects or problems with method use. Table 12-11 outlines health education points related to the use of the contraceptive ring.

| Table 12-11 | Educational Content to Be Emphasized When Counseling Individuals Using the Intravaginal Contraceptive Ring[a] |
|---|---|

Remove the ring from its packaging, and insert it into the vagina by compressing the sides.

The ring must be completely inserted into the vagina.

Insert only one ring at any time. Use of multiple rings is likely to increase side/adverse effects with no corresponding increase in effectiveness.

Rings usually are best removed by the individual slipping their index finger under the rim of the ring and guiding it down and out of the vagina.

Because rings are typically removed every 21 days, an individual may benefit from some type of reminder system, such as a calendar, app, or text service.

A used ring can be replaced inside its foil pouch or container and discarded in the trash, away from pets and children. Rings should never be flushed down a toilet.

[a] In addition to the information in Table 12-6.

Spontaneous expulsion occurs in fewer than 3% of individuals using the contraceptive ring. If the ring is outside of the individual's body for less than 3 hours, then it should simply be rinsed with tepid water and reinserted. If it has been out of the vagina for more than 3 hours, then the individual may not be protected from pregnancy and needs to use a back-up method for 7 consecutive days in addition to reinserting the ring.[14]

If the individual fails to remove the ring and no more than 28 days has passed since they first inserted this ring, they should remove it and insert a new ring. They may or may not experience a withdrawal bleed, but contraceptive protection is maintained.

Like the patch, the ring may retain some residual active agent and should be carefully discarded away from children and pets. If more than 28 days has passed since a NuvaRing was initially inserted, the individual may not be protected from pregnancy. They should perform a pregnancy test. If the test is negative, they should insert a new ring and use a back-up method for 7 days.

## Injectable Depot Medroxyprogesterone Acetate Contraceptives

Depot medroxyprogesterone acetate (DMPA) is an injectable hormonal method. Injectable contraception is highly effective, is reversible, does not require

partner participation, avoids daily need for intervention, and is not coital dependent.

### Mechanism of Action of Depot Medroxyprogesterone Acetate

DMPA is a derivative of progesterone. Its primary mechanism of action is inhibition of ovulation by prevention of follicular maturation. Secondary mechanisms of action include thickening of cervical mucus, which serves as a barrier to sperm, and induction of endometrial atrophy, which reduces the likelihood of implantation.[3] Like other steroidal hormones, DMPA is metabolized by the liver and excreted in the urine.[10]

Two formulations of DMPA are available, both of which require a prescription. The first is DMPA-IM 150 mg/mL (Depo-Provera), which is contained in a 1-mL vial or prefilled syringe and administered every 13 weeks intramuscularly. DMPA is detected in the serum within 30 minutes after an injection of 150 mg of this formulation. Serum concentrations vary, but gradually plateau for approximately 3 months, after which the serum concentration gradually declines.

The second formulation is DMPA-SC 104 (Depo-subQ Provera 104), an agent administered subcutaneously every 13 weeks that has been found to be equally effective in inhibiting ovulation. The Depo-subQ Provera 104-mg dose and serum levels are approximately 30% lower than those found with the standard DMPA-IM 150-mg dose. This formulation has been shown to have equal, if not improved, tolerability, as side effects of DMPA are dose dependent.[99]

### Special Considerations for Use of Depot Medroxyprogesterone Acetate

The major and most common side effects of DMPA are menstrual changes, irregular bleeding, weight gain, headaches, and delayed return of fertility. The overall incidence of irregular bleeding experienced by individuals using DMPA can be as high as 70% in the first year of use.[100] Variations usually begin as episodes of unpredictable irregular bleeding and spotting that may last as long as 7 days or more or may be heavy during the first few months. These episodes gradually become less frequent and of shorter duration until the individual has amenorrhea. Approximately 10% to 30% of individuals experience amenorrhea after one injection, and 40% to 50% do so by the fourth injection. The rates of irregular bleeding and amenorrhea are similar for the subcutaneous and intramuscular formulations.[2]

Weight gain is often noted as a concern among individuals using DMPA. Studies of weight gain in users of DMPA have yielded variable results. The largest systematic review failed to find a consistent association of DMPA with significant increase in weight among users.[101] Nevertheless, in some observational trials individuals who are obese have gained additional weight, suggesting special attention should be given to counseling for these individuals.[102]

The use of progestins may cause fluid retention. Certain conditions may, in turn, be exacerbated by this fluid retention, such as headache. Perhaps not surprisingly, then, headaches have been reported among users of DMPA contraceptives. Individuals who develop migraines with aura should stop using DMPA (U.S. MEC Category 3) because aura is a specific risk for stroke.[15] However, studies examining the use of natural progesterone or progestin use have found these agents to be associated with a decreased frequency of migraines.[103] Therefore, a history of headaches is not necessarily a contraindication to initiation of DMPA,[15] but individuals should be counseled to report the development of headaches to their healthcare provider. If an individual develops severe headaches while using DMPA, they should have a thorough evaluation to diagnose the type of headache they experience.

Long-term users of DMPA may develop temporary, but usually reversible, decreased bone density, with declines ranging from 5% to 7% in the hip and spine.[104–106] DMPA suppresses gonadotropin secretion, which in turn suppresses ovarian estradiol production. In this hypoestrogenic state, bone resorption outpaces bone formation, resulting in a decline in bone mineral density. Based on studies of adolescents, bone loss appears to be greatest during the first 2 years of use, but then slows dramatically.[107] Bone density has been shown to return to baseline following discontinuation of DMPA in individuals of all ages, with this effect being seen as early as 24 weeks after stopping therapy.[108] Observational studies have suggested a possible increased fracture risk among DMPA users, but study designs limit a fuller understanding of causation.[25] Given these findings, individuals with conditions that place them at high risk for osteoporosis and fracture, such as chronic corticosteroid use, disorders of bone metabolism, a strong family history of osteoporosis, or anorexia nervosa, may not be well suited for long-term DMPA use. Likewise, individuals who have other risk factors that may contribute to lower bone mineral density, such as low calcium intake, high alcohol intake, and lower BMI, should be evaluated carefully to assess suitability of DMPA use.

Concerns regarding bone loss caused the FDA to mandate a black box warning be placed on the label for DMPA. This warning includes the recommendation that DMPA be limited to a 2-year period of use. However, concerns regarding bone mass density alone should not prevent providers from prescribing DMPA for longer periods of time.[25]

Studies have been inconsistent regarding the effects of DMPA on mood changes.[100] Administration of DMPA in the immediate postpartum period does not appear to predispose individuals to postpartum depression.[109]

DMPA was thought to cause changes within the vaginal environment and cervical ectopy that could increase susceptibility to STIs, but recent data collected in sub-Saharan Africa show no changes in broad inflammatory or microbiota changes among DMPA users.[110] DMPA is therefore a safe method to offer individuals at increased risk for STIs and HIV, even though the evidence of the just-mentioned physiologic changes remains inconclusive. Other potential side effects include nervousness, decreased libido, breast discomfort, dizziness, hair loss, and bloating.[100] Among those individuals using the subcutaneous formulation, some report an indentation or induration at the injection site (granuloma or atrophy) or other minor skin reactions.

Return to fertility for individuals using DMPA tends to take longer than for individuals using other hormonal methods. The median time to conception is 9 to 10 months after the last injection.[2] A systematic review indicated that resumption of ovulation can occur anywhere from 15 to 49 weeks after the last injection, making it difficult to predict when pregnancy could occur for an individual who may wish to become pregnant.[111]

Detectable amounts of the drug have been found in the human milk of individuals receiving DMPA; however, no adverse changes in milk composition, quality, or amount have been identified. There is much concern about postpartum administration of DMPA interfering with lactation, given that the decline of natural progesterone triggers milk synthesis. However, this hypothesis is not supported by data on postpartum DMPA administration and lactation.[31]

## Care of Individuals Requesting Depot Medroxyprogesterone Acetate

DMPA can be administered at any time in a menstrual cycle if the individual is reasonably certain that they are not pregnant. However, if it is given later than the seventh day in the menstrual cycle, the individual should use back-up contraception for 7 days and receive a follow-up pregnancy test several weeks later to confirm the absence of an early pregnancy prior to a second dose of DMPA. If DMPA is initiated within the first 5 to 7 days of the menstrual cycle, a pregnancy test is unnecessary; however, a pregnancy test is warranted if DMPA is initiated outside of this period. Individuals can safely continue to use DMPA until menopause.

Fewer absolute (U.S. MEC Category 4) contraindications exist for DMPA compared to COCs, but the relative contraindications (U.S. MEC Criteria for Contraceptive Use Category 3) include several major conditions as well as unexplained vaginal bleeding. The complete list of contraindications is available through the U.S. MEC.[15]

DMPA is injected either subcutaneously or intramuscularly, depending on the formulation. Massaging the injection site can lower the effectiveness of the DMPA.[2] Ovulation does not occur for at least 14 weeks post injection. If the individual is more than 2 weeks late for their subsequent dose, a pregnancy test is recommended prior to administration to assure they are not pregnant.[7] Various methods of appointment reminders are available.

Starting at 13 weeks post injection, use of a secondary contraceptive method is recommended until the next dose is given. Conversely, subsequent injections may be administered up to 10 weeks after the previous DMPA injection without adverse effects. Table 12-12 provides important information for individuals regarding DMPA injections.

## Long-Acting Reversible Contraceptives

LARCs include implants and IUDs. Once inserted, these methods confer contraceptive protection for years. Although these methods have a higher initial expense, their long-term use tends to make them cost-effective. These methods require no regular dosing by the individual, which means they are very effective at preventing pregnancy.

## Subdermal Implants

Implantable contraceptives consist of one or more matchstick-sized rods or tubes containing progestin. These implants are inserted beneath the top layers of skin, on the inner aspect of the upper arm. Depending on the model of implant, subdermal devices can provide contraception for up to 7 years.

The first subdermal implant available in the United States was Norplant, which consists of six plastic tubes containing the progestin levonorgestrel. In 2002, the manufacturer removed Norplant from the U.S. market, citing limited availability of

| Table 12-12 | Educational Content to Be Emphasized When Counseling Individuals Using Depot Medroxyprogesterone Acetate[a,b] |
|---|---|

Individuals should eat a diet high in calcium and vitamin D to support bone health. Risks related to bone health for an individual at low risk for osteoporosis or fractures should not be a reason to discontinue DMPA after 2 years.

Although such outcomes are rare, an individual should be aware of and report any signs or symptoms of infection at the injection site, such as a fever, or changes at the insertion site, including drainage, redness, and warmth.

Irregular spotting is common after the first injection and decreases with subsequent injections.

Other conditions that should be reported to a healthcare provider:
- Significant headaches
- Menorrhagia
- Depression
- Severe lower abnormal pain or any other signs or symptoms that may suggest pregnancy

[a] In addition to the information in Table 12-6.
[b] Education counseling is primarily based on expert opinion and common practice. Little strong evidence exists in this area.

product components. Although Norplant is not currently available in the United States, it continues to be used internationally. An individual may have Norplant inserted outside the country; it may be retained up to 7 years.[112]

Although more implants may be available in the future, the only subdermal implant currently available in the United States is an etonogestrel-containing, single-rod device.[113] Nexplanon entered the U.S. market in 2012, replacing its predecessor Implanon. Implanon and Nexplanon are biologically equivalent.

### Mechanism of Action of Subdermal Implants

Nexplanon is a polyethylene vinyl rod, 4 cm in length and 2 mm in diameter, that is impregnated with 68 mg of etonogestrel, a progestin analogue, and 12 mg of barium sulfate. This latter substance makes the device detectable by X ray. Nexplanon works by continuously releasing etonogestrel to suppress ovulation. Although Nexplanon is approved for 3 years of use, data suggest it is effective to use a single rod for up to 5 years.[114]

### Special Considerations for Use of Subdermal Contraceptive Implants

As with most long-acting contraceptive devices, the initial costs of subdermal implants are significantly higher when compared to the costs of SARCs. However, when averaged over 3 to 5 years of use, the total costs of subdermal implants usually make these options less expensive than COCs, POPs, or DMPA. At the time of implant removal, a new device can be reinserted in the same site, thereby providing continuing contraception if desired.

### Care of the Individual Requesting a Subdermal Contraceptive Implant

Based on an agreement between the manufacturer of Nexplanon and the FDA, implants are available for dispensing only to providers who have completed a 3-hour training session focusing on identifying individuals who are candidates for the implant as well as health counseling, insertion, and removal. Individuals who have completed Implanon training previously can update their training online. This chapter does not address the specifics of Implanon insertion or removal (see the *Implant Insertion and Removal* appendix).

Contraindications for implants can be found in the U.S. MEC.[15] No specific physical or laboratory assessment is recommended before insertion, with the exception of being reasonably certain that the individual is not pregnant. Monitoring for detrimental side effects, menstrual pattern, blood pressure, and user satisfaction can be done at a follow-up visit approximately 3 months following insertion. Limited data are available regarding the use of implants by lactating individuals; small amounts of etonogestrel have been observed in human milk.[32] Table 12-13 lists health education topics for individuals using the subdermal implant.

| Table 12-13 | Educational Content to Be Emphasized When Counseling Individuals Using Subdermal Contraceptive Implants[a] |
|---|---|

Although rare, an individual should be aware of and report the following:

- Signs or symptoms of infection at the insertion site, such as a fever
- Changes at the insertion site, including drainage, redness, and warmth

[a] In addition to the information in Table 12-6.

When an individual wishes to discontinue use of this contraceptive method, removal of the implant is usually performed easily during an office visit. Often this is scheduled at the 3- to 5-year mark, but some individuals may desire to continue with the method. In that case, a new implant can be placed into the small incision created for removal.

Providers may occasionally find it difficult to remove an implant. Removal, however, is never an emergency. The first action should be to verify placement by ultrasound imaging to confirm that the implant is still present as well as to determine its location.

On rare occasions, the implant may inadvertently be placed very deep (in muscle or fascia). Should such a situation occur, providers are encouraged to consult with, or refer the individual to, a specialist, especially a specialist at one of the Family Planning Fellowship training sites around the country. At these sites, the contraceptive specialist will collaborate with an interventional radiologist to remove the implant, and a surgeon if needed.

## Hormonal Intrauterine Devices

Two types of IUDs exist: nonhormonal and hormonal. The *Nonhormonal Contraception* chapter provides general information and explains use of intrauterine contraceptive devices. Most adverse effects, timing for insertion, and removal are the same for both types of IUDs, and are described in the *Intrauterine Device Insertion and Removal* appendix. This chapter focuses on details specific to the levonorgestrel-releasing IUD, the hormonal device.

### Mechanism of Action of Levonorgestrel-Releasing Intrauterine Device

The levonorgestrel-releasing IUD (LNG-IUD) is a T-shaped, flexible polyethylene device widely marketed in the United States. The body of the device includes a reservoir that contains levonorgestrel, a progestin. The LNG-IUD provides for continuous release of levonorgestrel, which is absorbed locally by the endometrium and results in increased viscosity of cervical mucus, remodeling of the endometrial lining, and impaired tubal motility.[3] As a result of these localized effects, sperm motility is impaired, thereby inhibiting fertilization of the ovum. A possible secondary mechanism of action is suppression of ovulation.

The LNG-IUD is a long-acting contraceptive method, which is cost-effective when used over a period of years. Individuals who have an aversion to checking for the device strings regularly may not desire this method. A few individuals experience IUD-associated side effects such as bleeding changes or pain, and others simply do not like the idea of having a foreign object inside their body.[115]

In 2000, the FDA approved the first LNG-IUD, which is marketed with the brand name Mirena. The Mirena IUD releases an average of 20 mcg of levonorgestrel per day and provides contraception for up to 5 years. This device measures 33 mm long by 32 mm wide. The FDA approved an additional indication for use of this device as a therapeutic agent for individuals with menorrhagia in 2009. Subsequent studies have found that the LNG-IUD is more effective than oral therapy and, although not as effective in reducing bleeding as a hysterectomy, more cost-effective than the surgery.[116] As compared to the copper IUD (see the *Nonhormonal Contraception* chapter), the LNG-IUD is associated with decreased bleeding, decreased dysmenorrhea, and a greater likelihood of amenorrhea. Commonly accepted contraindications for this type of IUD include uterine anomalies, acute pelvic inflammatory disease, pregnancy, breast cancer, and unexplained vaginal bleeding.[15]

Today, four different LNG-IUDs are available in the United States (**Table 12-14**). These devices contain different amounts of levonorgestrel and have different FDA-approved durations (i.e., years of use). No specific guidelines exist regarding matching an individual with a particular IUD. Mirena and Liletta are approximately 4 mm wider and 2 mm longer than the other devices and might be more easily tolerated by a parous individual. These two LNG-IUDs release higher levels of daily levonorgestrel, and are more likely to be associated with amenorrhea, which may or may not be desired. Because of the dosing, they may be indicated for individuals with heavier

bleeding. Mirena provides the longest duration of action, with Liletta offering the second longest duration. As with all methods, cost, availability, and personal desires of the individuals seeking contraception must be considered when selecting an LNG-IUD.

## Special Considerations for Use of Levonorgestrel-Releasing Intrauterine Device

The IUD insertion and removal procedures carry some risks, even though they are only minimally invasive. Bleeding, infection, perforation of the uterus, and pain can occur, although serious complications are rare. While IUDs do not cause ectopic pregnancy, if fertilization occurs with an IUD in place, there is a greater risk of ectopic implantation. It is important to underscore, however, that the overall risk of ectopic pregnancy for an individual with any IUD is lower than the risk of ectopic pregnancy for an individual not using contraception.

The *Intrauterine Device Insertion and Removal* appendix provides detailed information on the insertion and removal of both nonhormonal (copper) IUDs as well as the four types of LNG-IUDs. Information about pre-insertion medication, STI screening, timing of insertion, and immediate adverse effects may also be found in this appendix. Management of an individual with a pregnancy and an IUD in situ, expulsion of the device, and associated ectopic pregnancies are the same for copper IUDs and LNG-IUDs and are discussed in detail in the *Nonhormonal Contraception* chapter.

## Care of the Individual Requesting a Levonorgestrel-Releasing Intrauterine Device

Most individuals, including adolescents and nulliparous individuals, are good candidates for intrauterine contraception.[7] Category 3 and 4 contraindications

| Table 12-14 | Intrauterine Devices Containing Levonorgestrel | | | |
|---|---|---|---|---|
| Brand Name | Total Dose of LNG in Device (mg) | Initial Release of LNG (mcg/day) | Size | Years of FDA Approval[a] |
| Liletta | 52 | 18.6 | 32 mm horizontal and vertical | 6 |
| Kyleena | 19.5 | 17.5 | 28 mm horizontal and 30 mm vertical | 5 |
| Mirena | 52 | 20 | 32 mm horizontal and vertical | 8 |
| Skyla | 13.5 | 14 | 28 mm horizontal and 30 mm vertical | 3 |

Abbreviations: FDA, Food and Drug Administration; LNG, levonorgestrel.
[a] FDA approval may change, given that ongoing studies tend to suggest longer-term use is effective.

| Table 12-15 | Educational Content to Be Emphasized When Counseling Individuals Using an LNG-IUD[a] |
|---|---|

Individuals should verify that the device is in situ by feeling for the strings at least monthly.

The mnemonic PAINS can be used to remind individuals of conditions that should be reported to the provider:

**P**eriod—late or abnormal bleeding (although this is relatively common for these individuals)

**A**bdominal pain or dyspareunia

**I**nfection, especially associated with exposure to sexually transmitted infection or an abnormal vaginal discharge

**N**ot feeling well, especially if the individual experiences fever, chills, or generalized malaise

**S**trings missing or inability to feel the plastic thread of the device

[a] In addition to the information in Table 12-6.

are outlined in the U.S. MEC, and include current pelvic inflammatory disease, breast cancer, endometrial cancer, severe cirrhosis, suspicion of intrauterine disease including chlamydia, gonorrhea, and tuberculosis.[15] Individuals should not have an IUD inserted immediately postpartum or post abortion if sepsis is present.

Table 12-15 lists information to be reviewed when counseling individuals using an LNG-IUD.

# Emergency Contraception

Misnamed as postcoital or morning-after contraception, this contraceptive method is more appropriately termed *emergency contraception*. This form of contraception is not intended as a regular method of birth control unless the individual has infrequent sexual intercourse. It is recommended either when there has been a method failure, such as condom breakage, or after unintended unprotected intercourse. Emergency contraception may be used anytime in the first 3 to 5 days after unprotected intercourse depending on the method chosen. Individuals seeking contraceptive services should be counseled about the availability and correct use of emergency contraception.

Four methods of emergency contraception are currently available in the United States: (1) the Yuzpe method; (2) LNG oral formulations (Plan B One Step, Next Choice One Dose, Take Action); (3) selective progesterone receptor modulators

(ulipristal acetate [UPA; ella]); and (4) the copper IUD. The dose, efficacy, timing, availability, U.S. MEC rating, and clinical conditions for these methods are summarized in Table 12-16. The LNG-IUD is also being tested as emergency contraception and will likely become a more commonly used method of emergency contraception over the next few years.[117,118] Additionally, 10 mg of mifepristone taken within 120 hours of unprotected intercourse is highly effective and available internationally. Because of laws restricting and limiting access to abortion, however, it is not used for these purposes in the United States.[2]

## Hormonal Emergency Contraception: Mechanisms of Action

The mechanism of action of hormonal emergency contraception methods is inhibition and/or delay of ovulation secondary to suppression, delaying, or blunting the LH surge, depending on when in the menstrual cycle the contraceptive pill is ingested.[119] Oral contraceptive and LNG formulations for pregnancy prevention do not effectively prevent follicular rupture if used in the late preovulatory stage; thus, these two methods are most effective if used prior to ovulation and as soon as possible after unprotected intercourse. UPA does prevent follicular rupture if taken before the onset of the LH surge and reduces endometrial thickness, thereby making the endometrium less hospitable for implantation of an embryo.[119] Hormonal emergency contraception methods do not interfere with a conceptus that has already implanted and present no risk to that embryo.[119]

Calculating effectiveness rates for emergency contraception is complex because accurately estimating when ovulation occurs relative to the timing of sexual intercourse is difficult, and some research reports use different statistics to report estimated efficacy. In general, emergency contraception is most effective when the interval between intercourse and use is short. Longer intervals result in decreased effectiveness.[120]

## The Yuzpe Method

The Yuzpe method, an eponymous regimen that was first published by a Canadian scientist in the 1970s, is the oldest of the current emergency contraception methods. This method involves the ingestion of high doses of estrogen and progestin, which is accomplished by administering several COC pills in a single dose to inhibit ovulation. More than 25 brands of COCs can be used with this method.

| Table 12-16 | Emergency Contraception in the United States | | | | |
|---|---|---|---|---|---|
| Brand Name | Estimated Efficacy[a] | Timing After Intercourse[b] | Availability | U.S. MEC | Clinical Considerations |
| **FDA-Approved Emergency Contraception** | | | | | |
| Plan B One Step<br>Next Choice One Dose<br>Take Action<br>My Way<br>Other generics | 1.2–2.1% failure rate | Within 72 hours | No prescription No age restriction | 1 or 2 | May be less effective for individuals with BMI ≥ 26, may consider double dose with BMI ≥ 30.<br>Avoid use of CYP3A4 inducers at same time. |
| ella (Ulipristal acetate [UPA]) (1 pill) | 1.2% failure rate | Within 120 hours | Prescription only | 1 or 2 | May reduce contraceptive action of progestin-containing hormonal contraceptive methods because of its affinity for binding to the progesterone receptor; SPR recommends hormonal contraception delay for 5 days with abstinence for 7 days post UPA, although depot medroxyprogesterone acetate can be started simultaneously with UPA.<br>Avoid use of CYP3A4 inducers at same time.<br>Discard breast milk for 24 hours after administration due to higher concentrations in milk. |
| **Not FDA-Approved Emergency Contraception But Available** | | | | | |
| Combined oral contraceptives | 1.3–1.5% failure rate | Within 72 hours | Prescription only | 1–2 | Also known as the Yuzpe method. More than 25 brands can be used. |
| ParaGard copper IUD | < 1% failure rate | Within 120 hours | Prescription only | 1–3[c] | U.S. MEC level varies based on risk of sexually transmitted diseases. |

Abbreviations: BMI, body mass index; FDA, Food and Drug Administration; IUD, intrauterine device; SPR, *U.S. Selected Practice Recommendations for Contraceptive Use, 2016*; U.S. MEC, *U.S. Medical Eligibility Criteria for Contraceptive Use, 2016*.

[a] Studies report different metrics regarding efficacy.

[b] Per package insert/manufacturer's guide. Some methods have been studied only up the time noted but may be effective longer.

[c] For use as emergency contraception. For use as an intrauterine device, other rare conditions, such as a distorted uterine cavity, may also preclude use. See https://www.cdc.gov/reproductivehealth/contraception/pdf/summary-chart-us-medical-eligibility-criteria_508tagged.pdf.

Based on Curtis KM, Tepper NK, Jatlaoui TC, et al. U.S. medical eligibility criteria for contraceptive use, 2016. *MMWR Recomm Rep.* 2016;65(3):1-103; Curtis KM, Jatlaoui TC, Tepper NK, et al. U.S. selected practice recommendations for contraceptive use, 2016. *MMWR Recomm Rep.* 2016;65(4):1-66; Haeger KO, Lamme J, Cleland K. State of emergency contraception in the U.S., 2018. *Contracept Reprod Med.* 2018;3:20. doi:10.1186/s40834-018-0067-8.

Studies of the Yuzpe method have focused on pills containing 100 to 120 mg ethinyl estradiol and either norgestrel or levonorgestrel. No published studies have been conducted using combined pills that include gestodene, etonorgestrel, or other progestins, so pills containing these ingredients are not recommended as emergency contraception.[2]

This contraceptive method frequently causes nausea, vomiting, headache, vertigo, and breast tenderness. The individual may also experience irregular bleeding or spotting in the 3 to 4 weeks following treatment. Because of the dosing regimen and the frequency of bothersome side effects, this method is not recommended unless no other method is available.[120] However, the Yuzpe method may be a good choice if an individual has difficulty obtaining other dedicated emergency contraception methods because of age or lack of availability of these methods in the geographic area, or already has pills on hand that can be easily taken.

## Levonorgestrel: Plan B One Step and Next Choice One Dose

Single-dose LNG is the most widely used method of emergency contraception in the United States. The LNG formulations are more effective and have fewer side effects than those that contain both estrogen and progestins. LNG primarily inhibits or delays ovulation by preventing the LH surge if taken before the surge occurs. If taken close to or during the LH surge, it blunts and delays the surge and makes the ovum resistant to fertilization.[119]

LNG for emergency contraception is formulated under the brand name Plan B One Step as well as a variety of other brand and generic names. When using a one-dose product, according to the package insert, a single dose of 1.5 mg LNG is taken within 72 hours following unprotected intercourse, although some research suggests this method may still be somewhat effective up to 120 hours post intercourse.[121] If vomiting occurs within 3 hours of taking a single-dose LNG, a repeat dose should be considered.[7]

Recent data suggest that obesity interferes with the pharmacokinetics of LNG emergency contraception, resulting in lower total and bioavailable amounts of LNG.[122,123] Therefore, among individuals with a BMI of 30 or greater, doubling the dose or using another method, such as ella, may be prudent.

## Ulipristal Acetate

In 2010, UPA, a selective progesterone receptor modulator marketed under the brand name ella, received FDA approval for use as emergency contraception. Thus, UPA is the first—and to date only—selective progesterone receptor modulator agent available for emergency contraception in the United States. Selective progesterone receptor modulators bind to progesterone receptors and inhibit or delay ovulation, depending on when the agent is taken during the menstrual cycle. If used during the midfollicular phase, UPA prevents follicular rupture. When this agent is taken in the late follicular phase, it delays the normal LH surge, thereby delaying ovulation.[119]

UPA appears to be more effective as emergency contraception than either the Yuzpe method or single-dose LNG, and can be effective up to 120 hours after unprotected intercourse—an effect attributed to its ability to prevent follicular rupture, although its effectiveness does decrease with time.[124] Side effects are the same as those reported for the Yuzpe method and LNG, but occur less frequently. Because most of these side effects are also symptoms of pregnancy, it is not clear exactly which ones occur secondary to administration of the drug. This method is more effective, can be taken longer after coitus occurs, and is highly effective regardless of body weight when compared to LNG emergency contraception; however, it is currently available only by prescription, so it is less commonly used.[120]

## Contraindications to Hormonal Emergency Contraception

The major contraindication to the use of any method of emergency contraception is a known pregnancy. Oral formulations of emergency contraception are contraindicated in pregnancy because they are ineffective; the contraindication is not related to concerns about teratogenicity.[43] Because these hormones are taken in low doses for a short period of time, individuals with health conditions for which oral contraceptives are contraindicated can use emergency contraception safely.

Although adverse drug–drug interactions have not been reported by individuals using oral emergency contraception, adverse drug interactions are possible. Anticonvulsants such as phenobarbital (Luminal), carbamazepine (Tegretol), and phenytoin (Dilantin) activate the CYP450 system and could decrease effectiveness of the contraceptive. Other drugs that interfere with the metabolism of oral contraceptive agents include rifampin (Rifadin), topiramate (Topamax), and St. John's wort.[125]

## Copper Intrauterine Device

The copper IUD (ParaGard) can be used as emergency contraception when inserted within 120 hours (5 days) following intercourse and is the most effective emergency contraception method currently available.[120] The IUD is not effective for emergency contraception if inserted after the fertilized egg has implanted in the uterus, which normally occurs 6 to 12 days after ovulation. The technique for insertion is described in the *Intrauterine Device Insertion and Removal* appendix.

The pregnancy rate following insertion of a copper IUD is approximately 0.1%.[126] The copper IUD alters tubal transport, is toxic to the ovum, and incapacitates sperm, thereby preventing fertilization.[119] Unlike oral formulations of emergency contraception, the copper IUD also creates an inhospitable uterine environment for implantation.[119] If an individual is a candidate for intrauterine contraception, placement of a copper IUD for emergency contraception offers the additional advantage of establishing an ongoing contraceptive method. Note that the LNG-IUD is not currently indicated for emergency contraception, but may be soon.

### Contraindications to Use of the Copper IUD for Emergency Contraception

General contraindications to use of a copper IUD are reviewed in detail in the *Nonhormonal Contraception* chapter. Insertion of a copper IUD for emergency contraception after rape is an important topic to review. The U.S. MEC category for insertion of a copper IUD for emergency contraception is 3 if the individual has a high risk for being exposed to an STI, but is 1 if they have a low risk for being exposed to an STI.[15] There are no agreed-upon definitions for what constitutes high risk versus low risk for STI. In addition, the U.S. MEC category 3 means that the theoretical risks generally outweigh the advantages.

### Special Considerations for Dispensing Emergency Contraception

Some pharmacies may opt out of dispensing emergency contraception methods, and a number of states protect their right to do so, as well as the rights of providers and other professionals who do not choose to provide contraception.[127] In such cases, the Yuzpe regimen may be recommended. Many healthcare professionals regularly and proactively prescribe emergency contraception for individuals using a SARC method in case of missing COCs, breakage of a condom, or other circumstances.[83]

Many national women's health organizations recommend that all individuals who are victims of sexual assault be offered emergency contraception.[128] Some states mandate that individuals must be offered emergency contraception after rape. State laws can change, however, so the provider should determine the specific state laws that apply. In any case, the provider who may care for an individual post assault should discuss whether they have either received appropriate information or been treated with emergency contraception.

### Follow-Up Care

Individuals who need emergency contraception should also be offered screening for STIs including HIV infection. Individuals using emergency contraception may be counseled to return for evaluation 1 to 3 weeks following use of this treatment, specifically to assess the result of emergency contraception and discuss ongoing contraceptive needs, although this follow-up visit is not considered a necessary component of emergency contraception care by all professional organizations.

In most situations, a suitable method of contraception can be started as soon as possible after the individual has used an emergency contraception method. Individuals who use hormonal emergency contraception can initiate any contraceptive method immediately, but are advised to use a barrier method or abstinence for the next 7 days.[7] Because UPA has a unique mechanism of action, using a hormonal contraceptive simultaneously can decrease the effectiveness of both methods. Therefore, individuals using UPA should also use a barrier method or abstinence until the next menses, although they can begin a hormonal contraceptive method 5 days after ingestion of UPA.[7] Individuals using a copper IUD have both immediate and continuing contraceptive protection.

### Health Education

Individuals using emergency contraception should be advised that the next menses may be delayed after using an oral regimen. It is important to be evaluated for pregnancy if menses does not occur within 3 weeks after emergency contraception use.[7] Individuals should also be counseled about signs of ectopic pregnancy and advised to contact a healthcare provider as soon as possible if they develop severe abdominal pain at any point after using the emergency contraception method.

## Conclusion

Over the last half-century, hormonal contraceptives have expanded from a drug category that included only combined pills to a repertoire of effective methods such as progestin-only pills, transdermal patches, intrauterine devices, vaginal rings, and implants. Hormonal contraception, like nonhormonal methods, is not a "one size fits all" situation: Individuals should choose the option that best fits their unique circumstances. An individual's decision should consider their desires and priorities, their own eligibility, the conceptive method's effectiveness, noncontraceptive benefits, and the individual's ability to use the method correctly and consistently.

### Resources

| Organization | Description |
|---|---|
| Centers for Disease Control and Prevention (CDC) | *U.S. Medical Eligibility Criteria for Contraceptive Use* (U.S. MEC)<br><br>*U.S. Selected Practice Recommendations for Contraceptive Use* (U.S. SPR) |
| Monthly Prescribing Reference (MPR) | Monographs, charts, and app that list all current oral contraceptives by brand name and their components |

## References

1. Liao PV, Dollin J. Half a century of the oral contraceptive pill: historical review and view to the future. *Can Fam Physician*. 2012;58(12):e757-760.

2. Hatcher RA. *Contraceptive Technology*. 21st ed. New York, NY: Managing Contraception, LLC; 2018.

3. Rivera R, Yacobson I, Grimes D. The mechanism of action of hormonal contraceptives and intrauterine contraceptive devices. *Am J Obstet Gynecol*. 1999;181(5):1263-1269. doi:10.1016/S0002-9378(99)70120-1.

4. Brucker MC, King TL. *Pharmacology for Women's Health*. 2nd ed. Burlington, MA: Jones & Bartlett Learning; 2017.

5. Yu Q, Zhou Y, Suturina L, et al. Efficacy and safety of estradiol valerate/dienogest for the management of heavy menstrual bleeding: a multicenter, double-blind, randomized, placebo-controlled, Phase III clinical trial. *J Womens Health (Larchmt)*. 2018;27(10):1225-1232. doi:10.1089/jwh.2017.6522.

6. Westhoff CL, Eisenberger A, Tang R, et al. Clotting factor changes during the first cycle of oral contraceptive use. *Contraception*. 2016;93(1):70-76. doi:10.1016/j.contraception.2015.09.015.

7. Curtis KM, Jatlaoui TC, Tepper NK, et al. U.S. Selected practice recommendations for contraceptive use, 2016. *MMWR Recomm Rep*. 2016;65. doi:10.15585/mmwr.rr6504a1.

8. Regidor PA. The clinical relevance of progestogens in hormonal contraception: present status and future developments. *Oncotarget*. 2018;9(77):34628-34638. doi:10.18632/oncotarget.26015.

9. Girum T, Wasie A. Return of fertility after discontinuation of contraception: a systematic review and meta-analysis. *Contracept Reprod Med*. 2018;3:9. doi:10.1186/s40834-018-0064-y.

10. Food and Drug Administration. Depo-Provera prescribing information. https://www.accessdata.fda.gov/drugsatfda_docs/label/2010/020246s036lbl.pdf. Revised October 2010. Accessed March 12, 2023.

11. Yland JJ, Bresnick KA, Hatch EE, et al. Pregravid contraceptive use and fecundability: prospective cohort study. *BMJ*. 2020;371:m3966. doi:10.1136/bmj.m3966.

12. Raidoo S, Kaneshiro B. Contraception counseling for adolescents. *Curr Opin Obstet Gynecol*. 2017;29(5):310-315. doi:10.1097/GCO.0000000000000390.

13. Long ME, Faubion SS, MacLaughlin KL, et al. Contraception and hormonal management in the perimenopause. *J Womens Health (Larchmt)*. 2015;24(1):3-10. doi:10.1089/jwh.2013.4544.

14. Jin P, Xie Y. Treatment strategies for women with polycystic ovary syndrome. *Gynecol Endocrinol*. 2018;34(4):272-277. doi:10.1080/09513590.2017.1395841.

15. Curtis KM, Tepper N, Jatlaoui T. U.S. medical eligibility criteria for contraceptive use, 2016. *MMWR Recomm Rep*. 2016;65. doi:10.15585/mmwr.rr6503a1.

16. Shenfield GM, Griffin JM. Clinical pharmacokinetics of contraceptive steroids: an update. *Clin Pharmacokinet*. 1991;20(1):15-37. doi:10.2165/00003088-199120010-00002.

17. Lopez LM, Chen M, Mullins Long S, et al. Steroidal contraceptives and bone fractures in women: evidence from observational studies. *Cochrane Database Syst Rev*. 2015;7:CD009849. doi:10.1002/14651858.CD009849.pub3.

18. Skovlund CW, Mørch LS, Kessing LV, Lidegaard Ø. Association of hormonal contraception with depression. *JAMA Psychiatry*. 2016;73(11):1154-1162. doi:10.1001/jamapsychiatry.2016.2387.

19. Roos-Hesselink JW, Cornette J, Sliwa K, et al. Contraception and cardiovascular disease. *Eur Heart J*. 2015;36(27):1728-1734, 1734a-1734b. doi:10.1093/eurheartj/ehv141.

20. Mørch LS, Skovlund CW, Hannaford PC, et al. Contemporary hormonal contraception and the risk of breast cancer. *N Engl J Med*. 2017;377(23):2228-2239. doi:10.1056/NEJMoa1700732.

21. Karlsson T, Johansson T, Höglund J, et al. Time-dependent effects of oral contraceptive use on breast, ovarian and endometrial cancers. *Cancer Res*. December 2020. doi:10.1158/0008-5472.CAN-20-2476.

22. de Bastos M, Stegeman BH, Rosendaal FR, et al. Combined oral contraceptives: venous thrombosis. *Cochrane Database Syst Rev*. 2014;3:CD010813. doi:10.1002/14651858.CD010813.pub2.

23. Nicolussi S, Drewe J, Butterweck V, et al. Clinical relevance of St. John's wort drug interactions revisited. *Br J Pharmacol*. 2020;177(6):1212-1226. doi:10.1111/bph.14936.

24. Berry-Bibee EN, Kim MJ, Tepper NK, et al. Co-administration of St. John's wort and hormonal contraceptives: a systematic review. *Contraception*. 2016;94(6):668-677. doi:10.1016/j.contraception.2016.07.010.

25. Committee Opinion No. 602: depot medroxyprogesterone acetate and bone effects. *Obstet Gynecol*. 2014;123(6):1398-1402. doi:10.1097/01.AOG.0000450758.95422.c8.

26. Apter D. Contraception options: aspects unique to adolescent and young adult. *Best Pract Res Clin Obstet Gynaecol*. 2018;48:115-127. doi:10.1016/j.bpobgyn.2017.09.010.

27. Committee Opinion No 699: adolescent pregnancy, contraception, and sexual activity. *Obstet Gynecol*. 2017;129(5):e142-e149. doi:10.1097/AOG.0000000000002045.

28. Carpenter E. "The health system just wasn't built for us": queer cisgender women and gender expansive

individuals' strategies for navigating reproductive health care. *Womens Health Issues.* 2021;31(5): 478-484. doi:10.1016/j.whi.2021.06.004.

29. Greene MZ, Carpenter E, Hendrick CE, et al. Sexual minority women's experiences with sexual identity disclosure in contraceptive care. *Obstet Gynecol.* 2019;133(5):1012-1023. doi:10.1097/AOG .0000000000003222.

30. Boudreau D, Mukerjee R. Contraception care for transmasculine individuals on testosterone therapy. *J Midwifery Womens Health.* 2019;64(4):395-402. doi:10.1111/jmwh.12962.

31. Lopez LM, Grey TW, Stuebe AM, et al. Combined hormonal versus nonhormonal versus progestin-only contraception in lactation. *Cochrane Database Syst Rev.* 2015;3:CD003988. doi:10.1002/14651858. CD003988.pub2.

32. Phillips SJ, Tepper NK, Kapp N, et al. Progestogen-only contraceptive use among breastfeeding women: a systematic review. *Contraception.* 2016;94(3): 226-252. doi:10.1016/j.contraception.2015.09.010.

33. Stanton TA, Blumenthal PD. Postpartum hormonal contraception in breastfeeding women. *Curr Opin Obstet Gynecol.* 2019;31(6):441-446. doi:10.1097 /GCO.0000000000000571.

34. Committee Opinion No. 670: immediate postpartum long-acting reversible contraception. *Obstet Gynecol.* 2016;128(2):e32-e37. doi:10.1097/ AOG.0000000000001587.

35. Averbach SH, Ermias Y, Jeng G, et al. Expulsion of intrauterine devices after postpartum placement by timing of placement, delivery type, and intrauterine device type: a systematic review and meta-analysis. *Am J Obstet Gynecol.* 2020;223(2):177-188. doi:10.1016/j.ajog.2020.02.045.

36. Cameron S. Postabortal and postpartum contraception. *Best Pract Res Clin Obstet Gynaecol.* 2014;28(6): 871-880. doi:10.1016/j.bpobgyn.2014.05.007.

37. Somefun O, Constant D, Endler M. Immediate IUD insertion after second trimester abortion: implications for service delivery. *BMC Health Serv Res.* 2021;21(1):1304. doi:10.1186/s12913-021-07306-2.

38. Dragoman MV, Simmons KB, Paulen ME, Curtis KM. Combined hormonal contraceptive (CHC) use among obese women and contraceptive effectiveness: a systematic review. *Contraception.* 2017;95(2): 117-129. doi:10.1016/j.contraception.2016.10.010.

39. Simmons KB, Edelman AB. Hormonal contraception and obesity. *Fertil Steril.* 2016;106(6):1282-1288. doi:10.1016/j.fertnstert.2016.07.1094.

40. Viatris. Xulane safety information. https://www .xulane.com/. Accessed February 14, 2022.

41. Yamazaki M, Dwyer K, Sobhan M, et al. Effect of obesity on the effectiveness of hormonal contraceptives:

an individual participant data meta-analysis. *Contraception.* 2015;92(5):445-452. doi:10.1016/j .contraception.2015.07.016.

42. Zieman M, Guillebaud J, Weisberg E, et al. Contraceptive efficacy and cycle control with the Ortho Evra/Evra transdermal system: the analysis of pooled data. *Fertil Steril.* 2002;77(2 suppl 2):S13-S18. doi:10.1016/s0015-0282(01)03275-7.

43. Jatlaoui TC, Curtis KM. Safety and effectiveness data for emergency contraceptive pills among women with obesity: a systematic review. *Contraception.* 2016;94(6):605-611. doi:10.1016/j .contraception.2016.05.002.

44. Kardos L. Levonorgestrel emergency contraception and bodyweight: are current recommendations consistent with historic data? *J Drug Assess.* 2020;9(1): 37-42. doi:10.1080/21556660.2020.1725524.

45. Kardos L, Magyar G, Schváb E, Luczai E. Levonorgestrel emergency contraception and bodyweight. *Curr Med Res Opin.* 2019;35(7):1149-1155. doi:10. 1080/03007995.2018.1560250.

46. Gemzell-Danielsson K, Kardos L, von Hertzen H. Impact of bodyweight/body mass index on the effectiveness of emergency contraception with levonorgestrel: a pooled-analysis of three randomized controlled trials. *Curr Med Res Opin.* 2015;31(12):2241-2248. doi:10.1185/03007995.2015.1094455.

47. World Health Organization. *Contraceptive Eligibility for Women at High Risk of HIV.* Geneva, Switzerland: World Health Organization; 2021. https:// apps.who.int/iris/handle/10665/346345. Accessed February 14, 2022.

48. HIV incidence among women using intramuscular depot medroxyprogesterone acetate, a copper intrauterine device, or a levonorgestrel implant for contraception: a randomised, multicentre, open-label trial. *Lancet.* 2019;394(10195):303-313. doi:10.1016 /S0140-6736(19)31288-7.

49. Haynes RM, Boulet SL, Fox MH, et al. Contraceptive use at last intercourse among reproductive-aged women with disabilities: an analysis of population-based data from seven states. *Contraception.* 2018;97(6): 538-545. doi:10.1016/j.contraception.2017.12.008.

50. Wu JP, McKee MM, McKee KS, et al. Female sterilization is more common among women with physical and/or sensory disabilities than women without disabilities in the United States. *Disability Health J.* 2017;10(3):400-405. doi:10.1016/j.dhjo.2016.12.020.

51. Wu J, Braunschweig Y, Harris LH, et al. Looking back while moving forward: a justice-based, intersectional approach to research on contraception and disability. *Contraception.* 2019;99(5):267-271. doi:10.1016/j.contraception.2019.01.006.

52. McGilloway C, Smith D, Galvin R. Barriers faced by adults with intellectual disabilities who experience sexual assault: a systematic review and

meta-synthesis. *J Appl Res Intellect Disabil.* 2020;33(1):51-66. doi:10.1111/jar.12445.

53. Hillard PJA. Contraception for women with intellectual and developmental disabilities: reproductive justice. *Obstet Gynecol.* 2018;132(3):555-558. doi:10.1097/AOG.0000000000002814.

54. Sonalkar S, Chavez V, McClusky J, et al. Gynecologic care for women with physical disabilities: a qualitative study of patients and providers. *Womens Health Issues.* 2020;30(2):136-141. doi:10.1016/j.whi.2019.10.002.

55. Committee Opinion No. 668: menstrual manipulation for adolescents with physical and developmental disabilities. *Obstet Gynecol.* 2016;128(2):e20-e25. doi:10.1097/AOG.0000000000001585.

56. Seymour JW, Fix L, Grossman D, Grindlay K. Facilitators and barriers to contraceptive use among U.S. servicewomen who had an abortion. *Mil Med.* 2019;184(5-6):e417-e423. doi:10.1093/milmed/usy340.

57. Harrington LA, Shaw KA, Shaw JG. Contraception in US servicewomen: emerging knowledge, considerations, and needs. *Curr Opin Obstet Gynecol.* 2017;29(6):431-436. doi:10.1097/GCO.0000000000000414.

58. American College of Obstetricians and Gynecologists' Committee on Health Care for Underserved Women. Reproductive health care for incarcerated pregnant, postpartum, and nonpregnant individuals: ACOG Committee Opinion, Number 830. *Obstet Gynecol.* 2021;138(1):e24-e34. doi:10.1097/AOG.0000000000004429.

59. Peart MS, Knittel AK. Contraception need and available services among incarcerated women in the United States: a systematic review. *Contracept Reprod Med.* 2020;5:2. doi:10.1186/s40834-020-00105-w.

60. Hayes CM, Sufrin C, Perritt JB. Reproductive justice disrupted: mass incarceration as a driver of reproductive oppression. *Am J Public Health.* 2020;110(S1):S21-S24. doi:10.2105/AJPH.2019.305407.

61. McCormick E. Survivors of California's forced sterilizations: "It's like my life wasn't worth anything." *The Guardian.* https://www.theguardian.com/us-news/2021/jul/19/california-forced-sterilization-prison-survivors-reparations. Published July 19, 2021. Accessed February 15, 2022.

62. ICE, a whistleblower and forced sterilization. *NPR.* https://www.npr.org/2020/09/18/914465793/ice-a-whistleblower-and-forced-sterilization. Published September 22, 2020. Accessed February 15, 2022.

63. Alspaugh A, Im EO, D Reibel M, Barroso J. The reproductive health priorities, concerns, and needs of women in midlife: a feminist poststructuralist qualitative analysis. *Qual Health Res.* November 2020:1049732320970491. doi:10.1177/1049732320970491.

64. Alspaugh A, Reibel MD, Im EO, Barroso J. "Since I'm a little bit more mature": contraception and the arc of time for women in midlife. *Womens Midlife Health.* 2021;7(1):3. doi:10.1186/s40695-021-00062-7.

65. Miller TA, Allen RH, Kaunitz AM, Cwiak CA. Contraception for midlife women: a review. *Menopause.* 2018;25(7):817-827. doi:10.1097/GME.0000000000001073.

66. Lethaby A, Wise MR, Weterings MA, et al. Combined hormonal contraceptives for heavy menstrual bleeding. *Cochrane Database Syst Rev.* 2019;2:CD000154. doi:10.1002/14651858.CD000154.pub3.

67. Dayal M, Barnhart KT. Noncontraceptive benefits and therapeutic uses of the oral contraceptive pill. *Semin Reprod Med.* 2001;19(4):295-303. doi:10.1055/s-2001-18637.

68. Schrager S, Larson M, Carlson J, et al. Beyond birth control: noncontraceptive benefits of hormonal methods and their key role in the general medical care of women. *J Womens Health (Larchmt).* 2020;29(7):937-943. doi:10.1089/jwh.2019.7731.

69. Grandi G, Barra F, Ferrero S, et al. Hormonal contraception in women with endometriosis: a systematic review. *Eur J Contracept Reprod Health Care.* 2019;24(1):61-70. doi:10.1080/13625187.2018.1550576.

70. Morgante G, Massaro MG, Di Sabatino A, et al. Therapeutic approach for metabolic disorders and infertility in women with PCOS. *Gynecol Endocrinol.* 2018;34(1):4-9. doi:10.1080/09513590.2017.1370644.

71. Westhoff C, Kerns J, Morroni C, et al. Quick start: novel oral contraceptive initiation method. *Contraception.* 2002;66(3):141-145. doi:10.1016/s0010-7824(02)00351-7.

72. Cramer JA. Compliance with contraceptives and other treatments. *Obstet Gynecol.* 1996;88(3suppl):4S-12S.doi:10.1016/0029-7844(96)00248-7.

73. Ernst A, Lauridsen LLB, Brix N, et al. Pubertal development after unintended intrauterine exposure to oral contraceptives: a nationwide cohort study. *Fertil Steril.* 2019;112(3):552-561.e2. doi:10.1016/j.fertnstert.2019.05.011.

74. Westhoff C, Heartwell S, Edwards S, et al. Initiation of oral contraceptives using a quick start compared with a conventional start: a randomized controlled trial. *Obstet Gynecol.* 2007;109(6):1270-1276. doi:10.1097/01.AOG.0000264550.41242.f2.

75. Lopez LM, Newmann SJ, Grimes DA, et al. Immediate start of hormonal contraceptives for contraception. *Cochrane Database Syst Rev.* 2012;12:CD006260. doi:10.1002/14651858.CD006260.pub3.

76. Glasier A. Starting hormonal contraception after using emergency contraception: what should we recommend? *Hum Reprod.* 2015;30(12):2708-2710. doi:10.1093/humrep/dev242.

77. Richards M, Teal SB, Sheeder J. Risk of luteal phase pregnancy with any-cycle-day initiation of subdermal contraceptive implants. *Contraception.* 2017;95(4):364-370. doi:10.1016/j.contraception.2017.01.010.

78. Littlejohn KE. Hormonal contraceptive use and discontinuation because of dissatisfaction: differences by race and education. *Demography*. 2012;49(4):1433-1452. doi:10.1007/s13524-012-0127-7.

79. Villavicencio J, Allen RH. Unscheduled bleeding and contraceptive choice: increasing satisfaction and continuation rates. *Open Access J Contracept*. 2016;7:43-52. doi:10.2147/OAJC.S85565.

80. Higgins JA, Kramer RD, Ryder KM. Provider bias in long-acting reversible contraception (LARC) promotion and removal: perceptions of young adult women. *Am J Public Health*. 2016;106(11):1932-1937. doi:10.2105/AJPH.2016.303393.

81. Amico JR, Stimmel S, Hudson S, Gold M. "$231 … to pull a string!!!": American IUD users' reasons for IUD self-removal: an analysis of Internet forums. *Contraception*. 2020;101(6):393-398. doi:10.1016/j.contraception.2020.02.005.

82. Biggs MA, Tome L, Mays A, et al. The fine line between informing and coercing: community health center clinicians' approaches to counseling young people about IUDs. *Perspect Sex Reprod Health*. 2020;52(4):245-252. doi:10.1363/psrh.12161.

83. Polis CB, Hussain R, Berry A. There might be blood: a scoping review on women's responses to contraceptive-induced menstrual bleeding changes. *Reprod Health*. 2018;15(1):114. doi:10.1186/s12978-018-0561-0.

84. Coffee AL, Sulak PJ, Hill AJ, et al. Extended cycle combined oral contraceptives and prophylactic frovatriptan during the hormone-free interval in women with menstrual-related migraines. *J Womens Health (Larchmt)*. 2014;23(4):310-317. doi:10.1089/jwh.2013.4485.

85. Lopez LM, Grimes DA, Gallo MF, et al. Skin patch and vaginal ring versus combined oral contraceptives for contraception. *Cochrane Database Syst Rev*. 2013;4:CD003552. doi:10.1002/14651858.CD003552.pub4.

86. Van Vliet HAAM, Grimes DA, Lopez LM, et al. Triphasic versus monophasic oral contraceptives for contraception. *Cochrane Database Syst Rev*. 2011;11:CD003553. doi:10.1002/14651858.CD003553.pub3.

87. Edelman A, Micks E, Gallo MF, et al. Continuous or extended cycle vs. cyclic use of combined hormonal contraceptives for contraception. *Cochrane Database Syst Rev*. 2014;7:CD004695. doi:10.1002/14651858.CD004695.pub3.

88. Nelson AL. Extended-cycle oral contraceptive pills with 10 microg ethinyl estradiol pills in place of placebo pills. *Womens Health (Lond)*. 2007;3(5):529-535. doi:10.2217/17455057.3.5.529.

89. Raine TR, Foster-Rosales A, Upadhyay UD, et al. One-year contraceptive continuation and pregnancy in adolescent girls and women initiating hormonal contraceptives. *Obstet Gynecol*. 2011;117(2 pt 1):363-371. doi:10.1097/AOG.0b013e31820563d3.

90. Dutton C, Kim R, Janiak E. Prevalence of contraindications to progestin-only contraceptive pills in a multi-institution patient database. *Contraception*. 2021;103(5):367-370. doi:10.1016/j.contraception.2021.01.010.

91. Drospirenone (Slynd): a new progestin-only oral contraceptive. *JAMA*. 2020;323(19):1963-1964. doi:10.1001/jama.2020.1603.

92. Tepper NK, Whiteman MK, Marchbanks PA, et al. Progestin-only contraception and thromboembolism: a systematic review. *Contraception*. 2016;94(6):678-700. doi:10.1016/j.contraception.2016.04.014.

93. Brooks M. FDA approves weekly contraceptive patch Twirla. *OB GYN News*. 2020;55(2):4-5.

94. Jacobson JC, Likis FE, Murphy PA. Extended and continuous combined contraceptive regimens for menstrual suppression. *J Midwifery Womens Health*. 2012;57(6):585-592. doi:10.1111/j.1542-2011.2012.00250.x.

95. Galzote RM, Rafie S, Teal R, Mody SK. Transdermal delivery of combined hormonal contraception: a review of the current literature. *Int J Womens Health*. 2017;9:315-321. doi:10.2147/IJWH.S102306

96. NuvaRing® (etonogestrel/ethinyl estradiol vaginal ring). https://www.nuvaring.com/. Accessed May 10, 2022.

97. Annovera® contraceptive (segesterone acetate and ethinyl estradiol vaginal system). https://annovera.com/. Accessed May 10, 2022.

98. Britton LE, Alspaugh A, Greene MZ, McLemore MR. CE: an evidence-based update on contraception. *Am J Nurs*. 2020;120(2):22-33. doi:10.1097/01.NAJ.0000654304.29632.a7.

99. Taylor DJ, Halpern V, Brache V, et al. Ovulation suppression following subcutaneous administration of depot medroxyprogesterone acetate. *Contracept X*. 2022;4:100073. doi:10.1016/j.conx.2022.100073.

100. Dianat S, Fox E, Ahrens KA, et al. Side effects and health benefits of depot medroxyprogesterone acetate: a systematic review. *Obstet Gynecol*. 2019;133(2):332-341. doi:10.1097/AOG.0000000000003089.

101. Lopez LM, Ramesh S, Chen M, et al. Progestin-only contraceptives: effects on weight. *Cochrane Database Syst Rev*. 2016;8:CD008815. doi:10.1002/14651858.CD008815.pub4.

102. Sims J, Lutz E, Wallace K, et al. Depo-medroxyprogesterone acetate, weight gain and amenorrhea among obese adolescent and adult women. *Eur J Contracept Reprod Health Care*. 2020;25(1):54-59. doi:10.1080/13625187.2019.1709963.

103. Martin VT, Behbehani M. Ovarian hormones and migraine headache: understanding mechanisms and pathogenesis—part 2. *Headache*. 2006;46(3):365-386. doi:10.1111/j.1526-4610.2006.00370.x.

104. Cromer BA, Bonny AE, Stager M, et al. Bone mineral density in adolescent females using injectable or

oral contraceptives: a 24-month prospective study. *Fertil Steril.* 2008;90(6):2060-2067. doi:10.1016/j.fertnstert.2007.10.070.

105. Lara-Torre E, Edwards CP, Perlman S, Hertweck SP. Bone mineral density in adolescent females using depot medroxyprogesterone acetate. *J Pediatr Adolesc Gynecol.* 2004;17(1):17-21. doi:10.1016/j.jpag.2003.11.017.

106. Walsh JS, Eastell R, Peel NFA. Effects of depot medroxyprogesterone acetate on bone density and bone metabolism before and after peak bone mass: a case-control study. *J Clin Endocrinol Metab.* 2008;93(4):1317-1323. doi:10.1210/jc.2007-2201.

107. Bachrach LK. Hormonal contraception and bone health in adolescents. *Front Endocrinol (Lausanne).* 2020;11:603. doi:10.3389/fendo.2020.00603.

108. Harel Z, Johnson CC, Gold MA, et al. Recovery of bone mineral density in adolescents following the use of depot medroxyprogesterone acetate contraceptive injections. *Contraception.* 2010;81(4):281-291. doi:10.1016/j.contraception.2009.11.003.

109. Worly BL, Gur TL, Schaffir J. The relationship between progestin hormonal contraception and depression: a systematic review. *Contraception.* 2018;97(6):478-489. doi:10.1016/j.contraception.2018.01.010.

110. Dabee S, Tanko RF, Brown BP, et al. Comparison of female genital tract cytokine and microbiota signatures induced by initiation of intramuscular DMPA and NET-EN hormonal contraceptives: a prospective cohort analysis. *Front Immunol.* 2021;12:760504. doi:10.3389/fimmu.2021.760504.

111. Paulen ME, Curtis KM. When can a woman have repeat progestogen-only injectables: depot medroxyprogesterone acetate or norethisterone enantate? *Contraception.* 2009;80(4):391-408. doi:10.1016/j.contraception.2009.03.023.

112. Gu S, Sivin I, Du M, et al. Effectiveness of Norplant implants through seven years: a large-scale study in China. *Contraception.* 1995;52(2):99-103. doi:10.1016/s0010-7824(95)00141-7.

113. Nexplanon prescribing information. https://www.organon.com/product/usa/pi_circulars/n/nexplanon/nexplanon_pi.pdf.

114. Ali M, Akin A, Bahamondes L, et al. Extended use up to 5 years of the etonogestrel-releasing subdermal contraceptive implant: comparison to levonorgestrel-releasing subdermal implant. *Hum Reprod.* 2016;31(11):2491-2498. doi:10.1093/humrep/dew222.

115. Dickerson LM, Diaz VA, Jordon J, et al. Satisfaction, early removal, and side effects associated with long-acting reversible contraception. *Fam Med.* 2013;45(10):701-707.

116. Bofill Rodriguez M, Lethaby A, Jordan V. Progestogen-releasing intrauterine systems for heavy menstrual bleeding. *Cochrane Database Syst Rev.* 2020;6:CD002126. doi:10.1002/14651858.CD002126.pub4.

117. Boraas CM, Sanders JN, Schwarz EB, et al. Risk of pregnancy with levonorgestrel-releasing intrauterine system placement 6–14 days after unprotected sexual intercourse. *Obstet Gynecol.* 2021;137(4):623-625. doi:10.1097/AOG.0000000000004118.

118. BakenRa A, Gero A, Sanders J, et al. Pregnancy risk by frequency and timing of unprotected intercourse before intrauterine device placement for emergency contraception. *Obstet Gynecol.* 2021;138(1):79-84. doi:10.1097/AOG.0000000000004433.

119. Gemzell-Danielsson K, Berger C, Lalitkumar PGL. Emergency contraception: mechanisms of action. *Contraception.* 2013;87(3):300-308. doi:10.1016/j.contraception.2012.08.021.

120. Haeger KO, Lamme J, Cleland K. State of emergency contraception in the U.S., 2018. *Contracept Reprod Med.* 2018;3:20. doi:10.1186/s40834-018-0067-8.

121. Piaggio G, Kapp N, von Hertzen H. Effect on pregnancy rates of the delay in the administration of levonorgestrel for emergency contraception: a combined analysis of four WHO trials. *Contraception.* 2011;84(1):35-39. doi:10.1016/j.contraception.2010.11.010.

122. Natavio M, Stanczyk FZ, Molins EAG, et al. Pharmacokinetics of the 1.5 mg levonorgestrel emergency contraceptive in women with normal, obese and extremely obese body mass index. *Contraception.* 2019;99(5):306-311. doi:10.1016/j.contraception.2019.01.003.

123. Edelman AB, Cherala G, Blue SW, et al. Impact of obesity on the pharmacokinetics of levonorgestrel-based emergency contraception: single and double dosing. *Contraception.* 2016;94(1):52-57. doi:10.1016/j.contraception.2016.03.006.

124. Glasier AF, Cameron ST, Fine PM, et al. Ulipristal acetate versus levonorgestrel for emergency contraception: a randomised non-inferiority trial and meta-analysis. *Lancet.* 2010;375(9714):555-562. doi:10.1016/S0140-6736(10)60101-8.

125. Le Corvaisier C, Capelle A, France M, et al. Drug interactions between emergency contraceptive drugs and cytochrome inducers: literature review and quantitative prediction. *Fundam Clin Pharmacol.* 2021;35(2):208-216. doi:10.1111/fcp.12601.

126. Turok DK, Godfrey EM, Wojdyla D, et al. Copper T380 intrauterine device for emergency contraception: highly effective at any time in the menstrual cycle. *Hum Reprod.* 2013;28(10):2672-2676. doi:10.1093/humrep/det330.

127. Moore A, Ryan S, Stamm C. Seeking emergency contraception in the United States: a review of access and barriers. *Women Health.* 2019;59(4):364-374. doi:10.1080/03630242.2018.1487905.

128. Ensuring access to emergency contraception after rape. American Civil Liberties Union. https://www.aclu.org/other/ensuring-access-emergency-contraception-after-rape. Published February 2007. Accessed May 13, 2022.

APPENDIX

# 12A

# Intrauterine Device Insertion and Removal

MELICIA ESCOBAR

## Introduction

Intrauterine devices are long-acting reversible contraceptive (LARC) agents that require little, if any action, by the patient after they are inserted, resulting in a very effective contraceptive method. Intrauterine devices can be referred to by several different terms and abbreviations: intrauterine device (IUD), intrauterine contraceptive device (IUCD), intrauterine contraception (UC), and intrauterine system (IUS). For the purposes of this appendix, the terms "intrauterine device" and "IUD" will be used throughout.

Five different brands of IUDs are currently available in the United States, one of which is wrapped in copper (copper IUD) and four of which are impregnated with levonorgestrel (LNG-IUD). More information about the effectiveness and use of these devices is found in the *Fertility, Family Building, and Contraception*; *Nonhormonal Contraception*; and *Hormonal Contraception* chapters. For more information on IUD insertion during the postplacental period, see the *Postplacental IUD Insertion* appendix.

This appendix can be used as a guide for any of the current IUDs discussed within these chapters. In addition to its use as a contraceptive, the LNG-IUD can be used in the treatment of individuals with menorrhagia; more information about this noncontraceptive usage is found in the *Menstrual Cycle Abnormalities* chapter.

## Advancing Reproductive Justice

In advance of IUD insertion, the clinician should examine personal biases toward contraceptive options, which is essential to providing evidence-based information that is free of judgment.[1] See the *Context of Individuals Seeking Midwifery Care* chapter for further considerations.

## Health Counseling for Individuals Considering an Intrauterine Device

A thorough reproductive life plan and health history, health education, contraindications, risks, contraceptive and noncontraceptive benefits, side effects, and adverse effects are reviewed as part of the shared decision-making process between the midwife and the client.[1-7] These topics are presented briefly in this appendix. The reader is referred to the *Hormonal Contraception* chapter, resources, and references for a more detailed description of health counseling prior to IUD insertion.

A written consent form granting permission to the clinician for IUD insertion, signed by the patient either on paper or by electronic means, is part of the shared decision making and legal informed consent. Health education should include the costs involved with IUD insertion. Although the initial cost may be higher than for other contraceptive methods, the IUD becomes cost neutral after 3 years of continuous use and has an added cost savings associated with reduction in unintended pregnancies.[6,7] For those individuals without health insurance coverage, some financial support for IUD use may be available directly through the pharmaceutical companies or their associated philanthropic programs.

### Contraindications for Intrauterine Device Insertion

The initial step prior to consideration of an IUD is to determine if the patient has any contraindications. Alternatives should also be considered as

508

appropriate based on patient desires and health history. Once an IUD has been selected as a method, health counseling, prior to insertion or on the day of insertion, should be conducted. This counseling should include a thorough discussion of risks and benefits, potential side effects, and complications related to insertion. To better inform this discussion, see the IUD-related content in the *Nonhormonal Contraception* and *Hormonal Contraception* chapters.

## Risks and Benefits Associated with Intrauterine Devices

Benefits of IUDs include ease of use—that is, these devices are non-coital dependent, long-acting reversible methods, with a limited number of side effects.[5,8] For more information about the risks and benefits associated with IUD use, see the *Nonhormonal Contraception* and *Hormonal Contraception* chapters. Two specific risks related to insertion include vasovagal response and uterine perforation.

### Vasovagal Response

During IUD insertion, some patients may experience a vasovagal reaction secondary to cervical manipulation. Common symptoms include syncope, vertigo, dyspnea, nausea, and diaphoresis. This response usually resolves spontaneously if the clinician stops any manipulation and waits for the symptoms to resolve. At that point, insertion can usually be resumed without incident. It is rare that an IUD cannot be inserted due to a vasovagal reaction.

### Uterine Perforation

Perforation of the uterus at the time of IUD insertion is always a risk, but it is a rare event with an estimated incidence of 1 to 2 cases per 1000 insertions. The benefits of prevention of unintended pregnancies outweigh this risk.[9] If uterine perforation occurs during placement of the IUD, the clinician may find that during fundal placement, the IUD continues to travel beyond the original uterine depth and the threads begin to travel upward. Patients most at risk for perforation are those who are lactating, who have recently given birth, or both.[10,11] When perforation is suspected, the IUD should be removed and the patient should be evaluated closely. Most perforations are small and require little treatment.[11] Any patient demonstrating symptoms of bleeding or shock post insertion should be transferred to an appropriate care facility for prompt treatment.

## Side Effects and Adverse Effects Associated with Intrauterine Devices

Many myths and misconceptions exist regarding IUDs that can be addressed during preinsertion counseling.[5] IUDs are not associated with an increased risk for infertility, ectopic pregnancy, or infections such as pelvic inflammatory disease (PID) or human immunodeficiency virus (HIV). Side effects include primarily changed vaginal bleeding patterns. The copper-containing IUD is associated with increased menstrual flow and menstrual cramping. In contrast, the LNG-IUD gradually induces amenorrhea, which is associated with insertion.

### Choice of an Intrauterine Device

Several IUDs are currently available in the United States. Both the copper and LNG-releasing IUDs provide highly effective contraception, can be identified on ultrasound if needed, and are easily reversible. Nevertheless, certain differences between them must be taken into consideration—patient preference around the use of a hormonal method, duration of use, and menstrual bleeding pattern. The immediate need for emergency contraception should also be considered. See the IUD-related content in *Nonhormonal Contraception* and *Hormonal Contraception* chapters for more information about IUD options.

### Timing of the Intrauterine Device Insertion

IUDs may be inserted at any time if the clinician is reasonably sure that the patient is not pregnant, including postpartum (including after cesarean birth) and post abortion (either spontaneous or induced).[3] In both cases, sepsis precludes use of the method until resolution of any infection. Insertion in the immediate postpartum period (postplacental) or early postpartum period is becoming more common in the United States, despite an increased rate of expulsion associated with this timing, in an effort to reduce unplanned pregnancies (see the *Postplacental IUD Insertion* appendix).[8,12] Postabortion insertion remains a common practice and has been found to be safe and effective.[3] The copper IUD also can be used as a type of emergency contraception; its use for that indication is discussed in the *Hormonal Contraception* chapter.

In years past, IUDs for contraceptive use were almost exclusively inserted during menses in an attempt to provide additional assurance that the patient was not pregnant as well as based on the belief that insertion would be easier during menses. A theory existed that the cervix might be slightly open and softer at this time. In reality, little evidence exists to support this timing.[13] Current guidelines state that insertion can occur at any time for individuals without preexisting contraindications to the method, assuming there is reliable evidence that they are not currently pregnant.

For a patient who already is using a hormonal contraceptive method such as a combined oral contraceptive, the IUD can be inserted at any time during the cycle and no secondary method of contraception is needed.[3] This seamless transition also can occur when a patient has one IUD removed and then replaced with another IUD.

### Screening for Sexually Transmitted Infections

According to national screening guidelines, risk assessment for sexually transmitted infections (STIs) and HIV should be conducted routinely and screening conducted accordingly.[14] However, requiring that negative results of recent STI screening be available prior to IUD insertion imposes an unnecessary barrier to access for this method. Studies have found that the rate of PID is no different in women who screen positive for chlamydia infection or gonorrhea at the time of insertion versus those for whom IUD insertion is deferred.[15] An exception is those individuals who have active disease or signs and symptoms of purulent cervicitis, chlamydia, or gonorrhea infection; in these individuals, insertion should be deferred until the infection is resolved.[3] Screening for human papillomavirus infection or cervical cancer prior to IUD insertion is not beneficial and, therefore, is not required.[16] If an individual is due for routine cervical cancer screening, this can be optionally completed at the time of IUD insertion.

## Day of Intrauterine Device Insertion

The insertion procedures for copper IUDs and LNG-containing IUDs have minor differences based on the configuration of both the inserter and the device. In all cases, the intention is to place the IUD in the fundus of the uterus. If the IUD placement is not fundal, there is a higher likelihood of unintended pregnancy as well as expulsion of the IUD.

Several training programs are available in which clinicians can learn how to insert an IUD. Most of these programs are sponsored by the manufacturers of the devices, and these vendors may restrict use of their products until such education is completed. Multiple resources for IUD insertion procedures exist online, including video recordings that help the clinician review the process. In addition, the Food and Drug Administration (FDA)–approved prescribing information and package label for each device include insertion instructions and images. The following steps for insertion are general guidelines and cannot replace hands-on experiences.

### Premedication

It is common practice to administer a prophylactic nonsteroidal anti-inflammatory drug (NSAID) such as ibuprofen to patients prior to insertion of an IUD. These drugs effectively treat the pain associated with IUD use, such as copper IUD–associated dysmenorrhea, although no evidence suggests that they diminish discomfort at the time of IUD insertion.[12] Anesthesia such as topical lidocaine may or may not decrease pain, but published studies on this topic lack enough rigor to draw any conclusion.[3,17] By comparison, lidocaine, when delivered as a paracervical nerve block, may reduce pain with tenaculum placement or insertion.[12] Only limited evidence supports the use of nitrous oxide as a possibly effective analgesia option for patients during an IUD insertion; however, high satisfaction rates among users were noted.[12]

Using misoprostol (Cytotec) as a cervical softening agent does not significantly improve ease of IUD insertion and may even increase pain.[12] Thus, misoprostol is not recommended for regular use as part of the insertion procedure. However, this agent may offer some benefit when attempting a second insertion after a previous failed attempt.[18]

The use of antimicrobial agents has been shown to have limited effectiveness in reducing infection, including PID and endocarditis, despite a theoretical risk of these complications.[15,19] Although the overall risk of IUD-related infection is low, one systematic review found a small, but significant, reduction in infections among patients receiving such treatment; the authors cautioned that the number of participants in the studies was small and routine use was likely not to be cost-effective.[17]

### Required Equipment for Intrauterine Device Insertion

*General equipment* includes the following items that are clean, albeit not necessarily sterile:

- Clean, nonsterile gloves for a bimanual examination.
- Lubricant for a bimanual exam.
- Adequate lighting for visualization.
- Speculum of appropriate shape and size.
- Sharp, long, curved scissors to cut the IUD threads after insertion.

- Antiseptic solution (povidone–iodine or 4% chlorhexidine gluconate).
- Cotton-tipped swab (drumstick swab) and/or a cotton ball or 4 × 4 gauze pads. These may be used to apply the antiseptic to the cervix. The swab may also be inserted to the level of the cervix against the uterine sound and then removed simultaneously for easy visualization of the measurement.
- Ring forceps to hold the 4 × 4 gauze pads if utilized, to remove the IUD if needed, or to remove the cut strings from the vaginal vault.
- A sanitary pad for the patient in the event of postprocedure spotting or bleeding.

A *sterile field* includes use of sterile equipment:

- Uterine sound to verify the depth of the uterine cavity and the appropriateness of a specific size of IUD.
- Tenaculum (single tooth) to grasp the cervix, straighten the cervical canal, and stabilize the uterus during insertion. An Allis clamp may be equally effective and reduce the risk of tenaculum-related bleeding.[20]
- Sterile gloves of appropriate size.

### Optional Equipment for Intrauterine Device Insertion

- Os finder or other such dilator
- Monsel's solution or silver nitrate sticks to control tenaculum-related bleeding
- Supplies for administering a paracervical block, including trumpet, needle, syringe, and anesthesia
- 1% lidocaine, to be injected 3 to 5 minutes prior to IUD insertion
- 10-cc syringe with 22-gauge needle with extender or a spinal needle for the lidocaine

The IUD of choice may be placed on the field or handed to the clinician by an assistant. At some sites, a secondary IUD may be available should contamination occur with the first one. At other sites, consumers must purchase their own IUD. In those situations, it is likely that only one device will be available.

### Key Points for Insertion of Any Intrauterine Device

1. Optimally the clinician should have another individual available to assist with the procedure.

2. A bimanual pelvic examination should be carefully performed to ascertain the position of the uterus and rule out any gross abnormalities. Although a patient who is postpartum or lactating may have a softer uterus, and therefore a higher risk of perforation, these conditions are not contraindications to the procedure.

3. After engaging in shared decision making, the patient should have signed legal consent for documentation and verification of understanding of the procedure.

4. The patient should be in a physical position that prioritizes their comfort and safety during the procedure.

5. The clinician should have good visualization of the vagina and cervix.

6. The patient should be reassured that the procedure can be stopped at any time should they make this request.

7. The insertion is begun using sterile technique.

8. The cervix and vagina can be swabbed with the antiseptic if desired; similarly, anesthesia can be administered as appropriate.

9. Use the tenaculum to grasp the anterior lip of the cervix, with the teeth placed parallel to the plane of the speculum blades, or perpendicular if an Allis clamp is used. If the uterus is retroverted, it may be more effective to place the tenaculum or Allis clamp on the posterior lip. Gentle traction is exerted toward the clinician to straighten the cervical canal in alignment with the uterine cavity. Usually the clinician uses the nondominant hand to hold the tenaculum or Allis clamp.

10. While performing these actions, the clinician should observe for a vasovagal response caused by manipulation of the cervix. If the patient feels faint or very nauseated, the clinician should stop the procedure and wait. Usually the second attempt at insertion is successful, assuming several minutes have elapsed.

11. While the clinician's nondominant hand holds the tenaculum or Allis clamp in place, the dominant hand slides the uterine sound into the uterus to measure the depth of the uterine cavity (**Figure 12A-1**). Caution must be taken not to aggressively force the sound. Most of the currently available IUDs are designed for a uterine cavity that sounds between 6 and 9 cm,

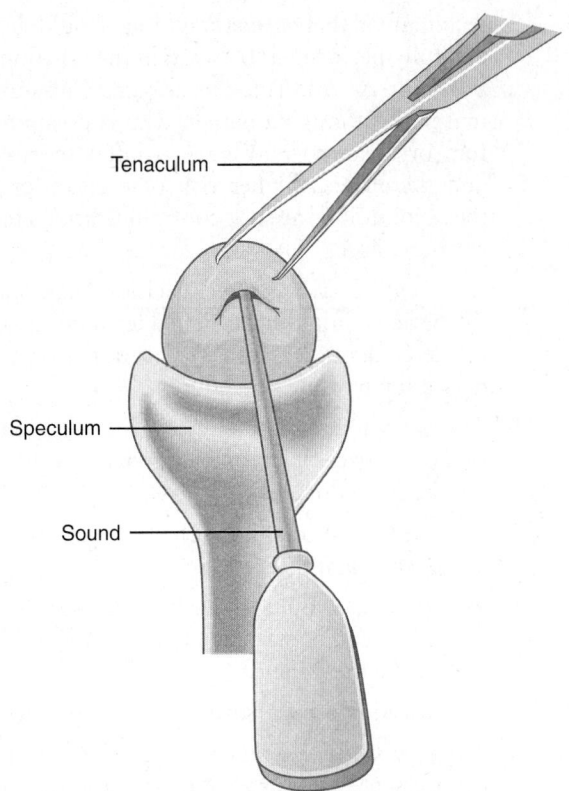

**Figure 12A-1** Cervix with tenaculum and uterine sound.

although the sounding threshold for Liletta is lower, 5.5 cm. Skyla and Kyleena are physically smaller and may be appropriate for the uterine cavities of nulliparous individuals, which are typically smaller than the uterine cavity in a multiparous individual. The depth of the uterus in centimeters should be noted. If the sound does not confirm a depth within the acceptable range, the insertion procedure should be discontinued and an alternative method of contraception discussed.

12. At this point, the steps for the insertion vary based on the device. However, for all IUDs, the clinician must maintain scrupulous sterile technique. The device is not opened until it has been deemed appropriate for immediate insertion.

### Insertion of an LNG-IUD

The Mirena, Skyla, Kyleena, and Liletta IUDs are inserted in a similar manner. However, the anatomy of the Liletta device differs, particularly the loading mechanism and slider.

1. The IUD package is opened, usually by the assistant, and the clinician reaches for the device in a sterile manner. Alternatively, the entire package can be opened by the clinician, who then dons sterile gloves and proceeds with the insertion. **Figure 12A-2** provides an illustration of the device in the packaging and the anatomy of the various LNG devices.

2. The threads of the Mirena, Skyla, and Kyleena IUDs are self-contained within the device. The threads of the Liletta IUD are secured on the handle of the inserter and are ultimately released from the groove so they can hang freely.

3. Placement of the clinician's thumb or forefinger on the slider will stabilize the inserter and should be maintained until the insertion is complete. The slider should *not* be moved downward at this time, as this action may prematurely release the threads of the IUD. This is particularly relevant to the Mirena, Skyla, and Kyleena IUDs: Once the slider is moved below the mark, the IUD cannot be reloaded. The Liletta, however, may be reloaded.

4. The arms of the device should be in a horizontal position. If they are not, they can be realigned on a flat sterile area, such as the inside of the sterile package (**Figure 12A-3**).

5. To load the strings into the Mirena, Skyla, and Kyleena IUDs, push the slider forward until a "click" is heard or felt, indicating it is in place, while maintaining forward pressure on the slider. For the Liletta IUD, while continuing forward pressure on the blue slider, pull both strings straight back toward the clinician until a hard stop is achieved. This two-handed action retracts the IUD arms in the tubing (**Figure 12A-4**). The Liletta IUD may be reloaded by releasing the thread from the cleft and pulling back on the blue slider until the groove becomes aligned with the green. By returning the blue slider to the forward position, the loading steps can be repeated. Do not load the IUD too far in advance of insertion so as to allow the device to retain its memory and allow optimal expansion of the arms to occur; prolonged time in the inserter may cause the device to lose structural memory.

6. Based on the uterine size determined by the sound, the flange on the insertion device is set at that number by sliding the flange over the marked increments on the IUD insertion

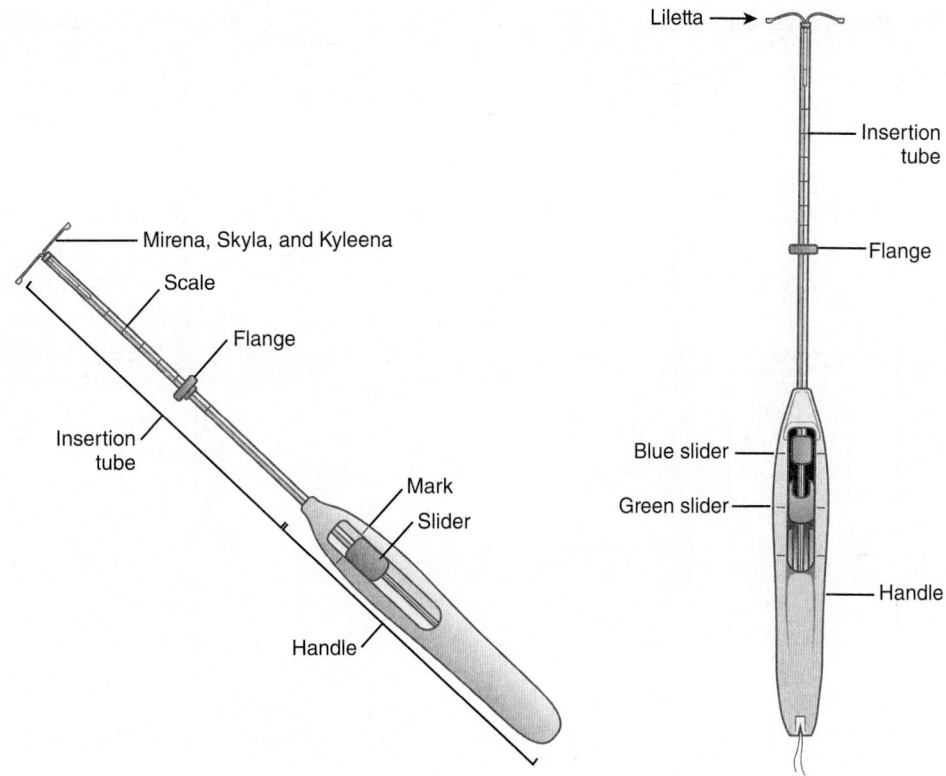

**Figure 12A-2** Anatomy of LNG-IUDs: Mirena, Skyla, Kyleena, and Liletta.

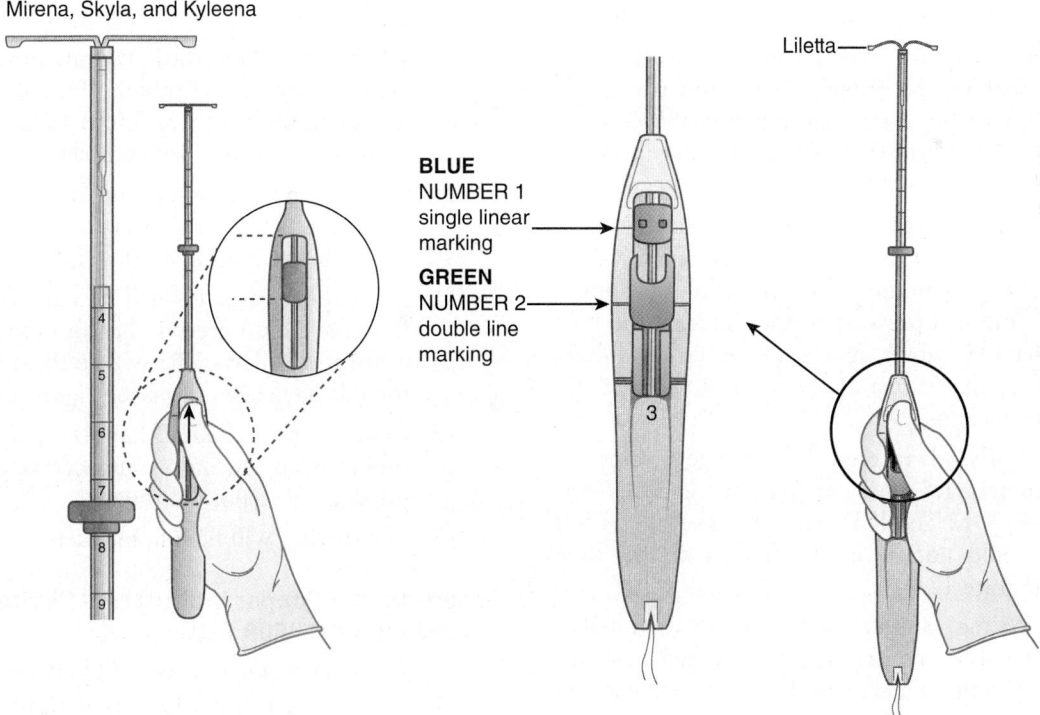

**Figure 12A-3** Stabilization of the slider and verification of the position of the IUD.

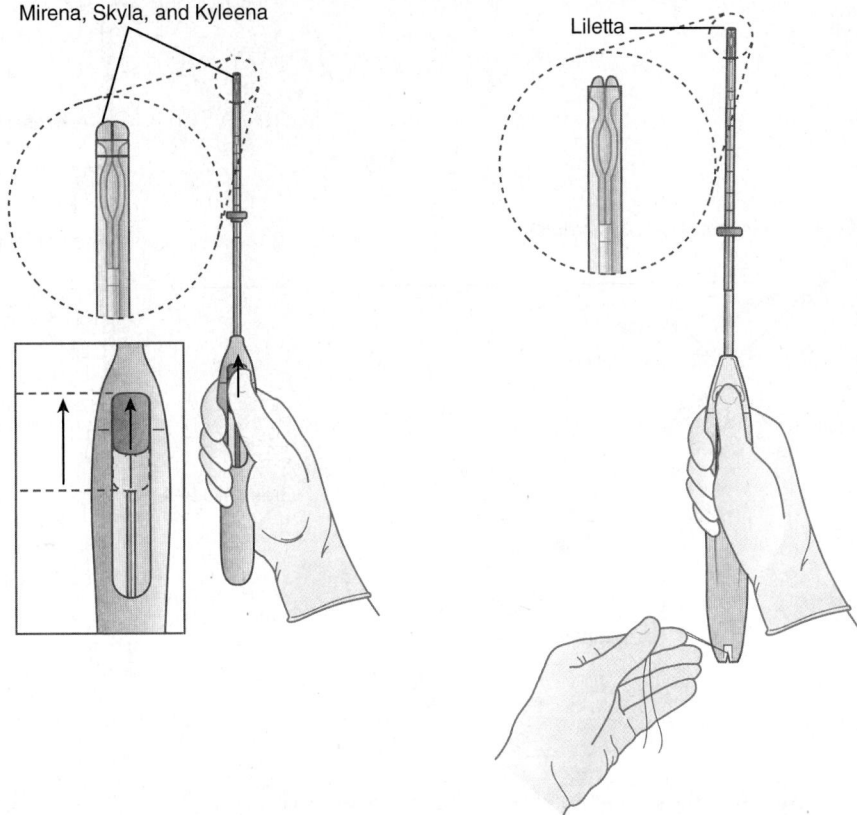

**Figure 12A-4** Retraction of the LNG-IUD into the tubing.

tube. Sterile gloves must be used when touching the flange. The Liletta packaging has a built-in tray notch that enables the clinician to adjust the flange without touching it (Figure 12A-5).

7. The clinician's nondominant hand exerts gentle traction on the tenaculum or Allis clamp. Simultaneously, the clinician applies continued pressure to the slider on the IUD handle, which places the insertion tubing into the vagina at the level of the external cervical os.

8. Gently advance until the flange is approximately 1.5 to 2 cm from the external cervical os. The IUD will be in the uterus but should not be in the fundus at this time (Figure 12A-6).

9. For the Mirena, Skyla, and Kyleena IUDs, the slider on the handle is pulled back toward the clinician until the level of the raised mark on the insertion handle is reached. For the Liletta IUD, pull the blue slider back until resistance is reached; a common thumb recess is created once merged with the green

slider. At that time, the IUD arms are expelled from the insertion tubing (Figure 12A-7). The clinician must wait 10 to 15 seconds to allow the arms to open completely.

10. Advance the insertion tubing until the flange is at the external cervical os. At that point, the IUD is in the uterine fundus (Figure 12A-8).

11. Move the slider(s) toward the clinician to release the IUD. A green indicator in the thread cleft of the Liletta IUD will confirm that the threads have been released (Figure 12A-9).

12. Gently remove the IUD handle and insertion tubing from the uterus and cervix and appropriately dispose of them.

13. The threads will remain in place.

### Insertion of a Copper Intrauterine Device (ParaGard T CU 380A IUD)

1. The IUD package (Figure 12A-10) is opened in the same manner for any IUD, usually by the assistant, and the clinician reaches for the device in a sterile manner. The clinician should be aware of the components of this IUD (Figure 12A-11).

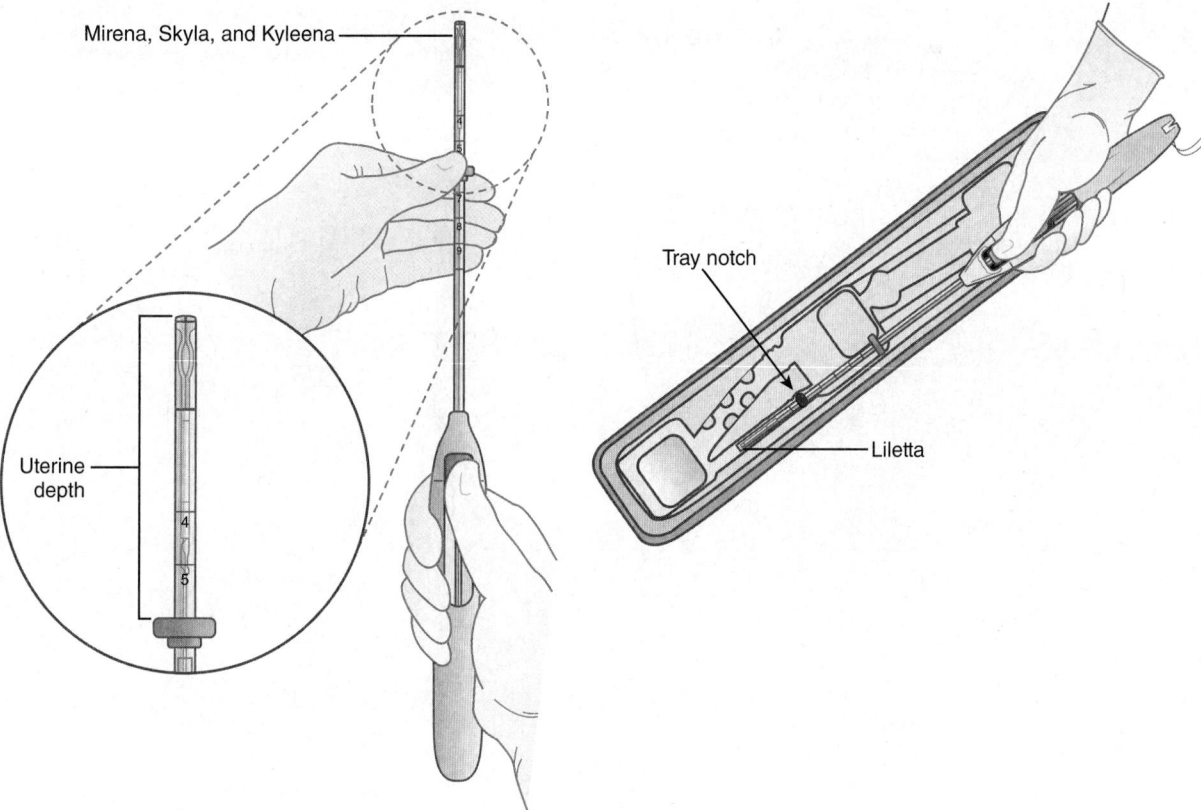

**Figure 12A-5** LNG-IUD flange moved to uterine depth.

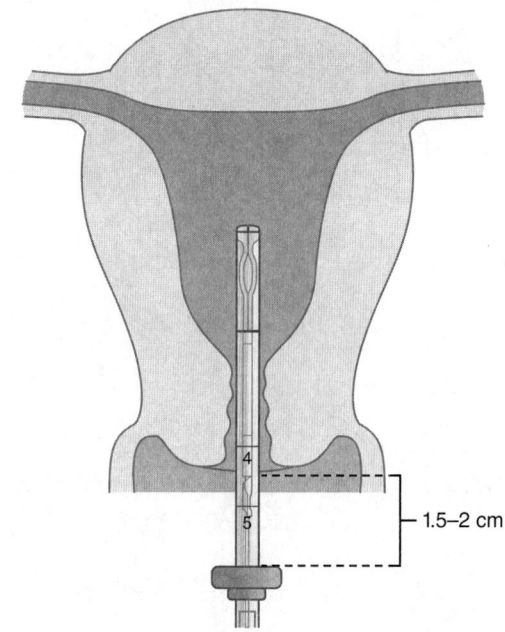

**Figure 12A-6** LNG-IUD inserter guided through the cervix.

2. Load the IUD into the insertion tubing by slightly withdrawing the insertion tubing and folding the horizontal arms of the IUD down along the vertical arm using the thumb and

forefinger. This can be accomplished through the packaging (**Figure 12A-12**) or by using an open sterile technique (**Figure 12A-13**). Take precautions to ensure that the arms are not bent into the tubing until immediately before insertion. If the arms are folded for more than 5 minutes, the device may lose its memory and may not completely unfold in the uterus.

3. Advance the insertion tubing so that the horizontal arms sit securely within the insertion tubing.

4. Place the solid white rod into the bottom of the insertion tubing, advancing it until it touches the bottom of the IUD.

5. Grasp the insertion tube at the open end, and set the flange to the centimeter level predetermined by sounding the uterus.

6. Rotate the insertion tubing so that the horizontal arms of the IUD are parallel to the long axis of the flange.

7. Use a tenaculum or Allis clamp to stabilize the cervix. This stabilization usually is accomplished by the clinician's nondominant hand holding the tenaculum or Allis clamp as

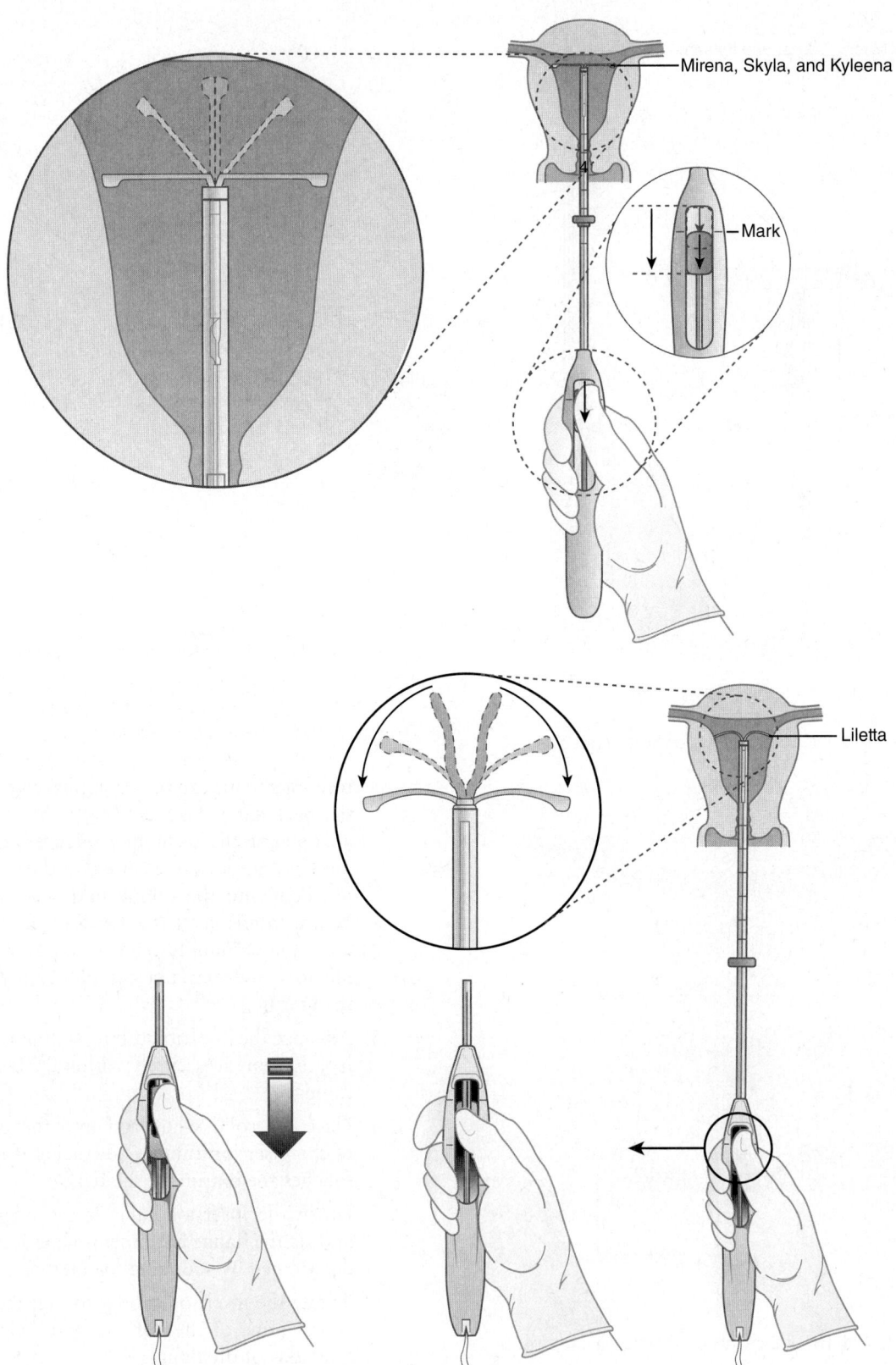

**Figure 12A-7** Opening of the LNG-IUD arms via moving the slider to the preset mark.

the loaded insertion tube is passed through the cervical canal guided by the dominant hand. When resistance is met at the uterine fundus, the flange should be at the external cervical os (Figure 12A-14).

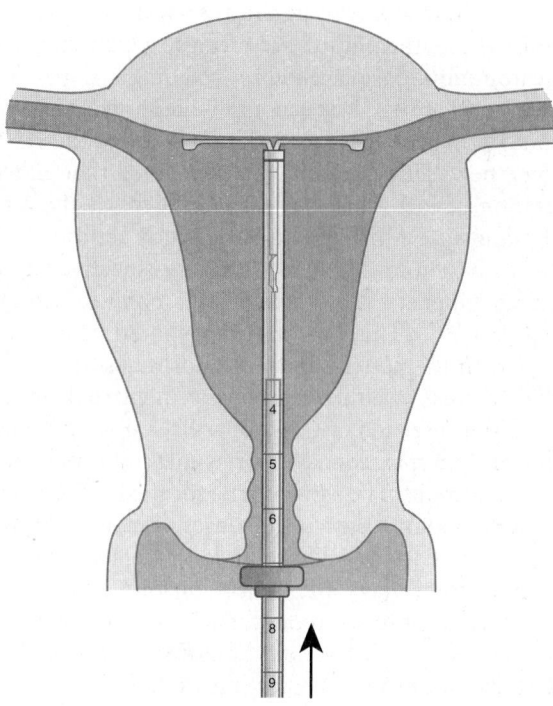

**Figure 12A-8** LNG-IUD in the fundus with the flange at the level of the external cervical os.

8. While the clinician's nondominant hand stabilizes the solid white rod, withdraw the insertion tubing with the clinician's other hand for a distance of approximately 1 cm. At this time, the IUD is released from the inserter.

9. Gently advance the insertion tube to ensure the IUD is placed in the fundus (Figure 12A-15).

10. Gently withdraw the insertion tubing (Figure 12A-16 and Figure 12A-17), and appropriately dispose of both the rod and the tubing.

## Postinsertion Care

The clinician should be able to visualize the IUD threads or strings in the vagina after IUD insertion is complete and the inserter materials have been removed. Using sharp scissors, the threads may be trimmed to the recommended length of approximately 3 cm from the external os so that they fall within the vagina. If cut too short, the threads may migrate into the os, whereas longer strings can be shortened at a subsequent visit for the comfort of the patient (Figure 12A-18). The patient's unique context should also be considered. For example, if the patient's body size and habitus or physical mobility warrant it, the clinician may cut the IUD threads longer than 3 cm to assure that the patient

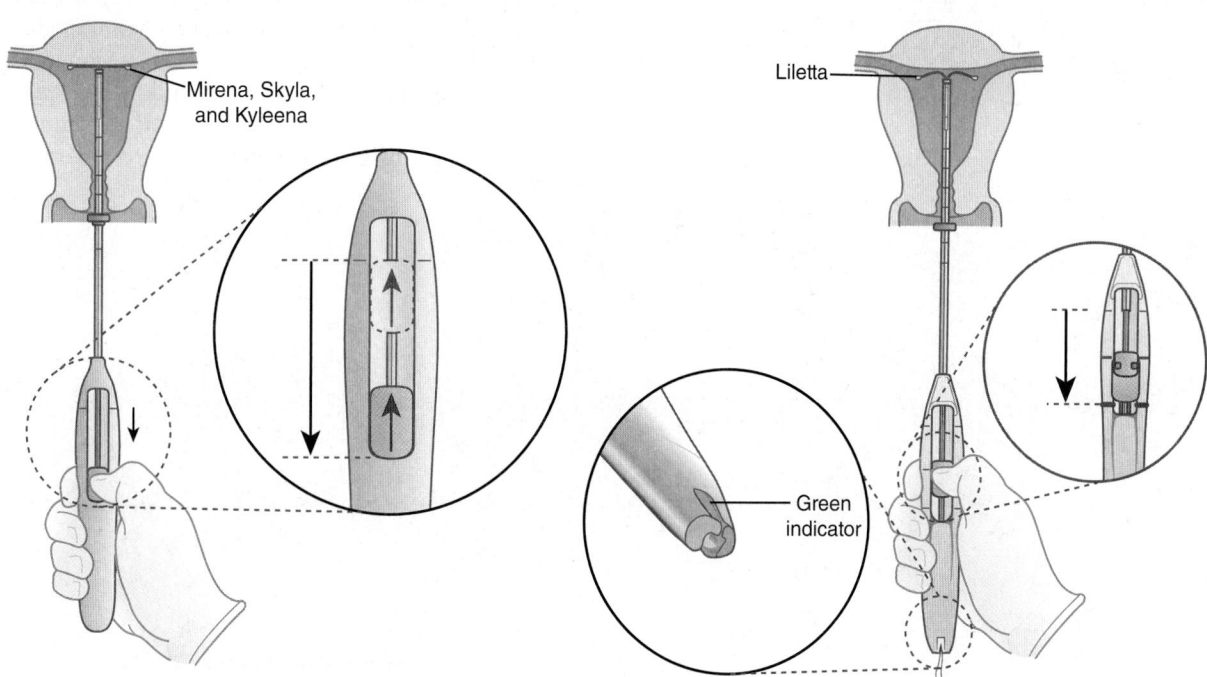

**Figure 12A-9** Release of the LNG-IUD slider.

can easily feel them. Conversely, for patients experiencing reproductive coercion, cutting the string length such that it is not visible outside of the cervical os is recommended.[21]

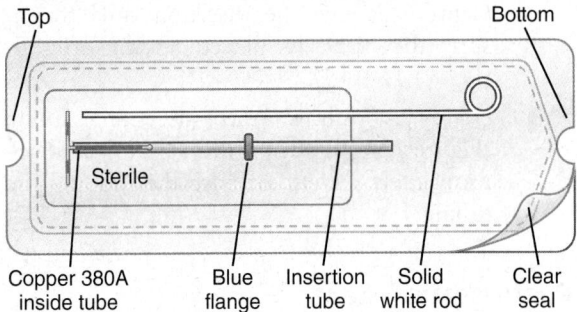

**Figure 12A-10** Packaging of a copper IUD.

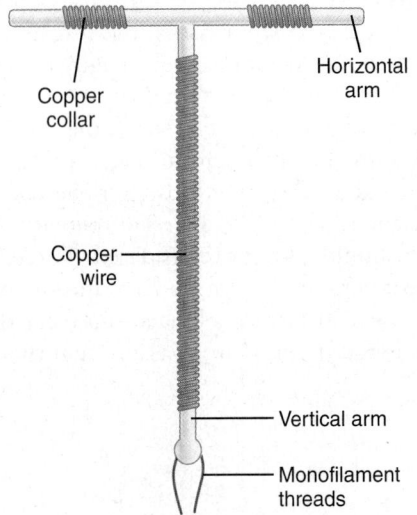

**Figure 12A-11** Anatomy of a copper IUD.

## Health Education

After insertion of an IUD, health education includes teaching about how to feel for and identify the threads in the vagina (Figure 12A-19). A sample IUD with strings the patient can feel may be used as a teaching aid. Any significant variations such as unusual lengthening of the strings, which may indicate nonfundal placement, or feeling any part of the plastic of the device should be reported, as these findings may suggest partial expulsion of the IUD. Some new IUD users may be concerned that either tampon or menstrual cup use will increase the rate of expulsion. Although an early study did not find this to be the case, a more recent prospective study detected higher rates of expulsion among menstrual cup users.[22,23] This potential risk should be considered with the patient and need not necessarily preclude the use of either tampons or menstrual cups.

After insertion of the copper IUD, no additional contraception is required, as this method is immediately effective.[3] The same is true for the LNG-IUD if inserted within 7 days of the onset of menses. However, abstinence or additional contraception should be used for 7 days after initiation of LNG-IUD if this device is inserted more than 7 days after the onset of menses.[3] All patients should be counseled that IUDs do not provide protection from STIs.

The mnemonic "PAINS" is often shared after IUD insertion as an easy-to-use reminder of potentially significant deviations that should be reported (see Table 15 in the *Hormonal Contraception* chapter). In all cases, patients should be encouraged to contact their provider with questions or concerns, although most people using an IUD do not experience major side effects. Among the most common side effects of all IUDs are menstrual irregularities.

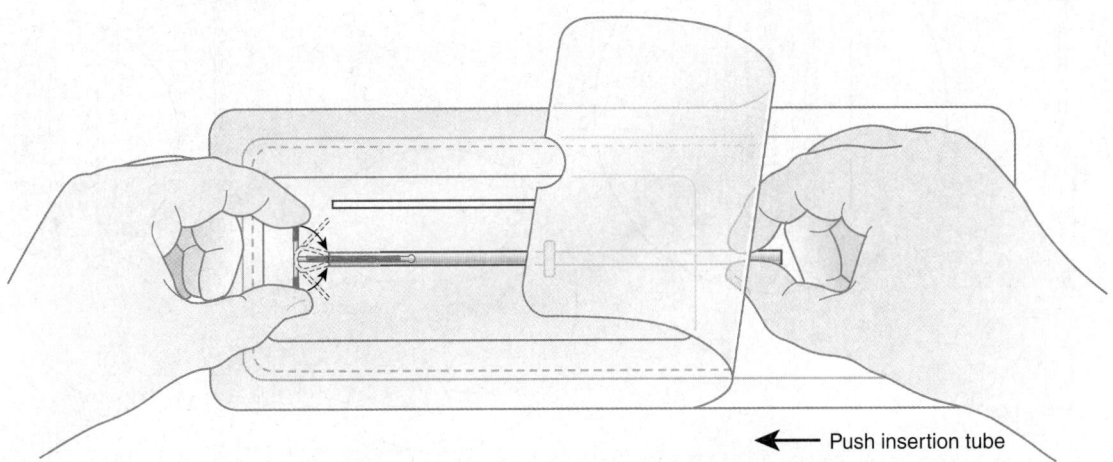

← Push insertion tube

**Figure 12A-12** Placement of the arms of a copper IUD into the tubing through the packaging.

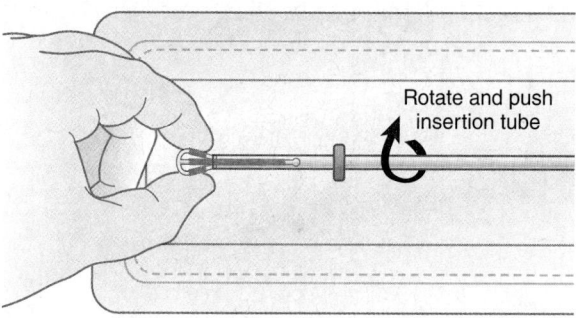

**Figure 12A-13** Placement of the arms of a copper IUD into the tubing by open sterile technique.

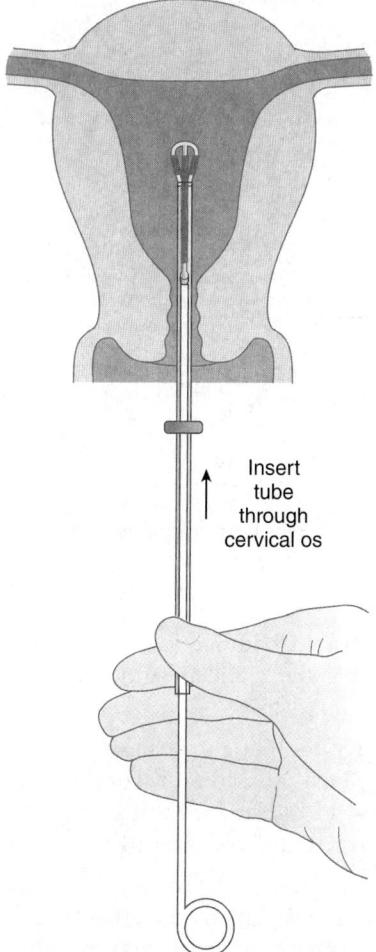

**Figure 12A-14** Insertion of a copper IUD and inserter through the cervical os.

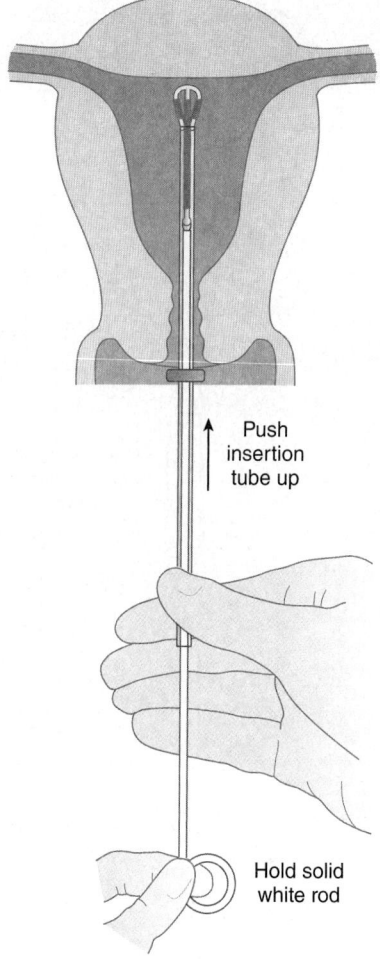

**Figure 12A-15** Placement of a copper IUD through the inserter in the fundus.

In some patients, especially those using a copper IUD, dysmenorrhea or heavy bleeding may occur; the use of NSAIDs provides relief from either or both of these symptoms. Conversely, those individuals using an LNG-IUD may experience decreased menstrual flow or amenorrhea. However, sudden amenorrhea for any person with an IUD may be suggestive of pregnancy, and they should be evaluated for this condition.

### Follow-Up Care

Although a dedicated postinsertion visit is not indicated, it may be beneficial to conduct a thorough risk-assessment or to be responsive to the unique needs of the patient.[3] If a follow-up visit is conducted, typically 4 to 6 weeks post IUD insertion, any concerns patients may have can be addressed at this time. A speculum exam may be performed to confirm that the threads are visible if there is suspicion for expulsion or malposition. After the initial postinsertion visit, future appointments should be made based on routine screening intervals or other risk factors. The patient should be reminded that the IUD can be removed at any point that they desire including at the time of the IUD expiration (e.g., Skyla at 3 years). Once expired, a new device can

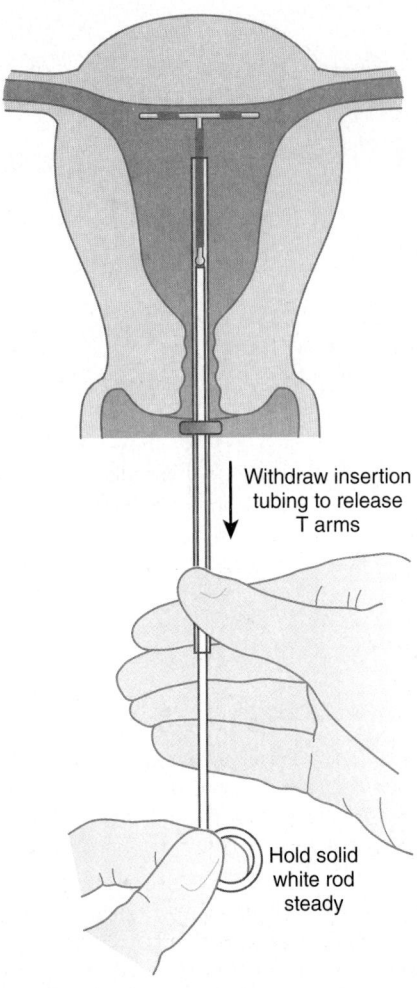

**Figure 12A-16** Withdrawal of insertion tubing to release the arms for a copper IUD.

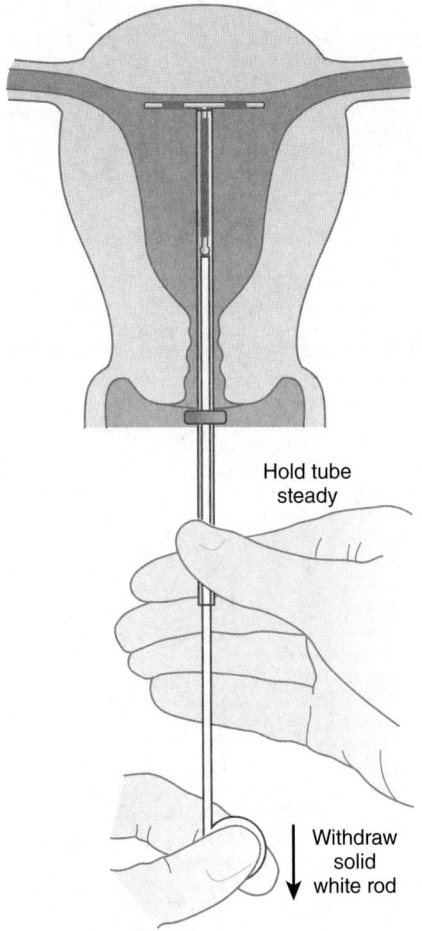

**Figure 12A-17** Withdrawal of rod and insertion tubing for a copper IUD.

be inserted at that time if continuity of IUD use is desired.

## Removal of an Intrauterine Device

Common reasons cited for requesting removal of an IUD include desire for a pregnancy, unnecessary troublesome side effects of menstrual irregularities, establishment of menopause, or end of the duration of effectiveness. The removal procedure is the same for all of the IUDs.

### Procedure for Removing an Intrauterine Device

1. Removal of an IUD requires clean, but not sterile technique.

2. Removal is a rapid procedure. A visit in the office takes approximately the same amount of time as a visit for a Pap test.

3. Constant communication should occur between the clinician and the patient during the removal.

4. After the patient positions themselves in a reclined position of comfort, a speculum may be inserted with their consent. It may be warmed and/or lubricated prior to insertion.

5. Visualize the IUD threads, if possible, and use an instrument (e.g., ring forceps) to grasp the threads. If the strings are not visualized, ultrasound can be used to guide removal.

6. Guide the IUD threads downward toward the clinician until the IUD emerges through the cervix and vagina. Some patients may feel a sharp cramp as the device passes the cervix, but most report no discomfort or little sensation. Most research on pain with IUDs has focused on insertion, with relatively little research being published on IUD removal.

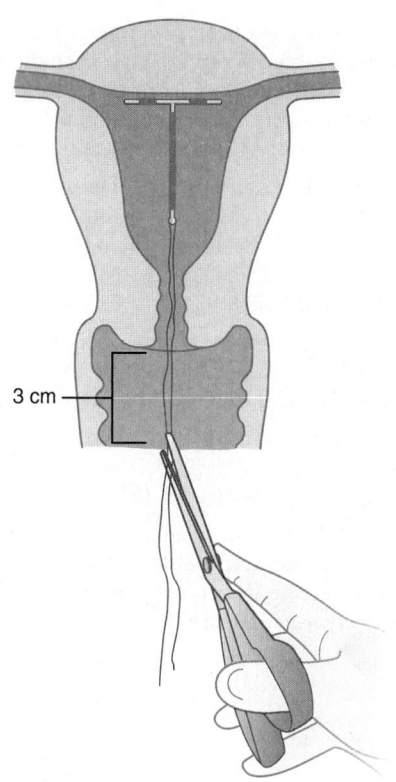

**Figure 12A-18** Cutting threads for any IUD.

3 cm

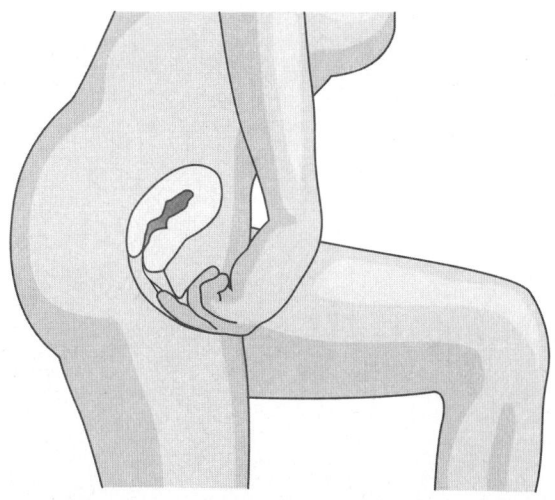

**Figure 12A-19** How to feel for IUD threads or strings.

7. The device may be shown to the patient to reassure them it has been removed.

8. The removal is now complete. If the patient desires a new device, it can be immediately placed by following the procedure presented earlier in this appendix.

### References

1. Dole DM, Martin J. What nurses need to know about immediate postpartum initiation of long-acting reversible contraception. *Nurs Womens Health*. 2017;21(3):186-195.

2. Callegari LS, Aiken AR, Dehlendorf C, et al. Addressing potential pitfalls of reproductive life planning with patient-centered counseling. *Am J Obstet Gynecol*. 2017;216(2):129-134.

3. Curtis KM, Jatlaoui TC, Tepper NK, et al. U.S. selected practice recommendations for contraceptive use, 2016. *MMWR Recomm Rep*. 2016;65(RR-4):1-66.

4. Curtis KM, Tepper NK, Jatlaoui TC, et al. U.S. medical eligibility criteria for contraceptive use, 2016. *MMWR Recomm Rep*. 2016;65(RR-3):1-104.

5. American College of Obstetricians and Gynecologists. Adolescents and long-acting reversible contraception: implants and intrauterine devices. ACOG Committee Opinion No. 735. *Obstet Gynecol*. 2018, reaffirmed 2021;131;e130-e139.

6. Trussell J, Hassan F, Lowin J, et al. Achieving cost-neutrality with long-acting reversible contraceptive methods. *Contraception*. 2015;91(1):49-56.

7. Bearak JM, Finer LB, Jerman J, Kavanaugh ML. Changes in out-of-pocket costs for hormonal IUDs after implementation of the Affordable Care Act: an analysis of insurance benefit inquiries. *Contraception*. 2016;93(2):139-144.

8. Committee on Practice Bulletins—Gynecology, Long-Acting Reversible Contraception Work Group. Practice Bulletin No. 186: long-acting reversible contraception: implants and intrauterine devices. *Obstet Gynecol*. 2017;130(5):e251-e269. https://www.ncbi.nlm.nih.gov/pubmed/29064972. doi:10.1097/AOG.0000000000002400.

9. Barnett C, Moehner S, Do Minh T, Heinemann K. Perforation risk and intra-uterine devices: results of the EURAS-IUD 5-year extension study. *Eur J Contracept Reprod Health Care*. 2017;22(6):424-428.

10. Heinemann K, Barnett C, Reed S, et al. IUD use among parous women and risk of uterine perforation: a secondary analysis. *Contraception*. 2017;95(6):605-607.

11. O'Brien PA, Pillai S. Uterine perforation by intra-uterine devices: a 16-year review. *J Fam Plan Reprod Health Care*. 2017;43(4):289-295.

12. Lopez LM, Bernholc A, Hubacher D, et al. Immediate postpartum insertion of intrauterine device for contraception. *Cochrane Database Syst Rev*. 2015;6:CD003036. doi:10.1002/14651858.CD003036.pub3.

13. Whiteman MK, Tyler CP, Folger SG, et al. When can a woman have an intrauterine device inserted? A systematic review. *Contraception*. 2013;87(5):666-673.

14. Workowski KA, Buchman LH, Chan PA, et al. Sexually transmitted diseases treatment guidelines, 2021. *MMWR Recomm Rep.* 2021;70(4):1-192.

15. Esposito CP. Intrauterine devices in the context of gonococcal infection, chlamydial infection, and pelvic inflammatory disease: not mutually exclusive. *J Midwifery Womens Health.* 2020;65(4):562-566.

16. Tepper NK, Steenland MW, Marchbanks PA, Curtis KM. Laboratory screening prior to initiating contraception: a systematic review. *Contraception.* 2013;87:645-649.

17. Grimes DA, Lopez LM, Schulz KF. Antibiotic prophylaxis for intrauterine contraceptive device insertion. *Cochrane Database Syst Rev.* 1999;3:CD001327. doi:10.1002/14651858.CD001327.

18. Bahamondes MV, Espejo-Arce X, Bahamondes L. Effect of vaginal administration of misoprostol before intrauterine contraceptive insertion following previous insertion failure: a double blind RCT. *Hum Reprod.* 2015;30:1861-1866.

19. Baddour LM, Wilson WR, Bayer AS, et al. Infective endocarditis in adults: diagnosis, antimicrobial therapy, and management of complications: a scientific statement for healthcare professionals from the American Heart Association. *Circulation.* 2015;132(15):1435-1486. https://www.ncbi.nlm.nih.gov/pubmed/26373316. doi:10.1161/CIR.0000000000000296.

20. Johnson LT, Johnson IM, Heineck RJ, Lara-Torre E. Allis compared with tenaculum for stabilization of the cervix during IUD placement. *Obstet Gynecol.* 2015;125. doi:10.1097/01.AOG.0000463550.01588.fd.

21. Grace KT. Caring for women experiencing reproductive coercion. *J Midwifery Womens Health.* 2016;61(1):112-115. doi:10.1111/jmwh.12369.

22. Wiebe ER, Trouton KJ. Does using tampons or menstrual cups increase early IUD insertion rates? *Contraception.* 2012;86(2):119-121.

23. Long J, Schreiber C, Creinin MD, et al. Menstrual cup use and intrauterine device expulsion in a copper intrauterine device contraceptive efficacy trial. *Obstet Gynecol.* 2020;135:1S.

A P P E N D I X

# 12B

# Implant Insertion and Removal

AMY ALSPAUGH

## Introduction

Subdermal contraceptive implants have been available in the United States since 1990 and are the most effective Food and Drug Administration (FDA)–approved method of contraception. Currently, only Nexplanon is available in the United States. The Nexplanon implant is a single-rod implant containing 68 mg of etonogestrel, a synthetic progestin. Clinicians who work internationally or care for individuals who have lived abroad may encounter other types of implants with distinctive characteristics.

## Timing of the Implant Insertion

Implants may be inserted at any time if the clinician is reasonably sure that the individual is not pregnant, including postpartum and post abortion (either spontaneous or induced).[1] Notably, the implant will not harm a pregnant individual or a fetus, so placement or continuation in the presence of pregnancy is not a cause for concern.[2]

Insertion in the immediate postpartum period may be appealing to some individuals and does not appear to have any effect on breastfeeding initiation or continuation. A Cochrane review found that immediate postpartum placement was associated with more bleeding days and more reports of side effects within the first 6 weeks compared to delayed postpartum placement, but no difference was observed in bleeding profile or side effects at 12 months.[3] The clinician and individual should weigh the advantages and disadvantages of immediate postpartum placement. Postabortion insertion continues to be a common practice, with research suggesting this option may be especially appealing for adolescents.[4]

For an individual who is already using a hormonal contraceptive method such as combined oral contraceptives, the implant can be inserted at any time during the cycle and no secondary method of contraception is needed.[2] This seamless transition also can occur when an individual has one implant removed and another implant inserted. If the individual is not using hormonal contraception and the insertion is 5 days or more after the first day of menses, a back-up method of contraception should be used for 7 days when engaging in sexual activity that could result in pregnancy.[2] Current data suggest there is no negative impact on breastfeeding/chestfeeding[5,6] and no increased risk of venous thromboembolism with immediate postpartum insertion.[7] As with any contraceptive method, an individual should be engaged in shared decision making and the decision should be made prior to labor if possible.

Importantly, clinicians may encounter many instances where it is unclear whether an individual may be pregnant. In these cases, the benefits of starting the implant likely exceed the risk; therefore, the implant may be considered for placement at any time.[2] Performing a pregnancy test 2 to 4 weeks after insertion is important in these instances, and can be done by the patient at home or in the clinic.

## Day of Implant Insertion

Unlike the case of other long-acting reversible contraceptives, all individuals who may place or remove the Nexplanon implant are required to receive formal instruction and training from the manufacturer.[1] In addition, the FDA-approved prescribing information and package label for each device include insertion instructions and images. The following steps for insertion are general guidelines and cannot replace hands-on experience.

Prior to insertion, confirm that the individual does not have allergies to the antiseptic or anesthetic used during insertion.

### Required Equipment for Implant Insertion

*General equipment* includes the following items that are clean, as most items do not need to be sterile for implant insertion:

- Clean, nonsterile gloves
- Sterile gloves of appropriate size
- Examination table for the individual to lie on
- Sterile surgical drape
- Antiseptic solution
- Surgical marker
- Local anesthetic
- 2-mL syringe
- 18-gauge needle for drawing up the anesthetic
- 25-gauge, 1.5-cm needle for injecting the anesthetic
- Sterile gauze
- Adhesive bandage
- Pressure bandage
- Medical tape
- Implant inside its applicator, either placed on the field or handed to the clinician by an assistant

### Key Points Related to Insertion of the Nexplanon Implant

1. Optimally, the clinician should have another individual available to assist with the procedure, but it can easily be done alone.

2. The individual should have previously signed a legal consent form for documentation and verification of their understanding of the procedure.

3. The individual should be reassured that the procedure can be stopped at any time should they make this request.

4. To help make sure the implant is inserted just under the skin, the healthcare professional should be positioned to observe the advancement of the needle by viewing the applicator from the side and not from above the arm. From the side view, the insertion

site and the movement of the needle just under the skin can be clearly visualized.

5. Among healthy individuals, no specific examinations or tests are needed before insertion of an implant. A baseline weight and body mass index (BMI) may be useful information in case an individual reports concerns about weight changes while using the implant.[2]

### Step-by-Step Insertion of an Implant

1. The individual should be in a physical position so that they are comfortable for the procedure and the clinician has good visualization. Typically, the individual is lying back on the examination table with their nondominant arm flexed at the elbow and externally rotated so that their nondominant hand is under or near their head (Figure 12B-1). The individual may also elect to have the insertion in their dominant arm.

2. While wearing clean gloves, locate the insertion site, which should be at the inner side of the upper arm, overlying the triceps muscle about 3 to 4 inches from the medial epicondyle of the humerus and 1.25 inches posterior to the sulcus (groove) between the biceps and triceps muscles (Figure 12B-2 and Figure 12B-3). This site is intended to

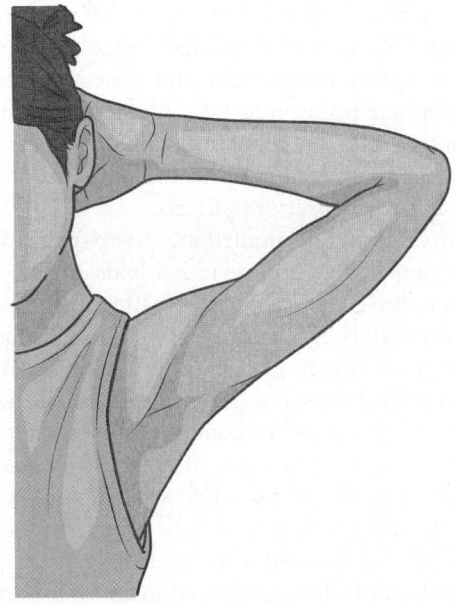

**Figure 12B-1** Positioning for implant insertion.

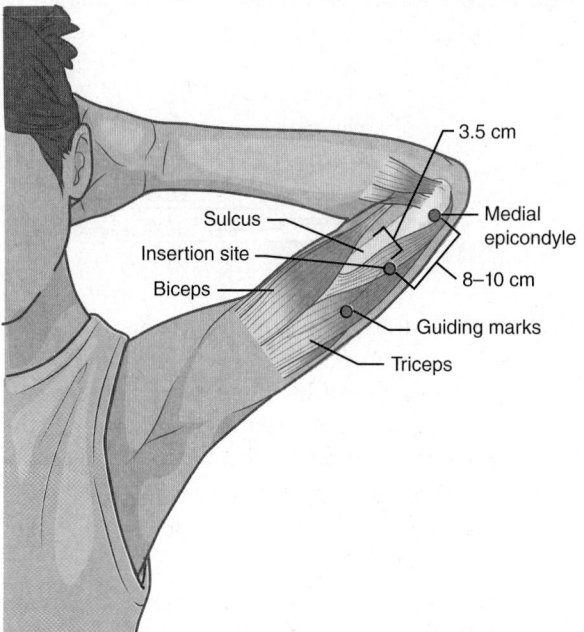

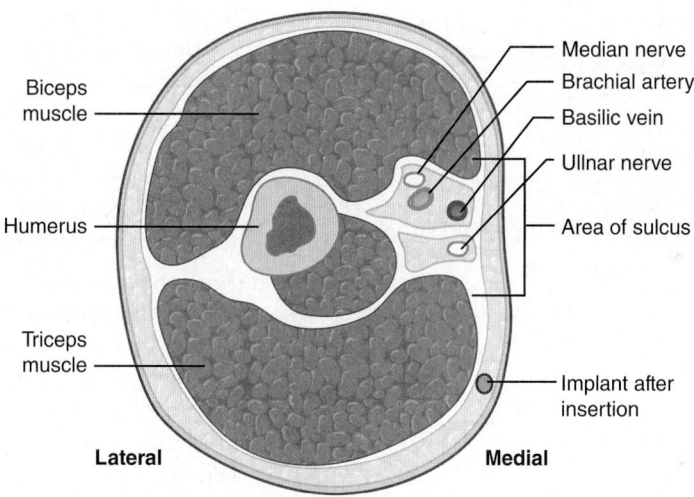

avoid damage to the large blood vessels and
nerves lying within and surrounding the sulcus. If it is not possible to use this location,
in the instance of a very thin arm the implant
should be inserted as far posterior from the
sulcus as possible.

3. Using a surgical marker, mark two spots.
Place a mark first on the insertion site, then
mark a spot 2 inches proximal (toward the

**Figure 12B-2** Location of the implant insertion site and underlying
anatomy.

shoulder) from the first mark (Figure 12B-4).
This second mark serves as a guiding mark
used during insertion.

4. Check that the site of insertion is in the correct location on the inner side of the arm.

5. Clean the skin around the insertion site to
the guiding mark with antiseptic solution.

6. Anesthetize the insertion area using 2 mL of
1% lidocaine just under the skin along the
planned insertion tunnel. Lidocaine with
epinephrine can be used to decrease bleeding, if available.

7. Open the paper backing on the implant applicator and ensure sterile gauze, adhesive
bandage, and pressure bandage are accessible to the clinician.

8. Put on sterile gloves. Remove the sterile pre-
loaded implant applicator from the package.

9. Holding the applicator just above the needle with your fingers gripping the textured
surface area, remove the transparent protective cap by sliding it horizontally in the direction of the arrow away from the needle
(Figure 12B-5). Make sure that the white tip
of the implant is visible from the applicator
needle. *Do not touch the purple slider* at this
point.

10. Using your free hand, lightly stretch the skin
around the insertion site toward the elbow
(Figure 12B-6).

11. Position yourself at the level of the arm to
ensure that the implant is inserted just under

**Figure 12B-3** Cross-sectional view of a properly inserted implant.

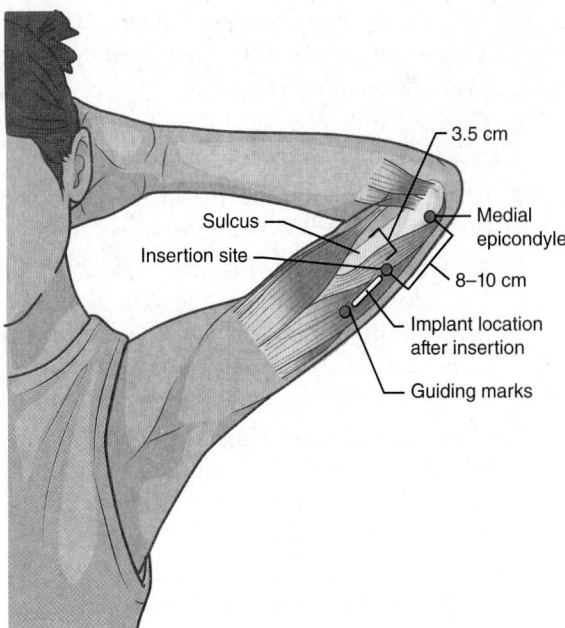

**Figure 12B-4** Marking the insertion site and guiding mark.

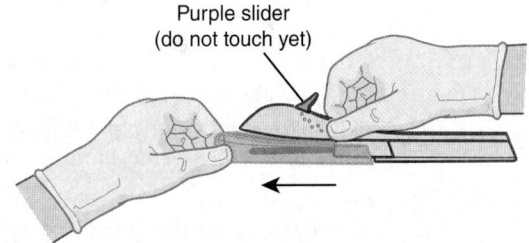

**Figure 12B-5** Removing the protective cap from the applicator.

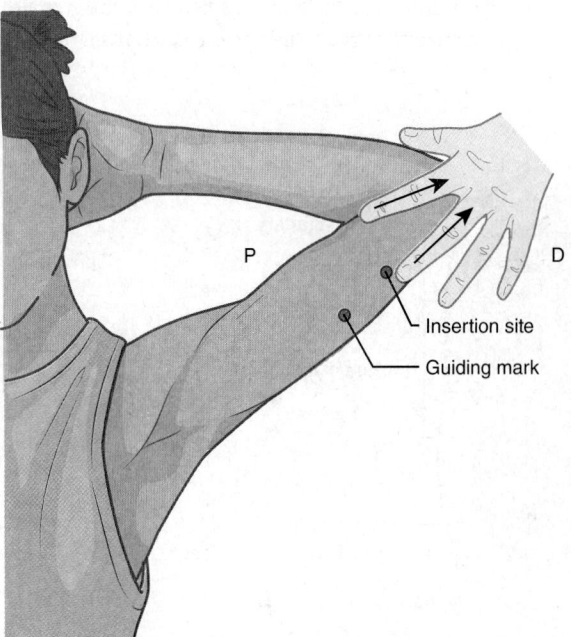

**Figure 12B-6** Stretching the skin with the free hand.

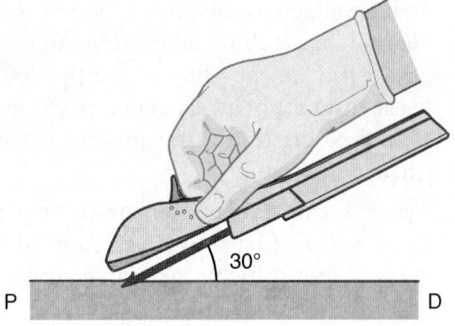

**Figure 12B-7** Puncture the skin with the needle at an angle.

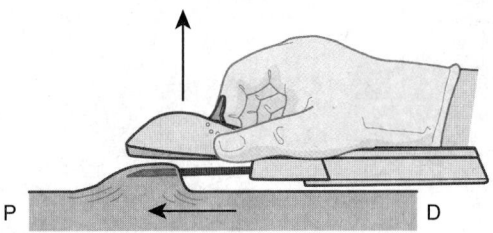

**Figure 12B-8** Inserting the needle while lifting the skin.

the skin. From this side view, you should be able to clearly see the insertion site and the movement of the needle just under the skin.

12. With the tip of the needle angled slightly less than 30 degrees, puncture the skin (Figure 12B-7).

13. Slowly insert the needle until the bevel (slanted opening) is just under the skin and no farther. At this point, lower the applicator to a nearly horizontal position. Then, to enable the subdermal placement, lift the skin slightly with the needle to form a small tent. Continuing to lift slightly, slide the needle to its *full length* (Figure 12B-8). While you may encounter slight resistance, do not use excessive force.

If the needle tip emerges from the skin before the needle insertion is complete, pull the needle back and readjust to a slightly different subdermal position before completing the insertion procedure.

14. With the applicator inserted to its full length, unlock the purple slider by pushing it slightly down. You can use your free hand to stabilize the applicator if needed. Move the slider fully back until it stops, but *do not move the applicator while moving the purple slider* (Figure 12B-9). The implant is now in its subdermal position and the needle is locked inside the body of the applicator, which can

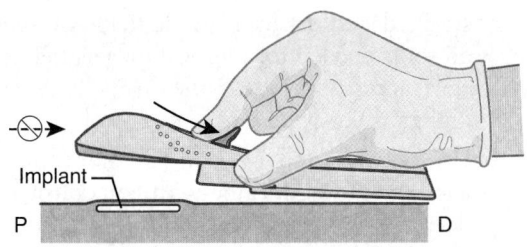

Implant

P                    D

**Figure 12B-9** Retracting the slider.

now be removed from the individual's arm by gently sliding the applicator away from the insertion site.

15. Clean the insertion site with sterile gauze as needed, and place a small adhesive bandage over the insertion site.

16. Verify the presence of the implant by palpation. Palpate both ends of the implant, and have the individual palpate their implant at this point as well. If you cannot feel the implant or are in doubt of its insertion, see the package insert for next steps.

17. Apply the pressure bandage to minimize bruising, using medical tape as needed to secure the bandage.

18. Complete the User Card and give it to the patient. Complete the Patient Chart Label and affix it to the medical record, if using paper records.

## Postinsertion Care

The pressure bandage should be removed by the patient 24 hours after insertion, and the small adhesive bandage may be removed 3 to 5 days after insertion. If the original adhesive bandage falls off prior to 3 days post insertion, instruct the patient to replace the bandage and keep the site covered for at least 3 days.

### Health Education

After insertion of an implant, health education should include a discussion of back-up contraception, if indicated. Postinsertion complications are rare with the implant, but could include pain, paresthesia, bleeding from the insertion site, hematoma, scarring, or infection. Anticipatory guidance should review these complications, next steps that can be taken, and how the patient can easily reach a clinician with questions. It is especially important to review the likelihood of irregular bleeding with the implant, which is usually lighter and shorter than a normal menses but will likely occur at irregular intervals.[8] Nonsteroidal anti-inflammatory drugs (NSAIDs) can help with any postinsertion pain and, at higher doses, decrease any irregular vaginal bleeding that can occur with implant use. All individuals should be counseled that implants do not provide protection from sexually transmitted infections.

### Follow-Up Care

No routine follow-up is needed for most individuals who receive the implant, although adolescents and those with multiple medical conditions may benefit from more frequent follow-up.[2] Advise the individual that they should return at any point to discuss side effects or other problems, if they want to change methods, or when they desire implant removal. At other routine health visits, the clinician should assess for the individual's satisfaction with the method and determine whether they have any concerns about using the method.

## Implant Removal

Common reasons for requesting removal of an implant include desire for a pregnancy, bothersome side effects such as irregular bleeding, and end of duration of effectiveness. It is essential that the clinician minimize impediments to removal in the same way that they minimize barriers to placement, thereby centering bodily autonomy of the patient through prompt support of their request for same-day removal. Resistance to removal by the provider for any reason is a barrier to the patient's right of bodily autonomy and can harm the provider–patient relationship in both the long and short terms.[9] Additionally, it is important to consider the problematic ways in which contraception has caused harm to communities of color and other marginalized groups and center the individual patient's needs and desires above all else.[10,11]

Prior to removal, confirm that the individual does not have allergies to the antiseptic or anesthetic used during insertion.

### Required Equipment for Implant Removal

*General equipment* includes the following items that are clean, as most items do not need to be sterile for this procedure:

- Clean, nonsterile gloves
- Sterile gloves of appropriate size
- Examination table for the individual to lie on

- Sterile surgical drape
- Antiseptic solution
- Surgical marker
- Local anesthetic
- 2-mL syringe
- 18-gauge needle for drawing up the anesthetic
- 25-gauge, 1.5-cm needle for injecting the anesthetic
- Sterile scalpel, forceps (straight and curved mosquito)
- Skin closure bandage
- Sterile gauze
- Adhesive bandage
- Pressure bandage

### Procedure for Removing an Implant

1. Position the individual in a similar manner as for insertion, lying back on an exam table with the elbow of the arm with the implant flexed and the hand underneath or near their head.

2. Wearing clean gloves, palpate the inner arm to locate the implant. Push down gently on the end of the implant closest to the shoulder to stabilize it; the other tip of the implant closest to the elbow should create a slight bulge (Figure 12B-10). Mark the distal end (closest to the elbow) with a surgical marker. If the tip of the implant does not pop up, removal may be more challenging and should be performed by clinicians with experience removing deeper implants.

3. Clean the marked site with antiseptic solution. Change into sterile gloves. Using a

sterile drape, set up a sterile field and place all tools needed for removal on this field for easy access, including the scalpel, forceps, and gauze to wipe away any blood.

4. Use between 0.5 to 1 mL of lidocaine; if available, use lidocaine with epinephrine to decrease the bleeding at the insertion site, thereby improving visualization. Be careful to inject the local anesthetic *under the tip of the implant* to keep the implant close to the surface of the skin, making removal easier (Figure 12B-11).

5. While pushing downward gently on the proximal (closest to the shoulder) end of the implant, make a 2-mm longitudinal incision *parallel to the implant* toward the elbow. Do not cut the tip of the implant.

6. In some cases, the tip of the implant will pop out of the incision with gentle pressure on the proximal end. In other cases, gently push the proximal end of the implant toward the incision until the tip is visualized at the incision. Grasp the implant with whichever style of forceps works best for that particular removal, as conditions will change.

   Unless the implant was placed recently, it may be necessary to use the scalpel to gently remove adherent tissues from the implant while holding the tip with the forceps.

7. If the implant is not visualized after gentle pressure, there are two ways to attempt removal. The clinician may (1) extend the incision into the tissue sheath and remove the implant with forceps or (2) insert forceps (generally a curved mosquito forceps with

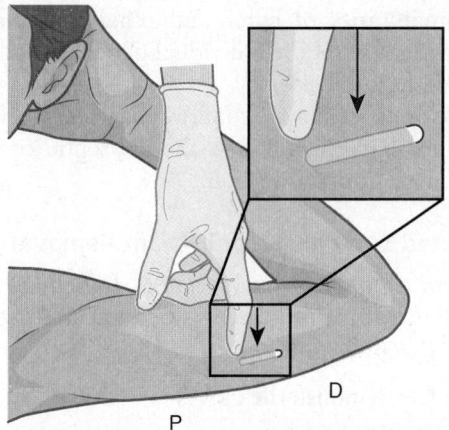

**Figure 12B-10** Palpating the implant to identify the distal end.

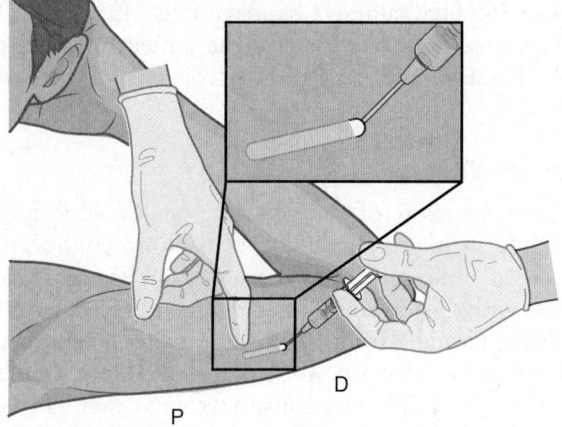

**Figure 12B-11** Injection of lidocaine underneath the tip of the implant.

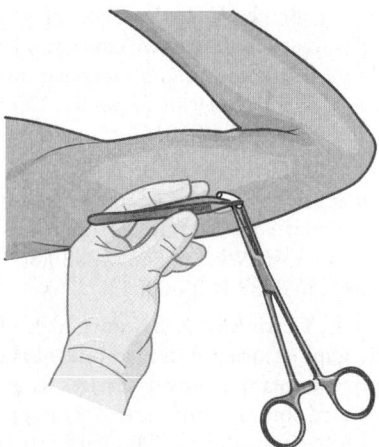

**Figure 12B-12** Grasping the implant for removal.

the tip pointed up yields the best results) superficially into the incision to attempt to grasp the implant. Pass this set of forceps to the nondominant hand, and then grasp the implant with a second set of forceps to gently remove it (Figure 12B-12). If both of these attempts fail, stop the procedure and refer the patient to a clinician with experience in complex removals or check the package insert for further information on referrals.

8. Confirm that the entire implant has been removed by inspecting the implant and ensuring all 4 cm is present and intact.

9. Close the incision site with sterile adhesive wound closures, and apply gauze and a pressure bandage to minimize bruising. Encourage the patient to remove the pressure bandage after 24 hours and the adhesive bandage in 3 to 5 days.

## Concurrent Removal and Reinsertion

Much like an intrauterine device, a new implant may be placed once an expired implant is removed if the individual desires to continue using the implant method. Simply insert the applicator into the same incision once the old implant has been removed. Bandage and review the patient education topics as you would during an initial insertion.

## Other Types of Implants

Although Nexplanon is the only FDA-approved implant in the United States, several different types of implants are available worldwide. A clinician may encounter these while working internationally or while caring for people who had implants placed in other countries. The original six-rod implant was phased out worldwide in 2007, but some individuals may still have them in place. As these implants are more difficult to remove, they should be referred to a clinician experienced in Norplant or difficult implant removal. Two other types of implants currently in production worldwide are the Jadelle and Sino-Implant (II) options. Both implants are composed of two rods instead of one, and contain the hormone levonorgestrel. Jadelle is labeled for 5 years of use, while Sino-Implant (II) is labeled for 3 years of use.[12]

Efforts are under way to create an implant that would biodegrade naturally, thereby eliminating implant removal as a barrier to implant use in more underserved or rural communities where reliable access to health care is limited.[13,14] Both the Jadelle and Sino-Implant (II) implants can be removed with the same procedure as the Nexplanon implant, although depending on migration of the rods, removal may require making two incisions at the distal ends of the rods instead of one.

## References

1. Nexplanon prescribing information. https://www.organon.com/product/usa/pi_circulars/n/nexplanon/nexplanon_pi.pdf. Revised July 2021. Accessed March 13, 2023.

2. Curtis KM, Jatlaoui TC, Tepper NK, et al. U.S. selected practice recommendations for contraceptive use, 2016. *MMWR Recomm Rep*. 2016;65. doi:10.15585/mmwr.rr6504a1.

3. Grimes DA, Lopez LM, O'Brien PA, Raymond E. Progestin-only pills for contraception. *Cochrane Database Syst Rev*. 2013;11. doi:10.1002/14651858.CD007541.pub3.

4. Roe AH, Fortin J, Janiak E, et al. Prevalence and predictors of initiation of intrauterine devices and subdermal implants immediately after surgical abortion. *Contraception*. 2019;100(2):89-95. doi:10.1016/j.contraception.2019.05.001.

5. Lopez LM, Grey TW, Stuebe AM, et al. Combined hormonal versus nonhormonal versus progestin-only contraception in lactation. *Cochrane Database Syst Rev*. 2015;3:CD003988. doi:10.1002/14651858.CD003988.pub2.

6. Phillips SJ, Tepper NK, Kapp N, et al. Progestogen-only contraceptive use among breastfeeding women: a systematic review. *Contraception*. 2016;94(3):226-252. doi:10.1016/j.contraception.2015.09.010.

7. Floyd JL, Beasley AD, Swaim LS, et al. Association of immediate postpartum etonogestrel implant insertion and venous thromboembolism. *Obstet Gynecol*. 2020;135(6):1275-1280. doi:10.1097/AOG.0000000000003760.

8. Zigler RE, McNicholas C. Unscheduled vaginal bleeding with progestin-only contraceptive use. *Am J Obstet Gynecol.* 2017;216(5):443-450. doi:10.1016/j.ajog.2016.12.008.

9. Amico JR, Bennett AH, Karasz A, Gold M. "She just told me to leave it": women's experiences discussing early elective IUD removal. *Contraception.* 2016;94(4): 357-361. doi:10.1016/j.contraception.2016.04.012.

10. Ross LJ, Solinger R. *Reproductive Justice.* Oakland, CA: University of California Press; 2017.

11. Higgins JA. Celebration meets caution: LARC's boons, potential busts, and the benefits of a reproductive justice approach. *Contraception.* 2014;89(4):237-241. doi:10.1016/j.contraception.2014.01.027.

12. Steiner MJ, Brache V, Taylor D, et al. Randomized trial to evaluate contraceptive efficacy, safety and acceptability of a two-rod contraceptive implant over 4 years in the Dominican Republic. *Contracept X.* 2019;1:100006. doi:10.1016/j.conx.2019.100006.

13. Callahan R, Lebetkin E, Brennan C, et al. What goes in must come out: a mixed-method study of access to contraceptive implant removal services in Ghana. *Glob Health Sci Pract.* 2020;8(2):220-238. doi:10.9745/GHSP-D-20-00013.

14. Howett R, Gertz AM, Kgaswanyane T, et al. Closing the gap: ensuring access to and quality of contraceptive implant removal services is essential to rights-based contraceptive care. *Afr J Reprod Health.* 2019;23(4):19-26. doi:10.29063/ajrh2019/v23i4.3.

CHAPTER

# 13

# Gender-Affirming Care

SIGNEY OLSON AND KATIE DEPALMA

## Introduction: Care of Transgender and Nonbinary Individuals

The care that midwives and advanced practice registered nurses (APRNs) are educated to provide, such as primary care, reproductive and sexual health care, gynecologic care, pregnancy and birth care, is essentially the same for the transgender and nonbinary (TGNB) clients whom they serve. Midwifery care should be easily accessible to anyone who desires it, including TGNB individuals, who do not have inherently more complex healthcare needs than cisgender individuals.

Midwives and APRNs seek to understand individuals by adopting a broad and holistic view, provide a therapeutic presence, actively listen, support what is physiologic and normal, identify and address any abnormalities, discuss and offer options, partner with families and communities, understand disparities and issues of equity, provide informed consent, and shift the paternalistic power dynamics of the healthcare system back to their clients. However, due to a history of anti-transgender bias in health care, TGNB individuals may need more individualized care and consideration than someone who has never been marginalized due to their gender identity. The unique aspects of this care are discussed in this chapter. The authors' hope is that within our lifetimes, parts of this chapter will no longer be necessary, as there will be no binary assumptions that dictate the provision of care. We hope that only a holistic approach for clients, the organs they possess, and the goals they share remains. For now, midwives must move forward with determination that the profession will be at the forefront of breaking down systems of oppression that hinder everyone's humanity.

## Prevalence

Determining the number of individuals who identify as trans and nonbinary is challenging due to the limiting nature of terminology as well as the possible lack of safety in disclosing one's identity. Best estimates are that 0.5% to 0.6% of the U.S. adult population is transgender or nonbinary, although many experts believe this number is higher due to some individuals being unable to safely use these terms to self-identify.[1] Higher rates of TGNB individuals are seen with each new generation, such as the 1.8% of Generation Z (those born 1997 and later) who are TGNB.[2] This increase has not occurred because there are suddenly more TGNB individuals, but rather is a representation of the enhanced visibility of TGNB people and improved language to describe the ways in which people experience their gender.[3]

## Concepts of Gender

Gender-expansive individuals have always existed and, prior to colonialist structures, were revered and celebrated community members in numerous cultures.[4] The gender binary is relatively new in the history of humanity, but is a deeply rooted structure that dominates our culture, creates anti-trans bias, and causes harm to many individuals.[5] This binary often begins to become engrained even before an individual is born and affirms the belief that a person is either male or female, masculine or feminine, with specific attributes, traits, and expectations based on that designation. These traits are viewed as inherent and immutable, and are often the foundation of social and political violence. Humans often prefer things to be categorized and labeled, but the reality of gender is that it cannot be neatly compartmentalized. While categorization may not always be inherently harmful, the world around an individual will immediately begin to demonstrate gender expectations based on that assigned category. A binary fails to address the fact that gender does not need to exist in a defined box and may look different for all individuals, often evolving over the course of a person's life.

Gender typically begins to emerge as an internally recognized concept around age 3, with most people further solidifying their gender identity by their mid-teens.[6] Recent research shows that 94% of transgender youth younger than age 18 continue to identify as the gender to which they had transitioned after an average time frame of 5 years.[7]

The use of the terms *transgender* and *nonbinary* and the acronym *TGNB* in this chapter is done with the acknowledgment that gender is an individualized constellation and not always able to be contained within labels. The authors also acknowledge that because TGNB people are not a monolith, there is no one best practice or generalizable way to care for all gender-expansive clients. Midwives offer this same reverence of individualized care to our cisgender clients; liberation from the binary is intertwined and beneficial to all.

## Personal Reflection

An important aspect of providing gender-inclusive care is personal reflection. Clinicians are recommended to reflect on their own lived experiences of gender bias and ways that gender norms harm all individuals, not just TGNB people (Table 13-1).[8]

## Approach to Terminology

As a general rule, it is recommended that providers use gender-neutral language when speaking in generalities so as to be inclusive and minimize harm.[9] Clients may not always share their gender identity, and many cisgender clients also prefer gender-inclusive language. Clinicians may find it easiest to default to gender-neutral language, which helps to avoid othering of clients. For discussions with a client, it is best to ask which words or language affirms them and to use those words when speaking directly with them as well as in scenarios where the client is not present.[10] Additionally, reclamation of words is always an individual or community choice, so a client may decide to use words that other individuals recommend to avoid. Table 13-2 provides recommended terms to use when communicating on sex and gender.[11–15]

## State Laws and Scope of Practice Complexities

The American College of Nurse-Midwives (ACNM) established a Gender Equity Task Force to specifically address questions regarding the provision of midwifery care for TGNB individuals. As of 2021, affirming care of TGNB individuals is included in both ACNM's Core Competencies for Basic Midwifery Practice and the ACNM Definition of Midwifery and Scope of Practice of Certified Nurse-Midwives and Certified Midwives (CNM/CM).[16,17] While certain aspects of this care, such as gender-affirming hormone care, were previously considered part of an expanded scope of practice, this is no longer the case. Historically, there has been discussion regarding whether midwives were qualified to care for trans women. As affirmed repeatedly through the revisions of the previously mentioned documents, ACNM includes care of trans women in its explanation of both midwifery core competencies and CNM/CM scope of practice.

| Table 13-1 | Reflective Questions for Clinicians to Explore Individual Biases |
|---|---|
| Why do you choose to present, behave, speak, and dress in the ways you do? How are those things representative of your gender? | |
| What are ways that you have been treated differently because of your gender in your childhood, adolescence, or adulthood? | |
| Why does society have certain expectations of men? Who benefits? Who is harmed? | |
| Why does society have certain expectations of women? Who benefits? Who is harmed? | |
| Does it cause you discomfort to observe men engaging in activities considered traditionally feminine? Does it cause you discomfort to observe women engaging in activities considered traditionally masculine? | |
| What is the origin of the various cultural narratives regarding gender? | |
| Why do various cultures continue to buy into those narratives? | |
| What would it look like if our current understanding of rigid gender categories shifted? | |

| Table 13-2 | Appropriate Gender-Affirming Terminology and Definitions[a] |
|---|---|
| **Term** | **Definition** |
| Sex | Often thought of as a biologic construct consisting of chromosomes, reproductive organs, genitalia, and hormones. Historically, sex has had only two options—male or female; this is not accurate, as sex characteristics exist on a spectrum and definitions of binary sex are typically socially constructed rather than solely biologic. |
| Sex assigned at birth | The sex category to which individuals are assigned at the time of birth, typically based on perception of external genitalia. However, this term does not provide the person's current identity or anatomy, only what sex they were presumed to be at the time of birth.<br>This language is intentional, as it puts the onus of the potential "misassignment" on the provider or system rather than the individual. Some TGNB individuals think of their sex assigned at birth as the clinician "getting it wrong." |
| Assigned female at birth (AFAB) | Individuals who were assigned a female gender at the time of birth, typically by a birth attendant, based on the appearance of external genitalia. |
| Assigned male at birth (AMAB) | Individuals who were assigned a male gender at the time of birth, typically by a birth attendant, based on the appearance of external genitalia. |
| Intersex | Refers to individuals born with physical and/or biologic sex characteristics that do not neatly fall into categories of male or female.[11] Intersex people can have internal or external features that appear stereotypically male, stereotypically female, or androgynous, as there are many types of intersex traits based on variations in chromosomal patterns, internal reproductive organs, genitalia, secondary sex characteristics, and hormones. It is estimated that approximately 1.7% of the population is intersex, although the actual percentage may be higher, given that most individuals have not had a chromosomal analysis.[11] Of note, this term does not have a universally agreed-upon definition within the medical community and prevalence may vary slightly depending on exclusion criteria.<br>Many national and global medical organizations oppose medically unnecessary surgeries on intersex infants and children due to the potential risk for physical and psychological harm.[12,13]<br>It is important to understand that intersex is not a gender identity or sexual orientation. Diversity in sex chromosomes is shown throughout various species and provides additional evidence that many animals have more than two biologic sexes.[14,15] |
| Gender | A social, rather than biologic, construct, which refers to norms, social expectations, and roles that individuals play in society. These roles and norms vary within any given culture and may be influenced by life stage. |
| Gender identity | The ways in which a person experiences their gender internally. It may be a feeling of being female, male, both, neither, or another gender. |
| Gender expression or gender presentation | The ways in which a person expresses themself and their gender externally. It may include things such as clothing choices, hairstyle, makeup, jewelry, and other appearance-related choices. |
| Transgender (or trans) | An adjective that refers to an individual who has a gender identity other than the sex or gender they were assigned at birth. The opposite of cisgender. |
| Cisgender (or cis) | An adjective that refers to an individual who has a gender identity congruent with the sex they were assigned at birth. The opposite of transgender. |
| Gender binary | The classification of gender into two distinct, opposite categories of either male/masculine or female/feminine. Some trans individuals who identify entirely as a man or a woman will fall within the binary. |
| Nonbinary | An adjective that refers to an individual whose gender identity exists outside of a gender binary and does not identify as entirely male or entirely female but often somewhere in between, in fluctuation, or outside of the binary. This may also be similar to other terms such as genderqueer, genderfluid, gender nonconforming, agender, and bigender. |
| Trans woman | A woman who was assigned male at birth. |
| Trans man | A man who was assigned female at birth. |

*(continues)*

| Table 13-2 | Appropriate Gender-Affirming Terminology and Definitions[a] *(continued)* |
|---|---|
| **Term** | **Definition** |
| Trans feminine | Typically used to describe an individual on the feminine side of the gender spectrum (but who does not necessarily identify as entirely female) who was assigned male at birth. Often shortened to *trans femme* or *trans fem*. |
| Trans masculine | Typically used to describe an individual on the masculine side of the gender spectrum (but who does not necessarily identify as entirely male) who was assigned female at birth. Often shortened to *trans masc*. |
| Two-Spirit | A modern Pan-Indian term coined in 1990 but rooted in older U.S. Native American and Canadian First Nations communities to describe tribe members who embodied physical and emotional traits of both men and women. Often, these individuals were considered a "third gender" and not assigned a male or female category. Of note, this term is used as a form of self-identification only by individuals with Indigenous heritage, often as a way of remaining connected to important ancestral history. |
| Gender dysphoria | Clinically significant distress related to an incongruence between gender identity and sex assigned at birth, often with a strong desire to be another gender. Not all TGNB individuals experience gender dysphoria, and some experts believe gender dysphoria to be primarily caused by harmful gender norms and expectations in society. |
| Gender euphoria | The experience of feeling joy, happiness, and contentedness as a result of moving away from one's birth-assigned gender and toward one's affirmed gender identity. |
| Top surgery | Umbrella term for surgery performed on the chest as part of gender affirmation. This could be a masculinizing procedure to flatten the chest and remove breast tissue, such as during a bilateral double mastectomy. It could also be a feminizing procedure to increase breast mass/volume such as during a bilateral breast augmentation. |
| Bottom surgery | Umbrella term for surgery performed on the reproductive organs as part of gender affirmation. In both masculinizing and feminizing procedures, this often includes several surgeries, sometimes over a certain time frame. In trans masculine individuals, it may refer to the surgical creation of a phallus, testicular implants, or a hysterectomy. In trans feminine individuals, it may refer to the creation of a neovagina, orchiectomy, or vulvar/labial construction. |
| **Words and Phrases to Avoid** | |
| Transsexual | Generally considered derogatory or a slur in modern discussions of gender, although some individuals may choose to self-identify as transsexual. Additionally, some research, particularly from Europe, may continue to utilize this term. |
| A transgender | Because the word *transgender* is an adjective, not a noun, this phrase would not be an appropriate way to refer to a transgender person. |
| Transman or transwoman | Writing *trans man* or *trans woman* is the correct way to phrase these terms. Using these words without a space is not recommended because this implies a separateness between trans men and cis men and between trans women and cis women. Though the slight is often unintentional, these terms may exclude or degrade trans people. |
| **Examples of Microaggressions** | |

Assumption of gender and/or pronouns
Acting offended if someone thinks you are trans
Staring at individuals in public whose gender expression confuses you
Use of the term *real man* or *real woman*
"This person used to be a man, but now he's a woman"
Using a person's former name (*dead-naming*) or pronouns (*misgendering*)
"Wow, I would never have known you used to be a girl!"
"You're so beautiful for a trans person!"

[a] This list is not comprehensive and is ever-evolving; some individuals may interpret these terms through a slightly different lens.

This is particularly impactful because many individual states base their nursing scope of practice laws on ACNM documents. However, each state's CNM/CM scope of practice legislation is unique, and some contain antiquated gendered language. Thus, it remains the responsibility of each midwife to confirm their state laws (this is recommended for all types of care and midwifery skills, not just gender-affirming care).

Appropriately, the majority of midwifery educational programs now include specific content regarding care of TGNB individuals. At a minimum, midwives graduate with foundational knowledge, as defined in the ACNM Core Competencies, about these communities and strategies to provide respectful care.[17] As with other areas of care, such as menopause and primary care, individual midwives may need to develop and strengthen their knowledge in any given area as they gain experience following their midwifery education. However, it is important to note that care of TGNB individuals is not to be considered an expanded scope that requires documentation of competency.

### Feminism, Midwifery, and Gender

Feminism has been a powerful driving force in the field of midwifery and has set the profession apart from others in health care. Feminism that is inclusive and intersectional must be prioritized. The authors recommend approaching patient care with the following principles:

- Cisgender women and TGNB individuals should have rights equal to cisgender men.
- There are more than two biologic sexes.
- There are infinite genders and gender expressions.
- Healthcare providers can affirm TGNB people without erasing cisgender women.
- The gender binary harms both TGNB and cisgender people.

The term *trans-exclusionary radical feminist (TERF)* refers to a small, but vocal group of cisgender women who intentionally engage in transphobia by excluding trans women in their efforts for women's rights and assert that being assigned female at birth is the only way to define womanhood.[18] TERF ideology has been responsible for significant harms to the TGNB community, including the dissemination of inaccurate information, engaging in hate speech, and committing or endorsing violent crimes, causing damage ranging from loss of employment to loss of community, trauma, and death.[18,19]

While the midwifery philosophy of care is inconsistent with that of TERFs, it is also important to acknowledge harm caused by the midwifery profession, as the narrative within midwifery about noncisgender identity has been a source of damaging dialogue regarding the inclusion of care for trans men and, more explicitly, trans women. It is crucial that the profession of midwifery denounce any narrative that excludes vulnerable populations from life-saving care. Midwifery moves forward with a clear voice for inclusive and intersectional feminism—examples include the decision to include trans-affirming care in ACNM's Core Competencies in 2020 and ACNM's 2021 position statement "Health Care for Transgender and Gender Non-Binary People."[17,20]

### Creating a More Inclusive Space

Table 13-3 identifies challenges and opportunities for making clinical spaces and interactions more inclusive for all genders.

## Providing Affirming Care

A clinician who is knowledgeable about trauma-sensitive and consent-based care is someone who can affirm a client's multidimensional existence. The initial steps in providing this type of affirming care are described next.

### Identify and Evaluate Personal Implicit Bias

Do personal biases stem from lack of exposure? Lack of experience? Lack of knowledge? Something else? An honest and common answer is "yes," but clinicians will need to address their own bias before they can create a space with the safety deserved by clients who could be harmed by those biases.[21] Advertising care as safe or inclusive before addressing personal biases is never appropriate. It is best to reflect on this internally first, and then with someone who is cisgender and/or a professional resource. It can be harmful to TGNB people for clinicians to process that bias with them. If someone volunteers, it is okay to accept and be sure to negotiate boundaries for the conversations and check in periodically to be sure they are okay.

### Commit to Learning or Relearning Language

This step is important when discussing anatomic parts of the body. Ask clients which terms they are comfortable with, and then use those. Remove gendered language from discussions regarding health. This is and will continue to be a challenge due to

| Table 13-3 | Creating a More Inclusive Space |
| --- | --- |
| **Touchpoints with Higher Potential to Provoke Gender Dysphoria** | **Examples of Harmful Interactions** |
| Scheduling an appointment | A receptionist equates voice tone and pitch with a certain gender and may use gendered honorifics with the client. |
| Checking in for a visit | A traditionally masculine-appearing individual is asked if they are sure they're in the correct office or a client has to state their name or reason for visit audibly in the waiting room. |
| Being called from the waiting area | A staff member calls out the patient's legal name or using the incorrect honorific. |
| Clinician discomfort during history-taking discussion | The clinician avoids conversations due to lack of awareness or embarrassment. The clinician asks inappropriate questions that are not relevant to the care being provided. |
| **Examples of Inclusive Practices** | |
| Gender-neutral office decor and waiting room materials | |
| Staff trained in use of affirming language and office etiquette Remind staff that not using a person's stated pronouns or name is a form of discrimination and harassment | |
| Gender-neutral bathrooms | |
| Forms need spots for the client's chosen name and pronouns, at a minimum | |
| Normalizing staff adding their own pronouns (email signature and badges) | |
| Consider a hired "secret shopper" experience in your office in which a paid professional helps to evaluate the process of what patients experience. | |

the history of unnecessary, yet engrained, gendering in healthcare education, practice, publication, and media. For example, the term *well-woman exams* becomes more specific and gender-inclusive when changed to *periodic* or *wellness GYN exams*. Remember to document in the health record with the same terminology agreed upon with the client. If that is not possible, be sure to discuss with the client why the words may differ in their health record, as unexpected incongruences can dissolve trust and cause harm as clients gain access to their electronic health records and notes. It can be helpful to create note templates with gender-neutral terminology to use for all clients.

### Seek Education Outside of the Exam Room

One important aspect of cultural humility is to seek out educational experiences and opportunities.[22] While clients may voluntarily share some information about their personhood, a clinician should not expect to be educated by their clients. Showing up to the visit as a provider who has done their own work is an important step in creating safety for clients.

It is recommended to seek opportunities from gender-expansive educators, especially Black, Indigenous, and people of color (BIPOC) educators who are compensated for their time, emotional labor, and expertise. Additionally, clinicians must remember that BIPOC and TGNB people are not monoliths, and that no one person or resource can possibly convey the breadth of experiences of a community.

It is inappropriate for the clinician to ask questions out of curiosity that are not clinically relevant to the care they are providing. For example, if a client discloses a history of top surgery, it is appropriate to ask about the timing and type of procedure done, as it potentially relates to care that may be considered or provided. It would not be acceptable to inquire whether the client missed having breasts after a mastectomy. Ideally, the clinician is also able to convey to the client their intention behind asking questions. It's important that the clinician recalls that being TGNB does not require hormonal or surgical treatments—plenty of TGNB people do not have a desire or access to those types of care.[23] Similarly, it's recommended that providers avoid any and all comments about a client's appearance or experience that do not relate to the care they are providing. Education and understanding aside, an individual's gender is whatever they say it is—believe them.

### Choose Humility and Respect over Defensiveness

Best clinical practice is ever-changing, as it represents improvements in the delivery of care. Language seems to change even more frequently.[24] Even the best-intentioned providers can feel intimidated when engaging with clients with different or historically oppressed identities for fear of misspeaking and causing harm. Given that best practices and inclusive language are not universal among all clients, it is fair to assume that mistakes will be made. It is important for the clinician to receive any feedback with humility, be okay with getting it wrong, apologize quickly, center the client's experience (not the clinician's shame), and move on with the conversation if the client is comfortable doing so.[9]

### Review Health Disparities That Affect the TGNB Community

To provide culturally humble care, clinicians must understand the historical context that has led to current rates of health disparities disproportionately affecting the TGNB community. These disparities are compounded by other forms of systemic oppression, and BIPOC individuals who are also TGNB frequently face intersectional issues of oppression.[25,26] These disparities are reviewed in more depth in the *Context of Individuals Seeking Midwifery Care* chapter.

### Avoid Gatekeeping

Clinicians have the ability to remove unnecessary barriers to care, such as requiring all clients to provide documentation from mental health providers prior to prescribing hormone therapy.

### Appreciate the Whole Person

It is important to consider aspects of intersectionality such as race, ethnicity, age, body size, disability, neurodiversity, socioeconomic status, class, financial security, access to systems of support and safety, immigration or migration status, primary language, health literacy, culture, spirituality, religious health beliefs, access to food and clean water, exposure to environmental toxins, and access or desire for non-Western modalities of care. While this chapter focuses on gender diversity, clinicians must recognize and acknowledge any other identities the client has and honor the intersectionality of them all.[26] The client has lived their whole life in their body and is an expert on their experience—when a clinician acknowledges the value and beauty in that, affirming care becomes truly possible.

## Psychosocial Considerations and Mental Health

It is well established that TGNB identity itself is not a psychological condition. More formally, gender identity disorder was removed as a diagnosis from the *Diagnostic and Statistical Manual of Mental Disorders* (DSM) in 2013.[27] However, TGNB individuals do experience a higher rate of mental health conditions such as depression, anxiety, post-traumatic stress disorder (PTSD), eating disorders, and substance use disorders.[28–30] Increased rates of these diagnoses are not due to a client's gender identity, but rather stem from the pervasiveness of anti-trans bias and experiences of microaggressions in society, communities, and the media.[28] While historically oppressed groups often exhibit remarkably high rates of resiliency, it is the responsibility of those in power to unlearn biased behaviors that result in the need for resiliency in the first place.

The risk of attempted and completed suicide is higher in TGNB groups than in most other marginalized groups in the United States, with some studies showing 86% of transgender individuals have contemplated suicide.[31,32] This is likely due to systemic oppression and underlying anti-trans bias that feeds into systemic inequities. Many TGNB individuals have experienced mental health concerns and suicidal ideation prior to accessing affirming care. Passive suicidal thoughts are not a contraindication to gender-affirming hormone (GAH) therapy, but should be considered thoughtfully. External support systems have been shown to be one of the more impactful factors in all mental health risks, especially for trans youth younger than the age of 18.[31] Some studies show that among trans youth who do not have parental support or accepting adults in their lives, nearly 80% have attempted suicide.[33] With parental and/or other accepting adult support, this risk drops to 35%. Parental support is also the most significant factor in preventing homelessness in trans youth.[33] The queer community in general has always placed a high importance on the role of nonbiologic chosen family and community in maintaining safety and resiliency.[34,35]

Mental health risks increase with the intersectionality of other oppressed identities such as race, disability, class, and immigration status.[26] TGNB individuals are also at increased risk of experiencing physical violence and trauma from their communities, close contacts, and intimate partners.[36] In particular, BIPOC trans women are victims of homicide at higher rates than other members of the TGNB community.[37] Again, systems of oppression and the harms of gender norms contribute to these risks, not the person's gender identity itself.[8] Awareness of the rates of violence can be taxing and result in increased allostatic load and hypervigilance.[38]

Increased rates of eating disorders and body dysmorphia have been reported in the TGNB community, specifically in the trans masculine, trans feminine, and nonbinary communities.[39] Some research suggests that individuals with nonbinary identities may experience the highest rate of disordered eating and other mental health concerns, possibly due to societal discomfort with less frequently acknowledged gender identities.[40] For example, trans masculine individuals may experience dysphoria around their chest, hips, and body curvature and desire a reduction in these areas. Trans feminine individuals may experience dysphoria related to muscle mass and seek to reduce overall body size. It is important that clinicians be sensitive to this risk and use a weight-neutral approach to care as well as incorporate routine eating disorder screening into their history taking, regardless of body size. See the *Skillful Communication to Mitigate Clinician Bias* appendix for additional information on weight-neutral care, and the *Common Conditions in Primary Care* chapter for additional information on eating disorders.

Mental health improves with use of an individual's correct name, pronouns, and increased access to gender-affirming care.[29,33] Some individuals may find that treatment of gender dysphoria through GAH therapy decreases the need for other mental health interventions, although it is important to recognize that not all depression and anxiety stem from gender dysphoria.[28] Thus, clinical judgment and shared decision making are recommended when deciding on a mental health plan of care. Testosterone and estrogen have been shown to strongly improve mental health for nearly all individuals, despite the known potential side effects of mood changes when used in other contexts.[28,41] However, the route of administration can influence these medications' mental health effects (as discussed further in the "Gender-Affirming Hormones" section of this chapter). If a client opts to initiate GAH therapy

without seeking mental health care and finds their mental health concerns are still present, offering mental health medication and a referral to a therapist, as with any client, is recommended. There are no contraindications to mental health medications with concurrent use of GAH therapy.[23]

## Physical and Appearance Changes

### Nonpharmacologic Options

It is recommended that clinicians use a harm-reduction approach to gender-affirming body modifications, keeping in mind education, access to care, hormones, surgery, clothing, device sizing, and accessibility of body work.

### Gender-Affirming Presentation Changes

Clothing, makeup, jewelry, and hairstyles can all be easily modified to affirm one's gender. This may be done only in private or in both private and public, depending on an individual's level of safety and support.

### Voice Coaching

Some trans feminine individuals work to alter voice tone and pitch, as estrogen does not have a significant effect on the vocal cords.[23] This can lead to increased tightness and tension in the scalene and sternocleidomastoid muscles, and cause headaches and muscle pain.[42]

### Hair Modifications or Treatments

Change in hair style or appearance may be desired by assigned male at birth (AMAB) or assigned female at birth (AFAB) clients to reach their goals. Treatments could include one or more of the following options: over-the-counter medications or supplements, use of wigs or extensions, and hair removal (shaving, waxing, electrolysis, laser hair removal).

### Packing

Packing refers to the use of a wearable prosthesis that may create the appearance and/or sensation of having a penis and/or scrotum. A packer is typically inserted into or clipped onto underwear or may have a harness to hold in place. Some packers can be used to aid in urination while standing, called an STP (or stand-to-pee). Other prostheses can be used for packing, urination, and insertive sex, commonly called a 3-in-1.

| Table 13-4 | Possible Sequelae of Tucking |
|---|---|
| Musculoskeletal | Inguinal canal and ligament stretching leading to decreased elasticity/structural integrity Inguinal hernia |
| Urinary | Urine retention, increased risk of urinary tract infections |
| Reproductive | Decreased sperm count Testicular torsion |
| Integumentary | Skin irritation or damage with use of adhesives |

Based on UCSF Gender Affirming Health Program, Department of Family and Community Medicine, University of California San Francisco. *Guidelines for the Primary and Gender-Affirming Care of Transgender and Gender Nonbinary People.* 2nd ed. Deutsch MB, ed. June 2016. https://transcare.ucsf.edu/guidelines.

| Table 13-5 | Possible Sequelae of Chest Binding |
|---|---|
| Integumentary | Erythema, swelling, rash, skin infections, acne, scarring, itching |
| Musculoskeletal | Back pain, shoulder pain, rib pain, rib fracture, rib or spine misalignment, change in posture, muscle wasting, weakness |
| Respiratory | Restricted lung capacity, shortness of breath, respiratory infections, cough |
| Neurologic | Pain, numbness, headache, dizziness |
| Gastrointestinal | Heartburn, digestive issues |
| Other | Fatigue, overheating, change in breast appearance or shape |

Based on Jarrett BA, Corbet al, Gardner IH, et al. Chest binding and care seeking among transmasculine adults: a cross-sectional study. *Transgend Health.* 2018;3(1):170-178. doi:10.1089/trgh.2018.0017; Reed F. Bodywork techniques for transgender clients who wear chest binders. Published online March 2, 2021. https://www.freedbodyworks.com/frances.

## Tucking

Tucking refers to a technique used by AMAB individuals that helps to minimize or hide the visible outline or bulge of the penis and testes, particularly when wearing tight clothing.[43] This may be desired due to gender dysphoria and/or as a safety measure taken in public. Typically, it involves tucking the external genitalia posteriorly between the legs, often held in place with garments (such as a gaffe), tapes, or other methods. Unintended consequences of tucking are described in Table 13-4.

## Chest Binding

Chest binding refers to the use of compression to mechanically create a flatter chest appearance. It can be done with strategic or tight clothing, bandages, tape, or a fabric binder.[44,45] A binder, created for this purpose, is generally the safest approach and can help avoid or minimize injury when sized and worn appropriately.[45] It is recommended that binding safety be discussed with clients; safety considerations include using breathable materials, proper sizing of garments, taking days off from use and avoiding binding while sleeping, being aware of potential side effects, and considering accessible body work such as massage and physical therapy.[45] Some harmful sequelae occur quickly; others, such as pain, tend to increase over time (Table 13-5). While binding too tightly or too frequently may increase their incidence, the listed sequelae can occur even when proper precautions are taken.

## Gender-Affirming Hormones

Historically, there have been numerous barriers to care for TGNB individuals who want to utilize GAH for the purpose of medically transitioning. Today, there are no legal or regulatory requirements for an adult to begin GAH therapy. The only requirement for a clinician to prescribe GAH is their documentation of persistent gender dysphoria or incongruence.[46] Medical interventions include options such as hormones and surgery. No specific approach is more valid than any other, and many TGNB individuals never opt to utilize hormones or surgery, regardless of access or cost issues. However, access to clinicians who are educated in these interventions, or are willing to be educated, remains a significant issue. Trans and nonbinary BIPOC individuals often experience additional barriers to accessing safe and respectful care, continuing systemic patterns of inequity.[47]

Transitioning refers to internal and external processes that some TGNB individuals choose to undergo when desiring a shift from living as their assigned sex at birth to their affirmed gender. This process may include nonmedical approaches such as clothing and/or hairstyle changes, as well as social changes such as name, pronoun, and legal document changes. Individuals do not need to have presented in their affirmed gender, to have provided letters of support or medical necessity, or to have undergone a legal name or gender change prior to hormone initiation.[46] Because regional requirements may apply and some clinicians may support the use of a letter, occasionally a client may present with a letter of support from a therapist.

While GAH may or may not be a desired aspect of an individual's gender expression, the therapy has been well documented as a life-saving treatment for TGNB individuals who desire these hormones.[10,46] Studies of both trans youth and trans adults have shown that access to and receiving hormone therapy contributes to less self-reported depression and fewer suicide attempts compared to those who wanted but could not receive hormone therapy.[33,48]

## Clinician Scope

Gender-affirming hormones can safely be prescribed and managed by various primary care clinicians and specialty clinicians, including CNMs/CMs, nurse practitioners, physician assistants, obstetrician-gynecologists, and endocrinologists.[23] It is vital that providers and educators do not perpetuate the view of provision of GAH as specialty or complex care. GAH is a component of primary care, and it is recommended that all primary and gender-focused care providers be prepared in basic provision of this care.[10] Hormones are commonly utilized for contraception, menopause, menstrual concerns, hirsutism, and other types of care. Therefore, the majority of providers are already well versed in these medications' use and effects.[10,23] Many medical, midwifery, and nursing education programs are standardizing GAH information in their curricula as part of the full range of care that clinicians need to know, bringing equity to historically oppressed populations. In addition to ethical considerations, healthcare students expect programs to provide them with the tools and resources to become proficient in this care.

## Risk Factors

Risk factors that may be a contraindication to GAH in another healthcare scenario are also evaluated in the context of gender dysphoria and gender euphoria.[10,49] This assessment is necessary because while the same risk factor(s) might exist for TGNB individuals as for non-TGNB individuals, there is no reasonable alternative to hormonal medications.[10] For example, a cisgender woman with migraines with aura would be counseled that combined oral contraceptives are contraindicated and offered other contraceptive methods not containing estrogen. However, a broader range of criteria are considered for TGNB individuals desiring estrogen-containing medications. The case study in Table 13-6 describes

a clinical scenario in which an individual with multiple chronic health concerns presents to a clinic seeking initiation of estrogen therapy.

In a clinical encounter like the one described in the case study, it is not appropriate to withhold a client's estrogen treatment, as there is no reasonable alternative to treat her gender dysphoria.[10] It is appropriate to focus care on counseling and shared decision making, but it must also incorporate harm reduction and recognize the significant risk of self-harm or suicide in the TGNB community, especially when members of that community lack access to gender-affirming care. When they have limited means of acquiring GAH or lack access to a safe practitioner, individuals may choose to obtain hormones outside of the healthcare system or from non-U.S. sources.[10] While obtaining medication this way may carry health risks if care is not monitored, the clinician should acknowledge their client's choices in a nonjudgmental way, understanding this choice as the best way the client knows how to meet their healthcare needs.

## Hormone Ranges

Some clinicians may inquire about the range of normal hormone levels. It is important to acknowledge the wide range of average hormonal lab values. All bodies, regardless of sex or gender, produce all sex hormones, albeit usually in different ratios.[50] While these sex-specific hormones tend to exist in common ranges for AFAB and AMAB bodies, there can be significant variations for some people (Table 13-7). Because gender, sex, and hormonal composition are all separate aspects of a person, many cisgender women have bodies that naturally produce higher levels of testosterone, and some cisgender men have bodies that naturally produce higher levels of estrogen. Viewing bodies through a lens of a hormonal binary is not recommended and can be harmful—both from a broad view (as described in earlier sections of the chapter) and on a cellular level related to individual hormone metabolism. Additionally, a specific dosage given to one individual may produce different effects in another individual.[49]

While clinicians may not be able to predict how any given person will respond, variability in response is thought to be related to individual hormone receptor sensitivity, genetics, and body composition.[10] This variability also illustrates the need for clinicians to adjust medication dosage based on client reports of achieving desired effects. *Supraphysiologic levels* of hormones are defined as serum blood test results that are significantly higher than typically expected physiologically. This outcome usually occurs in the context of an individual

| Table 13-6 | Case Study: Prescribing Estrogen Therapy to a Client with Chronic Health Concerns |
|---|---|

**Encounter 1: Initial visit**

A 49-year-old trans woman (she/her pronouns) presents to the reproductive healthcare clinic. She desires initiation of gender-affirming hormones (GAH) today and agrees to completing recommended lab work. In her past medical history, she describes a 5-year history of hyperlipidemia, which she manages with 20 mg simvastatin daily, and a 10-year history of moderately well-controlled hypertension, which she manages with exercise and stress management. She reports her blood pressures (BPs) are typically in the range of 130–140/82–95. She also reports she smokes a half a pack of cigarettes per day and has been trying to cut back for the past few years. Her family history is positive for diabetes mellitus type 2 in several extended family members. She has previously engaged in regular exercise but is not currently engaging in regular physical activity. She reports being married to her wife for 20 years and they have two adult children together, all of whom are very supportive. She states she has struggled with mild to moderate depressive symptoms for most of her life, some of which are tied to experiencing anti-trans bias. She declines being weighed today and notes an altered relationship with her body. She has been working with a therapist for the past 2 years and is excited to discuss beginning GAH.

Current medications and supplements she takes include fish oil, vitamin D 125 mcg, and 20 mg simvastatin.

Vital signs from today include:

- BP: 140/84 mm Hg
- Respiratory rate: 16 bpm
- Temperature: 98.5°F
- Weight: declined by client

Clinical considerations and plan:

- Ensure the clinician understands the client's goals related to the physical and psychological effects of GAH
- Screen for suicide and self-harm risk
- Assess the client's level of motivation for change related to cigarette smoking
- Screen for disordered eating and chronic dieting
- Obtain informed consent from the client, answer questions, and discuss individual goals in the context of the expected effects
- Draw baseline blood work
- Recommend that client return to office in 1–2 weeks

Appropriate blood tests for this client include:

- Comprehensive metabolic panel (CMP)
- Fasting lipid panel
- Hemoglobin A1c
- Total testosterone
- Free testosterone
- Sexually transmitted infection (STI) panel

**Encounter 2: Follow-up visit**

Clinical considerations and plan:

- Review results of lab work from the first visit
  - Refer to a primary care clinician or specialist as needed for any abnormal findings, although abnormal findings are unlikely to be a contraindication to initiation of hormones (see Tables 13-9 and 13-14 later in this chapter). However, through shared decision making, a client may decide to postpone GAH initiation while addressing another health concern.
- Review informed consent with the client and answer questions
- Prescribe the medication route and dosage as discussed through shared decision making
- Develop a follow-up plan, and identify any symptoms to report to the provider

| Table 13-7 | Physiologic Estrogen and Testosterone Ranges |
|---|---|

Average physiologic estrogen range for cisgender women not on hormonal contraceptives: varies by age and menstrual cycle phase

- Follicular: 12.5−166.0 pg/mL
- Ovulation: 150−350 pg/mL
- Luteal: 43.8−211.0 pg/mL
- Postmenopausal: <6.0−54.7 pg/mL

Average testosterone range for cisgender men: 400–950 ng/dL

Optimal estrogen range for transgender women: 150−500 pg/mL

Optimal testosterone range for transgender men: 500–1000 ng/dL

Based on Olson S. A person-centered approach to prescribing gender-affirming hormones, part one. Presented at Virtual Clinician Course: Gender-Affirming Hormones. March 3, 2022; Ellis S, Sherley C, Gromko L. Transgender health care toolkit: resources for transgender health care. Cedar River Clinic. http://www.cedarriverclinics.org/transtoolkit/. Published 2021. Accessed December 1, 2021; Testosterone, total. Labcorp. https://www.labcorp.com/tests/004226/testosterone-total. Accessed March 23, 2023; Estradiol. Labcorp. https://www.labcorp.com/tests/004515/estradiol. Accessed March 23, 2023.

accidentally administering a higher dose of their medication. Levels below physiologic ranges may also occur, and clinicians should address these in the context of a client's physical goals to avoid incidental underdosing.[10,49]

Guidelines for recommended interval blood tests vary, but it is generally advisable to offer hormone testing every 3 to 6 months in the first 1 to 2 years of hormone initiation.[10,49] Testing is also recommended when clients notice any adverse effects such as mood changes, vaginal bleeding, or change in energy levels.[10,49] Client-reported feelings of gender euphoria or decrease in gender dysphoria should drive the hormonal medication protocol, with blood tests being used primarily to ensure serum blood levels have not reached supraphysiologic levels.[10,49] This can be done by testing the peak of the hormonal curve, which is likely to occur 2 to 3 days post injection for those administering weekly doses.[10,49] For those clients taking a daily medication, testing can be done at any time. Hormone levels should also be confirmed when a person reports not experiencing the level of masculinization or feminization desired.[10] Counseling regarding realistic expectations is part of complete care, and creating a trusting therapeutic relationship will allow clients to feel able to express themselves if they feel dissatisfaction with the progress of their physical effects.[10,49]

## Passing

The goal of all hormone care is individualized, and clients may want to focus on external physical changes, internal psychological changes, or both.[10] Some TGNB individuals may seek hormone care with the desire of *passing*—that is, when a TGNB person is perceived by others to be cisgender instead of the sex they were assigned at birth.[51] For example, when walking in public, a transgender man may easily *pass* as a cisgender man due to having a masculine appearance. However, the duality of passing can be both limiting and life-saving in certain cases.[52] For some people, passing allows them to feel affirmed within their gender identity, creating a sense of gender euphoria. Other individuals may have the goal of passing to be accepted or validated by those in their lives. Individuals who do not conform to traditional gender expression, norms, or roles may be the targets of anti-trans bias, discrimination, and violence. Therefore, some individuals view passing as a way to increase their own safety and reduce the risk of anti-trans violence when navigating a society in which TGNB identities may not be respected.[52] Thus, when making decisions regarding gender expression, some individuals may choose to present externally as more masculine or more feminine than they would like. This scenario demonstrates the responsibility that cisgender individuals have to deconstruct their own gender biases, as ultimately reducing societal bias increases the safety of TGNB individuals.[52]

## Individualizing Care

Before initiating hormone care, the clinician engages in a thorough discussion with the client to understand their individual treatment goals for physical change to avoid making assumptions about the client's desires.[10] For example, some clients may primarily desire a lowered voice and facial hair but feel ambivalent about clitoral/phallus growth. It is important for the clinician to discuss with the client any or all possible effects of the medication that may occur, not just the client-desired effect(s).[10,49]

The majority of clinicians who assist adult clients in initiating GAH utilize the *informed consent model of care*, in which the clinician conducts a thorough history, assesses for a history of gender dysphoria, and reviews possible short- and long-term effects of the medications.[10,49] This approach minimizes medical gatekeeping and allows for discussion with the client regarding gaps in research and expected benefits.

| Table 13-8 | Clinician-Specific GAH Resources |
|---|---|
| Cedar River Clinic Transgender Toolkit[49] | Created by Cedar River Clinics and led by CNM Simon Adriane Ellis, this toolkit is a straightforward clinical guide for clinicians looking to reference dosages, protocols, and lab monitoring schedules. |
| Guidelines for the Primary and Gender-Affirming Care of Transgender and Gender Nonbinary People[23] | Created through University of California San Francisco's Center for Excellence, this comprehensive guideline assists clinicians in troubleshooting clinical scenarios and reviews current research regarding GAH effects. |
| The World Professional Association for Transgender Health (WPATH), Standards of Care, Version 8[46] | Published first in 1979, this evolving document seeks to provide clinicians with a general outline of clinical guidance in caring for transgender and gender-diverse individuals. This document also sets forth criteria and recommendations for clinicians writing letters of support for clients seeking gender-affirming surgeries. |
| TransLine Consultation Service | Consult services free to clinicians |

Abbreviation: GAH, gender-affirming hormones.

The use of GAH is typically lifelong, although harm is unlikely if individuals decide to discontinue the medication at some point in time.[10,49] Experts have discussed whether there should be a recommendation to discontinue GAH at a specific age or near menopause, but there is no evidence on which to base such a recommendation.[10]

TGNB individuals have been utilizing hormones for many decades. However, previous perceptions and discussions within the healthcare community were often based on supraphysiologic doses of hormones, which carry additional risks compared to the approaches recommended today. While there is no universal approach to prescribing GAH and long-term research is still somewhat limited, guidelines do exist to assist clinicians interested in learning more about providing this type of care. Resources for clinicians prescribing GAH are detailed in **Table 13-8**.

| Table 13-9 | Risk Considerations for Estrogen Use |
|---|---|

Absolute contraindications:
- Inability to obtain informed consent
- Active estrogen-sensitive cancer

Factors associated with increased risk of adverse events:
- Personal or family history of estrogen-sensitive cancer
- History of thromboembolic events
- Age > 40
- Smoking
- Diabetes
- Uncontrolled hypertension
- Uncontrolled hyperlipidemia
- Renal insufficiency

Based on UCSF Gender Affirming Health Program, Department of Family and Community Medicine, University of California San Francisco. *Guidelines for the Primary and Gender-Affirming Care of Transgender and Gender Nonbinary People.* 2nd ed. Deutsch MB, ed. June 2016. https://transcare.ucsf.edu/guidelines; Ellis S, Sherley C, Gromko L. Transgender health care toolkit: resources for transgender health care. Cedar River Clinic. http://www.cedarriverclinics.org/transtoolkit/. Published 2021. Accessed December 1, 2021.

## Estrogen-Dominant Protocols (Feminizing)

Typically, the goal of feminizing hormone protocols is to increase the development of secondary sex characteristics associated with estrogen while simultaneously decreasing levels of androgens, resulting in reduced secondary sex characteristics associated with testosterone.[10,23,49] Estradiol is the primary hormone utilized in feminizing protocols for AMAB individuals, commonly in conjunction with an androgen blocker and/or progestin.[10,23,49] Conjugated equine estrogen and ethinyl estradiol are not utilized due to the associated increased thrombogenicity risks.[10,23,49]

### Effects and Risks

Risk considerations and reversible and irreversible side effects to estrogen use are described in Table 13-9, Table 13-10, and Table 13-11.

### Administration

Estrogen can be administered via an oral or sublingual tablet, transdermal patch, injection (estradiol valerate or estradiol cypionate), subdermal pellet, or—more rarely—topical gel or cream.[10,23,49] The route of administration is chosen through shared decision making with the client and incorporates considerations such as cost, insurance coverage, desired physical effects, ability to take a daily medication,

| Table 13-10 | Reversible Effects of Estrogen Therapy |
|---|---|
| Effect | Typical Timing of Onset and Peak |
| Softening and thinning of skin, decreased oil production/increased dryness, decreased pore size | Often noticed within weeks |
| Redistribution of facial and body subcutaneous fat | 3–6 months, with peak at 2–5 years |
| Changes in emotional and social patterns | Often noticed within weeks, in combination with normal physiologic ongoing changes |
| Changes or shifts in libido, arousal, erectile ability, orgasm, and ejaculation | Often noticed within 1–2 months, in combination with normal physiologic ongoing changes |
| Decreased sweat, change in body odor patterns, hot flashes | Often noticed within weeks |
| Nausea | Variable, typically only experienced with initiation or with supraphysiologic dosage |
| Increased headaches or migraines (possible) | Variable |
| Reduction of muscle mass | 3–6 months, with peak at 1–2 years |
| Reduction of body hair, possible reduction in facial hair, and possible reversal of scalp hair loss | 6–12 months, with peak at 3–5 years |
| Increased risk of blood clots | Ongoing, likely higher during initiation of therapy or with supraphysiologic levels |

Based on UCSF Gender Affirming Health Program, Department of Family and Community Medicine, University of California San Francisco. *Guidelines for the Primary and Gender-Affirming Care of Transgender and Gender Nonbinary People.* 2nd ed. Deutsch MB, ed. June 2016. https://transcare.ucsf.edu/guidelines; Ellis S, Sherley C, Gromko L. Transgender health care toolkit: resources for transgender health care. Cedar River Clinic. http://www.cedarriverclinics.org/transtoolkit/. Published 2021. Accessed December 1, 2021.

| Table 13-11 | Irreversible Effects of Estrogen |
|---|---|
| Effect | Typical Timing of Onset and Peak |
| Breast tissue development (most commonly to Tanner stage 2 or 3) | Breast buds often noticed within weeks; more significant tissue increases noticed within 3–6 months, with a peak at 2–5 years |
| Reduced or absent sperm count and ejaculatory fluid (possible) | Variable |
| Reduced testicular size (possible) | Variable |
| Weight gain (possible, may be reversible) | Variable |

Based on UCSF Gender Affirming Health Program, Department of Family and Community Medicine, University of California San Francisco. *Guidelines for the Primary and Gender-Affirming Care of Transgender and Gender Nonbinary People.* 2nd ed. Deutsch MB, ed. June 2016. https://transcare.ucsf.edu/guidelines; Ellis S, Sherley C, Gromko L. Transgender health care toolkit: resources for transgender health care. Cedar River Clinic. http://www.cedarriverclinics.org/transtoolkit/. Published 2021. Accessed December 1, 2021.

fear of injections, age, dermatologic concerns, thrombosis risk, and efficacy of any prior medications.[10] Oral tablets are typically taken daily or twice daily.[10,49] Injections are typically self-administered weekly.[10] Considerations for different routes of administration are provided in Table 13-12.[10,49,53–60]

There is a well-documented increased thrombosis risk in cisgender women who utilize various forms of estrogen in contraception or menopausal treatment. Similarly, a question has arisen regarding whether this same thrombosis risk exists for AMAB individuals utilizing gender-affirming estrogen.[53,54] While age remains the factor most closely correlated with thrombosis, some research suggests that thrombosis risk may be elevated with use of oral estradiol.[53,61] This relationship may be due to increased metabolism of oral tablets into estrone ($E_1$) and the first-pass effect, which increase the release of clotting factors by the liver.[61] For this reason, many clinicians encourage older clients to utilize transdermal estradiol patches, which bypass the liver, do not increase sex hormone–binding globulin (SHBG), and result in lower estrone levels than oral estradiol—all of which may lower thrombosis risk.[55,61] Clients who begin medical transition after the typical age of menopause in their cisgender peers may still desire standard dosages of estrogen. While informed

| Table 13-12 | Estrogen Routes | |
|---|---|---|
| **Available Formulations of Estradiol** | | |
| **Route of Administration** | **Pros** | **Cons** |
| Oral estradiol tablet (frequently recommended to be taken sublingually to minimize stress on the liver[10,49]) | Lowest cost<br>Usually covered by insurance<br>Sublingual administration may result in higher absorption and avoidance of the first-pass effect | While oral estradiol tablets are commonly recommended to be taken sublingually, these tablets are not formulated to be taken this way and thus may have varying rates of oral dissolution.[10]<br>Compared to other methods, oral tablets may increase thrombosis risk by increasing estrone ($E_1$) and increasing production of SHBG via the first-pass effect in the liver. This risk is possibly lowered slightly by use of sublingual administration.[53–60] |
| Transdermal estradiol patch<br>Topical estradiol gel or cream | Considered to have the lowest risk of thrombosis due to avoidance of the first-pass effect and neutral effect on SHBG; thus, it is likely the safest approach for those with significant cardiovascular risk factors.[56,60] | Possible skin irritation with patch adhesives<br>More gradual physical effects<br>Patches may have decreased adhesive efficacy, leading to early patch removal<br>Possible increased documentation steps required for insurance coverage |
| Injectable estradiol valerate or estradiol cypionate | Possible lower risk of thrombosis as compared to oral estradiol due to avoidance of the first-pass effect and lower rates of estrone ($E_1$) production<br>Physical effects produced more quickly than with other routes due to increased rate of absorption | Patient discomfort with or inability to self-inject<br>Possible skin irritation with injection technique and/or sensitivity to carrier oil<br>Additional documentation steps may be required for insurance coverage<br>Occasional shortages of medication nationally; consider alternative specialty pharmacy options<br>Multiple strengths of medication available; increased likelihood of accidental supraphysiologic levels if incorrect dosage injected<br>Accompanying needles require separate prescription |
| Estradiol pellet | Continuous absorption of estradiol with fewer peaks and troughs | Few trained clinicians in pellet insertion, resulting in low availability<br>High cost and infrequent insurance coverage<br>Possible discomfort with insertion procedure |

Abbreviation: SHBG, sex hormone–binding globulin.

consent discussions regarding risk are essential in these cases, it is important that the clinicians discuss all options regardless of age to avoid underdosing.[10]

### Dosages

Many protocols recommend titrating the estrogen dosage to cisgender female levels. However, cisgender women experience a wide range of estrogen levels throughout a normal menstrual cycle. Therefore, this recommendation may be better interpreted as titrating to average peak ovulatory estrogen levels.[10] Additionally, client-reported efficacy may be more useful in management than specific numbers, though it is best for levels to stay below a supraphysiologic but near-ovulatory range.[10] While endogenous estrogen release in cisgender women occurs in a pulsatile manner, this pattern is not typically possible with exogenous estrogen administration, nor has it been shown to have beneficial effects.[10] Additionally, no benefit has been shown with use of supraphysiologic dosages, which may also increase thrombosis risk.[10,49] Dose adjustments are appropriate when the clinical response is inadequate, the client desires additional physical effects within the ability of the medication, and there are no risk factors to contraindicate an increase.[10,23,49] Initiation and follow-up care for estrogen provision are described in Table 13-13.

| Table 13-13 | Estrogen Initiation Process |
|---|---|
| Initial visit | • Thorough history of presenting illness (HPI); assess risk factors<br>• Documentation of gender dysphoria or gender incongruence<br>• Assess desire for fertility preservation, referral as needed<br>• Physical exam not needed<br>• Order blood work:<br>  ♦ Comprehensive metabolic panel<br>  ♦ Lipid panel<br>  ♦ HbA1c (if indicated)<br>  ♦ STI testing (if indicated)<br>  ♦ Testosterone (not required but may be helpful to obtain a baseline level to monitor gradual decrease) |
| Follow-up visit | • Review results of blood work<br>• Answer patient questions since previous visit<br>• Provide referral(s) if indicated<br>• Prescribe estradiol, possibly antiandrogen<br>  ♦ Example:<br>    ○ Estradiol 2 mg tablet, #60, 1 tab PO BID, 3 refills<br>    ○ Spironolactone 50 mg #30, 1 tab PO in morning, 3 refills |
| 3-month follow-up | • Assess patient experience on medications, affirm normalcy if minimal effects have occurred after this time frame<br>• Assess need for dosage change<br>  ♦ Estradiol should be increasing, testosterone should be decreasing<br>• Address any concerns<br>• Order blood work:<br>  ♦ Estradiol<br>  ♦ Testosterone |
| 6-month follow-up | • Assess patient experience on medications, affirm normalcy if mild effects have occurred after this time frame<br>• Assess need for dosage change<br>  ♦ Estradiol should be increasing, testosterone should be decreasing<br>• Address any concerns<br>• Order blood work:<br>  ♦ Estradiol<br>  ♦ Testosterone |
| 12-month follow-up | • Assess patient experience on medications<br>• Assess need for dosage change<br>  ♦ Estradiol should be increasing to peak of 150–350 pg/mL, testosterone should be < 50 ng/dL<br>• Address any concerns<br>• Order blood work:<br>  ♦ Estradiol<br>  ♦ Testosterone<br>  ♦ Comprehensive metabolic panel<br>  ♦ Lipid panel<br>  ♦ HbA1c (if indicated)<br>  ♦ STI testing (if indicated) |

| 18-month follow-up | • Assess patient experience on medications |
| | • Assess need for dosage change |
| | • Address any concerns |
| | • Order blood work: |
| |     ◆ Estradiol |
| |     ◆ Testosterone |
| 24-month follow-up | • Assess patient experience on medications |
| | • Assess need for dosage change |
| | • Address any concerns |
| | • Order blood work: |
| |     ◆ Estradiol |
| |     ◆ Testosterone |
| |     ◆ Comprehensive metabolic panel |
| |     ◆ HbA1c (if indicated) |
| |     ◆ STI testing (if indicated) |
| Annual follow-up, ongoing | • Assess patient experience on medications |
| | • Assess for change in risk factors |
| | • Assess need for dosage change |
| | • Address any concerns |
| | • Order blood work: |
| |     ◆ Estradiol |
| |     ◆ Testosterone |
| |     ◆ Comprehensive metabolic panel |
| |     ◆ HbA1c (if indicated) |
| |     ◆ STI testing (if indicated) |

Abbreviations: BID, twice daily; HBA1c, hemoglobin $A_{1c}$; PO, per oral; STI, sexually transmitted infection.

Based on Olson S. A person-centered approach to prescribing gender-affirming hormones, part one. Presented at Virtual Clinician Course: Gender-Affirming Hormones. March 3, 2022; UCSF Gender Affirming Health Program, Department of Family and Community Medicine, University of California San Francisco. *Guidelines for the Primary and Gender-Affirming Care of Transgender and Gender Nonbinary People.* 2nd ed. Deutsch MB, ed. June 2016. https://transcare.ucsf.edu/guidelines; Ellis S, Sherley C, Gromko L. Transgender health care toolkit: resources for transgender health care. Cedar River Clinic. http://www.cedarriverclinics.org/transtoolkit/. Published 2021. Accessed December 1, 2021.

## Antiandrogens

Antiandrogens are used in conjunction with estrogen in many cases to assist in efficient lowering of endogenous testosterone production.[10,23,49] In the United States, the primary antiandrogen utilized is spironolactone, a potassium-sparing diuretic that also inhibits androgen-receptor activity and reduces testosterone production.[23] A secondary effect of spironolactone is slight breast tissue development, which is considered irreversible.[23] Although this effect is often desired in trans feminine clients, it creates a contraindication for the medication in cisgender men.[62] Other side effects related to diuretic effects include polyuria, risk for hyperkalemia (this effect is rare except in patients with kidney disease), hypotension, headache, and dizziness.[10,23,49] While

not recommended in most current guidelines, some clinicians may use bicalutamide as an alternative to spironolactone.[10]

Estrogen-containing medications are also inherently antiandrogenic on their own, given the inverse relationship between estrogen and testosterone levels. In addition to occurring in the GAH setting, this clinical effect can be seen when combined oral contraceptives are utilized to decrease acne in cisgender women.[63] Because of this relationship, estrogen administered alone will also lower testosterone without the use of an antiandrogen such as spironolactone.[10] While estrogen alone may produce more gradual effects, some clients and/or clinicians may prefer this approach.[10,49] While spironolactone has only mild side effects in most cases, some anecdotal reports recommend delaying the initiation of spironolactone for a minimum of 6 to 12 months to allow for evaluating the effect of estradiol on individual testosterone levels with the goal of avoiding the use of spironolactone.[10,49] Additionally, some research suggests that spironolactone may cause initial growth of breast tissue but ultimately induce premature closure of breast buds, limiting long-term breast tissue growth, an effect often desired by trans feminine individuals.[10,49]

### Administration and Dosages

Antiandrogens are administered as an oral tablet taken once or twice daily.[10,49] A low dose may initially be used, such as spironolactone 50 mg, and then the dosage titrated upward as needed. Average maintenance dosages of spironolactone are typically 100 to 200 mg, dependent on the testosterone levels and noticed effects by the client.[10,49] Through shared decision making, the client may also opt to wait to start an antiandrogen until stable on an estrogen-only protocol for a mutually agreed-upon length of time.[10,49] Some clients may opt to never use an antiandrogen.[10]

### Progestins

Progesterone receptors are densely clustered in the uterine muscle for those persons with a uterus and secondarily in the chest or breast tissue in both AFAB and AMAB individuals.[10,64] The effect of progesterone during the luteal phase for an individual with a uterus is typically to support the endometrium, often resulting in menstrual-related symptoms such as bloating, breast tenderness and swelling, and mood fluctuations.[10,64] While current research has not shown a clear benefit from the use of progestins in most individuals, some trans feminine individuals report increased breast tissue and improved mood when taking these medications.[10,64] Other individuals may find that this class of medication worsens mental health symptoms; thus, it is best to employ shared decision making when contemplating the potential use of progestins.[10,64] Some research suggests that increased breast tissue may be temporary when progestins are used in this manner, reflective of the bloating effect.[10,64] Despite the lack of research, there are no known harms from the use of progestins in this context, and many clients may opt for a trial to determine if they will experience the desired effects.[10,64]

### Administration and Dosages

Progestins are available in capsule form, but can also be administered orally or rectally, with a decrease in side effects sometimes being noted when using the rectal route.[10,64] Lab monitoring is typically undertaken every 3 months for the first year, and occasionally more frequently if troubleshooting a clinical concern.[10,49] In subsequent years, blood work monitoring can typically be safely moved to every 6 to 12 months.[10,49] Timing of hormonal blood levels results depends on the route of administration and expected time of peak and trough.

## Other Medications Used in Feminizing Protocols
### Finasteride (Propecia or Proscar)

This medication can be used to modestly decrease dihydrotestosterone (DHT) levels to prevent or halt "male-pattern baldness."[10,23,49]

### Sildenafil (Viagra)

This medication is commonly prescribed for trans women with a penis who experience diminished capacity for erection and desire erection.[10,23,49]

## Testosterone-Dominant Protocols (Masculinizing)
### Testosterone

Typically the goal of masculinizing hormone protocols is to increase the development of secondary sex characteristics associated with testosterone while simultaneously decreasing levels of estrogen, resulting in reduced secondary sex characteristics associated with estrogen.[10,23,49] Unlike estrogen-dominant protocols, which may combine several medications, testosterone-dominant protocols primarily rely on only testosterone, which is available in several forms.[10,23,49] When reviewing informed consent and risks of using testosterone for gender affirmation, clinicians should discuss a client's individual and family histories in the setting of available data about risks (Table 13-14). It is important to inform clients that while treatment protocols may exist, care should be individualized based on a person's goals and their response to medication.[10] Clients should understand that responses are based heavily on nonmodifiable factors such as genetics and age.[10,23,49] While many effects of hormone therapy have predictable timing and courses, those courses may be shorter or longer for some clients. Table 13-15 and Table 13-16 describe the effects of testosterone.

| Table 13-14 | Considerations for Testosterone Hormone Therapy |
|---|---|
| **Absolute Contraindications** | |
| Inability to obtain informed consent<br>Active hormone-sensitive cancer<br>Current pregnancy | |
| **Conditions Associated with Increased Risk of Adverse Events** | |
| Personal or family history of a hormone-sensitive cancer<br>Uncontrolled hypertension<br>Uncontrolled hyperlipidemia<br>Liver disease<br>Polycythemia<br>Smoking<br>Personal history of venous thromboembolism<br>Family history of heart disease | |

Based on Olson S. A person-centered approach to prescribing gender-affirming hormones, part one. Presented at Virtual Clinician Course: Gender-Affirming Hormones. March 3, 2022; UCSF Gender Affirming Health Program, Department of Family and Community Medicine, University of California San Francisco. *Guidelines for the Primary and Gender-Affirming Care of Transgender and Gender Non-binary People.* 2nd ed. Deutsch MB, ed. June 2016. https://transcare.ucsf.edu/guidelines; Ellis S, Sherley C, Gromko L. Transgender health care toolkit: resources for transgender health care. Cedar River Clinic. http://www.cedarriverclinics.org/transtoolkit/. Published 2021. Accessed December 1, 2021.

| Table 13-15 | Reversible Effects of Testosterone Therapy | |
|---|---|---|
| **Effect** | **Typical Timing of Onset and Peak** | **Considerations** |
| Cessation of menses | Onset: within 6 months, may be longer when using a low dose | Anovulation is possible but ovulation status is typically unknown even with amenorrhea; thus, pregnancy is possible and it is recommended to address the need for contraception as usual |
| Vaginal dryness | Onset: within 6 months; variable based on genetics, age at initiation, and body makeup; most commonly occurs after more than 12 months<br>Peak: 2–5 years and likely to persist without intervention | Dryness results from atrophic changes due to suppressed estrogen. If nonpharmacologic methods are not effective, it can be treated with topical hormones, which have not been shown to interfere with systemic hormone therapy.<br>Pain and itching are evaluated independent of dryness. Conditions with different etiologies (e.g., vaginismus, hormonally mediated vestibulodynia, and lichen sclerosus) can be overlooked when pain or itching is attributed to only dryness. |
| Acne | Onset: soon after initiation<br>Peak: around 1 year, then tends to decline | |
| Increased muscle mass | Onset: 6–12 months, but variable based on genetics, age at initiation, and body makeup<br>Peak: 2–5 years | |

Based on Olson S. A person-centered approach to prescribing gender-affirming hormones, part one. Presented at Virtual Clinician Course: Gender-Affirming Hormones. March 3, 2022; UCSF Gender Affirming Health Program, Department of Family and Community Medicine, University of California San Francisco. *Guidelines for the Primary and Gender-Affirming Care of Transgender and Gender Non-binary People.* 2nd ed. Deutsch MB, ed. June 2016. https://transcare.ucsf.edu/guidelines; Ellis S, Sherley C, Gromko L. Transgender health care toolkit: resources for transgender health care. Cedar River Clinic. http://www.cedarriverclinics.org/transtoolkit/. Published 2021. Accessed December 1, 2021.

| Table 13-16 | Irreversible Effects of Testosterone | |
|---|---|---|
| **Effect** | **Typical Timing of Onset and Peak** | **Considerations** |
| Polycythemia | Onset: variable based on genetics, age at initiation, and body makeup. Peak: not applicable; assessed annually and as needed | Important to utilize the cisgender male lab values range if the patient is amenorrheic. Can be managed by dose adjustment. Recommend evaluating for elevated estradiol, as testosterone can aromatize into estrogen in the body. Regular blood donation or therapeutic phlebotomy (having blood drawn and discarded instead of donated) can decrease hematocrit without adjusting the dose of testosterone. Important to rule out other causes of polycythemia such as obstructive sleep apnea, tobacco use, cardiopulmonary dysfunction, and malignancy. |
| Development of facial and body hair | Onset: 6–12 months, but variable based on genetics, age at initiation, and body makeup Peak: 2–5 years | Likely partially reversible |
| Deepening of vocal tone and pitch | Onset: 6–12 months, but variable based on genetics, age at initiation, and body makeup Peak: 2–5 years | |
| Clitoral growth | Onset: within 6 months, but variable based on genetics, age at initiation, and body makeup Peak: 2–5 years | |
| Frontal and temporal hairline recession, hair thinning on the crown | Onset: 6–12 months, but variable based on genetics, age at initiation, and body makeup Peak: progressive | |
| Increase in libido and arousal, change in orgasm | Onset: shortly after initiation Peak: not applicable | |
| Redistribution of facial and body subcutaneous fat | Onset: within 6 months, but variable based on genetics, age at initiation, and body makeup Peak: 2–5 years | |
| Change in sweat and odor patterns | Onset: variable based on genetics, age at initiation, and body makeup Peak: 2–5 years | |
| Changes in emotional and social pattern | Onset: shortly after initiation Peak: not applicable; mental health assessed annually at minimum and as needed | |

Based on Olson S. A person-centered approach to prescribing gender-affirming hormones, part one. Presented at Virtual Clinician Course: Gender-Affirming Hormones. March 3, 2022; UCSF Gender Affirming Health Program, Department of Family and Community Medicine, University of California San Francisco. *Guidelines for the Primary and Gender-Affirming Care of Transgender and Gender Non-binary People.* 2nd ed. Deutsch MB, ed. June 2016. https://transcare.ucsf.edu/guidelines; Ellis S, Sherley C, Gromko L. Transgender health care toolkit: resources for transgender health care. Cedar River Clinic. http://www.cedarriverclinics.org/transtoolkit/. Published 2021. Accessed December 1, 2021.

| Table 13-17 | Testosterone Routes | |
|---|---|---|
| **Available Formulations of Testosterone** | | |
| **Route of Administration** | **Pros** | **Cons** |
| Injectable testosterone cypionate (most commonly utilized) | Physical effects produced more quickly compared to other routes | Patient discomfort with or inability to self-inject<br>Possible skin irritation with injection technique and/or sensitivity to carrier oil<br>May require prior authorization of insurance, though typically covered<br>Multiple strengths of medication available; increased likelihood of accidental supraphysiologic levels if incorrect dosage injected<br>Accompanying needles require separate prescription |
| Transdermal testosterone patch<br>Topical testosterone gel or cream | Ease of administration, less potential transfer to other individuals with patches | Possible skin irritation with patch adhesives<br>More gradual physical effects<br>Patches may have decreased adhesive efficacy, leading to early patch removal<br>Possible increased documentation steps required for insurance coverage<br>Topical testosterone cream or gel should be used with caution by clients who interact with children or pets, as transfer from topical methods may affect the hormone levels and subsequent effects for other humans and pets |
| Testosterone pellet | Continuous absorption of testosterone, with fewer peaks and troughs | Few trained clinicians in pellet insertion, resulting in low availability<br>High cost and infrequent insurance coverage<br>Possible discomfort with insertion procedure |

Based on Olson S. A person-centered approach to prescribing gender-affirming hormones, part one. Presented at Virtual Clinician Course: Gender-Affirming Hormones. March 3, 2022; UCSF Gender Affirming Health Program, Department of Family and Community Medicine, University of California San Francisco. *Guidelines for the Primary and Gender-Affirming Care of Transgender and Gender Non-binary People.* 2nd ed. Deutsch MB, ed. June 2016. https://transcare.ucsf.edu/guidelines; Ellis S, Sherley C, Gromko L. Transgender health care toolkit: resources for transgender health care. Cedar River Clinic. http://www.cedarriverclinics.org/transtoolkit/. Published 2021. Accessed December 1, 2021.

**Administration.** Testosterone can be administered via a transdermal patch, injection, subcutaneous pellet, or topical gel or cream (**Table 13-17**). Of note, while some countries may offer oral preparations of testosterone, these are not recommended due to suboptimal absorption and predictability of serum levels.[65] The route of administration is chosen through shared decision making with the client and incorporates considerations such as cost, insurance coverage, desired physical effects, ability to take daily medication, fear of injections, age, dermatologic concerns, and efficacy of any prior medications.

**Dosages.** Most protocols recommend titrating the testosterone dosage to average cisgender male levels.[10,49] Because normal fluctuations in these values may occur, it is important to base management on client-reported efficacy rather than specific numbers while keeping levels out of a supraphysiologic range.[10,49] In cisgender men, testosterone is released in a relatively consistent pulsatile manner over a 24-hour period, but this pattern is not typically possible with exogenous testosterone administration, nor has it been shown to have beneficial effects.[10] Additionally, no benefit has been shown with use of supraphysiologic serum testosterone levels, which are likely to result in aromatization of exogenous testosterone into estrogen. This process of aromatization may also result in unscheduled uterine bleeding and undesired mood changes.[10,23,49] Initiation and follow-up care for testosterone provision are described in Table 13-18.

### Other Medications Used in Masculinizing Protocols

**Finasteride.** Finasteride may be prescribed for trans men with significant concerns regarding hair loss with use of testosterone. However, considering that the mechanism of action of finasteride is to block the conversion of testosterone to dihydrotestosterone (DHT), the antiandrogenic effects may not be desired by the client.[10,23,49]

| Table 13-18 | Testosterone Initiation Process |
|---|---|
| Initial visit | • Thorough history of present illness (HPI); assess risk factors<br>• Documentation of gender dysphoria or gender incongruence<br>• Assess desire for fertility preservation, referral as needed<br>• Physical exam not needed<br>• Order blood work:<br>  ♦ Complete blood count<br>  ♦ HbA1c (if indicated)<br>  ♦ STI testing (if indicated)<br>  ♦ Testosterone (not required but may be helpful to obtain baseline) |
| Follow-up visit | • Review results of blood work<br>• Answer patient questions since previous visit<br>• Referral if indicated<br>• Prescribe testosterone<br>  ♦ Example:<br>    ○ Testosterone cypionate 200 mg/mL 10-mL vial, inject 0.3 mL IM once weekly, 1 refill<br>    ○ 1-mL syringes #12<br>    ○ 18-gauge needle cap #12, used to draw up medication<br>    ○ 22-gauge or 23-gauge needle cap #12, used to inject medication |
| 3-month follow-up | • Assess patient experience on medications, affirm normalcy if minimal effects have occurred after this time frame<br>• Assess need for dosage change<br>  ♦ Testosterone should be increasing<br>• Address any concerns<br>• Order blood work:<br>  ♦ Testosterone |
| 6-month follow-up | • Assess patient experience on medications, affirm normalcy if mild effects have occurred after this time frame<br>• Menses cessation expected if the patient experienced menses before testosterone initiation<br>• Assess need for dosage change<br>  ♦ Testosterone should be increasing, estradiol should be decreasing<br>• Address any concerns<br>• Order blood work:<br>  ♦ Estradiol<br>  ♦ Testosterone<br>  ♦ Complete blood count |
| 12-month follow-up | • Assess patient experience on medications<br>• Assess need for dosage change<br>  ♦ Testosterone should be increasing to peak of 600–800 ng/dL, estradiol should be < 50 pg/mL<br>• Address any concerns<br>• Order blood work:<br>  ♦ Estradiol<br>  ♦ Testosterone<br>  ♦ Complete blood count<br>  ♦ HbA1c (if indicated)<br>  ♦ STI testing (if indicated) |

| 18-month follow-up | • Assess patient experience on medications<br>• Assess need for dosage change<br>• Address any concerns<br>• Order blood work:<br>  ◆ Estradiol<br>  ◆ Testosterone<br>  ◆ Complete blood count |
|---|---|
| 24-month follow-up | • Assess patient experience on medications<br>• Assess need for dosage change<br>• Address any concerns<br>• Order blood work:<br>  ◆ Estradiol<br>  ◆ Testosterone<br>  ◆ Complete blood count<br>  ◆ HbA1c (if indicated)<br>  ◆ STI testing (if indicated) |
| Annual follow-up, ongoing | • Assess patient experience on medications<br>• Assess for change in risk factors<br>• Assess need for dosage change<br>• Address any concerns<br>• Order blood work:<br>  ◆ Estradiol<br>  ◆ Testosterone<br>  ◆ Complete blood count<br>  ◆ HbA1c (if indicated)<br>  ◆ STI testing (if indicated) |

Abbreviations: HbA1c, hemoglobin $A_{1c}$; IM, intramuscular; STI, sexually transmitted infection.

Based on Olson S. A person-centered approach to prescribing gender-affirming hormones, part one. Presented at Virtual Clinician Course: Gender-Affirming Hormones. March 3, 2022; UCSF Gender Affirming Health Program, Department of Family and Community Medicine, University of California San Francisco. *Guidelines for the Primary and Gender-Affirming Care of Transgender and Gender Nonbinary People.* 2nd ed. Deutsch MB, ed. June 2016. https://transcare.ucsf.edu/guidelines; Ellis S, Sherley C, Gromko L. Transgender health care toolkit: resources for transgender health care. Cedar River Clinic. http://www.cedarriverclinics.org/transtoolkit/. Published 2021. Accessed December 1, 2021.

***Compounded Testosterone.*** A topical cream, gel, or lotion may be considered by some clinicians.[10] While most are not regulated by the Food and Drug Administration (FDA), these preparations may be considered for local effects such as application to the clitoris for potential bottom growth or to the face for potential hair growth. Additionally, compounded products may be more cost-effective for those individuals without insurance coverage.[10]

***Minoxidil.*** Minoxidil is an over-the-counter topical treatment to address or prevent hair loss, which typically has modest effects.[10,49]

### GAH for Nonbinary Individuals

Many nonbinary and genderqueer individuals desire GAH therapy, which may entail a slightly different approach than the traditional feminizing or masculinizing protocols.[10,49] Such therapy might be desired for an array of reasons, including voice deepening, skin changes, cessation of menses, and changes in muscle and fat distribution. While hormone dosages cannot be chosen based purely on identity, many nonbinary individuals prefer low-dose hormones.[10] This approach, sometimes called *microdosing*, uses either the estrogen or testosterone in a lower and/or more gradual protocol and is based on individual

| Table 13-19 | Clinician-Specific Resources: Gender-Affirming Hormone Therapy for Youth |
| --- | --- |
| U.S. Department of Health and Human Services, Office of the Assistant Secretary for Health: "Gender-Affirming Care and Young People" | |
| *Journal of Adolescent Health* | |
| Endocrine Society | |

goals.[10] The clinician may use creativity in choosing the route and dosing so as to achieve the client's desired outcome. These low-dose regimens are likely to result in less prominent, more gradual effects, and clients can decide if they would like to titrate their dosage at any time.[10,23,49] Some clients may opt to utilize GAH for a certain amount of time before discontinuing the treatment. For example, an individual whose priority is achieving a lower voice pitch may opt to take testosterone for 2 years to achieve the desired effect.

### GAH in Trans Youth

Administration of GAH to persons younger than age 18 is an important aspect of care and is considered life-saving care for many.[7] Although a comprehensive discussion is beyond the scope of this chapter, Table 13-19 provides resources for those interested in furthering their education. One question that commonly arises is whether trans youth have the legal right to initiate hormone therapy prior to age 18 with or without parental consent. With parental consent, some U.S. states allow the provision of gender-affirming medications, whereas other states have passed legislation that explicitly prohibits prescribing GAH to persons younger than age 18. The gender identity of youth under age 18 is more likely to shift over the course of childhood or adolescence when compared to adult gender identity, though a stated shift in gender identity is most likely to persist, even in childhood.[7] Access to affirming discussions which center bodily autonomy are essential and allow youth to be empowered. Questions regarding risk of regret have been used to justify withholding care, though the risk of worsening mental health and/or suicide is typically a higher risk.[7,31]

The form of GAH used in youth typically consists of gonadotrophin-releasing hormone agonists (GnRHa), also referred to as *puberty blockers*, which are initiated prior to or near the time of puberty

(Tanner stage 2) to suppress the development of secondary sex characteristics.[23,66] These medications suppress the release of gonadotropins, reduce luteinizing hormone (LH) and follicle-stimulating hormone (FSH) production in AFAB individuals, and reduce testosterone production in AMAB individuals.[66] Puberty blockers can be valuable in temporarily halting or slowly bodily changes, especially for a child who is exploring their gender.[10,66] Particularly in AMAB individuals, many secondary sex characteristics are permanent upon completion of puberty and may cause significant dysphoria.[10,66] While puberty blockers do have potential associated physiologic risks, such as decreased bone density, the intentional choice to forgo all GAH treatment is not benign, but also comes with significant psychological risks such as increased mental health disorders and risk for suicide.[10,31,33,66] Because estrogen and testosterone are less prominent in childhood, puberty-blocking medications are less commonly prescribed before puberty.[10,66] Given that there is limited research on the long-term effects of puberty blockers, it is recommended that individuals and families seek care with a pediatric provider familiar with weighing the risks and benefits of the various approaches to childhood gender incongruence.

Sex-specific hormones such as estrogen and testosterone are typically added through the routes identified earlier after the age at which puberty would normally occur.[66] Therapy is typically initiated using lower dosages and more gradually over months and years for adolescents as compared to adult dosages, though the final dosage may be similar.[66] Some adolescents may remain on GnRHa instead of spironolactone for a period of time. Currently, most states require parental consent for the prescription of adolescent GAH; during this process, the clinician may note differences in opinion between the child and parent(s), which can create challenges in clinical communication.[66]

## Surgical Care of TGNB Clients

### Gender-Affirming Surgery

While some clients may desire gender-affirming surgical intervention, other trans or nonbinary individuals do not desire such surgery.[10] This does not in any way invalidate their lived experience of their gender. For TGNB individuals who pursue gender-affirming surgery (GAS), the plan may include several individual procedures or a single surgery.

Some clients may opt to pursue surgical procedures in countries other than the United States for cost and accessibility reasons.[67] Because of the logistics of travel, clients may not have easy access to return to the surgeon who performed their surgery, so it is recommended that primary care, plastic surgeons, and gynecologic clinicians in the United States be familiar with these procedures and their potential complications.[10]

Midwives may see clients who schedule visits specifically to obtain a referral to a specialized plastic surgeon or a letter of support for obtaining surgery. In these situations, the midwife's responsibility is to document an accurate, respectful history in the client's health record and provide appropriate referrals. Many clients may desire a referral to a surgeon in a different state than their residence based on desired technique or clinician reputation. Additionally, it is recommended that clinicians maintain a working list of regional and national referral sources.

## Documentation Prior to Surgery

Individual surgeons may differ in which types of documentation they require from clients prior to scheduling a gender-affirming procedure. If a client plans to utilize insurance benefits, most plans will require documentation in the form of two letters of support, one from a healthcare clinician and one from a mental health specialist, both of which should reference the most updated World Professional Association for Transgender Health (WPATH) guidance regarding criteria for obtaining GAS.[10] Before writing these letters, the clinician should confirm with the client the diagnoses and the language they are comfortable using. For example, many insurance companies may require labeling of the client as either *male-to-female (MtF)* or *female-to-male (FtM)*, which may not feel appropriate or acceptable to a nonbinary patient who does not view their gender within a narrow perspective or as binary. Table 13-20 provides an example of support letter language.

| Table 13-20 | Example Letter of Support for Gender-Affirming Surgery |
|---|---|

[on letterhead]

[date]

Re: [patient name on insurance card], [patient's chosen name], [patient date of birth]

Dear [Surgeon's name],

[Patient name] is a patient in my care at [your practice name]. They have been a patient here since [date]. They identify as [gender identity] and go by [pronouns]. They note that they first knew their gender identity differed from their assigned sex at age [age]. They have socially transitioned by [list how—change name, pronoun, dress, makeup, hair, tuck, pack, binding, coming out, etc.). They have been successfully and consistently living in a gender role congruent with their affirmed gender since [date]. They have been consistently on hormone therapy since [date] (if contraindicated or has chosen not to take hormones, state that here). Despite these interventions, they report significant anxiety, depression, and distress due to their experience of dysphoria. By my independent evaluation of [patient name], I diagnosed them with gender dysphoria (ICD-10 F64.1). They have expressed a persistent desire for [surgery]. Their goals of surgery are [goals]. Surgery will address their gender dysphoria in these ways: [explain].

[Patient name] is physically healthy to undergo this surgery. [List any medical and mental health diagnoses that may be relevant to having surgery]. Their current medications include [medications]. Their surgical history includes [surgical history]. They are stably housed and have prepared for their post-op recovery (if this is true, if not, state plan for postoperative recovery). They have no issues with illicit drug use or abuse (if this is true; if not, explain the plan of care for stabilization).

[Patient name] has more than met the WPATH criteria for [surgery]. I have explained the risks, benefits, and alternatives of this surgery and believe they have an excellent understanding of them. They are capable of making an informed decision about undertaking surgery. I believe that the next appropriate step for them is to undergo [surgery], and I believe this will help them make significant progress in further treating their gender dysphoria. Therefore, I hereby recommend and refer [patient name] to have this surgery.

If you have any questions or concerns please do not hesitate to contact myself or my office.

Sincerely,

[your name], [credentials]

[your license number]

Based on Mosser S. Writing a letter of support for gender affirming surgeries. https://www.genderconfirmation.com/wp-content/uploads/2022/04/How-to-Write-a-Letter-of-Support_New.pdf. Accessed October 2, 2022; Sample surgery letter. TransLine: Transgender Medical Consultation Service. https://transline.zendesk.com/hc/en-us. Accessed October 2, 2022. Transgender Medical Benefits. World Professional Association for Transgender Health. https://www.wpath.org/media/cms/Documents/Public%20Policies/2018/6_June/Transgender%20Medical%20Benefits.pdf. Accessed October 2, 2022.

## Gender-Affirming Surgical Options

Surgical options may be pursued by clients so as to change their genitals, the contour of the body, or both (Table 13-21). Creation of a vagina, or *neovagina*, and vulva can be achieved through surgery. Advancements have been slower in general regarding bottom surgery for AFAB individuals desiring phallus construction, but multiple options do exist. Face, chest, and body contour alteration can also be achieved via surgical means. Considerations for individual clients include goals, benefits of the procedure, potential risks, cost and insurance coverage, access to an experienced surgeon, recovery time, and need for ongoing maintenance or therapies.[67]

## Routine Reproductive and Gynecologic Care for TGNB Individuals

Inclusive and comprehensive history taking prior to a physical examination is of particular importance when providing reproductive and gynecologic care to TGNB individuals.[68] As with any client, the provider will explain the components of a physical exam, describe why each component may be indicated, and obtain consent for each recommended portion, with an explicit option to decline that part of the exam (Table 13-22). For TGNB clients, discussing these issues is especially important, as some individuals may experience dysphoria with care of

| Table 13-21 | Gender-Affirming Surgery Options |
|---|---|
| **Top Surgery: Chest or Breast Alteration** | |
| Bilateral mastectomy (chest reconstruction) | Typically desired by trans masculine individuals; refers to removal of all breast tissue, creating a flatter, more masculine-appearing contour. Possible surgical techniques depend primarily on chest size and skin elasticity, and are addressed during a surgical consultation. Hormone therapy is not required before top surgery, although testosterone use may create some chest muscle growth. Typically, a small amount of chest or breast tissue remains regardless of the surgical technique. Therefore, individuals require counseling regarding the risks and benefits of continuing routine chest/breast cancer screening, with specific attention to family history of cancer. |
| Bilateral breast augmentation | Typically desired by trans feminine individuals; refers to augmentation of existing breast tissue, creating a more prominent, more feminine-appearing contour. Estrogen may increase breast tissue size; therefore, many individuals may utilize hormones several years prior to surgery, though it is not a requirement. |
| Nonbinary top surgery | Could refer to either significant breast or chest tissue reduction or limited breast augmentation, depending on client preferences. |
| **Bottom Surgery: Vagina or Phallus Creation** | |
| Orchiectomy | Gonadectomy or removal of the testes and scrotum. Sometimes done to avoid use of antiandrogen medications. |
| Vaginoplasty | Chosen by some trans feminine individuals; refers to the surgical creation of a *neovagina*, most frequently through a technique involving penile inversion. Some individuals may purposefully opt to have a no-depth neovagina that does not include a full vaginal canal. |
| Hysterectomy | Previously recommended for AFAB individuals, but no longer routinely recommended without reason, although clients may choose this due to gender dysphoria or genetic risk. The decision to retain one's cervix, ovaries, or vaginal canal is individualized. |
| Metoidioplasty | Pursued by some trans masculine individuals; refers to the surgical creation of a small phallus using the tissue from an enlarged clitoris post use of testosterone, which causes clitoromegaly. Advantages include increased preservation of sensation and being able to urinate while standing. |
| Phalloplasty | Pursued by some trans masculine individuals; refers to the surgical creation of a phallus, which tends to be larger than the smaller phallus created in a metoidioplasty. Uses skin grafts and muscle from other places in the body, such as the forearm, thigh, or back, to create the penis. |

| Scrotoplasty and testicular implants | Pursued by some trans masculine individuals; refers to the surgical creation of a scrotum and sometimes testes using testicular prostheses. |
|---|---|
| **Other Gender-Affirming Medical/Surgical Options** | |
| Tracheal shave (chondrolaryngoplasty) | Procedure pursued by some trans feminine individuals, in which the thyroid cartilage/Adam's apple is reduced in size by shaving down the cartilage through a small incision in the throat. |
| Facial feminization or contouring surgery | A combination of procedures with the goal of softening facial features and reducing masculine facial features. Procedures may include rhinoplasty, forehead recontouring, brow lift, chin surgery, lip lift, hairline recontouring, lipofilling of cheeks, jaw-angle reduction, and/or eyelid lift. |
| Hair treatments | Many individuals begin with shaving, waxing, and tweezing, frequently moving to more permanent methods. Large areas of application are to be avoided, but clinicians may want to offer a prescription of compounded numbing cream for clients preparing for hair removal.<br>Hair implants are another option for those with more significant hair loss.<br>Some individuals also choose medications to reduce or prevent hair loss. |
| Vocal cord surgery | Some trans feminine individuals may choose voice feminization surgery to raise voice pitch in addition to nonsurgical voice training and coaching. Surgical techniques may include shortening the length of or tightening the vocal cords.<br>While voice masculinization is possible with surgery, desired voice changes are frequently achieved to a satisfactory level utilizing testosterone to affect the vocal fold mucosa. |

Based on UCSF Gender Affirming Health Program, Department of Family and Community Medicine, University of California San Francisco. *Guidelines for the Primary and Gender-Affirming Care of Transgender and Gender Nonbinary People.* 2nd ed. Deutsch MB, ed. June 2016. https://transcare.ucsf.edu/guidelines; Pariser JJ, Kim N. Transgender vaginoplasty: techniques and outcomes. *Transl Androl Urol.* 2019;8(3):241-247. doi:10.21037/tau.2019.06.03; Djordjevic ML, Stojanovic B, Bizic M. Metoidioplasty: techniques and outcomes. *Transl Androl Urol.* 2019;8(3):248-253. doi:10.21037/tau.2019.06.12; Kim HT. Vocal feminization for transgender women: current strategies and patient perspectives. *Int J Gen Med.* 2020;13:43-52. doi:10.2147/IJGM.S205102.

| Table 13-22 | Overview and Steps of a Physical Exam |
|---|---|

1. Agree on the parts of the exam to be done that day (e.g., visual exam, palpation, use of speculum, bimanual, sonography, Pap testing, cultures, biopsies).
2. Review the option to withdraw consent any time (i.e., the client holds the power in the exam versus the clinician).
3. Offer the option of having a support person present and ask for any accommodations needed.
4. Allow the client to undress or change privately.
5. Ask permission and wait for a response before each time you touch a client or move to another part of the exam.
6. Use the client's stated language for their anatomy.
7. Complete the exam with periodic verbal check-ins with the client.
8. Allow the client to dress privately before finishing the review of the plan and next steps.
9. Continue any applicable discussions or planning with the client fully dressed.
10. When applicable, thank the client for any explanation they have shared, and inquire if any aspects of the visit could be improved.

Based on Olson S. A person-centered approach to prescribing gender-affirming hormones, part one. Presented at Virtual Clinician Course: Gender-Affirming Hormones. March 3, 2022; Fuzzell L, Fedesco HN, Alexander SC, et al. "I just think that doctors need to ask more questions": sexual minority and majority adolescents' experiences talking about sexuality with healthcare providers. *Patient Educ Counsel.* 2016;99(9):1467-1472. doi:10.1016/j.pec.2016.06.004.

their chest and genitals (some may not have any dysphoria). In all individuals, there may be increased pelvic floor dysfunction when gender-neutral bathrooms are not available, resulting in increased pressure and urinary retention.

### Breast/Chest Assessment

Some clients may have opted for gender-affirming chest or breast surgery and/or may have visible changes to their anatomy related to hormone use. Family history considerations remain the same as for any client, regardless of gender. For example, if a 30-year-old transmasculine client who had top surgery/bilateral mastectomy 10 years ago (and still possesses ovaries and a uterus) recently found out that his mother is a BRCA1 carrier, his clinician would consider the anatomy he has and his reproductive plans when assessing his risks, screening recommendations, and prophylactic options. Assessment considerations are provided in Table 13-23.

### External and Internal Genitalia

For pelvic care, consider options and recommendations based on the anatomy a client has and their personal history and risk factors. As with all clients, perform physical exams only as medically indicated and previously agreed upon with the client. When appropriate, offer for the client to return to the office another day for their physical exam and complete only the verbal history portion of the visit at their initial appointment. Considerations for genital or pelvic exams are provided in Table 13-24, Table 13-25, and Table 13-26.

### Potential Gynecologic Concerns

#### Dyspareunia

Vaginal tissue can be impacted by the use of testosterone, which decreases estrogen production, which in turn increases vaginal pH and may potentially induce vaginal atrophy. There is an increased risk of tearing vaginal tissue with testosterone therapy, so it is recommended to counsel clients on the regular use of lubricant to prevent tissue damage. As when treating cisgender women with dyspareunia, application of topical testosterone or a compounded combination of topical testosterone/estrogen to the introitus and labia may help to decrease hormonally mediated dyspareunia. As when treating

| Table 13-23 | Breast/Chest Assessment |
| --- | --- |
| **History** | **Recommendation** |
| **AFAB Individuals** | |
| History of chest/breast reduction | Offer routine screening and diagnostic care per guidelines due to retained mammary tissue. |
| History of bilateral mastectomy (chest reconstruction) | Offer a clinical chest/breast exam to assess for skin changes, lymphadenopathy, and nipple changes or discharge (if nipple-sparing surgery). Counseling should be completed regarding the potential risk of gender dysphoria versus the potential benefits of routine screening mammography/imaging, as some mammary tissue is retained. Recommend diagnostic imaging based on abnormal clinical findings. |
| No history of chest/breast surgery | Offer a routine clinical chest/breast exam. Screening mammography or diagnostic imaging per current guidelines. Note: Some individuals notice atrophic changes of mammary tissue with long-term use of testosterone. |
| Current chest/breast binding | Offer a routine clinical chest/breast exam as well as screening or diagnostic imaging, when applicable. Assess for injury that may be related to inappropriate sizing or overuse of compression (see Table 13-5). |
| **AMAB Individuals** | |
| History of chest/breast augmentation | Offer routine clinical chest/breast exam, screening mammography, and diagnostic imaging per current guidelines. |

Abbreviations: AFAB, assigned female at birth; AMAB, assigned male at birth.

Based on Olson S. A person-centered approach to prescribing gender-affirming hormones, part one. Presented at Virtual Clinician Course: Gender-Affirming Hormones. March 3, 2022; Ellis S, Sherley C, Gromko L. Transgender health care toolkit: resources for transgender health care. Cedar River Clinic. http://www.cedarriverclinics.org/transtoolkit/. Published 2021. Accessed December 1, 2021; Parikh U, Mausner E, Chhor CM, et al. Breast imaging in transgender patients: what the radiologist should know. *RadioGraphics*. 2020;40(1):13-27. doi:10.1148/rg.2020190044.

| Table 13-24 | Pelvic Examination of AFAB TGNB Clients |
|---|---|
| No history of bottom surgery | External genitalia<br><br>• Increased clitoral size may be noted.<br><br>• Atrophic changes may be present with long-term testosterone use.<br><br>Internal genitalia assessed via (1) speculum and/or (2) manual or bimanual exam<br><br>• As with cisgender clients, this exam is based on current guidelines, client risk factors, concerns, and consent. |
| History of bottom surgery<br>Bottom surgery may encompass a wide range of possible surgeries—for example, removal of the vagina, uterus, ovaries, or some combination of these organs. Additionally, the creation of a phallus and/or testicular implants may be present. | Counseling includes discussion of the risks and benefits of a pelvic exam, including risk for gender dysphoria, pain, and/or medical trauma. Recommending an exam is approached based on the client's surgical history and current organs present, so a detailed history and review of systems is essential. Discussion includes visual exam, internal speculum exam and bimanual exam (and consent or declination and considerations for each of these). Routine cervical cytology screening guidelines are followed for clients who have a cervix and/or vagina. |

Abbreviations: AFAB, assigned female at birth; TGNB, transgender and nonbinary.

Based on Olson S. A person-centered approach to prescribing gender-affirming hormones, part one. Presented at Virtual Clinician Course: Gender-Affirming Hormones. March 3, 2022; Ellis S, Sherley C, Gromko L. Transgender health care toolkit: resources for transgender health care. Cedar River Clinic. http://www.cedarriverclinics.org/transtoolkit/. Published 2021. Accessed December 1, 2021.

| Table 13-25 | Cervical Cytology Screening Collection Considerations |
|---|---|
| Tissue atrophy | Given the atrophic effect that testosterone can have on vulvar and vaginal tissue, it is important for the clinician to use slow, gradual movements for pelvic and/or speculum exams to avoid tissue injury. Communication via frequent verbal check-ins and explicit discussion around ability to stop is essential. |
| Insufficient sample | AFAB individuals on testosterone experience higher rates of unsatisfactory Pap results related to the atrophy that can be seen with testosterone use.<br>Vaginal (topical) estrogen can be used for 2 weeks prior to a planned Pap specimen collection and has been shown to decrease rates of unsatisfactory cytologic samples related to atrophy. This limited use of estrogen does not interfere with other testosterone-related changes and can be used concurrently.<br>The provider should inform the client of the potential for unsatisfactory results and offer the treatment prior to a collection attempt, if desired. Some clients would rather opt for this and reschedule, whereas others some may prefer to collect the Pap specimen and consider topical estrogen only if needed subsequently. |
| Declination | Use respectful language that is supportive of client choices and includes all options in a shared decision-making approach. The provider's role is to provide the information, recommendations, and rationale as well as to discuss the risks, benefits, and alternatives of all options.<br>For example, clinicians should understand potential reasons why clients may want to decline Pap smears (or pelvic exams) altogether. A client's risk of dysphoria-related stress or trauma may be significantly higher than their risk of cervical dysplasia, and it is up to them to make an informed decision. |
| Self-collection | From a lens of harm reduction, if clients decline exams, it is recommended that clinicians offer, but not require, alternatives such as self-collection of cervical cytology screening samples or self-collection of HPV screening. |

Abbreviations: AFAB, assigned female at birth; HPV, human papillomavirus.

Based on Olson S. A person-centered approach to prescribing gender-affirming hormones, part one. Presented at Virtual Clinician Course: Gender-Affirming Hormones. March 3, 2022; Ellis S, Sherley C, Gromko L. Transgender health care toolkit: resources for transgender health care. Cedar River Clinic. http://www.cedarriverclinics.org/transtoolkit/. Published 2021. Accessed December 1, 2021.

| Table 13-26 | Pelvic Examination of AMAB TGNB Clients |
|---|---|
| No history of bottom surgery | Reasons for exam may include penile pain, concern for dermatologic changes<br>Possible discussion of tucking practice, use of gaffe |
| Status post vaginoplasty | Slightly different vaginal pH, minimal self-lubrication, and flora differences leading to decreased incidence of *Candida* infection and bacterial vaginosis[69-71]<br>For some individuals, a pelvic exam may be affirming in certain contexts or not preferred; consider offering use of a mirror during the exam<br>No recommendation for cervical cytology screening because a cervix is not typically created during surgery<br>Discuss regular vaginal dilation to maintain tissue integrity and decrease the chance of vaginal stenosis or closure of the vaginal canal (unless zero-depth vaginoplasty was performed)<br>Potential for scar tissue, pain with sex<br>Douching with gentle soap and water is recommended several weeks after surgery<br>Multidisciplinary approach; recommend collaborating with:<br>• Pelvic physical therapy<br>• Plastic surgeon specializing in gender-affirming surgery<br>• Urogynecologist<br>Additional recommendations for postoperative care can be found through UCSF Center for Excellence's Transgender Care and Treatment Guidelines[23] |
| Prostate care | Prostate remains in AMAB individuals, even status post vaginoplasty.<br>Usage of estrogen and removal of testes is likely to result in a decreased risk for prostate cancer and benign prostatic hypertrophy<br>It is recommended that prostate cancer screening be approached through shared decision making and based on guidelines for cisgender men. If a prostate exam is indicated, both rectal and neovaginal approaches may be considered.<br>• Transgender women who have undergone vaginoplasty have a prostate anterior to the vaginal wall, and a digital neovaginal exam examination may be more effective |

Abbreviations: AMAB, assigned male at birth; TGNB, transgender and nonbinary; UCSF, University of California San Francisco.

Based on Olson S. A person-centered approach to prescribing gender-affirming hormones, part one. Presented at Virtual Clinician Course: Gender-Affirming Hormones. March 3, 2022; Ellis S, Sherley C, Gromko L. Transgender health care toolkit: resources for transgender health care. Cedar River Clinic. http://www.cedarriverclinics.org/transtoolkit/. Published 2021. Accessed December 1, 2021; UCSF Gender Affirming Health Program, Department of Family and Community Medicine, University of California San Francisco. *Guidelines for the Primary and Gender-Affirming Care of Transgender and Gender Nonbinary People.* 2nd ed. Deutsch MB, ed. June 2016. https://transcare.ucsf.edu/guidelines; van der Sluis WB, de Haseth KB, Elfering L, et al. Neovaginal discharge in transgender women after vaginoplasty: a diagnostic and treatment algorithm. *Int J Transgend Health.* 2020;21(4):367-372. doi:10.1080/26895269.2020.1725710.

cisgender women, clinicians should consider recommending increased lubrication use during insertion of anything vaginally, pelvic floor therapy with an affirming physical therapist, and/or the use of premenstrual dysphoric disorder (PMDD)–targeted antidepressants or gabapentin.

### Pelvic Pain

Pelvic pain, with or without gastrointestinal symptoms, is assessed in the typical manner, as GAH typically does not cause or increase pain beyond changes associated with atrophy.[10,23] Similar to the case for many individuals with chronic pain, there may be a delay in TGNB clients seeking care for pelvic pain, due to fear, anxiety, and body or genital dysphoria.

Differential diagnoses include atrophic or infectious vaginitis, sexually transmitted infections (STIs), cystitis or bladder dysfunction, adnexal masses, cervicitis, endometriosis, and pelvic floor muscle dysfunction. For individuals with endometriosis, there is no current research to recommend for or against use of gonadotropin-releasing hormone antagonists such as elagolix (Orilissa). If the patient has recently undergone surgery, postsurgical adhesions or complications may contribute to pelvic pain. Psychosomatic etiologies such as a history of trauma, PTSD, and other mental health concerns may also be explored and considered, though should not be assumed by the clinician.

### Other Reproductive and Sexual Health Concerns

*Post-Phalloplasty.* Consider the capacity for erection/insertion and possibility of nerve damage; surgery may create scar tissue and/or adhesions.

*STI Screening, Treatment, and Prophylaxis.* Dysphoria may prevent individuals from seeking regular screening. Rates of STI transmission may be increased in individuals with atrophic or friable tissue.

*Abnormal Uterine Bleeding.* All abnormal uterine bleeding (AUB) is evaluated as usual, regardless of testosterone use, although testosterone use itself may trigger AUB during the initial 3 to 6 months as the endometrium undergoes atrophy. AUB may be ongoing for individuals on low-dose testosterone. Typically, a standard dosage is necessary to achieve amenorrhea. For individuals on testosterone, missed doses may trigger episodes of AUB that are not pathologic, but other etiologies should not be disregarded.

*Contraceptive Needs.* Individuals not taking testosterone may desire contraception use for cycle suppression as a primary goal, as experiencing menses can increase gender dysphoria for many. Additionally, the frequent gendering of menstrual products may contribute to these feelings.[72] Testosterone is not indicated for use as birth control and individuals may still ovulate, even in the absence of menses.[73] There are no contraindications to any types of hormonal or nonhormonal contraception associated with testosterone therapy. Increased chance of unplanned pregnancy may occur, as individuals may assume they are at lower risk for pregnancy and missed doses may contribute to this belief.

*Abortion Care.* TGNB individuals require the same care as cisgender individuals, but potentially may have even more limited access to abortion care.

## Fertility Considerations for TGNB Individuals

TGNB individuals have similar rates of desiring parenthood as their cisgender peers. Therefore, the clinician should ask about reproductive goals in the same way as with any other client. Initial conversations regarding fertility include a discussion of short-term and long-term reproductive goals, including clarification of whether the client desires to become pregnant.

Prior to beginning GAH, it is important that all clients be offered the chance to engage in a discussion regarding their reproductive life plans and desire for parenthood, although this does not always occur for a variety of reasons. While it is preferred that these conversations take place before GAH begins, desire for pregnancy and parenthood should be assessed even after initiating GAH and post surgery. Although long-term research is pending, expert opinion is that the baseline fecundity of most individuals is unlikely to be altered permanently by prior use of hormones. Thus, if an individual utilizes GAH and later experiences difficulty conceiving, current understanding is that this scenario is less likely to be related to use of GAH and more likely to indicate that the individual falls into the 15% of people who experience infertility in general.[10]

In discussions of baseline fertility, some research suggests that sperm-producing individuals may have lower sperm counts prior to initiation of hormones, although the reason for this finding is unclear.[74] These lower sperm counts may be suboptimal for conception and may require assisted reproductive technologies such as intrauterine insemination (IUI) or in vitro fertilization (IVF) to achieve conception.[10] Earlier research suggested that the prevalence of polycystic ovarian syndrome (PCOS) is higher in AFAB individuals who identify as TGNB, although more recent research is needed to clarify this potential relationship.[75] Ideally, PCOS will be identified prior to initiation of hormones because of the association with altered baseline fertility, so to differentiate the possible effects that can be attributed to PCOS versus GAH. Nevertheless, the clinician and client should understand that GAH does not cause PCOS.[76]

### Timing of Discontinuation of GAH

There are no formal recommendations regarding the timing of discontinuing GAH therapy so as to plan for conception. Many individuals or couples may conceive immediately, whereas others may take longer to conceive. However, it is difficult to determine whether hormones contribute to the length of time until conception versus baseline hormonal variance. There are typically two approaches for AFAB individuals wishing to time ovulation with sperm contact: (1) waiting for return of menses or (2) utilizing ovulation-induction medications such as clomiphene citrate (Clomid) or letrozole (Femara) to quicken the process. Although menses may return immediately for some clients, on average it takes three to six cycles for menses to resume if an individual experienced regular cycles prior to use of testosterone. For those persons with a history of irregular menses (such as occurs with PCOS) prior to use of testosterone, return of menses is likely to revert back to an irregular pattern, in which case the use of an ovulation-induction medication may be more strongly recommended.

For sperm-producing individuals, the return of sperm production may take 72 days, which is the typical sperm life cycle.[10,77,78] However, as noted earlier, some research suggests that baseline sperm count may be lowered even prior to initiation of GAH and sperm counts may be suboptimal for conception.[74,77,79]

### Fertility Preservation

Discussions about fertility preservation are routinely offered to all clients considering GAH care, as this therapy may impact future fertility or the ability to family-build biologically.[10] This discussion is not unique to TGNB people, but also applies to clients with high-risk conditions such as genetic susceptibility to cancer, diagnosed cancer, some pelvic masses, endometriosis, and reproductive structural anomalies. Counseling for clients receiving GAH therapy should include their individual risks, potential impacts on future fertility, and options for fertility preservation.[10,80] While being TGNB is not a health problem, clients considering GAH and/ or surgeries have historically been offered fertility preservation less frequently than individuals with high-risk health conditions, demonstrating the need for improved provider education, bias identification, and advocacy.[10]

As discussed in the *Fertility, Family Building, and Contraception* chapter, access to fertility treatment is not covered by many insurance plans.[81] This is most evident when considering cryopreservation, which is commonly considered an elective procedure. Lack of insurance coverage exacerbates existing health disparities for people with historically oppressed identities by leaving them with the choice to either forgo biologic family building or take on significant debt to access the needed care.[81] The expense associated with fertility preservation is a significant equity issue for the TGNB community, and providers must be aware of their local limitations, have informed conversations with clients, and advocate for inclusive and equitable care at the local and national levels.[10,81] Aside from the barrier of cost, some individuals may forgo fertility preservation because of the potential to experience increased gender dysphoria during the treatment.[81]

The medically necessary focus on frequently gendered organs and hormones on an almost daily basis can pose a significant challenge to one's sense of self and gender.[10] Additionally, other types of affirming care may be delayed during the preservation process. For oocyte collection, per FDA guidelines, cervical cytology screening and STI results must be current and frequent internal ultrasounds are often recommended or necessary.[10] For sperm freezing, the intimate nature of sperm collection may be prohibitive to someone who has dysphoria regarding their genitals, self-touch, or ejaculation. These challenges are related to societal constructs of gender that have impacted the self-embodiment of some TGNB individuals, and are not due to illness or failure on the client's part.[10]

Midwives and APRNs often have a unique ability to use a trauma-sensitive approach to conversations with clients who are contemplating this type of care. If a client elects to proceed with fertility preservation, their clinicians must be aware of which clinics and providers are affirming of a client's intersectional identities.

### Oocyte/Egg Freezing

Oocyte/egg freezing has not been considered experimental since 2012, but it is still widely considered optional care.[10,77,80] Due to the more invasive nature of this treatment, oocyte preservation is much costlier than sperm freezing. Depending on an individual's health history, menstrual cycle, and insurance coverage, some medications used for this care may be covered. For example, if a transgender man has PCOS with irregular cycles or anovulation, stimulation medication and cycle monitoring expenses may be considered medically necessary. This would reduce the cost, but still leaves the client to bear the cost of the procedure, anesthesia, lab, and cryopreservation fees. Another difficult consideration is that this treatment could require multiple cycles and does not guarantee a certain number of eggs or that they will thaw properly and create viable embryos in the future.[10,77,80]

### Sperm Freezing

Sperm freezing is also rarely covered by insurance, but is a less expensive, less invasive option for fertility cryopreservation.[10,77,80] To complete this procedure, individuals are typically scheduled for several appointments in which they provide a semen sample, either at home or in a collection room at a clinic or cryobank.[10] Semen is made up of many components—sperm cells, water, protein, sugars, plasma, lactic acid, and small amounts of essential nutrients such as zinc, calcium, magnesium, and potassium. While semen volume can be normal, if the count is low, an individual may need to schedule a larger number of freezing appointments.[10] If the count is average or high, one semen sample can typically be divided into multiple vials for use in future intrauterine insemination or in vitro fertilization cycles.

When working with a fertility specialist or cryobank, specific designation of these vials as appropriate for use in vaginal insemination, intrauterine insemination, or in vitro fertilization is typically documented.[10] If an individual plans to conceive in the future with a partner or co-parent as the gestational parent, the cost tends to be lower. If an individual plans to conceive in the future with a gestational carrier or surrogate, it is usually necessary to follow an FDA-guided freezing process, which will add to the cost.[10]

## Pregnancy, Birth, and Postpartum Care for TGNB Individuals

Perinatal care for TGNB clients and families is no different than the care for cisgender clients and families from a clinical standpoint. Some differences do arise, however, in regard to cultural, psychosocial, and equity considerations for this population (Table 13-27 and Table 13-28). It is important that clinicians proactively become familiar with local and national resources that are available for perinatal TGNB clients. Understanding of TGNB identities and use of inclusive language is at the core of this care.

| Table 13-27 | Perinatal Considerations for TGNB Clients |
| --- | --- |
| Birth setting | Many TGNB clients opt for community birth (birth center or home birth), due to personal preference as well as to limit potentially harmful interactions with more staff in hospitals.[82] Community birth options also allow for a greater sense of control and autonomy for the client as well as increased trust and understanding between client and clinician. Conversations regarding the birth setting ideally start early in pregnancy, so that clients and families have time to decide the safe options for themselves. It may be helpful for clients to share birth preferences surrounding planned or unplanned hospital admission so as to discuss and prioritize any planning that may be needed. |
| Documentation | Many health record templates and diagnoses have inappropriate gendered language that may or may not be able to be edited by the clinician. If editable, the recommendation is to use accurate and gender-neutral language for all clients. If a field cannot be changed—for example, a field stating "maternal blood pressure" or "advanced maternal age"—the client should be informed that they would see this terminology in their record. This would be an opportunity to inform the client that the language is wrong and unable to be changed at that moment, preserving trust that the clinician is not ignoring their gender identity. See Table 13-28 for terminology suggestions. |
| Fetal sex | Clarify the client's preferences about discussion, disclosure, and documentation of fetal sex chromosomes or genitalia that may result from screening or diagnostic testing in pregnancy. |
| Route of birth | Risks and benefits of vaginal and operative birth do not differ for TGNB clients. However, it is reasonable to inquire about the approach to labor and birth that feels safest to the client and to provide any information they may need in their decision-making process. If the thought of labor or vaginal birth causes distress or dysphoria, a client may consider a planned cesarean birth in some cases.[82,83] In other cases, validation of fears and emphasis on autonomy may allow a client to feel safe with a planned vaginal birth. For example, if the thought of cervical exams causes distress, ensuring that no procedures or exams will be performed without consent may be reassuring and allay those concerns. |
| Lactation[84] | Both AFAB and AMAB parents can breastfeed/chestfeed.[85] Lactation can be induced in nongestational parents under the guidance and support of knowledgeable clinicians and lactation specialists, although it often requires a period of medication use (hormones and/or galactogogues) as well as diligent pumping efforts before lactation is established.[86] See the *Infant Feeding and Lactation* chapter. |

*(continues)*

| Table 13-27 | Perinatal Considerations for TGNB Clients (*continued*) |
|---|---|
| | The success of lactation depends on the availability of support, genetics, and chest anatomy, as well as the medical and procedural history of the individual.[86] Parents may produce very little milk or enough to sustain an infant and should be advised on feeding per current guidelines and recommendations. Keep in mind that feeding an infant in any amount may increase bonding and satisfaction for the entire family unit. |
| Contraceptive needs | TGNB clients are offered contraception if they are at risk for unwanted pregnancy. As with all clients, these options are best discussed antenatally so that options can be considered and planned for, if needed. |
| Hormone therapy | For TGNB clients who plan to resume or start testosterone therapy after a pregnancy, care is individualized based on the person's plans and priorities.<br>No detailed guidelines currently exist regarding restarting testosterone postpartum, but many anecdotal reports describe individuals restarting this therapy within days to weeks without incident.[10]<br>Shared decision making guides this discussion, including an assessment of thrombosis risk, desire for breastfeeding/chestfeeding, and discussion of dysphoria.[10]<br>The route of administration is discussed, while noting that it is generally advisable to avoid topical testosterone due to potential for skin transfer to the newborn. Low- or average-dose testosterone is unlikely to cause elevated serum testosterone levels in breast milk, but high-dose testosterone may potentially decrease prolactin levels.[87] |
| Collaboration | Ensuring any referrals are inclusive and competent is important to avoid causing harm and dissolving trust. If it is not known if a referral clinician is trans-knowledgeable, be sure to inform the client so they may decide how to proceed.<br>Some common examples of collaborators include radiology centers, specialists (e.g., gastroenterology, maternal–fetal medicine, physical therapy, mental health), doulas, childbirth educators, places of birth (with attention to staff and policies), lactation support, massage therapists, chiropractors, acupuncturists, group care, in-home care, and infant care. |

Abbreviations: AFAB, assigned female at birth; AMAB, assigned male at birth; TGNB, transgender and nonbinary.

| Table 13-28 | Replacing Historically Gendered Phrases | |
|---|---|---|
| **Avoid** | **Consider** | |
| Well-woman exam | Periodic, wellness, or preventive gynecologic exam | |
| Female genitourinary exam | Pelvic exam | |
| Normal external female genitalia (NEFG) | Healthy external genitalia (What is "normal"?) | |
| Breast … (exam, concerns, feeding, etc.) | Chest …<br>Breast or chest …<br>• "Do you have any questions about breastfeeding or chestfeeding?"<br>• "Based on your concerns, I recommend we do a chest exam today. Does that sound OK to you?" | |
| "Do you know what you're having?" (in reference to assumption of fetal sex) | Avoid the question. Try connecting with clients in another way.<br>• "What time of day does your baby move most?"<br>• "Have you chosen a name for your baby?"<br>It's OK to say "they," "the baby," or other gender-neutral terms in conversation. If the client uses pronouns or words for their fetus, it's also OK to follow their lead. | |
| "Baby's gender is a surprise" | Accurate, but likely not what the author intended.<br>• "Cell-free fetal DNA done, does not wish to know fetal sex chromosomes." | |

| Avoid | Consider |
| --- | --- |
| Vulva<br>Labia<br>Penis<br>Scrotum | External genitalia<br>• "When talking about genitals, I usually use the terms external and/or internal genitalia. Are there any words that you prefer I use or not use?"<br>Clients will have their own affirming words for their body parts, so ask their preference for the words you use as their provider. It is OK to refer to anatomic landmarks in documentation. Best practice is to inform clients of the words you use in documentation, as they have access to their charts and should not be surprised by your language.<br>• "When discussing your health or any exams, I'd like to use words that feel most comfortable for you if you feel comfortable sharing them. When I document today's visit, I may be limited by some options in our system or need to choose from words or diagnoses that are outdated or wrong, and I'm sorry for that." |
| Clitoris | Ask the client; clitoris may be acceptable, or the client may prefer phallus, penis, etc. |
| Penis | Ask the client; penis may be acceptable, or the client may prefer clitoris or something else. |
| Vagina* | Internal genitalia<br>Ask the client; they may use another term like "front hole." |
| Pre-op, preoperative | Non-op, nonoperative (post-op or postoperative is OK)<br>• "Client had lower libido which she attributes to past dysphoria about nonoperative genitalia. Over the last 6 months, libido has improved and she is working with a pelvic floor PT and using dilators for postoperative care." |
| Mom and baby | Client and infant |
| Male infant<br>Female infant | Assigned male infant<br>Assigned female infant<br>(Acknowledges the provider's role in this designation as opposed to the actual identity of the newborn) |
| Starting a family | Family building or expanding |

* The issue is not that a word like *vagina* is wrong or inappropriate. The issue is that through centuries of patriarchal systems that led to the current culture and gender binary, anatomic terms have been ascribed genders that are not necessarily congruent with the people who have them. For example, if society did not consider a vagina to be "female" and it was understood that it was a genderless and powerful body part, there might be less dysphoria for men or nonbinary individuals who had vaginas. This example serves only for a simple perspective, and is extremely limited and not inclusive of other feminist ideals or acknowledgment of other systems of oppression that have contributed a toxic binary.

Based on Rossi AL, Lopez EJ. Contextualizing competence: language and LGBT-based competency in health care. *J Homosex.* 2017;64(10):1330-1349. doi:10.1080/00918369.2017.1321361; Olson S. A person-centered approach to prescribing gender-affirming hormones, part one. Presented at Virtual Clinician Course: Gender-Affirming Hormones. March 3, 2022.

## References

1. Herman JL, Flores AR, O'Neil KK. How many adults and youth identify as transgender in the United States? Williams Institute; 2022. https://williamsinstitute.law.ucla.edu/publications/trans-adults-united-states/. Accessed October 12, 2022.

2. Jones J. LGBT identification rises to 5.6% in latest U.S. Estimate. Gallup; 2021. https://news.gallup.com/poll/329708/lgbt-identification-rises-latest-estimate.aspx. Accessed October 1, 2022.

3. Ghorayshi A. Report reveals sharp rise in transgender young people in the U.S. *New York Times*, June 10, 2022. https://www.nytimes.com/2022/06/10/science/transgender-teenagers-national-survey.html. Accessed October 1, 2022.

4. Janssen DF. Transgenderism before gender: nosology from the sixteenth through mid-twentieth century. *Arch Sex Behav.* 2020;49:1415-1425. https://doi.org/10.1007/s10508-020-01715-w.

5. Crockett C, Cooper B. Gender norms as health harms: reclaiming a life course perspective on sexual and reproductive health and rights. *Reprod Health Matt.* 2016;24(48):6-13. doi:10.1016/j.rhm.2016.11.003.

6. Fausto-Sterling A. A dynamic systems framework for gender/sex development: from sensory input in infancy to subjective certainty in toddlerhood. *Front Hum Neurosci.* 2021;15:613789. doi:10.3389/fnhum.2021.613789.

7. Olson KR, Durwood L, Horton R, et al. Gender identity 5 years after social transition. *Pediatrics*, May 4, 2022. doi:10.1542/peds.2021-056082.

8. Chandra-Mouli V, Plesons M, Amin A. Addressing harmful and unequal gender norms in early adolescence. *Nat Hum Behav.* 2018;2(4):239-240. doi:10.1038/s41562-018-0318-3.

9. Rossi AL, Lopez EJ. Contextualizing competence: language and LGBT-based competency in health care. *J Homosex.* 2017;64(10):1330-1349. doi: 10.1080/00918369.2017.1321361.

10. Olson S. A person-centered approach to prescribing gender-affirming hormones, part one. Presented at Virtual Clinician Course: Gender-Affirming Hormones, March 3, 2022.

11. Intersex Society of North America. What is intersex? https://isna.org/faq/what_is_intersex/. Published 2019. Accessed March 23, 2023.

12. Policies supporting intersex youth. interACT: Advocates for Intersex Youth. https://interactadvocates.org/policies-supporting-intersex-youth/. Accessed June 6, 2022.

13. US medical association stands against unnecessary intersex surgeries. Human Rights Watch. https://www.hrw.org/news/2018/09/17/us-medical-association-stands-against-unnecessary-intersex-surgeries. Published September 17, 2018. Accessed July 10, 2022.

14. Mastromonaco GF, Houck ML, Bergfelt DR. Disorders of sexual development in wild and captive exotic animals. *Sex Develop.* 2012;6(1-3):84-95. doi:10.1159/000332203.

15. Grilo TF, Rosa R. Intersexuality in aquatic invertebrates: prevalence and causes. *Sci Total Environ.* 2017;592:714-728. doi:10.1016/j.scitotenv.2017.02.099.

16. American College of Nurse-Midwives. Definition of midwifery and scope of practice of certified nurse-midwives and certified midwives. https://www.midwife.org/acnm/files/acnmlibrarydata/uploadfilename/000000000266/Definition%20Midwifery%20Scope%20of%20Practice_2021.pdf. Published December, 2021. Accessed August 10, 2022.

17. American College of Nurse-Midwives. ACNM core competencies for basic midwifery practice. https://www.midwife.org/acnm/files/acnmlibrarydata/uploadfilename/000000000050/ACNMCoreCompetenciesMar2020_final.pdf. Published March 20, 2020. Accessed April 13, 2021.

18. Carrera-Fernández MV, DePalma R. Feminism will be trans-inclusive or it will not be: why do two cis-hetero woman educators support transfeminism? *Sociol Rev.* 2020;68(4):745-762.doi:10.1177/0038026120934686.

19. Williams C. The ontological woman: a history of deauthentication, dehumanization, and violence. *Sociol Rev.* 2020;68(4):718-734. doi:10.1177/0038026120938292.

20. American College of Nurse-Midwives. Health care for transgender and gender non-binary people. https://www.midwife.org/acnm/files/acnmlibrarydata/uploadfilename/000000000326/ACNM--PS--Care%20for%20TGNB%20People-%20Final_1.pdf. Published March 2021. Accessed December 2, 2021.

21. Ogungbe O, Mitra AK, Roberts JK. A systematic review of implicit bias in health care: a call for intersectionality. *IMC J Med Sci.* 2019;13(1):5. doi:10.3329/imcjms.v13i1.42050.

22. Anakwe A, Green J, BeLue R. Perceptions of cultural competence and utilization of advanced practice providers. *J Allied Health.* 2021;50(1):54-62.

23. UCSF Gender Affirming Health Program, Department of Family and Community Medicine, University of California San Francisco. *Guidelines for the Primary and Gender-Affirming Care of Transgender and Gender Nonbinary People.* 2nd ed. Deutsch MB, ed. June 2016. https://transcare.ucsf.edu/guidelines.

24. Schreuder MC. Safe spaces, agency, and resistance: a metasynthesis of LGBTQ language use. *J LGBT Youth.* 2019:1-17. doi:10.1080/19361653.2019.1706685.

25. Jaffee KD, Shires DA, Stroumsa D. Discrimination and delayed health care among transgender women and men: implications for improving medical education and health care delivery. *Med Care.* 2016;54(11):1010-1016. doi:10.1097/MLR.0000000000000583.

26. Crenshaw, K. Demarginalizing the intersection of race and sex: a Black feminist critique of antidiscrimination doctrine, feminist theory and antiracist politics. *Univ Chicago Legal Forum.* 1989;1(8):139-167. http://chicagounbound.uchicago.edu/uclf/vol1989/iss1/8.

27. Davy Z, Toze M. What is gender dysphoria? A critical systematic narrative review. *Transgend Health.* 2018;3(1):159-169. doi:10.1089/trgh.2018.0014.

28. Valente PK, Schrimshaw EW, Dolezal C, et al. Stigmatization, resilience, and mental health among a diverse community sample of transgender and gender nonbinary individuals in the U.S. *Arch Sex Behav.* 2020;49(7):2649-2660. doi:10.1007/s10508-020-01761-4.

29. Bränström R, Pachankis JE. Reduction in mental health treatment utilization among transgender individuals after gender-affirming surgeries: a total population study. *Am J Psychiatry.* 2020;177(8):727-734. doi:10.1176/appi.ajp.2019.19010080.

30. Wanta JW, Niforatos JD, Durbak E, et al. Mental health diagnoses among transgender patients in the clinical setting: an all-payer electronic health record study. *Transgend Health.* 2019;4(1):313-315. doi:10.1089/trgh.2019.0029.

31. Austin A, Craig SL, D'Souza S, McInroy LB. Suicidality among transgender youth: elucidating the role of interpersonal risk factors. *J Interpers Violence*. 2022;37(5-6):NP2696-NP2718. doi:10.1177/0886260520915554. [Published correction appears in *J Interpers Violence*. 2020:886260520946128.]

32. Wolford-Clevenger C, Cannon CJ, Flores LY, et al. Suicide risk among transgender people: a prevalent problem in critical need of empirical and theoretical research. *Violence Gender*. 2017;4(3):69-72. doi:10.1089/vio.2017.0006.

33. Accepting adults reduce suicide attempts among LGBTQ youth. The Trevor Project. https://www.thetrevorproject.org/research-briefs/accepting-adults-reduce-suicide-attempts-among-lgbtq-youth/. Published October 5, 2021. Accessed October 13, 2022.

34. Follins LD, Garrett-Walker JJ, Lewis MK. Resilience in Black lesbian, gay, bisexual, and transgender individuals: a critical review of the literature. *J Gay Lesbian Mental Health*. 2014;18(2):190-212. doi:10.1080/19359705.2013.828343.

35. Furstenberg FF, Harris LE, Pesando LM, Reed MN. Kinship practices among alternative family forms in Western industrialized societies. *J Marriage Fam*. 2020;82(5):1403-1430. doi:10.1111/jomf.12712.

36. Dowd R. Transgender people over four times more likely than cisgender people to be victims of violent crime. Williams Institute. https://williamsinstitute.law.ucla.edu/press/ncvs-trans-press-release/. Published March 31, 2021. Accessed December 30, 2021.

37. Dinno A. Homicide rates of transgender individuals in the United States: 2010–2014. *Am J Public Health*. 2017;107(9):1441-1447. doi:10.2105/AJPH.2017.303878.

38. Smith NA, Voisin DR, Yang JP, Tung EL. Keeping your guard up: hypervigilance among urban residents affected by community and police violence. *Health Aff (Millwood)*. 2019;38(10):1662-1669. doi:10.1377/hlthaff.2019.00560.

39. Nagata JM, Ganson KT, Austin SB. Emerging trends in eating disorders among sexual and gender minorities. *Curr Opin Psychiatry*. 2020;33(6):562-567. doi:10.1097/YCO.0000000000000645.

40. Diemer EW, White Hughto JM, Gordon AR, et al. Beyond the binary: differences in eating disorder prevalence by gender identity in a transgender sample. *Transgender Heal*. 2018;3(1):17-23. http://www.ncbi.nlm.nih.gov/pubmed/29359198.

41. Davis SA, Meier SC. Effects of testosterone treatment and chest reconstruction surgery on mental health and sexuality in female-to-male transgender people. *Int J Sex Health*. 2014;26(2):113-128. doi:10.1080/19317611.2013.833152.

42. Schneider S, Courey M. Transgender voice and communication: vocal health and considerations. https://transcare.ucsf.edu/guidelines/vocal-health. Published online June 17, 2016. Accessed April 14, 2023.

43. Trussler JT, Carrasquillo RJ. Cryptozoospermia associated with genital tucking behavior in a transwoman. *Rev Urol*. 2020;22(4):170-173.

44. Jarrett BA, Corbet AL, Gardner IH, et al. Chest binding and care seeking among transmasculine adults: a cross-sectional study. *Transgend Health*. 2018;3(1):170-178. doi:10.1089/trgh.2018.0017.

45. Peitzmeier S, Gardner I, Weinand J, Corbet A, Acevedo K. Health impact of chest binding among transgender adults: a community-engaged, cross-sectional study. *Cult Health Sex*. 2017;19(1):64-75. doi:10.1080/13691058.2016.1191675.

46. World Professional Association for Transgender Health. Standards of care for the health of transgender and gender diverse people, version 8. https://wpath.org/publications/soc. Published 2022. Accessed November 1, 2022.

47. Mirza SA, Rooney C. Discrimination prevents LGBTQ people from accessing health care. Center for American Progress. https://www.americanprogress.org/issues/lgbt/news/2018/01/18/445130/discrimination-prevents-lgbtq-people-accessing-health-care/. Published August 23, 2022. Accessed October 30, 2022.

48. Tordoff DM, Wanta JW, Collin A, et al. Mental health outcomes in transgender and nonbinary youths receiving gender-affirming care. *JAMA Netw Open*. 2022;5(2):e220978. doi:10.1001/jamanetworkopen.2022.0978.

49. Ellis S, Sherley C, Gromko L. Transgender health care toolkit: resources for transgender health care. Cedar River Clinic. http://www.cedarriverclinics.org/transtoolkit/. Published 2021. Accessed December 1, 2021.

50. Campbell M, Jialal I. Physiology, endocrine hormones. In: *StatPearls*. Treasure Island, FL: StatPearls Publishing; September 26, 2022. https://www.ncbi.nlm.nih.gov/books/NBK538498/.

51. Anderson AD, Irwin JA, Brown AM, Gela CL. "Your picture looks the same as my picture": an examination of passing in transgender communities. *Gend Issues*. 2020;37(1):44-60. https://doi.org/10.1007/s12147-019-09239-x.

52. Billard TJ. "Passing" and the politics of deception: transgender bodies, cisgender aesthetics, and the policing of inconspicuous marginal identities. In: *The Palgrave Handbook of Deceptive Communication*. Cham, Switzerland: Springer International Publishing; 2019:463-477. https://doi.org/10.1007/978-3-319-96334-1_24.

53. Gialeraki A, Valsami S, Pittaras T, et al. Oral contraceptives and HRT risk of thrombosis. *Clin Appl Thromb Hemost*. 2018;24(2):217-225. doi:10.1177/1076029616683802.

54. Vinogradova Y, Coupland C, Hippisley-Cox J. Use of hormone replacement therapy and risk of venous thromboembolism: nested case-control studies using the QResearch and CPRD databases. *BMJ.* 2019. doi:10.1136/bmj.k4810.

55. Bergendal A, Bremme K, Hedenmalm K, et al. Risk factors for venous thromboembolism in pre- and postmenopausal women. *Thromb Res.* 2012;130(4):596-601. doi:10.1016/j.thromres.2012.05.024.

56. Başbuğ M, Aygen E, Tayyar M, et al. Twenty two weeks of transdermal estradiol increases sex hormone-binding globulin in surgical menopausal women. *Eur J Obstet Gynecol Reprod Biol.* 1997;73(2):149-152. doi:10.1016/s0301-2115(97)02706-1.

57. Scheres LJJ, van Hylckama Vlieg A, Ballieux BEPB, et al. Endogenous sex hormones and risk of venous thromboembolism in young women. *J Thromb Haemost.* 2019;17(8):1297-1304. doi:10.1111/jth.14474.

58. Bozkurt M. The impact of sex hormone-binding globulin levels on thromboembolic events at patients with advanced stage adenocarcinoma. *Turk J Oncol.* 2022;37(2):187-191. doi:10.5505/tjo.2022.3466.

59. The 2017 hormone therapy position statement of the North American Menopause Society. *Menopause.* 2017;24(7):728-753. doi:10.1097/gme.0000000000000921.

60. Hugon-Rodin J, Alhenc-Gelas M, Hemker HC, et al. Sex hormone-binding globulin and thrombin generation in women using hormonal contraception. *Biomarkers.* 2016;22(1):81-85. doi:10.1080/1354750x.2016.1204010.

61. Bagot CN, Marsh MS, Whitehead M, et al. The effect of estrone on thrombin generation may explain the different thrombotic risk between oral and transdermal hormone replacement therapy. *J Thromb Haemost.* 2010;8(8):1736-1744.

62. Stripp B, Taylor AA, Bartter FC, et al. Effect of spironolactone on sex hormones in man. *J Clin Endocrinol Metab.* 1975;41(4):777-781. doi:10.1210/jcem-41-4-777.

63. Zimmerman Y, Eijkemans MJ, Coelingh Bennink HJ, et al. The effect of combined oral contraception on testosterone levels in healthy women: a systematic review and meta-analysis. *Hum Reprod Update.* 2014;20(1):76-105. doi:10.1093/humupd/dmt038.

64. Milionis C, Ilias I, Koukkou E. Progesterone in gender-affirming therapy of trans women. *World J Biol Chem.* 2022;13(3):66-71. doi:10.4331/wjbc.v13.i3.66.

65. Moravek MB, Kinnear HM, George J, et al. Impact of exogenous testosterone on reproduction in transgender men. *Endocrinology.* 2020;161(3):bqaa014. doi:10.1210/endocr/bqaa014.

66. Nokoff NJ. Medical interventions for transgender youth. In: Feingold KR, Anawalt B, Boyce A, et al., eds. *Endotext.* South Dartmouth, MA: MDText.com, Inc.; January 19, 2022.

67. Bosworth A, Turrini G, Pyda S, et al. *Health Insurance Coverage and Access to Care for LGBTQ+ Individuals.* Issue Brief No. HP-2021-14. Washington, DC: Office of the Assistant Secretary for Planning and Evaluation, U.S. Department of Health and Human Services; June 2021. https://aspe.hhs.gov/sites/default/files/2021-07/lgbt-health-ib.pdf.

68. Fuzzell L, Fedesco HN, Alexander SC, et al. "I just think that doctors need to ask more questions": sexual minority and majority adolescents' experiences talking about sexuality with healthcare providers. *Patient Educ Counsel.* 2016;99(9):1467-1472. doi:10.1016/j.pec.2016.06.004.

69. van der Sluis WB, de Haseth KB, Elfering L, et al. Neovaginal discharge in transgender women after vaginoplasty: a diagnostic and treatment algorithm. *Int J Transgend Health.* 2020;21(4):367-372. doi:10.1080/26895269.2020.1725710.

70. Birse KD, Kratzer K, Zuend CF, et al. The neovaginal microbiome of transgender women post-gender reassignment surgery. *Microbiome.* 2020;8(1):61. doi:10.1186/s40168-020-00804-1.

71. Krakowsky Y, Potter E, Hallarn J, et al. The effect of gender-affirming medical care on the vaginal and neovaginal microbiomes of transgender and gender-diverse people. *Front Cell Infect Microbiol.* 2022;11:769950. doi:10.3389/fcimb.2021.769950.

72. Atkins C. For transgender men, pain of menstruation is more than just physical. NBCNews.com. https://www.nbcnews.com/feature/nbc-out/transgender-men-pain-menstruation-more-just-physical-n1113961. Published January 11, 2020. Accessed December 30, 2021.

73. Taub RL, Ellis SA, Neal-Perry G, et al. The effect of testosterone on ovulatory function in transmasculine individuals. *Am J Obstet Gynecol.* 2020;223(2):229.e1-229.e8. doi:10.1016/j.ajog.2020.01.059.

74. Rodriguez-Wallberg KA, Häljestig J, Arver S, Johansson ALV, Lundberg FE. Sperm quality in transgender women before or after gender affirming hormone therapy: a prospective cohort study. *Andrology.* 2021;9(6):1773-1780. doi:10.1111/andr.12999.

75. Liu M, Murthi S, Poretsky L. Polycystic ovary syndrome and gender identity. *Yale J Biol Med.* 2020;93(4):529-537.

76. Chan KJ, Liang JJ, Jolly D, Weinand JD, Safer JD. Exogenous testosterone does not induce or exacerbate the metabolic features associated with PCOS among transgender men. *Endocr Pract.* 2018;24(6):565-572. doi:10.4158/EP-2017-0247.

77. Sterling J, Garcia MM. Fertility preservation options for transgender individuals. *Transl Androl*

*Urol.* 2020;9(Suppl 2):S215-S226. doi:10.21037/tau.2019.09.28.

78. Griswold MD. Spermatogenesis: the commitment to meiosis. *Physiol Rev.* 2016;96(1):1-17. doi:10.1152/physrev.00013.2015.

79. McCracken M, Nangia AK, Roby K, McLaren H, Gray M, Marsh CA. Total motile sperm in transgender women seeking hormone therapy: a case-control study. *Fertil Steril.* 2018;110(4):e22. doi:10.1016/j.fertnstert.2018.07.078.

80. Abern L, Maguire K. Fertility preservation among transgender individuals. *Fertil Steril.* 2018;110(4):e281.

81. Estevez SL, Ghofranian A, Brownridge SR, Abittan B, Goldman RH. Insurance coverage for LGBTQ patients seeking infertility care. *Fertil Steril.* 2020;113(4):e44. doi:10.1016/j.fertnstert.2020.02.095.

82. Besse M, Lampe NM, Mann ES. Experiences with achieving pregnancy and giving birth among transgender men: a narrative literature review. *Yale J Biol Med.* 2020;93(4):517-528.

83. Obedin-Maliver J, Makadon HJ. Transgender men and pregnancy. *Obstet Med.* 2016;9(1):4-8. doi:10.1177/1753495X15612658.

84. Trautner E, McCool-Myers M, Joyner AB. Knowledge and practice of induction of lactation in trans women among professionals working in trans health. *Int Breastfeed J.* 2020;15(1). doi:10.1186/s13006-020-00308-6.

85. Reisman T, Goldstein Z. Case report: induced lactation in a transgender woman. *Transgend Health.* 2018;3(1):24-26. doi:10.1089/trgh.2017.0044.

86. García-Acosta JM, Juan-Valdivia RMS, Fernández-Martínez AD, Lorenzo-Rocha ND, Castro-Peraza ME. Trans* pregnancy and lactation: a literature review from a nursing perspective. *Int J Environ Res Public Health.* 2020;17(1):44. doi:10.3390/ijerph17010044.

87. Testosterone. Drugs and Lactation Database (LactMed) [Internet]. Bethesda, MD: National Library of Medicine. https://www.ncbi.nlm.nih.gov/books/NBK501721/. Published 2006. Revised May 15, 2022.

CHAPTER

# 14

# Menopause

RUTH ZIELINSKI AND EVA FRIED

*The editors acknowledge Julia Lange Kessler, who was the author of this chapter in the previous edition.*

## Introduction

Menopause care is positioned at the intersection of overmedicalization, under-recognition, and societal constructs of womanhood, personhood, and aging. Most scientific literature and many healthcare settings continue to frame menopause as a disease of estrogen deficiency that can only be fixed by replacing hormones.[1] In other spaces, including from a feminist perspective, menopause is framed as a normal phase of life. It *is* normal to experience menopause, of course, yet over-normalization can lead healthcare providers and people experiencing menopause to discount the experience. Like menarche, menopause includes changes in physical and psychological systems, as well as relational experiences, that deserve attention. Some individuals need to name and share their experience, while others may have a need to treat bothersome symptoms.

Menopause is defined as a one-time event that marks permanent cessation of ovulation and menstruation, diagnosed by 12 months of amenorrhea with no other identified cause. Although menopause is a universal experience, it may be influenced by diet, environment, cultural beliefs, and genetics. While the median age of menopause in North America is 51 years, a wide age range—40 to 58 years—is considered normal for physiologic menopause.[2] The experience of physiologic menopause varies widely, from no symptoms to troublesome symptoms that can last for a decade or more. Menopause induced by surgery, chemotherapy, or radiation therapy often results in a more dramatic transition, with symptoms more likely to be bothersome for these individuals.[2] The experience of menopausal symptoms is culturally determined to a great degree. Generalizing from the experiences of one group of

people to other groups can lead to misunderstandings and suboptimal care.[3]

While permanent cessation of menses can be diagnosed only retrospectively, the symptoms of menopause can start many years prior. Therefore, unlike menarche and pregnancy, there is no clear test, or moment in time, to determine that a person's symptoms are due to the menopausal transition. There is inadequate space in public discourse for conversations about menopause and aging in general. Furthermore, changes in body image and reproductive processes are deeply stigmatized and often cloaked in shame. These forces intersect with cultural norms about privacy and trust or mistrust of healthcare professionals.[4,5] Midwives can help to bridge these gaps by asking thoughtful questions and providing anticipatory guidance about the menopause transition. This approach, in turn, can help foster the knowledge and personal agency that midwives value in all stages of life.[6]

## Terms and Definitions for Menopause

Table 14-1 identifies terms and definitions frequently used to describe aspects of the menopausal period.[2,7,8] While terms are often used interchangeably, some are imprecise or have negative connotations of pathology or failure or are not the preferred terms.

## Physiology of Menopause

### Ovarian Changes

The physiologic changes associated with menopause actually begin at birth and continue over the course of a lifetime. During fetal life, the ovaries contain approximately 1 to 2 million follicles—the maximum

**571**

| Table 14-1 | Definitions Related to Menopause | |
|---|---|---|
| **Preferred Term** | **Other Terms** | **Definition** |
| Early menopause | Premature menopause | Menopause that occurs earlier than 2 standard deviations below the mean estimated age for the reference population. The age frequently used as a benchmark is 40 years. Early menopause can be physiologic or induced. |
| Estrogen therapy | Estrogen replacement therapy | Treatment with estrogen for menopausal symptoms such as vasomotor conditions or vulvovaginal atrophy. *Replacement* is no longer used because it connotes an unnatural deficiency state when the changed endogenous hormone levels that occur with menopause are physiologic and expected. |
| Estrogen plus progestin therapy | Combination therapy | Similar to *estrogen therapy* but with added progestin to decrease the risk of endometrial hyperplasia or cancer. |
| Final menstrual period (FMP) | | The last menstrual period of a person's life; it is recognized after 12 months of amenorrhea has passed. The average age at FMP in the global north is 51 years (range: 40–58 years). |
| Hormone therapy | Menopausal hormone therapy Hormone replacement therapy | Primarily use of estrogen with or without an added progestin. *Replacement* is no longer used because it connotes an unnatural deficiency state when the changed endogenous hormone levels that occur with menopause are physiologic and expected. |
| Induced menopause | Surgical menopause | Cessation of menstruation due to surgical removal of the ovaries or ablation of ovarian function from chemotherapy or pelvic radiation therapy. |
| Menopause | | A one-time event that marks permanent cessation of ovulation and menstruation. It is diagnosed after 12 months of amenorrhea with no other identified cause. |
| Menopause transition | Perimenopause, climacteric | Often used synonymously with *perimenopause*, this term describes the time of variation in cycle length and/or symptoms. However, unlike perimenopause, it does not include the 12 months following the FMP. |
| Perimenopause | Climacteric | A time of menstrual and endocrine changes, beginning with variation in cycle length or symptoms attributable to those changes and extending to the 12 months following the FMP. Average age at onset is 46 years (range: 39–51 years). Average duration of perimenopause is 5 years (range: 2–8 years). |
| Postmenopause | | The period of time after the final menstrual period. |
| Primary ovarian insufficiency | Premature ovarian failure | Ovarian insufficiency leading to amenorrhea age younger than 40 years. Cessation of ovarian function is not always permanent. |
| Progesterone | | A steroid hormone secreted by the corpus luteum and by the placenta. This term is most commonly used to describe the naturally occurring progestational hormone. |
| Progestin | | A natural or synthetic substance that mimics the actions of progesterone. This term is most commonly used to describe the progestational hormone used for contraception and menopausal hormone therapy. |

Abbreviation: FMP, final menstrual period.

Based on North American Menopause Society, ed. *Menopause Practice: A Clinician's Guide.* 6th ed. Pepper Pike, OH: North American Menopause Society; 2021; Fritz MA, Speroff L. Menopause and perimenopausal transition. In: *Clinical Gynecologic Endocrinology and Infertility.* 8th ed. Philadelphia, PA: Lippincott Williams & Wilkins; 2011:673-748; Harlow SD, Gass M, Hall JE, et al. Executive summary of the Stages of Reproductive Aging Workshop + 10: addressing the unfinished agenda of staging reproductive aging. *Fertil Steril.* 2012;97:843-851.

number of follicles during a lifetime.[2] Most individuals will ovulate fewer than 500 times during their reproductive years, with the majority of follicles being lost through ovarian follicular depletion, or atresia of follicles.[9] Follicles begin a physiologic depletion process even before birth, with the loss increasing exponentially and eventually leading to nearly all follicles being depleted, which results in menopause.

As the number of follicles diminishes, the ovaries become more resistant to the action of follicle-stimulating hormone (FSH).[2] The ovaries also decrease production of estrogen, androgen, and progesterone. Loss of the negative feedback from ovarian estrogen production means that gonadotropin production is no longer inhibited. Subsequently, levels of FSH and luteinizing hormone (LH) rise markedly, to the point that the FSH level exceeds the LH level. Secretion of the ovarian glycoprotein inhibin, which selectively inhibits FSH, also decreases. The decreased release of inhibin eventually results in sustained elevation of FSH. Elevated FSH levels stabilize approximately 24 months after the final menstrual period. Although FSH and LH levels generally trend upward over time throughout this process, they fluctuate widely and unpredictably. These variations are why routine testing of hormone levels as a method of diagnosing menopause or perimenopause is not recommended.[2]

After menopause, the ovaries change considerably both in physical appearance and in function. Despite the absence of functional follicles, both the remaining corticostromal cells and the hilar cells are steroidogenic; therefore, they contribute to androgen production and continue to provide significant amounts of androstenedione and testosterone for several years.[9] These hormones influence muscle strength and sexual desire.[7]

Following menopause, the ovaries decrease in size and are typically not palpable on bimanual examination. Thus, if an ovary is palpated in a postmenopausal person, an ovarian neoplasm must be ruled out.[2] During the postmenopausal period, the cervix gradually decreases in size and produces less mucus, which can contribute to vaginal dryness and dyspareunia. Progressive atrophy of the cervical epithelium creates an increasingly sparse capillary bed and makes the surface of the cervix appear smooth, shiny, and pale.[2]

After ovarian follicular activity ceases, hormonal stimulation of the endometrium and myometrium also dissipates. Endometrial tissue, regardless of its location, becomes atrophic and inactive after menopause. Thus, not only does the uterine lining become atrophic, but small to moderate-size fibroids, which are highly sensitive to estrogen stimulation, usually shrink after menopause, as do the cyst-like invasions of the myometrium characteristic of adenomyosis.[10]

### Hormonal Changes

The three main human estrogens are estrone ($E_1$), estradiol ($E_2$), and estriol ($E_3$). After menopause, estrone accounts for the majority of circulating estrogen; it is derived principally from the metabolism of estradiol and from the conversion of androstenedione in adipose tissue. In contrast, estradiol—the most potent of the three estrogens—accounts for 95% of the circulatory estrogen in the premenopausal phase of life. The dominant follicle and the corpus luteum both excrete large amounts of estradiol during the reproductive phase of life.[2] Estriol, a weak estrogen, is secreted from the placenta but can also be metabolized in small amounts from estrone.[7] Postmenopausal serum estradiol levels are lower than 37 pg/mL (picograms/milliliter) and mean estrone levels are between 6 and 63 pg/mL. By comparison, premenopausal estradiol levels range from 10 to 100 pg/mL in the early follicular phase, 200 to 800 pg/mL at midcycle, and 200 to 340 pg/mL during the luteal phase, with estrone levels ranging from 30 to 180 pg/mL.

Although 95% of postmenopausal androstenedione production occurs in the adrenal gland and 5% occurs in the ovaries, the ovarian stroma continues to produce androstenedione and testosterone under the influence of LH. These hormones, along with the androstenedione produced by the adrenal glands, are converted to estrone in peripheral adipose tissue. Thus, increased conversion to estrone is associated with a higher body mass index (BMI) or increasing weight postmenopausally.[2] Some estradiol continues to be produced, albeit to a significantly less extent than occurs during the reproductive phase of life.[2]

## Diagnosing Menopause

As noted earlier, no single laboratory test can predict or confirm menopause. Instead, the diagnosis of menopause is based on menstrual and medical history and on reported symptoms.[2] Thus, a diagnosis of menopause is generally assured if a patient has been amenorrheic for 12 months and if there is no reason to suspect an underlying alternative cause of the symptoms. Hormone testing to predict menopause or help manage symptoms is not usually of clinical value. Even on the rare occasion when hormonal testing is indicated, challenges arise in interpreting the results. As with any test, hormone testing should be ordered only if the results can affect the treatment options offered. Table 14-2 lists potential indications for obtaining hormone levels and associated problems.

## Stages of Reproductive Aging

On their own, chronologic age, symptoms, and hormonal levels are not accurate predictors of menopause, a reality that can make diagnosis of

| Table 14-2 | Hormone Testing During Perimenopause and Menopause | |
|---|---|---|
| **Hormone** | **Possible Indications** | **Problems Associated with Test** |
| Estrogen levels | To assess absorption of estrogen in patients taking hormone therapy who experience persistent vasomotor symptoms | Estradiol and estrone levels are erratic; isolated levels are unlikely to give meaningful information |
| Progesterone | To document ovulation in perimenopausal patients who are trying to conceive | Levels are likely to be low in anovulatory cycles; isolated levels are unlikely to give meaningful information |
| Follicle-stimulating hormone (FSH) | Multiple FSH levels demonstrating sustained elevation > 30 mIU/mL, or months of amenorrhea and FSH > 40 mIU/mL, can provide a reasonably sound diagnosis of menopause | Highly variable during perimenopause; even elevated FSH levels (> 30 mIU/mL) can return to the premenopausal range days, weeks, or months later |
| Luteinizing hormone (LH) | In a patient taking hormonal contraceptives, a serum FSH:LH ratio greater than 1 on the seventh pill-free day can provide a reasonably sound diagnosis of menopause | LH elevation occurs late in perimenopause—much later than FSH elevation; minimal or no utility in confirming perimenopause or menopause |
| Prolactin | To rule out a pituitary cause for oligomenorrhea or amenorrhea, particularly in the presence of galactorrhea | |
| Thyroid-stimulating hormone (TSH) | To rule out thyroid dysfunction as a cause for symptoms otherwise attributed to perimenopause and menopause (e.g., abnormal uterine bleeding, hot flashes, sleep difficulties, fatigue, weight gain) | |
| Testosterone | To rule out a state of testosterone excess from testosterone treatment or endogenous excess | Levels change little from 4 years before to 2 years after menopause; little value in diagnosing testosterone insufficiency because testosterone levels are only one part of total androgen status |

Abbreviations: FSH, follicle stimulating hormone; LH, luteinizing hormone.

Based on North American Menopause Society. *Menopause Practice: A Clinician's Guide*. 6th ed. Mayfield Heights, OH: North American Menopause Society; 2021; Taylor HS, Pal LSE. *Speroff 's Clinical Endocrinological Gynecology and Infertility*. Philadelphia, PA: Walter Kluwer; 2020.

menopause challenging for patients and clinicians alike. Named after the workshop in 2001 where it was developed, the *Stages of Reproductive Aging Workshop* (STRAW) model uses menstrual cycle changes and FSH levels to describe reproductive aging through menopause.[11] This system, which became the gold standard, was updated to include anti-Müllerian hormone (AMH), inhibin B, and estradiol levels in 2012, when it was renamed the STRAW + 10 system.[11] The stages progress from the reproductive years toward the final menstrual period and beyond, and can be used regardless of demographics, age, BMI, or sociocultural factors. Use of this staging system can aid clinicians and patients in understanding the expected physiologic changes that occur during the menopausal transition. STRAW + 10 staging is not as useful in patients with primary ovarian insufficiency, and menstrual-cycle criteria cannot be used if patients do not have regular menstrual cycles or if they have undergone surgical removal of their uterus or endometrial ablation. **Figure 14-1** provides a graphic representation of the STRAW + 10 stages.

### Late Reproductive Stage (Stage –3b)

During the late reproductive stage, there are frequently changes in the amount of menstrual flow (may be more variable, lighter, or heavier) and in cycle length (often shorter). FSH levels typically increase, but can vary from one cycle to the next. Importantly, even irregular or long cycles can still be ovulatory. Ovulation occurs in as many as 25% of late reproductive stage cycles[7]; thus, conception is possible during this phase.[11]

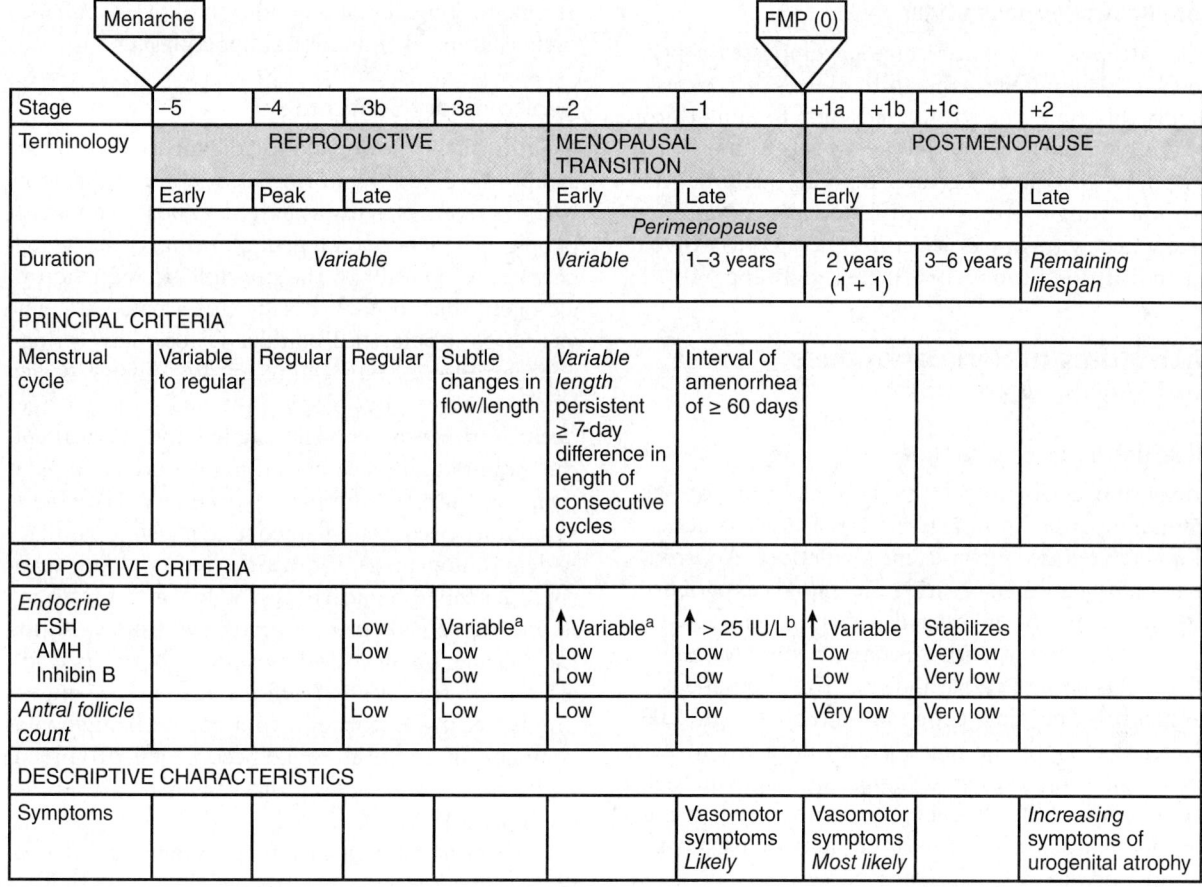

| Stage | −5 | −4 | −3b | −3a | −2 | −1 | +1a | +1b | +1c | +2 |
|---|---|---|---|---|---|---|---|---|---|---|
| Terminology | REPRODUCTIVE | | | | MENOPAUSAL TRANSITION | | POSTMENOPAUSE | | | |
| | Early | Peak | Late | | Early | Late | Early | | | Late |
| | | | | | *Perimenopause* | | | | | |
| Duration | *Variable* | | | | *Variable* | 1–3 years | 2 years (1 + 1) | | 3–6 years | *Remaining lifespan* |
| **PRINCIPAL CRITERIA** | | | | | | | | | | |
| Menstrual cycle | Variable to regular | Regular | Regular | Subtle changes in flow/length | *Variable length* persistent ≥ 7-day difference in length of consecutive cycles | Interval of amenorrhea of ≥ 60 days | | | | |
| **SUPPORTIVE CRITERIA** | | | | | | | | | | |
| *Endocrine* FSH AMH Inhibin B | | | Low Low Low | Variable[a] Low Low | ↑ Variable[a] Low Low | ↑ > 25 IU/L[b] Low Low | ↑ Variable Low Low | Stabilizes Very low Very low | | |
| *Antral follicle count* | | | Low | Low | Low | Low | Very low | Very low | | |
| **DESCRIPTIVE CHARACTERISTICS** | | | | | | | | | | |
| Symptoms | | | | | | Vasomotor symptoms *Likely* | Vasomotor symptoms *Most likely* | | *Increasing symptoms of urogenital atrophy* | |

**Figure 14-1** The Stages of Reproductive Aging Workshop + 10 staging system.
Abbreviations: ↑, elevated; AMH, anti-Müllerian hormone; FMP, final menstrual period; FSH, follicle-stimulating hormone.
[a] Blood draw on cycle days 2–5.
[b] Approximate expected level based on assays using current international pituitary standard.
Reproduced with permission from Harlow SD, Gass M, Hall JE, et al. Executive summary of the Stages of Reproductive Aging Workshop + 10: addressing the unfinished agenda of staging reproductive aging. *Fertil Steril*. 2012;97:843-851. Used with permission of Elsevier, Ltd.

## Early Menopausal Transition (Stage −2)

As the final menstrual period approaches, cycle-length variability increases, often with a difference of 7 days or more in cycle length. FSH levels remain elevated and highly variable. Estradiol levels remain in the normal range or slightly elevated until approximately 1 year before the cessation of follicular development. This finding is contrary to earlier research indicating that estradiol levels gradually waned in the years before menopause.[11]

## Late Menopausal Transition (Stage −1)

During the late menopausal transition stage, cycle length remains variable, with episodes of amenorrhea lasting 60 days or longer, wide deviations in cycle length, and marked fluctuations in FSH levels. In addition, cycles become increasingly anovulatory. In this stage, which usually lasts 1 to 3 years, vasomotor symptoms are often experienced. The conclusion of the late menopausal transition phase is the final menstrual period (FMP).[11]

## Early Postmenopause (Stages +1a, +1b, and +1c)

FSH level continues to increase with estradiol levels decreasing until approximately 2 years after the FMP. Early postmenopause is subdivided into three stages: *Stage +1a* usually lasts 1 year, and its end marks the 12-month period required to make the retrospective diagnosis of spontaneous menopause. *Stage +1b* lasts approximately 1 year and is characterized by rapid changes in FSH and estradiol levels. Symptoms such as hot flashes are most likely to occur in this stage. *Stage +1c* lasts approximately 3 to 6 years, during which time hormonal levels stabilize with high FSH and low estradiol levels.[11]

### Late Postmenopause (Stage +2)

The late postmenopause stage encompasses a person's remaining lifespan; with today's life expectancy, this time period may account for one-third of the total lifespan. Hormone levels remain stable, with FSH consistently greater than 20 mIU/mL and estradiol ranging from 10 to 25 pg/mL. Symptoms associated with low estrogen levels, such as vulvovaginal atrophy, can become increasingly apparent.[11]

## Symptoms of Perimenopause and Menopause

### Bleeding Pattern Changes

Menstrual cycle irregularity is a hallmark of the perimenopause, resulting from hormonal fluctuations related to inconsistent ovulation. Approximately 90% of menstruating individuals experience 4 to 8 years of menstrual changes before their FMP.[2,12] Exactly what those changes entail for an individual is unpredictable and can differ from menses to menses. The most common pattern is a gradual decrease in both the amount and duration of the menstrual flow, leading to vaginal spotting and then to cessation of bleeding. However, more frequent or heavier periods occur for some individuals during perimenopause, which can be troublesome. This type of abnormal uterine bleeding (AUB) is discussed in detail in the *Menstrual Cycle Abnormalities* chapter. Table 14-3 compares normal and potentially abnormal bleeding patterns during the perimenopause phase. Any bleeding that occurs after menopause (i.e., after 12 months of amenorrhea) requires investigation for a pathologic cause. Bleeding after menopause may be an indication of endometrial or uterine malignancy or a condition of premalignancy such as atypical endometrial hyperplasia.[2,7]

### Genitourinary Syndrome

Genitourinary syndrome is diagnosed when the symptoms described in this section are bothersome to the person. As many as half of all postmenopausal people experience some genital, urinary, and sexual changes as a result of the physiologic reduction of estrogen that occurs during menopause.[2,13] The vagina, vestibule, and bladder trigone have a high concentration of estrogen receptors. When estrogen levels change, physiologic and anatomic changes occur in these tissues. The vaginal and cervical epithelium gradually becomes thinner, dryer, and paler compared with the premenopausal body. The tissue sometimes becomes inflamed, and a visible capillary bed may appear as a diffusely red appearance or small petechial hemorrhages. Vulvovaginal atrophy is one element of genitourinary syndrome. During the perimenopausal and postmenopausal periods, the vagina transitions from an acidic environment dominated by lactobacilli to a more alkaline environment. In addition, rugae become less prominent and sometimes disappear and vaginal secretions decrease (Table 14-4).

All perimenopausal and postmenopausal people should be verbally screened for symptoms of genitourinary changes. It is common to underreport discomfort with these symptoms and simply assume that having them is a normal part of aging. Unlike vasomotor symptoms, genitourinary symptoms are unlikely to improve with time. Therefore, screening and anticipatory guidance should be standard components of care for all people experiencing perimenopause and menopause.

| Table 14-3 | Physiologic Versus Potentially Abnormal Bleeding Patterns During Perimenopause |
|---|---|
| **Common Perimenopausal Menstrual Changes** | **Potentially Abnormal Perimenopausal Bleeding Patterns** |
| Shorter intervals between periods (but at least 21 days) | Very heavy bleeding, especially with clots |
| Longer intervals between periods | Long bleeding duration (> 7 days or ≥ 2 days longer than usual) |
| Lighter bleeding | |
| Heavier bleeding than normal (difficult to quantify; consider evaluation if significant change) | Very short cycles (< 21 days from beginning of one period to beginning of next period) |
| Shorter duration of bleeding | Irregular bleeding: spotting or bleeding between periods |
| Longer duration of bleeding (up to 1–2 days longer than usual) | Bleeding after vaginal penetration |
| Skipped periods | Any bleeding that occurs following menopause (12 months of amenorrhea) is abnormal |
| No changes | |

Based on North American Menopause Society. *Menopause Practice: A Clinician's Guide.* 5th ed. Mayfield Heights, OH: North American Menopause Society; 2017.

| Table 14-4 | Signs and Symptoms Associated with Genitourinary Syndrome of Menopause | |
|---|---|---|
| | **Genitalia** | **Bladder and Urethra** |
| Physiologic changes | Labia: atrophy and labia minora absorbed, loss of hymeneal remnants, introitus retracts | Prominence of urethral meatus |
| | Vagina: reduced secretions, decreased elasticity in vagina, loss of rugae, pallor, petechiae or erythema, friability | Reduced blood flow to vestibule and bladder trigone |
| Signs and symptoms | Vaginal pain | Dysuria |
| | Alkaline pH | Urinary frequency or urgency |
| | Genital dryness | Nocturia |
| | Bleeding during or after penetration | Postvoid dribbling |
| | Vulvar or vaginal burning or itching | Recurrent urinary tract infections |
| | Vaginal or introital stenosis | Urinary incontinence |
| | Pale and/or thin vaginal mucosa | Pelvic organ prolapse |

Data from Gandhi J, Chen A, Dagur G, et al. Genitourinary syndrome of menopause: an overview of clinical manifestations, pathophysiology, etiology, evaluation, and management. *Am J Obstet Gynecol*. 2016;215(6):704-711.

Sexual arousal and touching improve blood supply to the pelvis and the vaginal tissues. Consequently, experiencing sexual arousal and stimulation of the genital area may decrease the amount of atrophy experienced.[2] The *Sexuality* chapter discusses approaches to assessment and treatment of sexual dysfunction. People troubled by genitourinary syndrome symptoms may also report dryness or itching of the vulva and vagina and pain upon insertion of a penis, fingers, or sex toy into the vagina. In such cases, the midwife may observe micro-abrasions and few or absent vaginal rugae. Urinary changes can include prominence of the urethral meatus, urinary frequency, dysuria, nocturia, and incontinence. Urinary incontinence is discussed in the *Malignant and Chronic Gynecologic Disorders* chapter.

## Vasomotor Symptoms

Vasomotor symptoms are common during the perimenopausal period. For a subset of people experiencing these symptoms, they are disruptive to activities of daily living. Estimates of the percentage of participants in studies reporting hot flashes in the literature vary significantly, as it is difficult to control for confounding factors and symptom severity. Regardless of the precise rate of occurrence, hot flashes, like changes in the pattern of bleeding, are so common that they are considered a hallmark of perimenopause and menopause. Diet, climate, sociocultural factors, and attitudes about aging all influence the experience of vasomotor symptoms. People who undergo induced menopause (bilateral oophorectomy with or without hysterectomy) have a more abrupt change in hormones and, in turn,

report more abrupt and bothersome symptom onset and duration if not treated with hormone therapy.[2] In addition, the criteria for and duration of hormone therapy differ significantly for people undergoing induced menopause prior to age 51.[14]

The physiology of vasomotor symptoms likely includes hormonal changes (including changes in estrogen, LH, and cortisol levels), changes in thermoregulation, and changes in regulation of the hypothalamic–pituitary–adrenal axis.[2,15] The terms *vasomotor symptoms*, *hot flashes*, *hot flushes*, and *night sweats* all refer to the manifestations of similar experiences. This phenomenon is characterized by recurrent, transient periods of flushing, sweating, and a sensation of heat, often accompanied by palpitations and a feeling of anxiety, and sometimes followed by chills. These flashes can occur during sleep, causing disruption.

A single hot flash usually lasts 1 to 5 minutes, during which time the person experiences a sudden wave of heat that soon spreads over the body, particularly over the face and upper torso. Elevations in skin temperature, heart rate, blood flow to the skin, and metabolic rate follow quickly. As the hot flash ends, skin temperature begins to gradually return to normal and the person sometimes feels chilled, often due to heat loss from sweating and continued peripheral vasodilation.

Although the precise chance of experiencing vasomotor symptoms cannot be predicted, some associated factors have been identified. Numerous studies have linked current cigarette smoking with increased risk of hot flashes.[16] In contrast, the literature contains conflicting evidence on the role of body weight in predicting vasomotor symptom frequency and severity. In one study, higher weight relative to height was associated with more vasomotor symptoms perimenopausally, yet had a protective effect postmenopausally.[16] There is no consistent evidence regarding the amount or distribution of weight in relation to vasomotor symptoms.

The highest prevalence of vasomotor symptoms occurs within the first 1 to 2 years of menopause. The percentage of menopausal people reporting hot flashes declines after 2 years, then declines again at 5 and 10 years post menopause. However, some people report having hot flashes for decades after menopause.[14] Some individuals experience relatively few hot flashes, whereas others have very frequent hot flashes. Moreover, some people describe these symptoms as easily managed, whereas others report that hot flashes are disrupting their lives. Hot flashes that occur during sleep (often called night sweats) can cause sleep disruption and, in turn, a whole host of issues associated with interrupted sleep.

## Mood Symptoms

Experts disagree about whether changes in hormone levels during the perimenopausal and postmenopausal periods actually *cause* mood symptoms. Individuals with a history of depression or premenstrual syndrome seem to be more vulnerable to depression around the time of menopause.[17] However, interactions between hormones and mood are complex, as are the interactions among the symptom clusters—including pain, vasomotor symptoms, and sleep disruption—experienced during perimenopause/menopause.[18] It is difficult to determine whether the mood changes are due to hormonal fluctuations or are the result of the vasomotor symptoms causing lack of sleep. Moreover, coexisting stressors during this time may be caused or exacerbated by family changes, including children leaving home, caring for both children and elderly family members, and health changes in a spouse or partner.[2]

## Weight Changes

Midlife is often associated with weight gain, with the average weight gain during perimenopause and menopause being approximately 5 pounds. However, evidence does not support a causal relationship: Neither menopause nor hormone therapy appears to *cause* weight gain.[2] Instead, aging and changes in lifestyle are more likely to cause an increase in weight.[19] Lean muscle mass decreases with age, lowering the metabolic rate; combined with a more sedentary lifestyle, this factor can result in

weight gain if caloric intake is not reduced.[20] Regular exercise, which may include walking and biking, is important to overall health and can assist in controlling weight gain. Strength training can reduce loss of muscle mass, increase strength and metabolic rate, and even reduce the risk of falls.[21]

The health consequences of living in a society with strong biases against people with larger bodies cannot be ignored. Studies have consistently shown that many healthcare providers have implicit or even explicit weight bias, which leads to suboptimal care and feelings of shame and embarrassment for clients with higher weights.[22] In addition, the experiences that people with larger bodies have with providers can lead to reluctance to seek health care.[22]

Small changes in weight and small increases in activity can significantly improve overall health versus achieving an ideal BMI, which can be very difficult for patients to achieve and maintain.[23] In fact, more than 80% of weight lost through diet is regained within 5 years.[24] For these reasons, it is extremely important for midwives explore their own biases and approach the issue of weight with patients in a way that is thoughtful, evidence based, and focused on meaningful and achievable goals.

## Hair and Skin Changes

Sun damage, redistributed or decreased subcutaneous fat, skin laxity from weight changes, and decreased underlying muscle tissue cause most of the skin changes that people may notice during the midlife years. Other potential midlife skin changes include dryness, acne, hair loss, brittle and slow-growing nails, and decreased wound healing, all of which may contribute to psychological distress or altered body image.[2] A comprehensive assessment of the skin is very important, as skin cancer and other disorders become increasingly common as people age. Endocrine and autoimmune disorders such as hypothyroidism can also contribute to skin complaints. Therapies include limiting the time and temperature when bathing, avoiding harsh soaps and chemicals, and use of moisturizing lotions to reduce dryness.

# Therapeutic Approaches for Menopause and Perimenopause Symptoms

## Nonpharmacologic Therapies for Genitourinary Symptoms

Sexual activity including entering the vagina with a penis, fingers, or sex toy, as well as arousal through partnered or self-pleasuring, can help to maintain

| Table 14-5 | Nonpharmacologic Therapies for Genitourinary Symptoms | |
|---|---|---|
| **Intervention** | **Mechanism of Action** | **Comments** |
| Sexual arousal and orgasm | Blood flow to the genitals and natural secretions | People may need instruction regarding nonpenetrative intimacy alone or with a partner. It may also be helpful to provide person-centered resources for self-pleasuring and procurement of lubricants, moisturizers, and sex toys. |
| Objects in the vagina | Maintenance of vaginal size and tone | This can include fingers, a penis, sex toys, and other objects. |
| Vaginal lubricant | Reduce friction | Short-acting; should be applied to the vagina or to object of insertion just prior to insertion |
| Vaginal moisturizer | Adhere to the vaginal mucosa | Apply every 1–3 days |
| Pelvic floor therapy | Individualized exercises and treatments including biofeedback and weights | Often appropriate as an adjunct therapy along with localized hormones<br><br>May include the use of vaginal dilators |

Data from: North American Menopause Society. *Menopause Practice: A Clinician's Guide*. 6th ed. Pepper Pike, OH: North American Menopause Society, 2021; Gandhi J, Chen A, Dagur G, et al. Genitourinary syndrome of menopause: an overview of clinical manifestations, pathophysiology, etiology, evaluation, and management. *Am J Obstet Gynecol.* 2016;215(6):704-711.

vaginal health.[2] Vaginal lubricants can be used specifically during sexual activity, whereas vaginal moisturizers are longer-lasting products that can maintain moisture over time and beneficially lower the vaginal pH.[2] Water-based lubricants can be used to increase comfort when something is placed in the vagina. Oil-based products coat the vaginal lining, thereby preventing the release of natural secretions, and should be avoided. Oil-based products can also cause condom breakage. If possible, it is best to avoid over-the-counter products that have drying effects, as well as douches, sprays, and colored or perfumed toilet paper and soaps. See the *Sexuality* chapter for more information on lubricants. Pelvic floor physical therapy can be effective for treating pelvic pain and dysfunction including incontinence and is often an appropriate adjunct to localized hormone therapy.[2] Nonpharmacologic therapies for genitourinary symptoms are summarized in Table 14-5.

## Nonpharmacologic Therapies for Vasomotor Symptoms

Many perimenopausal and menopausal people try nonpharmacologic therapies, yet most of them will not initiate a discussion about this topic with their healthcare provider.[25] These therapies typically lack robust evidence regarding their efficacy. Therefore, providers can start with knowledge of safety when helping patients decide whether to try any of these measures. People who have mild vasomotor symptoms may find adequate relief from the nonpharmacologic approaches described in Table 14-6. However, it is important to note that insufficient evidence exists to support use of most of these measures as compared to placebo. Therefore, people should not be expected to first try and fail to experience relief with lifestyle measures prior to being offered appropriate pharmacologic treatment for their symptoms.

## Nonhormonal Pharmacologic Therapies for Vasomotor Symptoms

Although some evidence supports the effectiveness of some nonhormonal methods, none is as effective as systemic hormone therapy in treating hot flashes, and all of these medications have varying side-effect profiles. The anticonvulsant gabapentin has been found to be moderately effective for treatment of hot flashes, but its common side effect of somnolence may be problematic; thus, initial dosing should be at bedtime.[26] Selective serotonin reuptake inhibitors (SSRIs) and serotonin–norepinephrine reuptake inhibitors (SNRIs) have moderate effectiveness in providing relief from hot flashes and may be especially useful for people with coexisting mood disorders. At this time, paroxetine is the only SSRI with a Food and Drug Administration (FDA) indication for treatment of vasomotor symptoms. Note that SSRIs and SNRIs can both contribute to weight gain and decrease libido, which may counter their desirability in menopausal people.[2] Nonhormonal pharmacologic therapies for vasomotor symptoms are summarized in Table 14-7.

| Table 14-6 | Nonpharmacologic Therapies for Vasomotor Symptoms |
|---|---|
| **Intervention** | **Comments** |
| Identification and avoidance of hot flash triggers | A symptom diary to identify triggers, and thereby help the person avoid them, and to increase personal feelings of control may be of value. Triggers may include hot beverages, spicy food or beverages, and alcohol. |
| Tobacco use | People who smoke tend to have more frequent and more severe vasomotor symptoms than people who do not smoke. |
| Weight | One study showed that higher body weight relative to height was a predictor of more bothersome vasomotor symptoms in perimenopause, but was associated with fewer vasomotor symptoms in postmenopause. |
| Exercise | A 2014 Cochrane review found no association between exercise or yoga and incidence or severity of vasomotor symptoms. |
| Diet | There is insufficient evidence to promote or reject soy foods as therapy for vasomotor symptoms. |
| Herbs and supplements | There is insufficient evidence to promote or reject herbs and supplements for menopause. In addition, there is a dearth of knowledge regarding formulation, route, and dosing. Once lack of potential for harm can be determined, there is evidence for a positive placebo effect with the use of some herbs. |
| Homeopathy | There is no evidence of efficacy greater than that of the placebo effect. Generally recognized as safe. |
| Aromatherapy | Several studies have examined lavender essential oil as a therapy for vasomotor symptoms, with some studies showing positive effects on symptoms. There are no guidelines for formulation, amount, or technique for use. General safety guidelines for use of essential oils should be followed. |
| Ambient temperature and dressing | Anecdotal reports of cooler room temperatures, cooling bedding and pillows, and dressing in layers of breathable clothing such as cotton suggest these interventions may help some people cope with hot flashes. |
| Acupuncture | No statistically significant findings; likely has a higher cost than other lifestyle interventions. |
| Cognitive-behavioral therapy (CBT)/management of concurrent depression and/or anxiety | There is some evidence for efficacy of CBT as a treatment for vasomotor symptoms. Efficacy was demonstrated with both individual and group therapy. |
| Relaxation techniques such as meditation, deep breathing, guided imagery, stretching, massage, mindfulness, and prayer | There is insufficient evidence to recommend or refute any of these practices during menopause, as methodologic challenges limit the ability to evaluate the effectiveness of these strategies, but there is little likelihood of harm and most of these techniques have little cost. |

Data from Anderson DJ, Chung HF, Seib CA, et al. Obesity, smoking, and risk of vasomotor menopausal symptoms: a pooled analysis of eight cohort studies. *Am J Obstet Gynecol*. 2020;222(5):478.e1-478.e17. doi:10.1016/j.ajog.2019.10.103; Daley A, Stokes-Lampard H, Thomas A, et al. Exercise for vasomotor menopausal symptoms. *Cochrane Database Syst Rev*. 2014;11:1-43. doi:10.1002/14651858. CD006108.pub4; Gracia CR, Freeman EW. Onset of the menopause transition: the earliest signs and symptoms. *Obstet Gynecol Clin North Am*. 2018;45(4):585-597. doi:10.1016/J.OGC.2018.07.002; Johnson A, Roberts L, Elkins G, et al. Complementary and alternative medicine for menopause. *J Evidence-Based Integr Med*. 2019;24. doi:10.1177/2515690X19829380; Liu Z, Ai Y, Wang W, et al. Acupuncture for symptoms in menopause transition: a randomized controlled trial. *Am J Obstet Gynecol*. 2018;219(4):373.e1-373. e10. doi:10.1016/j.ajog.2018.08.019; Liu ZM, Ho SC, Woo J, et al. Randomized controlled trial of whole soy and isoflavone daidzein on menopausal symptoms in equol-producing Chinese postmenopausal women. *Menopause*. 2014;21(6):653-660; Minkin MJ. Menopause: hormones, lifestyle, and optomizing aging. *Obstet Gynecol Clin North Am*. 2019;46(2019):501-514; Moore TR, Franks RB, Fox C. Review of efficacy of complementary and alternative medicine treatments for menopausal symptoms. *J Midwifery Womens Health*. 2017;62(3):286-297. doi:10.1111/jmwh.12628; North American Menopause Society, ed. *Menopause Practice: A Clinician's Guide*. 6th ed. Pepper Pike, OH: North American Menopause Society; 2021; Salehi-Pourmehr H, Ostadrahimi A, Ebrahimpour-Mirzarezaei M, et al. Does aromatherapy with lavender affect physical and psychological symptoms of menopausal women? A systematic review and meta-analysis. *Complement Therap Clin Pract*. 2020;39:101150. doi:10.1016/j.ctcp.2020.101150.

| Table 14-7 | Nonhormonal Pharmacologic Therapies for Vasomotor Symptoms |
|---|---|
| **Intervention** | **Comments** |
| Selective serotonin reuptake inhibitors | Paroxetine 7.5 mg is FDA approved for treatment of hot flashes |
| | Consider weight and libido side effects when prescribing SSRIs to people in menopause |
| Selective norepinephrine reuptake inhibitors | Venlafaxine 37.5–150 mg (off label) |
| Gabapentin | 300–900 mg dosing in clinical trials |
| | Reduction of vasomotor symptoms in several studies; not FDA approved for this indication |
| | Consider bedtime dosing due to potential for sedating effects |
| | Less effective than estrogen, more effective than placebo, equally effective as SSRIs and SNRIs |

Abbreviations: FDA, Food and Drug Administration; SNRIs, serotonin–norepinephrine reuptake inhibitors; SSRIs, selective serotonin reuptake inhibitors.

Data from North American Menopause Society, ed. *Menopause Practice: A Clinician's Guide.* 6th ed. Pepper Pike, OH: North American Menopause Society; 2021; Shan D, Zou L, Liu X, et al. Efficacy and safety of gabapentin and pregabalin in patients with vasomotor symptoms: a systematic review and meta-analysis. *Am J Obstet Gynecol.* 2020;222(6):564-579. doi:10.1016/j.ajog.2019.12.011.

## Hormone Therapy

Hormone therapy (HT) either with estrogen (ET) or estrogen and progestin in combination (EPT) remains the most effective evidence-based treatment for vasomotor symptoms and vulvovaginal atrophy related to menopause. It significantly reduces the severity of vasomotor symptoms and, on average, reduces their frequency by 75%. HT for menopausal symptoms was first introduced in 1941 as Premarin, a pill derived from pregnant mares' urine containing estrogen only.[2] Following the discovery that unopposed estrogen significantly increased the risk of endometrial cancer, estrogen doses were decreased and formulations with added progestins were developed for use in patients who had a uterus.[27] In 1986, the FDA added osteoporosis prevention to the indications for HT.[2,28] Subsequent observational studies suggested HT was also useful in prevention of conditions such as cardiovascular disease, stroke, dementia, and urinary incontinence.[2,12]

Then, in 2002, reports emerged from the Women's Health Initiative (WHI) study that initiated a rapid change in the recommendations for the use of HT during perimenopause and menopause.[29] In this large longitudinal study, participants aged 50 to 79 years were randomized to HT (estrogen or estrogen plus progestin for participants with a uterus) or placebo. Although the full longitudinal study was intended to continue for 9 years, it was discontinued early because the interim analysis found an *increased*—rather than decreased—risk of coronary heart disease among women in the EPT cohort. In addition, participants had small but statistically significant increased risks of breast cancer (in the EPT group), stroke, and pulmonary embolism. The WHI study did show decreased risks of colorectal cancer and bone fracture with use of HT.[29] Its findings were disseminated widely, including in consumer publications. Although the absolute number of adverse events was low, both consumers and healthcare providers were concerned enough that prescriptions for menopausal HT rapidly declined.

Results of the WHI study must be interpreted in context. The average age of participants was more than a decade older than the average age at which menopause occurs. Subsequent studies have found a trend toward lower rates of cardiovascular mortality in participants ages 50 to 59 years who start HT within the first 10 years of experiencing menopause. In patients with early menopause (younger than age 40) early initiation of HT may reduce the risk of atherosclerosis, cardiovascular disease, and dementia. Another limitation of the WHI study is that a single specific progesterone (medroxyprogesterone acetate [Provera]) and a single specific estrogen (conjugated equine estrogen) were used. Subsequent studies with different estrogens and progestins have yielded slightly different statistical findings, although the majority of reports are congruent with the original WHI reports.[2,30]

A meta-analysis of the long-term effects (more than 1 year) of HT, published in the Cochrane Library in 2017, included 22 randomized, double-blinded studies involving 43,627 primarily postmenopausal participants.[31] The average age of the participants was 60. The researchers identified an increased risk of some health events, including coronary events, venous thromboembolism, and stroke, with long-term HT use. The risks for breast cancer and death from lung cancer were slightly increased with estrogen and progesterone combination therapy, but not with estrogen alone. Dementia risk increased with combination therapy but only in participants age 65 and older. Clinical fracture risk decreased with all HT use. The results of this Cochrane review meta-analysis are summarized in Table 14-8.

Contraindications for HT include undiagnosed abnormal vaginal bleeding; known, suspected, or history of breast cancer; known or suspected estrogen-dependent cancer; current or history of deep vein thrombosis or pulmonary embolism; current or recent (within the last year) stroke or myocardial infarction; liver disease; known or suspected pregnancy; and known hypersensitivity to HT. Smoking is not a contraindication to HT, although it is a contraindication for combined hormonal contraceptive use after age 35 years.[2]

Side effects can occur with HT—although similar to hormonal contraceptives, these will often subside on their own within the first 1 to 2 months of use or with adjusting or reducing the estrogen and progestin doses. The most common side effect of EPT is uterine bleeding, although the risk is lower with lower-dose formulations and most often the bleeding stops over time.[2,12] Weight gain often occurs at this time of life, but HT does not increase the risk of weight gain.[32] Clinicians should be aware that systemic HT has been associated with worsening

of preexisting stress and urge urinary incontinence, and with increased incidence of new urinary incontinence.[33] In contrast, local vaginal estrogen topical therapy may improve continence.[34]

In summary, the current research suggests that the use of HT is appropriate for troublesome vasomotor or vulvovaginal symptoms in patients without contraindications, but HT should not be prescribed specifically for chronic disease prevention.[2,33] This therapy is considered a safe option for healthy individuals who are within 10 years of menopause, are younger than 60 years, and lack any contraindications. The risk of an adverse event from HT is very low (less than 1 event/1000 person-years) and even lower when initiated within 10 years of menopause.

The decision of whether to use HT requires thoughtful conversation and shared decision making. It must consider age at menopause, whether menopause was physiologic or induced, which symptoms the patient is experiencing, and the effects of those symptoms on the person's quality of life. Counseling about HT includes a discussion about the risks, benefits, side effects, contraindications, and alternatives tailored for the individual.[35] Table 14-9 is a decision-making guide that may be useful when providing care for patients.

| Table 14-8 | Effect of Hormone Therapy on Health Outcomes Reported in a Cochrane Review | |
|---|---|---|
| **Condition** | **Estrogen Therapy** | **Estrogen and Progestin Therapy** |
| Coronary event | No statistically significant difference | Increased from 2/1000 to 3–7/1000 over 1 year |
| Stroke | Increased from 24/1000 to 25–40/1000 over 7 years | Increased from 6/1000 to 6–12/1000 over 3 years |
| Venous thromboembolism | Increased from 1/1000 to 2–10/1000 over 1–2 years and from 16/1000 to 16–28/1000 over 7 years | Increased from 2/1000 to 4–11/1000 over 1 year |
| Death from lung cancer | No statistically significant difference | Increased from 5/1000 to 9/1000 over 8 years |
| Breast cancer | Decreased from 25/1000 to 15/1000 over 7 years | Increased from 19/1000 to 20–30/1000 over 5.6 years |
| Gallbladder disease | Increased from 27/1000 to 38–60/1000 over 7 years | Increased from 27/1000 to 38–60/1000 over 5.6 years |
| Clinical fracture | Decreased from 141/1000 to 92–113/1000 over 7 years | Decreased from 111/1000 to 79–96/1000 over 4 years |
| Probable dementia | No statistically significant difference | In participants older than age 65, increased from 9/1000 to 11–30/1000 over 4 years |

Data from Marjoribanks J, Farquhar C, Roberts H, et al. Long-term hormone therapy for perimenopausal and postmenopausal women (review). *Cochrane Database Syst Rev.* 2017;1(1):CD004143. doi:10.1002/14651858.CD004143.pub5.

| Table 14-9 | Decision-Making Guide for Hormone Therapy for Vasomotor Symptoms |
|---|---|

- Is the patient having bothersome vasomotor symptoms attributed to perimenopause/menopause?
  - No: Nothing further is needed, focus on anticipatory guidance and when to follow up.
  - Yes: Continue with queries.
- Is the patient interested in HT?
  - No: Discuss nonhormonal therapies for symptoms.
  - Yes: Continue with queries.
- Does the patient need contraception?
  - No: No need to consider unintended pregnancy.
  - Yes: Discuss low-dose contraceptives or other methods along with HT.
- Does the patient have any contraindications? [undiagnosed abnormal vaginal bleeding; known, suspected, or history of breast cancer; known or suspected estrogen-dependent cancer; current or history of deep vein thrombosis or pulmonary embolism; current or recent (within the last year) stroke or myocardial infarction; liver disease; known or suspected pregnancy; and known hypersensitivity to HT]
  - No: Continue with queries.
  - Yes: Discuss nonhormonal therapies.
- Does the patient have a uterus?
  - No: Combined therapy with progestins is not necessary.
  - Yes: Combined therapy with progestins is necessary.
- Does the patient choose to initiate HT?
  - Yes: Discuss routes of administration, risks and benefits, and potential side effects.
  - No: Discuss nonhormonal/nonpharmacologic therapies for symptoms.

Abbreviation: HT, hormone therapy.

## Hormone Therapy Options

Once a decision is made to initiate HT, the next decision is which type of formulation to prescribe. There is a dizzying array of HT options: estrogen alone, progesterone alone, and combination therapies. In addition, different types of estrogen and progesterone are used in HT. Some patients will prefer a non-oral systemic formulation. Available formulations in this category include skin patches that are replaced once or twice weekly and gels or spray that may be used daily. Combination therapy with added progesterone is indicated to decrease the risk of endometrial cancer in patients with a uterus, but within that guideline many options are available and no one product or formulation is superior to any of the others. Evidence supports starting with the lowest dose of estrogen that effectively treats the patient's symptoms. There is no evidence for serum hormone level testing as part of dosing.[2]

### Estrogen Therapy Versus Estrogen and Progesterone Therapy

Estrogen therapy (ET) is available in oral, transdermal, topical, and vaginal formulations; EPT

is available in oral and transdermal formulations. For patients with a uterus, a progestin is needed to protect from the endometrium-building effects of estrogen and the predisposition to endometrial hyperplasia.[32] Compounded topical therapies may be insufficient and should not be used for endometrial protection.[2] Conversely, patients who have undergone a hysterectomy do not usually need a progestin. Most menopause experts agree that patients with a uterus who use estrogen in *nonsystemic* doses (i.e., local vaginal therapy) do not need a progestin.[7] An exception is the vaginal ring Femring: It contains a dose of estrogen at the level intended for systemic therapy, which may lead to endometrial hyperplasia.[2]

### Hormone Therapy Formulations

While numerous types of estrogen and progestin are available, rarely does the specific estrogen or progestin determine the choice of product. None of the specific agents seems to be more effective than the others in relieving symptoms or minimizing side effects.[2] Most of these products are proprietary fixed-drug compositions and are usually prescribed by brand name.

Some estrogens are chemically manipulated to be conjugated or esterified so that they become more water soluble; those drugs are then administered orally or vaginally.[31] Patches, gels, rings, spray, and some creams generally contain 17ß-estradiol. Synthetic estrogens are available in some products.

Progestins also vary, with some products containing either drospirenone, levonorgestrel, norethindrone acetate, or norgestimate.[2] These products are also available in a range of doses. Medroxyprogesterone acetate (Provera) is one of the few progestins used without estrogen, although such use is uncommon. For patients who experience problematic side effects of systemic progestin, alternative approaches can be used, such as use of a levonorgestrel-containing intrauterine device (IUD) or regular endometrial biopsies or monitoring by transvaginal ultrasound.

Additional considerations arise when prescribing the proprietary drug Premarin and its combinations, such as Premphase and Prempro. These products contain conjugated equine estrogens (CEEs)—a complex blend of a number of steroids, including estrogens that are derived from pregnant mares' urine.[2] Some individuals may be uncomfortable receiving hormones from horses, and for these individuals, use of other estrogens can be recommended.

A drug combination that was previously on the market but is currently unavailable, and that includes conjugated estrogens and bazedoxifene, is Duavee, an estrogen antagonist and agonist (EAA) originally marketed for prevention of osteoporosis. This formulation is indicated for treatment of mild to severe hot flashes and to prevent osteoporosis. The package insert states that individuals who require only protection from osteoporosis should seek another formulation without estrogen, perhaps to reduce estrogen-related risks.[8]

When considering the optimal route of administration, an important first consideration is whether *systemic* or *local* vaginal therapy is indicated. If relief from vasomotor symptoms (e.g., hot flashes) is needed, then systemic-level dosing is indicated, which can be obtained with oral and transdermal formulations or the estradiol acetate vaginal ring (Femring). For urogenital concerns such as vulvovaginal atrophy, topical therapy or one of the vaginal rings (e.g., 17β-estradiol vaginal ring [Estring]) is appropriate.[36] With the exception of the estradiol acetate vaginal ring, the topical products do not result in systemic levels of hormone.[36] The decision to choose oral administration versus another route can be guided by individual preference, ability to use the method, and other factors such as avoidance of the first-pass effect with transdermal products. A recent meta-analysis

indicates that HT is below the willingness-to-pay threshold,[37] so factors that affect the cost of specific products—such as insurance coverage—must be taken into account when prescribing HT.

A variety of dosing regimens are available for estrogen plus progestin therapy. One of the oldest EPT regimens is *cyclic EPT*, in which estrogen is given for the first 25 days of each month. Progestin is added to the estrogen for the last 10 to 14 days, and no hormones are taken for the final 3 to 6 days of the month. This regimen is seldom used now because users tend to experience withdrawal bleeding and hot flashes on the hormone-free days.[2,31]

With *continuous-cyclic (sequential) EPT*, estrogen is included every day, with a progestin added for 10 to 14 days each month. This regimen provides predictable withdrawal bleeding but no hot flash–inducing estrogen-free days. Premphase is one brand-name product that uses this formulation; it is sometimes prescribed for patients during perimenopause, a time when HT-induced endometrial growth is likely. Continuous-cyclic (sequential) EPT creates a predictable pattern of bleeding during this transitional period.[2,31] Keep in mind that continuous-cyclic (sequential) EPT does not provide contraceptive benefits.

*Continuous-combined EPT*, in which estrogen and progestin are included every day, is currently the most commonly used formulation of HT. Several formulations and doses are available within this category. Within a few months of using this dosing option, for patients who had bleeding with EPT, the endometrium becomes thin and most patients will become amenorrheic.[2,31]

*Intermittent-combined EPT* (also called *pulsed progestin* or *continuous-pulsed EPT*) is available as well. In this regimen, estrogen is administered every day, with progestin given intermittently for 3 days on, 3 days off, repeated without interruption. This regimen (Prefest is the only current formulation) reduces the incidence of bleeding found in cyclic therapies, with 80% of patients developing amenorrhea after 1 year.[2,31]

Most HT products are also available in a variety of doses. The effective dose for symptom relief varies from individual to individual, so a certain amount of trial and error is often needed to determine the appropriate dose. Clinicians should prescribe the lowest dose of HT that effectively manages symptoms, increasing the dose or changing formulations if symptoms are not improved within 2 to 3 months of initiation of therapy. The guiding principle should be to start with a low dose and titrate upward, eventually selecting the lowest dose that accomplishes the HT goal.[38] Table 14-10

| Table 14-10 | Estrogen-Only Therapies | |
|---|---|---|
| **Composition** | **Brand Names** | **Doses** |
| **Oral Preparations** | | |
| Conjugated equine estrogen | Premarin | 0.3, 0.45, 0.625, 0.9, 1.25 mg/day |
| Conjugated estrogen | Cenestin | 0.3, 0.45, 0.625, 0.9, 1.25 mg/day |
| | Enjuvia | |
| Esterified estrogen | Menest | 0.3, 0.625, 1.25, 2.5 mg/day |
| Estropipate | Ortho-Est | 0.625, 1.25, 2.5, 5.0 mg/day |
| | Ogen | 0.625, 1.25, 2.5 mg/day |
| | Various generics | 0.625, 1.5, 5.0 mg/day |
| Estradiol acetate | Femtrace | 0.45, 0.9, 1.8 mg/day |
| **Transdermal Preparations** | | |
| 17β-estradiol (17β-e) matrix patch | Climara | Delivers 0.025, 0.0375, 0.05, 0.075, 0.1 mg/day |
| | | Apply twice weekly |
| | Esclim, Vivelle, Vivelle-Dot, Minivelle, Climara | Delivers 0.025, 0.0375, 0.05, 0.075, 0.1 mg/day |
| | | Apply once weekly |
| | FemPatch | Delivers 0.025 mg/day |
| | | Apply once weekly |
| | Various generics | Delivers 0.05, 0.05 mg/day |
| | | Apply once or twice weekly |
| 17β-estradiol (17β-e) transdermal gel | Estrogel | 0.75 mg/day |
| | Elestrin | 0.52 mg/day |
| | Divigel | 0.003, 0.009, 0.027 mg/day |
| 17β-estradiol (17β-e) topical emulsion | Estrasorb | 0.05 mg/day |
| 17β-estradiol (17β-e) transdermal spray | Evamist | 1.53 mg/day |
| **Vaginal Preparations** | | |
| Conjugated equine estrogen (CEE) cream | Premarin vaginal cream | 0.5–2 g/day (0.625 mg CEE/g) |
| 17β-estradiol (17β-e) | Estrace vaginal cream | Initial: 2–4 g/day for 1–2 weeks |
| | | Maintenance: 1 g 1–3 times/week (0.1 mg 17β-e/g) |
| 17β-estradiol (17β-e) vaginal ring | Estring | Releases 7.5 mcg/day (90 days) |
| Estradiol acetate | Femring | Releases 0.05 or 0.10 mg/day (90 day ); systemic dosing |
| Estradiol vaginal insert | Imvexxy | 4, 10 mcg |
| | | 1 insert/day for 2 weeks, then 1 insert 2 times/week |
| Estradiol hemihydrate | Vagifem (Generic available) | 10 mcg |
| | | 1 insert/day for 2 weeks, then 1 insert 2 times/week |

Data from Ward K, Deneris A. An update on menopause management. *J Midwifery Women's Health*. 2018;63(2):168-177. doi:10.1111/jmwh.12737; North American Menopause Society, ed. *Menopause Practice: A Clinician's Guide*. 6th ed. Pepper Pike, OH: North American Menopause Society; 2021.

lists currently available estrogen-only formulations, **Table 14-11** lists EPT formulations, and **Table 14-12** lists progestin-only products.

## Androgen Therapy

While testosterone supplementation in menopausal patients may improve some aspects of sexual function, there are currently no androgen-containing HT products approved by the FDA for use in women. Some clinicians prescribe custom-compounded micronized testosterone or various other androgen-containing products on an off-label basis. Similar to other sex hormones, there is no serum androgen level that will determine whether an individual's sexual dysfunction is related to low testosterone.[2]

Many side effects are associated with androgen therapy, including acne, growth of facial and body hair, clitoral enlargement, permanent voice deepening, emotional volatility, and deleterious effects on lipids and liver function.[2,39] The effects on cardiovascular disease or breast cancer, as well as long-term consequences of androgen therapy, are poorly understood.

## Fertility in Perimenopause

Pregnancy is possible until 12 months after the final menstrual period. Individuals in the perimenopausal

| Table 14-11 | Estrogen Plus Progestin Combination Therapies | |
|---|---|---|
| **Composition** | **Brand Names** | **Dose** |
| **Oral Continuous Combined Estrogen Plus Progestin** | | |
| Conjugated equine estrogen + medroxyprogesterone acetate | Prempro | 0.3 mg CEE + 1.5 mg MPA, 1 tab/day |
| | | 0.45 mg CEE + 1.5 mg MPA, 1 tab/day |
| | | 0.625 mg CEE + 2.5 mg MPA, 1 tab/day |
| | | 0.625 mg CEE + 5 mg MPA, 1 tab/day |
| Ethinyl estradiol + norethindrone acetate | Femhrt | 2.5 mcg EE + 0.5 mg NETA, 1 tab/day |
| | | 5.0 mcg EE + 1 mg NETA, 1 tab/day |
| 17β-estradiol (17β-e) + norethindrone acetate | Activella | 0.5 mg 17β + 1 mg NETA, 1 tab/day |
| 17β-estradiol (17β-e) + drosperinone | Angeliq | 1 mg 17β-e + 0.5 mg DRSP, 1 tab/day |
| | | 1 mg 17β-e + 1 mg DRSP, 1 tab/day |
| **Oral Sequential Combined Estrogen Plus Progestin** | | |
| Conjugated equine estrogen + medroxyprogesterone acetate | Premphase | 0.625 mg CEE, 1 tab/day for 14 days |
| | | 0.625 mg CEE + 5 mg MPA, 1 tab/day for 14 days Repeat continuously |
| **Oral Intermittent/Sequential Combined Estrogen Plus Progestin** | | |
| 17β-estradiol (17β-e) + norgestimate | Prefest | 17β-e (1 mg), 1 tab/day for 3 days |
| | | 17β-e (1 mg) + NGM (0.09 mg), 1 tab/day for 3 days Repeat continuously |
| **Transdermal Combined Estrogen Plus Progestin** | | |
| 17β-estradiol (17β-e) + norethindrone acetate | Combipatch | 0.05 mg 17β + 0.14 mg NETA or 0.05 mg 17β + 0.25 mg NETA Apply twice weekly |
| 17β-estradiol (17β-e) + levonorgestrel | Climara Pro | 0.045 mg 17β-e + 0.015 mg LNG Apply once weekly |

Abbreviations: CEE, conjugated equine estrogen; DRSP, drosperinone; EE, ethinyl estradiol; LNG, levonorgestrel; MPA, medroxyprogesterone acetate; NETA, norethindrone acetate; NGM, norgestimate.

Data from Ward K, Deneris A. An update on menopause management. *J Midwifery Women's Health*. 2018;63(2):168-177. doi:10.1111/jmwh.12737; North American Menopause Society, ed. *Menopause Practice: A Clinician's Guide*. 6th ed. Pepper Pike, OH: North American Menopause Society; 2021.

| Table 14-12 | Progestin-Only Therapies | |
|---|---|---|
| **Composition** | **Brand Names** | **Dose** |
| **Oral Progestin Therapies** | | |
| Medroxyprogesterone acetate | Provera (Generic available) | 2.5, 5, 10 mg/day |
| Norethindrone acetate | Aygestin (Generic available) | 5 mg/day |
| Micronized progesterone | Prometrium | 100, 200 mg/day |
| Megestrol acetate | Megace (Generic available) | 40 mg/day |
| **Intrauterine Progestin Therapies** | | |
| Levonorgestrel | Mirena (5 year) | Releases approximately 20 mcg/day |
| | Skyla (3 year) | Releases approximately 6 mcg/day |
| | Liletta (5 year) | Releases approximately 17 mcg/day |
| | Kyleena (5 year) | Releases approximately 17.5 mcg/day |
| **Vaginal Preparations** | | |
| Progesterone | Crinone 4% gel | 45 mg, 1 applicator/day |
| | Endometrin tablet | 100 mg/day |

Data from Ward K, Deneris A. An update on menopause management. *J Midwifery Women's Health*. 2018;63(2):168-177. doi:10.1111/jmwh.12737; North American Menopause Society, ed. *Menopause Practice: A Clinician's Guide*. 6th ed. Pepper Pike, OH: North American Menopause Society; 2021.

period who wish to avoid pregnancy cannot rely on HT and need contraception to prevent pregnancy. Although both HT and combined hormonal contraceptives contain estrogen and progestin, the doses and formulations used for HT will not prevent pregnancy. Moreover, individuals whose ovaries are still functioning in a reproductive capacity are not likely to benefit from the doses of hormones found in HT because they are low in comparison to reproductive-age hormone levels. For patients who experience perimenopausal symptom relief with hormonal contraception use, experts recommend making the transition to HT, if desired and appropriate, at the age of 55 years, at which time 90% of individuals will have reached menopause.[2]

## Discontinuation of Hormone Therapy

The decision to discontinue therapy should be individualized. Notably, there does not seem to be any benefit from tapering versus immediate discontinuation.[40] For ET, a longer duration of use may be safer compared to EPT. In a longitudinal study conducted as part of the WHI, women using EPT for a median of 5.6 years and women using ET only for a median of 7.2 years were found to have no increase in all-cause, cardiovascular, or cancer mortality during 18 years of follow-up.[39] For this reason, 5 years is often used as a recommendation for discontinuing EPT, although 50% of patients will experience a return of vasomotor symptoms with discontinuation.[41] Extended duration of treatment is now considered a reasonable option for patients experiencing vasomotor symptoms that interfere with their quality of life. Consider decreasing the dose or switching to vaginal ET if the symptoms are primarily genitourinary. At least yearly visits with a provider are recommended for patients receiving HT.[2]

## Custom-Compounded Formulations

Some consumers, healthcare providers, and pharmacists use the term *bioidentical hormone* to describe formulations that are more accurately described as *custom-compounded*. Bioidentical hormones are plant-derived hormones that are chemically identical to the endogenous hormones (e.g., estrogen, progesterone) produced by the ovaries during the reproductive years.[2] Many bioidentical hormone therapies are available in FDA-approved formulations. Examples include 17ß-estradiol products, estradiol acetate products, and oral micronized progesterone.

Custom-compounding of HT involves individual mixing of preparations, usually by a compounding pharmacist. In an attempt to individualize therapy, such products may be specified to include one or more hormones, often delivered via nonstandard routes such as subdermal implants, sublingual tablets, rectal suppositories, or nasal sprays. Custom-compounded products were initially intended for use when standard FDA-approved products were ineffective, but post-WHI safety concerns caused an increasing number of patients and clinicians to explore options other than the commercial products used in the WHI study.[2]

A number of concerns have arisen regarding custom-compounded HT. Clinicians who prescribe custom-compounded hormones often base the dosing on salivary hormone testing, despite no evidence to support the claim that such testing can accurately guide HT doses.[2,12] Moreover, no evidence supports the contention that custom-compounded hormones are safer than traditional HT, and their effectiveness is an open question given the limited research conducted on these formulations.[42] Safety concerns stem from the lack of batch-to-batch testing for consistency, purity, or dose.[42] The FDA does not regulate compounded products. Instead, individual state agencies regulate compounding pharmacies, and the regulatory process varies widely from state to state. Topical progesterone, which is typically found in the custom-compounded HT gels, creams, and lotions, does not adequately raise serum levels to protect the endometrium against estrogen's stimulatory effects, which may ultimately lead to endometrial hyperplasia and endometrial cancer in some cases.[2] Custom-compounded hormones also may be substantially more expensive because they may not be covered by insurance.[42]

Consensus from several organizations, including the North American Menopause Society (NAMS), the FDA, the American Congress of Obstetricians and Gynecologists (ACOG), the Endocrine Society, the American Medical Association, and the American Cancer Society, is that custom-compounded therapy is no safer than traditional, commercially prepared and FDA-approved therapies, and that compounding may impart additional risks.[2]

## Bone Health, Osteopenia, and Osteoporosis

Humans build bone throughout childhood, adolescence, and young adulthood, with bone mass peaking by age 18 to 25 years. Genetic factors, and to a lesser extent nutrition, physical activity, and general health, determine the amount and quality of bone. Throughout the bone formation process, osteoclasts help to remove old bone and osteoblasts help to build new bone. Aging and the lower estrogen levels associated with menopause result in bone resorption, as osteoclasts outpace osteoblasts' ability to form new bone so that more bone is removed than is built. The result can be a fragile, weakened bone structure and decreased bone mass that is more prone to fracture even without significant trauma. The weakened structure and decreased mass in turn affect bone density, increasing the risk of osteopenia (low bone mass) and osteoporosis (disorder of low bone mass). Table 14-13 defines key terms related to osteoporosis.

Approximately 2 million osteoporosis-related fractures occur annually in the United States, which lead to significant morbidity.[43] Hip fracture is the most costly and dramatic type of fracture. While fractures associated with osteoporosis typically occur years after menopause, the rate of bone loss is highest at the time of menopause. Thus, preventing fracture—and particularly hip fracture—needs to begin years before the fracture may occur.

The U.S. Preventive Services Task Force (USPSTF) current recommendations are that all women be screened by age 65, and that patients with risk factors for low bone mineral density (BMD) be screened at menopause.[44] Certain risk factors predispose individuals to experience an even greater extent of bone loss and/or an even higher risk of fracture. Table 14-14 summarizes risk factors for osteoporosis and osteoporosis-related fractures. Understanding that race and sex are social constructs, midwives should be aware of the elements included in the table related to race and use clinical judgment and shared decision making when applying these risk factors to individuals.

Many commonly prescribed medications can cause bone loss and subsequent osteoporosis. Individuals taking these drugs, particularly in combination, should be offered earlier and more regular screening for osteopenia/osteoporosis (Table 14-15).

Clinicians usually diagnose and manage patients with low bone mass by measuring BMD with dual-energy X-ray absorptiometry (DXA), an enhanced type of X ray. Examples of indications for BMD are listed in Table 14-16. Although BMD is not a perfect surrogate for fracture risk, it is currently the best option for screening available.[45]

If bone mass is placed on a continuum in which normal bone mass is 1 standard deviation (SD) above and below 0, *osteopenia* represents the next finding on the continuum. Osteopenia is defined as decreased bone mass ranging from 1 SD below 0 to 2.5 SD below 0. This condition is three times more prevalent than osteoporosis. Moving even further away from normal bone mass on the continuum,

| Table 14-13 | Osteoporosis Definitions |
|---|---|
| **Term** | **Definition** |
| Bone mineral density (BMD) | Surrogate marker for bone strength and resistance to fracture<br>Measured by dual-energy X-ray absorptiometry<br>Usually measured and reported for the hip, femoral neck, and spine<br>Results reported as standard deviations from the mean of a reference population |
| Dual-energy X-ray absorptiometry | Gold-standard diagnostic technology for measuring BMD |
| Fracture risk assessment tool | Online fracture risk assessment tool to assist in clinical decision making for screening and treatment decisions<br>Calculates absolute fracture risk/estimate of risk for fracture in the next 10 years<br>Calculations include age, bone density, and risk factors |
| Osteopenia | Low bone mass<br>T-score between −1.0 and −2.5 |
| Osteoporosis | Skeletal disease of low bone mass and deterioration of bone micro-architecture<br>Resulting bone fragility increases the risk that bone will fracture<br>BMD T-score < −2.5 constitutes osteoporosis |
| T-score | Comparison with mean peak BMD of a young, same-sex population without additional risk factors<br>Number of standard deviations that a person's BMD differs from the mean peak BMD of a normal young adult of the same sex<br>Most commonly used measurement when making clinical decisions about midlife and older patients |
| Z-score | Comparison with a reference population of the same age, gender, and ethnicity<br>Not commonly used when evaluating midlife and older patients; can be misleading because bone density is often low in older adults<br>Used primarily for children, teens, and young adults |

Abbreviation: BMD, bone mineral density.

Data from Management of osteoporosis in postmenopausal women: the 2021 position statement of the North American Menopause Society. *Menopause*. 2021;28(9):973-997. doi:10.1097/GME.0000000000001831; Curry SJ, Krist AH, Owens DK, et al. Screening for osteoporosis to prevent fractures: US Preventive Services Task Force recommendation statement. *JAMA*. 2018;319(24):2521-2531. doi:10.1001/JAMA.2018.7498; North American Menopause Society, ed. *Menopause Practice: A Clinician's Guide*. 6th ed. Pepper Pike, OH: North American Menopause Society; 2021.

| Table 14-14 | Risk Factors for Osteoporosis and Osteoporotic Fractures |
|---|---|
| **Nonmodifiable Risk Factors** | **Potentially Modifiable Risk Factors** |
| Age ≥ 65 years<br>Sex<br>Personal history as an adult of fracture in the absence of substantial trauma<br>Family history of osteoporosis<br>Hip, spine, or wrist fracture without substantial trauma in a first-degree relative<br>Race: white and Asian race are greatest risk, followed by Hispanic and African American<br>Late menarche (> 15 years) or early menopause (< 45 years) | Smoking<br>Body mass index < 20 or weight < 127 pounds<br>Eating disorder or exercise-induced amenorrhea<br>Chronic glucocorticoid use (e.g., prednisone > 5 mg/day for > 3–6 months)<br>Multiple risk factors for falling (e.g., decreased leg or arm muscle strength, diminished vision, environmental hazards, impaired cognition)<br>Chronic illnesses: rheumatoid arthritis, hyperparathyroidism, impaired absorption syndromes<br>Heavy alcohol use (≥ 3 drinks/day) |

Data from Management of osteoporosis in postmenopausal women: the 2021 position statement of the North American Menopause Society. *Menopause*. 2021;28(9):973-997. doi:10.1097/GME.0000000000001831; Curry SJ, Krist AH, Owens DK, et al. Screening for osteoporosis to prevent fractures: US Preventive Services Task Force recommendation statement. *JAMA*. 2018;319(24):2521-2531. doi:10.1001/JAMA.2018.7498; North American Menopause Society, ed. *Menopause Practice: A Clinician's Guide*. 6th ed. Pepper Pike, OH: North American Menopause Society; 2021; Kanis JA, Harvey NC, Johansson H, et al. FRAX update. *J Clin Densitom*. 2017;20(3): 360-367. doi:10.1016/J.JOCD.2017.06.022.

| Table 14-15 | Potential Osteoporosis-Inducing Medications | |
|---|---|---|
| **Drug Classification** | **Examples** | **Comments** |
| Androgen deprivation therapy | Leuprolide (Lupron), Goserelin (Zoladex), Triptorelin (Trelstar) | Used for treatment of endometriosis and some types of cancer |
| Anticonvulsants | Phenytoin (Dilantin), phenobarbital, carbamazepine (Tegretol), valproate (Depakote) | All classes of anticonvulsants are associated with bone loss |
| Aromatase inhibitors | Anastrozole (Arimidex), letrozole (Femara), exemestane (Aromasin), testolactone (Teslac) | Used in the treatment of breast cancer |
| Calcineurin inhibitors | Cyclosporine, tacrolimus | Used for immunosuppression and atopic dermatitis |
| Chemotherapies | Cyclophosphamides, ifosfamide, high-dose methotrexate | Some cause direct bone loss; others are indirect causes |
| Glucocorticoids | Cortisone, prednisone, budesonide, triamcinolone | Bone loss is dose dependent, with the greatest risk associated with doses ≥ 20 mg/day |
| Heparin | Heparin | Associated with long-term heparin use |
| Depo-medroxyprogesterone acetate | Depo-Provera | DMPA-induced bone loss is reversible; MPA in OCs and EPT is not associated with bone loss |
| Proton pump inhibitors | Esomeprazole (Nexium), pantoprazole (Protonix), lansoprazole (Prevacid), omeprazole (Prilosec) | Bone loss with use > 1 year |
| Selective serotonin receptor inhibitors | Fluoxetine (Prozac), sertraline (Zoloft), paroxetine (Paxil), citalopram (Celexa) | Risk is highest post menopause |
| Thiazolidinediones | Rosiglitazone (Avandia), pioglitazone (Actos) | Increased risk for women all ages |

Source: Management of osteoporosis in postmenopausal women: the 2021 position statement of the North American Menopause Society. *Menopause*. 2021;28(9):973-997. doi:10.1097/GME.0000000000001831; Curry SJ, Krist AH, Owens DK, et al. Screening for osteoporosis to prevent fractures: US Preventive Services Task Force recommendation statement. *JAMA*. 2018;319(24):2521-2531. doi:10.1001/JAMA.2018.7498; North American Menopause Society, ed. *Menopause Practice: A Clinician's Guide*. 6th ed. Pepper Pike, OH: North American Menopause Society; 2021.

| Table 14-16 | Considerations for Ordering Bone Mineral Density Testing |
|---|---|
| At menopause: for patients with a history of fracture or with a parent who had a hip fracture or multiple vertebral or nonvertebral fragility fractures | |
| At age 65 for patients with no risk factors | |
| Before menopause or during perimenopause: patients with specific risk factors for increased fracture risk such as anorexia, long-term glucocorticoid use, metabolic bone disease, hyperthyroidism, low body weight, prior low-trauma fracture, or high-risk medication | |
| For treatment decisions: to monitor effects of osteoporosis therapy, if being considered for medications, or if evidence of bone loss would lead to treatment | |
| As indicated by FRAX (the World Health Organization's Fracture Risk Assessment Tool): clinicians can use FRAX to determine which patients younger than 65 years should have BMD testing; if FRAX indicates that a patient has a 9.3% or higher 10-year risk of major osteoporotic fracture, it is reasonable for that patient to have a DXA. Additional information on FRAX can be found in the "FRAX: The Fracture Risk Assessment Tool" section. | |
| To monitor effects of DMPA on bone density | |

Abbreviations: BMD, bone mineral density; DMPA, depot medroxyprogesterone acetate; DXA, dual-energy X-ray absorptiometry; FRAX, World Health Organization's Fracture Risk Assessment Tool.

Data from Curry SJ, Krist AH, Owens DK, et al. Screening for osteoporosis to prevent fractures: US Preventive Services Task Force recommendation statement. *JAMA*. 2018;319(24):2521-2531. https://doi.org/10.1001/JAMA.2018.7498; North American Menopause Society, ed. *Menopause Practice: A Clinician's Guide*. 6th ed. Pepper Pike, OH: North American Menopause Society; 2021.

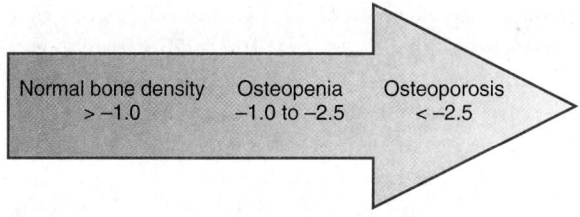

| Normal bone density > −1.0 | Osteopenia −1.0 to −2.5 | Osteoporosis < −2.5 |

**Figure 14-2** Bone mineral density continuum.
Data from National Osteoporosis Foundation. *Clinician's Guide to Prevention and Treatment of Osteoporosis.* Washington, DC: National Osteoporosis Foundation; 2014.

*osteoporosis* represents even more significantly decreased bone mass, 2.5 SD below 0 and lower (**Figure 14-2**). A T-score is the most commonly used reporting method for the results of the DXA measurements.[46] Generally, DXA measurements are taken at the femoral neck, at the posterior–anterior lumbar spine, and as a total hip measurement; the lowest of the three values determines the diagnostic category to which the individual is assigned.[46]

## FRAX: The Fracture Risk Assessment Tool

Clinically, the important goal related to bone health is *fracture prevention*, rather than simply promoting a specific BMD score. BMD is just one aspect of bone health, as other factors also influence fracture risk. The World Health Organization's Fracture Risk Assessment Tool (FRAX) was developed to assist clinicians in estimating the likelihood of a major (e.g., hip, spine, forearm) fracture in the next 10 years.[47] Economic modeling for cost-effectiveness determines the cutoffs for treatment recommendations. For the U.S. population, the National Osteoporosis Foundation recommends treatment for persons with a 3% or higher chance of breaking a hip in the next 10 years or a 20% or greater chance of breaking any major bone in the next 10 years.[46]

Risk factors in the FRAX algorithm include age, gender (sex), smoking, consumption of three or more alcoholic drinks per day, rheumatoid arthritis, low BMI, prolonged corticosteroid use, secondary osteoporosis, parent with a hip fracture, and lower BMD.[43] The algorithm does not take into account certain aspects of these risk factors, such as the amount of tobacco use or corticosteroid use, and it does not consider some risk factors at all (e.g., activity level; risk for falling; intake of caffeine).[43]

The National Osteoporosis Foundation has identified several clinical caveats to consider when using FRAX. When caring for patients in the United States, for example, clinicians should consider that FRAX is intended for postmenopausal patients and not for younger adults or children. For patients currently or previously taking osteoporosis medications,

clinicians should exercise caution in interpreting FRAX scores because FRAX has not been validated in this population. Moreover, while the intent of FRAX is to make clinical decisions more straightforward, all treatment decisions require careful clinical judgment of characteristics of the individuals. FRAX does not capture all risk factors; conversely, its recommendations do not mandate treatment.[43]

## Nonpharmacologic Strategies for Osteoporosis Prevention

Evidence supports nonpharmacologic strategies to promote bone health, but these strategies are not successful in replacing bone loss or treating osteoporosis.[2] For risk reduction in otherwise healthy individuals, these strategies are generally inexpensive, have minimal inherent risks, and can confer benefits for other aspects of a person's health. Exercise promoting strength and balance, for example, can reduce fall-related fractures.[48]

Muscle-strengthening and weight-bearing exercise has multiple benefits for bone health (and overall well-being). Improved strength, balance, agility, and posture can reduce the risk of falling; falling has the potential to bring significant negative sequelae, such as fractures, pain, disability, and death. Exercise also has a modest effect on bone density; that is, bone mass increases in response to activities that place stress on bones.[49] Body weight less than 127 pounds and a BMI less than 20 kg/mm$^2$ are risk factors for low bone mass and increased fracture risk.[32] The benefits of gaining weight should be discussed with very thin patients, with recommendations made for approaches that can be used to achieve a healthy weight.[46]

Of the various dietary nutrients, calcium and vitamin D are important for bone health, although calcium and vitamin D levels are not correlated with bone loss or fracture risk.[2] Major organizations such as the National Osteoporosis Foundation, the National Academy of Sciences, and the Institute of Medicine recommend 1200 mg of calcium for persons age 50 years and older and 600 IU of vitamin D from age 51 to 71 and 800 IU after 71 years of age.[2] The best sources of vitamin D and calcium are in foods. Vitamin D and calcium supplements for the purpose of improving bone health have not been shown to be effective and are not recommended for healthy adults.[2] Magnesium supplements are not beneficial except in the case of malabsorption issues. Vitamin K supplementation was shown to decrease factures in only one small study, and phytoestrogens showed inconsistent results and are not recommended to prevent or treat osteoporosis.[2]

In addition to their many other deleterious health effects, smoking and excessive alcohol intake have significant negative effects on bone health. Smokers have lower bone mass, lose bone more quickly, and have significantly higher fracture risk than nonsmokers.[32] While moderate alcohol intake does not have any recognized detrimental effects on bones, consuming three or more alcoholic drinks per day increases the risk of osteoporotic fracture and falling.[32,43]

## Pharmacologic Therapies for Osteoporosis Management

A focus on lifestyle strategies may be all that is necessary to promote bone health and minimize fracture risk for midlife and older patients at low risk for fracture. However, clinicians can offer pharmacologic therapy for patients with any of the following: osteoporosis (T-score of –2.5 or lower), history of a low-trauma hip or vertebral fracture, or osteopenia (T-score between –1 and –2.5) *if* FRAX indicates a 10-year probability of 3% or greater of a hip fracture or a 10-year probability of 20% or greater of a major osteoporosis-related fracture.[2,32,43]

Estrogen in the form of ET or EPT has long been an FDA-approved agent for *preventing* osteoporosis, but it is not approved as a *treatment* for this condition. Aside from estrogen, a variety of FDA-approved medications are available to prevent and/or treat osteoporosis, including bisphosphonates, raloxifene (Evista), calcitonin (Fortical), and teriparatide (Forteo). Table 14-17 summarizes the medications in each category, their doses, and

| Table 14-17 | Medications for Treatment of Osteoporosis | |
|---|---|---|
| **Medication Generic (Brand)** | **Dose** | **Comments** |
| **Bisphosphonates** | | |
| Alendronate (Fosamax) | Prevention: 5 mg daily or 35 mg weekly tablet or oral solution<br>Treatment: 10 mg daily or 70 mg weekly tablet or oral solution | Bisphosphonates are considered by many experts to be first-line therapy for osteoporosis |
| Ibandronate (Boniva) | Prevention: 2.5 mg daily or 150 mg monthly tablet<br>Treatment: 2.5 mg daily or 150 mg monthly tablet or 3 mg every 3 months IV | Choice of bisphosphonate is often made based on the desired dosing regimen<br>Take 30–60 minutes before eating in the morning, with 8 ounces water; sit/stand upright for 30–60 minutes |
| Risedronate (Actonel) | Prevention and treatment: 5 mg daily; 35 mg weekly; 35 mg weekly packaged with 6 tablets of 500 mg calcium carbonate; 75 mg on 2 consecutive days every month; and 150 mg monthly tablet | Side effects for all oral bisphosphonates: difficulty swallowing, esophageal inflammation, gastric ulcers |
| Zoledronic acid (Reclast) | Prevention: 5 mg IV every 2 years<br>Treatment: 5 mg IV annually | |
| **Calcitonin** | | |
| Salmon calcitonin (Miacalcin, Fortical) | Treatment (> 5 years post menopause): 200 IU daily nasal spray | FDA approved for treatment of patients with vertebral osteoporosis but not osteoporosis at nonvertebral sites (e.g., hip)<br>Other agents are more reliable at both vertebral and nonvertebral sites; calcitonin is not a first-tier therapy |
| **Estrogen Agonist/Antagonists (EAAs) [previously known as selective estrogen receptor modulators (SERMs)]** | | |
| Raloxifene (Evista) | Prevention and treatment: 60 mg daily | Not only inhibits bone resorption, but also decreases risk of breast and uterine cancers<br>Effective at reducing the risk of vertebral fractures but not hip or other nonvertebral fractures<br>Can cause hot flashes<br>Contraindicated in patients with venous thromboembolism history |

| Medication Generic (Brand) | Dose | Comments |
|---|---|---|
| **Parathyroid Hormone** | | |
| Teriparatide (Forteo) | Treatment (postmenopausal patients at very high fracture risk): 20 mcg daily SQ | Indicated for patients with established osteoporosis at very high risk of primary fracture |
| | | Indicated for patients with continued fractures despite use of other antiresorptive therapies |
| Abaloparatide (Tymlos) | Treatment of patients with a recent osteoporotic fracture: 80 mcg SQ daily | Increases risk of osteosarcoma |
| **RANK Ligand Inhibitor** | | |
| Denosumab (Xgeva) | 60 mg SQ every 6 months | Postmenopausal patients with osteoporosis; no limit to duration of therapy |

Abbreviations: FDA, U.S. Food and Drug Administration; IV, intravenous; SQ, subcutaneous.

Data from Management of osteoporosis in postmenopausal women: the 2021 position statement of the North American Menopause Society. *Menopause*. 2021;28(9):973-997. doi:10.1097/GME.0000000000001831.

basic prescribing issues. Adherence to pharmacologic osteoporosis treatment is often poor, with adherence rates in 6- to 12-month studies ranging from less than 25% to as high as 81%.[50] Thus, if indicated and agreed upon by the patient, it is important to thoroughly discuss the patient's individual fracture risk and the purpose of therapy, and then to identify and eliminate barriers to appropriate use of that agent.[32] Dosing frequency seems to affect adherence, such that weekly dosing enhances adherence for many patients as compared to daily dosing.[32,50] Additional reasons for nonadherence include older age, polypharmacy, and medication side effects, while patient education and follow-up have been shown to improve adherence.[51] There is no benefit to combining therapies. Guidelines recommend BMD testing after 1 to 2 years of treatment.[32]

## Conclusion

Menopause is a healthy, natural life process that, similar to menstruation and pregnancy, causes significant distress for some people. Midwives' skill in provision of holistic, person-centered health care translates well into caring for people experiencing perimenopause and menopause. This care includes provision of appropriate anticipatory guidance and development of an individualized plan for health promotion and disease prevention.

## Resources

| Organization | Description |
|---|---|
| North American Menopause Society (NAMS) | Organization focused on midlife and older |
| North American Menopause Society (NAMS): *Menopause Practice: A Clinician's Guide* | Publication available for download (for a fee) that includes background information, evidence for health care, and guidelines |
| World Health Organization: Fracture Risk Assessment Tool (FRAX) | Instrument for determining risk of bone fractures |
| National Center for Complementary and Integrative Health, National Institutes of Health | Information about complementary and integrative health care |
| American College of Cardiology and American Heart Association Task Force on Practice Guidelines | Heart risk calculator |
| National Cancer Institute | Breast cancer risk assessment tool |
| National Osteoporosis Foundation (NOF) | Information for professionals and patients |

## References

1. Voicu I. The social construction of menopause as disease: a literature review. *J Comp Res Anthropol Sociol.* 2018;9(2):11-21.

2. North American Menopause Society, ed. *Menopause Practice: A Clinician's Guide.* 6th ed. Pepper Pike, OH: North American Menopause Society; 2021.

3. Solomon DH, Ruppert K, Greendale GA, et al. Medication use by race and ethnicity in women transitioning through the menopause: a study of women's health across the national drug epidemiology study. *J Womens Health (Larchmt).* 2016;25(6):599-605. doi:10.1089/JWH.2015.5338.

4. Aririguzo C, Spencer BS, Freysteinson W. "You're acting womanish!" A qualitative descriptive study of the experiences of African American women in menopausal transition. *J Women Aging.* 2021;1-18. doi:10.1080/08952841.2021.1915095.

5. Felice MC, Sndergaard MLJ, Balaam M. Resisting the medicalisation of menopause: reclaiming the body through design. *Conf Hum Factors Comput Syst Proc.* May 6, 2021. doi:10.1145/3411764.3445153.

6. Alspaugh A, Im E, Reibel MD, Barroso J. The reproductive health priorities, concerns, and needs of women in midlife: a feminist poststructuralist qualitative analysis. *Qual Health Res.* 2021;31(4):643-653. doi:10.1177/1049732320970491.

7. Taylor HS, Pal LSE. *Speroff's Clinical Endocrinological Gynecology and Infertility.* Philadelphia, PA: Walter Kluwer; 2020.

8. Parish SJ, Gillespie JA. The evolving role of oral hormonal therapies and review of conjugated estrogens/bazedoxifene for the management of menopausal symptoms. *Postgrad Med.* 2017;129(3):340-351. doi:10.1080/00325481.2017.1281083/.

9. Louwers YV, Visser JA. Shared genetics between age at menopause, early menopause, POI and other traits. *Front Genet.* 2021;12. doi:10.3389/FGENE.2021.676546.

10. Imanaka S, Shigetomi H, Kawahara N, Kobayashi H. Clinicopathological characteristics and imaging findings to identify adenomyosis-related symptoms. *Reprod Med Biol.* 2021;20(4):435-443. doi:10.1002/RMB2.12409.

11. Harlow SD, Gass M, Hall JE, et al. Executive summary of the Stages of Reproductive Aging Workshop + 10: addressing the unfinished agenda of staging reproductive aging. *Fertil Steril.* 2012;97(4):843. doi:10.1016/J.FERTNSTERT.2012.01.128.

12. Ward K, Deneris A. An update on menopause management. *J Midwifery Women's Health.* 2018;63(2):168-177. doi:10.1111/jmwh.12737.

13. Angelou K, Grigoriadis T, Diakosavvas M, et al. The genitourinary syndrome of menopause: an overview of the recent data. *Cureus.* 2020;12(4). doi:10.7759/CUREUS.7586.

14. Minkin MJ. Menopause: hormones, lifestyle, and optomizing aging. *Obstet Gynecol Clin North Am.* 2019;46(2019):501-514.

15. Gracia C, Freeman E. Onset of the menopause transition: the earliest signs and symptoms. *Obstet Gynecol Clin North Am.* 2018;45(4):585-597. doi:10.1016/J.OGC.2018.07.002.

16. Anderson DJ, Chung HF, Seib CA, et al. Obesity, smoking, and risk of vasomotor menopausal symptoms: a pooled analysis of eight cohort studies. *Am J Obstet Gynecol.* 2020;222(5):478.e1-478.e17. doi:10.1016/j.ajog.2019.10.103.

17. Willi J, Ehlert U. Assessment of perimenopausal depression: a review. *J Affect Disord.* 2019;249:216-222. doi:10.1016/J.JAD.2019.02.029.

18. Cray LA, Woods NF, Herting JR, Mitchell ES. Symptom clusters during the late reproductive stage through the early postmenopause: observations from the Seattle Midlife Women's Health Study. *Menopause.* 2012;19(8):864-869. doi:10.1097/GME.0B013E31824790A6.

19. Varkevisser RDM, van Stralen MM, Kroeze W, et al. Determinants of weight loss maintenance: a systematic review. *Obes Rev.* 2019;20(2):171. doi:10.1111/OBR.12772.

20. Hirschberg AL. Sex hormones, appetite and eating behaviour in women. *Maturitas.* 2012;71(3):248-256. doi:10.1016/J.MATURITAS.2011.12.016.

21. Daley A, Stokes-Lampard H, Thomas A, MacArthur C. Exercise for vasomotor menopausal symptoms. *Cochrane Database Syst Rev.* 2014;11:1-43. doi:10.1002/14651858.CD006108.pub4.

22. Tomiyama AJ, Carr D, Granberg EM, et al. How and why weight stigma drives the obesity "epidemic" and harms health. *BMC Med.* 2018;16(1):1-6. doi:10.1186/S12916-018-1116-5/PEER-REVIEW.

23. Centers for Disease Control and Prevention. Healthy weight, nutrition, and physical activity: losing weight. https://www.cdc.gov/healthyweight/losing_weight/index.html. Last reviewed September 19, 2022. Accessed November 13, 2021.

24. Hall KD, Kahan S. Maintenance of lost weight and long-term management of obesity. *Med Clin North Am.* 2018;102(1):183. doi:10.1016/J.MCNA.2017.08.012.

25. Johnson A, Roberts L, Elkins G. Complementary and alternative medicine for menopause. *J Evidence-Based Integr Med.* 2019;24. doi:10.1177/2515690X19829380.

26. Shan D, Zou L, Liu X, et al. Efficacy and safety of gabapentin and pregabalin in patients with vasomotor symptoms: a systematic review and meta-analysis. *Am J Obstet Gynecol.* 2020;222(6):564-579. doi:10.1016/j.ajog.2019.12.011.

27. Ziel HK, Finkle WD. Increased risk of endometrial carcinoma among users of conjugated estrogens. *N*

*Engl J Med.* 1975;293(23):1167-1170. doi:10.1056/NEJM197512042932303.

28. Colman EG. The Food and Drug Administration's osteoporosis guidance document: past, present, and future. *J Bone Miner Res.* 2003;18(6):1125-1128. doi:10.1359/jbmr.2003.18.6.1125.

29. Rossouw JE, Anderson GL, Prentice RL, et al. Risks and benefits of estrogen plus progestin in healthy postmenopausal women: principal results from the Women's Health Initiative randomized controlled trial. *JAMA.* 2002;288(3):321-333. doi:10.1001/JAMA.288.3.321.

30. Anderson GL, Limacher M. Effects of conjugated equine estrogen in postmenopausal women with hysterectomy: the Women's Health Initiative randomized controlled trial. *JAMA.* 2004;291(14):1701-1712. doi:10.1001/JAMA.291.14.1701.

31. Marjoribanks J, Farquhar C, Roberts H, Lethaby A, Lee J. Long-term hormone therapy for perimenopausal and postmenopausal women. *Cochrane Database Syst Rev.* 2017;2017(1). doi:10.1002/14651858.CD004143.pub5.

32. Management of osteoporosis in postmenopausal women: the 2021 position statement of the North American Menopause Society. *Menopause.* 2021;28(9):973-997. doi:10.1097/GME.0000000000001831.

33. Gartlehner G, Patel SV, Feltner C, et al. Hormone therapy for the primary prevention of chronic conditions in postmenopausal women: evidence report and systematic review for the US Preventive Services Task Force. *JAMA.* 2017;318(22):2234-2249. doi:10.1001/jama.2017.16952.

34. Brubaker L. Identification and management of urinary incontinence in midlife women. *Menopause.* 2019;26(11):1324-1326. doi:10.1097/GME.0000000000001431.

35. Charbonneau DH. Health literacy and the readability of written information for hormone therapies. *J Midwifery Womens Health.* 2013;58(3):265-270. doi:10.1111/JMWH.12036.

36. Lethaby A, Ayeleke RO, Roberts H. Local oestrogen for vaginal atrophy in postmenopausal women. *Cochrane Database Syst Rev.* 2016;2016(8). doi:10.1002/14651858.CD001500.pub3.

37. Velentzis LS, Salagame U, Canfell K. Menopausal hormone therapy: a systematic review of cost-effectiveness evaluations. *BMC Health Serv Res.* 2017;17(1). doi:10.1186/S12913-017-2227-Y.

38. Lindh-Astrand L, Bixo M, Hirschberg AL, et al. A randomized controlled study of taper-down or abrupt discontinuation of hormone therapy in women treated for vasomotor symptoms. *Menopause.* 2010;17(1):72-79. doi:10.1097/GME.0B013E3181B397C7.

39. Davis SR, Baber R, Panay N, et al. Global consensus position statement on the use of testosterone therapy for women. *J Clin Endocrinol Metab.* 2019;104(10):4660-4666. doi:10.1210/JC.2019-01603.

40. Lindh-Åstrand L, Bixo M, Hirschberg AL, et al. A randomized controlled study of taper-down or abrupt discontinuation of hormone therapy in women treated for vasomotor symptoms. *Menopause.* 2010;17(1):72-79. doi:10.1097/GME.0B013E3181B397C7.

41. Ockene JK, Barad DH, Cochrane BB, et al. Symptom experience after discontinuing use of estrogen plus progestin. *JAMA.* 2005;294(2):183-193. doi:10.1001/JAMA.294.2.183.

42. Gaudard AMIS, Silva de Souza S, Puga MES, et al. Bioidentical hormones for women with vasomotor symptoms. *Cochrane Database Syst Rev.* 2016;2016(8). doi:10.1002/14651858.CD010407.pub2.

43. Kanis JA, Harvey NC, Johansson H, et al. FRAX update. *J Clin Densitom.* 2017;20(3):360-367. doi:10.1016/J.JOCD.2017.06.022.

44. Curry SJ, Krist AH, Owens DK, et al. Screening for osteoporosis to prevent fractures: US Preventive Services Task Force recommendation statement. *JAMA.* 2018;319(24):2521-2531. doi:10.1001/JAMA.2018.7498.

45. Hsieh C-I, Zheng K, Lin C, et al. Automated bone mineral density prediction and fracture risk assessment using plain radiographs via deep learning. doi:10.1038/s41467-021-25779-x. *Nat Commun.* 2021;12(1):5472. doi:10.1038/s41467-021-25779-x.

46. Cosman F, de Beur SJ, LeBoff MS, et al. Clinician's guide to prevention and treatment of osteoporosis. *Osteoporos Int.* 2014;25(10):2359-2381. doi:10.1007/S00198-014-2794-2.

47. Roux S, Cabana F, Carrier N, et al. The World Health Organization Fracture Risk Assessment Tool (FRAX) underestimates incident and recurrent fractures in consecutive patients with fragility fractures. *J Clin Endocrinol Metab.* 2014;99(7):2400-2408. doi:10.1210/JC.2013-4507.

48. U.S. Preventive Services Task Force. USPSTF bulletin: an independent, volunteer panel of national experts in prevention and evidence-based medicine. https://www.uspreventiveservicestaskforce.org/uspstf/. Accessed November 14, 2021.

49. Benedetti MG, Furlini G, Zati A, Mauro GL. The effectiveness of physical exercise on bone density in osteoporotic patients. *Biomed Res Int.* 2018;2018. doi:10.1155/2018/4840531.

50. Tomková S, Telepková D, Vaňuga P, et al. Therapeutic adherence to osteoporosis treatment. *Int J Clin Pharmacol Ther.* 2014;52(8):663-668. doi:10.5414/CP202072.

51. Cornelissen D, de Kunder S, Si L, et al. Interventions to improve adherence to anti-osteoporosis medications: an updated systematic review. *Osteoporos Int.* 2020;31(9):1645. doi:10.1007/S00198-020-05378-0.

CHAPTER

# 15

# Menstrual Cycle Abnormalities

DEBORA M. DOLE

## Introduction

Changes in the menstrual cycle can create a range of cultural, emotional, physical, and psychological concerns for individuals. Individual variation and experiences are important considerations when providing accurate and relevant information for shared decision making. Acknowledging the normalcy of variation in menstrual cycles provides a framework within which individuals and midwives can identify and address variations when they occur. This chapter addresses the complex condition of amenorrhea as well as the different bleeding patterns associated with atypical and abnormal uterine bleeding (AUB). It should be noted that reference to AUB as abnormal uterine bleeding is currently the recognized nomenclature and is used in this chapter based on the current literature. Use of the term *atypical* in reference to menstrual variations is intentional when distinguishing bleeding patterns associated with use of diagnostic criteria (PALM-COEIN) from variations that occur infrequently. Updates to the International Federation of Gynecology and Obstetrics (FIGO) classification systems are incorporated throughout the chapter. A discussion of dysmenorrhea, or painful menses, completes the chapter.

## Menstrual Health

Menstruation has an impact on the physical, mental and social well-being of individuals. How individuals experience menstruation is impacted by cultural norms, societal stigma, and medicalization of a normal physiologic process. Conversely, providers' attempts to normalize the impact of menstruation on people's everyday lives—including pain, heavy menstrual bleeding, and psychological stress—can increase barriers for those who would seek advice, support, or evaluation of other concerns from healthcare providers.[1,2]

Providers and patients possess varying levels of menstruation literacy. Individual provider biases contribute to furthering stereotypes and cultural insensitivity concerning menstruation. The combination of literacy, bias, and cultural insensitivity may create communication barriers impacting patients' level of comfort and trust in discussing menstrual concerns. The increased utilization of mobile health (mHealth) apps that address menstrual health and tracking has contributed to increasing health literacy in general. Increased menstrual literacy improves communication between provider and patient, creating a more trusting environment.[1] Continued efforts to eliminate stigma around menstruation through provider and organizational self-reflection on process and approach are necessary to reduce barriers and ensure equitable care for everyone.[3]

## The Menstrual Cycle and Variations

A wide variation in menstrual cycles exists, with only 15% of reproductive-age individuals reporting a cycle of 28 days.[4] The average range is 21 to 34 days and can vary between 2 and 20 days over a 12-month period.[4,5] The duration of bleeding is 4.5 to 8 days. The amount of blood loss considered normal during menses has been described as approximately 30 mL based on research conducted in the 1960s, with anything more than 80 mL deemed abnormal.[4] There are practical challenges with quantifying actual menstrual blood loss. More recent nomenclature has moved to describing heavy menstrual bleeding (HMB) as excessive menstrual blood loss that interferes with physical, social, or emotional quality of life.[2] However, it is common to either overestimate or underestimate the amount of menstrual bleeding that occurs on a monthly basis.[5] Additional information about the menstrual cycle is found in the *Anatomy and Physiology of the Reproductive System* chapter.

The onset of menstruation, termed *menarche*, usually occurs between 11 and 13 years (median age is 12.4 years), which is 2 to 3 years after thelarche (breast budding). The initial bleeding is usually related to anovulatory cycles and unpredictable.[4,5] Cycles become regular and occur with typical adult frequency by the third year after menarche.[5] By late adolescence, the typical ovulatory menstrual pattern is predictable in cycle regularity within a few days, and can be accompanied by dysmenorrhea. A few individuals also experience discomfort or a cramping sensation during ovulation, known as *mittelschmerz*.

Changes in menstrual cycle length are primarily due to differences in the follicular phase of the ovarian cycle; by comparison, the luteal phase tends to remain consistent. People in their late 30s typically experience slightly shorter and less variable menstrual cycles than younger people due to increases in follicle-stimulating hormone (FSH) levels and decreases in inhibin levels, which results in a shorter follicular phase.[4] Cycles typically lengthen again 2 to 4 years prior to menopause, followed by a complete cessation of menstruation. Menopause occurs at a median age of 51 years, with a range of 45 to 55 years.

Thus, the greatest fluctuation in duration of menstrual cycles occurs at either end of the reproductive spectrum, primarily due to an increase in anovulatory cycles among individuals younger than 20 years and those older than 40 years.[2] Because there can be a great deal of normal variation in the menstrual cycle in the early and later reproductive years, the initial steps in clinical evaluation of anyone who has menstrual irregularities differs for (1) adolescents, (2) people of reproductive age, and (3) individuals who are entering the menopausal transition. This distinction by age and proximity to menarche or menopause is always one of the initial considerations factored into the evaluation.[1-5]

Many people describe any vaginal bleeding as a period, and some automatically interpret any blood found in underwear or on toilet tissue as vaginal or uterine in origin. For example, withdrawal bleeding associated with combined oral contraceptives can be mischaracterized by users as a menses. Nevertheless, an important distinction should be made between menstrual bleeding that occurs as a component of the menstrual cycle, even if it may vary in timing and amount, and AUB, which occurs independently of the menstrual cycle. The adoption of more descriptive terms can also contribute to a better understanding of possible causes of menstrual variation or indicate possible pathology. Table 15-1

| Table 15-1 | Terminology for Menstrual Variations |
|---|---|
| **Description** | **Quantification** |
| **Frequency of Menses** | |
| Absent | Amenorrhea |
| Infrequent | > 38 days |
| Normal | Occurs between 24 and 38 days |
| Frequent | < 24 days |
| **Regularity: Variation in Cycle Length** | |
| Regular | 2–20 days[a] |
| Irregular | > 20 days[a] |
| **Duration of Menses** | |
| Prolonged | > 8 days |
| Normal | ≤ 8 days |
| **Flow Volume per Menses (as determined by the patient)** | |
| Heavy | Volume that interferes with one's physical, social, emotional and/or material quality of life |
| Normal | |
| Light | |

[a] Normal variation in menstrual cycle regularity depends on age.

Based on Munro MG, Critchley H, Fraser IS, et al. The two FIGO systems for normal and abnormal uterine bleeding symptoms and classification of causes of abnormal uterine bleeding in the reproductive years: 2018 revisions. *Int J Gynaecol Obstet.* 2018;143(3):393-408; Munro MG. Practical aspects of the two FIGO systems for management of abnormal uterine bleeding in the reproductive years. *Best Pract Res Clin Obstet Gynaecol.* 2017;40:3-22.

reviews menstrual cycle parameters, and Table 15-2 provides a glossary of terms used to describe forms of AUB.[3-6]

## Amenorrhea

*Amenorrhea* is the absence of menses or menstrual bleeding.[7,8] Amenorrhea is further categorized as *primary* or *secondary* based on its occurrence prior to or after menarche, respectively.[8,9] Although some causes of primary amenorrhea are distinct, most of the causes of secondary amenorrhea can also be the etiology of primary amenorrhea. Furthermore, amenorrhea can result from common events such

| Table 15-2 | Terminology for Menstrual Irregularities and Variations in Menstrual Bleeding |
|---|---|
| **Term** | **Description** |
| Abnormal uterine bleeding (AUB) | Any variation from the typical menstrual cycle. Changes include those in regularity, duration of flow, amount of flow, and frequency of flow |
| AUB: Acute | An episode of bleeding in an individual of reproductive age, who is not pregnant, of sufficient quantity to require immediate intervention to prevent further blood loss |
| AUB: Chronic | Bleeding that is atypical in duration, volume, and/or frequency that has been present for the majority of the last 6 months |
| AUB: Intermenstrual | Bleeding between clearly defined cyclically predictable menses |
| Amenorrhea | No menses for $\geq$ 3 previous consecutive months<br>Subclassified into primary (prior to menarche) or secondary (post menarche) |
| Heavy menstrual bleeding (HMB) | Excessive menstrual blood loss ($\geq$ 80 mL/cycle), which interferes with a person's physical, social, emotional, and/or quality of life |
| Prolonged menstrual bleeding | Menstrual blood loss that exceeds 8 days in duration |
| Heavy and prolonged menstrual bleeding (HPMB) | Heavy menstrual bleeding lasting > 8 days |
| Irregular menstrual bleeding | Range of varying lengths of bleeding-free intervals of > 20 days within one 90-day reference period |
| Infrequent menstrual bleeding | Bleeding at intervals > 38 days apart (1–2 episodes in a 90-day period) |
| Frequent menstrual bleeding | Bleeding at intervals < 24 days apart (> 4 episodes in a 90-day period) |
| Shortened menstrual bleeding | Menstrual bleeding < 3 days in duration |
| Irregular, nonmenstrual bleeding | Intermenstrual: Irregular episodes of bleeding, often light and short occurring between otherwise regular and predictable menstrual cycles<br>Postcoital: Bleeding after intercourse<br>Premenstrual and postmenstrual spotting: Bleeding that can occur on a regular basis for $\geq$ 1 days before or after the recognized menstrual period |
| Bleeding outside of reproductive age | Postmenopausal bleeding: Bleeding occurring > 1 year after the acknowledged menopause<br>Precocious menstruation: Bleeding occurring before the age of 9 years |

Based on Munro MG, Critchley H, Fraser IS, et al. The two FIGO systems for normal and abnormal uterine bleeding symptoms and classification of causes of abnormal uterine bleeding in the reproductive years: 2018 revisions. *Int J Gynaecol Obstet.* 2018;143(3): 393-408; Munro MG. Practical aspects of the two FIGO systems for management of abnormal uterine bleeding in the reproductive years. *Best Pract Res Clin Obstet Gynaecol.* 2017;40:3-22.

as pregnancy, lactation, menopause, and use of hormonal contraception, or it can be attributable to a pathologic condition. Common and potentially pathologic causes of amenorrhea involve a disruption of the hypothalamic–pituitary–ovarian (HPO) axis or anatomic anomaly within the outflow tract. Thus, it is helpful to consider five possible categories when evaluating causes of amenorrhea: (1) outflow tract abnormality, (2) ovarian disorder, (3) pituitary disorder, (4) hypothalamus disorder, or (5) endocrine disorder that interferes with the HPO axis.[8]

The list of differential diagnoses for amenorrhea is long. The majority of cases that are not related to a normal process (e.g., pregnancy, menopause, hormonal contraception, or lactation) can usually be attributed to one of the following four conditions: (1) polycystic ovary syndrome, (2) hypothalamic amenorrhea (i.e., amenorrhea without an organic cause secondary to an eating disorder, stress, or excessive exercise), (3) hyperprolactinemia, or (4) primary ovarian insufficiency (also referred to as premature ovarian failure, premature menopause, or gonadal dysgenesis).[8,9]

The etiologies unique to primary amenorrhea include anomalies of the outflow tract, genetic disorders that affect gonadal function such as Turner syndrome, and central anomalies of the HPO axis.[7,8,10] Approximately 30% to 40% of adolescents with primary amenorrhea are found to have Turner syndrome (45,XO karyotype).[8,10] The next most common causes of primary amenorrhea are structural abnormalities of the outflow tract (uterus, vagina, hymen) and central HPO axis anomalies.[8,10] Table 15-3 lists differential diagnoses associated with amenorrhea.

The definition of *primary amenorrhea* is not standardized. One definition is the absence of menses by age 15 years in individuals with developed secondary sex characteristics, within 5 years after breast development if breast development occurs before age 10 years, or if there is no pubertal

development by age 13 years.[4,8,10] Another definition is a more relative description based on time from appearance of secondary sexual characteristics. According to this definition, primary amenorrhea is lack of menarche within 3 to 5 years of thelarche (Tanner breast stage II development) or by the age of 15 to 16 years regardless of the presence of secondary sex characteristics. Age at menarche of other family members can be helpful in determining whether the initiation of menses is within expected parameters for the individual.

Secondary amenorrhea is defined as absence of menses for 3 months in a previously menstruating person or for 9 months in a someone who has experienced previous irregular menses with fewer than nine cycles in a year.[4,8]

## Evaluation for Amenorrhea

The evaluation of amenorrhea starts with, first, a determination of primary versus secondary amenorrhea and, second, consideration of the patient's age and proximity to menarche or menopause. These distinctions will direct the focus of the history and physical examination. The list of possible etiologies of amenorrhea is long, however, and multiple algorithms exist for evaluation of this condition. Figure 15-1 provides a representative example of the common steps involved in the initial evaluation.[8,10,11] Follow-up tests to assess for specific disorders are recommended after initial screening to identify the most likely category of etiologies.

### History and Physical Examination

When initiating an evaluation for amenorrhea, a thorough history and physical examination are required. A detailed menstrual and family history will establish primary versus secondary amenorrhea and can provide insight into any familial patterns of irregular menses or early menopause. The history should also inquire about use of hormonal contraception, any change in overall health status, current and past medications, galactorrhea, presence of premenopausal symptoms, increase in stress levels, eating and exercise patterns, and any physical or emotional trauma.

The physical examination includes an assessment of weight trends, including recent increase or decrease; breast development (an indicator of previous estrogenic influence); and presence of hirsutism or extensive muscle mass, both of which are suggestive of excessive testosterone levels. Thyroid palpation can detect possible thyroid dysfunction. External and internal genitalia should be

| Table 15-3 | Classification of Causes of Amenorrhea |
|---|---|
| **Category** | **Examples** |
| Expected physiologic findings | Pregnancy, lactation, hormonal contraceptive use, menopause |
| Outflow tract defects | Congenital: Müllerian agenesis, vaginal septum, imperforate hymen |
| | Acquired: Cervical stenosis, Asherman syndrome |
| Primary hypogonadism: ovarian insufficiency or ovarian failure | Congenital (e.g., Turner syndrome, Müllerian agenesis, gonadal dysgenesis) |
| | Acquired (e.g., chemotherapy, autoimmune disorder); primary ovarian insufficiency |
| Hypothalamic disorders | Functional hypothalamic amenorrhea (secondary to weight loss, disordered eating, excessive exercise, stress, rarely pseudocyesis), gonadotropin deficiency, infection, chronic debilitating disease, malabsorption, traumatic brain injury, tumor |
| Pituitary disorders | Prolactinomas, hormone-secreting pituitary tumor, autoimmune disease, Cushing's syndrome, medications, Sheehan syndrome |
| Endocrine disorders | Polycystic ovary syndrome,[a] thyroid dysfunction, adrenal disease (Cushing's syndrome), ovarian tumors |

[a] Polycystic ovary syndrome is sometimes categorized as a sixth category termed *multifactorial* because several abnormalities of the hypothalamic–pituitary–ovarian axis are involved in this disorder.

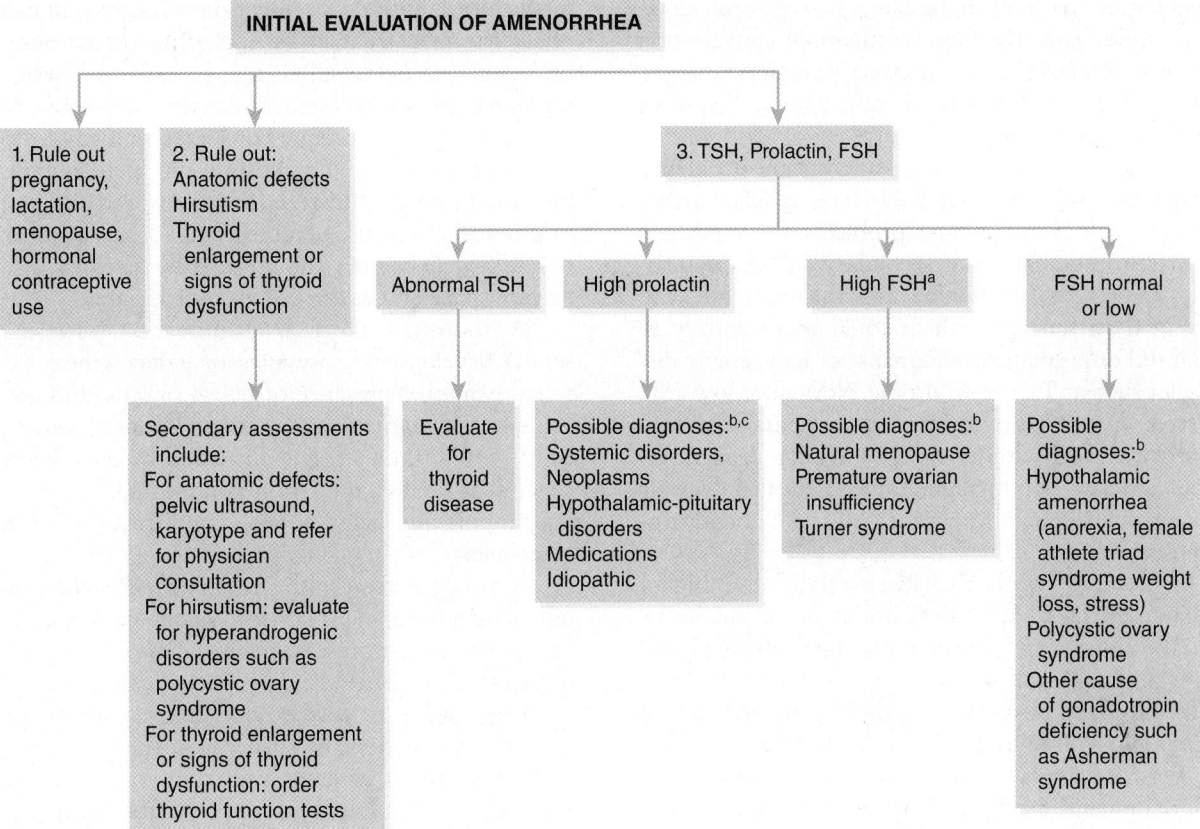

**Figure 15-1** Initial evaluation of amenorrhea and common etiologies.

Abbreviations: FSH, follicle-stimulating hormone; MRI, magnetic resonance imaging; TSH, thyroid-stimulating hormone.

[a] Some clinicians add a test for estradiol and/or luteinizing hormone to this initial evaluation.

[b] This list of diagnoses reflects common diagnoses and is not a complete list of the possible diagnoses.

[c] Hyperprolactinemia can occur secondary to many different disorders, including systemic disease, hypothalamic–pituitary disorders, medication use, or neoplasm. Hyperprolactinemia may also be idiopathic. Approximately 50–60% of those with a high prolactin level have a pituitary tumor.[13] The standard follow-up examination is an MRI.

Based on Klein DA, Paradise SL, Reeder RM. Amenorrhea: a systematic approach to diagnosis and management. *Am Fam Physician*. 2019;100(1):39-48. PMID: 31259490; Gibson ME, Fleming N, Zuijdwijk C, Dumont T. Where have the periods gone? The evaluation and management of functional hypothalamic amenorrhea. *J Clin Res Pediatr Endocrinol*. 2020;12(suppl 1):18-27. doi:10.4274/jcrpe. galenos.2019.2019.S0178; Huhmann K. Menses requires energy: a review of how disordered eating, excessive exercise, and high stress lead to menstrual irregularities. *Clin Ther*. 2020;42(3):401-407. doi:10.1016/j.clinthera.2020.01.016.

thoroughly assessed for structural anomalies such as a hypoplastic vagina, absent vagina, or imperforate hymen. Significant findings indicating anomalies in the genital tract are noted in an estimated 15% of individuals with amenorrhea.[8,10] Generally, the findings on physical examination will be normal, and the evaluation continues with an assessment of laboratory data.

### Laboratory Studies

If the history and physical examination do not detect signs of congenital abnormalities, the next step (unless the individual is postmenopausal) is to rule out pregnancy. Pregnancy remains the most common

reason for amenorrhea, and results of this test will directly influence the next steps in evaluation.

Once pregnancy is ruled out, initial laboratory testing assesses FSH level, thyroid-stimulating hormone (TSH), and prolactin level, with these results then guiding the rest of the evaluation. Other tests that can be indicated include pelvic ultrasound, especially in the event of nonpalpable ovaries. Such imaging provides information about structural and congenital anomalies and endometrial thickness. Magnetic resonance imaging (MRI) is indicated if a pituitary tumor is suspected. The complex relationship of the HPO axis to menstruation can be challenging to assess. The midwife can initiate the evaluation to establish the category of possible diagnoses, but after the initial evaluation, consultation with and referral to a reproductive endocrinologist is recommended to ensure appropriate diagnosis and management.

High FSH levels suggest ovarian problems, whereas low or normal FSH levels indicate either pituitary or hypothalamus problems. Elevated FSH levels in the absence of secondary sex characteristics indicate a functioning hypothalamus but lack of ovarian function, which could be secondary to natural or premature menopause or to a genetic disorder such as Turner syndrome. Normal or low FSH levels in persons with secondary sexual development (with or without signs of hyperandrogenism) can indicate hypothalamic amenorrhea, polycystic ovary syndrome, or other rare causes of gonadotropin deficiency.[8-10]

Elevated prolactin levels (typically higher than 100 ng/L) with or without headache or visual changes can indicate a pituitary adenoma and are an indication for imaging (MRI) to evaluate the pituitary. Prolactin suppresses the release of gonadotropin-releasing hormone (GnRH), and hyperprolactinemia can develop at any point of sexual development. Subclinical or overt hypothyroidism can also affect ovulatory function. Elevated TSH levels suppress GnRH release either directly or by causing increased prolactin release. Prolactin inhibits GnRH as part of a physiologic negative feedback mechanism.

### Hormonal Challenge Testing (Progesterone Challenge, Estrogen or Progestin Challenge)

Historically, a progesterone challenge test was included in the evaluation of patients with amenorrhea. However, current bioassays are sensitive tests, and withdrawal bleeding correlates poorly with estrogen status. Thus, many experts no longer use this test as part of an initial evaluation.[8-11]

### Evaluation of a Young Person with Primary Amenorrhea

The most common causes of primary amenorrhea can be identified by performing a physical examination to determine the presence of secondary sex characteristics or structural anomalies, rule out pregnancy, and assess the HPO axis through measurement of FSH, TSH, and prolactin levels.[10-12] The work-up begins with a thorough history, including review of any sexual activity, age at menarche for the adolescent's mother, and any underlying conditions,

medications, lifestyle, or nutritional deficits that can affect the menstrual cycle, including recent onset of headaches or visual disturbances.[4,9-12,14] When assessing adolescent sexual activity, the midwife should engage in a private conversation away from family or anyone who could prevent open communication or pose a threat. Issues of suspected sexual or physical abuse, use of recreational drugs, or other risk-taking behaviors should also be assessed in a private space and addressed as appropriate.

A thorough physical examination assessing sexual development, presence of galactorrhea, external genitalia, presence of pelvic organs, and any evidence of outflow tract anomalies is essential. Sensitivity to the fact that this could be the adolescent's first such examination is important in building rapport and being able to conduct a thorough assessment.

A young person with primary amenorrhea requires care from a specialist. If secondary sex characteristics are not present, bone age may need to be determined. Elevated FSH levels indicate the need for karyotyping to further investigate reasons for ovarian dysfunction. In such cases, the skills of a midwife can best be employed to interact with the adolescent and to initiate an appropriate referral for care.

Management of secondary amenorrhea largely focuses on treatment of the underlying etiology. Midwives are often involved in initial assessment and primary care for these individuals. The conditions seen most frequently in people of reproductive age are polycystic ovary syndrome and functional hypothalamic amenorrhea.[8,10,13,15,16]

### Polycystic Ovary Syndrome

Polycystic ovary syndrome (PCOS)—the most common diagnosis implicated in infertility related to ovarian dysfunction—is also the most common endocrine disorder, with a prevalence of approximately 6% to 10% depending on the population studied.[17-20] The incidence varies according to the criteria used to diagnose the condition. Historically, this condition was termed Stein–Leventhal syndrome, but later was renamed more descriptively as polycystic ovary syndrome.

PCOS is characterized by menstrual alterations, hyperandrogenism, and ovulatory disruption.[17-21] Its three classic features are hirsutism, irregular menstrual cycles, and central obesity. While amenorrhea is common in conjunction with this syndrome, menstrual cycle disruption is just one aspect of PCOS.

PCOS is often associated with insulin resistance and increases the individual's risk for type 2 diabetes. Acanthosis nigricans—a brown, velvety appearance to the skin in various folds, such as the back of the neck, in the axillae, under the breasts, or in the groin—is a marker of insulin resistance and appears in some individuals with PCOS.[17–21] Polycystic ovaries are common with PCOS but can be seen without this disorder, so by itself this finding is somewhat non-specific. PCOS also increases the risk for developing endometrial cancer, sleep apnea, steatohepatitis, and mood disorders.[18,19]

The cause of PCOS remains unknown, but recognition of the possible adverse long-term sequelae is emerging, resulting in greater attention to diagnosis and treatment.[20,21] For example, people with PCOS—even those without obesity—can have significant insulin resistance and, therefore, are at a higher lifetime risk for the development of both type 2 diabetes and cardiovascular disease.[4,20,21] Chronic anovulation associated with PCOS can result in unopposed estrogen stimulation of the endometrium and hyperplasia, increasing the risk of endometrial cancer.

### Diagnosis of Polycystic Ovary Syndrome

Criteria for diagnosis of PCOS continue to be debated by international experts.[17,19,20,22–24] The Rotterdam PCOS Consensus Group criteria, which are listed in Table 15-4, are still recognized as the consensus criteria for diagnosis and are currently recommended by the U.S. National Institutes of Health.[18–21] Some sources suggest that infrequent menses or episodes of amenorrhea must be present for at least 2 years after menarche or primary amenorrhea at 16 years to make this diagnosis.[21] Additionally, true hyperandrogenism should be documented through measurement of testosterone levels, rather than just signs of androgen excess such as acne.[18–21] The Rotterdam criteria recognize three distinct clinical phenotypes of PCOS:

- Frank PCOS: Oligomenorrhea, hyperandrogenism, and polycystic ovaries
- Ovulatory PCOS: Hyperandrogenism, polycystic ovaries, and regular menstrual cycles
- Nonpolycystic ovary PCOS: Oligomenorrhea, hyperandrogenism, and normal ovaries

The diagnostic criteria for PCOS are different for adolescents versus adults. Menstrual irregularities, multifollicular ovaries, and signs of androgen excess (e.g., acne) are common in adolescents.[21] Thus, the current diagnostic criteria for adolescents

| Table 15-4 | Rotterdam PCOS Consensus Group Criteria for Diagnosis of Polycystic Ovary Syndrome |
|---|---|
| Exclusion of other etiologies and two out of three of the following: | |
| Oligomenorrhea and/or amenorrhea | |
| Clinical and/or biochemical signs of hyperandrogenism | |
| Polycystic ovaries | |

Abbreviation: PCOS, polycystic ovary syndrome.

Based on National Institutes of Health. Evidence-based methodology workshop on polycystic ovary syndrome. December 3–5, 2012. Executive summary. https://prevention.nih.gov/sites/default/files/2018-06/FinalReport.pdf. Accessed April 17, 2023.

focus on evidence of ovulatory dysfunction and androgen excess.[21] Evidence of androgen excess in adolescents includes one or more of the following: moderate to severe hirsutism, persistent acne vulgaris that is resistant to topical treatments, and elevation of serum total and/or free testosterone level. The diagnosis of PCOS is not established until other causes of hyperandrogenism have been ruled out.

If the diagnosis is confirmed, assessment for diabetes or cardiovascular disease is warranted, including measurement of glucose, hemoglobin $A_{1c}$ (HbA1c), and lipid levels. Insulin resistance does not always reveal itself as elevated blood glucose levels or an elevated HbA1c value, but more typically results in blood sugar spikes and abdominal obesity prior to elevation of glucose levels. On examination, an assessment of body mass index (BMI), blood pressure, waist-to-hip circumference, and hirsutism should also be made. A waist-to-hip ratio of 0.85 or more indicates abdominal obesity and an increased risk for metabolic and cardiovascular conditions.[18–21]

### Treatment for Polycystic Ovary Syndrome

Treatment of PCOS varies and often depends on the degree of infertility or desire for conception. For some individuals, the alterations associated with PCOS can be treated with weight loss and lifestyle changes alone, with the aim of improving insulin sensitivity. Subsequent significant weight loss has been observed to result in more typical ovulatory and menstrual patterns as well as unassisted conception.[18,19] The use of the anti-hyperglycemic drug metformin (Glucophage) has increased in popularity in recent years, although the effectiveness of this medication in the treatment of PCOS is not clear.[18,19]

If conception is not desired immediately, ovarian function and continued enlargement of the ovaries can be suppressed with the use of combination hormonal contraceptives.[25] This temporary ovarian suppression will likely result in the initiation of normal ovarian function for a short time upon discontinuation of the hormonal contraceptive. Use of a hormonal contraceptive method will also protect the individual from the potential risks of unopposed estrogen stimulation of the endometrium, which might otherwise result in endometrial hyperplasia or even endometrial cancer. Additional information, including contraindications for the use of combined oral contraceptives, can be found in the *Hormonal Contraception* chapter.

Various medications, such as gonadotropin-releasing hormone (GnRH) agonists and the diuretic spironolactone (Aldactone), have also been employed as antiandrogens. Induction of ovulation, through administration of clomiphene citrate (Clomid), is a common strategy for the prompt treatment of individuals with infertility as a result of PCOS.[18,19] Individuals are best referred to a specialist for these treatments. Table 15-5 provides a sample of the critical elements in a referral note to the specialist.

Early diagnosis and intervention for PCOS, with respect to the health risks of hyperglycemia, abnormal cholesterol and lipid profiles, and reproductive cancer risk, can positively influence the affected individual's overall health. In addition, mental health disruptions that can result from a diminished sense

| Table 15-5 | Sample Critical Elements for a Referral Note for an Individual with Possible Polycystic Ovary Syndrome |
|---|---|
| Menstrual history, including duration of amenorrhea and irregular menses | |
| Signs and symptoms suggestive of PCOS (e.g., hirsutism, obesity) | |
| Laboratory results or if pending, including pregnancy test, TSH, HbA1c, and sonography | |
| Care provided before referral: procedures and results | |
| Assessment/diagnosis | |
| Summary of rationale for referral and request for information about treatment plan for follow-up | |

Abbreviations: HbA1c, hemoglobin $A_{1c}$; PCOS, polycystic ovary syndrome; TSH, thyroid-stimulating hormone.

of self-esteem due to physical appearance and infertility require the midwife's attention.[18]

## Functional Hypothalamic Amenorrhea

Functional hypothalamic amenorrhea (FHA) can occur when the HPO axis is disrupted by nutritional deficiency, extreme weight loss, exercise, and stress; it is characterized by a chronic low estrogen state along with low to normal FSH levels in the absence of organic disease.[10,15] FHA accounts for 25% to 35% of all cases of secondary amenorrhea and approximately 3% of all cases of primary amenorrhea.[11] People who experience FHA have a functional disruption in the normal pulsatile GnRH secretion. The decreased pulses mean that the midcycle LH surge does not occur, which then leads to anovulation and amenorrhea. The diagnosis of FHA is made after excluding other organic disorders that may potentially cause amenorrhea. Low serum FSH and low estradiol levels in combination with the presence of precipitating factors such as excessive exercise, disordered eating, stress, and weight loss are usually present. Limited energy availability is associated with hypothalamic dysfunction, leading to low estrogen levels, which adversely affects menstruation and bone health.[10,15]

### Disordered Eating and Excessive Exercise

People who are diagnosed with FHA should be assessed for disordered eating and excessive exercise. A positive energy balance is necessary for a properly functioning HPO axis. This is particularly important during puberty, when energy needs are high. Disordered eating, stress, and excessive exercise can all contribute to a negative energy balance. When adolescents and young adults who participate in physically demanding sports or have disordered eating do not maintain a positive energy balance, they are at risk for developing FHA.[11,12,14] Menstrual function can be restored when the energy imbalance is addressed.

Managing the complex condition of disordered eating requires an interdisciplinary team approach that includes nutritional support, mental health services, and family support.[12] Most importantly, the focus should center on the person and shared decision making about lifestyle choices. Treatment should include close monitoring for osteopenia or osteoporosis, as the hypo-estrogenic state can negatively influence bone density over time and should be monitored.[11,12,14]

### Hyperprolactinemia (Pituitary Adenoma)

Elevated prolactin levels can suppress the normal gonadotropin release necessary to stimulate ovulation, resulting in amenorrhea. Prolactin levels can be elevated by a number of conditions, including pituitary adenoma and prolonged hypothyroidism.[13,15] Other causes of elevated prolactin levels include use of medications that block dopamine receptors (e.g., tricyclic antidepressants and opioids. Dopamine normally inhibits prolactin secretion, so anything that blocks dopamine can result in increased prolactin levels.[13,15] Prolactin levels much higher than the maximum of the normal range, which is 20 ng/mL, which may or may not be accompanied by visual changes or headaches, can indicate the presence of a pituitary adenoma and require evaluation by MRI and an endocrinologist.[13,15] Management of suspected pituitary adenoma warrants consultation and referral.

### Rare Conditions Associated with Secondary Amenorrhea

Amenorrhea is also associated with premature ovarian insufficiency, autoimmune disorders, and ovarian tumors.[8,9,15,16] Premature ovarian insufficiency, defined as the inability of the ovary to respond to gonadotropin stimulation, is usually encountered in people 40 years or younger.[9,16] It affects 0.5% to 3.0% of reproductive-age people.[9,16] This condition can result from natural causes, chemotherapy, radiation, extreme stress, other medications, or autoimmune causes.[9,16] Autoimmune disorders that are associated with premature ovarian insufficiency include adrenal insufficiency (Addison's disease) and autoimmune thyroid disease (Graves' or Hashimoto disease); metabolic conditions (e.g., type 1 diabetes) can also cause secondary amenorrhea. Ovarian tumors can disrupt menstrual function by changing the responsiveness of the ovary to gonadotropins.

Less common conditions associated with amenorrhea include late-onset congenital adrenal hyperplasia, Cushing's syndrome, adrenal and androgen-secreting tumors, Asherman syndrome, and Sheehan syndrome. Congenital adrenal hyperplasia can present later in life as increased androgen production and observable androgenic effects that affect the normal menstrual cycle. Other hyperandrogenic states resulting from conditions such as Cushing's syndrome and adrenal tumors affect the menstrual cycle by suppressing normal ovarian function through overproduction of androgens. Ovulation and menstruation often return after correction of the hyperandrogenic state.

Asherman syndrome is the development of intrauterine adhesions and/or fibrosis of the endometrium as a result of trauma, excessive instrument manipulation, or evacuation of the uterus.[4] In this condition, the endometrium is not functional and does not respond to hormonal stimulation. The entire endometrium may not be affected, resulting in lighter than normal cyclical endometrial shedding versus complete amenorrhea.

Sheehan syndrome is ischemic necrosis of the pituitary gland, which usually occurs as a result of a profound postpartum hemorrhage.[4] Destruction of the pituitary gland results in amenorrhea, hypothyroidism, and impaired initiation of lactation.[4]

### Complementary Therapies for the Treatment of Amenorrhea

Herbalists may recommend blessed thistle or blue cohosh for the relief of amenorrhea, while acupuncture and homeopathic remedies have been suggested as other treatment modalities.[22] To date, no published, evidence-based investigations have addressed the safety of using these remedies, and their effectiveness has not been conclusively demonstrated.

## Abnormal or Atypical Uterine Bleeding

AUB is an overarching term for uterine bleeding that is atypical in frequency, duration, regularity, and/or volume.[6,7,24,26,27] AUB affects as many as 30% of menstruating individuals at some point between menarche and menopause.[7,24,26,27] This condition can be acute or chronic.

AUB is often subcategorized as demonstrating either an anovulatory or ovulatory pattern. Anovulatory AUB is associated with prolonged unopposed estrogen stimulation of the endometrium and subsequent irregular bleeding. PCOS, thyroid dysfunction, hyperprolactinemia, uncontrolled diabetes, and use of some medications are typical causes of anovulatory AUB. Anovulatory AUB is associated with an increased risk for endometrial cancer. Ovulatory AUB is associated with heavy menstrual bleeding and can be caused by thyroid dysfunction, coagulation defects, endometrial polyps, or submucosal uterine fibroids.[6,7,24,26-28]

In practice, AUB can present as a range of bleeding patterns that encompass more than one of these categories. For example, a person can experience heavy menstrual bleeding that is longer in duration and higher in volume than normal bleeding. Intermenstrual bleeding can be frequent and irregular. AUB also refers to any bleeding that occurs post menopause, as discussed in the *Menopause* chapter.

Similar to the causes associated with amenorrhea, the most common etiologies of AUB differ by age. In adolescents younger than 18 years, AUB is often the result of anovulation that occurs secondary to dysregulation of the HPO axis and can be a normal physiologic finding. The second most common cause of AUB in this age group is an inherited coagulopathy.[29] Between the ages of 19 and 39 years, pregnancy, leiomyomas, polyps, PCOS, and use of hormonal contraception are common causes of AUB.[30,31] In people 40 years and older, AUB can again be a symptom of the normal physiology of menopause, but can also be a symptom of endometrial hyperplasia, leiomyomas, or endometrial carcinoma.[26–28]

## A Newer Lexicon for Abnormal or Atypical Uterine Bleeding

Many terms have been used to define menstrual irregularities. The lack of a common nomenclature has hindered research and development of evidence-based treatments. In 2011, the International Federation of Gynecology and Obstetrics (FIGO) proposed a system, PALM-COEIN,[6,7,24] that recommended replacing the term "dysfunctional uterine bleeding" (DUB) with abnormal uterine bleeding (AUB), and

then adding a suffix to identify the proposed etiology. The PALM-COEIN nomenclature uses a classification system of structural and nonstructural causes followed by specific etiologies.[6,7,24] This terminology standardized the nomenclature and parameters for both normal uterine bleeding and AUB that occurs in reproductive-age individuals, based on the 5th to 95th percentiles identified in large epidemiologic studies.[6,7] System 1 of the FIGO recommendations describes the frequency, regularity, duration, and volume of uterine bleeding.[6] A recent update to the original work further categorizes the type of bleeding by including intermenstrual bleeding.[6] System 2 focuses on possible etiologies of uterine bleeding, with an update further clarifying and adding more diagnostic criteria to consider.[6] The PALM-COEIN nomenclature has been adopted as the standard, and outdated terms such as menorrhagia are no longer recommended to be used.[6,7,24,32] The widespread use of more precise language ultimately can facilitate both diagnostic efforts and health education/communication with patients. Table 15-6 summarizes the PALM-COEIN system.

| Table 15-6 | Abnormal Menstrual Bleeding Assessment Framework: PALM-COEIN | |
|---|---|---|
| **Terminology** | **Abbreviation** | **Description** |
| **PALM: Discrete Structural Entities Measurable Using Imaging Techniques and/or with Histopathology** | | |
| **P**olyp | AUB-P | Endometrial or endocervical polyps. |
| | | Categorized as present or absent, with no distinction regarding size or number. |
| **A**denomyosis | AUB-A | Disorder in which ectopic endometrial tissue (endometrial glands and stroma) are present in the uterine myometrium, which causes uterine myometrial hypertrophy and hyperplasia. |
| | | Clinical presentation is heavy menstrual bleeding and dysmenorrhea. |
| | | Adenomyosis is diagnosed via ultrasound or MRI. Subcategories based on diffuse versus focal or multifocal disease and volume have been proposed. |
| | | **Update: Refined ultrasound diagnostic criteria.** |
| **L**eiomyoma | AUB-L | Leiomyomatas (uterine fibroids) are fibromuscular tumors of the myometrium. |
| | | First subclassification: Present or absent. |
| | | Second subclassification: Submucosal (SM) or other (O). Submucosal is further categorized as 0: pedunculated intracavity; 1: < 50% intramural; 2: more than 50% intramural; 3: contacts endometrium, 100% intramural; 4: intramural; 5: subserosal > 50% intramural; 6: subserosal < 50% intramural; 7: subserosal pedunculated; and 8: cervical, parasitic, and other lesions not related to the myometrium. |
| | | Third subclassification: Used for hybrid lesions that describes the endometrial relationship first and the serosal relationship second, separated by a hyphen. |
| | | **Update: Further clarified types.** |
| **M**alignancy and hyperplasia | AUB-M | Endometrial intraepithelial neoplasia (atypical hyperplasia) and/or malignancy. |
| | | Subclassified by separate WHO and FIGO systems that stage malignancy based on histopathology and extent of the tumor. |

| Terminology | Abbreviation | Description |
|---|---|---|
| **COEI: Entities Not Defined by Imaging or Histopathology** | | |
| **C**oagulopathy | AUB-C | AUB secondary to a coagulopathy or systemic disorder that causes a coagulopathy. |
| | | Approximately 13% of individuals with heavy menstrual bleeding have von Willebrand's disease. |
| | | **Update: No longer includes pharmacologic agents that affect coagulation.** |
| **O**vulatory dysfunction | AUB-O | Disorders of ovulation can cause a spectrum of menstrual abnormalities that range from amenorrhea to heavy menstrual bleeding. Examples include PCOS, hypothyroidism, hyperprolactinemia, anorexia, extreme stress, gonadal steroids, and tricyclic antidepressants. |
| | | Otherwise unexplained ovulatory dysfunction can occur during adolescence and the menopause transition. |
| **E**ndometrial | AUB-E | AUB occurring within a predictable and cyclic menstrual cycle, such as prolonged bleeding. This indicates ovulation is occurring. If no other etiology is identified, the primary disorder is likely to be in the endometrium. |
| | | The etiology may be infection, or a combination of mechanisms that interfere with local production of vasoconstrictors (e.g., prostaglandin F), increased production of hormones that break down endometrial clots (e.g., plasminogen activator), and/or increased production of substances that promote vasodilation (e.g., prostacyclin). |
| **I**atrogenic | AUB-I | Many medical devices and medications can cause or contribute to AUB. Examples include intrauterine devices and warfarin (Coumadin). |
| | | AUB associated with estrogen and progestogen formulations administered continuously to induce amenorrhea is termed "break-through bleeding." |
| | | **Update: Now includes pharmacologic agents that affect coagulation.** |
| **Not Otherwise Classified** | | |
| **N**ot otherwise classified | AUB-N | Causes of AUB that are rare or whose role in causing AUB is not well defined. Examples include arteriovenous malformations and cesarean scar defects. |

Abbreviations: AUB, abnormal uterine bleeding; FIGO, International Organization of Gynecology and Obstetrics; MRI, magnetic resonance imaging; PCOS, polycystic ovary syndrome; WHO, World Health Organization.

Based on Munro MG, Critchley HO, Fraser IS, et al. The two FIGO systems for normal and abnormal uterine bleeding symptoms and classification of causes of abnormal uterine bleeding in the reproductive years: 2018 revisions. *Int J Gynaecol Obstet.* 2018;143(3):393-408.

## Evaluation of Abnormal and Atypical Uterine Bleeding

The initial steps in evaluating of AUB are listed in Table 15-7.[7,24,26,28,29,33] Medications associated with AUB are listed in **Table 15-8**. Because the list of differential diagnoses is extensive, the initial steps in the evaluation to assess for common etiologies of AUB first take into consideration three primary factors: (1) age (i.e., proximity to menarche or menopause), (2) whether the AUB pattern is indicative of ovulatory or anovulatory status, and (3) a priori risk for endometrial cancer.

For example, the physical examination for an adolescent will include assessment of sexual maturity and if the bleeding is heavy, signs of coagulopathy, but may not require a pelvic examination if the patient is not sexually active or is just recently past menarche. The risk of endometrial cancer is quite low in adolescence, whereas etiologies discernable via laboratory evaluation are more likely. In contrast, a pelvic ultrasound and possibly endometrial biopsy are always considered for postmenopausal individuals to rule out malignancy, which becomes much more likely as individuals age.

The choice of imaging studies or endometrial biopsy in the evaluation of AUB is also an example of how the evaluation of AUB differs on the basis of age, type of bleeding, and risk for endometrial cancer. Approximately 70% to 90% of those persons who develop endometrial cancer will have AUB. Risk factors for endometrial cancer that indicate a need for evaluation of the endometrium are

| Table 15-7 | Initial Evaluation of Abnormal Uterine Bleeding |
| --- | --- |

**A. Initial History and Assessment**

1. Determine if the bleeding is acute or chronic. Individuals who have acute vaginal bleeding or are hemodynamically unstable should be immediately referred for emergent care.

2. If chronic, establish the clinical impact that AUB has on activities of life.

   Assess for iron deficiency and symptoms of anemia

3. Assess for pregnancy: Pregnancy-related bleeding can present as any degree of bleeding, from light spotting to menstrual-like flow. The latter underscores the importance of considering pregnancy for all reproductive-age women who present with AUB.

4. Review health history using the PALM-COEIN system to focus on possible etiologies.

   Menstrual history:

   > Age of menarche and menopause

   > Detailed history of frequency, duration, predictability, amount of bleeding, interval, relation of AUB to normal menstrual cycle, associated symptoms

   Sexual and reproductive history: Assess use of contraception, STIs, infertility, possible pregnancy.

   Symptoms associated with a systemic cause of AUB, such as obesity, PCOS, hypothyroidism, hyperprolactinemia, or adrenal disorder

   Chronic medical illness that might cause a coagulopathy, such as liver disease, renal disease, inherited bleeding disorders, systemic lupus erythematosus

   Medication history: medications associated with AUB are listed in Table 15-8.

   Family history of bleeding disorders or individuals with "heavy periods," or thromboembolic disorders, or hormone-sensitive cancers

   Surgical history: especially obstetric or gynecologic surgery

**B. Physical Examination**

A complete physical examination with attention focused on the following components:

   Vital signs, body mass index, blood pressure

Skin should be assessed for signs of:

   Coagulation disorder: Pallor, bruising, bleeding gums, petechiae, swollen joints

   Hyperandrogenism: Hirsutism, acne, male-pattern baldness

   Insulin resistance: Acanthosis nigricans on neck

Thyroid examination

Abdominal assessment for tenderness, distention, and palpable masses

Gynecologic examination:

1. Origin of the bleeding: Bleeding that originates from the cervix, vagina, external genitalia, urinary tract, or rectum can appear different from uterine bleeding in volume, color, quality, and timing.

2. External genitalia should be examined for signs of trauma, lesions, hemorrhoids, or infection.

3. Speculum examination to identify sources of bleeding outside of the uterus such as a cervical polyp, cervicitis, or vaginal laceration.

4. A bimanual pelvic examination to assess the uterus and adnexa for tenderness, size, and/or palpable masses

**C. Laboratory Tests**

Initial laboratory testing for all types of AUB:

   Complete blood count with platelets

   Pregnancy test

   Thyroid-stimulating hormone

Transvaginal ultrasound to assess pelvic structures and endometrial thickness is usually included in a standard evaluation of reproductive-age and postmenopausal people, but may not be necessary for adolescents near menarche.

| **C. Laboratory Tests** |
| --- |
| Additional laboratory testing as indicated: |
|    Endocrine disorders: Follicle-stimulating hormone, luteinizing hormone, estradiol, progesterone level (obtained 22–24 days in menstrual cycle), free testosterone level, prolactin level |
|    Coagulation abnormalities: Coagulation profile or von Willebrand diagnostic panel |
|    STI: Chlamydia, wet mount of vaginal discharge, vaginal culture |
|    Cervical cancer screening |
| Additional tests as indicated: |
|    Endometrial biopsy to evaluate the endometrium |
|    Hysteroscopy |
|    Magnetic resonance imaging |

Abbreviations: AUB, abnormal uterine bleeding; PCOS, polycystic ovary syndrome; STI, sexually transmitted infection.

Based on Munro MG. Practical aspects of the two FIGO systems for management of abnormal uterine bleeding in the reproductive years. *Best Pract Res Clin Obstet Gynaecol.* 2017;40:3-22; Munro M, Critchley H, Fraser I. Research and clinical management for women with abnormal uterine bleeding in the reproductive years: more than PALM-COEIN. *BJOG.* 2017;124(2):185-189; Khafaga A, Goldstein SR. Abnormal uterine bleeding. *Obstet Gynecol Clin North Am.* 2019;46(4):595-605. doi:10.1016/j.ogc.2019.07.001; Marnach ML, Laughlin-Tommaso SK. Evaluation and management of abnormal uterine bleeding. *Mayo Clin Proc.* 2019;94(2):326-335. doi:10.1016/j.mayocp.2018.12.012; Wouk N, Helton M. Abnormal uterine bleeding in premenopausal women. *Am Fam Physician.* 2019;99(7):435-443; American College of Nurse-Midwives. Clinical Bulletin No. 15: abnormal uterine bleeding. *J Midwifery Womens Health.* 2016;61:522-527.

listed in Table 15-9.[34] Evidence of an endometrial stripe larger than 4.0 mm on ultrasound suggests the possibility of endometrial hyperplasia or carcinoma, and is an indication for further investigations such as endometrial biopsy and possibly surgical treatment such as endometrial curettage.[34–36] Endometrial biopsy is an office procedure that can be performed by midwives who have received training in the technique. This procedure is described in the *Endometrial Biopsy* appendix.

Trauma and subsequent bleeding from genital lacerations is one of the differential diagnoses to be considered with AUB. Intimate-partner violence or sexual assault requires a more extensive assessment, and should involve consultation or referral to a community center or a professional experienced in working with individuals who have experienced assault or abuse (e.g., a rape crisis center or a sexual assault nurse examiner [SANE]).[34] Depending on the local laws that govern such cases, the midwife may also be legally required to report suspicion, or confirmation, of abuse. Most importantly, the midwife should initiate safety and support mechanisms. Referral to a surgeon may be necessary if anatomic damage is identified that appears to require surgery or extensive treatment.

## Management of Abnormal or Atypical Uterine Bleeding

After common menstrual changes, pregnancy, infection, trauma, and malignancy have been ruled out,

interventions for AUB will vary based on the following initial considerations:

- Specific etiology
- Bleeding severity
- Associated symptoms such as pain or infertility
- Reproductive planning: desire for contraception and plans for pregnancy
- Medical comorbidities
- Individual preferences with consideration of side effects of possible treatments

Furthermore, effective treatments can be either surgical or medical. For example, infection can be treated with antibiotics and leiomyomata can be treated with hormonal contraceptives or surgical resection. Therefore, when offering treatment for AUB, the patient's age, desire for pregnancy, and degree of bleeding factor into the management plan. Individuals with heavy menstrual bleeding secondary to leiomyomata who want to become pregnant may choose surgical therapy to preserve fertility, whereas those who do not want to become pregnant can treat this condition with contraceptives that decrease menstrual bleeding.

In general, indications for treatment of AUB include heavy menstrual bleeding and AUB with ovulatory dysfunction (AUB-O). Anemia should be treated with iron supplementation regardless of the type of bleeding.

| Table 15-8 | Selected Drugs That Can Cause Abnormal or Atypical Uterine Bleeding |
|---|---|
| **Drug Category** | **Drugs: Generic (Brand)** |
| Analgesics | Aspirin |
| | Nonsteroidal anti-inflammatory drugs (NSAIDs) |
| Anticoagulants | Warfarin |
| | Heparin |
| Anticonvulsant | Valproic acid |
| Antibiotics | Rifampin |
| | Griseofulvin |
| Antidepressants | Selective serotonin reuptake inhibitors (SSRIs)[a] |
| Antiemetics | Metoclopramide (Reglan)[a] |
| | Prochlorperazine (Compazine)[a] |
| Antipsychotics | Phenothiazines (e.g., thioridazine, chlorpromazine, risperidone)[a] |
| | Tricyclic antidepressants (e.g., amitriptyline[a]) |
| Corticosteroids | Prednisone |
| | Dexamethasone |
| Herbal supplements | Ginseng, ginkgo, motherwort |
| Hormonal contraceptives | Combined oral contraceptives: transdermal, vaginal, injectable Progestin-only pills |
| | Levonorgestrel-releasing intrauterine device |
| Menopausal hormone therapy | Estrogen, progesterone, androgens and combination formulations |
| Opioids | Methadone[a] |
| | Morphine[a] |
| Selective estrogen receptor modulators | Tamoxifen |

Abbreviation: AUB, abnormal uterine bleeding.

[a] Prolactin secretion from the pituitary is normally suppressed by dopamine. Any drug that blocks dopamine receptors can cause hyperprolactinemia, which can then cause ovulatory dysfunction and AUB.

Based on Taylor HS, Pall L, Seli E. *Speroff's Clinical Gynecologic Endocrinology and Infertility*. 9th ed. Philadelphia, PA: Wolters Kluwer; 2020; Munro M, Critchley H, Fraser I. Research and clinical management for women with abnormal uterine bleeding in the reproductive years: more than PALM-COEIN. *BJOG*. 2017;124(2):185-18925; Munro MG, Critchley HO, Broder MS, Fraser IS. The FIGO classification system (PALM-COEIN) for causes of abnormal uterine bleeding in the non-gravid reproductive years including guidelines for clinical investigation. *Int J Gynaecol Obstet*. 2011;113:3-13; Munro MG. Practical aspects of the two FIGO systems for management of abnormal uterine bleeding in the reproductive years. *Best Pract Res Clin Obstet Gynaecol*. 2017;40:3-22.

| Table 15-9 | Risk Factors for Endometrial Cancer That Require Evaluation of the Endometrium[a] |
|---|---|
| **Age** | **Indication for Evaluation of the Endometrium** |
| Postmenopausal | Any bleeding, staining, or spotting |
| 45 years to menopause | Any AUB, including intermenstrual bleeding, heavy menstrual bleeding, prolonged bleeding |
| 19–45 years | Prolonged period of amenorrhea |
| | Any AUB with conditions associated with unopposed estrogen exposure |
| | AUB that is persistent in the presence of: |
| | Chronic anovulation |
| | Unsuccessful medical management of bleeding |
| | Lynch syndrome |

Abbreviation: AUB, abnormal uterine bleeding.

[a] Additional risk factors not related to AUB include abnormal cervical cytology results and monitoring of patients with endocervical hyperplasia.

Based on Munro MG. Practical aspects of the two FIGO systems for management of abnormal uterine bleeding in the reproductive years. *Best Pract Res Clin Obstet Gynaecol*. 2017;40:3-22; Khafaga A, Goldstein SR. Abnormal uterine bleeding. *Obstet Gynecol Clin North Am*. 2019;46(4):595-605. doi:10.1016/j.ogc.2019.07.001; Marnach ML, Laughlin-Tommaso SK. Evaluation and management of abnormal uterine bleeding. *Mayo Clin Proc*. 2019;94(2):326-335. doi:10.1016/j.mayocp.2018.12.012.

## Heavy Menstrual Bleeding

Heavy menstrual bleeding (HMB) is defined as excessive bleeding, either in amount or in duration, at the regular interval of normal menstruation and, by definition, presumes the person is ovulatory. HMB should be treated if it is interfering with the person's quality of life or when it causes anemia. The most common etiologies of HMB during the reproductive years are leiomyomata and adenomyosis. The goal of treatment is to reduce the volume of menstrual flow, correct anemia, and prevent cancer.

The first-line therapies for HMB are monophasic low-dose combined oral contraceptives or levonorgestrel-releasing intrauterine devices (LNG-IUD).[24,27,28,31,33,35,37] Combined oral contraceptives have been shown to reduce menstrual blood loss by 35% to 69%.[37]

The choice between combined oral contraceptives and the LNG-IUD is based on the presence or absence of contraindications to estrogens and personal preference. Combined oral contraceptives will induce a regular withdrawal bleed, while the LNG-IUD is associated with irregular bleeding in the first months that then progresses to amenorrhea.

While the typical treatment algorithm calls for combined oral contraceptives to be prescribed in the same manner as when they are used for contraception, evidence suggests that extended or continuous usage may be a more effective approach for treating HMB.[37] This approach facilitates stabilization of the endometrium and offers a brief respite from the previously experienced excessive bleeding. Injection of depot medroxyprogesterone acetate (DMPA) is also effective. The progesterone formulations are associated with irregular bleeding, headaches, and weight gain in some individuals, but ultimately these agents will result in amenorrhea. Amenorrhea or menstrual suppression can improve the quality of life for some individuals, especially trans men. Additional information about menstrual suppression can be found in the *Hormonal Contraception* chapter.

If combined oral contraceptives, the LNG-IUD, or DMPA are not acceptable or are contraindicated, physician consultation is generally recommended. Other effective treatments for HMB include progesterone, GnRH agonists, nonsteroidal anti-inflammatory drugs (NSAIDs), danazol, a synthetic steroid that suppresses HPO axis activity, and tranexamic acid. Progestin-only oral contraceptives and hormonal contraceptive implants are not effective for treating HMB. However, orally administered progesterone in higher doses can be effective if used continuously for 21 days.

GnRH agonists (e.g., leuprolide) affect the HPO axis, hindering the ability of the ovaries to release the hormones required for normal function of the menstrual cycle. Interfering with cyclic menstruation causes the person to enter a physiologic state resembling menopause. However, because of the bone mass loss associated with the decrease in estrogen levels and vasomotor menopausal symptoms, use of these medications tends to be limited to persons for whom other therapies have been unsuccessful, and may be best managed by a practitioner specializing in gynecologic disorders.[1] Prolonged treatment using GnRH agonists requires bone density monitoring.

Reduction of HMB occurs in those who are taking NSAIDs, due to the ability of these medications to block the synthesis of prostaglandins necessary for cyclic endometrial sloughing.[4] However, NSAID therapy is not always effective and can cause gastrointestinal bleeding with long-term use; in other individuals, NSAID use can result in increased vaginal bleeding due to inhibition of platelet aggregation and prolongation of bleeding time. When using combined oral contraceptives, NSAIDs may be taken at the time of menstruation, and patients may benefit from the combination of these medications.

Danazol, a synthetic steroid, has been successful in controlling HMB in some individuals, although it requires daily dosage for 3 to 6 months, given as 100 mg orally twice a day, during which time a state of amenorrhea is likely to occur. Significant androgenic side effects, including weight gain, acne, and seborrhea, are common with use of this medication, and the availability of other treatments has resulted in danazol no longer being the first choice of treatment for HMB.

### Complementary Therapies

Some observational studies have produced findings that support the treatment of HMB with traditional Chinese medicines and acupuncture, as well as with the use of herbal, homeopathic, and aromatherapy remedies. Nevertheless, there is insufficient evidence to support use of nonpharmacologic methods at this time.

### Treatment for Abnormal or Atypical Uterine Bleeding–Ovulatory Dysfunction

If AUB is not HMB but is suspected to result from an ovulatory dysfunction (AUB-O), the person can present with irregular erratic bleeding that can vary from light to heavy. The underlying etiology in this situation is that lack of ovulation prevents the development of a corpus luteum and the ovaries do not secrete progesterone. The lack of progesterone affects the uterine endometrium so that it continues to proliferate without progesterone withdrawal–induced shedding. Thus, the bleeding is irregular in timing and amount.

After malignancy has been ruled out, the choice of treatment with progestin, estrogen, or a combination of the two has historically depended on the type of bleeding. In general, infrequent menses has been treated first with progestin, while irregular bleeding has been treated initially with estrogen.[4] However, combination hormonal contraceptives are effective in controlling a number of menstrual disorders. Thus, many clinicians use combined oral contraceptives or another combined hormonal method as the first-line treatment, especially if there is no objection to the use of contraception. With each monthly withdrawal cycle while on the combined hormonal methods, bleeding and cramping should decrease.

# Dysmenorrhea

Painful menstruation, particularly with pain in the lower abdomen and back and typically of a cramping nature, is known as *dysmenorrhea*. Dysmenorrhea is usually associated with regular, predictable menses. In the United States, this condition is experienced by 60% to 91% of menstruating adults.[4,38] Dysmenorrhea that occurs in the absence of other disease is termed *primary dysmenorrhea*. Dysmenorrhea that is caused by a disorder such as endometriosis or leiomyomata is termed *secondary dysmenorrhea*.

In distinguishing dysmenorrhea from other causes of pelvic pain, it is important to establish this pain as cyclic in nature, coinciding with the onset of menses and resolving after cessation of the menstrual flow. Primary dysmenorrhea is typically recurrent, is crampy, and can radiate to the back or thighs. It can be accompanied by nausea, fatigue, and general malaise. Primary dysmenorrhea generally starts just before the onset of menses and lasts 2 or 3 days.

The principal cause of primary dysmenorrhea is the presence of prostaglandins that are released from the endometrium at the beginning of menses. These prostaglandins induce uterine contractions, which result in uterine ischemia and accumulation of metabolites that stimulate pain nerves (Figure 15-2).[36,38] Primary dysmenorrhea usually begins in adolescence after ovulatory cycles are established. Pain can be mild to severe and generally improves as the individual ages.

## Evaluation of Dysmenorrhea

The evaluation of dysmenorrhea focuses on excluding the presence of disorders that can cause cramping uterine pain.[38,39] Although endometriosis is the most common cause of secondary dysmenorrhea, other etiologies include pregnancy, an IUD in place, pelvic inflammatory disease, adenomyosis, ovarian cysts, pelvic adhesions, and cervical stenosis. Nongynecologic causes include inflammatory bowel disease and irritable bowel syndrome.

## Treatment of Primary Dysmenorrhea

The goal when treating primary dysmenorrhea is to relieve pain. Application of local heat to the abdomen has demonstrated effectiveness that in some individuals is equal to the relief achieved after taking ibuprofen.[38–40] The first-line pharmacologic agents recommended are NSAIDs because these drugs inhibit prostaglandin synthesis.[36,38] Given that no one NSAID is more effective than the others, the choice of agent depends on individual preference and tolerability, as these drugs are associated with some adverse effects. The medications should be taken for 2 to 3 days beginning on the first day of symptoms on a fixed schedule to maximize effectiveness.

The primary adverse effect of NSAIDs is gastrointestinal distress, but these agents are also (albeit less frequently) associated with peptic ulcer, renal injury, hepatotoxicity, and bronchospasm in persons with asthma. Furthermore, these agents induce several drug interactions. Therefore, before prescribing an NSAID that will be taken on a regular basis, a

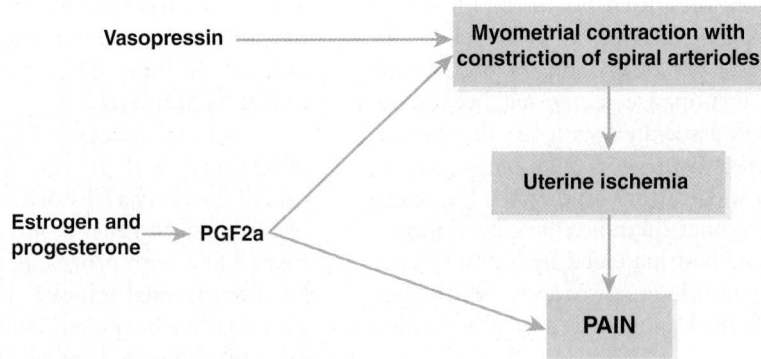

The prostaglandin PGF2a stimulates myometrial contraction and sensitizes the afferent nerves to pain, thereby contributing to dysmenorrhea in two ways.

**Figure 15-2** Pathophysiology of primary dysmenorrhea.
Reproduced from Durain D, McCool WF. Pelvic and menstrual disorders. In: Brucker MC, King TL. *Pharmacology for Women's Health*. 2nd ed. Burlington, MA: Jones & Bartlett Learning; 2017: 901-928.

review of the person's health and current medications is needed. Although acetylsalicylic acid (aspirin), another NSAID, has also been found to offer some relief from dysmenorrhea, there is no evidence that the non-NSAID analgesic acetaminophen is beneficial in eliminating menstrual pain.[36,38]

If dysmenorrhea persists, consideration of alternative therapies can become necessary. Because combined hormonal contraceptives decrease prostaglandin synthesis and menstrual flow, these drugs are frequently used on an off-label basis for the treatment of dysmenorrhea.[41] In addition, the various progestin-only methods of contraception (injectable DMPA, progestin-only oral contraceptives, LNG-IUDs, and etonogestrel-containing implants) often result in temporary states of amenorrhea due to decreased endometrial stimulation. In turn, these methods can result in less dysmenorrhea.[41,42]

Several nonpharmaceutical approaches to the treatment of dysmenorrhea have been widely advocated. Among them are the application of local heat in the form of small heat packs continuously applied to the abdomen, homeopathy (e.g., belladonna, chamomilla, cinnamon), acupuncture, biofeedback, dietary supplements, relaxation techniques, massage, exercise, aromatherapy (e.g., rose oil), and the use of certain herbs (e.g., black cohosh, raspberry leaf, shakuyaku-kanzo-to, semen coicis, and chaste berry).[43–49] Complementary therapies offer varying degrees of relief and can be included in a multimodal approach to relieving dysmenorrhea.

## Conclusion

Menstrual cycle alterations are a common reason for seeking healthcare services, and their assessment requires a sensitive and thorough approach. Exploring the individual's sense of reproductive or hormonal well-being or normalcy can often be achieved by taking a comprehensive history of the menstrual pattern and examining attitudes and beliefs about the significance of, and even need for, cyclic bleeding. Treatment of menstrual abnormalities can positively influence a person's long-term health well beyond the specific change appreciated by the person at the outset of care. This aspect of health care calls upon midwives' expertise as primary and gynecologic care clinicians who are concerned with the entirety of an individual's health.

## References

1. Critchley HOD, Babayev E, Bulun SE, et al. Menstruation: science and society. *Am J Obstet Gynecol.* 2020;223(5):624-664. doi:10.1016/j.ajog.2020.06.004.

2. Schoep ME, Nieboer TE, van der Zanden M, et al. The impact of menstrual symptoms on everyday life: a survey among 42,879 women. *Am J Obstet Gynecol.* 2019;220(6);569.e1-569.e7. doi:10.1016/j.ajog.2019.02.048.

3. Casola A, Kunes B, Jefferson K, Riley A. Menstrual health stigma in the United States: communication complexities and implications for theory and practice. *J Midwifery Womens Health.* 2021;66(6);725-728.

4. Taylor HS, Pall L, Seli, E. Speroff's *Clinical Gynecologic Endocrinology and Infertility.* 9th ed. Philadelphia, PA: Wolters Kluwer; 2020.

5. American College of Obstetricians and Gynecologists. Committee Opinion No. 651: menstruation in girls and adolescents: using the menstrual cycle as a vital sign. *Obstet Gynecol.* 2015;126:e143-e146. [Reaffirmed 2021].

6. Munro MG, Critchley HO, Fraser IS, et al. The two FIGO systems for normal and abnormal uterine bleeding symptoms and classification of causes of abnormal uterine bleeding in the reproductive years: 2018 revisions. *Int J Gynaecol Obstet.* 2018;143(3):393-408.

7. Munro MG. Practical aspects of the two FIGO systems for management of abnormal uterine bleeding in the reproductive years. *Best Pract Res Clin Obstet Gynaecol.* 2017;40:3-22.

8. Klein DA, Paradise SL, Reeder RM. Amenorrhea: a systematic approach to diagnosis and management. *Am Fam Physician.* 2019;100(1):39-48. PMID: 31259490.

9. American College of Obstetricians and Gynecologists. Committee Opinion 605: primary ovarian insufficiency in adolescents and young women. *Obstet Gynecol.* 2014;123:193-197. [Reaffirmed 2016].

10. Gibson ME, Fleming N, Zuijdwijk C, Dumont T. Where have the periods gone? The evaluation and management of functional hypothalamic amenorrhea. *J Clin Res Pediatr Endocrinol.* 2020;12(suppl 1):18-27. doi:10.4274/jcrpe.galenos.2019.2019.S0178.

11. Huhmann K. Menses requires energy: a review of how disordered eating, excessive exercise, and high stress lead to menstrual irregularities. *Clin Ther.* 2020;42(3):401-407. doi:10.1016/j.clinthera.2020.01.016.

12. Ackerman KE, Misra M. Amenorrhoea in adolescent female athletes. *Lancet Child Adolesc Health.* 2018;2(9):677-688. doi:10.1016/S2352-4642(18)30145-7.

13. Moltich M. Diagnosis and treatment of pituitary adenomas. *JAMA.* 2017;317(5):516-524.

14. Thein-Nussenbaum J, Hammer E. Treatment strategies for the female athlete triad in the adolescent athlete: current perspectives. *Open Access J Sports Med.* 2017;8:85-95.

15. Gordon CM, Ackerman KE, Berga SL, et al. Functional hypothalamic amenorrhea: an Endocrine Society clinical practice guideline. *J Clin Endocrinol Metab* 2017;102:1413.

16. Komorowska B. Autoimmune premature ovarian failure. *Menopause Rev.* 2016;15(4):210-214.

17. Ferreira SR, Motta AB. Uterine function: from normal to polycystic ovary syndrome alterations. *Curr Med Chem.* 2017. doi:10.2174/0929867325666171205144119.

18. Azziz R. Polycystic ovary syndrome. *Obstet Gynecol.* 2018;132(2):321-336. doi:10.1097/AOG.0000000000002698.

19. Hoeger KM, Dokras A, Piltonen T. Update on PCOS: consequences, challenges, and guiding treatment. *J Clin Endocrinol Metab.* 2021;106(3):e1071-e1083. doi:10.1210/clinem/dgaa839.

20. Dumesic DA, Oberfield SE, Stener-Victorin E, et al. Scientific statement on the diagnostic criteria, epidemiology, pathophysiology, and molecular genetics of polycystic ovary syndrome. *Endocr Rev.* 2015;36(5):487-525.

21. Rosenfield RL. The diagnosis of polycystic ovary syndrome in adolescents. *Pediatrics.* 2015;136:1154-1158.

22. Lim C, Ng RWC, Xu K, et al. Acupuncture for polycystic ovarian syndrome. *Cochrane Database Syst Rev.* 2016;5:CD007689. doi:10.1002/14651858.CD007689.pub3.

23. American College of Obstetricians and Gynecologists. Practice Bulletin No. 136: management of abnormal uterine bleeding associated with ovulatory dysfunction. *Obstet Gynecol.* 2013;122:176-185. [Reaffirmed 2016].

24. Munro M, Critchley H, Fraser I. Research and clinical management for women with abnormal uterine bleeding in the reproductive years: more than PALM-COEIN. *BJOG.* 2017;124(2):185-189.

25. Dokras A. Noncontraceptive use of oral combined hormonal contraceptives in polycystic ovary syndrome: risks versus benefits. *Fertil Steril.* 2016;106(7):1572-1579.

26. National Institute for Health and Care Excellence. Heavy menstrual bleeding: assessment and management (NG88). https:www.nice.org.uk/guidance/ng88. Last updated May 24, 2021. Accessed March 30, 2023.

27. Khafaga A, Goldstein SR. Abnormal uterine bleeding. *Obstet Gynecol Clin North Am.* 2019;46(4):595-605. doi:10.1016/j.ogc.2019.07.001.

28. Marnach ML, Laughlin-Tommaso SK. Evaluation and management of abnormal uterine bleeding. *Mayo Clin Proc.* 2019;94(2):326-335. doi:10.1016/j.mayocp.2018.12.012.

29. Borzutzky C, Jaffray J. Diagnosis and management of heavy menstrual bleeding and bleeding disorders in adolescents. *JAMA Pediatr.* 2020;174(2):186-194. doi:10.1001/jamapediatrics.2019.5040.

30. Wouk N, Helton M. Abnormal uterine bleeding in premenopausal women. *Am Fam Physician.* 2019;99(7):435-443.

31. Bacon JL. Abnormal uterine bleeding: current classification and clinical management. *Obstet Gynecol Clin North Am.* 2017;44(2):179-193.

32. Deneris A. PALM-COEIN nomenclature for abnormal uterine bleeding. *J Midwifery Womens Health.* 2016;61(3):376-379.

33. American College of Nurse-Midwives. Clinical Bulletin No. 15: abnormal uterine bleeding. *J Midwifery Womens Health.* 2016;61:522-527.

34. Adams P, Hulton L. The sexual assault nurse examiner's interactions within the sexual assault response team: a systematic review. *Adv Emerg Nurs J.* 2016;38(3):213-227.

35. Jewson M, Purohit P, Lumsden MA. Progesterone and abnormal uterine bleeding/menstrual disorders. *Best Pract Res Clin Obstet Gynaecol.* 2020;69:62e73. https://doi.org/10.1016/j.bpobgyn.2020.05.004.

36. Durain D, McCool WF. Pelvic and menstrual disorders. In: Brucker MC, King TL. *Pharmacology for Women's Health.* 2nd ed. Burlington, MA: Jones & Bartlett Learning; 2017:901-928.

37. Heikinheimo O, Fraser I. The current status of hormonal therapies for heavy menstrual bleeding. *Best Pract Res Clin Obstet Gynaecol.* 2017;40:111e-120e.

38. Ferries-Rowe E, Corey E, Archer J. Primary dysmenorrhea: diagnosis and therapy. *Obstet Gynecol,* 2020;136(5):1047-1058. doi:10.1097/AOG.0000000000004096.

39. Tsonis O, Gkrozou F, Barmpalia Z, et al. Integrating lifestyle focused approaches into the management of primary dysmenorrhea: impact on quality of life. *Int J Womens Health.* 2021;13:327-336. doi:10.2147/IJWH.S264023.

40. Song JA, Lee MK, Min E, et al. Effects of aromatherapy on dysmenorrhea: a systematic review and meta-analysis. *Int J Nurs Stud.* 2018;84:1-11. doi:10.1016/j.ijnurstu.2018.01.016.

41. Marjoribanks J, Ayeleke RO, Farquhar C, Proctor M. Nonsteroidal anti-inflammatory drugs for dysmenorrhea. *Cochrane Database Syst Rev.* 2015;7:CD001751. doi:10.1002/14651858.CD001751.pub3.

42. Yonkers KA, Simoni MK. Premenstrual disorders. *Am J Obstet Gynecol.* 2018;218(1):68-74. doi:10.1016/j.ajog.2017.05.045.

43. Jahangirifara M, Taebib M, Dolatianc M. The effect of cinnamon on primary dysmenorrhea: a randomized, double blind clinical trial. *Complement Ther Clin Pract.* 2018;33:56-60. https://doi.org/10.1016/j.ctcp.2018.08.001.

44. Pattanittum P, Kunyanone N, Brown J, et al. Dietary supplements for dysmenorrhea. *Cochrane Database Syst Rev.* 2016;3:CD002124. doi:10.1002/14651858.CD002124.pub2.

45. Uysal M, Doru HY, Sapmaz E, et al. Investigating the effect of rose essential oil in patients with primary dysmenorrhea. *Complement Ther Clin Pract.* 2016;24:45-49.

46. Hong GY, Shin BC, Park SN, et al. Randomized controlled trial of the efficacy and safety of self-adhesive low-level light therapy in women with primary dysmenorrhea. *Int J Gynecol Obstet.* 2016;133(1):37-42.

47. Lee HW, Jun JH, Kil K-J, et al. Herbal medicine (Danggui Shaoyao San) for treating primary dysmenorrhea: a systematic review and meta-analysis of randomized controlled trials. *Maturitas.* 2016;85:19-26.

48. Sut N, Kahyaoglu-Sut H. Effect of aromatherapy massage on pain in primary dysmenorrhea: a meta-analysis. *Complement Ther Clin Pract.* 2017;27:5-10.

49. Smith CA, Armour M, Zhu X, et al. Acupuncture for dysmenorrhea. *Cochrane Database Syst Rev.* 2016;4:CD007854. doi:10.1002/14651858.CD007854.pub3.

# APPENDIX

# 15A

# Endometrial Biopsy

AMI GOLDSTEIN

*The editors acknowledge Wendy Grube and William F. McCool, who were authors of this appendix in the previous edition.*

Endometrial biopsy (EMB) using a flexible plastic device is a cost-effective, safe, and simple method of collecting a histologic sample of the uterine endometrium. A number of clinical circumstances can require investigation of the endometrium, especially among individuals who experience abnormal uterine bleeding (AUB) that might be associated with premalignant hyperplasia or carcinoma. The risk of uterine perforation associated with EMB is less than the risk of uterine perforation associated with dilatation and curettage (D & C) (0.1–0.2% versus 0.3–2.6%, respectively.)[1] The diagnostic D & C is no longer considered the "gold standard" for this purpose due to the associated surgical risks, need for anesthesia, and cost.[1,2] The evolution of sampling devices such as the Pipelle has allowed EMB to be easily accomplished in an office setting by providers.

The specificity of EMB has been noted to be 100% for detection of endometrial carcinoma and hyperplasia in postmenopausal individuals, with sensitivities of 90% and 82%, respectively.[2] The sensitivity limitations are primarily due to the limited surface area of the uterine lining that is capable of being sampled via EMB devices. Combining transvaginal ultrasonography and sonohysterography with EMB can assist with the identification of structural abnormalities such as polyps as well as location of focal pathology. When evaluating postmenopausal individuals with bleeding, ultrasonography should be done prior to EMB to avoid artifacts on imaging.[2]

## Indications

1. Postmenopausal individuals with any uterine bleeding

2. AUB in individuals older than 45 years, or individuals at any age if AUB has not been controlled with appropriate medications

3. Thickened endometrium (> 4 mm) noted on transvaginal ultrasound of the uterus in the sagittal position

4. Atypical glandular cells (endometrial or other) found in cervical cytology sampling

5. Individuals at high risk for endometrial cancer, such as those on tamoxifen therapy, those with a history of Lynch syndrome, and those who have undergone treatment for endometrial cancer with uterus-sparing therapy

6. Assessment of adverse pregnancy outcomes that can be secondary to chronic subclinical endometritis

## Contraindications

1. Pregnancy

2. Known or suspected cervical cancer

3. Coagulopathy

4. Inability to visualize cervical os

5. Obstructing cervical lesion

## Relative Contraindications Requiring Consultation

1. Infection of the vagina, cervix, or uterus requires evaluation and treatment prior to EMB procedure

2. Use of medications that can alter clotting—requires consultation with a healthcare

provider who is knowledgeable in hematologic disorders

3. Fever (temperature > 38°C [100.4°F]) at the time of the procedure

4. Severe cervical stenosis or atypical uterine anatomy

## Potential Side Effects, Complications, and Preventive Measures

1. Cramping, uterine spasm, and vasovagal response are the most common side effects associated with this procedure. Prophylactic analgesia with 600–800 mg ibuprofen (Advil) administered 60 minutes prior to the procedure is recommended. In addition, individuals should be encouraged to eat prior to the procedure to avoid symptoms of hypoglycemia.

2. Uterine perforation. The following steps decrease the risk of uterine perforation:

   a. Make certain that the individual is not pregnant or has a well-involuted postpartum uterus.

   b. Perform a thorough pelvic examination prior to the procedure to note the uterine and cervical size, position, and angulation, as well as any structural abnormalities.

   c. Use a tenaculum to straighten the utero-cervical angle if the uterus is not close to axial in position. Tenaculum use can increase pain experience during this procedure and could be avoided by having the individual Valsalva during Pipelle insertion.[2–4]

3. Uterine infection, pelvic infection, and bacteremia.

4. Excessive uterine bleeding is rare but may occur if the individual has an undiagnosed coagulopathy.

## Procedure

1. Obtain informed consent.

2. If the purpose for obtaining the sample is confirmation of ovulation or diagnosis of luteal-phase defects, schedule the procedure for day 22 or 23 of the menstrual cycle. Timing is not important if the sampling is being performed to detect cancer or its precursors.

3. Gather equipment needed for the procedure:[1–3]

   a. Nonsterile and sterile gloves

   b. Vaginal speculum of appropriate size

   c. Ring forceps and cotton balls or large cotton swabs

   d. Antiseptic solution (such as Betadine or Hibiclens)

   e. Topical anesthetic such as Benzocaine gel 20% (Hurricane) or 2% lidocaine

   f. Scissors

   g. Labeled specimen containers with 10% formalin

   h. Endometrial sampling devices (make certain there are at least two available)

   i. Tenaculum

   A sample tray for endometrial biopsy is shown in **Figure 15A-1**.

4. Thoroughly review the individual's health history, including the date of last menses, contraception and possibility of pregnancy, risk of sexually transmitted infection (STI), known bleeding disorder, medication or supplement use, and allergies. Based on this information, contraindications can emerge that preclude performance of the procedure, or additional testing prior to the EMB can be necessary such as a pregnancy test, STI diagnostic testing, saline or potassium hydroxide (KOH) slide tests, or a complete blood count.

5. Provide education and instruction regarding the procedure, side effects, and possible adverse effects of EMB. Informed consent must be obtained before proceeding.

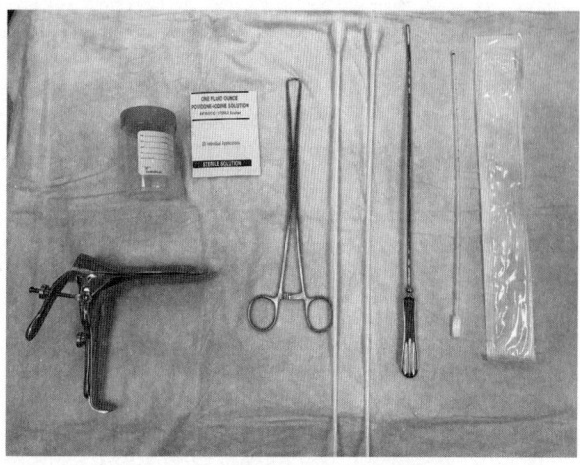

**Figure 15A-1** Sample tray for endometrial biopsy.

6. Offer a nonsteroidal anti-inflammatory drug (NSAID) as an oral agent to decrease cramping and uterine spasm associated with the procedure.

7. Assist the individual to assume a lithotomy position. Using nonsterile gloves, perform a bimanual and rectovaginal examination (if needed) to verify uterine and cervical position, angle, and structure to ensure that the curette can be placed in the appropriate direction and to minimize the risk of uterine perforation.

8. Insert the appropriately sized speculum.

9. Apply antiseptic solution to the cervix with a large cotton swab or cotton ball.

10. Apply topical anesthetic (e.g., Benzocaine gel 20%) to the anterior lip of the cervix and into the os with a small cotton swab to lessen the pain associated with the curette or tenaculum. If additional pain reduction is indicated, 5 mL of 2% lidocaine can be instilled into the endometrial cavity through a small catheter.[1,2]

11. If a tenaculum is needed, place the tenaculum on the anterior aspect of the cervix, and gently pull the device to straighten the utero-cervical angle. An assistant can be asked to hold the tenaculum and thereby maintain this angle.

12. Change to sterile gloves, and remove the curette (the outer sheath and inner piston) from the sterile package as instructed on the package insert.

13. With the piston fully inserted into the sheath, gently introduce the curette through the cervical os and into the uterine cavity until resistance is felt (**Figure 15A-2**). If strong resistance is encountered prior to reaching the fundus, stop the procedure.

14. If there is difficulty advancing the device through the inner os, the introduction of a small cervical dilator or a uterine sound by using steady, moderate pressure can be helpful. Another option is to discontinue the procedure and insert a 3-mm osmotic laminaria, which can be placed in the cervix on the morning of the day of the EMB and removed that afternoon prior to conducting the actual procedure.

15. Once resistance is felt, note the distance that the curette has entered the uterus, using the markings located on the sheath. On average, the length of the cervix from external to

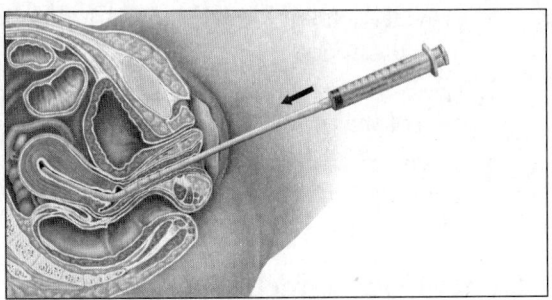

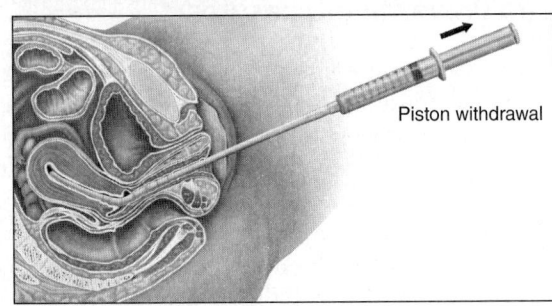

Piston withdrawal

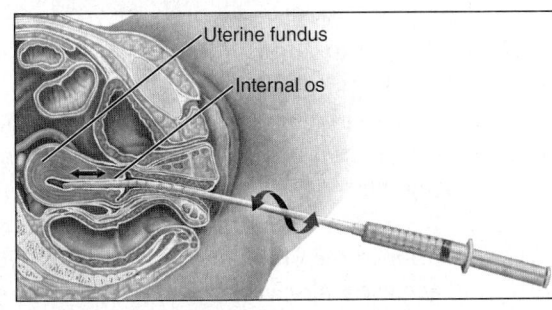

Uterine fundus

Internal os

**Figure 15A-2** Endometrial biopsy technique. **A.** Insert the device until resistance is felt or the uterine fundus is reached (Step 13). **B.** Withdraw the piston from the fully inserted device (Step 16). **C.** Rotate the device through 360 degrees while moving it back and forth between the fundus and the internal cervical os (Steps 17 and 18).

internal os is 2.5 cm, and the total distance from the external os to the wall of the fundus is approximately 6 to 9 cm. This information should be noted and recorded in the individual's health record.

16. With the tip of the device at the fundus, hold the curette securely, and slowly but consistently partially withdraw the inner piston. Withdrawal of the piston creates the suction, or negative pressure, at the tip needed to collect the tissue sample. It is not necessary to withdraw and replace the piston repeatedly; indeed, doing so is counterproductive. The piston should *not* be totally withdrawn or suction will be lost.

17. Move the sheath of the device back and forth, with the tip moving from fundus to

internal os, while simultaneously rolling it between the thumb and fingers to allow collection of cells from different levels of the endometrium as well as different locations. Avoid allowing the tip of the device to slip back out of the internal os into the cervical canal, as this will result in the loss of suction.

18. Complete the simultaneous moving and rolling of the sheath maneuver until the sheath is filled. Both tissue and some blood should be visible.

19. Remove the device. If only blood can be visibly identified within the sheath, after removing the entire curette, place the contents in formalin, and use another curette to attempt the procedure once or twice more depending on the individual's consent and how well the procedure is tolerated. The same curette can be reused if it has maintained sterility, including not touching the formalin.

20. Once the tissue has been adequately collected, the distal tip from the device can be cut and placed in the labeled formalin container. Cutting the tip from the device allows the sample to be removed intact, without causing the cell breakup that can occur when tissue is forced through the tip. Placing the tip of the catheter in the specimen container ensures that any tissue collected in this portion of the device will be analyzed with the remainder of the specimen.

21. Gently press the piston back into the sheath to expel the remaining specimen into the same labeled container.

22. Remove the tenaculum (if used) and speculum, and encourage the individual to remain supine for a few minutes to reduce the risk of a vasovagal response. It is common for an individual to experience some cramping either during the procedure or immediately afterward; anticipatory guidance is indicated on this possibility.

23. Instruct the individual to expect some light spotting during the next few days, but to contact the office if bright red blood or excessive bleeding or clotting, fever, vaginal discharge with a foul odor, pelvic cramping, or pain occurs. Counseling includes advising no vaginal penetration sexual intercourse for 2 to 3 days after the procedure.

24. Document the procedure, including any analgesic or anesthetic given, any abnormal findings during the examination or procedure, the sampling device used, the depth of insertion of the curette, adequacy of the specimen obtained, and the individual's toleration of the procedure.

## Results and Management

Laboratory findings can vary in language and presentation depending on the laboratory reporting system. In general, the provider will receive a histology report, with information that can contribute to making a diagnosis regarding the status of the endometrium. In communicating the findings to the individual, the provider should ensure that the individual understands the results and the possible courses of action to follow. The most common histologic reports received, with suggestions for follow-up, are listed in **Table 15A-1**.

| Table 15A-1 | Common Histologic Findings from Endometrial Biopsy Samples | | |
|---|---|---|---|
| **Histology** | **Probable Diagnosis** | **Suggested Management** | **Need for Referral** |
| Insufficient cells or unable to assess | Unable to assess | Dependent on clinical indication for EMB; may repeat EMB or potential referral for dilatation and curettage | Dependent upon specific clinical indication |
| Inactive endometrium | Hypoestrogenic state | Dependent on clinical presentation and indication for EMB | Dependent upon specific clinical indication |
| Proliferative (estrogen-influenced preovulation), disorganized proliferative endometrium or secretory (progesterone-influenced postovulation) | AUB | TVUS to rule out structural pathology<br>Hormonal therapy such as combined oral contraceptives, or cycling with progestins or a LNG-IUS if the individual is of reproductive age | Individuals with an abnormal TVUS, or those who do not respond to hormonal therapies as expected |
| Simple or complex nonatypical hyperplasia | Premenopausal or perimenopausal individual | Combined oral contraceptives, cycling with progestins, or insertion of a LNG-IUS<br>Repeat EMB in 6 months | No response to hormonal therapy |
| | Postmenopausal individual | No therapy, or hormonal therapy depending on amount of bleeding, age, and time lapsed from menopause (discussed in more detail in the *Menopause* chapter) | Continued irregular bleeding, or no response to hormonal therapy |
| Atypical hyperplasia (simple or complex)—suspicion of cancer | Rule out endometrial carcinoma | Refer to a specialist (e.g., collaborating physician or gynecologic oncologist) for probable surgery | Continued irregular bleeding, or no response to hormonal therapy |

Abbreviations: AUB, abnormal uterine bleeding; EMB, endometrial biopsy, LNG-IUS, levonorgestrel intrauterine system; TVUS, transvaginal ultrasound.

## References

1. American College of Nurse-Midwives. Clinical Bulletin No. 17: endometrial biopsy. *J Midwifery Womens Health*. 2017;62:502-506.

2. Williams PM, Gaddey HL. Endometrial biopsy: tips and pitfalls. *Am Fam Physician*. 2020;101(9):551-556.

3. Kucukgoz Gulec U, Khatib G, Guzel AB, et al. The necessity of using tenaculum for endometrial sampling procedure with Pipelle: a randomized controlled study. *Arch Gynecol Obstet*. 2014;289(2):349-356. doi:10.1007/s00404-013-3005-7.

4. Narin R, Uysal G, Baş S, et al. Is Valsalva maneuver an alternative to use tenaculum for endometrial sampling procedure in cases where the cervix cannot be passed spontaneously with Pipelle? A randomized study. *J Obstet Gynaecol Res*. 2021;47(2):529-532. doi:10.1111/jog.14546.

CHAPTER

# 16

# Malignant and Chronic Gynecologic Disorders

KATIE WARD

*The editors acknowledge Sharon Bond, William McCool, and Mary Brucker, who were the authors of this chapter in the previous edition.*

## Introduction

This chapter covers primarily malignant and structural problems commonly encountered in the care of nonpregnant patients. Certified nurse-midwives (CNM) and certified midwives (CMs) are ideal primary care providers, and most midwives provide routine gynecologic care.[1] While many conditions described in this chapter require referral to a specialist, a midwife may be the first point of contact an individual has with the healthcare system, and therefore the first provider to identify an abnormality.

## Screening for Malignancies

Breast, lung, and colon cancer—in that order—are the most common causes of cancer and cancer deaths among individuals assigned female at birth living in the United States.[2] Gender- and sexual-minority individuals may be at higher risk for a delayed cancer diagnosis, and therefore a worse outcome, due to a lack of culturally competent healthcare providers or a previous negative interaction with the healthcare system.[3] All cancer care is improved by early detection, and midwives should be familiar with current screening guidelines. The U.S. Preventive Services Task Force (USPSTF), American Cancer Society (ACS), and professional organizations including the American College of Obstetricians and Gynecologists (ACOG) publish and regularly update recommendations regarding screening intervals.

While screening tests are valuable for secondary prevention of disease, the practice of an annual or preventive physical examination has not been shown to reduce any morbidity or mortality, including cancer.[4] Likewise, routine pelvic examination in asymptomatic individuals has not been shown to reduce gynecologic cancers.[5] Controversy among professional organizations as to the value of a preventive care visit can make recommendations confusing for patients and clinicians alike.

## Cancer of the Uterine Cervix

Since the 1980s, it has been well recognized that virtually all cases of cervical cancer are caused by persistent infection with a high-risk type of human papillomavirus (HPV).[6] HPV is a small deoxyribonucleic acid (DNA) virus that is easily transmitted from one person to another via close skin-to-skin intimate contact. HPV enters the body through microscopic breaks in the skin and can be transmitted via any type of sexual contact.[7] While more than 150 genotypes of HPV have been identified, approximately 40 are known to infect the anogenital area. To date, 12 to 14 major HPV types have been linked to the development of anal, oral, and cervical cancer. HPV types 16 and 18 are responsible for approximately 70% of all cervical cancers, 90% of anal cancers, 65% of vaginal cancers, 50% of vulvar cancers, and greater than 45% of oropharyngeal cancers.[8]

The ability to identify high-risk HPV types with liquid-based cytology tests has changed cervical cancer screening practices. Cervical cancer can take years to develop, so population-based screening can be an effective means of identifying this cancer or its precursor lesions. Testing for high-risk HPV types can be performed singly, as a co-test with a cytology test, or as reflex testing (a test of residual cells from the primary sample, relieving patients of a follow-up visit) if the cytology test identifies abnormal cells.

## Cervical Cancer Screening Tests

Since the introduction of liquid-based cytology and the advent of testing for high-risk HPV DNA, liquid-based testing has replaced glass-slide techniques in well-resourced settings. Today, more than 90% of laboratories use liquid-based cytology testing because this technology assures improved quality of the sample, improved reproducibility, fewer false negatives, and the ability to test for HPV subtypes.

### Cytology Test

As described in the *Anatomy and Physiology of the Reproductive System* chapter, the external cervix (ectocervix) is covered with smooth, pink, squamous epithelial cells. The inner section of the cervical os is lined with columnar epithelial cells. The squamocolumnar junction is the site of active metaplasia, or conversion of one cell type (columnar epithelium) to another (squamous epithelium), although these changes are not grossly visible. The squamocolumnar junction is clinically important because the cells around it, called the *transformation zone*, tend to be the site of most abnormalities. For this reason, healthcare providers attempt to obtain cells from this area for a cytology test. When abnormalities occur in the cells within the transformation zone, they often are characterized as *dysplasia*—an umbrella term referring to abnormal cells that may signify a stage preceding the development of cancer.

In individuals who are pregnant or using hormonal contraception, the presence of pronounced eversion of the columnar epithelium, also known as *ectopy*, often enhances the possibility of obtaining satisfactory cells for a cytology test. Individuals who are in the postmenopausal period may lack any visual appearance of the endocervix, as the squamocolumnar junction migrates into the cervical canal. The procedure for performing a cytology test is described in the *Collecting Laboratory Specimens* appendix.

### Human Papillomavirus DNA Test

The U.S. Food and Drug Administration (FDA) has now approved several brands of HPV DNA tests as stand-alone screening tests for cervical cancer in individuals age 25 years and older. A large trial involving more than 42,000 individuals, conducted in the United States, demonstrated the effectiveness and sensitivity of HPV infection as a first-line screening test for cervical cancer, finding that it yielded fewer false-negative results when compared with cytology testing.[9] In 2020, the ACS endorsed use of HPV DNA testing alone for primary screening for cervical cancer beginning at age 25. In 2021, however, the American Society for Colposcopy and Cervical Pathology (ASCCP) endorsed the 2018 USPSTF guidelines, which rely on cytology as the primary screening methodology; in doing so, ASCCP cited the lack of inclusion of underrepresented minorities in the HPV screening trials as well as the implementation issues in practice. Table 16-1 summarizes the various organizations' guidelines for screening.[10–12]

## Cervical Cancer Screening Recommendations

Current age-based cervical cancer screening guidelines for all individuals with a cervix, including those who have been either fully or partially vaccinated against HPV, are summarized in Table 16-1. HPV vaccination does not negate the need for continued cervical cancer screening.

All professional organizations in the United States recommend against performing a cytology test for individuals with a cervix who are younger than 21 years, unless there is a history of an immunosuppressive condition (e.g., human immunodeficiency virus [HIV] infection).[13] Most HPV types, including 16 and 18, resolve spontaneously and do not increase the risk of cervical cancer later in life unless HPV infection remains persistent over time. If testing occurs inadvertently for a someone younger than 21 years, then guidelines for management for age 21- to 24-year-olds are followed.[13]

Cervical cancer screening is discontinued in individuals with a cervix who are age 65 years or older unless they meet the criteria noted in Table 16-1. Individuals at any age who have undergone a hysterectomy that included removal of the cervix and have no history of a past high-grade cervical lesion (cervical intraepithelial neoplasia [CIN] 2, 3, or greater) no longer need a cytology test.[12,13]

## Miscellaneous Organisms Identified on Cytology Tests

Cytology testing is a screening test designed to detect cervical cancer. However, when reviewing specimens, cytologists and pathologists can note the presence of incidental organisms unrelated to cervical cancer, such as *Trichomonas*, *Candida*, coccobacilli, or the

| Table 16-1 | Cervical Cancer Screening Guidelines | | |
|---|---|---|---|
| | **2020 American Cancer Society[a]** | **2018 U.S. Preventive Services Task Force and ASCCP[b]** | **2020 ACOG Practice Bulletin[c]** |
| Age 21–24 | No screening | Cytology alone every 3 years | Cytology alone every 3 years |
| Age 25–29 | HPV test (preferred) every 5 years OR Cytology with HPV co-test (acceptable) every 5 years OR Cytology alone every 3 years | Cytology every 3 years | Cytology every 3 years |
| Age 30–65 | HPV test (preferred) every 5 years OR Cytology with HPV co-test (acceptable) every 5 years OR Cytology alone every 3 years | Cytology with HPV co-test every 5 years OR Cytology alone every 3 years | Cytology with HPV co-test every 5 years OR Cytology alone every 3 years |
| Age 65 and older | No screening if a series of prior tests was normal | No screening if a series of prior tests was normal AND no CIN 2 in past | Can discontinue screening if a series of prior tests was normal AND no CIN 2 in past |
| Hysterectomy including cervix | No screening of individuals who do not have a history of high-grade lesions or cervical cancer | | |

Abbreviations: ACOG, American College of Obstetricians and Gynecologists; ASCCP, American Society for Colposcopy and Cervical Pathology; CIN, cervical intraepithelial neoplasia; HPV, human papillomavirus.

[a]Saslow D, Andrews KS, Manassaram-Baptiste D, Smith RA, Fontham ET, Group ACSGD. Human papillomavirus vaccination 2020 guideline update: American Cancer Society guideline adaptation. *CA Cancer J Clin*. 2020;70(4):274-280.

[b]Marcus JZ, Cason P, Downs Jr LS, Einstein MH, Flowers L. The ASCCP Cervical Cancer Screening Task Force endorsement and opinion on the American Cancer Society updated cervical cancer screening guidelines. *J Low Genit Tract Dis*. 2021;25(3):187-191.

[c]ACOG Practice Bulletin number 131: screening for cervical cancer. *Obstet Gynecol*. 2020;120(5):1222-1238.

presence of endometrial cells. When *Trichomonas* is identified on a cytology result, this finding is not considered diagnostic for infection that requires treatment because false positives are known to occur. In such a case, it is recommended that the midwife recall the patient for confirmatory testing by office-based examination of vaginal secretions via saline prep wet mount, or preferably via nucleic acid amplification testing (NAAT).[14]

Likewise, *Candida* found on a cytology test does not necessarily require treatment. *Candida* forms colonies intravaginally as a component of normal flora, and the presence of this organism on a cytology test report does not correlate well with the clinical presentation. If individuals report symptoms of vaginal candidiasis, signs of vulvovaginitis are present, fungal elements are confirmed on microscopic examination, and potassium hydroxide (KOH) testing is positive, then treatment is indicated.

Similarly, cytology tests can report cellular changes associated with the presence of herpes simplex virus (HSV). However, a cytology test is neither a screening nor a diagnostic test for herpes.[14]

Obtaining an HSV culture of a visible lesion and testing by polymerase chain reaction (PCR) remain the most accurate methods of identifying herpes. In asymptomatic individuals, type-specific serology will determine the presence of antibodies (evidence of past exposure) to herpes, but a positive serology result does not provide information about a current outbreak or when someone could have been exposed to herpes. The Centers for Disease Control and Prevention (CDC) recommends against routine serologic screening for herpes in the general population. If a cytology test result indicates the presence of HSV, the person should be notified, and a discussion regarding further diagnostic testing should occur.

Many laboratories report a predominance of coccobacilli consistent with a shift in vaginal flora. Some clinicians consider this finding suggestive of bacterial vaginosis. Bacterial vaginosis is multibacterial in origin and cannot be diagnosed via cytology. When coccobacilli are identified on a cytology report, the midwife can inquire whether the person is symptomatic, and offer an examination to assess for bacterial vaginosis. Current research findings are inconsistent concerning the value of screening asymptomatic individuals for bacterial vaginosis.[15]

A finding of *Actinomyces* on a cytology test result for someone who is using intrauterine contraception should be further evaluated. *Actinomyces* is a strain of bacteria found in the normal genital tract. In rare cases, its presence has been associated with the development of pelvic inflammatory disease and pelvic abscess in individuals using intrauterine contraception. If infection is likely or the person is symptomatic, the intrauterine device (IUD) should be removed and antibiotics initiated. If the person is asymptomatic, the device can be left in place, and antibiotic treatment is not indicated.[16,17]

To summarize, the purpose of cytology testing is to detect cervical cancer and categorize epithelial cell abnormalities. The cytology test is a *screening* measure, rather than a diagnostic test. If the clinician visualizes an unusual lesion or mass on the cervix, cytology testing can be performed as an initial step in evaluation. While a variety of incidental findings may be noted on a cytology report, these findings are not diagnostic. Additional follow-up may be needed depending on the report, the person's symptoms, and/or abnormal findings during the examination.

## Alternative Methods of Cervical Cancer Screening in Low-Resource Areas

In many countries without cytology test screening systems, cervical cancer is a significant cause of death among individuals with a cervix. An alternative method used for screening individuals in such circumstances is visual inspection with either a 5% solution of acetic acid or Lugol's iodine solution. This technique involves the application of the agent during a speculum examination and examination of the cervix with the naked eye to identify lesions that appear acetowhite when exposed to acetic acid, or bright yellow when exposed to Lugol's solution. This test is usually performed by trained lay health workers, making the technique cost-effective and accessible to large populations who might not otherwise be screened during their lifetime. Single-visit "screen and treat" programs would also reduce the burden of cervical cancer where resources are scarce.[18]

Another method of cervical cancer screening sometimes used in low-resource countries is cervicography. This method uses low-magnification photographs of the cervix, now available in digital format, which are interpreted by a cytopathologist, frequently at a different site and later in time. Women with abnormal cervigrams are referred for further evaluation and treatment. This method is not as sensitive or specific as colposcopy, but evidence shows that it has a high negative predictive value and serves an important role in cervical cancer screening in locations where cytology screening is unavailable.[19]

## Diagnosis and Treatment of Abnormal Cytology Test Results

The ASCCP's 2019 guidelines form the basis for patient care following cytology test findings, as well as the management guidelines proposed by ACOG for abnormal cervical cancer screening test results.[13] These guidelines have been endorsed by 25 other organizations, including the Society of Gynecologic Oncology.[20] The midwife's role once cytology test results are obtained can range from making an immediate referral to performing follow-up tests, including colposcopy, depending on the midwife's formal preparation, experience, institutional guidelines, and skill level. If the results of a cytology test include findings such as carcinoma in situ, squamous cell carcinoma, or adenocarcinoma, immediate referral to a gynecologic oncology specialist is indicated.

Factors such as age, HPV status, pregnancy, previous cytology tests, past treatments, and histologic results can affect abnormal cytology test management, making it very complex. The 2019 ASCCP guidelines moved from a test result–based strategy to a risk-based approach. This risk-based strategy is individualized based on the person's age, previous history and treatment, and other co-factors. For each abnormal result, the provider consults a table that calculates the risk and recommends next steps. To facilitate this individualized approach, the ASCCP guidelines are available free of charge on this organization's website (and for a small fee, on mobile apps). The ASCCP website and app are updated on a regular basis; information about accessing these guidelines is provided in the Resources section at the end of this chapter.

### Colposcopy

The primary diagnostic method for determining the presence of cervical cancer or precancerous cells is colposcopic examination. Although a detailed description of the procedure is beyond the scope of this chapter, an increasing number of midwives are receiving formal education in performing colposcopy and have formally incorporated this procedure into their clinical practices as congruent with Standard VIII in the *ACNM Standards for the Practice of Midwifery*.[21] Principles and standards of colposcopy education and practice for all clinicians are

| Table 16-2 | Common Indications for Colposcopic Examination of the Cervix |
|---|---|
| Grossly visible or palpable abnormality of the cervix | |
| Abnormal cervical cytology | |
| Positive screening test for cervical neoplasia (e.g., high-risk HPV DNA strain) | |
| Persistent unsatisfactory cervical cytology | |
| History of in utero DES exposure | |
| Unexplained cervicovaginal discharge | |
| Unexplained abnormal lower genital tract bleeding | |
| Conditions that increase risk for lower genital tract neoplasia (cervical, vaginal, vulvar) such as lichen sclerosus. | |
| Post–lower genital tract cancer treatment surveillance | |

Abbreviations: DES, diethylstilbestrol; DNA, deoxyribonucleic acid; HPV, human papillomavirus.

Based on American College of Obstetricians and Gynecologists. Practice Bulletin No. 168: cervical cancer screening and prevention: interim update. *Obstet Gynecol*. 2016;128:e111-e130; Ocque R, Austin M. Follow-up of women with negative Pap test results and abnormal clinical signs or symptoms. *Am J Clin Pathol*. 2016;145:560-567.

now established and endorsed by several women's health professional organizations.[22] ASCCP provides training, mentorship, and continuing education for clinicians wishing to become credentialed to perform colposcopy. Common indications for colposcopy are listed in Table 16-2.[23,24]

When lesions of the vulva, vagina, or ectocervix are identified during colposcopy, a biopsy is performed at the same time. Endocervical curettage is recommended in certain situations (e.g., no lesion is found during a satisfactory colposcopy examination) to evaluate tissue not easily visible on the ectocervix. The purpose of a tissue biopsy or endocervical curettage is to identify cancer or precancerous lesions, and to guide subsequent treatment.

The choice of treatment depends on the size, location, and significance of the abnormality (CIN 1, 2, 3, or cancer), the person's age, and their desire for future childbearing. As with any gynecologic procedure, it is important to engage in shared decision making and obtain informed consent.

## Cancer of the Uterine Endometrium

While a variety of carcinomas may be found in the uterus, including sarcomas and gestational trophoblastic tumors (e.g., hydatidiform mole), the endometrium is the source of approximately 90% of all cancers involving the corpus of the uterus.[25] When detected early in the disease process, the cure rate for endometrial cancer is high because tumors tend to be localized and well defined. Even so, the incidence of endometrial cancer results in more than 12,000 deaths per year in the United States—a mortality rate that, based on the ratio of deaths to new diagnoses (1 to 5.1), is comparable to that of breast cancer (1 to 5.2).[2,25]

Conditions associated with a prolonged exposure to unopposed estrogen are risk factors for development of endometrial cancer. Examples include early menarche and late menopause, polycystic ovary syndrome with anovulation, nulliparity, and use of unopposed estrogens or tamoxifen (Nolvadex). Factors that suggest an underlying prolonged exposure to estrogen may have occurred include unexplained vaginal bleeding in postmenopausal individuals, Lynch syndrome, infertility, obesity, and history of breast or ovarian cancer. The most common sign of endometrial cancer, which always requires diagnostic follow-up, is unexplained vaginal bleeding, especially when it is experienced by a postmenopausal individual. Thus, the most widely recommended screening approach for endometrial cancer is education of patients about the signs, symptoms, and risk factors associated with the disease. People who are seeking care from providers offering compounded hormone therapy should be carefully queried about any unscheduled vaginal bleeding.

The Women's Health Initiative (WHI) was a series of clinical trials designed to address morbidity and mortality in postmenopausal women. The hormone therapy arms of this trial were stopped early due to increased breast cancer in the treatment arms. This led to a significant decrease in the use of menopausal hormone treatment. Paradoxically, the incidence of endometrial cancer has increased in the years following the publication of the WHI data. This may reflect increased use of compounded bioidentical hormone therapy that began following the publication of the WHI trial results.[26]

Endometrial cancer is categorized into two types. Type I, commonly referred to as endometrioid adenocarcinoma, is the most common form, accounting for approximately three-fourths of all cases. Endometrioid adenocarcinoma usually occurs in the perimenopausal years, and if discovered in its early stages, is treatable. Type II, which is unrelated to the presence of estrogen, is less common and has a more dire prognosis than Type I. Some oncologists include a third subclassification, which is hereditary in nature and rarer than Types I and II. The most common cause of this third type of endometrial tumor is Lynch syndrome, also called hereditary nonpolyposis colorectal cancer. Lynch syndrome is caused by a genetic mutation that puts the individual at high risk for developing colorectal cancer as well as some other cancers (e.g., endometrial, ovarian, and gastrointestinal cancers).[27]

The first diagnostic test for endometrial cancer is endometrial biopsy (EMB), which will reveal normal tissue, hyperplasia, or possibly endometrial cancer depending on the sample obtained. The procedure for performing an endometrial biopsy is presented in the *Endometrial Biopsy* appendix. Traditionally, the other standard method used for preliminary diagnosis of endometrial cancer has been transvaginal ultrasound. The most effective method to definitively diagnose endometrial cancer following an EMB or transvaginal ultrasound is to perform hysteroscopy accompanied by a dilatation and curettage (D & C).[28]

For a postmenopausal individual, any vaginal bleeding, except that experienced as part of an expected withdrawal bleeding while on hormone therapy, is considered a possible sign of cancer requiring further evaluation (see the *Menstrual Cycle Abnormalities* chapter). Other signs and symptoms of endometrial cancer, such as pain, usually occur during late-stage disease, when the cancer has spread beyond the uterus.

### Other Uterine Cancers

While endometrial cancer is by far the most prevalent form of uterine cancer, two additional forms of abnormal growth are important to note: gestational trophoblastic tumors (e.g., hydatidiform mole) and uterine sarcoma. The most common of these tumors is hydatidiform mole, which comprises abnormal growth of placental tissue. In its beginning stages, this tumor is a benign growth. Women with hydatidiform mole present with a positive pregnancy test, usually with excessively elevated human chorionic gonadotropin (hCG) levels, and abnormal bleeding. The uterus is often found to be larger than expected based on the person's gestational dates, and confirmation of diagnosis is accomplished through ultrasonography. Treatment most frequently involves the use of suction curettage with the goal of preventing the development of metastatic disease.[29] Additional information on hydatidiform mole can be found in the *Early Pregnancy Loss and Abortion* chapter.

Uterine sarcomas are a rare form of gynecologic cancer (less than 1% of these cancers) that account for approximately 3% to 7% of all uterine carcinomas.[30] Generally occurring after menopause, these anomalies originate in the endometrium, the myometrial muscle, or the endometrial stroma. Risk factors include prior therapeutic radiation to the pelvic region, prolonged use of tamoxifen, and African Caribbean ancestry.[30] There is no recommended form of regular screening. The most common symptom or sign of uterine sarcomas is abnormal uterine bleeding. While sarcomas cannot be easily distinguished on physical examination from benign leiomyomas, it is important to remember that sarcomas usually are found in postmenopausal individuals, whereas uterine fibroids more commonly manifest prior to menopause, and begin to regress in size after menopause when estrogen stimulation diminishes.

If sarcoma is suspected, further assessment can include an endometrial biopsy or a hysteroscopic-guided D & C. However, these diagnostic modalities are less sensitive for sarcomas than they are for endometrial carcinomas. By comparison, more sensitive assessment is achieved with imaging studies, such as computed tomographic (CT) scans used to guide needle biopsy or magnetic resonance imagining (MRI). Employing ultrasound for the diagnosis of sarcoma is not very useful.

Generally, the midwife refers the person in whom uterine sarcoma is suspected to an appropriate specialist. Prognosis depends on the extent of the disease when the diagnosis is made. If the cancer is confined to the uterine corpus at the time of discovery, the 5-year survival rate is 50%; by comparison, the 5-year survival rate for individuals with sarcoma that has metastasized ranges from 0% to 20%.[30] Clearly, early discovery is vital to curtailing the spread of this disease—one reason why the significance of uterine bleeding in postmenopausal individuals should be stressed.

## Ovarian Cancer

Ovarian cancer is often found at a late stage and is the most common cause of gynecologic cancer–related death.[31] Ovarian cancer can occur in epithelial, germ cell, or sex cord stromal cell tissue, though the majority of these cancers are epithelial. The 5-year survival rate for individuals with ovarian cancer is markedly lower than that for individuals with other cancers, primarily because ovarian cancer is often first diagnosed at a late stage in the disease's progression.

The lifetime risk of being diagnosed with breast cancer is 1 in 8 women, whereas the comparable lifetime risk of being diagnosed with ovarian cancer is 1 to 2 per 100 women.[31] However, this risk varies among different populations. For example, the risk of developing ovarian cancer is greatly increased in individuals who have a mutation in breast cancer gene 1 (BRCA1) or breast cancer gene 2 (BRCA2). As with most cancers, the risk of developing ovarian cancer increases with age: This disease is most prevalent after age 45 years; the median age at diagnosis is 63 years.[32,33]

Known and possible risk factors for ovarian cancer include a history of breast, uterine, or colorectal cancer; postmenopausal status; evidence of mutations in the BRCA1 or BRCA2 genes; rarer mutations in more recently discovered genetically based cancers (e.g., the phosphatase and tensin homolog [PTEN] gene associated with Cowden disease that causes a form of thyroid cancer and breast cancer); Lynch syndrome; more than 40 years of active ovulation (e.g., nulliparous never-user of oral contraceptives); early menarche or late menopause; use of infertility drugs for longer than 1 year; and use of unopposed estrogen therapy.[33] Notably, repetitive stimulation of the epithelium of the ovary is theorized to result in the development of a malignant state. In contrast, conditions associated with decreased ovulation, such as high parity, use of oral contraceptives or injectable depot medroxyprogesterone acetate (DMPA), breastfeeding/chestfeeding, hysterectomy and salpingectomy, and prophylactic oophorectomy, are all associated with a decreased risk of developing ovarian cancer.[33]

Unfortunately, history and physical examination have not been predictive for the detection of ovarian cancer, particularly in its earlier stages. Although CA-125 levels are elevated in individuals with ovarian cancer, the specificity of this biomarker is limited: Elevated CA-125 levels are associated with many other conditions as well, and levels of this antigen are not consistently elevated in early-stage disease. Developing an effective screening method for ovarian cancer is an area of ongoing research.[34,35]

Approximately 10% to 20% of individuals who develop ovarian cancer have an inherited genetic mutation in BRCA1 or BRCA2. Risk factors that increase the chance of having a BRCA1 or BRCA2 mutation are presented in the *Breast and Chest Conditions* chapter. The term "hereditary breast and ovarian cancer syndrome" (HBOC) refers to persons who have a family history of multiple cases of breast, ovarian, and/or peritoneal cancers in first-degree relatives. Criteria for offering individuals screening for HBOC are reviewed in the *Breast and Chest Conditions* chapter. Persons at increased risk for having a BRCA1 or BRCA2 mutation should be offered genetic counseling.[36] In short, the current recommendation for ovarian cancer screening is that everyone should be screened for a family history that suggests they are at risk for HBOC, with those found to be at risk then being offered genetic counseling, which may include testing for BRCA mutations.

The lack of evidence regarding the exact etiology of ovarian cancer, definitive risk factors, and means of early detection make screening for this disease difficult for individuals and practitioners alike. Reminders about the signs and symptoms of ovarian cancer can potentially aid in detecting this carcinoma. These signs and symptoms include abdominal distension or bloating; flatulence, difficulty eating or easily feeling full when eating, and other persistent gastrointestinal disturbances, including either diarrhea or constipation; abdominal or pelvic pain; fatigue; urinary complaints, including urgency or frequency that occur more than 12 days per month;[34,35] and irregular vaginal bleeding.[33,36]

## Cancer of the Vulva and the Vagina

Cancer of the vulva and the vagina account for approximately 6% to 7% of all gynecologic malignancies. The relative 5-year survival rates for vulvar and vaginal cancers are approximately 72% and 49%, respectively.[37] The lower survival rate for individuals with vaginal cancer is in part due to the fact that this malignancy usually presents as a result of metastatic spreading of a cancer whose primary source of development was in another gynecologic organ, such as the vulva or the cervix. When vaginal cancer is discovered prior to spreading beyond the vagina, involving lymph nodes, or metastasizing, the 5-year survival rate is approximately 70%.[38] The vast majority of both forms of cancer are of the squamous cell type, and their incidence increases with age.

Both vulvar and vaginal cancer have been increasingly associated with HPV exposure.[39] Consequently, the CDC now emphasizes that receiving the HPV vaccine will protect individuals against not only cervical cancer, but also vulvar and vaginal cancer. A history of infection with a high-risk HPV type should be considered a risk factor for vulvar or vaginal cancer, though the incidence of these cancers is less than the incidence of cervical cancer. Other risk factors for vulvar and vaginal malignancies include smoking, multiple sex partners, other gynecologic cancers, lichen sclerosus, and immunosuppressive disorders (e.g., HIV infection).

A rarer form of vaginal cancer, found primarily in female offspring of women who took diethylstilbestrol (DES) during pregnancy, is clear cell adenocarcinoma. It first occurs in late adolescence and the early twenties, although most of the individuals affected directly by DES are now much older and no longer at risk for clear cell adenocarcinoma.[40]

Both screening for and diagnosis of vulvar and vaginal cancers include the identification of any growths in the genital area noted by the person or by the midwife during a pelvic examination. The most common site of vulvar cancer is the labia majora, while the most common location of vaginal cancer is the upper third of the vaginal wall.

Early symptoms of vulvar cancer can include persistent pruritus and the presence of condylomata, whereas vaginal disease can be accompanied by bleeding, unusual discharge, and pelvic discomfort. Depending on the extent of the disease process, pelvic examination can reveal a mass at the site of involvement, and possibly lymphadenopathy. Any suspicious lesion should be biopsied, either by a midwife with experience in collecting such samples or by the specialist to whom the referral was placed. Referral should occur if any of the following conditions are present: unexplained lymphadenopathy, an HPV lesion that does not improve with topical treatment, or a lesion with an unusual presentation or continued growth over time. As with other gynecologic malignancies, early detection of a vulvar or vaginal cancer can result in a high rate of survival.

## Benign Gynecologic Findings

### Disorders of the Vulva

Benign (noncancerous) conditions that affect the vulva include cysts, dermatoses, vulvodynia, and infections.

#### Greater Vestibular Gland Cysts

The greater vestibular glands (also called Bartholin's glands), are two mucus-secreting, nonpalpable structures located within the vaginal vestibule in the space between the hymenal ring and the labia minora at approximately the 4 o'clock and 8 o'clock positions (Figure 16-1). The vestibular glands can develop both cysts and abscesses.

Vestibular glands normally secrete a small amount of viscous fluid. If the gland openings become obstructed, a cyst will develop, resulting in a mass of variable size. Most vestibular gland cysts are asymptomatic and do not require treatment. However, if the fluid becomes infected, an abscess can develop.

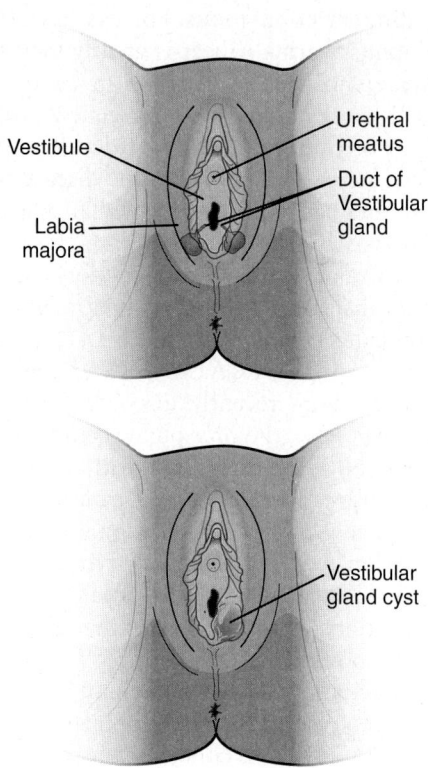

**Figure 16-1** Location of vestibular glands with vestibular gland cyst on the patient's left side.

Infected vestibular glands are usually erythematous and painful. The majority of abscesses in the vestibular glands contain multiple types of bacteria, some of which are part of the normal vaginal flora, including *Escherichia coli*, but there is a higher incidence of *Neisseria gonorrhea* or *Chlamydia trachomatis* in people with an abscess.[41] Methicillin-resistant *Staphylococcus aureus* (MRSA) has been found in vestibular gland abscesses in some studies, but not all. In general, cysts that exhibit induration, but no evidence of abscess, are treated with a course of antibiotics and warm compresses. First-line antibiotics include those effective against both aerobic and anaerobic organisms.[41] Individuals who are pregnant or otherwise immunocompromised require close follow-up. While the procedure for incision and drainage with placement of a Word catheter is beyond the scope of this text, midwives may add this procedure to their practices following completion of the process described in the *Standards for Practice of Midwifery*.[19]

The Infectious Diseases Society of America publishes guidelines for the treatment of skin and soft-tissue infections, classifying soft-tissue infections into three categories—mild, moderate, and severe.[42] Mild infections demonstrate only a local, mildly purulent lesion, while moderate infections involve systemic symptoms. A severe vestibular gland infection is one that has failed incision and drainage, has not responded to antibiotic therapy, or shows more significant systemic involvement.[42] Persons with recalcitrant or recurrent infections, as well as those requiring surgical intervention, are usually referred to a specialist.[43]

## Human Papillomavirus–Associated Lesions

In addition to causing condylomata on the cervix, infection with HPV can cause condylomata acuminata on the vulva, vagina, perineum, and anus. External genital warts are commonly caused by low-risk HPV types 6 and 11, and are not associated with cancer, but they often cause physical symptoms, carry a social stigma, and lead to multiple costly visits to healthcare providers. The care and treatment of vulvar condylomata acuminata are reviewed in more detail in the *Reproductive Tract and Sexually Transmitted Infections* chapter.

## Herpes Simplex Lesions

Within the HSV family of DNA viruses, eight are associated with human infection. Notably, HSV-1 and HSV-2 can cause both oral and genital infections.

Genital herpes is a chronic, recurrent condition of skin and mucosal surfaces caused by infection with HSV; it is transmitted by sexual contact. The initial infection with HSV typically manifests as painful blisters on the vulva, perineum, vagina, cervix, or anus, although the majority of individuals who carry and transmit genital herpes have never had an outbreak of painful blisters, are asymptomatic, and have not been diagnosed. Although both HSV-1 and HSV-2 can cause genital infection, their clinical courses are generally different: Specifically, HSV-2 causes more genital pain, and outbreaks are typically more frequent. Serologic testing capable of distinguishing HSV-1 versus HSV-2 (or the presence of both) is available. Diagnosis, counseling, and treatment of genital herpes, including its potential effects during the perinatal period, are addressed in the *Reproductive Tract and Sexually Transmitted Infections* chapter.

## Dermatologic Disorders

The vulva can develop a variety of benign and cancerous dermatologic conditions. Skin disorders of the vulva can be either chronic or acute. Vulvar disorders can also be a source of sexual pain and dysfunction. Most individuals with skin disorders of the vulva have itching, pain, or irritation that can be a cause of significant personal distress. Care of people with chronic vulvar conditions can be challenging relative to determining the correct diagnosis, and treatments may or may not be effective. When caring for individuals with vulvar skin disorders, thorough knowledge of vulvar anatomy and function will guide the evaluation. Skin conditions common in other body sites, such as eczema, psoriasis, and contact dermatitis, frequently appear on the vulva as well. Vulvar biopsies are the gold standard to differentiate among the various vulvar conditions. Midwives trained in this procedure may incorporate vulvar biopsies in their gynecologic practice depending on the practice setting and guidelines.

### Folliculitis

Folliculitis of the vulva is a common condition involving hair follicles and sebaceous glands of the vulva. It occurs in hair-bearing areas of the vulva. The typical appearance is that of yellow-white- or red-colored, pinhead-sized pustules with a central hair. Most folliculitis is noninfectious, but secondary skin infections can occur mostly from surface skin bacteria and trauma, such as from shaving, waxing, or use of depilatories. Folliculitis can extend to the buttocks and upper, inner thighs. Treatment consists of avoidance of trauma and treatment with antibiotic creams or ointments.[44]

### Hidradenitis Suppurativa or Acne Inversa

Hidradenitis suppurativa or acne inversa is a chronic skin disease involving a recurrent, inflammatory response in areas where apocrine (sweat) glands reside.[45] Problems with frequent or recurring boils on the skin can also be reported. Without a high index of suspicion, an accurate diagnosis can be inadvertently delayed, thereby allowing for progression of disease. This condition is painful and typically has a significant impact on the affected individual's quality of life.[46]

Hidradenitis suppurativa can first appear in adolescence, beginning as painful, nodular lesions or abscesses in the axillary or genital region. When lesions drain, sinus tracts often form, leading to scarring, pain, and deformity in severe cases. Areas most commonly affected by hidradenitis suppurativa are the groin, perineum, and axilla.

Hidradenitis suppurativa is estimated to affect 1% to 4% of the population. While men can also be affected, cases among women outnumber those among men by 3 to 1.[47] The etiology of this disease has not been established, but studies suggest it is a multifocal condition, possibly an inherited, inflammatory or immune system disorder involving atrophy of sebaceous or apocrine glands; these glands secrete sebum into hair follicles and produce inflammation, leading to hair follicle destruction. Smoking and obesity have been associated with more severe disease.[48]

No diagnostic testing exists for hidradenitis suppurativa. Depending on the clinical diagnosis and extent of disease, treatment can be topical or systemic. In extreme cases, immunosuppressive therapy, surgical treatments, or laser treatments are recommended.[48] Well-controlled clinical trials have not been published comparing modalities to help providers determine which treatments are most effective, and referral to a specialist is usually the best action.

## Vulvar Dermatosis

Vulvar dermatoses include lichen sclerosus, lichen planus, lichen simplex chronicus, psoriasis, dermatitis (allergic, contact, or atrophic), and seborrheic dermatitis. The lichens are so named because they share a rough texture, but have important distinctions in etiology and prognosis (Table 16-3). People with vulvar itching may try a number of self-treatments prior to seeking professional care, delaying diagnosis. Although vulvar intraepithelial neoplasia is not typically pruritic, vulvar biopsy is important to distinguish benign and malignant causes.[49]

### Lichen Sclerosus

Lichen sclerosus is a common, lifelong, benign condition that can occur at any age, but has two peaks of onset: in prepuberty and during perimenopause and postmenopause.[46] While its cause remains unclear, other conditions with an autoimmune component, such as thyroid disorders, systemic lupus erythematosus, and alopecia, are found among individuals with lichen sclerosus. Individuals with lichen sclerosus have itching and pain and can present with dyspareunia.[50] On examination, there are changes in the appearance of the vulvar skin and loss of vulvar architecture. The skin becomes thin, with white patches occurring in a figure-eight distribution around the vestibule and anus. Once the diagnosis is confirmed by biopsy, treatment includes topical steroids and surveillance for signs of vulvar cancer, as its risk is increased in persons with lichen sclerosus.[51] Referral to an expert in management of vulvar disorders is essential when diagnosis is uncertain or there is limited improvement in the person's symptoms.

### Lichen Planus

Lichen planus is an autoimmune disorder that affects the skin, mucocutaneous sites such as the mouth, the scalp, and most often, the vulva or vagina. Its etiology is unknown, but the disorder is thought to occur secondary to a T-cell–mediated autoimmune response to basal keratinocytes. Like lichen sclerosus, lichen planus primarily affects perimenopausal and postmenopausal individuals, and is associated with other autoimmune disorders. Symptoms are similar to those of lichen sclerosus, including vulvar soreness, burning, and intense pruritus.[52] Dyspareunia is common. Vulvar tissue can be more reddened with an erosive appearance and is extremely tender to touch. Architectural changes involving the vulva and vagina can also be present.

Once biopsy confirms lichen planus, referral to a provider who specializes in the management of vulvar disorders is advisable, as lichen planus can be refractory to treatment. Lichen planus is associated with a small increase in the risk of vulvar cancer.[52]

### Lichen Simplex Chronicus

Lichen simplex chronicus is another vulvar skin condition that can involve the entire perianal region. The most common symptom associated with lichen simplex chronicus is severe itching, leading to a cycle of itch–scratch–itch, with the itching often being severe enough to interrupt sleep.[53] A thickened, leathery-like skin texture results after long-term scratching, which ultimately damages the protective skin barrier, increasing the risk of secondary infection. Diagnosis is generally based on clinical appearance, as biopsy may be nonspecific. Treatment is directed at reducing the itch–scratch–itch cycle with topical steroids, restoring the normal protective skin barrier, and reducing or managing recurrences.[53]

### Psoriasis, Seborrhea, and Dermatitis

Psoriasis of the vulvar skin is not uncommon in people who have psoriasis elsewhere, but it can sometimes be isolated to the vulva. The skin shows well-demarcated erythematous plaques that can have a scaly appearance.[54] Seborrhea is another inflammatory condition that can affect the vulva, taking the form of erythematous plaques that itch more than might be expected based on their appearance.[55] Contact dermatitis is a common cause of vulvar irritation, burning, and itching. Irritants can include sources of moisture, such as sweat and urine, and topical products, fragrances, and lubricants. Topical applications can also cause allergic

| Table 16-3 | Differentiation of Lichenoid Disorders of the Vulva | | | |
|---|---|---|---|---|
| **Factor** | **Lichen Sclerosus** | **Lichen Planus** | **Lichen Simplex Chronicus** | **Psoriasis** |
| Etiology | Autoimmune, hereditary; hormone-receptor variant present<br><br>Inflammatory, possibly oxidative stress | Autoimmune, hereditary, inflammatory condition | Local variant of atopic dermatitis; spontaneous onset or response to chronic friction/scratch | Autoimmune, hereditary |
| Incidence | Approximately 2% | Rare (less than 1% of women) | 0.5% | Approximately 3%; most common autoimmune disorder |
| Age at onset | Bimodal age peak (prepuberty and early postmenopause); 20% of onset is in young adults | Most commonly midlife (ages 40 to 60) | Most common in mid- to late adulthood | Any age; peak onset is adolescence to young adulthood |
| Distribution | Primarily affects genitalia; anal and perineal involvement common; extragenital and vaginal involvement rare | Diverse; variant: oral, vulvar, and vaginal involvement | Vulva, particularly hair-growing areas, are most commonly affected, but can occur on any chronically irritated skin | Generally scattered (knees, elbows, scalp, nails, umbilicus, gluteal fold), but may be only vulvar |
| Symptoms | Asymptomatic to severe itching, burning, dysuria, dyspareunia, apareunia, constipation; chronic or remitting | Asymptomatic to severe pain; vulvar itching, dysuria, dyspareunia; chronic or remitting | Severe itching; temporary relief by scratching or rubbing; excoriations common because scratching offers relief | Asymptomatic or mild itch, burning, soreness; intermittent flares; common triggers: cold, dry climate, dry skin, stress; joint pain with related arthritis |
| Signs | Onset: Maculopapular coalescing plaques.<br><br>Advanced: Ivory, "cigarette paper" skin; pale figure-of-eight around vulva and anus; fissures, ecchymosis, erosion, phimosis, and atrophy; agglutination may obscure clitoris, introitus, and/or urethra; lichenification if scratching; postinflammatory hyperpigmentation common | Type 1 (classic): Pruritic papular lesions of vulva, perineum, perianus; may have white reticulation/striae or hyperpigmentation after lesions have resolved in darker-skinned women<br><br>Type 2 (hypertrophic): Rare; white hypertrophic, rough vulvar plaques, which may have ulcers<br><br>Type 3 (erosive): Pain; erythematous erosions; serosanguinous discharge; white striae; friable, eroded vagina; adhesions, stenosis, with vaginal and/or clitoral obliteration possible; may have oral involvement | Onset: Mild erythema<br><br>Advanced: Thickened patches, fissures, pallor, excoriations, hyperpigmentation; area may be denuded of pubic hair due to scratching | On vulva: Thin plaques, typically highly erythematous with scant scaling due to maceration; satellite lesions common<br><br>Inverse psoriasis: Predominantly in skin folds |
| Malignant potential | Less than 5% | Up to 3% | Not identified | Not identified |

(continues)

| Table 16-3 | Differentiation of Lichenoid Disorders of the Vulva (*continued*) | | | |
|---|---|---|---|---|
| **Factor** | **Lichen Sclerosus** | **Lichen Planus** | **Lichen Simplex Chronicus** | **Psoriasis** |
| Differentiating factors | Symmetrical depigmentation in a figure-of-eight of pale, tissue-paper thin tissue around vulva and perianal area<br><br>Loss of vulvar architecture with agglutination is common and supports the diagnosis | Vaginal (lesions and/or discharge) and/or oral involvement; can also affect scalp, skin, and nails<br><br>Other diagnostic criteria: Well-demarcated erosions; white, hyperkeratotic borders; pain, burning, scarring, loss of genital architecture<br><br>Association with other autoimmune disorders, including thyroid disease, is less common | Temporary relief with scratching; thickened keratinized skin; excoriations; lack of vaginal involvement; leathery quality to skin; vulvar architecture typically intact | Family or personal history; thick, pale red to white scaly plaques outside the genital area; typically, thin, bright red, well-demarcated plaques without scaling on genitals; milder itch typical, excoriations uncommon |
| Management | Rule out other autoimmune disorders (thyroid, anemia, vitiligo, diabetes)<br><br>Defer biopsy of symmetrical classic signs pending 3-month treatment trial<br><br>First-line: High- or very high-potency steroid ointment tapered (e.g., daily for 1 month, every other day the next month, then twice weekly); daily use for 3 months is also an accepted treatment schedule<br><br>Nonresponse warrants biopsy and/or referral<br><br>Maintenance therapy after successful treatment is often needed (continuous or intermittent) | Swab excoriated lesions to rule out secondary infection<br><br>Type 1: May resolve spontaneously or may use emollient and medium-potency topical steroid<br><br>Type 2: Superpotent topical steroid over 3 months or intralesional injection (triamcinolone) repeated in 6 to 8 weeks as needed<br><br>Type 3: Superpotent topical steroid for 3 months; taper as symptoms improve, then maintenance (once or twice weekly); second-line includes tacrolimus, pimecrolimus, intralesional corticosteroid injection, oral prednisolone, antibiotics, or immunosuppressive (e.g., azathioprine, cyclosporine)<br><br>Surgical repair of vaginal occlusion | Eliminate identifiable irritants<br><br>Rule out secondary infection (e.g., yeast culture)<br><br>Topical xylocaine and oral antihistamine/anxiolytic (e.g., hydroxyzine) to break nighttime itch–scratch–itch cycle<br><br>Superpotent topical steroid ointment, tapered over 3 to 4 months until lichenification is totally resolved<br><br>Cognitive behavioral therapy for concomitant mental illness | Biopsy seldom required for diagnosis<br><br>Keep skin moist with emollients; careful exposure to sunlight may be helpful; topical mid- or low-potency steroids |
| Other considerations | Ongoing yearly vulvar examination warranted to identify early skin changes due to the small increased risk of vulvar cancer | Specialist referral for erosive or vaginal disease because condition is highly debilitating<br><br>Early use of progressive vaginal dilators may improve and preserve vaginal integrity | Consider psychological component if resolution is atypical (e.g., obsessive–compulsive disorder) | Referral and online support groups may be helpful for women with extensive disease |

Information from Edwards SK, Bates CM, Lewis F, Sethi G, Grover D. 2014 UK national guideline on the management of vulval conditions. http://www.bashh.org; Schlosser BJ, Mirowski GW. Lichen sclerosus and lichen planus in women and girls. *Clin Obstet Gynecol.* 2015;58:125-142.

contact dermatitis, with resulting inflammation. When evaluating any symptoms of vulvar pruritis or inflammation, the midwife should inquire about detergents, cleansers, topical applications, and sources of prolonged moisture.[49]

## Complications of Genital Piercing and Genital Cosmetic Surgery

Though not a disorder, the practice of cosmetic procedures including genital piercing has increased dramatically among all segments of the population. People can choose genital piercing as a means of personal and sexual expression, and in some cases, it is perceived as a form of psychological healing following a traumatic event such as abuse or sexual assault.[55,56] When problems arise as a consequence of piercing, individuals may initially seek answers from the Internet rather than from their healthcare provider.[57]

Genital piercing is usually safe when performed by a licensed provider whose practice is regulated by state laws. Nevertheless, no national safety guidelines exist. Unless the individual performing the procedure is a licensed health professional, no anesthesia is used when performing piercings.

Health risks of genital piercings include local and systemic infection, scarring, infertility due to infection complications, and urethral scar formation.[58,56] Individuals considering pregnancy or who are pregnant are recommended to defer genital piercing to avoid the risk of blood-borne complications such as hepatitis.[58] The Association of Professional Piercers (listed in the Resources section at the end of this chapter) publishes a quarterly journal on piercing techniques, safety, anthropology, and legislative issues relating to body piercing.

The International Society for the Study of Vulvovaginal Disease warns that most procedures advertised as increasing sexual function, such as G-spot augmentation, hymenoplasty or labiaplasty, perianal bleaching, and vaginal tightening, are ineffective and carry significant risks.[55] Midwives can help educate patients about the range of normal anatomy and the risks associated with modification procedures.

## Vulvodynia

Vulvodynia is a chronic genital pain syndrome that is estimated to affect as many as 28% of reproductive-age women during their lifetimes.[59] In 2015, the International Society for the Study of Vulvovaginal Disease (ISSVD), the International Society for the Study of Women's Sexual Health (ISSWSH),

and the International Pelvic Pain Society (IPPS) revised terminology related to vulvar pain. With the new system, vulvar pain is classified into one of two categories: (1) vulvar pain that is associated with a specific disorder or (2) vulvodynia, which refers to persistent vulvar pain without an identified etiology. Examples of causes for vulvar pain that are not vulvodynia include recurrent *Candida* infections, inflammatory disorders such as lichen sclerosus, and trauma such as birth injury and female genital cutting.[60,61] The intent of the new terminology was to reflect the complexity of the disease, to distinguish vulvodynia from other pain or infectious syndromes with known causes, and to better guide diagnosis and treatment. The terminology includes *localization* (localized or generalized), *provocation* (provoked or spontaneous), *onset* (primary or secondary), and *temporality*. Patterns of vulvodynia can include mixed manifestation of these categories.[60,61] The current definition of vulvodynia is vulvar pain that has lasted at least 3 months and has no identifiable etiology.[59]

The cause of vulvodynia is believed to be multifactorial, and several elements—including pathophysiologic factors, psychological factors, and social and relational factors[62]—can influence either the development or subsequent consequences of this disorder. The presentation of vulvodynia includes symptoms that are either chronic and unrelenting or cyclic in nature, which makes the diagnosis of vulvodynia difficult and generally one of exclusion. Various algorithms have been published to aid the clinician in ruling out other potential conditions; Figure 16-2 shows one example.[61]

### Evaluation of Vulvodynia

The evaluation for vulvodynia starts with a comprehensive history of the onset and duration of symptoms using the OLDCARTS mnemonic (see the *Collecting a Health History* appendix). Other comorbid symptoms, such as interstitial cystitis, fibromyalgia, or irritable bowel, are frequently found among individuals with vulvodynia.[63] Physical and sexual abuse in childhood have been identified as possible risk factors for development of vulvodynia.[64]

Examination of the vulva includes evaluation of skin changes, vaginal secretions, presence of lesions, and changes in the vulvar architecture. It is useful to perform an evaluation of point-specific pain and sensitivity by using a cotton swab and gently proceeding in a clockwise fashion on the vulva. Particular areas of sensitivity may be noted, especially

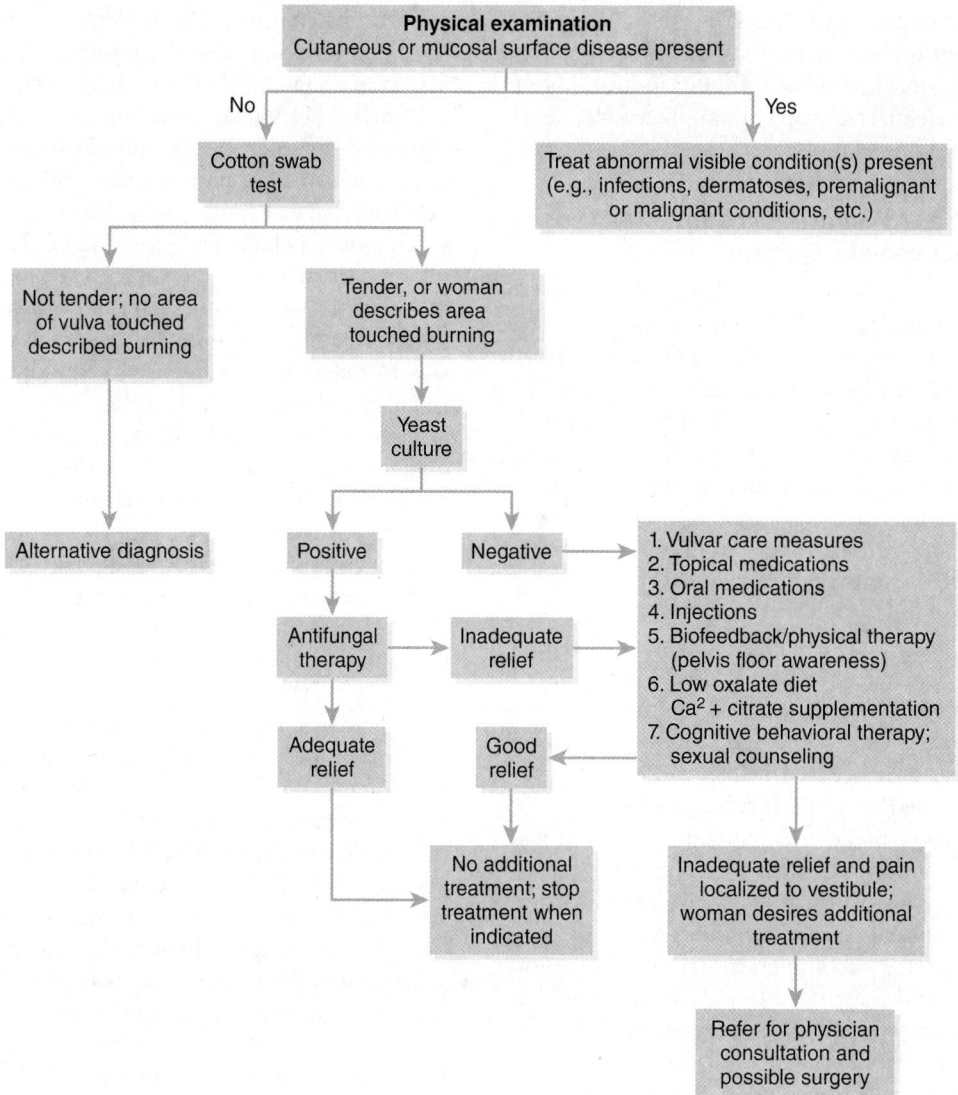

**Figure 16-2** Algorithm for the diagnosis and management of vulvodynia.
Modified with permission from Haefner HK, Collins ME, Davis GD, et al. The vulvodynia guideline. *J Low Genit Tract Dis.* 2005;9:40-51.

at the 11 to 1 o'clock points and the 5 to 7 o'clock points (Figure 16-3).[65] A pelvic examination presents the perfect opportunity to educate individuals about care and hygiene practices that protect the vulva, as outlined in Table 16-4.[53,66]

### Treatment of Vulvodynia

Treatments for vulvodynia are wide-ranging in scope, are highly individualized, and usually begin with avoidance of potential irritants. A person experiencing vulvar pain may have tried numerous over-the-counter treatments, including antifungal and topical steroid preparations. These treatments in themselves may have caused a dermatitis that

must be minimized before further evaluation can occur.[53] Use of unscented toilet tissue, loose cotton clothing, unscented soaps, and showers instead of baths is recommended. Avoidance of feminine hygiene products, fragranced baths, baby or personal wipes, over-the-counter anti-itch products, detergent additives, fabric softeners, dryer sheets, and latex products has been found to reduce vulvar pain for some individuals.[53,67]

Following these initial steps, recommendations for treatment may include psychological interventions, physical therapy, and pelvic floor physical therapy.[67,68] Antidepressants, particularly selective serotonin reuptake inhibitors (SSRIs)

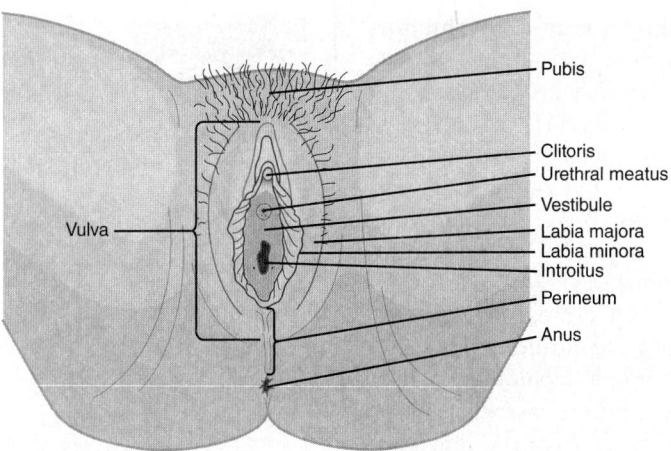

**Figure 16-3** Cotton swab test for specific location of vulvodynia.

| Table 16-4 | Measures to Minimize Vulvar Irritation | |
|---|---|---|
| | **Dos** | **Dont's** |
| **Clothing** | Wear loose, 100% cotton underwear | Wear girdles or thongs (any time) |
| | Remove sweaty, wet clothes and wet bathing suits as soon as possible | Wear underwear at night |
| | Use laundry detergents labeled as hypoallergenic or for sensitive skin (without perfumes or dyes) | Use bleach, stain removers, liquid fabric softeners, or dryer fabric softener sheets on underwear |
| **Bathing** | Use mild soaps without scents or perfumes for bathing | Apply soap directly to the vulva |
| | Clean or soak the vulva only with warm water; soak in warm bath or sitz bath in toilet | Use washcloths or bath sponges to clean or scratch the vulva |
| | Pat the vulva dry after bathing | Use bubble baths, bath salts, or scented oils |
| | | Use hair dryers on the vulvar area |
| **Toileting** | Use soft, white, unscented toilet paper | |
| | Rinse with plain water and pat the vulva dry after urination | |
| | Only wear pads when needed | |
| **Protection** | Use small amounts of vegetable oil, extra virgin olive oil, or solid oils (shortening or coconut oil) on the vulva to protect and hold in moisture | Use oils with condoms during sex |
| | Use adequate lubrication for vaginal penetration during sexual activity | |
| **Itching** | A cool compress or icepack/gel pack wrapped in a cloth or towel | Scratch the vulva |
| **Hygiene** | Trim pubic hair as desired | Shave the pubic hair or use depilatory creams |
| | | Use baby wipes, personal wipes, sprays, perfumes, douches, or other feminine hygiene products |
| **Menstruation** | Use unscented tampons, pads, and panty liners | Use panty liners or pads that retain moisture |
| | Wear pads or panty liners only when needed | |
| | Use 100% cotton menstrual pads if regular pads are irritating | |

Based on American College of Obstetricians and Gynecologists Committee Opinion No. 673: persistent vulvar pain. *Obstetr Gynecol.* 2016;128:378-384; Vulvar care. *J Midwifery Womens Health.* 2022;67(4):527-528. doi.org/10.1111/jmwh.13344.

or serotonin–norepinephrine reuptake inhibitors (SNRIs), also have been used and appear to have some value for relief of pelvic neuropathies.[67,68] A variety of complementary therapies have shown varying degrees of success, including biofeedback, pelvic floor exercises, cognitive group therapy, cognitive-behavioral therapy (CBT), acupuncture, transcutaneous nerve stimulation, hypnotherapy, and cannabis, although none of these is considered a first-line treatment.[69,70] When most or all of the aforementioned modalities are unsuccessful, clinicians may recommend surgery, including excision of nerve pathways or nerve injuries associated with specific locations of pain.[71]

## Pelvic Floor Dysfunction Disorders

The two most common findings related to pelvic floor changes are pelvic organ prolapse and urinary incontinence.[72] Both of these conditions can occur secondary to a number of structural abnormalities, physical trauma, or pathophysiologic conditions. Risk factors for both conditions include pregnancy (regardless of the mode of birth), older age, increasing parity, family history, obesity, smoking, constipation, a history of heavy lifting, prior lower abdominal or pelvic surgeries, a lower abdominal or pelvic mass, a history of chronic lung disease, and a history of a connective tissue disorder (e.g., Marfan syndrome).[72,73]

### Pelvic Organ Prolapse

Pelvic organ prolapse refers to herniation of pelvic organs to or beyond the vaginal walls. Common forms of pelvic organ prolapse include *cystocele* or *urethrocele* (bladder or urethral descent into the vagina), *rectocele* or *enterocele* (protrusion of the rectum into the vagina), and *uterine prolapse* (descent of the uterus into the vagina); see Table 16-5. Each of these conditions, or a combination of them, can cause abnormal bladder or rectal function, pelvic or lower back pain, and decreased pleasure with sexual activity.[74,75]

Although several instruments have been developed to describe the nature and extent of pelvic organ prolapse, the most widely supported is the Pelvic Organ Prolapse Quantification (POP-Q) system, which is endorsed by professional organizations, and used for both research and clinical care.[76–78] When using the POP-Q system, the hymen acts as a fixed point of reference and the prolapse is measured with regard to six anatomic locations. The potential range of measurements is indicated with

| Table 16-5 | Pelvic Organ Prolapse Conditions |
|---|---|
| **Term** | **Description and Findings** |
| Urethrocele | Prolapse of the urethra, evident as descent of the anterior vaginal wall |
| Uterine or cervical prolapse | Prolapse of the uterus, evident as descent of the uterus or uterine cervix into the vagina |
| Vaginal vault (cuff scar) prolapse | Descent of the vaginal vault or cuff scar into the vagina after hysterectomy |
| Cystocele | Prolapse of the bladder, evident as descent of the anterior vaginal wall |
| Rectocele | Prolapse of the rectum, evident as descent of the posterior vaginal wall |
| Enterocele | Hernia of peritoneal sac and small intestine into the rectovaginal space between the vagina and rectum |

each point. The results define one of four stages of prolapse as described in Table 16-6.

### Evaluation of Pelvic Floor Disorders

Evaluation of pelvic floor disorders includes obtaining a comprehensive history and visualizing the external genitalia, vagina, and cervix for signs of urinary leakage or organ displacement, or prolapse. Asking the person to perform a Valsalva maneuver or cough allows the midwife to visually assess the level of vaginal wall support. Some uterine prolapse is more readily apparent when the examination is done with the patient standing. In severe cases, the cervix can protrude through the vulva simply by the pull of gravity. A follow-up bimanual examination during which the person tightens vaginal muscles around the clinician's fingers will help gauge the strength of the pelvic muscles. This also presents an opportunity to teach the correct method for performing muscle tightening exercises. Two short survey instruments to help clinicians determine the nature and extent of prolapse—the Pelvic Floor Impact Questionnaire and the Pelvic Floor Distress Inventory—are also widely available and have been shown to guide treatment that improves quality of life.[79]

### Treatment for Pelvic Floor Disorders

In the absence of pelvic masses, treatment for pelvic floor relaxation may include pelvic floor muscle training. While some evidence indicates that pelvic

| Table 16-6 | Pelvic Organ Prolapse Quantification (POP-Q) System |
|---|---|
| **Point** | **Description** |
| Aa | Anterior vaginal wall 3 cm proximal to the hymen −3 cm to +3 cm |
| Ba | Most distal portion of the remaining upper anterior vaginal wall −3 cm to +3 cm |
| C | Most distal edge of the cervix or vaginal cuff scar |
| D | Posterior fornix (not applicable if posthysterectomy) |
| Ap | Posterior vaginal wall 3 cm proximal to the hymen −3 cm to +3 cm |
| Bp | Most distal position of the remaining upper posterior vaginal wall −3 cm to +3 cm |
| **Point** | **POP-Q Staging Criteria** |
| Stage 0 | Aa, Ap, Ba, Bp = −3 cm and C or D ≤ − (total vaginal length − 2) cm |
| Stage I | Most distal portion of the prolapse −1 cm (above the level of hymen) |
| Stage II | Most distal portion of the prolapse ≥ −1 cm but ≤ +1 cm (≤ 1 cm above or below the hymen) |
| Stage III | Most distal portion of the prolapse > +1 cm but < + (total vaginal length − 2) cm (beyond the hymen; protrudes no farther than 2 cm less than the total vaginal length) |
| Stage IV | Complete eversion; most distal portion of the prolapse ≥ + (total vaginal length − 2) cm |

Based on Haylen BT, De Ridder D, Freeman RM, et al. An International Urogynecological Association (IUGA)/International Continence Society (ICS) joint report on the terminology for female pelvic floor dysfunction. *Neurourol Urodyn.* 2010 Jan;29(1):4-2

floor muscle training alone can improve pelvic organ prolapse, patients often require specific instruction and feedback during a vaginal examination to learn how to perform these maneuvers correctly, and referral to a physiotherapist specializing in such training may be warranted.[80–82]

A variety of support devices or pessaries can be employed in the case of significant uterine prolapse.[83] In general, two types of pessaries (described in the *Fitting a Pessary* appendix) are used: those that offer support (e.g., ring pessary) and those that fill space in the vagina (e.g., cube pessary). The former is suited for patients at POP-Q Stage 1 or 2, while the latter is designed for patients at Stage 3 or 4. After the initial examination and placement of the pessary, the person returns for a follow-up visit in 1 to 2 weeks to assess comfort and normal urinary function. They return again in 3 to 6 months and at least semi-annually thereafter to assess proper use and effectiveness of the pessary. The midwife should teach the person to remove and clean the pessary weekly with soap and warm water. Those unable to change the pessary should be seen by the provider as needed to remove and clean the pessary and ensure proper fitting.[84]

The most important aspect of pessary fitting is ensuring patient comfort with the device.[85,86] Vaginal evaluation includes visual inspection to assess for lesions or bleeding due to tissue erosion caused by the pessary. A person with a pessary in place should be cautioned to report vaginal bleeding promptly, as this can be a sign of tissue damage or intrauterine bleeding indicative of the growth of a malignancy. Low-dose topical estrogen has not been shown to reduce vaginal irritation with pessary use.[87,88]

Several surgical procedures have been introduced in an attempt to repair or restore the lost muscle tone associated with pelvic organ prolapse. Despite these efforts, the long-term success rates of different surgical approaches vary, and the procedures can result in complications such as urinary incontinence.[89]

## Urinary Incontinence

Urinary incontinence is underreported for many reasons, including personal embarrassment, limited access to health care, and lack of proper screening by clinicians. Underreporting has made it difficult to identify how many individuals experience urinary incontinence, but reviews of the prevalence, identification, and treatment of this condition suggest that between 25% and 55% of adult women experience urinary incontinence at some point in their lives. The prevalence can be as high as 75% in older age groups.[90]

Urinary incontinence is often associated with significant diminishment of a person's quality of life. Effects of urinary incontinence can include impaired sleep, limitations on the ability to travel far from home or to engage in social activities, and difficulty in maintaining good hygiene to avoid skin irritation or breakdown. The role of the midwife in assessing and treating urinary incontinence is most often accomplished in consultation with colleagues who specialize in urogynecologic care.

Urinary incontinence is classified based on the presenting symptoms and signs, as summarized in **Table 16-7** The most common types of urinary incontinence are stress, urgency, and overflow incontinence. *Stress urinary incontinence* involves involuntary leakage of urine when intra-abdominal pressure increases, such as with a cough or sneeze. *Urgency urinary incontinence* is less common than stress urinary incontinence; it causes the person to experience a sudden urge to urinate and subsequent involuntary loss of urine if they are unable to empty their bladder immediately. This form of urinary incontinence can be due to a variety of neuropathies. *Overflow urinary incontinence* presents with continuous urine leakage and incomplete bladder emptying. A person with overflow urinary incontinence may also have frequency, nocturia, hesitancy, or a weak intermittent urinary stream. If the bladder is very full, stress leakage can cause symptoms that are similar to those of stress or urgency incontinence. The combination of stress and urgency urinary incontinence is termed *mixed urinary incontinence.*[88,91]

The need to void once or twice during the night is not necessarily indicative of urinary dysfunction, and an occasional episode of leaking urine does not meet the criteria for incontinence treatment. If the urinary incontinence is a side effect of a pharmacologic agent, change in mental status, mobility, or new onset of constipation, the condition may be temporary. Increasing age, obesity, smoking, pregnancy, and increased abdominal pressure due to constipation and occupational lifting also have been shown to contribute to urinary incontinence.

Certain disease states are associated with increased urination and incontinence, including diabetes, urinary tract infection or other renal disease, bladder mass, and pelvic masses such as fibroids and ovarian cancer. Surgery or pelvic trauma also can result in involuntary loss of urine. Vaginal birth does not appear to increase the risk of urinary incontinence compared with having a cesarean birth. A genetic disposition can increase the risk of urinary incontinence even if the person has never been pregnant. Urinary incontinence is not a normal part of aging and should not be attributed solely to advancing age.[92]

### Evaluation of Urinary Incontinence

In the absence of a urinary tract infection, a pelvic mass, pelvic organ prolapse, or some other extrinsic cause of incontinence, the diagnosis of incontinence

| Table 16-7 | Types of Urinary Incontinence |
|---|---|
| **Type of Incontinence** | **Definition and Description** |
| Stress urinary incontinence | Involuntary leakage caused by increases in abdominal pressure, effort, or exertion (e.g., sneezing or coughing) but no urge to urinate prior to leakage. |
| | Caused by urethral hypermobility, which causes the bladder neck and urethra to lose the ability to close. Can occur secondary to insufficient support from pelvic floor muscles, trauma from childbirth, or chronic pressure from obesity or chronic cough. |
| Urgency urinary incontinence | Urge to urinate is sudden, with involuntary leakage and frequent small-volume voids. |
| | The result of detrusor (muscle in bladder wall) overactivity. |
| | Can occur secondary to bladder abnormalities or neurologic disorders. |
| Neurogenic detrusor overactivity (overactive bladder) | Involuntary bladder contractions during the filling phase of the bladder, due to a defined neurologic condition. |
| | A form of urgency urinary incontinence. |
| Mixed urinary incontinence | Involuntary leakage associated with both urgency and stress incontinence. |
| Overflow incontinence | Frequent or constant dribbling or stress incontinence. Typically caused by an underactive detrusor muscle or outlet obstruction. Can occur secondary to detrusor underactivity, which may stem from a low estrogen state, peripheral neuropathy (e.g., diabetes, alcoholism), or spinal cord damage (e.g., muscular sclerosis). Urinary retention can also occur secondary to drug therapy. |
| Nongenitourinary incontinence | Variable leaking of urine caused by functional problems (e.g., neurologic, psychologic, cognitive), pharmacologic agents, environmental problems, or metabolic disorders. |

is made using a combination of history and a variety of urinary function tests.

Many clinical assessment instruments are available to aid making a diagnosis of urinary incontinence. Periodic screening should focus on whether people experience urinary incontinence and if so, whether it affects their activity or quality of life. The International Consultation on Incontinence (ICI) questionnaire has the strongest endorsement for initial screening, with more in-depth questioning becoming necessary when more details are needed.[93] A significant amount of diagnostic information can be shared with the provider by completing a daily urinary diary that includes the time and amount of oral intake, urine output, any urine leakage, and necessary pad changes. These validated questionnaires are often used to help establish a diagnosis and can be readily obtained from the sites listed in the Resources section at the end of this chapter.

Urinary function tests can range from simple to complex. Simple measures include the cough stress test, which can be performed in the office by asking the person to cough with a full bladder and subsequently observing for leaking from the urethra. More complex testing includes urodynamic testing, which involves the use of equipment that can evaluate urethral function, bladder capacity, bladder stability, and the ability to control voiding. The latter form of assessment can be expensive, is usually reserved as second-line testing, and is typically performed by a urologist or urogynecologist.[90,93]

### Treatment of Urinary Incontinence

For patients with stress urinary incontinence, initial treatment includes pelvic floor muscle exercises, behavioral modifications, and dietary changes. Weight loss can improve symptoms of stress urinary incontinence.[94] Some clinicians advocate use of the Knack maneuver, which involves contracting the pelvic muscles as deep into the vagina as possible and holding the contraction while doing other activities during which the person usually experiences incontinence, such as coughing or exercising in general.[95]

The successful use of pelvic floor muscle training can be enhanced by using provider *feedback* (i.e., giving instructions while performing a bimanual examination) or *biofeedback* (i.e., using a vaginal insertion device that offers feedback on the success of attempt with the exercises). Similarly, the promotion of healthy dietary changes, especially in individuals with obesity or constipation, can help reduce incontinence.

Pharmacologic treatments for stress urinary incontinence are generally considered ineffective,

and there are no FDA-approved drugs for treatment of stress urinary incontinence.[90] If a person is diagnosed with stress urinary incontinence combined with urgency or detrusor overactivity (overactive bladder), bladder training is recommended. This training involves either (1) encouraging the person to delay any initial urges to void by using the Knack technique and simultaneously using distracting mental exercises or (2) teaching them to empty their bladder before an urge occurs using timed voiding.

Two classes of drugs are used as first-line therapy to treat urgency urinary incontinence: beta-adrenergic drugs and antimuscarinic agents. The antimuscarinic agents are recommended as first- or second-line treatments for urge incontinence or overactive bladder.[90,93] Extended-release formulations can result in less dry mouth—a common side effect of the antimuscarinic medications. Medications should be combined with behavioral therapy such as timed voiding and fluid management for optimal results. The antimuscarinic and beta-adrenergic drugs should be not used (or used with caution) in elderly persons or in individuals with cognitive impairment, myasthenia gravis, narrow-angle glaucoma, or history of impaired gastric emptying or urinary retention.

Injections of botulinum toxin A (Botox A) into the bladder wall are another effective treatment for some individuals with detrusor overactivity or urgency urinary incontinence. This therapy appears to offer only short-term relief, so repeat injections may be necessary for continence to be maintained. The need to self-catheterize is a possible complication with botulinum toxin treatment.[90,93]

Estrogen was once thought to be a promising treatment for urinary incontinence, especially after menopause. While some evidence suggests that topical or vaginal application of estrogen can improve incontinence, oral systemic use of this agent has been associated with worsening symptoms.[90]

Mechanical devices for control of urinary incontinence include vaginal cones and pessaries in various sizes and shapes, with some reports indicating they are effective. Nevertheless, in population studies, their use has not been demonstrated to make a significant difference in bladder control,[96] and they appear to be most effective in conjunction with other treatments, such as pelvic floor muscle exercises and behavioral modifications.

When other treatments have been ineffective, the final approach to treatment of a person with urinary incontinence is surgery. Surgical options are limited to individuals with stress urinary incontinence, however—they are not applicable to persons

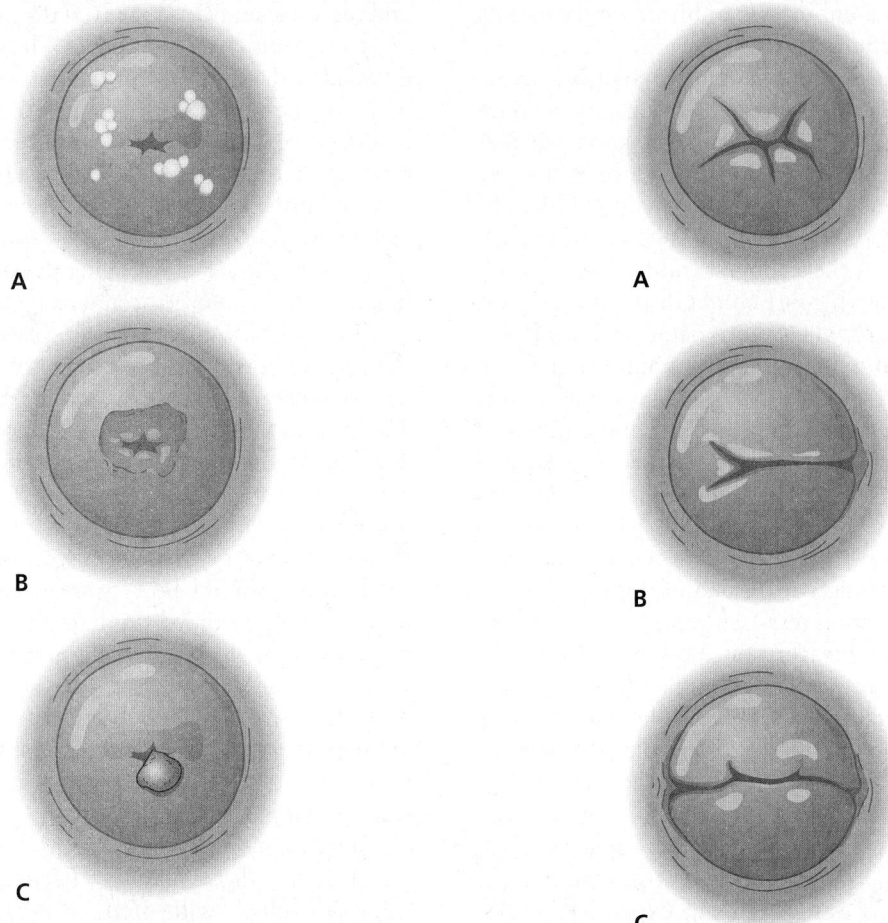

**Figure 16-4  A.** Nabothian cyst. **B.** Cervical ectopy. **C.** Endocervical polyp.

**Figure 16-5**  Cervical lacerations. **A.** Stellate. **B.** Unilateral transverse. **C.** Bilateral transverse.

with urgency urinary incontinence.[90] Clients with stress urinary incontinence considering surgery should be referred to appropriate specialists and informed of the multiple surgical procedures available and the related side effects associated with each respective approach.

## Uterine Cervical Variations and Disorders

The cervix undergoes cellular maturation and repair processes throughout the course of a person's lifetime.[97] Inspection of the cervix with the naked eye during the course of a pelvic examination can reveal several normal and abnormal features relative to the person's age; hormonal status; contraceptive method; stage of pregnancy; and presence or absence of inflammation, infection, or disease. The size and shape of the cervical os is largely determined by parity. Figure 16-4 and Figure 16-5 illustrate common variations noted when visualizing the

cervix—specifically, mucin (Nabothian) cysts, cervical ectopy, polyps, and cervical lacerations.

### Mucus Cysts

Mucus cysts, also referred to as Nabothian cysts or epithelial cysts, are often seen on the cervix during routine examination. They are a benign and normal feature of the adult cervix. Nabothian cysts arise from glandular, mucus-producing tissue, and are then superficially covered by squamous epithelium. They are typically raised with a yellow or white appearance and can range from a few millimeters to 3 to 4 centimeters in diameter. Most require no treatment unless excessively large.[98]

### Cervical Ectopy

Cervical ectopy can cause increased vaginal discharge and, in some cases, postcoital bleeding. While cervical ectopy is normal and is not cervical erosion, patients with excessive, symptomatic discharge or postcoital bleeding require further evaluation to rule out abnormalities.[99]

## Endocervical Polyps

Endocervical polyps often are an incidental finding during the course of a regular pelvic examination. Their typical appearance is that of a small, red, tongue-like growth protruding from the endocervical canal. An endocervical polyp can frequently be the reason patients report postcoital bleeding. The vast majority of polyps are benign and do not require removal unless they are a cause of bleeding, though their presence should be noted in the person's health record.[100]

## Cervical Lacerations

Parous individuals may have sustained a cervical laceration during a birth that was not repaired. If the laceration is extensive, it can be a risk for cervical insufficiency in a subsequent pregnancy. Cervical lacerations should be noted in the person's chart and consultation obtained if they are noted during pregnancy or in individuals planning a pregnancy.

## Condylomata Acuminata

Condylomata acuminata (condylomas) are the manifestation of genital infection with HPV. When found on the cervix, condylomas typically appear as bright white growths with a warty or cauliflower-like appearance. They may be seen in the vagina and on the vulva, perineum, or anus as external genital warts. When administered prior to any HPV exposure, the current HPV vaccine will prevent at least 90% of cases of external genital warts. The *Health Promotion Across the Lifespan* chapter provides additional information regarding vaccines, and additional discussion of condylomas can be found in the *Reproductive Tract and Sexually Transmitted Infections* chapter.

## Leukoplakia

Leukoplakia is a nonspecific term referring to a white spot on the external or internal genitalia. The midwife can use a cotton-tip applicator to verify if such a patch is adherent. The adherent discharge of candidiasis will wipe off with gentle pressure. Leukoplakia can indicate atrophy, lichen sclerosus, condyloma, psoriasis, or just hyperkeratotic areas. Because it is not possible to distinguish leukoplakia from CIN with the naked eye, further evaluation—for example, with a cytology test, colposcopy, or biopsy—is indicated.[101]

# Adnexal Masses During the Reproductive Years

When an adnexal mass is detected, the differential diagnosis includes a functional (as in related to the function of the ovary) physiologic cyst (e.g., follicular or corpus luteum), ectopic pregnancy, benign ovarian neoplasms (e.g., dermoid cyst), ovarian cancer, tubo-ovarian abscess, endometriosis, and ruptured cyst.[102] Adnexal masses can be found in both premenopausal and postmenopausal individuals. Some individuals may be asymptomatic; others may present with symptoms of pelvic pressure, pain, or dyspareunia. Some symptoms associated with ovarian cysts can be vague, such as abdominal bloating, a sensation of fullness, or, possibly, urinary frequency or retention.

Pelvic examinations are often inadequate to determine the size, location, and characteristics of an adnexal mass. Such examinations are especially inadequate for identifying ovarian cysts in individuals with obesity. Ultrasound and MRI are the most commonly used imaging modalities for assessment of the size, character, and malignant characteristics of adnexal masses.[103]

## Corpus Luteum Cysts

Corpus luteum (hemorrhagic) cysts develop following hemorrhage of the corpus luteum, most often during days 20–26 of the menstrual cycle. These cysts can become heavy, causing ovarian torsion. Ultrasound or imaging can confirm the diagnosis. In the absence of bleeding, the cyst will regress spontaneously. In the event of significant bleeding, or with acute pain secondary to the bleeding, a negative pregnancy test can assist in differentiating a ruptured corpus luteum cyst from an ectopic pregnancy. If bleeding continues, surgical intervention can become necessary.[104]

## Ectopic Pregnancy

Ectopic pregnancy is any pregnancy implanted outside the endometrial cavity. An ectopic pregnancy is considered a life-threatening emergency, even if the individual appears stable and asymptomatic. Thus, ectopic pregnancy is one of the first differential diagnoses to be considered in any reproductive-age person. Suspicion for an ectopic pregnancy should be high if an individual reports amenorrhea or intermittent abdominal or pelvic pain of varying duration and intensity. Furthermore, patients who present with any of these symptoms in addition to shoulder pain (i.e., referred pain secondary to the presence of blood in the abdominal cavity, fever, tachycardia, or low blood pressure) must be evaluated for shock and emergency referral even in the absence of vaginal bleeding. The person with an ectopic pregnancy may have not suspected they were pregnant and may be required to integrate a great deal of information at a very stressful moment. More discussion of ectopic pregnancy is found in the *Early Pregnancy Loss and Abortion* chapter.

## Ovarian Cysts

The management of individuals with ovarian cysts is based on the presence of symptoms, imaging results, age, medical history, physical examination, and blood test results. The cyst is first classified as simple or malignant based on features identified on ultrasound.[102] Cysts that have both benign and malignant features require further evaluation to determine the risk for malignancy. Simple ovarian cysts that are thin walled, unilocular, and small are usually benign, but may best be followed with periodic ultrasound assessment. The Society of Radiologists in Ultrasound has published guidelines for management of asymptomatic ovarian cysts detected on ultrasound; these guidelines are based on the person's premenopausal or postmenopausal status, size, and characteristics.[105]

## Dermoid Cysts

Dermoid cysts and cystic teratomas are asymptomatic, unilateral ovarian masses that arise from all three germ cell layers (ectoderm, endoderm, and mesoderm) and, therefore, can contain skin, bone, hair, and teeth. Dermoid cysts are generally asymptomatic and first identified during a pelvic examination or ultrasound. Such cysts do not regress and have a small chance of becoming malignant; therefore, the treatment is surgical removal.[106]

## Ovarian Torsion

An uncommon cause of acute pelvic pain is ovarian torsion, also referred to as adnexal torsion. While causes of torsion include previous adnexal surgical manipulation (especially tubal ligation), an adnexal structural anomaly, or pregnancy, the majority of cases are related to ovarian or adnexal masses. The person can present with specific pain or more generalized unilateral pelvic or flank pain, as well as nausea and vomiting.[107] This condition is often confused with gastrointestinal disorders.

The treatment for a person with ovarian torsion is surgery, during which the ovary is fixed in

place or removed depending on the etiology, if evident, and the presence of tissue damage or necrosis. False-positive diagnoses of ovarian torsion based on ultrasound are not uncommon, and the presence of blood flow to the ovary ascertained by Doppler sonography does not completely exclude torsion.[108] In such a case, the pain can be due to endometriosis, ovarian enlargement without torsion, or unknown causes not readily apparent.

## Disorders of Uterine Origin

The most common disorders associated with the uterus include endometriosis and uterine fibroids. A less common disorder is adenomyosis.

### Endometriosis

Endometriosis is the presence of endometrial tissue outside of the uterine cavity. Although gauging the prevalence of this condition is difficult, it is estimated to affect 5% to 15% of people of childbearing age.[109] The incidence is higher in individuals who present with infertility and chronic pelvic pain. Associated risk factors include a family history, early age at menarche, frequent menses, nulliparity, a history of other pain syndromes (e.g., interstitial cystitis, bladder pain syndrome), inflammatory bowel disease, and a diagnosis of immunologically impaired conditions (including asthma and allergies).[109]

The American Society for Reproductive Medicine (ASRM) categorizes endometriosis into one of four stages depending on the location(s) of the endometrial tissue, depth of the endometrial lesions (implants), extent of the implants, presence of adhesions, and presence of ovarian endometriomas (a type of ovarian cyst):[110]

- Stage I: Minimal; characterized by few implants and no adhesions
- Stage II: Mild; characterized by superficial implants, and no significant adhesions
- Stage III: Moderate; characterized by the presence of both superficial and deep implants, as well as notable adhesions
- Stage IV: Severe; characterized by multiple implants, dense adhesions, and an association with infertility

Unfortunately, these stages do not correlate with the severity of symptoms or infertility.[111] Despite the limitations of the ASRM system, it is helpful as a uniform classification of surgical findings.

| Table 16-8 | Proposed Etiologies of Endometriosis |
| --- | --- |
| **Proposed Etiology** | **Rationale** |
| Retrograde menstruation | During menses, endometrial tissue migrates into the peritoneal cavity, via the oviducts, attaching itself onto pelvic organs. |
| Deviations in cellular physiology | Peritoneal tissue is spontaneously transformed into endometrial tissue. |
| Deviations in lymphatic system | Endometrial tissue is transported to other organs via the lymphatic pathways. |
| Deviations in immune system | Menstrual tissue found outside the uterus is normally cleared by the immune system, which appears unable to do so in individuals found to have endometriosis. |
| Deviations in hormonal system | Unlike in intrauterine endometrial tissue, the estrogenic effects of extrauterine endometrial tissue are not influenced by the antagonistic action of progesterone. |
| Genetics | A 3 to 9 times increased incidence is found among first-degree relatives of affected individuals (i.e., mothers or siblings) compared to the incidence found in the general population. |
| Environmental influences | Dioxin-like compounds discovered in industrial waste by-products can alter gene development or estrogen–progesterone balance in a manner that leads to extrauterine development of endometrial tissue. |

Based on Koninckx PR, Ussia A, Adamyan L, Wattiez A, Gomel V, Martin DC. Pathogenesis of endometriosis: the genetic/epigenetic theory. *Fertil Steril.* 2019 Feb 1;111(2):327-340; Wang Y, Nicholes K, Shih IM. The origin and pathogenesis of endometriosis. *Annu Rev Pathol Mechanisms Dis.* 2020 Jan 24;15:71-95; Saunders PT, Horne AW. Endometriosis: Etiology, pathobiology, and therapeutic prospects. *Cell.* 2021 May 27;184(11):2807-2824

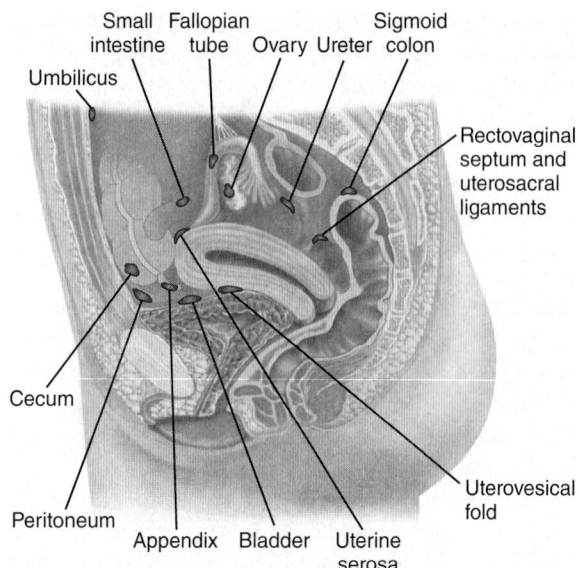

**Figure 16-6** Possible locations in which extrauterine endometrial tissue may be found.

The cause of endometriosis remains elusive, and multiple etiologic theories have been proposed (Table 16-8).[112–115] Retrograde menstruation followed by extrauterine implantation remains the oldest and most widely accepted theory, although findings of endometriosis implants in pre-menarche adolescents suggest more than one etiology might exist. Findings during laparoscopy have revealed that during menses, endometrial tissue migrates into the peritoneal cavity via the oviducts, attaching itself to the pelvic organs. However, this finding does not explain all cases of endometriosis that have been documented. Indeed, retrograde menstruation is even more prevalent than endometriosis. Thus, there is support for theories suggesting that additional factors—such as hormonal, inflammatory, or immunologic conditions—contribute to the actual development of endometriosis in a subpopulation of individuals.[114]

Endometriosis is associated with a number of symptoms—most commonly pelvic pain (particularly dysmenorrhea), dyspareunia, and infertility. However, because endometrial tissue can be found in or proximate to a dozen extrauterine sites (Figure 16-6), symptoms can also include lower back pain, heavy menstrual bleeding, irregular menses, pain between menstrual cycles, dysuria, constipation or diarrhea, postcoital bleeding, lower abdominal pain associated with ovarian cysts, and chronic fatigue. Surgeons sometimes discover endometriosis among asymptomatic patients incidental to an unrelated pelvic surgery or procedure. For this reason, some researchers suggest endometriosis is a syndrome rather than a disease.[114]

Pelvic or lower abdominal pain due to endometriosis can be related to the menstrual cycle, typically appearing at ovulation or intermittently in the time between ovulation and menses. The pain can continue throughout the menses. Pain associated with endometriosis can also occur in patterns unrelated to the menstrual cycle. For example, pain during or after coitus can be so severe as to preclude sexual activities.

Physical examination findings in individuals with endometriosis can be normal, with no significant tenderness associated with organ palpation or movement. In other cases, the exam may reveal cervical motion tenderness, bilateral or unilateral adnexal tenderness, tender nodules on the uterosacral ligaments, ovarian enlargement, or a fixed, retroverted uterus. Definitive diagnosis requires visualization of endometrial implants during surgery. Confirmation of the diagnosis requires biopsy and guides the direction of future treatment. The use of imaging, such as MRI and transvaginal ultrasonography, can provide diagnostic information in individuals with advanced endometriosis; however, these imaging techniques are not useful to identify small or early lesions.

Treatments for endometriosis have shown mixed success. Providers may select a combination of pharmacologic and surgical therapy, including complete hysterectomy and oophorectomy. Pharmacologic treatments include hormonal contraception (either combined or progestin-only), which improves both dysmenorrhea and dyspareunia. Additionally, with extended use of combined oral contraception, people can reduce the number of withdrawal bleeds to a few per year. Depo-medroxyprogesterone acetate (DMPA, Depo-Provera) and the levonorgestrel-releasing IUDs also reduce menstrual pain. Gonadotropin-releasing hormone (GnRH) agonists such as leuprolide acetate (Lupron), with or without add-back estrogen therapy, have been effective, but are expensive and pain relief is not superior to oral contraceptive pills. Elagolix (Orlissa), is non-peptide GnRH antagonist that has fewer hypoestrogenic side effects than leuprolide acetate. Elagolix can be used for 6 months at a high dose or 2 years at a lower dose.[116] Pain relief measures such as use of nonsteroidal anti-inflammatory drugs (NSAIDs) are also helpful. Surgical procedures can be performed to remove lesions.

The treatment employed depends on the wishes of the affected person, including their desire for future childbearing, the degree of pain, the effects of endometriosis on their quality of life, the degree to which their fertility is affected, and their age. A multidisciplinary approach is recommended. Small lesions can be removed during the diagnostic laparoscopy, followed by hormonal treatment to suppress further growth of the excess endometrial tissue, and the use of individually tailored pain management strategies.[117]

## Leiomyomas (Uterine Fibroids)

Leiomyomas, also known as uterine fibroids or fibromyomas, are benign tumors that develop from uterine smooth muscle. They are very common, with a prevalence that ranges from approximately 60% in white people to 80% in Black people. As many as 50% of patients with fibroids have symptoms, including heavy menstrual bleeding, pelvic pain, dyspareunia, or urinary frequency if the tumor presses anteriorly on the bladder.[118] Thus, half of people with fibroids may never know of the tumors' presence and remain asymptomatic across their lifespan.

Estrogen and progesterone promote fibroid growth and theoretically could facilitate growth of leiomyomas in size during pregnancy, although most research has found that fibroids visualized on ultrasound either remain the same size or decrease in size during pregnancy. Generally, fibroids regress after menopause. While these tumors are rarely associated with the development of cancer, any postmenopausal growth of a fibroid or accompanying symptoms, particularly uterine bleeding, warrants evaluation for possible leiomyosarcomas.[119]

Leiomyomas are described on the basis of their anatomic location.

- *Subserosal fibroids* exist just under the uterine serosa and are located outside of the uterus. These growths are attached to the uterus by a large or small base and can be easily palpated on abdominal examination.
- *Intramural* or *myometrial fibroids* are located within the uterine myometrium and can give the uterus an irregular contour.
- *Submucosal fibroids* are located in the uterine endometrium and are usually palpable only as an enlarged uterus.
- *Pedunculated fibroids* present either outside or within the uterine cavity.

When fibroids are present, the uterus will feel firm and irregularly shaped during palpation. If fibroids are suspected during an examination, this finding is shared with the person and confirmed via an ultrasound examination. The benign nature of fibroids is reviewed, as fears of cancer may arise whenever a person is told they may have an unexpected mass. Figure 16-7 depicts fibroids in relation to the uterus as determined by diagnostic imaging or at the time of surgery.

Individuals with slow-growing fibroids can gradually become accustomed to feelings of pelvic fullness and report few symptoms or little pain, even though the fibroids can be large. Other patients can

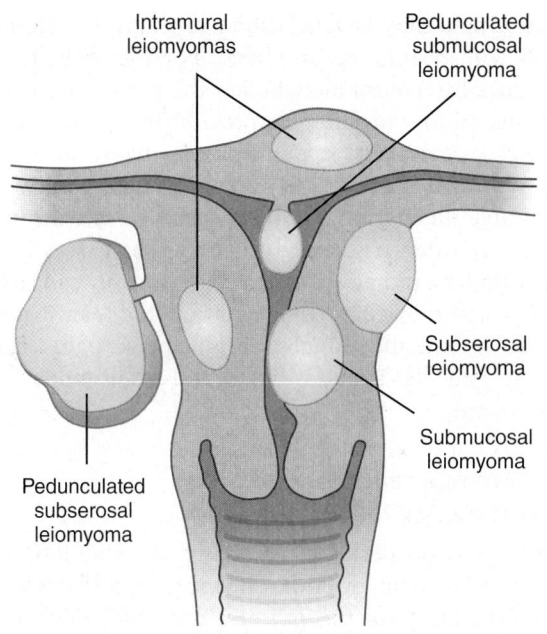

Intramural
leiomyomas

Pedunculated
submucosal
leiomyoma

Subserosal
leiomyoma

Submucosal
leiomyoma

Pedunculated
subserosal
leiomyoma

**Figure 16-7** Classification of fibroids (leiomyomas) by location in relation to the uterus.

present with chronic pelvic pain, lower abdominal pressure, or abnormal uterine bleeding. Fibroids can cause urinary frequency, rectal pressure, interference with sexual activity, and dyspareunia. Depending on their location, these masses can cause infertility, miscarriage, premature labor, malpresentation of a fetus during pregnancy or labor, or abnormal labor progress.[120] Fibroids can also be implicated in abnormal uterine bleeding, especially during the perimenopausal stage of a person's life. The presence of large fibroids or the degeneration of fibroids can cause pain, including during pregnancy.

Treatment of individuals with fibroid-related pain depends on the situation and severity of symptoms. Expectant management is recommended for most individuals, as many fibroids may never be associated with symptoms and most regress after menopause.[118,119] Careful documentation of fibroid size and shape at each annual examination, along with a review of any change in symptoms, is an acceptable management plan.

When intervention is necessary, a variety of nonsurgical interventions, including pharmacologic agents, can be employed to preserve the uterus.[121] Pharmacologic treatments for fibroids include GnRH agonists (e.g., leuprolide acetate [Lupron]) as well as the levonorgestrel-releasing IUD. Success rates in diminishing the size or symptoms of fibroids vary considerably with these methods. While the use of GnRH agonists can be most effective, significant

side effects preclude their first-line use because they induce menopausal symptoms.[122] However, if surgery is deemed appropriate, a GnRH agonist may be used preoperatively to shrink the fibroid(s). Smaller fibroids are easier to remove, and any reduction in size prior to surgery may provide the option of a vaginal versus an abdominal hysterectomy procedure.

Myomectomy is recommended to patients with pain or other indications for fibroid removal who also wish to maintain fertility. While a variety of surgical techniques have emerged in recent years, including uterine artery embolization (UAE) and ultrasonography ablation, each method requires individualization depending on the preference of the person and the characteristics of the fibroid. In the case of large fibroids, persistent heavy vaginal bleeding, or refractory anemia, hysterectomy remains a common treatment option. Midwives should collaborate with specialists in the care of patients who are experiencing fibroid-related pain during pregnancy, as a myomectomy during pregnancy may be needed.[122]

## Adenomyosis

Whereas fibroids are composed of uterine smooth muscle, adenomyosis results from the growth of endometrial tissue in the myometrium layer of the uterus, typically causing uterine enlargement. Because adenomyosis involves growth of endometrial tissue, some sources consider this condition to be a form of endometriosis.[123] Two forms of adenomyosis have been identified: (1) diffuse adenomyosis, in which endometrial tissue is found throughout the myometrium; and (2) focal adenomyosis, in which one or more nodular lesions, known as adenomyomas, are located in specific areas of the uterine myometrium. Diffuse adenomyosis is the more common of the two forms, and is found in approximately two-thirds of diagnosed cases.[13]

Due to difficulty in diagnosing adenomyosis, reports of the incidence of this disorder vary widely—between 20% and 35% of individuals.[124] While many individuals with adenomyosis are asymptomatic, one-third of persons with this diagnosis report heavy menstrual bleeding, dysmenorrhea, and dyspareunia. In general, most individuals with adenomyosis have given birth and typically develop the condition in their fourth or fifth decade of life. Transvaginal sonography can be helpful in diagnosing adenomyosis, although the more definitive diagnostic tool is MRI.

Because the symptoms most commonly associated with adenomyosis are heavy menstrual bleeding and dysmenorrhea, traditional pharmacologic treatments include NSAIDs and combined oral contraceptives. However, greater success is reported with use of progestin-only agents, GnRH agonists, tranexamic acid (Lysteda), and the levonorgestrel-releasing IUD. The reduction of symptoms achieved with these approaches varies, and the clinician should be familiar with the risks, benefits, and contraindications of each approach before making a recommendation. For example, tranexamic acid, a blood-clotting agent, is contraindicated for individuals with a history of venous thromboembolism or individuals who are using a combined hormonal contraceptive method because tranexamic acid increases the risk of thrombosis. Other therapeutic approaches include UAE and radiofrequency ablation (RFA)—techniques also used to treat fibroids.[54] However, if various therapies have been attempted with few positive results, the definitive treatment for adenomyosis is hysterectomy.[125]

## Evaluation of Pelvic Pain

Reports of abdominal and/or pelvic pain are a common motivation for seeking gynecologic care and account for a significant number of visits to healthcare providers. This section introduces the initial gynecologic evaluation and common differential diagnoses for gynecologic pain.

### Acute Pain

Acute abdominal or pelvic pain is a medical emergency. The ability to provide safe care for someone experiencing acute pain requires that the midwife have relationships with surgical and nongynecologic providers and a system for referral. Careful screening and triage must be done to determine the optimal setting for evaluation of acute pain to ensure appropriate management; this setting may be an emergency department or a targeted visit in an office setting, depending on how stable the person is and which other resources are available or needed for a thorough evaluation. Immediate consultation or referral is indicated for a person with acute pain, especially if their pain is accompanied by fever, tachycardia, significant changes in blood pressure, signs of shock, vomiting, unstable vital signs, or evidence of significant blood loss.

### Chronic Pain

Chronic pelvic pain can arise secondary to one or several underlying disorders, and it can be very difficult to evaluate and treat.[117] People with chronic pelvic pain may have a history of multiple encounters with healthcare providers. For the midwife, it is crucial to determine whether the person has been evaluated for chronic pain previously and to clarify their expectations for midwifery involvement in care. Because chronic pelvic pain is associated with multiple underlying etiologies, people with chronic pain are often best cared for by specialists. A general understanding of chronic pelvic pain can help a midwife participate in evaluation and team-based care for these individuals. Chronic pelvic pain treatment benefits from a biopsychosocial model of treatment.[126]

### Differential Diagnoses Associated with Pelvic Pain

Multiple disorders are associated with abdominal pain, pelvic pain, or both. The list of candidates varies depending on the person's age (e.g., premenopausal or postmenopausal) and other demographic characteristics. Table 16-9 lists common differential diagnoses to be considered for reproductive-age individuals who present with acute or chronic abdominal or pelvic pain. This list suggests which components should be included in the physical examination. Because the list of differential diagnoses is large, the following assessments will help focus the direction of the evaluation:

1. Is the person premenopausal or postmenopausal?
2. Could they be pregnant or attempting pregnancy?
3. What are the characteristics of the pain and associated symptoms?
4. Is the pain cyclic or throughout the cycle?

### Evaluation of Abdominal/Pelvic Pain

In all settings, the role of midwives when evaluating a person with abdominal or pelvic pain includes taking a thorough history, performing a physical examination, implementing the initial laboratory evaluation, and providing a referral for specialist care as needed.

A helpful tool in the evaluation of any symptom, including pain, is the OLD CARTS system (see the *Collecting a Health History* appendix).[127] Use of validated questionnaires is also recommended when assessing chronic pelvic pain. Some patients will respond to questionnaires in detail and provide a wealth of information; others, who may have not considered their pain in a comprehensive manner, may need to return for a future visit after completing

| Table 16-9 | Selected Differential Diagnoses for Acute or Chronic Abdominal and/or Pelvic Pain[a] |
|---|---|
| **System** | **Differential Diagnoses** |
| Gastrointestinal | Appendicitis<br>Bowel obstruction<br>Crohn's disease<br>Constipation<br>Diverticulitis<br>Gallbladder obstruction<br>Inflammatory bowel disease or irritable bowel disease<br>Pancreatitis |
| Musculoskeletal | Fibromyalgia<br>Herniated disc<br>Hernia<br>Pelvic pain syndrome<br>Sprain or strain<br>Pelvic floor muscle spasm or injury |
| Gynecologic, acute pain in nonpregnant individuals, not at risk for pregnancy | Endometriosis (rupture of endometrioma)<br>Dysmenorrhea<br>Intrauterine device perforation<br>Mittelschmerz<br>Ovarian cyst<br>Pelvic inflammatory disease<br>Torsion or degeneration of uterine fibroids |
| Gynecologic, chronic pain in nonpregnant persons, not at risk for pregnancy | Adenomyosis<br>Adhesions<br>Endometriosis<br>Malignancy<br>Prior pelvic inflammatory disease<br>Ovarian cancer<br>Uterine fibroid |
| Gynecologic, fertility treatment | Ectopic pregnancy<br>Ovarian hyperstimulation syndrome<br>Ovarian cyst<br>Ovarian torsion |
| Pregnancy-related | Corpus luteal cyst<br>Ectopic pregnancy<br>Normal pregnancy nausea and vomiting<br>Ovarian torsion<br>Miscarriage<br>Preterm labor or placental abruption |
| Postmenopausal | Malignancy |
| Urologic | Interstitial cystitis<br>Pyelonephritis<br>Urinary retention/obstruction<br>Urinary tract infection |
| Neuropathic | Fibromyalgia<br>Trigger points<br>Nerve damage<br>Pudendal neuralgia |

[a]This list is not comprehensive. These disorders are included here because they are either commonly encountered or not common but associated with severe morbidity and, therefore, essential considerations during an evaluation.

a pain diary or history. Many causes of acute pain can become causes of chronic pain, as pain spreads through the central nervous system.[35]

In addition, it is always important to ask two initial questions: (1) What does the individual think is causing the pain? and (2) How is the pain affecting their quality of life? If the initial history results in an inability to diagnose the cause of pain and the person wishes to continue investigation with the midwife, a more detailed history of the pain can be suggested. Assessment modalities may include use of anatomic drawings to locate the pain; use of a pain diary with a pain severity scale; or use of a journal to chart the pain in relation to daily activities, menstrual cycle, bowel habits, sexual activity, and diet. The International Pelvic Pain Society publishes a detailed assessment form available to members.

### Physical Examination

Examination of a person presenting with pelvic pain may require a complete physical examination. Many gynecologic disorders will manifest in different ways, including pain in the abdomen, in the pelvis, or both. If a more narrowly focused examination is indicated, vital signs and both abdominal and pelvic examinations should be performed. In the absence of an acute presentation, a complete examination of systems is appropriate. The person's demeanor and presentation are included in this evaluation. Evaluation of the back and lower extremities is necessary to rule out a musculoskeletal injury, such as a muscle strain or stress fracture, or an anatomic variation, such as scoliosis.

### Abdominal Examination

The goal with palpation of the abdomen is to identify organ enlargement, displacement, masses, or enlarged lymph nodes as well as to ascertain if and where the pain can be elicited. The midwife can ask the person if they can elicit the pain themselves. If not, it is advisable to focus on the unaffected side or area first. Communicating findings and letting the person know which part of the examination is next can help maintain an atmosphere of trust and caring. Special attention should be paid to any area of tension or guarding, and knowledge of patterns of referred pain points is useful as well.

### Pelvic Examination

During the visual inspection of the vulva and vagina, signs of swelling, lesions, trauma, or other skin changes can be assessed. The person's ability to tolerate a speculum insertion with or without pain is an important observation, especially if they report pain with sexual activity. After speculum insertion, a sample of vaginal discharge is collected for a saline or KOH examination or cultures, and subsequent testing for sexually transmitted infections (STIs) if indicated. The introitus can be examined with a cotton swab, noting any point-specific tenderness.

After the speculum examination is complete, a gentle bimanual examination enables the midwife to observe whether the person exhibits discomfort at the introitus versus deep in the vagina or pelvis. Any cervical, adnexal, or uterine motion tenderness elicited provides further information in addition to signs of organ displacement. Attention should be paid to pain specific to the pelvic floor and abdominal wall muscles.[128]

Palpation for any masses, uterine fibroids (leiomyomata), or uterine or adnexal enlargement indicative of pregnancy is the next step. Assessment of pelvic muscle tone is performed, and the presence of a cystocele, a rectocele, or uterine prolapse is ascertained. Confirmation of findings can be accomplished with a rectal examination as well as assessment for hemorrhoids, polyps, or masses, in rare situations.

Documentation of a mass or enlarged organ should include description of the size, shape, location, consistency, mobility, tenderness, and relationship of the mass to other organs. Additionally, if pain is elicited, its intensity and location should be noted. If the person's pain limits the midwife's ability to perform full palpation and/or pelvic examination, that finding should be documented as well.

Acute pelvic pain should yield a specific, treatable diagnosis. Pain that lasts for more than 6 months and that has cognitive, behavioral, sexual, or emotional consequences in the person's life constitutes chronic pelvic pain; in such a case, the individual should be referred to a specialist in pelvic pain management.

### Laboratory/Screening/Diagnostic Tests

Only tests that will generate results that could directly influence management should be performed. A pregnancy test is inexpensive and generally indicated for any pregnancy-capable individual at risk of pregnancy, regardless of contraceptive use. A complete blood count is often ordered as a standard test; however, in the absence of heavy vaginal bleeding, an infectious process, or concerns about anemia, it may not be useful. If the cause of the pain is considered urologic in nature, a urinalysis or urine culture can be informative. Tests for STIs or vaginitis may be indicated by history and examination. A fecal occult blood test can aid in the assessment of any abdominal mass or gastrointestinal condition. Any fecal occult blood test that is positive should result in referral to a specialist for further evaluation and possible colonoscopy or sigmoidoscopy testing.

Pelvic or abdominal ultrasound is commonly used to aid in the diagnosis of uterine or adnexal abnormalities. If ultrasonography is ordered, a transvaginal ultrasound may be more accurate than a transabdominal approach. For individuals who have never experienced vaginal penetration, people who have cultural prohibitions with regard to pelvic procedures, or those with a personal history of sexual assault trauma, this part of the test can be distressing. Anticipatory guidance includes an explanation of the reason for using ultrasound and shared decision making. If the individual wishes to have the ultrasound performed, it is important to alert staff that this is an initial transvaginal pelvic ultrasound and that additional patience and time may be necessary.

## Sexual and Gender-Based Violence

A person who has experienced gender-based violence, sexual abuse, or trauma may have unique gynecologic care needs.[129,130] When caring for individuals who have been sexually abused or assaulted, it is essential for the midwife to provide care that addresses the person's needs in a manner that does not increase physical discomfort, emotional distress, or trauma. An objective and straightforward explanation of the examination should occur before the individual takes off their clothes. Patience and use of skills in facilitating relaxation are indispensable. If abuse is known or revealed during the visit, the midwife should offer the presence of a support person or other staff member for the examination, in an effort to give the person a sense of control over the procedure. Consent is necessary for the initiation and continuation of any pelvic examination.

If the physical examination proves difficult for the client, it can be conducted in smaller steps, over more frequent encounters when possible, unless an acute or emergent problem is suspected. If the problem appears to be acute, the midwife should assess which type of examination other providers may need to do and limit the current examination to only those elements that are absolutely necessary for consultation or referral. For example, if a person has been recently assaulted, it may be necessary to ask a Sexual Assault Nurse Examiner (SANE) to conduct the examination. Some midwives are SANE certified and may perform a complete forensic examination, including collection of evidence.

Regardless of the reason for the visit, the midwife should clearly acknowledge the person's experience and offer the office as a safe haven for exploration and healing.[129] Suspicion or evidence of physical or sexual abuse or assault or gender-based violence requires the midwife to follow institutional guidelines and the laws of the jurisdiction where the midwife is practicing, including those that dictate the legal authority to which the midwife must report any suspicion or evidence of abuse or assault.

## Conclusion

The scope of practice of midwives involves care for people across the lifespan. Both historically and currently, that care includes the management of gynecologic health. This chapter summarizes some of the chronic and malignant conditions most commonly encountered by midwives, such as pelvic organ prolapse, urinary incontinence, and cervical cancer.

Essential to all midwifery care, for every element of practice, and for every situation are good listening skills. Indeed, the key to excellent care is listening to what a person says about their personal symptoms or conditions. All midwives should have a working knowledge of the information presented in this chapter regarding the diagnosis and management of common gynecologic problems, and the need for screening for more complicated conditions. Knowing how and when to access resources and expert collaborators is a lifelong skill for practicing midwives.

## Resources

| Organization | Description |
|---|---|
| Agency for Healthcare Research and Quality (AHRQ) | Federal agency that publishes multiple guidelines, including guidelines from other groups such as the U.S. Preventive Services Task Force. Among the publications available online are those dealing with cervical screening, management of urinary incontinence, cancer and contraception, and vulvar carcinoma. |

| Organization | Description |
| --- | --- |
| American College of Nurse-Midwives (ACNM) | Midwifery organization that provides information about standards and scope of practice as well as a number of position statements. These position statements include *Collaborative Management in Midwifery Practice for Medical, Gynecologic, and Obstetric Conditions* and *Joint Statement of Practice Relations Between Obstetrician-Gynecologists and Certified Nurse-Midwives/Certified Midwives*, along with *Standards for the Practice of Midwifery*, all of which address how to incorporate new procedures into practice. |
| American College of Obstetricians and Gynecologists (ACOG) | Organization that issues multiple guidelines and recommendations regarding women's health care. Although large parts of its website are behind a firewall, ACOG Committee Opinions and Practice Bulletins are usually published in the journal *Obstetrics & Gynecology*. Toolkits on female sexual dysfunction and HPV vaccinations also are available. |
| American Society for Colposcopy and Cervical Pathology (ASCCP) | Organization that provides algorithms essential for managing abnormal cytology results and positive high-risk HPV tests. A free website helps provide individualized patient care using a risk-based calculator. A smartphone app is available for a small fee. |
| American Society for Reproductive Medicine (ASRM) | Practice guidelines on this website include recommended algorithms for evaluating female and male infertility. |
| American Urogynecologic Society (AUGS) | Source for bladder diaries and patient handouts on incontinence and prolapse. |
| Association of Professional Piercers (APP) | An international nonprofit organization dedicated to the dissemination of vital health and safety information about body piercing to piercers, healthcare professionals, legislators, and the general public. |
| Centers for Disease Control and Prevention (CDC) | Consumer-focused page on selected bibliographies related to diethylstilbestrol exposure. |
| International Society for the Study of Vulvovaginal Disease (ISSVD) | Provides a document, in outline form, describing vulvar lesions by color and shape, to help with diagnosis and treatment. A downloadable app is available for a nominal fee. |
| National Cancer Institute (NCI) | Federal agency that includes professional information about a variety of cancers, including cervical, ovarian, peritoneal, vaginal, and vulvar cancer. Clinical databases detailing research in the area as well as clinical trials are available. |
| Our Bodies Ourselves (OBOS) | Provides information about diethylstilbestrol exposure, health risks, and other gynecologic conditions. |
| Practicing Physician Education in Geriatrics Project (PPE) | Urinary incontinence toolkit. It also offers the Questionnaire for female Urinary Incontinence Diagnosis (QUID) and other bladder diary tools as well as professional resources. |

## References

1. American Midwifery Certification Board. 2017 task analysis: a report of midwifery practice. https://www.amcbmidwife.org/docs/default-source/task-analysis/2017-task-analysis-report.pdf. Published 2017. Accessed January 17, 2023.

2. American Cancer Society. *Cancer Facts and Figures.* Atlanta, GA: American Cancer Society. https://www.cancer.org/content/dam/cancer-org/research/cancer-facts-and-statistics/annual-cancer-facts-and-figures/2022/2022-cancer-facts-and-figures.pdf. Published 2022.

3. Margolies L, Brown CG. Current state of knowledge about cancer in lesbians, gay, bisexual, and transgender (LGBT) people. *Semin Oncol Nurs.* 2018;34(1):3-11. doi:10.1016/j.soncn.2017.11.003.

4. Krogsbøll LT, Jørgensen KJ, Larsen CG, Gøtzsche PC. General health checks in adults for reducing morbidity and mortality from disease. *Cochrane Database Syst Rev.* 2019;1(1):CD009009. doi:10.1002/14651858.CD009009.pub3.

5. Guirguis-Blake JM, Henderson JT, Perdue LA. Periodic screening pelvic examination: evidence report and systematic review for the US Preventive Services Task Force. *JAMA.* 2017;317(9):954-966.

6. Arbyn M, Weiderpass E, Bruni L, et al. Estimates of incidence and mortality of cervical cancer in 2018: a worldwide analysis. *Lancet Global Health.* 2020;8(2):e191-e203.

7. Petca A, Borislavschi A, Zvanca ME, et al. Non-sexual HPV transmission and role of vaccination for a better future. *Exp Ther Med.* 2020;20(6):1-1.

8. La Rosa G. Papillomavirus. In: *Global Water Pathogen Project.* Rose JB, Jiménez-Cisneros B, eds. *Part 3: Specific Excreted Pathogens: Environmental and Epidemiology Aspects, Section 1: Viruses.* East Lansing, MI: Michigan State University, UNESCO; 2016. https://www.waterpathogens.org/book/papillomavirus.

9. Wright TC, Stoler MH, Behrens CM, et al. Primary cervical cancer screening with human papillomavirus: end of study results from the ATHENA study using HPV as the first-line screening test. *Gynecol Oncol.* 2015;136(2):189-197.

10. Marcus JZ, Cason P, Downs LS Jr, et al. The ASCCP Cervical Cancer Screening Task Force endorsement and opinion on the American Cancer Society updated cervical cancer screening guidelines. *J Low Genit Tract Dis.* 2021;25(3):187-191.

11. Saslow D, Andrews KS, Manassaram-Baptiste D, et al. Human papillomavirus vaccination 2020 guideline update: American Cancer Society guideline adaptation. *CA Cancer J Clin.* 2020;70(4):274-280.

12. American College of Obstetricians and Gynecologists. ACOG Practice Bulletin Number 131: screening for cervical cancer. *Obstet Gynecol.* 2020;120(5):1222-1238.

13. Perkins RB, Guido RS, Castle PE, et al. 2019 ASCCP risk-based management consensus guidelines for abnormal cervical cancer screening tests and cancer precursors. *J Low Genit Tract Dis.* 2020;24(2):102.

14. Workowski KA, Bachmann LH, Chan PA, et al. Sexually transmitted infections treatment guidelines, 2021. *MMWR Recomm Rep.* 2021;70(4):1.

15. Muzny CA, Schwebke JR. Asymptomatic bacterial vaginosis: to treat or not to treat? *Curr Infect Dis Rep.* 2020;22(12):1-9.

16. American College of Obstetricians and Gynecologists' Committee on Gynecologic Practice. Committee Opinion No. 672: clinical challenges of long-acting reversible contraceptive methods. *Obstet Gynecol.* 2016;128(3):e69-e77.

17. Shimoni N, Bishop IJ, Westhoff CL. Intrauterine contraception. In: Shoupe D, ed. *The Handbook of Contraception.* Cham, Switzerland: Springer; 2020:141-161.

18. Vu M, Yu J, Awolude OA, Chuang L. Cervical cancer worldwide. *Curr Probl Cancer.* 2018;42(5):457-465.

19. Cholli P, Bradford L, Manga S, et al. Screening for cervical cancer among HIV-positive and HIV-negative women in Cameroon using simultaneous co-testing with careHPV DNA testing and visual inspection enhanced by digital cervicography: findings of initial screening and one-year follow-up. *Gynecol Oncol.* 2018;148(1):118-125.

20. Huh WK, Ault KA, Chelmow D, et al. Use of primary high-risk human papillomavirus testing for cervical cancer screening: interim clinical guidance. *Obstet Gynecol.* 2015;125(2):330-337. doi:10.1097/AOG.0000000000000669.

21. American College of Nurse-Midwives. *Standards for the Practice of Midwifery.* Silver Spring, MD: American College of Nurse-Midwives; 2011. https://www.midwife.org/acnm/files/ACNMLibraryData/UPLOADFILENAME/000000000051/Standards_for_Practice_of_Midwifery_Sept_2011.pdf. Accessed January 17, 2023.

22. Wentzensen N, Massad LS, Mayeaux EJ Jr, et al. Evidence-based consensus recommendations for colposcopy practice for cervical cancer prevention in the United States. *J Low Genit Tract Dis.* 2017;21(4):216-222.

23. Ocque R, Austin RM. Follow-up of women with negative Pap test results and abnormal clinical signs or symptoms. *Am J Clin Pathol.* 2016;145(4):560-567.

24. Practice Bulletin No. 168: cervical cancer screening and prevention. *Obstet Gynecol.* 2016;128(4):e111-e130.

25. American Cancer Society. Key statistics for endometrial cancer. https://www.cancer.org/cancer/endometrial-cancer/about/key-statistics.html. Last revised January 12, 2023. Accessed January 17, 2023.

26. Constantine GD, Kessler G, Graham S, Goldstein SR. Increased incidence of endometrial cancer following the Women's Health Initiative: an assessment of risk factors. *J Womens Health.* 2019;28(2):237-243.

27. Practice Bulletin No. 149: endometrial cancer. *Obstet Gynecol.* 2015;125(4):1006-1026. doi:10.1097/01.AOG.0000462977.61229.de.

28. Trojano G, Damiani GR, Casavola VC, et al. The role of hysteroscopy in evaluating postmenopausal asymptomatic women with thickened endometrium. *Gynecol Minimally Invasive Ther.* 2018;7(1):6.

29. Ghadeer H, AlJulaih GH, Muzio MR. Gestational trophoblastic neoplasia. [Updated 2022 Nov 6]. In: *StatPearls* [Internet]. Treasure Island (FL): StatPearls Publishing; 2022 Jan. https://www.ncbi.nlm.nih.gov/books/NBK562225/.

30. Benson C, Miah AB. Uterine sarcoma: current perspectives. *Int J Womens Health.* 2017;9:597.

31. Torre LA, Trabert B, DeSantis CE, et al. Ovarian cancer statistics, 2018. *CA Cancer J Clin.* 2018;68(4):284-296.

32. Kurian AW, Ward KC, Howlader N, et al. Genetic testing and results in a population-based cohort of breast cancer patients and ovarian cancer patients. *J Clin Oncol.* 2019;37(15):1305.

33. Stewart C, Ralyea C, Lockwood S. Ovarian cancer: an integrated review. *Semin Oncol Nurs.* 2019;35(2):151-156. doi:10.1016/j.soncn.2019.02.001. Epub 2019 Mar 11.

34. Goff BA, Mandel LS, Drescher CW, et al. Development of an ovarian cancer symptom index: possibilities for earlier detection. *Cancer.* 2007;109(2):221-227.

35. Baker DE, Simpson LR. Medical and surgical management of chronic pelvic pain. *Obstet Gynaecol Reprod Med.* 2019;29(10):273-280.

36. Grossman DC, Curry SJ, Owens DK, et al. Screening for ovarian cancer: US Preventive Services Task Force recommendation statement. *JAMA.* 2018;319(6):588-594.

37. Yue Y, Zhou W, Pei D. Rising and falling trends in incidence rates of vulvar and vaginal cancers in the United States, 2000–2016. *Research Square;* 2020. Preprint. doi:10.21203/rs.3.rs-60446/v1.

38. Bhat R. Vaginal cancer: epidemiology and risk factors. In: Mehta S, Singla A, eds. *Preventive Oncology for the Gynecologist.* Singapore: Springer; 2019:309-314.

39. Bray F, Laversanne M, Weiderpass E, Arbyn M. Geographic and temporal variations in the incidence of vulvar and vaginal cancers. *Int J Cancer.* 2020;147(10):2764-2771.

40. Goodman A, Schorge J, Greene MF. The long-term effects of in utero exposures: the DES story. *N Engl J Med.* 2011;364(22):2083-2084.

41. Elkins JM, Hamid OS, Simon LV, Sheele JM. Association of Bartholin cysts and abscesses and sexually transmitted infections. *Am J Emerg Med.* 2021;44:323-327.

42. Stevens DL, Bisno AL, Chambers HF, et al. Practice guidelines for the diagnosis and management of skin and soft tissue infections: 2014 update by the Infectious Diseases Society of America. *Clin Infect Dis.* 2014;59(2):e10-e52.

43. Illingworth B, Stocking K, Showell M, et al. Evaluation of treatments for Bartholin's cyst or abscess: a systematic review. *BJOG.* 2020;127(6):671-678.

44. Selk A, Wood S. Folliculitis. In: Bornstein J, ed. *Vulvar Disease.* Cham, Switzerland: Springer; 2019:215-218.

45. Zouboulis CC, Bechara FG, Dickinson-Blok JL, et al. Hidradenitis suppurativa/acne inversa: a practical framework for treatment optimization: systematic review and recommendations from the HS Alliance working group. *J Eur Acad Dermatol Venereol.* 2019;33(1):19-31.

46. Fergus KB, Lee AW, Baradaran N, et al. Pathophysiology, clinical manifestations, and treatment of lichen sclerosus: a systematic review. *Urology.* 2020;135:11-19.

47. Goldburg SR, Strober BE, Payette MJ. Hidradenitis suppurativa: epidemiology, clinical presentation, and pathogenesis. *J Am Acad Dermatol.* 2020;82(5):1045-1058.

48. Seyed Jafari SM, Hunger RE, Schlapbach C. Hidradenitis suppurativa: current understanding of pathogenic mechanisms and suggestion for treatment algorithm. *Front Med.* 2020;7:68.

49. American College of Obstetricians and Gynecologists' Committee on Practice Bulletins—Gynecology. Diagnosis and management of vulvar skin disorders: ACOG Practice Bulletin, Number 224. *Obstet Gynecol.* 2020;136(1):e1-e14. doi:10.1097/AOG .0000000000003944.

50. Sadownik LA, Koert E, Maher C, Smith KB. A qualitative exploration of women's experiences of living with chronic vulvar dermatoses. *J Sex Med.* 2020;17(9):1740-1750.

51. Wijaya M, Lee G, Fischer G, Lee A. Quality of life in vulvar lichen sclerosus patients treated with long-term topical corticosteroids. *J Low Genit Tract Dis.* 2021;25(2):158-165.

52. Day T, Weigner J, Scurry J. Classic and hypertrophic vulvar lichen planus. *J Low Genit Tract Dis.* 2018;22(4):387.

53. Stockdale CK, Boardman L. Diagnosis and treatment of vulvar dermatoses. *Obstet Gynecol.* 2018;131(2):371-386.

54. Raef HS, Elmariah SB. Vulvar pruritus: a review of clinical associations, pathophysiology and therapeutic management. *Front Med (Lausanne).* 2021;8:649402. doi:10.3389/fmed.2021.649402.

55. Vieira-Baptista P, Almeida G, Bogliatto F, et al. International Society for the Study of Vulvovaginal Disease recommendations regarding female cosmetic genital surgery. *J Low Genit Tract Dis.* 2018;22(4):415-434.

56. Young C, Armstrong ML, Roberts AE, et al. A triad of evidence for care of women with genital piercings. *J Am Acad Nurse Pract.* 2010;22(2):70-80.

57. Holbrook J, Minocha J, Laumann A. Body piercing. *Am J Clin Dermatol.* 2012;13(1):1-17.

58. Van Hoover C, Rademayer CA, Farley CL. Body piercing: motivations and implications for health. *J Midwifery Womens Health.* 2017;62(5):521-530.

59. Bornstein J, Bogliatto F, Haefner HK, et al. The 2015 International Society for the Study of Vulvovaginal Disease (ISSVD) terminology of vulvar squamous intraepithelial lesions. *Obstet Gynecol.* 2016;127(2):264-268.

60. Haefner HK, Collins ME, Davis GD, et al. The vulvodynia guideline. *J Low Genit Tract Dis.* 2005;9(1):40-51.

61. Stockdale CK, Lawson HW. 2013 vulvodynia guideline update. *J Low Genit Tract Dis.* 2014;18(2):93-100.

62. Vieira-Baptista P, Lima-Silva J, Pérez-López FR, et al. Vulvodynia: a disease commonly hidden in plain sight. *Case Rep Womens Health.* 2018;20:e00079.

63. Bergeron S, Rosen NO. Psychosocial factors in vulvodynia. In: Goldstein AT, Pukall CF, Goldstein I, Krapf JM, Goldstein SW, Goldstein G, eds. *Female Sexual Pain Disorders: Evaluation and Management.* Hoboken, NJ: John Wiley & Sons; 2020:87-95.

64. Arbel A, Lev-Sagie A. Generalized unprovoked vulvodynia. In: Goldstein AT, Pukall CF, Goldstein I, Krapf JM, Goldstein SW, Goldstein G, eds. *Female Sexual Pain Disorders: Evaluation and Management.* Hoboken, NJ: John Wiley & Sons; 2020:381-386.

65. Bergeron S, Reed BD, Wesselmann U, Bohm-Starke N. Vulvodynia. *Nat Rev Dis Primers.* 2020; 6(1):1-21.

66. American College of Obstetricians and Gynecologists. Committee Opinion No. 673: persistent vulvar pain. *Obstet Gynecol.* 2016;128(3):e78-e84.

67. Rosen NO, Dawson SJ, Brooks M, Kellogg-Spadt S. Treatment of vulvodynia: pharmacological and non-pharmacological approaches. *Drugs.* 2019; 79(5):483-493.

68. Ventegodt S. New trends in the treatment of vulvodynia and other chronic female disorders: a review. *J Pain Manag.* 2020;13(1):19-25.

69. Spadt SK, Fariello JY. Complementary and alternative treatments for female sexual pain. In: Bartlik B, Espinosa G, Mindes J, eds. *Integrative Sexual Health.* Oxford, England: Oxford University Press; 2018:395-407.

70. Barach E, Slavin MN, Earleywine M. Cannabis and vulvodynia symptoms: a preliminary report. *Cannabis (Res Soc Marijuana).* 2020;3(2):139-147.

71. Lyra J, Lima-Silva J, Vieira-Baptista P, et al. Surgical treatment for provoked vulvodynia: where do we stand? A narrative review. *Pelviperineology.* 2021;40(3):120-128.

72. Rogers RG, Pauls RN, Thakar R, et al. An International Urogynecological Association (IUGA)/ International Continence Society (ICS) joint report on the terminology for the assessment of sexual health of women with pelvic floor dysfunction. *Int Urogynecol J.* 2018;29(5):647-666.

73. Billecocq S, Bo K, Dumoulin C, et al. An International Urogynecological Association (IUGA)/International Continence Society (ICS) joint report on the terminology for the conservative and non-pharmacological management of female pelvic floor dysfunction. *Progres en urologie: Journal de l'Association francaise d'urologie et de la Societe francaise d'urologie.* 2019;29(4):183-208.

74. Verbeek M, Hayward L. Pelvic floor dysfunction and its effect on quality of sexual life. *Sex Med Rev.* 2019;7(4):559-564.

75. American College of Obstetricians and Gynecologists. Pelvic organ prolapse. *Female Pelvic Med Reconstr Surg.* 2019;25(6):397-408.

76. Madhu C, Swift S, Moloney-Geany S, Drake MJ. How to use the Pelvic Organ Prolapse Quantification (POP-Q) system? *Neurourol Urodyn.* 2018;37(S6):S39-S43.

77. Haylen BT, De Ridder D, Freeman RM, et al. An International Urogynecological Association (IUGA)/ International Continence Society (ICS) joint report on the terminology for female pelvic floor dysfunction. *Neurourol Urodyn.* 2010;29(1):4-20.

78. Tulikangas P. Pelvic organ prolapse: ACOG Practice Bulletin Summary, Number 214. *Obstet Gynecol.* 2019;134(5):1124-1127.

79. Radzimińska A, Strączyńska A, Weber-Rajek M, et al. The impact of pelvic floor muscle training on the quality of life of women with urinary incontinence: a systematic literature review. *Clin Interv Aging.* 2018;13:957.

80. Basow SA. The hairless ideal: women and their body hair. *Psychol Women Q.* 1991;15(1):83-96.

81. Basnet R. Impact of pelvic floor muscle training in pelvic organ prolapse. *Int Urogynecol J.* 2021;32(6):1351-1360. doi:10.1007/s00192-020-04613-w.

82. Maxwell M, Berry K, Wane S, et al. Pelvic floor muscle training for women with pelvic organ prolapse: the PROPEL realist evaluation. *Health Serv Delivery Res.* 2020;8(47).

83. Bugge C, Adams EJ, Gopinath D, et al. Pessaries (mechanical devices) for managing pelvic organ prolapse in women. *Cochrane Database Syst Rev.* 2020;11(11):CD004010. doi:10.1002/14651858 .CD004010.pub4.

84. Barnes H, Pham T. Pessary fitting trial. In: Tam T, Davies M, eds. *Vaginal Pessaries.* Boca Raton, FL: CRC Press; 2019:33-40.

85. Radnia N, Hajhashemi M, Eftekhar T, et al. Patient satisfaction and symptoms improvement in women using a vginal pessary for the treatment of pelvic organ prolapse. *J Med Life.* 2019;12(3):271.

86. Vasconcelos CTM, Gomes MLS, Geoffrion R, et al. Pessary evaluation for genital prolapse treatment: from acceptance to successful fitting. *Neurourol Urodyn.* 2020;39(8):2344-2352.

87. Chiengthong K, Ruanphoo P, Chatsuwan T, Bunyavejchevin S. Effect of vaginal estrogen in postmenopausal women using vaginal pessary for pelvic organ prolapse treatment: a randomized controlled trial. *Int Urogynecol J.* 2022;33(7):1833-1838. doi:10.1007/s00192-021-04821-y.

88. de Albuquerque Coelho SC, Giraldo PC, Brito LGO, Juliato CRT. ESTROgen use for complications in women treating pelvic organ prolapse with vaginal PESSaries (ESTRO-PESS): a randomized clinical trial. *Int Urogynecol J.* 2021;32(6):1571-1578. doi:10.1007/s00192-020-04654-1.

89. Baessler K, Christmann-Schmid C, Maher C, et al. Surgery for women with pelvic organ prolapse with or without stress urinary incontinence. *Cochrane Database Syst Rev.* 2018;8(8):CD013108. doi:10.1002/14651858.CD013108.

90. ACOG Practice Bulletin No. 155: Urinary incontinence in women. *Obstet Gynecol.* 2015;126(5):e66-e81. doi:10.1097/AOG.0000000000001148.

91. O'Reilly N, Nelson HD, Conry JM, et al. Screening for urinary incontinence in women: a recommendation from the Women's Preventive Services Initiative. *Ann Intern Med.* 2018;169(5):320-328.

92. Vaughan CP, Markland AD. Urinary incontinence in women. *Ann Intern Med.* 2020;172(3):itc17-itc32.

93. Sussman RD, Syan R, Brucker BM. Guideline of guidelines: urinary incontinence in women. *BJU Int.* 2020;125(5):638-655.

94. Cacciari LP, Dumoulin C, Hay-Smith EJ. Pelvic floor muscle training versus no treatment, or inactive control treatments, for urinary incontinence in women: a Cochrane systematic review abridged republication. *Brazil J Phys Ther.* 2019;23(2):93-107.

95. Miller JM, Sampselle C, Ashton-Miller J, et al. Clarification and confirmation of the Knack maneuver: the effect of volitional pelvic floor muscle contraction to preempt expected stress incontinence. *Int Urogynecol J.* 2008;19(6):773-782.

96. Dumoulin C, Hay-Smith J, Habée-Séguin GM, Mercier J. Pelvic floor muscle training versus no treatment, or inactive control treatments, for urinary incontinence in women: a short version Cochrane systematic review with meta-analysis. *Neurourol Urodyn.* 2015;34(4):300-308.

97. Casey PM, Long ME, Marnach ML. Abnormal cervical appearance: what to do, when to worry? *Mayo Clin Proc.* 2011;86(2):147-150; quiz 151. doi:10.4065/mcp.2010.0512.

98. Barrigón A, Ziadi S, Jacot-Guillarmod M, et al. Nabothian cyst content: a potential pitfall for the diagnosis of invasive cancer on Pap test cytology. *Diagn Cytopathol.* 2019;47(2):127-129.

99. Aggarwal P, Amor AB. Cervical ectropion. [Updated 2022 Nov 7]. In: *StatPearls* [Internet]. Treasure Island (FL): StatPearls Publishing; 2022 Jan. https://www.ncbi.nlm.nih.gov/books/NBK560709/.

100. Alkilani YG, Apodaca-Ramos I. Cervical polyps. [Updated 2022 Sep 5]. In: *StatPearls* [Internet]. Treasure Island (FL): StatPearls Publishing; 2022 Jan. https://www.ncbi.nlm.nih.gov/books/NBK562185/.

101. Yordanov A, Tantchev L, Kostov S, et al. Vulvar leukoplakia: therapeutic options. *Przegląd Menopauzalny [Menopause Review].* 2020;19(3):135.

102. Ross E, Fortin C. Ovarian cysts. Cleveland Clinic. 2016. https://my.clevelandclinic.org/health/diseases/9133-ovarian-cysts.

103. Graham L. ACOG releases guidelines on management of adnexal masses. *Am Fam Physician.* 2008;77(9):1320.

104. Khati NJ, Kim T, Riess J. Imaging of benign adnexal disease. *Radiol Clin.* 2020;58(2):257-273.

105. Andreotti RF, Timmerman D, Strachowski LM, et al. O-RADS US risk stratification and management system: a consensus guideline from the ACR Ovarian-Adnexal Reporting and Data System Committee. *Radiology.* 2020;294(1):168-185.

106. Hamad Morcy HM, L. Alanazi FA, Oqla Alanazi WM, et al. An overview on etiology, diagnosis and management of ovarian dermoid cyst: simple review article. *J Pharm Res Int.* 2021;33(48B):335-340. doi:10.9734/jpri/2021/v33i48B33291.

107. Sasaki KJ, Miller CE. Adnexal torsion: review of the literature. *J Minim Invasive Gynecol.* 2014;21(2):196-202.

108. Ssi-Yan-Kai G, Rivain A-L, Trichot C, et al. What every radiologist should know about adnexal torsion. *Emerg Radiol.* 2018;25(1):51-59.

109. Parasar P, Ozcan P, Terry KL. Endometriosis: epidemiology, diagnosis and clinical management. *Curr Obstet Gynecol Rep.* 2017;6(1):34-41.

110. Hoeger KM, Guzick DS. Classification of endometriosis. *Obstet Gynecol Clin North Am.* 1997;24(2):347-359.

111. Andres MP, Borrelli GM, Abrão MS. Endometriosis classification according to pain symptoms: can the ASRM classification be improved? *Best Pract Res Clin Obstet Gynaecol.* 2018;51:111-118.

112. Brown J, Farquhar C. Endometriosis: an overview of Cochrane reviews. *Cochrane Database Syst Rev.* 2014;2014(3):CD009590. doi:10.1002/14651858.CD009590.pub2.

113. Koninckx PR, Ussia A, Adamyan L, et al. Pathogenesis of endometriosis: the genetic/epigenetic theory. *Fertil Steril.* 2019;111(2):327-340.

114. Saunders PT, Horne AW. Endometriosis: etiology, pathobiology, and therapeutic prospects. *Cell.* 2021;184(11):2807-2824.

115. Wang Y, Nicholes K, Shih I-M. The origin and pathogenesis of endometriosis. *Annu Rev Pathol Mechanisms Dis.* 2020;15:71-95.

116. Vercellini P, Buggio L, Frattaruolo MP, et al. Medical treatment of endometriosis-related pain. *Best Pract Res Clin Obstet Gynaecol.* 2018;51:68-91.

117. ACOG Practice Bulletin No. 218: chronic pelvic pain. *Obstet Gynecol.* 2020;e98-e109.

118. Marsh EE, Al-Hendy A, Kappus D, et al. Burden, prevalence, and treatment of uterine

fibroids: a survey of US women. *J Womens Health*. 2018;27(11):1359-1367.

119. Pérez-López FR, Ornat L, Ceausu I, et al. EMAS position statement: management of uterine fibroids. *Maturitas*. 2014;79(1):106-116.

120. Coutinho LM, Assis WA, Spagnuolo-Souza A, Reis FM. Uterine fibroids and pregnancy: how do they affect each other? *Reprod Sci*. 2021;(8):1-7.

121. Martínez-Perez O, Vouga M, Cruz Melguizo S, et al. Association between mode of delivery among pregnant women with COVID-19 and maternal and neonatal outcomes in Spain. *JAMA*. 2020;324(3):296-299.

122. Riggan KA, Stewart EA, Balls-Berry JE, et al. Patient recommendations for shared decision-making in uterine fibroid treatment decisions. *J Patient Exper*. 2021;8:23743735211049655.

123. García-Solares J, Donnez J, Donnez O, Dolmans M-M. Pathogenesis of uterine adenomyosis: invagination or metaplasia? *Fertil Steril*. 2018;109(3):371-379.

124. Vannuccini S, Luisi S, Tosti C, et al. Role of medical therapy in the management of uterine adenomyosis. *Fertil Steril*. 2018;109(3):398-405.

125. Oliveira MAP, Crispi CP, Brollo LC, De Wilde RL. Surgery in adenomyosis. *Arch Gynecol Obstet*. 2018;297(3):581-589.

126. Rachin S, Sharov M, Zaitsev A, et al. Chronic pelvic pain: from correct diagnosis to adequate therapy. *Neurol Neuropsychiatry Psychosomatics*. 2020;12(2):12-16.

127. Ball JW, Dains JE, Flynn JA, et al. *Seidel's Guide to Physical Examination E-Book: An Interprofessional Approach*. St. Louis, MO: Elsevier Health Sciences; 2022.

128. Arnold MJ, Osgood AT, Aust A. Chronic pelvic pain in women: ACOG updates recommendations. *Am Fam Physician*. 2021;103(3):186-188.

129. Ades V, Wu SX, Rabinowitz E, et al. An integrated, trauma-informed care model for female survivors of sexual violence: the engage, motivate, protect, organize, self-worth, educate, respect (EMPOWER) clinic. *Obstet Gynecol*. 2019;133(4):803-809.

130. Hillard A, Paula J. Why and how to perform trauma-informed care. *Contemp OB/GYN*. 2019; 64(8):15-17.

APPENDIX

# 16A

# Fitting a Pessary

KATHRYN OSBORNE

Pelvic organ prolapse (POP) occurs with the descent of one or more of the pelvic organs and resulting herniation of the vaginal wall. This herniation can occur in the anterior vaginal wall (cystocele and urethrocele), the vaginal apex (uterine prolapse), or the posterior vaginal wall (rectocele or enterocele).[1] The most common type of POP is cystocele, which results from descent of the bladder.[1] The peak occurrence of POP symptoms is in individuals ages 70 to 79 years.[2] An estimated 41% to 50% of women in the United States have been diagnosed with some degree of POP.[3]

The symptoms of POP differ according to the severity and type of prolapse, and often result in reduced health-related quality of life as a result of bulging in the vagina, sexual dysfunction, and varying degrees of urinary and fecal incontinence.[1] Current recommendations are to consider treatment for those persons who experience discomfort associated with vaginal pressure or bulging, sexual dysfunction, or alterations in urinary or defecatory function, and to offer vaginal pessary as a first-line treatment alternative to surgery.[2] Evaluation and management of POP are described in the *Malignant and Chronic Gynecologic Disorders* chapter; fitting a ring pessary is described in this appendix.

## Types of Pessaries

When shared decision making results in identification of a vaginal pessary as the best approach to treating POP, the first step is to determine which type of pessary to use. Two types of pessaries are available: *space-occupying pessaries* (such as the Gellhorn or cube) and *support pessaries* (such as the ring or the ring with support) (Figure 16A-1). The choice of pessary type has traditionally been made based on the degree of prolapse: Support pessaries have been used to treat Stage I and Stage II prolapse, whereas

Stage III and IV prolapse have typically been treated with space-occupying pessaries.[1,4] However, recent research has identified that individuals with Stage III and IV prolapse can achieve adequate symptom relief with pelvic floor exercises in conjunction with support pessaries,[5,6] which are easier to remove and replace, and which are associated with less discharge and irritation compared to space-occupying pessaries.[1,4] The most commonly used pessary is the ring pessary with support, which is also associated with high rates of symptom relief.[1,4,5]

## Fitting the Pessary

1. Obtain the necessary supplies: nonsterile gloves, set of fitting rings, and lubricant.

2. Offer the patient an opportunity to empty their bladder.

3. Assist the patient onto an examination table and into the same position used for a pelvic examination; provide draping for privacy and comfort.

4. Inform the patient that you will be conducting a pelvic examination to obtain the internal measurements necessary to fit the pessary, and to let you know if they become uncomfortable at any time. After obtaining consent, proceed with the examination.

5. Put on gloves. Insert a middle finger and forefinger into the vagina. Place your middle finger behind the cervix in the posterior fornix and note where the posterior pubic notch rests against your index finger; in the absence of a cervix, gently place the middle finger against the posterior vaginal wall. You will use the distance between the end of your middle finger and the location on your index finger that marked the posterior pubic notch

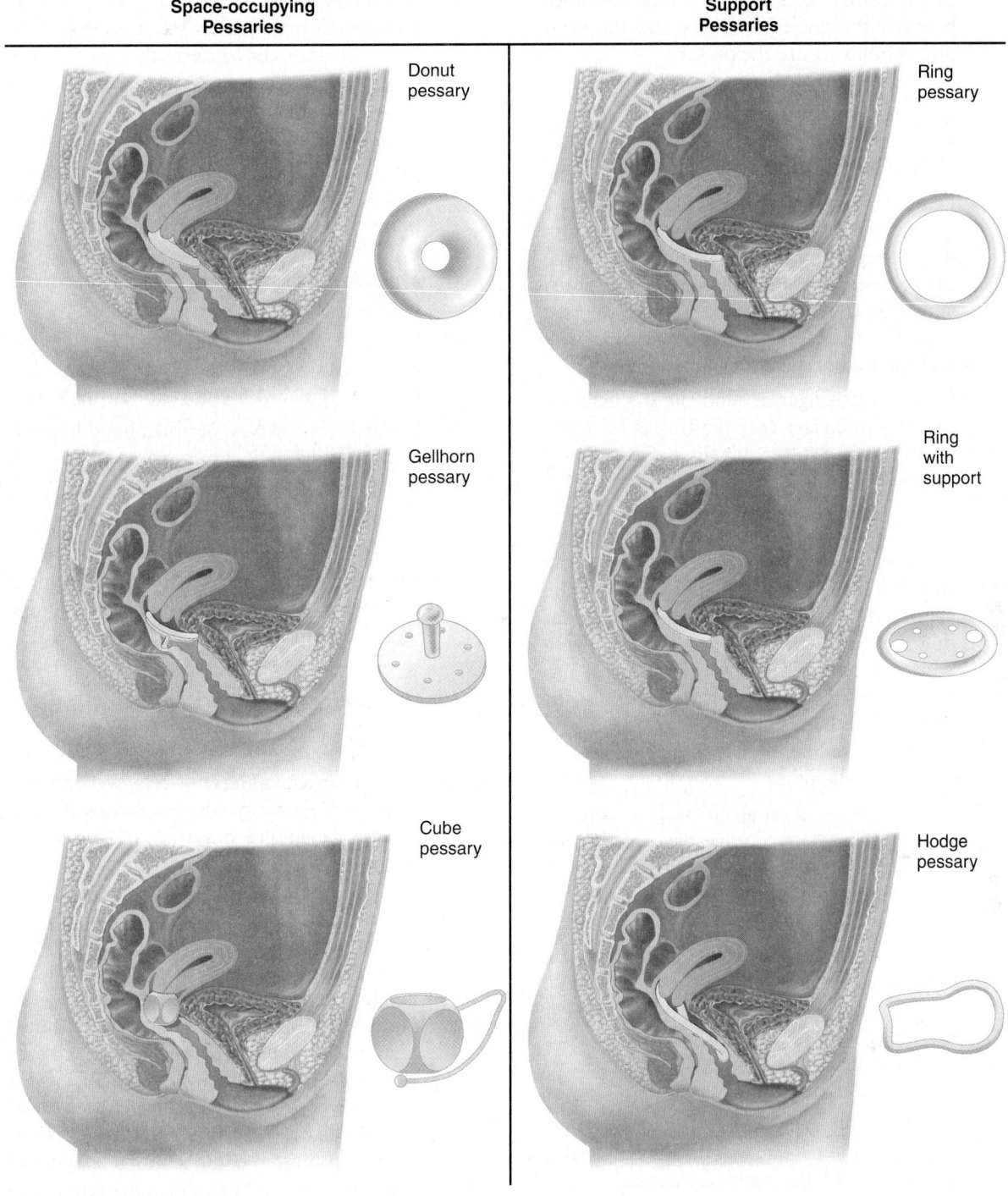

**Figure 16A-1** Types of pessaries.

as the initial measurement of the distance between the posterior fornix and the symphysis pubis to size the pessary.

6. Remove your fingers and choose the fitting ring with the diameter that most closely approximates the distance between your middle and index fingers.

7. Fold the ring in half and apply lubricant to the end that will be inserted; insert the ring into the vagina so that the ring rests behind the cervix posteriorly and behind the pubic notch anteriorly. In the absence of a cervix, the ring should rest posteriorly against the vaginal wall and anteriorly behind the pubic notch.

8. Sweep your finger around the diameter of the ring to ensure that the ring is fully unfolded and comfortably in place without undue pressure against the posterior, anterior, or lateral vaginal walls. Ask the patient to bear down and check for movement of the ring while bearing down. If the ring slides over the cervix or downward in the vagina, or is visible at the introitus, repeat this test with a larger ring. A smaller ring will be necessary if the pessary cannot unfold completely or if you are unable to fit your finger between the vaginal wall and the ring; use the largest pessary that retains a comfortable fit.

9. Ask the patient to get up and walk around for several minutes, encourage them to void or defecate if possible. Remove gloves and perform hand hygiene while the patient is moving around.

10. When they return, assist the patient onto the examination table and put on new gloves. Reassess the placement of the pessary. If it remained in place, remove and discard your gloves before teaching about self-care. Assist the patient to a sitting position.

11. Explain to the patient that they may remove and clean the pessary as often as they feel it is necessary (daily, weekly, or monthly). Also explain that you will offer an opportunity to practice removing and replacing the pessary before leaving the clinic.

12. Using a diagram, show the patient how to insert their index finger to locate the pessary (behind the pubic notch) and remove it. Step out of the room to provide a private space to remove the pessary.

13. When you return to the room, ask if they felt comfortable removing the pessary and respond to any questions or concerns they may have.

14. Demonstrate how to fold the pessary in half, apply lubricant, and (using a diagram) demonstrate how the pessary is inserted. Explain that placing one foot on the examining table's step stool may make insertion (and removal) easier. Ask if they have any questions before you leave the room to provide a private space to practice insertion of the pessary.

15. Upon returning to the room, apply gloves and check to see that the fitting ring has been properly replaced. Remove the fitting ring.

16. Remove your gloves, perform hand hygiene, and assist the patient to a sitting position.

17. Provide the patient with cleansing tissue and exit the room so that they may get dressed for the remainder of the visit.

18. Return to the room to discuss any questions or concerns the patient has and review ongoing follow-up care.

## Ongoing Follow-Up and Management

The recommended frequency of follow-up visits following pessary placement has not been well studied. However, experts generally advise a follow-up visit 1 month after beginning pessary use to evaluate symptom improvement and satisfaction with the pessary.[4-6] Most patients can safely perform pessary self-care and management of a vaginal pessary, removing and cleaning the pessary with soap and water as often as desired.[1,4] Those who perform self-care should return to the clinic every 6 to 12 months for an examination and assessment of the vaginal wall.[1,4] Patients who do not engage in self-care of the pessary should return to the clinic every 3 months to have the pessary removed and cleaned and for an examination of the vaginal wall.[1,5,6]

The most common complications associated with pessary use are a malodorous vaginal discharge, vaginal irritation and ulceration, pain, and vaginal bleeding.[1] Most of these complications appear to occur less frequently in those persons who engage in at least monthly removal and self-care of the pessary.[7] Any patient with an intact uterus who reports vaginal bleeding should be referred for further evaluation. In addition, patients who do not achieve adequate symptom relief with a pessary should be referred to a gynecologic or urologic specialist for more extensive evaluation and a discussion of treatment options.

## References

1. Iglesia CB, Smithling KR. Pelvic organ prolapse. *Am Fam Physician.* 2017;96(3):179-185.

2. American College of Obstetricians and Gynecologists. ACOG practice bulletin summary: pelvic organ prolapse. *Obstet Gynecol.* 2019;134(5):1124-1127.

3. American College of Obstetricians and Gynecologists, American Urogynecologic Society. Pelvic organ prolapse. *Female Pelvic Med Reconstruct Surg.* 2019;25(6):397-408.

4. Ding J, Chen C, Song X, et al. Changes in prolapse and urinary symptoms after successful fitting of a ring pessary with support in women with advanced pelvic organ prolapse: a prospective study. *Urology.* 2016;87(C):70-75.

5. Gold RS, Baruch Y, Amir H, et al. A tailored flexible vaginal pessary treatment for pelvic organ prolapse in older women. *J Am Geriatr Soc.* 2021;69(9):2518-2523.

6. Li B, Chen Q, Zhang J, et al. A prospective study of pessary use for severe pelvic organ prolapse: 3-year follow-up outcomes. *Arch Gynecol Obstet.* 2020;301:1213-1218.

7. Daneel L, West N, Moore KH. Does monthly self-removal of vaginal ring pessaries for stress urinary incontinence/prolapse reduce complication rates? A 5 year audit. *Austral NZ Continence J.* 2016;22(4):105-106.

APPENDIX

# 16B

# Punch Biopsy

MELISSA G. DAVIS

## Introduction

A skin biopsy is used in many clinical scenarios to diagnose and treat skin conditions and lesions. Common techniques include shave, punch, and incisional biopsies, with the technique chosen based on the biopsy site and the characteristics of the area to be biopsied. These characteristics include the size of the area being evaluated, if a minimum depth or size is needed for evaluation, and the differential diagnoses being considered. Skin biopsies are used to determine the cause of chronic or acute skin disorders and lesions as well as to diagnose precancerous and cancerous lesions.

Punch biopsy is a type of biopsy that uses a cylindrical tool with a round stainless-steel blade called a skin or surgical punch. It is a cost-effective, safe, and simple procedure for collecting tissue samples for evaluation. It can be done in outpatient clinics and is generally well tolerated. Punches come in 2- to 6-mm sizes, although the 3- and 4-mm sizes are most common. Numerous clinical scenarios can require the histopathologic evaluation of skin abnormalities. New or chronic lesions, rashes, lesions not responding to treatment, and previously diagnosed skin disorders such as lichen sclerosus may all need confirmation by histologic examination.

If there is a high suspicion of malignancy, a punch biopsy is not recommended. In these instances, an experienced clinician needs to choose the proper biopsy method to ensure that the appropriate depth and size are obtained so that the entire lesion and its margins are removed. A referral to a dermatologist or general surgeon is warranted.

Injectable lidocaine should be used to reduce the pain of the punch biopsy. While topical creams have been shown to be more effective than injectable lidocaine for a punch biopsy on an area with no hair, it has not been studied adequately in areas with hair.[1] Providers should discuss both options with the individual and make the decision based on patient preference. For patients reporting anxiety prior to the procedure, topical lidocaine–prilocaine could be applied 10 minutes before the use of injectable lidocaine.[1] The risks of punch biopsy are minimal and related to infection at the biopsy site, bleeding, scarring, and obtaining an inadequate sample.[2]

## Indications for Punch Biopsy[2,3]

- Benign tumors (such as dermatofibroma)
- General rashes
- Small lesions with concern for malignancy (such as nevi or small melanomas)
- Papulosquamous disease
- Atypical lesions (hyperpigmented, indurated, bleeding, ulcerated)
- Lesions in immunocompromised individuals

## Contraindications to Punch Biopsy

- Infection at the biopsy site
- Presence of superficial vessel or nerve at the site
- Lesion is larger than 6 mm in diameter and/or larger than the punches available to the clinician

## Potential Side Effects/Complications and Preventive Measures

- Pain, infection, and bleeding at biopsy site
- Scarring at biopsy site

Preventive measures:

- Clean technique
- Use of petroleum ointment to minimalize scarring

## Supplies

Gather the equipment needed for the procedure:

- Nonsterile gloves
- Punch biopsy of appropriate size
- Labeled specimen cup with formalin
- Antiseptic solution (such as alcohol or chlorhexidine)
- Anesthetic such as lidocaine–prilocaine cream or lidocaine for injection[1]
- Scissors and/or scalpel
- Sterile sponges or gauze pads
- Pickup forceps
- Supplies for suturing: needle drivers, monofilament nonabsorbable suture appropriate for thickness of skin and biopsy site (4-0 black nylon on a P-12 is useful for most)[2]
- Petroleum-based ointment such as Vaseline or Aquaphor
- Adhesive bandage of appropriate size

A sample tray for punch biopsy is shown in Figure 16B-1.

## Procedure

1. Thoroughly review the individual's health history (paying attention to any known bleeding disorders), medication or supplement use, and allergies.

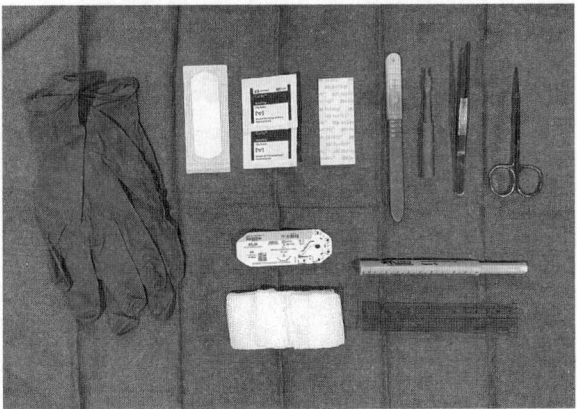

**Figure 16B-1** Sample tray for punch biopsy.

2. Provide education and instruction regarding the procedure, side effects, and possible adverse effects of punch biopsy.
3. Obtain informed consent after reviewing the risks, benefits, and alternatives to the procedure.
   - Informed consent form
   - Witness if required by protocol
4. Assist the individual to a comfortable position based on the site being biopsied. If collecting a vulvar sample, assist the individual to assume a lithotomy position.
5. Apply antiseptic solution to the area with a large cotton swab or cotton ball.
6. Apply an anesthetic to the area being sampled.
7. Using the gloved, nondominant hand, stretch the skin perpendicular to the relaxed skin lines.[2]
8. With the gloved, dominant hand, place the punch over the lesion and apply gentle downward pressure while twisting the punch. You will feel a slight "pop" as the tissue releases and the punch goes through the dermis.
9. Retract the punch. Gently grasp the freed lesion with pickups, and use a scalpel or scissor to free the base of the lesion from the subcutaneous layer.
10. Place the lesion in the labeled specimen cup.
11. Blot the biopsy site with gauze. Apply direct pressure until hemostatic, then close the defect in the usual fashion using interrupted sutures. Larger defects nay require a deep cuticular absorbable suture to prevent dead space at the base of the defect.[2]
12. Apply a petroleum-based ointment and adhesive dressing.

The procedure for punch biopsy is shown in Figure 16B-2.

## Results and Management

Laboratory findings can vary in their language and presentation depending on the laboratory reporting system. In general, the provider will receive a histology report, with information that can confirm a diagnosis. In communicating the findings to the individual, the provider should ensure that the person understands the results and the possible courses of action to follow.

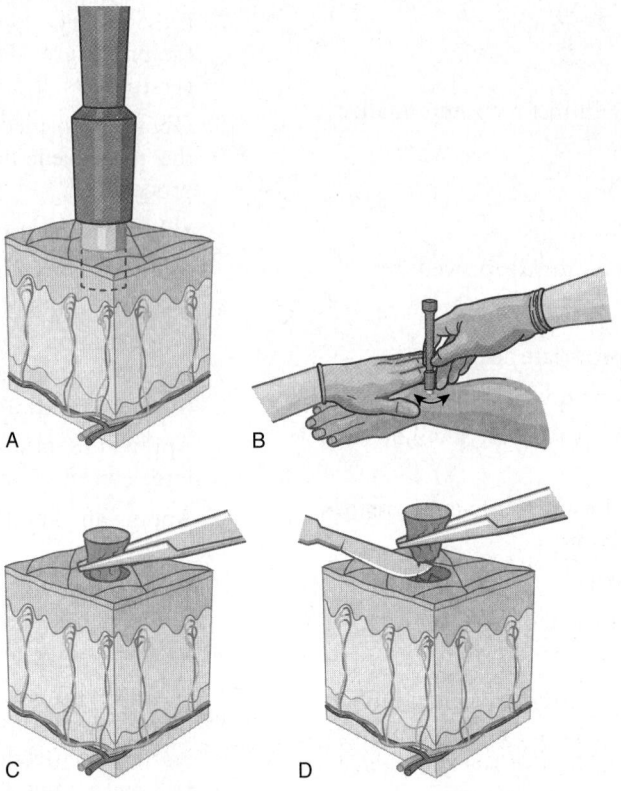

**Figure 16B-2** Punch biopsy technique. **A.** Insert the device to the designated depth. **B.** Gently but firmly rotate the punch to release the tissue. **C.** Gently grasp the top of the core of tissue with forceps. **D.** Cut or snip the tissue at the base of the sample.

## References

1. Williams LK, Weber JM, Pieper C, et al. Lidocaine–prilocaine cream compared with injected lidocaine for vulvar biopsy: a randomized controlled trial. *Obstet Gynecol.* 2020;135(2):311-318.

2. Bobonich M, Nolen M, Honaker J, DiRuggiero D. *Dermatology for Advanced Practice Clinicians: A Comprehensive Guide to Diagnosis and Treatment.* 2nd ed. Philadelphia, PA: Wolters Kluwer; 2021.

3. American College of Obstetricians and Gynecologists. Diagnosis and management of vulvar skin disorders: ACOG Practice Bulletin, Number 224. *Obstet Gynecol.* 2020;136(1):e1-e14.

CHAPTER

# 17

# Breast and Chest Conditions

MIRIAM E. LEVI

*The editors acknowledge Joyce L. King, who was the author of this chapter in the previous edition.*

## Introduction

Breast and chest health are essential as part of primary care management for individuals assigned female at birth. Conditions of the breast or chest encompass a broad range of diagnoses, from benign disorders such as fibroadenomas to life-threatening malignancies. Midwives provide expert care in this aspect of gynecology and must have depth to their knowledge base. This chapter reviews normal development of the breast, current recommendations for breast and chest examination, and common benign breast disorders. It also provides an overview of breast cancer, including risk factors, the impact of health disparities, diagnosis, and treatment options. Considerations for transgender individuals, surgical procedures, and maintenance care are discussed as well.

## Breast Development

The anatomy and embryonic development of the breast are discussed in detail in the *Anatomy and Physiology of the Reproductive System* chapter. The process of development of secondary sex characteristics takes place in an orderly and predictable sequence. Tanner's classification of sexual maturity is a scale used to evaluate breast and pubic hair growth as a way of assessing normal growth and development. Often the first sign of puberty is thelarche, the onset of breast development. On average, breast development is initiated between 8 and 10 years old.[1]

Both estrogen and progesterone influence breast development, with estrogen stimulating the ductal portion of the glandular system and progesterone stimulating the alveolar or milk-producing components of the system.[2] These two hormones are not sufficient to achieve optimal growth and development; therefore, breast stimulation from insulin, cortisol, thyroxine, prolactin, and insulin-like growth factor is also required. The complete development of the alveolus into a mature milk-producing gland occurs with the increases in estrogen and progesterone levels that occur during pregnancy.[2]

It is not uncommon for the breasts to develop asymmetrically. By the end of puberty, the breasts are approximately the same size in most women, although many have persistent visible breast asymmetry.[2] Significant asymmetry is modifiable through breast surgery. Hormone therapy is ineffective for treatment of this chest condition.

As an individual ages, their breast tissue changes from a highly dense state during adolescence to predominantly glandular tissue later in life. Breast changes that occur during pregnancy and lactation (i.e., mammogenesis and lactogenesis) are discussed in the *Anatomy and Physiology of Pregnancy* and *Anatomy and Physiology of Postpartum* chapters. After lactation is complete, glandular tissue in the breast regresses, with associated tissue remodeling. The breasts become less dense with age, converting into fat and fibrous tissue through the transition to menopause.[2]

Patients assigned male at birth can experience a period of breast enlargement similar to thelarche called gynecomastia. Approximately 50% of adolescent individuals assigned male at birth will experience physiologic gynecomastia during early puberty around age 13, which usually resolves within 6 months to 2 years after onset.[3] This chest condition can also be physiologic, caused by the decrease in testosterone during the aging process later in life. Alternatively, gynecomastia may be associated

663

with specific diseases such as Klinefelter syndrome, hyperthyroidism, and liver failure, or it may result from an unexpected side effect of a chronic medication (including spironolactone and digoxin). If symptoms persist after 2 years or continue past 17 years of age, further evaluation is needed.[3]

## Evaluation of Breast Symptoms

A systematic approach to breast examination is critical to evaluate new-onset patient-reported breast symptoms. According to the American Cancer Society (ACS), the most common symptom of breast cancer is a new lump or mass.[1] Many benign breast conditions can present in a similar manner, but an expedited evaluation must be completed to determine the risk of malignancy whenever a new breast mass is palpated. Midwives are often the first healthcare contact for a patient with breast symptoms and are responsible for completing a comprehensive work-up, including evaluation for breast cancer, for these patients.

### History

The history of present illness portion of the clinical assessment should include the items noted in Table 17-1 for any patient who is evaluated for new breast symptoms. The midwife documents these components in the health record with pertinent negative symptoms as well as important positive findings.

A standard clinical assessment should also be completed, including exacerbating and alleviating factors, medications or treatments tried with clinical response, and any history of similar symptoms in the past.

In addition to the history of present illness information collected, a pertinent health history must be obtained to determine patient risk factors that might indicate breast cancer or another breast/chest condition. When evaluating a patient with breast symptoms, factors that increase or decrease their risk for breast cancer should be identified and documented in the health record as described Table 17-2. Factors that are known to be protective against breast cancer include breastfeeding/chestfeeding, physical activity, and avoidance or limiting alcohol intake.

### Physical Examination

A comprehensive evaluation of the breasts during the physical examination portion of a clinical visit includes assessment of the neck, breasts, nipples, chest wall, and axillae. The technique for

| Table 17-1 | Breast Symptom Evaluation and Documentation |
|---|---|

Change in overall appearance of the breast(s) over specified time, especially in relation to the menstrual cycle

Skin changes such as thickening of skin (*peau d'orange*), which may indicate inflammatory cancer

New-onset nipple inversion

Nipple discharge, including the following information:
- Bilateral or unilateral
- Color
- Timing
- Frequency
- Spontaneous or elicited

Cyclic or noncyclic pain (mastalgia), including pain characteristics

New-onset breast mass or a change in previously stable breast mass, including the following descriptive details:
- Location on the breast
- Consistency
- Size
- Border characteristics
- Tenderness to palpation, especially with relationship to menstrual cycle

examination of the breast is detailed in the *Breast and Chest Examination* appendix.

When abnormalities are noted during the exam, further evaluation should ensue. Breast findings characteristic of nonmalignant breast disorders include painful or even tender, firm, mobile, well-defined masses that may fluctuate in size and tenderness with menstrual-cycle changes. A breast mass is considered a dominant mass if it is a three-dimensional lesion that cannot be replicated in the same location on the other breast. The classic sign of a breast lesion suspicious for breast cancer is a hard, rocky, immobile mass with irregular or ill-defined borders.

Breast masses should be measured in centimeters and noted in the patient's health record if palpated. The location, consistency, symmetry, tenderness, and mobility are noted, as are any skin or nipple changes. The location should be recorded by distance in centimeters from the areola. Directionally, the location should be described by comparing the breast to a clock, with the nipple at the center

| Table 17-2 | Risk Factors for Breast Cancer |
|---|---|
| **Risk Factor** | **Description** |
| Age | • Advancing age<br>  ◆ Most breast cancer is diagnosed at 55 years of age or older. |
| Sex | • Assigned female at birth |
| Race | • Incidence of breast cancer is higher among African American individuals than among white individuals younger than age 45.<br>• Incidence of breast cancer is higher in white individuals than in African American individuals between 60 and 84 years of age.<br>• African American individuals are more likely to die from breast cancer at any age than members of other racial and ethnic groups. |
| Height | • Taller women (unknown etiology) |
| Weight | • Overweight or obese body mass index after menopause<br>  ◆ Often associated with higher insulin levels |
| Family history | • First-degree relative with breast cancer doubles the risk<br>  ◆ Two first-degree relatives with breast cancer triples the risk<br>• Jewish ancestry of Ashkenazi (Eastern European) descent<br>• Breast cancer in a patient assigned male at birth<br>• One or more first-degree relatives with ovarian cancer<br>• Multiple relatives with any type of cancer, especially hereditary breast, and ovarian syndrome–associated cancer (e.g., prostate, pancreatic)<br>• Known inherited genetic mutations, including BRCA1 or BRCA2 |
| Health history | • Personal history of invasive breast cancer, ductal carcinoma in situ, or lobular carcinoma in situ<br>• Biopsy-confirmed proliferative breast lesions with atypia<br>• High-dose radiation to chest as a teenager or young adult when breasts are still developing<br>• Never breastfed<br>• Previous cancer of the endometrium, ovary, or colon<br>• High bone density if postmenopausal<br>• Known inherited genetic mutations, including BRCA1 or BRCA2 |
| Reproductive history | • Early menarche, before 12 years of age<br>• Nulliparity<br>• Older than age 30 years at time of first birth<br>• Onset of menopause after 55 years of age<br>• Personal or in utero exposure to diethylstilbestrol (DES) |
| Medications | • Current use of oral contraceptives that contain both estrogen and progesterone<br>• Hormone therapy with estrogen and progesterone for 5–9 years of use[a] |
| Alcohol | • Alcohol consumption<br>  ◆ Risk increases in relation to intake amount |
| Breast density | • Dense breasts on mammogram increase breast cancer risk by 1.5–2 times compared to average breast density |

[a]The increased risk of breast cancer is no longer present if more than 5 years has passed since discontinuation of menopausal hormone therapy.

Based on American Cancer Society. *Cancer facts & figures 2022*. American Cancer Society; 2022:1-78. https://www.cancer.org/content/dam/cancer-org/research/cancer-facts-and-statistics/annual-cancer-facts-and-figures/2022/2022-cancer-facts-and-figures.pdf. Accessed April 13, 2023; U.S. Preventive Services Task Force. Screening for breast cancer: U.S. Preventive Services Task Force recommendation statement. *Ann Intern Med*. 2016;164(4):279-296; Hoffman B, Schorge J, Bradshaw K, et al. Breast diseases. In: Hoffman B, Schorge J, Bradshaw K, Halvorson LM, et al., eds. *Williams Gynecology*. 3rd ed. New York, NY: McGraw-Hill; 2016:275-286; Britt KL, Cuzick J, Phillips KA. Key steps for effective breast cancer prevention. *Nat Rev Cancer*. 2020;20(8):417-436. doi:10.1038/s41568-020-0266-x; Yedjou CG, Sims JN, Miele L, et al. Health and racial disparity in breast cancer. *Adv Experim Med Biol*. 2019;1152;31-49. https://doi.org/10.1007/978-3-030-20301-6_3.

| Table 17-3 | Sample Clinical Note Documentation for Breast Symptom Evaluation |
|---|---|
| Subjective | Chief Concern: new breast lump |
| | History of Present Illness: Patient reports new breast lump palpated 2 weeks ago. Patient states lump has grown slightly since she first noticed it. Lump is felt above the nipple on the right breast. Firm, mobile, about 2 centimeters in diameter, with distinct borders and tender to patient self-palpation. Patient denies changes on breast skin, nipple discharge, or nipple inversion on both breasts. Patient reports the breast lump pain is worse at the end of the day and resolves with ibuprofen (Advil) administration. Patient states this has never happened to her before. |
| Objective | Chest/Breasts: Breasts are symmetric without erythema, dimpling or thickening of skin. 2.5-centimeter mass palpated at 12 o'clock on right breast. Mild tenderness to palpation. No mass palpated on left breast. No nipple cracking, inversion, discharge, tenderness, or ulceration bilaterally. No axillary lymphadenopathy. |

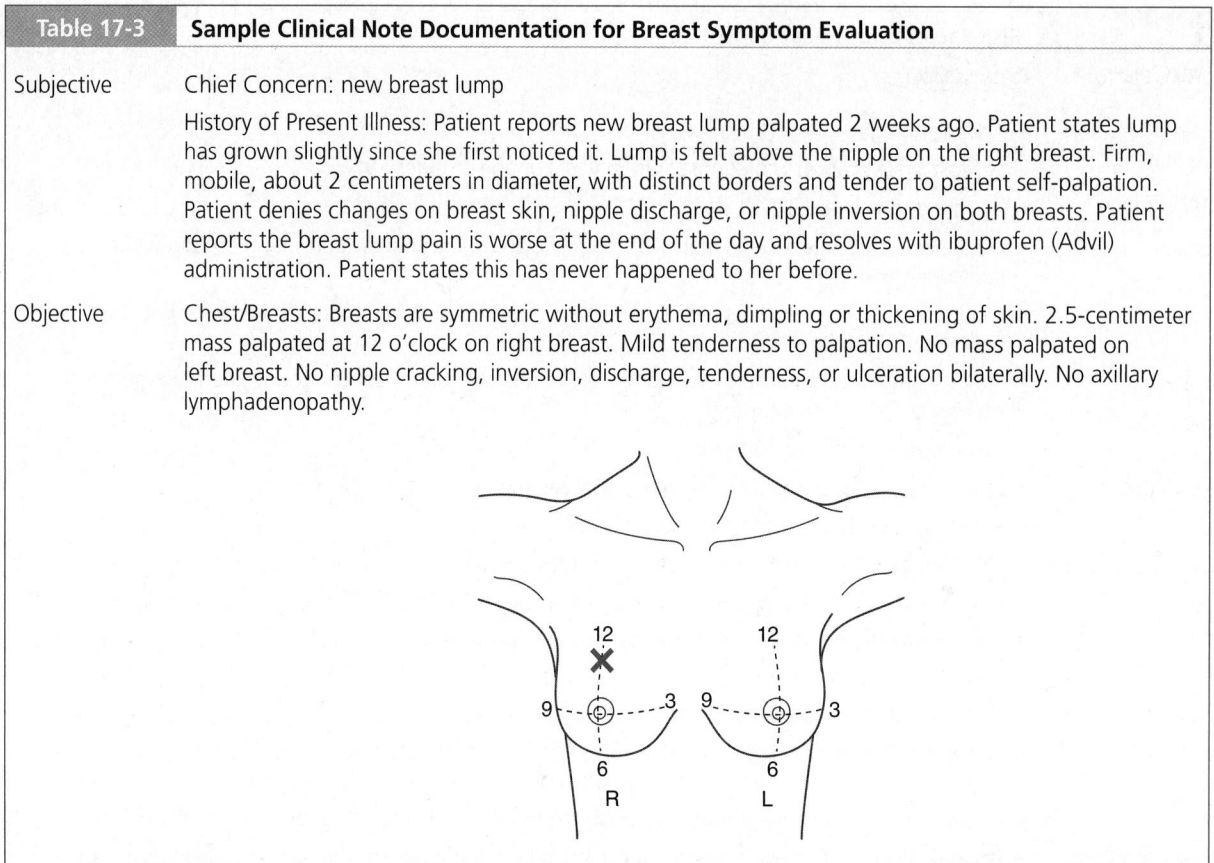

of the clock face. A sample documentation for a breast mass noted on exam includes the following information: "2 × 3 cm firm, discrete, smooth, mobile, nontender mass 3 cm from the areola in the 4 o'clock position." Negative findings should also be recorded in the patient's health record. Physical examination cannot distinguish between malignant and nonmalignant masses; therefore, any palpable mass should be evaluated by the use of diagnostic breast assessment modalities to rule out malignancy.

Table 17-3 provides an example documentation for the subjective and objective portions of a breast exam for the midwife's clinical note. A full physical examination may also be indicated based on the patient's needs.

## Breast Assessment Modalities

Several instruments are available to assess breast health and provide diagnostic imaging for breast masses. Some of these modalities are meant for screening only, whereas other clinical tools can provide diagnostic determinations as well. Table 17-4 summarizes the available options;

additional information is provided in subsequent sections of this chapter.

Several algorithms have been developed for evaluation of dominant breast masses.[3-5] Some recommend a fine-needle biopsy as the first step, whereas others recommend ultrasound or mammography first. Variations depend on local radiology, pathology, and surgical resources; the person's age; and their preferences. Ultrasound is generally recommended for people younger than 30 years. Diagnostic mammography is recommended for people older than 30 years, because breast tissue has usually decreased in density by this time of life, making it easier to view clear mammogram images.

Table 17-5 lists components that could be included in a note for consultation or transfer of care to a specialist in the area.

## Benign Breast Disorders

Benign breast disorders are common and encompass all nonmalignant conditions of the breast and chest, including breast pain, nipple discharge, and noncancerous breast tumors. Benign breast disorders

| Table 17-4 | Common Breast Assessment Methods | |
|---|---|---|
| **Method** | **Description** | **Comments** |
| Self-breast awareness or breast self-examination | Ongoing self-breast assessment utilizing the patient's own knowledge about their breasts. May or may not include breast self-examination. | General screening for any breast-related disorder, most often breast masses. Patients are encouraged to become familiar with their breasts so they can notice if there is an abnormality, and to report any abnormality to their healthcare provider right away. |
| Provider-led clinical breast examination (CBE) | Examination by a provider as outlined in the *Breast and Chest Examination* appendix | An essential component of the physical examination for diagnostic breast symptom evaluation. No longer recommended as a component of routine breast cancer screening for patients at average risk. |
| Mammogram[a] | Standard mammogram uses X rays to assess abnormalities of the breast, including masses, density, and changes in architecture | Regular mammograms are the gold-standard screening technique for breast cancer. Also used as part of the diagnostic evaluation indicated when breast masses are palpated. |
| | Digital breast tomosynthesis: a newer type of mammography that provides three-dimensional views | Although FDA approved, in most areas this modality is reserved for patients at high risk for breast cancer because of cost and specificity issues. |
| Ultrasound | Sonographic assessment of the breast | May be used for screening patients with dense breasts at high risk for breast cancer. Indicated for people with palpable masses, especially those that are not identifiable on mammogram. |
| Magnetic resonance imaging (MRI) | Method using radio waves and magnetic field to assess the breasts | Primarily used in conjunction with mammography or ultrasound to evaluate the extent of cancer of the breast. Can be used to screen individuals at high risk for breast cancer. Due to the lack of ionizing radiation, MRI is the preferred method to determine whether silicone implants have ruptured. |
| Biopsy of breast mass | Fine-needle biopsy: a commonly performed outpatient procedure to provide cells for cytologic study and identification of malignancy. Core biopsy, using a larger needle, and open biopsy may be indicated based on size of the mass. | Performed by a physician under guided ultrasound or mammogram. |
| | Biopsy at the time of surgery (e.g., lumpectomy, mastectomy) | Most commonly combined with biopsy of nodes. Provides staging of cancer. |

Abbreviation: FDA, U.S. Food and Drug Administration.

[a]A palpable mass with a normal mammogram may indicate the need for referral and additional diagnostic evaluation if there is a high level of suspicion for breast cancer.

are often classified as nonproliferative, proliferative without atypia, or atypical hyperplasia, with the risk level depending on the classification. Nonproliferative disorders, which include fibrocystic changes and breast cysts, are not associated with a risk of malignancy. Proliferative without atypia disorders, which include intraductal papillomas, are associated with a modest increase in risk for malignancy.

| Table 17-5 | Critical Elements for a Consultation or Transfer Note for a Patient with a Breast Mass |
|---|---|

Risk factors for breast cancer, including genetic history, family history, and personal past history

Current and past use of hormone therapy, including hormonal contraception

Discovery of breast mass: by breast self-examination and/or clinical breast examination

Description of breast mass: location, size, shape, mobility, tenderness, and consistency

Any breast, nipple, and/or skin changes

Care provided before transfer: procedures and results; laboratory results or pending status, including pregnancy test, mammogram, and/or ultrasound

Assessment/diagnosis of the situation

Summary of rationale for transfer and request for information about the treatment plan for follow-up

Atypical ductal hyperplasia and atypical lobular hyperplasia are associated with a significant increased risk for malignancy. These lesions usually require surgical excision for treatment and regular follow-up for 10 years after the diagnosis.[4-6]

## Mastalgia

Breast pain, more formally known as mastalgia, affects many individuals, with approximately two-thirds of people assigned female at birth developing this pain and seeking clinical attention at some point during their reproductive years.[7] Mastalgia can range from mild to severe, and can demonstrate cyclic or noncyclic incidence.

Cyclic breast pain generally occurs bilaterally during the luteal phase of the menstrual cycle and resolves after the onset of menses. It is often described as sharp, shooting, deep aching, or throbbing pain.

Noncyclic breast pain is sometimes idiopathic. Alternatively, it can be caused by mastitis, cysts, or tumors; be related to a history of breast surgery; or arise as a side effect of medication. Some studies indicate that caffeine, foods high in fat, smoking, and anxiety may be contributing factors to mastalgia, although this link has not been definitively proven.[8] Noncyclic mastalgia tends to be localized, subareolar, or medial, and is often characterized as tender, burning, stabbing, pulling, or pinching pain.

Mastalgia can also be extramammary, meaning that the pain is not specifically related to the breast. A wide variety of differential diagnoses must be considered in these cases, including cardiopulmonary, gastrointestinal, or musculoskeletal sources.[8]

Approximately 15% of patients with mastalgia require treatment to relieve breast pain symptoms. A well-fitting bra may relieve some degree of cyclical and noncyclical mastalgia if the breasts were not previously well supported (70% of patients report a decrease in pain with this intervention[8]). Application of heat or cold, relaxation techniques including meditation, and increased physical activity can be helpful. Other beneficial lifestyle changes include reducing caffeine, consuming a low-fat diet, and increasing vitamin and fiber intake. Studies show conflicting results from decreasing caffeine intake as well as use of several other nutritional supplements (vitamin E, vitamin B, flaxseed, *Vitex agnus*, and evening primrose oil). Patients can be advised that they may experience an improvement with these agents.[8]

Over-the-counter medications can be used to manage the symptoms of moderate to severe mastalgia. Nonsteroidal anti-inflammatory drugs (NSAIDs) are the recommended first-line pharmacologic treatment for temporary pain relief.[8] Oral agents such as naproxen sodium or ibuprofen can be prescribed according to standard medication dosing. Topical nonsteroidal anti-inflammatory agents such as a diclofenac patch or gel can also be considered.[8] Acetaminophen can be used as a second-line agent for patients who do not respond to NSAIDs or require additional pain management.

Physician consultation may be indicated for patients whose pain is not controlled with over-the-counter medication and nonpharmacologic pain therapies. For patients with more severe mastalgia, tamoxifen (Nolvadex) and danazol (Danocrine) can be prescribed to treat symptoms. Low-dose tamoxifen, taken as a 10 mg oral tablet daily dose, is the first-line prescription treatment.[2] Tamoxifen is administered during the luteal phase of the menstrual cycle to avoid side effects, but can cause headache, nausea, vaginal dryness, hot flashes, and joint pain. This medication should be discontinued if symptom relief is not achieved after 4 months of administration. Use of tamoxifen has also been associated with an increased risk of endometrial cancer.[9]

Danazol is the only Food and Drug Administration (FDA)–approved drug for the treatment of mastalgia.[8] Danazol, dosed as a 50 to 200 mg oral tablet twice a day, has been found to relieve breast pain but can cause voice changes, weight gain, hot flashes, menstrual irregularity, acne, and hirsutism. Patients often discontinue danazol treatment due to its side-effect profile.

## Nipple Discharge

Nipple discharge is common in reproductive-age people assigned female at birth and is generally benign. However, 10.2% of patients with nipple discharge will have a breast cancer diagnosis.[10] Benign discharge is generally bilateral, multiductal, milky or green in color, and occurs with breast manipulation.[5,11] Bilateral milky nipple discharge may occur during pregnancy and lactation. It may continue for several months or even years after childbirth or cessation of breastfeeding. In contrast, nipple discharge that is unilateral and occurs spontaneously is more likely to be associated with a malignancy. Such discharge is often clear, serous, or bloody. Patients at the highest risk for breast cancer are those who are 40 years or older and present with one-sided nipple discharge and an accompanying breast mass.[11]

*Galactorrhea* is defined as bilateral nipple discharge occurring in patients who have not been pregnant or lactating within the past 12 months. Galactorrhea is most often idiopathic and not caused by breast disease. It can be associated with prolactin-secreting pituitary adenomas, hypothyroidism, breast stimulation, trauma, herpes zoster, and medications that inhibit dopamine (e.g., some psychotropic medications, combined oral contraceptives, metoclopramide [Reglan], and phenothiazines).[2,5,11] More information about pituitary tumors can be found in the *Menstrual Cycle Abnormalities* chapter.

Uniductal, bloody discharge may be associated with intraductal papilloma, a benign tumor of the lactiferous ducts that is generally managed with surgical excision. With spontaneous unilateral, uniductal discharge (clear, serous, or bloody), a diagnostic mammogram and ultrasound are indicated. Patient care typically requires management by a breast specialist.[2]

## Fibrocystic Breast Changes

Fibrocystic breast changes (previously called fibrocystic disease) are benign masses, commonly found in individuals assigned female at birth, that cause the breasts to appear dense. These normal breast lumps are generally associated with hormonal changes during the menstrual cycle, so they rarely affect postmenopausal patients. Fibrocystic breast changes can manifest as pain or discomfort in both breasts or under the arms, which fluctuates with the menstrual cycle. Breast lumps can be palpated by the patient and can intermittently change in size in relation to the hormonal phases of the menstrual cycle. Clinical findings include symmetrical nodularity, usually more prominent in the upper outer region of the breast. Fibrocystic breast changes are described as feeling similar to a bag of beans. The fibrous tissue may feel firm or rubbery, while the cystic portion can feel like grapes.

There is no evidence that fibrocystic breast changes increase the risk for developing breast cancer.[2,4,5] Management options include expectant watchful waiting, aspiration of large or painful cysts, and prescription of combined oral contraceptives to decrease the risk of additional fibrocystic breast changes. Minimal evidence exists to suggest that changes in dietary practices, use of vitamins such as vitamin E, herbal preparations including evening primrose oil, or avoidance of methylxanthines decreases the symptomology associated with fibrocystic changes.[8] Additionally, if the clinical presentation does not fully support a diagnosis of fibrocystic breast changes, the patient should be evaluated further with a mammogram and/or ultrasound diagnostics to rule out breast cancer.

## Breast Cysts

Breast cysts can occur individually or diffusely throughout the breasts as an aspect of fibrocystic changes. Breast cysts are usually smooth, mobile, fluid-filled, round, or oval masses with well-described borders that develop from terminal breast lobules. They may be painful, tender, swollen, or painless. Similar to fibrocystic changes, these cysts are hormonally influenced and typically appear during menstrual changes in premenopausal or perimenopausal women.

Breast cysts are classified as simple, complex, or complicated based on ultrasonographic evidence of the thickness of the cyst wall and the presence of echogenic material within the cyst. Malignancy in simple and complicated cysts is rare, but this risk increases with complex cysts and cysts that have thickened walls or thick internal septations.[5]

Simple cysts are diagnosed via ultrasound or fine-needle biopsy. Nonbloody fluid can be aspirated, and the cyst usually resolves as a result of the biopsy procedure. Because the risk of malignancy is very low, a simple cyst generally does not require treatment or ongoing follow-up, although it can be aspirated if it is very large or painful. Some experts recommend a follow-up clinical breast examination or ultrasound in 2 to 4 months to document that the cyst has not changed or recurred after aspiration.

Complex or complicated cysts can have various etiologies, so multiple differential diagnoses—abscess, breast cancer, hematoma, fat necrosis, and galactocele—should be considered. These cysts require a fine-needle biopsy, core biopsy, or excisional biopsy to establish the diagnosis. Care for a patient with a complex or complicated breast cyst is best provided by a specialist physician.

### Fibroadenomas

Fibroadenomas are breast masses that most frequently occur in adolescent and young people assigned female at birth, although they can occur at any age until menopause. These masses tend to be solitary findings, with multiple fibroadenomas noted in only 10% to 15% of patients.[12] On examination, the tumors are nontender, mobile, and well circumscribed, and have a firm or rubbery consistency. Mammogram or ultrasound is utilized for the initial differentiation between a solid or fluid-filled (cystic) mass. The final diagnosis is confirmed through either core-needle or open breast mass biopsy. Diagnosis on the basis of the clinical examination only is inadequate.

If the biopsy indicates that the tumor is a fibroadenoma, it does not need to be removed. Instead, the tumor can be followed clinically and removed only if it becomes enlarged or visibly distorts the breast. If the pathology is unclear, the tumor should be surgically excised.[4,5] Fibroadenomas can increase rapidly during pregnancy or estrogen therapy and may regress after menopause. They are not associated with an increased risk of breast cancer.[2,4,5]

### Atypical Hyperplasia and Lobular Carcinoma in Situ

Atypical hyperplasia includes ductal and lobular hyperplasia, which are often incidental findings from a core-needle biopsy performed as part of the evaluation of another breast mass. Atypical hyperplasia is a pathologic diagnosis that describes abnormal cells of the breast that are associated with an increased risk of breast cancer. This condition is generally treated with surgery such as wide-excision biopsy or lumpectomy to remove all the affected tissue. More frequent screening for breast cancer and strategies to reduce breast cancer risk, including preventive medications such as tamoxifen and anastrozole, may be utilized in such cases. Additional information can be found in Table 17-9 later in this chapter.[4]

Lobular carcinoma in situ (LCIS) is an area of abnormal cell growth. LCIS is a histologic diagnosis, and the disorder is associated with an increased risk for breast cancer, in both the affected breast and the contralateral breast. There are no breast masses associated with LCIS. Since LCIS is not a precursor lesion for breast cancer, complete excision is not indicated. LCIS is not a true breast cancer despite the inclusion of "carcinoma" in its name. To decrease the potential for confusion, some oncologists prefer to use the term "lobular neoplasia" to describe this finding. Increased surveillance for breast cancer and risk-reduction medication should be strongly recommended when a patient is diagnosed with LCIS.[4]

## Breast and Chest Conditions During Pregnancy and Lactation

Pregnancy and lactation status are not independent risk factors for breast and chest disorders. The rate of breast cancer diagnosis in pregnancy is approximately 1 in 3000, making it the second most common cancer in pregnant patients after melanoma.[13] Breast examination can be more difficult when examining a pregnant person secondary to engorgement and proliferation of breast tissue. Notably, small breast masses can be more difficult to detect, potentially delaying diagnosis. Fibroadenomas can also grow during pregnancy, and occasionally they may infarct and become painful. In addition, a few types of benign lesions are unique in pregnancy and lactation. The most common of these disorders are lactation adenomas, galactoceles, mastitis, and breast abscess. The diagnosis and management of mastitis and breast abscess are reviewed in the *Infant Feeding and Lactation* chapter.

Lactation adenomas usually occur during the third trimester or during lactation.[14] These painless, soft, mobile masses can appear similar to fibroadenomas when viewed on ultrasound. They are not associated with an increased risk for malignancy.

A galactocele is a mammary duct that becomes distended due to milk retention; hence, it is also known as a milk retention cyst. Galactoceles almost always present during lactation or after cessation of breastfeeding.[15] They are typically round, soft, painless masses that may be associated with nipple discharge. Risk factors for galactocele include poor latch and abrupt cessation of breastfeeding. They usually regress spontaneously and do not require aspiration.

Breast ultrasound should be utilized for the initial evaluation of breast masses detected during pregnancy and lactation. If the ultrasound imaging is suspicious for breast cancer, breast magnetic resonance imaging (MRI) and/or mammogram can be considered for further evaluation. Biopsy can be performed in pregnancy if needed since determination of possible malignancy is of utmost importance.

When breast cancer is diagnosed in pregnancy, referral to a breast oncologist for immediate treatment management is required. Certain treatments, such as chemotherapy and surgery, can be administered during pregnancy but must be individualized based on patient circumstances.

## Considerations for Transgender Individuals

Transgender and nonbinary individuals may choose to undergo treatment to alter their breasts to increase their sense of gender congruence and body satisfaction. These treatments may include hormone therapy, breast augmentation, and chest reconstruction.

Transgender women most often choose to take estrogen hormone therapy to foster the development of female secondary sex characteristics and to minimize male secondary sex characteristics (see the *Gender-Affirming Care* chapter for additional information). Breast development in transgender women on hormone therapy, also called secondary puberty, is rarely as complete as in individuals who experienced breast growth during primary puberty; therefore, some transgender women may consider breast augmentation to add breast volume. The risks versus benefits of using estrogen should be carefully evaluated for each individual. Only the presence or a history of estrogen-sensitive cancer is an absolute contraindication to feminizing hormone therapy. Standard mammography guidelines are recommended for this population due to the lack of research regarding breast cancer risk in trans women.[16–18]

Transgender men often perceive that breasts are incongruent with their gender and may choose to either use a breast binder or pursue chest reconstruction. Chest reconstruction is not equivalent to mastectomy, and a variety of techniques are used depending on the preoperative anatomy. If reconstruction has not been performed, recommended mammography screening is indicated. Although the risk for breast cancer after chest reconstruction is reduced, the ACS recommends that individuals who have had mastectomies undergo clinical breast examination annually to evaluate the chest wall, skin, and incision. These guidelines can be extrapolated to transgender individuals, even though the recommendations do not specifically identify their applicability.[16–18]

Chest reconstruction for transgender men is more complex than a standard mastectomy. It involves reduction of the chest wall, aesthetic contouring, and scar minimization techniques. Nipple and areolar positioning must also be considered, with nipple-sparing or nipple-grafting options being considered depending on the size of the breasts prior to surgery. Post surgery, drains are placed where the breasts were removed to avoid fluid accumulation, and patients are advised to wear a compression wrap for several weeks. Scar tissue and nerve damage during the surgery will result in an initial loss of sensation to the breast and nipple structures; however, non-erotic sensation can return several months or years later as the nerves regrow. In some cases, multiple surgeries are needed to achieve optimal results. Nonetheless, research indicates that transgender men are usually happy with the results after surgery and feel more gender congruence in their bodies.[19]

Routine breast cancer screening with mammography is not needed for transgender men who have undergone complete chest reconstruction. However, breast self-examination is advised, as chest reconstruction surgery may not remove all breast tissue, leaving a small potential risk for breast cancer development throughout the lifespan.[18,20]

## Breast Cancer

Breast cancer is the most commonly diagnosed cancer worldwide and a leading cause of death among individuals assigned female at birth from ages 40 to 55 years in the United States. The incidence of breast cancer is higher in Black patients younger than 45 years, with a higher mortality rate observed for Black patients at any age.[21] White patients have a higher rate of breast cancer diagnosis after age 45 years, and Asian, Hispanic, and Native American patients have a lower incidence and mortality risk for breast cancer overall.[22] The divergence in mortality rates between white and Black patients is multifactorial, but includes health inequities such as low rates of breast cancer screening, late-stage diagnoses, and inadequate or disparate treatment due to systemic racism.[23]

Black patients have historically been underrepresented in epidemiologic studies of breast cancer, resulting in limited evidence-based data to inform prevention and treatment options in this population. Breast cancer risk prediction models are not specific to the Black community, so there are fewer recommendations for early or more frequent screening for Black patients at a higher risk of developing breast cancer.[24] Inadequate access to breast cancer screening in this population often leads to late-stage diagnosis of breast cancer and ultimately increased mortality among Black patients assigned female at birth.[25] Moreover, Black patients are often diagnosed with more aggressive, difficult-to-treat types of breast cancer.[25] The U.S. Preventive Services Task Force (USPSTF) provides a broad recommendation for breast cancer screening that does not take racial disparities into account. Consideration should be given to the higher-risk status of Black patients and the use of shared decision making to determine the appropriate timing at which to begin annual mammography screening, usually between the ages of 40 and 50.[4]

In addition to the previously mentioned factors, Black patients experience breast health inequity due to their increased allostatic load, defined as the biologic impact of chronic environmental challenges that trigger stress signals, leading to heightened neuroendocrine response and epigenetic changes due to systemic racism.[26] Higher unemployment rates in the Black community, increased incidence of obesity and poor diet, and difficulty accessing care due to geography, transportation, and childcare concerns all contribute to disparities in mortality.[26] Clinical trial enrollment and germline genetic differences between white and Black patients further impact survival rates.[26]

Individuals assigned female at birth have approximately a 1 in 8 chance of developing breast cancer over the course of their lifetime.[27] The risk of developing breast cancer increases as an individual ages. Conversely, mortality rates have decreased in recent years. Between 1989 and 2012, death rates due to breast cancer declined by 36% overall—a trend attributed to earlier detection, improved treatment modalities, and decreasing use of hormone therapy after menopause.

Cancer may develop in any of the tissues present in the breast, including epithelial, muscle, and connective tissues, or fat. The majority of breast cancers are carcinomas that appear in the epithelial cells that line other tissues. Breast carcinomas are categorized as invasive (infiltrating) or noninvasive (in situ).

## Factors Affecting Breast Cancer Risk

Several personal characteristics that increase or decrease an individual's risk for breast cancer have been identified and are listed in Table 17-2. For example, breastfeeding decreases a person's risk for breast cancer, whereas alcohol use can increase the risk. The National Cancer Institute provides a tool

on its website that calculates an individual's risk of developing breast cancer (see the Resources section at the end of this chapter). The variables used to calculate risk include a history of ductal carcinoma in situ or LCIS, presence of BRCA1 or BRCA2 gene mutations, current age, age at menarche, age at first live birth, number of previous breast biopsies, number of first-degree relatives with breast cancer, and the patient's race and ethnicity.[28] The National Cancer Institute's interactive program is based on the Gail model, the most commonly accepted program to calculate risk. This assessment tool and other similar models provide a framework for identifying a patient's individual risk.[28]

A meta-analysis of prospective studies regarding soy isoflavones consumption and risk of breast cancer suggests that soy isoflavones intake is associated with a significant reduction in the risk of breast cancer in Asian populations.[29] This benefit is not found in Western populations, although further studies are needed to confirm this finding. Other factors that may be associated with lowering of breast cancer risk include breastfeeding, 3 to 5 hours of moderate to vigorous physical exercise per week, limiting alcohol intake, and maintaining a healthy body weight.[30]

## Hereditary Breast and Ovarian Cancer Syndrome

Although most women with breast cancer do not have a family history of the disease, approximately 5% to 10% have inherited gene mutations that place them at increased risk for developing this disease. Hereditary breast and ovarian cancer syndrome (HBOC) refers to a genetically driven, inherited risk for cancer. HBOC may be present in people who have multiple cases of breast, ovarian, pancreatic, or prostate cancer within their family. The majority of people with HBOC have mutations in breast cancer susceptibility gene 1 (BRCA1), which is located on chromosome 17q21.3, or breast cancer susceptibility gene 2 (BRCA2), which is located on chromosome 13q12-13. These genes are associated with tumor suppression. Mutations of BRCA1 and BRCA2 are inherited in an autosomal dominant pattern, so offspring have a 50% chance of inheriting this mutation from a parent.

The prevalence of BRCA1 or BRCA2 in the general population is approximately 1 in every 300 to 800 people, whereas approximately 1 in 40 individuals who are of Ashkenazi Jewish background carry the mutation. Black and white patients have a similar level of risk for having a breast cancer–related genetic mutation.[31] Among patients with breast cancer who are age 50 years or younger, 12.4% of Black patients have a BRCA1 or BRCA2 mutation, with more than 40% of those patients reporting no family history of breast or ovarian cancer.[32]

When one of these gene mutations is present, the risk for developing breast or ovarian cancer is greatly increased. The cumulative lifetime risk of developing breast cancer in a patient with a BRCA1 or BRCA2 mutation is 38% to 87%, while the lifetime risk for ovarian cancer is 39% to 63% for BRCA1 carriers and 16.5% to 27% for BRCA2 carriers.[33] BRCA mutations are also associated with an increased risk for pancreatic cancer and melanoma.

In addition to BRCA1 and BRCA2 mutations, several other genetic mutations increase a person's risk for developing breast cancer. Genetic testing should include evaluation for a full panel of mutations, including the TP53, PTEN, CDH1, ATM, CHEK2, and PALB2 genes. Referral to a genetic counselor for discussion of genetic testing options and follow-up after the results are received can be beneficial for patients with a family history of breast cancer who are considering testing for HBOC.

### Screening for Hereditary Breast and Ovarian Cancer Syndrome

It is recommended that all patients be screened for possible inherited cancer gene mutations. If risk factors are present (Table 17-6),[34,35] they should receive genetic counseling and be offered genetic testing. Knowing their genetic status may allow the patient to seek out preventive measures such as prophylactic removal of the breasts, uterine tubes, or ovaries, or the use of medications to lower their risk for breast cancer. Several screening tools approved by the USPSTF are listed in the Resources section at the end of this chapter.

### Breast Cancer Screening Options

#### Individuals with a High Risk of Breast Cancer

Patients who have HBOC mutations, have a personal or family history of breast cancer, or are deemed a high risk for the development of breast cancer for other reasons should practice self-breast examination monthly, have ongoing self-breast awareness, and obtain an annual provider-performed clinical breast examination. In addition, breast cancer surveillance for these high-risk individuals should include an annual mammogram and annual breast MRI. These imaging tests are often scheduled on an alternating basis to ensure that the patient is being evaluated every 6 months with a different

| Table 17-6 | Risk Factors for Hereditary Breast and Ovarian Cancer Syndrome |
|---|---|
| **Medical History for an Individual Assigned Female at Birth** | |
| Breast cancer diagnosis at ≤ 50 years | |
| Breast cancer at any age and Ashkenazi Jewish ancestry | |
| Breast cancer and close relative[a] with breast cancer that developed at age ≤ 50 years or close relative with epithelial ovarian, tubal, or peritoneal cancer at any age | |
| Breast cancer diagnosis with two or more close relatives[a] with breast cancer at any age | |
| Breast cancer diagnosis at ≤ 50 years with limited or unknown family history | |
| Triple-negative breast cancer diagnosed at ≤ 60 years | |
| Two or more primary breast cancers with first diagnosed at ≤ 50 years | |
| Epithelial ovarian, tubal, or peritoneal cancer | |
| Pancreatic cancer and two or more close relatives[a] with breast, ovarian, tubal, or peritoneal, pancreatic, or aggressive prostate cancer | |
| **Family History** | |
| Close relative who meets any of the above criteria | |
| Close relative who is a known carrier for BRCA1 or BRCA2 | |
| Close relative[a] with breast cancer in an individual assigned male at birth | |

[a]"Close relative" refers to a first-, second-, or third-degree relative.

Based on American College of Obstetricians and Gynecologists. Practice Bulletin No. 182: hereditary breast and ovarian cancer syndrome. *Obstet Gynecol.* 2017;130e110-130e116; US Preventive Services Task Force. Risk assessment, genetic counseling, and genetic testing for BRCA-related cancer: US Preventive Services Task Force recommendation statement. *JAMA.* 2019;322(7): 652-665. doi:10.1001/jama.2019.10987.

modality. High-risk screening should start by age 30 or 10 years prior to when a family member may have died from cancer.

HBOC mutation carriers are also at risk for developing ovarian cancer at an earlier age than the general population. Early screening is offered that includes a serum CA-125 lab test with transvaginal pelvic ultrasound every 6 months and an annual provider-performed pelvic examination. Additional information about hereditary ovarian cancer screening and detection is reviewed in the *Malignant and Chronic Gynecologic Disorders* chapter.

### Individuals with an Average Risk of Breast Cancer

Widespread use of breast cancer screening modalities as well as advances in treatment have significantly reduced mortality due to breast cancer in recent years. A systematic review demonstrated that for patients of all ages at average risk, screening reduced breast cancer mortality by approximately 20%.[36] Regular breast screening for cancer has become standard practice in the United States. Nevertheless, controversies regarding the best type of screening and the ideal frequency of screening persist. Organizations focused on cancer prevention, such as the ACS, tend to advocate more-frequent screening. In contrast, other population-based groups, such as the USPSTF, have published guidelines that recommend delaying initiation and extending the interval between screenings. Although all groups have access to the same evidence, interpretation of those data depends on the particular lens of the organization. Due to the discrepancies between the national associations' recommendations, a shared decision-making model is required when considering breast cancer screening for patients at average risk, including a risk–benefit analysis discussion.

#### Breast Self-Examination.

Historically, monthly breast self-examination (BSE) was a standard part of routine screening in an attempt to diagnose a new malignant tumor at an early stage. However, this recommendation has been withdrawn due to a lack of evidence supporting it.[37]

Today, several organizations, including the USPSTF and ACS, recommend that patients utilize self-breast awareness techniques to watch for breast changes that may need evaluation.[37] No standard definition exists for self-breast awareness, but the general consensus is that individuals can be taught to be aware of the normal shape and consistency of their breasts over time. Any changes in how their breasts feel or look should be an impetus for a visit with a healthcare provider. The majority of breast lumps and resulting cancers are first identified by patients and then confirmed by a provider through clinical breast examination (CBE).[37] Thus, BSE and CBE continue to play important roles in breast cancer diagnosis.

For those patients who perform BSE, the technique that is recognized by the ACS includes both inspection and palpation using the vertical stripe technique described in the *Breast and Chest Examination* appendix. Some evidence indicates that the up-and-down pattern of examining the breast decreases the likelihood that breast tissue will be missed.[38]

#### Clinical Breast Examination.

Regular examination of the breasts by a healthcare professional is also no longer routinely recommended by national association guidelines.[37] CBE is an important tool for patients who present for evaluation of a palpable mass as well as for patients at high risk of developing breast cancer. CBE technique should be systematic and consistent. Initial visual breast inspection is completed with the patient in a seated position. Visualization of the breasts while the patient places their hands on their hips, raises their arms above their head, and flexes their pectoral muscles with hands on their hips is required.[38] Clinician palpation of the breasts is then completed with the patient in a supine position.

There are several techniques for palpating the breasts, including the radial wagon wheel or spoke method, the vertical strip method, and the concentric circles method.[38] Light, medium, and deep pressure with palpation is necessary to increase the chance of palpating a suspicious mass.[38] After palpation of the breasts, the axilla and the supraclavicular area should be palpated to rule out a concerning lump in the breast tissue or lymph system in this area.[38]

#### Mammography.

Mammography, which uses X rays to image breast tissue, can be done as either a screening modality or a diagnostic test. A standard screening mammogram involves four images that are evaluated for changes suspicious for cancer. A diagnostic mammogram is used to further examine areas of concern that are seen on the screening mammogram. Mammography can often detect early-stage breast cancers for which treatment may be more effective, resulting in disease cure. Numerous studies have shown that routine mammography may reduce breast cancer mortality by as much as 30%.[39] Mammography can detect an estimated 80% to 90% of breast cancers in asymptomatic persons assigned female at birth.[39]

Similar to the case for BSE and CBE, controversy exists regarding the use of routine screening for the average-risk population. Screening mammograms can lead to false-positive test results with subsequent unnecessary biopsies.[40] This can cause significant anxiety and distress for patients. Mammograms are also uncomfortable, often causing pain for many patients. Overdiagnosis and overtreatment are potential concerns that patients need to understand and consider when deciding when to start screening mammography.[40]

Mammographic findings are reported using the Breast Imaging Reporting and Data System (BI-RADS),[41] as described in Table 17-7. Based on these

| Table 17-7 | Breast Imaging Reporting and Data System Classification |
| --- | --- |
| **BI-RADS Assessment Category** | **Likelihood of Malignancy** |
| 0: Incomplete | Unknown; need additional imaging evaluation |
| 1: Negative | Essentially 0% |
| 2: Benign | Essentially 0%; may be affected by breast density |
| 3: Probably benign | > 0% to ≤ 2% |
| 4: Suspicious | 4A (low): >2% to ≤ 10% <br> 4B (moderate): >10% to ≤ 50% <br> 4C (high): >50% to < 95% |
| 5: Highly suggestive of malignancy | ≥ 95% |
| 6: Known biopsy-proven malignancy | Only used for findings on a mammogram, ultrasound, or magnetic resonance imaging that has already been diagnosed as cancer from a previous biopsy |

Abbreviation: BI-RADS, Breast Imaging Reporting and Data System.

Based on American College of Radiology. Mammography reporting. https://www.acr.org/-/media/ACR/Files/RADS/BI-RADS/Mammography-Reporting.pdf. Published 2013. Accessed October 26, 2022.

findings, further imaging studies or a tissue diagnosis may be indicated if a suspicious mass is noted.

Debate exists particularly regarding the point at which to initiate mammography screening, the frequency of screening, and the age at which it can be discontinued for individuals who are not at high risk for breast cancer (see Table 17-8 later in this section). Studies indicate that the sensitivity of mammography is highest among patients assigned female at birth who are 50 years or older, since they tend to have reduced breast density due to increased fatty tissue within the breast. Conversely, sensitivity is lowest among patients younger than 50 years due to their increased breast density, although rapid tumor growth is more likely to occur in this younger population.[42] Under the USPSTF's 2016 guideline, biennial screening mammography is recommended for patients assigned female at birth aged 50 to 74 years.[43] In contrast, the updated ACS screening guidelines recommend the choice of annual mammography for individuals 40 to 44 years of age, annual mammography at ages 45 to 54, and biennial or annual mammography for those 55 and older who are healthy with a life expectancy of 10 years or more.[43,44]

In 2017, the American College of Obstetricians and Gynecologists (ACOG) issued a position paper with screening recommendations for patients at average risk.[45] Similar to the ACS, ACOG now recommends offering the option of a screening mammogram regimen (annual or biennial) starting at age 40 and strongly encourages beginning mammography by age 50 at a minimum.

Similar to the controversy about when to initiate and the frequency of screening, there is debate about the appropriate age to discontinue screening mammograms. The USPSTF has stated there is insufficient evidence to recommend when to discontinue screening, while ACS and National Comprehensive Cancer Network (NCCN) recommend discontinuation if life expectancy is less than 10 years.

Table 17-8 provides a brief summary of the current recommendations for screening individuals who are not at high risk for breast cancer. The variations in these guidelines present a challenge for a midwife in practice. Ideally, healthcare providers should use one guideline instead of alternating among them.

***Digital Breast Tomosynthesis.*** A newer mammographic technique, known as digital breast tomosynthesis (DBT), provides a three-dimensional picture of the breast using X rays. This more detailed mammographic technique is approved by the FDA but is not yet considered the standard of care for breast cancer screening. Several studies have shown benefits of DBT, including lower recall rates and faster diagnosis due to shorter time to biopsy, in diagnostic imaging for breast cancer.[45,46] Newer research indicates that DBT in combination with standard two-dimensional (2-D) or digital mammography is superior to any of these imaging modalities alone in the breast cancer screening population.[46] To minimize the radiation dose, growing evidence supports imaging via DBT plus standard 2-D mammography for optimal breast cancer detection.[46] Nonetheless, this screening modality has not yet become a mainstream recommendation and may not be routinely covered by health insurance coverage, limiting patient access to DBT.

***Magnetic Resonance Imaging.*** MRI is the most sensitive test for breast cancer. Nevertheless, due to its high expense, it is recommended only for

| Table 17-8 | Breast Screening Recommendations for Patients at Average Risk | | | |
|---|---|---|---|---|
| Age | U.S. Preventive Services Task Force (2016) | American College of Obstetricians Gynecologists (2017) | American Cancer Society (2022) | National Comprehensive Cancer Network (2022) |
| **Clinical Breast Examination** | | | | |
| 25–39 years | Insufficient evidence to recommend for or against | May offer every 1–3 years | No recommendation | Recommend every 1–3 years |
| ≥ 40 years | Insufficient evidence to recommend for or against | Recommend annually | No recommendation | Recommend annually |
| **Mammogram Initiation Age and Frequency** | | | | |
| 40–44 years | Screening at age 40 years; decision made on an individual basis | Offer annual or biennial screening starting at 40 years | Offer optional annual screening | Recommend annual screening at age ≥ 40 years |
| 45–49 years | Screening at age 40 years; decision made on an individual basis | Initiate annual or biennial screening after counseling if the individual desires screening | Recommend annual screening | Recommend annual screening at age ≥ 40 years |
| ≥ 50 years | Every 2 years until age 75 years | Recommend annual or biennial screening if not already initiated | 50–54: recommend annual screening  ≥ 55: recommend biennial screening with option to continue annual screening | Recommend annual screening at age ≥ 40 years |
| **Mammogram Discontinuation** | | | | |
| | Insufficient evidence to recommend for or against at 75 years; decision to be based on shared decision making | Insufficient evidence to recommend for or against at 75 years; decision to be based on shared decision making | When life expectancy is < 10 years | When severe comorbidities limit life expectancy to ≤ 10 years |

Based on U.S. Preventive Services Task Force. Breast cancer: screening. 2016. https://www.uspreventiveservicestaskforce.org/uspstf/recommendation/breast-cancer-screening. Accessed October 2, 2021; American College of Obstetricians and Gynecologists. ACOG Practice Bulletin No 179: breast cancer risk assessment and screening in average-risk women. *Obstet Gynecol.* 2017;130(1):e1-e16. doi:10.1097/AOG.0000000000002158; American Cancer Society. *Cancer facts & figures 2022.* American Cancer Society; 2022:1-78. https://www.cancer.org/content/dam/cancer-org/research/cancer-facts-and-statistics/annual-cancer-facts-and-figures/2022/2022-cancer-facts-and-figures.pdf. Accessed April 14, 2023; National Comprehensive Cancer Network Foundation. Breast cancer screening and diagnosis. https://www.nccn.org/patients/guidelines/content/PDF/breastcancerscreening-patient.pdf. Published 2022. Accessed April 14, 2023.

screening of patients who are at very high risk for breast cancer, such as those who are positive for the BRCA gene mutations. MRI is recommended for use in conjunction with mammography as indicated.[47]

***Ultrasonography.*** Ultrasonography is employed to screen the breast tissue of younger patients at increased risk for breast cancer, diagnostically to differentiate between solid and cystic breast masses, and to guide fine-needle biopsies. The performance of this test is not affected by breast density. The American College of Radiology Imaging Network's randomized trial showed that adding ultrasound to mammography screening in high-risk patients with dense breasts improved the sensitivity of the screening, but also increased the rate of false-positive examinations.[48] Patients at high risk for breast cancer most likely are more fearful of a delayed diagnosis of breast cancer than of a false-positive result.[49]

## Breast Cancer Diagnosis

In the majority of cases, breast cancer screening results are negative without suspicious masses seen or malignancies found. When abnormalities are found, however, diagnostic testing is required. In many situations, these tests are performed at specialty or tertiary care facilities in the region to ensure diagnostic accuracy.

The definitive diagnosis of breast cancer is generally made through tissue sampling. This can be accomplished through fine-needle aspiration, ultrasound-guided core-needle biopsy, or excisional breast biopsy. The tissue sample obtained through the selected modality is then sent for histologic examination. If cancer is present, the histology report will state whether the tumor is ductal or lobular in origin. When the diagnosis of cancer has been made, it is also necessary to assess the lungs, abdomen, brain, and bone for metastasis.

A commonly used diagnostic test is fine-needle aspiration, also called fine-needle aspiration biopsy or fine-needle aspiration cytology. In this test, a physician inserts a thin (23–25 gauge), hollow needle into the breast mass and uses it to withdraw cells. Placement of the needle is performed under ultrasonic guidance and as an outpatient procedure. The cells obtained via fine-needle aspiration are subsequently evaluated specifically for malignancies.

Once breast cancer has been diagnosed, the malignancy is staged using the TNM system, which describes characteristics of the tumor (T), involvement of regional lymph nodes (N), and presence or absence of distant metastasis (M). Each cancer type has its own classification system, so use of the lexicon for breast cancer may be necessary.[50] The TNM system is used in conjunction with staging, an essential delineation applied to determine the appropriate treatment options.[51]

An essential component of staging is investigation of the axillary nodes. This is accomplished by injection of radioisotope dye into the breast tissue surrounding the cancer site to locate the axillary node to which the dye initially spreads. The tissue from this node is then examined intraoperatively for cancer cells. In patients with Stage I or II breast cancer, sentinel lymph node biopsy is performed. If the sentinel node is positive for breast cancer, additional axillary nodes will be removed for evaluation. If the level of acuity is Stage III or greater, an axillary node dissection of at least 10 nodes from the first two levels of lymph drainage in the breast is indicated.

In addition to staging, the receptor status of the tumor is assessed. This evaluation provides information for treatment options and serves as an indicator of breast cancer prognosis. For example, the presence of estrogen and progesterone receptors improves prognosis, whereas over-expression of the growth factor receptor coded by the oncogene Her2/neu confers a poorer prognosis.[52]

## Skin Cancer of the Nipple and Inflammatory Breast Cancer

Although most breast cancer is associated with breast masses, cancer can also occur on the skin of the nipple. This type of disease was originally described by nineteenth-century British doctor Sir James Paget and has been colloquially called Paget's disease. Cancer on the skin of the nipple is a rare form of cancer that most often occurs on the areolar area. Women may report burning or itching of the nipple as a reason for a visit to a healthcare provider. The skin may have the appearance of eczema. Skin cells become malignant and are pathognomonic for the cancer. Most women with this disorder will be found to have ductal carcinoma in situ or invasive breast cancer.[53] Several other diseases bear similar names, such as Paget's disease of the bone, but are distinct diseases that share only the name of the physician who first described them.

Inflammatory breast cancer affects only a small number of patients with breast cancer and without discrete masses. It often presents with a clinical picture similar to mastitis. This aggressive carcinoma involves the lymphatic system, and care for individuals with this cancer is best managed by a specialist provider in the area.

## Breast Cancer Treatment

Breast cancer treatment can include surgery, radiation, chemotherapy, hormone therapy, or immunotherapy. Radiation therapy or systemic therapies can be administered prior to surgery (neoadjuvant) with the goal of shrinking tumor size, or after surgery (adjuvant) to prevent recurrence. Treatment regimens are determined by the breast oncologist, often at a regional center of excellence, and then implemented at a local cancer clinic. Telehealth can be utilized to connect patients to specialists for a treatment plan or second-opinion discussions to help direct care.

Surgical options for breast cancer include lumpectomy, mastectomy, and reconstruction.[51,54] Lumpectomy is a breast-conserving surgery in which only the tumor and a few nearby lymph nodes are removed. It is the least invasive option but has the highest rate of recurrence. When combined with radiation post surgery, the rate of recurrence is significantly decreased.[51] Mastectomy involves removal of the breast tissue and the nipple–areolar complex with conservation of the pectoralis muscle. This surgical procedure can be completed on the affected breast with inclusion of the contralateral breast for prophylaxis if desired by the patient. There is a benefit to completing a bilateral mastectomy to avoid contralateral breast cancer especially in patients at higher risk, although it does not completely eliminate the risk of recurrence.[51,55] For patients with HBOC mutations, prophylactic bilateral mastectomy should be considered to significantly reduce their risk of developing breast cancer. Risk-reducing options should be discussed with a genetic counselor and a high-risk breast specialist to aid the patient in the decision-making process.[55]

Breast reconstruction is an option for patients who undergo mastectomy either for treatment of breast cancer or as prophylaxis. The reconstructive surgery can be performed immediately post mastectomy or as a subsequent surgery based on patient desire and clinical presentation. Several surgical options for reconstruction are available, including silicone or saline implants, autologous or "flap" reconstruction, and fat grafting surgery.[51,54] In some cases, nipple-sparing mastectomy can be performed to conserve parts of the nipple–areolar complex.[51,54] Breast reconstruction does not impact breast cancer recurrence or survival rates. Therefore, breast reconstruction can be completed based on patient preference.

Patients who choose breast reconstruction with implants need to be informed of the possible need for subsequent surgery because of implant leak, rupture, or other complications.[56] Implants are also at risk of rupture prior to swapping, and patients must be monitored through clinical breast exam and periodic imaging for early symptoms that might indicate a rupture. Particular types of breast implants have also been associated with anaplastic large-cell lymphoma, a rare type of cancer unrelated to breast cancer. The lymphoma occurs around the implant, especially if the implant has a textured surface.[54]

No matter the surgical or reconstructive method, patients must be taught breast self-awareness techniques. They should be advised to contact their care team if they note any new lumps or changes in their breasts.

Adjuvant (systemic) therapy is used to treat all stages of breast cancer. It includes chemotherapeutic agents, hormonal therapies that are estrogen

antagonists (e.g., aromatase inhibitors for estrogen receptor–positive cancer), and immunotherapy (including a monoclonal antibody treatment for cancer that overexpresses the Her2/neu protein).[57] After the patient completes the treatment phase and the cancer enters remission, oral antiestrogen therapy is often initiated to prevent recurrence of the cancer.[58] Primary care providers such as midwives often see patients for their routine health care when they are taking these protective medications. All of these therapies are associated with a number of side effects, which the patient should discuss with their oncologist prior to the start of treatment.[59] Common side effects of adjuvant and preventive therapies are listed in Table 17-9.

Treatment options for breast cancer during pregnancy are the same as for nonpregnant patients, except for radiation therapy, which is considered to be unsafe for the embryo or fetus throughout all stages of gestation. It is also recommended that chemotherapy be delayed until after the first trimester of pregnancy due to an increase in miscarriages and a possible increase in the risk for major fetal malformations secondary to exposure to chemotherapeutic agents. Chemotherapy in the second and third trimesters, while not associated with major malformations, may cause fetal growth restriction. Termination of pregnancy does not improve survival rates and is generally not recommended.[60]

### Follow-Up

During the first 2 years after breast cancer treatment is completed, follow-up appointments generally occur every 3 to 6 months and include physical examination and mammography. Routine laboratory evaluation for metastasis, including liver function tests, and bone scans are not recommended unless specifically indicated clinically.[61] Ovarian dysfunction is common in women of reproductive age who are treated for breast cancer, and reflects their age, ovarian function at the time of treatment, and the specific chemotherapy agents used. In patients of childbearing age, it can take as long as 2 years for menses to return, necessitating contraception if pregnancy is not desired.[62] For postmenopausal patients, menstruation may not resume after chemotherapy treatment.[59]

### Contraceptive and Pregnancy Considerations Following Breast Cancer

Breast cancer is a hormonally sensitive tumor, so hormonal contraception is contraindicated for patients with current or past history of breast cancer.

| Table 17-9 | Side Effects of Selected Adjuvant and Preventive Therapies for Breast Cancer | | |
|---|---|---|---|
| **Agent**<br>**Generic (Brand)** | **Route** | **Side Effects and Toxicities** | |
| **Antiestrogens** | | | |
| Tamoxifen (Nolvadex) | Oral | The most common side effects are hot flashes, vaginal discharge or bleeding, nausea, fatigue, depression, alopecia, and loss of libido. Significant adverse events can include blood clots, stroke, and endometrial cancer. | |
| Raloxifene (Evista) | Oral | The most common side effects are hot flashes, vaginal discharge, joint/muscle pain, depression, gastrointestinal upset, weight gain, and insomnia. Raloxifene does not increase the risk for endometrial cancer. It should not be used in individuals who are premenopausal. | |
| **Aromatase inhibitors** | | These medications are recommended for individuals who are postmenopausal. They have a lower incidence of serious short-term side effects such as blood clots, stroke, and endometrial cancer as compared to tamoxifen. However, they have a higher risk of cardiac disease, osteoporosis, and joint pain or stiffness. | |
| Anastrozole (Arimidex) | Oral | The most common side effects are mild hot flashes, vaginal dryness, musculoskeletal pain, and headache. Serious side effects can include hives, swelling, flu-like symptoms, and skin lesions. | |
| Letrozole (Femara) | Oral | The most common side effects are musculoskeletal pain, nausea, fatigue, nausea, and hot flashes. Serious side effects can include worsening of osteoporosis and allergic reaction to the medication. | |
| Exemestane (Aromasin) | Oral | The most common side effects are fatigue, nausea, hot flashes, depression/anxiety, and weight gain. A significant side effect is decrease in bone mineral density, which can lead to osteoporosis. | |
| **Monoclonal Antibody** | | | |
| Trastuzumab (Herceptin) | Intravenous | Used to treat HER2-positive breast cancer. The most common side effects are nausea, insomnia, headache, diarrhea, and rash. Significant side effects include cardiac damage that can lead to ventricular dysfunction and heart failure. Many individuals experience flu-like symptoms during the first infusion. Infrequently, patients may have a serious hypersensitivity reaction. Trastuzumab does not cause bone marrow suppression or hair loss. | |

Based on Jahan N, Jones C, Rahman RL. Endocrine prevention of breast cancer. *Mol Cell Endocrinol*. 2021;530. https://doi.org/10.1016/j.mce.2021.111284; National Institutes of Health, National Cancer Institute. Hormone therapy for breast cancer. https://www.cancer.gov/types/breast/breast-hormone-therapy-fact-sheet. Published 2022. Accessed April 13, 2023.

Copper-containing intrauterine devices, tubal ligation, and vasectomy are considered to be best practice for contraceptive management in these patients. The safety of the progesterone-only intrauterine device in this population remains unknown. Further research is needed on contraceptive implants and injectables for patients with a history of breast cancer, but initial evaluation demonstrated no increased risk. Other benefits of hormonal contraceptive use should also be considered during the shared decision-making process with the patient.[63,64] Barrier contraceptive methods such as condoms, or concomitant use of spermicide and a diaphragm/cervical cap, can be utilized as well as natural family planning tracking methods with midwife-provided patient education.

Premenopausal patients may be interested in carrying a pregnancy once remission has been achieved. Experts recommend waiting to conceive for at least 1 year after completion of breast cancer treatment to allow time for cancer medications to clear from the body.[65] Chemotherapy can also cause genetic mutations in the oocyte that may lead to illness in the newborn. Ovarian reserves damaged by chemotherapy can be cleared from the body without intervention within 1 year of treatment completion.

When patients choose to become pregnant following breast cancer, both patient and provider must watch carefully for a recurrence. If the patient does develop a new malignant breast mass during pregnancy, treatment will be limited and individualized due to the risk of exposure for the fetus.

## Postmenopausal Hormone Therapy After Breast Cancer

Many patients experience menopausal symptoms during or after breast cancer treatment. Hormone therapies necessary for cancer treatment (e.g., tamoxifen), ovarian suppression treatment, and chemotherapy can cause menopausal symptoms that must be managed. The safety of estrogen-containing hormone therapy for menopausal symptoms in patients with a history of breast cancer is not well established, and such therapy is generally avoided. Nonhormonal treatments, such as selective serotonin reuptake inhibitors or gabapentin (Neurontin), are effective alternatives for the treatment of individuals with vasomotor symptoms. Clonidine, a blood pressure medication, and oxybutynin, a drug used to treat overactive bladder, have also been associated with a reduction in hot flashes in this patient population.[66,67] Nonpharmacologic approaches such as weight loss, exercise, meditation, dietary changes, and acupuncture are encouraged. Symptoms of vaginal dryness can be treated with nonhormonal vaginal moisturizers, lubricants, and gels, although low-dose hormonal medication can be considered after a risk–benefit analysis discussion with the patient. If used, these medications must be applied directly to the vaginal tissue to avoid systemic exposure.[68]

## Conclusion

The midwife may be the first healthcare provider consulted for breast-related concerns and must be familiar with breast and chest conditions that affect patients assigned female at birth. Breast cancer is one of the most frequently diagnosed cancers worldwide, and screening and early detection of this condition are essential components of primary care services provided by midwives. Midwives are important members of multidisciplinary teams caring for patients with a diagnosis of breast cancer and fulfill this role by providing accurate information and support as the patient is making decisions regarding breast cancer treatment and management of symptoms. Several hereditary genetic mutations increase the risk for breast cancer; thus, patients with a family history of breast, ovarian, pancreatic, or prostate cancer should meet with a genetic counselor to discuss testing for high-risk breast cancer mutations such as BRCA1 and BRCA2. Special considerations may be needed for patients diagnosed with cancer during pregnancy and individuals who identify as transgender.

## Resources

| Organization | Description |
| --- | --- |
| American Cancer Society (ACS) | Nonprofit organization that provides updated statistics regarding all types of cancers, including breast cancer. |
| Cochrane Nordic Mammogram Leaflet | Pamphlet available in multiple languages discussing components of shared decision making for an individual considering mammogram screening. |
| Susan G. Komen Breast Cancer Foundation | Nonprofit organization named for an individual who died of breast cancer; its website includes support resources for women with the disease. |
| Facing Our Risk of Cancer Empowered (FORCE) | Nonprofit organization supporting individuals and families facing hereditary breast, ovarian, pancreatic, prostate, colorectal, and endometrial cancers. |
| **Mobile Apps** | |
| Becca | Support app to aid patents after breast cancer treatment. |
| Breast Cancer @Point of Care | Evidence-based tool for clinicians to support diagnosis, treatment, and care management decisions. |
| Know Your Lemons | Patient app that offers education and tracking of self-breast examination. |
| Mammography Assistant | Literature-based tool for radiologists to help with diagnosis and report completion. |

| Organization | Description |
|---|---|
| **Mobile Apps** | |
| OWise | Created by medical professionals in the Netherlands. App provides practical support and guidance for patients with a breast cancer diagnosis. |
| Touch Surgery | Free surgical simulator app. It offers full-color illustrations of the breast, including surgical procedures, which can be used when educating patients about expected care. |
| **Breast Cancer Screening Tools** | |
| National Cancer Institute (NCI) | The Breast Care Risk Tool is an interactive risk calculator based on the Gail model, which is used to estimate an individual's risk of developing breast cancer. |
| National Comprehensive Cancer Network (NCCN) | Guidelines for breast cancer screening, breast cancer risk reduction, and guidelines for women with hereditary breast and ovarian cancer syndrome. |
| U.S. Preventive Services Task Force (USPSTF) | Its final recommendation statement, "BRCA-Related Cancer: Risk Assessment, Genetic Counseling, and Genetic Testing, is a summary document that provides several validated screening tools for familial cancer risk, including the Ontario Family History Assessment Tool, Manchester Scoring System, and Referral Screening Tool. |

## References

1. Smith CE, Biro FM. Pubertal development: what's normal/what's not. *Clin Obstet Gynecol*. 2020;63(3): 491-503. doi:10.1097/GRF.0000000000000537.

2. De Silva NK. Breast development and disorders in the adolescent female. *Best Pract Res Clin Obstet Gynaecol*. 2018;48:40-50. doi:10.1016/j.bpobgyn .2017.08.009.

3. Soliman AT, De Sanctis V, Yassin M. Management of adolescent gynecomastia: an update. *Acta Bio-medica Atenei Parmensis*. 2017;88(2):204-213. https://doi.org/10.23750/abm.v88i2.6665.

4. American College of Obstetricians and Gynecologists. Practice Bulletin No. 164: diagnosis and management of benign breast disorders. *Obstet Gynecol*. 2021;127(6):e141-e156.

5. Latronico A, Nicosia L, Faggian A, et al. Atypical ductal hyperplasia: our experience in the management and long term clinical follow-up in 71 patients. *Breast*. 2018;37:1-5. https://doi.org/10.1016/j.breast .2017.10.003.

6. Bahl M. Management of high-risk breast lesions. *Radiol Clin North Am*. 2021;59(1):29-40.

7. Tahir MT, Shamsudeen S. Mastalgia. In: *StatPearls*. https://www.ncbi.nlm.nih.gov/books/NBK562195. Updated November 1, 2022. Accessed April 13, 2023.

8. Salman B, Collins E, Hersh L. Common breast problems. *Am Fam Physician*. 2019;99(8):505-514.

9. Ignatov A, Ortmann O. Endocrine risk factors of endometrial cancer: polycystic ovary syndrome, oral contraceptives, infertility, tamoxifen. *Cancer*. 2020; 12(7):1766.

10. Leong A, Johnston A, Sugrue M. Variations in abnormal nipple discharge management in women: a systematic review and meta-analysis. *J Surg*. 2018. doi:10.29011/2575-9760. 001154.

11. Wong Chung JE, Jeuriens-van de Ven SA, van Helmond N, et al. Does nipple discharge color predict (pre-)malignant breast pathology? *Breast J*. 2016; 22(2):202-208.

12. Hoffman B, Schorge J, Bradshaw K, et al. Breast diseases. In: Hoffman B, Schorge J, Bradshaw K, et al., eds. *Williams Gynecology*. 3rd ed. New York, NY: McGraw-Hill; 2016:275-286.

13. Durrani S, Akbar S, Heena H. Breast cancer during pregnancy. *Cureus*. 2018;10(7):e2941. https://doi.org /10.7759/cureus.2941.

14. Ravikanth R, Kamalasekar K. Imaging of lactating adenoma: differential diagnosis of solid mass lesion in a lactating woman. *J Med Ultrasound*. 2019;27(4): 208-210. https://doi.org/10.4103/JMU.JMU_3_19.

15. Varshney B, Bharti JN, Saha S, et al. Crystallising galactocele of the breast: a rare cytological diagnosis. *BMJ Case Rep*. 2021;14(e242888):1-2.

16. Bond Maycock L, Powell Kennedy H. Breast care in the transgender individual. *J Midwifery Womens Health*. 2014;59:74-81.

17. Selix NW, Rowniak S. Provision of patient-centered transgender care. *J Midwifery Womens Health*. 2016; 00:1-8.

18. Clarke CN, Cortina CS, Fayanju OM, et al. Breast cancer risk and screening in transgender persons: a call for inclusive care. *Ann Surg Oncol*. 2022;29:2176-2180. https://doi.org/10.1245/s10434-021-10217-5.

19. Bustos VP, Bustos SS, Mascaro A, et al. Transgender and gender-nonbinary patient satisfaction after transmasculine chest surgery. *Plast Reconstr Surg Glob Open*. 2021;9(3):e3479. doi:10.1097/GOX.000000 0000003479.

20. de Blok CJM, Wiepjes CM, Nota NM, et al. Breast cancer risk in transgender people receiving hormone treatment: nationwide cohort study in the Netherlands. *BMJ (Clin Res Ed)*. 2019;365:l1652. https://doi.org/10.1136/bmj.l1652.

21. Yedjou CG, Tchounwou PB, Payton M, et al. Assessing the racial and ethnic disparities in breast cancer mortality in the United States. Chakraborty J, ed. *Int J Environ Res Public Health*. 2017;14(5):486.

22. Sung H, Ferlay J, Siegel RL, et al. Global cancer statistics 2020: Globocan estimates of incidence and mortality worldwide for 36 cancers in 185 countries. *CA Cancer J Clin*. 2021;71:209-249. https://acsjournals.onlinelibrary.wiley.com/doi/full/10.3322/caac.21660. Accessed April 13, 2023.

23. Yedjou CG, Sims JN, Miele L, et al. Health and racial disparity in breast cancer. *Adv Experim Med Biol*. 2019;1152:31-49. https://doi.org/10.1007/978-3-030-20301-6_3.

24. Palmer JR, Zirpoli G, Bertrand KA, et al. A validated risk prediction model for breast cancer in US Black women. *J Clin Oncol*. 2021;39(34):3866-3877.

25. Chapman CH, Schechter CB, Cadham CJ, et al. Identifying equitable screening mammography strategies for Black women in the United States using simulation modeling. *Ann Intern Med*. 2021;175(12):1637-1646.

26. Stringer-Reasor EM. Disparities in breast cancer associated with African American identity. *Am Soc Clin Oncol Educational Book*. 2021;41:e29-e46. doi:10.1200/EDBK_319929.

27. Akram M, Iqbal M, Daniyal M, Khan AU. Awareness and current knowledge of breast cancer. *Biol Res*. 2017;50:33. doi:10.1186/s40659-017-0140-9.

28. National Cancer Institute. The Breast Cancer Risk Assessment Tool. National Institutes of Health. https://bcrisktool.cancer.gov/. Accessed March 25, 2022.

29. Youn HJ, Han W. A review of the epidemiology of breast cancer in Asia: focus on risk factors. *Asian Pac J Cancer Prev*. 2020;21(4):867-880. doi:10.31557/APJCP.2020.21.4.867.

30. Kolak A, Kamińska M, Sygit K, et al. Primary and secondary prevention of breast cancer. *Ann Agri Environ Med*. 2017;24(4):549-553.

31. Domchek SM, Yao S, Chen F, et al. Comparison of the prevalence of pathogenic variants in cancer susceptibility genes in Black women and non-Hispanic white women with breast cancer in the United States. *JAMA Oncol*. 2021;7(7):1045-1050. doi:10.1001/jamaoncol.2021.1492.

32. Bonner PT, Cragun D, Monteiro AN, et al. A high frequency of BRCA mutations in young Black women with breast cancer residing in Florida. *Cancer*. 2015; doi121:4173-4180. https://doi.org/10.1002/cncr.29645.

33. Yoshida R. Hereditary breast and ovarian cancer (HBOC): review of its molecular characteristics, screen, treatment, and prognosis. *Breast Cancer*. 2021;28:1167-1180. https://doi.org/10.1007/s12282-020-01148-2.

34. American College of Obstetricians and Gynecologists. Practice Bulletin No. 182: hereditary breast and ovarian cancer syndrome. *Obstet Gynecol*. 2017; 130e110-130e116.

35. U.S. Preventive Services Task Force. Risk assessment, genetic counseling, and genetic testing for BRCA-related cancer: US Preventive Services Task Force recommendation statement. *JAMA*. 2019;322(7):652-665. doi:10.1001/jama.2019.10987.

36. Myers ER, Moorman P, Gierisch JM, et al. Benefits and harms of breast cancer screening: a systematic review. *JAMA*. 2015;314(15):1615-1634.

37. Huang N, Chen L, He J, et al. The efficacy of clinical breast exams and breast self-exams in detecting malignancy or positive ultrasound findings. *Cureus*. 2022;14(2):e22464.

38. Henderson JA, Duffee D, Ferguson T. Breast examination techniques. In: *StatPearls*. 2022; https://www.ncbi.nlm.nih.gov/books/NBK459179/. Accessed April 13, 2023.

39. Welch HG, Prorok PC, O'Malley AJ, Kramer BS. Breast-cancer tumor size, overdiagnosis, and mammography screening effectiveness. *N Engl J Med*. 2016;375:1438-1447.

40. American College of Obstetricians and Gynecologists. ACOG Practice Bulletin No 179: breast cancer risk assessment and screening in average-risk women. *Obstet Gynecol*. 2017;130(1):e1-16. doi:10.1097/AOG.0000000000002158.

41. American College of Radiology. Mammography reporting. https://www.acr.org/-/media/ACR/Files/RADS/BI-RADS/Mammography-Reporting.pdf. Published 2013. Accessed April 13, 2023.

42. Yi M, Hunt KK. Optimizing mammography screening intervals. *JAMA*. 2015;314(15):1635-1636.

43. U.S. Preventive Services Task Force. Breast cancer: screening. https://www.uspreventiveservicestaskforce.org/uspstf/recommendation/breast-cancer-screening. Published January 11, 2016. Accessed October 2, 2021.

44. Bevers TB, Helvie M, Bonaccio E, et al. Breast cancer screening and diagnosis, version 3.2018, NCCN clinical practice guidelines in oncology. *J Natl Compr Canc Netw*. 2018;16(11):1362-1389. doi:10.6004/jnccn.2018.0083.

45. Chong A, Weinstein SP, McDonald ES, et al. Digital breast tomosynthesis: concepts and clinical practice. *Radiology*. 2019;292(1):1-14. https://doi.org/10.1148/radiol.2019180760.

46. Alabousi M, Wadera A, Kashif Al-Ghita M, et al. Performance of digital breast tomosynthesis, synthetic mammography, and digital mammography in breast cancer screening: a systematic review and meta-analysis. *J Natl Cancer Inst.* 2021;113(6):680-690. https://doi.org/10.1093/jnci/djaa205.

47. Narayan AK, Visvanathan K, Harvey SC. Comparative effectiveness of breast MRI and mammography in screening young women with elevated risk of developing breast cancer: a retrospective cohort study. *Breast Cancer Res Treat.* 2016;158(3):583-589.

48. Gundry KR. Breast ultrasound: indications and findings. *Clin Obstet Gynecol.* 2016;59(3):380-393

49. Mathioudakis AG, Salakari M, Pylkkanen L, et al. Systematic review on women's values and preferences concerning breast cancer screening and diagnostic services. *Psychooncology.* 2019;28(5):939-947. doi:10.1002/pon.5041.

50. Bond-Bero S. Filling the gap for early-stage breast cancer follow-up: an overview for primary care providers. *J Midwifery Womens Health.* 2016;61:166-176.

51. Moo TA, Sanford R, Dang C, Morrow M. Overview of breast cancer therapy. *PET Clin.* 2018;13(3):339-354. doi:10.1016/j.cpet.2018.02.006.

52. Hernandez-Blanquisett A, Touya D, Strasser-Weippl K, et al. Current and emerging therapies of *HER2*-positive metastatic breast cancer. *Breast.* 2016;20:170-177.

53. Sisti A, Huayllani MT, Restrepo DJ, et al. Paget disease of the breast: a national retrospective analysis of the US population. *Breast Dis.* 2020;39(3-4):119-126. doi:10.3233/BD-200439.

54. Frey J, Salibian A, Karp N, Choi M. Implant-based breast reconstruction: hot topics, controversies, and new directions. *Plast Reconstr Surg.* 2019;143(2):404e-416e. doi:10.1097/PRS.0000000000005290.

55. Franceschini G, Di Leone A, Terribile D, et al. Bilateral prophylactic mastectomy in BRCA mutation carriers: what surgeons need to know. *Ann Ital Chir.* 2019;90:1-2.

56. Schrager S, Lyon SM, Poore SO. Breast implants: common questions and answers. *Am Fam Physician.* 2021;104(5):500-508.

57. Eini M, Zainodini N, Montazeri H, et al. A review of therapeutic antibodies in breast cancer. *J Pharm Pharm Sci.* 2021;24:363-380. doi:10.18433/jpps31864.

58. Jahan N, Jones C, Rahman RL. Endocrine prevention of breast cancer. *Mol Cell Endocrinol.* 2021;530:111284. doi:10.1016/j.mce.2021.111284.

59. Koga C, Akiyoshi S, Ishida M, et al. Chemotherapy-induced amenorrhea and the resumption of menstruation in premenopausal women with hormone receptor–positive early breast cancer. *Breast Cancer.* 2017;24:714-719. https://doi.org/10.1007/s12282-017-0764-1.

60. Becker S. Breast cancer in pregnancy: a brief clinical review. *Best Pract Res Clin Ob.* 2016;33:79-85.

61. Sisler J, Chaput G, Sussman J, Ozokwelu E. Follow-up after treatment for breast cancer: practical guide to survivorship care for family physicians. *Can Fam Physician.* 2016;62:805-811.

62. Jacobson MH, Mertens AC, Spencer JB, et al. Menses resumption after cancer treatment-induced amenorrhea occurs early or not at all. *Fertil Steril.* 2016;105(3):765-772.

63. Centers for Disease Control and Prevention. U.S. medical eligibility criteria for contraceptive use, 2016. *MMWR.* 2016;65(15). https://www.cdc.gov/mmwr/volumes/65/rr/rr6503a1_appendix.htm. Accessed April 24, 2017.

64. Gompel A, Ramirez I, Bitzer J; European Society of Contraception Expert Group on Hormonal Contraception. Contraception in cancer survivors: an expert review. Part I. Breast and gynaecological cancers. *Eur J Contracept Reprod Health Care.* 2019;24(3):167-174. doi:10.1080/13625187.2019.1602721.

65. Hartnett KP, Mertens AC, Kramer MR, et al. Pregnancy after cancer: does timing of conception affect infant health? *Cancer.* 2018;124(22):4401-4407. doi:10.1002/cncr.31732.

66. Leon-Ferre RA, Novotny PJ, Wolfe EG, et al. Oxybutynin vs placebo for hot flashes in women with or without breast cancer: a randomized, double-blind clinical trial (ACCRU SC-1603). *JNCI Cancer Spectrum.* 2020;4(1):pkz088. https://doi.org/10.1093/jncics/pkz088.

67. McNeil MA, Merriam SB. Menopause. *Ann Intern Med.* 2021;74(7):ITC97-ITC112. doi:10.7326/AITC202107200.

68. Lubián López DM. Management of genitourinary syndrome of menopause in breast cancer survivors: an update. *World J Clin Oncol.* 2022;13(2):71-100. doi:10.5306/wjco.v13.i2.71.

CHAPTER

# 18

# Reproductive Tract and Sexually Transmitted Infections

BETHANY SANDERS AND MELISSA DAVIS

*The editors acknowledge Julia Phillippi, who was the author of this chapter in the previous edition.*

## Introduction

A person's overall well-being includes sexual and reproductive components. The healthy expression of sexuality and the ability to safely engage in sexual and reproductive behaviors is supported by national and international organizations such as the United Nations,[1] the World Health Organization (WHO),[2] and the *Healthy People* initiative in the United States.[3] Unfortunately, individuals across the globe continue to struggle to obtain services to improve their sexual and reproductive health. Midwives are ideal care providers for individuals' sexual health needs, which include screening, diagnosis, and treatment of infections in individuals and their partners. This chapter reviews midwifery care for individuals with reproductive tract and sexually transmitted infections (STIs), while sexuality is covered in the *Sexuality* chapter.

Sexually transmitted infections are diseases that are passed from one person to another through sexual contact and sometimes via genital contact. Some STIs, such as gonorrhea, are transmitted only via exchange of body fluids during sexual contact; this chapter primarily focuses on these diseases. However, it is possible to spread a wide variety of infections and parasites through sexual contact. Some conditions that are not traditional STIs but are easily transmitted during sexual contact are described in the final section of this chapter.

## Incidence of Sexually Transmitted Infections

STIs impact health across the lifespan, having both wide-ranging and persistent effects. According to WHO, more than 374 million cases of curable STIs occur annually.[2] The Centers for Disease Control and Prevention (CDC) reports that 26 million new STIs occur each year in the United States, with an immediate cost of more than $16 billion.[4] While immediate costs are easy to calculate, the long-term costs of STIs may be much higher, as such infections are associated with cancer, pelvic inflammatory disease, infertility, ectopic pregnancy, and lifelong malformations and blindness in infants born to individuals who have an STI during pregnancy or at the time of birth.[5]

Sexually transmitted infections vary greatly in incidence by geographic area, including within the United States. In addition, many variants or strains of an infection may occur, and the prevalence of these strains differs. If an individual and their partner are new to the geographic area or have recently traveled to another location, it can be useful to check treatment guidelines developed in the geographic area where the infection may have originated. For example, the antibiotic resistance profile of *Neisseria gonorrhoeae* varies by geographic region.[6] National and international organizations monitor the prevalence of infections and their susceptibility to treatment and produce reports to guide clinical management. However, with increasing global travel, persons may be infected with strains or subtypes not typical for their current location.

The prevalence of STIs also varies by personal risk factors. Individuals with a vagina have a disproportionate health burden from STIs, are more likely to contract an STI from a single sexual encounter, and are more likely to have long-term sequelae than other individuals.[5] Furthermore, accessing appropriate and affordable services related to STI care and prevention may be difficult for some persons. Stigma surrounding STIs, including within the healthcare realm, remains a barrier to reducing the incidence and effects of these infections.[7]

Research on the prevalence of STIs in marginalized groups, such as transgender persons, is limited primarily to human immunodeficiency virus (HIV) and transgender women. While some studies have found higher rates of STIs in this population, many of these studies took place outside of the United States and focused on infections among commercial sex workers. Disparities in STI prevalence by geographic region, racial and ethnic identity, age, socioeconomic status, education level, and immigration status are pervasive.[8] This is likely due to interacting elements of social determinants of health, sexual practices, access barriers to testing and treatment, and increased susceptibility to infection owing to biologic stress responses.[9] Historically, some STI research was founded in racism, as seen in the cases of Henrietta Lacks and the Tuskegee syphilis study.[10] Similarly, medical response to and public attitudes toward individuals with HIV historically have been negatively shaped by bias against individual sexual practices.[11] Understanding the effects of these events on modern community trust of the healthcare system as well as current systemic biases may enable clinicians to reduce disparities in transmission, screening, and treatment of STIs.[12,13]

In the United States, the CDC monitors reportable diseases, such as chlamydia, gonorrhea, and syphilis.[5] Current information about these conditions is maintained on the agency's website. The CDC also periodically updates guidelines for diagnosis and treatment of STIs; these guidelines, which were most recently updated in 2021, are extensively used in the United States.[5] The CDC guidelines can be downloaded, and paper copies can be printed as well. In addition, the CDC has free apps to assist clinicians in accessing guidelines quickly at the point of care (see the Resources section at the end of this chapter). The U.S. Preventive Services Task Force (USPSTF) also releases guidelines that address STI

screening based on current evidence. In addition, the Agency for Healthcare Research and Quality (AHRQ) has a mobile electronic device application that displays the USPSTF-recommended STI screenings based on the individual's age and risk factors.

While the CDC provides clear guidance for STI treatment in the United States, these guidelines are not always appropriate in other countries because treatment availability, drug names, and antibiotic resistance vary by geographic location. WHO and country-specific health organizations are the best source of current STI treatment information outside the United States.

## History and Physical Examination for Vaginal Symptoms and Sexually Transmitted Infections

Individuals may come to see a midwife with concerns about vaginitis or STIs or present for a comprehensive physical examination. Knowing an individual's previous and current anatomic parts will guide recommendations for preventive health screenings and anatomy-specific history questions. Begin any visit by asking the person, in an open and inviting tone, the reason for their clinic visit. If a person is concerned about their privacy, they may have not been completely forthcoming with other staff members. Give them a chance to talk without interruption, as listening patiently establishes rapport and provides important information.

### Problem-Focused Visit

Ideally, the individual will have already participated in a more comprehensive visit that included a complete history and physical examination. In these cases, a targeted but thorough history of the symptoms is important. The chief concern should be used to generate a list of differential diagnoses. It is helpful to use a systematic method to assess the problem. Many clinicians use the OLDCARTS technique to assess the Onset, Location/radiation, Duration, Character, and Aggravating factors, Relieving factors, Timing, and Severity of symptoms. After exploring the person's chief concern for the visit, ask them about additional STI-related symptoms, such as fever, sore throat, enlarged lymph nodes, sores in the mouth or genital area, dysuria, discharge, and dyspareunia.

### Sexual History

WHO recommends offering person-centered services in the care of individuals with STIs, focusing on communication, autonomy, individuality, and respect for dignity of the person.[7] Sex-positivity and trauma-informed care are important tools in the respectful care of persons. Obtaining an in-depth sexual history helps determine risk mitigation strategies and the need for screening during both preventive care and problem-based visits (see the *Sexuality* chapter). The individual is an essential partner in their health care, and listening to their concerns and history is one of the first steps in establishing a trusting relationship. It is important to be respectful when obtaining a thorough sexual history. While striving to put the person at ease, the clinician should not shy away from asking personal questions. It is crucial to know the extent and location of previous and current sexual contacts. For example, a vaginal test for gonorrhea would be useless if the person has engaged in only anal or oral intercourse.

A variety of approaches may be used when obtaining a thorough sexual history. Some midwives request that the person complete a paper form as a guide for discussion, whereas others talk through the entire history. It is important to provide privacy in which to complete the forms and a private space for discussion. A person may be less forthcoming when others are with them, especially their parents or children. While they may want their family or friends nearby for support, it is ideal to speak with the individual alone at some point during the visit. When discussing sensitive topics, it helps if the midwife and the individual are seated on equal levels without anything blocking their vision. While taking note of key items discussed, the focus should be on the person, rather than on the chart or computer.

A guide for obtaining a sexual history can be found in the *Collecting a Health History* appendix and the *Sexuality* chapter. It is important to ask questions (the 5 P's)[14] to obtain needed information without making assumptions about the person's sexuality or beliefs. Remain open and engaged no matter what the individual reveals, using open- and closed-ended questions as necessary. Focus on building rapport and obtaining the information needed to guide your assessment.

## Physical Examination for Vaginitis and Sexually Transmitted Infections

The physical examination for STIs includes evaluation of all systems that may be affected. These systems are included in a complete preventive examination but are examined individually during a targeted physical examination. Table 18-1 lists

| Table 18-1 | Physical Examination for Sexually Transmitted Infections |
|---|---|
| **Organ/System** | **Abnormal Findings Related to STIs** |
| Mouth | Lesions, pharyngitis |
| Cervical lymph nodes/chains | Palpable lymph nodes, possibly painful |
| Abdominal palpation | Abdominal tenderness |
| Inguinal lymph nodes | Palpable lymph nodes, which may be fluctuant or draining |
| Inspection of the pubis | Parasites, lesions, excoriations |
| Vulva, vagina, neovagina, and perineum | Lesions, warts, excoriations, edema, discharge |
|    Paraurethral glands | Enlarged glands, discharge on palpation |
|    Greater vestibular glands | Enlarged glands, discharge on palpation |
| Scrotum | Rashes, lesions, ulcerations, erythema, edema |
| Testes | Swelling, tenderness, masses |
| Epididymis | Tenderness, masses |
| Penis | Rashes, lesions, ulcerations, erythema |
| Shaft, foreskin | Condyloma, discharge |
| Glans | Balanitis |
| Urethra | Inflammation, swelling, discharge |
| Rectal area and anus | Lesions, warts, excoriations, signs of trauma |
| Prostate | Tenderness, enlargement, irregular surface |

*(continues)*

| Table 18-1 | Physical Examination for Sexually Transmitted Infections (*continued*) |
|---|---|
| **Organ/System** | **Abnormal Findings Related to STIs** |
| Speculum examination | |
|    Vaginal mucosa | Lesions, discharge, color, and character of vaginal walls |
|    Cervix | Petechiae, erythema, friability, lesions, discharge |
|    Obtain needed specimens | Wet mount, gonorrhea and chlamydia tests, cultures/testing of lesions, HPV testing with Pap test |
| Bimanual examination | |
|    Uterus | Enlarged uterus could indicate pregnancy; tenderness is a symptom of PID |
|    Cervix | Cervical motion tenderness is a sign of PID |
|    Adnexa | Adnexal tenderness is a sign of PID (and ectopic pregnancy) |
| Urine testing as indicated (nitrites, leukocytes, NAAT for gonorrhea and chlamydia) | Urinary tract infection signs include nitrites, leukocytes |
| | Urine test for chlamydia and gonorrhea is appropriate for screening and testing |
| Blood work as indicated (HIV, VDRL/RPR, HSV, hepatitis B, hepatitis C) | Blood testing can confirm or enhance physical examination findings |

Abbreviations: HIV, human immunodeficiency virus; HPV, human papillomavirus; HSV, herpes simplex virus; NAAT, nucleic acid amplification test; PID, pelvic inflammatory disease; RPR, rapid plasma reagin; STI, sexually transmitted infection; VDRL, Venereal Disease Research Laboratory test.

important systems to include in a targeted examination if the person or midwife has concerns about STIs. While looking closely for STIs, take a holistic approach to the examination and avoid ruling out non-STI-related diagnoses too soon. A comprehensive and gentle physical examination can reveal many non-infection-related abnormalities that may be causing symptoms. A chaperone for the physical exam may be requested by either the individual or the midwife. Although laboratory data can be very valuable in the diagnosis of an STI, the physical examination is important to help determine which laboratory tests are indicated. In addition, treatment may be initiated on the basis of physical findings without waiting for laboratory confirmation.

## Self-Care of the Reproductive Tract

Maintaining a healthy reproductive tract is an important component of sexual health and prevention of infection. The midwife can provide education about the individual's anatomy, helping to dispel stigma that some individuals may have about their body. Self-care of the reproductive tract includes both maintaining hygiene and avoiding unnecessary or harmful practices. The individual's age and culture may influence their attitudes and reproductive self-care practices, so the midwife should be open and nonjudgmental in taking a history.[15]

## Care of the Vulva and Vagina

Promoting vulvar and vaginal health includes decreasing contact with potential irritants, reducing moisture, and avoiding excessive friction. Perfumes and chemicals found in soaps, laundry detergents, and feminine hygiene products can cause vulvar and vaginal irritation. New clothing, especially undergarments or lingerie, should be washed and rinsed well prior to wearing. Fabric choice, rather than style of underwear, may play a greater role in risk of vulvar or vaginal irritation or infection; cotton fabric is recommended to promote better airflow.[16] Individuals with urinary or fecal incontinence should strive to keep the vulva dry and free of urine or stool, cleaning this area as needed with water and soft, nonabrasive wipes. Tight, constricting clothing can increase friction and result in vulvar irritation. Plain water is sufficient for washing without disrupting the normal bacterial flora and skin integrity.[17] Removal of pubic hair through waxing or shaving can lead to folliculitis, contact dermatitis, and, rarely, abscess formation.[18] Table 18-2 outlines some of the considerations for self-care of the vulva and vagina.

Personal lubricants can disrupt the vaginal pH and normal flora, resulting in vaginitis. Spermicides may irritate the vagina as well. Douching washes away beneficial bacteria and should be advised against. Vaginal irritation can also occur during

| Table 18-2 | Health Education for Prevention of Vulvar Irritation and Vaginitis |
|---|---|
| **General Health Measures That Support a Healthy Vaginal Microbiome** | |

Avoid cigarette smoking.

Avoid foods that have high dietary fat content and glycemic load.

**Cleaning the Vulva and Vagina**

Clean only the outside of the vagina with gentle, unscented soap.

Do not douche, as it eliminates helpful bacteria and increases risk of infection.

Use unscented, dye-free soaps, especially on the hands, anal areas, and genital areas.

Use a clean, previously dry washcloth or towel each time the vulva is cleaned or dried.

Wipe or pat the vulva gently after urinating; excessive wiping can damage the skin.

Cleaning with warm water after urinating and defecating can be helpful.

**Keeping the Vulva Dry**

Gently but thoroughly dry the vulva after bathing; a hair dryer is ideal for this purpose.

Sleep without underwear to increase air circulation.

Cotton underwear (with a cotton crotch) is the most breathable.

Avoid staying in a wet bathing suit.

**Avoiding Irritating Substances**

Individuals and their partners should use unscented and dye-free detergents for laundering underwear.

Double-rinse underwear to eliminate soap.

Avoid pads and panty liners unless needed, and try a variety of pads to find the least irritating.

Clean and gently dry the vulva as soon as possible after incontinence, as urine and stool are caustic to skin.

**Altering Sexual Practices**

Only clean objects should touch or enter the vagina (e.g., fingers, penis, sex toys).

Sexual contact should be gentle and nonpainful.

Use a water-based lubricant to prevent chafing during sexual activities.

Try a variety of pH-balanced lubricants to determine which is least irritating.

Clean objects (including fingers, penis, and sex toys) with soap and water after contact with the anus before they touch the vagina.

Consider condoms or nonvaginal ejaculation with recurrent infections, as semen may affect the pH of the vagina, especially when intercourse is frequent.

**Choosing Birth Control**

Spermicides may irritate the vagina.

Oral contraceptives alter the vaginal flora in some individuals, increasing their risk of vaginitis.

Reconsider use of these birth control method(s) for recurrent, severe vaginitis.

intercourse if the tissues do not have adequate lubrication or if the contact is rough or damaging; this finding might be indicative of relationship problems and needs further exploration. Sex toys should be washed after use. If sex toys are shared between partners, a condom should be used or the sex toy should be cleaned before each individual use. Avoiding anal insertion followed immediately by vaginal insertion during sex avoids introduction of enteric bacteria into the vagina. Fingernails should be trimmed and cleaned to prevent abrasions during sex.

Anything left within the vagina can also cause vaginitis—including tampons, pessaries, menstrual cups, or any other foreign body. Odor and irritation are often the presenting symptoms when a foreign object is retained in the vagina for longer than the recommended use. A speculum examination can identify the cause of the odor in this situation. On speculum examination, a tampon may at first appear to be a fleshy mass, as it may blend in with the surrounding tissue. Forgotten tampons have an extreme odor; thus, a plastic bag or container with water should be prepared before their removal and the tampon immediately submerged as soon as it is removed. Tampons can be removed with ring forceps or digitally. Pessaries, when left in the vagina for long time periods, can become irritating, especially if the individual has atrophic vaginal changes. While an increase in vaginal discharge is normal with pessary use, it is important to assess for vaginal infections and skin erosions if the person reports problems or discomfort.

### Care of the Neovagina

After vaginoplasty, individuals need to begin dilator use so as to maintain neovagina patency during healing. Instructions should include using the largest dilator that is comfortable for the individual, washing the dilator prior to use, applying a water-based lubricant, relaxing the pelvic floor with insertion, maintaining the dilator in place for approximately 15 to 20 minutes, and washing the dilator after removal.[19] Initially dilation is recommended multiple times daily, eventually decreasing to 1 to 2 times weekly unless regular insertive intercourse is ongoing.[19] Frequency and dilator size recommendations are specific to the individual and the vaginoplasty procedure and should be provided by a specialized healthcare provider, although general guidelines are available.[20] The tissue of the neovagina is keratinized, so it does not self-clean. Thus, douching is recommended every 1 to 2 days for the first 2 months postoperatively, then 1 to 2 times weekly thereafter to remove excess lubricant. Nonscented douches are recommended. Referral for electrolysis of residual pubic hair after some vaginoplasty procedures is recommended to avoid risk of infection or ingrown hair.[19]

### Care of the Penis and Foreskin

Regular care of the head of the penis and the foreskin can prevent complications such as phimosis, paraphimosis, and balanitis. While intact foreskin should never be forcibly retracted, the majority of individuals with a penis will experience retractability by age 10 years.[21] The head of the penis and foreskin should be washed regularly with water only or water and gentle soap if preferred, gently retracting the foreskin if present. Care must be taken to replace the foreskin after retracting it. In addition, reducing irritants from soaps and laundry detergent prevents penile irritation.

Cotton underwear also promotes airflow, and changing underwear daily can prevent accumulation of bacteria and moisture. Avoiding excessive friction from tight, constricting clothing also reduces irritation to the penis and foreskin. Individuals who practice tucking—that is, moving the scrotum, testicles, and penis to the perineum and securing them in place with tape or tight-fitting garments—should allow their anatomy to hang freely for some time every day to prevent urinary or testicular trauma.[20]

## Vaginitis

Vaginitis, or inflammation of the vagina, refers to a disruption of the normal healthy microbial environment within the vagina. It can be a common problem from menarche through menopause, with many causes and origins that are not fully understood. Vaginitis can be a symptom of an STI, a disruption of the normal vaginal flora, or simple transient irritation of the tissue. Recurrent vaginitis can have many causes and warrants a thorough sexual and lifestyle history that includes evaluation of the individual's overall health and well-being, including information about behaviors of the sexual partner. While partner transmission of noninfectious vaginitis is not common, partners may act as a bacterial reservoir, reinoculating susceptible individuals. Common vaginitis conditions include bacterial vaginosis, vulvovaginal candidiasis, and atrophic vaginitis.

### Bacterial Vaginosis

Bacterial vaginosis (BV) is the most common cause of vaginal infections in reproductive-age individuals with a vagina[22] (Figure 18-1). Formerly known as *Gardnerella vaginalis*, *Haemophilus vaginalis*, or *Corynebacterium vaginitis*, BV is a dysbiosis of vaginal bacteria.[22] In essence, this infection represents a non-inflammatory disturbance in the vaginal microflora—therefore the term *vaginosis*, rather than *vaginitis*, is used. Understanding of the pathogenesis of BV continues to evolve, with current research suggesting it has an incubation period of 4

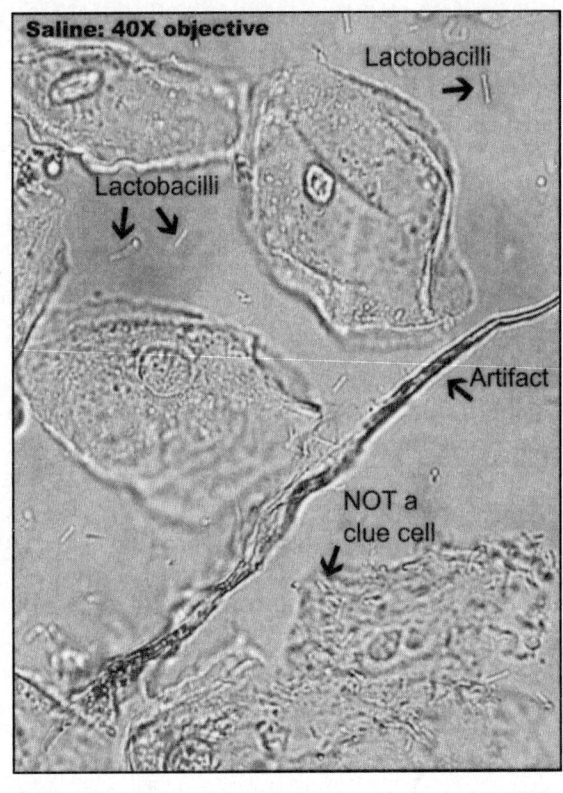

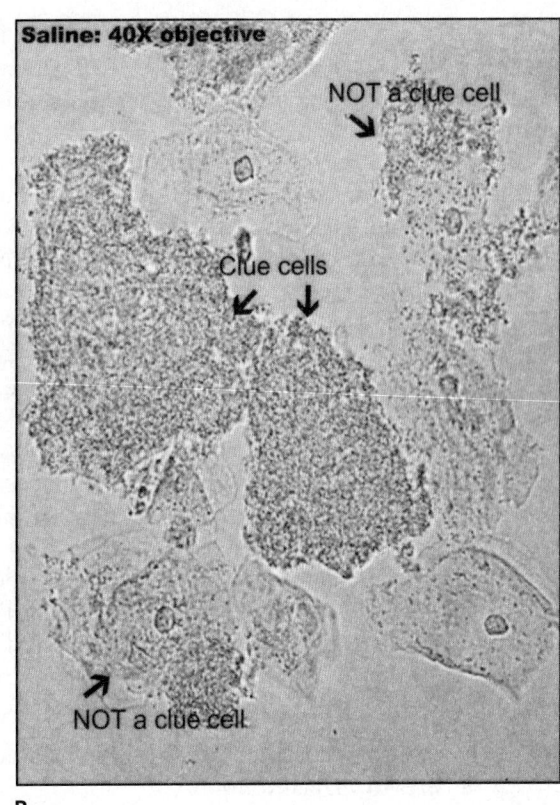

**Figure 18-1** Microscopic diagnosis of bacterial vaginosis (BV). **A.** No BV; note the normal epithelial cells and presence of lactobacilli. **B.** BV; note the clue cells and lack of lactobacilli.
Reproduced with permission from Seattle STD/HIV Prevention Training Center and Cindy Fennell, MS, MT, ASCP.

days after sexual transmission.[22] During episodes of BV, the vaginal flora is shifted toward a preponderance of anaerobic bacteria; these bacteria displace *Lactobacillus* and form a biofilm that adheres to vaginal epithelial cells.[22] During microscopic exam of vaginal discharge, these adherent bacteria can be seen covering the surface of the vaginal epithelial cells and are called clue cells. In addition, production of volatile amines increases, promoting a synergistic relationship with the causative bacterium and leading to breakdown of the protective mucus layer of the vaginal epithelium.[22] Disruption of this mucin layer increases the individual's susceptibility to STIs.[23]

Although the exact cause of bacterial vaginosis is not known, many factors are associated with its development, including smoking, menstruation, douching, sexual contact without a condom, low level of education, and engaging in oral or anal sex. At this time, BV is not generally considered an STI, but evidence has identified an association between sexual activity and risk of infection.[24] The alkaline properties of semen may facilitate the vaginal flora's shift toward a predominance of anaerobic

bacteria. Individuals with vaginas whose sexual partners also have vaginas have increased prevalence of BV, and coinfection is common. People of African descent have a higher prevalence of BV than individuals of other races, for unknown reasons.[24] Menopausal individuals have an increased risk for BV as a consequence of the decrease in healthy vaginal flora noted in menopause. Rates of BV infection are highest in the first week of the menstrual cycle.[24]

Bacterial vaginosis is associated with many adverse health outcomes, including preterm birth, postoperative infections, endometritis following pregnancy, and acquisition of other STIs.[24] However, this association is not fully understood, and treatment of BV does not prevent or mitigate the risk of associated adverse outcomes.[5]

### Diagnosis of Bacterial Vaginosis

Symptoms of BV include vaginal irritation and itching, dyspareunia, gray or white discharge, and a "fishy" odor that is often most noticeable after vaginal penetration during sexual activity. Nevertheless, BV is asymptomatic in 75% to 85% of individuals with vaginas.[24] On speculum examination, BV is usually evident as a thin white/gray homogenous discharge, irritated vaginal mucosa and introitus, and possibly cervicitis.

Gram stain with use of the Nugent scoring system is the gold standard for diagnosis of BV, but is rarely available in outpatient settings. To make the diagnosis via clinical microscopy, a sample of the vaginal discharge is collected with a swab, as described in the *Collecting Laboratory Specimens* appendix. The sample is first tested to determine the pH, and then samples of the discharge are placed on two slides. Normal saline is added to one slide, which is covered with a slide cover and set aside for microscopy. Potassium hydroxide (KOH) is added to the other slide, which is used immediately for the "whiff test."

Studies have confirmed the sensitivity and specificity of individual components of Amsel's criteria for diagnosis of BV.[25] Clinically, BV is diagnosed when three of four of Amsel's criteria are present:

1. Presence of a thin homogenous discharge that adheres to vaginal walls

2. Presence of clue cells on the normal saline–prepared slide

3. pH of the vagina or vaginal discharge is 4.5 or higher

4. Positive "whiff test," which signals the release of an amine "fishy" odor when vaginal discharge contacts alkaline KOH

Alternatively, BV can be diagnosed with commercially available tests such as a nucleic acid amplification test (NAAT), a DNA probe for *Gardnerella vaginalis*, or point-of-care testing, which detects an enzyme produced by common BV-related organisms. All of these types of tests are approved for use in making the diagnosis of BV.[5] While the sensitivity and specificity of these tests for diagnosing BV are better than that of Amsel's criteria alone, they are also more expensive.[5] Point-of-care testing allows for results to be obtained immediately, whereas NAAT results are typically available within 3 to 4 days.[26] Testing for BV with cervical cytology is not recommended due to its low sensitivity and specificity.[5]

### Screening and Treatment of Bacterial Vaginosis

Routine screening for BV is not recommended, but all individuals who are symptomatic should be tested and offered treatment if the diagnosis is confirmed. Table 18-3 outlines pharmacologic treatments for BV.[5,27] The choices for treatment include oral medications such as metronidazole (Flagyl), clindamycin (Cleocin), and tinidazole (Tindamax), as well as vaginal medications such as metronidazole gel and clindamycin cream or ovules. Selection of a specific agent should be part of the shared decision-making process, as the drugs have different side effects. For example, drinking alcohol during treatment with metronidazole and for 24 hours afterward can cause severe nausea and vomiting. Vaginal creams may be perceived as messy, and those containing clindamycin can weaken latex condoms and diaphragms. To ensure the treatment is compatible with the patient's lifestyle, the plan of care must be developed in partnership with the affected individual.

Some studies have shown that probiotics may have a role in the treatment of BV. However, the safety and effectiveness of these therapies have not been established.[28]

Health education includes the recommendations to abstain from vaginal intercourse during treatment and to wash all objects before they touch the vagina. More information related to maintaining healthy vulvar skin and the vaginal microbiome can be found in the *Malignant and Chronic Gynecologic Disorders* chapter. Receptive oral and anal sex may increase the risk for BV related to microbial inoculation. Condoms may reduce the risk of BV by preventing contact with alkaline semen.

Until a normal vaginal flora is reestablished, relapses are common. These relapses occur in part because the anaerobic bacteria involved in BV form a biofilm that resists treatment.[24] After initial treatment, follow-up with another evaluation is recommended only if symptoms persist or reoccur. Chronic reinfection warrants further investigation and more intense treatments as outlined by the CDC.

### Management of Bacterial Vaginosis During the Perinatal Period

Bacterial vaginosis is associated with an increased incidence of preterm birth.[24] However, treatment of BV during pregnancy with metronidazole (Flagyl) does not lower the incidence of preterm birth and, in fact, may increase the preterm birth rate via one of several mechanisms.[5] Therefore, as in nonpregnant individuals, routine screening for

| Table 18-3 | Treatment for Bacterial Vaginosis | | |
|---|---|---|---|
| **Recommended Treatments for Nonpregnant Individuals Generic (Brand)** | **Alternative Treatments for Nonpregnant Individuals Generic (Brand)** | **Recommended Treatments for Pregnant Individuals Generic (Brand)** | **Recommended Treatments for Lactating Individuals Generic (Brand)** |
| Metronidazole (Flagyl) 500 mg orally twice a day for 7 days | Tinidazole (Tindamax) 2 g orally for 2 days | Metronidazole (Flagyl) 500 mg orally twice a day for 7 days | Metronidazole (either oral or vaginal) is preferred. |
| Metronidazole gel (MetroGel) 0.75%, one full applicator per vagina at bedtime for 5 days | Tinidazole (Tindamax) 1 g orally for 5 days | Metronidazole (Flagyl) 250 mg orally 3 times a day for 7 days | Metronidazole (Flagyl) taken orally during lactation is excreted in human milk and has active metabolites, increasing infants' exposure, but has not been demonstrated to be harmful. Timing the dose after nursing may decrease infant exposure, or lactation may be discontinued for 12–24 hours after taking the medication. |
| Clindamycin (Cleocin) cream 2%, one full applicator per vagina at bedtime for 7 days | Clindamycin (Cleocin) 300 mg orally for 7 days | Clindamycin (Cleocin) 300 mg orally for 7 days | |
| | Clindamycin (Cleocin) ovules 100 mg intravaginally at bedtime for 3 days. May weaken latex or rubber condoms or diaphragms; avoid use for 72 hours after treatment. | Clindamycin (Cleocin) cream 2%, one full applicator per vagina at bedtime for 7 days | |
| | Secnidazole (Solosec) 2 g oral granules for one dose | | |

Based on Workowski KA, Bachmann LH, Chan PA, et al. Sexually transmitted infections treatment guidelines, 2021. *MMWR Recomm Rep.* 2021;70(4):1-187. doi:10.15585/mmwr.rr7004a1; U.S. National Library of Medicine. Drugs and Lactation Database (LactMed). https://www.ncbi.nlm.nih.gov/books/NBK501922. Published 2021. Accessed July 21, 2021.

BV is not recommended, but diagnosis and treatment are recommended for individuals who are symptomatic.

## Vulvovaginal Candidiasis

Candidiasis is an overgrowth of a *Candida* (yeast) species that affects the vagina, vulva, groin, and other moist areas of the body. The most common cause is *Candida albicans*, but other species may also cause this STI and are harder to treat. While candidiasis can be found in many locations on and in the body, this section focuses on infections in the female genital region. Approximately 75% of individuals with a vagina will have vulvovaginal candidiasis (VVC), commonly known as a yeast infection, at some point during their life.[5]

VVC is classified as uncomplicated or complicated. Uncomplicated VVC is a common condition that occurs sporadically throughout an individual's life and is associated with mild to moderate symptoms and manifestations. If infections occur more than four times per year, produce severe symptoms, or occur in individuals who are immunocompromised, VVC is classified as complicated and requires more intensive treatment.[29] Recurrent VVC is more likely to involve different *Candida* species, such as *C. glabrata*, that are not responsive to conventional antimycotic treatments.[5]

Several factors can make conditions favorable for *Candida* growth and increase an individual's risk of developing candidiasis, such as wearing non-breathable clothes or being in very humid or warm living conditions. The hormonal changes that occur during pregnancy and while taking oral contraceptive pills also increase this risk. In addition, diabetes is associated with increased incidence of candidiasis. Antibiotics administered to treat any infection may alter the vaginal flora, thereby facilitating proliferation of *Candida*. Immunosuppressed states, like those seen in persons with HIV and persons using

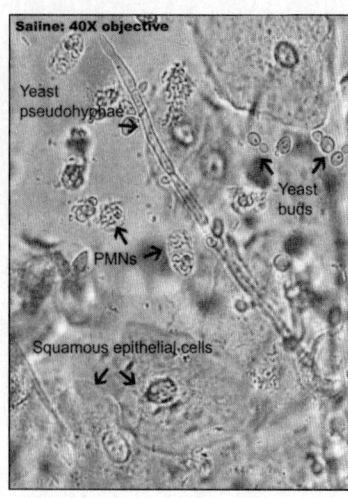
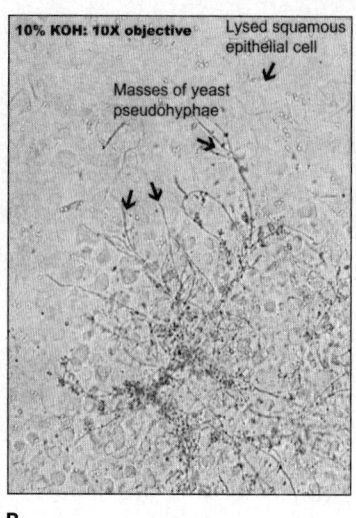
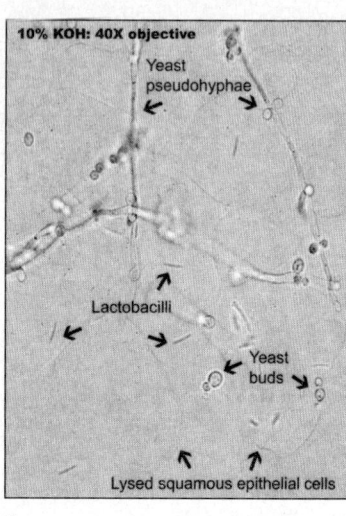

**A**          **B**          **C**

**Figure 18-2** *Candida* pseudohyphae and budding spores under microscopic examination. **A.** Saline, 40×. **B.** KOH, 10×. **C.** KOH, 40×.
Abbreviations: KOH, potassium hydroxide; PMNS, polymorphonuclear cells.
Reproduced with permission from Seattle STD/HIV Prevention Training Center and Cindy Fennell, MS, MT, ASCP.

corticosteroids, can also increase the risk of developing candidiasis in the vulvovaginal region and other moist areas of the body. Although species of *Candida* can be passed between sexual partners and can cause penile irritation or balanitis, candidiasis involves an overgrowth of normal flora and routine partner treatment is not recommended.[5]

### Diagnosis of Vulvovaginal Candidiasis

Symptoms of candidiasis include vaginal itching, burning, irritation, dyspareunia, and increased vaginal discharge. The vulva may be erythematous and slightly swollen, and have areas of redness with 1- to 2-mm "satellite" lesions extending from the affected area on external examination. The vagina is often red and slightly edematous. The vaginal discharge is usually thick, white, and curd-like, but can also be thin and watery, or adherent to the vaginal walls. Douching can complicate the physical examination by washing away discharge. Manifestations of severe candidiasis include widespread and severe erythema, skin fissures, edema, and excoriations.

A wet mount may reveal a lack of lactobacilli on a saline preparation or the presence of hyphae and pseudohyphae with a saline or KOH preparation (Figure 18-2). However, lack of hyphae does not rule out candidiasis, especially for individuals experiencing recurrent or severe symptoms, as the species of *Candida* implicated in recurrent and severe infection—*C. glabrata*—does not form hyphae. A culture can be performed in the absence of

hyphae to check for non-*albicans* varieties of yeast. Treatment can begin without waiting for culture results. While polymerase chain reaction (PCR) tests are available for *Candida*, not all are have received Food and Drug Administration (FDA) clearance for this indication.[5]

### Screening and Treatment of Vulvovaginal Candidiasis

Routine screening for VVC is not recommended. Treatment options for this condition are listed in Table 18-4. Many of these treatments are available without a prescription, and individuals may use the medications prior to a clinical diagnosis of candidiasis. There is no standard recommendation about being seen by a healthcare provider prior to initiating treatment. Use of over-the-counter medications can decrease costs for individuals if they have VVC, but can also mean that people delay seeking treatment for harder-to-treat or more serious vaginal infections.

The class of medications used to treat VVC comprises antifungal agents that work by interfering with the formation of fungal cell membranes. Options include oral treatments, vaginal creams and tablets, and topical preparations. The costs and side effects of these therapies vary. All locations of infection (vaginal and/or vulva) should be treated. The creams require vaginal insertion, and they may weaken condoms. The oral medication fluconazole (Diflucan) does not require handling of the

| Table 18-4 | Recommended Treatment for Uncomplicated Vulvovaginal Candidiasis | | | |
|---|---|---|---|---|
| **Agents** | **OTC or Rx** | **Brand Name** | **Dose** | **Duration** |
| **Intravaginal** | | | | |
| Butoconazole 2% cream (single-dose bioadhesive patch) | Rx | Gynazole-1 | 5 g intravaginally once at night | Single dose |
| Clotrimazole 1% cream | OTC | Gyne-Lotrimin-7 | 5 g intravaginally once at night | 7–14 days[a] |
| Clotrimazole 2% cream | OTC | Gyne-Lotrimin-3 or Clotrimazole-3 | 5 g intravaginally | 3 days |
| Miconazole 2% cream | OTC | Monistat-7 | 5 g intravaginally once at night | 7 days[a] |
| Miconazole 4% cream | OTC | Miconazole-3 | 5 g intravaginally | 3 days |
| Miconazole 100 mg suppository | OTC | Monistat-7 | 1 suppository intravaginally once at night | 7 days |
| Miconazole 200 mg suppository | OTC | Monistat-3 | 1 suppository intravaginally once at night | 3 days |
| Miconazole 1200 mg suppository | OTC | Monistat-1 | 1 suppository | Single dose |
| Tioconazole 6.5% cream (5 g) | OTC | | 5 g intravaginally once at night | Single dose |
| Terconazole 0.4% cream (45 g) | Rx | Terazol-7 | 5 g intravaginally once at night | 7 days |
| Terconazole 0.8% cream (30 g) | Rx | Terazol-3 | 5 g intravaginally once at night | 3 days |
| Terconazole 80 mg suppository | Rx | Terazol-3 | 1 suppository intravaginally once at night | 3 days |
| **Oral** | | | | |
| Fluconazole | Rx | Diflucan | 150 mg oral tablet once at night | Single |

Abbreviations: OTC, over-the-counter; Rx, prescription.

[a] A 7-day course is recommended during pregnancy.

Based on Workowski KA, Bachmann LH, Chan PA, et al. Sexually transmitted infections treatment guidelines, 2021. *MMWR Recomm Rep.* 2021;70(4):1-187. doi:10.15585/mmwr.rr7004a1.

genitals but has systemic side effects including alterations in hepatic function and several drug–drug interactions.[5]

Complicated VVC in nonpregnant individuals, which includes skin fissures, should be treated with a longer treatment course of either 7 to 14 days of a topical "azole" or two doses of 150 mg fluconazole, taken 72 hours apart.[5] If the vagina is very irritated, topical creams may aggravate the discomfort experienced by some people. For the midwife treating a client with candidiasis, it is important to involve the individual in choosing the route of administration and medication.

Probiotics, especially oral *Lactobacillus*, may help to restore normal vaginal flora, but conclusive evidence is lacking in part due to variations in probiotic composition.[30] Douching is not a recommended treatment. Health education includes methods to decrease yeast growth by reducing vulvar moisture

and eliminating irritants. Additional health information is found in Table 18-5 later in this chapter. Some complementary medicine sources recommend lifestyle changes, including decreasing consumption of refined sugars and yeast products. While these strategies have minimal potential for harm, they have not been substantiated as beneficial in otherwise healthy individuals. Alternative or complementary therapies such as vinegar washes, garlic, and tea tree oil have been the subject of only limited research into their safety or effectiveness.[31] There is no need for a test of cure if symptoms resolve; individuals should be rescreened only if they are symptomatic.

### Recurrent Candidiasis

Recurrent candidiasis is defined as three or more occurrences of candidiasis within one year.[5] If an individual has recurrent candidiasis, assess for contributing lifestyle factors, including those related to care of the vulva, and perform a culture to test for non-*albicans Candida* strains. Testing for underlying diabetes or HIV infection may be indicated depending on the individual's history and risk factors. If the person has severe, recurrent infections, they may consider changing their sexual practices or (if applicable) changing their birth control method to avoid spermicides and oral contraceptive pills.

A variety of treatment regimens for recurrent candidiasis are available. For recurrence of infection with *C. albicans* strains, longer duration of topical treatment combined with sequential oral treatment may be considered.[5] For non-*albicans* yeast, pharmaceutical-grade boric acid is approximately 70% effective when administered as a gelatin capsule that contains 600 mg; this capsule is inserted into the vagina once daily for 2 weeks.[5] Alternatively, a 7- to 14-day course of treatment with a non-fluconazole agent administered either topically or orally is acceptable.[5] Consultation with a specialist may be necessary for continued recurrences or complicated infections.

## Atrophic Vaginitis

Atrophic vaginitis is a collection of inflammatory vaginal symptoms related to low estrogen levels.[32] Lower estrogen levels can cause vaginal changes, including decreased elasticity, dryness, and thinning of the mucosal layer of the vaginal epithelium.[32] These changes make the vagina more friable and prone to irritation, and increase the risk of vaginal infections. Low estrogen levels can occur with natural menopause or cycle cessation during lactation, chemotherapy, treatment with anti-estrogenic medications, oophorectomy, and premature ovarian failure. While not an infection, these changes put individuals at increased risk for other infections such as BV, candidiasis, and STIs.

Vaginal changes in menopause are normal and do not require intervention unless they adversely impact the individual's functioning or quality of life. Some individuals may be reluctant to disclose such problems, so questions about vaginal dryness, irritation, and dyspareunia are important history components in patients assigned female at birth who are menopausal or not having regular menses. Vaginal dryness is the most frequent symptom of atrophic vaginitis, occurring in as many as 47% of postmenopausal individuals.[32] Other symptoms may include frequent vaginal infections, dyspareunia, and lack of lubrication with sexual activity.

Diagnosis of atrophic vaginitis is made via physical examination. Factors that suggest this diagnosis include thinning of the vulvar skin; decreasing prominence of the inner labia; small, non-elastic vaginal introitus; few vaginal rugae; pale pink vaginal walls; shortening of the vagina; and a lack of vaginal moisture. Wet mount may reveal parabasal cells with a negative whiff test. The vaginal pH may be higher than 4.5.[32]

Over-the-counter, water-based vaginal moisturizers that contain polycarbophil and are mildly acidic, such as Replens, can decrease symptoms when used daily and are appropriate for most individuals. Use of water-based lubricant products such as Astroglide, K-Y Jelly, or K-Y Liquibeads during sexual activity can decrease discomfort. Regular sexual arousal, and sexual intercourse, can be helpful in improving vaginal blood flow to increase tissue health.

Estrogen can also be used to alleviate symptoms of atrophic vaginitis. Topical estrogen administration via vaginal ring, tablet, or cream is preferable to oral administration as a first-line pharmacologic treatment.[33] When used topically, estrogen does not need to be paired with progesterone in individuals with an intact uterus. However, long-term data on the safety of topical estrogens are not available. Some research indicates elevated serum estrogen levels can occur with topical estrogen administration.[34] If an individual has a history of cancer, they should consult a cancer specialist before using any estrogen-containing therapies.

Non-estrogen treatment options for atrophic vaginitis include ospemifene oral tablets and dehydroepiandrosterone (Prasterone) vaginal inserts.[35] Ospemifene is an estrogen agonist/antagonist, so it carries a theoretical risk of inducing thromboembolic events and endometrial hyperplasia, although short-term safety data are reassuring.[36] Dehydroepiandrosterone (Prasterone) is converted in the body to androgens and estrogen; it is not associated with changes in serum levels of steroids.[37]

### Other Causes of Vaginitis

The skin of the vulva and vagina can become inflamed in response to many substances. For example, exposure to urine or stool, such as occurs with even mild incontinence, can cause chronic irritation and vaginitis. Perfumes and chemicals found in soaps, laundry detergents, and feminine hygiene products can also cause irritation. Personal lubricants can disrupt vaginal pH and normal flora, resulting in vaginitis. Spermicides may irritate the vagina as well. Douching washes away beneficial bacteria and irritates the vaginal mucosa, increasing the risk for vaginitis. A thorough exploration of all substances that contact the vulva and vagina is warranted for individuals who have unexplained or recurrent vaginitis. Individuals with urinary or fecal incontinence should strive to keep the vulva dry and free of urine or stool, cleaning this area as needed with water and soft, nonabrasive wipes.

As noted earlier, anything left within the vagina can also cause vaginitis—including tampons, pessaries, menstrual cups, or any other foreign body. Odor and irritation are often the presenting symptoms when a foreign object is retained in the vagina for longer than the recommended use. Vaginal irritation can also occur during intercourse if the individual does not have adequate lubrication or if the contact is rough or damaging. This finding might be indicative of relationship problems and needs further exploration.

## Epididymitis, Prostatitis, and Balanitis

Acute epididymitis lasts less than 6 weeks and is characterized by pain, swelling, and inflammation of the epididymis. It is commonly caused by STIs, such as *Chlamydia trachomatis*, *Neisseria gonorrhoeae*, or *Mycoplasma genitalium*, or by enteric bacteria such as *Escherichia coli*.[5]

Individuals with prostatitis may present with acute onset of systemic symptoms such as fever, chills, nausea and vomiting, in addition to urinary symptoms of frequency, urgency, or hesitancy. Prostatitis is most commonly caused by *E. coli* but may also result from infection with *C. trachomatis*, *N. gonorrhoeae*, or *Trichomonas vaginalis*.[38]

Balanitis is most common in uncircumcised individuals as a result of inadequate hygiene, but may also be due to chlamydia, gonorrhea, trichomoniasis, human papillomavirus, syphilis, or *Candida* infections.[39] Signs and symptoms of balanitis include redness, irritation, itching, odor, swelling, sores on the glans, or inability of the foreskin to retract.

## Sexually Transmitted Infections

Because sexual contact involves close bodily proximity, many microbes are shared between partners, most of which are nonpathogenic. The close contact of mucous membranes and the sharing of body fluids during such contact allow several pathogenic organisms the opportunity to find a new host. STIs may be caused by bacterial, viral, protozoal, or parasitic organisms, as described in Table 18-5. Some clinicians, however, prefer to organize their list of differential diagnoses according to the person's chief concern, as shown in Table 18-6. Many STIs are asymptomatic even while causing bodily damage.

| Table 18-5 | Causes of Sexually Transmitted Infections | |
|---|---|---|
| **Bacterial Disease (Organism)** | **Virus (Abbreviation)** | **Protozoal and Parasitic Disease (Organism)** |
| Chlamydia (*Chlamydia trachomatis*) | Human papillomavirus (HPV) | Trichomoniasis (*Trichomonas vaginalis*) |
| Gonorrhea (*Neisseria gonorrhoeae*) | Herpes simplex virus (HSV-1 and HSV-2) | Pubic lice/crabs (*Phthirus pubis*) |
| Syphilis (*Treponema pallidum*) | Human immunodeficiency virus (HIV) | Scabies (*Sarcoptes scabiei*) |
| Chancroid (*Haemophilus ducreyi*) | Zika virus | |
| Lymphogranuloma venereum (*Chlamydia trachomatis* serovars L1, L2, and L3) | *Molluscum contagiosum* | |
| Granuloma inguinale (*Klebsiella granulomatis*) | | |

| Table 18-6 | Common Presenting Concerns for Sexually Transmitted Infections | |
|---|---|---|
| **Vaginal/Urethral Discharge (Organism)** | **Sores (Organism or Virus)** | **Lesions (Organism or Virus)** |
| Chlamydia (*Chlamydia trachomatis*) | Herpes (herpes simplex virus [HSV-1 and HSV-2]) | Genital warts (human papillomavirus) |
| Gonorrhea (*Neisseria gonorrhoeae*) | Syphilis (*Treponema pallidum*) | Condyloma acuminata (human papillomavirus) |
| Trichomoniasis (*Trichomonas vaginalis*) | Chancroid (*Haemophilus ducreyi*) | Condylomata lata (*Treponema pallidum*) |
| | Lymphogranuloma venereum (*Chlamydia trachomatis* serovars L1, L2, and L3) | Mollusca (*Molluscum contagiosum*) |
| | Granuloma inguinale (*Klebsiella granulomatis*) | |

Anyone at risk for STIs should be screened according to CDC guidelines to prevent health sequelae and transmission to others. Pre-exposure prophylaxis for HIV or vaccination against hepatitis B may also be indicated.

## General Management Considerations Specific to Sexually Transmitted Infections

When individuals have symptoms of an STI or possible exposure to an STI, management includes some unique approaches and special considerations.

### Screening Strategies: Opt-in Versus Opt-out

Screening for any disorder can be offered in one of two ways. "*Opt-in*" (voluntary) refers to the individual being counseled about a test and then choosing or agreeing to have that screening test performed. "*Opt-out*" (universal) is a strategy in which the test is presented as part of standard care and unless the person declines, the test is performed. Midwives using an "opt-in" approach ask individuals about STI tests individually and obtain consent to screen for each infection. This approach presents STI screening as routine, thereby normalizing testing, but results in much lower rates of STI screening, as individuals are more likely to decline testing. By comparison, the opt-out approach, which has been studied with regard to HIV screening, greatly increases screening rates both during pregnancy and when people enter the hospital for care.[5]

The CDC advises clinicians to use an opt-out approach that presents individuals with a consent form that lists all of the common tests and allows them to opt out of any tests if they wish. Individuals should be informed of recommended tests and allowed to "opt out" of testing that is routinely recommended.[5] An opt-out approach to STI testing decreases barriers and presents these screening tests as tests that are routinely offered to all people.

### Reportable Diseases

Most states in the United States require healthcare providers to notify the local health department when a person is diagnosed with certain communicable STIs, as shown in Table 18-7.[5] Notifiable diseases are those for which obtaining information regarding individual cases is important for prevention and control of that disease. Reporting usually involves revealing the individual's name to the local health department and indicating whether the sexual partner was treated. The individuals should be told that this report will take place. This information is used to notify and treat sexual partners and to monitor

| Table 18-7 | Sexually Transmitted Infections Reportable for National Surveillance |
|---|---|
| Chancroid | |
| *Chlamydia trachomatis* | |
| Gonorrhea | |
| Hepatitis B | |
| Hepatitis C | |
| Human immunodeficiency virus (HIV) | |
| Syphilis | |
| Syphilis, congenital | |

prevalence of STIs on the local, state, and national levels.[40] U.S. law requires that the spouse (current or within the past 10 years) of a person who is positive for HIV be notified, and the health department can assist in this endeavor.[41] Midwives should be aware of the laws concerning partner notification in their state or legal jurisdiction.

### Test of Cure, Test for Reinfection, and Pre-exposure or Postexposure Prophylaxis

*Test of cure* refers to the practice of reculturing a specimen from the site of initial infection to confirm that the infection is no longer present. A test of cure is recommended for some vaginal infections and STIs when the risk of therapy failure is well known and adverse outcomes are significant. A test of cure is performed shortly after the completion of therapy. In contrast, a *test for reinfection* is recommended when the therapy is known to be highly effective but the partner may not be adequately treated. A test for reinfection is often performed a few months after completion of therapy.

*Pre-exposure prophylaxis* and *postexposure prophylaxis* may be recommended for individuals who are at risk for contracting HIV. These management strategies are reviewed in more detail in the section on HIV.

### Expedited Partner Therapy

Treatment of the individual's sexual partner for STIs is within the scope of midwifery practice.[42] Partner treatment may involve examination and testing of the sexual partner or presumptive treatment without a clinic visit depending on the diagnosed STI. It is acceptable to treat sexual partners for STIs without a physical examination—a practice known as *expedited partner therapy* (EPT).[43] EPT allows for rapid treatment of sexual partners, thereby reducing the risk of reinfection and decreasing healthcare costs. To prevent adverse outcomes from drug allergies, the clinician should provide information with the prescription about potential side effects and an allergy warning.

Evidence to support the practice of EPT has largely been obtained from studies of heterosexual individuals diagnosed with gonorrhea and/or chlamydia and their partners who engage in penile–vaginal sex.[44] Although there is limited research to support EPT to prevent reinfection with trichomoniasis, midwives may provide EPT in such cases using shared decision making. The use of EPT for adolescents is supported by the American Academy of Pediatrics and the Society for Adolescent Medicine. EPT should not be used to treat syphilis or long-term, chronic STIs such as herpes or HIV.[44]

For individuals diagnosed with chlamydia, sexual partners from the previous 60 days who are unlikely to receive timely evaluation are eligible for EPT.[5] A multiday treatment with doxycycline for nonpregnant individuals is more effective than single-dose azithromycin for rectal chlamydia. Adherence to multiday treatment may be a consideration in the choice of antibiotic for EPT. If this option is available, providing packaged oral medication is preferred rather than a written prescription. For individuals diagnosed with gonorrhea, the preferred antibiotic for EPT is a single dose of intramuscular ceftriaxone.[44] For partners who are unlikely to seek timely evaluation and treatment, a single dose of oral cefixime is an acceptable alternative. EPT for gonorrhea and chlamydia infection may be provided at the same time, and the CDC recommends treatment for chlamydia for individuals with gonorrhea infection unless a negative test result is available. The midwife should also provide written educational information with the EPT, as well as treatment instructions, medication warnings, general health counseling, and directions to seek evaluation for HIV testing and STI symptoms, particularly pelvic inflammatory disease (PID).

EPT is permissible in 46 states, the District of Columbia, and the Commonwealth of the Northern Mariana Islands. EPT is potentially allowable in four states, Puerto Rico, and Guam.[45] Partner treatment is included in the American College of Nurse-Midwives' *Core Competencies for Basic Midwifery Practice*.[46] However, while a state may legally allow EPT, some state licensure boards, such as boards of nursing, prohibit writing prescriptions for individuals who have not been evaluated or who do not have a chart within the clinic of the prescribing provider.

The CDC maintains an interactive database of state statutes concerning EPT that can provide guidance on pertinent state regulations.[45]

## Indications for Sexually Transmitted Infection Screening

If a person is concerned that they may have been exposed to a STI, they should be offered tests for all STIs that are common in the geographic area, including those deemed most likely to occur based on their own or their partners' sexual behaviors.[5] Local and regional prevalence rates are used to determine which infections are prevalent in the region or in the individual's or partner's area of origin.[47] The CDC provides a list of groups at increased risk for specific STIs.[5] The STI tests recommended by the CDC for asymptomatic individuals (pregnant or nonpregnant) are reviewed in **Table 18-8**.[5]

Recommended screening tests for STIs, for individuals of all ages, are discussed in greater detail in the *Health Promotion Across the Lifespan* and *Prenatal Care* chapters. Individuals who are unable to conceive due to known infertility, menopause, or sterilization may neglect STI precautions. *Any* person at *any* age who has a new or nonmonogamous sexual partner is at risk for STIs and should be offered testing. It is important to guard against age bias in the decision to offer STI tests; rates of STIs among people older than 50 years have been increasing.[48]

Any individual with symptoms of an STI, including urethritis, proctitis, epididymitis, abnormal vaginal or penile discharge, dysuria, cervicitis, or cervical motion tenderness, should be evaluated with a thorough history, targeted physical examination, and indicated laboratory tests. If a person has one STI, they are at risk for having another and should be offered tests for HIV and all common STIs.[5]

Half of all STIs occur in persons younger than 25 years.[49] The CDC recommends all sexually active individuals with a vagina younger than 25 years be offered screening tests for chlamydia and gonorrhea annually.[5] In addition, they should be offered HIV screening (although the screening interval for HIV testing has not been determined) and other diagnostic tests if they are symptomatic. Cervical cytology testing with human papillomavirus (HPV) testing should begin at age 21 years, regardless of the number of sexual partners or the age when the person first became sexually active.

Adolescents can receive tests for STIs without parental notification or consent in all 50 states and the District of Columbia.[5] However, if an individual

| Table 18-8 | CDC Screening Test Recommendations for STIs Among Asymptomatic Individuals[a] | | |
|---|---|---|---|
| **Infection** | **Nonpregnant Individuals with a Vagina** | **Individuals with a Penis** | **Pregnant Individuals** |
| Chlamydia | Sexually active individuals younger than 25 years<br><br>Use shared decision making about rectal screening based on sexual practices and exposure<br><br>Sexually active individuals ≥ 25 years with new partners, more than one sex partner, a sex partner with concurrent partners, or a sex partner with a STI<br><br>Individuals < 35 years living in a correctional facility<br><br>Rescreen for reinfection approximately 3 months after original treatment | Consider screening for adolescents in correctional facilities or presenting at STI clinics<br><br>Urethral, rectal, and pharyngeal screening offered annually for adolescent individuals engaging in oral sex or receptive anal sex<br><br>Urethral and rectal screening offered annually for individuals engaging in oral sex or receptive anal sex<br><br>Individuals < 30 years living in a correctional facility | All pregnant individuals < 25 years<br><br>Pregnant individuals ≥ 25 years if new partners, more than one sex partner, a sex partner with concurrent partners, or a sex partner with a STI<br><br>Rescreen for reinfection approximately 3 months after original treatment<br><br>Test of cure 3–4 weeks after treatment<br><br>Consider rescreening for reinfection during third trimester |
| Gonorrhea | Sexually active individuals < 25 years<br><br>Use shared decision making about rectal screening based on sexual practices and exposure<br><br>Sexually active individuals ≥ 25 years with new partners, more than one sex partner, a sex partner with concurrent partners, or a sex partner with STI<br><br>Individuals < 35 years living in a correctional facility<br><br>Rescreen for reinfection approximately 3 months after original treatment | Urethral, rectal, and pharyngeal screening offered annually to individuals engaging in oral sex or receptive anal sex<br><br>Consult with the local health department for guidance in identifying communities with higher incidence of infection acquisition<br><br>Individuals < 30 years living in a correctional facility | All pregnant individuals < 25 years<br><br>Pregnant individuals ≥ 25 years with new partners, more than one sex partner, a sex partner with concurrent partners, or a sex partner with STI<br><br>Rescreen for reinfection approximately 3 months after original treatment<br><br>Rescreen for reinfection in third trimester for individuals at risk |
| Hepatitis B | Recommended for individuals with multiple sex partners, individuals seeking care at STI clinics, individuals who engage in transactional sex, individuals with drug misuse, and individuals with history of STI<br><br>Individuals living in a correctional facility<br><br>More frequent screening for individuals taking pre-exposure prophylaxis (PrEP) | Recommended for individuals engaging in oral sex or receptive anal sex<br><br>More frequent screening for individuals taking pre-exposure prophylaxis (PrEP)<br><br>Individuals living in a correctional facility | Test for HBsAG at first prenatal visit regardless of prior testing or vaccination<br><br>Rescreen for reinfection during intrapartum if at high risk and those with clinical hepatitis |
| Hepatitis C | At least once for all individuals unless local infection rate is < 0.1%<br><br>Individuals living in a correctional facility | At least once for all individuals unless local infection rate is < 0.1%<br><br>Individuals living in a correctional facility | All pregnant individuals unless local infection rate is < 0.1%<br><br>Consider for pregnant individuals with multiple sex partners, individuals who engage in transactional sex, individuals with drug misuse, and individuals with history of STI risk |

| Infection | Nonpregnant Individuals with a Vagina | Individuals with a Penis | Pregnant Individuals |
|---|---|---|---|
| HIV | All individuals seeking STI evaluation<br>At least once for all individuals, with opt-out option<br>Individuals living in a correctional facility, with opt-out option | At least once for all individuals, with opt-out option<br>Individuals living in a correctional facility, with opt-out option | All pregnant individuals at the first prenatal visit, with opt-out option<br>Rescreen for reinfection during third trimester and during intrapartum if at high risk |
| HSV | Genital swabs and serologic screening in asymptomatic individuals are not recommended<br>Consider type-specific HSV serologic testing for women in high-prevalence settings (e.g., STI clinics) and those at risk (e.g., multiple sex partners)[a] | Genital swabs and serologic screening in asymptomatic individuals are not recommended | Routine serologic screening is not recommended<br>Type-specific test may be considered for individuals with a sex partner with known HSV[a] |
| Syphilis | Consider for individuals seeking care at STI clinics, individuals with multiple sex partners, individuals who engage in transactional sex, individuals with drug misuse, and individuals with history of STI | Consider for individuals seeking care at STI clinics, individuals with multiple sex partners, individuals who engage in transactional sex, individuals with drug misuse, and individuals with history of STI | All pregnant individuals at the first prenatal visit<br>Rescreen for reinfection during third trimester and during intrapartum if at high risk |
| *Trichomonas* | Individuals < 35 years living in a correctional facility, with opt-out option<br>Consider for individuals seeking care at STI clinics, individuals with multiple sex partners, individuals who engage in transactional sex, individuals with drug misuse, and individuals with history of STI<br>Consider for individuals engaging in oral sex or sharing sex toys with partners with vaginas<br>Annual screening for individuals with HIV | No recommendation for routine screening | Consider for individuals living in correctional facilities, individuals with multiple sex partners, individuals who engage in transactional sex, individuals with drug misuse, individuals with history of STI, and individuals at high risk[a] |

Abbreviations: CDC, Centers for Disease Control and Prevention; HBsAG, hepatitis B surface antigen; HIV, human immunodeficiency virus; HSV, herpes simplex virus; STI, sexually transmitted infection.

[a]Consideration based on evidence but not a CDC recommendation.

Based on Workowski KA, Bachmann LH, Chan PA, et al. Sexually transmitted infections treatment guidelines, 2021. *MMWR Recomm Rep*. 2021;70(4):1-187. doi:10.15585/mmwr.rr7004a1.

uses health insurance for payment, the services provided will be included on the insurance explanation of benefits, which could breach confidentiality.[5] Adolescents and young adults, especially those using parental insurance, should be informed about insurance reports. If the individual wants to use parental insurance, it may be helpful to forewarn their parents that they were screened for STIs as a component of a recent healthcare visit. If this is not acceptable, it may be best to refer the person to local resources for free or low-cost STI testing.

### Gender-Diverse Persons

STIs can be transmitted in numerous ways through direct contact with body fluids as well as through fomites such as sex toys. While the prevalence of specific infections can vary in different populations, all sexually active individuals are at risk of infection. Midwives should provide unbiased STI counseling and appropriate screening to all individuals based on their anatomy and their sexual practices.

### Sexually Transmitted Infections During Pregnancy

Sexually transmitted infections can adversely affect the embryo or fetus, causing a wide range of complications, including lifelong morbidity and intrauterine death. Early screening and treatment for STIs can prevent complications in the pregnant individual, the fetus, and the neonate. For this reason, comprehensive STI testing should be performed during the first visit for pregnancy or as soon as possible. States often mandate the provision of these services within a set time frame. As a consequence, STI tests should not be delayed to coincide with other testing, such as routine second trimester bloodwork. Pregnant individuals who have multiple sexual partners or individuals who are diagnosed with an STI during pregnancy should be rescreened in the third trimester or in labor if indicated. Individuals are rescreened during each pregnancy, regardless of interconceptional spacing.[5]

All pregnant individuals are offered testing for chlamydia and HIV using an opt-out approach in the first trimester, and individuals at high risk should be offered repeat screening tests in the third trimester. High-risk groups for chlamydia include persons who have tested positive for chlamydia during the current pregnancy, who are younger than 25 years, or who have new, multiple, or nonmonogamous sexual partners. High-risk status for HIV is conferred by the following factors: living in a high-prevalence area, drug misuse, diagnosis of an STI during pregnancy, and new, multiple, nonmonogamous, or HIV-positive sexual partner(s). Even if screened earlier during pregnancy, individuals at risk for STIs should be rescreened in the third trimester or at the time of admission in labor. Some states mandate third trimester testing for STIs unless the person specifically declines such tests.[5]

The CDC recommends hepatitis B screening for all pregnant individuals, and individuals at high risk of infection may have repeat screening. In addition, unless local rates of hepatitis C are less than 0.1%, hepatitis C screening should be recommended at the first prenatal visit.[5] High-risk categories for hepatitis C include current or previous use of injected or intranasal drugs, obtaining an unregulated tattoo, and a history of blood transfusion or organ transplantation prior to 1992.

Pregnant individuals who are considered to be at risk for gonorrhea should be routinely screened for this STI. At-risk groups for gonorrhea include individuals who have the following characteristics: living in an area with a high prevalence of gonorrhea, such as the southern United States; age younger than 25 years; a history of STIs; new or multiple sex partners; transactional sex; drug misuse; and irregular condom use, which is common among pregnant individuals who may not consider the use of condoms for protection against STIs. Persons who are at continued risk and those who acquire a risk factor over the course of pregnancy should be rescreened in the third trimester.

Regardless of their risk status, asymptomatic individuals do not need to be routinely screened for trichomoniasis or bacterial vaginosis during pregnancy. The degree to which identification and treatment of persons with these conditions decreases adverse health outcomes and reduces the risk of preterm birth remains a controversial topic. However, individuals should be tested if they have symptoms; if positive, they should be offered treatment following informed decision making based on health education about potential risks of preterm birth.[5]

### Individuals Who Are Incarcerated

Individuals entering correctional facilities are a particularly vulnerable population, as the rates of STIs in this population are high.[50] Persons who are incarcerated are more likely than those who are not incarcerated to have been abused or exchanged sexual contact for food, housing, or money.[51] The CDC recommends that on intake to a correctional facility and following consent, all individuals younger than 35 years be screened for gonorrhea, chlamydia, and HIV.[5] Syphilis screening in this population is based on local prevalence.[5]

### Communicating Information About Sexually Transmitted Infections

Telling a person that they have an STI is often difficult for both novice and experienced practitioners. The CDC advises clinicians to discuss positive HIV testing in person.[5] However, for STIs other than HIV, discussion of the diagnosis and planning for treatment may occur via the phone if an in-person visit is not feasible. Phone consultations are acceptable, but not ideal, as it is more difficult for the midwife to gauge how the person is responding to the diagnosis. However, phone visits can facilitate prompt treatment and decrease the chance that the individual is unable to receive treatment. Prior to phoning a person with STI results, make sure they have consented to be contacted by phone. Once they answer, ask if they are in an acceptable location to have a discussion before beginning the conversation.

Maintaining a normal tone of voice without judgment is helpful in being present for the person. It may take time for the individual to adjust to the news that they have a STI. Openly discuss the fact that the infection is sexually transmitted and address whether it is possible for the infection to be transmitted in other ways, such as through common contact. While nonsexual transmission is possible with some infections, such as scabies, it is very unlikely for others, such as gonorrhea. Some infections produce symptoms soon after initial infection, whereas others, such as HPV, may not manifest for months or years. Avoid assumptions about the origin of the STI, and use open- and closed-ended questions to further explore the person's feelings and needs. Always assess for the possibility of intimate partner violence if the diagnosis is shared with a sexual partner.

While health education to avoid future infections is needed, it can be difficult for an individual to concentrate on such health-promoting messages immediately after receiving an STI diagnosis. Written materials that the person can take home will allow them to review the information when they are more receptive to it. A well-placed follow-up visit in person or by phone may be a better time for additional health education if the person seems overwhelmed at the time of diagnosis.

### Relationship Stressors and Violence

STIs can be associated with intimate-partner relationship difficulties. Although many STIs are acquired from a new partner who was previously infected, a new STI diagnosis may reveal infidelity of a long-term sexual partner or may be an indicator that the individual has been forced to have sex. Screening for human trafficking is warranted if the person has more than one STI, an advanced case of the infection, or other risk factors for nonconsensual sex.[52] Individuals who experience interpersonal violence are at an increased risk of acquiring an STI, but partner notification and treatment have not been shown to greatly increase the rate of violence.[53]

### Psychosocial Needs

Individuals with STIs are more likely to be members of vulnerable social groups. Being young, being poor, and misusing drugs are all risks for STI

acquisition.[47] Sometimes sexual activity is one of many risk-taking behaviors. In other cases, the person did not have a choice about engaging in sexual contact. Individuals who are abused or forced into sexual encounters may not be able to advocate for condom use. Negotiating for safer sexual practices requires self-confidence and power within the relationship. Obtaining condoms requires money or access to services, which may be difficult to obtain for persons of low socioeconomic status and those who do not have a support network. Individuals who trade sex for food, housing, drugs, or money or who are victims of trafficking are more likely to acquire STIs, as they often have multiple sexual partners who have little concern for the person's health.[54] Individuals often enter care for one reason but have other needs besides the chief concern and can benefit from a holistic approach that provides them with needed information or referrals beyond their presenting diagnosis.

### Contraception

Individuals with a uterus engaging in penile–vaginal sex are at risk for pregnancy. The time at which the person is diagnosed with an STI presents an excellent opportunity to discuss their reproductive life plan. A critical first step in this discussion is to determine the individual's intentions regarding pregnancy. Straightforward questioning about whether they are planning a pregnancy in the near future can provide the midwife with answers that guide the discussion. For individuals who are planning a pregnancy, the midwife can use this opportunity to discuss the importance of pregnancy prevention until STI treatment is complete and returning for a test of cure if one is indicated.

When a person is not planning a pregnancy in the near future, it is essential to review their contraceptive options and allow them to choose a method that provides prevention of unintended pregnancy as well as protection from STIs. Whereas both internal and external condoms are part of safer sex practices, other birth control methods offer little protection from STI acquisition. However, condoms have a fairly high failure rate for pregnancy prevention and may be an inadequate primary contraceptive method. A person may need to use condoms in addition to other contraceptive methods to prevent STIs, and may need to be reminded of the importance of safer sexual practices even when they are not concerned about pregnancy prevention. Some individuals need guidance on how to negotiate for safer sexual practices even if they are protected from pregnancy.

### Evaluation of the Need for Immediate Intervention, Consultation, or Collaboration

The treatment of individuals with STIs often involves interprofessional collaboration. Local pharmacists, physicians, and health department staff may be involved in this process. If the person has a disseminated or advanced STI, hospitalization and consultation with physicians, pharmacists, and infectious disease specialists may be appropriate. Treatment failures may necessitate consultation with regional health departments or the CDC. Pediatric care providers need to know about any STIs in the pregnant or laboring person that may affect their newborn or infant. Judicious use of other members of the interprofessional healthcare team can improve the quality of the care received while protecting a person's rights and dignity. Although consultation may involve disclosing the individual's name and diagnosis, this should be done in ways that respect their rights and maintain their confidentiality. Care provider communication can facilitate quick and effective treatment, thereby preventing morbidity and mortality.[55]

Suspected sexual abuse of minors must be reported to local authorities for further investigation. In addition, reporting of STIs to local health departments is a responsibility that does not violate confidentiality. While local health departments should not reveal the name of the index patient, there is the chance that someone could guess which partner had an STI, and this recognition could have wide-ranging implications for the individual, including violence. Therefore, the CDC advises all health departments to ask individuals, without coercion, to provide information about previous sexual partners so they can be notified and treated.[14]

### Development of a Comprehensive Plan of Care That Is Supported by a Valid Rationale

It is important to ensure that individuals are treated appropriately for STIs to prevent short- and long-term morbidity and to reduce transmission. Treatment options can be presented to the person and a plan of care developed to meet their needs. Effectiveness, cost, and convenience are chief considerations in choosing a treatment. Dosing frequency, privacy, and ability to apply or wash off the medicine may also be important in the decision-making process.

Follow-up after STI diagnosis and treatment differs according to the specific infection. While it can sometimes be difficult for individuals to return to the clinic, appropriate and well-timed follow-up is important to decrease infection-related morbidity,

prevent transmission, and detect drug-resistant strains early.[5]

### Chlamydia

*Chlamydia trachomatis* is a small, gram-negative bacterium that is an obligate intracellular organism. Chlamydia is the most common reportable STI, with more than 1.7 million new cases occurring each year in the United States.[47] The majority of these infections occur in individuals 24 years or younger, although any sexually active person is at risk.[5] Because most cases of chlamydia are asymptomatic, the CDC recommends screening for this infection in all individuals who have a new sexual partner, and annual screening for individuals 25 years or younger.[5]

If left untreated, chlamydia can ascend into the upper reproductive tract and cause pelvic inflammatory disease (PID). Ascending infections increase the risk of subsequent ectopic pregnancy and infertility. Urogenital transmission is the most common way in which this infection is spread, but sexual transmission to the oropharynx and rectum is also possible. Vertical transmission can occur during vaginal birth, causing conjunctivitis or pneumonia in affected neonates.

Although chlamydial infection in individuals is usually asymptomatic, increased vaginal discharge, dysuria, or greater vestibular (Bartholin) gland infection can be presenting symptoms. Some individuals are initially diagnosed when they present with salpingitis (infection in the uterine tubes) or PID.

### Screening and Diagnosis of Chlamydia

All individuals who are younger than 25 years, have new or multiple sex partners, have a sex partner with a concurrent partner or a sex partner with STI, have receptive anal intercourse, have a history of inconsistent condom use if not in a mutually monogamous relationship, engage in drug use, engage in sex work, have a history of a previous STI, or live in a geographic area with a high prevalence of gonorrhea (i.e., the southeastern United States) should be screened for chlamydia annually.

Physical examination may reveal cervicitis, mucopurulent discharge, or cervical motion tenderness. Although an increased number of white blood cells may be detected on a wet prep, the diagnosis of chlamydia is made based on laboratory tests. NAAT is the most commonly used diagnostic test for chlamydia; it can be performed on urine, cervical, vaginal, or liquid cytology specimens.[5] Individuals can self-collect vaginal or urethral meatus NAAT cultures if desired; the rates of sensitivity with such samples are similar to those for provider-collected samples.[5] NAAT may also be used with rectal and oral samples, depending on the manufacturer and laboratory. Pharyngeal and rectal infections with *C. trachomatis* can occur in persons who engage in receptive oral or anal intercourse. NAAT can be utilized at the anatomic exposure site with similar rates of detection as in urine samples.

Individuals with a surgically constructed vagina who are having vaginal intercourse should be screened for chlamydial infection per standard testing guidelines. Testing should be done regardless of type of tissue grafted during the surgical procedure.

NAAT detects small amounts of gene sequences in bacterial DNA and replicates those sequences so that a large amount is present. Most samples sent to the laboratory for STI diagnosis are tested using NAAT technology. Urine testing is the least invasive option and has high sensitivity rates.[5] NAAT on liquid cytology (liquid Pap test) may have a lower sensitivity for detecting infection. Point-of-care NAAT-based testing is becoming more widely available and can reduce unnecessary presumptive antibiotic treatment.[5]

### Treatment and Follow-up for Chlamydia

Pharmacologic treatments for chlamydia are listed in Table 18-9. Single-dose treatment is preferable. Ensure treatment of all sexual partners from the last 60 days.[5] Individuals with chlamydia should abstain from intercourse until partners are treated and for 7 days after single-dose treatment or until the multidose treatment is completed. Most treatment failures are related to reinfections due to inadequate treatment of partners.[5]

The medications listed in Table 18-9 are recommended, but others can be considered in the first trimester for pregnant individuals diagnosed with chlamydia. For example, levofloxacin (Levaquin) poses a low risk to the fetus and could be used in case of drug allergies. Always consult the CDC for

| Table 18-9 | Treatments for Chlamydia in Adolescents and Adults | | |
|---|---|---|---|
| Recommended Treatments for Nonpregnant Individuals Generic (Brand) | Alternative Treatments for Nonpregnant Individuals Generic (Brand) | Recommended Treatments for Pregnant Individuals Generic (Brand) | Considerations for Lactating Individuals |
| Doxycycline (Vibramycin) 100 mg orally twice a day for 7 days | Azithromycin (Zithromax, Z-Pak) 1 g orally once<br><br>Levofloxacin (Levaquin) 500 mg orally daily for 7 days | Azithromycin (Zithromax, Z-Pak) 1 g orally once<br><br>Alternative treatment: Amoxicillin 500 mg three times per day for 7 days | There is a theoretical potential that an infant's forming teeth will become stained if doxycycline is used by a lactating person. However, its levels in human milk are low and short courses of doxycycline are acceptable. If doxycycline is needed, consider strategies to minimize its transfer to the milk.<br><br>Azithromycin is compatible with lactation.<br><br>There are limited data on the use of levofloxacin during lactation but amounts in human milk appear to be lower than the infant dose and not expected to cause harm.<br><br>Amoxicillin is compatible with lactation. |

Based on Workowski KA, Bachmann LH, Chan PA, et al. Sexually transmitted infections treatment guidelines, 2021. *MMWR Recomm Rep.* Jul 23 2021;70(4):1-187. doi:10.15585/mmwr.rr7004a1; U.S. National Library of Medicine. Drugs and Lactation Database (Lactmed). https://www.ncbi.nlm.nih.gov/books/NBK501922. Published 2021. Accessed July 26, 2021.

the most appropriate treatment regimen, as this is the most likely area for change.

Individuals who have a positive test for chlamydia should be tested for all common STIs, as coinfections frequently occur.[5] It is not necessary to repeat testing (test of cure) in nonpregnant individuals treated with the recommended regimens unless treatment compliance is in question, reinfection is suspected, or the patient reports continued symptoms.

### Management of Chlamydia During the Perinatal Period

Individuals with a history of chlamydial infection are at increased risk for ectopic pregnancy. The CDC recommends routine screening for chlamydia for all pregnant individuals as early as possible during pregnancy. Pregnant individuals at increased risk for STIs (e.g., those younger than 25 years, those with a new or nonmonogamous sexual partner during pregnancy) may be rescreened in the third trimester.[5] Treatment should occur as soon as possible after diagnosis, using a treatment regimen compatible with pregnancy. Pregnant individuals should be retested no sooner than 3 weeks after treatment, and then rescreened again 3 months later or in the third trimester, whichever comes first.[5]

Chlamydial ophthalmia can cause ocular scarring and blindness and/or life-threatening pneumonia.[5] Because routine neonatal ocular prophylaxis is only 80% effective against chlamydia, infants born to individuals who are infected with chlamydia should be closely observed for symptoms but not routinely treated.[5] Additional information about eye prophylaxis for newborns to prevent chlamydial and gonorrheal ophthalmia can be found in the *Neonatal Care* chapter.

## Gonorrhea

*Neisseria gonorrhoeae* is a gram-negative intracellular diplococcus that exclusively affects humans. This bacterium primarily infects the mucocutaneous surfaces of the genitourinary tract, pharynx, conjunctiva, and rectum. Gonorrhea is the second most common reportable communicable disease in the United States, with 710,151 cases reported in 2021.[56] In recent years, there has been a surge in antibiotic resistance to this organism, and the organism has the potential to become resistant to all currently available antibiotics.[57] The CDC and WHO monitor infectious disease resistance

patterns and release updates as needed. Clinicians are advised to use the most current guidelines for the geographic location of infection acquisition and treatment.

Transmission of gonorrhea occurs through oral, anal, and vaginal sex and via contact with secretions from the source individual's urogenital tract. Vertical infection is possible during vaginal birth. Individuals infected with gonorrhea can be asymptomatic, or they may experience a variety of symptoms. Individuals may have dysuria, abnormal vaginal discharge, or bleeding if infected vaginally. Oral infection can result in a sore throat. Anal infection can cause anal itching, soreness, bleeding, discharge, or painful bowel movements.[5] Disseminated gonorrhea is a rare, life-threatening condition characterized by symptoms of joint pain and a rash. Gonorrhea can increase the risk of HIV acquisition and is associated with PID, infertility, and ectopic pregnancy.[5] Individuals with PID that is caused by gonorrhea can have fever, vaginal discharge, and abdominal pain (see the section on Pelvic Inflammatory Disease later in this chapter).

### Screening and Diagnosis of Gonorrhea

Individuals at risk for gonorrhea include all sexually active individuals younger than 25 years and individuals with new sexual partners, engaging in transactional sex, with more than one sex partner, with a sex partner with concurrent partners, or with a sex partner who has an STI. Individuals at risk should be screened for gonorrhea annually. Asymptomatic screening in low-risk populations, such as heterosexual people older than age 25 without other risk factors, is not recommended.

The physical examination may be unremarkable in persons with gonorrhea. Conversely, lymph nodes surrounding the affected area may be enlarged. Urethritis and inflammation and discharge from the periurethral (Skene's) and greater vestibular (Bartholin) glands may be present. Cervicitis is common. If the person has mucopurulent discharge from the cervix and uterine or adnexal tenderness, or cervical motion tenderness, PID is a likely diagnosis.

Diagnosis of gonorrhea is based on laboratory tests. However, if this infection is considered a likely diagnosis based on clinical findings, treatment can begin prior to receiving the results of testing. NAAT samples can be collected by the provider or the patient, with the testing being performed on endocervical, rectal, urethral, vaginal, ororpharyngeal, or urine samples. NAAT products on the market have differing collection methods and sample requirements, so it is important to be familiar with the manufacturer's guidelines for each product. Cultures require an endocervical or urethral sample. If rectal, oropharyngeal, or ophthalmic testing is needed, ensure that the laboratory has tests that are specific to *N. gonorrhoeae*, as common bacteria present in these areas may cause false-positive results.

Oropharyngeal infections can be more difficult to eradicate than infections at other sites, and there are no reliable alternative treatments for oropharyngeal infection. For persons with a severe cephalosporin allergy such as anaphylaxis or Stevens-Johnson syndrome, providers will need to consult an infectious disease specialist for an alternative regimen. Pharyngeal infections need to have a test of cure by either culture or NAAT in 7 to 14 days; repeat testing at 7 days may lead to more false positives. Positive cultures will need to be sent for sensitivity testing to ensure appropriate treatment.

### Treatment and Follow-up for Gonorrhea

Table 18-10 lists the recommended treatment regimens for uncomplicated gonorrhea infection. Ideally, treatment is provided on site and observed.[5] Individuals with gonorrhea are also frequently coinfected with chlamydia, so all CDC-approved treatments for gonorrhea include dual therapy treatment

| Table 18-10 | Treatments for Uncomplicated Gonorrhea of the Cervix, Urethra, Rectum, or Pharynx in Adolescents and Adults | | | |
|---|---|---|---|---|
| **Recommended Treatments for Nonpregnant Individuals Generic (Brand)** | **Alternative Treatments for Nonpregnant Individuals[a] Generic (Brand)** | **Recommended Treatments for Pregnant Individuals Generic (Brand)** | **Considerations for Lactating Individuals** |
| Ceftriaxone (Rocephin) 500 mg in one intramuscular dose if weighing < 150 kg (if > 150 kg, 1 g IM in one dose), regardless of site of infection AND Doxycycline 100 mg orally twice a day for 7 days *if chlamydia has not been excluded* | Gentamicin 240 mg IM in a single dose PLUS Azithromycin 2 g orally in a single dose OR Cefixime 800 mg orally in a single dose AND Doxycycline 100 mg orally twice a day for 7 days *if chlamydia has not been excluded* | Ceftriaxone (Rocephin) 500 mg in one intramuscular dose if weighing < 150 kg (if > 150 kg, 1 g IM in one dose) regardless of site of infection; if significant cephalosporin allergy is present, consult an infectious disease specialist for a management plan AND Azithromycin 1 g orally one time if chlamydia has not been excluded There are no alternative treatments in pregnancy. | Ceftriaxone (Rocephin) is compatible with lactation There is a theoretical potential that an infant's forming teeth will become stained if doycycline is used by a lactating person. However, its levels in human milk are low and short courses of doxycycline are acceptable. If doxycycline is needed, consider strategies to minimize its transfer to the milk. Azithromycin is compatible with lactation. Although there are no data on cefixime use in lactation, cephalosporins are compatible with lactation. Diarrhea and thrush are theoretical risks to the nursing infant. Gentamicin is poorly excreted into human milk and infants serum levels are far below those attained when infants are treated for infections. Infants should be monitored for gastrointestinal effects (diarrhea, candidiasis, or blood in stool). |

Abbreviation: IM, intramuscularly.

[a]Alternative treatments are not reliable for pharyngeal gonorrhea.

Based on Workowski KA, Bachmann LH, Chan PA, et al. Sexually transmitted infections treatment guidelines, 2021. *MMWR Recomm Rep.* 2021;70(4):1-187. doi:10.15585/mmwr.rr7004a1; U.S. National Library of Medicine. Drugs and Lactation Database (LactMed). https://www.ncbi.nlm.nih.gov/books/NBK501922. Published 2021. Accessed July 26, 2021.

for chlamydia if this infection cannot be excluded at time of the gonorrhea diagnosis. This strategy is intended both to reduce the incidence of PID and to combat increasing antibiotic resistance.[5]

Alternative regimens are recommended only if ceftriaxone (Rocephin) is not available or if the person is severely allergic to penicillin or cephalosporins. In such a case, an infectious disease consultation should be obtained because the choice of cephalosporin needs to be individualized. The CDC website provides further guidance for unusual or complicated cases, such as treatment failure or disseminated gonorrhea.

Individuals receiving treatment for gonorrhea should be screened for other STIs, including syphilis, chlamydia, and HIV. They should abstain from sexual contact for 7 days after treatment and until all sexual partners are screened and treated. Otherwise, healthy nonpregnant adults with uncomplicated urogenital or rectal gonorrhea do not need a test of cure if treated with the ceftriaxone/doxycycline (Vibramycin) regimen. If treatment with ceftriaxone was not possible the individual will need a test of cure 2 weeks after finishing treatment using either NAAT or culture for the repeat test.

The CDC recommends retesting for gonorrhea 3 months after treatment to test for reinfection in individuals who have been treated for multiple lifetime gonococcal infections.[5] If a 3-month rescreening is not possible, the individual should be screened the next time they present for health care. Most positive tests after treatment reflect reinfection; if treatment failure is suspected, a culture should be obtained, an infectious disease specialist or the CDC should be contacted, and the individual and partner(s) should be immediately treated using current CDC guidelines for treatment failures.

### Management of Gonorrhea During the Perinatal Period

All pregnant individuals should be tested for gonorrheal infection. Individuals with a history of possible exposure to gonorrhea can be offered treatment before the test results are available. Pregnant individuals should receive a test of cure following treatment and should be tested for reinfection in 3 months or during the third trimester.[5] If the pregnant person is allergic to the recommended treatments, consultation with an infectious disease specialist is recommended.[5]

Gonorrhea can be transmitted during birth and cause ophthalmia, localized infections of mucosa, abscesses at the site of a placed fetal heart rate electrode, or disseminated infection in the neonate. Because gonococcal ophthalmia can result in permanent blindness, the CDC advises ophthalmia neonatorum prophylaxis using erythromycin ophthalmic ointment for *all* newborns, regardless of maternal testing status or route of birth; this prophylaxis is reviewed in more detail in the *Neonatal Care* chapter.[5] Many state laws mandate such treatment, and a parent must sign a waiver to opt out of treatment. Infants born to individuals with untreated gonorrhea or suspected gonorrhea should also receive parenteral antibiotics presumptively to prevent more severe infections.[5] Pediatric care providers should be notified at the time of birth if there is a concern the newborn has been exposed to gonorrhea.

### Pelvic Inflammatory Disease

*Pelvic inflammatory disease* (PID) is the term used to refer to a spectrum of disorders that are characterized by inflammation in the cervix, uterus, oviducts, and ovum; these disorders include endometritis, salpingitis, tubo-ovarian abscess, and pelvic peritonitis. PID can result from any of a variety of organisms that ascend from the vagina into the upper urogenital tract, where they induce an inflammatory response.[58] *N. gonorrhoeae* and *C. trachomatis* are common causative organisms of PID. Abnormal vaginal microflora, such as BV, may increase the risk that pathogens will ascend into the uterus and uterine tubes, causing PID. The onset of PID symptoms often occurs after menses, as the transient change in vaginal microflora during menstruation facilitates pathogen ascension into the uterus.[23] A slight increase in the risk of PID is also noted in the first 4 weeks following insertion of an intrauterine device (IUD), as pathogenic bacteria may be deposited in the uterus as the cervical mucus barrier is broken during the IUD's placement.[59] Any sexual activity is a risk factor for developing PID, as is age younger than 24 years, HIV infection, and multiple or new sexual partners.

PID has many adverse short- and long-term sequelae for individuals. The inflammation from even mild cases of PID can cause scarring and permanent damage to tubal cilia, thereby impairing fertility and greatly increasing the risk of ectopic pregnancy throughout the reproductive years. Individuals may also develop chronic pelvic pain from PID-related adhesions.[58] Tubo-ovarian abscesses are immediate, severe risks of untreated PID, which cause severe abdominal pain. This condition warrants referral for specialized care and likely hospitalization.[5] Because PID has severe, long-term outcomes, the threshold for diagnosis and treatment is low.[5]

### Diagnosis of Pelvic Inflammatory Disease

To make the diagnosis of PID, the individual must have pelvic or lower abdominal pain, no other cause for the illness can be apparent, and at least one of the following must be present: (1) cervical motion tenderness, (2) uterine tenderness, or (3) adnexal tenderness. Additional symptoms, such as fever and mucopurulent vaginal or cervical discharge, increase the specificity of the diagnosis. Invasive tests are rarely warranted, as definitive diagnosis is not necessary before treatment is recommended. However, ultrasound and laparoscopy can be useful to rule out other diagnoses, such as ectopic pregnancy or acute appendicitis.[58] Table 18-11 provides the full diagnostic criteria for PID. A physical examination is needed to rule out other causes of abdominal pain, including gastrointestinal problems, ovarian cysts, and appendicitis or other surgical emergencies.

When an individual presents with symptoms of PID, NAAT should be performed for gonorrhea and chlamydia; HIV testing is also recommended. A wide range of additional tests may be performed depending on the individual's clinical situation and the likelihood of other diagnoses. A wet mount that shows many white blood cells is suggestive of PID. Clue cells, a positive whiff test, and altered pH may be present. Blood tests may reveal an elevated white blood cell count and erythrocyte sedimentation rate. A urine or blood test for human chorionic gonadotropin (hCG) might be needed to rule out ectopic pregnancy.

Diagnosis of PID is based on clinical presentation alone. The CDC advises a low threshold for diagnosis, as PID may have minimal symptoms but still cause tubal damage.[5] Laboratory tests for gonorrhea and chlamydia should be performed, but treatment should not be delayed while awaiting their results.

### Treatment of Pelvic Inflammatory Disease

Individuals with PID are treated with antibiotics that provide a broad spectrum of coverage for both aerobic and anaerobic organisms. A client with PID should be presumptively treated for both gonorrhea and chlamydia because a negative endocervical culture for one of these organisms does not rule out their presence in the upper genital tract (Table 18-12). Metronidazole (Flagyl) should be strongly considered to treat possible anaerobic organisms that may cause PID.[5] Oral treatment is acceptable unless the individual has not responded to oral treatment or is acutely ill. If an individual has an IUD in place, they should be treated as usual and the IUD does not need to be removed.[59] That said, if the person does not improve between 48 and 72 hours, the IUD should be removed.[5] Consider other bacteria such as E. coli and group B Streptococcus (GBS) in individuals with IUDs.[60]

The symptoms of PID should improve dramatically within 72 hours after initiation of treatment. If no improvement is evident within this time frame, the individual should be reevaluated, and hospitalized for intravenous antibiotics and supportive therapy. Hospitalization should also be considered if the person is pregnant; if oral treatment is not possible; when the PID appears to be severe, such as in the presence of a high fever or nausea and vomiting; and when emergencies such as appendicitis, tubo-ovarian abscess, or other conditions cannot be excluded.[5,59]

| Table 18-11 | Diagnostic Criteria for Pelvic Inflammatory Disease |
|---|---|
| **Minimum Criteria (pelvic or abdominal pain AND one or more of the following criteria needed for diagnosis)** | |
| Cervical motion tenderness OR | |
| Uterine tenderness OR | |
| Adnexal tenderness | |
| **Additional Criteria (increase the specificity of the diagnosis)** | |
| Fever > 38.3°C (101°F) | |
| Mucopurulent cervical or vaginal discharge | |
| Numerous white blood cells on saline wet prep | |
| Elevated C-reactive protein | |
| Elevated erythrocyte sedimentation rate | |
| Documented infection with C. trachomatis or N. gonorrhoeae | |
| **Definitive Criteria (not needed to begin treatment, but beneficial to rule out other diagnoses)** | |
| Transvaginal ultrasound, magnetic resonance imaging, or Doppler studies showing thickened and fluid-filled tubes | |
| Laparoscopic visualization of pelvic inflammatory disease–related abnormalities | |
| Endometrial biopsy showing histopathologic evidence of endometritis | |

Based on Workowski KA, Bachmann LH, Chan PA, et al. Sexually transmitted infections treatment guidelines, 2021. *MMWR Recomm Rep.* 2021;70(4):1-187. doi:10.15585/mmwr.rr7004a1.

| Table 18-12 | Outpatient Treatments for Pelvic Inflammatory Diseases | | |
|---|---|---|---|
| **Recommended Treatments for Nonpregnant Individuals Generic (Brand)** | **Alternative Treatments for Nonpregnant Individuals Generic (Brand)** | **Recommended Treatments for Pregnant Individuals Generic (Brand)** | **Considerations for Lactating Individuals** |
| Ceftriaxone (Rocephin) 500 mg IM once (1 g in individuals weighing ≥ 150 kg)<br>AND<br>Doxycycline (Vibramycin) 100 mg orally twice a day for 14 days<br>WITH<br>Metronidazole (Flagyl) 500 mg orally for 14 days (for parenteral or inpatient treatment, refer to CDC guidelines) | If person has a severe cephalosporin allergy:<br>Levofloxacin (Levaquin) 500 mg orally daily<br>WITH<br>Metronidazole (Flagyl) 500 mg twice daily for 14 days<br>OR<br>Moxifloxacin (Vigamox) 400 mg orally daily | Pregnant individuals with suspected PID should be hospitalized for evaluation and treatment by an infectious disease specialist | Doxycycline (Vibramycin) is generally considered to be safe with lactation, but longer courses of the drug have the potential to stain infants' teeth. Consider methods to decrease infant ingestion or an alternative regimen.<br><br>Metronidazole (Flagyl) administered orally to the lactating individual is excreted in human milk and has active metabolites in the infant. While no harm has been shown in infants, the potential amount ingested by the infant should be considered. |
| Cefoxitin (Mefoxin) 2 g IM once<br>AND<br>Probenecid (Benemid) 1 g orally administered as a single dose<br>AND<br>Doxycycline (Vibramycin) 100 mg orally twice a day for 14 days<br>WITH<br>Metronidazole (Flagyl) 500 mg orally for 14 days | | | Probenecid (Benemid) may increase the excretion of cimetidine into human milk.<br><br>Ceftriaxone is compatible with lactation.<br><br>Cefoxitin is compatible with lactation.<br><br>There are limited data on the use of levofloxacin during lactation but amounts in human milk appear to be lower than the infant dose and not expected to cause harm.<br><br>There are no data on the use of moxifloxacin during lactation. It is preferable to use alternative medications with available safety information. Use is acceptable with monitoring of infant for gastrointestinal effects such as diarrhea and candidiasis. |

Abbreviations: CDC, Centers for Disease Control and Prevention; IM, intramuscular; IV, intravenous; PID, pelvic inflammatory disease.

aFor inpatient treatments, see the CDC guidelines.

Based on Workowski KA, Bachmann LH, Chan PA, et al. Sexually transmitted infections treatment guidelines, 2021. *MMWR Recomm Rep.* 2021;70(4):1-187. doi:10.15585/mmwr.rr7004a1; U.S. National Library of Medicine. Drugs and Lactation Database (LactMed). https://www.ncbi.nlm.nih.gov/books/NBK501922. Published 2021. Accessed July 26, 2021.

Sexual partners from the 60 days preceding the onset of symptoms of PID should be treated presumptively for gonorrhea and chlamydia.[5] Health education includes recommending abstinence from sexual intercourse until therapy is completed and sexual partners have been treated, use of condoms, and other practices to decrease STI transmission, including HIV pre-exposure prophylaxis (PrEP) if indicated. If tests were positive for gonorrhea or chlamydia, the individual should be retested at 3 months or the next time health care is sought.

### Management of Pelvic Inflammatory Disease During the Perinatal Period

Individuals with a history of PID are at increased risk for ectopic pregnancy, and can benefit from early prenatal care. Although PID is rare during pregnancy, likely due to the protective effects of cervical mucus, pregnant individuals with PID are at high risk for preterm labor and maternal morbidity. Pregnant individuals should be hospitalized for evaluation and treatment.[5]

### Syphilis

Caused by a spiral-shaped spirochete (*Treponema pallidum*), syphilis is known as the "Great Pretender" because it may be asymptomatic or present with a variety of symptoms mimicking other conditions. Transmission occurs through oral, anal, or vaginal sexual contact. The incidence of syphilis has been increasing in recent years, with a 27% increase in reported cases in women who reside in the United States between 2014 and 2015 alone.[47] In 2019, the CDC reported 129,813 new diagnoses of syphilis, of which 38,992 were cases of primary or secondary syphilis.[61] While rates of syphilis are increasing among all sexually active people, nearly half of new cases in 2019 were in individuals with penises engaging in receptive anal sex.[47] Globally, 18 million people are infected with syphilis.[2]

Approximately 50% of individuals exposed to *T. pallidum* will develop infection if not treated. The systemic disease progresses through three primary phases: primary syphilis (chancre and regional lymphadenopathy), secondary syphilis (disseminated skin eruptions and generalized lymphadenopathy), and tertiary syphilis (cardiovascular syphilis, neurologic symptoms and gummas [granulomatous lesions in skin and bone]).[62] A latent form of syphilis can develop between the secondary and tertiary phases. The three phases can overlap somewhat, and neurologic manifestations of syphilis can occur at any time in the disease process. Ocular syphilis and otosyphilis more commonly occur in early stages of syphilis infection and can present without symptoms of additional nervous system involvement.[5] In addition, a newborn may present with congenital syphilis, as the *T. pallidum* organism readily crosses the placenta.

Primary syphilis is characterized by a chancre that appears at the site of inoculation. On average,

chancres appear 21 days after exposure, although their emergence can range from 10 to 90 days after infection transmission. The chancre is a nontender indurated ulcerous lesion. It is usually a single lesion, filled with spirochete-laden purulent discharge, and is highly infectious. The chancre begins as a papule that erodes into a well-demarcated area, with induration of the base and circumference. Because the chancre is usually painless and heals spontaneously without treatment in 3 to 6 weeks, it may not be noticed, especially if it is inside the vagina or rectum. The chancre is an open wound, so it increases the risk of the person developing other infections to which they might be exposed, including HIV and herpes. In addition, secondary infections may occur within the chancre.

Secondary syphilis marks the change from local to systemic infection. The manifestations of secondary syphilis usually appear 4 to 10 weeks after infection, and can reappear following periods of latency. The most characteristic symptom of this stage of syphilis is a rash that appears on the palms of the hands, soles of the feet, and trunk; this rash can be macular, papular, or psoriasiform. Other symptoms include patchy alopecia, condylomata lata, lesions of the mucous membranes, and symptoms of a systemic illness such as low-grade fever, sore throat, hoarseness, malaise, headache, anorexia, and generalized lymphadenopathy. Condylomata lata can also occur; these highly contagious, flat, moist, wart-like lesions usually appear in body folds such as the vulva and perianal area.[5]

After the symptoms of secondary syphilis resolve, some affected individuals convert to early or late latent syphilis before the symptoms of tertiary syphilis appear. Persons with latent syphilis have no clinical manifestations, but their infection can be detected with blood serology tests. Syphilis is not transmitted sexually during latent stages; however, treatment is important to prevent disease progression. Vertical transmission from pregnant person to fetus can occur during the early and late latent syphilis stages. According to the CDC, individuals with latent syphilis who have been infected within the past year are classified as having early latent syphilis.[5] Individuals infected for a year or more are classified by the CDC as having late latent syphilis and will need a longer course of treatment. WHO, however, uses infection within the past 2 years as the definition for early latent infection.[62]

Tertiary syphilis can appear anywhere from 1 to 2 years after infection to 30 or more years later. Today, this form of the disease is rare in the developed world. Associated with high morbidity and mortality, tertiary syphilis takes two forms: gumma and cardiovascular syphilis.[62] Gumma are soft-tissue granuloma tumors, which occur in tissues throughout the body. These masses cause extensive damage within the body and are difficult to distinguish from carcinomas. Cardiovascular syphilis may result in aortic valve disease, aortic aneurysm, and coronary artery disease.[63]

Neurosyphilis can occur during any stage of syphilis. For individuals in the United States, clinical symptoms of central nervous system disease in the presence of positive serologic evidence of syphilis warrant examination of the cerebrospinal fluid.[5] The disease may also present as acute syphilitic meningitis, syphilis of the spinal cord, or vascular neurosyphilis.[62]

From 2012 to 2019, the rate of congenital syphilis in the United States increased 477% to 48.5 cases per 100,000 live births.[5] This recent increase demonstrates the need for increased attention to screening and prevention of syphilis.

### Screening and Diagnosis of Syphilis

Serologic laboratory testing for syphilis is categorized as non-treponemal and treponemal. Diagnosis of syphilis through serologic testing requires both types of testing to avoid false negatives in individuals with primary syphilis and false positives in individuals with previously treated syphilis or without syphilis.

Non-treponemal tests, known as VDRL (Venereal Disease Research Laboratory) and RPR (rapid plasma reagent) tests, have high false-positive rates. Pregnancy, autoimmune disorders, recent vaccination, and acute bacterial or viral infections, for example, can cause a false-positive result on these tests. Non-treponemal antibody titers can be useful for monitoring treatment response and identifying disease activity. Serial titers should be performed using the same test, as the results of the VDRL and RPR tests are not equivalent. A four-fold decrease in titers is considered to be an adequate response to syphilis treatment. Non-treponemal titers may eventually become nonreactive.

Treponemal tests such as fluorescent treponemal antibody absorption test (FTA-ABS), passive particle agglutination (TP-PA) assay, enzyme immunoassays (EIAs), and chemiluminescent immunoassays (CLIAs) detect antibodies specific for *T. pallidum*.[5] Most individuals will continue to have reactive treponemal tests throughout their lives after receiving treatment for syphilis.

Screening for syphilis may begin with either type of serologic testing. The traditional approach is to perform a non-treponemal test; if the test is positive, treponemal testing is then conducted on the same sample. An alternative approach to syphilis screening is to initiate treponemal testing first, a practice referred to as reverse sequence testing. A quantitative non-treponemal test should be ordered after an initial positive treponemal test result. If the non-treponemal test is negative, then a second type of treponemal test using a different antigen is recommended to help differentiate between late latent syphilis, syphilis of unknown duration, and reinfection.[5] Further guidance on testing algorithms and interpretation of results is provided by local health departments as well as the CDC. Syphilis is a reportable disease in all states.

Positive results on dark-field microscopy of exudate from the chancre lesion provide a definitive diagnosis and are considered the gold standard for testing; however, dark-field microscopy is not available in all settings.[5] If serologic tests are discordant with the patient's clinical symptoms, treatment with biopsy including histology, PCR, and immunostaining is recommended. Symptoms of neurosyphilis, ocular syphilis or otosyphilis warrant referral to a specialist, as evaluation of cerebrospinal fluid may be necessary for definitive diagnosis and more intensive treatment.

### Treatment of Syphilis

Parenteral penicillin G is the best treatment for syphilis. Other forms of penicillin are not as effective because they do not adequately penetrate into sequestered sites such as the central nervous system. Clinicians should take care to order the correct penicillin preparation, as multiple preparations of benzathine penicillin with similar names are available. Table 18-13 identifies the recommended doses and routes of treatment based on stage of infection. While alternative treatments are provided for non-pregnant individuals, their efficacy has not been studied in depth. If a person has a penicillin allergy, consider skin testing for verification, especially for late latent syphilis or syphilis of unknown duration.[5] Referral to a specialist for treatment of tertiary, neurosyphilis, ocular syphilis, and otosyphilis is appropriate.

Within 24 hours of treatment, some individuals may experience a Jarisch-Herxheimer reaction with symptoms such as fever, headache, and myalgia. This reaction is a response to lipoproteins from the spirochete, which induce a systemic inflammatory response.[64] Individuals with early syphilis are more likely to experience this reaction than those

| Table 18-13 | Outpatient Treatments for Syphilis in Adolescents and Adults | | | |
|---|---|---|---|---|
| Stage of Syphilis | Recommended Treatments for Nonpregnant Individuals Generic (Brand) | Alternative Treatments for Persons with Penicillin Allergy | Recommended Treatments for Pregnant Individuals Generic (Brand) | Considerations for Lactating Individuals |
| Primary, secondary, and early latent syphilis | Benzathine penicillin G (Bicillin LA) 2.4 million units IM in a single dose<br><br>If the person is allergic to penicillin, refer for penicillin skin testing or challenge unless history of Stevens-Johnson syndrome or hemolytic anemia | Refer for penicillin skin testing or challenge unless history of Stevens-Johnson syndrome or hemolytic anemia<br><br>Doxycycline and tetracycline are alternatives | Benzathine penicillin G (Bicillin LA) 2.4 million units IM in a single dose<br><br>If the person is allergic to penicillin, desensitize per CDC guidelines | Benzathine penicillin is safe during lactation.<br><br>Doxycycline and tetracycline have the theoretical risk of staining forming teeth; however, courses of treatment less than 21 days are acceptable. Avoid repeat courses of treatment.[27] |
| Late latent syphilis, syphilis of unknown duration | Benzathine penicillin G (Bicillin LA) 7.2 million units IM total administered as 2.4 million units IM once a week for 3 weeks | Refer for penicillin skin testing or challenge unless history of Stevens-Johnson syndrome or hemolytic anemia<br><br>Doxycycline, tetracycline, and ceftriaxone are alternatives | Benzathine penicillin G (Bicillin LA) 7.2 million units IM once a week for 3 doses | |

Based on Workowski KA, Bachmann LH, Chan PA, et al. Sexually transmitted infections treatment guidelines, 2021. *MMWR Recomm Rep.* 2021;70(4):1-187. doi:10.15585/mmwr.rr7004a1; U.S. National Library of Medicine. Drugs and Lactation Database (LactMed). https://www.ncbi.nlm.nih.gov/books/NBK501922.

in other stages of infection. Antipyretic agents may alleviate symptoms of the reaction, and individuals can be reassured that the symptoms are not an allergic reaction to penicillin. A Jarisch-Herxheimer reaction in pregnant individuals may cause preterm labor or fetal distress. Nevertheless, prompt treatment is still recommended, and additional monitoring may be considered in pregnant individuals with a viable fetus.[65]

Clinical assessment and a non-treponemal test (VDRL or RPR) should be performed 6 months and 1 year following treatment to test for treatment effectiveness. A third reassessment at 2 years for individuals diagnosed with latent syphilis is also recommended.[5] With adequate treatment, titers usually decline four-fold (e.g., from 1:128 to 1:32); however, in 15% of treated individuals, the titer does not decline. An increase in titers by four-fold following treatment is indicative of treatment failure or reinfection.

All individuals who have a positive test for syphilis should be offered HIV screening. Also, all of the person's sexual partners from within the past 90 days should be treated presumptively for syphilis. Presumptive treatment may also be offered to sexual partners of individuals when contact occurred more than 90 days before diagnosis if serologic test results are not readily available or follow-up is uncertain. Recommendations for partner testing and presumptive treatment may vary based on geographic location; local or state-level health departments may be able to assist in this process as well as with notification of individuals.

### Management of Syphilis During the Perinatal Period

Syphilis readily crosses the placenta after 9 weeks' gestation. Transmission of the pathogen to the fetus usually occurs between the 16th and 28th weeks of pregnancy.[43] Treatment of syphilis in pregnant individuals prior to 20 weeks' gestation is uniformly successful and therefore critical in reducing the incidence of congenital syphilis.[65] As many as 40% of pregnant individuals with untreated syphilis will miscarry. As many as 80% of infants born to individuals with primary syphilis will have congenital syphilis, including congenital malformation, but the risk of vertical transmission decreases with the length of time the individual has been infected.[65] Syphilis is also associated with preterm birth, low birth weight, and congenital malformations. Thus, screening for syphilis is recommended for all pregnant individuals at their first prenatal visit; rescreening is recommended again at 28 weeks' gestation and at labor onset for individuals with higher risk of syphilis, such as those having multiple sex partners, transactional sex, incarceration, and housing instability or homelessness. Prenatal screening may also include an assessment of the partner's risk of infection. Serologic screening for syphilis may involve either non-treponemal testing first or the reverse testing sequence. Individuals without documented syphilis testing during pregnancy should be screened for syphilis during the intrapartum period and delayed hospital discharge of the newborn may considered.[5] Screening for syphilis is also appropriate for all pregnant individuals following intrauterine fetal death.

Penicillin G is the only acceptable treatment for syphilis during pregnancy. A repeated dose of penicillin administered 1 week after the first dose may reduce the risk of congenital syphilis for individuals with primary, secondary, or early latent syphilis. If an individual is allergic to penicillin, they should be desensitized prior to treatment.[5] Desensitization is a procedure that works to alter a person's immune reaction so that the body does not react to the antigenic agent. It is accomplished by administering sub-threshold doses of the medication that cause immunoglobulin E (IgE) to bind to basophils and mast cells, thereby making them unresponsive to higher doses of the drug.[66] An oral protocol for penicillin desensitization is recommended by the CDC.[5] Note that this procedure should be performed only in a setting where resuscitative equipment is readily available.

Follow-up after treatment consists of repeated serologic titers. A baseline titer at the time of treatment allows for monitoring of the treatment response over time, with the caveat that this result may differ from the titer at the time of diagnosis.[65] Pregnant individuals often will not demonstrate the four-fold decrease in titers that is seen in nonpregnant individuals, but this response does not indicate treatment failure. Those persons diagnosed and treated prior to 24 weeks' gestation are recommended to have repeat titers at 8 weeks post treatment and again at birth. Persons diagnosed and treated after 24 weeks' gestation are recommended to have titers at birth.

Management of syphilis in pregnancy includes fetal sonographic evaluation for congenital syphilis, particularly when the infection is diagnosed after 20 weeks' gestation. The risk of treatment failure may be higher when signs of fetal or placental involvement are sonographically detected; these signs include hepatomegaly, ascites, hydrops, and placental thickening. Although consultation with a specialist is appropriate for all pregnant individuals diagnosed with syphilis, treatment should not be delayed until that consult is obtained.

If the pregnant individual is treated for syphilis less than 4 weeks before giving birth, the newborn will need additional testing and treatment as outlined by the CDC.[5]

In 2019, 1,870 cases of congenital syphilis were reported in the United States.[5] Congenital malformations are common in infants born to birthing people with untreated syphilis during pregnancy, and include deafness, hepatomegaly, and bone abnormalities. Even when treatment for syphilis is provided during pregnancy, it may come too late in gestation to prevent such congenital abnormalities.[65] Notify the infant's care provider of syphilis exposure to facilitate appropriate neonatal care.

Treponemal serologic testing in infants is complicated by passive transfer of antibodies across the placenta, so non-treponemal testing is recommended in newborns. Umbilical cord blood testing is not acceptable due to false-positive results from contamination from the birthing person's blood at birth and false-negative results from Wharton's jelly. Infants born to individuals with positive serologic tests need in-depth evaluation, including testing of the placenta and dark-field microscopy testing of suspicious body lesions.[5] Abnormal results warrant treatment and more invasive testing per CDC guidelines.[5] Penicillin is the only acceptable treatment for congenital syphilis, as alternative treatments have not been shown effective.

## Genital Lesions with Bacterial Etiology

Clinicians are most likely to encounter genital lesions resulting from infection with herpes simplex virus, syphilis, or HPV. However, bacterial pathogens can also be transmitted via sexual contact, resulting in symptomatic infection. Differentiation of genital lesions based on the presence or absence

| Table 18-14 | Differentiation of Genital Lesions by Symptoms | |
| --- | --- |
| **Typically Painless** | **Typically Painful** |
| Genital warts/condyloma acuminata | Herpetic vesicles and open lesions |
| Syphilis chancre | Chancroid |
| Condylomata lata | Lymphogranuloma venereum |
| | Lymphadenopathy and lesions |

of pain is presented in **Table 18-14**. In the United States, declining rates of these bacterial infections have coincided with the increased use of antibiotics.[67] Nevertheless, given the prevalence of global travel and commercial sex work, isolated outbreaks in high-resource countries have occurred and remain possible.

### Chancroid

In 2019, 8 cases of chancroid were reported in the United States.[67] Chancroid is characterized by non-indurated painful lesions caused by a gram-negative anaerobic bacillus, *Haemophilus ducreyi*. The infection is transmitted through sexual contact with mucous membranes. Lymph node abscess can lead to rupture, spreading infection and leading to permanent scarring. Culture of the causative organism is difficult due to limited availability of commercial tests and low sensitivity; therefore, diagnosis is often based on clinical findings.[5] Symptomatic improvement should occur within 3 days of antibiotic treatment and single-dose treatment is generally preferred. Guidelines for acceptable antibiotic choices are available from the CDC. All individuals diagnosed with chancroid should be offered HIV screening.

### Lymphogranuloma Venereum

Lymphogranuloma venereum (LGV) is a rare disease caused by *C. trachomatis* that is transmitted via genital or rectal mucosal contact. LGV is primarily an infection of the lymphatic system and lymph nodes. Although this infection is caused by *C. trachomatis*, serovars (subtypes) of the bacterium involved in LGV are different than those that cause chlamydial infection of the vagina or upper reproductive tract. LGV is not reportable in all states, and limited information about its incidence is available from the CDC.[68]

The physical examination of an individual with LGV will be remarkable for unilateral, painful, inguinal lymphadenopathy. Lymph nodes may be fluctuant and rupture on compression. Rectal infection has been more common in recent years, and presenting symptoms can include constipation, anal pain, tenesmus, and bloody and mucoid anal discharge.[5] Treatment with antibiotics may be initiated based on clinical presentation alone. Very large and fluctuant lymph nodes may require needle aspiration and drainage to prevent ulcerations. All sexual partners within the 60 days prior to onset should be evaluated, tested, and receive prophylactic antibiotic treatment and HIV prophylaxis if seronegative.[5]

### Granuloma Inguinale

Granuloma inguinale is rare in the United States, but is more common in low-resource tropical areas around the world. This infection is predominately transmitted through sexual contact, although non-sexual transmission may be possible. Caused by a gram-negative bacterium (*Klebsiella granulomatis*), granuloma inguinale infection begins with painless, beefy-red lesions that bleed on contact. These genital lesions are progressive, and lymphadenopathy and subcutaneous granulomas can occur.

Antibiotic treatment can be initiated based on clinical presentation and should be accompanied by HIV screening. Treatment also includes basic wound management to treat or prevent secondary infections. Sexual partners within the previous 60 days should be evaluated and offered treatment, but the value of treatment for asymptomatic individuals has not been established.[5]

### Human Papillomavirus

HPV is estimated to be the most common STI; as many as half of all sexually active adults will be infected with one or more subtypes of HPV in their lifetime.[47] More than 100 subtypes of HPV have been identified to date, of which more than 40 subtypes infect the genital and potentially oropharyngeal areas. Papillomaviruses infect the surface epithelia and mucous membranes, where they cause variable cellular changes depending on the virus subtype.

Most HPV infections are asymptomatic, and 90% are eliminated by the immune system within 2 years following infection. However, certain subtypes are associated with persistent infection, leading to symptoms such as genital warts or cancers of the genitals, cervix, rectum, and oropharynx. Symptoms can appear years after the initial infection. HPV subtypes 6 and 11 cause 90% of genital warts, although subtypes 18, 31, and 33 are also found in warts. HPV subtypes 16 and 18 cause 60% to 80%

of anogenital cancers, but subtype 31 is associated with anogenital cancers as well. Subtype 16 has been strongly associated with oropharyngeal cancer.[69] Warts caused by HPV subtypes 6 and 11 can also be found on mucous membranes of the mouth, nose, and eyes. This section focuses on HPV infection manifesting as growths or warts on the vulva, perineum, or anus, or within the vagina.

The path from HPV acquisition to oncogenic cell changes is complex and may be related to the individual's overall health status. Smoking increases the risk of cellular persistence of HPV and later both genital and oropharyngeal cancers.[70,71] Prolonged alcohol use is another risk factor for oropharyngeal cancer following HPV infection.[72] People with diabetes are more likely to develop genital warts than people without a diagnosis of diabetes.[73]

Genital warts are common in the United States, accounting for hundreds of millions of dollars in healthcare expenditures annually. Among adults ages 18 to 59, 4.4% report a diagnosis of genital warts by a healthcare provider, with one-third of those diagnoses occurring before age 26.[74] Prevalence of anogenital warts in the United States has decreased since the introduction of HPV vaccination.[5] Although the U.S. Advisory Committee on Immunization Practices first recommended routine vaccination against HPV in 2007, uptake of HPV vaccines has fallen short of the targets, with only approximately 50% of adolescents completing the series.[75] Since 2016, the HPV vaccine formulation has included coverage of nine HPV serotypes.[75]

The virus that causes genital warts is transmitted through skin and mucous membrane contact with the genitals, vulva, perineum, rectum, and—for some subtypes—oropharynx. Condoms do not thoroughly protect from genital HPV; female condoms offer some additional protection for the vulva when compared with male condoms, but do not completely eliminate the risk of infection.

### Screening and Diagnosis of Human Papillomavirus Infection and Genital Warts

Screening for cervical HPV infection and cancer is part of routine health promotion, as reviewed in the *Health Promotion Across the Lifespan* chapter. Although HPV is an STI, it is impossible to determine the time of its acquisition. The onset of genital warts is not a reliable indicator of either recent infection or reinfection, as it may be months or years after sexual contact before a lesion appears. Individuals with subclinical infection may still be able to transmit the virus to sexual partners. Treatment of genital

warts is targeted toward the physical symptoms of infection, rather than focusing on the virus itself.

Diagnosis of HPV-related genital warts occurs via physical examination, which will reveal fleshy papules or pedunculated warty lesions on the vulva, introitus, perineum, anus, cervix, and vaginal walls. Biopsy of lesions, including those atypical in appearance, is diagnostic for HPV. Large warts, known as condylomata acuminata, may have a cauliflower-like appearance and may bleed when abraded. These lesions may appear similar to the condylomata lata associated with syphilis, but condylomata lata are usually flat. Warts caused by HPV turn white when exposed to acetic acid, although this test is not recommended due to its lack of relevance for clinical management.[5] Serologic testing for syphilis can be useful to differentiate condylomata acuminata from condylomata lata if needed.

### Treatment of Genital Warts

Many genital warts resolve spontaneously within 1 year and may not need treatment. Available treatments recommended by the CDC are presented in Table 18-15. All treatments for warts have localized side effects, including irritation, pain, and burning. While treatment may diminish the size and number of genital warts, it may not affect transmission rates. The CDC advises individuals to abstain from intercourse with new partners until the warts have resolved, but notes that the person may remain contagious even after treatment. Sexual partners should be treated only if they are symptomatic and desire treatment. Treatment can be self-applied, clinician-applied, or a combination of both, although the efficacy and risks of complications with combination treatment are unknown. Decisions about treatment should be made in partnership with the person.

Podophyllin resin, as opposed to solution or gel, is no longer recommended by the CDC for treatment of genital warts. While other alternative treatments have been proposed, a lack of data on their safety or efficacy limits their use.

The number, size, location of warts, cost, availability of treatments, and experience of the healthcare provider are important considerations in shared decision making related to management of genital warts.[5] Treatment plans recommended by the CDC based on the location of the genital warts are presented in Table 18-16. Treatment of genital warts with laser, electrocautery, or ultrasonic devices may cause aerosolization of viral particles and put healthcare providers at risk for

| Table 18-15 | Treatments for Genital Warts Caused by Human Papillomavirus |
|---|---|
| **Treatments**<br>**Generic (Brand)** | **Clinical Considerations** |
| Podofilox 0.5% solution or gel (Condylox, Podofilox) | Applied by the person twice a day for 3 days, then no treatment for 4 days<br>Useful when warts are smaller than 10 cm × 10 cm<br>Maximum dose of 0.5 mL of the solution per day<br>Demonstrate application in the office for instruction<br>Contraindicated during pregnancy |
| Imiquimod 3.75% or 5% cream (Aldara) | May worsen autoimmune or inflammatory disorders<br>Low risk for use during pregnancy but data are limited; not recommended for use during pregnancy<br>Applied by the person at bedtime—for 3.75% strength, apply every night for up to 16 weeks; for 5% strength, use 3 times a week for up to 16 weeks<br>Wash off the cream with soap and water after 6–10 hours<br>May cause a local inflammatory response<br>The cream may weaken latex condoms and diaphragms |
| Sinecatechins 15% ointment (Veregen) | Contraindicated for individuals who have herpes or HIV, or who are immunocompromised<br>No safety data for use during pregnancy; not recommended during pregnancy<br>Applied by the person in a thin film over the affected area using a finger, 3 times a day for up to 16 weeks<br>Do not wash the film off the affected area<br>Avoid touching the skin with applied ointment to other genital, anal, or oral tissues |
| TCA or BCA 80–90%[a] | Applied by the provider<br>Protect areas surrounding the wart with petroleum jelly<br>Apply acid sparingly and allow to dry, forming a white frosting<br>Excessive acid can be neutralized with sodium bicarbonate or liquid soap<br>Treatment can be repeated once a week<br>Can be used during pregnancy |
| Cryotherapy with liquid nitrogen | Consider local anesthetic if the area treated is large<br>Can cause scarring<br>Requires specialized training and equipment<br>Performed by the provider<br>Can be repeated every 1–2 weeks |
| Surgical excision | May be done with scissors excision, shave excision, curettage, laser, or electrosurgery<br>Requires specialized training and equipment<br>Suturing is rarely indicated for hemostasis<br>Laser removal can be used for large warts or those unresponsive to previous treatment<br>May cause hyperpigmentation or hypopigmentation in affected area |

Abbreviations: BCA, bichloroacetic acid; HIV, human immunodeficiency virus; TCA, trichloroacetic acid.

Based on Workowski KA, Bachmann LH, Chan PA, et al. Sexually transmitted infections treatment guidelines, 2021. *MMWR Recomm Rep.* 2021;70(4):1-187. doi:10.15585/mmwr.rr7004a1.

HPV-related oropharyngeal disease. Providers performing such procedures may consider obtaining HPV vaccination due to this potential occupational exposure.[76]

The need for follow-up visits is influenced by the size of lesions and the response to treatment. Typically, improvement occurs within 3 months of treatment. Warts may return following treatment,

| Table 18-16 | Pharmacologic Treatments for Genital Warts Caused by Human Papillomavirus Based on Location of Lesions | |
|---|---|---|
| **Location of Genital Warts** | **Recommended Treatment** | **Clinical Considerations** |
| Penis, groin, scrotum, perineum, vulva, external anus, perianus | Imiquimod Podofilox Sinecatechins Cryotherapy Surgical removal TCA | |
| Urinary meatus | Cryotherapy Surgical excision | |
| Vagina | Cryotherapy Surgical excision TCA | Avoid use of the cryoprobe in the vagina due to the risk of vaginal perforation and formulation of vaginal fistulas |
| Cervix | Cryotherapy Surgical excision TCA | Consult a specialist; may need biopsy prior to removal to rule out high-grade squamous intraepithelial lesion (HGSIL) |
| Intra-anus | Cryotherapy Surgical excision TCA | Consult colorectal specialist |

Abbreviation: TCA, trichloroacetic acid.

Based on Workowski KA, Bolan GA. Sexually transmitted diseases treatment guidelines, 2015. MMWR Recomm Rep. 2015;64(3):1-137. Available at: https://www.cdc.gov/std/tg2015/tg-2015-print.pdf. Accessed March 31, 20177; U.S. National Library of Medicine. Drugs and lactation database (LactMed). 2016. Available at: https://toxnet.nlm.nih.gov/newtoxnet/lactmed.htm. Accessed June 6, 2017.

however, and can be retreated with the same agent used for treating the initial infection. Regular cervical cytology screening according to current guidelines is important to evaluate for cervical cancer in individuals with cervices, but a diagnosis of genital warts does not change regular screening frequency. People with genital warts should be offered screening tests for common STIs.

## Management of Genital Warts During the Perinatal Period

Warts may initially appear or increase in size during pregnancy. Treatment with trichloroacetic acid (TCA) or bichloroacetic acid (BCA) is safe during pregnancy, but other medications used to treat HPV, such as podophyllin, are not recommended for use in pregnancy. It may be difficult to fully eliminate warts during pregnancy, and they may regress spontaneously postpartum. Surgical treatment is indicated if the warts might complicate vaginal birth.

Genital warts are highly vascularized and may bleed excessively if torn or cut during birth. Care should be taken to avoid warts during suturing of perineal lacerations following vaginal birth. Cesarean birth is indicated only if extensive warts obstruct the vaginal opening or are expected to bleed uncontrollably during birth.[5]

Infants born to individuals with genital warts caused by HPV subtypes 6 and 11 may develop respiratory papillomatosis—that is, warts within their airway—during the neonatal period or beyond. The mode of transmission to the fetus or neonate is not clear, and cesarean birth may not decrease the incidence of papillomatosis.[5] Some research suggests that prenatal vaccination may reduce intrapartum fetal transmission due to antibody transfer to the fetus.[77] The infant's healthcare provider should be alerted about the potential for respiratory papillomatosis.[5]

## Special Considerations

Individuals with immunosuppression are more likely to develop anogenital warts. In addition, immunosuppression is associated with recurrence of warts after treatment, larger and greater number of anogenital warts, and incomplete or failed response to treatment of warts.[5] Treatment of anogenital warts in this population does not differ from that in individuals without immunosuppression. Squamous cell carcinomas may occur more frequently in individuals with immunosuppression and may mimic anogenital warts in appearance. Clinicians may consider biopsy of atypical warts.

The tissues utilized in surgical creation of a neovagina are susceptible to HPV infection. Individuals may present with dyspareunia, postcoital bleeding, or lesions.[78] Currently, guidelines for diagnosis and treatment of anogenital warts in individuals with a neovagina are not available, so clinicians may approach care for these individuals in the same way as with other populations. Case reports indicate successful treatment with imiquimod, laser ablation, and podophyllin.[78,79]

## Herpes Simplex Virus

A variety of herpesviruses affects humans. Sexually transmitted herpes infection is caused by one of two subtypes of herpes simplex virus: HSV-1 or HSV-2. These two viruses are not completely cleared from the body after the initial infection and can cause recurrent symptoms throughout life. Recurrent genital herpes is most commonly caused by HSV-2. The prevalence in the United States of both HSV-1 and HSV-2 declined between 2000 and 2016 to 47.8% and 11.9%, respectively, in individuals ages 14 to 49.[80] Prevalence of HSV-2 is highest in non-Hispanic Black individuals, whereas prevalence of HSV-1 is highest in Mexican American individuals.[80] Persons with vaginas are more vulnerable to HSV infection and have higher baseline rates of infection compared to persons with penises, in part due to prolonged contact with semen during vaginal intercourse.

HSV-1 and HSV-2 can cause painful ulcerations of the anogenital region and the mucous membranes of the mouth and nose. HSV-1 is commonly acquired in childhood through oral contact but can also be sexually transmitted, especially through orogenital sex. In some populations, this virus is the major cause of genital herpes.[7] HSV-1 usually has a milder clinical presentation than HSV-2, both during the first infection and in subsequent outbreaks. In addition, HSV-1 is associated with lower rates of asymptomatic viral shedding.[5] HSV-2 is more often sexually transmitted and is associated with more severe symptoms and more frequent recurrences compared to HSV-1 infection.[5] Genital herpes infection increases the risk of acquiring HIV by four-fold, in part due to its tendency to cause skin breaks and open lesions.

Herpes is a lifelong infection that retains its potential for transmission throughout the lifespan. Individuals can have HSV for many years before becoming symptomatic. Although an outbreak of HSV in an individual is caused by a virus that is sexually transmitted, the timing between infection and appearance of symptoms is highly variable. Furthermore, most infections involving HVS-1 and HSV-2 are asymptomatic. Because HSV can be shed from asymptomatic lesions, the disorder may be transmitted to a sexual partner unknowingly. These characteristics of the viral infection can greatly complicate health education and partner counseling.

Outbreaks of HSV are commonly categorized as primary versus recurrent. The first episode of HSV (primary outbreak) is usually more severe than subsequent outbreaks. Prodromal symptoms may occur before the appearance of painful lesions, including tingling and burning. Constitutional symptoms can include fever, malaise, headache, and myalgia. The primary sign or symptom of the outbreak is painful lesions at the affected site. Primary outbreaks may include lesions that present in a wide swath or in multiple body locations; in contrast, recurrent outbreaks are usually more localized. Dysuria may also occur when urine comes in contact with an open lesion(s). All primary outbreaks should be treated to prevent prolonged or severe illness.[7] The focus of HSV management should be the chronic nature of the virus rather than episodic acute symptoms.

### Diagnosis of Herpes Simplex Virus

An individual having an HSV outbreak usually presents with small, very painful vesicles or open lesions on the mouth, vulva, perineum, or anus. The lesions typically appear in small groups and are disproportionately painful in comparison to their size and depth. They may be fluid-filled vesicles—that is, small skin splits that are covered, oozing, crusted, or nearly healed. Edema, diffuse inflammation, and vaginal or urethral discharge may be present as well. A speculum examination may be excessively painful and is not required for diagnosis. Tender inguinal lymphadenopathy may also be present.

Diagnosis of herpes is based on physical examination and confirmed with viral testing, serologic testing, or both, depending on the presence or absence of lesions. When genital lesions are present, HSV NAAT collected from the ulcerated site is preferred due to the high specificity of this test.[5] Viral culture is also acceptable for testing lesions but is limited by low sensitivity, especially if the area is crusted over or healing.[5] Note that a negative NAAT or viral culture does not rule out the possibility of HSV infection, as viral shedding occurs intermittently. Type-specific testing is recommended when the virus is isolated by either NAAT or culture. Viral testing of asymptomatic individuals is not recommended, and negative testing does not rule out the possibility of HSV infection.

When genital lesions are not present or if viral testing is negative, type-specific immunoglobulin G (IgG)–based assay blood testing can be used to diagnose herpes. Given that false negatives are possible when serologic testing is performed at early stages of HSV infection, repeat testing 3 months after suspected exposure may be recommended. Confirmatory testing should be performed on positive tests due to the low sensitivity and specificity of available tests. Immunoglobulin M (IgM) testing does not differentiate the findings by HSV type, so it is not recommended.

As infection with HSV-2 is nearly always sexually transmitted, a positive serologic test implies anogenital infection. Serologic testing for HSV-1 is more difficult to interpret, as it does not differentiate between oral or anogenital lesions. Individuals may have positive HSV-1 serologic testing from asymptomatic oral infection. Serologic screening for HSV-2 in individuals without a history of anogenital herpes symptoms is not recommended.[5] The person who has an initial herpes diagnosis should be offered testing for HIV as well as other common STIs.

### Treatment of Herpes Simplex Virus

While the clinical presentation of the two HSV subtypes is indistinguishable, the CDC recommends typing via blood testing to guide health education and treatment decisions, as HSV-2 has more virulent recurrences and a higher rate of transmission.[5] Serologic and viral test results are not needed to begin treatment for HSV with antiviral therapy.

Treatments for initial outbreaks, episodic outbreak, and suppressive therapy are presented in Table 18-17.[5,81] All initial outbreaks should be treated.[5] For episodic outbreaks, medication should be started when the first prodromal symptoms are noted for best effectiveness, but treatment can still offer benefits even if delayed until the outbreak of lesions.[5] Individuals may prefer suppressive treatment

to episodic treatment. Suppressive treatment can reduce the frequency of recurrences by 70% to 80% and reduces the risk of asymptomatic shedding and sexual partner transmission.[5] Viral shedding of HSV-1 decreases in the first year after infection and this type tends to have fewer recurrences, so the choice of whether to pursue suppressive therapy for genital HSV-1 should be made through shared decision making between the individual and the provider. A person's need for suppressive therapy may change over time and should be reevaluated annually.[5] Laboratory monitoring is not necessary for continuation of suppressive treatment.

Cost and frequency of dosing are considerations when choosing a treatment for the person with HSV-1 or HSV-2 infection. Famciclovir (Famvir) and valacyclovir (Valtrex) have greater oral bioavailability than acyclovir (Zovirax) but are more expensive. Topical treatments are not very effective for management of initial or subsequent outbreaks. Support includes non-opioid pain management. The individual can use a peri-bottle or urinate while sitting in water in a bowl or the bathtub to decrease symptoms of dysuria during outbreaks where lesions may be contact with urine.

There is limited definitive research on complementary suppressive therapies, although L-lysine has been found not to be effective for this indication.[82] While a variety of herbs, essential oils, dietary

| Table 18-17 | Pharmacologic Treatments for Herpes Simplex Virus in Adolescents and Adults | | |
|---|---|---|---|
| **Diagnosis** | **Recommended Treatments for Nonpregnant Individuals Generic (Brand)** | **Recommended Treatments During Pregnancy Generic (Brand)** | **Considerations for Lactating Individuals** |
| Initial outbreak of HSV in an adult | Acyclovir (Zovirax) 400 mg by mouth 3 times a day for 7–10 days OR Acyclovir (Zovirax) 200 mg by mouth 5 times a day for 7–10 days OR Famciclovir (Famvir) 250 mg by mouth 3 times a day for 7–10 days OR Valacyclovir (Valtrex) 1 g by mouth 2 times a day for 7–10 days | Acyclovir has more data supporting its benefits without risks to the fetus and is preferred by the CDC. ACOG supports the use of acyclovir or valacyclovir. Severe infections should be treated with intravenous acyclovir. Acyclovir (Zovirax) 400 mg by mouth 3 times a day for 7–10 days OR Acyclovir (Zovirax) 200 mg orally 5 times a day for 7–10 days OR Valacyclovir (Valtrex) 1 g by mouth 2 times a day for 7–10 days | Acyclovir (Zovirax) is considered safe in lactation, with the amount of drug that passes to the infant being much less than the newborn therapeutic doses. Lower dosages may decrease maternal serum levels, resulting in lower human milk concentrations. Valacyclovir (Valtrex) is acceptable for use during lactation, as it is converted to acyclovir prior to excretion in very low amounts into human milk. Famciclovir (Famvir) is not recommended during lactation due to a lack of data. |

| Diagnosis | Recommended Treatments for Nonpregnant Individuals Generic (Brand) | Recommended Treatments During Pregnancy Generic (Brand) | Considerations for Lactating Individuals |
|---|---|---|---|
| Recurrent episodic outbreak treatment | Acyclovir (Zovirax) 800 mg by mouth 2 times a day for 5 days OR Acyclovir (Zovirax) 800 mg by mouth 3 times a day for 2 days OR Famciclovir (Famvir) 125 mg by mouth 2 times a day for 5 days OR Famciclovir (Famvir) 1 g by mouth 2 times a day for 1 day OR Famciclovir (Famvir) 500 mg by mouth once, then 250 mg 2 times a day for 2 days OR Valacyclovir (Valtrex) 500 mg by mouth 2 times a day for 3 days OR Valacyclovir (Valtrex) 1 g by mouth once a day for 5 days | The CDC states that acyclovir has a better safety profile during pregnancy. ACOG supports the use of valacyclovir if needed. Acyclovir (Zovirax) 400 mg by mouth 3 times a day for 5 days OR Acyclovir (Zovirax) 800 mg 2 times a day for 5 days OR 3 times a day for 2 days OR Valacyclovir (Valtrex) 500 mg by mouth 2 times a day for 3 days OR Valacyclovir (Valtrex) 1 g by mouth daily for 5 days | |
| Suppression of HSV outbreaks | Acyclovir (Zovirax) 400 mg orally 2 times a day OR Famciclovir (Famvir) 250 mg orally 2 times a day OR Valacyclovir (Valtrex) 1 g orally once a day OR Valacyclovir (Valtrex) 500 mg orally once a day (may be less effective in persons with > 10 outbreaks yearly) | Acyclovir (Zovirax) 400 mg by mouth 3 times a day beginning at 36 weeks OR Valacyclovir (Valtrex) 500 mg orally 2 times a day beginning at 36 weeks | |

Abbreviations: ACOG, American College of Obstetricians and Gynecologists; CDC, Centers for Disease Control and Prevention; HSV, herpes simplex virus.

Based on Workowski KA, Bachmann LH, Chan PA, et al. Sexually transmitted infections treatment guidelines, 2021. *MMWR Recomm Rep*. 2021;70(4):1-187. doi:10.15585/mmwr.rr7004a1; U.S. National Library of Medicine. Drugs and Lactation Database (LactMed). https://www.ncbi.nlm.nih.gov/books/NBK501922. Published 2021. Accessed July 26, 2021.

supplements, and topical ointments containing bee products or aloe vera are used by individuals desiring alternative treatments for herpes lesions, there is a lack of clinical data to support their use.[83] The individual can decide if the costs and side effects of such treatments are worth the personal benefit. If the person's condition does not improve with treatment, they may have a strain of herpes resistant to standard antiviral treatments, and viral isolate testing is needed prior to specialist consultation for further treatment.[5]

Partner treatment is not needed when a person has HSV infection. Ideally, the affected individual will have an open conversation with their sexual partners about the risk of asymptomatic transmission and the need for safer sexual practices. Sexual contact with uninfected partners should be avoided while the affected individual is having prodromal or outbreak symptoms, as condoms do not provide full protection from transmission. A follow-up visit is best for health education about prevention when compared to the visit for the initial outbreak. When the individual is feeling better, they will be more prepared to understand the information.

### Management of Herpes During the Perinatal Period

All individuals should be asked if they have a history of herpes or genital lesions as part of their initial visit for pregnancy.[5] Recurrent infections during pregnancy pose little to no risk during the prenatal period, and the individual produces immunoglobulins that cross the placenta to protect the fetus from HSV. In contrast, primary outbreaks during pregnancy have been associated with a small increase in fetal abnormalities and a larger risk for intrapartum transmission.[84] Those individuals with a new diagnosis of herpes during the second half of pregnancy should be referred for maternal–fetal medicine consultation due to risk of fetal transmission.[5]

Individuals can be treated for herpes infections during pregnancy, as described in **Table 18-17**. Severe outbreaks with dissemination during pregnancy warrant hospitalization and treatment with intravenous acyclovir.[5] Prophylactic administration of acyclovir beginning at 36 gestational weeks has been shown to lower the incidence of asymptomatic shedding and outbreaks at term, the rate of cesarean birth for birthing persons with HSV lesions, and the neonatal incidence of HSV.[81] Routine administration of antiviral drugs beginning at 36 weeks' gestation for individuals with a history of genital HSV confirmed by serologic testing is currently recommended.[81] The extant data do not support routine use of antiviral agents in pregnant persons without a history of genital lesions but with positive serologic testing.

Pregnant persons without a history of herpes whose sexual partners have herpes should be encouraged to use safer sex practices and avoid sexual contact when the partner has prodromal symptoms and/or a visible lesion. This consideration is especially important when pregnant persons are close to term. In addition, individuals should not receive orogenital contact near their estimated date of birth if their partner has a history of oral herpes sores.

If an individual has a history of genital herpes, a careful perianal assessment is important at the first labor examination or prior to induction to rule out active infection. The greatest risk of intrapartum transmission to the infant occurs during a primary outbreak. Vaginal birth during a primary outbreak can have vertical transmission rates as high as 50%.[5] Vaginal birth during recurrent infections has a lower transmission rate (less than 1%), due in part to passage of maternal immunoglobulin to the fetus across the placenta.[5] However, because morbidity and mortality are high following neonatal infection, a cesarean birth should be offered as an option if the person has *any* active genital lesions or prodromal symptoms at the onset of labor in an area that could come in contact with the fetus during vaginal birth.[81]

If a person has nongenital lesions when they begin labor, vaginal birth may proceed normally. All nongenital lesions should be covered with an occlusive dressing to decrease the risk of transmission, especially when handling the newborn.[81] Occasionally, an individual will have a precipitous labor and give birth vaginally during a herpetic outbreak. In these cases, viral cultures of the newborn and prophylactic treatment with acyclovir may be considered, especially if this is the affected individual's first outbreak.[5]

The majority of newborns in the United States who develop neonatal herpes are born to persons with no known history of the disease; this is due in part to increased monitoring of individuals with a history of herpes.[81] Approximately 85% of newborns with HSV infection contracted the virus during birth through contact with maternal secretions, whereas 10% are infected after birth via contact with infected individuals.[84] In addition, ritual circumcision with suction of the baby's blood using the adult's mouth has been shown to transmit HSV.[85] Although rare (accounting for only 5% of all neonatal cases), HSV can be transmitted across the placenta. Manifestations of this condition are similar to intrauterine varicella infection and include skin lesions, malformations of the eyes, and central nervous system dysfunction.[84]

Regardless of the route of transmission or subtype involved, HSV infection is very risky for the newborn. Symptoms of neonatal herpes usually appear on days 5 to 12 of life and include respiratory distress, irritability, jaundice, and vesicular lesions around the site of infection. Late symptoms include seizures and shock. Although neonatal herpes can remain localized to one area, there is a high risk of disseminated infection and central nervous system involvement—a condition that can lead to mortality rates as high as 85% without treatment.[84] Early treatment with antiviral agents can reduce this risk of death to 29%.[84,86] The pediatric provider should be notified immediately following the birth if a newborn may have been exposed to HSV during the birth and intravenous administration of acyclovir may be considered

HSV is communicable only through contact with infected secretions from mucous membranes of the mouth or genitals. Individuals with HSV should be encouraged to breastfeed/chestfeed unless there is a herpetic lesion directly on the nipple.[81]

## Hepatitis

Hepatitis is a small double-stranded DNA hepadnavirus. Eight genotypes of hepatitis viruses (A–H) have been identified, all of which have been found in the United States. Nevertheless, hepatitis A, B, and C are the most prevalent types in the United States. The hepatitis viruses primarily attack the liver and cause acute and/or chronic hepatitis. Chronic infection can lead to cirrhosis, hepatocellular carcinoma, and death.

Hepatitis viruses can be acquired in different ways. Hepatitis A virus (HAV) is primarily transmitted via fecal–oral contact and is reviewed in the *Common Conditions in Primary Care* chapter. Hepatitis B (HBV), C (HCV), and D (HDV) are transmitted via blood and bodily secretions, including semen and (rarely) saliva. Such transmission may occur during sexual contact (genital and oral), during birth, through needle-sticks or sharing of needles, and with use of nonsterilized instruments. Thus, HBV, HCV, and HDV infections are considered STIs.

## Hepatitis B

More than 296 million people worldwide and 1.89 million people in the United States are chronically infected with the hepatitis B virus (HBV).[87,88] HBV can remain infectious outside the body for at least 7 days, even if dry, and is able to establish infection with very few initial organisms, making it highly infectious.[87] In addition, HBV has numerous components that are antigenic, including the surface antigen (HBsAg), core antigen (HBcAg), and e antigen (HBeAg). The chance of transmission of HBV depends on the infected individual's viral load and antigen status (a marker of high infectivity).

HBV can become a chronic infection that causes cirrhosis, liver cancer, and death. The chances of chronic infection vary by age at the time of initial infection. For example, 90% of infants who acquire HBV via vertical transmission at the time of birth will develop chronic infection, compared to 5% or fewer of persons who acquire the disease during adulthood.[87] Global rates of chronic infection are higher in part because of the impaired immune response associated with coinfection with HIV and tuberculosis.[87]

HBV infection is often asymptomatic, or symptoms may be vague enough to go unnoticed. This disease typically has an incubation period from exposure to symptom onset of 6 weeks to 6 months. The prodromal phase lasts 3 to 10 days, during which commonly noted symptoms include fatigue, nausea, and diffuse epigastric or right upper quadrant pain. This is followed by an icteric phase of 1 to 3 weeks, which is characterized by symptoms such as jaundice, dark urine, and gray stools. Convalescence can take weeks to months.

### Prevention of Hepatitis B

In the United States, the overall rate of HBV infection has declined more than 80% since 1991, when the CDC began a campaign to reduce HBV prevalence.[89] However, due to the opioid and heroin epidemic, HBV infection prevention measures have begun to stall in areas of the United States most impacted by substance use disorders.[90] The HBV vaccine is produced from derivatives of yeast, without the use of blood products, so it cannot cause hepatitis.[5] Vaccination is recommended for several at-risk groups, such as individuals with multiple sexual partners, men who have sex with men, and individuals who inject drugs. The vaccine dose varies based on the reason for vaccination, with immunocompromised adults receiving larger doses. Individuals should receive all doses from the same vaccine manufacturer.[5]

Routine screening of pregnant individuals and immunoprophylaxis of all newborns of infected persons have also been useful in decreasing the prevalence of chronic hepatitis in the United States.[91] Other preventive strategies include universal precautions, careful instrument sterilization, safer sex practices, and not sharing toothbrushes and razors with infected individuals.[92]

### Postexposure Immunoprophylaxis

Postexposure prophylaxis decreases rates of acute and chronic infection and is most useful if prophylaxis is administered within 24 hours of exposure.[5] If an individual who has not been previously vaccinated, or who is not fully vaccinated, is exposed to HBV, administration of the HBV vaccine at the same time (at different injection sites) as hepatitis B

| Table 18-18 | Interpretation of Hepatitis B Serology | | | | |
|---|---|---|---|---|---|
| Interpretation | | HBsAg | IgM Anti-HBc | Total Anti-HBc | Anti-HBs |
| Never infected (susceptible) | | − | − | − | − |
| Early acute or immediately after vaccination (≤ 18 days)[a] | | + | − | − | − |
| Acute infection | | + | + | + | − |
| Resolving acute infection | | − | + | + | − |
| Chronic infection | | + | − | + | − |
| Resolved (immune) and recovered from past infection | | − | − | + | + |
| Vaccinated (immune) | | − | − | − | + |
| Passive transfer to infant born to HBsAg-positive individual; past infection; low-level chronic infection; false positive[b] | | − | − | + | − |

Abbreviations: anti-HBs, antihepatitis B surface antibody; FDA, U.S. Food and Drug Administration; HBsAg, hepatitis B surface antigen; IgM anti-HBc, IgM antibody to hepatitis B core antigen; +, positive; −, negative.

[a]The HBsAg test can lead to false positives because it can react to other viral antigens. To ensure that a positive HBsAg is not a false positive, samples that are positive should be tested with an FDA-cleared test for HBsAg only.

[b]If the anti-HBc is positive and other hepatitis serologies are negative, it is unlikely the person is infected, except in case of previous blood transfusion or organ transplantation.

Based on Workowski KA, Bachmann LH, Chan PA, et al. Sexually transmitted infections treatment guidelines, 2021. *MMWR Recomm Rep*. 2021;70(4):1-187. doi:10.15585/mmwr.rr7004a.

immunoglobulin (HBIG) has been shown to reduce transmission.[5] The vaccine series should then be completed using the CDC-defined age-appropriate dose and schedule. Information about postexposure prophylaxis for viral blood-borne infections can be found on the CDC website.

### Screening and Diagnosis of Hepatitis B

Screening for HBV occurs via serologic testing for hepatitis B surface antigen (HBsAg). If the individual is HBsAg positive, a complete hepatitis panel can be obtained to determine acute versus chronic status. This panel may include the hepatitis B e antigen (HBeAg), which is a marker of a high degree of infectivity; the IgM anticore antibody (IgM anti-HBc), which is a marker of recent infection within the last 6 months and indicates acute infection; the IgG anticore antibody (IgG anti-HBc), which is a marker of past or current infection; the antihepatitis B surface antibody (anti-HBs), which is a marker of an immune response to HBV; the antihepatitis B e antigen (anti-HBe), which may be present in a person who is either infected or immune; and viral load, which reveals the concentration of the hepatitis B virus DNA within the blood.

Diagnosis is based on interpretation of hepatitis serology, as shown in Table 18-18[7,93] and Figure 18-3.[94] Physical examination findings during acute HBV infection include upper abdominal tenderness, hepatomegaly, and, occasionally, jaundice. Individuals with hepatitis may also exhibit other abnormal serum tests, including elevated aspartate aminotransferase (AST), elevated alanine aminotransferase (ALT), elevated bilirubin, and a prolonged prothrombin time.

### Treatment of Hepatitis B

All cases of newly diagnosed hepatitis B should be reported to the local health department. If an individual has hepatitis B, their household contacts should be vaccinated, and sexual partners tested and vaccinated if not infected.[91] There is no specific treatment for adults with acute hepatitis, other than a supportive lifestyle to assist the body in healing.[5] Individuals with chronic infection can receive treatment to decrease the risk of liver disease,[5] and should be referred to providers knowledgeable in the management of hepatitis and chronic liver disease.

### Management of Hepatitis B During the Perinatal Period

Serologic screening for HBsAg is routinely included as one of the initial laboratory tests for all pregnant individuals during each pregnancy.[95] Hepatitis B vaccination is safe during pregnancy. Pregnancy is a good time for vaccination of at-risk individuals, as they should already be in the clinic at the appropriate intervals.[96]

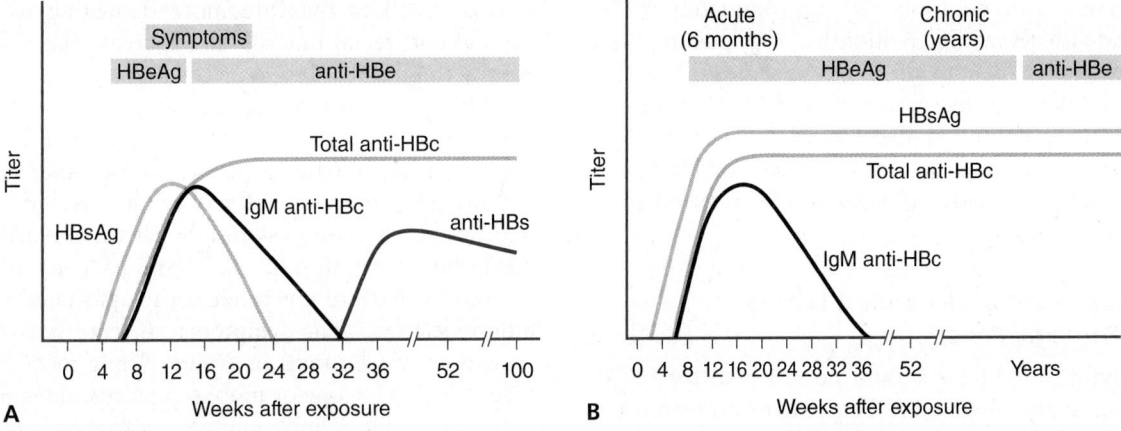

**Figure 18-3  A.** Acute hepatitis B virus infection with recovery types: serologic course. **B.** Chronic hepatitis B virus infection: serologic course.
Abbreviations: anti-HBc, antihepatitis B core antigen; anti-HBe, antihepatitis B e antigen; HBsAg, hepatitis B surface antigen; HBeAg, hepatitis B e antigen; IgM anti-HBc, IgM anticore antibody.
Reproduced from Weinbaum CM, Williams I, Mast EE, et al. Recommendations for identification and public health management of persons with chronic hepatitis B virus infection. *MMWR Recomm Rep.* 2008;57(RR08):1-20.

Individuals with hepatitis during pregnancy should be referred for specialist evaluation. Treatment of HBV during pregnancy is primarily directed toward decreasing the risk of vertical transmission. Viral load testing is used to determine which pregnant individuals are candidates for antiviral treatment.[91] Studies have shown that treatment of chronic HBV during pregnancy decreases the risk of vertical transmission.[97] The health record should note the pregnant individual's HBsAg status, and this information should be conveyed to the individual's chosen birth location to allow preparation for HBIG administration to the newborn following birth.

Intrapartum management of individuals infected with HBV is the same as that offered to persons who are not infected with HBV. Hepatitis status should not influence the preferred route of birth (vaginal or cesarean section). However, because fetal scalp electrodes may increase the risk of neonatal infection, an electrode should be applied only if the benefits outweigh the potential risks.

The CDC advises routine HBV vaccination of all infants weighing more than 2000 g, regardless of the birthing person's HBV status.[96] Newborns of individuals infected with HBV should be given HBIG and their first hepatitis vaccine within 12 hours of birth.[98] Removal of blood from the infant's skin or bathing of the infant soon after birth is also recommended to decrease infectious blood contact.[99] The CDC is an excellent resource for comprehensive information about prevention of perinatal transmission of hepatitis B and provides health education information in a variety of languages.

Hepatitis B is *not* transmitted through human milk, and individuals should be encouraged to breastfeed/chestfeed regardless of their hepatitis B status.[5] While transmission of HBV from breastfeeding/chestfeeding in the presence of cracked or bleeding nipples has raised some concerns, there is no conclusive evidence of transmission by this route. Breastfeeding/chestfeeding should not be interrupted for this reason.[5]

### Hepatitis C

Today, hepatitis C is the most common chronic blood-borne infection in the United States, with an estimated 2.4 million people now living with this chronic infection.[100,101] Risk factors for HCV include nonsterile tattooing, blood transfusion before 1987, organ transplant before 1992, HIV-positive status, current STI, history of injecting drugs or sharing of needles, multiple sexual partners, evidence of liver disease, and history of long-term hemodialysis.[102] The primary risk factors for HCV in the United States are use of blood products and intravenous drug use. Compared to HBV, HCV is much less likely to be transmitted via sexual contact or via parent-to-child transmission during birth, although transmission can occur through these routes.

The CDC recommends that all individuals older than age 18 be tested for HCV.[5] HCV RNA can be detected in the blood 1 to 3 weeks after exposure. Seroconversion occurs within 4 to 10 weeks, and anti-HCV can be found in approximately 97% of individuals within 6 months of exposure. Approximately 75% to 85% of persons with HCV will develop chronic infection, and HCV is one of the leading causes of liver cancer.[5] The FDA has approved several drugs for treatment of HCV. Individuals with acute HCV should be referred to a specialist for care.

### Management of Hepatitis C During the Perinatal Period

Pregnant individuals should be screened for HCV during every pregnancy. The risk of transmitting HCV to the fetus during birth is approximately 6%; at this time, there are no known treatments to prevent parent-to-child transmission during birth.[103] Treatment of acute HCV during pregnancy may require hospitalization and physician care, but there is no standard treatment for chronic HCV at this time. Midwives, in consultation with obstetric specialists, can manage care for pregnant individuals with chronic HCV. Mode of birth is not affected by HCV infection, but care should be taken to minimize interventions that increase the risk of fetal exposure to the birthing individual's blood and body fluids, including the use of fetal scalp electrodes and episiotomies. Delaying artificial rupture of membranes may also reduce exposure to body fluids. Individuals with chronic HCV may breastfeed/chestfeed.

### Human Immunodeficiency Virus

HIV is an RNA retrovirus (i.e., an RNA virus that replicates via production of DNA that is inserted into the host cell genome) that is transmitted through infected blood and bodily secretions. The CDC estimates that 50,000 individuals contract HIV in the United States every year, and 250,000 individuals have undiagnosed HIV infection. In the United States, HIV is most commonly transmitted through sexual intercourse. Exposure to infected blood through sharing of infected needles or accidental needle-sticks and other mechanisms are additional routes of transmission. Pre-exposure prophylaxis is available for those persons at high risk for HIV acquisition, and postexposure prophylaxis can be used within 72 hours of an exposure to prevent HIV acquisition.

The risk of acquisition of HIV during sex is greatly increased if a person has other STIs, such as herpes, gonorrhea, or STIs causing genital ulcers that facilitate the virus's access to the circulation. Sexual practices that are more damaging to the vaginal and rectal mucosa also increase the risk of contracting HIV.

HIV proceeds through several stages after infecting the immune system's CD4 cells (a type of T cell). The first stage, called acute retroviral syndrome, occurs within the first few weeks after infection. It is characterized by fever, malaise, a skin rash, nausea or diarrhea, headache, sore throat, and lymphadenopathy—symptoms that are much like those associated with mononucleosis.[5] The symptoms of acute retroviral syndrome can be mild or severe. While most individuals will have one or more symptoms, some individuals may be asymptomatic or not recognize any signs of illness. The infection then becomes asymptomatic during a period of clinical latency that can last a short time or up to 8 years or longer, depending on the individual. During this time, HIV reproduces at very low levels, although it is still active.

When the CD4 cell count falls below 200 cells/$mm^2$, symptoms of advanced infection or acquired immunodeficiency syndrome (AIDS) appear. Symptoms of AIDS include fever, weight loss, diarrhea, cough, shortness of breath, opportunistic infections, and more intense illnesses and infections that are more severe than would be expected for the individual's age or health status.

Initiation of effective antiretroviral therapy is associated with reduced morbidity, prevention of HIV transmission to sexual partners, and near-normal life expectancy.[5] Individuals newly diagnosed with HIV infection should receive prompt referral to a specialty clinic for antiretroviral therapy. Increased screening for HIV is a critical step toward achieving the public health goals of reducing viral transmission and decreasing AIDS-related complications.[104]

Rates of new HIV infections in the United States vary by race, with 41% of new HIV diagnoses in 2019 occurring in individuals who identify as Black. Issues such as racism, homophobia, HIV stigma, poverty, and access to health care contribute to this racial disparity.[105]

Two types of HIV viruses exist: HIV-1 and HIV-2. The vast majority of HIV infections in the United States and worldwide are caused by the HIV-1 virus. HIV-2 is predominately found in West Africa, but this subtype is now becoming more common globally.[7] Both types of HIV produce similar symptoms and effects within the body, but their infectivity and treatment vary. Initial screening tests for HIV are able to detect antibodies to both HIV-1 and HIV-2, and further tests can differentiate the viruses (see Figure 18-4 later in this section).

### Prevention of HIV Infection

Strategies to prevent HIV transmission range from behavioral to pharmacologic in nature. Methods to prevent transmission can be customized, based on HIV status and sexual behaviors, for the individual and their partner(s).[103,104] The CDC has developed an excellent, interactive risk-reduction tool that can be used for this purpose (see the Resources section at the end of this chapter). Individuals at high risk for HIV acquisition may also benefit from pre-exposure or postexposure prophylaxis.[106]

*Pre-exposure Prophylaxis.* Pre-exposure prophylaxis (PrEP) has been shown to reduce the risk of HIV acquisition by as much as 92%.[107] PrEP is appropriate for any sexually active person who is HIV negative, unless the last potential HIV exposure occurred within 72 hours, in which case postexposure prophylaxis may be more appropriate.[5] Individuals who use intravenous drugs, those having anal or vaginal sex with a partner with HIV infection, those with a history of bacterial STI infection in the previous 6 months, and those not using condoms consistently are considered to be at increased risk for HIV acquisition. Individuals living in Puerto Rico and persons identifying as Hispanic are less likely to be aware of the availability of PrEP or to receive this effective preventive measure.[108] Individuals engaging in penile–vaginal intercourse are also less likely to be offered PrEP.

Prior to beginning oral medications for PrEP, individuals should be tested for HIV, renal function, hepatitis B and C, and pregnancy if indicated.[107] If indicated, individuals should be offered vaccination for hepatitis B.[96] Contraception can also be offered to appropriate individuals while taking PrEP. All contraceptives can be used while taking antiviral medications.[109]

Once the person is appropriately screened, PrEP involves a once-daily oral combination of 300 mg tenofovir disoproxil fumarate and 200 mg emtricitabine (Truvada) or 200 mg tenofovir alafenamide and 25 mg emtricitabine (Descovy). These regimens decrease the chance of HIV acquisition, although individuals should continue to use safer sex practices. Adherence to daily dosing is necessary for prophylaxis efficacy.

Alternatively, cabotegravir 600 mg is available as an intramuscular injectable medication for PrEP for individuals with decreased renal function or inability to take daily oral medications, or by preference. Assessment of renal and liver function is not necessary prior to initiation of cabotegravir. After the initial dose, individuals should receive a second dose 4 weeks later, then every 8 weeks.

While receiving PrEP, the individual needs to visit their care provider every 3 months for HIV, other STIs, and pregnancy testing and continued health education on risk reduction; renal function should be tested at 3 months, and then every 6 months.[107] Alternative medication delivery systems and dosing regimens are under investigation. Specialist involvement may be appropriate, but should not delay access to PrEP when needed. The CDC regularly updates its PrEP clinical guidance documents for healthcare providers.

There are limited safety data on use of PrEP during pregnancy, but pregnancy is not a contraindication to use. Only the combination of tenofovir disoproxil fumarate and emtricitabine (Truvada) is currently approved for use in pregnancy, although cabotegravir is likely an acceptable alternative.[107] A discussion of the risks and benefits of PrEP during pregnancy should take place between the individual and the clinician.[110] Specialist referral is appropriate for individuals with a partner who is HIV positive who are planning pregnancy, as risk of HIV acquisition in pregnancy is related to the partner's viral load. Limited safety data on the use of PrEP in lactating individuals are available, but evidence suggests the risk of drug exposure through human milk is small.[111] Shared decision making about medication use in pregnancy and lactation is recommended.

*Postexposure Prophylaxis.* Postexposure prophylaxis (PEP) differs depending on the origin of the exposure: occupational or non-occupational. When a healthcare provider is exposed to potentially infectious fluids, HIV testing should ideally be performed on the source individual (with their consent), and then a plan for care quickly formulated using expert consultation or the current information on the CDC website.[112] PEP for HIV is time sensitive and should occur within 72 hours of exposure.[79]

Non-occupational exposure to HIV-infected fluids through sex, assault, or injection drugs also needs rapid attention (e.g., an expedited clinic appointment). Exposed individuals should receive a comprehensive assessment, including information on the exposure as well as the HIV status of the source individual. If the source individual is not known to be HIV positive, administration of PEP should be determined on an individual basis, with the person receiving health education about the risks and benefits of each approach so they can participate in shared decision making. The risk for

HIV acquisition depends on the source fluid (i.e., blood, semen, other body fluids) and the site of fluid contact. In addition to HIV counseling, the shared decision-making process should consider the person's risk for other STIs as well as hepatitis B and C acquisition.

The CDC provides comprehensive information on baseline testing and PEP regimens for HIV and other infections.[113] The usual PEP regimen is a 28-day course of three antiretroviral medications. PEP is appropriate only for intermittent use, and follow-up should include repeat HIV testing. Emergency contraception should also be offered when appropriate, as detailed in the *Fertility, Family Building, and Contraception* chapter.

### Screening and Diagnosis of HIV Infection

Midwives are often involved in screening and diagnosis of HIV infection. Such screening should be offered in the same manner as any test. Consent for HIV testing can be included within a larger consent for all health care; a special HIV testing consent form is not needed and may act as a barrier to screening. HIV testing should be presented as the norm, and individuals allowed to opt out without coercion if they do not wish to have testing.[5]

Routine HIV screening should be offered to all individuals ages 13 to 64 at risk for STIs, and more frequent screening may be provided to individuals at high risk. An algorithm for interpretation of HIV tests is found in Figure 18-4.[114] As many as 16% of persons who are HIV positive do not know their HIV status.[5] Pregnant individuals should be screened at least once during pregnancy using an opt-out approach, and another HIV test should be considered in the third trimester.[5] Many states require third trimester testing for all pregnant persons, unless they opt out of screening.[115] State requirements can be found on state health websites and as part of the CDC's HIV online resources.

Most of the commonly used screening tools detect antigens or antibodies to HIV, rather than the presence of the virus itself, and are appropriate first

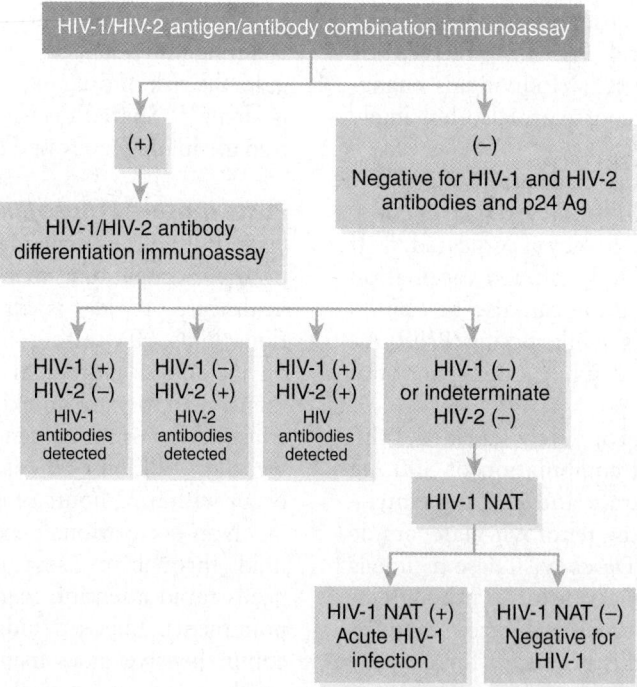

**Figure 18-4** Recommended laboratory HIV testing algorithm for serum or plasma specimens.

Abbreviations: HIV, human immunodeficiency disease; NAT, nucleic acid test; +, reactive test result; –, nonreactive test result.

Reproduced from Centers for Disease Control and Prevention. Laboratory testing for the diagnosis of HIV infection: updated recommendations. http://www.cdc.gov/hiv/pdf/guidelines_testing_recommendedlabtestingalgorithm.pdf. Published 2014. Accessed April 26, 2022.

tests for most individuals. Antibodies appear 2 to 12 weeks after infection occurs. Routine screening can be performed with in-office test kits using oral fluids, blood, or serum or with laboratory testing on blood specimens. In-office rapid testing can yield results in 20 minutes, although it is recommended that antigen/antibody screening be performed in most situations.[104] The most commonly used laboratory screening test is a conventional/rapid EIA. More rarely, a CLIA-waived test may be used. The provider should select a test that screens for both HIV-1 and HIV-2.[114] Note that if an individual is newly infected (as would be the case if a person presents with acute retroviral syndrome), these antigen/antibody tests can produce false-negative results, as they do not detect the actual virus. In this situation, an RNA test should be ordered.[5]

All HIV screening tests carry a risk of false-positive results. Therefore, if a screening test is positive, it is repeated. If both tests are positive, a diagnostic test is performed to ensure the person has HIV infection. Appropriate supplemental tests for confirmation of HIV-positive status include HIV-1/HIV-2 antibody differentiation, Western blot testing, and indirect immunofluorescence assay. A positive supplementary test, such as Western blot, indirect immunofluorescence assay, or HIV RNA assay, provides the definitive diagnosis of HIV infection. If the result of the confirmatory test is indeterminate, an HIV RNA test is performed.[114] Reporting to public health authorities is mandated when HIV infection is diagnosed, but not when a screening test is positive.[114]

Negative HIV test results can be conveyed by phone, but positive results should be given to the individual in person, if at all possible. Proper preparation prior to the visit can be helpful. Often, local or regional organizations offer specific behavioral and psychological services for HIV-positive individuals and can be contacted to provide information prior to meeting with the individual. The CDC recommends that a diagnosis of HIV infection be provided in conjunction with assessment of psychosocial support and prompt referral to specialty healthcare services, including mental health. The midwife should provide the individual with reference materials in case they are not able to remember the full details of the conversation (Table 18-19). Midwifery presence and therapeutic communication skills are useful in providing an honest diagnosis while remaining compassionate and adjusting the information to the person's needs. Similar to providing information about other STIs, the midwife should provide the individual with the diagnosis and allow them time to react and formulate questions.

| Table 18-19 | Health Education for a Person with HIV Diagnosis |
|---|---|
| **Essential Teaching at Time of Diagnosis (Verbally and Written Handouts)** ||
| Effectiveness of HIV treatments ||
| Potential for transmission to others, safer sex practices, risk-reduction strategies, and the availability of pre-exposure prophylaxis for partners ||
| Partner disclosure techniques and assistance ||
| Importance of early and ongoing health care ||
| Where to get health care for HIV infection (local clinic and provider name and phone number) ||
| What to expect with HIV care (daily medications even when well, preventive visits) ||
| Referrals to behavioral and psychosocial services designed for HIV-positive individuals ||
| **Additional Information to Provide When the Person Is Ready** ||
| Information on health insurance and healthcare provision for HIV-positive individuals ||
| Reproductive choices with HIV diagnosis, including need for birth control until ready to conceive ||
| Substance abuse screening and counseling if indicated ||

Abbreviation: HIV, human immunodeficiency virus.

Based on U.S. Public Health Service. *Preexposure Prophylaxis for the Prevention of HIV Infection in the United States—2014: A Clinical Practice Guideline*. Washington, DC: U.S. Public Health Service; 2014; Centers for Disease Control and Prevention. Recommendations for partner services programs for HIV infection, syphilis, gonorrhea, and chlamydial infection. *MMWR Recomm Rep*. 2008;57(RR-9):1-83; Centers for Disease Control and Prevention, Health Resources and Services Administration, National Institutes of Health, et al. Recommendations for HIV prevention with adults and adolescents with HIV in the United States, 2014: summary for clinical providers. https://stacks.cdc.gov/view/cdc/26063. Published 2014. Accessed April 16, 2023.

All individuals with a new diagnosis of HIV should also be screened for intimate partner violence and a discussion of how to disclose HIV status to sexual partners should be explored.[116,117] If the person is at risk for intimate partner violence, resources and ways to assure safety are a priority for this visit. Information about disclosure to a sexual partner, safer sex practices, risk reduction, PrEP, and PEP can be found on the CDC's website, and the state health department's partner services can be helpful as well. The information provided should be compatible with the individual's educational level, culture, and desire for knowledge; health education can be prioritized if the person appears to be overwhelmed or disinterested.

### Treatment of HIV Infection

Midwives should refer all individuals with a new HIV diagnosis to appropriate local or regional specialists and verify that care has been initiated. Early initiation of antiretroviral therapy following HIV diagnosis is recommended.[5] The specific treatment for HIV infection depends on the person's current health status, including their viral load and comorbid disorders.[118] Referral to an HIV specialist allows the individual to receive optimal care.

Although the majority of midwives in the United States do not routinely care for HIV-positive individuals, some do work in multidisciplinary teams to provide holistic and comprehensive care to HIV-positive individuals during pregnancy and across the lifespan. Midwives in these settings collaborate with, consult with, or refer patients to a variety of healthcare providers to ensure individuals with HIV infection receive care at facilities that are accessible, are acceptable, and provide evidence-based care.

Individuals who are HIV positive, who are sexually active, and who do not desire pregnancy need contraception. While condoms are an essential part of safer sex practices, their effectiveness in preventing pregnancy may not be adequate. The WHO and CDC eligibility criteria list a variety of contraceptives that are safe in individuals with HIV infection, and the CDC recommendations can be accessed via a smartphone app. All contraceptive methods, other than spermicides, are acceptable for clinically well individuals receiving antiretroviral treatment. If the person is not receiving treatment or is ill, an IUD may not be an ideal choice, but can be used.[109] Spermicides are implicated in STI acquisition and are not a highly effective method of pregnancy prevention; therefore, their use is not advised.[119] If an HIV-positive individual wishes to conceive, preconception planning is essential to optimize their own health, avoid birth defects from teratogenic medications, and prevent transmission of HIV to their partner and fetus.

Individuals with HIV infection face a wide range of potential sequelae from this infection. Treatment to prevent immune system depletion and opportunistic infections should be ongoing and requires close collaboration between the person and their healthcare team. Preventive care, including cervical cytology screening and physical examinations, should occur more frequently for HIV-positive individuals with a cervix due to their increased susceptibility to infections and cancer.[5]

### Management of HIV Infection During the Perinatal Period

All pregnant people should be offered screening for HIV early during pregnancy and, ideally, again in the third trimester. Repeat screening is recommended for pregnant people at increased risk of HIV acquisition, those receiving care in areas where HIV infections rates are high, and those receiving care in clinical settings where 1 or more pregnant people tests positive for HIV for every 1000 birthing people screened.[5] Pregnant people who have not received prenatal care should be screened upon hospital admission for birth. There are wide racial health disparities in vertical transmission of HIV in the United States, and ensuring pregnant people are tested and then welcomed into person-centered, affirming, and culturally appropriate care is essential in reducing these disparities.[120]

Early and consistent antiretroviral treatment is an essential component of HIV management during pregnancy and prevention of vertical transmission.[121] While pregnancy does not affect HIV progression to AIDS, HIV infection has been associated with poor perinatal outcomes, especially in low-resource areas of the world.[122]

Prenatal care for pregnant people with HIV infection should also involve practitioners skilled in HIV management and pregnancy care. Ideally, care will involve interprofessional collaboration between clinicians and behavioral and psychological health professionals. Midwives can be a component of this care, but the knowledge needed for HIV management is beyond the American College of Nurse-Midwives' Core Competencies. If advanced skills are practiced, they should be added using the procedures outlined in the Standards for the Practice of Midwifery.[123] The CDC provides regularly updated guidelines for the treatment of HIV for pregnant people. The National Perinatal HIV Hotline is a resource for free clinical consultation for healthcare providers within the United States if guidance is needed.[121] Notably, the combination of antiretroviral medications and cesarean birth for individuals with a high viral load has reduced vertical transmission from rates as high as 25% to 2% or less in the United States.

Newborns with perinatal exposure to HIV should be treated with antiretroviral therapy as soon as possible after birth, preferably within 6 hours of birth.[121] Consultation with pediatric care providers or infectious disease specialists is recommended. Newborns of birthing people treated with antiretroviral medications can develop a variety of problems, including anemia, jaundice, and birth defects, and need evaluation by clinicians experienced in HIV care.

Human milk of individuals with HIV infection can transmit the virus. In areas where safe human milk substitutes are consistently available, their use is recommended. This is the case in the United States and throughout the developed world; the CDC recommends that individuals who are HIV positive in the United States do not breastfeed/chestfeed their infants.[5]

Worldwide, however, the majority of cases of HIV/AIDs occur in areas where safe human milk substitutes are not reliably available. Infants and children fed human milk substitutes in these areas may have higher rates of morbidity and mortality as compared to their breastfed/chestfed peers. In these circumstances, the risk of death from other infections, especially diarrheal illness, is higher than the risk of HIV acquisition from breastfeeding/chestfeeding, especially if the individual is taking antiretroviral medication.[124] Local or country-level health officials should decide whether the breastfeeding/chestfeeding benefits outweigh the risks in their particular area.

If a child is already known to be HIV positive, they may be breastfed/chestfed as long as the parent and infant desire. However, if the infant is HIV negative or has an unknown HIV status, the risk of HIV acquisition through human milk feeding accumulates as the infant ages. The individual's viral load and CD4 count play a role in transmission of the virus to the child, and antiretroviral therapy decreases transmission through human milk, although it does not eliminate it.[121] The individuals' personal health, their environment, and the availability of safe feeding alternatives influence the decision of when to wean the infant.

### Zika Virus

Zika is a single-stranded RNA arbovirus related to yellow fever and dengue. The virus is transmitted by the bite of the *Aedes* genus of mosquitos, gestational parent-to-child transmission, blood transfusion, or sexual contact. Zika is endemic in some regions of the world, but became more widely recognized in the United States following a small outbreak in Florida in 2016.[125] Symptoms of Zika virus infection are generally mild and self-limited. While the rate of vertical transmission during pregnancy is low, perinatal infection is associated with microcephaly, ventriculomegaly, ophthalmologic abnormalities, fetal growth restriction, and stillbirth.[126] Guidance about travel to Zika-endemic areas for individuals planning a pregnancy or during pregnancy is available from the CDC. Pregnant individuals may also be asked about their recent travel history as well as that of their partner(s) at the first prenatal visit to assess risk of infection.[127]

Testing for Zika infection is recommended for symptomatic individuals who may have had exposure through sex, pregnant persons with symptoms of infection and recent exposure, pregnant persons without symptoms of infection with ongoing exposure, and pregnant persons with a fetus with birth defects suspected to be associated with Zika infection.[128] Treatment of Zika virus disease is supportive. In pregnant persons, care focuses on surveillance for vertical transmission and fetal effects. Healthcare workers should follow universal precautions to protect against exposure to body fluids.[129] More information can be found on the CDC website listed in the Resources section at the end of this chapter.

### Mpox

Mpox (formerly known as monkeypox) is in the same virus family as smallpox. First identified in the 1970s, this virus is endemic in some African countries but gained worldwide attention following an outbreak in 2022.[130] Initial cases in this outbreak were identified in individuals with a penis who engaged in anal sex with other individuals with a penis, raising concern for infection-related stigma.[131] Infection is possible without sexual contact, however, and occurs within 21 days of viral exposure. Viral transmission typically occurs through contact with body fluids or lesion exudate, including through fomites such as bedsheets or towels.[130] Less commonly, transmission of the mpox virus can occur through respiratory droplets. Individuals with mpox can transmit the virus until the scabs are completely healed and new skin has formed, a process that can take 2 to 4 weeks.[132]

Symptoms of mpox infection include fever, malaise, lymphadenopathy, headache, sore throat, cough, and rash. The rash characteristic of the virus may cause pain and pruritus; it progresses from macule, to papule, to vesicle and then to pustule before forming a scab.[130] This rash may be centrifugal in distribution, occurring on the arms, face, and legs, but has also been described as localized and scattered in other cases. Guidance about distinguishing mpox virus rash from other infections associated with rashes is available on the CDC website and includes color photographs.[130]

Testing for mpox is performed by swabbing the lesions. Preferably more than one swab is collected from a lesion, and multiple lesions from different body locations should be swabbed.[130] The clinician should take care to wear appropriate personal protective equipment while collecting samples to prevent viral exposure.

Currently both an attenuated vaccine and a live vaccine for mpox are available. Immunization is recommended for selected individuals at high risk for occupational exposure[130] as well as for individuals with recent exposure or at high risk of exposure. Live virus vaccination is contraindicated during pregnancy and human lactation, although attenuated virus vaccination may be considered. Treatment of individuals with complications from vaccination is available through antibody infusion. PEP is available with the antiviral medication tecovirimat, which may be administered either in oral capsules or as an intravenous infusion.[130] Individuals who are pregnant or lactating are considered at increased risk of severe disease and may be offered treatment after consultation with the CDC. Distribution of vaccines, PEP, and treatment are currently only available through requests to state health departments.

Infection with mpox during pregnancy can cause miscarriage, intrauterine fetal demise, preterm labor, and neonatal transmission.[133] No human safety data about the use of tecovirimat during pregnancy or lactation are available, although animal studies have not demonstrated harm from this medication. Alternative medications for treatment of mpox are teratogenic and should not be used during pregnancy. No data are available about the safety of mpox antibody infusions during pregnancy or lactation, but other antibody infusions have been used without negative effects. Shared decision making between the individual, the healthcare provider, and consultation with infectious disease experts is recommended.

## Protozoal and Parasitic Infections

Several organisms classified as protozoans or parasites can cause reproductive tract infections. Trichomoniasis is the most common protozoan-related STI. Lice are parasitic organisms that can infect the head, body, or pubic area depending on the type of louse. Specifically, *Pthirus pubis* is the type of louse that infects the pubic area. Although *P. pubis* is commonly spread via sexual contact, this organism can be transmitted via contact with linens or other objects. Although infections with the scabies parasite and *Molluscum contagiosum* are not traditional STIs, these organisms are often transmitted via sexual contact.

## Trichomoniasis

Trichomoniasis, commonly known as "trich," is a vaginal or urethral infection caused by the protozoa *Trichomonas vaginalis* (Figure 18-5). The

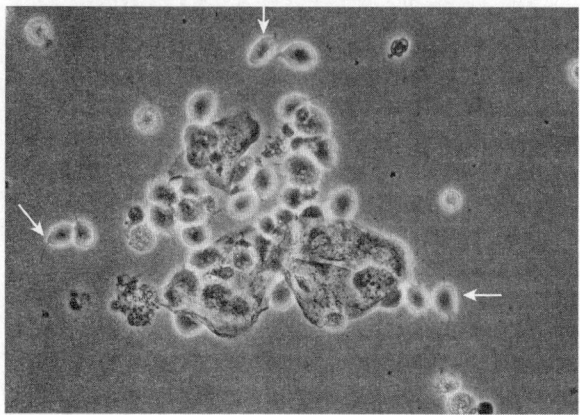

**Figure 18-5** Trichomonas.
Courtesy of Centers for Disease Control and Prevention/Joe Miller.

pear-shaped protozoa have five flagella and are highly motile. They are transmitted through sexual contact, which transfers infected secretions to the urethra and vagina. Fomites are a possible, albeit unlikely, mechanism of infection, as trichomonads must be kept moist and warm.

Approximately 3.7 million persons in the United States have trichomoniasis at any given time; in some populations, as many as 9.6% of persons with a uterus are infected.[5] *Trichomonas* infection is not required to be reported; therefore, incidence and prevalence estimates lack precision. Additionally, it is difficult to track trichomoniasis in individuals identifying as male due to the possibility of spontaneous resolution (there are no data available for trans individuals).[134]

Trichomoniasis is frequently asymptomatic. Symptoms, when present, include vaginal itching, irritation, and malodorous vaginal discharge. Abdominal discomfort may also be present. Trichomoniasis is associated with increased risk for preterm birth and a 1.5-fold increase in risk of HIV acquisition.[5]

### Screening and Diagnosis of Trichomoniasis

Routine screening for trichomoniasis is recommended only for individuals who are HIV positive because this coinfection is associated with an increased risk for PID. This recommendation applies to both nonpregnant and pregnant individuals. Routine screening and treatment in HIV-negative persons have not been shown to lower risks of other adverse outcomes.

Symptomatic individuals can be evaluated via physical examination and one of several laboratory tests. Although the person may be asymptomatic, common physical examination findings include an inflamed and irritated vulva with minor excoriations, and possibly a malodorous, frothy, thin, yellow-green vaginal discharge. The cervix may be deep red or pink, a condition known as "strawberry cervix," although this it typically more visible on colposcopy than routine physical examination.[5]

For diagnosis of this infection, the CDC recommends the use of tests specific for detection of *T. vaginalis*. A variety of very sensitive NAATs are available and can be used on clinician-collected endocervical or vaginal swabs, urine specimens from persons assigned female at birth, and certain liquid Pap smear specimens. In addition, several brands of FDA-cleared rapid tests are available for use in individuals with a vagina. These tests can be performed in clinic laboratories for on-site diagnosis. While these tests are expensive, they provide greater diagnostic certainty. Clinicians should review the type of test offered in their clinical environment and become familiar with the testing capabilities.

A saline wet-mount microscopic evaluation has historically been used to diagnose trichomoniasis and is still commonly employed for this purpose. However, this method has low sensitivity (44% to 68%) as compared to culture.[5] Detection can be improved by evaluating slides immediately after collecting the sample, because sensitivity decreases to 20% within an hour of collection.[5] Trichomonads quickly become immobile and will be difficult to distinguish from other cells. The CDC advises clinicians to move toward more sensitive and specific tests when possible.[5]

While the presence of *T. vaginalis* may be reported as part of cervical cytology screening results, this finding should not be used for diagnosis due to high rates of false-positive and false-negative findings. Individuals with *T. vaginalis* detected on a Pap test should be offered retesting with a more sensitive diagnostic test and treated upon confirmation of infection.

### Treatment of Trichomoniasis

Treatment options for trichomoniasis are listed in Table 18-20.[27,134] Oral therapies are required, as topical treatment with metronidazole is not effective in eradicating this infection. Counseling includes avoidance of alcohol for 24 hours after treatment with metronidazole (Flagyl) and for 72 hours after treatment with tinidazole (Tindamax).[5] Current

| Table 18-20 | Treatments for Trichomoniasis in Adolescents and Adults | | | | |
|---|---|---|---|---|---|
| **Recommended Treatment for Vaginal/Urethral Infection in Nonpregnant Individuals Generic (Brand)** | **Recommended Treatment for Penile (Urethral) Infection Generic (Brand)** | **Alternative Treatment for All Nonpregnant Individuals Generic (Brand)** | **Recommended Treatment for Pregnant Individuals Generic (Brand)** | **Considerations for Lactating Individuals** | |
| Metronidazole (Flagyl) 500 mg 2 times per day for 7 days | Metronidazole (Flagyl) 2 g orally once | Tinidazole (Tindamax) 2 g orally in a single dose | Metronidazole (Flagyl) 500 mg 2 times per day for 7 days OR 2 g orally once | Metronidazole (Flagyl) 500 mg 2 times per day for 7 days may be associated with lower concentration in human milk. | |
| | | | Animal data suggest that tinidazole (Tindamax) poses moderate risk during pregnancy; avoid using this therapy in pregnant individuals. | Metronidazole is preferred secondary to the higher maternal plasma levels that occur with the tinidazole 2 g single dose. | |
| | | | | Individuals should not breastfeed/chestfeed for 72 hours after taking tinidazole (Tindamax). | |

Based on Workowski KA, Bachmann LH, Chan PA, et al. Sexually transmitted infections treatment guidelines, 2021. *MMWR Recomm Rep.* 2021;70(4):1-187. doi:10.15585/mmwr.rr7004a1; U.S. National Library of Medicine. Drugs and Lactation Database (LactMed). https://www.ncbi.nlm.nih.gov/books/NBK501922.

sexual partner(s) should be treated, even if they are asymptomatic. Both partners should abstain from sexual contact until after treatment is completed and symptoms have resolved. If the initial treatment fails to eliminate the symptoms and trichomonads, consider tinidazole or a longer course of metronidazole. For strains resistant to both of these drugs, contact the CDC for susceptibility tests and additional treatments.[5] The CDC recommends that individuals with a vagina should be rescreened 3 months after treatment, if possible, to test for reinfection.

### Management of Trichomoniasis During the Perinatal Period

Only persons with symptoms of trichomoniasis or those who are HIV positive need to be screened for this infection during pregnancy. Infection with *Trichomonas* has been associated with an increased risk for prelabor rupture of membranes, preterm birth, and low birth weight as well as greater vertical transmission of HIV. However, treatment with metronidazole does not appear to decrease preterm birth rates.[135] Metronidazole was previously thought to contribute to preterm birth, stillbirth, and low birth weight when used during pregnancy, but that has been shown to be untrue. Thus, metronidazole is considered safe for use in pregnancy.[134] Until they are treated, the patient can still transmit the infection. Partner treatment can occur at any time but may need to be repeated when the patient is treated to prevent reinfection.[5]

Transfer of trichomoniasis to a fetus or newborn during vaginal birth is rare. The newborn may present with fever and either respiratory or genital infection.

### Pubic Lice (Pthiriasis)

Pubic lice (*Pthirus pubis*; Figure 18-6), also known as "crabs," are found on coarse body hairs, including pubic, axillary, and occasionally facial hair (eyebrows, eyelashes, or beard). Individuals usually present with itching and a report of visible lice or nits. Sexual transmission is most common, as parasites are pushed onto a new host's hair. However, pubic lice can live for as long as 44 hours off the body, so transmission via fomites such as towels, linens, and other objects is possible. Scalp infestations are not common but can occur, especially in advanced cases. Head lice (*Pediculus humanus capitis*; Figure 18-7) and pubic lice can be differentiated by their appearance, as pubic lice have a characteristic crab-like appearance and a lower length-to-width ratio than head lice.

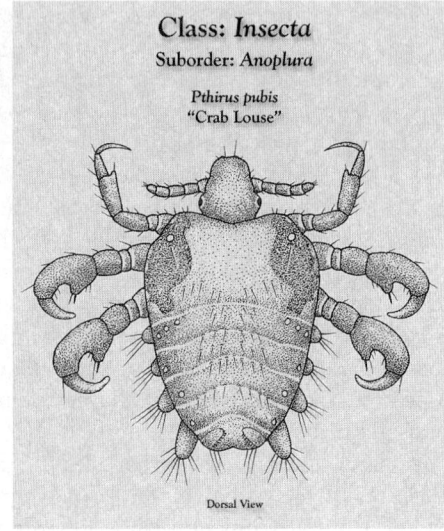

**Figure 18-6** Pubic lice.
Courtesy of Centers for Disease Control and Prevention.

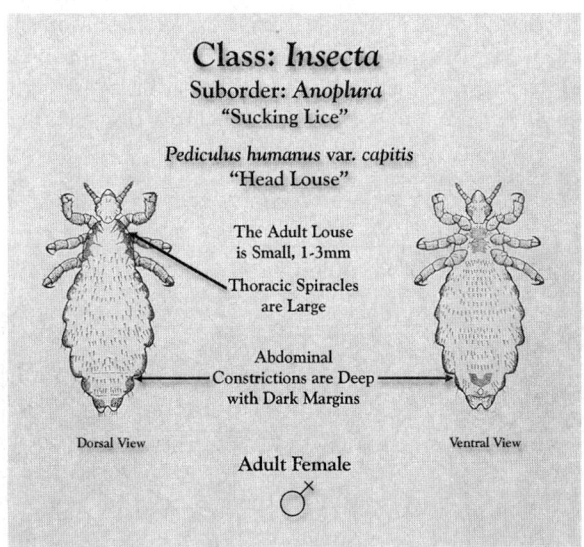

**Figure 18-7** Head lice.
Courtesy of Centers for Disease Control and Prevention.

### Diagnosis of Pubic Lice

All hairy or shaved areas of the body are inspected to differentiate the type of infection. Lice and nits are visible on hairs in one or more body area(s), with coarse hairs being more frequently infested than scalp hairs. Small punctuate lesions and bluish macules may also be seen. Lice can be viewed under the microscopic for confirmation, but the physical examination is all that is needed for diagnosis.

### Treatment of Pubic Lice

Table 18-21 lists the CDC-recommended treatments for pubic lice in all body areas except the eyes. Pubic

| Table 18-21 | Treatments for Pthiriasis in Adolescents and Adults | | |
| --- | --- | --- | --- |
| Recommended Treatments for Nonpregnant Individuals Generic (Brand) | Alternative Treatments for Nonpregnant Individuals Generic (Brand) | Recommended Treatments for Pregnant Individuals Generic (Brand) | Considerations for Lactating Individuals |
| Permethrin 1% cream (Nix) rinse applied to affected area and washed off after 10 minutes OR Pyrethrins with piperonyl butoxide (RID) applied to area and then washed off after 10 minutes | Malathion 0.5% (Ovide) lotion applied for 8–12 hours and washed off (has a strong odor but is useful for resistant cases) OR Ivermectin (Stromectol) 250 mcg/kg orally with food, repeated in 1–2 weeks | Permethrin 1% cream (Nix) rinse applied to affected area and washed off after 10 minutes OR Pyrethrins with piperonyl butoxide (RID) applied to area and then washed off after 10 minutes Second-line treatment: Ivermectin (Stromectol) 250 mcg/kg orally with food, repeated in 2 weeks; data suggest low risk to fetus during pregnancy Malathion (Ovide) is contraindicated during pregnancy | Data suggest that ivermectin is probably compatible with lactation. Avoid direct application to the breast/chest. Malathion (Ovide) is contraindicated during lactation |

Based on Workowski KA, Bachmann LH, Chan PA, et al. Sexually transmitted infections treatment guidelines, 2021. *MMWR Recomm Rep.* 2021;70(4):1-187. doi:10.15585/mmwr.rr7004a1; U.S. National Library of Medicine. Drugs and Lactation Database (LactMed). https://www.ncbi.nlm.nih.gov/books/NBK501922. Published 2021. Accessed July 26, 2021.

lice infestation of the eyelashes should be treated with an occlusive ophthalmic ointment twice a day for 10 days.[5] All clothing and bedding should be washed and dried on a hot setting, dry cleaned, or kept from body contact for 72 hours. Bagging items may be more affordable for individuals who do not have a washer or dryer.

The CDC advises treatment for all sexual partners from the previous month. Household contacts should be examined and treated as needed.[5] Individuals with pubic lice should be counseled that screening for HIV, syphilis, chlamydia, and gonorrhea is recommended. Retreatment is necessary if no improvement occurs in 1 week. Resistance to treatment is common, and malathion (Ovide) is recommended for retreatment of those who are not pregnant in cases where resistance is suspected.[5]

## Other Infectious Agents Spread by Sexual Contact

In addition to the STIs reviewed in this chapter, a wide variety of other infections may be spread through sexual contact. For example, viruses such as cytomegalovirus (CMV) and Epstein-Barr virus

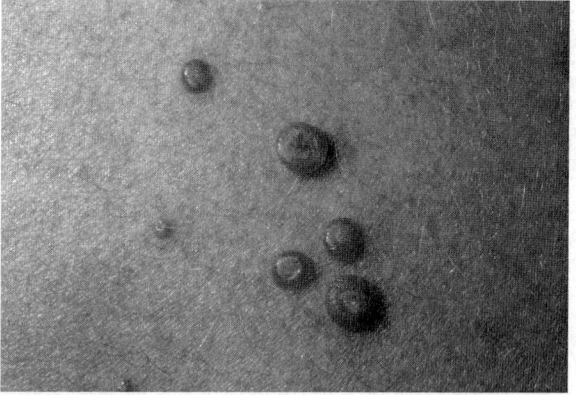

**Figure 18-8** *Molluscum contagiosum.*
© Dr P. Marazzi/Science Source.

can be transmitted through sharing of body fluids. *Molluscum contagiosum* is a pox virus spread through skin-to-skin contact and, in adults, is most often seen on the genitals, upper thighs, and abdomen with sexual transmission (**Figure 18-8**).[136]

Parasites commonly seen in primary care can also be transmitted sexually. Scabies mites (**Figure 18-9**) can be easily transmitted through

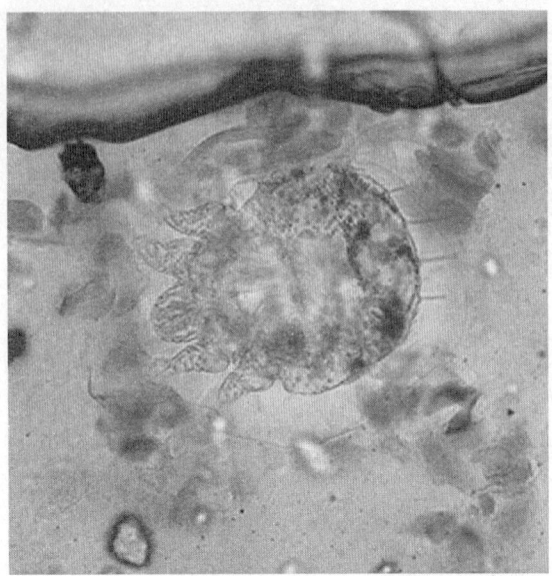

**Figure 18-9** Scabies.
Courtesy of Centers for Disease Control and Prevention. https://www.cdc.gov/dpdx/scabies/index.html. Accessed October 21, 2022.

close genital contact; a papular rash with itching can be found in the webbing between fingers and on the wrist, buttocks, elbows, knees, breast, and shoulder blades. Permethrin and ivermectin are first-line treatments for all adults, although permethrin is preferred for pregnant and lactating individuals.[5] The scabies-related itching and rash typically persist for as long as 2 weeks, but treatment failures are common due to inadequate treatment or resistance.[5] Alternative treatment regimens may be needed for resistant cases.

Intestinal infections and parasites, such as shigellosis and *Giardia*, can be transmitted sexually, especially when there is contact with the anus or mouth. The CDC provides excellent resources for treatment of individuals with these and other infectious conditions and provides guidance on the need for sexual-partner and household-contact treatment for conditions spread through sexual or close physical contact. Selected conditions that can be transmitted through sexual contact are described in Table 18-22.

| **Table 18-22** | **Selected Parasitic Infections Spread by Sexual Contact** | | | |
|---|---|---|---|---|
| **Parasitic Infection** | **Symptoms** | **Physical Examination** | **Treatment** | **Follow-Up** |
| Scabies (*Sarcoptes scabiei*) | Severe itching of the groin, between fingers, and in body folds. Itching is bilateral and often occurs more at night. | Excoriations surrounding papules, consisting of small linear or curved burrows, may be present. Definitive diagnosis is based on microscopic visualization of the mite obtained from skin scrapings. Secondary infections are common. | Permethrin 5% applied to the body from the neck down and washed off after 8–14 hours (safe during pregnancy and lactation) OR Ivermectin (Stromectol) 200 mcg/kg orally, repeated in 14 days (This treatment is preferred for outbreaks at residential facilities.) Household linens need to be dried using the hot setting or isolated for 72 hours. | Itching may persist for 2–4 weeks. If treatment fails, lindane is recommended as a second treatment in otherwise well, nonpregnant and nonlactating persons. |
| *Molluscum contagiosum* | Lesions can be found on any part of the body. With sexual transmission, they are more common on the legs, abdomen, and genital area. | Multiple 2- to 5-mm, shiny white or flesh-colored papules with an indented (umbilicated) center. A thick white discharge can be expressed from the center of the lesion. Large and extensive lesions are more common in HIV-positive adults. | Symptoms are usually self-limiting and resolve without scarring in more than 90% of otherwise healthy adults. Treatments are not usually recommended but can decrease the spread of the infection. Treatments include cryotherapy, excision, oral cimetidine, and topical creams. Transmission can be decreased by covering lesions and not sharing towels or clothing. | None needed; lesions usually heal within 6–12 months. |

Abbreviation: HIV, human immunodeficiency virus.

Workowski KA, Bachmann LH, Chan PA, et al. Sexually transmitted infections treatment guidelines, 2021. *MMWR Recomm Rep.* 2021;70(4):1-187. doi:10.15585/mmwr.rr7004a1.

| Table 18-23 | Diagnoses That May Mimic Sexually Transmitted Infections That Are Not Sexually Transmitted | | |
|---|---|---|---|
| **Diagnosis** | **Presenting Concerns and History** | **Physical Examination** | **Treatment Generic (Brand)** |
| Chiggers (*Trombicula* mite bites) | Severe itching usually 3–24 hours after outdoor activity in hot, humid weather. | Small, grouped, excoriated papules along the panty line or in the folds of the groin, often found along a line of clothing constriction. | Irritation is self-limiting. Topical antihistamines and corticosteroids may provide relief. Oral antihistamines can be used in severe cases. |
| Herpes zoster ("shingles") | Open lesions that are painful superficially and have a deeper nerve pain component. Often occurs in elderly or immunosuppressed persons assigned female at birth. Approximately 10–15% of affected individuals will have postherpetic neuralgia following an initial outbreak. | Painful papules, or vesicles that rupture and crust over. Lesions may be in various stages of forming and healing. Found on the L5 and S1 dermatomes. Indistinguishable from herpes by examination. Serologic tests will be negative for HSV infection. | Treatment within 72 hours is ideal to decrease incidence of postherpetic neuralgia:<br>• Acyclovir (Zovirax) 800 mg, 5 times a day<br>• Famciclovir (Famvir) 500 mg, 3 times a day<br>• Valacyclovir (Valtrex) 100 mg, 3 times a day<br>• Appropriate pain control medications<br>Lesions are contagious via the air and physical contact, and can cause varicella in previously uninfected individuals. Covering the lesions reduces transmission risk. |

Abbreviation: HSV, herpes simplex virus.

## Infections That Mimic Sexually Transmitted Infections in Genital Areas

Many primary care conditions produce symptoms in the groin region that can mimic STIs. For example, herpes zoster (commonly known as shingles) looks identical to HSV, except that the lesions occur along one or more dermatomes. *Trombica* mite bites, commonly known as chiggers, cause itchy, uncomfortable lesions in the groin that may be a presenting concern. Other conditions, such as tinea cruris and other forms of dermatitis, can manifest on and around the vulva. While targeting the examination to the patient's chief concern, the clinician should not prematurely rule out a primary care diagnosis that may have genital manifestations. Table 18-23 lists some conditions that are not STIs, but may appear as such and should be considered in a differential diagnosis.

## Resources

| Organization | Description |
|---|---|
| **Sexually Transmitted Infections** | |
| Centers for Disease Control and Prevention (CDC) | 2021 sexually transmitted infection treatment guidelines. |
| | Laboratory reporting of pregnancy status for hepatitis B–positive pregnant persons. |
| | HIV risk reduction tool. This tool allows individuals to explore their risk in detail and learn about risk-reduction strategies. |
| U.S. Library of Medicine: Medline Plus | This website includes resources for consumers and providers on diagnosis and treatment of STIs. |

| Organization | Description |
|---|---|
| **Postexposure Prophylaxis and Occupational Exposure** | |
| Clinician Consultation Center (CCC) | Postexposure prophylaxis (PEPline). Website provides clinician consultation and expert guidance for managing healthcare-related exposure to HIV. |
| Centers for Disease Control and Prevention (CDC) | Guidelines for occupational postexposure prophylaxis. |
| **Zika Virus** | |
| Centers for Disease Control and Prevention (CDC) | Information for healthcare providers about screening and testing for Zika virus. Includes considerations for healthcare workers and occupational exposure. |
| ZikaCare Connect | In collaboration with the March of Dimes, this website provides resources and referrals to healthcare providers who are actively involved in caring for persons exposed to Zika virus during pregnancy. |
| **Apps** | |
| Centers for Disease Control and Prevention (CDC) | 2015 sexually transmitted infection treatment guidelines. |
| Agency for Healthcare Research and Quality (AHRQ) | ePSS is a mobile app that allows the user to find U.S. Preventive Services Task Force recommendations for screening and treatment. |

## References

1. United Nations Population Fund. Sexual & reproductive health. https://www.unfpa.org/sexual-reproductive-health. Published 2022. Accessed April 21, 2022.

2. World Health Organization. Sexually transmitted infections (STIs). https://www.who.int/news-room/fact-sheets/detail/sexually-transmitted-infections-(stis)#:~:text=STIs%20have%20a%20profound%20impact,and%20trichomoniasis%20(156%20million). Published 2022. Accessed April 21, 2022.

3. Office of Disease Prevention and Health Promotion. Sexually transmitted infections. https://health.gov/healthypeople/objectives-and-data/browse-objectives/sexually-transmitted-infections. Accessed April 21, 2022.

4. Weinstock HS, Kreisel KM, Spicknall IH, et al. STI prevalence, incidence, and costs in the United States: new estimates, new approach. *Sex Transm Dis.* 2021;48(4):207. doi:10.1097/olq.0000000000001368.

5. Workowski KA, Bachmann LH, Chan PA, et al. Sexually transmitted infections treatment guidelines, 2021. *MMWR Recomm Rep.* 2021;70(4):1-187. doi:10.15585/mmwr.rr7004a1.

6. Wi T, Lahra MM, Ndowa F, et al. Antimicrobial resistance in *Neisseria gonorrhoeae*: global surveillance and a call for international collaborative action. *PLoS Med.* 2017;14(7):e1002344. doi:10.1371/journal.pmed.1002344.

7. Garcia PJ, Miranda AE, Gupta S, et al. The role of sexually transmitted infections (STI) prevention and control programs in reducing gender, sexual and STI-related stigma. *EClinicalMedicine.* 2021;33: 100764. doi:10.1016/j.eclinm.2021.100764.

8. Centers for Disease Control and Prevention. STD health equity. https://www.cdc.gov/std/health-disparities/default.htm. Accessed April 23, 2022,

9. Sales JM, Newton-Levinson A, Swartzendruber AL. Racial disparities in STIs among adolescents in the USA. In: Hussen SA, ed. *Sexually Transmitted Infections in Adolescence and Young Adulthood: A Practical Guide for Clinicians.* Cham, Switzerland: Springer International Publishing; 2020:31-42.

10. Bajaj SS, Stanford FC. Beyond Tuskegee: vaccine distrust and everyday racism. *N Engl J Med.* 2021;384(5):e12. doi:10.1056/NEJMpv2035827.

11. Andrasik M, Broder G, Oseso L, et al. Stigma, implicit bias, and long-lasting prevention interventions to end the domestic HIV/AIDS epidemic. *Am J Public Health.* 2020;110(1):67-68. doi:10.2105/ajph.2019.305454.

12. McDowell MJ, Goldhammer H, Potter JE, Keuroghlian AS. Strategies to mitigate clinician implicit bias against sexual and gender minority patients. *Psychosomatics.* 2020;61(6):655-661. doi:10.1016/j.psym.2020.04.021.

13. Bailey ZD, Feldman JM, Bassett MT. How structural racism works: racist policies as a root cause of U.S. racial health inequities. *N Engl J Med.* 2021;384(8): 768-773. doi:10.1056/NEJMms2025396.

14. Centers for Disease Control and Prevention. A guide to taking a sexual history. https://www.cdc.gov/std

/treatment/sexualhistory.htm. Updated January 14, 2022. Accessed April 21, 2022.

15. Murina PF, Graziottin A, Bagot O, et al. Real-world practices and attitudes towards intimate self- care: results from an international women's survey. *J Gynecol Obstet Hum Reprod*. 2021;50(10):102192. https://doi.org/10.1016/j.jogoh.2021.102192.

16. Hamlin AA, Sheeder J, Muffly TM. Brief versus Thong Hygiene in Obstetrics and Gynecology (B-THONG): a survey study. *J Obstet Gynaecol Res*. 2019;45(6):1190-1196.

17. Banga L. The microbiota of the vulva and vagina: ways of washing to optimise the protective function of the vulvo-vaginal microbiota during pregnancy. *N Z Coll Midwives J*. 2021;57:34-40.

18. Stenson AL, Leclair C. To shave or not to shave? A series of periclitoral masses associated with depilatory techniques and a review of the literature. *J Low Genit Tract Dis*. 2018;22(4):412-414.

19. Grimstad F, McLaren H, Gray M. The gynecologic examination of the transfeminine person after penile inversion vaginoplasty. *Am J Obstet Gynecol*. 2021;224(3):266-273.

20. University of California San Francisco. Guidelines for the primary and gender-affirming care of transgender and non-binary people. https://transcare.ucsf.edu/guidelines. Published June 17, 2016. Accessed April 27, 2022.

21. Wodwaski N, Munyan K. Self-care promotion of the intact (non-circumcised) patient: a review of available recommendations. *J Spec Pediatr Nurs*. 2020;25(4):e12297.

22. Muzny CA, Taylor CM, Swords WE, et al. An updated conceptual model on the pathogenesis of bacterial vaginosis. *J Infect Dis*. 2019;220(9):1399-1405.

23. Dabee S, Passmore J-AS, Heffron R, et al. The complex link between the female genital microbiota, genital infections, and inflammation. *Infect Immun*. 2021;89(5):e00487-20. doi:10.1128/IAI.00487-20.

24. Coudray MS, Madhivanan P. Bacterial vaginosis: a brief synopsis of the literature. *Eur J Obstet Gynecol Reprod Biol*. 2020;245:143-148.

25. Schwebke JR, Hillier SL, Sobel JD, et al. Validity of the vaginal Gram stain for the diagnosis of bacterial vaginosis. *Obstet Gynecol*. 1996;88(4 pt 1):573-576. https://doi.org/10.1016/0029-7844(96)00233-5.

26. LabCorp. Bacterial vaginosis, NAA. https://www.labcorp.com/tests/180060/bacterial-vaginosis-naa. Accessed August 24, 2022.

27. National Library of Medicine. Drugs and Lactation Database (LactMed). https://www.ncbi.nlm.nih.gov/books/NBK501922/. Accessed April 15, 2023.

28. Li C, Wang T, Li Y, et al. Probiotics for the treatment of women with bacterial vaginosis: a systematic review and meta-analysis of randomized clinical trials. *Eur J Pharmacol*. 2019;864:172660.

29. Denning DW, Kneale M, Sobel JD, Rautemaa-Richardson R. Global burden of recurrent vulvovaginal candidiasis: a systematic review. *Lancet Infect Dis*. 2018;18(11):e339-e347.

30. Buggio L, Somigliana E, Borghi A, Vercellini P. Probiotics and vaginal microecology: fact or fancy? *BMC Womens Health*. 2019;19(1):1-6.

31. Felix TC, de Brito Röder DVD, dos Santos Pedroso R. Alternative and complementary therapies for vulvovaginal candidiasis. *Folia Microbiol (Praha)*. 2019; 64(2):133-141.

32. Neal CM, Kus LH, Eckert LO, Peipert JF. Noncandidal vaginitis: a comprehensive approach to diagnosis and management. *Am J Obstet Gynecol*. 2020; 222(2):114-122.

33. ACOG Practice Bulletin No. 141: management of menopausal symptoms. *Obstet Gynecol*. 2014; 123(1):202-216. doi:10.1097/01.Aog.0000441353.20693.78.

34. Rioux JE, Devlin MC, Gelfand MM, et al. 17β-Estradiol vaginal tablet versus conjugated equine estrogen vaginal cream to relieve menopausal atrophic vaginitis. *Menopause*. 2018;25(11):1208-1213.

35. Crandall CJ. Treatment of vulvovaginal atrophy. *JAMA*. 2019;322(19):1910-1911.

36. Bachmann GA, Komi JO, Group OS. Ospemifene effectively treats vulvovaginal atrophy in postmenopausal women: results from a pivotal phase 3 study. *Menopause*. 2010;17(3):480-486.

37. Labrie F, Archer D, Bouchard C, et al. Intravaginal dehydroepiandrosterone (Prasterone), a physiological and highly efficient treatment of vaginal atrophy. *Menopause*. 2009;16(5):907-922.

38. Domachowske J, Suryadevara M. Prostatitis, epididymitis, orchitis. In: *Clinical Infectious Diseases Study Guide: A Problem-Based Approach*. Cham, Switzerland: Springer International Publishing; 2020: 149-153.

39. Wray AA, Velasquez J, Khetarpal S. *Balanitis*. Treasure Island, FL: StatPearls Publishing; 2021.

40. Centers for Disease Control and Prevention. What is case surveillance? https://www.cdc.gov/nndss/about/index.html. Accessed April 21, 2022.

41. The Ryan White Care Act: implementation of the spousal notification requirement (1999). https://oig.hhs.gov/oei/reports/oei-05-98-00391.pdf.

42. American College of Nurse-Midwives. Definition of midwifery and scope of practice of certified nurse-midwives and certified midwives. http://www.midwife.org/acnm/files/acnmlibrarydata/uploadfilename/000000000266/Definition%20Midwifery%20Scope%20of%20Practice_2021.pdf. Accessed April 21, 2022.

43. Nelson T, Nandwani J, Johnson D. Gonorrhea and chlamydia cases are rising in the United States: expedited partner therapy might help. *Sex Transm Dis.* 2022;49(1):e1-e3.

44. Centers for Disease Control and Prevention. Expedited partner therapy in the management of sexually transmitted diseases: review and guidance. https://www.cdc.gov/std/treatment/eptfinalreport2006.pdf. Accessed April 21, 2022.

45. Centers for Disease Control and Prevention. Legal status of expedited partner therapy (EPT). https://www.cdc.gov/std/ept/legal/default.htm. Accessed April 21, 2022.

46. American College of Nurse-Midwives. ACNM core competencies for midwifery practice. http://www.midwife.org/acnm/files/acnmlibrarydata/uploadfilename/000000000050/ACNMCoreCompetenciesMar2020_final.pdf. Accessed April 21, 2022.

47. Centers for Disease Control and Prevention. About NCHHSTP AtlasPlus. https://www.cdc.gov/nchhstp/atlas/about-atlas.html. Accessed April 21, 2022.

48. Centers for Disease Control and Prevention. Chlamydia: reported cases and rates of reported cases by age group and sex, United States, 2017–2021. https://www.cdc.gov/std/statistics/2021/tables/4.htm. Updated April 12, 2022. Accessed April 22, 2022.

49. Centers for Disease Control and Prevention. Sexually transmitted disease: adolescents and young adults. https://www.cdc.gov/std/life-stages-populations/adolescents-youngadults.htm. Accessed April 22, 2022.

50. Kouyoumdjian FG, Leto D, John S, et al. A systematic review and meta-analysis of the prevalence of chlamydia, gonorrhoea and syphilis in incarcerated persons. *Int J STD AIDS.* 2012;23(4):248-254. doi:10.1258/ijsa.2011.011194.

51. Tromble E, Bachmann L. Screening and treatment of chlamydia, gonorrhea, and syphilis in correctional settings. In: Greifinger RB, ed. *Public Health Behind Bars: From Prisons to Communities.* New York, NY: Springer US; 2022:195-205.

52. Dovydaitis T. Human trafficking: the role of the health care provider. *J Midwifery Womens Health.* 2010;55(5):462-467. https://doi.org/10.1016/j.jmwh.2009.12.017.

53. Garrett NJ, Osman F, Maharaj B, et al. Beyond syndromic management: opportunities for diagnosis-based treatment of sexually transmitted infections in low-and middle-income countries. *PLoS One.* 2018;13(4):e0196209.

54. Deshpande NA, Nour NM. Sex trafficking of women and girls. *Rev Obstet Gynecol.* 2013;6(1):e22.

55. American College of Obstetricians and Gynecologists. Executive summary: collaboration in practice: implementing team-based care: report of the American College of Obstetricians and Gynecologists' Task Force on Collaborative Practice. *Obstet Gynecol.* 2016;127(3):612-617. doi:10.1097/aog.0000000000001304.

56. Centers for Disease Control and Prevention. Sexually transmitted disease surveillance 2021. https://www.cdc.gov/std/statistics/2021/default.htm. Accessed August 24, 2022.

57. Schlanger K, Kirkcaldy RD. Rising to meet the programmatic public health challenges of emerging *Neisseria gonorrhoeae* antimicrobial resistance: strengthening the United States response to resistant gonorrhea. *Sex Transm Dis.* 2021;48(12S): S91-S92.

58. Savaris RF, Fuhrich DG, Maissiat J, et al. Antibiotic therapy for pelvic inflammatory disease. *Cochrane Database Syst Rev.* 2020;8(8):Cd010285. doi:10.1002/14651858.CD010285.pub3.

59. Levin G, Dior UP, Gilad R, et al. Pelvic inflammatory disease among users and non-users of an intrauterine device. *J Obstet Gynaecol.* 2021;41(1):118-123.

60. Ravel J, Moreno I, Simón C. Bacterial vaginosis and its association with infertility, endometritis, and pelvic inflammatory disease. *Am J Obstet Gynecol.* 2021; 224(3):251-257.

61. Centers for Disease Control and Prevention. Syphilis: CDC detailed fact sheet. https://www.cdc.gov/std/syphilis/stdfact-syphilis-detailed.htm. Accessed April 23, 2022.

62. World Health Organization. World Health Organization treatment guidelines for *Treponema pallidum* (syphilis). https://www.who.int/publications/i/item/9789241549714. Accessed April 23, 2022.

63. Ghanem KG, Ram S, Rice PA. The modern epidemic of syphilis. *N Engl J Med.* 2020;382(9):845-854.

64. Butler T. The Jarisch–Herxheimer reaction after antibiotic treatment of spirochetal infections: a review of recent cases and our understanding of pathogenesis. *Am J Trop Med Hygiene.* 2017;96(1):46.

65. Rac MW, Revell PA, Eppes CS. Syphilis during pregnancy: a preventable threat to maternal–fetal health. *Am J Obstet Gynecol.* 2017;216(4):352-363.

66. Furness A, Kalicinsky C, Rosenfield L, et al. Penicillin skin testing, challenge, and desensitization in pregnancy: a systematic review. *J Obstet Gynaecol Can.* 2020;42(10):1254-1261.

67. Centers for Disease Control and Prevention. Table 1. Sexually transmitted diseases—reported cases and rates of reported cases, United States, 1941–2020. https://www.cdc.gov/std/statistics/2021/tables/1.htm. Accessed April 23, 2022.

68. Rawla P, Thandra KC, Limaiem F. Lymphogranuloma venereum. In: *StatPearls.* Treasure Island, FL: StatPearls Publishing; 2021. https://www.ncbi.nlm.nih.gov/books/NBK537362.

69. You E, Henry M, Zeitouni A. Human papillomavirus–associated oropharyngeal cancer: review of current evidence and management. *Curr Oncol*. 2019;26(2):119-123.

70. Nagelhout G, Ebisch RM, Van Der Hel O, et al. Is smoking an independent risk factor for developing cervical intra-epithelial neoplasia and cervical cancer? A systematic review and meta-analysis. *Expert Rev Anticancer Ther*. 2021;21(7):781-794.

71. Chen SY, Massa S, Mazul AL, et al. The association of smoking and outcomes in HPV-positive oropharyngeal cancer: a systematic review. *Am J Otolaryngol*. 2020;41(5):102592.

72. Laprise C, Madathil SA, Schlecht NF, et al. Increased risk of oropharyngeal cancers mediated by oral human papillomavirus infection: results from a Canadian study. *Head Neck*. 2019;41(3):678-685.

73. Reinholdt K, Munk C, Thomsen LT, et al. Increased incidence of genital warts among women and men with type 1 diabetes compared with the general population: results from a nationwide registry-based, cohort study. *Acta Diabetol*. 2022;59(1):105-112. doi:10.1007/s00592-021-01786-8.

74. Singh P, Zumpf KB, Liszewski W. Rates of genital warts after the age of 26: an analysis of the National Health and Nutrition Examination Survey. *Int J Womens Dermatol*. 2020;6(5):429-430. doi:10.1016/j.ijwd.2020.06.003.

75. Saslow D, Andrews KS, Manassaram-Baptiste D, et al. Human papillomavirus vaccination 2020 guideline update: American Cancer Society guideline adaptation. *CA Cancer J Clin*. 2020;70(4):274-280.

76. Harrison R, Huh W. Occupational exposure to human papillomavirus and vaccination for health care workers. *Obstet Gynecol*. 2020;136(4):663-665.

77. Shah KV. A case for immunization of human papillomavirus (HPV) 6/11–infected pregnant women with the quadrivalent HPV vaccine to prevent juvenile-onset laryngeal papilloma. *J Infect Dis*. 2014;209(9):1307-1309.

78. van der Sluis WB, Buncamper ME, Bouman M-B, et al. Symptomatic HPV-related neovaginal lesions in transgender women: case series and review of literature. *Sex Transm Infect*. 2016;92(7):499-501.

79. Matsuki S, Kusatake K, Hein KZ, et al. Condylomata acuminata in the neovagina after male-to-female reassignment treated with $CO_2$ laser and imiquimod. *Int J STD AIDS*. 2015;26(7):509-511.

80. McQuillan GM, Kruszon-Moran D, Flagg EW, Paulose-Ram R. Prevalence of herpes simplex virus type 1 and type 2 in persons aged 14–49: United States, 2015–2016. *NCHS Data Brief*. 2018;(304):1-8.

81. Management of genital herpes in pregnancy: ACOG Practice Bulletin Summary, Number 220. *Obstet Gynecol*. 2020;135(5):1236-1238. https://doi.org/10.1097/AOG.0000000000003841.

82. Chi CC, Wang SH, Delamere FM, et al. Interventions for prevention of herpes simplex labialis (cold sores on the lips). *Cochrane Database Syst Rev*. 2015;8. CD010095. Published 2015 Aug 7. doi:10.1002/14651858.CD010095.pub2.

83. Perfect MM, Bourne N, Ebel C, Rosenthal SL. Use of complementary and alternative medicine for the treatment of genital herpes. *Herpes (Cambr)*. 2005;12(2):38.

84. Pinninti SG, Kimberlin DW. Neonatal herpes simplex virus infections. 2018:168-175. doi:10.1053/j.semperi.2018.02.004.

85. Centers for Disease Control and Prevention. Neonatal herpes simplex virus infection following Jewish ritual circumcisions that included direct orogenital suction—New York City, 2000–2011. *MMWR*. 2012;61(22):405-409.

86. Cogan R, Spinnato JA. Social support during premature labor: effects on labor and the newborn. *J Psychosomat Obstet & Gynecol*. 1988;8(3):209-216.

87. World Health Organization. Hepatitis B. https://www.who.int/news-room/fact-sheets/detail/hepatitis-b. Published June 24, 2022. Accessed April 15, 2023.

88. Roberts H, Ly KN, Yin S, et al. Prevalence of HBV infection, vaccine-induced immunity, and susceptibility among at-risk populations: US households, 2013–2018. *Hepatology*. 2021;74(5):2353-2365.

89. Kruszon-Moran D, Paulose-Ram R, Martin CB, et al. Prevalence and trends in hepatitis B virus infection in the United States, 2015–2018. *NCHS Data Brief*. 2020;(361):1-8.

90. Kushner T, Chen Z, Tressler S, et al. Trends in hepatitis B infection and immunity among women of childbearing age in the United States. *Clin Infect Dis*. 2020;71(3):586-592.

91. Terrault NA, Lok AS, McMahon BJ, et al. Update on prevention, diagnosis, and treatment of chronic hepatitis B: AASLD 2018 hepatitis B guidance. *Hepatology*. 2018;67(4):1560-1599.

92. World Health Organization. *Global Health Sector Strategy on Viral Hepatitis 2016–2021: Towards Ending Viral Hepatitis*. Geneva, Switzerland: World Health Organization; 2016.

93. Song JE. Diagnosis of hepatitis B. *Ann Transl Med*. 2016;4(18). doi:10.21037/atm.2016.09.11.

94. Weinbaum CM, Williams I, Mast EE, et al. Recommendations for identification and public health management of persons with chronic hepatitis B virus infection. *Hepatology*. 2009;49(5 Suppl):S35-S44. doi:10.1002/hep.22882.

95. Owens DK, Davidson KW, Krist AH, et al. Screening for hepatitis B virus infection in pregnant women: US Preventive Services Task Force reaffirmation recommendation statement. *JAMA*. 2019;322(4):349-354.

96. Schillie S, Vellozzi C, Reingold A, et al. Prevention of hepatitis B virus infection in the United States: recommendations of the Advisory Committee on Immunization Practices. *MMWR Recomm Rep*. 2018; 67(1):1.

97. [Profile. Mrs. Masako Okumura: an experience in natural childbirth by Bradley's method and cooperation by her husband]. *Kangogaku Zasshi*. 1979; 43(5):545.

98. Byington CL, Maldonado YA, Barnett ED, et al. Elimination of perinatal hepatitis B: providing the first vaccine dose within 24 hours of birth. *Pediatrics*. 2017;140(3). doi:10.1542/peds.2017-1870.

99. Kilpatrick SJ. *Guidelines for Perinatal Care*. Elk Grove Village, IL: American Academy of Pediatrics; 2017.

100. Ryerson AB, Schillie S, Barker LK, et al. Vital signs: newly reported acute and chronic hepatitis C cases—United States, 2009–2018. *MMWR*. 2020;69(14):399.

101. Hofmeister MG, Rosenthal EM, Barker LK, et al. Estimating prevalence of hepatitis C virus infection in the United States, 2013–2016. *Hepatology*. 2019;69(3):1020-1031.

102. Centers for Disease Control and Prevention. Viral hepatitis surveillance report 2019: hepatitis C. https://www.cdc.gov/hepatitis/statistics/2019surveillance/HepC.htm. Accessed April 24, 2022.

103. Koneru A, Nelson N, Hariri S, et al. Increased hepatitis C virus (HCV) detection in women of childbearing age and potential risk for vertical transmission—United States and Kentucky, 2011–2014. *MMWR*. 2016;65(28):705-710.

104. Chou R, Dana T, Grusing S, Bougatsos C. Screening for HIV infection in asymptomatic, nonpregnant adolescents and adults: updated evidence report and systematic review for the US Preventive Services Task Force. *JAMA*. 2019;321(23):2337-2348.

105. Centers for Disease Control and Prevention. HIV and African American people. https://www.cdc.gov/hiv/group/racialethnic/africanamericans/index.html. Last reviewed February 16, 2023. Accessed April 15, 2023.

106. Chou R, Evans C, Hoverman A, et al. Preexposure prophylaxis for the prevention of HIV infection: evidence report and systematic review for the US Preventive Services Task Force. *JAMA*. 2019; 321(22):2214-2230.

107. Centers for Disease Control and Prevention. Preexposure prophylaxis for the prevention of HIV Infection in the US: 2021 update clinical practice guideline. https://www.cdc.gov/hiv/pdf/risk/prep/cdc-hiv-prep-guidelines-2021.pdf. Accessed April 26, 2022.

108. Baugher AR, Trujillo L, Kanny D, et al. Racial, ethnic, and gender disparities in awareness of preexposure prophylaxis among HIV-negative heterosexually active adults at increased risk for hiv infection—23 urban areas, United States, 2019. *MMWR*. 2021;70(47):1635.

109. Tepper NK, Curtis KM, Cox S, Whiteman MK. Update to US medical eligibility criteria for contraceptive use, 2016: updated recommendations for the use of contraception among women at high risk for HIV infection. *MMWR*. 2020;69(14):405.

110. Riddell J, Amico KR, Mayer KH. HIV preexposure prophylaxis: a review. *JAMA*. 2018;319(12): 1261-1268.

111. Joseph Davey DL, Pintye J, Baeten JM, et al. Emerging evidence from a systematic review of safety of pre-exposure prophylaxis for pregnant and postpartum women: where are we now and where are we heading? *J Int AIDS Soc*. 2020;23(1):e25426.

112. Kuhar DT, Henderson DK, Struble KA, et al. Updated U.S. Public Health Service Guidelines for the Management of Occupational Exposures to HIV and Recommendations for Postexposure Prophylaxis [Pamphlet 25/2013]. Updated May 23, 2018.

113. Dominguez KL, Smith DK, Vasavi T, et al. Updated guidelines for antiretroviral postexposure prophylaxis after sexual, injection drug use, or other nonoccupational exposure to HIV—United States, 2016. https://www.cdc.gov/hiv/pdf/programresources/cdc-hiv-npep-guidelines.pdf.

114. Branson BM, Owen SM, Wesolowski LG, et al. Laboratory testing for the diagnosis of HIV infection: updated recommendations. 2014. https://stacks.cdc.gov/view/cdc/23447.

115. Centers for Disease Control and Prevention. An Opt-Out Approach to HIV Screening. https://www.cdc.gov/hiv/group/gender/pregnantwomen/opt-out.html. Accessed April 26, 2022.

116. Dooley SW, Dubose OT, Fletcher JF, et al. Recommendations for partner services programs for HIV infection, syphilis, gonorrhea, and chlamydial infection. *MMWR Recomm Rep*. 2008;57(RR-9): 1-CE4.

117. Curry SJ, Krist AH, Owens DK, et al. Screening for intimate partner violence, elder abuse, and abuse of vulnerable adults: US Preventive Services Task Force final recommendation statement. *JAMA*. 2018; 320(16):1678-1687.

118. Centers for Disease Control and Prevention. Guidelines for the use of antiretroviral agents in adults and adolescents living with HIV. https://clinicalinfo.hiv.gov/en/guidelines/adult-and-adolescent-arv/whats-new-guidelines. Accessed April 26, 2022.

119. Wilkinson D, Ramjee G, Tholandi M, Rutherford G. Nonoxynol-9 for preventing vaginal acquisition of HIV infection by women from men. *Cochrane Database Syst Rev*. 2002;4:Cd003936. doi:10.1002/14651858.Cd003936.

120. Anderson LM, Adeney KL, Shinn C, et al. Community coalition-driven interventions to reduce health disparities among racial and ethnic minority populations. *Cochrane Database Syst Rev*. 2015;6: Cd009905. doi:10.1002/14651858.CD009905.pub2.

121. Centers for Disease Control and Prevention. Recommendations for the use of antiretroviral drugs during pregnancy and interventions to reduce perinatal HIV transmission in the United States. https://clinicalinfo.hiv.gov/en/guidelines/perinatal/whats-new-guidelines. Accessed April 26, 2022.

122. Calvert C, Ronsmans C. The contribution of HIV to pregnancy-related mortality: a systematic review and meta-analysis. *AIDS*. 2013;27(10):1631.

123. American College of Nurse-Midwives. Standards for the practice of midwifery. https://www.midwife.org/acnm/files/ACNMLibraryData/UPLOADFILENAME/000000000051/Standards_for_Practice_of_Midwifery_Sept_2011.pdf. Accessed April 26, 2022.

124. World Health Organization. *Updates on HIV and Infant Feeding*. Geneva, Switzerland: World Health Organization; 2016.

125. Baud D, Gubler DJ, Schaub B, et al. An update on Zika virus infection. *Lancet*. 2017;390(10107): 2099-2109.

126. Roth NM, Reynolds MR, Lewis EL, et al. Zika-associated birth defects reported in pregnancies with laboratory evidence of confirmed or possible Zika virus infection—US Zika Pregnancy and Infant Registry, December 1, 2015–March 31, 2018. *MMWR*. 2022;71(3):73.

127. Centers for Disease Control and Prevention. Zika and pregnancy: couples trying to conceive. https://www.cdc.gov/pregnancy/zika/testing-follow-up/couples-trying-to-conceive.html. Accessed April 26, 2022.

128. Centers for Disease Control and Prevention. Clinical guidance for healthcare providers for prevention of sexual transmission of Zika virus. https://www.cdc.gov/zika/hc-providers/clinical-guidance/sexual transmission.html. Accessed April 26, 2022.

129. Zorrilla CD, Mosquera AM, Rabionet S, Rivera-Viñas J. HIV and Zika in pregnancy: parallel stories and new challenges. *Obstet Gynecol Int J*. 2016;5(6):180. doi:10.15406/ogij.2016.05.00180.

130. Centers for Disease Control and Prevention. Monkeypox in the United States: what clinicians need to know. https://www.cdc.gov/poxvirus/mpox/pdf/What-Clinicians-Need-to-Know-about-mpox-6-21-2022.pdf. Published June 2022. Accessed August 24, 2022.

131. Centers for Disease Control and Prevention. Mpox equity and anti-stigma toolket. https://www.cdc.gov/poxvirus/mpox/resources/toolkits/equity.html?CDC_AA_refVal=https%3A%2F%2Fwww.cdc.gov%2Fpoxvirus%2Fmpox%2Fresources%2Ftoolkits%2Fvaccine-equity.html. Published March 16, 2023. Accessed April 15, 2023.

132. Centers for Disease Control and Prevention. Mpox: signs and symptoms. https://www.cdc.gov/poxvirus/mpox/symptoms/index.html. Updated February 2, 2023. Accessed April 15, 2023.

133. Centers for Disease Control and Prevention. Clinical considerations for mpox in people who are pregnant or breastfeeding. https://www.cdc.gov/poxvirus/mpox/clinicians/pregnancy.html. Published March 27, 2023. Accessed April 15, 2023.

134. Muzny CA, Van Gerwen OT, Kissinger P. Updates in trichomonas treatment including persistent infection and 5-nitroimidazole hypersensitivity. *Curr Opin Infect Dis*. 2020;33(1):73.

135. Ajiji P, Uzunali A, Ripoche E, Vittaz E, Vial T, Maison P. Investigating the efficacy and safety of metronidazole during pregnancy; A systematic review and meta-analysis. *Eur J Obstet Gynecol Reprod Biol*. 2021;11:100128.

136. Meza-Romero R, Navarrete-Dechent C, Downey C. *Molluscum contagiosum*: an update and review of new perspectives in etiology, diagnosis, and treatment. *Clin Cosmet Investig Dermatol*. 2019;12:373.

# IV

P A R T

# Antepartum

CHAPTER

# 19

# Anatomy and Physiology of Pregnancy

KATHLEEN DANHAUSEN AND TEKOA L. KING

## Introduction

Pregnancy is a period of profound anatomic and physiologic change. Not just the reproductive organs are affected—all maternal physiologic systems undergo adaptions to support the developing fetus and maintain maternal homeostasis. A thorough understanding of these changes is an essential foundation for all healthcare providers, including midwives, who care for individuals during pregnancy. This chapter provides an overview of changes in the reproductive organs, the effects of the major hormones of pregnancy, fetal development, maternal physiologic adaptations of pregnancy, and fetopelvic relationships.

## Duration of Pregnancy and Gestational Age Terminology

Fertilization takes place during or shortly after ovulation, which is usually approximately 14 days before the next menstrual period, assuming a 28-day menstrual cycle. A normal pregnancy lasts approximately 266 days (38 weeks) between fertilization and birth.

Pregnant people are not usually aware of the date of fertilization, but they typically do know the date when their last menstrual period started. Thus, historically, a person's due date has been calculated as 40 weeks (280 days) after the first day of their last menstrual period. This translates into 10 lunar months (4 weeks between moon phases) or 9 calendar months (some calendar months include part of a fifth week). When pregnancy dating is counted from the last normal menstrual period, the duration of human pregnancy is approximately 280 days or 40 completed weeks' gestation.

The terms "gestational age" and "weeks' gestation" are used to refer to the number of weeks

subsequent to the last menstrual period. The mean gestational age (i.e., menstrual age) for spontaneous labor in primigravid individuals is 41 weeks from the last menstrual period (287 days), or 40 weeks 3 days (283 days) for the multiparous person.[1] Estimates based on pooled data are consistent with this finding and suggest that the mean duration of pregnancy using menstrual dating is 283 to 284 days. When counting gestation in weeks after the last menstrual period, it is important to remember that the number changes after the week is completed. Therefore 23 5/7 weeks' gestation is 23 completed weeks since the last menstrual period and an additional 5 days. This translates into 21 completed weeks and 5 days since conception.

The field of embryology prefers language referring to "embryonic age," "postconceptional age," or "ovulation age," which more precisely reflects the age of the embryo or fetus. An embryonic age differs from a gestational age by 2 weeks, because fertilization occurs approximately 2 weeks after menses begins. This text generally uses menstrual age to denote gestational age because it is the method of timing the duration of pregnancy most commonly encountered in clinical practice. However, in this chapter, when reviewing information about embryonic development or exposure to teratogenic agents, embryonic age is more specific. Therefore, the method used to denote gestational age of the fetus, postmenstrual or embryonic, is noted to avoid confusion.

### Trimesters

The prenatal period is divided into three trimesters, each consisting of 12 to 13 weeks or 3 calendar months. In practice, the first trimester is considered to be gestational weeks 1 to 12 (12 weeks) because organogenesis is completed at the end of 12 weeks and the risk for spontaneous abortion is significantly reduced at this time. Historically, the second trimester was considered to be gestational weeks 13 to 28 because prior to the introduction of modern neonatal intensive care techniques, 28 weeks' gestation was the lower limit of viability of the fetus. The third trimester extends from weeks 28 to birth.

Fetal maturation is a continuum.[1] Historically, fetal development was considered complete by "term," or 37 weeks 0 days *estimated gestational age* (37.0 weeks EGA). Significant morbidity and mortality are often experienced by infants who are born "preterm" or before 37.0 weeks' gestation, with fetal and infant outcomes improving with increasing gestational age. Term pregnancy is from 37.0 weeks to 41 weeks 6 days (41.6 weeks EGA). A greater number of adverse outcomes are experienced at either end of the term pregnancy continuum, with increased respiratory and other complications occurring more frequently at "early term," or before 39.0 weeks, compared with 39.0 to 40.6 weeks EGA. A greater number of complications also occur at "late term" or between 41.0 and 41.6 weeks, with morbidity and mortality further increasing "post term," or after 42 completed gestational weeks. The definitions of pregnancy dating shown in Table 19-1 are based on neonatal clinical presentation, associated medical complications, and the risks associated with earlier birth throughout gestation.[1]

## Fetal–Maternal Interface: Ontology of the Embryo and Placenta

The processes that make it possible for the single cell that results from the fusion of the ovum and the sperm to develop and mature into a fetus and then a newborn within the course of months are the subject of many fields of study, including genetics, embryology, and fetology. It is beyond the scope of this chapter and this text to cover these topics in detail. Instead, this chapter presents an overview of the knowledge needed by a practicing midwife with regard to the milestones of embryologic and fetal development and the intricate and vulnerable steps that create organs and organ systems. This understanding will help the midwife discuss embryonic and fetal development with the pregnant person and their family and also provides general knowledge regarding the causes of early pregnancy loss, congenital malformations, and health problems that can be experienced by a pregnant person or a fetus in utero.

## Fertilization

Fertilization is the process in which two haploid (containing 23 chromosomes) cells—a sperm and an ovum—fuse to form a diploid (containing 46 chromosomes) cell or zygote. Once a sperm cell binds to receptors on the oocyte membrane, its nucleus is pulled into the cytoplasm of the oocyte and the oocyte membrane depolarizes, causing destruction of other sperm cells. This prevents the binding of other sperm cells and, therefore, polyspermy. Once the sperm enters the ovum, the oocyte, which was arrested in the metaphase of the second meiotic division, completes metaphase. Fertilization occurs as the nuclei of the ovum and the sperm swell, the nuclear membranes disappear, and the chromosomes combine to create the diploid zygote (Figure 19-1).

| Table 19-1 | Clinical Definitions of Fetal Gestational Ages | |
|---|---|---|
| | **Definition** | **Gestational Age Range** |
| **Preterm pregnancy (before 37 weeks' gestation)** | Extremely preterm | Before 28 weeks 0 days |
| | Very preterm | 28 weeks 0 day to 31 weeks 6 days |
| | Moderately preterm | 32 weeks 0 days to 33 weeks 6 days |
| | Late preterm | 34 weeks 0 days to 36 weeks 6 days |
| **Term pregnancy (37–41 6/7 weeks' gestation)** | Early term | 37 weeks 0 days to 38 weeks 6 days |
| | Full term | 39 weeks 0 days to 40 weeks 6 days |
| | Late term | 41 weeks 0 days to 41 weeks 6 days |
| **Post-term pregnancy** | Post term | 42 weeks 0 days and beyond |

Data from Spong CY. Defining "term" pregnancy: recommendations from the Defining "Term" Pregnancy Workgroup. *JAMA.* 2013;309(23):2445–2446. doi:10.1001/jama.2013.6235.

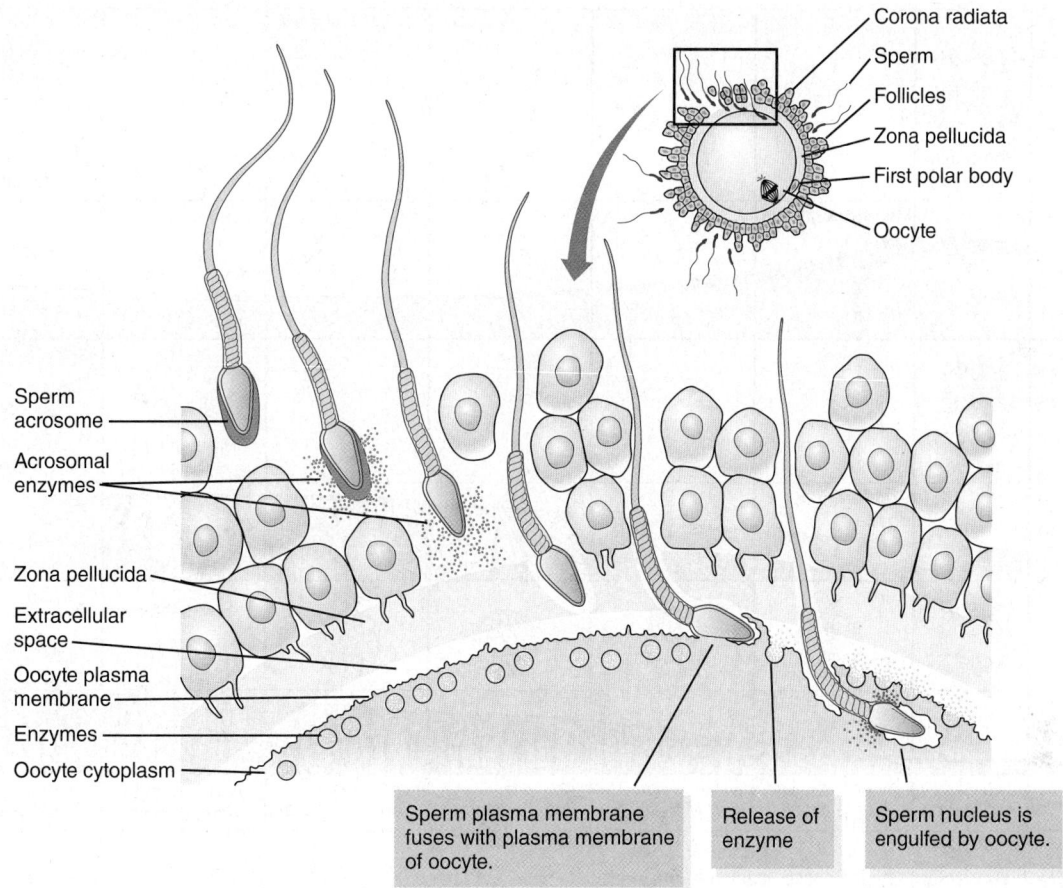

Corona radiata
Sperm
Follicles
Zona pellucida
First polar body
Oocyte

Sperm
acrosome
Acrosomal
enzymes
Zona pellucida
Extracellular
space
Oocyte plasma
membrane
Enzymes
Oocyte cytoplasm

Sperm plasma membrane
fuses with plasma membrane
of oocyte.

Release of
enzyme

Sperm nucleus is
engulfed by oocyte.

**Figure 19-1** The process of fertilization.

Fertilization usually occurs in the oviduct and takes approximately 18 to 24 hours. The fertilized oocyte becomes known as a *zygote*. The zygote begins as a single cell that contains 46 chromosomes: 23 from the ovum and 23 from the sperm. At this stage, the genetic code for that individual is formed. The 23rd pair of chromosomes determines the fetus's genetic sex. The ovum contains only an X chromosome, so the X or Y chromosome that pairs with the maternal X chromosome is donated by the sperm. Genetic patterns of inheritance are discussed in more detail in the *Assessment for Genetic and Fetal Abnormalities* chapter.

### Morula and Blastocyst

As the zygote moves through the oviduct into the uterine cavity, the cells divide rapidly, creating additional cells. These cells, known as blastomeres, are held together by the zona pellucida (an extracellular glycoprotein matrix) and form a solid ball of 12 to 16 cells known as the *morula.*

Approximately 4 days after fertilization, the morula enters the uterus, and a central fluid-filled

cavity forms within this bundle of cells. The zygote is now called a *blastocyst*. The blastocyst is composed of four components: (1) the zona pellucida; (2) an inner cell mass that will become the embryo and amnion; (3) an outer layer of cells called the trophoblast, which are in direct contact with the decidual tissue and will become the placenta and chorion; and (4) a fluid-filled cavity.[2] Figure 19-2 depicts the progression and growth of the zygote as it traverses the oviducts and implants in the uterus).

### Transformation of the Endometrium into the Decidua

The uterus consists of three layers: an inner secretory mucosal layer called the endometrium, which is surrounded by several layers of muscle called the myometrium, and a thin serous outer layer called the perimetrium. The secretory endometrium, which goes through a series of monthly transformations as part of the menstrual cycle, contains columnar epithelium, epithelial cells, nonresident or migratory immune cells, and spiral arteries. Uterine blood vessels branch into smaller vessels as they extend

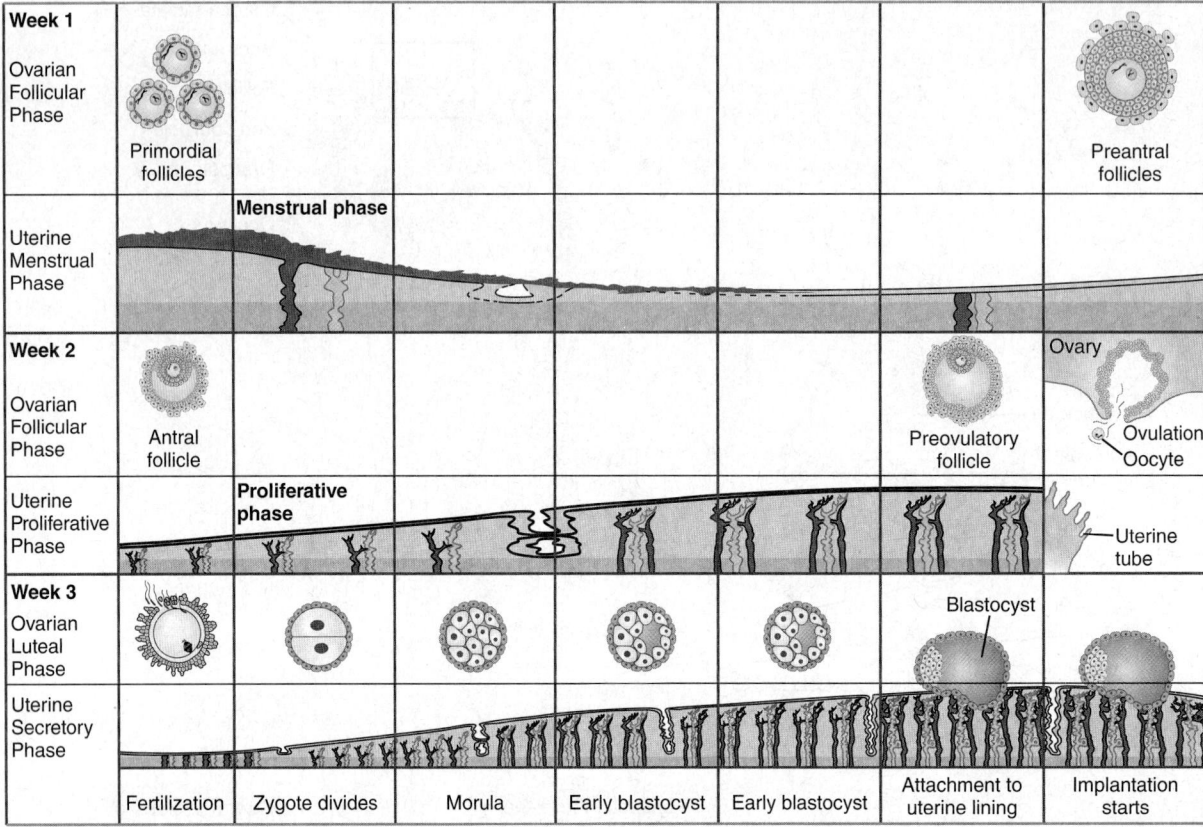

**Figure 19-2** Ovarian and Uterine phases leading to pregnancy are shown including development of the follicle and uterine lining as well as ovulation. Ovulation usually occurs around day 14 and is followed by fertilization, cleavage of the zygote, and implantation of the blastocyst.

through the layers of the uterus: The radial arteries that supply the myometrium branch into basal arteries, which become the spiral arteries that supply part of the myometrium and the endometrium.[3]

The secretory phase of the menstrual cycle first prepares the uterus for implantation, as described in the *Anatomy and Physiology of the Reproductive System* chapter. These changes in the endometrium become more substantial after fertilization, as the uterus prepares for implantation. The endometrial changes that allow and facilitate implantation are collectively termed the *decidual reaction*. The name "decidua" was chosen for this process because, like the leaves on deciduous trees, the transformed tissue is shed after birth.[4]

The decidual reaction, in which endometrial cells differentiate into specialized decidual cells, occurs in response to estrogen, progesterone, and a complex dance or "cross-talk" of locally produced chemicals generated by the blastocyst and maternal endometrium. The decidual cells become part of the synchronized process that prepares the uterine blood vessels for implantation, and they play a key role in

directing trophoblastic cells (which will become the placenta) as these cells grow and move into the endometrium. The decidua also provides nutrition to the embryo in the early stages before the placenta is developed. The portion of the decidua that interacts with the developing placenta is named the *decidua basalis*. It is subdivided into a *zona compacta* and a *zona spongiosa*; the latter is the site of detachment of the placenta in the third stage of labor.

The decidual reaction starts once the blastocyst is present at the endometrial site of implantation. Approximately 8 days after ovulation, the secretory endometrium provides a 4- to 5-day "window of implantation."[5] During this short span of time, the endometrium is optimally prepared for implantation; hence, this time is referred to as the period of *endometrial receptivity*. A surge of chemical "cross-talk" between the decidual cells and blastocyst facilitates adhesion and implantation of the blastocyst. Immune cells congregate, the endometrial glands become more secretory and rich with vacuoles containing the lipids and glycogen needed to nourish an early pregnancy, and the epithelial surface develops

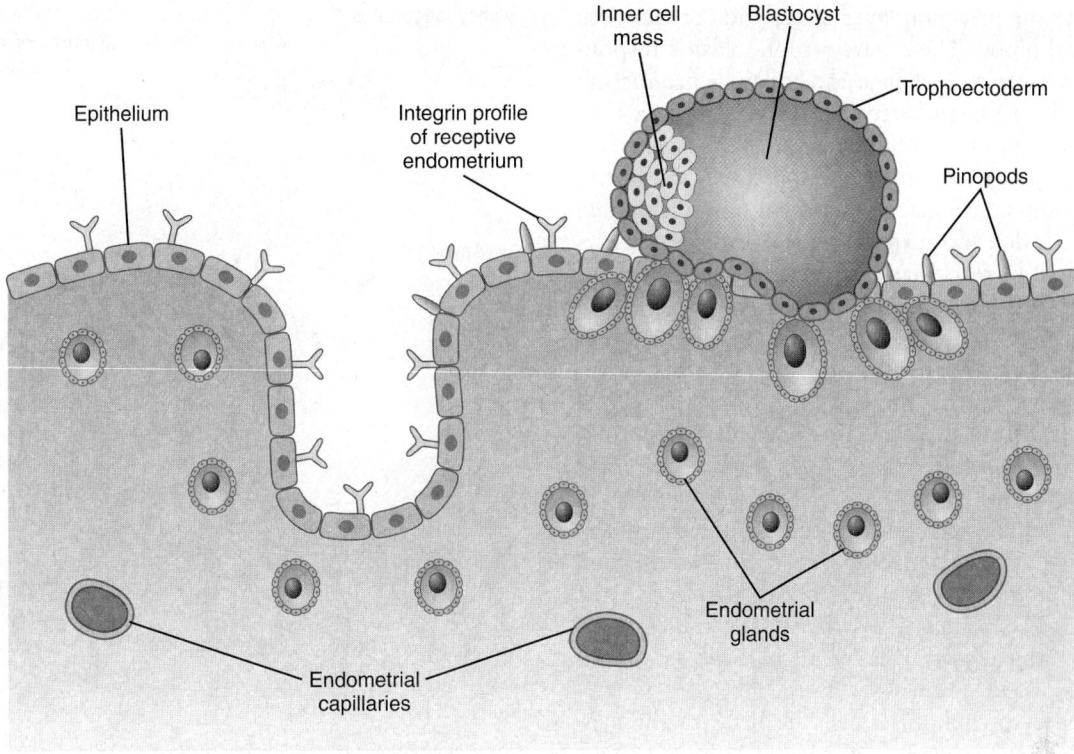

**Figure 19-3** Implantation of the blastocyst.

small protrusions called pinopods and cell-adhesion molecules.[6] The pinopods absorb fluid from the uterine cavity and likely play key roles in attracting the blastocyst. Once the blastocyst is in contact with the decidualized endometrium, the decidual pinopods and blastocyst trophoblastic protrusions interact to facilitate implantation (**Figure 19-3**).[7]

As soon as the blastocyst adheres to the endometrium, the embryonic tissue begins to produce human chorionic gonadotropin (hCG), a hormone that further prepares the endometrium for implantation and may help suppress the maternal immune response to invading tissue.[8] It is thought that physiologic variations in the development of the endometrial "window of implantation" could result in failure of implantation; this hypothesis is currently a subject of infertility research.

### Implantation and Initial Fetal–Maternal Interface

The blastocyst is said to "hatch" when it sheds the zona pellucida. At approximately 10 to 12 days post conception or 1 to 2 weeks' gestation, the blastocyst implants in the decidua.[7] By the first missed menstrual period, the blastocyst is embedded in the decidua and covered by surface epithelium. The implantation process can result in light

vaginal bleeding or spotting, referred to as "implantation bleeding," which can be mistaken for a light menses.

The blastocyst typically implants in a portion of the uterine fundus. Thus, the placenta will ultimately be found in either the anterior or posterior portion of the uterine fundus. Occasionally the blastocyst implants lower in the uterus. If this occurs, the placenta may grow such that it crosses over or touches the cervical os, which is called a placenta previa. Placental location can be detected on ultrasound. A placenta previa detected in early pregnancy may resolve as the uterus becomes more distended and the placental site shifts up and away from the cervix. Individuals who have a placenta previa at the time of birth require a cesarean birth.

### Trophoblastic Differentiation

The trophoblast is a unique tissue that plays an essential role in pregnancy as it develops into the mature placenta and chorion. During the implantation process, the trophoblast, in contact with the endometrium, differentiates into two distinct tissues: syncytiotrophoblast and cytotrophoblast.[9] The syncytiotrophoblast is formed by the fusion of cells into a mass of protoplasm with many nuclei, and becomes the placental layer directly in contact with maternal blood. The syncytiotrophoblast is responsible for nutrient exchange and hormone production and is the primary source of hCG, which signals the corpus luteum to continue producing progesterone until the placenta is fully developed.[9,10] The syncytiotrophoblast evades the maternal immune system because it does not express typical antigen markers that might be recognized as foreign (non-self) tissue.

As the syncytiotrophoblast moves deeper into the endometrium, it disrupts and engulfs maternal endometrial capillaries. This process initiates the lacunar stage, which is marked by the growth of small vacuoles within the syncytiotrophoblast that multiply and eventually fuse to form a system of *lacunae*, or fluid-filled spaces. Initially, these lacunae fill with glandular secretions of the endometrium and a filtrate of maternal blood that diffuses through the trophoblastic tissue and serves to nourish the embryo. The lacunar networks enlarge and communicate with each other as they evolve into the intervillous space.

The cytotrophoblast cells lie beneath the syncytiotrophoblast, and grow rapidly to form projections that push through into the decidua and act to anchor the blastocyst. These projections, called villi, consist of a cytotrophoblast core with an outer layer of syncytiotrophoblast. Their formation and growth is termed the villous stage of development. As the cytotrophoblast rapidly multiplies, it differentiates into *villous cytotrophoblasts* and *extravillous cytotrophoblasts*. Villous trophoblasts form finger-like columns of cells that project into the endometrium and become the anchoring villi of the placenta, progressively branching into a system of villous trees, with lacuna becoming the intervillous space that bathes the villi in maternal blood (Figure 19-4).[9,11] Fetal capillaries emerge within the villi by day 18 following fertilization. Extravillous cytotrophoblasts migrate from the chorionic villi and invade the uterus, extending into the inner third of the myometrium, and remodel the spiral arteries to promote placental development and adequate perfusion. At the same time, cytotrophoblasts interact with maternal immune cells to promote and regulate immunologic acceptance of placental formation and uterine invasion.[12]

## Initial Uteroplacental Blood Flow, Spiral Artery Invasion, and Deinnervation of the Uterus

The cytotrophoblastic invasion of the spiral arteries occurs in two waves: first into the spiral arteries of the decidua, and second into the spiral arteries

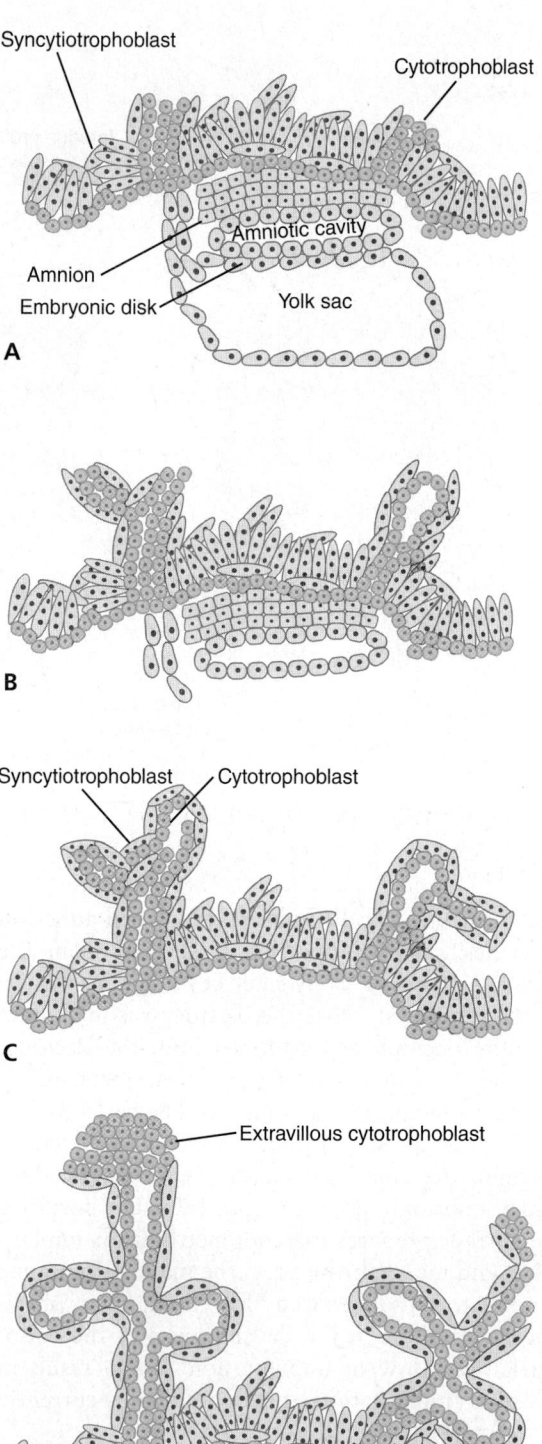

**Figure 19-4  A.** Cytotrophoblast columns in early implanted embryo. **B.** Extension of columns and differentiation of peripheral cells. **C.** Folding of extensions caused by shape of syncytiotrophoblast cells. **D.** Formation of trophoblastic villi.
Reproduced with permission from Cole LA. hCG, the wonder of today's science. *Reprod Biol Endocrinol.* 2012;10:24-28. Published by BioMed Central.

of the myometrium. The first wave takes place in the first weeks following implantation, as cytotrophoblast cells move down the endothelial lining of the spiral arteries in the decidua, destroying their muscular lining to transform these spiral arteries into low-resistance, deinnervated, open vessels that will allow a markedly increased blood flow to the intervillous space to adequately perfuse the placenta.[9,13,14] This transformation is an essential component of a healthy pregnancy.

Throughout the first trimester, cytotrophoblast cells accumulate in the lumens of the spiral arteries and form plugs that block maternal blood flow so that only maternal plasma seeps into the intervillous space. These plugs are thought to maintain the appropriate oxygen gradient for early fetal development and protect the fetus from oxidative stress.[15] By the end of the first trimester, the trophoblastic plugs disintegrate and maternal blood flow to the fetus increases dramatically.

Prior to the onset of uterine blood flow to the placenta, endometrial glands in the decidua are remodeled so they open into the intervillous space and nourish the fetus with "uterine milk": lipids, carbohydrates, proteins, growth factor, and immunosuppressive factors (to protect the "foreign" fetal tissue from the maternal immune system). These glandular secretions play an important role in early placental formation, and animal studies indicate that the trophoblast can communicate with the decidua to upregulate the glandular expression of growth factor to promote its own development.[16] A failure of this dialogue may inhibit adequate invasion of the spiral arteries and lay the foundation for pregnancy complications.

As maternal blood flow is fully established at the beginning of the second trimester, the second wave of cytotrophoblastic invasion occurs.[17] During this wave, the cytotrophoblast remodels the spiral arteries of the myometrium into large, high-volume, low-pressure vessels (Figure 19-5).[9,13,14,17,18] The changed spiral artery architecture accommodates a remarkable change in uterine blood flow. Prior to pregnancy, uterine blood flow is approximately 50 mL per minute; by comparison, at the end of pregnancy, uterine blood flow is approximately 750 mL per minute.

Complications of pregnancy can occur if cytotrophoblast cells fail to fully invade into the uterus or deinnervate the spiral arteries.[9,13,16] While the causes of preeclampsia and other hypertensive disorders of pregnancy are multifactorial and poorly understood, preeclampsia is known to be a placental disorder (and often resolves with birth of the

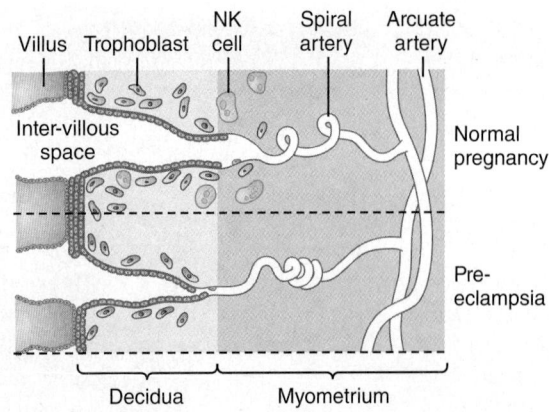

**Figure 19-5** Spiral artery invasion in normal and preeclamptic pregnancies.
Based on Jain A. Endothelin-1: a key pathological factor in preeclampsia. *Reprod BioMed Online.* 2012;25:443-449.

placenta, not the fetus).[16] Preeclampsia is considered part of the "Great Obstetrical Syndromes," which also include fetal growth restriction, unexplained stillbirth, placental abruption, and preterm labor.[13] The origins of these related disorders are thought to lie with inadequate cytotrophoblast invasion, such that uterine invasion is shallow and/or the spiral arteries retain all or some of their muscular lining so they remain small, high-resistance vessels.[9,13,18,19] Conversely, when the trophoblastic tissue invades in an uncontrolled manner and deep into the myometrium, without the normal complex immunologic checks and balances that occur between the maternal and trophoblastic tissues, placenta accreta can develop.

## The Mature Placenta

The placenta has been recognized as an important organ for centuries and has been imbued with many different meanings. In some cultures, the placenta is considered the alter ego or "secondary self."[20] In early Egypt, the placenta was described as the "external soul." In other cultures, it is referred to as "the tree of life," because the vessels that branch out from their insertion points on the maternal surface of the placenta look like the branches of a tree.

At term, the placenta weighs approximately 500 grams, is 18 to 22 centimeters in diameter, and is approximately 2 to 2.5 centimeters thick.[21] This organ consists of a network of as many as 40 *cotyledons* with a surface area of approximately 1.8 m[2] at term. Each cotyledon comprises a series of lobules containing a single anchoring chorionic villus that branches into other villi (**Figure 19-6**). The center of each villus

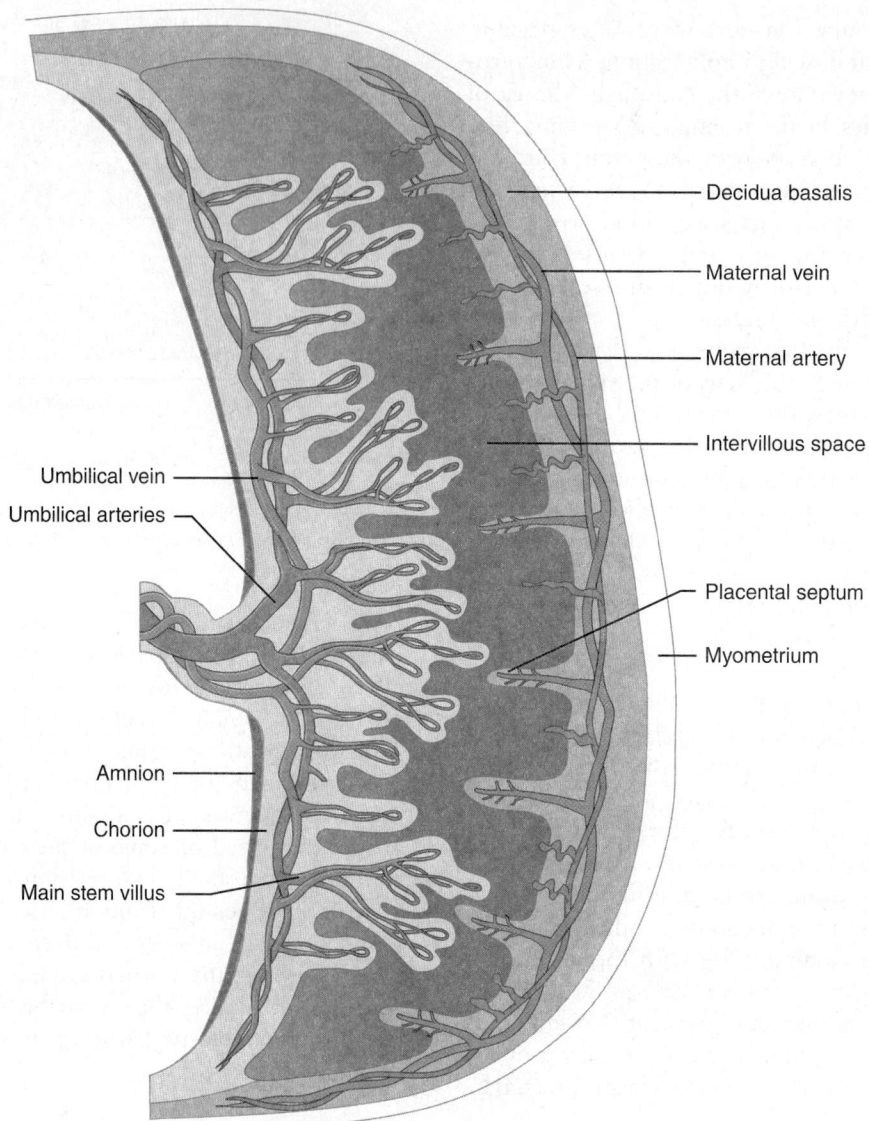

Decidua basalis

Maternal vein

Maternal artery

Intervillous space

Umbilical vein

Umbilical arteries

Placental septum

Myometrium

Amnion

Chorion

Main stem villus

**Figure 19-6** Transverse view of a placenta at a full-term pregnancy. Maternal blood flows into the intervillous spaces in spurts from the spiral arteries, and exchange of nutrients and gases occurs with the fetal blood as the maternal blood flows around the branch villi. The two umbilical arteries carry poorly oxygenated fetal blood away from the fetal heart to the placenta; the single umbilical vein carries oxygenated blood to the fetus. The placental cotyledons are separated from each other by septa projections of the decidua basalis. Each cotyledon consists of two or more main stem villi and branches.

contains fetal blood vessels, which are covered by mesoderm, cytotrophoblast cells, and an outer layer of syncytiotrophoblast. The villi are bathed by maternal blood in the lacunar spaces, and nutrients, gases, and wastes are exchanged across its layers. Maternal and fetal blood do not mix unless there is a defect in the interface. The clinical implications of common variations in placental gross anatomy and systematic evaluation of the placenta following birth are reviewed in the *Third Stage of Labor* chapter.

The placenta has four primary functions, which overlap:

- Produces hormones critical for maintenance of pregnancy, and other bioactive substances
- Transports substances between the maternal and fetal circulations, including acting as the respiratory organ for gas exchange
- Metabolizes and synthesizes agents necessary for sustaining pregnancy

- Provides an immunologic barrier between the maternal and fetal systems

Normal fetal growth is dependent on placental function. Adequate trophoblast invasion and uteroplacental blood flow, the transport of nutrients, and the production of growth-regulating hormones are critical components of fetal growth. Recent research regarding placental function suggests that the placenta may also play a more complex role during pregnancy. Instead of being just a passive filter or barrier, which has historically been its perceived role, this amazing organ integrates a wide range of chemical messages produced by the fetal and maternal systems and actively adapts to different conditions.[9,13] For example, the placenta signals when particular hormones or nutrients are needed by the fetus, and the maternal system responds. The

hormones synthesized by the placenta orchestrate the maternal physiologic adaptations necessary to support pregnancy. In short, the placenta plays an active and independent role in fetal growth and development.

## Hormones of Pregnancy

The placenta is an endocrine organ, and the central mediator for chemical messages between the fetus and the pregnant woman. The primary hormones of pregnancy produced by the placenta are estrogen, progesterone, human chorionic gonadotropin, and human placental lactogen.[22] Each of these hormones plays a major role in supporting pregnancy, and collectively they signal other maternal endocrine glands to drive maternal physiologic adaptations (Table 19-2). In addition, the placenta and

**Table 19-2    Major Hormones and Functions During Pregnancy**

| Hormone | Source | Selected Functions During Pregnancy | Associated Pregnancy Signs or Symptoms |
|---|---|---|---|
| Human chorionic gonadotropin (hCG) | Blastocyst Syncytiotrophoblast Placenta | Secreted by the blastocyst to prepare the endometrium for implantation | Nausea and vomiting of pregnancy |
| | | Suppresses maternal immune response to foreign placental/fetal tissue | Increases duration of sleep and rest |
| | | Stimulates production of progesterone from the corpus luteum, and prevents degeneration of the corpus luteum, ensuring ongoing estrogen and progesterone production | Stimulates heightened sense of smell, which can affect food preferences |
| | | Promotes formation of syncytiotrophoblasts during trophoblastic invasion | Stimulates thyroid to increase production of thyroid hormone |
| | | Aids spiral artery remodeling during the process of trophoblastic invasion | |
| | | Promotes angiogenesis in the uterine vasculature | |
| | | Stimulates thyroid production of thyroxine in the first trimester | |
| | | Involved with fetal organ growth and differentiation, and development of the umbilical cord | |
| | | Suppresses myometrial contractions | |
| Human placental lactogen (hPL) | Placenta | Increases insulin resistance in conjunction with human placental growth hormone (hPGH) | May stimulate nurturing and nesting behavior |
| | | Stimulates production of growth hormones | |
| | | Regulates maternal metabolism of carbohydrates and lipids | |
| | | Enhances insulin secretion | |
| | | Involved in facilitating development of mammary tissue | |
| | | May play a role in regulating the volume and composition of amniotic fluid | |

(continues)

| Table 19-2 | Major Hormones and Functions During Pregnancy (*continued*) | | |
|---|---|---|---|
| **Hormone** | **Source** | **Selected Functions During Pregnancy** | **Associated Pregnancy Signs or Symptoms** |
| Progesterone | Corpus luteum<br>Placenta | Supports decidualization within the endometrium | Conditions related to relaxed smooth muscle: |
| | | Has anti-inflammatory actions to protect the trophoblast from being rejected; promotes tolerance of the fetal allograft | • Constipation |
| | | Promotes systemic vasodilation | • Heartburn |
| | | Prevents myometrial contractility | • Varicose veins |
| | | Increases basal temperature | Increased flatulence |
| | | Increases hunger, fat storage, and insulin resistance | Insensitivity to heat |
| | | Inhibits uterine production of prostaglandins | Nasal congestion (rhinitis of pregnancy) |
| | | Hyperemia and edema of mucosal surfaces | Respiratory alkalosis |
| | | Dilates respiratory airways | |
| | | Increases respiratory center sensitivity to carbon dioxide, which results in mild respiratory alkalosis; maternal alkalosis facilitates transport of oxygen and carbon dioxide from the fetus to the maternal circulation across the placenta | |
| | | Supports mammary growth for lactation | |
| | | Withdrawal (or decreased receptivity to) at term leads to uterine contractions | |
| Estrogen | Ovaries<br>Corpus luteum<br>Placenta<br>Fetus | Softens collagen fibers in the cervix and ligaments | Edema of hands and feet |
| | | Stimulates placental angiogenesis and increases uterine blood flow through vasodilation of uterine and placental arteries | Gingivitis |
| | | Increases sodium retention and renal renin production, which increases fluid (water) volume within the body | Swollen nasal passages and rhinitis of pregnancy |
| | | Promotes endometrial growth and differentiation | Nosebleeds |
| | | Promotes growth of the uterus and breast glandular tissue | Chloasma, linea nigra, darkening of moles |
| | | Increases size and activity of the anterior pituitary gland | |
| | | Increases production of insulin-like growth factors | |
| | | Promotes fat storage | |
| | | Enhances myometrial contractility | |
| | | Plays a role in labor initiation: increases myometrial sensitivity to oxytocin, may upregulate oxytocin and prostaglandin receptors | |

the fetus synthesize other chemical mediators that act both locally and systemically to support growth and development of the fetus and placenta itself; many of these mediators are still being discovered.

### Human Chorionic Gonadotropin

Human chorionic gonadotropin (hCG) is a glycoprotein with both alpha and beta subunits. The alpha subunit is structurally the same as luteinizing hormone (LH), follicle-stimulating hormone (FSH), and thyroid-stimulating hormone (TSH). The beta unit of hCG can have various forms depending on which tissue produces it. Beta-hCG is the basis of modern qualitative pregnancy tests.[23,24]

hCG is secreted by the syncytiotrophoblast tissue within the blastocyst; this secretion starts before implantation occurs, and continues as the syncytio-trophoblast develops into the placenta. The first role of hCG is to sustain estrogen and progesterone production in early pregnancy by preventing degeneration of the corpus luteum. This hormone also plays a role in promoting maternal immunotolerance of the developing placenta and fetus.

The plasma level of the free beta unit of hCG (beta-hCG) rises in early pregnancy and is first detectable approximately 8 to 10 days after ovulation, or shortly before the first missed menses. This timing coincides with implantation of the fertilized ovum.[23] The beta-hCG level doubles approximately every 48 to 72 hours in 85% of individuals with normal pregnancies, maintaining this rate of increase until it reaches a peak of approximately 100,000 mIU/mL at 8 to 11 gestational weeks. At this point, the plasma level of beta-hCG slowly decreases to a stable level of approximately 20,000 mIU/mL (Figure 19-7).[23] Serial plasma levels of beta-hCG are used to diagnose and monitor development of the early conceptus and to help detect miscarriage, ectopic pregnancy, and molar pregnancies, as described in the *Prenatal Care* and *Medical Complications in Pregnancy* chapters.

The natural rise and fall of hCG levels occurs in parallel with the common symptoms of nausea and vomiting that are typically experienced in the first trimester. Although the direct etiology of nausea and vomiting in pregnancy is not known, it has been postulated that hCG may play a role. However, studies that have linked hCG levels to nausea symptoms have not consistently shown a direct correlation between the two.

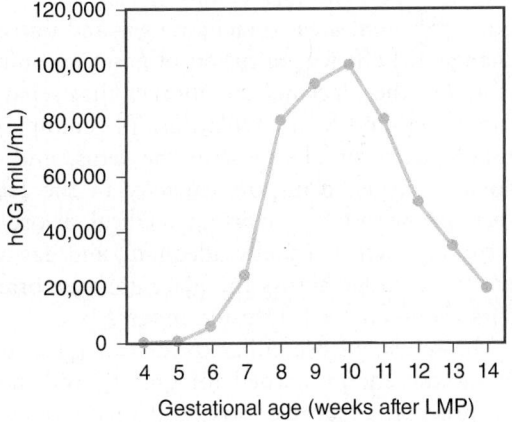

**Figure 19-7** Human chorionic gonadotropin values in the first trimester of pregnancy.
Abbreviations: hCG, human chorionic gonadotropin; LMP, last menstrual period.

hCG also affects production of thyroid hormone. The alpha unit of hCG is the same as TSH, so hCG can stimulate the thyroid gland to produce thyroid hormone, causing a transient hyperthyroidism. Most people demonstrate a change in measured thyroid hormone values but no actual change in thyroid function, because levels of thyroid binding globulin are also increased during pregnancy. Thyroid binding globulin binds to thyroid hormone, so that it cannot diffuse into tissue and become metabolically active.

Although there is a clear association between transient hyperthyroidism and nausea and vomiting, hyperthyroidism alone rarely causes vomiting, which supports the theory that hCG plays a part in this pregnancy-related condition.[25] Nausea and vomiting are typically worse with multiple and molar gestations, both of which are marked by higher levels of hCG.

### Human Placental Lactogen

Human placental lactogen (hPL), which is structurally similar to the hormones prolactin, growth hormone, and placental growth hormone, plays a role in fetal nutrition by altering maternal glucose metabolism so that glucose is available for fetal uptake. This transformation is achieved primarily by mobilizing fatty acids from lipids to provide an alternative fuel for the pregnant individual, while sparing glucose for the fetus. hPL also increases maternal insulin resistance, thereby assuring consistent blood levels of glucose for fetal use.[26]

The hPL-induced insulin resistance results in an increase in maternal insulin levels. This, in turn, stimulates amino acid production, thereby ensuring that amino acids are also available for fetal growth and development. Glucose is transported across the placenta via facilitated diffusion and is the primary source of nutrition for the fetus.

Like most essential pregnancy hormones, hPL is secreted by the placental syncytiotrophoblast. This hormone is detectable in maternal circulation at 6 to 8 gestational weeks, with levels increasing in direct proportion to placental growth. Much is unknown about the role of hPL during pregnancy. For example, levels of hPL are decreased by greater than 40% in pregnant persons with obesity as well as those with peripartum depression as compared to those persons without obesity or depression; disrupted levels of hPL (both elevated and decreased) have been noted in persons with diabetes.[27] Whether these disruptions in the secretion of hPL are a cause or an effect of the associated condition is unknown, but they have also been linked to fetal growth abnormalities, including both fetal growth restriction and macrosomia. In addition, high serum levels of hPL have been linked to placenta previa and accreta.[28]

### Progesterone

Progesterone and estrogen act as intracellular chemical messengers by binding to intracellular receptors. These steroid hormones influence many aspects of DNA transcription and cellular activities.

Progesterone is essential for maintenance of pregnancy in all mammals, and its name is derived from this function: "pro-gestational steroidal ketone." This hormone acts upon smooth muscle to relax it, which maintains the uterine myometrium in a quiescent (or inactive) state throughout most of pregnancy. Progesterone is also involved in suppressing the maternal immune response to fetal antigens so that the fetal tissue is not rejected. Progesterone is initially produced by the corpus luteum in early pregnancy. The placenta then assumes the progesterone production at some point during gestational weeks 7 to 9, an event called the "luteal–placental shift." Additional functions of progesterone during pregnancy are listed in Table 19-1.

Low levels of progesterone in pregnancy are associated with an increased risk of miscarriage. Individuals with luteal-phase defects can have progesterone levels that drop in early pregnancy, leading to spontaneous abortions. Some studies have shown progesterone supplementation is effective for preventing miscarriage in individuals who have a history of recurrent pregnancy loss.[29] Alternatively, administration of mifepristone, a progesterone receptor antagonist, will cause miscarriage (or therapeutic abortion). There is conflicting evidence about the use of progesterone to prevent preterm birth in singleton pregnancies.[29-32]

### Estrogen

Three types of naturally occurring estrogen have been identified: estrone, estradiol, and estriol. Estriol (E3) is the primary estrogen of pregnancy.

Estrogen production during pregnancy entails a three-part interplay between the pregnant individual, fetus, and placenta; each of these three separate but interrelated factors completes part of estrogen synthesis but not all of it. Estrogen is initially synthesized in the corpus luteum until the 8th or 9th week of gestation. At that point, the fetal adrenal glands are mature enough to produce the necessary estrogen precursors, and the placenta is able to produce and excrete the active forms of estrogen. Placental estrogen production depends on input from both the fetal and maternal adrenal cortex because the placenta cannot produce the androgenic C19 steroid dehydroepiandrosterone (DHEA), and its sulfoconjuate, DHEA-S, which are essential substrates of estriol.

Selected effects of estrogen during pregnancy are listed in Table 19-1. Estrogen encourages growth of breast tissue, stimulates uterine contractility, and increases uterine receptiveness to oxytocin and prostaglandins. For most of pregnancy, however, the uterus remains refractory to the effects of estrogen, a consequence of the influence of progesterone, which ensures that the uterine myometrium has very few estrogen receptors.

### Transport Across the Placenta

Transport from the maternal circulation to the fetal circulation involves traversing four layers of cells: (1) syncytiotrophoblast, (2) cytotrophoblast, (3) fetal connective tissue that supports the fetal blood vessels, and (4) the endothelial cells surrounding the fetal blood vessels (**Figure 19-8**).[33p14]

The syncytiotrophoblast is packed with receptors for nutrients, growth factor, hormones, and immunoglobulins. Placental transport involves multiple mechanisms, including facilitated diffusion, passive diffusion, active transport, pinocytosis, endocytosis, bulk flow, solvent drag, accidental capillary breaks, and independent movement.[34,35] These mechanisms are described in **Table 19-3**.

The optimal transfer of oxygen, carbon dioxide, and nutrients from the maternal circulation to the fetal circulation can occur only when the following five components function well: (1) adequate blood flow into the intervillous space, (2) a large enough placental area to facilitate gas and nutrient exchange, (3) efficient diffusion of gases and nutrients across the placental membranes that separate the maternal and fetal circulations, (4) unimpaired umbilical vein circulation into the fetus, and (5) adequate oxygen transport capacity in the fetus. In persons without preexisting medical disorders, placental growth is usually adequate, and gas and nutrient exchange across the placental membranes occurs via an efficient diffusion process.

The fetus can use either oxygen or glucose to produce the energy needed for growth and metabolic processes. Carbon dioxide ($CO_2$) and water ($H_2O$) are the end products of using oxygen for aerobic metabolism. When the fetus does not have sufficient oxygen, glucose is used to create adenosine triphosphate (ATP) for energy. This process is called

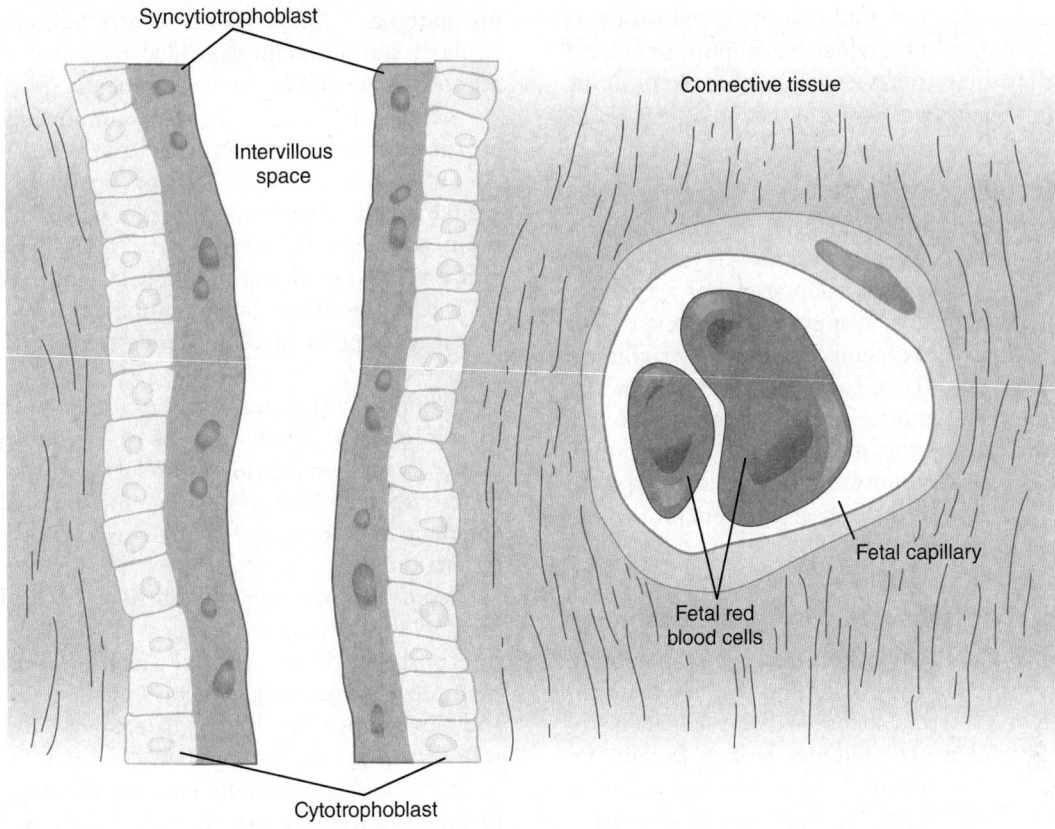

**Figure 19-8** The four cell layers between the maternal and fetal circulations.
Reproduced from Parer JT, King TL, Ikeda T. *Electronic Fetal Heart Rate Monitoring: The 5-Tier System*. 3rd ed. Burlington, MA: Jones & Bartlett Learning; 2018.

| Table 19-3 | Placental Transport Mechanisms | |
|---|---|---|
| **Transport Mechanism** | **Description of Mechanism** | **Examples of Substances Transported via This Mechanism** |
| Simple diffusion | Transfer of substances across a membrane down a concentration gradient (from an area of higher concentration of the substance to an area of lower concentration of the substance) | Oxygen, carbon dioxide, electrolytes, water, certain medications including analgesic and anesthetic agents |
| Facilitated diffusion | Transfer of substances across a membrane down a concentration gradient (such as diffusion), but in a manner that allows for more rapid or more specific transfer | Substances such as glucose that are essential for rapid fetal growth but are present in low concentrations in the maternal blood |
| Active transport | Transport against a concentration gradient, which requires energy | Transfer to the fetus of substances that are present in higher concentrations in the fetus than in the pregnant woman, such as iron and ascorbic acid |
| Pinocytosis | A form of endocytosis that allows small particles to be brought into a cell. The cell membrane folds around the particle and becomes an intracellular membrane. | Immunoglobulin G (IgG) maternal antibodies, phospholipids used to make cell membranes, lipoproteins used to transport cholesterol |
| Breaks between cells | Active capillary breaks allow fetal and maternal cells to mix | Cell migration across different tissues may play a role in fetal immunity and in maintaining maternal tolerance to the fetal allograft |
| Bulk flow | Movement of water and some solutes in water via aqueous pores | Free movement of water and some solutes maintains equal osmolality in the fetal and maternal compartments |

anaerobic metabolism, and one of its end products is lactic acid ($C_3H_6O_3$), which has important clinical implications that are reviewed in more detail in the *Fetal Assessment During Labor* chapter.

### Gas Exchange

Gas exchange across the placenta occurs via diffusion. The intervillous space is a low-oxygen setting, and maternal physiologic adaptations of pregnancy include a state of mild respiratory alkalosis (lower than normal level of carbon dioxide). This facilitates the diffusion of oxygen from the maternal circulation to the fetus, and the return of carbon dioxide from the fetus to the mother. Fetal hemoglobin, which has a high affinity for oxygen compared to adult hemoglobin, is the primary protein for oxygen transport in the developing fetus.[36,37]

### Transport of Essential Nutrients and Hormones

The supply of carbohydrates, fatty acids, and amino acids from the uterine circulation is a key determinant of fetal growth. Glucose is the principal energy source for fetal growth and metabolism. Because fetal production of glucose either does not occur or is undetectable, placental transport of glucose from maternal blood provides the essential supply of this substrate.[38] Glucose transport occurs via facilitated diffusion, a process that requires a higher glucose concentration in the maternal circulation relative to the fetal circulation—which is why a slight insulin resistance develops in pregnancy.

Glucose transport across the placenta is a highly complex and dynamic process. Glucose metabolism within the placenta, the density of glucose transporters, and the maternal supply of glucose all influence the amount of glucose received by the fetus. Several different types of glucose transporters exist, which adapt throughout pregnancy as individual cell requirements for glucose change.[39] Although there is a direct association between maternal serum glucose concentration and newborn size, the roles of various types of glucose transporters are complicated and not fully understood. Alterations in the number and type of glucose transporters is associated with gestational diabetes, fetal growth restriction, and preeclampsia.[39]

Fatty acids can cross the lipid bilayers of the placenta via simple diffusion; however, the placenta preferentially transports several types of fatty acids via fatty acid binding proteins. The mix of fatty acids transferred to the fetus is largely dependent on which fatty acids are available in the maternal circulation. However, the placenta may regulate its own supply through hormonal messengers acting on maternal adipose tissue.[40] Fatty acids are particularly important in the third trimester for fetal adipose tissue and brain development.

Cholesterol is an essential component in the creation of cell membranes and the production of steroid hormones. This hormone plays a role in regulating the development of the neural tube and brain, among other organs. The fetus begins creating its own cholesterol supply at approximately 20 weeks' gestation, but continues to rely on placental transfer of maternal cholesterol throughout pregnancy.[41]

Amino acids require active transport to cross the placenta, as concentrations of amino acids are higher in the fetal circulation relative to the maternal circulation. Alterations in amino acid transport and fetal uptake are seen in fetuses with growth restriction.[42]

Iron, another essential nutrient for cell function, plays a role in oxygen delivery, electron transport, and DNA synthesis. Iron also influences brain development and function in the fetal period and throughout the life span; fetal iron deficiency can result in abnormal neurocognitive development.[43] Iron requirements increase dramatically in pregnancy: Rapidly growing fetal cells with high metabolic rates have increased iron requirements, especially the fetal brain; the pregnant person's expanding blood volume necessitates additional iron; and the metabolically active placenta has its own iron requirements. Pregnancy is thus a "condition of impending or existing iron deficiency," and fetal iron stores are directly related to the maternal iron status.[35,43]

Fetal thyroid hormone production does not start until mid-gestation and is not fully functional until birth. Thus, the fetus is dependent on maternally produced thyroid hormone that crosses the placenta to support fetal thyroid function in utero. Maternal thyroid hormone is transferred across the placenta by placental transporters, with this flow peaking at the 34th week of gestation.[44] Thyroid hormones play a role in the development of the fetal–maternal vasculature and proliferation of trophoblastic tissue in early pregnancy; in facilitating placental hormone secretion; and in activating fetal gene expression. Thyroid hormone is also essential for fetal brain and skeletal development. Hypothyroidism during pregnancies is associated with an increased risk for miscarriage, preeclampsia, preterm labor, and fetal growth restriction.[44] Significant hypothyroidism during pregnancy is also associated with impaired fetal cognitive-neurodevelopment.

### Transport of Drugs and Other Substances

Distribution of drugs and other substances is complex during pregnancy, as four separate compartments exist: (1) the fetus, (2) the amniotic fluid, (3) the placenta, and (4) the mother. Each of the compartments affects the movement of drugs, and occasionally one compartment will have a higher concentration of drug than another.[45]

Drug transfer across the placenta is affected by various characteristics of the drug, including its size (molecular weight), lipid solubility, plasma protein binding, and acid versus basic properties.[45,46] Most drugs have a small molecular weight, usually less than 500 daltons (Da), so they easily cross the placenta and may transfer to the fetus. Drugs with a molecular weight greater than 500 Da transfer incompletely; those that have a molecular weight greater than 1000 Da, such as heparin and insulin, transfer very poorly. Drugs that are more lipophilic cross the placenta more readily than those that are hydrophilic, as the placenta is lipoid in character. A non-ionized state facilitates transfer. In addition, substances such as alcohol, tobacco, and opioids can cross the placenta and cause subsequent alterations in fetal development More details about placental transport of drugs and their effects on the fetus can be found in the *Prenatal Care* chapter.

Once a drug enters the fetal circulation, it is free to bind with proteins in the fetal plasma. Notably, albumin concentrations in the fetal compartment are higher than those in the maternal compartment. As a consequence, some highly protein-bound drugs may have an increased fetal effect when compared with their maternal effects.[47,48]

### Placental Metabolism

The placenta has its own significant energy requirements that must be met if it is to synthesize and transport hormones, nutrients, and oxygen for the embryo and growing fetus, and to deliver fetal waste products (e.g., carbon dioxide) back into maternal circulation. Placental metabolism uses approximately 40% to 60% of the oxygen and glucose that is delivered into the intervillous spaces, and has higher oxygen requirements than either the fetus or the pregnant person.[36] The placenta can also alter its metabolism in the presence of stressors such as hypoxia or nutrient scarcity.

### Immunology of the Placenta

The immune system of the pregnant person has two primary functions in supporting a healthy pregnancy: to tolerate foreign tissue (the fetus and fetal components of the placental unit), and to protect this tissue from infection.[49] The fetus is considered a semi-allogenic graft, meaning that the fetus consists of foreign tissue from the same species but has different (paternal) antigens compared to the mother. This foreign tissue is in direct contact with maternal blood and tissues, yet the maternal immune system not only accepts but also protects the fetus.[50,51] The processes that ensure the pregnant person's body does not reject the fetus have not been fully identified.

In addition to hormonally mediated immunologic adaptations, there appears to be more cellular traffic between the fetus and the pregnant woman than was originally hypothesized.[52] Fetal cells can be found in many maternal tissues and may play a role in fetal–maternal signaling; these cells can persist in a mother for decades. Similarly, maternal cells enter the fetal circulation via mechanisms that have not been fully elucidated and may support the development of fetal immunity. The full implications of this microchimerism are unknown.

### Immunologic Acceptance of Fetus

Pregnancy can be thought of as a period of both immunosuppression and immunotolerance. The populations of immune cells promoting immunotolerance (to foreign antigens) are increased, as are cells that interfere with or deactivate maternal immune cells that might be harmful to pregnancy.[51] The interplay of hormones with pregnancy-specific immune cells results in an adaptive system that regulates the maternal immune system and adjusts its response to microbial challenge.

The primary players at the maternal–fetal interface are the endometrial decidua, the fetal trophoblast, and maternal immune cells. Endometrial immune cells change in number and type with pregnancy, and a successful pregnancy depends on the appropriate number and type of these immune cells, which are pro-placentation: They support implantation, trophoblast migration and invasion, and remodeling of the uterine spiral arteries.[50,52] Indeed, dysregulation in the maternal immune response has been linked to pregnancy loss, preeclampsia, fetal growth restriction, and preterm birth.[53]

Several aspects of the placenta allow it to function as an "immunologic shield" for the fetus and evade maternal immune cells that may be harmful.[49] Most importantly, the syncytiotrophoblast, which is in direct contact with maternal tissues, does not express the cell surface antigens that are the usual targets for maternal antibodies. In fact, the antigens expressed by the syncytiotrophoblast are thought to moderate the maternal immune system by activating pathways that interfere with the killer function of immune cells.[49] These pregnancy-specific immune cells that promote immunotolerance and diminish the fetotoxic immune response are also hormonally mediated by progesterone, prostaglandins, and hCG, which alter the maternal immune response in ways that enable maternal tissue to have tolerance to the contact with the syncytiotrophoblast and cytotrophoblast.

### Placental Protection from Infection

While the fetal immune system does not act independently until at least the third trimester, the placenta is able to identify infectious triggers and mount an immune-like response. Immune cells of fetal origin, called Hofbauer cells, are placental macrophages that are present throughout pregnancy. These cells can mount a strong response to infection and are thought to engulf danger-signaling molecules to limit placental inflammation.[54] Hofbauer cells are also thought to contribute to placental growth and vascular development. Alterations of Hofbauer cells have been noted in pregnancy complications such as chorioamnionitis and preeclampsia.[55] However, these cells may be easily exploited by viral infection, which may partly explain why some viruses are dangerous to developing fetuses.

Immunoglobulin G (IgG) is an immune system antibody that persists and protects against infections a person has either had or been vaccinated for. This small molecule can transfer across the placenta to the fetus starting in the second trimester, with the majority of the IgG crossing the placenta in the third trimester. Generally, maternal antibodies are protective of the fetus (and neonate) and provide passive immunity, although certain unusual IgG antibodies can cause neonatal pathology—for example, in the case of Rh incompatibility between the mother and fetus. Rh incompatibility is described further in the *Prenatal Care* chapter.

### Placental Aging

Aging of the human body is a risk factor for many diseases, and similarly aging can affect a placenta's ability to function effectively. The risk of unexplained fetal death (stillbirth) rises as a pregnancy progresses into the late-term gestational weeks. In such cases, it has been theorized that oxidative damage to placental tissue, similar to the oxidative damage caused by aging in other organs, adversely affects the supply of nutrients and amniotic fluid required by the fetus. The risk of stillbirth starts to increase after 38 gestational weeks, with the rate of increase accelerating after 41 weeks and rising dramatically after 42 weeks.[56]

### Amnion, Chorion, Amnionic Fluid, and Umbilical Cord

The placental unit also includes the amnion, chorion, and umbilical cord. The fetus and amniotic fluid are surrounded by two membranes. The outer layer, the chorion, serves to separate the inner membrane, the amnion, from the uterine lining. The amnion contains the fetus, umbilical cord, and amniotic fluid, the pressure of which causes the amnion to be passively pushed against and attached to the chorion. The umbilical cord contains the umbilical arteries and umbilical vein that connect the placental unit to the fetal circulation.

### Amnionic Fluid

Amniotic fluid serves multiple functions during pregnancy, including cushioning and protecting the fetus, providing space for fetal movement and growth, and maintaining consistent temperature and pressure.[57] Amniotic fluid is also necessary for fetal lung development. Substances found in amniotic fluid include electrolytes, urea, creatinine, bile pigments, renin, glucose, hormones, fetal cells, lanugo, and vernix caseosa. Prostaglandin levels in amniotic fluid are elevated in preterm labor, intra-amniotic infection, and, to a lesser degree, term labor.[58] The fluid's osmolality and composition evolve throughout the course of the pregnancy and are similar to the characteristics of dilute fetal urine in a term gestation.

In the latter half of pregnancy, amniotic fluid is primarily produced by the fetus in the form of urine and lung fluid. The average amount of amniotic fluid at term is 700 to 800 mL.[59] Amniotic fluid is removed via fetal swallowing and diffusion across the placenta. The fluid secretions from the fetus's lungs contain phospholipids, including lecithin and sphingomyelin, which are components of surfactant, a substance essential for the function of the neonatal lungs. As pregnancy advances, the absolute and relative amounts of lecithin in amniotic fluid increase. The ratio of lecithin to sphingomyelin is used as means of assessing fetal lung maturity to help guide decisions about delivery prior to term. While the amount of fluid varies in the third trimester and begins to decrease after 40 gestational weeks, the amount of fluid that is cycled via production and removal remains relatively constant, at approximately 1000 mL per day.

Amniotic fluid is essential for normal fetal growth, and abnormalities of amniotic fluid volume can indicate fetal disease, maternal disease, or both. *Oligohydramnios* refers to an abnormally low amount of amniotic fluid. Oligohydramnios in the second trimester can inhibit normal fetal lung and musculoskeletal development. At term, oligohydramnios is associated with low birth weight, fetal heart rate decelerations during labor, and increased perinatal mortality and morbidity. Causes of this disorder include fetal urinary obstruction or renal abnormalities, heart disease, and fetal growth restriction. Maternal conditions that can cause oligohydramnios include dehydration, severe hypertension, and renal disorders.[59]

*Polyhydramnios* refers to an abnormally large amount of amniotic fluid. Polyhydramnios is caused by too much production or too little removal of amniotic fluid. Conditions that can cause polyhydramnios include maternal hyperglycemia (diabetes), obstructed fetal swallowing, fetal cardiac failure, and severe fetal anemia.[59] Modest polyhydramnios can be idiopathic, whereas oligohydramnios is most likely to be associated with an abnormal condition in the fetus or the pregnant woman.

### Umbilical Cord

The umbilical cord contains two arteries and one vein, which are surrounded by a gelatinous collagen material called *Wharton jelly*. The maximum length of the cord averages 55 to 60 centimeters. The cord epithelium, which is formed by the amnion, typically inserts into the placenta centrally but may insert at any portion of the placenta. A *marginal cord insertion* occurs when the cord inserts at or near the placental edge; it may be noted as an incidental finding on ultrasound but is not associated with complications of pregnancy.[60] A *velamentous cord insertion* occurs when the cord inserts into the placental membranes and not the placenta itself. With a velamentous cord insertion, fetal vessels run through the amniotic membranes unprotected by Wharton's jelly. Velamentous cord insertion is associated with increased rates of fetal growth restriction, perinatal death, and cesarean section.

Vasa previa occurs when the unprotected vessels of a velamentous cord run across or near the internal os of the cervix. Although vasa previa is very rare, when rupture of membranes occurs and fetal blood vessels subsequently rupture and hemorrhage, the fetus can lose a great deal of blood quickly. In consequence, this condition can result in fetal/neonatal death. With prenatal diagnosis and planned cesarean, a 100% neonatal survival rate is possible.[61]

The blood vessels within the umbilical cord are longer than the cord itself, so they coil in a spiral fashion as the cord lengthens. This coiling may protect the blood flow within the cord if it is subjected to tension or compression. Evidence is mixed regarding whether hypocoiling of the cord is associated with poor obstetric outcomes, probably due to hypoxia related to umbilical cord compression.[62,63]

Abnormalities of the umbilical cord that cause stillbirth are typically called "cord accidents." They include vasa previa; cord entrapment (umbilical cord wrapped around the fetus's neck, body, or shoulder); umbilical knots, torsions, and strictures; cord prolapse (umbilical cord slips in front of the presenting fetal part and is compressed); and compromised fetal microcirculation (e.g., a thrombosis of the cord). While a "nuchal cord" (e.g., cord wrapped around the fetal neck) is a common presentation at birth, as are "true knots" in the cord, they can also can be associated with poor obstetric outcomes.

## Fetal Programming and Epigenetics

Prior to a review of normal embryonic and fetal development, it is important to consider the effects of genetics. The intrauterine environment can affect how various fetal genes are expressed, or turned on or off. The term *epigenetics* refers to any process that causes an alteration in gene activity that is not a change in the individual's actual DNA sequencing and that can result in modifications, which can then be heritable. A number of different epigenetic mechanisms exist, but the most well researched is DNA methylation or demethylation. The addition of a methyl group to part of a DNA molecule (usually cytosine) blocks a gene on that DNA strand from becoming active.[64] Fetal exposure to stress within the uterus—such as the stress related to nutrient scarcity, hypoxia, or high levels of cortisol—can affect patterns of DNA methylation, which in turn can affect a fetus's lifetime risk for disease.[65,66]

In the 1990s, physician and researcher David Barker published a theory about *fetal programming*, which is now typically referred to as the "developmental origins of health and disease" (DOHaD). Fetal programing, or "developmental plasticity," is the ability of a fetus to alter development based on the fetal environment.[67] Barker's initial work linked birth records with later health and death records in the United Kingdom, and credited the meticulous and complete records of midwives, without whom he would not have had adequate data.[68] His major finding was that infant birth weights were inversely proportional to rates of adult hypertension, obesity, and diabetes. In other words, as birth weight increased (across the normal range), lifetime rates of chronic disease decreased. Barker theorized that in infants with lower birth weights, the fetal response to nutrient scarcity was slowed growth and altered metabolism, which subsequently affects their lifetime risk for disease.[67]

This finding has now been replicated in multiple studies across the globe: Poor in utero nutrient supply related to maternal malnutrition or placental dysfunction has been found to create epigenetic adaptations that result in altered metabolic processes and increased rates of certain diseases in the offspring later in life including, but not limited to, heart disease, diabetes, obesity, and certain cancers.[66,69] In times of stress or scarcity, the fetus prioritizes the development and survival of the brain over other organs such as the kidney, liver, and pancreas, and redirects blood flow to the brain. This altered resource allocation has its trade-offs, however: As less-vital organs receive decreased oxygen and nutrients, their growth and function are altered. These adaptations affect the set-points of hormones as well as the development and function of endocrine and metabolic processes, and they ultimately make the fetus more vulnerable to adverse influences in later life, especially if the fetus already has a genetic predisposition for metabolic or vascular disease.

Maternal overnutrition or hyperglycemia can also contribute to epigenetic alterations. Altered maternal metabolic function, such as occurs with maternal obesity, accelerated weight gain during pregnancy, or diabetes, can cause fetal growth abnormalities and changes in metabolic programming, which are then associated with increased lifetime risks of diseases such as diabetes, heart disease, stroke, obesity, and asthma.[70,71] A fetal environment characterized by elevated levels of circulating lipids and glucose leads to cellular changes, inflammation, and oxidative stress, all of which can affect the delivery of oxygen and nutrients to the fetus.[72]

Current research suggests many types of prenatal stresses—including maternally generated stress hormones, environmental toxins, and nutrient scarcity or excess—can affect fetal physiology and infant development. For example, high levels of maternal psychosocial stress are theorized to alter the development of fetal brain structures and program a more reactive stress response system in the newborn, contributing to an increased risk of emotional dysregulation and psychosocial disorders in later life.[73]

The fetal stress response system (the hypothalamus, pituitary gland, and adrenal gland, collectively known as the HPA axis) is the subject of a great deal of epigenetic research. The fetal HPA axis is functional and responsive to levels of circulating stress hormones, utilizing a negative feedback loop to maintain levels of circulating cortisol. If maternal cortisol levels remain elevated for prolonged periods of time, the fetal stress response system may be altered to become more reactive. This prolonged stress exposure likely also plays a role in growth restriction.[74]

In short, although the epigenetic changes and genomic plasticity that occur during fetal development are the subject of a great deal of research, individual variations are significant yet largely uncharted. Thus, the clinical implications of this field of study are not fully known. Nonetheless, the work surrounding fetal programming and the developmental origins of chronic disease is of particular relevance to midwifery because it underscores the importance and complexity of preconceptional and prenatal care.

## Fetal Development

### Embryo to Fetus

Several excellent textbooks detail embryonic and fetal development, and it is beyond the scope of this chapter to review this fascinating physiology; rather, highlights as they pertain to clinical practice will be discussed here.

### Embryonic Period

Returning to the blastocyst, the *embryonic period*, which is the period of organogenesis, occurs between 2 and 8 weeks following fertilization. The *fetal period*, marked by growth and tissue differentiation, starts at 8 weeks after fertilization and extends to birth. This section of the chapter uses the embryonic age or weeks post fertilization in references to fetal growth and development. Because some developmental milestones are used clinically to evaluate fetal health, the menstrual age weeks' gestation is noted where necessary.

### Germ Layers and Organogenesis

The embryonic disc within the blastocyst gives rise to three germ layers: (1) the endoderm, (2) the mesoderm, and (3) the ectoderm. The third week of embryo development is marked by a period of rapid growth, during which the mesoderm, ectoderm, and endoderm begin to undergo the dramatic

| Table 19-4 | Differentiation of Embryonic Germ Layers | |
|---|---|---|
| **Ectoderm** | **Mesoderm** | **Endoderm** |
| Central and peripheral nervous system | Connective tissues | Epithelium of the digestive system (except the mouth and anus, which are involutions of the ectoderm) |
| Epidermis including hair, nails, and sebaceous glands | Muscle tissue | |
| | Skeleton (bone) | Liver and pancreas |
| Epithelium of sensory organs | Cardiovascular | Respiratory system, including alveolar cells of the lung |
| Nasal and oral cavities | Lymphatics | |
| Salivary glands | Urogenital structures (gonads and kidney) | Thymus, thyroid, parathyroid, and pancreas |
| Adrenal medulla | Serous lining of body cavities (peritoneum, pleural, and pericardium) | |
| Parts of the pituitary gland | | |

transformations that form specific embryonic structures (Table 19-4). Most functional organs and organ systems are formed from all three embryonic germ layers. Each germ layer contributes a specific feature, but the germ layers do not produce specific structures separately from each other.

## Morphogenesis

The genetically controlled process during which cells and cell groups take on a specific form, shape, and function is known as *morphogenesis*. Initially, the cells in the embryoblast are all the same; that is, they are stem cells, which are capable of becoming any type of body cell. These unspecialized cells must proceed through two distinct phases: (1) determination, which restricts the cell to a specific type, and (2) differentiation, in which the morphologic and functional characteristics specific to that cell type develop.

Cell differentiation often involves a process called induction, in which cells in a local environment signal one another to develop in a specific manner. The signaling cell is called the inductor, and the cells that respond to induction are called the inducers. If any of the differentiation sequences is disrupted, the next step in the process will not proceed in the usual fashion, and an abnormality will develop. Notably, organ agenesis may occur when the process is disturbed at an early stage. For example, anencephaly is a form of organ agenesis in which the brain does not form. Some disruptions in differentiation sequences will result in miscarriage or fetal demise, whereas others may produce a fetal defect that can range from undetectable to minor to clinically significant.

In addition to cell differentiation and induction, several other cellular mechanics are involved in morphogenesis, including proliferation, migration, adhesion, and folding. Examples of these processes are summarized in Table 19-5.

## Teratogenic Mechanisms

Pregnant individuals may sometimes be exposed to or take medications or other agents that are teratogenic. *Teratology* refers to the study of congenital anomalies and teratogens; the latter include any agent that irreversibly alters structure or function in a developing embryo or fetus. Teratogens include alcohol, viruses such as rubella, chemicals such as mercury, and drugs such as isotretinoin (Accutane).[75] The term *fetotoxic* is used to describe agents, such as tobacco, that have toxic effects on the fetus that adversely affect growth or development. Teratogenic agents can cause the most harm in the first trimester, whereas fetotoxic agents generally cause more harm in the second and third trimesters.

Overall, birth defects occur in approximately 3% to 5% of all births.[76,77] This percentage is often called the "background risk" against which additional risks are calculated based on family history, past history, and environmental exposure including medication exposure. Chromosomal and genetic abnormalities and environmental exposures are known causes of birth defects, but most birth defects are thought to have multifactorial causes. Only 20% of birth defects typically have a known cause.[78] Exposure to teratogenic medications alone is estimated to account for only a very small fraction of all birth defects.[79]

The unique fact about teratogenic agents is that avoiding the teratogen can prevent the associated congenital anomaly. For this reason, knowledge of teratogenic drugs is essential for the practicing midwife. Fortunately, the number of teratogenic agents is relatively small, and even fewer are in common use. Drugs that are known to have teratogenic or

| Table 19-5 | Selected Cellular Mechanisms Involved in Morphogenesis | |
|---|---|---|
| **Cell Mechanism** | **Description** | **Congenital Defects That May Result from a Faulty Mechanism** |
| Cell proliferation (hypertrophy) | A rapid increase in the number of cells by cell division and growth | Inhibition of cell proliferation can occur when there is a lack of space. A diaphragmatic hernia will allow abdominal contents to be in the thoracic cavity; pulmonary hypoplasia occurs when the lungs are not allowed to continue cell proliferation. |
| Cell differentiation | Process by which pluripotent cells become more specialized cells | Prenatal exposure to high levels of methylmercury is thought to result in failure of cell differentiation in the central nervous system, causing neurologic and developmental defects. |
| Apoptosis | A genetically determined process of cell self-destruction; cells produce enzymes that lead to their dissolution | Excessive enzymatic release can lead to excessive cellular destruction and result in defects such as limb shortening; deficient enzymatic release can lead to defects such as bowel atresia, syndactyly, or imperforate anus. |
| Migration | A dynamic and cyclical process in which layers migrate to a strategic location along the developing embryo. The cell extends protrusions at its front and attaches to the substratum on which the cell is migrating. | Central nervous system abnormalities, such as lissencephaly (lack of grooves on the brain) |
| Adhesion | The interaction of specific mechanisms on one cell and complementary adhesion molecules on the membrane of another cell | Cleft palate and neural tube defects occur as a result of alterations in cell recognition and the adhesion process. |
| Folding | As new cells form, the embryo is forced to conform to the available space. The embryo folds in both the transverse and longitudinal planes. Structures within the embryo also must fold to conform to the space available to them. | Congenital heart defects<br>Diverticula |

fetotoxic effects are discussed in more detail in the *Prenatal Care* chapter.

The preimplantation period is considered the "all or nothing" period with regard to teratogenic effects. If a small number of cells are damaged during this period, the fetus usually compensates without any damage. Conversely, if a large number of cells are damaged, the embryo will be unable to form, and a miscarriage will occur. The period of organogenesis, between 2 and 8 weeks post fertilization (4 to 10 gestational weeks), is the most critical period in which teratogenic exposures can cause fetal malformations (**Figure 19-9**).[2] Interestingly, this is also the time when incidence of nausea peaks in pregnant individuals; there is perhaps an evolutionary advantage to food aversions and the subsequent avoidance of potential teratogens.

## Fetal Period

All major organs have formed by the beginning of the fetal period, which begins at 8 weeks post fertilization. During the fetal period, the fetus grows and organs develop to become functional. Fetal growth involves both hyperplasia (cellular division that yields a significant increase in cell numbers) and hypertrophy (an increase in cell size). At approximately 32 weeks' gestation, hypertrophy dominates.[42]

The rate and amount of fetal growth are determined by many factors, including genetics, placental metabolism, maternal conditions, maternal behavior, and environmental factors. For example, there is a well-known correlation between maternal smoking and impaired fetal growth.[80] Adequate fetal growth is also directly associated with optimal function of the placenta and the uterine vascular

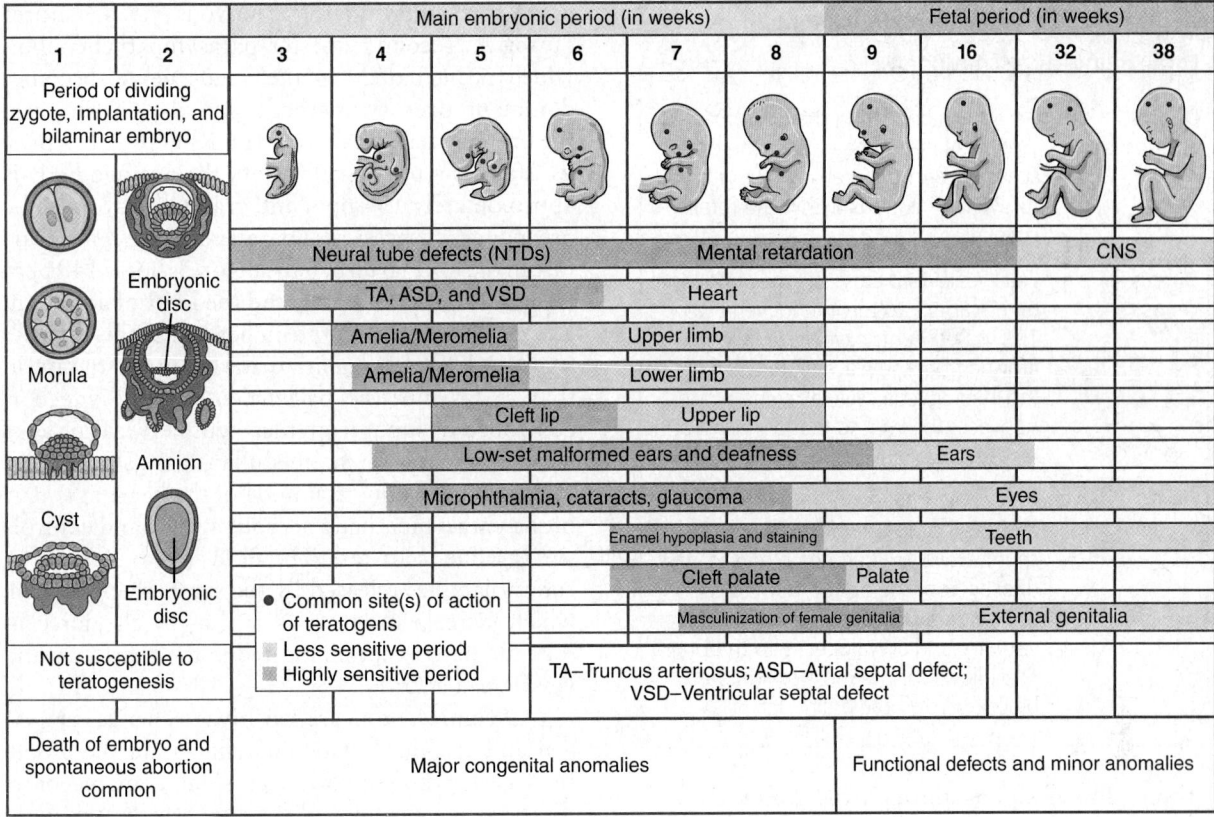

**Figure 19-9** Early stages of fetal development.
Reproduced with permission from Moore KL, Persaud TVN, Torchia MG. *The Developing Human: Clinically Oriented Embryology.* 11th ed. Philadelphia, PA: Elsevier; 2018.

system. Alterations in the trophoblastic invasion of the maternal spiral arterioles as well as inadequate development of the chorionic villus can result in impaired fetal growth as well as a number of other pregnancy complications.

### Fetal Cardio-Respiratory Physiology

Fetal oxygenation depends on adequate blood flow and placental function, as well as sufficient capacity in the fetus to transport oxygen. Crucially, the fetus has enhanced oxygen-carrying capability relative to an adult owing to several physiologic mechanisms. These differences allow the fetus to remain well oxygenated at a relatively low partial pressure of oxygen ($PO_2$), approximately 35 mm Hg, which is the same as the $PO_2$ in the maternal venous system. They include the following:

- Fetal hemoglobin has a higher affinity for oxygen than does maternal hemoglobin, which favors transfer of oxygen from the uterine circulation to the fetal circulation.

- The fetus has more hemoglobin in circulation than do adults (the average fetal hematocrit ranges from 43% to 63%).

- The fetus has a higher cardiac output and heart rate for an overall faster circulation.

- Organs that need oxygen such as the heart and brain are over-perfused in the fetus.

**Cardiovascular System.** The fetal cardiac output is approximately 1000 mL per minute.[40] The fetal lungs are not fully functional prior to birth, and three circulatory shunts exist to allow fetal blood (oxygenated via the placenta) to bypass the lungs and adequately perfuse developing tissue and organs: the ductus arteriosus, ductus venosus, and foramen ovale (**Table 19-6**).

Oxygen diffuses across the placenta to enter the umbilical vein. It travels through the umbilical cord and enters the fetus near the liver. The majority of oxygenated blood shunts away from the liver directly to the heart, moving through the *ductus venosus* to the inferior vena cava and into the right

| Table 19-6 | Fetal Circulatory Shunts |
|---|---|
| **Fetal Shunt** | **Description** |
| Ductus arteriosus | An artery connecting the pulmonary artery exiting the heart with the descending aorta, thereby allowing blood to bypass the lungs within the fetal circulation. |
| Ductus venosus | Fetal vessel that connects the abdominal umbilical vein to the inferior vena cava. This vessel shunts oxygenated blood arriving from the placenta directly into the inferior vena cava, allowing blood to bypass the liver, so that the heart and lungs receive oxygen first. |
| Foramen ovale | An opening between the right atrium and the left atrium of the heart. This shunt allows oxygen-rich blood to pass directly from the right atrium to the left atrium, then out through the left ventricle and aorta directly to the brain. This allows for the most oxygenated blood to go to the brain first. |

atrium. Blood shunts through the *foramen ovale* from the right atrium into the left atrium, and then into the left ventricle; there, it enters the aorta and is sent to the heart and brain. This shunt allows for the preferential oxygenation of the fetal heart and brain. After the blood oxygenates the brain, it returns to the right atrium (where a small amount of the now deoxygenated blood mixes with oxygenated blood) and into the right ventricle. This less-oxygenated blood is sent through the pulmonary artery and bypasses the lungs via the *ductus arteriosus* to the descending aorta where it travels to the lower half of the fetal body. This less-oxygenated blood also travels back to the placenta to return carbon dioxide and wastes into maternal circulation and gather additional oxygen and nutrients for the fetus.

### Control of the Fetal Heart Rate

The heart is one of the first fetal organs to function during embryonic development. The initial heartbeat occurs at approximately 22 days after fertilization, and blood begins to circulate by approximately 4 weeks after fertilization.[81] The fetal heart begins to contract at its fastest rate in early pregnancy, with an average heart rate of 170 beats per minute (bpm) at its peak in the first trimester. A slow embryonic heart rate (less than 100 bpm) at 6 to 7 weeks' gestation is associated with an increased risk of miscarriage.

As the parasympathetic nervous system matures during the second trimester, parasympathetic input, which is mediated via the vagus nerve, becomes dominant over sympathetic stimulation; in turn, the baseline fetal heart rate (FHR) gradually slows. At 20 weeks post fertilization, the average FHR is approximately 155 bpm and gradually drops as the pregnancy progresses. The average baseline heart rate in the normal term fetus before labor is 140 bpm (range: 120 to 160 bpm), and the FHR of a preterm fetus is likely to be on the higher end of this range.[33]

The FHR is similar to the adult heart rate in that it has intrinsic pacemaker activity, which is controlled by input from the vagus nerve. The vagus nerve originates in the medulla oblongata and terminates in the sinoatrial node of the heart; it is part of the parasympathetic nervous system and controls the baseline heart rate. The FHR is also affected by catecholamines released by the sympathetic system, which increase the rate, as well as by chemoreceptors and baroreceptors located in the heart's carotid vessels and aorta.

Chemoreceptors are sensitive to changes in oxygen and carbon dioxide content within the blood. Increased carbon dioxide causes the chemoreceptors to signal the medulla oblongata, which stimulates the vagus nerve and slows the FHR. The responses to chemoreceptor stimulation in the fetus are not totally understood, but the result of transient hypercarbia is clearly a slowing of the FHR. Baroreceptors in the aortic and carotid arches rapidly detect changes in blood pressure. When blood pressure rises, a quick reflex occurs (via the vagal nerve) to slow the FHR.

### Respiratory Function in the Fetus

Because the fetal lungs are not involved in the exchange of oxygen and carbon dioxide, only about 10% of fetal blood passes through the pulmonary circulation. Fetal lung growth and development depend on the presence of adequate fetal lung fluid (and amniotic fluid). The fetus's closed vocal cords allow fetal lung secretions to accumulate within the developing airway structures, which causes a passive pressure in the lungs that keeps them open. Fetal lung secretions also contribute to the elevated pulmonary vascular resistance that directs fetal blood through the circulatory shunts.

Glucocorticoid hormones play an important role in fetal lung development. Glucocorticoids stimulate surfactant production, which is critical for normal lung function. Surfactant decreases the surface tension of the lung alveoli so that they do not collapse with exhalation and the work of breathing is decreased. Glucocorticoids also inhibit the secretion of fetal lung fluid while promoting its reabsorption; this increase in surfactant and decrease in lung fluid helps prepare the fetus for birth.

The fetal lungs do not fully mature until the final weeks of pregnancy. Increasing glucocorticoid (cortisol) production at term helps prepare the fetal lungs for the extrauterine world.[82] While these processes begin prior to labor, the work of labor (and resultant increases in fetal cortisol production) plays an important final role in fetal lung development. In the setting of an increased risk of preterm birth, it is recommended that the pregnant person receive betamethasone or dexamethasone; both are glucocorticoids that can expedite fetal lung development in preparation for birth.

Breathing movements begin in utero, and the stretching of lung tissue through breathing plays an important role in the growth and development of the fetal lungs and respiratory muscles. Fetal breathing patterns are often episodic and include various forms: rapid, regular breathing; sighs; pauses while swallowing; and intermittent slow breaths during sleep cycles.[83] Fetuses typically have at least one 30-second episode of breathing movements within 30 minutes, and in the continuum of fetal distress, fetal breathing movements are the first thing to stop. Fetal breathing is therefore a component of the biophysical profile, a sonographic evaluation of fetal well-being.

### Gastrointestinal System and Liver

The development of the fetal gastrointestinal (GI) system is complex, involving rotation, retraction, herniation, and replacement, as well as some margin for error. Normally, all fetal abdominal contents are contained and fixed within the abdomen by 12 weeks after fertilization. By 20 weeks' gestation (22 postmenstrual weeks) the fetal GI tract is structurally similar to that of a term neonate, and by 32 to 34 weeks' gestation a fetus generally has the capacity to process enteral nutrition. Abnormalities in the GI tract are associated with reduced fetal growth.

While the placenta provides nutritional building blocks for the fetus, the fetal gut plays a major role in maintaining amniotic fluid volume and homeostasis. Fetuses begin swallowing amniotic fluid as early as 10 weeks after fertilization. In the latter part of pregnancy, fetuses may swallow as much as 1 liter of amniotic fluid each day. Amniotic fluid contains growth factors, nutrients, and hormones that stimulate the growth and development of the

GI tract, as well as providing as much as 10% of a fetus's protein intake.

The fetal liver remains immature until after birth. During pregnancy, unconjugated bilirubin that is transferred to the fetus from the maternal circulation remains unconjugated due to the immature fetal liver and intestines, and bilirubin clearance occurs via the placenta. Some neonates may develop hyperbilirubinemia when their immature liver assumes responsibility for bilirubin metabolism following birth.

Bile enters the fetal hepatic circulation by postfertilization week 13, which stimulates the production of meconium. Meconium moves from the bile ducts into the colon a few weeks later, and small amounts may enter the amniotic fluid before anal sphincter function develops. Mixed evidence exists whether bacteria and bacterial products are present in fetal meconium, amniotic fluid, and placenta.

### Fetal Nutrition and Metabolism

The fetus, the placenta, and the pregnant person all have their own metabolisms. Thus, fetal nutrition is dependent upon maternal diet, caloric intake, metabolic function, and adequate placental function. The placenta plays an important role in supporting fetal access to nutrients. For example, the placenta produces and releases hormones that stimulate maternal metabolism and increase the uptake of necessary nutrients. Adequate maternal nutrition during the first part of pregnancy has an effect on birth weight, and increased caloric intake is required during the second half of pregnancy to meet the metabolic and nutritional demands of the placenta and fetus.

Glucose is the primary energy source of the fetus, but fatty acids, amino acids, iron, folate, iodine, vitamin D, and calcium are also critical nutrients for fetal growth and development. Most fetal needs for vitamins and minerals can be met with an adequate maternal diet and/or supplementation with a prenatal vitamin.

### Glucose Metabolism and Anerobic Metabolism

Glucose is the primary source of energy for the fetus. The fetus cannot synthesize glucose and relies on glucose transported across the placenta from the maternal circulation, with almost half of the transferred glucose being used by the placenta for its own metabolic needs. In times of scarcity, however, the placenta will reduce its glucose utilization so that the fetus is less affected. Maternal fat stores will be metabolized to meet glucose requirements as necessary. If fetal needs cannot be met, hypoglycemia in both mother and fetus will occur.

The fetus releases insulin in response to glucose, which stimulates the release of growth factors, the synthesis of fatty acids and protein, and the continued placental uptake of glucose and other nutrients. The fetal liver receives the largest amount of glucose, as blood returning from the placenta moves first through the liver. The fetal liver contains enzymes that work in concert with glucocorticoids and insulin both to turn glucose into glycogen for storage and to catabolize glycogen into glucose for use. Glycogen is stored in the fetal liver as well as in the skeleton, heart, kidneys, intestines, and brain.

During normal aerobic metabolism, the fetus produces carbonic acid ($H_2CO_3$), which dissociates into water and carbon dioxide ($CO_2$) and diffuses across the placenta quickly. However, the fetus also uses anaerobic metabolism. Anaerobic metabolism utilizes glucose and glycogen to produce energy, with the final dissociation product being lactic acid ($C_3H_6O_3$). Lactate can serve as fuel for the fetus. However, unlike water and $CO_2$, lactic acid does not cross the placenta quickly. When anaerobic metabolism persists (e.g., under hypoxic conditions), the accumulating lactic acid will overwhelm the buffering capacity within the fetal circulation and lower the pH, resulting in a state of metabolic acidosis. This condition is discussed in further detail in the *Fetal Assessment During Labor* chapter.

### Fetal Brain Development

The architecture of the brain and major neurotransmitter systems is established early in pregnancy.[84] The size of the fetal brain in relation to the body is significantly greater in infants than in adults, and more so in humans than in any other mammal. During the second half of pregnancy, the fetal brain grows 10-fold in size.[40] The fetal circulation allows for preferential oxygenation of the brain. Notably, in the event of fetal growth restriction, brain growth is less affected than any other organ—a phenomenon referred to as "brain sparing."

The development of the brain and central nervous system begins with the development of the neural tube, between weeks 2 to 3 post fertilization. By week 5, neurons have begun to form and the first synapse has connected, forming a primitive cortical circuit. The fetal sensory system also begins forming in the embryonic period and is complete by the end of the second trimester: First the sense of touch and reflex to stimuli, then the sense of smell and taste, then the auditory system, and finally the visual system develop. By the third trimester, the sensory systems are integrated and functioning, so that fetuses can recognize and react to stimuli. For example,

after birth, neonates can recognize familiar voices and the smell of their amniotic fluid.[85,86]

Myelin is a fatty sheath surrounding a nerve that allows nerve impulses to move rapidly and efficiently. While mature myelin is noted as early as 20 weeks' gestation, myelination of the brain and spinal tract is an important part of central nervous system development during the third trimester and will not be completed until approximately age 3 years. During the third trimester, synaptic connections become more stable, and fetal behavior becomes organized into rapid eye movement (REM) and non-REM sleep states, suggesting neuronal connection in the thalamus and brain stem.[84]

Fetal brain development is shaped by genetics, epigenetic influences from the environment, spontaneous neural activity, and physical and chemical stimuli affecting the fetus. The complex interplay between maternal and fetal hormones and neurotransmitters affects neurodevelopment as well. For example, it appears that sustained high levels of maternal cortisol can affect fetal neurotransmitters and the fetal HPA axis system; it has also been shown that regular maternal exercise during pregnancy may facilitate fetal brain development.[87,88]

### Fetal Movement

Fetal movement can be seen on ultrasound by post-fertilization week 7, and by week 16 the full range of fetal movement is present. Limb movement develops at 9 weeks, with reflective leg movements occurring at 14 weeks. Hand-to-face movements become apparent by 12 to 13 weeks, while limb, head, and torso movements develop by 12 to 16 weeks. Fetuses begin to suck on their fingers by 15 weeks and develop more complex movement patterns after 24 weeks, when respiratory movements occur.[89] By 26 weeks' gestation, fetal movement is observed in response to sound, which corresponds to development of the sensory systems. Fetal movement increases until approximately 30 weeks post fertilization or 32 weeks menstrual age, and then begins to decrease. By term, there is not much room within the uterus, and fetal movement is typically limited to smaller movements, joint rotation, and spine extension. In addition, the fetus develops discrete cycles of quiet and active states close to term, which may affect maternal perception of movement. Fetal movement is linked to neurologic status and is an important measure of fetal health.[84]

### Fetal Behavior and Fetal States

Discrete fetal behavior states involving sleep–wake and other behavioral patterns begin to occur by

32 weeks' gestation menstrual age. Eye movement, gross body movement, and quiet states have been catalogued.[90,91] The average time the fetus spends in the quiet state ranges from 20 to 40 minutes.[89,90] The quiet state is associated with reduced variability in the interval between each fetal heartbeat—a phenomenon that can be observed during electronic FHR monitoring.

## Physiologic Adaptations to Pregnancy

Pregnant people experience a wide range of anatomic and physiologic alterations over the course of pregnancy and postpartum. While many of these changes cause normal symptoms of pregnancy, others herald the onset of abnormal processes. A thorough knowledge of the maternal anatomic and physiologic adaptations that occur during pregnancy is, therefore, an essential foundation for midwifery practice. This section presents an overview of some of the clinically important anatomic and physiologic pregnancy adaptations. Management of pregnancy symptoms is described in the *Prenatal Care*, *Pregnancy-Related Conditions*, and *Medical Complications in Pregnancy* chapters.

### The Reproductive Organs: Breast, Uterus, Cervix, and Vagina

Over the course of pregnancy, a woman's breasts grow and prepare for lactation. The uterus increases to approximately 5 times its normal size; at 38 gestational weeks, the uterus measures approximately 32 centimeters long, 22 centimeters across, and 24 centimeters wide. The cervix must first act as a barrier maintaining the uterine contents. However, at the end of pregnancy, the cervix becomes soft and short, opening to allow passage of the fetus during birth. These remarkable changes are the result of a complex interplay of hormonal stimulation that has important clinical implications for all pregnant people, but especially those who have congenital uterine anomalies, as well as those who experience miscarriage, preterm labor, preeclampsia, and other pregnancy complications.

### The Breast

The breast consists of adipose tissue, connective tissue, and glandular tissue. This glandular tissue, which makes up the primary functional unit of the breast, consists of 15 to 20 lobes. Each lobe comprises 20 to 40 lobules, and each lobule contains 10 to 100 alveoli. Breast alveoli are hollow cavities, each a few millimeters in size. These alveoli are lined with epithelial cells capable of creating the protein and lipid components of breast milk, and contracting to express this milk. Each lobe drains into a lactiferous duct; the lactiferous ducts expand into a lactiferous sinus, which then drains to the nipple.[92]

Under the direction of several different pregnancy hormones, the breast undergoes two distinct developmental changes to prepare for lactation during pregnancy. Both stages—mammogenesis and lactogenesis I—include hyperplasia and hypertrophy.[92] Hyperplasia refers to an increase in the number of cells, or cellular proliferation. Hypertrophy refers to enlargement of the cells; that is, cells grow in size.

Mammogenesis begins early in pregnancy. Breasts enlarge via cellular hyperplasia, and the breast lobules increase in size. The nipples become erectile, the areola becomes proportionately larger and darker, and superficial veins can become visible. During this process, an individual may feel the breasts are tender or even painful. Alveoli expand and proliferate at the end of breast lobules; the lobules proliferate as well. While these changes typically result in breast enlargement, the size of the breast does not correspond to its capacity for milk production.

Toward the middle of pregnancy, the alveoli epithelial cells change into secretory epithelium, which is the first stage of lactogenesis. By mid-gestation, the breasts are capable of producing milk components. Toward the end of pregnancy, the alveoli secrete colostrum but are primarily quiescent secondary to inhibition by progesterone, one of the primary pregnancy hormones. After birth of the placenta, the influence of progesterone abruptly ceases and lactogenesis II—that is, the onset of milk production—begins. A more detailed description of lactogenesis II and clinical implications is presented in the *Anatomy and Physiology of Postpartum* and *Infant Feeding and Lactation* chapters.

### The Uterus

The three layers of the uterus (endometrium, myometrium, and perimetrium) become clearly defined over the course of pregnancy. The uterus grows at a steady, predictable rate during pregnancy, with its expansion first becoming detectable at approximately 5 weeks' gestation. The initial uterine growth occurs in the anteroposterior diameter, while the isthmus or lower segment of the uterus can become very soft. This softening results in marked compressibility in the lower uterine segment that is present for a short period of time at approximately 4 to 6 weeks after the first day that the woman's last menstrual period started, and approximately 2 weeks after conception. This unusual compressibility, called *Hegar's sign*, is a probable sign of pregnancy. As seen in Figure 19-10, during a bimanual examination, the lower segment of the uterus is so soft that it can be easily compressed between the fingers of the examiner's two hands (one on the abdomen and the other gloved hand in the posterior fornix of the vagina). While it is a known sign of pregnancy, this is not a component of a standard physical exam.

The uterine shape changes from the nonpregnant pear shape to a ball or sphere in the first trimester, and then expands to an elongated cylinder. The anatomic location of the uterus in relation to maternal anatomy is illustrated in Figure 19-11.

The uterine round ligaments attach on either side of the uterus just below and in front of the insertion of the oviducts; they then cross the broad ligament in a fold of peritoneum, pass through the inguinal canal, and insert in the anterior (upper) portion of the labia majora on either side of the perineum. These ligaments are composed largely of smooth muscle that is continuous with the smooth muscle of the uterus. The round ligaments hypertrophy during pregnancy and stretch as the uterus enlarges. During periods of rapid uterine growth, individuals may feel stretching or sharp pain in the inguinal area when moving or turning. This effect occurs secondary to additional torsion or stretching of the round ligament and, therefore, is called "round ligament pain."

Growth of the uterus is due to two processes: (1) estrogen- and progesterone-induced hyperplasia of uterine smooth muscle cells within the myometrium during early pregnancy and (2) hypertrophy of the uterine muscles later in pregnancy. The muscles increase their content of actin, myosin, sarcoplasmic reticulum, and mitochondria, which collectively serve as the machinery used to contract the muscles during labor and birth, as described in the *Anatomy and Physiology of Labor and Birth* chapter. The myometrium thus has properties of both contractility and elasticity. Contractility allows for lengthening and shortening, whereas elasticity refers to the ability to stretch.

The uterus contracts irregularly throughout pregnancy. These generally sporadic and nonrhythmic contractions are called "Braxton Hicks contractions" after the nineteenth-century physician who first described them. At term, uterine contractions generally become more frequent, synchronized, and intense, with synchrony developing faster in multiparous individuals as compared to nulliparous persons.[93] Uterine contractions may or may not be perceived by the pregnant person. While they may be uncomfortable, they are generally not painful. They can be differentiated from true labor contractions by the fact that they do not progress in frequency, duration, or intensity within the same episode, and they do not result in cervical changes.

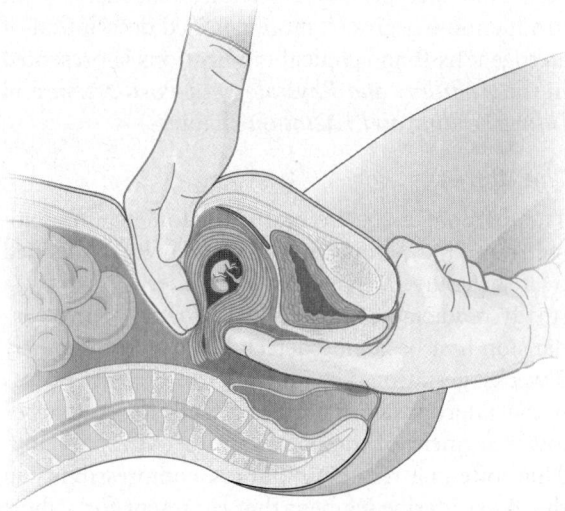

**Figure 19-10** Hegar's sign.

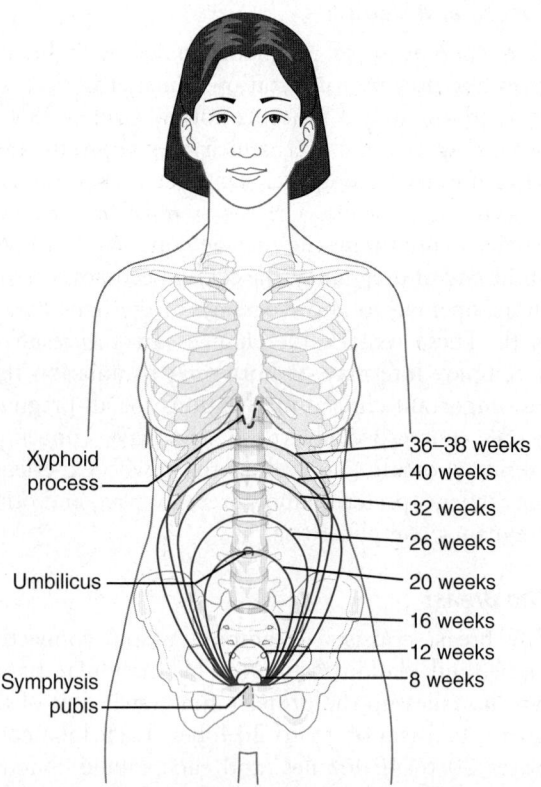

**Figure 19-11** Approximate normal fundal heights during pregnancy.

At term, approximately 500 to 900 mL of maternal blood flows through the uterus each minute. The majority of this blood enters the uterine spiral arteries, which run perpendicular through the myometrium to the intervillous space.[94,95] These remodeled arteries are large, flaccid vessels that do not have the ability to constrict, which facilitates maximized blood flow into the intervillous space of the placenta. Because the uterine arteries flow perpendicular to the myometrial muscle groups, they are compressed when the uterine muscles contract. The clinical relevance of this anatomy is described in more detail in the *Anatomy and Physiology of Labor and Birth* and *Anatomy and Physiology of Postpartum* chapters.

### The Cervix

In nonpregnant people, the cervix is, on average, approximately 3 centimeters, or 30 millimeters, long.[96,97] Usually the cervix remains between 30 and 40 millimeters in length throughout gestation. Those persons whose cervix shortens to less than 20 millimeters in the first half of pregnancy are at increased risk for preterm labor.

The cervix is composed primarily of extracellular connective tissue with some glandular tissue interspersed throughout it—a combination called the *extracellular matrix*. The glandular tissue in the cervix produces thick, tenacious mucus, which forms the mucus plug that seals the endocervical canal during pregnancy. This mucus plug helps prevent ascending bacteria or pathogens from entering the uterine cavity. The connective tissue is made of fibromuscular collagen and ground substance (an amorphous gelatinous material). The fibromuscular collagen includes protein in the form of collagen, elastin, and proteoglycans; the last are primarily hyaluronic acid and decorin.

The extracellular matrix is covered by a thin layer of smooth muscle, which is in turn covered with squamous and columnar epithelial cells at the internal os and external os. Approximately 80% of the cervix consists of extracellular matrix and 15% is smooth muscle, but the distribution is quite heterogeneous.[98–100] The area closest to the internal os has more smooth muscle, which is arranged in a circular sphincter-like pattern, whereas the area closer to the external os contains more extracellular matrix. The texture and strength of the collagen tissue depend on the type and number of cross-links between the collagen microfibrils.

Over the course of pregnancy, labor, birth, and the postpartum period, the cervix normally undergoes four distinct phases: (1) softening, also called *remodeling*; (2) accelerated softening at the end of pregnancy, referred to as *ripening*; (3) dilatation; and (4) repair.[99] Under the influence of estrogen, the cervix first begins to soften approximately 4 weeks after the first day of a woman's last menstrual period. This cervical softening, called *Goodell's sign*, is one sign of pregnancy. As vascularization increases, a cyanosis or bluish-purple discoloration called *Chadwick's sign* develops. Chadwick's sign is usually first evident at 6 to 8 weeks' gestation menstrual age. Following the initial relatively rapid softening, the cervix continues to soften throughout the pregnancy, albeit at a slower rate. The collagen becomes more soluble and compliant, but does not lose its structural integrity.

Cervical remodeling and activation of uterine contractions are the two primary physiologic events that are associated with the initiation of parturition or labor. Cervical ripening results from a series of interactions between hormonal and mechanical factors that have not been fully elucidated.[101] As progesterone levels fall and estrogen levels rise, the water content and vascularization of the cervix increase and the collagen cells become disorganized.

Several hormones are involved in the process of cervical remodeling. Prostaglandins, which are produced by cells in the uterus and cervix, affect nearby tissues locally and are referred to as paracrine agents. These prostaglandins initiate and facilitate the processes of both cervical ripening and the onset of labor. Production of pro-inflammatory cytokines leads to infiltration of the cervix by leukocytes and macrophages. These cells release enzymes that facilitate alterations in extracellular matrix proteins, loosening of collagen fibers, and a reduction in collagen content.

Toward the end of gestation and extending into early labor, the cervix shortens or thins so that there is no discernable length between the external os and the internal os. This process, which occurs in response to uterine contractions, is referred to as *effacement*. The cervix also begins to *dilate* as the process continues. Effacement and dilation generally occur during early labor in nulliparous people but may occur prior to progressive labor in multiparas. However, the onset of labor is not often a discrete event. There is significant variability between individuals with regard to the degree of effacement and dilatation that has occurred when labor begins.

### The Vagina

Pregnancy is a time marked by increased vascularity and vasocongestion, and these changes are particularly apparent in the vagina. The increased vascularity results in Chadwick's sign, which is detectable at approximately by 6 to 8 weeks' gestation menstrual age. The vaginal walls undergo significant change to prepare for the vaginal stretching that accompanies childbirth. These changes include epithelial thickening, connective tissue softening, and hypertrophy of smooth muscle. The vasocongestion, increased vascularity, and hypertrophy of pregnancy cause perineal structures to enlarge and may result in increased sensitivity or discomfort. Some pregnant people experience decreased or increased sexual arousal and pleasure owing to these changes.

Many people notice a small in increase in vaginal secretions (*leukorrhea*) during pregnancy. In addition to the normal vaginal secretions produced by epithelial cells, the cervical glands secrete an increased amount of mucus, which forms the cervical mucus plug as described earlier. These cervical and vaginal secretions likely form the basis of the physiological discharge of leukorrhea. The vaginal pH becomes more acidic in pregnancy, which is thought to protect against ascending infection that can contribute to preterm labor. Hormonal changes and an increase in vaginal glycogen stores contribute to a small increase in the risk for vulvovaginal candidiasis infections in pregnancy.[102]

## Cardiovascular System

Cardiovascular changes in the pregnant person begin early in the first trimester.[103] Blood volume increases by 40% to 50% over the course of pregnancy, reaching a maximum by 32 weeks' gestation. Plasma accounts for 75% of this increase. In addition to a significant increase in blood volume, there is a redistribution of fluid, with more extracellular fluid in intravascular spaces. The decrease in systemic vascular resistance, in combination with pressure on the vena cava from the growing uterus, is responsible for the dependent edema that most people experience in the third trimester and contributes to the development of varicosities, hemorrhoids, labial varicosities, and increased risk for venous thrombosis.

During pregnancy, cardiac output increases 30% to 50% to approximately 4 to 6 L per minute, primarily as a result of increased stroke volume.[37,94] The increase in cardiac output begins in the first trimester and peaks at approximately 25 to 30 weeks' gestation, when the total blood volume is approximately 5000 to 6000 mL. Heart rate increases by approximately 10 bpm, and blood pressure decreases gradually from prepregnancy values as early as 7 weeks' gestation. The decrease in blood pressure is presumed to occur in concert with expansion of the low-pressure placental compartment, as well as the lower systemic vascular resistance induced by progesterone. After blood pressure reaches a nadir in the second trimester, it begins to increase, and by term it typically has met or exceeded prepregnancy levels.

Anatomically, the heart is displaced upward (cephalad) and rotated to the left as the uterus enlarges. Mild pulmonic or tricuspid regurgitation often occurs. Several common signs and symptoms are related to these changes. Systolic ejection murmur that is loudest along the left sternal border and a third heart sound are common findings in pregnancy and attributed to the dramatic increase in cardiac output. These murmurs are clinically benign.[104] The third heart sound is a brief dull sound that may be audible at the end of diastole and just before the first sound occurs.

Careful monitoring of cardiovascular changes can facilitate early detection of abnormalities. For example, if a person's blood pressure fails to decrease during the second trimester, they may have chronic hypertension or be at risk for developing preeclampsia. Normal cardiovascular changes associated with pregnancy can also increase the risk for adverse outcomes in persons who have preexisting cardiomyopathies; these individuals should be referred promptly to a physician.[95] More information on these conditions is in the chapter on *Medical Complications in Pregnancy*.

## Hematologic Indices

Two aspects of hematologic changes in pregnancy have important clinical implications. First, pregnancy is a hypercoagulable state, due to an increase in clotting factors, a decrease in fibrinolytic factors, and decreased anticoagulant activity in pregnant individuals. Clotting factors I, II, VII, VIII, IX, and XII are produced in more abundance during pregnancy, whereas protein S levels and activated protein C levels fall. These alterations in the coagulation cascade are likely protective, and help prevent hemorrhage following birth of the placenta. Nevertheless, they also increase an individual's risk for venous thromboembolism in the prenatal and postnatal periods.

The second clinically important hematologic change in pregnancy relates to hemodilution, iron metabolism, and iron-deficiency anemia. During pregnancy, the increase in maternal plasma volume exceeds the increase in red cell mass, which results in a physiologic hemodilution. This physiologic hemodilution has a positive effect on placental perfusion, with blood becoming less viscous.[105] In addition, the maternal hemoglobin (Hgb) concentration decreases by approximately 2% to 10%. This drop in hemoglobin level occurs because the fetal uptake of iron is usually more than the maternal intestinal absorption of iron can replace. The net result of these two processes is a decrease in the maternal hematocrit of approximately 3% to 5%, reaching a nadir late in the second trimester or early in the third trimester.

Because iron is not easily absorbed, fetal uptake can drain a pregnant person's iron reserves, despite the fact that iron absorption in the second and third trimesters increases more than fivefold.[19] Thus, iron stores can be easily depleted in pregnancy and, in turn, iron-deficiency anemia is common in pregnancy. Additional hematologic changes include a decrease in the concentration of plasma proteins, especially albumin. Lower albumin results in lower colloid oncotic pressure, which, in tandem with decreased venous resistance, facilitates the development of dependent edema.

## Respiratory System

During pregnancy, oxygen consumption increases by 30%. Pregnancy is also associated with increases in minute ventilation (i.e., the volume of air inhaled and exhaled in a minute) and in blood volume within the pulmonary circulation. An increase in thoracic diameter and an upward displacement of the diaphragm (as much as 4 centimeters) changes the pregnant woman's lung capacity. Tidal volume (the amount of air that moves in and out of the lungs with each normal breath) increases by 30% to 40%, and vital capacity (the total amount of air that can be displaced from the lung with maximal expiratory effort) increases slightly (**Figure 19-12**).[94,106]

Progesterone causes an increase in minute ventilation that places the woman in a state of compensated respiratory alkalosis (lower than normal levels of carbon dioxide). This respiratory alkalosis promotes the diffusion of oxygen across the placenta to the fetus, and the return of carbon dioxide from the fetus. Pregnant women often report a sensation of dyspnea, which can occur secondary to the progesterone-induced hyperventilation, although the exact mechanism has not been fully elucidated.

Pregnant people commonly experience dyspnea even when at rest. The actual etiology of this condition is in part due to progesterone, but also arises secondary to an increased awareness of the sensitivity to carbon dioxide and respiratory drive in combination with added respiratory effort once the diaphragm is displaced upward.[94] Physiologic dyspnea can be distinguished from pathologic dyspnea by the respiratory rate. Tachypnea is a sign of possible respiratory compromise.

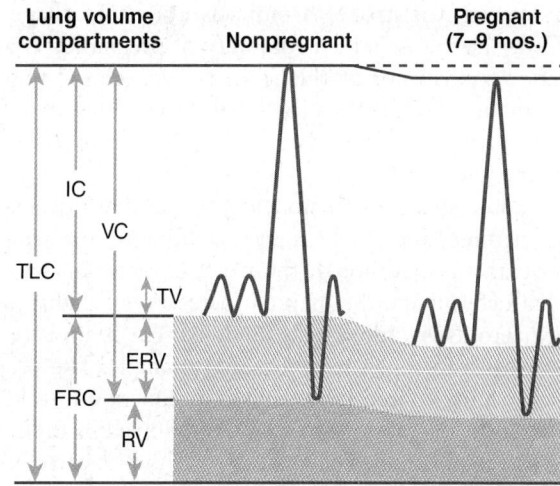

**Figure 19-12** Changes in lung volumes in persons who are 7–9 months pregnant compared with lung volumes in nonpregnant individuals.
Abbreviations: ERV, expiratory reserve volume; FRC, functional residual capacity; IC, inspiratory capacity; RV, residual volume; TLC, total lung capacity; TV, tidal volume; VC, vital capacity.

Under the influence of estrogen, progesterone, and increased blood volume, nasal passages become edematous and hyperemic in pregnancy. Pregnant individuals often report more congestion and/or rhinitis, sometimes confusing these symptoms with an upper respiratory infection or allergies.

## Cerebrum and Neurocognitive Adaptations

The brain undergoes both anatomic and functional changes during pregnancy that are just beginning to be identified and understood. Anatomically, the brain has a limited capacity to withstand significant increases in blood flow, in large part due to the constraints of the rigid skull. Thus, the primary adaptation of the brain during pregnancy is to maintain vascular homeostasis in the face of a 40% to 50% increase in blood volume and decreased systemic vascular resistance. Cerebral arteries adapt to withstand the chemical signals that cause the vasoconstriction of blood vessels in other organ systems, through either a decreased sensitivity to vasoconstrictors or an increased sensitivity to vasodilators.[107] Pregnancy also appears to tighten the regulation of cerebral blood flow so that it is less affected by acute changes in blood pressure.[108] Meanwhile, the blood–brain barrier, which serves to limit nonselective transport of solutes and chemicals into the brain, is normally unchanged during pregnancy.

Approximately 70% of the cerebral blood circulation is venous (as opposed to arterial), and pregnancy is a period of increased risk for cerebral vascular complications associated with the venous system, such as stroke, thrombosis, and hemorrhage. While the increased coagulability of pregnancy is a major contributor to this risk, it is speculated that pregnancy could affect the cerebral vascular structure in a way that increases the risk for cerebral vascular accidents.[109]

Some structural remodeling of the brain occurs during pregnancy, including the creation of new neural pathways. Although the exact etiology has not been determined, the marked increased exposure to sex steroids is undoubtedly involved. The brain is replete with estrogen receptors, for example. The primary change noted in humans is a reduction in gray matter during pregnancy, which is followed by an increase postpartum. The areas of gray matter affected govern motivation, somatosensory information, and social processes. Preliminary evidence indicates that these changes in brain plasticity facilitate "mothering" behaviors and recognition of infant cues.[110]

The placental hormones also signal several neuroactive hormones to act upon the maternal brain, including oxytocin, melatonin, serotonin, and thyrotropin-releasing hormone. Oxytocin stimulates nesting and nursing behaviors, serotonin and melatonin affect mood during pregnancy and postpartum, and thyrotropin-releasing hormone stimulates excess release of thyrotropin, which is thought to increase the secretion of prolactin.[111] Prolactin likely plays a key role in coordinating neuroendocrine and behavioral adaptations in the pregnant person, including appetite, oxytocin secretion, and the stress response.[112] Hormonally driven changes in the number and expression of neurons promote the establishment of parental caregiving behaviors.[113] The most profound hormonal shift that drives maternal behavior occurs at birth, when the progesterone level drops and the estradiol and oxytocin levels rise.

The dynamic changes that stimulate behavioral adaptations for caregiving and nurturing may also increase the risk of mental health disorders. For example, the incidence of mood disorders is higher during the peripartum period as compared to non-childbearing eras of a person's life.[110]

## Metabolic Changes

Among the many important endocrine and metabolic changes in pregnancy are changes that occur in the function of several organs that control metabolism, such as the hypothalamus, pituitary, thyroid, and adrenal glands; these organs often work in an interrelated manner. Calcium metabolism and the renin–angiotensin system also undergo significant alterations in ways that facilitate fetal growth and development.

## Thyroid Metabolism

Although all endocrine organs undergo changes in pregnancy, thyroid changes are particularly of note. Because both hypothyroid and hyperthyroid states can adversely affect the fetus, it is critical that a euthyroid state be maintained throughout pregnancy and is especially important during organogenesis.[114]

A person's thyroid gland slightly increases in size early in pregnancy and may be palpable on an initial prenatal visit as a smooth, regular-shaped mass. The basal metabolic rate also increases by 20% to 25% during pregnancy. Several changes occur in the production and transport of thyroxine during pregnancy. The alpha unit of hCG, which is molecularly very similar to TSH, thus stimulates the thyroid in the same manner as TSH. This causes an increase in thyroxine ($T_4$) levels (i.e., subclinical hyperthyroidism). Sensing the increase in $T_4$, the pituitary reduces its production of TSH. At the same time, higher levels of plasma albumin and thyroxine-binding globulin (TBG) bind more $T_4$ in serum. Thus, the individual remains euthyroid because the level of free thyroxine ($FT_4$) is normal, despite lower levels of TSH and higher levels of $T_4$. Free thyroxine is the form of the hormone that is able to become metabolically active by moving out of the circulation into cells (**Figure 19-13**). The higher levels of $T_4$ are thought to stimulate the pituitary gland to release other hormones necessary during pregnancy.[111] The TSH level reaches a nadir at approximately 10 gestational weeks.[115] Subsequently, as hCG levels

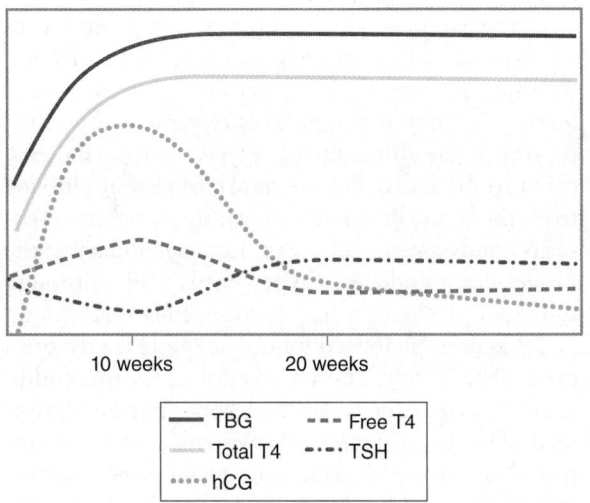

| TBG | Free T4 |
| Total T4 | TSH |
| hCG | |

**Figure 19-13** The pattern of changes in serum concentrations of thyroid function studies and hCG according to gestational age. While TSH physiologically decreases within the first trimester, it typically stays within the normal adult range.

decline, TSH levels rise to reach the nonpregnant level by the third trimester, and total thyroxine levels decline to a normal value.

Plasma values for thyroid function are trimester specific and cannot be determined via one measurement. In general, an assessment of TSH and either free $T_4$ or total $T_4$ is needed to interpret thyroid function during pregnancy.[116,117] Typically, persons with preexisting hypothyroidism need to increase their dose of synthetic thyroid hormone (levothyroxine) during pregnancy to account for the increased metabolic demand.[117]

### Glucose and Lipid Metabolism

Glucose metabolism is significantly altered in pregnancy. Glucose is transferred across the placenta via facilitated diffusion. Glucose delivery to the fetus depends on a concentration gradient between the maternal and fetal circulations, necessitating higher maternal glucose levels. Placental and maternal hormones, including estrogen, progesterone, leptin, cortisol, placental lactogen, and placental growth hormone, stimulate maternal insulin resistance, resulting in elevated blood glucose. This mild state of insulin resistance results in an increase in maternal glucose production of as much as 30% in the third trimester.

Because of the ongoing fetal use of glucose, a pregnant person will experience fasting glucose levels lower than in the nonpregnant state, yet because of insulin resistance, postprandial glucose levels can be higher than in nonpregnant individuals consuming a similar glycemic load.[118] Lower fasting blood glucose levels can worsen nausea and vomiting in early pregnancy but may also contribute to the pregnant person's enhanced appetite and their need to eat more often. As the placenta increases in size and function, maternal hyperinsulinemia likewise increases to keep pace. Individuals who are unable to sufficiently raise their insulin production will develop gestational diabetes in the latter half of pregnancy.

Lipid metabolism is also altered significantly during pregnancy, in part due to the lipolytic effects of increased insulin.[119] Body fat accumulates during the first two-thirds of pregnancy, but this growth then stops or declines during the last third of pregnancy. Thus, the pregnant woman is first in an *anabolic* state and then later in a *catabolic* state. During the period of rapid lipolysis, free fatty acids and glycerol are generated. Free fatty acids are converted to ketones, and glycerol is converted to glucose. The free fatty acids are used to synthesize triglycerides, which causes triglyceride levels to increase.[120]

### Immunologic Adaptations

Pregnancy is essentially an immunologic paradox: First, how does the pregnant woman avoid rejecting the fetus given that fetal cells and maternal cells are in direct contact in the maternal spiral arteries and intervillous space? Second, how do the immunologic changes that take place to accommodate the fetus, a semi-allograft, affect the maternal immune response? Immunologic changes in pregnancy are implicated in several important clinical disorders, including recurrent miscarriage, Rh sensitization, and preeclampsia.

The body's immune response is subclassified as either innate immunity or adaptive immunity; the latter is subdivided into cell-mediated immunity and antibody-mediated immunity. The innate immune response is the first line of defense against "non-self" invaders; it includes inflammation and phagocytosis. *Cell-mediated immunity* is responsible for elimination of intracellular microbes and involves several immune lymphocytes, including natural killer (NK) cells and T cells. *Antibody-mediated immunity* involves the production of antibodies by B cells; these antibodies then target extracellular microbes or antigens.

In general, innate immunity is enhanced during pregnancy, whereas adaptive immunity is less functional. In particular, cell-mediated (T helper 1) responses are somewhat suppressed compared to antibody-mediated (T helper 2) responses, which are more responsive. This change in the cell-mediated and antibody-mediated responses is referred to as a *Th1 to Th2 shift*.[121,122] These changes increase the risk of maternal infection, especially with regard to viral infections such as influenza or varicella. At the same time, the Th1 to Th2 shift results in improvement of some autoimmune disorders such as rheumatoid arthritis.

Chemotaxis is delayed in the pregnant woman, which can delay the maternal response to some infections. The total white blood cell count is elevated in pregnancy largely due to increased numbers of polymorphonuclear neutrophils, monocytes, and granulocytes. Many of the bioactive agents produced by the fetus and placenta effect subtle shifts in maternal immunity (Table 19-7).[120–122]

Although little overall change occurs in the maternal immune response, subtle changes in each of the three types of immunity have important clinical implications. There is a small increase in the risk for developing infections caused by gram-negative organisms as well as by mycotic agents and fungi. Pregnant individuals also have increased morbidity from gram-negative infections, H1N1 flu virus, and

| Table 19-7 | Changes in the Immune System During Pregnancy |
|---|---|
| **Type of Immune Response** | **Maternal Adaptations** |
| Primary host defense mechanisms | Increased number of white blood cells (primarily polymorphonuclear leukocytes), which enhances the pregnant woman's nonspecific immune response. |
| | Delayed chemotaxis (the movement of phagocytes to the site of foreign invasion), which may delay the maternal response to infection. |
| | Decreased number of natural killer cells, which may delay the maternal response to infection. |
| | Reduced levels of plasma IgG—the hemodilution of pregnancy and passive transfer of Ig antibody to the fetus reduces maternal blood levels of IgG. |
| Cell-mediated immunity | Although the overall number of lymphocytes remains unchanged, there is a decreased number of T-helper cells (CD4 cells) relative to the number of T-suppressor cells (CD8 cells). |
| | With fewer CD4 cells, B-cell function may be slightly impaired. |
| Antibody-mediated immunity | Overall unchanged. |

varicella if infections occur. In addition, pregnant persons are more likely to become infected when exposed to certain pathogens, such as herpes simplex virus, poliovirus, cytomegalovirus, malaria, and hepatitis. Some autoimmune disorders such as rheumatoid arthritis are likely to improve during pregnancy, whereas others, such as systemic lupus erythematosus, are more likely to flare.

## Renal System

Two different aspects of renal adaptations in pregnancy are responsible for symptoms that must be carefully evaluated to differentiate normal from abnormal alterations. First, a marked increase in renal plasma flow is the natural consequence of arterial vasodilation and increased cardiac output. Renal blood flow increases 60% to 80% above prepregnant levels in the first and second trimesters, and 50% above prepregnant levels in the third

trimester. The glomerular filtration rate (GFR) increases by 50% over prepregnant levels, peaking at 12 gestational weeks.[123] The obvious physiologic consequences of these changes are the commonly reported symptoms of urinary frequency and nocturia that frequently occur at two different times during the prenatal period. Frequency during the first trimester is due to hormonal changes affecting levels of renal function and bladder compression within the pelvis due to uterine growth. Bladder compression resolves as the uterus moves out of the pelvis and becomes an abdominal organ in the second trimester. Urinary frequency during the third trimester occurs most often among primiparous individuals, after engagement has occurred and the presenting part descends into the pelvis, causing direct pressure against the bladder.

Nocturia also can be caused by increased urine production at night. Venous return from the extremities is facilitated when the woman lies in a recumbent lateral position while sleeping. In this position, the uterus is not pressing against the pelvic vessels and inferior vena cava, and urinary output increases. Additionally, pregnant individuals have an increase in sodium excretion at night, with an associated increase in fluid excretion, which may also explain nocturia.

The increased flow through the kidneys may be great enough that the descending tubule is unable to reabsorb all glucose. This resultant physiologic glycosuria is usually intermittent, but it affects as many as 20% of pregnant individuals. Similarly, protein reabsorption is not as efficient as it is in the nonpregnant state. A small amount of urinary protein in a sample of concentrated urine can cause a dipstick test to be positive, which may be falsely interpreted as a urinary tract infection or even proteinuria associated with preeclampsia. Serum creatinine likewise falls; thus, plasma values for creatinine that would be considered normal in a nonpregnant woman may actually reflect renal dysfunction in a pregnant woman.

The smooth muscle found in the ureters, urethra, and bladder dilates under the influence of progesterone during pregnancy—a physiologic renal dilation known as hydroureter and/or hydronephrosis.[124] While this renal dilation is normal in pregnancy, it presents an increased risk for urinary tract infections, as well as ascending infections including pyelonephritis. In addition, the bladder becomes hyperemic and urinary stasis can occur, which occasionally results in stress incontinence.

Thus, physiologic changes in pregnancy cause symptoms that may be normal, or a sign of urinary tract infection or renal dysfunction. Urinary tract infections are also associated with preterm labor. Therefore, careful attention to the history, physical examination, and adjunct measures of urinary function are necessary to adequately care for individuals with urinary symptoms.

## Gastrointestinal System

Several physiologic changes of pregnancy predispose the pregnant woman to heartburn (pyrosis). The smooth muscle of the lower esophageal sphincter is relaxed, gastrointestinal motility is slower, esophageal function and peristalsis change, and the angle of the gastroesophageal junction is altered as the stomach is displaced by the enlarging uterus. Individuals with preexisting gastroesophageal reflux disorder may find this condition to be aggravated throughout pregnancy. Flatulence and gas pain are more common during pregnancy due to decreased motility from the effect of progesterone relaxing smooth muscle and from the displacement of and pressure on the intestines by the enlarging uterus.

During pregnancy, the effects of progesterone on smooth muscle also cause a decreased peristalsis of the large bowel, a decrease in gastric motility, and delayed emptying time. These alterations, in addition to changes in fluid reabsorption, increase the risk of constipation. Moreover, the displacement and compression of the bowel by the enlarging uterus or presenting part may contribute to decreased motility in the GI tract and increase constipation. Specifically, the stomach is moved upward and the intestines are displaced laterally. Thus, constipation is common in pregnant individuals, especially in the first trimester when the growing uterus places pressure on the descending colon. Constipation, prolonged straining, and venous engorgement in rectal veins secondary to pressure on the vena cava from the enlarging uterus also contribute to the increased incidence of hemorrhoids that is common in pregnant people.[125]

### Changes in the Oral Cavity

During pregnancy, bleeding gums (gingivitis), especially after brushing teeth, are related to estrogen- and progesterone-mediated inflammation and hyperemia. Elevated levels of estrogen create a favorable environment for the growth of bacteria that can cause gingivitis and gingival inflammation. Periodontal disease has been associated with adverse pregnancy outcomes.[126]

## Musculoskeletal Changes

The musculoskeletal changes that occur during pregnancy are primarily related to weight gain, the growing uterus, the softening effects of progesterone

on cartilage in joints, and the laxity of ligaments induced by estrogen and relaxin.[91] These changes result in lordosis, kyphosis, and altered gait that gradually increase as pregnancy progresses.[127]

Changes within the pelvic girdle are the most profound. The sacroiliac joint widens and has more mobility. The symphysis also widens, and the pelvis develops an anterior tilt. Many of the common discomforts of pregnancy can be attributed to these anatomic changes, including pelvic pain, sciatica, back pain, and carpal tunnel syndrome. A careful history and physical examination is needed to rule out more serious problems for which pregnant people are at increased risk, such as herniated discs and peripheral nerve injury.

## Integumentary Changes

Pregnancy is associated with many changes in the integument. Hyperpigmentation occurs as estrogen, progesterone, and melanocyte-stimulating hormone induce melanocytes to make and deposit pigment. This phenomenon results in darkening of the areola, the change of the linea alba to the *linea nigra*, and *melasma* or *chloasma* (irregular areas of pigmentation on the cheeks), also called the "mask of pregnancy."[128,129] Intertriginous areas such as the axillae, genitalia, perianal region, and inner thighs may also become darker during pregnancy.

Thinning of the elastin fibers in connective tissue under the skin predisposes pregnant people to striae gravidarum (stretch marks). As the sizes of the abdomen and breasts increase, elastin fibers at the dermal–epidermal junction stretch and shift from perpendicular to parallel, which can create striae.

Vascular nevi called spider angiomas are common as blood vessels dilate and proliferate. These small red lesions have a central puncta and branches that extend from the center and disappear after birth. Edema of the lower extremities, as well as the hands and face, is caused by increased blood volume and increased venous hydrostatic pressure. This increased venous pressure, in combination with the compression of the pelvic blood vessels and femoral vein increase can cause varicose veins in the legs and vagina.

## Effects of Pregnancy on Drug Absorption, Distribution, and Elimination

The many physiologic changes that occur during pregnancy affect the pharmacokinetics of any drugs or other agents used by the pregnant person. Pregnancy-related changes in pharmacokinetics with some clinical examples are summarized in Table 19-8.[48,130]

| Table 19-8 | Pregnancy-Related Changes in Pharmacokinetics | |
|---|---|---|
| **Pharmacokinetic Phase** | **Pregnancy Changes** | **Clinical Implications** |
| **Absorption** | Increased progesterone production causes decreased intestinal motility and 30–50% increase in gastric emptying time | Gestational nausea and vomiting may impair absorption |
| | | Slower gastric emptying time may delay onset of drug response |
| | Gastric pH increases at mid-gestation | Increased exposure to bacteria in the intestines may decrease bioavailability of some drugs |
| | | Calcium and iron bind when ingested concurrently, thereby decreasing absorption of both minerals |
| Lung absorption | Respiratory minute volume increases approximately 50% | Dose requirements for inhaled drugs are decreased |
| Transdermal, subcutaneous absorption | Skin perfusion and skin hydration are both increased | Both lipophilic drugs and hydrophilic drugs are more rapidly absorbed transcutaneously |
| | Enhanced perfusion to muscles | Intramuscular absorption of drugs is more rapid and complete compared to absorption in non-pregnant individuals |
| **Distribution** | Plasma volume is expanded by approximately 50% | Hydrophilic drugs have reduced plasma concentration and need to be given in higher doses |
| | Body fat stores increase by 3–4 kg | Lipophilic drugs that concentrate in body fat may accumulate; prolonged effects could be seen following long-term use |
| Protein binding | Plasma albumin concentrations are reduced secondary to increased plasma volume | Increased free drug is available for pharmacologic effects |
| | | Drugs that are highly protein bound will have more pharmacologic activity in a pregnant person |
| Fetal–maternal distribution | Fetal compartment available for distribution of drugs | Highly lipophilic, low-molecular-weight drugs that have low protein binding can accumulate in the fetal compartment |
| | The fetal circulation is more acidic than the maternal circulation | Basic drugs such as meperidine (Demerol) can have higher concentrations in the fetal compartment than in the maternal circulation secondary to "ion trapping" |
| | Fetal albumin concentration in plasma increases throughout pregnancy and is 20% higher than maternal concentrations at term | Drugs that are highly bound to albumin can concentrate in the fetus at term |
| | | Most drugs in the fetal compartment tend to be 50–100% of the concentration in the maternal compartment |
| **Metabolism** | Changes in estrogen and progesterone affect cytochrome P-450 enzyme activity | Metabolism of caffeine and theophylline (Theo-Dur) is inhibited or slower |
| | CYP1A2 is inhibited | Metabolism of sertraline (Zoloft) and metoprolol (Lopressor) is enhanced or faster |
| | CYP3A4 and CYP2C9 are increased | |
| **Elimination** | Glomerular filtration rate increases by 50% throughout pregnancy | More rapid clearance of drugs that are eliminated renally |

## Fetopelvic Relationships During Pregnancy

During labor and birth, the fetus passes through the bony cavity that is formed by the two innominate pelvic bones. The pelvic architecture, diameters of the fetal skull, and position of the fetal head are all important factors that affect how the fetus passes through the maternal pelvis during labor and birth. This section reviews aspects of the pelvic architecture and fetal anatomy that can be assessed during pregnancy to identify persons who have a risk for cephalopelvic disproportion or unusual fetal presentation; these data are used to provide best care to individuals during pregnancy, labor, and birth.

The bony portion of the pelvis traversed by the fetus during labor and birth is a curved tube. The iliac fossa and iliac crest, which are above the pelvic canal, have been historically referred to as the "false pelvis" because this area of the pelvis has little obstetric significance yet defines the lower border of the abdominal cavity.

The pelvic bony passageway that must be traversed by the fetus during vaginal birth is historically referred to as the "true pelvis." The linea terminalis—an invisible line that runs along the pelvic brim from the superior part of the symphysis pubis around to the sacral promontory (Figure 19-14)—demarcates the inlet or superior plane of this bony canal. This passageway has a shallow anterior wall made of the symphysis pubis, which is approximately 5 centimeters in length, and a concave (curved) posterior wall made of the sacrum, which is approximately 10 centimeters in length. The ability of the fetal head to pass through the pelvic bones is determined in part by the architecture of the sacrum, sacrosciatic notch, sidewalls, ischial spines, and subpubic arch.

For the purposes of clinical practice, four aspects of the shape of the pelvic canal are particularly relevant: (1) three planes called the inlet, midpelvis, and outlet; (2) the curvature of the sacrum; (3) the shape of the forepelvis, which is based on the angulation of the pelvic sidewalls between the greater sciatic arch and pubic arch; and (4) the angle of the pubic arch, which is created by the symphysis pubis and inferior rami of the ischial tuberosities.[131,132] Clinical assessment of the shape and size of the pelvic canal may be performed prenatally during a vaginal examination when indicated. This assessment is also performed during labor as one component of an evaluation of the '3 P's'—that is, the passageway (pelvis), passenger (position of the fetal presenting part), and powers (strength, duration, and frequency of uterine contractions). (Other 'P's' may be added to assessment that are beyond anatomy and physiology.)

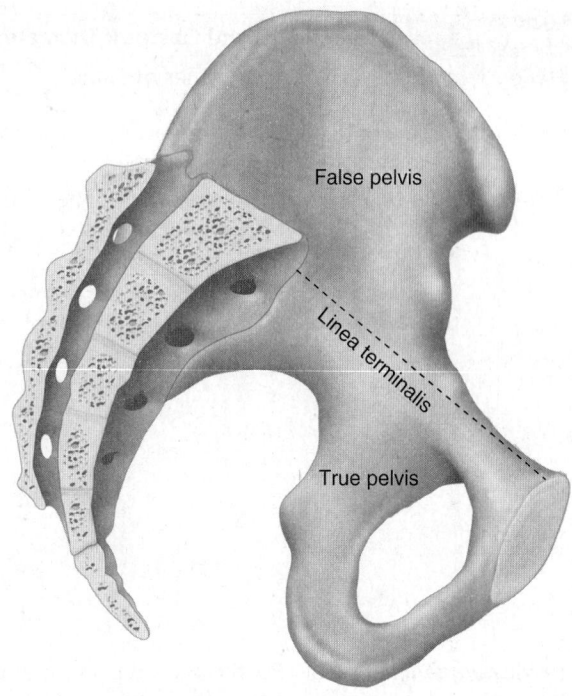

**Figure 19-14** The linea terminalis is a plane that separates the true pelvis and false pelvis. The linea terminalis consists of the superior posterior border of the symphysis pubis, iliopectineal (arcuate) line, and sacral promontory.

### Pelvic Planes and Obstetric Diameters

The pelvic canal has three planes of obstetric significance: the inlet, the midplane, and the outlet (Table 19-9). Each of these planes has anteroposterior and transverse diameters that are measured clinically when evaluating the shape and contour of the pelvis. The diameters of clinical importance are the diagonal conjugate (anterior–posterior diameter of the pelvic inlet) and the interspinous diameter of the midplane (transverse diameter of the midplane).

If the diagonal conjugate is easily palpated during a vaginal examination, the individual has an increased risk for the fetus being unable to engage in the pelvis. The interspinous diameter is the narrowest diameter that the fetal presenting part negotiates. The fetal skull is typically approximately 9.5 centimeters in diameter and the interspinous diameter is typically about 10 centimeters in diameter. Thus, prominent ischial spines that are easily palpable and a narrow interspinous diameter suggest that the fetal

| Plane | Boundaries of Plane | Significant Obstetric Diameters |
|---|---|---|
| **Pelvic *inlet*** (superior strait): upper entry into the true pelvis | **Posterior:** sacral promontory<br>**Lateral:** iliopectineal (arcuate) line that extends to the horizontal rami superior posterior edge of the pubic bones<br>**Anterior:** superior posterior border of the symphysis of the symphysis pubis | **Anteroposterior diameters:**<br>1. *Obstetric conjugate of the inlet:* This measurement is the true anterior–posterior diameter of the pelvic inlet. It extends backward from the middle of the posterior symphysis pubis to the middle of the sacral promontory. The pelvis is considered contracted if the obstetric conjugate measures less than 10 cm.<br>2. *Diagonal conjugate of the inlet:* This measurement can be assessed clinically as a proxy for the obstetric conjugate. The diagonal conjugate extends backward from the lower margin of the symphysis pubis to the middle of the sacral promontory. A typical clinical measurement is considered to be 11.5 cm or more.<br>**Transverse diameter:** greatest distance between the linea terminalis on either side of the pelvis; this distance is approximately 13.5 cm. |
| **Pelvic *midplane*:** plane of least dimensions | **Posterior:** sacrum at the junction of the fourth and fifth sacral vertebrae<br>**Lateral:** ischial spines<br>**Anterior:** inferior border of pubic symphysis | **Anteroposterior diameter:** extends from the middle of the inferior margin of the symphysis pubis through the middle of the transverse diameter and to the sacrum. This diameter is typically 11.5 cm or more.<br>**Transverse diameter (*interspinous diameter*):** distance between the ischial spines. Typically measures approximately 10 cm. This is the smallest diameter of the pelvis that the fetal presenting part must accommodate during the process of labor and birth. |
| **Pelvic *outlet*:** can be thought of as composed of two triangles, with the transverse diameter of the outlet serving as the common base of these two triangles | **Posterior:** sacrococcygeal joint<br>**Lateral:** inner surface of ischial tuberosities<br>**Anterior:** lower border of pubic symphysis | **Anteroposterior diameter:** Extends from the middle of the inferior margin of the symphysis pubis to the sacrococcygeal joint. This measurement is typically 11.5 cm or more.<br>**Transverse diameter (*intertuberous*, or *biischial*, diameter):** The distance between the inner aspect of the lowermost part of ischial tuberosities. This diameter has a measurement of approximately 10 cm. |

head may not be able to successfully rotate and descend from an occiput transverse or oblique position into an occiput anterior or posterior position during labor. This inability to rotate fully and/or descend beyond the midplane is called deep transverse arrest.

### Sacral Curvature

The posterior aspect of the pelvis is largely defined by the length and curvature of the sacrum. The curvature of the sacrum determines the amount of room in the posterior portion of the pelvis. The degree of sacral curvature can play a role in how easily the fetal head rotates to an anterior or posterior position during labor.

### Forepelvis

The forepelvis is defined by the pelvic sidewalls of the inner aspect of the ischium. The pelvic sidewalls extend from the upper anterior angle of the sacrosciatic notch at the point of the widest transverse diameter of the pelvic inlet in a downward and forward line to the ischial tuberosities; this is the transverse diameter of the pelvic outlet. The sidewalls are normally slightly convergent in that, if the lines of their angles were extended beyond the pelvis, the two lines would meet at about the level of the knees; however, when palpated, they feel generally straight.

The obstetric importance of the pelvic sidewalls hinges on the angle of the sidewalls. *Divergence or convergence* is based on whether the point of origin of the sidewall at the inlet and the ending point of the sidewall at the ischial tuberosities are essentially equidistant from the anteroposterior diameter of the pelvis. Convergent sidewalls usually decrease the angle of the pubic arch and may be accompanied by more prominent ischial spines. Divergent sidewalls are rare and indicate a very wide angle of the pubic arch.

## Pubic Arch

The descending rami of the pubic bones and the inferior margin of the symphysis pubis form the pubic arch. The angle of this arch is approximately 90 degrees, as the descending rami flare outward below the symphysis pubis. An arch that is narrower than 90 degrees decreases the space available to the fetal presenting part in the anteroposterior diameter of the pelvic outlet. In a typical vertex presentation, this means the fetal head comes out from under the pubic arch lower along the descending rami, which can put increased pressure on the soft tissue of the perineum that stretches across the descending rami. A narrow pubic arch is also associated with birth in the occiput posterior position.[133]

## Overall Pelvic Shape

In the 1930s, Caldwell and Molloy conducted X-ray studies of pregnant women to describe the morphology of the pelvis. The purpose of these studies was to determine if X-ray measurements of pelvic diameters could predict cephalopelvic disproportion. In addition to identification of persons who would require a cesarean birth, Caldwell and Molloy subdivided pelvic shapes into four types based on the shape of the pelvic inlet: *gynecoid, android, anthropoid,* and *platypelloid.*[134]

Although these four pelvic types have long been taught in medical, nursing, and midwifery education, there are multiple problems with the original work and nomenclature. First, modern measurement techniques have shown the four classic types to be inaccurate and not reflective of the true diversity in pelvic shape and size. Furthermore, the original classification was based on a racist belief system that is reflected in the nomenclature. In addition, the measurements obtained by Caldwell and Molloy did not accurately predict obstructed labor.[132] This is in part because the bony pelvis can expand slightly at joints, and because the size and position of the fetal head are important aspects of fetopelvic relationships and can adjust to the pelvic shape during the course of labor.

In this text, the original Caldwell and Molloy pelvic types are referred to as round, triangular, oval,

and kidney shape. Although pelvises can be categorized into basic shapes, there is a wide diversity of shapes, and the most clinical meaningful assessment considers the size of the pelvis and the position of the fetus together. By convention, the pelvis is initially categorized on the basis of the characteristics of the pelvic inlet (Table 19-10).

## Fetopelvic Relationships

The fetus can lie in numerous orientations in relationship to the maternal abdomen and pelvis. A few of these orientations preclude a vaginal birth; others are associated with protracted labor. For this reason, it is important to know all possible fetopelvic relationships and their clinical significance. The terminology used to describe fetopelvic relationships is listed in Table 19-11.

## The Fetal Skull

The fetal skull is composed of five bones—two frontal bones, two parietal bones, and one occipital bone. The fetal skull bones may be palpated during labor to identify the position of the cephalic fetus and assess labor progress. In addition, the two temporal bones are located inferior to the parietal bones on each side but are not anatomic markers of import during labor assessment (Figure 19-15). The five skull bones meet at the frontal suture, located between the two frontal bones; at the sagittal suture, located between the two parietal bones; at the two coronal sutures, where the parietal and frontal bones meet on either side of the head; and at the two lambdoid sutures, where the parietal bones and the upper margin of the occipital bone meet on either side of the head.

Two fontanels—that is, areas formed by the meeting of sutures—are found on either end of the sagittal suture. The anterior fontanel is the largest. This diamond-shaped fontanel is formed where the frontal, sagittal, and two coronal sutures come together. The posterior fontanel is more triangular shaped; it is formed where the sagittal suture meets the lambdoid sutures that separate the occiput from the parietal bones. The fetal head also has several diameters of importance in providing perinatal care, which are shown in Figure 19-11 and Figure 19-16.

## Lie, Presentation, Denominator, and Position

Determination of the lie, presentation, and position of the fetus requires an understanding of terms and the anatomic landmarks of the fetal skull in relation to the maternal pelvis.

| Table 19-10 | Pelvic Shapes and Their Identifying Characteristics | |
|---|---|---|
| **Pelvic Type and Description** | **Identifying Characteristics** | **Image** |
| **Round** | | |
| Common shape in females | *Inlet:* rounded. The transverse diameter approximately greater than or equal to the anteroposterior diameter. The posterior sagittal diameter only a little shorter than the anterior sagittal diameter.<br><br>*Sacrum:* parallel with the symphysis pubis.<br><br>*Sacrosciatic notch:* rounded with an approximate distance of 2½ to 3 fingerbreadths along the sacrospinous ligament.<br><br>*Sidewalls:* straight pelvic sidewalls.<br><br>*Ischial spines:* blunt and neither prominent nor encroaching.<br><br>*Pubic arch:* a wide arch (≥ 90 degrees). | |
| **Triangular or Heart Shape** | | |
| This shape is unusual and may make vaginal birth more difficult because the midplane and outlet contracture increases the incidence of fetopelvic disproportion | *Inlet:* heart shaped. Posterior segment is wedge shaped; anterior segment (forepelvis) is narrow and triangular. The posterior sagittal diameter is short in comparison to the anterior sagittal diameter. Limited space in the posterior portion of the pelvis for accommodating the fetal head.<br><br>*Sacrum:* anteriorly inclined and flat.<br><br>*Sacrosciatic notch:* highly arched and narrow, with an approximate distance of 1½ to 2 fingerbreadths along the sacrospinous ligament.<br><br>*Sidewalls:* pelvic sidewalls usually convergent.<br><br>*Ischial spines:* prominent and frequently encroaching, thereby decreasing the transverse (interspinous) diameter of the midplane.<br><br>*Pubic arch:* narrow, with an acute angle of much less than 90 degrees. | |

| Pelvic Type and Description | Identifying Characteristics | Image |
|---|---|---|
| **Oval** | | |
| The oval pelvis is characterized by a long sacrum. This shape favors a posterior position of the fetus. | *Inlet:* oval. The anteroposterior diameter is much larger than the transverse diameter. The anterior segment of the pelvis (forepelvis) is pointed and narrower than the posterior segment.<br><br>*Sacrum:* posteriorly inclined, so the posterior sagittal diameters are long throughout the pelvis. This allows more space in the posterior portion of the pelvis for accommodating the fetal head.<br><br>*Sacrosciatic notch:* of average height but quite wide; has an approximate distance of 4 finger-breadths along the sacrospinous ligament between the ischial spine and the sacrum.<br><br>*Sidewalls:* somewhat convergent.<br><br>*Ischial spines:* usually prominent but not encroaching. Transverse (interspinous) diameter of the midplane is generally less than that of the round pelvis but not as contracted as the triangular pelvis.<br><br>*Pubic arch:* somewhat narrow. | |
| **Kidney Shape** | | |
| This type of pelvic shape is rare. It is the widest of all pelvic types yet also shallow. These characteristics can make engagement, rotation, and descent of the fetal head difficult. | *Inlet:* flat. Short anteroposterior diameter and a wide transverse diameter. The anterior segment of the pelvis (forepelvis) is quite wide.<br><br>*Sacrum:* inclined posteriorly and quite hollow.<br><br>*Sacrosciatic notch:* wide and flat, with an acute angle between the ischial spines and the sacrum.<br><br>*Sidewalls:* slightly convergent.<br><br>*Ischial spines:* somewhat prominent but, because of wide transverse diameters throughout the pelvis, this prominence has no effect.<br><br>*Pubic arch:* quite wide. This pelvis is the widest of all the pelvic types. | |

| Table 19-11 | Fetopelvic Relationships |
|---|---|
| **Term** | **Definition** |
| Asynclitism | Oblique presentation of the fetal head. When the fetal head is tilted laterally toward the fetal shoulder, the biparietal diameter is not parallel to the planes of the pelvis. The sagittal suture will not be palpable as midway between the front and back of the pelvis. Asynclitism is called anterior when the anterior parietal bone is the point of presentation; it is called posterior when the posterior parietal bone is the presenting part of the fetal head. |
| Attitude | Relation of the fetal parts to each other. The basic attitudes are flexion and extension. The fetal head is flexed when the chin is close to the chest; it is extended when the occiput is closer to the cervical spine. |
| Cephalic prominence | Fetal part of head most easily felt (prominent) during Leopold's maneuvers and used to determine attitude. When the cephalic prominence is felt on the same side as the fetal small parts, the head is flexed; when it is on the same side as the fetal back, the head is extended. When the cephalic prominence is not palpable on one side or the other, it is often called a military attitude. |
| Denominator | An arbitrarily chosen point on the presenting part of the fetus that is used to describe fetal position. The denominator for a vertex presentation is the occiput; for a breech presentation, it is the sacrum. The denominator for a face presentation is the mentum or chin. |
| Engagement | The point at which the widest diameter of the presenting part is at or below the pelvic inlet. |
| Lie | Relationship of the long axis of the fetus to the long axis of the pregnant woman. The three possible lies are longitudinal, transverse, or oblique. |
| Position | Relationship of the denominator to the front, back, or sides of the maternal pelvis. To make this term easier to remember; the most common position is left occiput anterior. |
| Presentation | The part of the fetus that presents first to the maternal pelvis. The three possible presentations are cephalic, shoulder, and breech. Cephalic presentations are subcategorized by the portion of the fetal head that is presenting. Breech presentations are further subcategorized as presentation of the buttocks or feet. To make this term easier to remember; the most common presentation is vertex. |
| Presenting part | The most dependent part of the fetus that is closest to the maternal cervix. |
| Station | The number of centimeters above or below the plane between the ischial spines of the presenting part. The ischial spines are designated as 0 station; the centimeters above the spines are −1, −2, −3, −4, and −5 (pronounced as minus 1, minus 2, etc); and the centimeters below the ischial spines are +1, +2, +3, +4, and +5, when the fetal presenting part is visible at the vaginal introitus. |

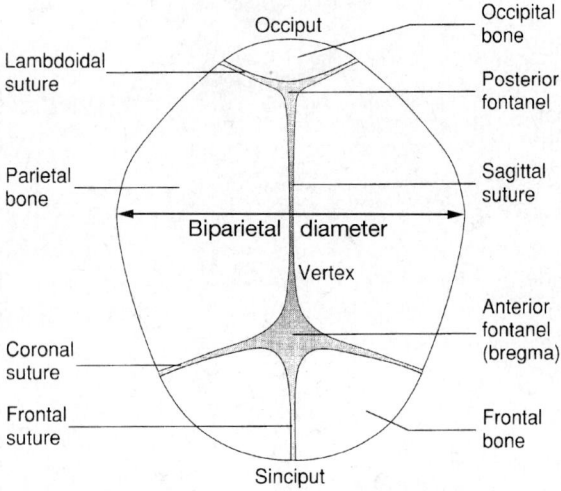

**Figure 19-15** Fetal skull: landmarks, bones, fontanels, sutures, and biparietal diameter.

*Lie* is the relationship of the long axis of the fetus to the long axis of the pregnant person. Three possible lies are longitudinal (vertex or breech), transverse, and oblique (**Figure 19-17**). Transverse and oblique lies in labor are abnormal conditions requiring collaboration with or referral to a physician because they will likely necessitate cesarean section.

*Presentation* is determined by the presenting part—that is, the part of the fetus that first enters the pelvic inlet. The three possible presentations are cephalic, breech, and shoulder. Cephalic and breech presentations are each further subdivided: A cephalic presentation can be vertex, median/military, brow, or face (**Figure 19-18**). A compound presentation occurs when the fetus has a hand (or rarely a foot) resting along the head such that the fingers are part of the presenting part. A breech presentation can be

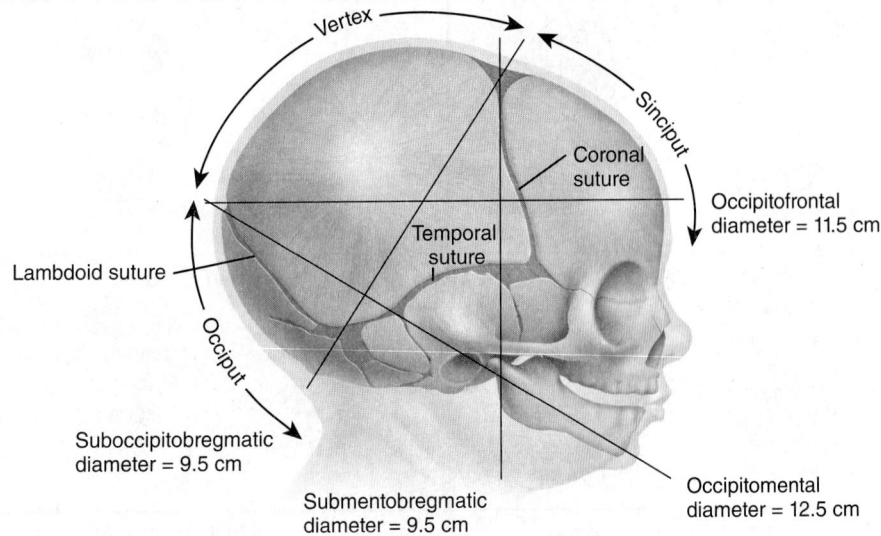

**Figure 19-16** Average diameters of the full-term fetal head.

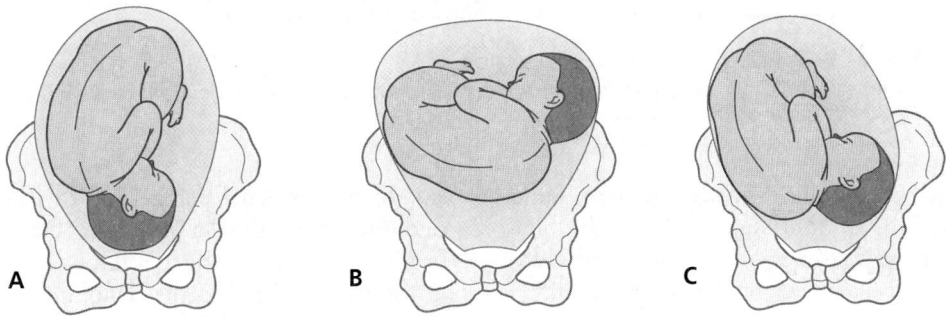

**Figure 19-17** Lies. **A.** Longitudinal. **B.** Transverse. **C.** Oblique.

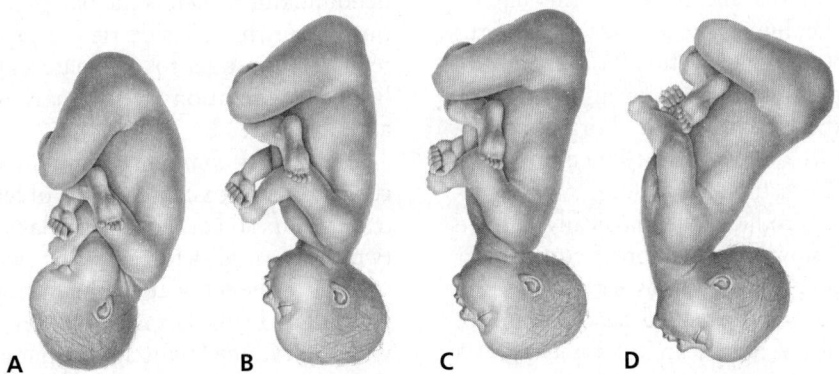

**Figure 19-18** Attitude of the fetus in various presentations. **A.** Vertex. **B.** Median/Military. **C.** Brow. **D.** Face.

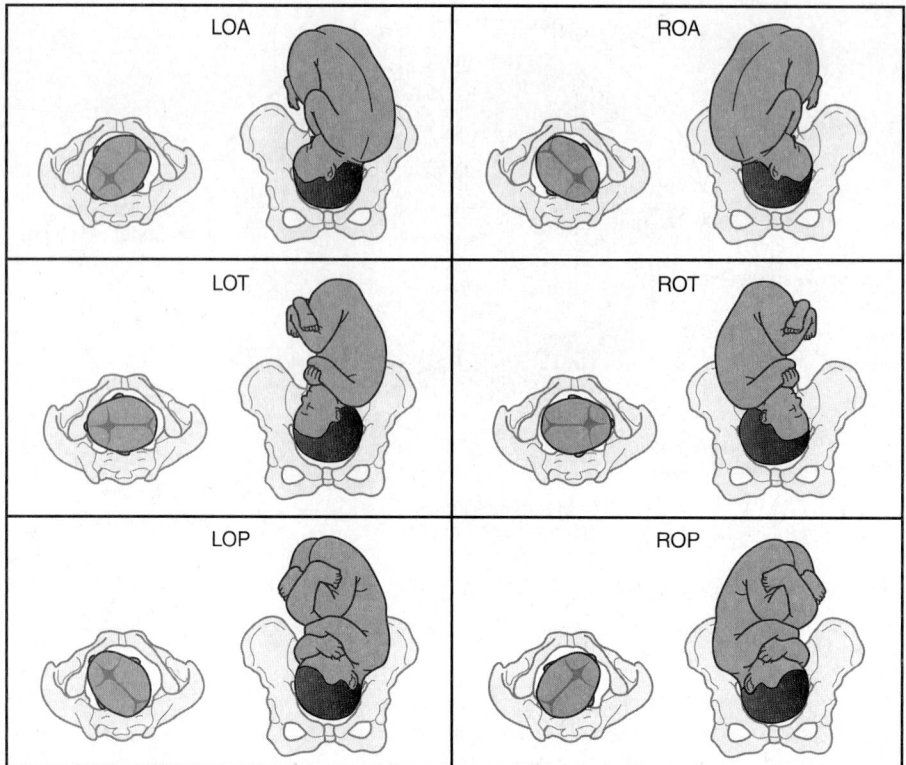

**Figure 19-19** Fetal position for occiput presentations.
Abbreviations: LOA, left occiput anterior; LOP, left occiput posterior; LOT, left occiput transverse; ROA, right occiput anterior; ROP, right occiput posterior; ROT, right occiput transverse.

frank (legs extended), full/complete (legs flexed and possibly crossed), or footling (single or double). Approximately 3.0% to 3.5% of pregnant individuals enter labor with a breech presentation and 0.5% with a face presentation. Approximately 0.5% enter labor with a shoulder presentation. The midwife collaborates with a physician in the management of women with a noncephalic presentations.

The *attitude* of the fetus is its characteristic posture, determined by the relationship of the fetal parts to one another and the effect this has on the fetal vertebral column. The attitude of the fetus varies according to its presentation. For example, a fetus in a vertex presentation has a well-flexed head, flexion of the extremities over the thorax and abdomen, and a convex curved back. By comparison, the straight upright attitude of a fetus with a sinciput presentation produces the classically defined military attitude, now known more frequently as the median attitude. Finally, a fetus with a face presentation has an acutely extended head, flexion of the extremities on the thorax and abdomen, and a vertebral column that is arched to some degree.

Fetal *position* is named using three letters in the following order: The first reference identifies the

side of the maternal pelvis (**L**eft or **R**ight); the second reference is the denominator (**O**cciput, **S**acrum, or **M**entum); and the third reference indicates where in the maternal pelvis the denominator lies (**A**nterior, **T**ransverse, or **P**osterior). These designations serve as a shorthand description for describing the lie, presentation, and position of the denominator within the circle of the pelvis (**Figure 19-19**). For example, the designation LOA indicates that the lie is longitudinal, the presentation is cephalic, and the denominator, which is the occiput, is in the anterior portion of the left side of the pelvis. The possible fetal relationships to the maternal pelvis for each lie and presentation are summarized in **Table 19-12** and **Table 19-13**.

The most common longitudinal lie is vertex or cephalic—approximately 95% of fetuses are in a vertex presentation at the onset of labor. Approximately two-thirds of all fetuses will be positioned with the occiput in the left side of the maternal pelvis (LOA, LOT, LOP) by the last month of pregnancy; one-third will be positioned with the occiput in the right side of the maternal pelvis (ROA, ROT, ROP). Because the head usually enters the inlet with the occiput directed to the transverse portion of the maternal pelvis, the

**Table 19-12    Possible Fetal Relationships to the Maternal Pelvis for Cephalic Presentations**

| Attitude | Description | Presenting Part | Denominator | Fetal Cephalic Diameter That Presents to the Maternal Pelvis | Designation for Position | Clinical Significance |
|---|---|---|---|---|---|---|
| Vertex | Complete flexion of head | Posterior portion of vertex. Fetal chin is on chest | Occiput | Suboccipitobregmatic | ROA, LOA, ROT, LOT, ROP, LOP | This position allows the smallest cephalic diameter to transverse the maternal pelvis |
| Median/Military (sometimes called sinciput) | Midway between flexion and extension of fetal head | Median portion of vertex. Fetal head is in neutral position neither flexed nor extended. | Occiput | Occipitofrontal | Unstable lie that converts to a vertex or face presentation as a fetus engages in the pelvis in most cases | Examiner will palpate frontal and parietal bones. Some obstetric classifications do not list the military position and consider this presentation to be a variation of the brow presentation |
| Brow | Partial extension of head | Portion of fetal head between orbital ridge (brow) and anterior fontanel. Face and chin not included. | Frontal bones (frontum or forehead) | Verticomental | Unstable lie that converts to a vertex or face presentation as a fetus engages in the pelvis in most cases | Examiner can palpate anterior fontanel but not sagittal suture, forehead, orbital ridge, and orbits; and possibly saddle of the nose, but not mouth or chin. If persistent, vaginal birth is not usually possible as the largest diameter of the fetal head does not enter the pelvis |
| Face | Hyperextension | Fetal neck sharply deflexed such that the occiput may touch the back | Mentum (chin) | Submentobregmatic | RMA, LMA, RMT, LMT, RMP, LMP | If there is adequate room in the maternal pelvis, the fetus may be born in this presentation, as mentum anterior. Examiner will palpate fetal facial area between orbital ridges and chin |

Abbreviations: LMA, left mentum anterior; LMP, left mentum posterior; LMT, left mentum transverse; LOA, left occiput anterior; LOP, left occiput posterior; LOT, left occiput transverse; RMA, right mentum anterior; RMP, right mentum posterior; RMT, right mentum transverse; ROA, right occiput anterior; ROP, right occiput posterior; ROT, right occiput transverse.

| Table 19-13 | Possible Fetal Relationships to the Maternal Pelvis for Breech, Transverse, and Oblique Presentations | |
|---|---|---|
| **Lie/Presentation** | **Denominator** | **Designation for Position** |
| Longitudinal/frank breech | Sacrum | RSA, LSA, RST, LST, RSP, or LSP |
| Longitudinal/full/complete breech | Sacrum | Same as frank presentation |
| Longitudinal/footling breech | Sacrum | Same as frank presentation |
| Transverse lie | | No presenting part |
| Oblique/shoulder | Acromion | RAA, LAA, RAP, LAP |

Abbreviations: LAA, left acromion anterior; LAP, left acromion posterior; LSA, left sacrum anterior; LST, left sacrum transverse; RAA, right acromion anterior; RAP, right acromion posterior; RSA, right sacrum anterior; RSP, right sacrum posterior; RST, right sacrum transverse.

most common position of the fetus at the onset of labor is left occiput transverse (LOT).

### Fetal Position and Engagement: Transition from Pregnancy to Labor

Lightening—that is, the descent of the fetus into the true pelvis—may occur as early as 4 weeks prior to the onset of labor. The movement of the fetus into a lower position in the true pelvis, referred to as *engagement*, is more common among nulliparous individuals than multiparous people. The anatomic change in fetal position, which may be measured objectively by a decrease in fundal height, is accompanied by characteristic signs and symptoms in the pregnant person, including partial relief of pressure on the diaphragm, leading to greater ease of breathing and decreased reflux. In turn, pressure on structures adjacent to the pelvis increases, with symptoms such as urinary frequency, pelvic pressure, leg cramps, and dependent edema in the lower extremities becoming more evident. Partial obstruction of the femoral veins caused by pressure of the fetal presenting part reduces venous return to the maternal heart, particularly when the pregnant person is standing. As blood pools in the lower leg veins, increased intravascular pressure promotes fluid movement out of the vessels and into the surrounding interstitial tissues, resulting in edema. When the person is supine, venous return is enhanced and intravascular pressure is reduced, resulting in improvement of lower extremity edema. Tilting the person to their left side further improves venous return by reducing pressure on the inferior vena cava, which lies slightly to the right of center. The reduced capacity of the maternal bladder due to anatomic pressure of the engaged fetal presenting part, coupled with increased venous return when recumbent, contributes to increased frequency of urination, which can lead to interrupted sleep in the last weeks of pregnancy.

In a vertex presentation, the fetal head usually enters the pelvis with the biparietal diameter parallel to the plane of the pelvis. If the fetal head is tilted laterally toward the fetal shoulder, the head will enter the pelvis at an oblique angle, referred to as *asynclitism*. The characteristic movements of the fetus through the pelvis during labor, called cardinal movements, are discussed in the *Anatomy and Physiology of Labor and Birth* chapter.

## Conclusion

Remarkable physiologic changes occur during pregnancy. Knowledge of the pregnancy-related changes that are physiologic in nature must inform every aspect of pregnancy care. A deep understanding of this unique physiology will allow midwives to interpret signs and symptoms accurately, enabling them to provide reassurance and guidance to help individuals manage common pregnancy discomforts and initiate assessment for pathology when indicated. These are essential steps in the provision of quality perinatal health care.

### References

1. Spong CY. Defining "term" pregnancy: recommendations from the Defining "Term" Pregnancy Workgroup. *JAMA*. 2013;309(23):2445-2446.
2. Moore KL, Persaud TVN, Torchia MG. *The Developing Human: Clinically Oriented Embryology*. 11th ed. Philadelphia, PA: Elsevier; 2018.
3. Cañumil VA, Bogetti E, de la Cruz Borthiry FL, et al. Steroid hormones and first trimester vascular remodeling. *Vitamins Hormones*. 2021;116;363-387.
4. Damjanov I. Vesalius and Hunter were right: decidua is a membrane [Editorial]. *Lab Invest*. 1985;53:597.

5. Craciunas L, Gallos I, Chu J, et al. Conventional and modern markers of endometrial receptivity: a systematic review and meta-analysis. *Hum Reprod Update*. 2019;25(2):202-223.

6. Achache H, Revel A. Endometrial receptivity markers, the journey to successful embryo implantation. *Hum Reprod Update*. 2006;12(6):731-746.

7. Quinn KE, Matson BC, Wetendorf M, Caron KM. Pinopodes: recent advancements, current perspectives, and future directions. *Mol Cell Endocrinol*. 2020;501:110644.

8. Schumacher A, Zenclussen AC. Human chorionic gonadotropin-mediated immune responses that facilitate embryo implantation and placentation. *Front Immunol*. 2019;10:2896.

9. Turco MY, Moffett A. Development of the human placenta. *Development*. 2019;146(22):dev163428.

10. Roberts RM, Ezashi T, Schulz LC, et al. Syncytins expressed in human placental trophoblast. *Placenta*. 2021;113:8-14.

11. Cole LA. hCG, the wonder of today's science. *Reprod Biol Endocrinol*. 2012;10:24-28.

12. Knöfler M, Haider S, Saleh L, et al. Human placenta and trophoblast development: key molecular mechanisms and model systems. *Cell Mol Life Sci*. 2019;76(18):3479-3496.

13. Brosens I, Puttemans P, Benagiano G. Placental bed research: I. The placental bed: from spiral arteries remodeling to the great obstetrical syndromes. *Am J Obstet Gynecol*. 2019;221(5):437-456.

14. Staud F, Karahoda R. Trophoblast: the central unit of fetal growth, protection and programming. *Int J Biochem Cell Biol*. 2018;105:35-40.

15. Weiss G, Sundl M, Glasner A, et al. The trophoblast plug during early pregnancy: a deeper insight. *Histochem Cell Biol*. 2016;146(6):749-756.

16. Burton GJ, Redman CW, Roberts JM, Moffett A. Pre-eclampsia: pathophysiology and clinical implications. *BMJ*. 2019;366:l2381.

17. Brosens I, Pijnenborg R, Vercruysse L, Romero R. The "Great Obstetrical Syndromes" are associated with disorders of deep placentation. *Am J Obstet Gynecol*. 2011;204(3):193-201.

18. Jain A. Endothelin-1: a key pathological factor in preeclampsia. *Reprod BioMed Online*. 2012;25:443-449.

19. Fisher AL, Nemeth E. Iron homeostasis during pregnancy. *Am J Clin Nutr*. 2017;106(suppl 6):1567S-1574S.

20. Longo LD, Reynolds LP. Some historical aspects of understanding placental development, structure, and function. *Int J Dev Biol*. 2010;54:237-255.

21. Schuler-Maloney D. Placental triage of the singleton placenta. *J Midwifery Womens Health*. 2000;45:104-113.

22. Costa MA. The endocrine function of human placenta: an overview. *Reprod Biomed Online*. 2016;32(1):14-43.

23. Fournier T. Human chorionic gonadotropin: different glycoforms and biological activity depending on its source of production. *Ann Endocrinol (Paris)*. 2016;77(2):75-81.

24. Brady PC, Farland LV, Racowsky C, Ginsburg ES. Hyperglycosylated human chorionic gonadotropin as a predictor of ongoing pregnancy. *Am J Obstet Gynecol*. 2020;222(1):68.e1-68.e12.

25. Erick M, Cox JT, Mogensen KM. ACOG Practice Bulletin 189: nausea and vomiting of pregnancy. *Obstet Gynecol*. 2018;131(5):935.

26. Handwerger S, Freemark M. The roles of placental growth hormone and placental lactogen in the regulation of human fetal growth and development. *J Pediatr Endocrinol Metab*. 2000;13(4):343-356.

27. Sibiak R, Jankowski M, Gutaj P, et al. Placental lactogen as a marker of maternal obesity, diabetes, and fetal growth abnormalities: current knowledge and clinical perspectives. *J Clin Med*. 2020;9(4):1142.

28. Li J, Zhang N, Zhang Y, et al. Human placental lactogen mRNA in maternal plasma plays a role in prenatal diagnosis of abnormally invasive placenta: yes or no? *Gynecol Endocrinol*. 2019;35(7):631-634.

29. Coomarasamy A, Devall AJ, Brosens JJ, et al. Micronized vaginal progesterone to prevent miscarriage: a critical evaluation of randomized evidence. *Am J Obstet Gynecol*. 2020;223(2):167-176.

30. American College of Obstetricians and Gynecologists' Committee on Practice Bulletins—Obstetrics. Prediction and prevention of spontaneous preterm birth: ACOG Practice Bulletin, Number 234. *Obstet Gynecol*. 2021;138(2):e65-e90.

31. Norman JE. Progesterone and preterm birth. *Int J Gynaecol Obstet*. 2020;150(1):24-30. [Published correction appears in *Int J Gynaecol Obstet*. 2020;151(3):487.]

32. Romero R, Conde-Agudelo A, Da Fonseca E, et al. Vaginal progesterone for preventing preterm birth and adverse perinatal outcomes in singleton gestations with a short cervix: a meta-analysis of individual patient data. *Am J Obstet Gynecol*. 2018;218(2):161-180.

33. Parer JT, King TL, Ikeda T. *Electronic Fetal Heart Rate Monitoring: The 5-Tier System*. 3rd edition. Burlington, MA: Jones & Bartlett Learning; 2018.

34. Maltepe E, Fisher SJ. Placenta: the forgotten organ. *Annu Rev Cell Dev Biol*. 2015;31:523-552.

35. Sangkhae V, Nemeth E. Placental iron transport: the mechanism and regulatory circuits. *Free Radic Biol Med*. 2019;133:254-261.

36. Carter AM. Placental gas exchange and the oxygen supply to the fetus. *Compr Physiol*. 2015;5(3):1381-1403.

37. Troiano NH. Physiologic and hemodynamic changes during pregnancy. *AACN Adv Crit Care*. 2018;29(3):273-283. doi:10.4037/aacnacc2018911.

38. Lager S, Powell TL. Regulation of nutrient transport across the placenta. *J Preg*. 2012;2012:179827.

39. Joshi NP, Mane AR, Sahay AS, et al. Role of placental glucose transporters in determining fetal growth. *Reprod Sci*. 2021. doi:10.1007/s43032-021-00699-9.

40. Pardi G, Cetin I. Human fetal growth and organ development: 50 years of discoveries. *Am J Obstet Gynecol*. 2006;194(4):1088-1099.

41. Horne H, Holme AM, Roland MCP, et al. Maternal–fetal cholesterol transfer in human term pregnancies. *Placenta*. 2019;87:23-29.

42. Murphy VE, Smith R, Giles WB, Clifton VL. Endocrine regulation of human fetal growth: the role of the mother, placenta, and fetus. *Endocrine Rev*. 2006;27:141-169.

43. Georgieff MK. Iron deficiency in pregnancy. *Am J Obstet Gynecol*. 2020;223(4):516-524.

44. Adu-Gyamfi EA, Wang YX, Ding YB. The interplay between thyroid hormones and the placenta: a comprehensive review. *Biol Reprod*. 2020;102(1):8-17.

45. Lassiter NT, Manns-James L. Pregnancy. In: Brucker M, King TL, eds. *Pharmacology for Women's Health*. Burlington, MA: Jones & Bartlett Publishers; 2017:1025-1065.

46. Zhao Y, Hebert MF, Venkataramanan R. Basic obstetric pharmacology. *Semin Perinatol*. 2014;38(8):475-486.

47. Tasnif Y, Morado J, Herbert. Pregnancy-related pharmacokinetic changes. *Clin Pharm Therap*. 2016;100(1):53-62.

48. Frederiksen MC. Physiologic changes in pregnancy and their effect on drug disposition. *Semin Perinatol*. 2001;25:120-123.

49. Tong M, Abrahams VM. Immunology of the placenta. *Obstet Gynecol Clin North Am*. 2020;47(1):49-63.

50. Ferreira LMR, Meissner TB, Tilburgs T, Strominger JL. HLA-G: at the interface of maternal–fetal tolerance. *Trends Immunol*. 2017;38(4):272-286.

51. Liu S, Diao L, Huang C, et al. The role of decidual immune cells on human pregnancy. *J Reprod Immunol*. 2017;124:44-53.

52. Gregori S, Amodio G, Quattrone F, Panina-Bordignon P. HLA-G orchestrates the early interaction of human trophoblasts with the maternal niche. *Front Immunol*. 2015;6:128.

53. Li H, Ouyang Y, Sadovsky E, et al. Unique microRNA signals in plasma exosomes from pregnancies complicated by preeclampsia. *Hypertension*. 2020;75(3):762-771.

54. Reyes L, Wolfe B, Golos T. Hofbauer cells: placental macrophages of fetal origin. *Results Probl Cell Differ*. 2017;62:45-60.

55. Reyes L, Golos TG. Hofbauer cells: their role in healthy and complicated pregnancy. *Front Immunol*. 2018;9:2628. doi:10.3389/fimmu.2018.02628.

56. MacDorman MF, Gregory EC. Fetal and perinatal mortality: United States, 2013. *Natl Vital Stat Rep*. 2015;64(8):1-24.

57. Dubil EA, Magann EF. Amniotic fluid as a vital sign for fetal wellbeing. *Australas J Ultrasound Med*. 2013;16(2):62-70.

58. Peiris HN, Romero R, Vaswani K, et al. Prostaglandin and prostamide concentrations in amniotic fluid of women with spontaneous labor at term with and without clinical chorioamnionitis. *Prostaglandins Leukot Essent Fatty Acids*. 2020;163:102195.

59. Moore TR. Amniotic fluid dynamics reflect fetal and maternal health and disease. *Obstet Gynecol*. 2010;116(3):757-763.

60. O'Quinn C, Cooper S, Tang S, Wood S. Antenatal diagnosis of marginal and velamentous placental cord insertion and pregnancy outcomes. *Obstet Gynecol*. 2020;135(4):953-959.

61. Melcer Y, Maymon R, Jauniaux E. Vasa previa: prenatal diagnosis and management. *Curr Opin Obstet Gynecol*. 2018;30(6):385-391.

62. Hammad IA, Blue NR, Allshouse AA, et al. Umbilical cord abnormalities and stillbirth. *Obstet Gynecol*. 2020;135(3):644-652.

63. Jessop FA, Lees CC, Pathak S, et al. Umbilical cord coiling: clinical outcomes in an unselected population and systematic review. *Virchows Arch*. 2014;464(1):105-112.

64. Zhang L, Lu Q, Chang C. Epigenetics in health and disease. *Adv Exp Med Biol*. 2020;1253:3-55.

65. DeSocio JE. Epigenetics, maternal prenatal psychosocial stress, and infant mental health. *Arch Psychiatr Nurs*. 2018;32(6):901-906. doi:10.1016/j.apnu.2018.09.001.

66. Hoffman DJ, Powell TL, Barrett ES, Hardy DB. Developmental origins of metabolic diseases. *Physiol Rev*. 2021;101(3):739-795.

67. Barker DJ, Thornburg KL. The obstetric origins of health for a lifetime. *Clin Obstet Gynecol*. 2013;56(3):511-519.

68. Barker D. The midwife, the coincidence, and the hypothesis. *BMJ*. 2003;327(7429):1428-1430.

69. Bar J, Weiner E, Levy M, Gilboa Y. The thrifty phenotype hypothesis: the association between ultrasound and Doppler studies in fetal growth restriction and the development of adult disease. *Am J Obstet Gynecol MFM*. 2021;3(6):100473.

70. Agarwal P, Morriseau TS, Kereliuk SM, et al. Maternal obesity, diabetes during pregnancy and epigenetic mechanisms that influence the developmental origins of cardiometabolic disease in the offspring. *Crit Rev Clin Lab Sci*. 2018;55(2):71-101.

71. Godfrey KM, Reynolds RM, Prescott SL, et al. Influence of maternal obesity on the long-term health of offspring. *Lancet Diab Endocrinol.* 2017;5(1):53-64.

72. Latendresse G, Founds S. The fascinating and complex role of the placenta in pregnancy and fetal well-being. *J Midwifery Womens Health.* 2015;60(4):360-370.

73. Shonkoff JP, Boyce WT, McEwen BS. Neuroscience, molecular biology, and the childhood roots of health disparities: building a new framework for health promotion and disease prevention. *JAMA.* 2009;301(21):2252-2259.

74. Lewis AJ, Galbally M, Gannon T, Symeonides C. Early life programming as a target for prevention of child and adolescent mental disorders. *BMC Med.* 2014;12:33.

75. Shroukh WA, Steinke DT, Willis SC. Risk management of teratogenic medicines: a systematic review. *Birth Defects Res.* 2020;112(20):1755-1786.

76. Mai CT, Isenburg JL, Canfield MA, et al. National population-based estimates for major birth defects, 2010–2014. *Birth Defects Res.* 2019;111(18):1420-1435.

77. Harris BS, Bishop KC, Kemeny HR, et al. Risk factors for birth defects. *Obstet Gynecol Surv.* 2017;72(2):123-135.

78. Toufaily MH, Westgate MN, Lin AE, Holmes LB. Causes of congenital malformations. *Birth Defects Res.* 2018;110(2):87-91. doi:10.1002/bdr2.1105.

79. Van Gelder MM, de Jong-van Berg LT, Roeleveld N. Drugs associated with teratogenic mechanism. Part II: a literature review of the evidence of human risks. *Hum Reprod.* 2014;29(1):168-183.

80. Abraham M, Alramadhan S, Iniguez C, et al. A systematic review of maternal smoking during pregnancy and fetal measurements with meta-analysis. *PLoS One.* 2017;12(2):e0170946.

81. Tan CMJ, Lewandowski AJ. The transitional heart: from early embryonic and fetal development to neonatal life. *Fetal Diagn Ther.* 2020;47(5):373-386.

82. Swanson JR, Sinkin RA. Transition from fetus to newborn. *Pediatr Clin North Am.* 2015;62(2):329-343.

83. Sapoval J, Singh V, Carter RE. Ultrasound biophysical profile. In: *StatPearls.* Treasure Island, FL: StatPearls Publishing; August 11, 2021.

84. Kadic AS, Kurjak A. Cognitive functions of the fetus. *Ultraschall Med.* 2018;39(2):181-189.

85. Schaal B, Marlier L, Soussignan R. Olfactory function in the human fetus: evidence from selective neonatal responsiveness to the odor of amniotic fluid. *Behav Neurosci.* 1998;112(6):1438-1449. doi:10.1037//0735-7044.112.6.1438.

86. Krueger C, Garvan C. Emergence and retention of learning in early fetal development. *Infant Behav Dev.* 2014;37(2):162-173.

87. Fatima M, Srivastav S, Mondal AC. Prenatal stress and depression associated neuronal development in neonates. *Int J Dev Neurosci.* 2017;60:1-7.

88. Labonte-Lemoyne E, Curnier D, Ellemberg D. Exercise during pregnancy enhances cerebral maturation in the newborn: a randomized controlled trial. *J Clin Exp Neuropsychol.* 2017;39(4):347-354.

89. de Vries JIP, Fong BF. Normal fetal motility: an overview. *Ultrasound Obstet Gynecol.* 2006;27:701-711.

90. Martin CB. Normal fetal physiology and behavior, and adaptive responses with hypoxemia. *Semin Perinatol.* 2008;32:239-242.

91. Borg-Stein J, Duagn S, Gruber J. Musculoskeletal aspects of pregnancy. *Am J Phys Med Rehabil.* 2005;84:180-192.

92. Alex A, Bhandary E, McGuire KP. Anatomy and physiology of the breast during pregnancy and lactation. *Adv Exp Med Biol.* 2020;1252:3-7.

93. Govindan RB, Siegel E, McKelvey S, et al. Tracking the changes in synchrony of the electrophysiological activity as the uterus approaches labor using magnetomyographic technique. *Reprod Sci.* 2015;22(5):595-601.

94. Kazma JM, van den Anker J, Allegaert K, et al. Anatomical and physiological alterations of pregnancy. *J Pharmacokinet Pharmacodyn.* 2020;47(4):271-285.

95. Ozuounian JG, Elkayam U. Physiologic changes during normal pregnancy and delivery. *Cardiol Clin.* 2012;30:317-329.

96. Ludmir J, Sehdev H. Anatomy and physiology of the uterine cervix. *Clin Obstet Gynecol.* 2000;43(3):433-439.

97. Myers KM, Feltovich H, Mazza E, et al. The mechanical role of the cervix in pregnancy. *J Biomech.* 2015;48(9):1511-1523.

98. Nott JP, Bonney EA, Pickering JD, Simpson NAB. Structure and function of the cervix during pregnancy. *Translational Res Anat.* 2016;2:1-7.

99. Vink J, Feltovich H. Cervical etiology of spontaneous preterm birth. *Semin Fetal Neonatal Med.* 2016;21(2):106-112.

100. Yao W, Gan Y, Myers KM, et al. Collagen fiber orientation and dispersion in the upper cervix of non-pregnant and pregnant women. *PLoS One.* 2016;11(11):e0166709.

101. Levine LD. Cervical ripening: why we do what we do. *Semin Perinatol.* 2020;44(2):151216.

102. Aguin TJ, Sobel JD. Vulvovaginal candidiasis in pregnancy. *Curr Infect Dis Rep.* 2015;17(6):462. doi:10.1007/s11908-015-0462-0.

103. Morton A. Physiological changes and cardiovascular investigations in pregnancy. *Heart Lung Circ.* 2021;30(1):e6-e15.

104. Tan EK, Tan EL. Alterations in physiology and anatomy during pregnancy. *Best Pract Res Clin Obstet Gynaecol*. 2013;27(6):791-802.

105. Stangret A, Skoda M, Whuk A, et al. Mild anemia during pregnancy upregulates placental vascularity development. *Med Hypoth*. 2017;102:37-40.

106. Elkus R, Popovich J. Respiratory physiology in pregnancy. *Clin Chest Med*. 1992;12:555-565.

107. Johnson AC. Physiology of the cerebrovascular adaptation to pregnancy. *Handb Clin Neurol*. 2020;171:85-96.

108. Chapman AC, Cipolla MJ, Chan SL. Effect of pregnancy and nitric oxide on the myogenic vasodilation of posterior cerebral arteries and the lower limit of cerebral blood flow autoregulation. *Reprod Sci*. 2013;20(9):1046-1054.

109. Bushnell C, McCullough LD, Awad IA, et al. Guidelines for the prevention of stroke in women: a statement for healthcare professionals from the American Heart Association/American Stroke Association. *Stroke*. 2014;45(5):1545-1588. doi:10.1161/01.str.0000442009.06663.48. [Published correction appears in *Stroke*. 2014;45(5):e95.] [Published correction appears in *Stroke*. 2014;45(10);e214.]

110. Barba-Müller E, Craddock S, Carmona S, Hoekzema E. Brain plasticity in pregnancy and the postpartum period: links to maternal caregiving and mental health. *Arch Womens Ment Health*. 2019;22(2):289-299.

111. Behura SK, Dhakal P, Kelleher AM, et al. The brain–placental axis: therapeutic and pharmacological relevancy to pregnancy. *Pharmacol Res*. 2019;149:104468.

112. Grattan DR. The actions of prolactin in the brain during pregnancy and lactation. *Prog Brain Res*. 2001;133:153-171. doi:10.1016/s0079-6123(01)33012-1.

113. Keller M, Vandenberg LN, Charlier TD. The parental brain and behavior: a target for endocrine disruption. *Front Neuroendocrinol*. 2019;54:100765.

114. Springer D, Jiskra J, Limanova Z, et al. Thyroid in pregnancy: from physiology to screening. *Crit Rev Clin Lab Sci*. 2017;54(2):102-116.

115. Casey MB, Leveno K. Thyroid disease in pregnancy. *Obstet Gynecol*. 2006;108:1283-1292.

116. Alemu A, Terefe B, Abebe M, Biadgo B. Thyroid hormone dysfunction during pregnancy: a review. *Int J Reprod Biomed*. 2016;14(11):677-686.

117. Thyroid disease in pregnancy: ACOG Practice Bulletin, Number 223. *Obstet Gynecol*. 2020;135(6):e261-e274.

118. Baeyens L, Hindi S, Sorenson RL, German MS. β-cell adaptation in pregnancy. *Diab Obes Metab*. 2016;18(suppl 1):63-70.

119. Kampmann U, Knorr S, Fuglsang J, Ovesen P. Determinants of maternal insulin resistance during pregnancy: an updated overview. *J Diab Res*. 2019;2019:5320156.

120. Zeng Z, Liu F, Li S. Metabolic adaptations in pregnancy. *Ann Nutr Metab*. 2017;70:59-65.

121. Munoz-Suano A, Hamilton AB, Betz AG. Gimme shelter: the immune system during pregnancy. *Immunol Rev*. 2011;241:20-38.

122. Morelli SS, Mandal M, Goldsmith LT, et al. The maternal immune system during pregnancy and its influence on fetal development. *Res Reports Biol*. 2015;6:171-189.

123. Beers K, Patel N. Kidney physiology in pregnancy. *Adv Chronic Kidney Dis*. 2020;27(6):449-454. doi:10.1053/j.ackd.2020.07.006.

124. Calimag-Loyola APP, Lerma EV. Renal complications during pregnancy: in the hypertension spectrum. *Dis Monit*. 2019;65(2):25-44.

125. Vazquez JC. Constipation, haemorrhoids, and heartburn in pregnancy. *BMJ Clin Evid*. 2008;2008:1411.

126. Iheozor-Ejiofor Z, Middleton P, Esposito M, Glenny AM. Treating periodontal disease for preventing adverse birth outcomes in pregnant women. *Cochrane Database Syst Rev*. 2017;6:CD005297. doi:10.1002/14651858.CD005297.pub3.

127. Anselmo DS, Love E, Tango DN, Robinson L. Musculoskeletal effects of pregnancy on the lower extremity: a literature review. *J Am Podiatr Med Assoc*. 2017;107(1):60-64. doi:10.7547/15-061.

128. Motosko CC, Bieber AK, Pomeranz MK, et al. Physiologic changes of pregnancy: a review of the literature. *Int J Womens Dermatol*. 2017;3(4):219-224.

129. Bieber AK, Martires KJ, Stein JA, et al. Pigmentation and pregnancy: knowing what is normal. *Obstet Gynecol*. 2017;129(1):168-173.

130. Tasnif Y, Morado J, Herbert MF. Pregnancy-related pharmacokinetic changes. *Clin Pharm Therap*. 2016;100(1):53-62.

131. Frémondière P, Thollon L, Adalian P, et al. Which foetal-pelvic variables are useful for predicting caesarean section and instrumental assistance? *Med Princ Pract*. 2017;26(4):359-367.

132. Maharaj D. Assessing cephalopelvic disproportion: back to the basics. *Obstet Gynecol Surv*. 2010;65(6):387-395.

133. Ghi T, Youssef A, Martelli F, et al. Narrow subpubic arch angle is associated with higher risk of persistent occiput posterior position at delivery. *Ultrasound Obstet Gynecol*. 2016;48:511-515.

134. Caldwell WE, Moloy HC. Anatomical variations in the female pelvis: their classification and obstetrical significance. *Proc R Soc Med*. 1938;32(1):1-30.

CHAPTER

# 20

# Assessment for Genetic and Fetal Abnormalities

GWEN LATENDRESSE AND JULIE KNUTSON

## Introduction

Essentially all health and disease conditions have a genetic component, and the provision of midwifery care increasingly will include genetics within the context of prevention, screening, diagnosis, and treatment selection. Furthermore, genetic disorders are not rare occurrences. Approximately 3% to 7% of the population will be identified with a genetic disorder at some point in life.[1] Chromosomal abnormalities occur in 20% of all pregnancy losses.[2] Approximately 2% to 3% of all newborns have a major congenital malformation; a majority of these conditions are multifactorial in etiology (i.e., involve multiple genetic and environmental components), with the cause of most remaining largely unknown.[2,3] Thus, genetic effects are a substantial contributor to newborn/infant mortality.

A solid understanding of genetics and available technology, as well as essential skills necessary for genetic risk assessment, screening, diagnostic testing, basic counseling, and appropriate referral, are needed for clinical midwifery practice. However, because genetic science and technology is evolving rapidly, it can be challenging to stay current with the knowledge necessary for clinical practice.[4] This chapter reviews basic genetics and contemporary approaches to genetic testing for individuals contemplating pregnancy and during pregnancy.

## Financial, Ethical, Legal, and Social Issues in Genetics

Along with the rapid increase in genetic knowledge and technology has come the urgent need to address a myriad of financial, ethical, legal, and social issues, collectively referred to as FELSI. The World Health Organization (WHO) has proposed international guidelines regarding ethical considerations in genetic testing, including in developed countries.[5] These guidelines include respect for the autonomy of individuals, beneficence, nonmaleficence, and justice in the provision of genetics-related services. The WHO guidelines are clear that genetic testing can have a profound impact on pregnant people and their families. Thus, confidentiality and privacy, the right for persons to receive sufficient information about testing and treatment, and individual autonomy to make decisions about testing and treatment, regardless of geographic area, socioeconomic status, ethnic background, religion, or belief system, are emphasized. Midwives have an obligation to understand and act on the principles related to FELSI, including a duty to fully inform clients, offer appropriate testing when available, and refer individuals and families to additional resources such as genetic counselors or geneticists when their own professional or personal limitations have been reached. Some of the more common FELSI concerns and questions are listed in Table 20-1.[6]

## Foundations in Genetics

The foundations of molecular genetics and heredity provide the basis for understanding perinatal genetics specifically. This section reviews basic principles in molecular genetics, as well as inheritance patterns and the meaning of genetic mutations, gene expression, and chromosomal structure. Table 20-2 provides a glossary of commonly used genetics-related terms.[7–10]

| Table 20-1 | Common Financial, Ethical, Social, and Legal Concerns in Genetic Testing |
|---|---|

**Financial**

Disparities in access to genetic resources due to lack of health insurance coverage, inability to pay, low-income economy, other competing priorities in healthcare needs, or geographic location

Cost-effectiveness: the high cost of genetic testing versus the possibility of improved health outcomes

**Ethical**

Distributive injustice (some populations benefit but not others), including racial and ethnic discrimination

Denial of health insurance or employment based on genetic test results[a]

The negative effects of false-positive test results

The ethics of testing for disorders that have no cure or treatment

Eugenics

**Social**

Religious and cultural beliefs and perceptions about genetic risk, decision making, health and disease, family, privacy, authority, invasive procedures, childbearing, influence over life events, and use of alternatives to Western medicine

Cultural factors that may impact the accuracy or interpretation of family history information

Discrimination or stigmatization by others based on genetic information

When or if relatives (who may not want to know) should be informed about an individual's genetic testing results

Implications of sensitive issues encountered, such as previously undisclosed adoption, rape, incest, misattributed paternity, substance abuse, mental illness, and ethnic origins

**Legal**

Privacy and confidentiality

Stigma and legality of consanguinity

Induced abortion

[a] The Genetic Information Nondiscrimination Act of 2008 (GINA) is a U.S. federal law that prohibits discrimination in health coverage and employment on the basis of genetic information including genetic test results.

Based on The New York – Mid-Atlantic Guide for Patients and Health Professionals. Ethical, legal, and social issues. In: *Understanding Genetics: A New York, Mid-Atlantic Guide for Patients and Health Professionals*. Washington, DC: Genetic Alliance; July 8, 2009. https://www.ncbi.nlm.nih.gov/books/NBK115574/. Accessed August 19, 2021.

Readers are also encouraged to access the many excellent genetics resources currently available for more in-depth information. A selected list of online resources can be found at the end of this chapter.

## Genes, Genome, DNA, and Chromosomes

*Genes*—the basic unit of inheritance—consist of *deoxyribonucleic acid (DNA)* that is found within the cell nucleus. Genes are contained within the 46 chromosomes found in every cell in the human body, except ova and sperm cells, which contain 23 chromosomes. *Chromosomes* consist of long segments of DNA that are tightly wrapped around proteins (Figure 20-1).[11] The human cell normally contains 46 chromosomes that are organized in 23 paired sets. In each of these sets, one chromosome is contributed by the egg and one chromosome is contributed by the sperm. Twenty-two of those pairs are called *autosomes* and are present in all individuals. The 23rd pair consists of the sex chromosomes: individuals usually assigned female at birth have two X chromosomes and individuals usually assigned male at birth have an X chromosome and a Y chromosome.

An individual's gender identity or expression does not necessarily correlate with their inherited X or Y chromosomes, as gender identity has cultural and personal components. People who are intersex (having disorders of sexual differentiation) can have a variety of chromosomal and genetic configurations resulting in a continuum of phenotypes. An individual's gender identity can differ from the sex they were assigned at birth.[12] Similarly, there are many ways in which people build families. Thus, to be inclusive of all gender and parental identities, this chapter uses terms such as XX and XY individuals in describing the genetic contributions to offspring.

The entire collection of genes in an individual, referred to as the *genome*, provides a complete set of "instructions" for directing all biologic functions within the living organism. The end product of gene instruction is the production of a protein, via the processes of *transcription* and *translation* of the DNA that occur as the instructions are used to construct actual proteins.[13] Every gene is composed of a sequence of nitrogenous base pairs—molecules of cytosine, thymine, adenine, and guanine—that form the double-stranded DNA molecule, and each genetic sequence encodes for a specific protein with a specific function. The single-stranded *ribonucleic acid (RNA)* contributes to this process by providing

| Table 20-2 | Genetics Glossary |
|---|---|
| **Term** | **Definition/Description** |
| Allele | One of the two or more versions of a genetic sequence that encodes for the same protein or function at a specific location on a chromosome. An individual normally inherits one allele from each gamete (sperm and egg), and these matching alleles contain the genes that code for the same characteristic. |
| Aneuploidy | A chromosomal condition in which there is an abnormal number of chromosomes in the complement of 23 pairs, secondary to either a deletion or an addition of a chromosome. |
| Autosome | A chromosome that is not a sex chromosome. Autosomes appear in pairs. |
| Base pair | Two nitrogenous bases paired together in double-stranded DNA (i.e., adenine paired with thymine, and guanine paired with cytosine). Sequences of various lengths of base pairs make up the various genes. |
| Cell-free fetal DNA | Fetal genetic material (DNA) that is not contained within cells and that circulates freely in the blood of a pregnant person. Cell-free fetal DNA is derived primarily from the placenta and can be used to test for aneuploidy in pregnant individuals. |
| Chromosomal abnormality | An alteration in the number or structure of a chromosome. Chromosomal abnormalities can be inherited or occur de novo. Most common chromosomal abnormalities, such as trisomy 21, are not heritable. |
| Chromosomal microarray analysis (CMA) | A technique for identifying chromosomal abnormalities, including those that are too small (i.e., microdeletions) to be detected by conventional karyotyping. CMA requires direct testing of fetal tissue, so it can be offered when chorionic villus sampling (CVS) or amniocentesis is performed, or via neonatal peripheral blood samples. |
| Chromosomal microdeletion | A very small deletion of a part of a chromosome or sequence of DNA, which results in a loss of genetic material. These microdeletions are usually not fatal, but they frequently result in physical and mental abnormalities depending on the genetic material that is lost. Conventional karyotyping is not able to identify microdeletions. Cri-du-chat syndrome is caused by a microdeletion on the short arm of chromosome 5. |
| Chromosomal translocation | A rearrangement of chromosomal segments between different chromosomes. These can be *balanced* (even exchange of material) or *unbalanced* (unequal exchange of material, resulting in extra or missing genetic material). Although there is frequently no effect on phenotype, an individual with chromosomal translocation may have an increased risk of a nonviable conception and a fetus with trisomy 21. |
| Cystic fibrosis transmembrane conductance regulator (CFTR) | The gene that encodes for chloride channel transmembrane regulation. Several variations of mutations in this gene are known, including those that directly cause cystic fibrosis. |
| Deoxyribonucleic acid (DNA) | The double-stranded helix of nitrogenous base pairs within cells that provides instructions for all cell activity, and is passed on from generation to generation. The DNA strand comprises the collection of genes within a chromosome. |
| Dominant allele | An allele that, if present, leads to expression of the phenotype associated with that allele. Dominant alleles can mask the presence of a recessive allele. |
| Epigenetics | Changes in the regulation of gene expression that occur due to modifications in DNA, rather than changes in DNA sequence. Methylation—the attachment of methyl groups to DNA at cytosine bases—is one example of a DNA modification that alters gene expression. |
| Exon | The segment of the gene that codes for specific amino acids. By comparison, introns are generally considered noncoding segments of DNA and are normally spliced out of the RNA sequence prior to formation of amino acids. |
| Expressivity | Phenotypic variation (severity) among persons who have a specific genotype. |

*(continues)*

| Table 20-2 | Genetics Glossary (*continued*) |
|---|---|
| **Term** | **Definition/Description** |
| Gene | The fundamental unit of heredity. An ordered sequence of DNA constitutes a gene; it is found on a specific location on a specific chromosome. Each gene encodes for a specific functional protein. |
| Gene expression | The process by which information from a gene is used to produce a functional gene product (usually a protein); it is how a genotype results in a particular phenotype. Not all genes are expressed. |
| Genetic disorder | Alterations in genes that code for a particular protein, which results in a heritable disorder. |
| Genome | The entire DNA sequence and set of genetic instructions found within each cell. The genome is different for each organism. The Human Genome Project documented the entire DNA sequence of the approximately 25,000 genes held within the 23 pairs of chromosomes in humans. |
| Genotype | A person's complete collection of specific genes. A person's genotype is largely responsible for determining the phenotype. |
| Heterozygous | Referring to an individual who has a mutant allele on only one of a pair of specific genes. A specific phenotype in a heterozygous individual is the result of a dominant gene mutation, requiring only one mutant allele. Conversely, a heterozygous individual with a recessive gene mutation is referred to as a "carrier" and does not exhibit the phenotype. |
| Homozygous | Referring to an individual who has a mutant allele on both genes in a specific gene pair (one from each parent). Autosomal recessive inheritance of a trait, condition, or disease occurs only when an individual is homozygous for the specific gene. Cystic fibrosis and sickle cell anemia, for example, occur only in individuals who are homozygous for the specific disease gene. |
| Incomplete penetrance | Genetic mutation that does not always result in the phenotype associated with that mutation. Often the expression of a gene with incomplete penetrance depends on the presence of other environmental factors. |
| Karyotype | An individual's full set of chromosomes. Also, the standardized laboratory result or visual display (i.e., a photograph) of an individual's set of chromosomes. |
| Meiosis | Cell division that results in sperm or ova. The products of meiosis contain only half the original number of chromosomes. |
| Monosomy | A chromosomal condition in which there is a single chromosome when there should be a chromosome pair. These mutations are almost always lethal when found in autosomal chromosomes. |
| Mosaicism | Occurs when cells in the body contain two or more genomes, as the result of spontaneous mutation after fertilization (postzygotic), or when a cell does not divide evenly into two cells. Manifestations of mosaicism vary widely, from normal phenotype to severe/lethal impact. |
| Multifactorial disease | A condition caused by the interactions between several genes and several environmental factors. Cancer, type 2 diabetes mellitus, and heart disease are all multifactorial conditions. |
| Mutation | A change in DNA sequence that may or may not result in a change in the protein product. Mutations may affect only one base pair or a larger segment in the DNA sequence via deletion, insertion, repetition, or duplication. Genetic mutations cause disorders such as cystic fibrosis, Tay-Sachs disease, and sickle cell anemia. |
| Nondisjunction | Failure of chromosome pairs to separate properly during meiosis. |
| Penetrance | The proportion of persons with a specific genotype who also express the expected phenotype. For example, if a particular gene mutation has 95% penetrance, then 95% of persons with that mutation will have the associated phenotype. |

| Term | Definition/Description |
|---|---|
| Phenotype | The observable traits or physical expression of an individual's genotype, which is also influenced by environmental factors. |
| Recessive allele | An allele that expresses a particular phenotype only if both alleles in the pair are recessive. |
| Ribonucleic acid (RNA) | A single-stranded nitrogenous molecule that mirrors the DNA sequence. RNA is essential for moving DNA instructions out of the nucleus (via transcription and translation) and into the cell cytoplasm, and for subsequent construction of amino acids into final protein products. |
| Single-nucleotide polymorphism (SNP) | Pronounced "snip"; any of the common variations found in a single nucleotide of genomic DNA sequence between individuals, as well as between different populations. |
| Transcription | The synthesis of an RNA strand from a sequence of DNA; the first step in gene expression. |
| Translation | During protein synthesis, the process through which the sequence of bases in a molecule of messenger RNA is read to create a sequence of amino acids. |
| Trisomy | A chromosomal condition in which three chromosomes occur where there should be only a pair. Trisomy is a form of aneuploidy. The occurrence of trisomy increases in infants born to older pregnant individuals. A common trisomy condition is trisomy 21 (Down syndrome). |
| X-Y linked (also called sex-linked) | A gene that is located on an X or Y sex chromosome. |

Based on Feero WG, Guttmacher AE, Collins FS. Genomic medicine: an updated primer. *N Engl J Med*. 2010;362:2001-2011; National Cancer Institute. NCI dictionary of genetics terms. https://www.cancer.gov/publications/dictionaries/genetics-dictionary. Accessed August 18, 2021; Elston R, Satagopan J, Sun S. Genetic terminology. *Meth Molec Biol*. 2012;850:1-9; American College of Obstetricians and Gynecologists. ACOG technology assessment in obstetrics and gynecology No. 14: modern genetics in obstetrics and gynecology. *Obstet Gynecol*. 2018;132(3):e143-e168. doi:10.1097/AOG.0000000000002831.

a template for the eventual assembly of amino acids into proteins within the cell's cytoplasm.

The human genome has approximately 20,000 genes in chromosomes and 37 genes in the mitochondria of each nucleated cell. Approximately 1% of these genes are translated into proteins. The rest are involved in regulation or repression of the protein-coding genes.[14]

Mitochondria are the components of cells responsible for aerobic respiration, or energy utilization. Mitochondria contain their own genome and replication systems. They are inherited exclusively from the egg's contribution to the genome. It is possible to inherit some normal mitochondria and some mutated mitochondria, leading to mitochondrial heteroplasmy, a state that can result in related diseases depending on the extent of the mutated component.[10]

*Gene expression* refers to the eventual production of a gene product, although not all genes are expressed in every cell or in precisely the same way. For example, an epithelial cell (a skin cell) does not look or function the same way as a myocyte (a muscle cell). Although both cell types contain the exact same set of genetic instructions, only those genes that are expressed will contribute to the unique structure and function of the specific cell type.[14] Gene expression is regulated by a complex set of signals within an organism. This signaling system allows undifferentiated cells (i.e., fetal stem cells) to evolve into a wide variety of cells with differing structures and functions. The term *epigenetic* refers to the regulation of gene expression via modifications of the DNA structure (i.e., histones or chromatin, as noted in Figure 20-1), but not modification of the DNA sequence itself.[15] Environmental signals, both internal and external to an organism, are now known to make tremendous contributions to the regulation of gene expression.[14–16]

### Genetic Mutations

*Mutation* refers to a permanent alteration in the DNA sequence within a gene, by either deletion, insertion, repetition, or duplication of a single base pair or larger segments of the DNA strand, entire genes, or pieces of chromosomes. Mutations occur rather frequently, and are often repaired by the cell; a large number of them do not result in any clinical effect or disease.[1,14] However, a genetic mutation that causes a change in the protein product can

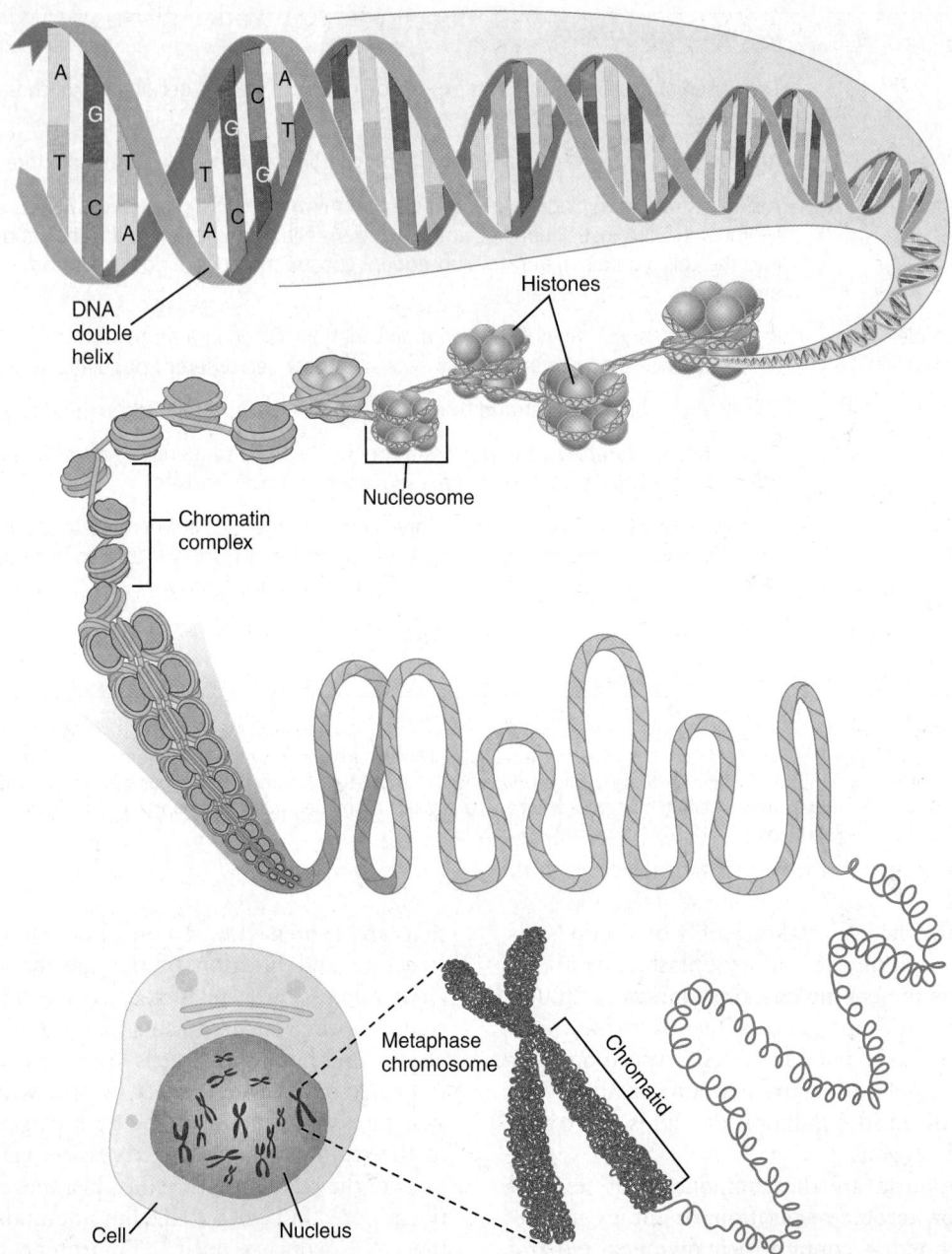

**Figure 20-1** Patterns of DNA coiling. DNA is wound around eight histone cores (proteins) to form nucleosomes. Nucleosomes make up the chromatin complex, which is tightly coiled into a chromatid. The chromosome is made up of chromatids, which are held together by a centromere.

subsequently alter the function of the cell. Such a change creates the disease *phenotype*, which refers to clinically or physically observed signs or symptoms that are reflective of the *genotype* within the individual. Genetic mutations can occur spontaneously or can be transmitted from gamete to child.

### Alleles and Penetrance

All of the genes on any specific inherited chromosome from the egg correspond to the same genes in the same location (*allele*) from the sperm's chromosome counterpart. Individuals with a mutant allele on only one of the pair of genes are referred to as "heterozygous," while those with a mutant allele on both genes in the pair are referred to as "homozygous."

*Penetrance* refers to the percentage of individuals with a specific disease genotype who also express the expected phenotype (the observable characteristics of the genotype). For example, a genetic mutation that is not associated with an expected phenotype 100% of the time has "incomplete penetrance," whereas a penetrance of 50% indicates that only half of the individuals with a specific disease genotype will exhibit the phenotype. The variation in phenotype (i.e., severity) of a particular genetic disorder, which is called *expressivity*, can be influenced by modifier genes, and perhaps by aging or the environment. Expressivity contributes to the wide range of abilities that are observed among individuals with Down syndrome, for example. Knowledge about penetrance and expressivity helps to answer the question of why all individuals with the same genotype do not have the same phenotypic characteristics or severity of the genetic disorder.

## Inheritance Patterns of Genetic Mutations

Genes, as the basic unit of inheritance, contribute significantly to an individual's characteristics, including disposition for health and disease in addition to aspects of physical appearance, such as height, eye color, and hair color. Mutations that occur in somatic cells are called acquired mutations and are significant when they lead to malignant transformation of the cell such as occurs in cancer. Genetic mutations that occur in sperm or eggs can be inherited, and several different patterns of inheritance are possible.

Patterns of inheritance are either *autosomal*, which means the inherited genes are located on the first 22 pairs of chromosomes, or *X-Y linked* (also known as *sex-linked*), which means the inherited genes are located on either the X or Y chromosome.[17] In addition, inheritance is either dominant or recessive. Many well-known heritable genetic disorders are caused by a mutation in a single gene. These conditions are referred to as classic *Mendelian* disorders, after the early geneticist Gregor Mendel. Mendel was an Austrian monk who was one of the first scientists to clearly establish that physical traits are heritable from one generation to the next.[1,17] The classic Mendelian patterns of inheritance are autosomal dominant, autosomal recessive, X-linked dominant, X-linked recessive, and Y-linked.

In contrast, most chromosomal abnormalities are not heritable. This clinical distinction is important because tests for chromosomal abnormalities are often inaccurately referred to as "genetic tests." Use of the word "genetics" when referring to tests for both genetic disorders and chromosomal abnormalities can mistakenly convey the idea that chromosomal abnormalities are inherited. Thus, when a midwife discusses genetic testing with individuals and their families, inheritance is an important concept to include in the discussion.

### Autosomal Dominant Inheritance

Disease phenotypes expressed in *heterozygous* individuals (i.e., those persons with one mutant allele in a specific gene pair) reflect an autosomal dominant inheritance pattern.[1,17] Only one copy of the mutant allele is required for expression of such a disorder. Examples of autosomal dominant disorders include achondroplasia (commonly known as dwarfism), neurofibromatosis, Marfan syndrome, and Huntington disease. Individuals of any sex who have an autosomal dominant condition have a 50% probability of having a child with the same disease-causing mutation. The existence of an autosomal dominant condition is usually well known to the affected family because it is commonly observed within all generations of the family tree, unlike autosomal recessive disorders.

The occurrence of spontaneous mutations in either the egg or the sperm explains why autosomal dominant disorders can occur in individuals with no family history of the condition. Since the mutation has not been inherited from the parents, the affected individual is the first in the family to experience the disorder. Although the disorder has not been inherited from the individual's parents, the affected individual will now have a 50% probability of transmitting the mutation to their offspring. The parents of an individual who has an autosomal dominant disorder resulting from a spontaneous mutation have a low risk of having another child with the mutation.[2]

A diagram referred to as a Punnett square is often used to demonstrate the probability of inheritance in the offspring of affected and unaffected parents, as shown in Figure 20-2A. A typical corresponding pedigree reflective of autosomal dominant inheritance is shown in Figure 20-2B.

### Autosomal Recessive Inheritance

Disease phenotypes expressed only in homozygous individuals (i.e., those persons with two mutant alleles in the specific gene pair) demonstrate an autosomal recessive inheritance pattern.[17] Individuals who are heterozygous for an autosomal recessive inheritance pattern are considered "carriers" and are largely unaffected by the disease. However, these carriers can pass the genetic mutation to their offspring. A carrier's single working gene is sufficient for normal function. Cystic fibrosis (CF), Tay-Sachs disease, and sickle cell anemia are examples of autosomal recessive disorders.

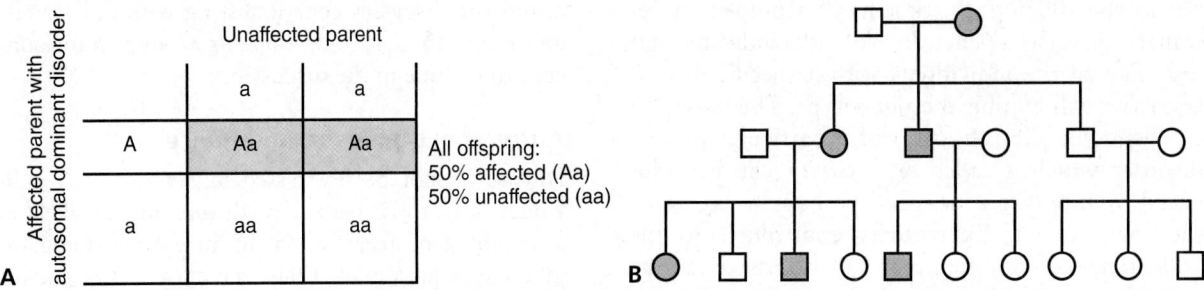

**Figure 20-2 A.** Probability of offspring inheriting an autosomal dominant disorder. This diagram demonstrates the probability of offspring inheriting an autosomal dominant disorder from a heterozygous (affected) parent and an unaffected parent. Shading indicates affected individuals. **B.** The corresponding dominant pedigree pattern. Pedigree showing the inheritance pattern of an autosomal dominant disorder. Both XX and XY individuals are equally affected. Solid shapes represent affected individuals and open shapes represent unaffected individuals. Circles represent XX individuals/individuals assigned female at birth and squares represent XY individuals/individuals assigned male at birth.
Abbreviations: A, chromosome with a dominant disease allele; a, chromosome with a normal allele.

| Table 20-3 | Autosomal Recessive Carrier Frequency in Specific Populations and Associated Incidence in Newborns | | |
|---|---|---|---|
| **Genetic Disease** | **Genetic Heritage** | **Carrier Frequency** | **Newborn Incidence** |
| Tay-Sachs disease | Ashkenazi Jewish | 1/30 | 1/3600 |
| Sickle cell disease | African | 1/12 | 1/600 |
| Cystic fibrosis | Northern European | 1/25 | 1/2500 |
| Beta-thalassemia | Greek/Italian | 1/30 | 1/3600 |
| Alpha-thalassemia | Southeast Asian, Chinese | 1/25 | 1/2500 |

While commonly used, location of genetic ancestors alone is not a reliable indicator of genetic risk.

Two individuals who have the same autosomal recessive mutation will have a 25% probability that any pregnancy they conceive will result in a child who is affected with the disorder—that is, a child who is homozygous for the mutation (two mutant alleles). Additionally, any child of these same individuals has a 25% probability of being an unaffected noncarrier (no mutant alleles) of the mutation and a 50% probability of being an unaffected carrier (one mutant allele). Since autosomal recessive mutations have an inheritance pattern that results in less frequent occurrence of the disorder (frequently skipping generations in which the condition is observed), families are often unaware that the disease mutation exists. No one in the immediate family may have the disorder, so families may not be aware of the possibility of the heritable disorder until an affected child is born.

The number of persons who are carriers for a specific autosomal recessive disorder varies greatly by genetic heritage. Although carrier status for some autosomal recessive disorders is quite common among some populations, the incidence of newborns being affected with the disorder actually

is much lower as noted in Table 20-3. Figure 20-3A demonstrates the probability of inheritance in the offspring of parents who are carriers of an autosomal recessive disorder, and Figure 20-3B shows a typical corresponding pedigree. Screening based on heritage becomes less sensitive with increasing genetic diversity, so this type of risk identification may become obsolete as populations become more multicultural worldwide.

## X-Y-Linked Inheritance

The terms *male* and *female* can have a range of meanings that encompass genetics, anatomy, and gender expression. The terms *XY individual* as well as *male/father/son* describe those persons with an X and a Y chromosome, who are usually born with a penis, while *female/mother/daughter* describe individuals who have XX chromosomes and are usually born with a vulva. Other common terminology includes ASAB (assigned sex at birth), where AFAB is a person assigned female at birth and AMAB is a person assigned male at birth. We acknowledge that the phenotype of genitals do not always reflect individuals' genetics and so this terminology

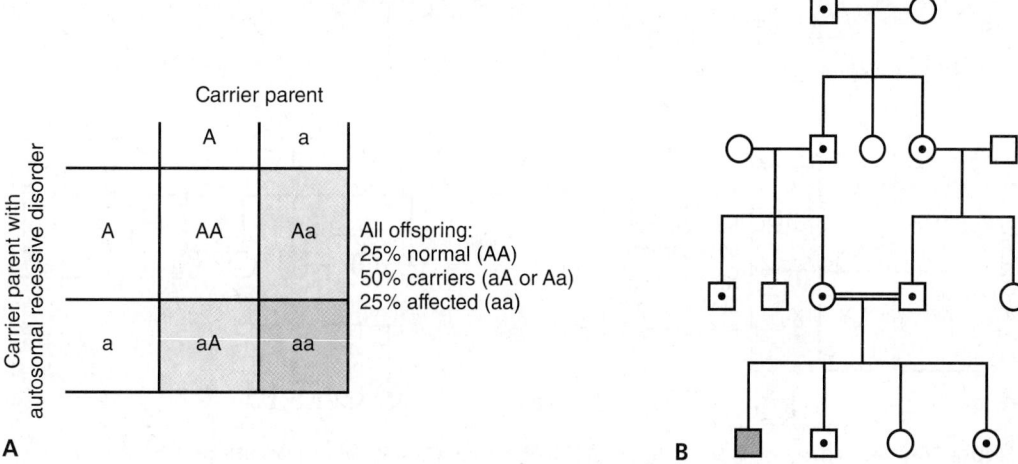

**Figure 20-3 A.** Probability of offspring inheriting an autosomal recessive disorder. Diagram demonstrating the probability of offspring inheriting an autosomal recessive disorder from two heterozygous (carrier) parents. Light shading indicates carrier status and heavy shading indicates affected individuals. **B.** The corresponding autosomal recessive pedigree pattern. Pedigree showing the inheritance pattern of an autosomal recessive disorder. Consanguinity is denoted as a double line in this figure, but should not be interpreted as a requirement for individual inheritance (i.e., inheritance does not depend on consanguinity). Solid shapes represent affected individuals and open shapes represent unaffected individuals. Circles represent XX individuals and squares represent XY individuals. Shapes containing a dot represent carriers of an autosomal recessive mutation. Abbreviations: A, chromosome with a normal allele; a, chromosome with the disease allele.

is imprecise. Gender identity is not described in this section.

Disorders caused by mutations on the sex chromosomes are inherited differently than disorders inherited via autosomal mutations. Since individuals who are XX do not have a Y chromosome, Y-linked disorders rarely occur in these individuals. The Y chromosome also contains far fewer genes than the X chromosome, creating far fewer opportunities for mutation among individuals who are XY. Therefore, Y-linked disorders are extremely rare. In contrast, X-linked disorders are more common and predominantly affect XY individuals, who do not have the paired X chromosome that XX individuals have. A paired X chromosome could contribute a normally functioning allele to compensate for a mutant allele. The inheritance pattern of X-linked mutations results in unaffected XX carriers of the mutation and affected XY individuals with a Y chromosome that cannot compensate for the mutation occurring on the X chromosome. In the XY individual, the single mutation on the X chromosome is sufficient to cause the disorder.

An XX individual who is a carrier for an X-linked recessive mutation has four possible pregnancy outcomes (assuming an XY partner without an X-linked disorder): a 25% chance for an unaffected, carrier XX offspring (one mutant X allele and one normal X allele); a 25% chance for an unaffected, noncarrier XX offspring (two normal X alleles); a 25% chance for an affected XY offspring

(one mutant X allele and one normal Y allele unable to compensate); and a 25% chance for an unaffected, noncarrier XY offspring (normal X and Y alleles).[17] An affected XY individual has two possible outcomes for offspring (assuming an XX partner who is not a carrier for an X-linked disorder): an XX child who is a carrier (one mutant X allele and one normal X allele) and an unaffected, noncarrier XY child (XY parents contribute a Y chromosome to their offspring who are XY). **Figure 20-4A** illustrates the inheritance probabilities for X-linked disorders among offspring of a carrier XX individual and an unaffected XY person—by far the most common occurrence. **Figure 20-4B** shows a typical corresponding pedigree.

Hemophilia A and Duchenne muscular dystrophy are among the more common X-linked disorders. One way to distinguish X-linked from autosomal dominant conditions when analyzing a pedigree is to determine whether affected XY individuals have affected XY offspring. Transmission from an XY individual to their XY offspring is observed with autosomal dominant conditions but not with X-linked recessive traits.

X-linked dominant disorders exist, but appear rarely in the population. These conditions also affect heterozygous XX individuals. Upon pedigree analysis, none of the XY offspring but all of the XX offspring of affected XY individuals will be affected.

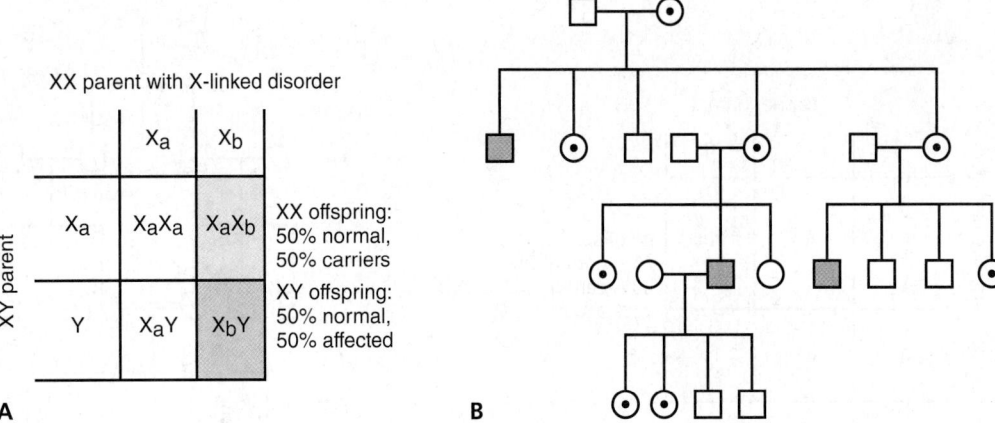

XX parent with X-linked disorder

| XY parent | | Xa | Xb | |
|---|---|---|---|---|
| | Xa | XaXa | XaXb | XX offspring: 50% normal, 50% carriers |
| | Y | XaY | XbY | XY offspring: 50% normal, 50% affected |

**A**

**B**

**Figure 20-4 A.** Probability of offspring inheriting an X-linked recessive disorder. Diagram demonstrating the probability of offspring inheriting an X-linked recessive disorder from a heterozygous (carrier) XX parent and an unaffected, noncarrier XY parent. Light shading indicates carrier status. Heavy shading indicates an affected individual. **B.** The corresponding X-linked recessive pedigree pattern. Pedigree showing inheritance pattern of an X-linked recessive disorder. Only XY individuals are affected. Only XX individuals are carriers. For offspring of a carrier XX parent and a normal XY parent, in each pregnancy there is an independent chance that for XY offspring there is a 50% chance the child will be affected and a 50% chance the child will be unaffected. For XX offspring, there is a 50% chance the child will be a carrier and a 50% chance the child will be unaffected. For offspring of affected XY individuals, 100% of XX offspring are carriers and 100% of XY offspring are normal. Solid shapes represent affected individuals and open shapes represent unaffected individuals. Circles represent individuals assigned female at birth (usually XX) and squares represent individuals assigned male at birth (usually XY). There is no standardized nomenclature to denote individuals with disorders of sex differentiation or trans individuals in a pedigree. Shapes containing a dot represent carriers of an autosomal recessive mutation.
Abbreviations: Xa, chromosome with a normal allele; Xb, chromosome with the disease allele.

## Multifactorial Inheritance

Many common conditions and disorders occur due to multifactorial inheritance, meaning that they are caused by the combined effects of several genes (genetic predisposition) and several environmental factors.[1] It is also generally accepted that a "threshold" must be reached for the disease or condition to become manifest. In other words, an additive effect of genetic predisposition and increasing environmental "load" will cause an individual to reach a certain "tipping point" when the disease phenotype will occur. Gender, age, socioeconomic status, lifestyle, nutritional status, geographic area, and ethnic background frequently influence the occurrence of a multifactorial condition or disease. Neural tube defects (e.g., spina bifida and anencephaly) and congenital pyloric stenosis are common examples of multifactorial conditions that are present at birth. Cancer, type 2 diabetes mellitus, and heart disease are multifactorial conditions that usually manifest in adulthood.

### Neural Tube Defects

Neural tube defects (NTDs) are examples of multifactorial conditions that contribute significantly to adverse birth outcomes. NTDs occur when the neural tube fails to develop and close properly during very early embryonic life (2–6 weeks' gestational age).[16] Multiple genes—particularly those associated with folate metabolism—contribute to a genetic predisposition for NTDs; environmental factors, such as the pregnant person's age, diet, geographic area, drug exposure, and socioeconomic status, are associated with these defects as well.[16] Spina bifida (protrusion of the spinal tissue through the vertebral column) and anencephaly (partial or complete absence of the cranial vault and partial or complete absence of the cerebral hemispheres) are the most commonly observed NTDs.[18] These two conditions are also referred to as open neural tube defects to differentiate them from the rarer closed neural tube defects, in which skin covers the spinal abnormality.

The prevalence of NTDs varies widely among different populations, from 1 to 2 persons per 1000 live births, to as high as 6 persons per 1000 live births in populations with a genetic heritage from northern China. While the pathophysiologic basis of NTDs is complex and not well understood, it is known that folic acid supplementation can reduce the occurrence of NTDs by 60% to 70%. This recognition led to widespread recommendations for folic acid fortification of enriched cereal products and supplementation (400–800 mcg per day) both prior to conception and during the first 8 weeks of pregnancy.[18] Hispanic populations (the phrasing used in the research) are at increased risk for folate-sensitive NTDs, and food fortification has not completely eliminated the disparity.[18,19] Although pregnant persons who have had an affected child have a risk of recurrence in subsequent children of approximately 2% to 5%, 95% of all NTDs occur in previously unaffected families.[20]

Individuals with spina bifida—the most common NTD—have varying degrees of physical and mental challenges, including hydrocephalus (which is independently associated with increased risk for physical and intellectual disability). The severity of disability increases with the severity of the defect. Surgical repair of the defect is the approach usually undertaken for improving prognosis.

Anencephaly has an extremely high level of mortality. The majority of infants with anencephaly are stillborn, and those who are born alive die soon after birth.[21]

## Chromosomal Disorders

Chromosomal disorders are not the result of single-gene mutations, such as the autosomal dominant and recessive disorders, but rather reflect changes in the number or structure of the chromosomes.[2] Chromosomal abnormalities are relatively common, occurring in an estimated 1 in 150 live births and approximately 50% of first trimester miscarriages.[2] Such abnormalities frequently are associated with common phenotypic and physical characteristics, thereby aiding in their early identification, including during fetal ultrasound examination. However, chromosomal evaluation via a *karyotype* (a visual display of the full complement of an individual's chromosomes) or *chromosomal microarray analysis* provides the definitive diagnosis.

The most common numerical chromosomal aberrations are caused by *aneuploidy*—the addition or deletion of an entire chromosome in a normal set of 23 pairs of chromosomes. Aneuploidy most often occurs due to nondisjunction during cell division in the egg or sperm.[22] The resulting absence of one chromosome (monosomy) in a set is almost always lethal, so such a mutation is rarely observed in live-born children. An exception is monosomy X, also called Turner syndrome.

In contrast, the addition of a chromosome (trisomy) leads to one of several disorders depending on which chromosome pair receives the extra genetic material. The most common trisomy is trisomy 21 (Down syndrome), which is caused by an extra

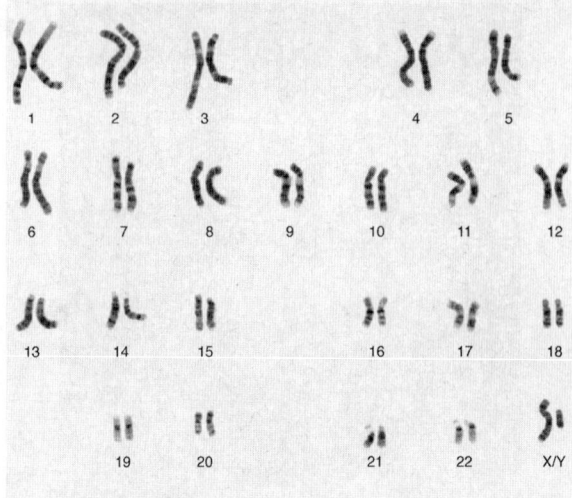

**A**

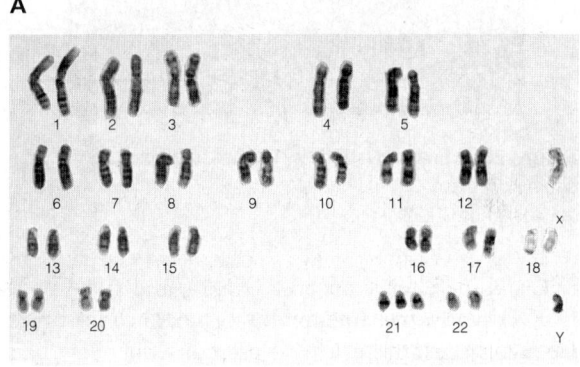

**B**

**Figure 20-5** Karyotype. **A.** A full complement of 23 pairs of chromosomes in an XX individual. **B.** An extra chromosome is observed in this XX individual with trisomy 21 (Down syndrome).
**A:** Courtesy of Darryl Leja/National Human Genome Research Institute. **B:** © Jens Goepfert/Shutterstock.

chromosome added to the 21st pair of chromosomes. Figures 20-5A and 20-5B contrast the 21st chromosomes in a normal XX karyotype and one with trisomy 21. Phenotypic characteristics of individuals with trisomy 21 include specific facial features, such as small upturned eyes, small flat nose, small mouth with large tongue, and small ears (Figure 20-6). Intellectual and physical disabilities of varying severity are also observed. Congenital heart defects, obstructions of the gastrointestinal tract, and frequent respiratory infections are associated with trisomy 21. Trisomy 18 (Edwards' syndrome) and trisomy 13 (Patau syndrome) are less frequently encountered aneuploidies, but both result in severe physical and intellectual disability in offspring, and are usually lethal during gestation or shortly after birth.[2,23]

Other common aneuploid disorders include sex chromosomal aberrations, such as Turner syndrome

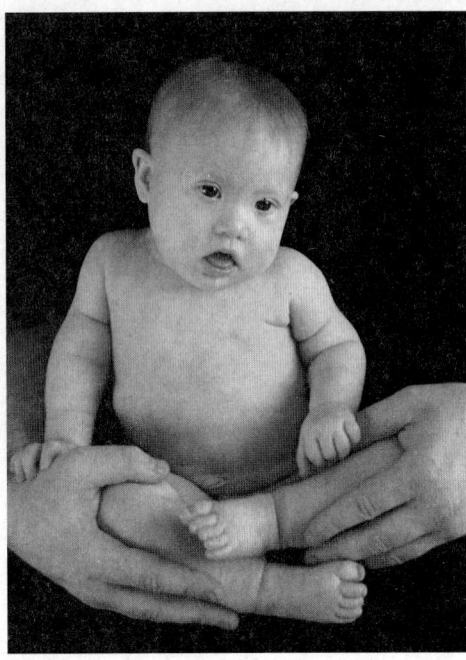

**Figure 20-6** Infant with trisomy 21 (Down syndrome) chromosomal disorder.
© iStockphoto/Thinkstock.

(XO), Klinefelter syndrome (XXY), and trisomy X (XXX) syndrome. Aneuploidy of sex chromosomes frequently results in less severe consequences than does autosomal aneuploidy, but the resulting conditions are associated with sex characteristic effects (including sterility, feminization, or virilization), and frequently with minor physical changes specific to the disorder.[23] Many individuals who are mildly affected are not identified as having a chromosome abnormality for much of their lives unless health care is sought for a seemingly unrelated condition (e.g., infertility) and a karyotype is performed to identify the potential genetic etiology of the condition.[2,24,25] Modern karyotyping has also found that as many as one-third of individuals previously thought to have Turner syndrome actually have mosaicism (discussed in the next section).[25] The gain of an entire haploid set of chromosomes (e.g., 69, XXY) also occurs in a partial hydatidiform mole, which is incompatible with life; this disorder often leads to miscarriage and other first trimester complications.

Rearrangements, inversions, small deletions, or microdeletions of portions of a chromosome are considered structural abnormalities. They contribute to infrequently occurring genetic conditions, such as cri-du-chat syndrome, the result of a deletion of a portion of chromosome 5; Wolf-Hirschhorn syndrome, the result of a deletion of a portion of

chromosome 4; Prader-Willi syndrome, a microdeletion of a portion of chromosome 15; and Williams syndrome, a microdeletion of a portion of chromosome 7.[26] Each abnormality has phenotypic characteristics specific to the condition.

## Mosaicism

Mosaicism occurs when cells in the body contain two or more cell lines (genomes).[27,28] Mosaicism was initially thought to be rare, but is now recognized as occurring in most humans at an unnoticeable level. It is not an inherited condition, but rather occurs after fertilization (postzygotic) from spontaneous mutations or, more commonly, when a cell does not divide evenly into two cells.[27] The fact that mosaicism is a postzygotic event means that there is no increased risk of recurrence of the same disorder in future offspring for parents with a child affected with mosaicism.

When mosaicism occurs during embryonic or fetal development, somatic or germline (gonadic) cells may be adversely affected. Individuals with mosaicism may be either phenotypically normal or profoundly affected; mutations can occur throughout the entire body or in specific regions and tissues (e.g., the placenta or skin—a frequent manifestation site for mosaicism). The severity of the condition depends on when the mutation or cell division occurs along the developmental timeline (earlier in development typically has broader impact), and whether it affects a single nucleotide base, a section of DNA, or an entire chromosome.[29] The mutation may result in a neutral, deleterious, or advantageous function. Mosaicism is an established cause of spontaneous abortion, birth defects, stillbirth, a wide variety of genomic disorders, and cancer.[27]

There is no way to predict mosaicism, given the spontaneous nature of mutations and the variance in aberrant cell division that contributes to this condition. Mosaicism can be complex and result in enormously divergent phenotypes. It is suspected when the results from standard diagnostic genetic or chromosomal testing are unexpected or unexplained, given a specific phenotype. Further testing beyond karyotyping, direct DNA testing, or chromosomal microarray analysis is necessary and may include next-generation sequencing (NGS).[28] However, because mosaicism can be tissue-specific and the clinical implications unpredictable, significant testing limitations exist. Mosaicism is typically not detected in blood, but only in affected tissue.

A known example of the complexity in diagnosis is found in relation to preimplantation genetic testing for aneuploidies; such testing is increasingly being conducted given the widespread use of reproductive technologies. The conduct of NGS is an improvement over previous types of testing for mosaic aneuploidies, but is often accompanied by diagnoses of uncertain clinical significance—that is, mosaicism can result in phenotypes ranging from normal to profoundly affected to lethal.[30] When confined to specific tissue, such as the placenta or skin, the effects will be localized rather than affecting all cells of the body. Mosaic neurofibromatosis, asymmetric growth disorders, developmental disorders, focal brain malformations, and cancer are some of the more common conditions that can be caused by mosaicism.[27]

## Birth Defects, Incidence, and Risk Identification

Genetic disorders and chromosomal disorders are not rare occurrences. An individual's risk for a genetic disorder is based on several factors, including age, gender, and ethnic background of those contributing the person's genetic components. For example, cystic fibrosis has a prevalence of 1 case per 2500 persons among individuals who are white and of Northern European descent, while sickle cell disease has a prevalence of 1 case per 400 to 600 persons among individuals who are Black and of African descent. Another example of a factor affecting the risk for fetal/neonatal chromosomal disorders is the age of the person who contributes the egg.[31]

Table 20-4, Table 20-5, and Table 20-6 list several conditions and diseases with a genetic component, along with their prevalence in specific populations. Understanding particular risks among specific populations and groups can prompt the midwife to probe further when obtaining a medical and family history, provide accurate patient education, recommend specific testing to individuals and families, or make a referral to a genetic counselor, as appropriate.

### Age

There is a well-documented increase in the risk for a chromosomal abnormality, particularly for aneuploidies such as trisomy 21 (Down syndrome), when the person providing the egg is older than 35 years of age.[32] The graph in Figure 20-7 demonstrates the escalating risk of a pregnancy being affected by a chromosomal anomaly as the age of the person providing the egg increases. By 45 years of age, the risk for any chromosomal disorder at birth is approximately 5.3% (with the majority being trisomy 21), compared to approximately 0.25% for pregnancies with an egg from a person younger than age

| Table 20-4 | Selected Chromosomal Disorders with Approximate Prevalence |
|---|---|
| **Chromosome Abnormality** | **Approximate Prevalence (per 10,000 live births)** |
| Klinefelter syndrome (XXY) | 10 - for individuals assigned male at birth |
| Trisomy 13 | 1 |
| Trisomy 18 | 3 |
| Trisomy 21 (Down syndrome) | 14 |
| Turner syndrome (XO) | 4 - for individuals assigned female at birth |

Data from Mai CT, Isenburg JL, Canfield MA, et al. National population-based estimates for major birth defects, 2010-2014. *Birth Defects Res*. 2019;111(18):1420-1435. doi:10.1002/bdr2 .1589; Rare disease database. National Organization for Rare Disorders, Inc. https://rarediseases.org/for-patients-and-families /information-resources/rare-disease-information/. Accessed September 18, 2022.

30 years. Presented another way, Table 20-7 shows that 1 in 30 infants born to people age 45 years will have trisomy 21, compared to 1 in 1250 infants born to people age 25 years.[31] The risk for any chromosomal disorder for infants born to pregnant people age 45 years is 1 in 20.

Although a few studies have shown a very slight increase in the risk of genetic disorders for children born to older XY parents (primarily autosomal dominant disorders such as achondroplasia and neurofibromatosis), most research has not found that pregnancies generated with sperm from older XY individuals is associated with an increased risk for chromosomal anomalies.[33,34] Furthermore, unlike the risk associated with advanced age of the pregnant person, no clear consensus exists for when an XY individual is considered to be of advanced age. A commonly used criterion is age 40 years, but there are no specific recommendations for couples in whom the individual contributing the sperm is of advanced age.

### Individual Conditions Associated with Teratogenicity

*Teratology* is the study of *teratogens*, or agents that irreversibly alter growth, structure, or function in a developing embryo or fetus.[35] Teratogens include viruses such as rubella, chemicals such as mercury, and drugs such as warfarin.[35] The term *fetotoxic* is used to describe agents, such as tobacco, that have toxic effects on the fetus and adversely affect growth or

| Table 20-5 | Single-Gene Genetic Disorders That Meet Screening Thresholds |
|---|---|
| **Examples of Single-Gene Disorders That Meet Evidence-Based Thresholds for Screening*** | **Screening Should Be Offered to Individuals with the Following History (personal, family, or genetic heritage).*** |
| Cystic fibrosis | All individuals |
| Spinal muscular atrophy | All individuals |
| Alpha thalassemia | CBC with RBC indices for all pregnant individuals to screen for hemoglobin-opathy; consider automatic hemoglobin electrophoresis for those with African, Mediterranean, Middle Eastern, Southeast Asian, or West Indian descent |
| Beta chain hemoglobinopathies including sickle cell disease | |
| Canavan disease | Ashkenazi Jewish |
| Familia dysautonomia | Ashkenazi Jewish |
| Tay–Sachs disease | Ashkenazi Jewish, French–Canadian, or Cajun descent and those with a family history of Tay–Sachs |
| Fragile X syndrome | Pregnant people with family history of fragile X-related disorders or intellectual disability suggesting fragile X syndrome, and those with unexplained ovarian insufficiency or elevated FSH before age 40 |

* Screening recommended in this column is based on American College of Obstetricians and Gynecologists (ACOG) guidance. Location of genetic ancestors is not a reliable indicator of genetic risk. However, widespread screening in a population at low risk for the disease can have a high rate of false positives. To decrease the rate of false positives and provide more cost-effective care, national organizations such as ACOG recommend targeted screening for these conditions based on genetic risk factors. For these conditions, testing should be offered to an individual with any family history of the condition or if one parent is from an at-risk group. The American College of Medical Genetics and Genomics (ACMG) recommends pan-ethnic screening for more than 100 conditions. Expanded carrier screening panels are created by the companies who offer these tests, while the conditions they screen for are informed by recommendations by national organizations such as ACOG and ACMG. Pregnant families should be provided information about carrier screening options and supported in their choices for targeted screening, expanded screening, or no screening.

Based on: Johansen Taber K, Ben-Shachar R, Torres R, et al. A guidelines-consistent carrier screening panel that supports equity across diverse populations. *Genet Med.* 2022;24(1):201-213. doi:10.1016/j.gim.2021.09.009; American College of Obstetricians and Gynecologists. Committee opinion no. 691: carrier screening for genetic conditions. *Obstet Gynecol.* 2017;129(3):e41-e55; Scotet V, L'Hostis C, Ferec C. The changing epidemiology of cystic fibrosis: incidence, survival and impact of the *CFTR* gene discovery. *Genes (Basel).* 2020;11(6):589. doi:10.3390/genes11060589.

| Table 20-6 | Selected Multifactorial Disorders with Approximate Prevalence |
|---|---|
| **Congenital Malformation** | **Approximate Prevalence (per 10,000 live births)** |
| Central nervous system defects | 7 |
| Cleft lip with or without cleft palate | 10 |
| Club foot | 17 |
| Congenital heart defects | 20 |
| Gastroschisis | 5 |

Based on Mai CT, Isenburg JL, Canfield MA, et al. National population-based estimates for major birth defects, 2010-2014. *Birth Defects Res.* 2019;111(18):1420-1435. doi:10.1002/bdr2.1589.

development. Exposure to teratogens may be a risk factor for birth defects depending on the level and type of exposure (i.e., duration, strength, potency).[36] Birth defects occur in approximately 3% to 5% of all births but cause one-fifth of total infant mortality.[37,38] This baseline percentage of birth defects is often called the "background risk" upon which additional risks are calculated based on family history, past history, and environmental exposure.[38] Teratogens cause approximately 10% of birth defects.[37] Selected conditions that are known or highly suspected contributors to birth defects are listed in Table 20-8.[38]

### Teratogenic and Fetotoxic Effects of Drugs

Most people take at least one medication during pregnancy.[39] Teratogenic medications are those that cause structural abnormalities in the fetus.[40] Fewer than 10% of congenital anomalies are associated with a particular drug exposure; however, little is known about fetal safety for most marketed

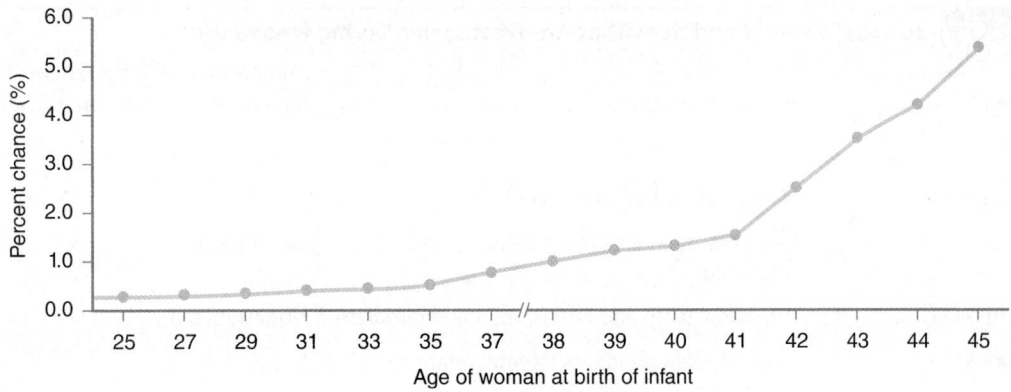

**Figure 20-7** Age during pregnancy and risk of chromosomal abnormality.
Data from Hook EB. Rates of chromosomal abnormalities. *Obstet Gynecol.* 1981;58(3):282-285

| Table 20-7 | Age During Pregnancy and Risk of Chromosomal Disorders (Among Live Births) | |
|---|---|---|
| **Age (years)** | **Risk for Trisomy 21** | **Risk for Any Chromosomal Disorder** |
| 20 | 1 in 1667 | 1 in 526 |
| 25 | 1 in 1250 | 1 in 476 |
| 30 | 1 in 952 | 1 in 384 |
| 35 | 1 in 385 | 1 in 204 |
| 40 | 1 in 106 | 1 in 65 |
| 45 | 1 in 30 | 1 in 20 |
| 49 | 1 in 11 | 1 in 7 |

Data from Arnold KM, Self ZB. Genetic screening and counseling: family medicine obstetrics. *Prim Care.* 2012;39:55-70.

drugs.[35,41] In 2015, the U.S. Food and Drug Administration implemented the Pregnancy and Lactation Labeling Rule (PLLR), which replaced the former alphabetic risk stratification system. Unfortunately, a majority of the data on effects associated with pregnancy and lactation is based on animal studies.[42] Knowledge of common teratogens and trustworthy resources for assessment of medications is important for the practicing midwife. More information can be found in the *Anatomy and Physiology of Pregnancy* chapter.

Avoiding teratogens during critical periods of pregnancy can prevent associated congenital anomalies. During the preimplantation period, if a small number of cells are damaged, the zygote usually compensates without any damage. Conversely, if a large number of cells are damaged, the embryo will be lost and a spontaneous abortion will occur. The period of organogenesis—between 2 and 8 weeks post fertilization, or 4 to 10 gestational weeks—is the most critical period in which teratogenic exposures can cause fetal malformations.[35] (See Table 20-8.) The susceptibility to a teratogenic agent can also be dose dependent, with implications for counseling patients requiring certain medications in pregnancy.[40,43] Table 20-8 lists drugs that are known to have teratogenic or fetotoxic effects.[35,38,44]

## Environmental Teratogens

A number of environmental chemicals, such as mercury, polychlorinated biphenyls (PCBs), some paints, and phthalates, have been linked to teratogenic or fetotoxic effects.[45] Most of these agents have suspected adverse effects on fertility, spontaneous abortion, and impaired neurodevelopment. Although the evidence that establishes some of these compounds as teratogens varies, these associations are the subject of current research. Increased exposure to environmental chemicals can contribute to health inequities of people from marginalized populations/identities. Discrimination results in individuals with demographic characteristics (such race/ethnicity/religion) being relegated to dangerous work environments or housing with exposure to toxins, causing persistent health implications. Adverse reproductive outcomes associated with specific environmental toxins and pollutants are discussed in more detail in the *Preconception Care* appendix of the *Health Promotion Across the Lifespan* chapter.

Teratogens may cause genetic mutations, but it is thought that an alteration in gene expression during critical embryonic and fetal developmental periods is the more likely mechanism contributing to genetic disorders that occur secondary to teratogen exposure.[46]

| Table 20-8 | Selected Health Conditions That Are Teratogenic During Pregnancy | |
|---|---|---|
| **Teratogen** | **Associated Defects** | **Percentage of Pregnancies Affected, Given Presence of the Condition** |
| **Infections** | | |
| Cytomegalovirus | Mental retardation, microcephaly | 10–15% |
| Rubella | Deafness, cataracts, heart defects, mental retardation | Up to 85% |
| Syphilis (untreated) | Abnormal teeth and bones, mental retardation | Not established |
| Toxoplasmosis | Hydrocephaly, blindness, mental retardation | 5–6% |
| Varicella | Limb reduction defects, skin scarring, muscle atrophy, chorioretinitis | 1% |
| Zika | Microcephaly, decreased brain tissue, joints with limited range of motion, restrictive muscle tone, damage to back of the eye | 6% overall<br>11% for exposure during first trimester |
| **Individual Conditions** | | |
| Active alcoholism | Miscarriage, fetal alcohol syndrome (minor facial changes, heart defects), fetal growth restriction, developmental delay | Up to 50% |
| Pregestational diabetes mellitus (type 1) | Heart defects, microcephaly, neural tube defects, skeletal defects, and defects in the urinary, reproductive, and digestive systems | HbA1c < 7.9%: 3.2%<br>HbA1c 8.0–9.9%: 8.1%<br>HbA1c > 10%: 23.5% |
| Hyperthermia (fever); early pregnancy only | Neural tube defects, heart and abdominal wall defects, oral cleft | Not established |
| Seizure disorder (treated) | Cleft lip with or without cleft palate, heart defects | 6–8% |
| Systemic lupus erythematosus (uncontrolled) | Miscarriage, stillbirth, congenital heart block, fetal growth restriction, prematurity | Not established |

Abbreviation: HbA1c, hemoglobin A1c.

Based on The Organization of Teratology Information Specialists (OTIS): MotherToBaby fact sheets. https://mothertobaby.org/fact-sheets/. Accessed January 12, 2022.

This is an important distinction because epigenetic regulation of gene expression is an increasingly documented and plausible mechanism that may explain some of the links between environmental exposures and birth.[46] For example, epigenetic regulation of gene expression may be the mechanism underlying the link between chronic hyperglycemia, a condition found among individuals with poorly managed diabetes (gestational or otherwise), and an increased risk of birth defects, such as heart defects and NTDs.[47,48] Moreover, epigenetic modifications may endure and confer risk for more than one generation.[49]

The major concern is for exposures to pregnant individuals affecting fetal development, particularly during the first trimester. Little to no evidence has been published suggesting that exposures to the nonpregnant biologic parent are associated with increased occurrence of birth defects, although there may be some association with adverse health outcomes during childhood.[50]

## Family History and Pedigree Evaluation as Risk Assessment Tools

One of the most effective, low-cost approaches to genetics risk assessment is to obtain a thorough personal health and family history that includes evaluation of a three-generation pedigree. A personal

| Table 20-9 | Drugs That Have Teratogenic or Fetotoxic Effects | |
|---|---|---|
| **Drug Category Name (Brand Name)** | **Teratogenic or Fetotoxic Effects** | **Clinical Implications** |
| Androgens and testosterone derivatives:<br>Danocrine (Danazol) | Virilization of XX individuals<br>Advanced genital development of XY individuals | Dose dependent; effects are more likely during a critical period. Before 9 weeks' gestation, labioscrotal fusion is common. Incidental, brief exposure usually has minimal risk. Recommend contraception during use. |
| Antibiotics:<br>Tetracyclines:<br>Tetracycline (Terramycin)<br>Doxycycline (Adoxa) | Abnormalities of teeth discoloration | Critical period is after the first trimester. Discoloration of permanent teeth is possible if exposure occurs after 24 weeks' gestation.<br>No well-controlled human studies of doxycycline have been performed. Recommend that doxycycline be used only if it is the sole effective agent available. |
| Sulfonamides:<br>Sulfamethoxazole (Bactrim, Septra) | Hyperbilirubinemia in neonates | Contraindicated after 32 weeks' gestation. |
| Chloramphenicol | "Gray baby syndrome" and possible cardiovascular collapse in neonates 2–9 days after therapy is administered near term | Oral chloramphenicol is contraindicated in pregnancy. |
| Aminoglycosides:<br>Gentamicin<br>Streptomycin<br>Kanamycin | Neonatal ototoxicity | Streptomycin and kanamycin when administered in high doses pose a clear risk of congenital deafness. Neonates of pregnant persons receiving antepartum gentamicin dosing may need serum concentrations drawn prior to postpartum therapy. |
| Anticonvulsants:<br>Carbamazepine (Tegretol)<br>Phenytoin (Dilantin)<br>Trimethadione (Tridione)<br>Valproic acid (Depakene)<br>Valproate (Depacon) | Neural tube defects (1%), cardiovascular defects, cleft lip, developmental delays, fetal growth restriction, neonatal seizures and/or respiratory depression<br>Phenytoin is specifically associated with cardiac defects, cleft palate, and fetal hydantoin syndrome (dysmorphic facial features, nail and digit hypoplasia, microcephaly, cognitive deficits) | Critical period is all trimesters. Risk of neural tube defects (NTDs) is increased with use of anticonvulsants, especially when they are used with other antiepileptic drugs.<br>Risk of NTDs can be decreased with increased folic acid supplementation prior to and during pregnancy.<br>Neonatal vitamin K prophylaxis is needed to decrease risk of bleeding.<br>Fetal risk from newer anticonvulsants such as gabapentin (Neurontin) cannot be ruled out due to the lack of human data; however, pregnancy registries do not demonstrate increased risk of major congenital anomalies. |
| Angiotensin-converting enzyme (ACE) inhibitors:<br>Captopril (Capoten)<br>Enalapril (Vasotec)<br>Lisinopril (Prinivil) | Fetal growth restriction<br>Oligohydramnios, leading to lung hypoplasia, skeletal deformities<br>Renal failure<br>Decreased skull ossification<br>Renal tubular dysgenesis | Discontinue as soon as possible in pregnancy. Risk of growth restriction is approximately 25%, with fetal morbidity of approximately 30%. Risk of adverse effects increases in the second and third trimesters.<br>Beta blockers such as labetalol (Trandate) are safe in pregnancy. |

*(continues)*

| Table 20-9 | Drugs That Have Teratogenic or Fetotoxic Effects (*continued*) | |
|---|---|---|
| **Drug Category Name (Brand Name)** | **Teratogenic or Fetotoxic Effects** | **Clinical Implications** |
| Antidepressants: Fluoxetine (Prozac) Paroxetine (Paxil) Sertraline (Zoloft) | Paroxetine increases the risk of cardiac defects (2%); the other selective serotonin reuptake inhibitor–type antidepressants do not appear to have teratogenic effects<br><br>Exposure in the third trimester is associated with neonatal withdrawal (irritability, jittery, unusual sleep patterns, trouble eating), which typically resolves within weeks<br><br>Persistent pulmonary hypertension noted in case reports | Overall, risks of teratogenic and fetotoxic effects are low. Antidepressants generally should not be discontinued during pregnancy; if using paroxetine, transition to another antidepressant. If starting antidepressant therapy during pregnancy, avoid paroxetine. |
| Antineoplastic drugs: Cyclophosphamide (Cytoxan) Methotrexate (Rheumatrex) | Multiple birth defects and spontaneous abortion if used in the first trimester | If one of these drugs is needed, consult with maternal–fetal medicine specialists and oncologists.<br><br>Methotrexate is used to treat ectopic pregnancy. |
| Angiotensin II receptor blockers: Losartan (Cozaar) | Prolonged renal failure and hypotension in the newborn, decreased skull ossification, and renal tubular agenesis | Critical period is all trimesters. Discontinue immediately when pregnancy is detected. |
| Antithyroid drugs: Propylthiouracil (PTU) Methimazole (Tapazole) | Fetal and neonatal goiter and fetal hypothyroidism with methimazole in the first trimester. Rarely, aplasia cutis, esophageal atresia, and choanal atresia. Conflicting evidence of birth defects from PTU. | Greatest risk of congenital malformations with methimazole in the first trimester. Individuals who need to take antithyroid drugs in the first trimester will generally be counseled to use PTU. Untreated hyperthyroidism is associated with maternal heart failure, stillbirth, and fetal hyperthyroidism. |
| Aspirin | More than 150 mg/day is associated with prolonged gestation, prolonged labor, bleeding complications in the neonate, premature closure of the ductus arteriosus, and fetal growth restriction | Critical period is all trimesters.<br><br>Low-dose aspirin (81 mg/day) is not associated with birth defects and reduces risk of preeclampsia in those pregnant persons at increased risk. |
| Benzodiazepines: Alprazolam (Xanax) Chlordiazepoxide (Librium) Diazepam (Valium) | Increased risk of neonatal withdrawal/neonatal abstinence syndrome<br><br>Some studies show increased risk of oral clefts with first trimester exposure to diazepam | Benzodiazepines are highly lipophilic and have a long half-life in the neonate. Neonatal withdrawal starts soon after birth and may last several days. |
| Coumadin (Warfarin) | Bone defects<br><br>Fetal growth restriction<br><br>Central nervous system defects<br><br>Developmental delays | 15–25% risk when anticoagulants that impair vitamin K are used, especially between 6 and 10 weeks of gestation. Later use in pregnancy is associated with abruption, central nervous system defects, stillbirth, and hemorrhage of the fetus/newborn. |
| Ergot alkaloids: Ergotamine (Cafergot) | Spontaneous abortion<br>Mobius syndrome<br>Intestinal atresia<br>Cerebral developmental abnormalities<br>Low birth weight and preterm birth<br>No studies in humans | Critical period is all trimesters.<br><br>Sumatriptan (Imitrex) is an alternative to ergotamine for acute migraine treatment. |

| Drug Category Name (Brand Name) | Teratogenic or Fetotoxic Effects | Clinical Implications |
|---|---|---|
| Folic acid antagonists:<br><br>Methotrexate (Rheumatrex)<br>Carbamazepine (Tegretol)<br>Phenytoin (Dilantin)<br>Phenobarbital (Solfoton)<br>Primidone (Mysoline)<br>Trimethoprim (Trimpex) | Spontaneous abortion<br>Neural tube defects<br>Cardiovascular defects<br>Urinary tract defects<br>Developmental delay | Drugs in many different drug categories are folic acid antagonists.<br>Some sources suggest that the risks can be decreased with folic acid supplementation.<br>Trimethoprim is a component of trimethoprim–sulfamethoxazole (Septra), which is commonly used to treat urinary tract infections. This drug should not be given in the first and third trimesters. |
| Lithium (Lithobid) | Cardiac defects<br>Epstein's anomaly | Absolute risk is small, but alternative drugs should be recommended if possible. |
| Mifepristone (RU-486) | Antiprogestogen; used as an abortifacient<br>Human data are limited | Primarily used for abortion in combination with misoprostol. Less effective when used alone. |
| Misoprostol (Cytotec) | Abortion<br>Potential for skull defects, cranial nerve palsies, facial malformations, limb defects if used during the first trimester | Potent uterostimulant capable of initiating uterine contractions at all gestational ages. |
| Nonsteroidal anti-inflammatory drugs:<br>Ibuprofen (Advil)<br>Naproxen (Aleve) | Theorized premature closure of the ductus arteriosus<br>Necrotizing enterocolitis<br>If taken after 20 weeks, may affect fetal kidneys<br>Conflicting evidence on risk for gastroschisis or heart defects if used in the first trimester | Contraindicated in general but especially in the third trimester. |
| Retinoids:<br>Isotretinoin (Accutane) | Multiple birth defects, including central nervous system, cardiac, and endocrine damage | Oral isotretinoin causes birth defects in 35% of exposed infants. It is contraindicated in pregnancy. Topical preparations are unlikely to have serious teratogenic effects but are still contraindicated because other agents can be used. |
| Statins:<br>Atorvastatin (Lipitor)<br>Lovastatin (Mevacor) | Interfere with cholesterol production<br>Primarily have theoretical adverse effects on the fetus | Contraindicated in pregnancy due to lack of safety information and no proof of medical benefit with treatment. |
| Other:<br>Thalidomide | Limb deficiencies<br>Cardiac and gastrointestinal abnormalities | 20–30% risk during critical period (very potent). Used to treat nausea/vomiting in pregnancy before its teratogenic effects became obvious.<br>On market for treatment of oral lesions in HIV infection, Hansen's disease (leprosy), and multiple myeloma.<br>A risk evaluation and mitigation strategy (REMS) is available online from the manufacturer. Users should use two effective birth control methods. |

Abbreviation: HIV, human immunodeficiency virus.

Based on Buhimschi CS, Weiner CP. Medications in pregnancy and lactation: part 1. teratology. *Obstet Gynecol*. 2009;113(1):166-188. doi:10.1097/AOG.0b013e31818d6788; Teratology Society: Organization of Teratology Information Specialists. MotherToBaby fact sheets. https://mothertobaby.org/fact-sheets/. Accessed January 12, 2022; *Micromedex*® [Electronic version]. IBM Watson Health, Greenwood Village, CA. https://www.micromedexsolutions.com/home/dispatch/. Accessed January 16, 2022.

and family history is a free, personalized tool that aids families in making informed choices regarding testing options or referral to a genetic counselor (Table 20-10).[51–53] A number of consumer-completed family genetics history tools are available, both in print and online, to facilitate collection of personal and family histories. (See the Resources section at the end of this chapter.) Such participation tools can be completed by an individual prior to prenatal care and as an effective and efficient way to identify genetic risk.

Constructing and evaluating a three-generation pedigree for genetic risk is a basic skill for all healthcare professionals, including midwives. Instructions for how to obtain a three-generation pedigree can be found in Appendix 20-A.

| Table 20-10 | Personal and Family History That May Warrant Genetic Testing and/or Referral to Genetic Counseling |
|---|---|

Age of the person providing the egg (ovum)

High-risk ethnic heritage

Consanguinity (blood relationship of parents)

Family history (of either biologic parent) of a known or suspected genetic condition

Multiple affected family members (of either biologic parent) with the same or related disorders

Any major malformations (e.g., heart, kidney, brain) or other birth defects occurring in the biologic parents, grandparents, offspring, or close relatives (brothers/sisters)

Congenital blindness or deafness in family members

Extremely tall or short stature of the biologic parents or their relatives

Developmental delays or intellectual disability occurring in the biologic parents, offspring, or close relatives

Recurrent pregnancy losses (two or more) in the pregnant person or first-degree family members

Environmental exposure to known or suspected teratogens

Infertility or premature ovarian failure

Based on The New York – Mid-Atlantic Guide for Patients and Health Professionals. Indications for a genetic referral. In: *Understanding Genetics: A New York, Mid-Atlantic Guide for Patients and Health Professionals*. Washington, DC: Genetic Alliance; 2009. http://www.geneticalliance.org/sites/default/files/publicationsarchive/UnderstandingGeneticsNYMA.pdf. Accessed August 19, 2021.

## Screening Tests Versus Diagnostic Tests

Screening tests separate those persons who "might" from those persons who "probably don't" have the specific condition being tested for. Diagnostic tests provide a definitive answer to whether an individual has a particular disorder. Screening tests are *not* diagnostic. Screening results usually aid in determining the level of risk for a specific disorder, and they identify individuals who might be advised to undergo further, definitive diagnostic testing.

For example, the results of a serum screening test for trisomy 21 during the first trimester are not simply reported as "normal" or "abnormal." Instead, the results will indicate the chance (e.g., 1 in 40, 1 in 400, 1 in 4000) of having a fetus with trisomy 21. This chance is based on the level of pregnancy-associated plasma protein A (PAPP-A) and human chorionic gonadotropin (hCG) in the serum in conjunction with a nuchal translucency measurement identified on ultrasound performed at a specific gestational age. Such screening test results give the individual the information necessary to help decide whether diagnostic testing will be chosen as the next step.

Screening tests have six critical components: (1) sensitivity, (2) specificity, (3) false-positive rate, (4) false-negative rate, (5) positive predictive value, and (6) negative predictive value (Table 20-11). The *sensitivity* refers to the number of individuals with the disorder who have a screening test that is positive for that disorder. *Specificity* is the number of individuals without the disorder who have a negative screening test. Again, using first trimester serum screening (without adding nuchal translucency ultrasound) as an example, such screening has the demonstrated ability to detect approximately 70% of all fetuses who have trisomy 21.[54] Thus, approximately 30% of fetuses with trisomy 21 will not be detected with this screening test; this is the *false-negative rate*. In contrast, the *false-positive rate* reflects the chance of a positive test result indicating a high likelihood for trisomy 21 when a healthy fetus is actually present. The false-positive rate for first trimester screening for trisomy 21 is approximately 5%,[55] and is a significant contributor to unintended parental anxiety during the prenatal period and potentially unnecessary interventions.

Many factors can affect test results, including gestational age, age of the pregnant individual, presence of multifetal gestation, certain medical conditions such as diabetes, and other coexisting congenital or genetic disorders.[56] In addition, the prevalence of a disorder varies within different

| Table 20-11 | Sensitivity, Specificity, Positive Predictive Value, and Negative Predictive Value | | |
|---|---|---|---|
| **Test Results** | **Person Has the Condition** | **Person Does *Not* Have the Condition** | |
| Screening test is positive | A (true positive) | B (false positive) | A ÷ (A + B) Positive predictive value |
| Screening test is negative | C (false negative) | D (true negative) | D ÷ (C + D) Negative predictive value |
| | A ÷ (A + C) Sensitivity | D ÷ (B + D) Specificity | |

populations (e.g., based on ethnicity or geographic location). These differences must be considered to accurately interpret test results and determine the positive predictive value and negative predictive value, as illustrated in Figure 20-8.

Continuing the example of first trimester screening, the *positive predictive value* is the proportion of all positive tests that truly indicate a fetus *with* trisomy 21; it is calculated as the number of fetuses with the condition who tested positive, divided by the total number of fetuses tested who had positive results (includes those with and without the condition). In contrast, the *negative predictive value* is the proportion of all negative tests that truly indicate a fetus without trisomy 21, calculated as the number of fetuses without the condition who had negative results divided by the total number of fetuses tested who had negative results (includes those with and without the condition).

This type of multifactorial input into test results is also illustrated with the use of serum alpha-fetoprotein (AFP) test. AFP is a protein made by the fetal liver and found in the amniotic fluid. It passes through the placenta and circulates in the pregnant individual's blood, thereby enabling assessment of AFP through serum sampling of the pregnant individual. Serum AFP is a screening test for NTDs, but is also used to identify risk for trisomy 21. High levels of serum AFP are associated with increased risk of NTDs, whereas lower levels are associated with elevated risk for trisomy 21.[57] In this case, one of the additional factors influencing the interpretation of results is an accurate estimation of gestational age. The serum AFP test has different normative values at different gestational ages. Thus, if a pregnant person has the test done at 15 weeks' gestation, it will be interpreted based on 15-week norms. However, if the gestational age has not been accurately determined and the pregnancy is actually at 13 gestational weeks, the test results will appear abnormal because they have been interpreted incorrectly. Similarly, different normative values have been identified for people who have a multifetal gestation. This situation has prompted clinicians to use multiple biochemical markers as screening tests, rather than relying on a single marker, such as serum AFP.

## Factors That Influence Perinatal Decision Making

Individuals are faced with many difficult decisions in healthcare settings, and prenatal genetic screening and testing are no exception. Many factors, such as individual, family, religious, and cultural values, as well as cost, will play a role in how a person perceives screening and diagnostic testing for genetic defects. Midwives can ease this process by engaging in evidence-based, shared decision making when offering prenatal testing, interpreting test results, and discussing options. Pregnant people and their families should have their questions answered adequately and candidly, but with compassion and respect for individual values and wishes.

Prenatal tests can screen for some genetic disorders, chromosomal abnormalities, and structural differences. The aim of prenatal screening and diagnostic testing is to provide families with the information necessary to make well-informed reproductive health decisions. Information about the fetus can be used in planning for the pregnancy, birth and birth location, and early parenting. The clinical implications of test results can be complicated, so sharing information with pregnant people both before and after tests are performed is a necessary skill for midwives.

### Pretest and Post-Test Counseling When Screening for Genetic and Chromosomal Disorders

Genetic and genomic health care is changing rapidly as new technologies are incorporated into clinical

**Chart A: 25-year-old G1P0 individual.**

Sensitivity (87%), specificity (95%), and predictive value of first trimester screening (nuchal translucency and serum) for trisomy 21 when the prevalence rate is 1 per 1250, as it is among pregnant people age 25 years[a]

|  | Trisomy 21 Present | Trisomy 21 Absent | Interpretation (Predictive Value) |
|---|---|---|---|
| **Positive test result** | 87 will have a true-positive test | 6235 will have a false-positive test | A 25-year-old pregnant person with a positive test for trisomy 21 has a 1.4% chance of actually having a fetus with trisomy 21 (out of 6322 positive tests, 87 fetuses had trisomy 21 and 6235 tests were false alarms). This is the positive predictive value. |
| **Negative test result** | 13 will have a false-negative test | 118,665 will have a true-negative test | A pregnant person with a negative test result has a 99.9% chance of *not* having a fetus with trisomy 21 (out of 118,678 negative tests, 13 fetuses actually had trisomy 21). This is the negative predictive value. |
|  | 100 fetuses affected | 124,900 not affected | Out of 125,000 fetuses of individuals who are 25 years old, 100 will have trisomy 21 and 124,900 will not have trisomy 21. |

**Chart B: 45-year-old G2P1 individual.**

Sensitivity (87%), specificity (95%), and predictive value of first trimester screening (nuchal translucency and serum) for trisomy 21 when the prevalence rate is 1 per 30, as it is among pregnant people age 45 years[a]

|  | Trisomy 21 Present | Trisomy 21 Absent | Interpretation (Predictive Value) |
|---|---|---|---|
| **Positive test result** | 87 will have a true-positive test | 145 will have a false-positive test | A 45-year-old pregnant person with a positive test for trisomy 21 has a 37.5% chance of actually having a fetus with trisomy 21 (out of 232 positive tests, 87 fetuses had trisomy 21 and 145 tests were false alarms). This is the positive predictive value. |
| **Negative test result** | 13 will have a false-negative test | 2755 will have a true-negative test | A pregnant person with a negative test result has a 99.5% chance of *not* having a fetus with trisomy 21 (out of 2768 negative tests, 13 fetuses actually had trisomy 21). This is the negative predictive value. |
|  | 100 fetuses affected | 2900 fetuses not affected | Out of 3000 fetuses of 45-year-old pregnant people, 100 will have trisomy 21 and 2900 will not have this chromosomal abnormality. |

**Figure 20-8** The impact of prevalence on the predictive value and interpretation of first trimester screening for trisomy 21 among pregnant persons of differing ages.[a]
[a] Test performance (specificity and sensitivity) is the same in both charts. However, the positive predictive value and the negative predictive value are different in the two charts because the prevalence rate for trisomy 21 is different for pregnant people who are 25 years old (chart A) and those who are 45 years old (chart B). The interpretation is therefore different for pregnant people of different ages as represented in each of these charts.

practice. The number of tests and algorithms promoted as part of prenatal testing continues to increase, and best practices for incorporating new tests are being studied. A standard algorithm for prenatal testing based on professional guidelines and the tests commonly available today is presented in the *Prenatal Care* chapter. This chapter reviews the process of counseling clients about these tests and the characteristics of the screening and diagnostic tests that are currently in use.

Counseling as described in this section is the foundation of shared decision making related to genetic testing. Midwives provide comprehensive information during discussions regarding testing options, and clients decide whether to participate in testing. All pregnant clients will be offered pretest counseling to help them decide whether they will pursue testing. Pretest and post-test counseling is recommended for all people who undergo prenatal screening for genetic disorders. Individuals who might have an elevated risk for a genetic or chromosomal disorder (as indicated in Table 20-10) and any person who wants more detailed information should be referred for genetic counseling. Most healthcare settings offer genetic counseling to any person who has a positive screening test.

Table 20-12 provides an overview of common questions and key topics to address in pretest

| Table 20-12 | Key Topics for Pretest Counseling as a Component of Shared Decision Making |
|---|---|
| **Commonly Asked Questions** | **Essential Information for Pretest Counseling** |
| Why is this test offered? | Review the conditions being tested for, including common phenotype and variability in phenotype |
| | Type of testing offered (screening, carrier screening, diagnostic test) |
| | Alternative testing options, including the risks, benefits, and limitations of each alternative |
| How are the results communicated? | Review how test results are shared with the pregnant person and timing for getting results |
| What will I do with the information? | Discuss ways the results might affect planning surrounding pregnancy, birth, and parenting |
| What if there is a positive result? | Availability of genetic counseling to provide additional information and assist decision making |
| | Review that genetic counseling will address diagnosis of the condition, options for the pregnant person if a disorder is diagnosed, and treatments for the condition |
| How much does the test cost and will insurance cover the cost? | Discuss the cost of testing and insurance coverage |
| | Address the effect on health insurance if a disorder is diagnosed |
| When does the test have to be done? | Review timing for performing the test |
| Who will know about the results? | Review patient confidentiality and discuss implications of sharing information with a partner and family |

Based on Fonda Allen J, Stoll K, Bernhardt BA. Pre- and post-test genetic counseling for chromosomal and Mendelian disorders. *Semin Perinatol.* 2016;40(1):44-55.

counseling.[58–65] The most important question is, "What will I do with the information?" This question will need to be answered by the individual with support from their significant others and midwife. Answering this question can assist in making the ultimate decision as to whether a person will undergo screening tests, diagnostic tests, or both.[63] An individual can often arrive at an answer by addressing additional, very personal questions: "Do I want to know that my baby is affected before the baby is born?" "Would testing simply make me more anxious, rather than less anxious?" "Am I willing to accept the increased risk of miscarriage associated with a diagnostic test such as chorionic villus sampling or amniocentesis?" "Am I strongly opposed to pregnancy termination even if I have a baby affected with (fill in the blank)?" "Would I terminate this pregnancy if I know my baby is affected with (fill in the blank)?" "Would I change the planned location of birth if my baby had this condition?" "Why should I have screening or diagnostic tests if I am fine with any outcome the baby might have?" It often helps people to self-identify their stance when the midwife offers statements that begin with "Some people choose to have these tests because . . ." and "Some people choose not to have these tests because. . . ."

## Tests for Genetic and Chromosomal Disorders

The number and types of tests that screen for or diagnose genetic or chromosomal disorders have increased rapidly in the last several years. These tests can be applied to carrier screening, preimplantation testing, prenatal screening, diagnostic testing, or newborn screening. In general, these tests can be classified into one of three categories:

- *Biochemical tests* evaluate the proteins or enzymes produced by the genetic code, but not the genes themselves. Biochemical tests can be performed on the pregnant individual or fetal cells and may be used for screening or diagnosis purposes.

- *Cytogenic testing* examines the chromosomes to identify structural abnormalities. The traditional karyotype cultures cells and stains the chromosomes to detect changes in structure. Fluorescent in situ hybridization (FISH) targets specific chromosomes to detect aneuploidy or smaller abnormalities such as deletions.

- *Molecular testing* is a direct analysis of DNA that detects small DNA mutations. Molecular

DNA testing may use polymerase chain reaction (PCR)–based assays to amplify the DNA present. Chromosomal microarray analysis is a molecular DNA test applied to fetal cells to detect aberrations in chromosomal structure that may not be visible on a normal karyotype.

## Carrier Screening

The purpose of carrier screening (often called expanded carrier screening) is to detect individuals at risk for having a child with a genetic condition that is not evident in either of the parents. Carrier screening for autosomal dominant or autosomal recessive disorders is ideally performed preconceptionally, but often is first addressed during pregnancy.

Carrier screening can be performed for one disorder or multiple disorders at one time.[65] Specific carrier screening tests have traditionally been offered to individuals from genetic, racial, and ethnic populations that have an increased prevalence of the disorder, a form of screening referred to as *ethnic-specific screening*. An ethnic-based screening strategy has multiple problems. For example, in today's multiracial society, it may be difficult to determine ethnicity. Furthermore, ethnicity does not identify all persons with an elevated risk, so this screening strategy can miss many persons who would benefit from such testing. *Panethnic screening* refers to a strategy of offering carrier screening to all individuals regardless of race or ethnicity. Panethnic screening is an acceptable strategy.

New sequencing technologies have created the ability to screen for large numbers of conditions simultaneously. Nevertheless, such *expanded carrier screening* is also associated with several unresolved problems. Many of the conditions covered by expanded carrier screening panels vary greatly in the expressed phenotype or disability, so counseling people about results can be quite complex. In addition, some of the expanded carrier screening panels screen for conditions that are rare and for which diagnostic tests are not well established. Furthermore, different commercially marketed panels screen for different disorders.

Current professional association guidelines recommend ethnic-specific, panethnic, or expanded carrier screening. The American College of Medical Genetics and Genomics recommends population-neutral carrier screening paradigms organized into a tier-based system to promote screening equity. Specifically, it recommends screening for all conditions with a carrier frequency greater or equal to 1/200 in any ethnic group with reasonable representation in the United States.[64] Factors such as severity of condition, prevalence carrier frequency, detection rates, and residual risk following screening results, as described in Table 20-13, contribute to the choice of screening strategy.[65,66]

## Screening Tests

Specific screening and diagnostic tests can be performed at several time points—including prior to conception, preimplantation, and during pregnancy—so that the most accurate results can be obtained. The decision whether to engage in any testing is always the pregnant person's choice. The midwife's role is to provide as much information as needed to facilitate an individual's decision making about what is personally best, as well as best for the family. Table 20-14 provides a comprehensive list of both screening and diagnostic tests for the most common congenital disorders, including the appropriate timing for tests that are regularly offered in the United States, as well as some that are expected to be adopted soon.[67]

Currently, low-risk, reliable, noninvasive techniques are available to screen for fetal chromosomal abnormalities. A person's baseline risk for having a fetus with such abnormalities should not limit testing options—serum screening with or without nuchal translucency ultrasound or cell-free DNA screening as well as diagnostic testing should be offered to all pregnant people.[51,68] If a person does choose aneuploidy screening, only one screening approach should be used.[51] Factors that are associated with chromosomal abnormalities include increasing age of the person contributing the egg, a parental chromosomal abnormality, a previous pregnancy with chromosomal abnormality, and fetal abnormalities found by ultrasound.[51] Clients with negative screening test results should understand that such results do not ensure that the fetus is unaffected by the screened disorder, or that the fetus is not affected by other disorders not evaluated for by the test.[51]

### Aneuploidy Screening in Any Trimester

There are many options for screening for fetal aneuploidy. Table 20-15 reviews the detection and false-positive rates of currently available screening and diagnostic tests.[67]

Fetal cell-free DNA (cfDNA) testing, often referred to as noninvasive prenatal testing (NIPT), is a screening option for identification of trisomies 13, 18, and 21, and sex chromosome aneuploidy.

| Table 20-13 | Carrier Screening: Recommendations for Specific Conditions | |
|---|---|---|
| **Disorder** | **Indications** | **Clinical Considerations** |
| Cystic fibrosis | Offer screening to all people of reproductive age | If screening is positive, offer screening to the other genetic parent. Offer fetal screening if both biologic parents screen positive. |
| Hemoglobinopathies | Individuals with African, Mediterranean, Middle Eastern, Southeast Asian, or West Indian ancestry | A complete blood count with red cell indices offered to all pregnant people can assess hemoglobinopathy risk. If MCH or MCV is low, perform hemoglobin electrophoresis. Southeast Asian ancestry: If hemoglobin electrophoresis is normal, perform molecular testing for alpha-thalassemia. |
| Fragile X syndrome | Individuals with a family history of intellectual disability or unexplained developmental delay, autism, or primary ovarian insufficiency | Offer genetic counseling for persons with a family history. |
| Spinal muscular atrophy | Offer screening to all people considering pregnancy or currently pregnant | Offer genetic counseling for persons with a family history. |
| Tay-Sachs disease | Ashkenazi Jewish ancestry French Canadian ancestry Cajun ancestry Family history | Expanded carrier screening panels are not the best approach to screening with a family history of Tay-Sachs disease, unless the familial mutation is known to be part of the panel. |

Abbreviations: MCH, mean corpuscular hemoglobin; MCV, mean corpuscular volume.

Data from American College of Obstetricians and Gynecologists. Committee Opinion No. 691: carrier screening for genetic conditions. *Obstet Gynecol.* 2017;129:e41–55. doi:10.1097/AOG.0000000000001952.

| Table 20-14 | Prenatal Screening and Diagnostic Tests Currently Available | | | | |
|---|---|---|---|---|---|
| | | | **Testing Available for These Conditions** | | |
| **Gestational Age When Test Is Performed** | **Test** | **Aneuploidy** | **Neural Tube Defects** | **Genetic Mutation** | **Congenital Anomalies** |
| **At Any Time Prepregnancy or During Pregnancy (for biologic parents), Newborns, and Children** | | | | | |
| | Karyotype and/or direct DNA[b] and cytogenetic[c] testing | ✓ | | ✓ | |
| **First Trimester Screening** | | | | | |
| 10–14 weeks | Ultrasound: nuchal translucency (thickness) | ✓ | | | ✓ |
| 10–14 weeks | Serum: PAPP-A and hCG | ✓ | | | |
| 10+ weeks | cfDNA (serum)[a] | ✓ | | | |
| **Second Trimester Screening** | | | | | |
| 15–23 weeks (optimal at 18 weeks) | Ultrasound: anatomic examination | ✓ | ✓ | | ✓ |

*(continues)*

| Table 20-14 | Prenatal Screening and Diagnostic Tests Currently Available (*continued*) | | | | |
|---|---|---|---|---|---|
| 15–18 weeks | Serum: multiple marker (quad): AFP, hCG, uE3, and inhibin-A | ✓ | ✓ | | |
| Integrated screening | Combines first and second trimester screening as a comprehensive risk assessment | ✓ | ✓ | | ✓ |
| Sequential screening | First trimester screening, followed by second trimester screening, as desired, based on first trimester results | ✓ | ✓ | | ✓ |
| **Screening Acceptable in Any Trimester** | | | | | |
| Anytime after 9–10 weeks of pregnancy | cfDNA (serum)[a] | ✓ | | | |
| **First Trimester Diagnostic Tests** | | | | | |
| 10–14 weeks | CVS  For karyotype and/or direct DNA[b] and cytogenetic (chromosomal)[c] testing | ✓ | | ✓ | |
| **Second Trimester Diagnostic Tests** | | | | | |
| 15–22 weeks | Amniocentesis for karyotype and/or direct DNA[b] and cytogenetic[c] testing, and amniotic fluid AFP level | ✓ | ✓ | ✓ | |

Abbreviations: AFP, alpha-fetoprotein; cfDNA, cell-free DNA; CVS, chorionic villus sampling; DNA, deoxyribonucleic acid; hCG, human chorionic gonadotropin; PAPP-A, pregnancy-associated plasma protein A; uE3, unconjugated estriol.

[a] cfDNA, often referred to as noninvasive prenatal testing (NIPT), is the most recently developed screening test for trisomies 21, 18, and 13; sex chromosome aneuploidy; and some microdeletions.

[b] DNA testing for genetic deletions, insertions, rearrangements, duplications, and other mutations can be accomplished using laboratory techniques, such as polymerase chain reaction (PCR) DNA amplification, hybridization of labeled probes to DNA, and microarray analysis, among others.

[c] Cytogenetic (chromosomal) structural aberrations, including microdeletions and aneuploidy, can be identified by karyotyping, chromosomal banding, fluorescence in situ hybridization (FISH), chromosomal microarray, and comparative genomic hybridization (CGH).

This test has become widely available since its introduction in 2011 and is the most sensitive and specific screening option for the common aneuploidies.[51,69,70] Testing of cfDNA involves collection of the pregnant person's blood after 10 weeks' gestation; this blood contains fragments of circulating cell-free fetal DNA, whose quantity increases throughout gestation. The test amplifies the fetal DNA and makes it possible to identify the extra genetic material that exists when aneuploidy is present in the fetus.[63] This is the only screening option that identifies fetal sex and sex chromosome aneuploidies.[51] Because cfDNA is a screening test rather than a diagnostic test, it is recommended that any positive result be followed with chorionic villus sampling (CVS) or amniocentesis to confirm the diagnosis.[51]

Cell-free DNA is more than 99% sensitive for detecting fetal trisomy 21, 98% sensitive for trisomy 18, and 99% sensitive for trisomy 13, with a combined false-positive rate of 0.13%.[71] The positive predictive value (PPV), or the chance that a positive screen is a true positive result, varies according to the population prevalence for a particular disorder. Some laboratories report PPV as part of the results.[51] Because the quantity of the fetal fraction can impact the accuracy of the test results, sending the sample to a laboratory that reports the fetal fraction is preferable.[72] Additionally, ultrasound performance prior to screening can prevent confounding variables, such as inaccurate gestational age, number of fetuses, or presence of anomalies.[51] The cfDNA test does not screen for NTDs, so clients should be offered additional testing for this condition in the second trimester.

| Table 20-15 | Detection and False-Positive Rates for Currently Available Prenatal Tests for Aneuploidy[a] | |
| --- | --- | --- |
| **Test** | **Detection Rate[b]**<br>**(Trisomy Type)** | **False-Positive Rate[c]**<br>**(Trisomy or Abnormality Type)** |
| **Any Trimester Screening** | | |
| Fetal cell-free DNA[d] | 99% (trisomy 18 and 21)<br>92% (trisomy 13) | 0.3–1% (overall) |
| **First Trimester Screening** | | |
| NT alone | 68% (trisomy 21)<br>68% (trisomy 18)<br>72% (trisomy 13) | 5% (trisomy 21)<br>0.5% (trisomy 18) |
| Serum markers alone | 67% (trisomy 21)<br>80% (trisomy 18)<br>59% (trisomy 13) | 5% (trisomy 21)<br>0.5% (trisomy 13 and 18) |
| Combined NT measurement and serum markers | 90% (trisomy 21)<br>97% (trisomy 18)<br>84% (trisomy 13) | 5% (trisomy 21)<br>0.5% (trisomy 13 and 18) |
| **Second Trimester Screening** | | |
| Serum markers alone (quad) | 80% (trisomy 21)<br>70% (trisomy 18)<br>19% (trisomy 13)<br>75–90% (ONTD)<br>95% (anencephaly) | 5% (trisomy 21)<br>0.2% (trisomy 13 and 18)<br>2–5% (ONTD) |
| Anatomic US alone | 73% (trisomy 21)<br>93–100% (trisomy 18)<br>90–100% (trisomy 13) | 4% (trisomy 21)<br>4% (trisomy 18)<br>0.5% (trisomy 13) |
| Quad screen and US | 83% (trisomy 21)<br>100% (trisomy 18)<br>100% (trisomy 13) | 5% (trisomy 21)<br>0.4% (trisomy 18)<br>0.5% (trisomy 13) |
| **Integrated Screening** | | |
| First and second trimester serum *without* NT | 86% (trisomy 21)<br>86% (trisomy 18)<br>49% (trisomy 13) | 2% (trisomy 21)<br>0.5% (trisomy 13 and 18) |
| First and second trimester serum *with* NT | 95% (trisomy 21)<br>92% (trisomy 18)<br>72% (trisomy 13) | 4% (trisomy 21)<br>0.5% (trisomy 13 and 18) |
| **Chorionic Villus Sampling** | 98% (aneuploidy) | < 0.04% |
| **Amniocentesis** | 99.5% (aneuploidy)<br>96–99% (ONTD) | < 0.04%<br>2% (ONTD) |
| **Direct DNA Testing**<br>Saliva, blood, placental, or skin cell sample for identification of genetic mutation and carrier status | 99.9% | < 0.04% |

Abbreviations: DNA, deoxyribonucleic acid; NT, nuchal translucency (thickness); ONTD, open neural tube defects; US, ultrasound.

[a] Detection and false-positive rates can vary depending on population risk and the risk cutoff used in testing.

[b] Detection rate reflects test sensitivity—that is, the "accuracy" or ability of a test to correctly identify those who have the disorder.

[c] False-positive rate reflects test specificity—that is, the ability of a test to correctly identify those who do not have the disorder.

[d] Fetal cell-free DNA, frequently referred to as noninvasive prenatal testing (NIPT).

Some laboratories offer testing for microdeletions and genome-wide screening, though this testing has yet to be clinically validated.[51] Given the rapidly advancing technology, it is feasible that cfDNA will be used as a noninvasive diagnostic test in the not-too-distant future, and will likely include full genomic testing of the embryo/fetus for genetic mutations and all chromosomal abnormalities.[73]

### First Trimester Screening for Aneuploidy

First trimester screening is best performed between 10 and 14 weeks' gestation. Risk for aneuploidy can be determined by measuring serum levels of PAPP-A and hCG (expressed as multiples of the median) in relation to the pregnant person's weight/age and the gestational age. Generally, an increased risk of trisomy 21 is associated with lower PAPP-A levels and higher hCG levels.[57]

Increased risk for aneuploidy can also be calculated during ultrasound measurement of nuchal translucency between 10 and 13 6/7 weeks' gestation. More than 3 mm of fluid retention in the nuchal fold is associated with an increased risk of trisomy 21, other aneuploidies, and perhaps other defects, such as heart defects, diaphragmatic hernias, skeletal dysplasia, and a variety of genetic syndromes.[56,74] Absence of the fetal nasal bone is also associated with trisomy 21; thus, some facilities include ultrasound assessment of the nasal bone.[57]

### Second Trimester Screening for Aneuploidy

Screening for aneuploidy and NTDs in the second trimester currently includes measurement of several markers in serum. Commonly referred to as a maternal serum, multiple marker, or quad screen, this test includes the measurement of the pregnant person's serum levels of alpha-fetoprotein, unconjugated estriol (uE3), human chorionic gonadotropin, and inhibin-A. The last three of these markers are hormones produced by the placenta and secreted into the circulatory system. In contrast, AFP is a protein made by the fetus. The serum AFP test has been in use longer than the other tests included in the quad screen. Fetal cell-free DNA testing also can be conducted at any time during the second trimester.

Screening options over the past 20 years have moved rapidly from a single serum marker test (AFP) to the addition of other markers. Multiple markers have been recognized as more effective in detecting abnormalities; they also decrease the risk of false-negative results compared to a single marker.[75]

### Integrated, Combined, or Sequential Prenatal Testing for Aneuploidy

First and second trimester screening can be combined (ultrasound and serum markers) in an effort to improve the ability to detect trisomy 21 and other trisomies.[51,66] Results can be calculated and returned to the pregnant person either after all testing has been completed (i.e., integrated/combined) or after each trimester's results are known (i.e., sequentially). Calculation of the risk that the fetus has trisomy 21 after all test results are known, however, would preclude the choice to have a CVS, if diagnostic testing is indicated. In contrast, the sequential screen calculates risk based on first trimester screening tests and returns the results to the pregnant person before proceeding with further screening tests. One advantage of a sequential screen is that it gives the option to continue with the second trimester screening or to proceed with diagnostic testing (CVS or amniocentesis) if the first trimester results indicate high risk for chromosomal abnormalities.[57,76]

### Diagnostic Tests for Aneuploidy

Diagnostic procedures for aneuploidy and direct DNA genetic testing include CVS and amniocentesis. The screening and diagnostic tests performed on fetal cells following CVS or amniocentesis are briefly described in Table 20-16.

### First Trimester Diagnostic Testing

Chorionic villus sampling entails collection of placental tissue between 10 and 14 weeks' gestation, transcervically or transabdominally, and completion of karyotyping for detection of aneuploidy using the placental tissue. Other technologies besides the karyotype may be required to detect smaller chromosomal abnormalities, such as microdeletions and translocations in the fetal cells obtained via CVS. Techniques such as FISH, spectral karyotyping, and comparative genomic hybridization (CGH) can be used to examine chromosomal structure more thoroughly.

One advantage of CVS over amniocentesis is that it can be performed earlier in the pregnancy. This early testing allows more time to consider options and to make decisions including induced abortion, particularly if a client desires to make those decisions before the pregnancy becomes known to others. The disadvantage of CVS is that it does not obtain amniotic fluid, which can be tested to detect the presence of NTDs. The best screening for NTDs consists of serum AFP testing followed by measurement of AFP in amniotic fluid collected during an

| Table 20-16 | Screening and Diagnostic Tests Performed on Fetal Cells | | |
| --- | --- | --- | --- |
| **Test** | **Description** | **Results** | **Clinical Considerations** |
| Karyotype | Cytogenic test<br>Metaphase analysis of cultured cells | All aneuploidies and chromosome abnormalities that are larger than 5–10 megabases | Diagnostic test<br>Relies on culture so results are not available for 7–14 days<br>May not detect mosaicism |
| Fluorescence in situ hybridization (FISH) | Cytogenic test<br>Fluorescent-labeled probes identify specific chromosomes<br>Performed on uncultured cells | Tests chromosomes 13, 18, 21, X, and Y<br>May detect deletions if a probe for a specific deletion is requested | Considered a screening test because the test can be falsely positive or falsely negative<br>Results are available in 2–3 days |
| Chromosomal microarray (CMA) | Molecular DNA<br>Performed on cultured or uncultured cells to detect copy-number variants | Detects aneuploidy, unbalanced translocations, microdeletions, and microduplications | Results available in 3–5 days<br>Primary test for pregnant individuals who have amniocentesis following detection of structural anomaly on ultrasound; approximately 6% of fetuses that have a normal karyotype will have a chromosomal abnormality detected by CMA |
| Whole-exome sequencing | Molecular DNA<br>High-throughput sequencing | Sequencing of only the exons or protein-coding regions of the genome | May be used in selected circumstances when multiple congenital anomalies are present and targeted sequencing tests have failed to provide a diagnosis<br>Has low clinical utility given the high cost and long turnaround time |

amniocentesis. The best diagnostic test for NTDs is anatomic ultrasound examination of the fetus.

**Figure 20-9A** depicts collection of placental tissue for diagnostic testing, which should be performed by an obstetrician or maternal–fetal medicine specialist. A separate direct DNA test can be completed to identify genetic mutations (e.g., Tay-Sachs disease, cystic fibrosis, hemophilia A, Huntington disease).

CVS is an invasive procedure that is associated with an additional 0.2% risk for miscarriage above the baseline risk of approximately 15% for an average pregnant person at a similar gestation.[77] Furthermore, CVS is not performed prior to 10 weeks' gestation due to the documented risk of limb-reduction birth defects among infants born to individuals who had CVS testing at an earlier gestational age. Transabdominal CVS is considered safer, technically less difficult, and more accurate than transcervical CVS.

### Second Trimester Diagnostic Testing

Diagnostic testing in the second trimester can be accomplished via amniocentesis, which entails inserting a fine needle through the abdomen and into the uterus to collect a small sample of amniotic fluid (**Figure 20-9B**). Fetal cells are found in the fluid, separated, and usually grown in a culture medium until the chromosomes can be examined under a microscope. The final result is a fetal "G-banded" karyotype that is used to identify aneuploidies and other chromosomal derangements (Figure 20-5A provides an example of a karyotype display.) As with CVS diagnostic testing, other technologies besides the G-banded karyotype may be required to detect smaller chromosomal abnormalities, such as microdeletions and translocations in the fetal cells obtained via amniocentesis.

Amniocentesis is usually performed at 16 to 18 weeks' gestation and has an associated risk of pregnancy loss of approximately 1 in 1000 above the background risk for pregnancy loss less than 24 weeks' gestation.[77] Early amniocentesis (14–15 weeks' gestation) can be performed, but may be associated with a higher risk of pregnancy loss (approximately 1%) and congenital anomalies (talipes, also called club foot).[78]

During a CVS or amniocentesis, direct DNA testing can be completed if warranted to identify genetic mutations in the fetus (e.g., Tay-Sachs disease,

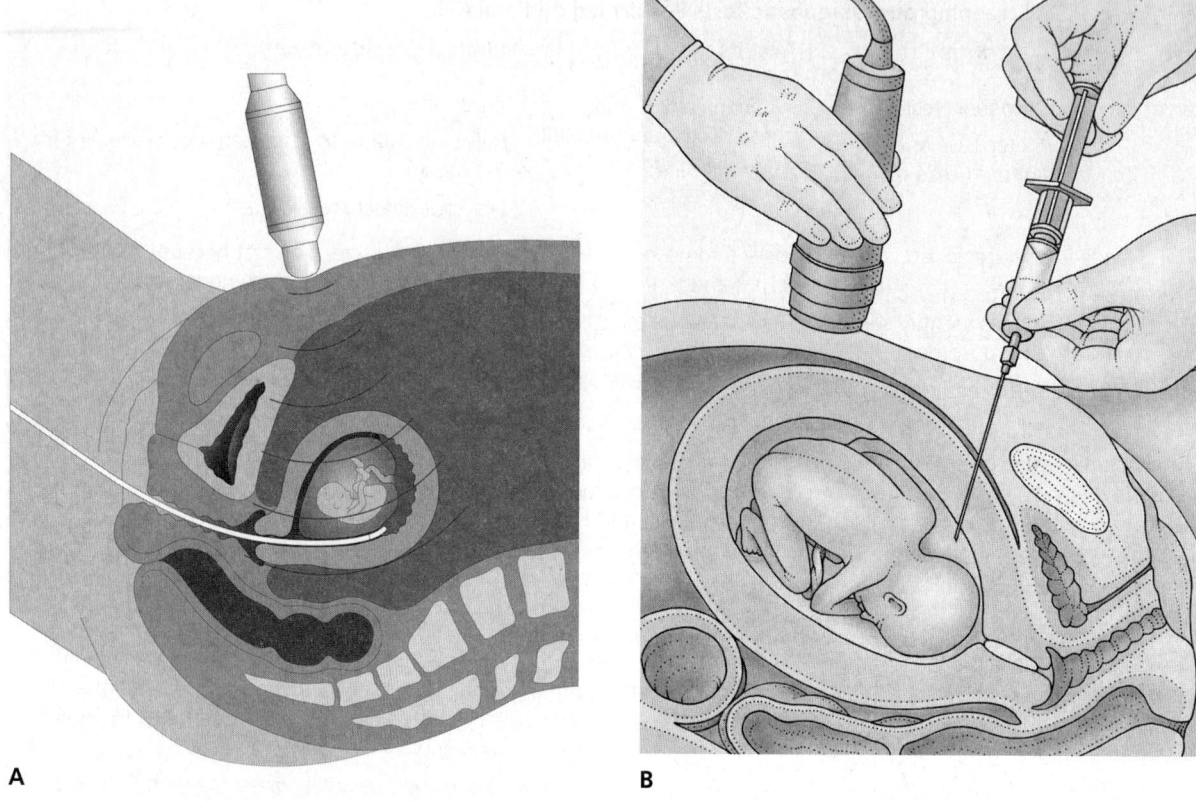

**A**

**B**

**Figure 20-9 A.** Transcervical chorionic villus sampling. **B.** Amniocentesis.
**A:** © Dorling Kindersley/Getty Images; **B:** © Halli Verrinder/Getty Images.

cystic fibrosis, hemophilia A, Huntington disease). If an individual chooses to have a diagnostic amniocentesis, an amniotic fluid AFP test can be completed at the same time to screen for NTDs.

## Ultrasound

Ultrasound examination of the fetus during the second trimester can establish gestational age and detect anatomic abnormalities such as NTDs and structural defects in the heart, kidneys, cranium/brain, and/or limbs. All clients should be offered this second trimester ultrasound, as structural defects may occur with or without aneuploidy.[51] However, certain physical characteristics are associated with aneuploidy phenotypes.[79,80] For example, ultrasound findings in a fetus that include an absent nasal bone, palmar creases, short femur, and echogenic bowel correspond to characteristics commonly found in the trisomy 21 phenotype.[79] Such findings would arouse suspicion for aneuploidy and prompt recommendations for further testing, such as diagnostic amniocentesis. Second trimester anatomic ultrasounds are usually performed at approximately 20 weeks' gestation for best results.

### Incidental Ultrasound Findings

Several anatomic variants in the fetus can be identified during second trimester ultrasounds. In the majority of cases, they are normal variations in fetal anatomy that are not associated with adverse effects. A few of these findings are more often seen in fetuses with trisomy 21 or trisomy 18, but studies have shown that most of these ultrasound markers do not modify the pretest risk for trisomy sufficiently to warrant further examination.

Table 20-17 reviews the prevalence of each variant and its association with aneuploidy or other fetal pathology.[79,81,82] Because the risk of trisomy 21 or trisomy 18 is generally low, even if the likelihood ratio increases that risk by 1.5- or even 5-fold, it rarely increases the absolute risk significantly. In addition, the risk of miscarriage associated with amniocentesis is generally higher than the post-test risk for aneuploidy following one of these ultrasound findings. Providing support and clarifying factual information can help minimize adverse psychological impacts following the detection of a soft marker on ultrasound.

| Table 20-17 | Incidental Ultrasound Findings | | |
|---|---|---|---|
| **Ultrasound Marker** | **Prevalence in General Population** | **Association with Aneuploidy** | **Description and Clinical Implications** |
| **Markers Not Significant in the Absence of Aneuploidy[a]** | | | |
| Choroid plexus cysts | 0.1–3.6% | 1% of identified cases are trisomy 18; no association with trisomy 21 | Small fluid-filled sacs in the neuroepithelial folds within the choroid plexus. Often transient and considered a normal developmental variant. |
| Echogenic intra-cardiac focus | 3–4%; as high as 30% in Asian women | LR 1.4–1.8 for trisomy 21 | Small echogenic brightness in the left ventricle thought to be a microcalcification. Usually disappears later in pregnancy, and has no association with cardiac dysfunction. Increases the risk of trisomy 21 by 1.5-fold, which usually leaves women in the low-risk category. Targeted ultrasound may be recommended if other risks for trisomy are present. |
| **Markers Associated with Other Fetal Pathologic Conditions** | | | |
| Echogenic bowel | 0.2–1.8% | LR 5.5–6.7 for trisomy 21 | Sonographic finding in which the fetal bowel appears bright. Associated with an increased risk for trisomy 21, cystic fibrosis, fetal growth restriction, and infection. Genetic counseling is recommended to recalculate the trisomy 21 risk; recommend parental screening for cystic fibrosis and evaluation for cytomegalovirus. |
| Pelviectasis | 0.5–5% | LR 1.5–1.8 for trisomy 21 | Mild hydronephrosis; most often a transient state but may indicate renal dysfunction. Consultation with a maternal–fetal medicine physician, comprehensive ultrasound to rule out other structural anomalies, and follow-up ultrasound at 32 weeks recommended. If still present, schedule a postnatal renal ultrasound. |
| Nuchal fold thickening | 0.5% | LR 8.6–49 for trisomy 21 | Measurement between the outer edge of the occiput and the outer margin of the skin. Present in 40% of fetuses with trisomy 21. Also associated with Noonan syndrome and cardiac defects. Genetic counseling and fetal echocardiogram recommended. |
| Shortened humerus and femur | 5% | LR 2.5–7.8 (shortened humerus) and 1.2–3.72 (shortened femur) for trisomy 21 | May be a normal genetic predisposition, or an early indicator of fetal growth restriction or skeletal dysplasia. Consultation with a maternal–fetal medicine physician recommended. LR for humerus only should be used to adjust the risk for trisomy 21, as it is more sensitive and specific than the LR for shortened femur. One follow-up ultrasound is recommended in the third trimester to assess fetal growth. |

*(continues)*

| Table 20-17 | Incidental Ultrasound Findings (*continued*) | | |
| --- | --- | --- | --- |
| **Markers Associated with Other Fetal Pathologic Conditions** | | | |
| Single umbilical artery | 0.2–1.9% in single gestation; 4.9% in twin gestation | 40% with trisomy 21 if other anomalies present | Single umbilical artery is an isolated finding associated with fetal growth restriction and increased risk of perinatal morbidity in some studies, though not all. More research is needed. |
| | | | Consultation with a maternal–fetal medicine physician for management plan if an isolated finding. |
| | | | Refer for genetic counseling and additional diagnostic testing if associated with other markers. |
| Ventriculomegaly | | | Larger than expected ventricles in the fetal brain, often idiopathic or a normal variant. |
| | | | May be associated with infection, hydrocephalus, or other chromosomal abnormalities. |
| | | | Consultation with a maternal–fetal medicine physician recommended; perform comprehensive ultrasound to look for other abnormalities. |

Abbreviation: LR, likelihood ratio.

[a] These findings are not clinically significant for an individual who has a low risk for aneuploidy according to the results of first and second trimester screening, or if the individual had a diagnostic test to rule out chromosomal abnormalities.

Based on Norton ME. Follow-up of sonographically detected soft markers for fetal aneuploidy. *Semin Perinatol.* 2013;37:365-369; American College of Obstetricians and Gynecologists. Practice Bulletin No. 175: ultrasound in pregnancy. *Obstet Gynecol.* 2016; 128:e241-e256; Rao R, Platt LD. Ultrasound screening: status of markers and efficacy of screening for structural abnormalities. *Semin Perinatol.* 2016;40(1):67-78.

## Genetic Disorder Prevention and Risk Reduction

There are currently no cures for genetic disorders. However, there are some options and preventive approaches that can improve the outcomes for many pregnant people and their infants, of which midwives will want to be aware.

Excellent nutrition, including folic acid supplementation, and avoidance of exposures to teratogens are two long-standing preventive strategies that are well known in most geographic areas of the world. Furthermore, many countries offer genetic risk assessment and genetic testing to those persons considering childbearing so that options can be considered before a pregnancy occurs. Indeed, some groups have taken it upon themselves to offer screening for carrier status of a genetic disorder specific to the population. One example is the Jewish Genetic Disease Consortium, which strongly encourages carrier status testing for Tay-Sachs disease prior to conception.[83]

Unfortunately, many parents learn of hereditary disorders only after the diagnosis of an affected child. In this situation, the midwife provides the family with accurate information and compassionate care. Preconception and postpartum testing for genetic disorders and carrier status can be obtained by families who already have a child with a birth defect. This testing often provides answers to the questions most families have. Testing may be able to identify the specific disorder, as well as predict the likelihood that subsequent children will be affected.

Moreover, options can be considered once a definitive answer is given. Options include the choice not to bear biologic children, addition of future children via adoption, sperm and/or egg donation, and, in some countries, preimplantation genetic testing as well as acceptance of the risk of future affected children. Preimplantation testing involves in vitro fertilization (often with the sperm and/or egg from the prospective parents), genetic testing of a cell collected from the eight-cell blastocyst, followed by selection of only normal embryos for transfer into the uterus.[84] This method assures that only embryos without genetic disease mutations will be implanted. Some couples are delighted with this choice, whereas others are strongly opposed to it for religious or personal reasons; still others find the use of such technology too complex, too expensive, or too reminiscent of eugenics to consider it.[85]

## When Genetic Disorders Are Identified

When a congenital anomaly is diagnosed prenatally, the pregnant individual and family may face a range of decisions, including induced abortion, carrying the pregnancy, accessing fetal therapy/fetal surgery, the degree of interventions desired in labor, and postdelivery care of the newborn (including perinatal hospice for lethal conditions). Depending on the condition of the newborn at birth, the pregnant individual and family may have continued decision making about parenting the child, placing the newborn in foster care, or relinquishing the child for adoption. In such circumstances, parents will undoubtedly have many questions and need resources to help them deal with the situation. Helpful resources will vary depending on the setting and geographic area, and cultural, societal, family, and personal beliefs. Individuals may choose to enlist their families, religious leaders, online support groups, or mental health counselors for direction and support, and may desire access to medical resources and options, where available.

Midwives can be a valuable resource in supporting families who need additional information and discussion of options, help in identifying important questions to ask, and referrals to other healthcare providers such as geneticists and genetics counselors. Some may desire referral to a maternal–fetal medicine physician or neonatologist. If the pregnant individual has an established relationship with a midwife, it may be helpful for them to meet again with the midwife after consultation with other providers.

Making decisions about how to proceed can be emotionally wrenching for affected individuals and their families.[86] It is important to provide time for the pregnant individual and their family during this process, and to recognize that information may need to be repeated. Nondirective counseling guided by professional ethics is difficult and may need to be practiced ahead of time so that the midwife can use this approach competently.[87] It is not uncommon for a pregnant individual with a fetus having an anatomic anomaly to request periodic reconfirmation that the anomaly still exists. A repeat ultrasound should be provided if requested.

Frequently, affected newborns will need additional antepartum monitoring or immediate pediatric attention after birth, and arrangements for this care will need to be made in advance, including the site for the birth and plans for types of interventions or supports desired surrounding birth. Fetal therapy may be an option for individuals who have a fetus with specific anomalies. The North American Fetal Therapy Network—a collaborative group of medical centers—provides specialized therapy for fetuses with NTDs, cardiac anomalies, dysrhythmias, ventral wall defects such as gastroschisis, and other anomalies as part of research protocols.

Perinatal palliative care is an option within a spectrum of care that includes induced abortion as well as full resuscitation and treatment.[88] Many people facing the birth of a child with a genetic or structural disorder can continue with midwifery care, in consultation or collaboration with other members of the healthcare team. Induced abortion may be desired and an option, depending on the pregnant person's preferences, the gestational age, and regulations and laws. It may be necessary to refer to specialists in states or areas where the desired services can be performed. Midwives can provide substantial assistance by offering nonjudgmental support and education about options and anticipatory planning. When induced abortion is chosen, the plan regarding procedures such as fetal heart rate monitoring and viewing the infant after birth can be detailed ahead of time. These options depend on gestational age and method of induced abortion. Other components of palliative care include prenatal and postpartum bereavement counseling.[88]

Many proponents of prenatal testing believe that the biggest value in testing lies in the ability for parents to access resources and make arrangements for the care of a special-needs child well in advance of the birth. In addition, many support networks exist to help families who have a child with a specific genetic disorder or birth defect, such as the National Down Syndrome Society. Whatever final decisions are made, the midwife can be instrumental in providing support and directing families to the best resources.

## Future Trends in Genetic Testing

Expanded carrier testing is an approach that can identify a greater number of diseases, and is applied across all ethnic groups, regardless of risk status.[89,90] The availability of expanded carrier testing is growing, with such testing increasingly being offered to individuals and couples in the preconception and early pregnancy periods. Testing for more than 100 autosomal recessive disorders is now readily available in the United States. Nevertheless, expanded carrier screening is not yet recommended for all people.

Direct-to-consumer (DTC) genetic testing is also widely available.[91] The harms and benefits of DTC genetic tests are the subject of debate. Proponents argue that provision of such testing options empowers people by increasing their knowledge about their own health and the genetic basis of their health. Others are concerned that many people have low health literacy, particularly regarding genetic information, and may not be able to interpret or emotionally process the results of these tests without the assistance of trained healthcare personnel.[76] Although some countries and locations have adopted an over-the-counter approach in making the tests freely available, others have banned DTC genetic testing.[92–94]

Where available, individuals can purchase noninvasive DTC tests, including expanded carrier testing from commercial enterprises if they would like to determine, for example, the presence of genetic mutations for heritable disorders, including those that indicate carrier status and susceptibility to multifactorial diseases. Some tests are targeted to pregnant people and couples who would like to determine carrier status for specific genetic and chromosomal disorders, paternity, or the sex of the fetus prenatally. Samples (usually saliva/cheek swab or blood spot via finger stick) are collected in the privacy of one's home and returned to the commercial testing facility. This step may not require the services of a healthcare intermediary, such as the midwife, obstetrician, or family practice provider, although some tests do. One advantage of DTC testing is that it enables potential parents to test for carrier status prior to making the decision to attempt pregnancy. This approach raises the prospect of increasing use of preventive options for couples who want to avoid having a child with specific heritable disorders.[93,94]

When fetal structural abnormalities are identified on ultrasound, pregnant individuals are offered amniocentesis or CVS for chromosomal microarray or karyotype; however, these tests identify a cause for the abnormality in approximately only 16% of cases. Prenatal whole-exome sequencing (WES) is a technique for improving the diagnosis of genetic variants that may cause structural abnormalities identified on ultrasound. In practice, WES can identify responsible genetic variants in as many as 80% of cases when standard genetic testing is normal.[95] Ethical issues include interpretation and disclosure of results and potential discrimination in the case of diagnosis.[95] Cost is another consideration, although a diagnosis is thought to be cost-effective.[95]

## Conclusion

The Human Genome Project, completed in 2003, mapped the more than 25,000 genes found in the entire genome of *Homo sapiens*. Knowledge gleaned from the Human Genome Project will continue to impact human genomics for the foreseeable future. In addition to knowledge being gleaned from the Human Genome Project, the body of information about non-Mendelian inheritance patterns continues to grow. For the midwife receiving a report of a CVS, amniocentesis, or direct DNA testing, the results usually are phrased in Mendelian terms (e.g., "autosomal recessive"). However, non-Mendelian inheritance patterns continue to emerge as important etiologies for some human genetic conditions; for example, genomic imprinting occurs when a child receives only one "working" copy from one parent (instead of both) due to gene "silencing" by epigenetic mechanisms. Research continues into the variety of inheritance patterns because they may be of significant clinical relevance in the future.[10]

This chapter has provided a foundation in genetics for midwives and described several approaches for the provision of genetics and phenotype-related healthcare services. The intention is to increase the confidence that midwives have when addressing prenatal genetic risk assessment, testing options, and decision making. Although genetics is considered a high-tech science, midwives have a talent for using low-tech tools to communicate potential risk, and screening and test results, to assist pregnant people and their families in shared decision making. Although most genetic disorders do not have a cure, prenatal genetic risk assessment, counseling, screening, and diagnosis have many potential benefits for individuals, including the ability to consider options, make well-informed decisions, access valuable resources, prepare for outcomes in advance, and ultimately optimize the health of pregnant people and newborns. Well-informed midwives can make valuable contributions to applications of genetic science.

Many excellent resources are available to assist midwives and individuals for whom they care in obtaining additional information related to genetics. A selected list is included in the Resources section.

## Resources

| Organization | Description |
|---|---|
| Genetic Alliance | A nonprofit health advocacy organization. The website has multiple resources, including current recommended genomics competencies for nurses, genetic counselors, and physicians. |
| *Understanding Genetics: A New York, Mid-Atlantic Guide for Patients and Health Professionals* | This e-book includes a basic review of genetic disorders and tests. The appendix lists the National Coalition for Health Professional Education in Genetics' (NCHPEG) Core Competencies in Genetics for Health Professionals. |
| National Human Genome Research Institute | For healthcare providers and educators of healthcare providers. |
| Online Mendelian Inheritance in Man (OMIM) | Comprehensive description of single-gene disorders |
| GeneReviews | Comprehensive list of all gene tests with a description of their characteristics |
| American Society of Human Genetics (ASHG) | Genetics basics; genetics and research; genetics and health; genetics and society |
| Genetics/Genomics Competency Center (G2C2) | Genetics/genomics education for your classroom or practice; genetic testing methods; education for genetic counselors, nurses, and pharmacists |
| Office of the Surgeon General and the National Human Genome Research Institute | My Family Health Portrait: a web-based, self-completed family history tool |
| Centers for Disease Control and Prevention | Genomics and precision public health |
| | Health equity and genetic disorders; family history; genetic testing |

[a] Interested readers are referred to the individual national organizations that have been formed for many genetic disorders, including Down syndrome, cystic fibrosis, hemophilia, Tay-Sachs disease, sickle cell disease, and thalassemia, and that have websites with educational material for providers and families.

## References

1. Jorde L, Carey J, Bamshad M. Background and history. In: Jorde L, Carey J, Bamshad M, eds. *Medical Genetics*. 5th ed. Philadelphia, PA: Elsevier; 2016:1-5.

2. Wojcik MH, Agrawal PB. Deciphering congenital anomalies for the next generation. *Cold Spring Harb Mol Case Stud*. 2020;6(5):a005504. doi:10.1101/mcs.a005504.

3. Jorde L, Carey J, Bamshad M. Multifactorial inheritance and common diseases. In: Jorde L, Carey J, Bamshad M, eds. *Medical Genetics*. 5th ed. Philadelphia, PA: Elsevier; 2016:239-264.

4. Crane MJ, Quinn Griffin MT, Andrews CM, Fitzpatrick JJ. The level of importance and level of confidence that midwives in the United States attach to using genetics in practice. *J Midwifery Womens Health*. 2012;57(2):114-119.

5. World Health Organization. *Medical Genetic Services in Developing Countries: The Ethical, Legal and Social Implications of Genetic Testing and Screening*. Geneva, Switzerland: World Health Organization; 2006.

6. New York–Mid-Atlantic Guide for Patients and Health Professionals. Ethical, legal, and social issues. In: *Understanding Genetics: A New York, Mid-Atlantic Guide for Patients and Health Professionals*. Washington, DC: Genetic Alliance; July 8, 2009. https://www.ncbi.nlm.nih.gov/books/NBK115574/. Accessed September 2, 2021.

7. Feero WG, Guttmacher AE, Collins FS. Genomic medicine: an updated primer. *N Engl J Med*. 2010;362(21):2001-2011.

8. National Cancer Institute. NCI dictionary of genetics terms. https://www.cancer.gov/publications/dictionaries/genetics-dictionary. Accessed August 30, 2021.

9. Elston R, Satagopan J, Sun S. Genetic terminology. *Meth Molec Biol*. 2012;850:1-9.

10. American College of Obstetricians and Gynecologists. ACOG Technology Assessment in Obstetrics and Gynecology No. 14: modern genetics in obstetrics and gynecology. *Obstet Gynecol*. 2018;132(3):E143-E168. doi:10.1097/Aog.0000000000002831.

11. Dorman JS, Schmella MJ, Wesmiller SW. Primer in genetics and genomics, Article 1: DNA, genes and chromosomes. *Biol Res Nurs*. 2017;19(1):7-17.

12. American College of Obstetricians and Gynecologists. ACOG Committee Opinion No. 823: health care for transgender and gender diverse individuals.

*Obstet Gynecol.* 2021;137(3):e75-e88. doi:10.1097 /AOG.0000000000004294.

13. Sakatani Y, Ischihashi N, Kazuta Y, Yomo T. A transcription and translation-coupled DNA replication system using rolling-circle replication. *Sci Rep.* 2015;5:10404.

14. Read CY. Primer in genetics and genomics. Article 3: explaining human diversity: the role of DNA. *Biol Res Nurs.* 2017;19(3):350-356.

15. Epigenetics. Learn.Genetics: Genetic Science Learning Center. 2015. http://learn.genetics.utah.edu /content/epigenetics/. Accessed February 21, 2017.

16. Krauss RS, Hong M. Gene–environment interactions and the etiology of birth defects. *Curr Topics Develop Biol.* 2016;116:569-580.

17. Aiello LB, Chiatti BD. Primer in genetics and genomics. Article 4: inheritance patterns. *Biol Res Nurs.* 2017;19(4):465-472.

18. Viswanathan M, Treiman KA, Doto JK, et al. *Folic Acid Supplementation: An Evidence Review for the U.S. Preventive Services Task Force.* Rockville, MD: Agency for Healthcare Research and Quality; 2017.

19. Wang A, Rose CE, Qi YP, et al. Impact of voluntary folic acid fortification of corn masa flour on RBC folate concentrations in the U.S. (NHANES 2011–2018). *Nutrients.* 2021;13(4):1325. doi:10.3390/nu1 3041325.

20. Agopian AJ, Tinker SC, Lupo PJ, et al. Proportion of neural tube defects attributable to known risk factors. *Birth Defects Res Part A Clin Molec Teratol.* 2013;97(1):42-46.

21. U.S. Department of Health and Human Services, National Institutes of Health. About neural tube defects (NTDs). https://www.nichd.nih.gov/health/topics/ntds /conditioninfo. Accessed August 30, 2021.

22. Webster A, Schuh M. Mechanisms of aneuploidy in human eggs. *Trends Cell Biol.* 2017;27(1):55-68.

23. Hutaff-Lee C, Cordeiro L, Tartaglia N. Cognitive and medical features of chromosomal aneuploidy. *Handb Clin Neurol.* 2013;111:273-279.

24. Nieschlag E. Klinefelter syndrome: the commonest form of hypogonadism, but often overlooked or untreated. *Deutsches Arzteblatt Int.* 2013;110(20):347-353.

25. Levitsky LL, Luria AH, Hayes FJ, Lin AE. Turner syndrome: update on biology and management across the life span. *Curr Opin Endocrin Diabet Obesity.* 2015;22(1):65-72.

26. Morin SJ, Eccles J, Iturriaga A, Zimmerman RS. Translocations, inversions, and other chromosomal rearrangements. *Fertil Steril.* 2017;107:19-26.

27. Moog U, Felbor U, Has C, Zirn B. Disorders caused by genetic mosaicism. *Dtsch Arztebl Int.* 2020;116(8): 119-125. doi:10.3238/arztebl.2020.0119.

28. Li X, Hao Y, Elshewy N, et al. The mechanisms and clinical application of mosaicism in preimplantation embryos. *J Assist Reprod Genet.* 2020;37(3):497-508. doi:10.1007/s10815-019-01656-x.

29. Levy B, Hoffmann ER, McCoy RC, Grati FR. Chromosomal mosaicism: origins and clinical implications in preimplantation and prenatal diagnosis. *Prenat Diagn.* 2021;41(5):631-641. doi:10.1002/pd.5931.

30. Popovic M, Dhaenens L, Boel A, et al. Chromosomal mosaicism in human blastocysts: the ultimate diagnostic dilemma. *Hum Reprod Update.* 2020;26(3):313-334. doi:10.1093/humupd/dmz050.

31. Arnold KM, Self ZB. Genetic screening and counseling: family medicine obstetrics. *Primary Care.* 2012;39:55-70.

32. Hook EB. Rates of chromosomal abnormalities. *Obstet Gynecol.* 1981;58(3):282-285.

33. Brandt JS, Cruz Ithier MA, Rosen T, Ashkinadze E. Advanced paternal age, infertility, and reproductive risks: a review of the literature. *Prenatal Diagnosis.* 2019;39(2):81-87. https://doi.org/10.1002/pd.5402.

34. Donate A, Estop AM, Giraldo J, Templado C. Paternal age and numerical chromosome abnormalities in human spermatozoa. *Cytogenet Genome Res.* 2016;148(4):241-248.

35. Buhimschi CS, Weiner CP. Medications in pregnancy and lactation: part 1. teratology. *Obstet Gynecol.* 2009;113(1):166-188. doi:10.1097/AOG .0b013e31818d6788.

36. Alwan S, Chambers CD. Identifying human teratogens: an update. *J Pediatr Genet.* 2015;4(2):39-41. doi:10.1055/s-0035-1556745.

37. Hansen WF, Yankowitz J. Pharmacologic therapy for medical disorders during pregnancy. *Clin Obstet Gynecol.* 2002;45(1):136-152. doi:10.1097/00003081 -200203000-00014.

38. Teratology Society: Organization of Teratology Information Specialists. MotherToBaby fact sheets. https:// mothertobaby.org/fact-sheets/. Accessed January 12, 2022.

39. Haas DM, Marsh DJ, Dang DT, et al. Prescription and other medication use in pregnancy. *Obstet Gynecol.* 2018;131(5):789-798. doi:10.1097/ AOG.0000000000002579.

40. Shroff S, McNeil M, Borrero S. An innovative framework to improve teratogenic medication risk counseling. *J Midwifery Womens Health.* 2017;62(3):353-357. doi:10.1111/jmwh.12604.

41. Mitchell AA. Research challenges for drug-induced birth defects. *Clin Pharmacol Ther.* 2016;100(1):26-28. doi:10.1002/cpt.374.

42. Byrne JJ, Saucedo AM, Spong CY. Evaluation of drug labels following the 2015 Pregnancy and Lactation Labeling Rule. *JAMA Netw Open.* 2020;3(8):e2015094. doi:10.1001/jamanetworkopen.2020.15094.

43. Koren G, Berkovitch M, Ornoy A. Dose-dependent teratology in humans: clinical implications for

prevention. *Paediatr Drugs*. 2018;20(4):331-335. doi:10.1007/s40272-018-0294-0.

44. *Micromedex®* [Electronic version]. Greenwood Village, CA: IBM Watson Health. https://www.micromedexsolutions.com/home/dispatch/. Accessed January 16, 2022.

45. Di Renzo GC, Conry JA, Blake J, et al. International Federation of Gynecology and Obstetrics opinion on reproductive health impacts of exposure to toxic environmental chemicals. *Int J Gynaecol Obstet*. 2015;131(3):219-225.

46. Honein MA, Dawson AL, Petersen EE, et al. Birth defects among fetuses and infants of US women with evidence of possible Zika virus infection during pregnancy. *JAMA*. 2017;317(1):59-68.

47. Ornoy A, Becker M, Weinstein-Fudim L, Ergaz Z. Diabetes during pregnancy: a maternal disease complicating the course of pregnancy with long-term deleterious effects on the offspring. *Int J Mol Sci*. 2021;22(6):2965. doi:10.3390/ijms22062965.

48. Balsells M, Garcia-Patterson A, Gich I, Corcoy R. Major congenital malformations in women with gestational diabetes mellitus: a systematic review and meta-analysis. *Diab Metab Res Rev*. 2012;28(3):252-257.

49. Duempelmann L, Skribbe M, Bühler M. Small RNAs in the transgenerational inheritance of epigenetic information. *Trends Genet*. 2020;36(3):203-214. doi:10.1016/j.tig.2019.12.001.

50. Lassi ZS, Imam AM, Dean SV, Bhutta ZA. Preconception care: caffeine, smoking, alcohol, drugs and other environmental chemical/radiation exposure. *Reprod Health*. 2014;11(suppl 3):S6.

51. American College of Obstetricians and Gynecologists. ACOG Practice Bulletin, Number 226: screening for fetal chromosomal abnormalities. *Obstet Gynecol*. 2020;136(4):e48-e69. doi:10.1097/AOG.0000000000004084.

52. New York–Mid-Atlantic Guide for Patients and Health Professionals. Indications for a genetic referral. In: *Understanding Genetics: A New York, Mid-Atlantic Guide for Patients and Health Professionals*. Washington, DC: Genetic Alliance; 2009. https://www.ncbi.nlm.nih.gov/books/NBK115563/pdf/Bookshelf _NBK115563.pdf. Accessed August 30, 2021.

53. American College of Obstetricians and Gynecologists. Committee Opinion No. 693: counseling about genetic testing and communication of genetic test results. *Obstet Gynecol*. 2017;129(4):e96-e101. doi:10.1097/AOG.0000000000002020.

54. Alldred SK, Takwoingi Y, Guo B, et al. First trimester serum tests for Down's syndrome screening. *Cochrane Database Syst Rev*. 2015;11:CD011975.

55. Dashe JS. Aneuploidy screening in pregnancy. *Obstet Gynecol*. 2016;128:181-194.

56. Lithner CU, Kublickas M, Ek S. Pregnancy outcome for fetuses with increased nuchal translucency but normal karyotype. *J Med Screen*. 2016;23(1):1-6.

57. Chitayat D, Langlois S, Wilson RD. No. 261: prenatal screening for fetal aneuploidy in singleton pregnancies. *J Obstet Gynaecol Can*. 2017;39(9):e380-e394. doi:10.1016/j.jogc.2017.06.013.

58. Allum N, Sibley E, Sturgis P, Stoneman P. Religious beliefs, knowledge about science and attitudes towards medical genetics. *Public Underst Sci*. 2014;23(7):833-849.

59. Di Mattei V, Ferrari F, Perego G, et al. Decision-making factors in prenatal testing: a systematic review. *Health Psychol Open*. 2021;8(1):2055102920987455. doi:10.1177/2055102920987455.

60. Hill M, Lewis C, Chitty LS. Stakeholder attitudes and needs regarding cell-free fetal DNA testing. *Curr Opin Obstet Gynecol*. 2016;28(2):125-131.

61. Minear MA, Alessi S, Allyse M, et al. Noninvasive prenatal genetic testing: current and emerging ethical, legal, and social issues. *Ann Rev Genomics Hum Genetics*. 2015;16:369-398.

62. Tekola-Ayele F, Rotimi CN. Translational genomics in low- and middle-income countries: opportunities and challenges. *Public Health Genomics*. 2015;18(4):242-247.

63. Fonda Allen J, Stoll K, Bernhardt BA. Pre- and post-test genetic counseling for chromosomal and Mendelian disorders. *Semin Perinatol*. 2016;40(1):44-55. doi:10.1053/j.semperi.2015.11.007.

64. Gregg AR, Aarabi M, Klugman S, et al. Screening for autosomal recessive and X-linked conditions during pregnancy and preconception: a practice resource of the American College of Medical Genetics and Genomics (ACMG). *Genet Med*. 2021. doi:10.1038/s41436-021-01203-z.

65. Edwards JG, Feldman G, Goldberg J, et al. Expanded carrier screening in reproductive medicine: points to consider: a joint statement of the American College of Medical Genetics and Genomics, American College of Obstetricians and Gynecologists, National Society of Genetic Counselors, Perinatal Quality Foundation, and Society for Maternal–Fetal Medicine. *Obstet Gynecol*. 2015;125(3):653-662.

66. American College of Obstetricians and Gynecologists. Committee Opinion No. 691: carrier screening for genetic conditions. *Obstet Gynecol*. 2017;129:e41-55. doi:10.1097/AOG.0000000000001952.

67. Latendresse G, Deneris A. An update on current prenatal testing options: first trimester and noninvasive prenatal testing. *J Midwifery Womens Health*. 2015;60(4):360-371.

68. Srebniak MI, Joosten M, Knapen MF, et al. Frequency of submicroscopic chromosomal aberrations in pregnancies without increased risk for structural chromosomal aberrations: systematic review and meta-analysis. *Ultrasound Obstet Gynecol*. 2018;51:445-452.

69. Norton ME, Wapner RJ. Cell-free DNA analysis for noninvasive examination of trisomy. *N Engl J Med.* 2015;373:2582.

70. Norton ME, Baer RJ, Wapner RJ, et al. Cell-free DNA vs sequential screening for the detection of fetal chromosomal abnormalities. *Am J Obstet Gynecol.* 2016;214(6):727.e1-727.e6.

71. Gil MM, Accurti V, Santacruz B, et al. Analysis of cell-free DNA in maternal blood in screening for aneuploidies: updated meta-analysis. *Ultrasound Obstet Gynecol.* 2017;50:302-314.

72. Gregg AR, Skotko BG, Benkendorf JL, et al. Noninvasive prenatal screening for fetal aneuploidy, 2016 update: a position statement of the American College of Medical Genetics and Genomics. *Genet Med.* 2016;18:1056-1065.

73. Tamminga S, van Maarle M, Henneman L, et al. Maternal plasma DNA and RNA sequencing for prenatal testing. *Ad Clin Chem.* 2016;74:63-102.

74. Christiansen M, Ekelund CK, Petersen OB, et al. Nuchal translucency distributions for different chromosomal anomalies in a large unselected population cohort. *Prenat Diag.* 2016;36(1):49-55.

75. Alldred SK, Takwoingi Y, Guo B, et al. First and second trimester serum tests with and without first trimester ultrasound tests for Down's syndrome screening. *Cochrane Database Syst Rev.* 2017;3(3):CD012599. doi:10.1002/14651858.CD012599.

76. Fisher J. Supporting patients after disclosure of abnormal first trimester screening results. *Curr Opin Obstest Gynecol.* 2012;24(2):109-113.

77. Salomon LJ, Sotiriadis A, Wulff CB, et al. Risk of miscarriage following amniocentesis or chorionic villus sampling: systematic review of literature and updated meta-analysis. *Ultrasound Obstet Gynecol.* 2019;54(4):442-451. doi:10.1002/uog.20353.

78. Alfirevic Z, Navaratnam K, Mujezinovic F. Amniocentesis and chorionic villus sampling for prenatal diagnosis. *Cochrane Database Syst Rev.* 2017;9(9):CD003252. doi:10.1002/14651858.CD003252.pub2.

79. Rao R, Platt LD. Ultrasound screening: status of markers and efficacy of screening for structural abnormalities. *Semin Perinatol.* 2016;40(1):67-78.

80. Rao RR, Valderramos SG, Silverman NS, et al. The value of the first trimester ultrasound in the era of cell free DNA screening. *Prenat Diag.* 2016;36(13):1192-1198.

81. Norton ME. Follow-up of sonographically detected soft markers for fetal aneuploidy. *Semin Perinatol.* 2013;37:365-369.

82. American College of Obstetricians and Gynecologists. Practice Bulletin No. 175: ultrasound in pregnancy. *Obstet Gynecol.* 2016;128:e241-e256. doi:10.1097/AOG.0000000000001815.

83. Jewish Genetic Disease Consortium. About the JGDC. https://www.jewishgeneticdiseases.org/about-the-jgdc/. Accessed October 20, 2021.

84. Dahdouh EM, Balayla J, Audibert F, et al. Technical update: preimplantation genetic diagnosis and screening. *JOGC.* 2015;37(5):451-463.

85. Londra L, Wallach E, Zhao Y. Assisted reproduction: ethical and legal issues. *Semin Fetal Neonatal Med.* 2014;19(5):264-271.

86. Reddy UM, Abuhamad AZ, Levine D, Saade GR. Fetal imaging: executive summary of a joint Eunice Kennedy Shriver National Institute of Child Health and Human Development, Society for Maternal–Fetal Medicine, American Institute of Ultrasound in Medicine, American College of Obstetricians and Gynecologists, American College of Radiology, Society for Pediatric Radiology, and Society of Radiologists in Ultrasound Fetal Imaging workshop. *Obstet Gynecol.* 2014;123(5):1070-1082.

87. Chervenak FA, McCullough LB. Professional ethics and decision making in perinatology. *Semin Perinatol.* 2021;151520. doi:10.1016/j.semperi.2021.151520.

88. American College of Obstetricians and Gynecologists. ACOG Committee Opinion No. 786: perinatal palliative care. *Obstet Gynecol.* 2019;134(3):e84-e89. doi:10.1097/AOG.0000000000003425.

89. Haque IS, Lazarin GA, Kang HP, et al. Modeled fetal risk of genetic diseases identified by expanded carrier screening. *JAMA.* 2016;316(7):734-742.

90. Lazarin GA, Haque IS. Expanded carrier screening: a review of early implementation and literature. *Semin Perinatol.* 2016;40(1):29-34.

91. Horton R, Crawford G, Freeman L, et al. Direct-to-consumer genetic testing. *BMJ.* 2019;367:l5688. doi:10.1136/bmj.l5688.

92. Borry P, van Hellemondt RE, Sprumont D, et al. Legislation on direct-to-consumer genetic testing in seven European countries. *Eur J Hum Genet.* 2012;20(7):715-721.

93. Covolo L, Rubinelli S, Ceretti E, Gelatti U. Internet-based direct-to-consumer genetic testing: a systematic review. *J Med Internet Res.* 2015;17(12):e279. doi:10.2196/jmir.4378.

94. American College of Obstetricians and Gynecologists. ACOG Committee Opinion No. 816: consumer testing for disease risk. *Obstet Gynecol.* 2021;137(1):e1-e6. doi:10.1097/AOG.0000000000004200.

95. Jelin AC, Vora N. Whole exome sequencing: applications in prenatal genetics. *Obstet Gynecol Clin North Am.* 2018;45(1):69-81. doi:10.1016/j.ogc.2017.10.003.

# APPENDIX

# 20A

## Steps in Constructing a Three-Generation Pedigree

GWEN A. LATENDRESSE

1. Use standard symbols and notation for building the pedigree (Figure 20A-1). However, there are not yet widely accepted symbols to note individuals who have a genital phenotype different from their genotype, and individuals whose gender expression is different than their sex assigned at birth.

2. Computer-generated pedigrees can be constructed, but a simple piece of paper works well.

3. For greater convenience, individuals can complete a genetic checklist or questionnaire or fill out a computer-generated (i.e., online) pedigree prior to the prenatal visit.

4. Collect information about the individual (often called the "proband") and their immediate family members (grandparents, parents, aunts and uncles, siblings, and any previous offspring).

5. Collect information from both biologic parents and their family members, including grandparents, parents, aunts and uncles, brothers and sisters, and any previous offspring.

6. Identify any genetic "red flags" and mark affected relatives (i.e., use shading of symbols as appropriate).

7. List any health or medical conditions, or cause of death (if known), for each relative, along with the current age or age at time of death (if known) next to each corresponding relative on the pedigree.

An example of a three-generation pedigree is shown in Figure 20A-2. In this example, the 34-year-old individual is the proband, who has a 2-year-old daughter. The individual and her partner, who is the biologic parent of their daughter, are healthy. The person has a sister who is healthy, one brother who has type 2 diabetes, and one brother who has a congenital heart defect. The person has an aunt who died of cystic fibrosis at the age of 12.

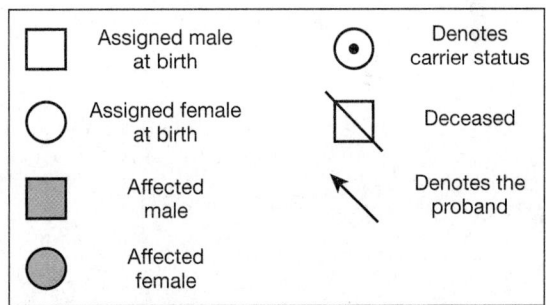

**Figure 20A-1** Symbols used in constructing a three-generation pedigree.

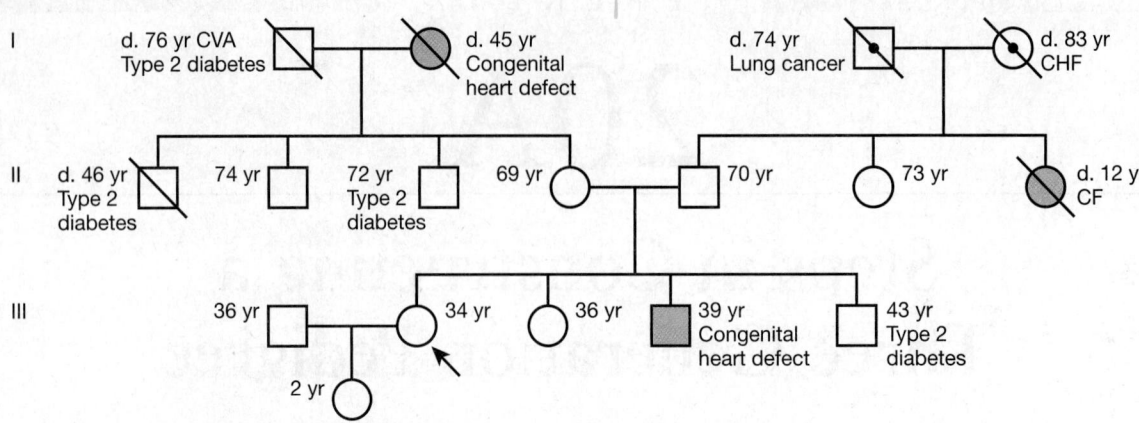

**Figure 20A-2** Example of a three generation pedigree.
Abbreviations: CF, cystic fibrosis; CHF, congestive heart failure; CVA, cardiovascular accident.

CHAPTER

# 21

# Prenatal Care

REBECCA H. BURPO, ANNE Z. COCKERHAM, AND ERIN E. SING

*The editors acknowledge Maria Openshaw, Cecilia M. Jevitt, and Tekoa
King, who were the authors of this chapter in the previous edition.*

## Introduction

Prenatal care is a foundational part of midwifery care. The partnership between pregnant individuals and midwives provides opportunities for person-centered facilitation of health.[1] Midwives around the world share a philosophy that delivering respectful care, supporting normal physiologic processes in pregnancy, and intervening only when indicated lead to optimal perinatal outcomes.[2,3] Worldwide, individuals partnering with midwives throughout pregnancy are less likely to experience pregnancy loss before 24 weeks' gestation and less likely to give birth to a preterm infant than those with other types of prenatal care providers.[4] In the United States, pregnant individuals cared for by a midwife are more likely to breastfeed/chestfeed longer, and less likely to supplement that feeding with human milk substitutes.[5] States in which more midwives provide care have lower rates of cesarean birth, preterm birth, babies born with low birth weights, and neonatal death compared with states where access to midwifery is limited.[6]

Data also suggest that the midwifery model, which emphasizes cultural congruency, has the potential to improve infant mortality rates for communities of color.[6] Pregnant individuals of color recommend relationship-building between the provider and pregnant person; individualized, person-centered care; and partnership in decision making as means to reduce health disparities due to racism.[7] Midwives who partner with members of historically under-resourced communities commit to providing person-centered care that values the experiences of all those seeking midwifery care,

humbly recognize past harms, and seek to move forward as leaders in improving prenatal care.

This chapter examines routine prenatal care, including the content and components of prenatal care and adaptations for special populations. It is divided into two parts. The first part focuses on the content of prenatal care, including relevant definitions, pregnancy diagnosis and dating, history and physical examination, physiologic and psychosocial screening, health promotion, and anticipatory guidance. In the second part of the chapter, prenatal care components are synthesized into a comprehensive organization of services across trimesters, with discussions of the traditional prenatal care schedule and the evolution of innovative models of prenatal care.

Detailed information about genetic counseling and screening tests can be found in the *Assessment for Genetic and Fetal Abnormalities* chapter. Management of the common discomforts of pregnancy and obstetric complications are reviewed in the *Pregnancy-Related Conditions* chapter. Medical complications of pregnancy are reviewed in the *Medical Complications in Pregnancy* chapter.

## The Content of Prenatal Care

Prenatal care content has expanded over the past decades, with wide variations in what constitutes these services. Midwives provide prenatal care that is based on clear and person-centered communication, accurate determination of pregnancy status, screening for potential complications, management of conditions that can occur, and health promotion with guidance to achieve optimal outcomes.

## Definitions and Acronyms

The prenatal period includes the time from the first day of the last normal menstrual period to the start of active labor, which marks the beginning of the intrapartum period. The anticipated date of birth was historically referred to as the estimated date of confinement (EDC). This terminology connotes illness, limitation, and a passive role, based on an archaic practice of isolating women in late pregnancy, rather than recognizing pregnancy as a normal event and healthy process, with active participation. While this term is still used in many settings, a number of healthcare professionals have changed to active, person-centered terms, such as the estimated date of delivery or estimated due date (EDD), or the estimated date of birth (EDB). Estimated due date (EDD) is used throughout this text.

Determining a pregnancy history focuses on how many pregnancies (gravida) and how many births (para) an individual has had. *Gravida* stems from the Latin word *gravidus*, which means "pregnant"; *para* derives from the Latin word *parous*, which means "bringing forth or producing." Para refers to the process of giving birth, not the number of fetuses, or the outcome of that birth. Sometimes confusion may occur regarding how to account for the various outcomes of pregnancy. Surveys of midwives and obstetricians reveal that documentation of parity remains inconsistent and there is a need for global standardization of the nomenclature.[8,9] In the United States, the reVITALize: Obstetrics Data Definitions are endorsed by American College of Nurse-Midwives (ACNM), Association of Women's Health, Obstetric, and Neonatal Nurses (AWHONN), and American College of Obstetricians and Gynecologists (ACOG). These Obstetrics Data Definitions define parity as the number of pregnancies reaching 20 weeks' gestation.[10]

The definitions listed in this chapter are those commonly in use the United States. Table 21-1 summarizes the nomenclature for documentation. A person who is pregnant for the first time is considered to be primigravid, whereas a person who has never given birth is considered to be nulliparous. The term for a person who has been pregnant more than once is multigravida, and a multiparous person has given birth more than once. It is important that these terms are used correctly with an accepted set of definitions. Because parity does not reflect all the possible outcomes of birth, a four-digit system, which encompasses term/premature/abortion/living (TPAL) outcomes, is used to better describe a person's birth history. The prenatal period is divided into three trimesters, each comprising 12–13 weeks or three calendar months. When the GTPAL system does not convey all the important information (e.g., when a person had a set of twins, one of whom is no longer living), a note can be used to provide more detail.

## Diagnosis of Pregnancy

An accurate diagnosis of pregnancy eliminates the possibility of other conditions that may manifest with similar symptoms and signs. Differentiating confirmatory information from suggestive data assures the provider and the individual of pregnancy status.

### Pregnancy Symptoms, Signs, and Confirmation

Several events raise a suspicion of pregnancy. Presumptive symptoms that an individual may report include amenorrhea, breast changes, fatigue, nausea and vomiting, perception of fetal movement (quickening), facial or abdominal skin pigmentation changes, elevated basal body temperature without infection, and urinary frequency.

Probable signs may be detected during the physical examination, leading the provider to conclude that the individual is probably pregnant. These include breast changes; abdominal or uterine enlargement; a bluish discoloration of the cervix, vagina, and labia; cervical softening; lower uterine segment softening; an asymmetrical bulge in the uterus; palpable fetal movement; palpable fetal outline; palpable uterine contractions; and a positive pregnancy test. However, these probable signs may be elicited with other conditions. Thus, they are unreliable for confirming pregnancy. Noting presumptive and probable changes of pregnancy is not a critical component of pregnancy diagnosis in the United States, but has value in under-resourced areas.

There are two positive or confirmatory signs of pregnancy to note: audible fetal heart tones and sonographic evidence of pregnancy. The reason pregnancy tests are considered probable, rather than positive, is because some conditions other than pregnancy can elevate human chorionic gonadotropin (hCG) levels (e.g., some tumors, hCG injections).

### Pregnancy Tests

The accuracy and reliability of pregnancy tests has increased since they were first introduced in the 1970s. With a sensitive test, the hormone can be detected as early as 8 days after conception.[11] Hormonal pregnancy tests are based on the presence of the beta subunit of human chorionic gonadotropin

| Table 21-1 | Nomenclature for Pregnancy History Documentation |
|---|---|
| Gravida (G) | Number of pregnancies |
| Para (P) | Number of preterm and term births |
| Term (T) | Number of pregnancies lasting at least 37 weeks |
| Preterm (P) | Number of pregnancies lasting between 20 and 36 6/7 weeks |
| Abortion (A) | Number of pregnancies ending before 20 weeks (includes miscarriages and induced abortions) |
| Living (L) | Number of currently living children. There is no universal consensus on whether this describes the number of pregnancies completed or the number of living individuals from the pregnancies. This text uses the number of living individuals from the pregnancies. |
| Gestational age (GA) | Number of weeks subsequent to the last menstrual period |
| Embryonic age (EA) | The age of the embryo or fetus. Synonyms are "postconceptional age" and "ovulation age." A postconceptional age differs from a gestational age by 2 weeks. When reviewing information about embryonic development or exposure to teratogenic agents, the type of calendar weeks being used—gestational or postconceptional—needs to be confirmed to avoid confusion. |
| Trimesters | The prenatal period is divided into three trimesters, or 3-month periods over 9 calendar months. Variations exist, depending on whether it is calculated from postconception or the last menstrual period. |

**Notation Systems for Pregnancy History**

| | |
|---|---|
| Gravida/para (two-digit notation) | Includes only the number of pregnancies and the number of term/preterm births.<br>Example: G2P1 indicates either a person who has been pregnant twice with one abortion and one birth after 20 weeks, or a person who is currently pregnant and who has had one prior birth after 20 weeks. |
| Gravida/para (four-digit notation) | Includes number of pregnancies, term births, abortions, preterm births, and living children.<br>Example: G4P2114 indicates a person who has had four pregnancies, two births after 37 weeks, one birth between 20 and 37 weeks of twins, one pregnancy ending before 20 weeks, four living children, and one multiple pregnancy. |

**Term-Related Definitions**

| | |
|---|---|
| Late preterm | 34 weeks and 0 days through 36 weeks and 6 days |
| Early term | 37 weeks and 0 days through 38 weeks and 6 days |
| Full term | 39 weeks and 0 days through 40 weeks and 6 days |
| Late term | 41 weeks and 0 days through 41 weeks and 6 days |
| Post term | Greater than or equal to 42 weeks and 0 days. |

Based on reVITALize. Obstetric Data Definitions. 2014; Version 1.0. https://www.acog.org/practice-management/health-it-and-clinical-informatics/revitalize-obstetrics-data-definitions. Accessed September 9, 2021.

(beta-hCG) in serum or in urine. Beta-hCG is produced by the syncytiotrophoblast of the placenta in increasing amounts in early pregnancy.

### Urine Pregnancy Tests

Different metabolites and subunits of hCG exist, which are used in pregnancy testing. Some of these are thought to lead to the rare occurrence of false-negative test results.[12–14] Commercially available urine pregnancy tests have varying sensitivity thresholds, but are usually intended to test positive when the beta-hCG level is approximately 20 to 50 mIU/L. This corresponds to approximately the date of the missed menses, at which time beta-hCG becomes detectable in urine. There is little difference between the commercially available home urine pregnancy tests and those performed in the clinical setting. However, independent studies report considerable difference in the usability and accuracy of the various tests.[11]

The concentration of beta-hCG in urine can vary within the same individual throughout the day depending on fluctuations in urine concentration. For some individuals, the first urine of the day will test positive, while subsequent voids test negative. Because many individuals have irregular periods, 10 to 20 pregnant individuals out of every 100 will have a negative pregnancy test on the first day of their missed period. Thus, the most common cause of a false-negative pregnancy test is testing too early.[15]

A positive pregnancy test does not confirm the viability of a pregnancy. The percentage of pregnancies that are detected very early and result in a miscarriage ranges between 20% and 62%.[16] Individuals who carefully track their menses and use highly sensitive home pregnancy tests may detect very early pregnancies that otherwise might be assumed to be a late or missed menses.

## Serum Pregnancy Tests

Serum pregnancy tests can detect the presence of beta-hCG either qualitatively or quantitatively.

However, as reviewed in the *Anatomy and Physiology of Pregnancy* chapter, individual blood values at specific gestational ages are highly variable, such that a single quantitative serum beta-hCG value does not provide reliable information about the gestational age or viability of the pregnancy. Instead, the clinical utility of quantitative beta-hCG measurement is based on following trends in these measurements in early pregnancy. When the serum beta-hCG is at least 1500 to 2000 mIU/L, the value is within the clinical "discriminatory zone" (Table 21-2). Approximately 91% of individuals with a beta-hCG level higher than this range will have an intrauterine gestational sac visible if transvaginal ultrasound is performed. Once the beta-hCG level reaches 3500 mIU/L, 99% of pregnancies are visible on ultrasound.[17]

Serum values of beta-hCG increase exponentially in early pregnancy, doubling every 1.4 to 2.0 days. Thus, a wide range of levels are possible, which increase from the day of implantation. The beta-hCG level peaks at 60 to 70 days' gestation. Thereafter, levels decline slowly to a plateau at approximately 16 weeks' gestation.[18]

## Dating of Pregnancy

Accurate determination of the expected date of birth informs decision making around the timing of screening diagnostics, intrauterine growth

| Table 21-2 | Discriminatory Levels of Human Chorionic Gonadotropin Levels and Ultrasound Findings by Gestational Age | |
|---|---|---|
| **Gestational Age in Weeks from Last Menstrual Period** | **Approximate beta-hCG Level (mIU/mL)[a]** | **Ultrasound Findings** |
| 3–4 weeks | 150–1000 | Decidual thickening |
| 4–5 weeks | > 1000–2000 | Gestational sac visible with TVUS when beta-hCG is approximately 1000 mIU/mL, and detectable on abdominal ultrasound when beta-hCG is approximately 1800 mIU/mL |
| 5–6 weeks | 1000–7200 | Yolk sac present when gestational sac is > 10 mm<br>Embryo present when gestational sac is > 18 mm<br>Cardiac activity present when crown–rump length is > 5 mm |
| 6–7 weeks | > 10,800 | Crown–rump length is 4–9 mm |

Abbreviations: beta-hCG, beta subunit of human chorionic gonadotropin; TVUS, transvaginal ultrasound.

[a] Beta-hCG values are approximate. Each ultrasound department will have institutionally specific values that can be used to guide management.

Data from Snell BJ. Assessment and management of bleeding in the first trimester of pregnancy. *J Midwifery Womens Health*. 2009;54:483-491.

assessments, risk assessments, the dividing line between preterm and term labor, possible induction, and other clinical judgments. Gestational age at the time of birth is the single most valuable predictor of newborn health. An accurate calculation of gestational age supports best practices in management of threatened preterm labor, evaluation of fetal growth, initiation of fetal surveillance, and decisions to induce labor. Conversely, incorrect estimation of the gestational age can lead to errors in screening, data interpretation, and interventions.

The opportunity for accurate assessment of gestational age decreases as the pregnancy progresses, and EDDs cannot be accurately recalculated after the second trimester. Several methods can be used to calculate the EDD, all of which have some variability. Appropriate management also requires clinicians to clearly communicate whether dates describe post-conceptional (embryonic) or post-menstrual (gestational) age. Table 21-1 defines embryonic age and gestational age. The *Anatomy and Physiology of Pregnancy* chapter discusses these concepts in more depth.

### Last Menstrual Period

The date of the first day of the last menstrual period (LMP) is used as the baseline for an initial determination of gestational age and the EDD. However, use of LMP to determine gestational age has several limitations. The normal menstrual cycle is 21 to 35 days, with the mean being 28.4 days. Many individuals with longer or shorter cycles, however, may not ovulate 14 days after their last menstrual period. Similarly, there is variation in the timing of implantation of the blastocyst, which can occur 5 to 14 days after the estimated time of ovulation.[19]

While many individuals can accurately recall the date of their LMP within 1 to 2 days,[20] the reported LMP can also be inaccurate. Some individuals do not keep a record of their menstrual periods, and others have a history of irregular cycles or amenorrhea, despite having ovulatory cycles. In addition, various medications, changes in weight, breastfeeding/chestfeeding, and shift work are examples of factors that can change menses frequency and the timing of ovulation.

Spotting in early pregnancy is common and may be perceived as a menstrual period. It is theorized that this bleeding or spotting, which occurs at the time of implantation of the blastocyst, results from the invasive activity of the chorionic villi in the endometrial lining.[21]

Given the inexact nature of menstrual frequency, it can help to establish the date of the last *normal* menstrual period (LNMP) before estimating gestational age. Compare the individual's description of the last menstrual period to a description of their usual menstrual periods with regard to timing, duration, and flow. Supplemental information that can be used in conjunction with LNMP to improve the accuracy of the EDD includes coital timing (inclusion or exclusion dates for exposure to conception), use (or not) of contraception (i.e., type, timing, consistency), and dates, types, and results of any home ovulation timing or pregnancy test that the individual has done prior to seeking prenatal care.

### Naegele's Rule

Traditionally the EDD is initially calculated using Naegele's rule, which is based on the assumption of a 28-day menstrual cycle. In 1812, Franz Karl Naegele, a German physician, authored a text that advised providers to estimate that a full-term pregnancy would end at approximately 40 weeks (280 days) after the first day of the last menstrual period.[22] Although this theory is not rooted in any modern concept of research and its accuracy has been questioned,[23] it remains widely used today and is the basis of many pregnancy calculators.

To use Naegele's rule, add 7 days to the LMP and then subtract 3 months to obtain the EDD. For LMPs that occur after the first 3 months of the year, an additional year is added. Thus, the formula is the first day of LMP + 7 days − 3 months = EDD.

Use the actual number of days in the month of the LMP if adding 7 days crosses over to the next month. This is illustrated in the following example of calculating the EDD by Naegele's rule: If the LMP is May 28, then May 28 + 7 days = June 4 (May has 31 days) − 3 months = an EDD of March 4 of the next year. Note that Naegele's rule does not account for the additional day in a leap year.

### Pregnancy Wheels and Apps

The pocket gestational wheel, which is traditionally used to calculate EDD and determine gestational age, calculates an EDD based on 280 days for the duration of gestation. Such gestational wheels are easy to use, but their calculated EDDs vary by 1 to 7 days.[24]

In many settings, the pocket wheel has largely been replaced by computer-based software. Most electronic health record systems used for prenatal care and obstetric ultrasonography include dating calculators, which allow the automatic calculation of an EDD. The electronic calculators that can be found on the Internet, or as a downloadable application (app), may remove most of the margin of error associated with pregnancy wheels and arithmetic calculations.[24]

## Ultrasound

Ultrasound technology is used in pregnancy to perform three types of evaluations: standard, limited, or specialized or targeted (described in Table 21-3). Ultrasonography is used throughout pregnancy for confirmation and gestational age estimation. Its findings and measurements vary by weeks and trimesters of pregnancy. Notably, this technology's accuracy for dating purposes declines as the pregnancy progresses. The midwife compares the timing of the ultrasound with the evidence related to its accuracy to determine the best estimate of gestational age. Midwives may acquire advanced skills in performing limited ultrasounds in accordance with ACNM guidelines.

## First Trimester

Calculation of gestational age and EDD based on ultrasound performed before 13 6/7 weeks is highly accurate for dating pregnancy.[25] In perinatal care, an ultrasound may be requested to provide a general or targeted assessment.

Serial measurements of quantitative serum beta-hCG values repeated every 48 to 72 hours are often used in conjunction with an early ultrasound and other clinical data. Serum beta-hCG levels are most useful prior to cardiac activity that is visible on ultrasound (typically at 6 weeks' gestation). These assessments assist the clinician in determining the presence and viability of an intrauterine pregnancy, in which serum beta-hCG levels usually double every 48 to 72 hours. With ectopic pregnancy, serum beta-hCG levels often rise more slowly than in an intrauterine pregnancy or levels may decline. Clinicians also monitor serum beta-hCG for the expected decline of levels when a miscarriage has occurred. The *Early Pregnancy Loss and Abortion* chapter reviews management of first

| Table 21-3 | Applications of Ultrasound in Pregnancy |
|---|---|
| **Type of Ultrasound** | **Description** |
| Standard ultrasound | Often referred to as an anatomy ultrasound, this examination provides fetal biometry needed to confirm gestational age and is simultaneously able to detect most major morphologic malformations prior to the time that the fetus would be viable if born. <br> A standard ultrasound identifies gestational age, fetal number, fetal biometry, amniotic fluid volume, cardiac activity, placental position, placental localization, and complete assessment of fetal anatomy. <br> Maternal adnexa and cervix including cervical length are usually included. <br> The standard ultrasound is offered to all pregnant women between 18 and 20 weeks' gestation. |
| Limited ultrasound | Performed for a specific indication, this evaluation is not considered a replacement for the routine standard ultrasound. <br> Components of a limited examination may include assessment of gestational age, embryonic or fetal viability, confirmation of fetal heart activity, identification of number of fetuses, confirmation of fetal presentation and position, determination of placental location, determination of amniotic fluid volume, fetal well-being, and cervical length. <br> A limited ultrasound may be done in any trimester and performed in the office setting. <br> A limited ultrasound with the specific purpose of assessing gestational age is often referred to as a dating ultrasound. |
| Specialized or targeted ultrasound | A specialized ultrasound is ordered when an anomaly is suspected based on the history, laboratory results, or abnormal findings on a standard ultrasound. <br> Additional technology can be utilized for specific purposes. For example, fetal echocardiogram can be used to accurately diagnose cardiac malformations. Fetal Doppler velocimetry is used to evaluate maternal–fetal blood flow, particularly in cases of fetal growth restriction, multifetal gestations, severe maternal hypertension, and placental abnormalities. <br> A specialized ultrasound is performed/reviewed by physicians trained in the technology—typically maternal–fetal medicine or specialist radiologists. |

trimester miscarriage, ectopic pregnancy, and *pregnancy of unknown location* (the diagnostic term for the clinical scenario in which the serum beta-hCG is positive but the ultrasound does not detect a pregnancy in the uterus).

First trimester ultrasound can be used to confirm LMP dating or to establish the gestational age for pregnant individuals without a known LMP. In the past decade, transvaginal sonography has become more widely used for confirming pregnancy and its location. A transvaginal ultrasound can detect a gestational sac, the first evidence of pregnancy, by 4 to 5 weeks of gestation. By the middle of the fifth week, a yolk sac within the gestational sac is considered to be confirmation of an intrauterine pregnancy. After 6 weeks, an embryo is seen as a linear structure immediately adjacent to the yolk sac, and cardiac motion is typically visible at this point. A fluid collection may also be noted with an ectopic pregnancy. Thus, further evaluation will be required if this is the only finding.[18]

At this time, the crown–rump length measurement remains the most accurate first trimester ultrasound measurement for determining gestational age.[26] This dating method can reduce the number of inductions of labor for post-dates pregnancies and has been shown to be cost-effective in most developed nations.[27,28] If the difference between the ultrasonographic and LMP due dates is more than 5 to 7 days, the ultrasound-calculated EDD will be used. The recommendations for changing due dates based on LMP and ultrasound dating discrepancies are presented in Table 21-4.

### Second Trimester

Second trimester ultrasound estimates of fetal age are based on composite measurements of the fetal head circumference, biparietal diameter, and femur length, as well as the abdominal circumference.[26] These estimates are slightly less accurate than first trimester ultrasound gestational age determinations because there is more individual variation in fetal growth and development as pregnancy progresses.

### Third Trimester

Third trimester ultrasound estimates of fetal age are the least reliable method for pregnancy dating. Table 21-4 describes the accuracy of this method of dating. This method typically is reserved for

| Table 21-4 | Guidelines for Establishing Estimated Due Date Based on Last Menstrual Period and Ultrasound Discrepancies |
|---|---|
| **Gestational Age in Weeks and Days Based on First Day of LMP** | **Discrepancy Between Ultrasound and Menstrual Dating That Supports Use of Ultrasound Dating** |
| ≤ 8 6/7 | > 5 days |
| 9 0/7 to 15 6/7 | > 7 days |
| 16 0/7 to 21 6/7 | > 10 days |
| 22 0/7 to 27 6/7 | > 14 days |
| 28 0/7 and beyond | > 21 days |

Abbreviations: LMP, last menstrual period.
Data from American College of Obstetricians and Gynecologists. Committee Opinion No. 700: methods for estimating the due date. *Obstet Gynecol*. 2017;129:e150-e154.

individuals who present late for care and requires clinical corroboration. Another ultrasound in 3 to 4 weeks can be helpful to confirm adequate fetal growth in a pregnancy with uncertain dating.

### Assisted Reproductive Technology

When a pregnancy is conceived through assisted reproductive technology (ART), the ART-derived gestational age is used, instead of the LMP. For example, with in vitro fertilization, the ART-derived date would be based on the age of the embryo and the date of the transfer.[26]

### Clinical Corroboration in Pregnancy Dating

Although uterine size correlates positively with gestational age, fundal measurement is a less reliable predictor of EDD than is the LMP.[29,30] Clinical assessment of uterine size may be affected by distension of the bladder (up to 7 cm), deposition of abdominal adipose tissue,[30] retroversion or retroflexion of the uterus, presence of fibroids, uterine anomaly, position and presentation of the fetus, amniotic fluid volume, and clinician experience.[29] Measurement of the uterine fundal height above the symphysis to monitor fetal growth is a standard component of prenatal care. The procedure of fundal height measurement is explained in detail in the *Abdominal Examination During Pregnancy* appendix.

Other indicators such as first fetal movement (quickening), along with the clinician's notation of first detection of fetal heart tones by ultrasound or fetoscope or the client's signs and symptoms of pregnancy, are poor predictors of gestational age but can be supportive data if reliable dating is not available. In addition, these observations can be of value in low-resource or disaster settings, and it is traditional practice to record the initial detection of the fetal heart tones and fetal movement in the pregnant individual's health record.

## Prenatal History

After the pregnancy is diagnosed and the individual's choice to pursue prenatal care has been confirmed, a complete history is obtained. This includes past medical and surgical history, along with family, genetic, social, menstrual, pregnancy, gynecologic, sexual, and contraceptive history. The midwife should inquire about all current and recently discontinued medications, including those that the pregnant individual stopped, with or without the recommendation of a provider. The midwife should review these medications for potential teratogenicity and discuss the risks and benefits of each, including treated and untreated conditions for which medications are intended. The components of the health history that can adversely affect the course of pregnancy are detailed in Table 21-5.

While extra time is typically allotted for the initial prenatal visit, the content of the visit may need to be divided between multiple visits. The scope of questions asked at the initial prenatal visit may seem intrusive. Sensitive subjects such as intimate partner violence, sexual abuse history, and substance use can be readdressed at subsequent visits when a trusting relationship has been established. Key lab tests, such as those for syphilis and human immunodeficiency virus (HIV), should be obtained as soon as possible after beginning prenatal care to expedite treatment, and timing of these tests in relation to the start of prenatal care may be mandated by state laws.

## Physical Examination

The midwife performs a physical examination at every prenatal visit. The focus of each examination depends on the type of visit and the concerns reported by the individual. The *Physical Examination*, *Breast and Chest Examination*, and *Pelvic Examination* appendices review the components of the physical examination.

### Initial Prenatal Visit

Traditionally, the purposes of the physical examination during the initial prenatal visit have been to verify the well-being of the pregnant person and the fetus, identify deviations from normal, and validate the gestational age of the fetus. Increasing use of technology, evolving practice guidelines,

| Table 21-5 | Components of the Health History That May Affect the Course of Pregnancy |
|---|---|
| **History Element** | **Clinical Implications** |
| Name, identities, and pronouns | Legal name and name used, pronouns, gender, and sexual identity are important elements for the midwife to respect as part of building trust and individualizing care. |
| Present pregnancy | Signs of pregnancy complications such as cramping, bleeding, or excessive vomiting in the first trimester; signs of preterm labor or preeclampsia in the late second and early third trimesters<br>Signs of medical complications such as fever, dysuria, or rash<br>Extreme discomforts of pregnancy<br>Exposures to teratogens such as drugs or medications, street drugs, alcohol, tobacco, X rays, environmental exposures, or occupational exposures |
| Oral health | Periodontal disease is common during pregnancy and, in some studies, has been associated with preterm birth. Individuals with poor oral health can transmit the bacteria that cause dental caries to their newborn, and studies have shown that their children are more likely to develop dental caries. Dental care during pregnancy can prevent this transmission. Midwives should ask about bleeding gums, tooth pain, and the date of last dental care. |
| Medical history | Medical conditions that are associated with increased risks for adverse maternal or fetal outcomes, such as diabetes or hypertension; they indicate a need for consultation, collaboration, co-management, or referral to a physician. |

| History Element | Clinical Implications |
|---|---|
| Surgical history | Uterine surgery such as cesarean birth or myomectomy, which may indicate a need for a physician consultation to evaluate the ability of the uterine scar to withstand a subsequent labor<br>Significant surgeries on vital organs such as the heart, lungs, or kidneys |
| Family history | Evidence of genetic disorders such as hemophilia, cystic fibrosis, or intellectual or developmental disability, which may suggest the need for specific genetic counseling or tests |
| Social history | Marital status has legal implications for birth certificates, especially if the person is married to someone other than their current partner. Holistic, person-centered assessment including languages spoken, individuals with whom the pregnant person shares a home, type of work, and children for whom they care.<br>Challenges that could indicate a need for additional visits, social services, psychology consultation, or referral:<br>• Barriers to accessing care such as transportation, work schedule, unemployment, homelessness, food insecurity<br>• Adolescent pregnancy<br>• History of substance use, alcohol use disorder<br>• Personal stressors: history of sexual, physical, or emotional abuse |
| Menstrual history | Irregular or regular cycles<br>Cycle length<br>Number of days between menses |
| Reproductive history | Gravidity, parity (TPAL)<br>Dates of previous births, as well as weights of newborns<br>Pregnancy complications such as mid-trimester loss, gestational diabetes, preterm labor, preterm premature rupture of membranes, fetal growth restriction, or preeclampsia[a]<br>Induction or augmentation of labor, prolonged stages of labor<br>Birth details including location of birth, coping and comfort strategies, positive and negative aspects of the birth<br>Previous birth complications: mode of birth, shoulder dystocia, birth lacerations, or episiotomies<br>Postpartum complications<br>Newborn health, feeding method, and complications such as injury, infection, or congenital defects |
| Gynecologic history | Past or current STIs, including herpes simplex virus, syphilis, gonorrhea, chlamydia, and HIV<br>Diagnosed malformations of the reproductive tract<br>History of female genital mutilation<br>Procedures for treatment of abnormal cervical cytology<br>Vulvovaginal disorders |
| Sexual history | Sexual and gender identity of pregnant individual<br>Sexual and gender identity(ies) of current partner(s)<br>Sexual activity: number of current partners and number of partners in the last year; gender of partners<br>Risks for STIs and use of barrier methods for prevention of STIs |
| Contraceptive history | What was the last form of contraception used and when was it discontinued?<br>Note any stated preferences for future contraception or reproductive life planning |
| Current medications | Current or recently discontinued medications, dose, and duration of treatment<br>Vitamins, supplements, or herbal remedies |
| Allergies | Allergies to medications<br>Allergies to foods or environmental exposures |

Abbreviations: HIV, human immunodeficiency virus; STI, sexually transmitted infection; TPAL, term birth, premature birth, abortion, living children.

[a] Refer to the chapters on each of these pregnancy complications for more information.

and questions about usefulness have altered some clinicians' approaches to selected elements of the traditional initial prenatal physical examination.

Weight and height assessments and calculation of a prepregnancy body mass index (BMI) are useful in guiding recommendations for weight gain throughout the pregnancy. An initial prenatal blood pressure measurement is beneficial to assess for chronic hypertension and to provide a baseline for comparison with later pregnancy measurements. A complete head-to-toe physical examination has traditionally been carried out at the initial prenatal visit, but some clinicians omit it if the pregnant person has recently undergone a physical examination. Oral health is particularly important during pregnancy but is frequently overlooked.[31]

The abdominal and pelvic portions of the examination can be particularly relevant in pregnancy. The techniques for abdominal examination are presented in the *Abdominal Examination During Pregnancy* appendix. Clinicians often assess uterine size with a bimanual examination, and this assessment can be helpful in validating gestational age. However, increasing use of ultrasound has resulted in a decreased reliance on uterine size assessment for pregnancy dating. Depending on the gestational age, the clinician auscultates fetal heart tones to assess fetal well-being. Cervical cytology testing guidelines have changed in recent years such that fewer individuals are recommended to undergo a cervical cytology test at the beginning of the pregnancy. If they do not need to collect cervical cytology, some clinicians may choose to forego the initial prenatal pelvic examination, which had previously been routine. Clinical pelvimetry, an assessment of pelvic architecture related to pelvic adequacy during labor, has traditionally been considered the standard of care at the initial prenatal visit. However, routine clinical pelvimetry in early pregnancy has questionable utility. Indeed, it is rare to identify an abnormality that changes clinical management prior to labor.[32]

Shared decision making, patient-centered care, and trauma-informed care frameworks all prompt clinicians to carefully consider their approaches to physical examination. Examinations, particularly the pelvic portion, can be difficult for patients. Undressing and exposure of genitals may be a trigger for individuals who have a history of abuse or those experiencing ongoing abuse. Some individuals may decline to have a pelvic examination for personal or cultural reasons. The midwife should explain the benefits of doing the examination and the information that can be obtained from the pelvic examination, but must respect the patient's autonomy in

declining or deferring the examination and must not cross the line into coercion once a patient declines the examination. Offering a chaperone is now recommended for all breast or chest, genital, and rectal examinations regardless of the gender of the examiner; patients have the right to decline the presence of a chaperone.[33,34]

## Interval Prenatal Visits

During interval prenatal visits, physical examination elements include blood pressure and weight. The clinician then assesses the interval weight gain and pattern of weight gain throughout the pregnancy. The clinician measures the fundal height in relation to the symphysis pubis and umbilicus prior to 20 weeks' gestation, but then uses a tape measure to determine this height (in centimeters) after 20 weeks' gestation. The clinician auscultates fetal heart tones, which can be heard as early as 12 weeks with a handheld Doppler and as early as 16 to 20 weeks with a fetoscope. The procedures of assessing fundal height and auscultating the fetal heart rate are described in the *Abdominal Examination During Pregnancy* appendix.

An entrenched practice that has been shown to be ineffective is routine assessment of the asymptomatic pregnant person's urine by dipstick at each interval prenatal visit. Primarily used in the past as a screen for preeclampsia, routine urine dipstick testing for proteinuria has been shown to provide no benefit.[35,36] Urine testing can be useful if the individual is experiencing problems such as hyperemesis or signs of a urinary tract infection that warrant further assessment.

## Additional Physical Examination Elements in Late Pregnancy

During late pregnancy visits, in addition to the interval prenatal visits described earlier, clinicians assess fetal presentation and, if clinically relevant, estimated fetal weight. Leopold's maneuvers to assess fetal presentation, lie, and position, and estimation of fetal weight are described in the *Abdominal Examination During Pregnancy* appendix.

During the last few weeks of pregnancy, some clinicians offer an examination of cervical dilation, effacement, and consistency, and an assessment of fetal station, position, and presentation. These examinations are sometimes performed to satisfy curiosity about the patient's cervical status or as an assessment to inform decisions about labor induction or other unique situations.[37] Shared decision making can be used to determine if a cervical examination is of value and desired by the individual.

## Physiologic Screening

This content focuses on the detection of potential physical problems that may not produce any symptoms of disease. The goal is early detection and lifestyle changes or surveillance either to reduce risk of disease or to detect and treat it. If such a condition is found, prompt consultation or referral for the appropriate type of care will ensure the best pregnancy outcome.

### Laboratory Tests

Laboratory tests may be performed for diagnosis or screening purposes. Screening tests are generally not considered diagnostic, but rather are used to identify a subset of the population who should have additional testing to determine the presence or absence of disease. Tests recommended or offered during pregnancy can be grouped into three categories:

- Laboratory tests that detect infection, immunity to infections known to have adverse perinatal effects, and certain pathologic processes are routinely performed in pregnancy. These screening tests may be recommended for all pregnancies or by risk profile (Table 21-6).
- Some tests are performed to screen for or diagnose fetal aneuploidy and chromosomal disorders. Screening tests are offered to pregnant individuals regardless of risk profile.[38]
- Carrier screening of either genetic parent to detect carrier status for inheritable autosomal disorders can be offered to expectant parents of any age.[39]

Most laboratory tests to detect infection, susceptibility to infection, and other pathologic processes that could result in risk to the pregnant individual or fetus are done at the first prenatal care visit, and may be repeated later in pregnancy, based on the individual's risk profile. Other laboratory tests in this category are performed at specific gestational ages (Table 21-6).

| Table 21-6 | Laboratory Screening Tests in Pregnancy | | |
|---|---|---|---|
| **Laboratory Test** | **Basis** | **Indication and Recommendations** | **Timing** |
| Urinalysis | Universal and risk-based | Baseline screen for protein to assess renal function | Entry to care |
| Urine culture | Universal | Recommended in all pregnancies to reduce perinatal complications | Entry to care |
| Blood type, Rhesus type | Universal | Rh (D)-negative individuals who do not have alloantibodies are offered prophylactic anti-D immune globulin at 28 weeks or to prevent alloimmunization | Entry to care. If Rh negative, repeat the antibody screen at 28 weeks prior to anti-D immune globulin administration. |
| Antibody screen | Universal | If antibodies are present, the baseline titer is used to monitor the condition as indicated by the type of positive titer. | Entry to care with follow-up individualized based on positive results |
| Complete blood count | Universal | Detects anemia and abnormal platelet levels. Follow-up based on individualized results. | Entry to care and early third trimester |
| Hepatitis B | Universal and risk-based | Recommended in all pregnancies to prevent perinatal transmission | Entry to care and again before giving birth if high risk |
| Hepatitis C | Universal | Recommended for all pregnant individuals | Entry to care |
| HIV | Universal and risk-based | Recommended in all pregnancies, as permitted by state regulations, to prevent perinatal transmission | Entry to care and again in the third trimester if high risk |
| Rubella | Universal | Individuals who are not immune are counseled to avoid exposure during pregnancy and offered vaccination postpartum. | Entry to care |

*(continues)*

| Table 21-6 | | Laboratory Screening Tests in Pregnancy (*continued*) | |
|---|---|---|---|
| **Laboratory Test** | **Basis** | **Indication and Recommendations** | **Timing** |
| Varicella | Risk-based | Recommended for individuals who do not report previous disease or vaccination | Entry to care |
| Tuberculosis | Risk-based | Recommended for all pregnant individuals at high risk of tuberculosis. Risk factors include:<br>• HIV infection<br>• Close contact with persons known or suspected to have TB<br>• Comorbidities and immune-suppression known to increase risk of sequelae from TB such as diabetes, lupus, cancer, renal disease, chronic steroid use, alcoholism, and substance use disorder<br>• Birth in or emigration from high-prevalence countries | Entry to care |
| Thyroid function (TSH) | Risk-based | Pregnant individuals who are taking thyroid medication or have signs or symptoms of thyroid disease | Entry to care |
| Syphilis (VDRL/RPR) | Universal and risk-based | Recommended in all pregnancies to prevent perinatal transmission | Entry to care and again in third trimester and at time of birth based on risk |
| Chlamydia (NAAT preferred) | Universal and risk-based | Recommended in all pregnancies to prevent perinatal transmission. Individuals at high risk of chlamydia should be retested in the third trimester. Risk factors include:<br>• Age younger than 25<br>• New sex partner<br>• Nonmonogamous relationship<br>• Sex partner with an STI | Entry to care and again in third trimester based on risk. If positive, repeat testing 3 to 4 weeks after treatment and again within 3 months. |
| Gonorrhea | Universal or risk-based | Recommended for all pregnant individuals at risk of gonorrhea. Risk factors include:<br>• Age younger than 25<br>• Living in a high-transmission area<br>• New or multiple partners<br>• Previous gonorrhea infection<br>• Other STI<br>• Inconsistent condom use<br>• Commercial sex work<br>• Drug use<br>If positive, repeat testing 3–6 months after treatment. | Entry to care and third trimester based on risk |
| Trichomoniasis | Risk-based | Recommended for all pregnant individuals with HIV | Entry to care |
| Gestational diabetes | Universal | Recommended in all pregnancies between 24 and 28 weeks | 24–28 weeks |

| Laboratory Test | Basis | Indication and Recommendations | Timing |
|---|---|---|---|
| Pregestational diabetes | Risk-based | Consider entry-to-care screening for individuals at higher risk for pregestational diabetes. Those at increased include those with:<br>• BMI ≥25<br>• Physical inactivity<br>• Previous GDM<br>• Previous infant weighing more than 4000 g<br>• First-degree relative with diabetes<br>• Polycystic ovarian syndrome or other condition associated with insulin resistance<br>• Ethnicity/race with high allostatic load (e.g., Black, Latinx, Native American, Asian American, Pacific Islander)<br>• History of cardiovascular disease<br>• Hypertension | First trimester/entry to care |
| Group B *Streptococcus* | Universal | Recommended in all pregnancies to prevent perinatal transmission, unless the individual has had GBS bacteriuria during the current pregnancy or a previously infected infant, in which case they should be given prophylactic antibiotics intrapartum. The midwife or the pregnant individual may collect the vaginal/rectal swab. | 36–37 weeks or earlier with symptoms of preterm labor |

Abbreviations: BMI, body mass index; GBS, group B *Streptococcus*; HIV, human immunodeficiency virus; NAAT, nucleic acid amplification test; STI, sexually transmitted infection; TB, tuberculosis; TSH, thyroid-stimulating hormone; VDRL/RPR, Venereal Disease Research Laboratory/rapid plasma reagin.

Based on American College of Obstetricians and Gynecologists, American Academy of Pediatrics. *Guidelines for Perinatal Care*. 8th ed. Washington, DC: American College of Obstetricians and Gynecologists; 2017. Published recommendations. https://www.acog.org /clinical-information/physician-faqs/-/media/3a22e153b67446a6b31fb051e469187c.ashx; Centers for Disease Control and Prevention. *Sexually Transmitted Diseases Treatment Guidelines, 2021*. Atlanta, GA: Centers for Disease Control and Prevention; 2021. https://www .cdc.gov/std/treatment-guidelines/STI-Guidelines-2021.pdf; U.S. Preventive Services Task Force. Published recommendations. https://www .uspreventiveservicestaskforce.org/BrowseRec/

## Genetic Screening and Testing

Carrier screening tests can be offered prior to conception or during pregnancy, and should be customized based on the individual's risks and preferences. Carrier screening tests are reviewed in the *Assessment for Genetic and Fetal Abnormalities* chapter, and frequently midwives refer patients to genetic counselors for more in-depth information. Multiple screening and diagnostic tests for fetal aneuploidy are available to pregnant individuals. Screening or diagnostic tests can be performed in the first or second trimester. Each test has different capabilities and limitations, which are reviewed in the *Assessment for Genetic and Fetal Abnormalities* chapter.

## Routine Fetal Ultrasound

Most pregnant individuals receive at least one ultrasound during pregnancy. In addition to determining gestational age, as described earlier in the chapter, ultrasound is routinely used to evaluate fetal cardiac activity, perform a fetal anatomic survey, measure fetal biometry, determine the number of fetuses, and check the location of the placenta.[25] Certified nurse-midwives and certified midwives may perform ultrasound evaluations with the proper training and certification.[40] When performed as recommended, ultrasound during all stages of pregnancy has been shown to be safe.[25]

### First Trimester Ultrasound Exam

In the first trimester, ultrasound is used to confirm the LMP dating or to establish the gestational age for those individuals without a known LMP. Other common reasons for conducting first trimester ultrasounds include determination of fetal viability, the location of the implantation or placenta, and the number of fetuses. Such evaluations can also be part of aneuploidy screening when conducted at a specific gestational age (see the *Assessment for Genetic and Fetal Abnormalities* chapter).[38] For low-risk individuals, the overall rate of detection for common anomalies using ultrasound is low in the first trimester, and this imaging is not routinely performed.[41]

### Second Trimester Ultrasound Exam

An ultrasound at 18 to 20 weeks' gestation has become a routine part of prenatal care offered to all pregnant individuals.[25] The primary purpose of this imaging is to detect structural fetal and placental anomalies.[41] The 18 to 20 weeks' gestational range is commonly used because by 18 weeks' gestation, enough amniotic fluid is present to support high-quality imaging and the fetal organs are formed and large enough that ultrasound can detect anatomic abnormalities.[25] It is important for midwives to be aware that many expectant parents view the mid-pregnancy ultrasound as simply the time they get to see their unborn child and find out if they are having a boy or a girl. When families are unprepared for the possibility that an abnormality could be discovered, they may react with stronger emotions than those families who are prepared for this outcome.[42] Midwives can counsel expectant parents prior to the ultrasound about the expected normal findings and possible abnormal findings, including the possibility of additional imaging being recommended.[42,43] Abnormal ultrasound findings are reviewed in the *Pregnancy-Related Conditions* chapter.

## Psychosocial Risk Screening

People who are pregnant may face multiple psychosocial challenges that have a negative impact on their personal health and pregnancy outcomes. At the same time, pregnancy is a profoundly significant period that is characterized by a shift in internal motivation. There are often feelings of self-efficacy and self-agency that result in a new capacity for self-care. In this context, fears of legal ramifications and retribution from child protective services may guide individuals to deny psychological challenges during their initial interactions with healthcare providers. However, they may be more motivated to confide and respond to assessments when they perceive that the provider is trustworthy.

Thus, midwives can impact the psychosocial aspects of prenatal health care by developing collaborative, empowering, goal-oriented communication skills that demonstrate acceptance, compassion, and partnership in a safe environment. For optimal effectiveness, midwives will engage in self-reflection and mindfulness regarding several factors, such as their implicit bias, the pervasiveness of psychosocial risk factors in the population and community, and the impact of social determinants on pregnancy outcomes. This foundation prepares midwives to approach their communication in a safe, person-centered manner. They may offer universal screening, knowing this may lead to immediate targeted, brief interventions, and specialty referrals that can ultimately effect change in morbidity and mortality outcomes. This section focuses on a variety of psychosocial screening and therapeutic communication techniques to assist the midwife with commonly encountered situations.

### Social and Structural Determinants of Health Screening

*Social determinants of health* (SDoH) refers to the social and environmental conditions in which people are born, grow, work, live, and age, as well as the wider set of forces and systems shaping the conditions of daily life.[44] Examples of social factors that may negatively affect pregnancy include housing, unemployment, food insecurity, exposure to environmental toxins, racism, poverty, and discrimination of all kinds. The World Health Organization (WHO) cites SDoH as one of the most important influences on health,[44] making this an excellent screening framework for exploring an individual's challenges during the pregnancy.

This is an evolving field of research, with emerging studies focusing on the association of racism and structural or systemic inequities with maternal mortality and severe morbidity, and evidence supporting the effects of race and ethnicity, insurance, and education on maternal mortality and severe morbidity.[45] However, such well-intentioned, problem-focused research conveys a "deficit discourse" that may affect the care provided by midwives. One strategy to counterbalance this deficit perspective is to explore the positive capabilities in the person's life. For example, there may be strong family engagement and a sense of community. Identifying these strengths provides a balanced approach that can reframe the context of the disadvantages faced by marginalized populations, and provides a sense of empowerment to the individual. A full discussion of SDoH can be found in the *Context of Individuals Seeking Midwifery Care* chapter.

### Trauma-Informed Screenings

People may endure multiple forms of violence and trauma. Sperlich et al.[46] conceptualized trauma as the occurrence of one or more specific events experienced by a person as harmful or life-threatening, which has lasting adverse effects on their functioning and well-being. Trauma may be acute (single incident), chronic (repeated or prolonged), or complex (varied and multiple events). Trauma is prevalent across all population groups, and is linked to adverse pregnancy outcomes.[47]

A landmark study conducted in the 1990s[45] revealed that adverse childhood experiences (ACEs) are potentially traumatic events that occur in childhood and exhibit a strong relationship between the breadth of the exposure and risk factors for several of the leading causes of death. Examples of additional health issues that are associated with ACEs include adolescent pregnancy, at-risk alcohol use, depression, intimate partner violence, suicide attempts, and substance use disorders. Beyond childhood, other forms of trauma, including post-traumatic stress disorder (PTSD) related to previous childbearing experiences, armed conflict, or mass-casualty violence, may occur.

Trauma occurs in all social contexts; however, marginalized individuals encounter fewer opportunities for recovery and more ongoing experiences.[46] Chronic traumatic exposures may also be a normalized experience for some people. For others, disclosure of traumatic exposures may be retraumatizing.

The pervasiveness of trauma exposure indicates a need for care provision that accounts for the impacts of trauma, recognizes its effects on people, integrates this knowledge into practice, and does not retraumatize the person. Figure 21-1 identifies the six principles that underscore trauma-informed care. Because of trauma's prevalence, the midwife should incorporate a universal trauma-informed approach to psychosocial screenings throughout pregnancy. Trauma-informed care is not a single technique or checklist; it is care that focuses on creating a safe, trustworthy environment that considers the person's social context. Trauma-informed care is provided through a stepped method of universal screening, targeted intervening, and specialized referral, as needed. The key to trauma-informed care is a trusting therapeutic relationship between the client and the midwife.[47]

It may take time for the client to view the provider as safe and trustworthy. To demonstrate that they meet these standards, and to tailor interventions to their practice population's needs, midwifery practices can determine the extent of trauma survivorship within their population. The PTSD Checklist (PCL) and the Trauma History Questionnaire are two validated, widely used screening tools. It may be easier for a person to complete the screening questionnaire in private and either submit it electronically or drop in a locked box at the clinic.[47] Midwifery clinics can demonstrate that they are safe spaces for trauma survivors by hanging posters or displaying resources that target the areas identified by their population. Some individuals do not choose to reveal their trauma, while others appreciate the opportunity to speak about it, as they feel it helps them to heal. A trauma-informed provider respects both approaches.[47]

## Intimate Partner Violence Screening

Intimate partner violence (IPV) significantly affects individuals of all gender identities. IPV is the most common form of violence against cisgender women.[48] In addition, transgender individuals experience a higher prevalence of IPV compared with cisgender individuals, regardless of sex assigned at birth.[48] Any person can encounter IPV, irrespective of race, ethnicity, socioeconomic status, profession, sexual orientation, or gender identity. The violence may manifest as threatened or actual physical, sexual, verbal, or psychological abuse, and is more likely to escalate during pregnancy. IPV requires a trauma-informed approach to screening. People may be more vulnerable to the effects of violence while pregnant, due to their physical condition or their financial and emotional dependence. When a pregnant individual is exposed to violence, child abuse is also more likely to occur. A trauma-informed practice is to recognize that people may need time to

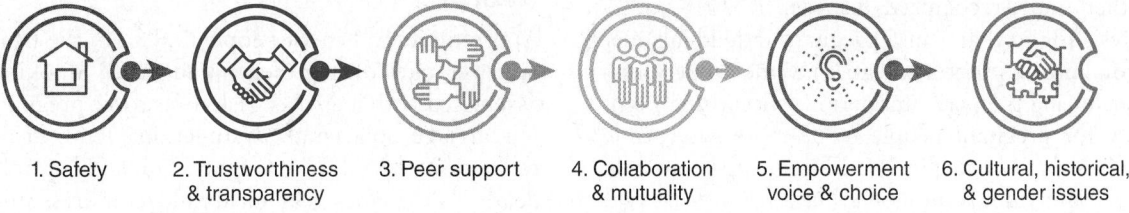

1. Safety   2. Trustworthiness & transparency   3. Peer support   4. Collaboration & mutuality   5. Empowerment voice & choice   6. Cultural, historical, & gender issues

**Figure 21-1** Six guiding principles to a trauma-informed approach.
From Centers for Disease Control and Prevention, Center for Preparedness and Response. 6 guiding principles to a trauma-informed approach. https://www.cdc.gov/cpr/infographics/6_principles_trauma_info.htm. Published 2020. Accessed August 25, 2021.

consider whether they want to reveal the violence during prenatal care.[49]

ACNM, ACOG, and the U.S. Preventive Services Task Force (USPSTF) recommend screening each trimester for IPV.[49] There is no single set of absolute indicators of IPV, but people who are exposed to violence are more likely to have the following characteristics: late entry to prenatal care or missed appointments, nonmedical or excessive use of substances, sexually transmitted infections, poor weight gain and nutrition, multiple somatic complaints or hospital visits, and undesired pregnancy.

A variety of screening tools for IPV can be used, though all such screening should be conducted in private.[50] There is no single screening method or tool that has demonstrated consistently high sensitivity and specificity in screening for IPV, especially in outpatient settings with diverse populations. Midwives may choose to screen for IPV in a face-to-face interview, using a self-administered questionnaire, or using a computer-assisted self-interview.[51] Some practices also have informational materials and ways to disclose IPV placed in the patient bathroom. Use of a variety of methods can give people multiple opportunities to disclose IPV.

Individuals experiencing IPV can be in grave danger; when it is revealed, the midwife has an ethical responsibility to provide needed resources and to follow up as indicated. The midwife's primary role in working with someone who screens positive for IPV is to assess their safety, assist the person in making a safety plan if needed, accurately document findings, and refer the individual to the appropriate resources. Midwives also need to be aware of legal reporting requirements. In particular, child abuse is reportable in all jurisdictions in the United States.

## Depression and Anxiety Screening

The perinatal period is a vulnerable time for the development of mental health disorders. A 2016 review of longitudinal studies reported an average prevalence of 17% for depression during pregnancy, with 39% of people continuing on to develop postpartum depression.[52] Anxiety in pregnancy is another under-recognized disorder. A 2019 meta-analysis found that 1 in 5 pregnant individuals met the diagnostic criteria for at least one anxiety disorder during the perinatal period, with a small tendency for pregnant people to be more susceptible than postpartum people. In addition, approximately 1 in 20 individuals met the criteria for at least two anxiety disorders.[53] Untreated depression has been associated with adverse perinatal outcomes, impaired maternal–infant attachment, and disordered family relationships.[54] Screening for depression and anxiety is recommended for all pregnant individuals, along with prompt treatment and/or referral.[55] For those pregnant individuals at high risk for developing depression, the USPSTF recommends providing or referring them for counseling interventions, such as cognitive-behavioral therapy or interpersonal therapy (B recommendation).[56] For individuals with moderate to severe depression, selective serotonin reuptake inhibitors (SSRIs) are an additional therapy for use in pregnancy.[57] The *Mental Health Conditions* chapter has more information on screening tools and evidence-based management.

## Substances Screening

Substance-use screening (tobacco, cannabis, alcohol, opioids, and other products) is part of the general health history. Use of substances or misuse of prescription drugs may cause fear of legal ramifications for the person and their unborn child, resulting in late presentation for care. It is the responsibility of the midwife and clinic staff to create an environment of respect and safety that allows a person to feel safe enough to disclose their use. The recognition of SDoH and trauma-informed care practices provide the foundation for effective midwifery screening practices. The National Harm Reduction Coalition has published a training guide for providers who work with people who are pregnant and using substances.[58] It recommends implementing a trauma-informed approach and focuses on positive regard, motivational interviewing, and person-first language that avoids stigmatizing the user. Figure 21-2 provides examples of motivational interview techniques. The *Skillful Communication to Mitigate Clinician Bias* appendix also contains strategies for improving therapeutic communication and decreasing bias within the clinical interaction. The *Mental Health Conditions* chapter provides an overview of substance use disorder and the *Health Promotion Across the Lifespan* chapter reviews screening and counseling related to substance use.

### Tobacco

Approximately 1 in 14 people (7.9%) in the United States smokes during their pregnancy.[59] Smoking is associated with increased risk for ectopic pregnancy, miscarriage, placental dysfunction, fetal growth restriction, low birth weight, and sudden infant death.[60] Pregnancy is an ideal time to address smoking cessation. Individuals have identified the following factors as motivators for smoking cessation in pregnancy: risk for infant health, encouragement

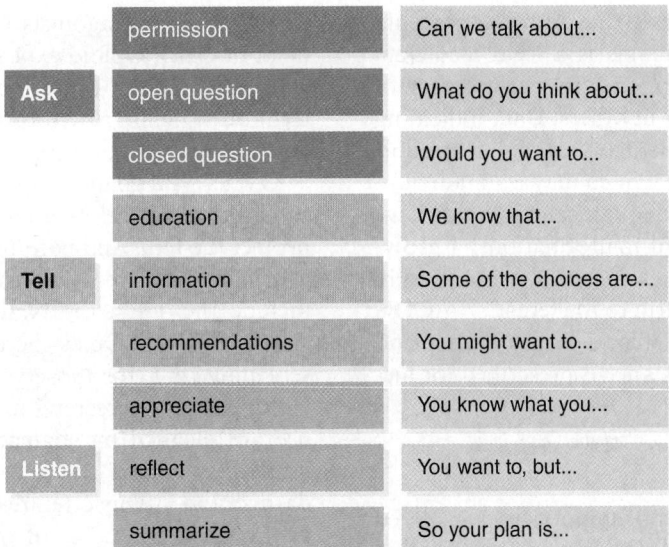

**Figure 21-2** Motivational Interview Methods.
Reproduced with permission from National Harm Reduction Coalition. Pregnancy and substance use: a harm reduction toolkit. https://harmreduction.org/issues/pregnancy-and-substance-use-a-harm-reduction-toolkit/. Published September 24, 2021. Accessed September 20, 2022.

and support from social network, access to behavioral and pharmacologic cessation treatments, increase in cigarette prices, and the warning labels on tobacco packages.[60] The USPSTF recommends that clinicians ask all pregnant persons about tobacco use, advise them to stop using tobacco, and provide behavioral interventions to encourage cessation to pregnant individuals who use tobacco (Recommendation A).[61] As many as 45% of people who smoke do stop during pregnancy, despite the metabolism of nicotine during pregnancy being faster, which can make smoking cessation more difficult.

Smoking-cessation interventions have been shown to lower the incidence of low-birth-weight infants and preterm birth.[62] Multiple options are available to help people to reduce or quit smoking. Nicotine patches, gum, lozenges, and e-cigarettes are available without a prescription, and are safe for use in pregnancy.[63] Insurance may cover the gum products, patches, or lozenges with a prescription from a healthcare provider. Smoking cessation counseling via use of the 5 A's prenatal smoking-cessation approach can be effective. Notably, a pilot study in West Virginia demonstrated a clear reduction in pregnant women's smoking after midwives were trained to use the 5 A's program.[64]

Behavioral interventions alone may be insufficient for the majority of individuals who attempt smoking cessation during pregnancy. However, research on the effects of smoking-cessation medications used during pregnancy is too limited to determine the harms and benefits.[61] The USPSTF has also concluded that the evidence on the use of e-cigarettes for tobacco smoking cessation in adults, including pregnant persons, is insufficient, and the balance of their benefits and harms cannot be determined. The USPSTF has identified the lack of well-designed, randomized clinical trials on e-cigarettes that report smoking abstinence or adverse events as a critical gap in the evidence.[61] A systematic review of vaping as a smoking-cessation modality during pregnancy also reported insufficient evidence to draw a conclusion on the effect of vaping in pregnancy; however, the limited evidence suggested it had little to no effect on infant birth weight.[65] Despite insufficient evidence on these products' use in pregnancy, many providers recommend nicotine sprays, inhaler, and medications such as bupropion (Wellbutrin) or varenicline (Chantix) to help people who are pregnant reduce or quit smoking. Tran et al. found no association with increased risk or adverse birth outcomes with the use of bupropion, varenicline, and nicotine replacement therapies.[66] However, these researchers concluded that there is still insufficient evidence to recommend their use.[66]

## Cannabis

Aside from tobacco and alcohol, cannabis is the most commonly used substance that leads to dependency.[67] It crosses the placenta, and chemoreceptors for cannabinoids are present in both the placenta and the fetal brain. Cannabis is a legal medicinal and recreational product in a growing number of states, but remains illegal in others. Data indicating safety or harm to the fetus from cannabis use during pregnancy are limited, which may lead individuals to believe it is safe. Although cannabinoids have not been linked with fetal malformations, a growing evidence base indicates that in utero exposure to cannabis may cause harm to the fetus.[68,69] ACOG advises cessation of cannabis use in pregnancy and lactation, even if this substance is prescribed for medicinal purposes.[70]

### Alcohol

No amount of alcohol consumption is considered safe in pregnancy. The dose–response relationship between alcohol intake and fetal effects is unknown. Alcohol freely crosses the placenta, and its elimination from both the maternal and fetal systems depends on the metabolism of the pregnant individual.

From 2015 to 2017, one in nine pregnant individuals (11.5%) reported drinking alcohol in the past 30 days. One-third of those (3.9%) reported binge drinking, with an average of 4.5 binges in the past 30 days.[71] A standard drink constitutes 5 ounces of wine (12% alcohol content), 12 ounces of beer (5% alcohol content), or 1.5 ounces of distilled liquor (40% alcohol content).

Alcohol consumption during pregnancy can cause miscarriage, stillbirth, and birth defects known as fetal alcohol syndrome disorders (lifelong physical, behavioral, and intellectual disabilities). Fetal alcohol syndrome is one of the most common preventable causes of mental disability in the United States. Universal screening and brief counseling, using motivational interviewing techniques, might potentially decrease the prevalence of drinking in pregnancy (See Figure 21-2 for motivational interviewing techniques.)

### Opioids

Opioid misuse in pregnancy continues to escalate, with an estimated 131% increase in opioid-related diagnoses at birth occurring from 2010 to 2017.[72] Opioid use disorder (OUD) refers to a problematic pattern of use that results in marked impairment or distress. Rates of OUD in pregnancy quadrupled from 1999 to 2014, from 1.5 to 6.5 per 1000 hospital births,[73] with rates of opioid misuse growing faster in rural areas.[74] Reasons for opioid use in pregnancy include prescribed pain management, misuse of prescribed opioids, use of illicit opioids, or use of opioid agonists or antagonists for treatment of OUD. Opioid exposure during pregnancy is associated with poor birth outcomes, including preterm birth, fetal growth restriction, stillbirths, birth defects, and neonatal opioid withdrawal syndrome (NOWS).[72] Pregnancy may be a motivational factor for a person to seek treatment, due to their desire to protect the fetus and become a responsible parent.[75]

Validated screening instruments for opioid use include the 4 P's, the National Institute on Drug Abuse (NIDA) Quick Screen, and the CRAFFT screening tool (for those younger than 26 years.)[76] Unfortunately, screening and treatment for opioid use are plagued by stigmatization, discrimination, limited supportive resources, and lack of care standardization.[77] This often results in those with OUD avoiding care because of guilt, shame, embarrassment, fear of judgment, criminalization, and fear of losing custody of their children.[77]

Midwives must first recognize their own contributions to the situation, acknowledging that there may be an intersection of socioeconomic status, race, and addiction that contributes to client mistrust in under-resourced environments.[77] The *Skillful Communication to Mitigate Clinician Bias* appendix provides strategies to approach conversations about sensitive topics with patients. Universal screening; targeted interventions focused on progression, rather than complete abstinence; medication therapy; and referral for supportive housing during recovery are the cornerstones to the treatment of OUD.

Integration of medication treatment with prenatal care is an important strategy to increase access to OUD treatment and reduce stigma.[77] ACOG supports the use of buprenorphine and methadone as best practice for the treatment of perinatal OUD.[76] Both have been shown to be safe and effective treatments for opioid use disorder during pregnancy.[74] Medication treatment of OUD during pregnancy is associated with decreased risk of opioid overdose, preterm birth, and low birth weight.[78] While NOWS can still occur in newborns whose mothers received these medications, it is less severe than in the absence of treatment.[74] Research does not support reducing medication doses to prevent NOWS, as doing so may lead to withdrawal symptoms and increased illicit drug use, resulting in greater risk to the fetus.[74]

### Use of Other Substances

The many other substances that have the potential for misuse challenge attempts to categorize them. Stimulants, inhalants, dissociative drugs, and hallucinogens are current categories in use.

Stimulants is an umbrella term for substances that increase the activity of the central nervous system and create a sense of euphoria. Although many everyday beverages fall into this category, the focus here is on the substances that may be prescribed or illicit, such as cocaine, methamphetamines, Ecstasy, prescription stimulants, and the herb ephedra. Stimulants are widely prescribed for mood disorders, attention-deficit disorders, sleep disorders, and obesity. Stimulant use in pregnancy is an under-recognized epidemic, with these agents constituting the second most widely used substances, behind cannabis.[79] Women exhibit increased vulnerability to developing a misuse disorder, and may progress faster from first exposure to addiction (known as "telescoping"), when compared to men.[79] Illicit use of stimulants in pregnancy has been associated with cardiovascular effects for the pregnant individual and negative neonatal outcomes including preterm birth, low birth weight, and small for gestational age, as well as vertical transmission of HIV, hepatitis, and syphilis.[79] Cocaine misuse is the leading cause of antepartum hospitalizations for substance use.[79]

Universal screening and brief interventions for stimulant use may produce positive responses in those persons who are at low to moderate risk for misuse. High-risk individuals (i.e., those meeting the criteria for a substance use disorder) generally require referral for specialized treatment.[80] There are no Food and Drug Administration (FDA)–approved medications for stimulant use disorder.[79]

Inhalant misuse is a global problem that occurs most frequently in adolescents. Indeed, more U.S. eighth-graders report use of inhalants than of any illicit drugs. Use spans all cultures and geographic areas.[81] Inhalants encompass a special group of drugs that are classified according to their shared administration route, rather than their similar pharmacologic properties. A wide variety of chemicals fall into this category. Some are gases; others become vapors at room temperature. The commonalities are that they are intentionally self-administered to achieve quick intoxication. In addition, these substances are legal, and are available in many commercial products. Toluene is the chemical most commonly used as an inhalant, and is readily available in such items as glue, paint thinners, and felt-tip markers.

To date, only very limited research has been done on inhalant agents. Animal studies suggest that the primary physiologic outcomes when used in pregnancy are low birth weight[82] and long-term neurotoxic effects on offspring.[83,84] Bowen reported on a sudden sniffing death and fetal solvent syndrome, similar to fetal alcohol syndrome.[84] Further research is needed to identify risks in individuals who are pregnant. Cruz and Bowen concluded that the effects depend on the duration of inhalation, number of repetitions, and length of prior use.[81,84]

### Summary of Substance Use

People who are pregnant may face multiple psychosocial challenges that have a negative impact on their personal health and pregnancy outcomes. Screening for substance use is recommended for all individuals early in pregnancy.[85] Several validated tools for substance use screening are available, as reviewed in the *Health Promotion Across the Lifespan* chapter. ACOG recommends universal screening, brief interventions, and referral for treatment for misuse of all substances discussed here, as well as dissociative drugs and hallucinogens.[86]

The pervasiveness of psychosocial risk factors in the population supports universal screening for substance use. Initial universal screening can lead to health interventions to improve outcomes or to specialty referrals. In addition to clinicians' reflection and mindfulness regarding their own biases and knowledge of social determinants, the development of person-centered communication skills may offer opportunities for the clinician to alleviate identified risks during the screening process (see the *Skillful Communication to Mitigate Clinician Bias* appendix). The care of an individual struggling with substance use also requires collaboration with professionals in multidisciplinary programs who have skills in treating substance misuse and addictions. Team-based care and referrals should be implemented to improve the person's health and experience of care. Unfortunately, care for substance use disorder can be difficult to obtain in pregnancy. Support in obtaining treatment and continued provision of prenatal care during treatment can improve both short- and long-term outcomes for the pregnant person and their child.

The factors that motivate recovery in a person who has been misusing substances are varied and unpredictable. Sometimes concern about a fetus during pregnancy may be the catalyst to begin the cycle of recovery. Insurance coverage during pregnancy may improve access to desired services. By providing ongoing care and support while recognizing the recovery/relapse pattern, the midwife can work to minimize maternal and fetal complications, encourage decreased substance use, and support the individual appropriately, depending on where they are in the cycle of recovery.

## Health Promotion During Pregnancy

Health promotion strategies are a core component of midwifery care for all people, as presented in the *Health Promotion Across the Lifespan* chapter. Nevertheless, many individuals do not access primary healthcare services until they are pregnant, and certain health promotion strategies are particularly important for fetal health. Thus, prenatal care is considered one of the most opportune periods to address these educational topics.

### Nutrition

A growing body of evidence indicates that nutrition in pregnancy can not only reduce the pregnant individual's risks of health problems in pregnancy, such as anemia and hypertensive disorders, but also has lifelong implications for the fetus.[87,88] Exposure to a high-quality diet in utero can reduce risk for chronic health conditions throughout their lifetime.[88] An optimal diet in pregnancy includes protein, whole grains, fruits, and vegetables. However, the quality of prenatal diets in the United States is generally poor, due in large part to excessive consumption of processed foods.[89] Food insecurity and disparities in nutrition during pregnancy may contribute to the higher rates of pregnancy-related death in the United States, especially for pregnant individuals of color and those who live in rural areas.[90]

The Special Supplemental Nutrition Program for Women, Infants, and Children (WIC) provided by the U.S. Department of Agriculture (USDA) has the goal of providing excellent nutrition to pregnant individuals, lactating parents, and young children up to age 5. Policy changes in 2009 made improvements in the dietary intakes of WIC participants by including farmer's markets as sources of nutrition and increasing access to fresh fruits and vegetables.[91] However, farmer's markets and even grocery stores with high-quality fresh produce are in short supply in many communities where WIC participants live. While multiple studies have found that pregnant participants have improved pregnancy outcomes when compared to pregnant individuals who do not participate in WIC, other studies have not shown any improvements.[92] Economic factors, based on the crops and food commodities subsidized by the USDA, may be a more powerful driver of consumable items covered by WIC than optimal nutrition from a largely plant-based diet.[93]

Most pregnant individuals are motivated to be healthy for their babies and want to receive positive advice on what to eat in pregnancy to promote health, rather than messages focusing on what not to do. Pregnancy can be a window of opportunity for individuals to make changes that improve their health.[94–96] Pregnant individuals who experience depression are at particular risk for poor diet quality and can benefit from additional nutritional counseling that is sensitive to their needs.[97] It is imperative that midwives and other prenatal care providers provide person-centered education on optimal nutrition in pregnancy that is individualized and sensitive to the person's access to food, cultural food preferences, and applicable social determinants of health, while also being free from weight bias.[95,96,98] A brief overview of dietary advice for pregnant individuals is found in Table 21-7. Detailed information on nutrition and the macronutrients needs in pregnancy is covered in the *Nutrition* chapter.

### Food Safety

Because a growing fetus can be particularly vulnerable to certain toxins and food-borne illnesses, it is important to give pregnant individuals information on foods to avoid. Such foods include:

- Soft cheeses, unless they clearly state they are made from pasteurized milk
- Pâtés and meat spreads, deli meats, and hot dogs (unless heated to steaming before eating)
- Raw sprouts, eggs, or mixtures containing raw eggs, such as unbaked cookie dough
- Raw or undercooked meats and fish, including smoked seafood
- Mercury-concentrating fish: king mackerel, marlin, orange roughy, shark, swordfish, tilefish (Gulf of Mexico), tuna (bigeye)[99]

### Vegetarians

The term *vegetarian* can encompass a number of subpopulations: individuals whose diets include dairy (lacto-vegetarians); those who eat eggs (ovo-vegetarians); and those who eat both dairy and eggs (lacto-ovo vegetarians). Pregnant individuals who eat any of the vegetarian diets can meet all their nutritional needs and have healthy birth outcomes,[100] although some modifications may be needed. In brief, a vegetarian diet during pregnancy may not provide the recommended daily amounts of iron, vitamin D, vitamin E, choline, and omega-3 fatty acids or docosahexaenoic acid (DHA).[101–103]

Individuals who strictly eat only foods from plant sources can be called vegans. Pregnant individuals consuming a vegan diet need to be certain that they are receiving vitamin $B_{12}$ and calcium.[101] See the *Nutrition* chapter for more detailed information.

| Table 21-7 | Overview of Positively Framed Nutritional Advice for All Pregnant Individuals |
|---|---|
| **Diet** | |
| Meals and snacks | Eat three meals a day and two snacks consisting of whole, unprocessed foods. Over each day, meals and snacks should ideally include: <br>• 5 servings of fiber-rich fruits and vegetables <br>• Other fiber-rich carbohydrates such as whole grains <br>• 60 g of lean protein from well-cooked, unprocessed meats, including fish and poultry, eggs, pasteurized cheese, or vegetable sources. <br>• 20% to 35% of daily calories from fats, with monosaturated fats as the primary type of fat consumed |
| Drinks | Water is the best hydration in pregnancy, and a person who is getting enough water will have pale urine, but other non-alcoholic drinks can be enjoyed. Safe, healthy choices include: <br>• Dairy milk and alternative/nut milks <br>• Tea of coffee containing up to 200 mg of caffeine a day <br>• Unsweetened, flavored sparkling waters |
| **Important Micronutrients, Vitamins, and Minerals** | |
| Folic acid | Getting adequate folic acid before conception and during the first trimester can prevent neural tube defects. Due to the widespread availability of foods fortified with folic acid in the United States, many individuals will get an adequate amount in their diets, but most pregnant individuals will still take a supplement of 400 mcg or more daily. |
| Iron | Foods from animal sources contain heme iron, which is easiest to absorb. Plant sources of iron include beans and lentils, tofu, cashews, and dark green leafy vegetables, and absorption is increased with concurrent ingestion of vitamin C. |
| Omega-3 fatty acid | Fish such as salmon, freshwater trout, shrimp, and canned, light tuna are good sources of omega-3 fatty acids, yet low in mercury. Pregnant individuals can also take an omega-3 fatty acid or docosahexaenoic acid (DHA) supplement. |
| Prenatal vitamins | Multivitamins can be important sources for additional vitamins and minerals needed in pregnancy, although there is not good evidence to say that all individuals need to take a prenatal vitamin. The typical composition of micronutrients in a prenatal vitamin and the percentage of the daily value recommended for pregnant and lactating individuals are as follows: <br><br>Vitamin A — 4000 IU as beta carotene (50%) <br>Vitamin $D_3$ — 400 IU as cholecalciferol (100%) <br>Vitamin E — 11 IU as DL-alpha-tocopherol acetate (37%) <br>Folic acid — 800 mcg (100%) <br>Niacin — 18 mg as niacinamide (90%) <br>Riboflavin — 1.7 mg as thiamine mononitrate (85%) <br>Thiamine — 1.5 mg (88%) <br>Vitamin $B_6$ — 2.6 mg as pyridoxine hydrochloride (104%) <br>Vitamin $B_{12}$ — 4 mg as cyanocobalamin (50%) <br>Vitamin C — 100 mg as ascorbic acid (167%) <br>Calcium — 150 mg as calcium carbonate (12%) <br>Iron — 27 mg as ferrous fumarate (150%) <br>Zinc — 25 mg as zinc oxide (167%) |

Based on Barger MK. Maternal nutrition and perinatal outcomes. *J Midwifery Womens Health*. 2010;55(6):502-511. doi:10.1016/j.jmwh.2010.02.017; Kominiarek MA, Rajan P. Nutrition recommendations in pregnancy and lactation. *Med Clin North Am*. 2016;100(6):1199-1215. doi:10.1016/j.mcna.2016.06.004.

### Medical Conditions That Affect Nutrition

Medical conditions that adversely impact nutrition during pregnancy include eating disorders, a history of bariatric surgery,[104] conditions associated with malabsorption, and need for medications, such as antiepileptic agents that affect folic acid metabolism. The most likely nutritional deficiencies in pregnant individuals with medical conditions that diminish their ability to absorb nutrients have been identified. Midwives caring for these individuals can consult with a maternal–fetal medicine specialist and/or a registered dietician to individualize their care. See the *Medical Complications in Pregnancy* chapter for more detailed pharmacotherapeutic information specific to a number of conditions.

### Multifetal Gestation

There are no national guidelines for the increases in other nutritional requirements for pregnant individuals carrying more than one fetus, but a systematic review suggests a higher risk for vitamin D and iron deficiencies.[105] The evidence for risk of other micronutrient deficiencies is inconclusive. When participating in the care of pregnant individuals carrying more than one fetus, collaboration with a nutrition expert will optimize outcomes.

### Pica

Pica is an unusual condition in which an individual purposefully ingests nonfood items. It is more common in pregnant individuals than in individuals who are not pregnant. The prevalence of pica varies by geographic region and culture, but has been noted to affect as many as 50% of women in some settings.[106] The most common substances eaten are earth, clay, or dirt; raw starches such as cornstarch; and ice and freezer frost. The etiology of pica is unknown, although several theories exist. There is a clear association between ice-ingestion pica and iron-deficiency anemia, but it is not clear whether pica causes anemia or whether anemia triggers pica. Pica can cause lead poisoning and may be associated with other micronutrient deficiencies. Management consists of diagnosis and treatment of nutritional deficiencies, assessment of hunger or eating disorders, and health education.

### Physical Activity

Ideally, pregnant individuals will engage in 30 minutes of moderate physical activity, including aerobic exercise and strength training, almost every day, for a total of 150 minutes of moderate-intensity exercise spread through the week.[89] Examples of exercise modalities that have been found to be both safe and beneficial in pregnancy are aerobic exercises such as walking, swimming and water aerobics, stationary cycling, and dancing; and strength training such as resistance with weights and bands, and yoga. Exercise programs may need to be modified for pregnant individuals, and midwives recommend individuals stay well hydrated, avoid prolonged exercise in the heat, and not to exert themselves to the point that they are too short of breath to talk. Although there are multiple barriers to remaining active in pregnancy, walking—the most common physical activity in pregnancy—appears to be more likely to be sustained in pregnancy.[107] An activity that a person enjoys is more likely to be continued than one that feels like a chore, so midwives can promote health by encouraging activities the individual likes rather than what may be a standard recommendation.

Pregnant individuals of any weight who exercise regularly are more likely to have a term baby at a healthy weight who is born vaginally, and are less likely to experience pregnancy complications such as excessive weight gain, gestational diabetes, and gestational hypertensive disorders.[108] Prenatal exercise may help reduce health disparities experienced by non-Hispanic Black pregnant individuals due to the stress of racism.[109] However, pregnant individuals living in under-resourced communities may have limited access to safe outdoor spaces or other places to gather for physical activity that are affordable.[110] Midwives should be aware of this dynamic and can use a shared decision-making approach to work with pregnant individuals to find a solution.

### Weight Gain

Weight gain recommendations during pregnancy are based on prepregnancy BMI (Table 21-8), and appropriate gestational weight gain can be a good indicator of sufficient nutritional intake.[111] For individuals whose prepregnancy BMI is less than 25, recommended weight gain is approximatively 1 pound per week in the third trimester. For individuals whose prepregnancy BMI is 25 or greater, the recommended weight gain drops to approximately 0.5 pounds per week. Inadequate pregnancy weight gain is associated with low-birth-weight infants and preterm birth, while excessive pregnancy weight gain also carries multiple risks.[111] These risks include hypertensive disorders in pregnancy, gestational diabetes, cesarean birth, postpartum weight retention, and development of chronic disease for the pregnant individual.[89,111] Motivational interviewing (Figure 21-2), in which the relationship between the provider and the individual allows them to work together to make an effective, person-centered

| Table 21-8 | Gestational Weight Gain Recommendations | |
|---|---|---|
| | Prepregnancy | Gestational Weight Gain Recommendations |
| Category | BMI, kg/m² | Total Weight Gain at Term, pounds |
| Underweight | <18.5 | 28–40 |
| Normal weight | 18.5–24.9 | 25–35 |
| Overweight | 25.0–29.9 | 15–25 |
| Obesity | ≥30 | 11–20 |

Abbreviation: BMI, body mass index.
Based on Institute of Medicine. *Weight Gain During Pregnancy: Reexamining the Guidelines*. Washington, DC: Institute of Medicine; 2009.

strategy, can be a useful tool enabling midwives to support positive diet and activity changes a pregnant person plans to make.[112]

It is important to note that BMI was not originally developed to be a tool applied to individuals, and it does not always correlate well with health or pregnancy outcomes, especially for individuals who identify as Black, Asian, or Hispanic.[113,114] Focusing on the quality of an individual's nutritional intake and activity level in pregnancy may be a better approach. Two-thirds of the U.S. population is overweight or obese, and discussing nutrition and weight gain with these pregnant individuals can be especially fraught.[115] In fact, although the word *obesity* is an accepted clinical term, many individuals regard it as pejorative. Midwives might consider using the phrase "person with a larger body" instead.

Incorporating a *Health at Every Size* (HAES) approach into midwifery practice encourages respect for the diversity of body types while focusing on healthy behaviors known to improve health. Because HAES takes an intersectional approach, recognizing the role that weight, racism, and economic status play in health disparities, it promotes a type of respectful care that may help reduce inequities in health care.[116]

## Medications and Supplements

Despite concerns about safety and a lack of research on the efficacy of most medications in pregnancy, use of medications in pregnancy is common.[117] A large national study of a diverse cohort of U.S. women in their first pregnancy found that, excluding vaccines, vitamins, and supplements, 73.4% of participants used at least one prescription or over-the-counter medication during pregnancy and 30.5% of women used five or more medications during their pregnancy. The most common types of medications taken in pregnancy were gastrointestinal agents and antiemetics, analgesics, and antibiotics.[118] The use

and dosing of medications in pregnancy is an area of ongoing research.[117,118]

Pregnant individuals need information and guidance about the risks and benefits of medications in pregnancies so that they can make informed choices. Midwives who maintain an up-to-date knowledge base regarding pharmacokinetics and pharmacogenomics are well positioned to provide this guidance.[117] Midwives should review all of the drugs, medications, and supplements taken by an individual, using a reliable source to determine their effects in pregnancy. A list of over-the-counter medications that are safe in pregnancy should also be given to individuals at their initial visit. Additional information on medications for specific conditions can be found in the *Pregnancy-Related Conditions* and *Medical Complications in Pregnancy* chapters.

## Occupational Health

Pregnant individuals contribute significantly to the U.S. workforce. Of the 23.5 million working mothers, 45% cite pregnancy as a reason for taking unpaid leave for more than 2 weeks.[119] (No data are currently available on the other individuals taking such leave.) Working during pregnancy is generally quite safe. Yet, some major issues are associated with working in pregnancy, such as pregnancy-related discrimination, work accommodations that allow for continued employment, job-protected leave, and wage replacement while on leave.[120] The Pregnancy Discrimination Act of 1964 protects pregnant persons from being fired secondary to being pregnant. It is also illegal to ban an individual from a particular job if they might become pregnant. Complaints about pregnancy discrimination based on the 1964 act are filed with the U.S. Equal Employment Opportunity Commission.

One in five pregnant individuals works in a low-paying job. Such jobs tend to be physically demanding and have reduced flexibility in work hours and conditions.[121] They are also occupied

| Table 21-9 | How to Write a Work Accommodation Note |
|---|---|

1. Only suggest a work restriction or modification when medically necessary. Start as small as possible and scale up to give the employer more flexibility for accommodations.

2. Try to determine whether the requested job modification limits an essential function (e.g., a typist must be able to type). Discuss possible accommodations to the request and the risks of requesting them (e.g., if an accommodation to an essential function is requested that cannot be provided, the employer may place the employee on medical leave. If the employee is not eligible for medical leave, they may be terminated).

3. Specifically state the work restriction (e.g., "Due to her pregnancy-related condition, it is medically advisable that Ms. Xyz not stand for prolonged periods [more than 2 hours continuously] without a break or without an opportunity to sit").

4. It is not necessary to suggest an accommodation, but doing so can be helpful to the employer and employee. Be as specific as possible (e.g., "I recommend the following reasonable accommodation: providing a stool or a 15-minute break every 2 hours"). Avoid general statements, such as "no physical activity" or "decreased stress." Do not request "light duty," as this has a specific legal definition, and not all employers have a light duty option. Asking for light duty may lead to a denial of the accommodation, leaving medical leave as the only option.

5. State that the person is able to continue to work (e.g., "Ms. Xyz is able to continue working with a reasonable accommodation").

6. State the expected duration of the modification (which can be extended).

Data from Jackson RA, Gardner S, Torres LN, Huchko MJ, Zlatnik MG, Williams JC. My obstetrician got me fired: how work notes can harm pregnant patients and what to do about it. *Obstet Gynecol.* 2015;126:250–254.

disproportionately by persons of color.[121] Accommodations like a stool to avoid prolonged standing, or a bottle of water to prevent dehydration, are simple changes that are short-term, inexpensive pregnancy adaptations that can enhance the individual's ability to actively support their family. Yet, the manner in which a midwife advocates for a pregnant individual to receive an accommodation can affect whether it is allowed by the employer. Table 21-9 describes the contents of a satisfactory accommodation note.

Multiple work hazards can affect the health of a pregnant individual, including stress, noise, heavy lifting, prolonged standing, prolonged sitting, shift work, or long work hours, as well as environmental exposures. Information about the most common workplace hazards is available from the Centers for Disease Control and Prevention (CDC).[122] Clinical guidelines for occupational lifting have been published and are shown in Figure 21-3.[122] Laws and eligibility requirements governing pregnancy-related disability for childbirth vary by state.

Parental leave benefits are usually a combination of short-term disability, sick leave, vacation, and unpaid leave. Not all jobs offer parental leave benefits. Although the federal Family Medical Leave Act (FMLA) mandates that individuals receive 12 weeks of unpaid leave for childrearing in a 12-month period, many women are not eligible for FMLA benefits.

Table 21-10 describes the role of the midwife in the preservation of occupational health in pregnancy.[123]

## Environmental Exposures

Environmental exposures may either improve or worsen prenatal health. Emerging evidence is finding that prenatal exposure to green spaces is associated with healthy birth weights, especially in individuals with lower socioeconomic status.[124] Conversely, toxic exposures are associated with miscarriage, preterm birth, low birth weight, and neurodevelopmental delays in the neonate and beyond. These exposures can be through chemicals, air pollution, or the climate. They can occur in the workplace, at home, or during recreation.[125] Table 21-11 summarizes the environmental exposures for which there is the most evidence of adverse pregnancy effects.[125] Several of these chemicals can be grouped into the category of endocrine disrupters that mimic or disrupt the effects of hormones.

Due to the breadth of possible exposures, it is unrealistic for the midwife to become an expert in all toxins. Instead, midwives should educate themselves on those environmental exposures that are prevalent within their specific communities and use evidence-based resources in case of other exposures. Health education focuses on exposure reduction and available resources if an exposure occurs. Environmental hazards affect everyone, but many toxic

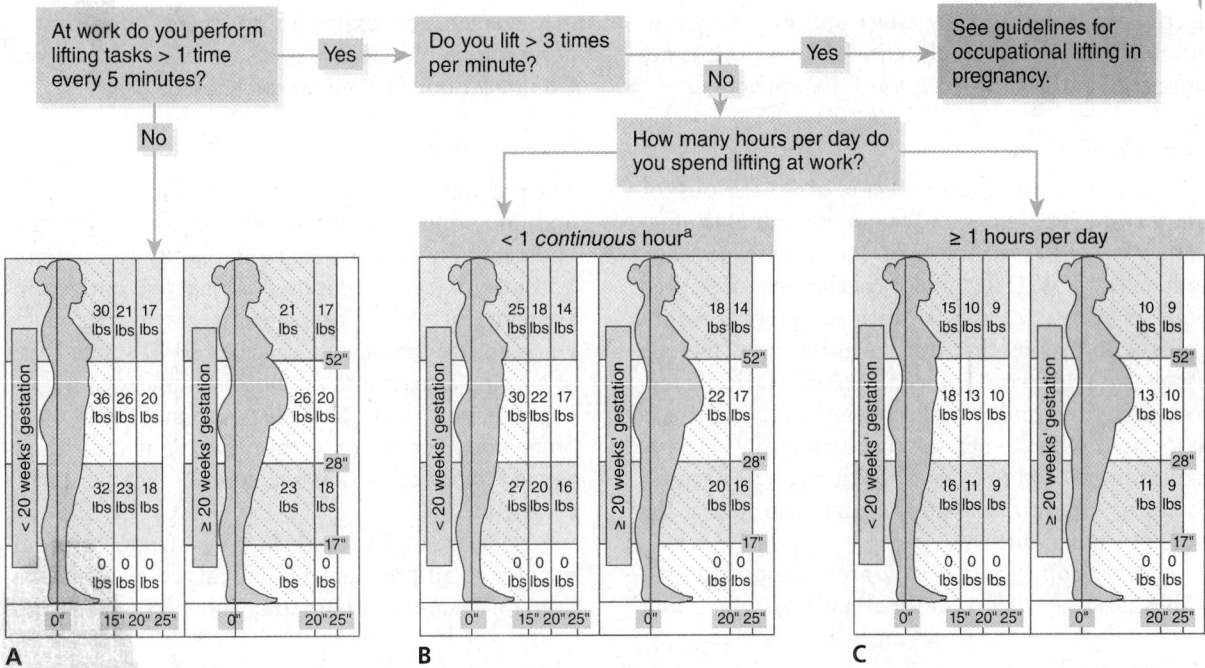

**Figure 21-3** Provisional recommended weight limits for lifting at work during pregnancy. **A.** Infrequent lifting. **B.** Repetitive short-duration lifting. **C.** Repetitive long-duration lifting.
ᵃ Repetitive short-duration lifting can encompass multiple hours of lifting per day; however, each continuous lifting period should be less than 1 hour and followed by a minimum of 1 hour of nonlifting activity before the next continuous lifting period is initiated.
Courtesy of National Institute for Occupational Safety and Health (NIOSH). https://www.cdc.gov/niosh/topics/repro/images/Lifting _guidelines_during_pregnancy_-_NIOSH.jpg.

| Table 21-10 | Midwifery Services Contributing to Occupational Health in Pregnancy |
|---|---|
| **Service** | **Benefit** |
| Reviewing workplace exposures and activities and discussing the effect of these on perinatal health | Provides the individual with information they can use to make decisions or changes about their workplace environment |
| Writing accommodation letters | Individual obtains accommodations; keeps working; guarantees paycheck, benefits, and job protection |
| Providing information on the limits of medical leave, and that it is often unpaid or partially paid | Information on the potential effects on income or job security allows lead time to make arrangements, especially if extended leave is needed |
| Providing resources to assist in understanding employment regulations | Resources empower the person to take legal action if job discrimination, accommodation denial, or extended medical leave is required |

| Table 21-11 | Environmental Exposures with Adverse Pregnancy Effects |
|---|---|
| **Potential Effect** | **Chemical or Pollutant** |
| Miscarriage | Antineoplastic drugs, bisphenol A (BPA), cigarette smoke, ethylene oxide, formaldehyde, polybrominated diphenyl ether (PBDE) flame retardant, solvents |
| Preterm birth and low birth weight | Air pollutants from fracking, ambient air pollutants, antineoplastic drugs, cigarette smoke, ethylene oxide, formaldehyde, perfluorochemicals (PFAS), pesticides, phthalates, PDBEs, toluene |
| Neurodevelopmental impairment | Ambient air pollutants, BPA, lead, mercury, pesticides, phthalates, PBDE flame retardants, polychlorinated biphenyls (PCBs) |

Data from ACOG Committee Opinion No. 832: reducing prenatal exposure to toxic environmental agents. *Obstet Gynecol.* 2021; 138(1):e40-e54.

agents disproportionately affect underserved populations.[125] Environmental toxins and teratogens are presented in the *Preconception Care* appendix.

## Infectious Diseases

Infectious disease exposure can cause serious or life-threatening illnesses when an individual is pregnant, as well as possibly harm the fetus or neonate. Influenza, COVID-19, and varicella are associated with an increased risk of death for pregnant individuals. Infections that can harm the fetus include listeriosis, parvovirus, rubella, syphilis, varicella, cytomegalovirus, and toxoplasmosis. The Zika virus is associated with congenital microcephaly.[126] Herpes and group B *Streptococcus* infection can be harmful to the newborn if the fetus becomes infected at the time of vaginal birth.

Prevention measures are described in Table 21-12.[127–132] Additional information about

management of exposure to these infections in nonimmune individuals is discussed in the *Medical Complications in Pregnancy* chapter.

## Vaccinations

The pregnant individual's immune antibodies of the immunoglobulin G (IgG) class cross the placenta and generally confer passive immunity to the fetus. Vaccines that are composed of inactive antigen ingredients or toxoid are safe for use in pregnancy, whereas live-attenuated vaccines have a small risk of causing disease and are not recommended for use in pregnancy. Table 21-13 lists vaccines that are recommended for all or certain pregnant individuals as well as vaccines that are contraindicated during pregnancy.

Both the CDC and ACNM strongly recommend that all pregnant individuals receive vaccination for tetanus, diphtheria, and pertussis (Tdap)

| Table 21-12 | Prevention of Infection During Pregnancy |
|---|---|
| **Infectious Agent** | **Prevention Measures** |
| Cytomegalovirus | Wash hands after changing a diaper or handling body fluids of an infant or toddler. |
| Herpes | Avoid sexual contact with persons who have active herpes lesions. |
| Listeriosis | Wash all fresh fruits and vegetables before eating them. Do not consume unpasteurized milk or soft cheeses made with unpasteurized milk. Do not eat raw meat and heat all meat, including precooked deli meats, before eating. Avoid smoked seafood and salads made in stores, as *Listeria* can grow slowly at refrigerator temperatures. |
| Parvovirus B19 (fifth disease or slap-cheek disease) | Teachers, childcare workers, and others who work with children are at risk. Avoid contact with a child who has this illness. |
| Pertussis (whooping cough) | Teachers, childcare workers, and others who work with children are at risk. Avoid contact with a child who has this illness unless immunity is known. Vaccination during each pregnancy is recommended. |
| Rubella | Avoid contact with a child who has this illness unless immunity is known. |
| Toxoplasmosis | Do not eat raw or uncooked meat. Thoroughly wash fresh fruits and vegetables. Wear gloves when working around cat feces or working with soil (dirt and sand). Avoid cleaning cat litter boxes. Wash hands after cleaning and working in soil. |
| Varicella (chickenpox) | Avoid contact with a child who has this illness unless immunity is known. |
| Zika virus | Protect oneself from mosquito bites. Avoid travel to areas known to have Zika outbreaks. Zika infection can be spread through sexual intercourse; use safer sexual practices if the partner is at risk. Insect repellant containing *N,N*-diethyl-meta-toluamide (DEET) is effective for prevention and is safe for use in pregnancy and breastfeeding.[127,128] |

Based on Centers for Disease Control and Prevention. Zika virus: Prevent mosquito bites. https://www.cdc.gov/zika/prevention/prevent-mosquito-bites.html. Published 2019. Accessed September 3, 2021; Centers for Disease Control and Prevention. Zika and pregnancy: Zika during pregnancy. https://www.cdc.gov/pregnancy/zika/protect-yourself.html. Published 2021. Accessed September 3, 2021; Madjunkoy M, Chaudhry S, Ito S. Listeriosis during pregnancy. *Arch Gynecol Obstet*. 2017;296(2):143-152; Sugishita Y, Akiba T, Sumitomo M, et al. Shedding of rubella virus among infants with congenital rubella syndrome born in Tokyo, Japan, 2013–2014. *Jpn J Infect Dis*. 2016;69(5):418-423; Neu N, Duchon J, Zachariah P. TORCH infections. *Clin Perinatol*. 2015;42(1):77-103; Feldman DM, Keller R, Borgida AF. Toxoplasmosis, parvovirus and cytomegalovirus in pregnancy. *Clin Lab Med*. 2016;36(2):407-419.

| Table 21-13 | Vaccination Recommendations During Pregnancy | |
|---|---|---|
| **Vaccinations Recommended for ALL Pregnant Individuals** | **Vaccinations Recommended for CERTAIN Pregnant Individuals** | **Vaccinations CONTRAINDICATED During Pregnancy** |
| Tetanus, diphtheria, pertussis (Tdap) Influenza inactivated COVID-19 | Hepatitis A Hepatitis B Meningococcal | Influenza live-attenuated Measles, mumps, rubella (MMR) Varicella (VAR) Human papillomavirus (HPV) |

Data from Freedman MS, Ault K, Bernstein H. Advisory Committee on Immunization Practices recommended immunization schedule for adults aged 19 years or older — United States, 2021. *MMWR Morb Mortal Wkly Rep.* 2021;70:193-196. http://dx.doi.org/10.15585/mmwr.mm7006a2

during pregnancy to protect the newborn from pertussis until infant vaccination is complete. Family members should be current on these vaccinations, according to the CDC schedule for their age group.[133] The ideal timing of the Tdap vaccination for a pregnant person is between weeks 27 and 36 of the pregnancy, with a preference for the earlier part of this period. Annual influenza vaccines are strongly encouraged for individuals who are in any trimester of pregnancy, as well as for members of their household, ideally by the end of October.[133] COVID-19 vaccination is recommended for all pregnant individuals because current data suggest that the benefits of vaccination outweigh any known or potential risks.[134]

Pregnant individuals at risk for hepatitis A or hepatitis B acquisition or for severe outcomes from infection may be candidates for vaccination for these diseases. Meningococcal vaccination should be considered for pregnant individuals at increased risk and for whom vaccination benefits outweigh potential risks. The CDC provides detailed information about risk factors. The live attenuated influenza; measles, mumps, rubella (MMR); varicella (VAR); and human papillomavirus (HPV) vaccines are contraindicated during pregnancy.

Midwives must be mindful of barriers to vaccination of pregnant individuals and employ harm reduction strategies to mitigate these barriers. Practical strategies that can address these barriers include addressing questions thoughtfully to build trust, providing clear statements about vaccines' safety and effectiveness, maintaining a respectful demeanor, considering family members' influence on the pregnant individuals' decisions, respecting the pregnant individual as the expert in their life, and maintaining a compassionate awareness of the individual's current place on the vaccine acceptance/hesitancy continuum.[135,136]

Midwives must also remain committed to reducing the longstanding and significant disparities in vaccination during pregnancy. Compared with white pregnant individuals, Black pregnant individuals report a lower rate of providers offering the influenza vaccine[137] and are less likely to receive Tdap and influenza vaccines.[138] The COVID-19 pandemic, with its marked inequities in vaccination rates between racial groups, has brought these disparities into even sharper focus. Improving access to prenatal care, offering vaccines in the prenatal care clinic, and increasing culturally congruent prenatal care may help mitigate these disparities.[139]

### Additional Topics of Interest

With their heightened interest in health, pregnant individuals may have a variety of questions about health-related issues. When a question arises about an unfamiliar topic or agent, the midwife can refer the person to the CDC for the most accurate information. Selected topics that are commonly solicited by pregnant individuals are summarized in Table 21-14.[140–147]

### Anticipatory Guidance

Anticipatory guidance is a crucial part of midwifery care. Midwives should strive to provide patients and families with the appropriate amount and type of information, at the appropriate time. This can support the pregnant individual and family in feeling empowered and prepared, without causing them to feel overwhelmed. Anticipatory guidance topics include warning signs for the pregnant individual to report (Table 21-15) and prenatal education topics to prepare for birth and the postpartum period (Table 21-16), and for infant care (Table 21-17). In addition to sharing the general and trimester-specific warning signs with pregnant individuals listed in Table 21-15, the midwife encourages the individual to report whenever they feel that something is not right.

| Table 21-14 | Selected Topics of Interest During Pregnancy |
|---|---|
| **Topic** | **Recommendations** |
| Air travel | Air travel is not associated with known risks for healthy people. Flying increases the risk for venous thromboembolism; pregnant individuals are encouraged to wear support hose and/ or move frequently if traveling a long distance.[141] Persons with conditions that increase the risk for hypoxia, such as cardiac disease or fetal growth restriction, may require supplemental oxygen, or avoid flying.[141] Pregnant individuals can be assured that it is safe to fly until 36 weeks' gestation, when the risk of spontaneous labor increases.[141] |
| Exercise and physical activity | Regular exercise is recommended in pregnancy (see the "Physical Activity" section). Activities for the pregnant individual to avoid are those that increase the risk for falls or abdominal injury (e.g., scuba diving and sky diving). |
| Hair treatments | No data support a relationship between hair dye and teratogenic effects. |
| Hot tubs and saunas | The pregnant individual should avoid hot tubs in the first trimester. Fever or increased core temperature (>102°F/38°C) in the pregnant individual is associated with an increased risk of neural tube defects (odds ratio: 1.62; 95% confidence interval: 1.10–2.17).[140] It takes approximately 10 minutes to raise the core temperature to more than 40°C (104°F) in water of 40°C (104°F) and 15 minutes if the water temperature is 39°C (102°F).[142] |
| Medication use | Although only a few medications are known teratogens, the safety of most medications for use in pregnancy has not been proven. Examples of common over-the-counter medications with a known safety profile in pregnancy include acetaminophen for pain relief; aluminum–magnesium hydroxide (Maalox), famotidine (Pepcid), and cimetidine (Tagamet) for digestive upsets; kaolin-pectin (kaopectate) for diarrhea; chlorpheniramine (Chlor-Trimetron), diphenhydramine (Benadryl), and saline nasal spray for nasal congestion or allergies; fiber agents like Metamucil for constipation; and Tucks pads for hemorrhoids. <br><br> For prescription medications, it is important to evaluate the risk and benefits of each. Stopping a medication can be more harmful for a person with asthma, epilepsy, hypertension, or depression. Thus, evaluating the medication, its dosage, and other options is imperative at the initial visit. |
| Radiographs | High levels of ionizing radiation from X rays during radiographic imaging can cause adverse fetal effects throughout pregnancy, depending on the dose. Exposure during the first 2 weeks after conception is an "all or none" effect—that is, either it is fatal or it has no adverse effects. Radiographs and computed tomography (CT) scans not involving the abdomen all have a predicted fetal dose of less than 10 mGy, and pose little fetal risk.[147] Refer the patient to a radiologist if significant exposure may have occurred, for dose calculation and counseling. Although CT scans and radiographs may be indicated in pregnancy for medical management, ultrasound and magnetic resonance imaging (MRI) are the imaging modalities of choice.[146] |
| Oral health | Pregnancy-associated changes increase a woman's risk of dental caries. Pregnancy-associated gingivitis increases the risk of developing periodontal disease. Recommend that the pregnant individual schedule a dental visit if it has been more than 6 months since the last dental examination, or if they are experiencing any dental problems.[145] Dental radiographs are safe, with abdomen and thyroid shielding. Most dental treatments can be performed during pregnancy. |
| Seat belts | Three-point seat belts are recommended. The lap belt is placed across the hips and below the uterus. The shoulder belt is placed between the breasts and lateral to the uterus.[144] |
| Sex during pregnancy | Sexuality during pregnancy is addressed in the *Sexuality* chapter. Sexual intercourse is not associated with adverse pregnancy outcomes, other than risk for sexually transmitted infections. Individuals with certain conditions may need to limit sexual behaviors because of risk of bleeding or contractions.[143] |

CHAPTER 21 Prenatal Care    **863**

| Table 21-15 | Warning Signs During Pregnancy |
|---|---|
| **Type and Timing** | **Warning Signs** |
| Medical complications that can occur throughout pregnancy | Thoughts of harming self or others<br>Fever > 100.4°F<br>Difficulty breathing<br>Chest pain<br>Swelling, redness, or pain in leg |
| First trimester pregnancy-specific complications | Painful uterine cramping<br>Vaginal bleeding<br>Severe nausea and vomiting |
| Second trimester pregnancy-specific complications | Uterine cramping or more than 4–6 contractions per hour<br>Vaginal bleeding<br>Leaking of fluid from the vagina<br>Absent fetal movement after quickening |
| Third trimester pregnancy-specific complications | Headache that is unrelieved by over-the-counter pain relievers or gets worse over time<br>Visual changes<br>Uterine cramping or more than 4–6 contractions per hour prior to 36 weeks' gestation<br>Vaginal bleeding<br>Leaking of fluid from the vagina<br>Decreased fetal movement |

Data from Council on Patient Safety in Women's Health Care. Urgent maternal warning signs. https://safehealthcareforeverywoman.org/urgentmaternalwarningsigns. Published 2020. Accessed November 9, 2022.

| Table 21-16 | Prenatal Education Topics to Prepare for Birth and the Postpartum Period |
|---|---|
| **Topic** | **Recommendations Appropriate to the Prenatal Period** |
| Planned place of birth | Individual choice and prenatal risk assessment can assist individuals in choosing a location for the birth: home, birth center, or hospital. Birth site arrangements are usually finalized in the third trimester. See the *Birth in the Home and Birth Center* chapter. |
| Symptoms of labor onset and when to notify the midwife and/or birth location staff | Midwives should share the expected and normal symptoms of labor onset, including contractions, increased pelvic pressure, bloody show, mucus discharge, gastrointestinal distress, rupture of membranes, and changes in energy levels. The pregnant individual should be given information about the specific symptoms that should prompt a call to the midwife and/or birth location staff, as well as suggestions for coping and self-care at home. (See the *First Stage of Labor* chapter for more information.) |
| Induction | Pregnant individuals might ask whether they should be or might be induced. The midwife should share that elective induction is not a routine part of midwifery care and is typically offered when indicated by pregnancy-related or medical complications. (See the *Complications During Labor and Birth* chapter for more information.) |
| Postpartum contraception | The midwife should support the pregnant individual in exploring intentions about future pregnancies and review the recommendation that the interval between birth and any subsequent pregnancy be at least 18 months.[148] Counseling for individuals who are at risk of pregnancy should include information about the timing of initiation and safety of contraceptive options and the expected return to fertility given the infant feeding method. (See the *Postpartum Care*, *Nonhormonal Contraception*, and *Hormonal Contraception* chapters, and the *Postplacental IUD Insertion* appendix for more information.) |

| Table 21-17 | Prenatal Education Topics to Prepare for Infant Care |
|---|---|
| **Topic** | **Recommendations Appropriate to the Prenatal Period** |
| Infant feeding | Breastfeeding/chestfeeding or human milk feeding is recommended unless medically contraindicated. Shared decision making is important when discussing infant feeding, as is an awareness that infant feeding can be a highly emotional and personal decision. Prenatal assessment for breastfeeding/chestfeeding should include self-efficacy and confidence in ability to breastfeed, medical conditions or medications that might affect breastfeeding or make breastfeeding contraindicated, history of breast surgery or breast disease, previous breastfeeding experiences, family members' attitudes toward breastfeeding, and a physical assessment of the breasts and nipples.[149] (See the *Infant Feeding and Lactation* chapter for more information.) |
| Newborn exams and tests | Some examinations, tests, and immunizations, such as eye prophylaxis, newborn hearing screening, and vitamin K administration, are offered to newborns in the first few days after birth. A review of these tests and their purpose during prenatal visits can help individuals prepare and make informed choices about the tests. |
| Circumcision | The American Academy of Pediatrics states that the health benefits of circumcision outweigh the risks of this procedure, but the benefits are not great enough to recommend routine circumcision of all male newborns. (See the *Neonatal Care* chapter for more information.) |
| Safe infant sleep | Families should make preparations prenatally concerning the American Academy of Pediatrics recommendation for safe infant sleep: Infants should sleep on their back in a separate crib or bassinet with a firm sleep surface, without any soft bedding, preferably in the same room with the parent for the first year of life.[150] |
| Car seats | Car seat use is required by state law in all states. Children younger than 12 months should always ride buckled into a rear-facing seat, and children should ride rear-facing as long as possible, ideally up to 3 years. The Insurance Institute for Highway Safety provides information about car seat safety. Local organizations often host car seat fittings to assist parents in making sure their seat is installed properly. |

## Childbirth Preparation Classes

Childbirth education in its broadest sense includes the wide variety of information that pregnant individuals receive from midwives and other healthcare professionals, family members, friends, electronic and social media, and books. As a subset of childbirth education, formal childbirth preparation classes align with a number of different philosophical approaches. Examples of formal childbirth education models include Lamaze Childbirth Education, with its goal of increasing confidence and teaching breathing techniques to cope with labor; the Bradley Method (also called husband-coached childbirth), with its goal of facilitating natural birth via breathing techniques and partner support; HypnoBirthing, with its focus on calm, peaceful, natural birth using relaxation techniques; Mindfulness-Based Childbirth Preparation (MBCP), which uses mindfulness techniques to help individuals and their support persons cope with labor; Birthing From Within, which is based on primordial knowing (knowledge of body) and modern knowing (knowledge of medical culture and how to give birth within this culture); and a wide variety of hospital-based classes, which often include a focus on institutional policies and procedures and medical procedures information.[151]

Determining the effectiveness of childbirth education and promoting equitable access are challenging. The goals and formats of the programs vary and the differences between pregnant individuals who are or are not willing and able to attend childbirth classes can affect outcomes.[152] Certain pregnant individuals can experience particular difficulties in accessing childbirth classes, including those from historically marginalized groups, those without health insurance or who work long hours, and those who are living in poverty.[153]

## The Delivery of Quality Prenatal Care

Earlier sections of this chapter provided detailed information about the components of prenatal care. This section takes a broader look at delivering quality prenatal care, including traditional, global, and newer schedules and models of prenatal care.

Despite significant societal changes, technological advances, and healthcare discoveries, the schedule of prenatal visits has remained largely unchanged since clinicians began providing formalized prenatal care in the early twentieth century. The schedule of 12 to 14 recommended visits (monthly until 28 weeks, biweekly until 36 weeks, and weekly until birth) has been in place since 1930, when the Children's Bureau published prenatal care guidance.[154] Table 21-18 depicts prenatal care activities that are commonly carried out at various points in pregnancy for an uncomplicated pregnancy. Note that variations in individual practice, community norms, and state laws may alter the specific timing and elements.

A major analysis of the structure and content of prenatal care occurred in 1989, when a U.S. Public Health Service Expert Panel reviewed the effectiveness

and efficiency of prenatal care. Concerning visit schedules, the panel concluded that data were lacking to clearly recommend a specific new prenatal care schedule, but raised the possibility of a reduced visit schedule with seven to nine encounters.[155,156] Decades passed before evidence began to accrue concerning prenatal visit schedules. A 2015 meta-analysis demonstrated that standard and reduced-frequency prenatal care schedules were associated with similar outcomes in high-resource countries.

A global perspective can provide additional insights into prenatal care norms and schedules. In its 2016 guidelines, WHO recommended eight prenatal contacts: one contact in the first trimester; two

| Table 21-18 | Traditional Prenatal Care Schedule Overview for Uncomplicated Pregnancy | | | |
|---|---|---|---|---|
| | **Prenatal Care Activities** | | | |
| Weeks' Gestation | Assessments | Laboratory Tests and Screenings | Health Promotion | Anticipatory Guidance |
| **First Trimester** | | | | |
| 6–8 | Pregnancy confirmation/diagnosis visit (separate visit prior to initial prenatal visit done in some practices) | Urine pregnancy test Dating ultrasound, if needed Counseling about genetic screening/testing options | Address immediate or high-priority health promotion needs | Pregnancy options counseling, as appropriate |
| 12 | Initial prenatal visit: History and physical examination using trauma-informed care approach Fetal heart tones with Doppler ultrasonography Determination of estimated date of birth, if not already done | Initial routine prenatal lab tests: blood group, Rh factor, antibody screen, CBC, RPR or VDRL, hepatitis B and C, rubella, HIV, urinalysis, urine C&S Individualized/risk or symptom-based lab tests: cervical cytology, gonorrhea, chlamydia, trichomonas, TSH, TB, HSV, varicella, pregestational diabetes Genetic screening/testing using shared decision making (e.g., cell-free DNA or nuchal translucency/serum analytes) Psychosocial: SDoH, IPV, substances, depression | Nutrition, activity, travel, oral health, vaccinations, occupational health, infectious disease prevention; food safety, medications and supplements use, environmental exposures | Pregnancy warning signs: pelvic or abdominal pain, vaginal bleeding, excessive nausea/vomiting Discussion about planned birth location |
| **Second Trimester** | | | | |
| Traditional schedule: prenatal visits every 4 weeks Assessment at each visit: common discomforts, fetal movement, BP, weight, fundal height, FHTs | | | | |
| 16 | Date of quickening | Genetic screening/testing using shared decision making (e.g., quad screen) | As appropriate for the individual: nutrition, activity, substance use, environmental and occupational exposures | Pregnancy warning signs: vaginal bleeding, cramping, PPROM, decreased or absent fetal movement after quickening Childbirth education classes |
| 20 | | Fetal anatomy ultrasound | | |
| 24 | | | | |

*(continues)*

| Table 21-18 | Traditional Prenatal Care Schedule Overview for Uncomplicated Pregnancy (*continued*) | | | | |
|---|---|---|---|---|---|
| | | **Prenatal Care Activities** | | | |
| Weeks' Gestation | Assessments | Laboratory Tests and Screenings | Health Promotion | Anticipatory Guidance | |

**Third Trimester**

Traditional schedule: prenatal visits every 2 weeks from 28 to 36 weeks, then every week from 36 weeks until birth
Assessment at each visit: common discomforts, fetal movement, BP, weight, fundal height, FHTs

| Weeks' Gestation | Assessments | Laboratory Tests and Screenings | Health Promotion | Anticipatory Guidance |
|---|---|---|---|---|
| 28 | | Glucose tolerance test and CBC Risk-based: chlamydia and GC, syphilis, TSH; repeat antibody screen if Rh negative | Tdap vaccine RhoGAM after antibody screen if Rh negative | Pregnancy warning signs: headache, visual changes, bleeding PROM, decreased fetal movements |
| 30 | | | | Planned place of birth (usually discussed earlier in pregnancy and finalized no later than the early third trimester) |
| 32 | Assess fetal presentation at each visit for the remainder of the pregnancy | | Reinforce fetal movement awareness at each visit for the remainder of the pregnancy | Desires for specific labor and birth choices and experiences |
| 34 | | | | Symptoms of labor onset and when to notify the clinician or birth location staff |
| 36 | | GBS vaginal/rectal swab (36 0/7 to 37 6/7 weeks' gestation) unless screening exception is present | | Wide range of early labor experiences, including challenges in determining the onset of active labor |
| 37 | | | | Self-care during early labor |
| 38 | | | | Postpartum contraception plan Infant feeding plan |
| 39 | | | | Newborn care elements such as eye prophylaxis, vitamin K, vaccinations, circumcision, safe sleep, and car seats |

Abbreviations: BP, blood pressure; CBC, complete blood count; C&S, culture and sensitivity; DNA, deoxyribonucleic acid; FHT, fetal heart tones; GBS, group B *Streptococcus*; GC, gonorrhea; HIV, human immunodeficiency virus; HSV, herpes simplex virus; IPV, intimate partner violence; PPROM, preterm premature rupture of membranes; PROM, premature rupture of membranes; Rh, Rhesus; RPR, rapid plasma reagin; SDoH, social determinants of health; TB, tuberculosis; TSH, thyroid-stimulating hormone; VDRL, Venereal Disease Research Laboratory.

contacts in the second trimester at 20 and 26 weeks; and five contacts in the third trimester at 30, 34, 36, 38, and 40 weeks. The word "contact" is preferred to "visit" in this model because contact emphasizes the active relationship and collaboration between the pregnant individual and care provider. The 2016 guidelines replace the previous schedule of four focused visits because Guidelines Development Group members concluded that four visits do not provide adequate contact with healthcare providers.[157]

Despite continued adherence to the traditional model and schedule of prenatal care, clinicians and the individuals they serve have long recognized the need for change. Innovative prenatal care models and schedules began to be introduced in the 1990s, and the COVID-19 pandemic compelled additional changes. Following is a discussion of a few examples of nontraditional models and schedules of prenatal care. It is likely that these represent just the beginning of the development of innovative models.

CenteringPregnancy (CP) is a model of group prenatal care that was developed in the 1990s by nurse-midwife Sharon Schindler Rising. In CP, 8 to 10 pregnant individuals who are due around the same time form a group. Prenatal care consists of approximately 10 visits, but unlike in the traditional model, each visit is 90 to 120 minutes long. Pregnant individuals measure and record their own weight and blood pressure and meet privately for a brief assessment with a provider. Then the group members gather together to engage in a facilitated discussion about timely health topics and their concerns and questions. The community that group members form can be a powerfully positive influence on their pregnancies and their lives beyond. Importantly, CP has been shown to improve outcomes in vulnerable populations and can promote health equity.[158] Since the initiation of CP, other models for group prenatal care have evolved, which do not require extensive training and costs.

More recently, researchers have investigated a variety of redesigns of prenatal care that are flexible and identify which services must be completed in person and which can be safely carried out remotely. One model, OB Nest, incorporates remote home monitoring devices and enhanced nursing support. OB Nest care consists of eight on-site visits with a provider; six virtual nurse visits consisting of phone or online communication, fetal Doppler ultrasonography, and blood pressure monitoring devices; and access to an online community of pregnant peers. OB Nest as a specific model will need to be studied further, but this trial provides support for safe and satisfying prenatal care models with fewer visits.[159]

Another promising new prenatal care model is the Michigan Plan for Appropriate Tailored Health Care (MiPATH). With this model, the pregnant individual's medical and social determinants of health inform an individualized prenatal plan. Services that cannot be offered remotely are delivered at four in-person visits: initial, 28 weeks, 36 weeks, and 39 weeks. Aside from those encounters, visit frequency and modality (in person or via telehealth) align with each person's needs. The model prioritizes support for SDoH, incorporates the pregnant individual's preferences, and requires that pregnant individuals have access to quality monitoring devices for use at home.[160] Table 21-19 depicts a possible MiPATH prenatal care plan for an example individual with an uncomplicated pregnancy.[161]

| Table 21-19 | MiPATH Example Schedule: Uncomplicated Pregnancy |
|---|---|
| Weeks' Gestation | Prenatal Care Activities |
| 6–8 | Initial visit, required in-person <br> • History and physical examination <br> • First trimester laboratory tests <br> • Genetic testing <br> • Influenza vaccine |
| 16 | In-person or telehealth visit, depending on the pregnant individual's preference <br> Blood pressure, weight, fetal heart tones, fundal height (via telehealth or office visit) |
| 22 | In-person or telehealth visit, depending on the pregnant individual's preference <br> Blood pressure, weight, fetal heart tones, fundal height (via telehealth or office visit) |
| 28 | Required in-person visit <br> • Third trimester laboratory tests (complete blood count, diabetes screen) <br> • Tdap vaccine <br> • Rho (D) immunoglobulin, if needed <br> • Blood pressure, weight, fetal heart tones, fundal height |
| 32 | In-person or telehealth visit, depending on the pregnant individual's preference <br> Blood pressure, weight, fetal heart tones, fundal height (via telehealth or office visit) |
| 36 | Required in-person visit <br> • Group B *Streptococcus* test <br> • Assessment of fetal presentation <br> • Blood pressure, weight, fetal heart tones, fundal height |
| 38 | In-person or telehealth visit, depending on the pregnant individual's preference <br> Blood pressure, weight, fetal heart tones, fundal height (via telehealth or office visit) |
| 39 | Required in-person visit <br> • Labor and birth planning <br> • Blood pressure, weight, fetal heart tones, fundal height |

## Conclusion

Regardless of the specific schedule or model, prenatal care is more than a series of visits with scripted interventions. Serving individuals during the prenatal period provides rich opportunities to develop relationships, promote normalcy, identify and address complications, provide health education and anticipatory guidance, and much more.

## References

1. Eri TS, Berg M, Dahl B, et al. Models for midwifery care: a mapping review. *Eur J Midwifery*. 2020;4:30. doi:10.18332/ejm/124110.

2. International Confederation of Midwives. *Philosphy and Model of Midwifery Care*. Prague: International Confederation of Midwives; 2014.

3. American College of Nurse Midwives. *Core Competencies for Basic Midwifery Practice*. Silver Springs, MD: American College of Nurse Midwives; 2020.

4. Ota E, da Silva Lopes K, Middleton P, et al. Antenatal interventions for preventing stillbirth, fetal loss and perinatal death: an overview of Cochrane systematic reviews. *Cochrane Database Syst Rev*. 2020;12(12):Cd009599. doi:10.1002/14651858. CD009599.pub2.

5. Wallenborn JT, Lu J, Perera RA, et al. The impact of the professional qualifications of the prenatal care provider on breastfeeding duration. *Breastfeed Med*. 2018;13(2):106-111. doi:10.1089/bfm.2017.0133.

6. Vedam S, Stoll K, MacDorman M, et al. Mapping integration of midwives across the United States: impact on access, equity, and outcomes. *PloS One*. 2018;13(2):e0192523. doi:10.1371/journal. pone.0192523.

7. Altman MR, McLemore MR, Oseguera T, et al. Listening to women: recommendations from women of color to improve experiences in pregnancy and birth care. *J Midwifery Womens Health*. 2020;65(4):466-473. doi:10.1111/jmwh.13102.

8. Opara EI, Zaidi J. The interpretation and clinical application of the word "parity": a survey. *BJOG*. 2007;114(10):1295-1297. doi:10.1111/j.1471-0528 .2007.01435.x.

9. Maraj H, Kumari S. No clarity on the definition of parity: a survey accessing interpretation of the word parity amongst obstetricians and midwives and a literature review. *Eur J Obstet Gynecol Reprod Biol*. 2021;263:15-19. doi:10.1016/j.ejogrb .2021.05.042.

10. reVITALize: obstetric data definitions. Version 1.0. https://www.acog.org/practice-management/health -it-and-clinical-informatics/revitalize-obstetrics-data -definitions. Published 2014. Accessed September 9, 2021.

11. Boxer J, Weddell S, Broomhead D, et al. Home pregnancy tests in the hands of the intended user. *J Immunoassay Iimmunochem*. 2019;40(6):642-652. doi:10.1080/15321819.2019.1671861.

12. Kleinschmidt S, Dugas JN, Nelson KP, Feldman JA. False negative point-of-care urine pregnancy tests in an urban academic emergency department: a retrospective cohort study. *J Am Coll Emerg Physicians Open*. 2021;2(3):e12427. doi:10.1002/emp2.12427.

13. Johnson S, Eapen S, Smith P, et al. Significance of pregnancy test false negative results due to elevated levels of β-core fragment hCG. *J Immunoassay Immunochem*. 2017;38(4):449-455. doi:10.1080 /15321819.2017.1329152.

14. Herskovits AZ, Chen Y, Latifi N, et al. False-negative urine human chorionic gonadotropin testing in the clinical laboratory. *Lab Med*. 2020;51(1):86-93. doi:10.1093/labmed/lmz039.

15. U.S. Food and Drug Administration. Pregnancy. https://www.fda.gov/medical-devices/home-use-tests /pregnancy. Published 2019. Accessed August 16, 2021.

16. Benagiano G, Farris M, Grudzinskas G. Fate of fertilized human oocytes. *Reprod Biomed Online*. 2010;21(6):732-741. doi:10.1016/j.rbmo .2010.08.011.

17. Connolly A, Ryan DH, Stuebe AM, Wolfe HM. Reevaluation of discriminatory and threshold levels for serum β-hCG in early pregnancy. *Obstet Gynecol*. 2013;121(1):65-70. doi:10.1097/aog .0b013e318278f421.

18. Cunningham FLK, Bloom SL, Dashe JS, et al, eds. *Williams Obstetrics*, 26th ed. New York, NY: McGraw-Hill; 2022.

19. Najmabadi S, Schliep KC, Simonsen SE, et al. Menstrual bleeding, cycle length, and follicular and luteal phase lengths in women without known subfertility: a pooled analysis of three cohorts. *Paediatr Perinatal Epidemiol*. 2020;34(3):318-327. doi:10.1111/ppe.12644.

20. Hunter LA. Issues in pregnancy dating: revisiting the evidence. *J Midwifery Womens Health*. 2009;54(3): 184-190. doi:10.1016/j.jmwh.2008.11.003.

21. Sapra KJ, Buck Louis GM, Sundaram R, et al. Signs and symptoms associated with early pregnancy loss: findings from a population-based preconception cohort. *Hum Reprod*. 2016;31(4):887-896. doi:10.1093/humrep/dew010.

22. Naegele FK. *Erfahrung und Abhandlungen des Weiblichen Geschlechtes*. Mannheim, Germany: Ben Lobias Loeffler; 1812.

23. Lawson GW. Naegele's rule and the length of pregnancy: a review. *Austral N Z J Obstet Gynaecol*. 2021;61(2):177-182. doi:10.1111/ajo.13253.

24. Chambliss LR, Clark SL. Paper gestational age wheels are generally inaccurate. *Am J Obstet Gynecol*.

2014;210(2):145.e141-145.e144. doi:10.1016/j.ajog.2013.09.013.

25. Practice Bulletin No. 175: ultrasound in pregnancy. *Obstet Gynecol.* 2016;128(6):e241-e256. doi:10.1097/aog.0000000000001815.

26. Committee Opinion No. 700: methods for estimating the due date. *Obstet Gynecol.* 2017;129(5):e150-e154. doi:10.1097/aog.0000000000002046.

27. Doubilet PM. Should a first trimester dating scan be routine for all pregnancies? *Semin Perinatol.* 2013;37(5):307-309. doi:10.1053/j.semperi.2013.06.006.

28. Whitworth M, Bricker L, Mullan C. Ultrasound for fetal assessment in early pregnancy. *Cochrane Database Syst Rev.* 2015;2015(7):Cd007058. doi:10.1002/14651858.CD007058.pub3.

29. Hertz RH, Sokol RJ, Knoke JD, et al. Clinical estimation of gestational age: rules for avoiding preterm delivery. *Am J Obstet Gynecol.* 1978;131(4):395-402. doi:10.1016/0002-9378(78)90414-3.

30. Neilson JP. Symphysis–fundal height measurement in pregnancy. *Cochrane Database Syst Rev.* 2000;1998(2):Cd000944. doi:10.1002/14651858.cd000944.

31. Hartnett E, Haber J, Krainovich-Miller B, et al. Oral health in pregnancy. *JOGNN NAACOG.* 2016;45(4):565-573. doi:10.1016/j.jogn.2016.04.005.

32. Pattinson RC, Cuthbert A, Vannevel V. Pelvimetry for fetal cephalic presentations at or near term for deciding on mode of delivery. *Cochrane Database Syst Rev.* 2017;3(3):Cd000161. doi:10.1002/14651858.CD000161.pub2.

33. Tillman S. Consent in pelvic care. *J Midwifery Womens Health.* 2020;65(6):749-758. doi:10.1111/jmwh.13189.

34. Sexual misconduct: ACOG Committee Opinion Number 796. *Obstet Gynecol.* 2020;135(1):e43-e50. doi:10.1097/aog.0000000000003608.

35. Bibbins-Domingo K, Grossman DC, Curry SJ, et al. Screening for preeclampsia: US Preventive Services Task Force recommendation statement. *J Am Med Assoc.* 2017;317(16):1661-1667. doi:10.1001/jama.2017.3439.

36. Fishel Bartal M, Lindheimer MD, Sibai BM. Proteinuria during pregnancy: definition, pathophysiology, methodology, and clinical significance. *Am J Obstet Gynecol.* 2020;226:S819-S834. doi:10.1016/j.ajog.2020.08.108.

37. Panelli DM, Robinson JN, Kaimal AJ, et al. Using cervical dilation to predict labor onset: a tool for elective labor induction counseling. *Am J Perinatol.* 2019;36(14):1485-1491. doi:10.1055/s-0039-1677866.

38. Screening for fetal chromosomal abnormalities: ACOG Practice Bulletin Number 226. *Obstet Gynecol.* 2020;136(4):e48-e69. doi:10.1097/aog.0000000000004084.

39. Committee Opinion No. 691: carrier screening for genetic conditions. *Obstet Gynecol.* 2017;129(3):e41-e55. doi:10.1097/aog.0000000000001952.

40. AIUM practice parameter for the performance of limited obstetric ultrasound examinations by advanced clinical providers. *J Ultrasound Med.* 2018;37(7):1587-1596. doi:10.1002/jum.14677.

41. Edwards L, Hui L. First and second trimester screening for fetal structural anomalies. *Semin Fetal Neonatal Med.* 2018;23(2):102-111. doi:10.1016/j.siny.2017.11.005.

42. Kaplan R, Adams S. Incidental fetal ultrasound findings: interpretation and management. *J Midwifery Womens Health.* 2018;63(3):323-329. doi:10.1111/jmwh.12754.

43. O'Brien K, Shainker SA, Modest AM, et al. Cost analysis of following up incomplete low-risk fetal anatomy ultrasounds. *Birth (Berkeley, CA).* 2017;44(1):35-40. doi:10.1111/birt.12262.

44. World Health Organization. Social determinants of health. https://www.who.int/health-topics/social-determinants-of-health#tab=tab_1. Accessed 8/22/2021.

45. Felitti VJ, Anda RF, Nordenberg D, et al. Relationship of childhood abuse and household dysfunction to many of the leading causes of death in adults: the Adverse Childhood Experiences (ACE) Study. *Am J Prevent Med.* 1998;14(4):245-258. doi:10.1016/s0749-3797(98)00017-8.

46. Sperlich M, Seng JS, Li Y, et al. Integrating trauma-informed care into maternity care practice: conceptual and practical issues. *J Midwifery Womens Health.* 2017;62(6):661-672. doi:10.1111/jmwh.12674.

47. Gokhale P, Young MR, Williams MN, et al. Refining trauma-informed perinatal care for urban prenatal care patients with multiple lifetime traumatic exposures: a qualitative study. *J Midwifery Womens Health.* 2020;65(2):224-230. doi:10.1111/jmwh.13063.

48. Peitzmeier SM, Malik M, Kattari SK, et al. Intimate partner violence in transgender populations: systematic review and meta-analysis of prevalence and correlates. *Am J Public Health.* 2020;110(9):e1-e14. doi:10.2105/ajph.2020.305774.

49. ACOG Committee Opinion No. 518: intimate partner violence. *Obstet Gynecol.* 2012;119(2 pt 1):412-417. doi:10.1097/AOG.0b013e318249ff74.

50. Chisholm CA, Bullock L, Ferguson JEJ 2nd. Intimate partner violence and pregnancy: screening and intervention. *Am J Obstet Gynecol.* 2017;217(2):145-149. doi:10.1016/j.ajog.2017.05.043.

51. Renker PR. Breaking the barriers: the promise of computer-assisted screening for intimate partner violence. *J Midwifery Womens Health.* 2008;53(6):496-503. doi:10.1016/j.jmwh.2008.07.017.

52. Underwood L, Waldie K, D'Souza S, et al. A review of longitudinal studies on antenatal and postnatal depression. *Arch Womens Mental Health*. 2016;19(5):711-720. doi:10.1007/s00737-016-0629-1.

53. Fawcett EJ, Fairbrother N, Cox ML, et al. The prevalence of anxiety disorders during pregnancy and the postpartum period: a multivariate Bayesian meta-analysis. *J Clin Psychiatry*. 2019;80(4). doi:10.4088/JCP.18r12527.

54. Breedlove G, Fryzelka D. Depression screening during pregnancy. *J Midwifery Womens Health*. 2011;56(1):18-25. doi:10.1111/j.1542-2011.2010.00002.x.

55. Rompala KS, Cirino N, Rosenberg KD, et al. Prenatal depression screening by certified nurse-midwives, Oregon. *J Midwifery Womens Health*. 2016;61(5):599-605. doi:10.1111/jmwh.12491.

56. Curry SJ, Krist AH, Owens DK, et al. Interventions to prevent perinatal depression: US Preventive Services Task Force recommendation statement. *J Am Med Assoc*. 2019;321(6):580-587. doi:10.1001/jama.2019.0007.

57. Latendresse G, Elmore C, Deneris A. Selective serotonin reuptake inhibitors as first-line antidepressant therapy for perinatal depression. *J Midwifery Womens Health*. 2017;62(3):317-328. doi:10.1111/jmwh.12607.

58. National Harm Reduction Coalition. Pregnancy and substance use: a harm reduction toolkit. https://harmreduction.org/issues/pregnancy-and-substance-use-a-harm-reduction-toolkit/. Published 2020. Accessed September 1, 2021.

59. Drake P, Driscoll AK, Mathews TJ. Cigarette smoking during pregnancy: United States, 2016. *NCHS Data Brief*. 2018(305):1-8.

60. Kedia SK, Ahuja NA, Carswell A, et al. Smoking cessation among pregnant and postpartum women from low-income groups in the United States. *J Midwifery Womens Health*. 2021;66(4):486-493. doi:10.1111/jmwh.13242.

61. Krist AH, Davidson KW, Mangione CM, et al. Interventions for tobacco smoking cessation in adults, including pregnant persons: US Preventive Services Task Force recommendation statement. *J Am Med Assoc*. 2021;325(3):265-279. doi:10.1001/jama.2020.25019.

62. Baraona LK, Lovelace D, Daniels JL, McDaniel L. Tobacco harms, nicotine pharmacology, and pharmacologic tobacco cessation interventions for women. *J Midwifery Womens Health*. 2017;62(3):253-269. doi:10.1111/jmwh.12616.

63. Claire R, Chamberlain C, Davey MA, et al. Pharmacological interventions for promoting smoking cessation during pregnancy. *Cochrane Database Syst Rev*. 2020;3(3):Cd010078. doi:10.1002/14651858.CD010078.pub3.

64. Chertok IR, Archer SH. Evaluation of a midwife- and nurse-delivered 5 A's prenatal smoking cessation program. *J Midwifery Womens Health*. 2015;60(2):175-181. doi:10.1111/jmwh.12220.

65. Calder R, Gant E, Bauld L, et al. Vaping in pregnancy: a systematic review. *Nicotine Tobacco Res*. 2021;23(9):1451-1458. doi:10.1093/ntr/ntab017.

66. Tran DT, Preen DB, Einarsdottir K, et al. Use of smoking cessation pharmacotherapies during pregnancy is not associated with increased risk of adverse pregnancy outcomes: a population-based cohort study. *BMC Med*. 2020;18(1):15. doi:10.1186/s12916-019-1472-9.

67. National Insitute on Drug Absuse. What is the scope of cannabis (marijuana) use in the United States? https://www.drugabuse.gov/publications/research-reports/marijuana/what-scope-marijuana-use-in-united-states. Published 2021. Accessed September 8, 2021.

68. Volkow ND, Compton WM, Wargo EM. The risks of marijuana use during pregnancy. *J Am Med Assoc*. 2017;317(2):129-130. doi:10.1001/jama.2016.18612.

69. Foeller ME, Lyell DJ. Marijuana use in pregnancy: concerns in an evolving era. *J Midwifery Womens Health*. 2017;62(3):363-367. doi:10.1111/jmwh.12631.

70. Braillon A, Bewley S. Committee Opinion No. 722: marijuana use during pregnancy and lactation. *Obstet Gynecol*. 2018;131(1):164. doi:10.1097/aog.0000000000002429.

71. Denny CH, Acero CS, Naimi TS, Kim SY. Consumption of alcohol beverages and binge drinking among pregnant women aged 18-44 years—United States, 2015–2017. *MMWR*. 2019;68(16):365-368. doi:10.15585/mmwr.mm6816a1.

72. Centers for Disease Control and Prevention. About opioid use in pregnancy. https://www.cdc.gov/pregnancy/opioids/basics.html. Published 2021. Accessed Ausust 27, 2021.

73. Haight SC, Ko JY, Tong VT, et al. Opioid use disorder documented at delivery hospitalization—United States, 1999–2014. *MMWR*. 2018;67(31):845-849. doi:10.15585/mmwr.mm6731a1.

74. National Insitute on Drug Abuse. Treating opioid use disorder during pregnancy. https://www.drugabuse.gov/publications/treating-opioid-use-disorder-during-pregnancy. Published 2021. Accessed September 9, 2021.

75. Goodman DJ, Saunders EC, Wolff KB. In their own words: a qualitative study of factors promoting resilience and recovery among postpartum women with opioid use disorders. *BMC Pregnancy Childbirth*. 2020;20(1):178. doi:10.1186/s12884-020-02872-5.

76. Committee Opinion No. 711: opioid use and opioid use disorder in pregnancy. *Obstet Gynecol*. 2017;130(2):e81-e94. doi:10.1097/aog.0000000000002235.

77. Busse MM, Kim J, Unite M, et al. Nurses' priorities for improving pregnancy and birth care for individuals with opioid use disorder. *J Midwifery Womens Health.* 2021;66:656-663. doi:10.1111/jmwh .13267.

78. Krans EE, Kim JY, Chen Q, et al. Outcomes associated with the use of medications for opioid use disorder during pregnancy. *Addiction.* 2021;116(12): 3504-3514. doi:10.1111/add.15582.

79. Smid MC, Metz TD, Gordon AJ. Stimulant use in pregnancy: an under-recognized epidemic among pregnant women. *Clin Obste Gynecol.* 2019;62(1): 168-184. doi:10.1097/grf.0000000000000418.

80. Wright TE, Terplan M, Ondersma SJ, et al. The role of screening, brief intervention, and referral to treatment in the perinatal period. *Am J Obstet Gynecol.* 2016;215(5):539-547. doi:10.1016/j.ajog .2016.06.038.

81. Cruz SL, Bowen SE. The last two decades on preclinical and clinical research on inhalant effects. *Neurotoxicol Teratol.* 2021;87:106999. doi:10.1016/j.ntt.2021.106999.

82. Callan SP, Kott JM, Cleary JP, et al. Changes in developmental body weight as a function of toluene exposure: a meta-analysis of animal studies. *Hum Exper Toxicol.* 2016;35(4):341-352. doi:10.1177/0960327115591377.

83. Malloul H, Mahdani FM, Bennis M, Ba-M'hamed S. Prenatal exposure to paint thinner alters postnatal development and behavior in mice. *Front Behav Neurosci.* 2017;11:171. doi:10.3389/fnbeh.2017.00171.

84. Bowen SE. Two serious and challenging medical complications associated with volatile substance misuse: sudden sniffing death and fetal solvent syndrome. *Substance Use Misuse.* 2011;46(suppl 1):68-72. doi: 10.3109/10826084.2011.580220.

85. Goodman DJ, Wolff KB. Screening for substance abuse in women's health: a public health imperative. *J Midwifery Womens Health.* 2013;58(3):278-287. doi:10.1111/jmwh.12035.

86. Committee Opinion No. 633: alcohol abuse and other substance use disorders: ethical issues in obstetric and gynecologic practice. *Obstet Gynecol.* 2015;125(6):1529-1537. doi:10.1097/01 .AOG.0000466371.86393.9b.

87. James-McAlpine JM, Vincze LJ, Vanderlelie JJ, Perkins AV. Influence of dietary intake and decision-making during pregnancy on birth outcomes. *Nutr.* 2020;77(3):323-330. doi:10.1111 /1747-0080.12610.

88. Koletzko B, Godfrey KM, Poston L, et al. Nutrition during pregnancy, lactation and early childhood and its implications for maternal and long-term child health: the Early Nutrition Project recommendations. *Ann Nutr Metab.* 2019;74(2):93-106. doi:10.1159/000496471.

89. Hoover EA, Louis JM. Optimizing health: weight, exercise, and nutrition in pregnancy and beyond. *Obstet Gynecol Clin North Am.* 2019;46(3):431-440. doi:10.1016/j.ogc.2019.04.003.

90. Kozhimannil KB, Interrante JD, Henning-Smith C, Admon LK. Rural–urban differences in severe maternal morbidity and mortality in the US, 2007–15. *Health Aff (Millwood).* 2019;38(12):2077-2085. doi:10.1377/hlthaff.2019.00805.

91. Landry MJ, Phan K, McGuirt JT, et al. USDA Special Supplemental Nutrition Program for Women, Infants and Children (WIC) vendor criteria: an examination of US administrative agency variations. *Int J Environ Res Public Health.* 2021;18(7). doi:10.3390 /ijerph18073545.

92. Parker HW, Tovar A, McCurdy K, Vadiveloo M. Socio-economic and racial prenatal diet quality disparities in a national US sample. *Public Health Nutr.* 2020;23(5):894-903. doi:10.1017 /s1368980019003240.

93. Freeman A. *Skimmed: Breastfeeding, Race, and Injustice.* Stanford, CA: Stanford University Press; 2019.

94. Whitaker KM, Wilcox S, Liu J, et al. Provider advice and women's intentions to meet weight gain, physical activity, and nutrition guidelines during pregnancy. *Matern Child Health J.* 2016;20(11):2309-2317. doi:10.1007/s10995-016-2054-5.

95. Abayomi JC, Charnley MS, Cassidy L, et al. A patient and public involvement investigation into healthy eating and weight management advice during pregnancy. *Int J Quality Health Care.* 2020;32(1):28-34. doi:10.1093/intqhc/mzz081.

96. Grenier LN, Atkinson SA, Mottola MF, et al. Be healthy in pregnancy: exploring factors that impact pregnant women's nutrition and exercise behaviours. *Matern Child Nutr.* 2021;17(1):e13068. doi:10.1111 /mcn.13068.

97. Avalos LA, Caan B, Nance N, et al. Prenatal depression and diet quality during pregnancy. *J Acad Nutr Dietetics.* 2020;120(6):972-984. doi:10.1016/j .jand.2019.12.011.

98. Kominiarek MA, Rajan P. Nutrition recommendations in pregnancy and lactation. *Med Clin North Am.* 2016;100(6):1199-1215. doi:10.1016/j.mcna .2016.06.004.

99. U.S. Food and Drug Administration: Food satfety for moms to be. https://www.fda.gov/food/people-risk -foodborne-illness/food-safety-moms-be. Accessed Spetember 7, 2021.

100. Penney DS, Miller KG. Nutritional counseling for vegetarians during pregnancy and lactation. *J Midwifery Womens Health.* 2008;53(1):37-44. doi:10.1016/j.jmwh.2007.07.003.

101. Britten P, Cleveland LE, Koegel KL, et al. Updated US Department of Agriculture food patterns meet

goals of the 2010 dietary guidelines. *J Acad Nutr Dietetics.* 2012;112(10):1648-1655. doi:10.1016/j .jand.2012.05.021.

102. Jordan RG. Prenatal omega-3 fatty acids: review and recommendations. *J Midwifery Womens Health.* 2010;55(6):520-528. doi:10.1016/j.jmwh .2010.02.018.

103. Middleton P, Gomersall JC, Gould JF, et al. Omega-3 fatty acid addition during pregnancy. *Cochrane Database Syst Rev.* 2018;11(11):Cd003402. doi:10.1002/14651858.CD003402.pub3.

104. Maslin K, James A, Brown A, et al. What is known about the nutritional intake of women during pregnancy following bariatric surgery? A scoping review. *Nutrients.* 2019;11(9). doi:10.3390 /nu11092116.

105. Zgliczynska M, Kosinska-Kaczynska K. Micronutrients in multiple pregnancies: the knowns and unknowns: a systematic review. *Nutrients.* 2021;13(2). doi:10.3390/nu13020386.

106. Fawcett EJ, Fawcett JM, Mazmanian D. A meta-analysis of the worldwide prevalence of pica during pregnancy and the postpartum period. *Int J Gynaecol Obstet.* 2016;133(3):277-283. doi:10.1016/j.ijgo.2015.10.012.

107. Connolly CP, Conger SA, Montoye AHK, et al. Walking for health during pregnancy: a literature review and considerations for future research. *J Sport Health Sci.* 2019;8(5):401-411. doi:10.1016/j .jshs.2018.11.004.

108. Physical activity and exercise during pregnancy and the postpartum period: ACOG Committee Opinion Summary Number 804. *Obstet Gynecol.* 2020;135(4):991-993. doi:10.1097/aog .0000000000003773.

109. Raper MJ, McDonald S, Johnston C, et al. The influence of exercise during pregnancy on racial/ ethnic health disparities and birth outcomes. *BMC Pregnancy Childbirth.* 2021;21(1):258. doi:10.1186 /s12884-021-03717-5.

110. Bantham A, Taverno Ross SE, Sebastião E, Hall G. Overcoming barriers to physical activity in underserved populations. *Prog Cardiovasc Dis.* 2021;64:64-71. doi:10.1016/j.pcad.2020.11.002.

111. Procter SB, Campbell CG. Position of the Academy of Nutrition and Dietetics: nutrition and lifestyle for a healthy pregnancy outcome. *J Acad Nutr Dietetics.* 2014;114(7):1099-1103. doi:10.1016/j .jand.2014.05.005.

112. McDowell M, Cain MA, Brumley J. Excessive gestational weight gain. *J Midwifery Womens Health.* 2019;64(1):46-54. doi:10.1111/jmwh.12927.

113. Boone-Heinonen J, Biel FM, Marshall NE, Snowden JM. Maternal prepregnancy BMI and size at birth: race/ethnicity-stratified, within-family associations in over 500,000 siblings. *Ann Epidemiol.* 2020;46:49.e45-56.e45. doi:10.1016/j .annepidem.2020.04.009.

114. Sorkin JD. BMI, age, and mortality: the slaying of a beautiful hypothesis by an ugly fact. *Am J Clin Nutr.* 2014;99(4):759-760. doi:10.3945/ajcn .114.084780.

115. Dieterich R, Demirci J. Communication practices of healthcare professionals when caring for overweight/obese pregnant women: a scoping review. *Patient Educ Couns.* 2020;103(10):1902-1912. doi:10.1016/j.pec.2020.05.011.

116. Rauchwerk A, Vipperman-Cohen A, Padmanabhan S, et al. The case for a health at every size approach for chronic disease risk reduction in women of color. *J Nutr Educ Behav.* 2020;52(11):1066-1072. doi:10.1016/j.jneb.2020.08.004.

117. Patil AS, Sheng J, Dotters-Katz SK, et al. Fundamentals of clinical pharmacology with application for pregnant women. *J Midwifery Womens Health.* 2017;62(3):298-307. doi:10.1111/jmwh.12621.

118. Haas DM, Marsh DJ, Dang DT, et al. Prescription and other medication use in pregnancy. *Obstet Gynecol.* 2018;131(5):789-798. doi:10.1097/aog .0000000000002579.

119. Christnacht C, Sullivan B. The choices working mothers make. United States Census Bureau. https://www .census.gov/library/stories/2020/05/the-choices -working-mothers-make.html. Published May 8, 2020. Accessed August 31, 2021.

120. ACOG Committee Opinion No. 733: employment considerations during pregnancy and the postpartum period. *Obstet Gynecol.* 2018;131(4): e115-e123. doi:10.1097/aog.0000000000002589.

121. Harwood M, Heydemann SD. By the numbers: where do pregnant women work? https://nwlc.org /wp-content/uploads/2019/08/Pregnant-Workers-by -the-Numbers-v3-1.pdf. Published 2019. Accessed November 8, 2022.

122. National Institute for Occupational Safety and Health. Reproductive health and the workplace. https://www.cdc.gov/niosh/topics/repro/default. html. Published 2019. Accessed September 9, 2021.

123. MacDonald LA, Waters TR, Napolitano PG, et al. Clinical guidelines for occupational lifting in pregnancy: evidence summary and provisional recommendations. *Am J Obstet Gynecol.* 2013;209(2):80-88. doi:10.1016/j .ajog.2013.02.047.

124. Torres Toda M, Miri M, Alonso L, et al. Exposure to greenspace and birth weight in a middle-income country. *Environ Res.* 2020;189:109866. doi:10.1016 /j.envres.2020.109866.

125. Reducing prenatal exposure to toxic environmental agents: ACOG Committee Opinion Number 832. *Obstet Gynecol.* 2021;138(1):e40-e54. doi:10.1097 /aog.0000000000004449.

126. Oduyebo T, Polen KD, Walke HT, et al. Update: interim guidance for health care providers caring for pregnant women with possible Zika virus exposure—United States (including U.S. territories), July 2017. *MMWR.* 2017;66(29):781-793. doi:10.15585/mmwr.mm6629e1.

127. Centers for Disease Control and Prevention. Zika virus: prevent mosquito bites. https://www.cdc.gov/zika/prevention/prevent-mosquito-bites.html. Published 2019. Accessed September 3, 2021.

128. Centers for Disease Control and Prevention. Zika during pregnancy. https://www.cdc.gov/pregnancy/zika/protect-yourself.html. Published 2021. Accessed September 3, 2021.

129. Feldman DM, Keller R, Borgida AF. Toxoplasmosis, parvovirus, and cytomegalovirus in pregnancy. *Clin Lab Med.* 2016;36(2):407-419. doi:10.1016/j.cll.2016.01.011.

130. Madjunkov M, Chaudhry S, Ito S. Listeriosis during pregnancy. *Arch Gynecol Obstet.* 2017;296(2):143-152. doi:10.1007/s00404-017-4401-1.

131. Neu N, Duchon J, Zachariah P. TORCH infections. *Clin Perinatol.* 2015;42(1):77-103, viii. doi:10.1016/j.clp.2014.11.001.

132. Sugishita Y, Akiba T, Sumitomo M, et al. Shedding of rubella virus among infants with congenital rubella syndrome born in Tokyo, Japan, 2013–2014. *Jpn J Infect Dis.* 2016;69(5):418-423. doi:10.7883/yoken.JJID.2015.316.

133. Cullen J, Stone S, Phipps MG, Cypher R. Immunization for pregnant women: a call to action. *J Midwifery Womens Health.* 2020;65(5):713-715. doi:10.1111/jmwh.13163.

134. Centers for Disease Control and Prevention. COVID-19 vaccines while pregnant or breastfeeding. https://www.cdc.gov/coronavirus/2019-ncov/vaccines/recommendations/pregnancy.html. Published 2021. Accessed September 9, 2021.

135. Castillo E, Patey A, MacDonald N. Vaccination in pregnancy: challenges and evidence-based solutions. *Best Pract Res Clin Obstet Gynaecol.* 2021;76:83-95. doi:10.1016/j.bpobgyn.2021.03.008.

136. Tharpe NL, McDaniel L. Using a harm reduction model to reduce barriers to vaccine administration. *J Midwifery Womens Health.* 2021;66(3):308-321. doi:10.1111/jmwh.13259.

137. Callahan AG, Coleman-Cowger VH, Schulkin J, Power ML. Racial disparities in influenza immunization during pregnancy in the United States: a narrative review of the evidence for disparities and potential interventions. *Vaccine.* 2021;39(35):4938-4948. doi:10.1016/j.vaccine.2021.07.028.

138. DiTosto JD, Weiss RE, Yee LM, Badreldin N. Association of Tdap vaccine guidelines with vaccine uptake during pregnancy. *PloS One.* 2021;16(7):e0254863. doi:10.1371/journal.pone.0254863.

139. Ojo A, Beckman AL, Weiseth A, Shah N. Ensuring racial equity in pregnancy care during the COVID-19 pandemic and beyond. *Matern Child Health J.* 2021:1-4. doi:10.1007/s10995-021-03194-4.

140. Duong HT, Shahrukh Hashmi S, Ramadhani T, et al. Maternal use of hot tub and major structural birth defects. *Birth Defects Res Pt A: Clin Molecul Teratol.* 2011;91(9):836-841. doi:10.1002/bdra.20831.

141. Freeman M, Ghidini A, Spong CY, et al. Does air travel affect pregnancy outcome? *Arch Gynecol Obstet.* 2004;269(4):274-277. doi:10.1007/s00404-003-0579-5.

142. Harvey MA, McRorie MM, Smith DW. Suggested limits to the use of the hot tub and sauna by pregnant women. *Can Med Assoc J.* 1981;125(1):50-53.

143. Sayle AE, Savitz DA, Thorp JM Jr, et al. Sexual activity during late pregnancy and risk of preterm delivery. *Obstet Gynecol.* 2001;97(2):283-289. doi:10.1016/s0029-7844(00)01147-9.

144. Schellenberg M, Ruiz NS, Cheng V, et al. The impact of seat belt use in pregnancy on injuries and outcomes after motor vehicle collisions. *J Surg Res.* 2020;254:96-101. doi:10.1016/j.jss.2020.04.012.

145. Steinberg BJ, Hilton IV, Iida H, Samelson R. Oral health and dental care during pregnancy. *Dental Clin North Am.* 2013;57(2):195-210. doi:10.1016/j.cden.2013.01.002.

146. Committee Opinion No. 723 summary: guidelines for diagnostic imaging during pregnancy and lactation. *Obstet Gynecol.* 2017;130(4):933-934. doi:10.1097/aog.0000000000002350.

147. Lowe S. Diagnostic imaging in pregnancy: making informed decisions. *Obstet Med.* 2019;12(3):116-122. doi:10.1177/1753495x19838658.

148. Goulding AN, Bauer AE, Muddana A, et al. Provider counseling and women's family planning decisions in the postpartum period. *J Womens Health.* 2020;29(6):847-853. doi:10.1089/jwh.2019.7872.

149. McKinley EM, Knol LL, Turner LW, et al. Enhancing patient–provider breastfeeding conversations: breastfeeding intention and prenatal breastfeeding self-efficacy among a sample of pregnant women. *South Med J.* 2021;114(4):223-230. doi:10.14423/smj.0000000000001238.

150. Moon RY. SIDS and other sleep-related infant deaths: evidence base for 2016 updated recommendations for a safe infant sleeping environment. *Pediatrics.* 2016;138(5). doi:10.1542/peds.2016-2940.

151. Walker DS, Visger JM, Rossie D. Contemporary childbirth education models. *J Midwifery Womens Health.* 2009;54(6):469-476. doi:10.1016/j.jmwh.2009.02.013.

152. Ricchi A, La Corte S, Molinazzi MT, et al. Study of childbirth education classes and evaluation of their effectiveness. *La Clinica Terapeutica.* 2020;170(1):e78-e86. doi:10.7417/ct.2020.2193.

153. Hetherington E, Tough S, McNeil D, et al. Vulnerable women's perceptions of individual versus group prenatal care: results of a cross-sectional survey. *Matern Child Health J.* 2018;22(11):1632-1638. doi:10.1007/s10995-018-2559-1.

154. Peahl AF, Howell JD. The evolution of prenatal care delivery guidelines in the United States. *Am J Obstet Gynecol.* 2021;224(4):339-347. doi:10.1016/j.ajog .2020.12.016.

155. Gregory KD, Johnson CT, Johnson TR, Entman SS. The content of prenatal care: update 2005. *Womens Health Issues.* 2006;16(4):198-215. doi:10.1016 /j.whi.2006.05.001.

156. Rosen MG, Merkatz IR, Hill JG. Caring for our future: a report by the expert panel on the content of prenatal care. *Obstet Gynecol.* 1991;77(5):782-787.

157. WHO Guidelines Approved by the Guidelines Review Committee. *WHO recommendations on antenatal care for a positive pregnancy experience.* Geneva, Switzerland: World Health Organization; 2016.

158. Carter EB, Mazzoni SE. A paradigm shift to address racial inequities in perinatal healthcare. *Am J Obstet Gynecol.* 2021;224(4):359-361. doi:10.1016/j.ajog .2020.11.040.

159. Butler Tobah YS, LeBlanc A, Branda ME, et al. Randomized comparison of a reduced-visit prenatal care model enhanced with remote monitoring. *Am J Obstet Gynecol.* 2019;221(6):638.e631-638.e638. doi:10.1016/j.ajog.2019.06.034.

160. Peahl AF, Zahn CM, Turrentine M, et al. The Michigan plan for appropriate tailored health care in pregnancy prenatal care recommendations. *Obstet Gynecol.* 2021;138:593-602. doi:10.1097 /aog.0000000000004531.

161. Peahl AF, Smith RD, Moniz MH. Prenatal care redesign: creating flexible maternity care models through virtual care. *Am J Obstet Gynecol.* 2020;223(3):389.e1-389.e10. doi:10.1016/j.ajog .2020.05.029.

# APPENDIX

# 21A

# Abdominal Examination During Pregnancy

MELAN J. SMITH-FRANCIS AND STEPHANIE DEVANE-JOHNSON

*The editors acknowledge Tekoa L. King and Cecilia M. Jevitt, who were the authors of this appendix in the previous edition.*

The components of the abdominal examination in pregnancy include (1) abdominal inspection and palpation; (2) measurement of fundal height; (3) abdominal maneuvers for determining fetal lie, presentation, position, attitude, and engagement; (4) estimation of fetal weight; and (5) detection of fetal heart tones.

While ultrasound can effectively be used to assess fetal growth and position—and should be used when discrepancies arise or assessment is challenging—being able to employ one's hands to gain information about the progress of a pregnancy is an invaluable skill. The standard descriptions in this appendix assume an individual of normal habitus and a singleton pregnancy. The pregnant individual's height and weight, uterine abnormalities, fetal growth pattern, and multiple pregnancies are all factors that can challenge interpretation of clinical findings, and their effects are discussed.

## Equipment

- Measuring tape with centimeter increments
- Pinard, Allen, DeLee, or Doppler fetoscope

## Preparation for Abdominal Examination During Pregnancy

1. The individual's bladder should be empty.
2. The individual's abdomen is typically exposed from just below the breasts to the symphysis pubis. Provide privacy and consider cultural variations in comfort with exposure of skin. Ask the individual to move their clothing instead of doing it for them. This allows the individual to control the extent and amount of skin exposure.
3. Relaxation of the abdominal muscles can be facilitated by:
   a. Placing a pillow under the individual's head and upper shoulders
   b. Asking them to place their arms by their sides or across their chest
   c. Having them bend their knees slightly
4. Before palpating, the midwife asks permission and lightly rests their hand on the individual's abdomen (Figure 21A-1). This action gives the individual an opportunity to adjust to the sensation of the midwife's touch and allows any initial muscle-tightening reaction to dissipate.

## Abdominal Inspection

**The following aspects of the abdomen are noted during inspection:**

1. Surgical scars. The scar of a previous cesarean birth is of particular importance; it may be either vertical or horizontal. It is useful to know if the individual has undergone an appendectomy so that appendicitis can be

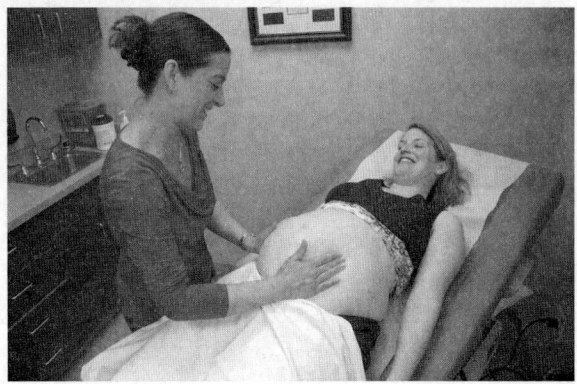

**Figure 21A-1** Midwife preparing to do an abdominal palpation. Reproduced with permission from Jenifer Fahey.

ruled out in the event of right-sided abdominal pain during the pregnancy.

2. Bruises or abrasions. Document a description and location of any bruises and discuss their origin with the individual, paying particular attention to the possibility of intimate partner violence and abuse.

3. Linea nigra. This hyperpigmented vertical line on the lower abdomen may be visible by approximately 20 weeks' gestation, or it may be faintly present from a previous pregnancy and begin to darken in the first trimester. The linea nigra will fade during the first 6 months postpartum.

4. Striae gravidarum. Many individuals develop these pink or red streaks during pregnancy as the dermis is stretched. Silvery white streaks may be present from previous weight changes or previous pregnancy.

5. Abdominal contours give some initial indication of the fetal lie, presentation, position, and attitude, although none of the following observations is diagnostic:

   a. Uterine shape is a longitudinal ovoid: Fundal height in the expected range suggests a longitudinal lie.

   b. Uterine shape is a transverse ovoid: Fundal height lower than expected for gestational age may indicate a transverse lie, fetal growth restriction, or oligohydramnios.

   c. A long, smooth curve prominent on one side of the abdomen suggests that the back of the fetus is on that side of the abdomen.

   d. A saucer-like depression appearing just below the umbilicus and a bulge like a full bladder appearing above the symphysis pubis suggests a possible occiput posterior position or a full bladder.

   e. Movement of fetal small parts seen all over the abdomen suggests an occiput posterior position.

## Abdominal Palpation

**The midwife may palpate these structures during physical examination:**

1. Diastasis recti (midline separation of the rectus abdominus muscle) presence and width are palpated by placing one or two fingers parallel to the abdominal midline, just below the epigastric region, and feeling the separation of the rectus abdominis muscle after asking the individual to lift their head while lying supine. This examination is routinely performed at the postpartum visit but may also be useful at the first prenatal visit, especially for a multiparous individual, as they may have a persistent diastasis recti.

2. Umbilical hernia (intestinal protrusion through a separation in the abdominal muscles behind the umbilicus) can be detected with palpation at any time during pregnancy.

3. Uterine muscle tone (hard versus soft), contractions (palpable or not palpable), and tenderness are evaluated to assess for signs of preterm labor in the second and third trimesters, for signs of labor after 37 weeks' gestation, and for signs of infection.

4. Amniotic fluid volume. When performing an abdominal examination, the midwife can estimate the quantity of amniotic fluid by placing one hand on each side of the uterus and gently pushing first on one side of the uterus, then the other. A fluid wave or thrill might be palpated depending on gestational age, size and position of the fetus, and amount of fluid present. If the individual has polyhydramnios, it will be difficult to palpate small parts of the fetus and may be difficult to determine fetal position. The opposite will be true in an individual with oligohydramnios.

## Abdominal Maneuvers to Assess Fetal Position

The process of evaluating fetal lie, position, and presentation with abdominal maneuvers, previously known as Leopold's maneuvers, also offers the opportunity to assess the abdomen for muscle tone, uterine tone and contractility, and palpable fetal movement, and to estimate fetal weight. The four abdominal maneuvers and the combined abdominal/fetal grip, also known as Pawlik's grip, are shown in **Figure 21A-2.**

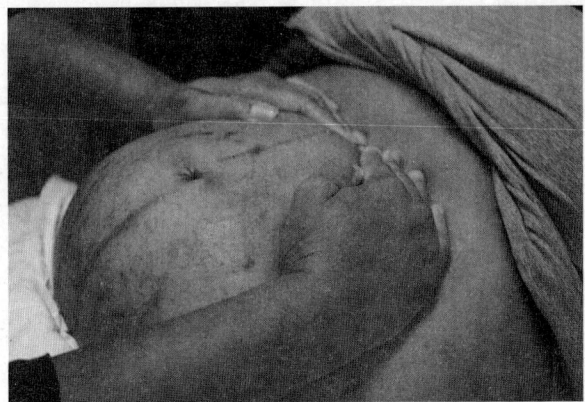
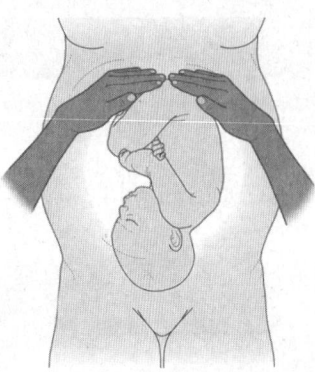

First maneuver. Identify the part of the fetus that resides in the fundus. Curve the fingers of both hands around the top of the fundus.

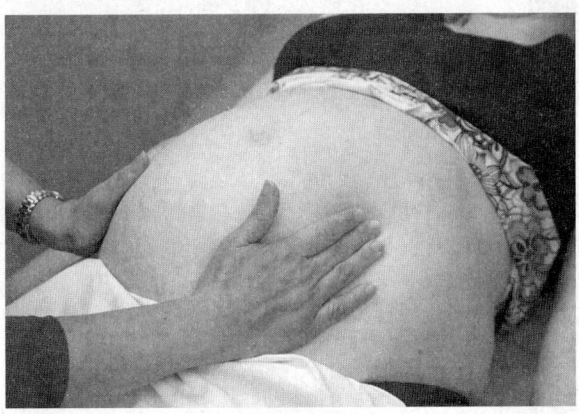
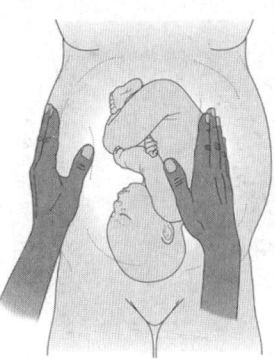

Second maneuver. Identify the location of the small parts and fetal back. Place both hands on the sides of the uterus.

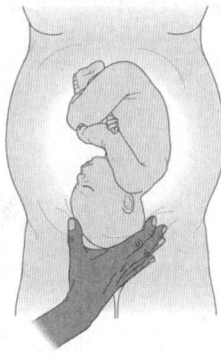

Third maneuver. Identify the presenting part. With the thumb and middle finger of one hand, press gently but deeply into the individual's abdomen immediately above the symphysis pubis and grasp the presenting part.

**Figure 21A-2** The four maneuvers and the combined abdominal/fetal (Pawlik's) grip.
Photos reproduced with permission from Jenifer Fahey, Melan Smith-Francis, and Stephanie DeVane-Johnson.

*(continues)*

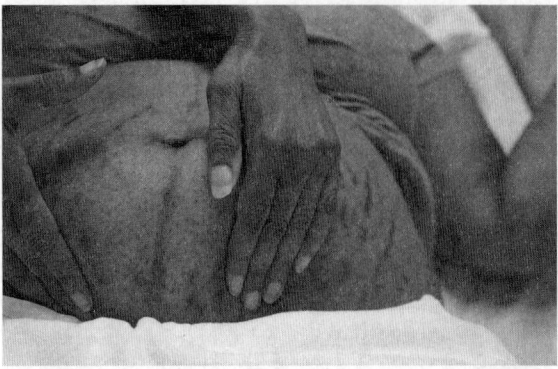
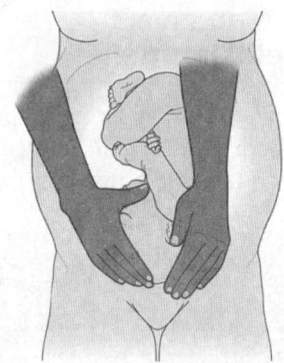

Fourth maneuver. Check whether the presenting part is engaged and the location of the cephalic prominence. Place both hands on the sides of the lower uterus, press deeply, and move the fingertips toward the pelvic inlet.

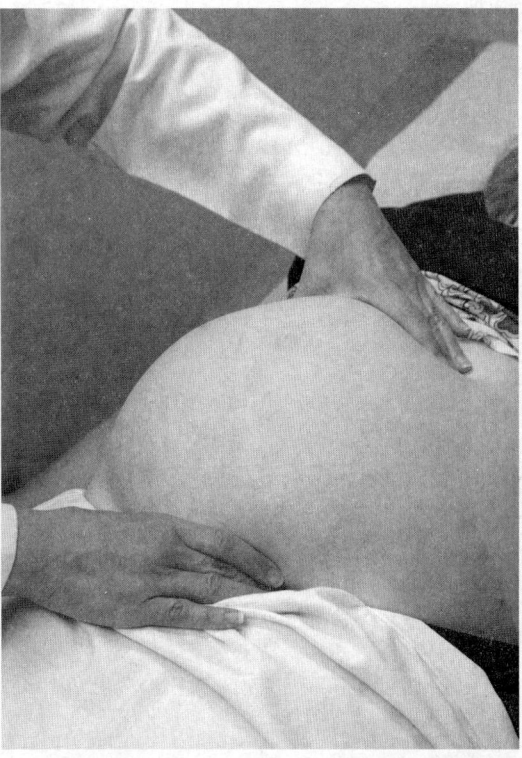
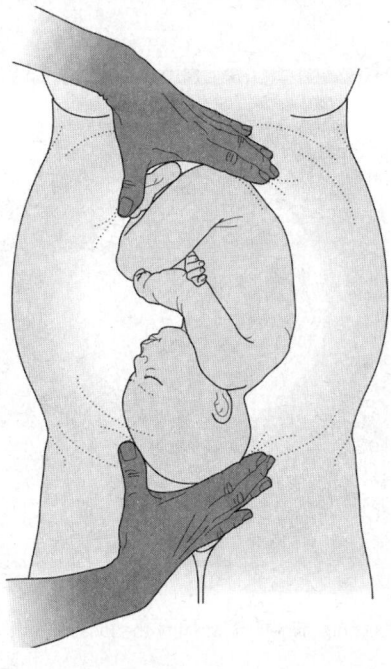

Combined abdominal/fetal (Pawlik's) grip. Combine the third abdominal maneuver with one hand and palpation of the fundus using the other hand. Compare the two poles for final determination of lie and presentation.

**Figure 21A-2** (continued)

## Procedure for Abdominal Maneuvers

### First Maneuver: Determine Fetal Lie and Presentation

Facing the individual's head, palpate the area of the uterine fundus, noting the shape of the fetal part in the fundus. A fetal part that feels round and hard, and that can be balloted between the midwife's fingers or hands, suggests a fetal head. The mobility arises from the head being able to move independently of the trunk. A fetal part that feels irregular, larger or bulkier, and less firm than a head, and that cannot be well delineated or readily moved or balloted, suggests the fetal breech. The breech cannot move independently of the trunk. In these cases, the lie is longitudinal. If neither of the preceding conditions is felt in the fundus, a transverse lie may be present.

### Second Maneuver: Determine the Location of the Fetal Back

1. Continue to face the individual's head. Place the hands on both sides of the uterus about midway between the symphysis pubis and the fundus.

2. Apply slight pressure with one stabilizing hand against the side of the uterus, thereby pushing the fetus to the other side of the abdomen against the examining hand. Maintain this pressure while the examining hand palpates the side of the uterus to identify fetal parts.

3. Palpate the entire area with the examining hand, from the abdominal midline to the lateral side, and from the fundus to the symphysis. Use firm, smooth pressure and rotary movement.

4. Reverse the procedure to examine the other side of the uterus.

5. The flat palmar surfaces of the fingers are used for palpating—*not* the fingertips. Smooth, deep pressure is used—as firm as is necessary to obtain accurate findings without causing pain or discomfort.

A firm, convex, continuously smooth, and resistant mass extending from the breech to the neck indicates the fetal back. The location of the back in the anterior, lateral, or posterior portion of the abdomen helps to determine the fetal position. Small, knobby, irregular masses that might move when pressed on suggest the fetal small parts—hands, feet, knees, elbows. When palpating the uterus, the fetal small parts should be opposite the fetal back. If the back is difficult to feel and seems to be just out of reach in the posterior portion of the abdomen, and small parts are palpable all over the abdomen, a posterior position may be present.

### Third Maneuver: Determine the Fetal Presentation and Engagement

The third maneuver is called abdominal/fetal (Pawlik's) grip. Clasp the lower abdomen immediately above the symphysis pubis between the thumb and middle finger of one hand, with the thumb and middle finger spread so they start the procedure as far laterally into the inguinal area as possible. It will be necessary to press gently but firmly into the abdomen to feel the presenting part between the thumb and finger. Abdominal/fetal grip can be uncomfortable and may be omitted, as the fetal presentation

can be determined with the fourth maneuver. A kicking motion palpated in the fundus during abdominal/fetal grip increases confidence that the presentation is cephalic, but does not provide certainty as the fetus may be frank breech.

If the fetal head is above the pelvic brim, it is readily movable and ballotable, as described for the first maneuver. A procedure that is sometimes added to this maneuver is called the combined abdominal/fetal grip, in which abdominal/fetal grip is utilized with one hand and the fundus is grasped in the same way with the other hand at the same time. This combination enables the simultaneous comparison of what is in the two poles for final determination of the fetal lie and presentation.

### Fourth Maneuver: Cephalic Prominence and Fetal Attitude

1. Turn and face the individual's feet.

2. Place both hands on the sides of the uterus with the palms just above the symphysis and iliac crest, with the fingers directed toward the symphysis pubis.

3. Press with the fingertips into the lower abdomen slowly but firmly, and move them toward the pelvic inlet to determine the *cephalic prominence*; note if it is on the side of the fetal back or fetal front. If the cephalic prominence is on the same side as the fetal small parts, the fetal *attitude* is flexed and the fetal head is tucked toward the chin. If the presentation is vertex and the cephalic prominence is on the same side as the fetal back, the fetus is in a face or brow presentation.

At the conclusion of the four maneuvers, share the findings with the individual. Offer to help them feel and identify various parts of their fetus if they would like and, if culturally appropriate, ask permission to let the partner or support person feel the fetus.

## Estimation of Fetal Weight

Estimated fetal weight (EFW) is used during the prenatal period, particularly after 30 weeks' gestation, as one clinical measurement in the overall evaluation of gestational age and progressive fetal growth. During abdominal maneuvers, the midwife can compare the palpated fetal size to known volumes such as a liter bag of IV fluid, a 5-pound bag of flour, or a gallon jug of milk to estimate size. Neither experienced hands nor an ultrasound is necessarily more accurate than the other method when assessing fetal weight in a full-term fetus. The EFW is important in the intrapartum period, when this estimation is compared with the clinical evaluation of the pelvis to assess the fetal–pelvic relationship. Estimating fetal weights and comparing those estimations to ultrasound estimations or birth weights for feedback sharpens a midwife's skill in estimating fetal weight.

## Auscultation of Fetal Heart

From 11 to 20 weeks, the fetal heart rate is best located by placing the Doppler above the symphysis pubis and slowly changing the angle until hearing the fetal heart. It may be necessary to move the transducer superiorly or laterally at later gestational ages. In the late second and third trimesters, the sound of the fetal heart is transmitted best through the convex portion of the fetus closest to the anterior uterine wall, which is usually the fetal back. Thus, if the position of the fetus is known, fetal heart tones can be readily located, allowing for some variation depending on how far the fetus has descended into the pelvis (Figure 21A-3). Location of the fetal heart is an additional piece of data that either confirms or calls into question the diagnosis of fetal presentation and position.

## Measuring Fundal Height

Fundal heights are measured at each prenatal visit. Serial fundal height measurements provide information about the enlargement of the uterus and, therefore, about the growth of the fetus. The height of the fundus, measured in centimeters from the top of the symphysis pubis to the top of the fundus, is used to monitor fetal growth and can be a screening tool for detection of multifetal gestation, fetal growth restriction, polyhydramnios, oligohydramnios, and other complications of fetal growth. Fundal height is of greatest value when it is measured the same way by the same midwife at successive prenatal visits.

The fundal height (measured in centimeters) and gestational age (expressed in weeks from the last menstrual period [LMP]) are closely correlated between 20 and 32 weeks' gestation, when the number of weeks' gestation is close to the number of centimeters measured between the symphysis and the

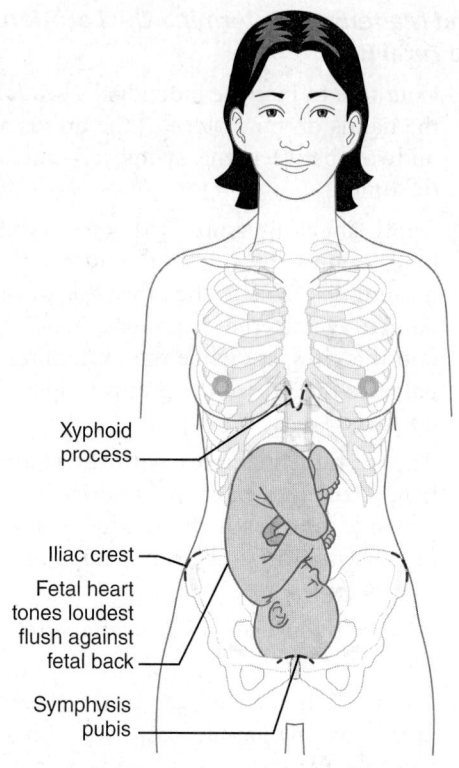

**Figure 21A-3** Location of the point of maximum intensity of auscultation of the fetal heart tones in the last trimester.

fundus.[1-6] However, the correlation between weeks' gestation and fundal heights depends on several factors, including maternal habitus and fetal lie. For example, an individual who is 5 feet (1.5 meters) tall may have different fundal measurements than a taller individual with a height of 6 feet (1.8 meters) at the same point in pregnancy. Similarly, individuals with a large deposition of abdominal adipose tissue may have a fundal height measurement that is larger than expected. Table 21A-1 lists the approximate expected location of the fundal height at different gestational ages for individuals with a normal body mass index (BMI) and singleton fetus in a longitudinal lie.

In clinical practice, it is common to use a rule of gestational age plus or minus 2 centimeters to diagnose adequate fetal growth. That is, during 20 to 32 weeks' gestation, an individual should have a fundal measurement in centimeters that is within 2 cm of the number of weeks' gestation. No strong evidence supports this approach, most likely because of the maternal and fetal variations noted earlier. Despite a lack of evidence, deviation from the 2-cm rule of thumb can be used as an alert to carefully assess for size–dates discrepancy. Assessment of size–dates discrepancies first includes

| Table 21A-1 | Approximate Expected Fundal Height at Specific Weeks' Gestation |
|---|---|
| **Weeks' Gestation** | **Approximate Expected Fundal Height** |
| 12 | Level of the symphysis pubis |
| 16 | Halfway between symphysis pubis and umbilicus |
| 20 | Within 1 fingerbreadth of umbilicus |
| 24 | 2–4 fingerbreadths above umbilicus |
| 28–30 | One-third of the way between umbilicus and xiphoid process (3 fingerbreadths above umbilicus) |
| 32 | Two-thirds of the way between umbilicus and xiphoid process (3–4 fingerbreadths below xiphoid process) |
| 36–38 | 1 fingerbreadth below xiphoid process |
| 40 | 2–3 fingerbreadths below xiphoid process if lightening has occurred |

remeasurement when the individual has an empty bladder, as a full bladder can elevate the uterus. Ultrasound is used to diagnose the etiology of a size–dates discrepancy.

### Key Points

1. Early in pregnancy, the uterus is contained within the pelvis. The uterine fundus can be palpated abdominally by 10 to 12 weeks' gestation just at or above the symphysis pubis. Prior to 18 to 20 weeks' gestation, the uterine size is best described in relation to the level of the uterine fundus between the symphysis pubis and the umbilicus, using the midwife's fingerbreadth (fb) as the measuring tool (e.g., 1 fb above symphysis, 4 fb below umbilicus). (For more information, see the *Anatomy and Physiology of Pregnancy* chapter.)

2. Between 20 and 32 weeks' gestation, the measurement should be within 2 cm of the number of weeks' gestation.

3. In the last few weeks of pregnancy, as the fetal presenting part moves into the pelvis, more variation is seen between measurements, and the absolute fundal height may remain stable or decrease slightly.

4. Used alone, the fundal height measurement may be specific, but lacks sensitivity. When a measurement is not within the expected value for the individual's gestational age:

    a. First assess for confounding factors such as a full bladder or abdominal adipose tissue.

    b. Refer the individual for ultrasound evaluation if the confounding factors do not sufficiently account for the size–dates discrepancy.

### Procedure for Measuring Fundal Height

Fundal height can be measured in a number of different ways. For an extensive review of fundal height measurement, the interested reader is referred to the classic series of articles written by Engstrom et al.[1–7]

1. Assessment of the fundal height should take place with the individual in a supine or semi-recumbent position.

2. Some midwives advocate turning the tape measure to hide the centimeter markings, thereby minimizing inadvertent bias by the midwife. Alterations in maternal position, a full urinary bladder, multiple examiners, and provider awareness of the weeks' gestation all create bias that can lead to inaccurate measurements.

3. Before measuring, the symphysis pubis and uterine fundus are identified (**Figure 21A-4**).

    a. The individual may need to partially remove their clothing to allow access to the symphysis and fundus. The abdomen is exposed from the xiphoid process to the top of the pelvis.

    b. Assessment is done with a gentle, firm touch using the palmar surface of the fingers.

    c. The midwife places the zero line of the tape measure on the uppermost border of the symphysis pubis and extends the tape in a smooth fashion straight to the uppermost border of the uterine fundus.[8] There is no strong evidence to show placing the tape under the cubital edge of the hand versus between the index and middle fingers alters the measurement.

    d. The uterine fundus is identified by walking one's hands up the sides of the uterus until they meet at the top. Smooth motions avoid the sensation of kneading or

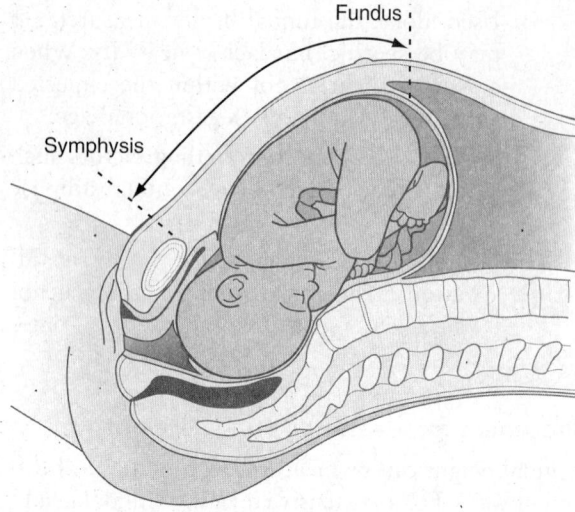

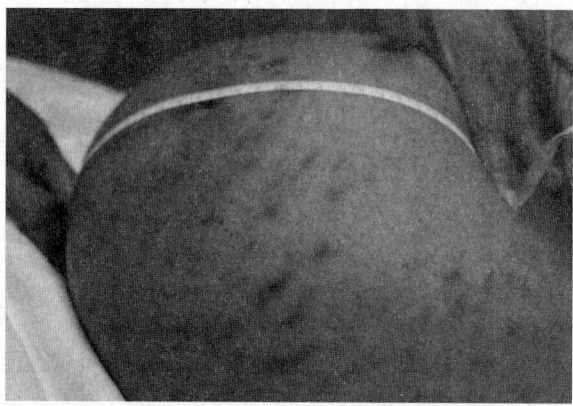

**Figure 21A-4** Measurement of fundal height.
Legend: Position of hand and tape for fundal height measurement. Photo reproduced with permission from Stephanie Devane-Johnson and Melan Smith-Francis.

poking and will decrease uterine contractility during the examination.

e. Measuring "over the top" of the fundus is a common error that can be avoided by paying attention to the curve of the uterus, the location of the fetal part highest in the uterus, and any laxity of the maternal abdomen.

4. Two techniques are commonly employed:

a. Place the zero line of the tape measure on the superior border of the symphysis and measure *upward* in a straight line, following the abdominal midline to the crest of the uterine fundus. Taking care not to cross over the top, begin to measure the posterior aspect of the uterus.

b. After identifying the fundus, place the tape at that point and measure *downward* to the superior border of the symphysis.

## References

1. Engstrom JL. Measurement of fundal height. *J Obstet Gynecol Neonatal Nurs.* 1988;17(3):172-178.

2. Engstrom JL, Ostrenga KG, Plass RV, Work BA. The effect of maternal bladder volume on fundal height measurements. *Br J Obstet Gynaecol.* 1989;96(8):987-991.

3. Engstrom JL, Sittler CP. Fundal height measurement. Part 1: techniques for measuring fundal height. *J Nurse-Midwifery.* 1993;38(1):5-16.

4. Engstrom JL, McFarlin BL, Sittler CP. Fundal height measurement. Part 2: intra- and interexaminer reliability of three measurement techniques. *J Nurse-Midwifery.* 1993;38(1):17-22.

5. Engstrom JL, Piscioneri LA, Low LK, et al. Fundal height measurement. Part 3: the effect of maternal position on fundal height measurements. *J Nurse-Midwifery.* 1993;38(1):23-27.

6. Engstrom JL, McFarlin BL, Sampson MB. Fundal height measurement. Part 4: accuracy of clinicians' identification of the uterine fundus during pregnancy. *J Nurse-Midwifery.* 1993;38(6):318-323.

7. Engstrom JL, Sittler CP, Swift KE. Fundal height measurement. Part 5: the effect of clinician bias on fundal height measurements. *J Nurse-Midwifery.* 1994;39(3):130-141.

8. Papageorghiou AT, Ohuma EO, Gravett MG, et al. International standards for symphysis–fundal height based on serial measurements from the Fetal Growth Longitudinal Study of the INTERGROWTH-21st Project: prospective cohort study in eight countries. *BMJ.* 2016;355:i5662. doi:10.1136/bmj.i5662.

CHAPTER

# 22

# Early Pregnancy Loss and Abortion Care

HANNAH DIAZ AND MEGHAN EAGEN-TORKKO

## Introduction

Early pregnancy loss and abortion care are critical aspects of midwifery practice. In each case, the management decisions focus on the well-being of the pregnant person, and as such the preferences and desires of the patient are central to care management. Both early pregnancy loss and abortion are common experiences for pregnancy-capable people, and both have a long history of midwifery management. In this chapter, we discuss the clinical management and social considerations of these two pregnancy outcomes.

A note about language: Both "induced abortion" and "spontaneous abortion" are terms used in the clinical literature, but patients will generally refer to a spontaneous abortion (pregnancy loss prior to 20 weeks' gestation) as a *miscarriage* or *loss* and will simply say *abortion* rather than refer to an induced or therapeutic abortion. These terms allow a clear differentiation of miscarriage from elective or induced abortion and may be more acceptable to patients dealing with loss. In this chapter, for clarity and to reflect the language patients use, we have chosen to use the terms *early pregnancy loss* and *miscarriage* to refer to spontaneous losses prior to 20 weeks' gestation, and *abortion* to refer to the intentional interruption of a pregnancy at any gestation. *Products of conception* refers to any tissues resulting from the fertilized ovum, including the embryo, fetus, chorionic villi, placenta, and membranes.

Many conditions can lead to pregnancy loss or increase the likelihood that an individual will select abortion for health reasons. It is important to understand the subtle differences in definitions (Table 22-1) and to know the warning signs and complications for each condition. Many of these conditions may cause vaginal bleeding during pregnancy.

## First Trimester Bleeding

Vaginal bleeding is one of the most common complications during the first trimester, occurring in approximately 25% of all pregnant patients.[1] In clinical practice, the management and evaluation of first trimester bleeding is a daily occurrence for midwives. Patients may report the bleeding as bright red (fresh), or dark brown (old), and as light and infrequent or persistent and heavy. The pattern and amount of bleeding are not predictive of early pregnancy loss. Most patients who have an episode of minor vaginal bleeding and documented normal fetal cardiac motion on ultrasound will remain pregnant. However, related pain or cramping and heavy bleeding are associated with a higher risk of early pregnancy loss. Regardless of the presentation, any patient reporting vaginal bleeding should be evaluated promptly. While the list of differential diagnoses is long, some of them are associated with significant morbidity, and it can take several days or even weeks to determine a conclusive diagnosis. Depending on the circumstances, the midwife may need to seek a physician consultation or referral early in the evaluation process.

### Differential Diagnoses

Vaginal bleeding in pregnancy may originate in the uterus, cervix, or vagina. Some causes of bleeding

| Table 22-1 | Definitions of Conditions Associated with Early Pregnancy Loss | |
|---|---|---|
| **Term** | **Definition** | **Clinical Presentation** |
| Ectopic pregnancy | Pregnancy that is implanted outside of the uterus

Most common is tubal pregnancy, in which the fertilized egg becomes implanted in the uterine tubes/oviducts

Ovarian and abdominal pregnancy are rare | May be asymptomatic initially and associated with irregular vaginal bleeding or no bleeding.

Pregnancy test (urine or serum beta-hCG) may or may not be positive.

Adnexal mass may be visible on TVUS; the mass may or may not be palpable on physical examination.

The uterus may be slightly enlarged due to hormonal stimulation of the endometrium.

If an ectopic pregnancy ruptures, the patient may experience hypotension, signs of shock, sharp severe pain that may be unilateral, CMT, bulging posterior vaginal fornix, and referred pain to the neck and shoulder if there is bleeding into the peritoneum. |
| Gestational trophoblastic disease (hydatidiform mole) | Complete: Haploid sperm fertilizes an ovum that has lost DNA; the sperm DNA replicates, resulting in a diploid genome. Fertilization of an ovum that has lost its DNA by two sperm can also result in a complete mole. Complete moles have a genotype of 46XX or 46XY.

Partial: Two haploid sperm fertilize a normal ovum; the resulting pregnancy is triploid (69XXY) or greater | The uterus can be larger than expected and hCG levels higher than expected for gestational age.

Significant NVP and uterine bleeding are present.

FHR is not detected.

May be associated with hypertension and early preeclampsia.

Ultrasound has diagnostic features including a cluster of grape-like material, a honeycomb effect, or a "snowstorm" on the screen.

Associated with choriocarcinoma (malignancy). |
| Pregnancy of uncertain viability | Ultrasound shows a gestational sac but no embryonic heartbeat | This diagnosis is based on findings on TVUS that do not definitively detect a viable fetus or a nonviable pregnancy. Examples:
• A gestational sac that is visible on TVUS days before a yolk sac or embryo appears
• Embryo with a crown–rump length greater than 7 mm but no FHR |
| Pregnancy of uncertain location (PUL) | Positive pregnancy test but pregnancy cannot be detected on TVUS | Neither ectopic pregnancy nor IUP is confirmed.

Patients with PUL are monitored carefully until an IUP is visualized, early pregnancy loss occurs, or ectopic pregnancy is diagnosed. |
| Subchorionic hemorrhage | Bleeding between the chorion and the myometrium, or between the chorion and the placenta | Irregular, slight vaginal bleeding may occur.

Subchorionic hemorrhage may result in early pregnancy loss if large enough to impede placental growth. Most often the hemorrhages are small and resolve spontaneously as the placenta grows.

Visible on ultrasound.

May be an incidental finding on early ultrasound. |
| Anembryonic gestation | Development of a gestational sac without development of an embryo

May also be referred to as blighted ovum or biochemical pregnancy | Gestational sac > 18 mm without an embryo, or > 13 mm without yolk sac.

Declining beta-hCG levels after beta-hCG level < 1000 mIU/mL is noted with a gestational sac visible on TVUS. |

| Term | Definition | Clinical Presentation |
|---|---|---|
| Missed miscarriage[a] | Nonviable products of conception are retained with or without vaginal bleeding | Irregularly shaped/collapsing gestational sac; no embryo, mean sac diameter of ≥ 25 mm. Crown-rump length ≥ 7 mm and lack of cardiac motion. Absence of embryo with heartbeat ≥ 2 weeks after an ultrasound showed a gestational sac without yolk sac or ≥ 11 days after ultrasound showed a gestational sac with a yolk sac. |
| Recurrent miscarriage | Spontaneous abortion that has terminated the course of ≥ 3 consecutive pregnancies | No specific diagnostic ultrasound findings. |
| Threatened miscarriage (abortion) | Painless vaginal bleeding at < 20 weeks' gestation without cervical dilation or effacement | May or may not show sonographic signs of abnormal sac or embryo. May show subchorionic bleeding. |
| Inevitable miscarriage (abortion) | < 20 weeks' gestation with cervical dilation and/or rupture of the membranes in addition to vaginal bleeding and lower abdominal or back pain but no passage of tissue | Embryo > 5 mm in size, without cardiac activity. Embryonic bradycardia after 8 weeks' gestation. Serum progesterone < 5 ng/mL. |
| Incomplete miscarriage (abortion) | Passage of some fetal or placental tissue through the cervix at < 20 weeks' gestation | Tissue visible in the uterus without evidence of viable gestation. |
| Complete miscarriage (abortion) | Spontaneous expulsion of fetal and placental tissue from the uterine cavity at < 20 weeks' gestation | Uterus empty on ultrasound; endometrial stripe may still be thickened. |
| Septic miscarriage (abortion) | Serious maternal infection that occurs after any abortion | May or may not show retained products of conception, which may include the gestational sac, fetal pole, or yolk sac on ultrasound. |

Abbreviations: Beta-hCG, beta human chorionic gonadotropin; CMT, cervical motion tenderness; FHR, fetal heart rate; IUP, intrauterine pregnancy; NVP, nausea and vomiting of pregnancy; PUL, pregnancy of unknown location; TVUS, transvaginal ultrasound.

[a] Findings that are suggestive but not diagnostic for early pregnancy loss include crown–rump length < 7 mm without a heartbeat; mean sac diameter of 16–24 mm without embryo; absence of embryo with heartbeat 7–13 days after ultrasound showed a gestational sac without a yolk sac or 7–10 days after an ultrasound showed a gestational sac with yolk sac; empty amnion; enlarged yolk sac > 7 mm; small gestational sac in relation to size of embryo; absence of embryo for ≥ 6 weeks after last menstrual period.

are pregnancy related, such as early pregnancy loss, subchorionic hemorrhage, and ectopic pregnancy. Non-pregnancy-related causes of vaginal bleeding include cervicitis, vaginitis, cervical lesions, cervical polyps, and postcoital bleeding.

### Evaluation of First Trimester Bleeding

The initial goal in evaluating a patient with first trimester bleeding is to rule out life-threatening conditions such as active hemorrhage or ectopic pregnancy. A patient reporting bleeding should be seen promptly for a physical exam, laboratory tests, and an ultrasound evaluation to determine potential causes of the bleeding and to provide management. Table 22-2 reviews the history and physical

components of the evaluation of a patient with first trimester bleeding. A midwife is frequently involved in the initial assessment of patients who have bleeding early in pregnancy. However, ectopic pregnancy requires physician care, and depending on the ultrasound and laboratory findings, close monitoring and repeat laboratory tests may be needed for several days before the diagnosis is clearly established. Figure 22-1 presents one algorithm for evaluation and management of first trimester bleeding that will help the midwife assess for the initial differential diagnoses, which include non-uterine source of bleeding, viable pregnancy, nonviable pregnancy, pregnancy of uncertain viability, pregnancy of uncertain location, and ectopic pregnancy.[2] Knowledge

| Table 22-2 | Evaluation of First Trimester Bleeding |
| --- | --- |
| **Data** | **Description and Differential Diagnosis** |
| **History** | |
| Pregnancy diagnosis | Obtain LMP, LNMP, result of pregnancy test, and ultrasound results. |
| | If IUP is identified, ectopic pregnancy is unlikely.[a] |
| Lifetime reproductive history | Risk of early pregnancy loss increases as the number of previous losses increases. |
| | Risk of ectopic pregnancy is increased in patients with previous ectopic pregnancies. |
| Bleeding pattern with this pregnancy and associated events | Profuse bleeding with clots suggests incomplete miscarriage or ectopic pregnancy. |
| | Intermittent spotting associated with intercourse or vaginal penetration indicates a cervical or vaginal source of bleeding. Chlamydia or gonorrhea can cause cervicitis that manifests as vaginal spotting. |
| | Intermittent bleeding can also suggest early pregnancy loss. |
| Tissue passage | Description of the tissue can assist in diagnosis (grape-like tissue is associated with gestational trophoblastic disease, and tissue that is much smaller than expected based on gestational age increases the suspicion of retained products of conception). |
| | Description of any changes in bleeding and pain after tissue passage. |
| | Passage of tissue suggests early pregnancy loss. |
| Pain | Abdominal pain and referred pain to the neck or shoulder suggest intra-abdominal bleeding from a ruptured ectopic pregnancy, or possibly an ovarian cyst (a nonpregnancy cause). |
| **Physical Examination** | |
| Vital signs and blood pressure | Determine if the patient is hemodynamically stable. |
| Abdominal examination | Palpate for tenderness/pain, fundal height, other masses, and rebound tenderness (appendicitis). |
| | Evaluate FHR using a Doppler device if gestational age is 10 weeks or greater (rule out ectopic pregnancy, hydatidiform mole, and missed miscarriage). |
| | Palpate for CVAT (pyelonephritis can present with referred pelvic pain). |
| Speculum examination | Inspect for lacerations, lesions, vaginitis, cervicitis, hemorrhoids, and varicosities. |
| | Perform a wet prep if indicated. |
| | Inspect the cervical os for polyps, dilation, presence of fluid, blood, clots, pus, or fetal parts or membranes. |
| Bimanual examination | Size of uterus. |
| | Cervical effacement, dilation, CMT. |
| | Adnexal masses or pain. |
| **Laboratory Tests and Ultrasound** | |
| | Obtain hemoglobin/hematocrit or CBC if indicated. |
| | Obtain ABO/Rh if unknown. |
| | Perform ultrasound if indicated. |
| | Consider serial serum quantitative beta-hCG or progesterone measurement. |

Abbreviations: Beta-hCG, beta human chorionic gonadotropin; CBC, complete blood count; CMT, cervical motion tenderness; CVAT, costovertebral angle tenderness; FHR, fetal heart rate; IUP, intrauterine pregnancy; LMP, last menstrual period; LNMP, last normal menstrual period.

[a] On rare occasions, a patient may have both an intrauterine and extrauterine pregnancy—a condition called a heterotopic pregnancy. Because of this, visualization of an intrauterine pregnancy does not absolutely rule out an ectopic pregnancy.

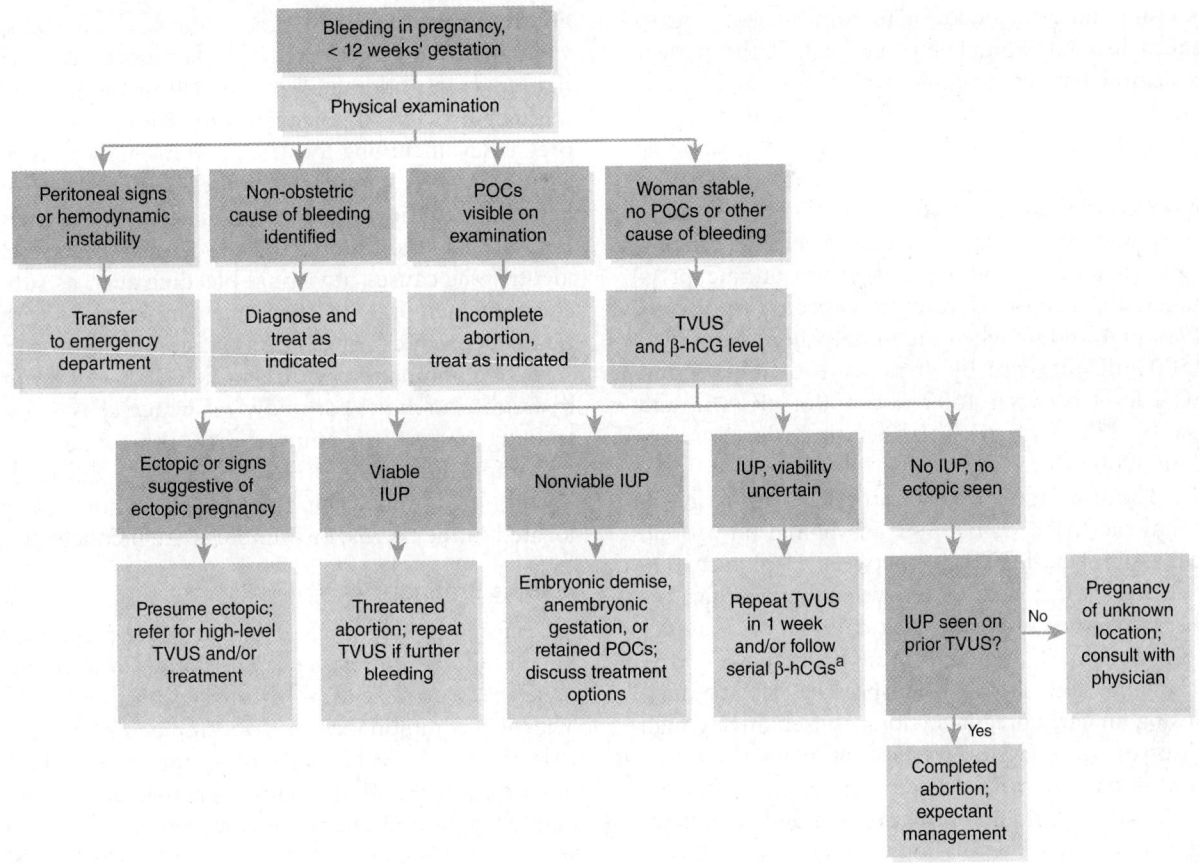

**Figure 22-1** First trimester bleeding algorithm.
Abbreviations: β-hCG, beta human chorionic gonadotropin; IUP, intrauterine pregnancy; POCs, products of conception; TVUS, transvaginal ultrasound.
[a] Care of a patient with a pregnancy of unknown location requires physician consultation for close supervision and monitoring of beta-hCG levels. Ectopic pregnancy cannot be ruled out. The patient's desire for continued pregnancy in combination with the assessment of the rise or fall in beta-hCG levels over several days will guide management.
Modified with permission from Reproductive Health Access Project. First trimester bleeding algorithm. https://www.reproductiveaccess.org /resource/first-trimester-bleeding-algorithm/. Accessed August 16, 2021.

of all possible diagnoses and likely progression of assessment and care allows the midwife to obtain physician consultation and referral at the appropriate time. Once a plan of management is established, the midwife can support the patient with anticipatory guidance as needed.

### Physical Examination

Performing a physical examination, including a pelvic examination, can sometimes determine the origin of the bleeding. Cervical polyps, cervicitis, hemorrhagic cystitis, perineal lesions, vulvar varicosities, and hemorrhoids are sources of bleeding that may be perceived as coming from the vagina. Thus, the initial evaluation is to rule out non-uterine sources of bleeding or to determine if a patient is actively

losing a pregnancy. For patients without bleeding or symptoms who present following ultrasound with a diagnosed pregnancy loss, a physical examination may be deferred depending on the midwife's clinical judgment and patient preference.

### Laboratory Tests

The beta subunit of human chorionic gonadotropin (beta-hCG) can be detected as early as 8 days after ovulation in the pregnant patient.[1] Normal values for beta-hCG in early pregnancy are described in more detail in the *Anatomy and Physiology of Pregnancy* and *Prenatal Care* chapters. Serial quantitative measurements of beta-hCG are frequently used to help establish the presence and viability of a pregnancy during the early period before a pregnancy is visible on ultrasound, or to confirm that a pregnancy loss has completely resolved. If the patient is hemodynamically stable, serum beta-hCG levels can be obtained every 48 to 72 hours. It is an old adage that beta-hCG levels are expected to double approximately every 48 hours in early pregnancy. With continuing research in diverse populations, we now know the data to be more varied and complex. In patients with a viable intrauterine pregnancy, the beta-hCG value is expected to rise by 49% in 48 hours when the initial value is less than 1500 mIU/mL, rise by 40% with an initial beta-hCG level between 1500 and 3000 mIU/mL, and rise by 33% with an initial beta-hCG level greater than 3000 mIU/mL.[3]

The discriminatory zone or level for a gestational sac to be visible by transvaginal ultrasound is a serum beta-hCG value between 1500 and 3000 mIU/mL.[1,4] If a beta-hCG level is higher than the discriminatory level and a gestational sac has not been visualized, then an ectopic pregnancy or early pregnancy loss should be suspected. Prior to diagnosing an early pregnancy loss, conservatively high levels of beta-hCG up to 3500 mIU/mL should be used in patients with desired pregnancy.[4] Other expected ultrasound findings have been linked to beta-hCG levels, albeit with significant variability: A yolk sac should be visible by ultrasound between 1094 and 17,716 mIU/mL, and a fetal pole is expected to be visualized with corresponding beta-hCG levels of 1295 to 47,685 mIU/mL.[5]

Progesterone levels can also be used to discriminate between a threatened early pregnancy loss and a viable intrauterine pregnancy. The primary limitation of this biomarker is that it does not help in determining the site of pregnancy. For this reason, assessment of a progesterone level is not a routine component of most clinical management protocols, but it may be of value in individual cases. Progesterone is produced by the corpus luteum in the first trimester of pregnancy. If the serum progesterone value is 20 ng/mL or greater, the pregnancy is likely viable. Similarly, a value of 6 ng/mL or less is consistent with a nonviable or possible ectopic pregnancy. When the serum progesterone level is between 6 and 20 ng/mL, further evaluation of the pregnancy is indicated.[1] Another potential problem with the use of progesterone as a biomarker for pregnancy is that some laboratories take several days to return results, which limits the clinical utility of this test as a timely diagnostic tool.

Ultrasound in the first trimester can be diagnostic for most of the uterine causes of first trimester bleeding and is a valuable evaluation tool.

For optimal views and precision, use of a transvaginal probe is preferred and far more accurate than a transabdominal probe. Ultrasound imaging can provide important information about the pregnancy, including location, gestational age, fetal cardiac activity, number of fetuses, and presence of abnormal findings such as adnexal masses, uterine fibroids, and fluid in the cul-de-sac. It can help identify the causes of vaginal bleeding such as subchorionic hemorrhage, incomplete miscarriage with retained products of conception, complete miscarriage in conjunction with beta-hCG lab values, or hydatidiform mole. For midwives who receive extra training to perform point-of-care ultrasound, it is still important to refer the patient for a full diagnostic ultrasound when a pregnancy is not clearly located in the uterus, or if findings are inconclusive.

## Ectopic Pregnancy

An ectopic pregnancy is defined as any pregnancy outside of the uterine cavity; it occurs in approximately 1% to 2% of all diagnosed pregnancies.[1,4] The most common location for ectopic implantation is in the uterine tube, accounting for at least 90% of cases. The remaining ectopic pregnancies are implanted in the abdomen (1%), the ovary (1% to 3%), the cervix (1%), or cesarean scars within the uterine muscle (1% to 3%). It is also possible to have an ectopic pregnancy concurrent with an intrauterine pregnancy, referred to as a heterotopic pregnancy.

More than half of patients diagnosed with ectopic pregnancy have no known risk factors, although having had a prior ectopic pregnancy does place a patient at higher risk of reoccurrence. Previous damage to uterine tubes, surgery leading to formation of scar tissue in the reproductive organs, past ascending pelvic infection, and pregnancy achieved with assisted reproductive technology are risk factors for ectopic pregnancy, and patients should be counseled on these risks.[4] Symptoms may include abdominal or pelvic pain (particularly one-sided) and vaginal bleeding. In the case of a ruptured ectopic pregnancy, a patient may also experience referred shoulder pain and dizziness.

Ectopic pregnancy will not result in a viable fetus and creates severe risks to the life and health of the pregnant individual. A patient with subjective symptoms or physical findings consistent with an ectopic pregnancy, or a patient with a positive pregnancy test and no intrauterine pregnancy on ultrasound (pregnancy of unknown location), needs immediate clinical assessment by a physician.

Once the diagnosis of ectopic pregnancy has been made and physician care has been established, management can be medical or surgical if the patient is hemodynamically stable. For patients who meet specific criteria, oral administration of methotrexate (Trexall) is safe and effective to resolve an ectopic pregnancy.[1,4] Methotrexate, which may also be administered intramuscularly, is a folate antagonist that inhibits DNA synthesis and cell replication. With this medication, a patient should be instructed to discontinue all vitamins, including prenatal vitamins and folic acid, as these may reduce the efficacy of the methotrexate treatment. After methotrexate administration, the body slowly resorbs all products of conception. Serial beta-hCG levels are monitored carefully to confirm that the medication was effective in stopping the pregnancy. If beta-hCG levels do not decrease as expected, methotrexate administration can be repeated if the patient remains stable; however, surgical management may be necessary when medication treatment is not successful. Surgical management is also a safe and effective first-line treatment as a patient-informed choice. Surgery is crucial if a patient exhibits signs of hemodynamic instability, intraperitoneal bleeding, or pelvic pain, which indicate a potential ruptured ectopic pregnancy.[4]

Most ectopic pregnancies that are detected early can be treated successfully without significant morbidity. In contrast, a ruptured ectopic pregnancy is a medical emergency and requires immediate intervention. Signs and symptoms of a ruptured ectopic pregnancy vary widely. In the classic presentation, the patient may or may not realize they are pregnant, and have no bleeding or slight irregular spotting. Sudden sharp, stabbing, severe, lower abdominal pain is followed by hypotension and signs of hypovolemic shock. Physical examination findings include tender abdomen, painful vaginal examination, cervical motion tenderness, and a possible adnexal mass. The cul-de-sac may be full of blood, causing the posterior vaginal fornix to bulge outward. Pain in the neck or shoulder, especially on inspiration, may be present as a result of diaphragmatic irritation from blood in the peritoneal cavity. A patient with this profile is experiencing a medical emergency and requires immediate care in a hospital.[4]

Ovarian, cervical, and abdominal pregnancies are rare forms of ectopic pregnancy. Abdominal pregnancy is the only form with any potential of survival and is usually the result of an early ectopic pregnancy that ruptured into the peritoneal cavity early enough that the embryo remained viable. In this scenario, the embryo implants in the abdomen. If the pregnancy continues to survive, it will be extremely high risk and necessitates care by a maternal–fetal medicine specialist.

## Pregnancy of Unknown Location

Approximately 8% to 31% of patients will have a positive pregnancy test, yet an intrauterine pregnancy cannot be seen during transvaginal ultrasound. In this situation, neither intrauterine nor ectopic pregnancy can be confirmed.[5] There are four potential outcomes in this situation: ectopic pregnancy, intrauterine pregnancy, spontaneous resolution to a nonpregnant state, or persistent pregnancy of unknown location. The most common outcome is spontaneous resolution of the pregnancy, with beta-hCG levels dropping to zero without intervention.[5] Although the site of pregnancy may never be determined, it is assumed that most of these patients experienced very early pregnancy losses.

Patients with a persistent pregnancy of unknown location (one in which no pregnancy is identified on ultrasound and hCG levels do not drop) may be managed expectantly or offered treatment once a viable intrauterine pregnancy has been reasonably excluded. A patient may be offered either uterine aspiration or an exploratory dilation and curettage (D & C) procedure to identify the presence or absence of chorionic villi in the uterus. Treatment with methotrexate may also be offered either before or after exploratory surgery.[4,5] Deciding between expectant management or interventions is based on multiple individual clinical factors and shared decision making between the patient and the provider.[5] Once a plan of management is made, typically with physician consultation or referral, midwives may participate in monitoring beta-hCG levels and ultrasound imaging to support the patient through the process.

## Pregnancy of Uncertain Viability

Management of a patient having an early pregnancy loss depends on a definitive diagnosis. A patient who has expelled products of conception and who has resolution of symptoms, an empty uterus on transvaginal ultrasound, and declining beta-hCG levels has had a completed miscarriage. Nevertheless, passage of tissue is not always noted, symptoms are not diagnostic, and beta-hCG values or transvaginal ultrasound findings can be inconclusive. Criteria that are diagnostic for pregnancy loss are listed in Table 22-3.[5–7]

## Subchorionic Hemorrhage

*Subchorionic hemorrhage (SCH)* is the term for bleeding that occurs between the chorion and the myometrium, or between the chorion and the placenta. It may also be referred to as *subchorionic*

| Table 22-3 | Diagnostic Criteria for Early Pregnancy Loss[a] |
|---|---|

Crown–rump length of 7 mm or greater without a fetal heartbeat

Mean sac diameter of 25 mm or greater without an embryo

Absence of an embryo with a heartbeat 2 weeks or more after an ultrasound that showed a gestational sac without a yolk sac

Absence of an embryo with a heartbeat 11 days or more after an ultrasound that showed a gestational sac with a yolk sac

[a] Other findings on transvaginal ultrasound may suggest the diagnosis of pregnancy loss but are not conclusive.

*hematoma* and in discussion with patients, the term *perigestational bleeding* may be preferred and easier to understand. This finding is noted in approximately 18% to 30% of patients who present with first trimester bleeding, appearing as a crescent-shaped hypoechoic area adjacent to the gestational sac on ultrasound.[1] The etiology of SCH is unclear, and no consensus exists regarding a specific course of treatment. Often, SCH is found incidentally on a first trimester ultrasound on an asymptomatic patient or may be diagnosed in a patient who presents with vaginal bleeding. While SCH can be very concerning to patients, such bleeding is very common and many of these hemorrhages resolve spontaneously without adverse pregnancy outcomes.

The volume of an SCH is difficult to measure because it is irregularly shaped. SCH is often described subjectively as small, moderate, or large, with a grading system being utilized by radiologists. Volume may also be calculated by ultrasound measurements, or as an estimate of hemorrhage size as a percentage in relation to gestational sac size. The risk to a viable pregnancy depends on the size of the hemorrhage. Studies have demonstrated that a small SCH, or one that encompasses less than 25% of the volume of the gestational sac, carries little to no risk of early pregnancy loss.[8] Larger subchorionic hemorrhages, or ones that encompass 50% or more volume in relation to the gestational sac, have been associated with early pregnancy loss.[8] The risk of loss increases with increasing hemorrhage size. For this reason, serial ultrasounds may decrease patient anxiety and allow for close monitoring especially with symptomatic patients. Individuals diagnosed

with SCH should be counseled that bleeding will continue until resolution; however, they should be encouraged to call or present for evaluation with an increase in their bleeding or passage of large clots with any cramping or pelvic pain.

## Gestational Trophoblastic Disease and Hydatidiform Mole

Gestational trophoblastic disease refers to a spectrum of conditions that develop from abnormal placental (trophoblastic) tissue, the most common of which is hydatidiform mole. Gestational trophoblastic neoplasms can develop from gestational trophoblastic disease and include gestational choriocarcinoma, invasive moles, and placental site trophoblastic tumor. All of these conditions can progress to become malignant and life-threatening.[5,9]

The term *hydatidiform mole* is derived from the combination of the Greek word *hydatisia*, which means "drop of water," and the Latin word *mola*, which means "false conception." A hydatidiform mole develops following an abnormal union of sperm and egg. No or limited fetal tissue develops, but abnormal trophoblastic tissue proliferates and fills the uterine space.

With this condition, placental villi become edematous grape-like structures that can be identified on ultrasound.[9] An ultrasound examination can be diagnostic for hydatidiform mole via the appearance of a cluster of grape-like material, a honeycomb effect, or a "snowstorm" on the screen. Hydatidiform mole occurs in approximately 1 in 15,000 pregnancies. Risk factors include pregnancy at a younger age (younger than 16 years) and older age (older than 40 years). The risk is higher for patients who have had a previous molar pregnancy.[5,9]

A molar pregnancy is classified as either complete or partial. A complete mole typically occurs when an ovum that has lost its DNA is fertilized by a sperm, and the resulting products of conception have sperm chromosomal DNA only, meaning that the haploid sperm DNA replicates and the resulting hydatidiform mole has a genotype of 46XX.[9] A complete mole can also develop from an empty ovum fertilized by two sperm; the resulting genome can be 46XX or 46XY. No embryonic tissue develops—only overgrowth of trophoblastic tissue. Complete molar pregnancy is characterized by marked enlargement of the uterus and extreme elevations of beta-hCG as the placental tissue synthesizes large amounts of this hormone. Symptoms include abnormal bleeding, uterine size greater than expected dates, absent fetal heart tones, hyperemesis, hyperthyroid symptoms, cystic enlargement of the ovaries, hypertension in the first trimester without previous diagnosis, and abnormally high beta-hCG levels for gestational dates.[5]

A partial mole occurs when two haploid sperm fertilize a normal ovum, and the result is usually a triploid chromosomal complement. Products of conception consist of nonviable fetal tissue and a smaller amount of abnormal trophoblastic tissue. Partial moles have a smaller amount of trophoblastic tissue compared to complete moles, and the patient's symptoms are correspondingly less severe.[5,9]

A patient with molar pregnancy needs referral to a consulting physician for care and follow-up. The plan of care usually includes suction dilation and evacuation (D & E) rather than dilation and curettage (D & C), because suction lessens the chance of uterine perforation and spread of trophoblastic tissue into the abdominal cavity. Hysterectomy is also an option. Medical abortion with methotrexate and misoprostol is not advised due to the rare but severe risk of trophoblastic embolism with uterine contractions.[5,9]

After resolution of molar pregnancy, a patient will be advised to avoid pregnancy for 6 to 12 months. This recommendation is made to facilitate ongoing surveillance of serial beta-hCG testing due to the increased risk of malignancy. A pregnant patient who has a history of a molar pregnancy is also at risk of malignancy and will be offered a first trimester ultrasound. Depending on the gestational age, they may be monitored with serial quantitative beta-hCG levels until a viable pregnancy is confirmed in a subsequent pregnancy.[5,9]

## Early Pregnancy Loss

*Early pregnancy loss* is defined as a nonviable intrauterine pregnancy in the first trimester that contains either an empty gestational sac or a gestational sac containing a fetus/embryo with no fetal cardiac activity.[6] As many as 10% to 25% of clinically recognized pregnancies end in loss, with the majority of those occurring in the first 10 weeks.[6,10] Most of these early losses are caused by random chromosomal abnormalities in the developing fetus.[10] In the majority of these cases, this means an abnormal fetal karyotype, with a single autosomal trisomy or an extra chromosome present. Other abnormal karyotypes associated with EPL are triploidy (i.e., three sets of chromosomes in each cell), monosomy X (e.g., Turner syndrome), chromosomal rearrangements, autosomal monosomy, sex chromosome trisomy, and tetraploidy.[11] Risk factors are thought to include having a prior early pregnancy loss, preexisting uncontrolled chronic disease, infection, substance use, exposure to toxins, reproductive tract abnormalities, and advanced maternal age.[7,10] It is important for patients to understand that beyond addressing modifiable risk factors, there is no treatment or intervention to prevent early pregnancy loss.

The diagnosis of early pregnancy loss is made with a combination of clinical, laboratory, and ultrasound findings. Patients may present with first trimester vaginal bleeding, after a routine dating or first trimester ultrasound with nonviable pregnancy findings, or with other clinical findings that lead to the diagnosis.[7] Once a diagnosis of early pregnancy loss is confirmed, the midwife should ensure the patient and their partner or other support people understand the findings, review all management options, provide resources for mental health support, and schedule close follow-up care.

### Early Pregnancy Loss Management

Management of early pregnancy loss involves consideration of a multitude of factors; it is performed best when all options are presented, and when a shared decision-making process takes place between patient and provider. Providers must discuss implications and management options in view of the patient's health status, symptoms, social support, and age. Options for management include expectant management, medical management, or surgical management with a physician. For clinically stable patients, all options should be discussed and offered.

Expectant management comprises watchful waiting for products of conception to pass on their own. The most conservative option, it does not involve any active intervention and is often recommended as first-line management by providers.[12] While many patients prefer this management option, it has the lowest effectiveness rates of all the options. Within 4 weeks of diagnosis, 90% of patients will spontaneously pass products following an incomplete early pregnancy loss.[1] This percentage is slightly lower for anembryonic gestations, of which only 66% will pass spontaneously, and is 76% for embryonic demises.[1]

If the patient decides to go the expectant management route, it is important to provide counseling that if products do not pass on their own after an agreed-upon length of time, the patient may need to choose a different management option. There is also no control over timing of when products of conception will pass. For patients with limited social support, work or family responsibilities, or limited access to transportation, this may not be a feasible choice.

The patient should be counseled to call their healthcare provider if they experience any signs of infection, including fever, chills, body aches, or foul odorous vaginal discharge. Strict bleeding precautions should also be given, and the patient educated to call or present for emergency care with heavy bleeding. This can be quantified by passing large clots frequently and/or soaking through a large sanitary pad in an hour or less for more than an hour. Patients should be offered nonsteroidal anti-inflammatory drugs (NSAIDs) or a short course of low-dose opioids for pain management.

For patients who have experienced two or more early pregnancy losses, genetic studies may be offered on the products of conception if testing is available at the facility. If a patient desires this optional testing, they should be provided with a container to collect products of conception to be brought to the lab or clinic.

Medication management of early pregnancy loss involves the prescription of misoprostol (Cytotec) or a combination of misoprostol and mifepristone (Mifeprex) to facilitate an expedited process of passing products of conception at home with strict bleeding precautions.[6,10] Mifepristone is a 19-nor steroid that prepares the myometrium and cervix for prostaglandin activity by acting as a competitive antagonist for progesterone receptors and glucocorticoid receptors, while misoprostol is a prostaglandin analogue.[13] While the combination medication regimen of mifepristone followed by misoprostol is preferred and more effective, mifepristone may not be available or difficult to prescribe in certain facilities. When it is not an option, the use of misoprostol alone should be considered as an alternative for medication management. The combination of mifepristone followed by misoprostol for medication management has been found to be as much as 95% effective, while misoprostol alone has an estimated success rate of 71% after a single dose and 84% after a second dose.[13]

Mifepristone has been approved by the Food and Drug Administration (FDA) and can be safely prescribed by clinicians up to 84 days' (12 weeks') gestational age with early pregnancy loss or up to 70 days' (10 weeks') gestational age with medication abortion.[14] The most commonly used regimen for medication management with mifepristone and misoprostol is as follows: 200 mg mifepristone administered to the patient in the clinic setting, with instructions to take 800 mcg misoprostol at home 24 to 48 hours later. The misoprostol may be taken buccally or vaginally depending on patient preference and comfort level. For early pregnancy loss,

| Table 22-4 | Medications for Early Pregnancy Loss | |
|---|---|---|
| **Medication** | **Timing** | **Repeat Dose** |
| Mifepristone 200 mg oral | Given in clinic setting due to FDA restrictions | Not applicable (one-time dosing) |
| Misoprostol 800 mcg buccal or vaginal | Taken at home 24 to 48 hours following mifepristone, or as a single medication when no access to mifepristone | Can receive second dose 12 to 24 hours after first dose |

Abbreviation: FDA, U.S. Food and Drug Administration.

either route is acceptable with comparable results, but patients should be counseled that the buccal route has a higher reported incidence of gastrointestinal symptoms. A second dose of 800 mcg misoprostol can be considered if bleeding or cramping do not occur within 12 to 24 hours of the initial dose (Table 22-4).[1,13,14]

When mifepristone is not available, misoprostol alone should be offered. The recommended regimen is the same: The patient takes 800 mcg misoprostol, either vaginally or buccally, at home; a repeat dose may be taken 12 to 24 hours later if the patient has no symptoms.[1,10]

Similar to the case with expectant management, patients who choose medication management should be thoroughly counseled on expectations, bleeding, and infection risks; given an option for pain management; and a follow-up plan made with their provider. For stable patients, it may be reasonable to repeat medication management for a second cycle; however, patients should be counseled that this treatment is not 100% effective and surgical intervention may be necessary.

With surgical management, a patient undergoes either a manual vacuum-aspiration/electric-aspiration procedure or D & C surgery to remove the failed pregnancy.[1] This management option should be used for patients with active hemorrhage (persistent heavy bleeding), hemodynamic instability, signs of infection, or other concerning medical comorbidities such as anemia or bleeding disorder.[6] Patients may also choose this option if they have limited support or access to transportation, or if they wish to complete the process as soon as possible. It allows for planning, clear expectations, and less follow-up. Traditionally, surgical management involves general anesthesia in the operating room and a D & C performed by an obstetrician-gynecologist. While D & C is still frequently performed with early pregnancy loss, the option of manual or electric vacuum aspiration (MVA) is the standard of care and thought to be superior to the use of sharp curettage; this procedure is performed by a physician in an outpatient clinical setting for stable patients.[6] MVA is not a core competency for midwives but may be part of their additional training depending on state regulations.

### RhoGAM

Regardless of loss type or management choice, the administration of Rho(D) immune globulin (Rho-GAM) after early pregnancy loss for patients who are Rh(D) negative is recommended. The risk of alloimmunization is low—1.5% to 2%—with early pregnancy loss, but it should still be given as consequences could be significant.[1] With losses or abortions prior to 8 weeks' gestational age, there is some debate over whether RhoGAM is needed. The National Abortion Federation (NAF) no longer recommends this treatment, while the American College of Obstetricians and Gynecologists (ACOG) states that it should still be considered, though not required. Rh(D)-negative patients who have surgical management should receive RhoGAM regardless of gestational age due to the higher risk of alloimmunization.[6] This medication should be given within 72 hours of the completed loss or abortion. The recommended dosage is 50 to 150 mcg prior to 12 weeks' and 300 mcg after 12 weeks' gestational age, though the higher dose can be used if a lower dose is not available.[1,6]

### Follow-Up Care After an Early Pregnancy Loss

To reduce risks of infection, it is generally recommended that patients abstain from vaginal intercourse for 1 to 2 weeks following completion of pregnancy loss.[6] Antibiotics are not indicated unless an infection is suspected for those individuals who choose expectant or medication management. It should also be noted that the use of misoprostol has been shown to cause a fever within 24 hours of administration, and this fever is not an indication of infection.[7] In-person follow-up should be arranged between 7 and 14 days following passage of tissue, at which time the beta-hCG level should be measured to confirm that the early pregnancy loss is complete. If the level is still elevated, serum beta-hCG levels should be repeated until they are less than 5mIU/mL, which is considered a negative

result. Ultrasound is not always necessary if the history and/or physical examination findings are normal and the beta-hCG level drops as expected, but may be employed to confirm the complete passage of products of conception.[11]

### Mental Health

There has long been a stigma surrounding early pregnancy loss despite its very frequent occurrence. This event can be traumatic for the patient and family members, whether or not the pregnancy was desired. Many patients may feel responsible for the loss or have feelings of guilt that they might have done something wrong to cause the pregnancy loss.[10] Providing patient-centered care can reduce the potential psychological complications following early pregnancy loss or abortion. Patients are at risk for depression, anxiety, low self-esteem, and grief following the termination or loss of a pregnancy.[12] Shared decision making and close communication throughout the process can make a tremendous difference to patients during this trying time. It is crucial to have close follow-up to assess mental health status in the weeks and months following any type of loss. Accessible mental health resources, counseling, and medication, when deemed appropriate, can all improve depression and other mental health disorders for these patients.

Racial disparities also exist in the diagnosis and treatment of mental health concerns following early pregnancy loss. While all patients are at high risk of developing major depression in the months following loss, Black patients have been found to be twice as likely to suffer from depression compared to non-Black patients.[15] Without stigmatizing them, extra care should be given to ensure Black patients receive identification of mental health disorders, appropriate follow-up, and support during this challenging time to improve health equity.[15]

### Contraception

A rapid return of fertility is expected after an early pregnancy loss, and patients should be counseled to anticipate ovulation and the ability to conceive again prior to their next menses.[10] For patients who are not ready to conceive immediately, or who do not desire pregnancy, contraceptive options should be reviewed and offered. Hormonal contraception or immediate intrauterine device (IUD) placement can be initiated immediately following a completed early pregnancy loss or abortion.[6] Note that for early pregnancy loss managed with medication only or for medication abortion, IUD placement should wait until after expulsion of the products of conception, while hormonal contraception or implant placement can occur prior to this event.

### Conception

There is no evidence that delaying conception after early pregnancy loss has benefits.[7] If a patient desires pregnancy right away, they should be counseled about its safety. There is no increased risk of subsequent loss with conception immediately, and most patients who experience a single early pregnancy loss can achieve a subsequent healthy pregnancy. Fewer than 5% of patients will experience a successive early pregnancy loss, although they are at higher risk of an early pregnancy loss than a patient who has never experienced such a loss.[10]

### Recurrent Miscarriage

When a patient has experienced three or more early pregnancy losses, genetic counseling and an endocrine evaluation should be considered. The standard evaluation for recurrent early pregnancy loss includes ultrasound to rule out congenital abnormalities of the genital tract (e.g., uterine septum, bicornuate uterus), genetic testing, and tests for coagulation disorders, autoimmune disorders, and thyroid abnormalities. Often no direct etiology can be determined. Progesterone is essential for the maintenance of a healthy pregnancy, and progesterone supplementation has been investigated as an intervention to prevent early pregnancy loss in patients with first trimester vaginal bleeding and/or recurrent pregnancy loss. Evidence is inconclusive regarding the benefits of this therapy.[16] In some settings, midwives may order initial laboratory tests before referring patients to fertility or perinatology specialists.

## Abortion

*Abortion* refers to the termination of a pregnancy, whether spontaneously or intentional, prior to 20 weeks after an individual's last menstrual period (LMP). However, in the United States and in many other places, this term is typically used to refer to the intentional termination of pregnancy before and after 20 weeks after LMP, and that language is used here. The political and social power of the word far outweigh the clinical and technical skills involved in its performance, and as midwives, the approach to patients seeking or considering abortion should reflect that complexity. Abortion is a common clinical procedure performed in the United States, with one in four pregnancy-capable people having an

abortion during their lifetime.[17] Nevertheless, it is rarely mentioned in many settings, including the clinical setting, and many midwives do not feel they have adequate information to discuss it.[18]

Abortion is considered to be within midwifery scope of care by the American College of Nurse-Midwives,[19] the International Confederation of Midwives,[20] and the World Health Organization (WHO).[21] Legal access to abortion varies widely both globally and within the United States,[19,22] as does the scope of midwifery practice within abortion care. The legal status of abortion globally varies dramatically, from being forbidden under all circumstances (e.g., Honduras, Egypt, Thailand) to being available on request (e.g., Sweden, Argentina, Australia). However, it is common for some restrictions or limitations to be placed on abortion access, such as gestational limits (e.g., United Kingdom, India, Japan), two concurring provider opinions (e.g., United Kingdom), or medical indications for mental or physical health (e.g., Poland, Algeria, Peru).[23] The United States has a variety of laws governing abortion by state, which creates a mosaic of restrictions on abortion that is somewhat unique: Globally, abortion access is usually determined at the national level.

### Historical and Current Context for Abortion in the United States

Abortion was commonly performed through "quickening" (first fetal movement) in the United States until the nineteenth century. Midwives were the primary abortion providers, as they were the primary pregnancy caregivers, and this procedure was considered part of pregnancy care, even if it was little discussed.[24] In the mid-1800s, an increasing number of abortion and contraceptive bans coincided with the shift in power to physician care during pregnancy and a generally restrictive legal context for women in the United States.[25] For the next century, abortion was illegal in every state, with varying case-by-case exceptions made for life, health, and fetal conditions such as exposure to rubella in the first trimester.[26]

Because abortion was illegal and reliable medication abortion was unavailable during this era, abortion was often unsafe, with providers who might have no healthcare training performing the procedure under unsterile conditions. Many organizations, including a group of clergy concerned with the risks of illegal abortion (Clergy Consultation Service on Abortion), the Association to Repeal Abortion Laws (now NARAL), and the American Medical Association, supported the decriminalization and/or legalization of abortion in the United States.[27] States slowly began to legalize abortion on request, beginning with Hawaii, New York, and Washington in 1970. A series of U.S. Supreme Court decisions beginning with *Connecticut v. Griswold* (1965) recognized a constitutional right to privacy, and in 1973 *Roe v. Wade* legalized abortion prior to viability in every state. Before this ruling, abortion was illegal in 30 states, and severely restricted in most others.

Almost immediately, abortion opponents sought to restrict access to the procedure. In 1976, the Hyde Amendment banned the use of federal funds for abortion care, limiting access for millions of people. Over the next 40 years, a series of antiabortion laws were passed, and had substantial support in the federal courts, including the U.S. Supreme Court. In 1992, *Planned Parenthood v. Casey* established an "undue burden" standard for abortion restrictions. Restrictions are deemed acceptable as long as they do not place an "undue burden" on the person seeking abortion. This has been interpreted as permitting parental consent laws, required waiting periods, and mandated counseling, although not spousal consent.

Violence against people providing abortion also became a significant problem. In March 1992, Dr. David Gunn, who provided abortion as part of his practice, was assassinated in the parking lot of his clinic in Pensacola, Florida. Since then, 11 clinic workers and providers have been killed, and in 2019 clinics reported more than 27,000 incidents of violence and threats of violence.[28] This violence contributed to the contraction of abortion availability; currently, 89% of U.S. counties have no known abortion provider.

In June 2022, the U.S. Supreme Court took the unprecedented step of removing a right it had previously recognized as located in the Constitution when *Dobbs v. Jackson Women's Health* was decided. This ruling overturned *Roe*, and the concurring opinion of Justice Clarence Thomas took aim at other rights, including LGBTQ+ rights and the right to use contraception, that had relied on the same constitutional interpretation as did *Roe*. As of January 2023, abortion was banned, effectively banned, or prohibited after certain gestational ages in 24 states.[30] By contrast, a number of states have changed their laws in recent years to codify the major findings of *Roe* into state law, anticipating a reversal by the Supreme Court, and/or to expand their state law beyond the requirements of *Roe*, including allowing advanced practice clinicians other than physicians to perform medical or procedural

abortions.[31] The post-*Dobbs* landscape is increasingly one of disparate access by race, geography, and income, and few signs of improving this situation.

## Abortion as a Clinical Procedure

### Values Clarification, Options Counseling, and Conscientious Objection

Abortions in the United States are performed in specialized clinics, in physician offices, in nonspecialized clinics, and in hospitals. In 2017, specialized abortion clinics represented only 16% of all abortion facilities, but performed 60% of all abortions.[32] Thus, many hospitals and other facilities do very few abortions annually, and their staff might especially benefit from values clarification work and other supportive services. This is particularly true for labor and delivery nurses, who often are the primary clinicians present for induction abortions and the aftercare that may be required, including bathing and dressing the fetus.

*Values clarification* refers to the active work to identify and clarify one's feelings about a topic, particularly in the context of potential moral or ethical objections, and to align those feelings or beliefs with actions. This clarification can assist midwives in delineating which aspects of care they are willing to participate in, as well as naming and exploring feelings about a topic of which they may not be consciously aware. Values clarification can be done as an individual exercise or as a group, using a formalized structure or not. Providers who participate in values clarification exercises may be more willing to participate in one or more aspects of abortion care in the future,[33] and report improved knowledge about abortion as well as more positive attitudes toward it.[34] The goal of values clarification, however, is not to change minds on ethical or moral issues, but rather to facilitate the individual assessment and understanding of the individual's own beliefs. Despite this utility for a number of complex issues, values clarification work is rarely taught in nursing or midwifery programs, and there exist relatively few data on its use in clinical practice for people other than physicians.

### Options Counseling

Options counseling presents patients with all options for an undesired, mistimed, or unexpected pregnancy, and facilitates their decision making as needed. It is an important skill for a provider caring for pregnant patients, since almost half of all pregnancies in the United States are mistimed or otherwise unintended,[35] although many patients

| Table 22-5 | Some Questions to Facilitate Options Counseling |
|---|---|

- How are you feeling about this pregnancy?
- Is there information that would be helpful to you in making your decision? What is it?
- Who is important to you in your life? Can you discuss your decision with them?
- How can I be most helpful to you in this decision?
- When you think about being pregnant, what are some of the feelings that come up? How about when you think about having an abortion? Parenting? Making an adoption plan?
- What values are important to you in making your decision?

will neither need nor desire options counseling. Options counseling involves information sharing, open-ended questions to help patients identify their desire, and nonjudgmental support of patients (Table 22-5). To adequately provide options counseling, midwives need to familiarize themselves with all options available to a pregnant person, and at a minimum have resources available for patients to explore further.

Ambivalence and mixed emotions regarding a pregnancy are common, regardless of the choice made about continuing the pregnancy. One important role of the midwife can be to normalize the complexity and nuances of an unintended pregnancy for patients, and to provide support for patients while they are making their decision. However, it is also important for the midwife to recognize that many responses to an unintended pregnancy are possible, and to avoid making assumptions about how best to support the patient. Patients may not want help making their decision, but may want assistance in locating prenatal care or an abortion provider, for example.

Midwives' responsibilities to their patients in this situation can be difficult to navigate when they object to participating in abortion. A delay in assisting a patient in locating a provider, however, can increase the risk to the patient or prevent them from accessing desired care. Because of these complexities, it is important for midwives and other healthcare providers to clarify their values around patient care in this situation ahead of time, and to plan for what they will do when the situation arises. However, in emergency situations, midwives have a clear responsibility for the patient's safety that outweighs

their own beliefs, and this should be considered as well.

Nondirective options counseling is an important part of informed decision making and consent, which is the responsibility of the provider. Without full and accurate knowledge of the risks and benefits of each option for an unintended pregnancy, decisions about care—including the decision to continue a pregnancy—cannot be considered fully informed consent. Patients may decline such a discussion, particularly if their decision is clear and unambivalent. However, that choice is the patient's to make, not the provider's.

### Conscientious Objection

Conscientious objection is the refusal by a healthcare provider to perform care that violates a sincerely held belief or value. Originally used by members of pacifist religious traditions to avoid participating in war as soldiers, conscientious objection has been applied to health care for almost a century.[36,37] The Church Amendments, passed in 1973, specifically protect the rights of U.S. providers not to participate in abortion care, and the Religious Freedom Restoration Act (RFRA) of 1992 has been used to bolster that right in U.S. courts and in practice.[38]

However, conscientious objection has obligations as well as rights. Specifically, the exercise of conscientious objection by a particular provider cannot prevent the patient from accessing the care they seek with a different provider. Additionally, the exercise of conscientious objection by a provider cannot constitute an undue burden, including delay of care, on the patient or the other members of the healthcare team. The difficulty many people experience in accessing abortion care in the United States has made this a higher bar for providers to meet.[39] While conscientious objection is legally protected, providers also should consider the ethical obligations contingent on its exercise.

### Abortion Timing and Safety

The timing, frequency, method, and safety of abortion vary widely according to the legal status of abortion in a given jurisdiction. For example, in 2015–2019, abortion rates per 1000 women aged 15 to 44 varied from a low of 15 in Australia and New Zealand to a high of 53 in Western Asia and Northern Africa,[40] with a global mean of 39 per 1000. Contrary to popular assumption, abortion frequency is not directly correlated with availability of legal abortion in a region. Safety of abortion is directly correlated with availability of legal abortion, however, and in 2014 between 4.7% and 13.2% of global pregnancy-related deaths were caused by unsafe illegal abortion,[41] almost half of which occurred in sub-Saharan Africa. By contrast, in the United States abortion is 12 to 14 times safer than childbirth.[42] Mortality and morbidity from unsafe abortion thus disproportionately harm Black, Indigenous, and other people of color (BIPOC) in low- and moderate-income countries; these individuals, because of systemic racism, lack of adequate health infrastructure, and the economic aftermath of white colonialism, are already at increased risk of pregnancy-related death and illness. This lack of access to safe abortion is considered to be a public health issue by WHO because of both the scope of the problem and its disparate impacts, and is prioritized even during times of crisis like the SARS-CoV-2 pandemic.[22]

Abortion access has been significantly limited in the United States in recent years because of restrictive laws known as "TRAP laws" ("targeted restrictions on abortion providers"), as well as because of long-standing funding limitations, provider shortages, and other issues in many areas. While Medicaid covers the pregnancy and birth costs for 48% of all U.S. births, since 1976 the Hyde Amendment has barred federal funds from paying for abortion care except under specific circumstances. Eleven states currently fund abortion care for people who are covered by their Medicaid programs, but Medicaid recipients in all other states, as well as federal employees, military members and veterans (and their families), Peace Corps volunteers, and individuals receiving care from the Indian Health Services, must pay for abortion costs out of pocket.[43]

The vast majority of abortions in the United States (92.2%) are performed at less than 13 weeks' gestation, with 77.7% performed at less than 9 weeks' gestation (measured from the LMP).[44] Almost all abortions (more than 99.9%) in the United States are performed using aspiration, medication, or D & E, and the discussion of the processes presented here focuses on these three methods for that reason (Table 22-6). The abortion rate has been falling in the United States since 2009, but the most recent monitoring data suggest a small (1% to 2%) increase since 2017.[43] This decrease is related to drops in pregnancy and birth rates overall, with a potential relationship to increased access to contraception, particularly long-acting reversible contraception (LARCs) such as IUDs.

Abortions after 20 weeks' gestation occur rarely in the United States,[44] but are often performed for

| Table 22-6 | Comparison of Medication, Aspiration, D & E, and Induction Abortion | |
| --- | --- | --- |
| **Type of Abortion** | **Considerations/Risks** | **Considerations/Benefits** |
| Medication | Outpatient use limited to ≤ 10 weeks 0 days' gestation (≤ 70 days LMP) | Privacy (resembles miscarriage, can be done at home) |
| | Risk of failed abortion—needing aspiration | Does not require a surgical procedure |
| | Hemorrhage and infection risk | Very effective |
| | Can be difficult to find a provider | Extremely safe |
| Aspiration (prior to 14 weeks' gestation) | Infection, perforation, hemorrhage risk | Highly effective—will leave the clinic no longer pregnant |
| | Can be difficult to find a provider | Immediate use of any contraception desired |
| | Requires a vaginal procedure | Extremely safe |
| D & E (≥14 weeks' gestation) | Infection, perforation, hemorrhage, possibly increased risk of cervical laceration | Highly effective—will leave the clinic no longer pregnant |
| | Requires vaginal procedure | Immediate use of all contraception |
| | Can be difficult to find a provider | Very safe |
| Induction | Increased risk of hemorrhage | Allows viewing/holding of the fetus if desired |
| | Longer procedure—can take several days | Very safe |
| | Inpatient | May support the grieving process if abortion is of an initially desired pregnancy |

Abbreviations: D & E, dilation and evacuation; LMP, last menstrual period.

fetal or maternal indications and may have different considerations than earlier abortions. When elective abortions occur after 20 weeks, they are strongly associated with restrictive abortion laws in the home state, including bans on Medicaid coverage,[45] and the proportion of post–20 weeks elective abortions is expected to grow post-*Dobbs* and the subsequent abortion bans. Later abortions carry significant stigma from both healthcare providers and the general public; as such, patients often need significant support from healthcare workers, including midwives. These abortions may also occur in less-common settings, such as labor and delivery units or in a general operating room, which means that staff may be less familiar with the needs of patients and families having later abortions.

### Medication Abortion

In 2000, the FDA approved the drug mifepristone, a progesterone antagonist that competes for progesterone receptors on the uterus (Table 22-7). Used in combination with misoprostol, a prostaglandin commonly used for cervical ripening, postpartum hemorrhage, and gastric ulcer treatment, mifepristone is 98% to 99% effective in terminating pregnancies up to 10 weeks 0 days' gestation. In 2016, the FDA guidelines for the use of mifepristone were changed to better reflect current evidence-based practice, and to allow advanced practice clinicians, including midwives, to order mifepristone. In January, 2023, the FDA removed the in-person dispensing requirement and established a process for certifying pharmacies to dispense mifepristone to patients who have a prescription from a certified prescriber. As of May 2023, the legitimacy of the FDA approval of mifepristone was being challenged in federal court.[46]

Medication abortion has been rapidly growing in popularity since the approval of mifepristone.

| Table 22-7 | Medication Abortion Mechanisms of Action |
|---|---|
| **Medication** | **Mechanism of Action** |
| Mifepristone (Mifeprex) | Competitively binds to progesterone receptors on the uterus and inhibits progesterone's action, including uterine quiescence |
| Misoprostol (Cytotec) | Prostaglandin; induces uterine contractions, softens and dilates the cervix |
| Oxytocin (Pitocin) | Induces uterine contractions |

In 2017, 60.0% of U.S. abortions performed at less than 10 weeks' gestation utilized medication.[32] The combination of mifepristone and misoprostol is the most commonly used drug protocol for medication abortion in the United States, but misoprostol is widely used alone in other countries for this purpose, and its use for self-managed abortion outside a clinical setting in the United States appears to be growing. This interest in and use of misoprostol outside the clinical setting may be related to dwindling access to clinical abortion care, or it may be a response to previous maltreatment or discrimination within the clinical healthcare system.[47]

The current FDA-approved drug protocol for mifepristone–misoprostol consists of (1) 200 mg of oral mifepristone administered in a clinical setting; (2) 24 to 48 hours later, 800 mcg of misoprostol administered buccally at home or in the clinic; and (3) follow-up with the provider in 7 to 14 days.[48] This regimen may be used through 10 weeks' gestation (70 days since the first day of the LMLP). It is very similar to the most common regimen used for early pregnancy loss; however, because mifepristone can be difficult to access, misoprostol alone is more often used for early pregnancy loss (Table 22-4). Within approximately 4 to 8 hours of misoprostol administration, the large majority of patients will complete the abortion. As with a miscarriage, bleeding and cramping can be significant, and teaching about the parameters of normal is important for the midwife to share (Table 22-8). For those patients who do not complete their abortion within 24 hours of the misoprostol dose and who are hemodynamically stable, options include a repeat dose of misoprostol or uterine aspiration. Follow-up for individuals without warning signs may be completed by phone, telehealth, or in person.

### Aspiration Abortion

Widely used in the United States, aspiration abortion uses suction from either a machine or a manual vacuum aspirator (MVA) to empty the uterus. Aspiration can also be used to manage early pregnancy loss/miscarriage, and is used from approximately 5 to 6 weeks after LMP until 12 to 14 weeks after LMP, when it is replaced with D & E. Regardless of the suction source, the procedure is the same. The cervix is dilated using tapered rods of increasing diameter to admit the cannula. A flexible or rigid cannula is attached to the source of suction and used to empty the uterus of the embryo or fetus and other products of conception. The products of conception are then inspected to ensure that the uterus has been emptied, and a second aspiration may be

| Table 22-8 | Expected Parameters for Medication Abortion | | |
|---|---|---|---|
| **Finding** | **Normal Parameters** | **Need for Urgent Evaluation?** | **Management** |
| Bleeding | Generally begins within 4 hours of misoprostol, like a menstrual period, then increases up to heavy bleeding, including clots, until pregnancy tissue is passed (may be hidden by clot).<br><br>Excessive bleeding is defined as (1) soaking one pad per hour for more than 2 hours, and/or (2) passing a clot larger than a lime. | The patient should discuss any concerning bleeding with the provider on call. Evaluation of the patient in the clinic, urgent care, or emergency department is indicated for bleeding outside the expected parameters, or with any signs of hemodynamic instability (e.g., weakness, syncope or near-syncope, decreased urine output). | If bleeding is within normal limits but concerning for the patient, reassurance can be helpful.<br><br>For excessive bleeding, management is determined by hemodynamic status. Misoprostol and uterine aspiration are common management strategies, along with fluid replacement as needed. |
| Cramping/pain | Generally begins prior to bleeding and can be significant. Excessive pain does not improve with analgesics or self-care strategies and needs evaluation. | Increasing pain in the context of little to no bleeding suggests the need for evaluation and possible uterine evacuation. | NSAIDs<br>Acetaminophen<br>Massage<br>Hot packs/shower<br>Emotional support<br>Position changes<br>Consider narcotics |
| Expected duration | Bleeding generally peaks within 24 hours of misoprostol administration and lessens rapidly afterward. Bleeding/spotting can continue for 1–2 weeks.<br><br>Pain should begin to resolve as bleeding does; failure to do so suggests the need for evaluation.<br><br>Fever should resolve within 24 hours of misoprostol administration. | Continued bleeding/cramping/fever or increased bleeding after initial resolution needs evaluation.<br><br>New vaginal discharge or odor, or pelvic/abdominal pain, needs evaluation. | Depends on cause |

Abbreviation: NSAIDs, nonsteroidal anti-inflammatory drugs.

performed. Bleeding is minimal and the procedure generally takes less than 5 minutes to complete. The patient can go home as soon as they are stable, or after recovery from anesthesia if it is used.

Variations of practice with aspiration abortion include the selection of cannula size, whether cervical dilation is done prior to the procedure, and pain management options. Generally speaking, cannula size will correspond to weeks' gestation, and cervical dilation prior to the procedure with osmotic cervical dilators is not required for abortions less than 13 weeks' gestation,[48] although this is a provider preference. Pain management options range from local anesthesia using a lidocaine cervical block to general anesthesia, usually in a hospital setting, as well as nonpharmacologic methods such as provision of support from abortion doulas. Common medication options include intravenous pain medication and moderate sedation, although availability of options depends on the site. Most patients report mild to moderate pain related to their abortion procedure, and may experience some cramping following the procedure. As with postpartum cramping, the amount of pain varies from person to person. This pain is generally manageable with NSAIDs, acetaminophen, and/or nonpharmacologic pain management strategies. Rarely, narcotics may be needed.

## Later Abortion (14 Weeks or More After LMP)

Later abortions are often more challenging, both logistically and clinically, for the patient and the provider. Many factors contribute to later timing of abortions, including lack of awareness of pregnancy, the need to save money for the procedure, difficulty finding an abortion provider, the need for parental notification or judicial bypass procedures, state-mandated waiting periods, and transportation issues.[45] Timing of abortion should not be considered evidence of ambivalence or lack of concern.

Later abortions can be further divided into pre- and post-viability. Post-viability abortions are performed in very few locations in the United States, and represent a vanishingly small proportion of all abortions. Periviable abortions, usually defined as those occurring at 20 weeks' gestation or later, usually include intrafetal injection of medication (often digoxin) to stop fetal cardiac motion prior to completion of the abortion. This addresses both the concern of delivery of a live fetus and concerns expressed by many patients and others about fetal pain. While the neurologic structures necessary to feel pain are not present until well after the timing of the vast majority of abortions,[49] intrafetal digoxin can reassure patients that the fetus will not experience pain during the abortion procedure.

### Dilation and Evacuation

For pregnancies beyond 12 to 14 weeks after LMP, D & E can be used for abortion. This procedure may require 1 to 2 days of cervical preparation with osmotic dilators (e.g., laminaria, Dilapan), misoprostol, or both. Osmotic dilators absorb fluid from the surrounding tissues and expand over many hours, which both gradually dilates the cervix and softens the tissues in preparation for any additional mechanical dilation needed. The intention with cervical preparation is to reduce the potential for cervical trauma, which may lead to future cervical insufficiency, by gradually dilating the cervix over a period of 24 to 48 hours. In some cases, cervical dilation itself can effectively end the pregnancy by initiating uterine contractions, and the patient should be counseled on this possibility as well as which symptoms to report. Cervical preparation can carry the risk of infection, particularly if the amniotic sac is inadvertently ruptured during the placement of osmotic dilators, or spontaneously ruptures. However, the risk of infection related to D & E remains low.[50]

As with first trimester aspiration abortion, the dilatation required increases with gestation, and can be augmented with mechanical dilation (using dilators similar to those used at earlier gestations) at the time of procedure. Following adequate dilation, the fetus and placental tissues are removed with ring forceps, and the uterus can be aspirated to ensure removal of all products of conception. Some providers will use a paracervical or intravenous injection of a uterotonic agent (oxytocin or vasopressin) to minimize risk of hemorrhage by avoiding uterine atony, while others will use uterotonics on an as-needed basis. These decisions are often partly related to access to follow-up care if needed, given the uneven status of abortion care in the United States, as well as the preferences of a given provider. The risks of D & E are the same as those of an aspiration abortion (i.e., infection, hemorrhage, perforation), but occur more frequently (in 0.5% to 4% of procedures).[50]

### Induction

Use of medication to end a pregnancy in the second or third trimester is more common outside the United States, but is frequently chosen by families ending a desired pregnancy for fetal or maternal indications, often because it allows the family to spend time with the fetus after birth or to document its birth. These abortions often take place in inpatient settings, commonly in labor and delivery units, and can be challenging for patients, families, and staff to negotiate. The care of patients with stillbirth and lethal fetal diagnoses is covered in the *Complications During Labor and Birth* Chapter.

Misoprostol alone will result in abortion of approximately 80% to 90% of second trimester pregnancies,[51,52] and has a long history of use for labor induction that may make it familiar and comfortable for clinicians, including nurses caring for the patient. However, if mifepristone is available, it may increase the efficacy of medication abortion for second trimester pregnancies.[52] Because of the difficulty in accessing mifepristone and its relatively high failure rate (7%),[52] a common practice when using medication for abortion in the second trimester is to administer misoprostol followed by induction of labor with oxytocin (Pitocin) in an inpatient setting. This is very similar to any induction of labor, and its familiarity, as well as the presence of staff for support and analgesia options, may make this option preferable from a patient perspective despite the relatively high cost compared to an outpatient procedure.

## Best Practices, Risks, and Considerations

The NAF—a professional group of abortion providers, clinics, and advocates—maintains evidence-based guidelines for safe abortion practice. Its recommendations are updated regularly. Midwives participating in abortion care should be familiar with the quality standards of NAF.

For early (less than 14 weeks' gestation) abortion, ultrasound to identify the location and gestational age of the pregnancy is commonly used in the United States.[48] If this imaging modality is not used for early abortion, the gestational age and location of pregnancy must be reasonably determined by the clinician, using the patient's history and physical examination as indicated.[48] For abortions at 14 weeks' gestation or later, ultrasound must be used to identify gestational age.[48] Early abortions prior to 7 weeks' gestation (56 days after LMP) do not require Rh typing or RhoGAM, although it may be used. Beyond 56 days after LMP, Rh type should be determined and RhoGAM administered as appropriate.[48] However, RhoGAM is not considered to be essential to medication abortion at less than 70 days after LMP.[48]

In all procedural abortions, the clinician should immediately inspect the tissue removed to ensure the abortion is complete.[48] If any doubt arises, ultrasound can be used to confirm the uterus is empty. This is not required for medication abortions unless there is reason to believe the abortion is incomplete (e.g., no noted passage of tissue, continued significant bleeding/cramping, continued pregnancy symptoms).[48] In those cases, ultrasound and/or serial beta-hCG measurements can guide clinical practice.

Pregnancy is possible immediately following abortion; if it is not desired, contraception should be started the day of the abortion procedure. For those individuals choosing medication abortion and desiring a LARC, the contraceptive can be placed either the same day that mifepristone is administered (for implants) or after confirmation of complete abortion (for IUDs).[48]

Patient counseling and consent are of paramount concern in abortion care, as in any midwifery care. This is sometimes complicated by state laws requiring providers to give non-evidence-based counseling on abortion. In every case, the provider must review risks, benefits, and alternatives, as with any procedure, and ensure that the patient's questions are answered. Because of the widespread misinformation about abortion, patients frequently have concerns about safety and health implications of the procedure, and may require significantly more time for counseling than with other similarly safe procedures. For midwives who do not provide abortion care as well as for those who do, it is important to be able to answer questions about abortion accurately.

## Risks

The primary risks of abortion at any gestational age are hemorrhage, infection, and (except for medication abortion) perforation. These risks are significantly lower than the risks associated with full-term pregnancy and birth, and their frequency increases with gestational age.[42,50] It is important to review postprocedure expectations with patients, including identifying bleeding parameters (more than one pad per hour for at least 2 hours and/or clots larger than lime size) and ensuring they know how to seek care. For patients choosing medication abortion, bleeding can be substantial (though not necessarily clinically significant) but should resolve to the previously mentioned parameters with passage of the products of conception. Reviewing signs and symptoms of infection (e.g., fever, chills, abdominal tenderness, foul-smelling discharge) is also important for appropriate follow-up. Pelvic rest after abortion is broadly recommended for 2 weeks, although the evidence for this recommendation is limited.

While some abortion opponents claim an association between abortion and future infertility, mental illness, and breast cancer, these claims are without merit.[50,53-55] However, they are frequently included in state-mandated counseling, and midwives can encounter patients with questions about them. Mental illness or harm is particularly concerning for many patients, and this narrative is widespread in popular culture as well as in the abortion debate. However, current research does not support a relationship between abortion and mental illness. For example, in a large-scale study of people who sought abortion, researchers found that people who were able to obtain an abortion were no more likely to experience mental health issues in the years following the undesired, mistimed, or unplanned pregnancy than those who were not. Rather, inability to access a desired abortion was associated with negative mental health outcomes in future years.[56] Other research over several decades has likewise shown no relationship between abortion and mental illness, abortion and infertility, and abortion and breast cancer.[50]

## Self-Managed Abortion

*Self-managed abortion* (SMA) refers to a medication or other abortion obtained outside the formal medical system.[57] In many countries and regions, there is a long tradition of inducing a miscarriage, "bringing down" a late period, or other informal ending of a confirmed or suspected pregnancy. Indeed, the medications used currently for SMA are often available over the counter or otherwise easily accessible in many countries. However, in the United States, a complex system of abortion regulation, including a 2021 Texas law that empowers any resident to report another person for assisting in abortion past 6 weeks after LMP, as well as fear of regulatory consequences, has made it more difficult for people to access SMA and for providers to appropriately assist in risk reduction.

Misoprostol, a prostaglandin analogue widely used in the United States for miscarriage management, ulcer treatment, cervical ripening for induction of labor, and medication abortion, is the most commonly used modality for SMA. It is available through websites, veterinary offices, pharmacies, and some gray-market routes such as importation from Central American countries, where it is widely available and used for SMA.

Midwifery support for SMA is very similar to that needed for a spontaneous early pregnancy loss, and the guidelines for bleeding and other complications are the same (Table 22-6). Midwives do not need to be aware of spontaneous versus induced EPL status to triage patient concerns, and can serve as a source of reassurance and clinical support for patients with an early pregnancy loss regardless of cause. Because misoprostol-induced abortions are indistinguishable clinically from miscarriage, people choosing SMA are often able to access medical care if it is needed. Midwifery support can potentially help patients manage their healthcare needs outside of the hospital system if such care is not clinically indicated, which can increase patient safety from a legal standpoint as well as limit potentially traumatizing interactions with law enforcement.

Laws banning SMA in a given jurisdiction, as well as the increasing prevalence of Catholic healthcare systems (which may decline to participate in abortion care or suspected abortion care), can make seeking care, particularly in an acute-care setting, legally hazardous. This is particularly true for BIPOC, low-income people, people with substance use disorders, and those with other children, who may come under increased scrutiny by the legal system to justify a miscarriage, whether self-induced or spontaneous. At least 22 people in the United States have been prosecuted for SMA, or for what is believed to be SMA, and the current legal climate increases the likelihood of more prosecutions in future.[58]

## Conclusion

Abortion and early pregnancy loss are part of midwifery practice, both in the United States and globally. The Core Competencies for Midwifery Practice include management of both undesired pregnancy and early pregnancy loss (ACNM, Core Competency V, section D, subsections 2–3). As such, the ability of the individual midwife to assess, provide, and/or refer to appropriate care as indicated is an expected skill and practice. Management of early pregnancy loss as part of midwifery practice enables provider continuity of care, and ensures that patient care is not delayed with pregnancy loss (a common event). The appropriate evaluation and management of early pregnancy loss reduces the risk of complications such as hemorrhage and infection, and includes the relational and emotional support that are hallmarks of holistic midwifery care.

Similarly, access to safe abortion is considered essential to improving pregnancy morbidity and mortality globally, and midwives are explicitly central to that goal. In the United States, abortion, whether medication or procedural, is a very common and extremely safe healthcare service, but there are significant barriers to access, particularly for young people, BIPOC, low-income people, and people living outside major urban areas. For the first time since 1973, abortion is illegal in broad swaths of the United States, and this trend is expected to expand over the coming years.[53] However, the legal status of abortion is irrelevant to whether it continues to occur, and midwives are responsible for providing comprehensive pregnancy care, including discussion of pregnancy options and referral as appropriate and possible, to fulfill their obligations to their patients.

Both abortion and early pregnancy loss are common events in the reproductive lifespan. As providers of comprehensive sexual and reproductive health care, midwives will encounter patients experiencing both of these events during their careers. Consistent with the midwifery model of care, midwives are obligated to provide individualized care that is centered on the patient's decision making and preferences, and that follows current evidence. For patients experiencing both unintended pregnancy and early pregnancy loss, social stigma and silence can create a sense of profound isolation, and midwives can help provide opportunities for community and connection during these common life events.

## References

1. Hendriks E, MacNaughton H, MacKenzie MC. First trimester bleeding: evaluation and management. *Am Fam Physician*. 2019;99(3):166-174.
2. Reproductive Health Access Project. First trimester bleeding algorithm. https://www.reproductiveaccess.org/resource/first-trimester-bleeding-algorithm/. Published November 1, 2017. Accessed April 14, 2023.

3. Barnhart KT, Guo W, Cary MS, et al. Differences in serum human chorionic gonadotropin rise in early pregnancy by race and value at presentation. *Obstet Gynecol*. 2016;128(3):504-511. PMID: 27500326.

4. ACOG Practice Bulletin Number 191: tubal ectopic pregnancy. *Obstet Gynecol*. 2018;131(2):e65-e77.

5. Fields L, Hathaway A. Key concepts in pregnancy of unknown location: identifying ectopic pregnancy and providing patient-centered care. *J Midwifery Womens Health*. 2017;62:172-179.

6. Soper J. Gestational trophoblastic disease. *Obstet Gynecol*. 2021;137(2):355-370. doi:10.1097/AOG.0000000000004240.

7. ACOG Practice Bulletin Number 200: early pregnancy loss. *Obstet Gynecol*. 2018;132(5):e197-e207.

8. Prine LW, MacNaughton H. Office management of early pregnancy loss. *Am Fam Physician*. 2011;84(1):75-82.

9. Heller HT, Asch EA, Durfee SM, et al. Subchorionic hematoma: correlation of grading techniques with first-trimester pregnancy outcome. *J Ultrasound Med*. 2018;37:1725-1732. doi:10.1002/jum.14524.

10. Monchek R, Wiedaseck S. Gestational trophoblastic disease: an overview. *J Midwifery Womens Health*. 2012;57:255-259.

11. Shorter JM, Atrio JM, Schreiber CA. Management of early pregnancy loss, with a focus on patient centered care. *Sem Perinatol*. 2019;43(2):84-94. https://doi.org/10.1053/j.semperi.2018.12.005.

12. Jackson T, Watkins E. Early pregnancy loss. *J Am Acad PAs*. 2021;34(3):22-27. doi:10.1097/01.JAA.0000733216.66078.ac.

13. Al Wattar BH, Murugesu N, Tobias A, et al. Management of first-trimester miscarriage: a systematic review and network meta-analysis. *Hum Reprod Update*. 2019;25(3):362-374. https://doi.org/10.1093/humupd/dmz002.

14. Schreiber CA, Creinin MD, Atrio J, et al. Mifepristone pretreatment for the medical management of early pregnancy loss. *N Engl J Med*. 2018;378(23):2161-2170. https://doi.org/10.1056/nejmao1715726.

15. MacNaughton H, Nothnagle M, Early J. Mifepristone and misoprostol for early pregnancy loss and medication abortion. *Am Fam Physician*. 2021;103(8):473-480.

16. Shorter JM, Koepler N, Sonalkar S, et al. Racial disparities in mental health outcomes among women with early pregnancy loss. *Obstet Gynecol*. 2021;137:156-163.

17. Coomarasamy A, Devall AJ, Cheed V, et al. A randomized trial of progesterone in women with bleeding in early pregnancy. *N Engl J Med*. 2019;380:1815-1824. doi:10.1056/NEJMoa1813730.

18. Jones RK, Jerman J. Population group abortion rates and lifetime incidence of abortion: United States, 2008–2014. *Am J Public Health*. 2017;107(12):1904-1909.

19. Coleman-Minahan K. Pregnancy options counseling and abortion referral practices among Colorado nurse practitioners, nurse-midwives, and physician assistants. *J Midwifery Womens Health*. 2021;66(4):470-477.

20. American College of Nurse-Midwives. Position statement: midwives as abortion providers. https://www.midwife.org/acnm/files/acnmlibrarydata/uploadfilename/000000000314/PS-Midwives-as-Abortion-Providers-FINAL-August-2019.pdf. Published 2019. Accessed August 22, 2021.

21. International Confederation of Midwives. Midwives' provision of abortion-related services. https://internationalmidwives.org/assets/files/statement-files/2018/04/midwives-provision-of-abortion-related-services-eng.pdf. Published 2014. Accessed April 14, 2023.

22. World Health Organization. Maintaining essential health services: operational guidance for the COVID-19 context: interim guidance, 1 June 2020. https://apps.who.int/iris/handle/10665/332240. Accessed April 14, 2023.

23. Guttmacher Institute. An overview of abortion laws. https://www.guttmacher.org/state-policy/explore/overview-abortion-laws. Published 2020. Accessed January 11, 2022.

24. Center for Reproductive Rights. The world's abortion laws. https://reproductiverights.org/maps/worlds-abortion-laws/?country=FIN&category[1351]=1351. Accessed November 11, 2021.

25. Acevedo Z. Abortion in early America. *Women Health*. 1979;4(2):159-167. doi:10.1300/j013v04n02_05.

26. Reagan LJ. *When Abortion Was a Crime: Women, Medicine, and Law in the United States, 1867–1973*. Berkeley, CA: University of California Press; 1997.

27. Joffe C. Abortion and medicine: a sociopolitical history. In: *Management of Unintended and Abnormal Pregnancy: Comprehensive Abortion Care*. Oxford, UK: Wiley-Blackwell; 2009:1-9.

28. Gold RB. Lessons from before *Roe*: will past be prologue? Guttmacher Institute. https://www.guttmacher.org/gpr/2003/03/lessons-roe-will-past-be-prologue. Published September 14, 2018. Accessed January 3, 2022.

29. National Abortion Federation. Provider security. https://prochoice.org/our-work/provider-security/. Accessed August 22, 2021.

30. Nash E, Cross L. Six months post-*Roe*, 24 US states have banned abortion or are likely to do so: a roundup. Guttmacher Institute. https://www.guttmacher.org/2023/01/six-months-post-roe-24-us-states-have-banned-abortion-or-are-likely-do-so-roundup. Published January10, 2023. Accessed May 24, 2023.

31. Taylor D, Safriet B, Kruse B, et al. State abortion laws and their relationship to scope of practice. AP Toolkit. https://aptoolkit.org/advancing-scope-of-practice-to-include-abortion-care/state-abortion-laws-and-their-relationship-to-scope-of-practice/. Published January 14, 2021. Accessed September 20, 2021.

32. Jones RK, Witwer E, Jerman J. Abortion incidence and service availability in the United States, 2017. Guttmacher Institute. https://www.guttmacher.org/report/abortion-incidence-service-availability-us-2017. Published 2017. Accessed August 22, 2022.

33. Guiahi M, Wilson C, Claymore E, et al. Influence of a values clarification workshop on residents training at Catholic hospital programs. *Contraception: X*. 2021;3:100054. doi:10.1016/j.conx.2021.100054.

34. Turner KL, Pearson E, George A, Andersen KL. Values clarification workshops to improve abortion knowledge, attitudes and intentions: a pre–post assessment in 12 countries. *Reprod Health*. 2018;15(1). doi:10.1186/s12978-018-0480-0.

35. Ahrens KA, Thoma ME, Copen CE, et al. Unintended pregnancy and interpregnancy interval by maternal age: National Survey of Family Growth. *Contraception*. 2018;98(1):52-55. doi:10.1016/j.contraception.2018.02.013.

36. Stahl RY, Emanuel EJ. Physicians, not conscripts: conscientious objection in health care. *N Engl J Med*. 2017;376(14):1380-1385.

37. Lamb C. Conscientious objection: understanding the right of conscience in health and healthcare practice. *New Bioeth*. 2016;22(1):33-44.

38. Religious Freedom Restoration Act of 1993. 42 USC §2000bb et seq. https://www.congress.gov/bill/103rd-congress/house-bill/1308/text. Accessed December 2, 2019.

39. Eagen-Torkko M, Levi AJ. The ethical justification for conscience clauses in nurse-midwifery practice: context, power, and a changing landscape. *J Midwifery Womens Health*. 2020;65(6):759-766. doi:10.1111/jmwh.13170.

40. Bearak J, Popinchalk A, Ganatra B, et al. Unintended pregnancy and abortion by income, region, and the legal status of abortion: estimates from a comprehensive model for 1990–2019. *Lancet Glob Health*. 2020;8(9). doi:10.1016/s2214-109x(20)30315-6.

41. Say L, Chou D, Gemmill A, et al. Global causes of maternal death: a WHO systematic analysis. *Lancet Glob Health*. 2014;2(6):e323-e333.

42. Raymond EG, Grimes DA. The comparative safety of legal induced abortion and childbirth in the United States. *Obstet Gynecol*. 2012;119(6):1271-1272. doi:10.1097/aog.0b013e318258c833.

43. Kaiser Family Foundation. State funding of abortions under Medicaid. https://www.kff.org/medicaid/state-indicator/abortion-under-medicaid/?currentTimeframe=0&sortModel=%7B%22colId%22%3A%22Location%22%2C%22sort%22%3A%22asc%22%7D. Published September 16, 2021. Accessed February 5, 2022.

44. Kortsmit K, Jatlaoui TC, Mandel MG, et al. Abortion surveillance—United States, 2018. *MMWR Surveill Summ*. 2020;69(SS-7):1-29. http://dx.doi.org/10.15585/mmwr.ss6907a1.

45. Upadhyay UD. Barriers push people into seeking abortion care later in pregnancy. *Am J Public Health*. 2022;112(9):1280-1281.

46. Simmonds KE, Beal MW, Eagen-Torkko MK. Updates to the US Food and Drug Administration regulations for mifepristone: implications for clinical practice and access to abortion. *J Midwifery Womens Health*. 2017;62(3):348-352. doi:10.1111/jmwh.12636.

47. Jelinska K, Yanow S. Putting abortion pills into women's hands: realizing the full potential of medical abortion. *Contraception*. 2018;97(2):86-89. doi:10.1016/j.contraception.2017.05.019.

48. National Abortion Federation. Clinical policy guidelines for abortion care. https://prochoice.org/wp-content/uploads/2020_cpgs_final.pdf. Published 2020. Accessed October 2, 2021.

49. Norton ME, Cassidy A, Ralston SJ, et al. Society for Maternal–Fetal Medicine Consult Series #59: the use of analgesia and anesthesia for maternal–fetal procedures. *Am J Obstet Gynecol*. 2021;225(6). doi:10.1016/j.ajog.2021.08.031.

50. National Academies of Science, Engineering, and Medicine. The safety and quality of abortion care in the United States. https://www.nap.edu/resource/24950/03162018AbortionCarehighlights.pdf. Published 2018. Accessed August 3, 2021.

51. Kalogiannidis I, Tsakiridis I, Dagklis T, et al. Comparison of the efficacy and safety of two combined misoprostol regimens for second trimester medical abortion. *Eur J Contraception Reprod Health Care*. 2020;26(1):42-47. doi:10.1080/13625187.2020.1830966.

52. Shay RL, Benson LS, Lokken EM, Micks EA. Same-day mifepristone prior to second-trimester induction termination with misoprostol: a retrospective cohort study. *Contraception*. 2021. doi:10.1016/j.contraception.2021.09.006.

53. Upadhyay UD, Desai S, Zlidar V, et al. Incidence of emergency department visits and complications after abortion. *Obstet Gynecol*. 2015;125(1):175-183. doi:10.1097/aog.0000000000000603.

54. Ralph LJ, Schwarz EB, Grossman D, Foster DG. Self-reported physical health of women who did and did not terminate pregnancy after seeking abortion services. *Ann Intern Med*. 2019;171(4):238. doi:10.7326/m18-1666.

55. Gerdts C, Dobkin L, Foster DG, Schwarz EB. Side effects, physical health consequences, and mortality associated with abortion and birth after an unwanted

pregnancy. *Womens Health Issues.* 2016;26(1): 55-59. doi:10.1016/j.whi.2015.10.001.

56. Foster DG. *The Turnaway Study: Ten Years, a Thousand Women, and the Consequences of Having—or Being Denied—an Abortion.* New York, NY: Simon and Schuster; June 2, 2020.

57. Jenkins J, Woodside F, Lipinsky K, et al. Abortion with pills: review of current options in the United States. *J Midwifery Womens Health.* 2021;66(6): 749-757. doi:10.1111/jmwh.13291.

58. Baker CN. Self-managed abortion is medically very safe. But is it legally safe? *Ms. Magazine.* April 2, 2020. https://msmagazine.com/2020/04/01/self-managed -abortion-is-medically-very-safe-but-is-it-legally -safe/. Accessed March 11, 2021.

CHAPTER

# 23

# Pregnancy-Related Conditions

ESTHER R. ELLSWORTH BOWERS AND MELISSA E. KITZMAN

*The editors acknowledge Nancy Jo Reedy and Tekoa King, who were past authors of this chapter.*

## Introduction

The majority of pregnant people experience healthy pregnancies, and midwifery care provides the appropriate support, monitoring, and interventions throughout. People with pregnancy-related complications and other medical needs can also benefit from midwifery care. This chapter addresses complications that are brought on by, or specifically related to, the condition of being pregnant. It also reviews management of common discomforts of pregnancy. Medical complications existing prior to pregnancy, or aggravated by pregnancy, are presented in the *Medical Complications in Pregnancy* chapter. Hypertensive diseases such as preeclampsia and gestational hypertension are presented together with chronic hypertension in the *Medical Complications in Pregnancy* chapter, although these conditions could be considered pregnancy-related. Similarly, gestational diabetes is presented together with prediabetes and type 2 diabetes in the *Medical Complications in Pregnancy* chapter.

## Overview of Midwifery Management for People With Pregnancy-Related Conditions

Assessment of the pregnant person for complications related to pregnancy begins preconception or with the first prenatal visit and continues throughout the gestation. The care that a midwife provides to a pregnant person with pregnancy-related conditions or complications depends on several factors, including the practice setting and institutional guidelines, the midwife's experience and education, the availability of collaboration with consultants from a variety of disciplines, and legal or regulatory statutes.[1] Table 23-1 lists examples of conditions that may arise during prenatal care that indicate a need for consultation or referral to a clinician who is specialized in the area of concern.

When an individual has a medical complication in pregnancy, the appropriate provider or care team and "level" of perinatal care facility must be determined (Table 23-2).[2] Given that perinatal risks change throughout a pregnancy, and transfer between care settings might be necessary, this conversation should be ongoing and use a shared decision-making approach. A pregnant person is often reassured to know that midwives provide care to pregnant people in a variety of settings.

## Common Discomforts of Pregnancy

The physiologic changes of pregnancy have wide-ranging effects on all body systems. These changes result in many symptoms, which, although not pathologic in nature, can disrupt a pregnant person's life to varying degrees. Discomforts of pregnancy are presented in this chapter because some—such as dyspnea, nausea and vomiting, or urinary frequency—may indicate a disorder that requires additional investigation, and possibly consultation with a specialist.

Differentiating normal from abnormal symptoms is the first task when these symptoms are evaluated during a prenatal care visit. A careful approach to differential diagnosis is recommended

| Table 23-1 | Selected Indications for Advanced Care, Collaboration, Consultation, or Referral During Pregnancy[a] |
|---|---|
| **Gynecologic or Reproductive History** | |

| | |
|---|---|
| Cervical insufficiency | Previous uterine surgery, including prior cesarean birth |
| Congenital uterine anomaly, such as bicornuate uterus | Prior unexplained third trimester fetal loss |
| Large uterine fibroids | |

**Medical Complications Prior to Pregnancy or That Worsen During Pregnancy**

| | |
|---|---|
| Anemia not responding to oral or intravenous iron therapy | Hypertension: chronic |
| Asthma requiring complex medication management | Infectious disease such as hepatitis, human immunodeficiency virus, syphilis, pneumonia, or tuberculosis |
| Autoimmune disorders such as systemic lupus erythematosus | Mental health conditions requiring complex medication management |
| Breast mass | Obesity: Class III or with metabolic complication |
| Cancer: recent history or current | Pelvic or spinal trauma |
| Cardiac disease such as arrhythmia, congenital heart disease, heart failure, valvular disorders: history or current | Persistent proteinuria |
| | Renal calculi |
| Cholestasis | Seizure disorder |
| Coagulopathies | Skin rashes or lesions without diagnosis |
| Deep vein thrombosis or pulmonary embolus: history, current, or suspected | Surgical history, including abdominal, bariatric, brain, cardiac, pelvic, and spine |
| Diabetes: pregestational | Suspected pneumonia |
| Gastrointestinal disease such as Crohn's disease | Syphilis |
| Headaches: severe or recurrent | Thyroid disorder: uncontrolled |
| Hemoglobinopathy | |

**Complications That Develop During Pregnancy**

| | |
|---|---|
| Abnormal genetic screening results, such as aneuploidy or single-gene disorders | Preeclampsia or gestational hypertension |
| Alloimmunization | Preterm labor |
| | Pyelonephritis |
| First trimester bleeding with pregnancy of unknown origin or suspected ectopic | Short cervix via transvaginal ultrasound or clinical examination |
| Gestational diabetes, White classification A2 | Ultrasound with abnormal findings such as fetal anomalies, fetal growth restriction, polyhydramnios, or unresolved size–dates discrepancy |
| Hypertensive disorders of pregnancy | |
| Malpresentation of the fetus after 36 weeks | Vaginal bleeding: persistent or heavy, not related to cervicitis, not bloody show |
| Molar pregnancy | Venous thrombosis |
| Multifetal gestation | |
| Nausea and vomiting that requires hospitalization | |
| Placenta previa: with significant bleeding, or persisting after 28 weeks | |
| Post-term pregnancy (beyond 42 0/7 weeks) | |

[a] This list is offered for consideration and is not absolute or all-inclusive. It is intended as an adjunct to clinical management based on the individual pregnant person, the midwife, the consulting physician, and institutional guidelines.

| Table 23-2 | Levels of Perinatal Care | | |
|---|---|---|---|
| **Level of Care** | **Capabilities** | **Services** | **Providers** |
| Birth center | Term, singleton, vertex low-risk pregnancy in spontaneous labor | Low risk, uncomplicated vaginal birth | Midwives and occasionally physicians |
| Level I | Term, low-risk pregnancy<br><br>Ability to manage unanticipated complications until transfer to a higher level of care | Induction and augmentation of labor<br><br>Ability to provide emergency cesarean and operative vaginal birth on a 24/7 basis | Midwives and physicians<br><br>Obstetric provider credentialed for cesarean birth |
| Level II | Pregnancy with complications that do not require subspecialty care | Medical and surgical consultants available to stabilize the pregnant person prior to transfer | Midwives<br><br>Anesthesia available on a 24/7 basis<br><br>Obstetrician-gynecologist available on a 24/7 basis<br><br>MFM available for consultation on site or by telemedicine 24/7 |
| Level III | Care of more complex medical, obstetric, and fetal conditions | Medical and surgical ICU with ability to collaborate with MFM<br><br>Subspecialists available for inpatient consultation | Midwives<br><br>Anesthesia available on a 24/7 basis<br><br>Obstetrician-gynecologist on site on a 24/7 basis<br><br>MFM available on site or by telemedicine with inpatient privileges |
| Level IV (regional perinatal health center) | Care of most complex medical conditions and critically ill pregnant persons | On-site obstetric ICU<br><br>Medical and surgical ICU<br><br>Medical and surgical subspecialists available on site on a 24/7 basis, including transplant specialists, cardiac surgery, and advanced neurosurgery | Midwives<br><br>Obstetrician-gynecologist on site on a 24/7 basis<br><br>MFM available on site on a 24/7 basis<br><br>MFM with expertise in critical care obstetrics<br><br>Anesthesia with special training in obstetrics |

Abbreviations: ICU, intensive care unit; MFM, maternal–fetal medicine specialist

Based on American College of Obstetricians and Gynecologists. Obstetric Care Consensus No. 2: levels of maternal care. *Obstet Gynecol.* 2015:125:502-515.

every time for every patient, to avoid assuming the discomfort is a normal physiologic change of pregnancy. Table 23-3 presents common discomforts of pregnancy by body system, highlighting "red flag" warning signs associated with each presenting sign and symptom.

Most of the common discomforts of pregnancy are not associated with adverse outcomes. However, some can be initial symptoms of a complication that requires evaluation and treatment. The rest of this chapter reviews complications that are a result of pregnancy.

## Nausea and Vomiting

Nausea occurs in as many as 85% of pregnancies.[3] The peak prevalence is at 11 weeks' gestation, with the average time of onset between 5 and 6 weeks. Typically, nausea and vomiting in pregnancy (NVP) will resolve by 14 to 16 weeks' gestation, although a small percentage of pregnant persons will have NVP that persists beyond 20 weeks' gestation. Hyperemesis gravidarum (HG)—a severe form of NVP—occurs in approximately 3% of pregnancies[3] and is one of the most common causes of hospitalization during pregnancy.[4]

Nausea, either with or without vomiting, can occur at any time of day. It is more severe when the stomach is empty, which may explain why some pregnant persons notice it more in the morning. A person with severe NVP or HG often requires hospitalization to break the cycle of vomiting and establish adequate rehydration.

| Table 23-3a | Common Discomforts of Pregnancy: Cardiovascular and Respiratory | | |
|---|---|---|---|
| **Physiology and Onset** | **Differential Diagnosis** | **Red Flags** | **Strategies to Decrease Discomfort** |
| **Dyspnea** | | | |
| Etiology is unclear but may be secondary to altered respiratory center sensitivity and diaphragm displacement.<br><br>May appear at any time in pregnancy. | Dyspnea with tachycardia: may suggest anxiety or panic attack<br><br>Respiratory infection<br><br>Cardiac disorder<br><br>Pulmonary embolism | Fever<br><br>Vital signs outside normal range<br><br>Abnormal findings on lung auscultation<br><br>Signs/symptoms of preeclampsia | Explain the physiologic basis for shortness of breath.<br><br>Deliberately regulate the speed and depth of respirations when aware of hyperventilation.<br><br>Use diaphragmatic or intercostal breathing as opposed to abdominal breathing. |
| **Dependent Edema** | | | |
| Occurs secondary to impaired venous circulation and increased venous pressure in the lower extremities from the enlarged uterus.<br><br>Typically appears in the third trimester. | DVT<br><br>Preeclampsia | Unilateral limb edema<br><br>Nondependent edema (face/neck)<br><br>Excessive/sudden weight gain | Regular exercise and avoiding prolonged sitting or standing may help.<br><br>Elevate legs periodically and position on the side when lying down. Keep legs uncrossed when sitting.<br><br>Graduated compression or support hose can reduce venous pooling in the lower extremities. |
| **"Heart Palpitations" or Short Period of Sinus Tachycardia** | | | |
| Etiology may be pregnancy-induced increase in blood volume, given that a physiologically enlarged heart is more arrhythmogenic.<br><br>Occurs at any time in pregnancy. | Anxiety<br><br>Cardiac disorder<br><br>Arrhythmia<br><br>Thyroid disorder | Extended period with elevated heart rate (> 120 beats/min)<br><br>Frequent events of arrhythmia | Avoid aggravating factors: dehydration, stress, strenuous physical activity, caffeine, tobacco, alcohol use.<br><br>No specific relief measures for short, benign arrhythmias. Reassurance and education that this is a normal symptom of pregnancy are usually sufficient.<br><br>To interrupt sinus tachycardia, perform the Valsalva maneuver. |
| **Syncope or Near-Syncope** | | | |
| The enlarged uterus impairs venous return and causes hypotension.<br><br>Typically appears in the third trimester. | Hypoglycemia<br><br>Seizure disorder | Frequent syncopal events | For prevention:<br>• Avoid lying flat on back<br>• Rise slowly from sitting to standing position<br>• Avoid standing in one position for extended period<br><br>If transient and no loss of consciousness, sit down with the head lowered or lie on the side. |

| Physiology and Onset | Differential Diagnosis | Red Flags | Strategies to Decrease Discomfort |
|---|---|---|---|
| **Varicosities** | | | |
| Occurs secondary to venous distention from increased venous pressure and vasodilation. Familial tendency may increase risk. <br><br> Most common in the legs and/or vulva. <br><br> Appears in the second or third trimester. | DVT <br><br> Peripheral arterial or venous disease | Unilateral limb swelling | Rest the affected extremity. <br><br> Wear compression stockings. <br><br> Wear a pregnancy support belt or vulvar varicosity garment. |

Abbreviation: DVT, deep vein thrombosis.

| Table 23-3b | Common Discomforts of Pregnancy: Gastrointestinal | | |
|---|---|---|---|
| **Physiology and Onset** | **Differential Diagnosis** | **Red Flags** | **Strategies to Decrease Discomfort** |
| **Constipation** | | | |
| Effect of progesterone slowing motility of the GI tract, as well as pressure on the GI tract from the enlarging uterus. May be exacerbated by iron supplements. <br><br> Occurs in the first trimester and resolves by the second trimester. | GI disorder such as IBS <br><br> Fecal impaction | Severe abdominal pain | Increase fluids and change the diet. <br><br> Warm liquids before drinking, so as to stimulate peristalsis. <br><br> Consume foods that contain roughage, bulk, and natural fiber. <br><br> Mild bulk-forming laxatives, stool softeners, and glycerin suppositories are safe for use in pregnancy. <br><br> Stimulant laxatives such as senna are not associated with congenital anomalies but are not recommended for use during pregnancy. These agents directly increase peristalsis and may cause dehydration or electrolyte imbalance. <br><br> Castor oil should be avoided, as it can cause uterine contractions. |
| **Flatulence and Gas Pain** | | | |
| Decreased GI motility and uterine displacement of intestines. <br><br> Usually develops in the first trimester but may occur at any time in pregnancy. | Dietary sensitivities <br><br> IBS <br><br> Appendicitis | Severe abdominal pain <br><br> Fever | Exercise can aid in improving GI motility. <br><br> Use of caffeine can stimulate GI motility. Note that caffeine may increase the risk of heartburn and accentuate insomnia. Caffeine metabolism slows during pregnancy, and a standard dose will be present in higher plasma concentrations compared to a nonpregnant person. <br><br> The knee–chest position may help with discomfort from unexpelled gas. |

*(continues)*

| Table 23-3b | Common Discomforts of Pregnancy: Gastrointestinal (*continued*) | | |
|---|---|---|---|
| **Physiology and Onset** | **Differential Diagnosis** | **Red Flags** | **Strategies to Decrease Discomfort** |
| **Heartburn** | | | |
| Reflux of acidic gastric contents into the lower esophagus.<br><br>Progesterone-induced relaxation of the LES, slower emptying of gastric contents, reduced stomach capacity.<br><br>Appears in the third trimester. | GERD<br>Peptic ulcer disease<br>Hiatal hernia<br>Cholecystitis<br>Pancreatitis<br>Preeclampsia | Symptoms unrelieved by stepwise treatment<br><br>Fever<br><br>Signs/symptoms of preeclampsia | Eat small, frequent meals.<br><br>Avoid foods that make heartburn worse. Elevate the head of the bed, and avoid lying down after eating.<br><br>Begin with antacids, then move as necessary to $H_2$ receptor antagonists and lastly to proton pump inhibitors. |
| **Hemorrhoids** | | | |
| Progesterone-induced relaxation of veins in the rectum, along with the enlarged uterus, causes pelvic venous congestion.<br><br>Appears at any time but is most likely in the third trimester. | Thrombosed hemorrhoid<br>Anal fissure<br>Cancer | Persistent rectal bleeding | Avoid constipation and straining during defecation.<br><br>Use witch hazel compresses or Epsom salt soak.<br><br>Topical anesthetics and topical cortisone creams or suppositories are safe for use in pregnancy. |
| **Nausea and Vomiting** | | | |
| Exact etiology is unknown.<br>Peaks in the first trimester. | Hyperemesis gravidarum<br>GERD<br>GI infection (viral or bacterial, such as listeriosis)<br>Bulimia<br>Cannabinoid hyperemesis | Fever<br><br>See the chapter text for an extended discussion of nausea and vomiting | Consume small, frequent meals. Avoid fried fatty foods and foods with strong odors.<br><br>Temporarily discontinue prenatal vitamins that contain iron, but continue folic acid supplementation.<br><br>Ginger, acupressure bands, and vitamin $B_6$ may help persons with mild to moderate symptoms.<br><br>Antiemetic medications are recommended in a stepwise fashion, depending on the severity of symptoms. |
| **Ptyalism** | | | |
| Etiology unknown. | Hyperemesis | Warning signs associated with nausea and vomiting of pregnancy | Ptyalism usually resolves spontaneously, although the condition may not disappear until after the pregnancy is over.<br><br>Some pregnant persons obtain temporary relief from gum chewing or sucking on hard candies. |

Abbreviations: GERD, gastroesophageal reflux disease; GI, gastrointestinal; IBS, irritable bowel syndrome; LES, lower esophageal sphincter.

| Table 23-3c | Common Discomforts of Pregnancy: Musculoskeletal | | |
|---|---|---|---|
| **Physiology and Onset** | **Differential Diagnosis** | **Red Flags** | **Strategies to Decrease Discomfort** |
| **Back Pain** | | | |
| Upper backache develops during the first trimester from increased size of the breasts.

Low back pain typically occurs in the last half of pregnancy, secondary to the increasing weight of the uterus and relaxation of the sacroiliac ligaments. The exaggerated lordosis of pregnancy strains the back muscles and causes pain. | Sciatica

Sprain/strain

Early labor

Pyelonephritis

Kidney stone

Spinal dysfunction

Cancer (bone metastasis)

Referred pain from pelvic or abdominal disease

Chronic back pain | Intense localized pain

Fever

History of traumatic injury

Progressive neurologic deficit (including incontinence)

Opioid or steroid use to manage pain

Unexplained weight loss or cancer history | For upper back pain: Wear a well-fitting and supportive bra.

For lower back pain: Proper body mechanics for lifting, pelvic rock/pelvic tilt exercises, external abdominal support (maternity support belt/band, sacroiliac belt).

Heat or ice packs.

A supportive mattress or positioning with pillows to straighten the back.

Cognitive-behavioral therapy, physical therapy, spinal manipulation/chiropractic care, acupuncture, massage, and yoga.

Pharmacologic therapy:

• Acetaminophen for acute pain

• Short-term use of a muscle relaxant for sprain/strain

• Caution with opioid therapy (benefit usually outweighed by potential for dependence)

• Tricyclic antidepressants for chronic low back pain |
| **Leg Cramps** | | | |
| May be linked to changes in calcium, magnesium, and phosphorus levels or the ability of calcium to enter the muscles, but causes have not been proven.

Occurs in the second and third trimesters. | DVT or phlebitis

Electrolyte imbalances

Peripheral neuropathy

Restless legs syndrome (may be associated with anemia) | Unilateral limb edema

Signs/symptoms of electrolyte imbalance | Straighten the affected leg and dorsiflex the ankle.

Magnesium supplementation at bedtime, to bowel tolerance. |
| **Sciatica** | | | |
| Pressure on the sciatic nerve from joint laxity, often elicited by twisting, lifting, or moving the leg.

Typically appears in the third trimester and is usually unilateral. | Cauda equina syndrome

Herniated disc | Progressive neurologic deficit (including incontinence) | Rest in a side-lying position on the contralateral side from the affected leg.

Heat packs, ice, or an abdominal support girdle may offer some relief.

Avoid twisting the torso. Use careful body mechanics when lifting.

Acetaminophen: Maximum daily dose is 4000 mg/day.

Referral to chiropractic care or physical therapy may be indicated. |

Abbreviations: DVT, deep vein thrombosis

| Table 23-3d | Common Discomforts of Pregnancy: Reproductive and Urinary | | |
|---|---|---|---|
| **Physiology and Onset** | **Differential Diagnosis** | **Red Flags** | **Strategies to Decrease Discomfort** |
| **Breast Tenderness** | | | |
| Associated with estrogen- and progesterone-caused breast changes. Appears in the first trimester and discomfort resolves in the second trimester, but enlarged size remains. | Fibrocystic breast changes Benign breast mass Breast cancer Mastitis | Breast mass palpable on clinical exam Fever or symptoms of systemic illness | Wear a correctly fitted and supportive bra. |
| **Dyspareunia** | | | |
| Progesterone-induced relaxation of veins in the pelvis, along with the enlarged uterus, causes pelvic/vaginal venous congestion. Most likely to appear in the second half of pregnancy. | Vaginitis Preexisting dyspareunia Vulvar varicosities Rectocele Sexual abuse (current or historical) | Abnormal findings on pelvic exam | May resolve with positional changes to accommodate the larger uterus or avoid pain from deep penetration. Use of water-based vaginal lubricants may be helpful. Treat vaginitis as indicated. Counseling referral may be appropriate for a person with history of sexual abuse. If current abuse is suspected, offer support and referral, and assess safety. |
| **Leukorrhea** | | | |
| Profuse white or clear vaginal secretions caused by high estrogen level. Typically appears in the second trimester. | STI Bacterial vaginosis Candida Prelabor rupture of membranes | Signs/symptoms of vaginitis Report of persistent, clear "leaking" | Avoid douching or using feminine hygiene sprays; clean the perineal and vaginal areas only with water. Reassurance and education that this is a normal symptom of pregnancy are usually sufficient. |
| **Round Ligament Pain** | | | |
| Round ligaments gradually increase in length as the uterus rises in the abdomen. Pain stems from sudden ligament stretching. Appears early in the second trimester. | Preterm labor Appendicitis Constipation Gas pain Abdominal muscle strain or sprain | Rhythmic backache or uterine contractions Fever Persistent or severe pain | Wear an abdominal support belt. Review movements that place less tension on the round ligament (such as supporting the abdomen while turning over or moving to a standing position). |
| **Urinary Frequency and Nocturia** | | | |
| Mechanical pressure from the enlarging uterus results in decreased bladder capacity. Increasing blood volume and glomerular filtration rate increases urine production. Frequently occurs in the first and third trimesters. | Urinary tract infection Pyelonephritis | Pain or foul odor with urination Fever Flank pain | Decreasing fluid intake at night may offer some relief, but pregnant people should not restrict fluids in general. Provide counseling regarding increased renal activity during pregnancy, normalcy of frequent urination. |

Abbreviations: STI, sexually transmitted infection.

| Table 23-3e | Common Discomforts of Pregnancy: Other | | |
|---|---|---|---|
| **Physiology and Onset** | **Differential Diagnosis** | **Red Flags** | **Strategies to Decrease Discomfort** |
| **Fatigue** | | | |
| Disrupted sleep, increased energy requirements of pregnancy, and progesterone contribute to fatigue. Common during the first and third trimesters. | Anemia Depression Cardiac conditions Sleep apnea Thyroid dysfunction Viral or other systemic infection | Vital signs outside normal range Positive sleep apnea screening Positive depression screening Fever | Treat any other condition contributing to fatigue. Regular exercise may help improve sleep patterns if fatigue is related to disrupted sleep. |
| **Gingivitis** | | | |
| Pregnancy changes in oral mucosa increase the likelihood of gingivitis. Appears in the second trimester. | Epulis (pregnancy tumor or benign overgrowth of gingiva) Periodontal disease | Persistent gingivitis even after dental cleaning and improved oral hygiene | Increase the frequency of home oral hygiene. Refer for dental care. |
| **Insomnia** | | | |
| Difficulty sleeping may be related to frequent waking from back pain, heartburn, or nocturia. | Sleep disorder Sleep apnea Anxiety Restless legs syndrome (may be associated with anemia) | Positive sleep apnea screening Positive mental health screening (especially depression or mania) | If no signs of pathology: Take warm baths, reduce stimulation prior to bedtime, and avoid caffeine. Regular exercise and regulation of temperature in the bedroom may improve sleep. Antihistamines such as diphenhydramine (Benadryl) 50–100 mg or doxylamine succinate (Unisom) 25 mg may help some pregnant persons, but discuss the risks and benefits if using a sleep aid regularly. Refer to a sleep therapist for cognitive-behavioral therapy for insomnia. |
| **Nasal Congestion and Epistaxis** | | | |
| Caused by hyperemia and increased blood flow in nasal passages (estrogen effect during pregnancy). Occurs at any time during pregnancy. | URI Sinusitis Hypertension Substance use disorder | Vital signs outside normal range Positive substance use screening | Use a humidifier to generate cool mist at night. Avoid blowing the nose hard. Nasal sprays with epinephrine may provide temporary relief but can be habit forming and result in rebound congestion (especially long-acting formulations). For epistaxis, elevate the head and compress the nose against the midline septum continuously for 5–10 minutes. |

*(continues)*

| Table 23-3e | Common Discomforts of Pregnancy: Other (*continued*) | | | |
|---|---|---|---|---|
| **Physiology and Onset** | **Differential Diagnosis** | **Red Flags** | **Strategies to Decrease Discomfort** | |
| **Tingling and Numbness of Fingers** | | | | |
| Kyphosis places pressure or traction on nerves in the arm, which can cause tingling and numbness of the fingers. Edema in the wrists/hands can cause temporary carpal tunnel syndrome symptoms. Often occurs at night. Is exacerbated by edema in the arms and hands. | Carpal tunnel syndrome | Neurologic symptoms do not resolve with position change  Progressive neurologic deficit | Move arms at the level of the shoulder to decrease pressure on the nerves when tingling starts.  Wrist splints that keep the wrist in a neutral position may be worn while sleeping or during work or other activities. | |

Abbreviation: URI, upper respiratory infection.

The cause of NVP is not fully known. Likely causes include the interplay between hormonal changes of pregnancy (e.g., human chorionic gonadotropin, estrogen, progesterone, placental prostaglandin $E_2$), slowed peristalsis, and genetic factors. Pathophysiologic factors such as preexisting gastroesophageal reflux disease (GERD) or *Helicobacter pylori* infection also contribute to the occurrence of NVP.

Little evidence supports an older theory that NVP reflects the transformation of psychological distress into physical symptoms. Nevertheless, a person's experience of NVP does have psychological and sociocultural components. Severe NVP can be associated with severe psychological distress, and depression may result.[5,6] These symptoms are accentuated for pregnant persons with minimal social support or persons who feel removed from their native culture.[7]

### Assessment of Nausea and Vomiting

Midwives and physicians frequently collaborate in the care of pregnant persons with NVP, with midwives initiating outpatient management or conducting initial assessment and treatment following hospital admission. Maternal–fetal medicine specialist (MFM) or obstetrician consultation or referral is recommended for a person with severe symptoms that are not relieved by first- and second-line treatment.

When evaluating a person with NVP, it is essential to rule out differential diagnoses, including thyroid dysfunction, GERD, peptic ulcer disease, cholecystitis, and eating disorder (Table 23-4). Next, the midwife should assess how the symptoms interfere with the person's ability to maintain

and engage in daily activities. Finally, the midwife should establish the severity of the disorder (i.e. mild, moderate, or severe). Several tools to measure the severity of NVP have been validated for use in clinical practice.[3,8,9] One of the most commonly used is the PUQE index, which is based on three questions, highly correlated with scores on the more detailed Rhodes index, and easily incorporated into clinical practice.[8] Critical components of the evaluation are the frequency of vomiting or dry heaves and the duration of nausea.

If the assessment yields a diagnosis of severe NVP, the midwife should also consider the diagnosis of HG. There is no standard definition for HG, but most diagnostic criteria include the following items:

- Persistent vomiting, onset before 9 weeks' gestation
- Dehydration and/or ketonuria
- Weight loss greater than 5% of initial body weight
- Electrolyte imbalance[10]

### Treatment of Nausea and Vomiting

Treatments for mild, moderate, and severe NVP are presented in Table 23-5.[11] First-line treatments for mild NVP begin with dietary changes, acupressure bands, ginger products, and vitamin $B_6$. A midwife can then advise the client about taking nonprescription or prescription antihistamines. A person with moderate NVP likely needs second-line treatments, which begin with prescription antihistamines and proceed to other categories of anti-emetics.

If a person with NVP needs rehydration therapy, the recommended IV solution is normal saline,

| Table 23-4 | Evaluation of Nausea and Vomiting in Pregnancy |
|---|---|

**History**

Abdominal pain (GI disorder)

Blood in vomitus (peptic ulcer or esophagitis from repeated vomiting)

Frequency of nausea, vomiting, and retching episodes (PUQE score to determine severity)

Dietary history (determine severity of NVP)

Elimination (frequency, amount, constipation, diarrhea)

Exposures to viral infection or contaminated food

History of eating disorders

History of chronic disease associated with nausea/vomiting

Medications (e.g., medications that cause nausea such as iron supplements)

**Physical Examination**

Weight (compare to previous weights to determine severity of NVP)

Vital signs with blood pressure (signs of infection and hypovolemia)

Skin turgor, moistness of mucous membranes (signs of dehydration to determine severity of NVP)

Abdominal palpation for organomegaly, tenderness, distention (GI disorders)

Bowel sounds (GI disorders)

Assessment of uterine size (rule out multiple pregnancy or hydatidiform mole)

**Laboratory Tests**

Complete blood count (signs of dehydration or infection)

Urinalysis and urine dipstick for specific gravity and ketones (dehydration indicates increased severity of NVP)

Blood urea nitrogen (BUN) and electrolytes (electrolyte imbalance indicates increased severity of NVP)

Liver function tests (rule out hepatitis, pancreatitis, and cholestasis)

Thyroid-stimulating hormone (TSH) and free $T_4$ (thyroxine) (rule out thyroid disease)

**Ultrasound**

Confirm pregnancy and rule out multiple pregnancy and/or hydatidiform mole

Abbreviations: GI, gastrointestinal; NVP, nausea and vomiting of pregnancy; PUQE, Pregnancy-Unique Quantification of Emesis/Nausea.

which helps prevent hyponatremia. Potassium chloride can be added as needed, and thiamine (vitamin $B_1$) or a multivitamin solution that includes thiamine should be added at least once a day. Thiamine supplementation reduces the risk of Wernicke's encephalopathy, a condition in malnourished individuals that presents with a classic triad of ocular abnormalities, ataxia, and confusion.[12]

For a person with a diagnosis of severe NVP or HG, hospitalization and MFM or obstetrician consultation are recommended. Intravenous or intramuscular administration of antiemetics such as metoclopramide (Reglan) or ondansetron (Zofran) is commonly used to break the initial cycle of vomiting. Of these medications, ondansetron is particularly effective at controlling vomiting. However, treatment of hyperemesis is an off-label use for ondansetron, and many providers prescribe ondansetron only after other medications have been tried.[13]

Following hospitalization, a person with severe NVP or HG may need multiple agents to manage their symptoms. While the outpatient treatment plan is often established by a physician colleague, a midwife can monitor the plan for effectiveness. This team approach requires ongoing consultation between the midwife and the obstetrician or MFM.

As marijuana gains legal status in many states, an increasing number of pregnant persons are using cannabis to manage NVP.[14] While individual reports of improved symptoms must be acknowledged, the effectiveness of cannabis as a treatment has not been established by clinical trials, and fetal cannabis exposure raises significant safety concerns. While it is difficult to isolate the health impacts of marijuana due to confounding factors such as polysubstance abuse, psychiatric comorbidity, and socioeconomic status, research has associated marijuana use with risks of preterm birth, low birth weight, exaggerated startle response, high-pitched cry, and sleep cycle changes in the newborn.[15]

Midwives should also be aware of a counterintuitive response to marijuana that can be mistaken for HG, called cannabinoid hyperemesis. Cannabinoid hyperemesis occurs following heavy marijuana use and is a response to saturated cannabinoid type 1 receptors in the gastrointestinal system.[16] With this condition, a person may present with symptoms of nausea and vomiting unresponsive to antiemetic treatment. If cannabinoid hyperemesis is suspected, treatment requires rehydration therapy during 24 to 48 hours of abstinence from marijuana. Symptoms will resolve if cannabinoid hyperemesis is the correct diagnosis.

| Table 23-5 | Selected Treatments for Nausea and Vomiting in Pregnancy | |
| --- | --- | --- |
| Treatment | Drug Dosage | Clinical Considerations |
| **Mild NVP (*May use multiple modalities.*)** | | |
| Temporarily discontinue prenatal vitamins with iron but continue folic acid supplementation | | Iron can increase gastrointestinal distress |
| Acupressure bands | | |
| Ginger | 250 mg every 6 hours | May cause acid reflux |
| Pyridoxine (vitamin B$_6$) | 10–25 mg every 8 hours | |
| **If no improvement, add one of the following agents:** | | |
| Doxylamine | 12.5 mg 2–4 times/day | May cause drowsiness; anticholinergic |
| Diphenhydramine (Benadryl) | 50–100 mg every 4–6 hours orally or rectally if vomiting frequently | May cause drowsiness; can offset the anxiety caused by metoclopramide |
| Prochlorperazine (Compazine) | 5–10 mg every 6–8 hours orally/IM/IV/rectally | Sedation, anticholinergic effects, dry mouth, dystonic reaction; hypotension if given IV too quickly. |
| Promethazine (Phenergan) | 12.5–25 mg every 4–6 hours orally/IM/rectally | Sedation, anticholinergic effects, dry mouth, dystonic reaction; hypotension if given IV too quickly |
| **Moderate NVP (*Start with one; add an additional agent if symptoms persist. Use caution because of cumulative side effects.*)** | | |
| Doxylamine/pyridoxine (Diclegis) | Combination, slow-release product containing 10 mg of pyridoxine hydrochloride and 10 mg doxylamine succinate<br>2 tablets at night<br>Maximum dose: 4 tablets/day | May cause drowsiness; anticholinergic |
| Promethazine (Phenergan) | 12.5–25 mg every 4–6 hours orally/IM/rectally | Sedation, anticholinergic effects, dry mouth, dystonic reaction; hypotension if given IV too quickly |
| Metoclopramide (Reglan) | 5–10 mg every 6–8 hours orally | FDA black box warning about agitation, anxiety, and acute dystonic reactions |
| Ondansetron (Zofran) | 4–8 mg every 6–8 hours orally or sublingual | Headache; FDA black box warning regarding QT prolongation and concern for cardiac arrhythmia |
| **If moderate NVP with dehydration, initiate:** | | |
| Non-dextrose IV fluid with multivitamins and electrolytes | | Multivitamin supplement is needed with IV fluids to prevent Wernicke's encephalopathy, which can develop secondary to thiamine deficiency |

| Treatment | Drug Dosage | Clinical Considerations |
|---|---|---|
| **Severe NVP/HG** | | |
| Maternal–fetal medicine specialist or obstetrician-gynecologist consultation | | Plan may include:<br>• NPO status<br>• IV fluid (non-dextrose, should contain multivitamins and electrolytes)<br>• IV administration of medications in the moderate NVP category<br>• IV/IM antipsychotics such as droperidol or chlorpromazine<br>• IV/oral steroids such as methylprednisolone |

Abbreviations: FDA, U.S. Food and Drug Administration; HG, hyperemesis gravidarum; IM, intramuscular; IV, intravenous; NPO, nothing by mouth; NVP, nausea and vomiting of pregnancy.

Based on King TL, Murphy PA. Evidence-based approaches to managing nausea and vomiting in early pregnancy. *J Midwifery Womens Health*. 2009;54(6):430-449; ACOG. Practice Bulletin No. 189: nausea and vomiting in pregnancy. *Obstet Gynecol*. 2018;131(1):e15-e30.

## Fetal Conditions

Today, genetic testing in the first trimester and the standard anatomy ultrasound in mid-pregnancy provide information about fetal abnormalities that could not be detected antenatally in the past. Fetal abnormalities range from relatively mild (e.g., cleft lip) to lethal (e.g., anencephaly) and are often first diagnosed in the first or early second trimester. An in-depth exploration of fetal screening can be found in the *Assessment for Genetic and Fetal Abnormalities* chapter. When these disorders are discovered, midwives often collaborate with or refer to interdisciplinary colleagues including obstetricians, MFMs, and genetic counselors.

### Fetal Growth Discrepancy

Serial measurement of fundal height is used to monitor fetal growth and as an initial screen for excessive growth or fetal growth restriction. After 20 weeks' gestation, the fundal height is expected to be within 2 cm of the weeks of pregnancy.[17] When the midwife identifies a discrepancy between fundal height and gestational weeks, a growth ultrasound should be ordered. If the pregnant person has persistent size–dates discrepancy, the standard timing of serial growth ultrasounds is every 4 weeks.

Primary factors influencing fundal height include the number of fetuses, size of fetus(es), and amount of amniotic fluid. Fundal height can also reflect extremes of body weight, especially if excess body weight is distributed to the pregnant person's abdomen. Ultrasound can easily determine the number of fetuses and amount of amniotic fluid present. This technology can also provide accurate measurements of each fetal parameter assessed (e.g., biparietal diameter, abdominal circumference). From there, an estimated fetal weight (EFW) is calculated using a formula selected from the ultrasound software menu. However, ultrasound estimates of fetal weight at term have limited accuracy, with an error rate as high as 20%.[18] This imprecision is rooted in EFW formulas' attempt to estimate three-dimensional size and density using two-dimensional measurements.

Once a fetal weight is calculated, the EFW is reported in grams or pounds and ounces and with a growth percentile. This growth percentile compares the fetus to a standard group of fetuses of the same age, in which the smallest fetus registers at less than the 1st percentile, the mid-size fetus at the 50th percentile, and the largest fetus at greater than the 99th percentile. Growth percentiles are used to guide clinical management decisions, because morbidity is increased for fetuses and newborns at the extremes of growth curves. However, the accuracy of growth percentiles is also limited—by the accuracy of the initial EFW calculation, and by population congruence between the fetus being assessed and the comparison group.[19] Many widely used growth curves (e.g., Hadlock) were not standardized in an ethnically or socioeconomically diverse population. Efforts have been made to develop population-specific fetal growth curves and growth curves reflecting diverse populations (WHO Fetal Growth Chart,[20] National Institute of Child Health and Human Development Fetal Growth Calculator[21]), but no single tool clearly outperforms all others.

### Fetal Growth: Large for Gestational Age

The intrauterine diagnosis for a fetus growing more rapidly than expected is *large for gestational age* (LGA). This describes a fetus whose estimated weight is greater than the 90th percentile for gestational age. A fetus can also receive the diagnosis of *suspected macrosomia* or *risk of macrosomia* if it is estimated to weigh more than 4000 or 4500 grams, regardless of gestational age. The research is unclear on which of these values should be used in decision making because of the limits of ultrasonography in predicting birth weight. However, a formal diagnosis of macrosomia cannot be made until newborn weight is measured after birth.

Risk factors for a fetus being LGA include gestational or pregestational diabetes, pre-pregnancy obesity, excess gestational weight gain, and multiparity. Additional risk factors for suspected macrosomia include post-term gestation and macrosomia in a prior pregnancy.[18]

A prenatal diagnosis of LGA is most clinically significant in pregnancies impacted by diabetes, because an LGA growth pattern can indicate exposure to excess glucose. A prenatal diagnosis of suspected macrosomia is clinically important because macrosomia carries increased risks for shoulder dystocia, birth trauma to either the fetus or the pregnant person, cesarean birth, and postpartum hemorrhage. In pregnancies impacted by diabetes, the risk for shoulder dystocia is particularly notable, because these fetuses develop more body fat centered in the shoulders and chest.[18]

Induction of labor is not recommended for the sole indication of LGA or suspected macrosomia. However, the provider team at birth should be thoroughly prepared for the possibility of shoulder dystocia, laceration, and postpartum hemorrhage. In addition, if the EFW is more than 4500 grams in a pregnancy impacted by diabetes (or 5000 grams in a pregnancy not impacted by diabetes), birth planning should include the option of planned cesarean birth because of the increased risk of birth complications.[18]

### Fetal Growth: Fetal Growth Restriction

Fetal growth restriction (FGR) is diagnosed when the fetus has an estimated weight or abdominal circumference less than the 10th percentile for gestational age.[22] Historically, researchers have also explored defining FGR according to fetal growth trajectory, hoping to provide a means of distinguishing fetuses that are constitutionally small but growing appropriately, from those with a pathology that impedes normal growth. However, in prospective studies this definition has not led to improved clinical outcomes. Therefore, the Society for Maternal–Fetal Medicine recommends FGR be defined by the 10th percentile cutoff.

Growth restriction is an area in which terminology continues to change. In the past, fetuses who were more than two standard deviations smaller than average were called "intrauterine growth retarded." This term was successively changed to "intrauterine growth restriction" (IUGR), and finally to the current "fetal growth restriction." The term "small for gestational age" (SGA) should not be used until after birth; it describes a newborn who is below the 10th percentile for weight for its gestational age.[23]

When FGR is related to a pathophysiologic condition, as opposed to reflecting parental genetics, perinatal morbidity and mortality are significantly increased. Pathologic conditions leading to FGR can be categorized as being related to the fetus, the placenta, or the health history of the pregnant person (Table 23-6).[24]

The presentation of FGR falls into two growth patterns identified during ultrasound: symmetrical or asymmetrical. A fetus with symmetrical growth restriction will have both its body and head smaller than expected. The most common cause of symmetrical growth restriction that occurs early in gestation and is progressively severe—that is, the discrepancy from gestational age becomes more pronounced as pregnancy continues—is congenital anomalies (including aneuploidy). Symmetrical growth restriction can also be associated with severe malnutrition of the pregnant person, low pre-pregnancy weight or no weight gain, multifetal gestation, perinatal infections, and exposure to drugs or environmental teratogens.

With asymmetrical growth restriction, the fetus's estimated weight or abdominal circumference is below the 10th percentile, but its head circumference is larger than the 10th percentile. Asymmetrical growth restriction can be caused by any condition that causes decreased placental blood flow or decreased oxygenation of the fetus. Under these conditions, blood flow (and thus oxygen) is preferentially directed to the fetal head and brain. Health conditions of the pregnant person that are associated with asymmetrical fetal growth restriction include

| Table 23-6 | Etiology of Fetal Growth Restriction | |
|---|---|---|
| **Fetus** | **Placenta** | **Health History of Pregnant Person** |
| Chromosome abnormalities<br><br>Genetic syndromes<br><br>Intrauterine infections: particularly viral<br><br>Multifetal gestation | Abnormal placental attachment to the uterus<br><br>Placental pathology (clotting)<br><br>Umbilical cord abnormalities | Extremes of age (< 18 years or ≥ 34 years)<br><br>Chronic disease impacting perfusion of the uterus and placenta (e.g., hypertension, pregestational diabetes, cardiovascular disease, renal insufficiency, sickle cell anemia, systemic lupus erythematosus)<br><br>Chronic respiratory disease (e.g., asthma)<br><br>Malnutrition<br><br>Previous history of fetal growth restriction<br><br>Substance use<br><br>Stress, depression<br><br>Teratogen exposure<br><br>Uterine malformation |

Based on Nardozza LM, Caetano ACR, Zamarian AC, et al. Fetal growth restriction: current knowledge. *Arch Gynecol Obstet.* 2017;295:1061-1077.

hypertension, renal disease, diabetes, heart disease, hemoglobinopathies, and severe asthma.

The most clinically relevant categorization of FGR is based on timing of onset, either before ("early onset") or after ("late onset") 32 weeks' gestation.[22] Early-onset FGR is strongly associated with progressive growth restriction, demonstrated by decreasing growth percentiles across successive ultrasounds. It is also associated with severe placental dysfunction, demonstrated by abnormal Doppler indices during pregnancy and abnormal placental pathology after birth. The most common etiologies of early-onset FGR are genetic anomaly in the fetus or hypertension in the pregnant person.

Late-onset FGR is associated with less severe growth restriction, lower incidence of abnormal Doppler flow during pregnancy, and fewer findings on placental pathology after birth. The etiologies of late-onset FGR are diverse. Late-onset FGR represents approximately 70% to 80% of cases of FGR.

Another clinically significant categorization of FGR is "severe" growth restriction, defined as estimated fetal weight at or less than the 3rd percentile.[22] Fetuses with severe growth restriction have an increased risk of abnormal Doppler indices and stillbirth, as well as an increased risk of neonatal morbidity and mortality, compared to fetuses with less severe FGR.

Perinatal complications for fetuses with growth restriction are generally associated with the etiology. For example, if FGR develops because chronic hypertension has decreased placental perfusion, a fetus is at risk for stillbirth, hypoxic injury, and intolerance of labor. However, if FGR develops because of severe malnutrition, risks related to placental dysfunction are fewer. Risk for neonatal complications depends on the gestational age at birth, birth weight, and etiology of growth restriction. Common neonatal complications following FGR diagnosis include hypothermia, hypoglycemia, and polycythemia.

Once fetal growth restriction is identified on ultrasound, prompt MFM consultation is required. Detailed anatomy ultrasound is recommended, if not already completed. Screening for chromosomal abnormalities and assessment for perinatal infections may also be advised. The timing for birth of a fetus with FGR and stable Doppler indices is between 37 and 39 weeks' gestation, but determination of the best time for induction of labor will depend on the underlying etiology, gestational age, pattern of fetal growth, and results of fetal surveillance tests.[22,25]

## Multifetal Gestation

Multifetal gestation refers to a pregnancy in which two or more fetuses are present. The most common type of multifetal gestation is twin pregnancy. The incidence of twin pregnancy in the United States increased 76% between 1980 and 2009,[26] largely because of the use of assisted reproductive technologies. It has since fallen slightly, with the most recent aggregate data showing a rate of 32.1 twins per 1000 total births in 2019.[27]

Twin pregnancies can develop secondary to implantation of two fertilized ova (called *dizygotic*, or fraternal twins), or when one fertilized ovum cleaves and develops into two fetuses (called *monozygotic*, or identical twins) (Figure 23-1). Monozygotic twins may be monochorionic or dichorionic, referring to whether they do or do not share a placenta, respectively. Monochorionic twins can be further categorized as monoamniotic or diamniotic, referring to whether they do or do not share an amniotic sac, respectively. Chorionicity and amnionicity in monozygotic twins depend on when, during the early gestational period, the zygote splits. It includes the following possibilities:

- Dichorionic/diamniotic: Cleavage happens by day 3 after fertilization.
- Monochorionic/diamniotic: The zygote splits between days 4 and 8.
- Monochorionic/monoamniotic: Cleavage happens between days 8 and 13.
- Monochorionic/monoamniotic conjoined twins: Partial cleavage happens after day 13.

Dizygotic twins will always be dichorionic and, therefore, diamniotic.

It is common for a pregnant person with a multifetal gestation to have an initial uterine size that is consistent with dates. The uterus starts to become larger than expected in the early second trimester. Diagnosis of multifetal gestation is confirmed via ultrasound, which will determine fetal number, fetal anatomy, and chorionicity of placentation. Chorionicity is an important part of the diagnostic ultrasound, because perinatal risks vary based on whether fetuses share a placenta and/or amniotic sac. If possible, an ultrasound examination should occur before 16 weeks for the most accurate determination of chorionicity.[28]

Once the diagnosis of multifetal gestation is made, obstetrician or MFM consultation or referral is recommended. For a twin pregnancy, a midwife may continue to serve as the primary perinatal provider, in the context of an interdisciplinary care team. For higher-order multifetal gestation, obstetrician or MFM referral is necessary. Prenatal care for all persons with multifetal gestation includes

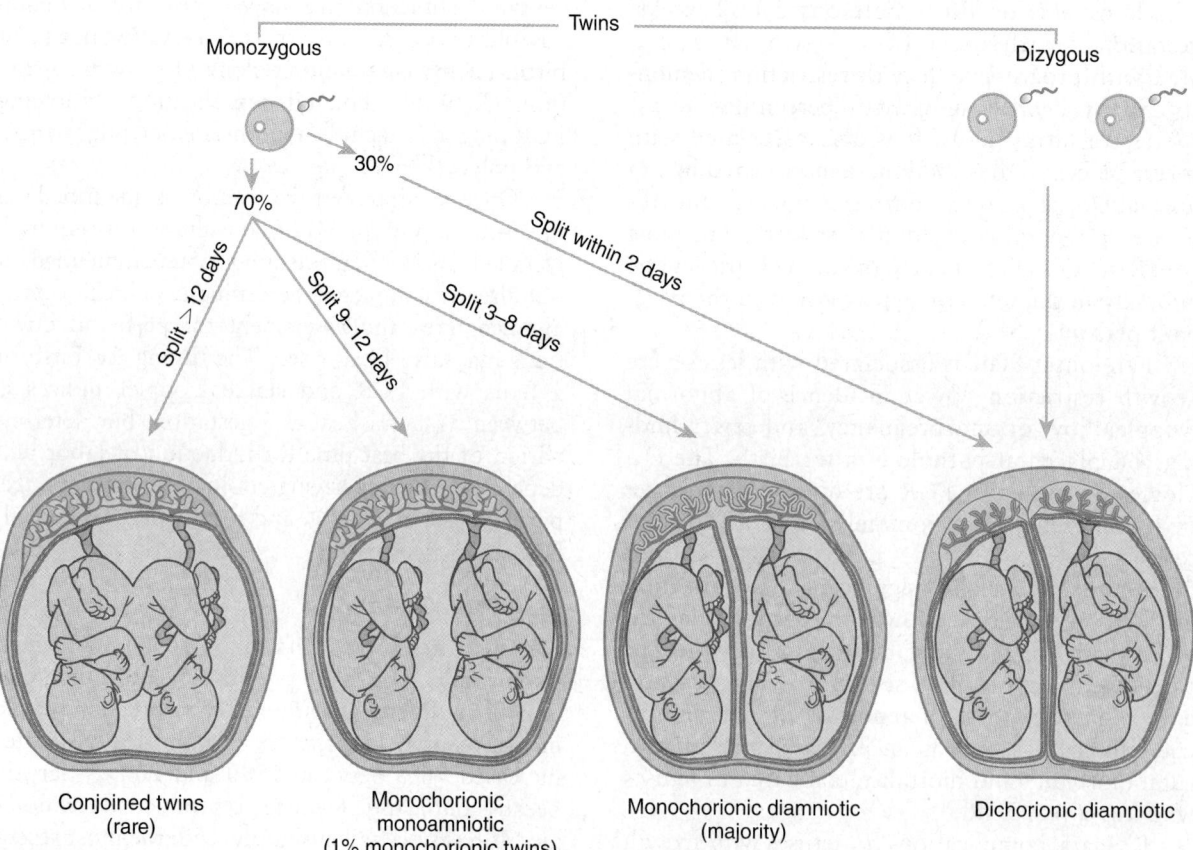

**Figure 23-1** Zygosity of twin gestations.

more frequent prenatal visits, increased surveillance for complications, serial ultrasounds to monitor fetal growth, dietary counseling, and counseling regarding changes in home and work responsibilities (to minimize pregnancy discomforts and chronic stress).

A pregnant person with a twin gestation may benefit from early nutritional counseling. For example, a person who is pregnant with twins needs more protein and calories. The recommended weight gain for a twin gestation is 40–45 pounds for a person with normal pre-pregnancy body mass index (BMI), 42–50 pounds for a person underweight prior to pregnancy, and 30–35 pounds for a person overweight prior to pregnancy. Outcomes are significantly improved when approximately half this weight is gained early in the pregnancy (24 pounds by 24 weeks).[29] A daily prenatal vitamin can provide needed micronutrients, including 30 mg of elemental iron, but the prenatal vitamin should be increased to two tablets daily in the second and third trimesters for sufficient iron supplementation. Supplementation with calcium and vitamin D is also recommended, and docosahexaenoic acid (DHA) supplementation should be considered. Folic acid supplementation is recommended at 1 mg daily.[29]

Multifetal growth and development are monitored with ultrasound examinations that are performed every 3 to 4 weeks from 20 weeks' gestation until term. Discordant growth among the fetuses or growth restriction in any individual fetus requires urgent MFM evaluation. One of the major concerns associated with discordant growth is the risk of twin-to-twin transfusion syndrome (TTTS), a complication associated with monochorionic placentation. This can also impact higher-order multifetal gestations. TTTS occurs when abnormal blood vessels form in the single placenta, such that blood returning to the placenta from one fetus flows directly into the placental vessels of the other fetus, without an opportunity for nutrient/gas exchange with the pregnant person. This results in one twin receiving an excess of blood volume (recipient) and the other twin having too little blood volume (donor). The donor twin may become significantly anemic and growth restricted, and frequently develops oligohydramnios. The recipient twin may develop polycythemia, as well as volume overload leading to cardiomegaly and cardiac failure. The recipient twin also may develop polyhydramnios. The development of discordant growth in monochorionic twins, with oligohydramnios in one twin and polyhydramnios in the other, is diagnostic for TTTS. Management of TTTS requires transfer of care to an MFM, with strategies ranging from monitoring (for mild cases) to laser ablation of anastomosing vessels (for moderate or severe cases).

For all persons with multifetal gestations, major fetal risks include preterm birth and fetal growth restriction. Complications for the pregnant person may include placenta previa, gestational diabetes, preeclampsia, malpresentation, and dysfunctional labor.

Prevention of preterm labor is a major priority in caring for a person with multifetal gestation. Lifestyle modifications such as smoking cessation and adjusting nutrition to meet weight gain milestones are evidence-based interventions for decreasing the risk of preterm birth in multifetal gestation.[29] Management may also include limiting activity and increasing daily rest periods. However, strict bedrest and pelvic rest are not effective means of preventing preterm labor in multifetal gestations. Likewise, prophylactic cerclage and progesterone therapy are not effective in preventing preterm birth in multiple gestations.[28]

Careful attention to signs of hypertension, preeclampsia, and gestational diabetes is especially important for a person with multifetal gestation, and development of these signs warrants early assessment. Medical complications for the pregnant person may become a medical indication for preterm birth, in addition to posing risks associated with the complication alone.

Plans should be made for an obstetrician or MFM physician to be present at the birth, and the mode of birth will depend on the number and position of fetuses, their chorionicity, and clinician experience. The most common presentation of twins at term is vertex/vertex. Vaginal birth is possible with this presentation, and in many settings a midwife–obstetrician team attends the birth. The next most common presentation of twins is a first twin presenting breech and a second twin presenting either vertex or breech. Breech/vertex presentation creates the risk of fetal heads becoming "locked," when the chin of one twin hooks under the chin of the other. Therefore, a cesarean birth is recommended for cases in which a first twin presents breech. The third most common presentation of twins is vertex/breech. Vaginal birth is possible with this presentation, depending on the breech birth skills of the obstetrician. It is also possible for a midwife–obstetrician team to attend this type of birth.

## Fetal Malpresentations at Term

The three possible fetal presentations, as reviewed in the *Anatomy and Physiology of Pregnancy* chapter, are cephalic, breech, and shoulder. Subcategories of cephalic presentation include face, brow, and occiput; the last is further categorized as occiput anterior, occiput transverse, or occiput posterior positioning. The breech presentation can present as a complete breech, frank breech, or footling breech.

### Cephalic Malpresentations

Cephalic malpresentations are diagnosed during labor and, therefore, are reviewed in more detail in the *Complications During Labor and Birth* chapter. Fetuses that are in a brow or face presentation usually convert to an occiput presentation during labor and birth, but the fetus may be born in one of these positions if the fetus is very small. Risk factors for brow and face presentation include prematurity, grand multiparity, polyhydramnios, multiple nuchal cords, and congenital anomalies such as anencephaly or hydrocephalus.

### Breech Presentation

By 35 to 36 weeks' gestation, the majority of fetuses will spontaneously settle into a cephalic presentation. In approximately 3% to 4% of pregnancies, however, at term the fetus will be in a breech presentation with the buttocks or feet presenting.[30] Three types of breech presentation are possible: frank, complete, or footling. In a *frank* breech presentation, the hips are flexed and the knees extended, with the infant's feet near the head. The buttocks (breech) are presenting at the pelvic inlet. A *complete* breech is similar, with the buttocks as the presenting part in the pelvis. The lower knees are flexed, however, and the infant is in a crossed-legged position. If one or both feet are extended down below the buttocks, this is referred to as a single or double *footling* breech. When assessing the position of a fetus in a breech presentation, the fetal sacrum is used as the point of reference—for example, *left sacrum anterior (LSA)* (Figure 23-2).

Prematurity, multifetal gestation, multiparity with lax uterine tone, polyhydramnios or oligohydramnios, previous breech presentation, and placenta previa have all been associated with an increased risk of breech presentation. In addition, uterine anomalies such as a bicornuate uterus or the presence of large fibroids in the lower uterine segment may impede a normal vertex presentation.

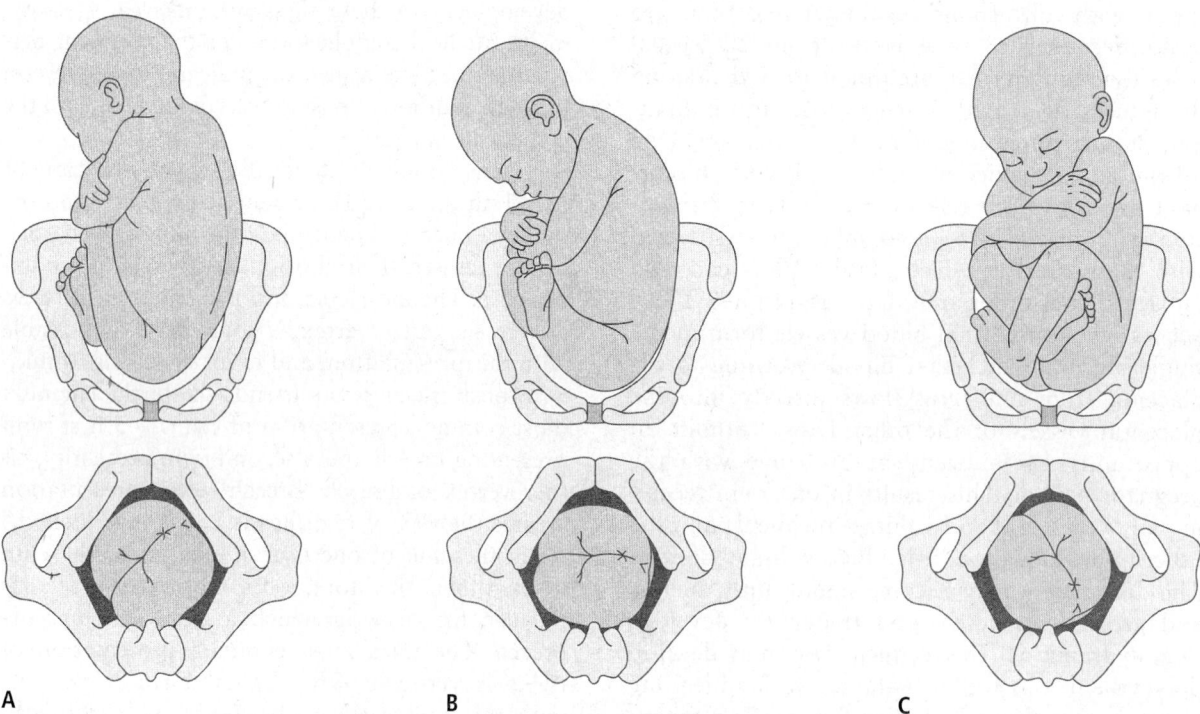

A                        B                        C

**Figure 23-2** Breech positions. **A.** Left sacrum anterior. **B.** Left sacrum transverse. **C.** Left sacrum posterior.

Breech presentation is also associated with an increased incidence of fetal anomalies such as hydrocephaly or anencephaly.[30]

A breech presentation is often identified during a prenatal visit using Leopold's maneuvers when the firm ballotable vertex is palpated in the upper fundal region. The pregnant person may report feeling increased movement in the lower pelvic area, and the fetal heart tones may be found in the upper abdomen. Prior to 35 weeks' gestation, this finding is normal but should be noted in the prenatal chart, especially if the pregnant person has any of the known predisposing risk factors. Approximately 10% of breech fetuses will spontaneously revert to vertex presentation after 36 weeks' gestation.[31]

Vaginal birth of a fetus in a breech position is associated with increased risks for perinatal morbidity and mortality. Although the risk of morbidity and mortality from planned vaginal breech birth remains a topic of debate, many health systems are not prepared to assist with planned vaginal breech birth. If a breech presentation is diagnosed after 35 weeks' gestation but before the onset of labor, the midwife should consult with a physician to determine whether the pregnant person is a candidate for an external cephalic version (ECV). During this procedure, external pressure is manually exerted on the person's abdomen to physically rotate the fetus to a vertex presentation. ECV is successful in approximately 58% of cases.[32] Factors that decrease the success of ECV include oligohydramnios, anterior placenta, breech engaged in the pelvis, fetal back located posteriorly ("back down"), and obesity in the pregnant person. ECV should not be performed if the pregnant person has any contraindication to vaginal birth (e.g., placenta previa) or if any of the following conditions are present: ruptured membranes, fetal or uterine anomalies, nonreassuring fetal heart rate patterns, hyperextended fetal head, placental abruption, or multifetal gestation.[32]

ECV is performed only in a hospital setting, at or after 37 weeks' gestation.[32] A prerequisite is a reassuring fetal heart rate assessment. After this assessment, the pregnant person is typically given a dose of subcutaneous terbutaline to induce uterine relaxation before the procedure is attempted. ECV is done under direct ultrasound guidance with continuous monitoring of the fetal heart rate (by an assistant). Because pregnant people can experience considerable discomfort during this procedure,

ECV can be attempted with intravenous analgesia or epidural or spinal anesthesia, and some evidence indicates that anesthesia improves the likelihood of success.[32] The most common fetal side effect of ECV is a transient nonreassuring fetal heart rate pattern, such as a prolonged deceleration. In rare circumstances, ECV has been reported to cause vaginal bleeding, placental abruption, fetal compromise, fracture of fetal limbs, and fetal death.[32] An emergency cesarean may be required if fetal compromise is noted. Midwives often assist during ECV by providing ultrasound guidance during the procedure and/or offering emotional support and comfort to the pregnant person. After the procedure, fetal heart rate and contraction monitoring should continue for at least 1 hour depending on institutional policies.

Various position change exercises by the pregnant person have been proposed as means to turn breech presentations to vertex (e.g., resting with hips elevated and knee–chest positions). However, research has not shown these methods to be successful.[33] Also proposed is the acupuncture process of moxibustion, for which evidence in scientific literature is positive but limited.[34] A person with persistent breech presentation after 37 weeks' gestation needs referral to an obstetrician or MFM for birth planning (either cesarean birth or planned vaginal breech birth). The approach to care when breech presentation is diagnosed during labor is reviewed in more detail in the *Complications During Labor and Birth* chapter.

## Umbilical Cord, Placental, and Amniotic Fluid Abnormalities

### Umbilical Cord Abnormalities

Umbilical cord variations include unusual insertions and single umbilical artery.

### *Umbilical Cord Insertion*

The umbilical cord is normally inserted centrally on the fetal side of the placenta. *Marginal insertion*, also called *battledore placenta*, refers to insertion of the umbilical cord near the edge of the placental mass. Fewer than 10% of placentas exhibit a marginal insertion. This morphologic variation is not associated with adverse effects.[35]

In *velamentous cord insertion*, the cord inserts into the amniotic membrane some distance from the placental tissue, leaving a span of vessels that traverse the membrane before being integrated into the placenta. These vessels traversing the membrane are not protected with Wharton's jelly. Prenatal ultrasound may or may not identify a velamentous cord insertion; indeed, this diagnosis is often made at birth. Risk factors for a velamentous cord insertion and vasa previa include placenta previa, multifetal gestation, history of assisted reproductive technology, obesity, and smoking.[36]

Any umbilical cord vessels that are not protected within the structure of the umbilical cord are vulnerable to rupture and compression during labor and birth.[36] Rupture of the velamentous vessels can cause rapid fetal exsanguination. Velamentous cord insertion is also associated with an increased risk for preterm birth, fetal growth restriction, and perinatal morbidity/mortality, although the absolute risk for these events is low. Obstetrician or MFM consultation is indicated when a velamentous cord insertion is diagnosed prenatally. Additional fetal growth ultrasounds or antepartum surveillance may be recommended. A note should be made in the person's health record where the intrapartum care providers can see it, because delivery of the placenta needs to be performed gently to avoid tearing the cord off.

If the velamentous vessels cross the internal cervical os, the condition is referred to as *vasa previa*. Labor and cervical dilation in the presence of vasa previa pose a risk for life-threatening fetal hemorrhage, due to the likelihood of rupturing the fetal vessels crossing the internal cervical os. Pregnant people with a vasa previa require obstetrician management, and they may need care in a Level III or Level IV facility. Recommendations for care include weekly fetal surveillance, administration of corticosteroids to stimulate fetal lung maturity, and planned preterm cesarean birth to reduce the risk of spontaneous onset of labor. Cesarean birth is typically scheduled for 34 to 36 weeks' gestation.[25]

### Single Umbilical Artery

The umbilical cord usually has two arteries and one larger vein. Occasionally, a fetus will have only one artery and one vein. The developmental mechanism in such a case is either agenesis or atrophy of one of the arteries. The prevalence of one umbilical artery is less than 1%. However, the prevalence is higher in fetuses with congenital anomalies (excluding aneuploidy) and in multifetal gestation. When this finding is noted, a detailed ultrasound

may be recommended to assess for other anatomic abnormalities—in particular, cardiac, gastrointestinal, and renal abnormalities.

If the fetus does not have other abnormalities, a single umbilical artery is associated with a slightly increased risk of FGR and stillbirth. Other complications such as preeclampsia and preterm birth have been reported, but studies are generally inconclusive regarding these outcomes. Current recommendations include antenatal fetal surveillance from 36 weeks forward. Most patients with this isolated finding can be reassured that there are no additional risks for the fetus.

## Placental Abnormalities

Placental abnormalities fall into three categories: (1) abnormal placental structure, (2) abnormal placement within the uterus, and (3) abnormal attachment.

### Circumvallate Placenta

Abnormal placental configurations are shown in Figure 23-3. A circumvallate placenta is a placenta with a double layer of membrane (chorion and amnion) that circles the edge of the placenta and appears as a whitish ring. The fetal vessels do not extend beyond this ring, but extrachorionic placental tissue does. This results in a decreased area of the placenta available for perfusion. The etiology of circumvallate placenta is not well known. Retrospective studies have found an association between

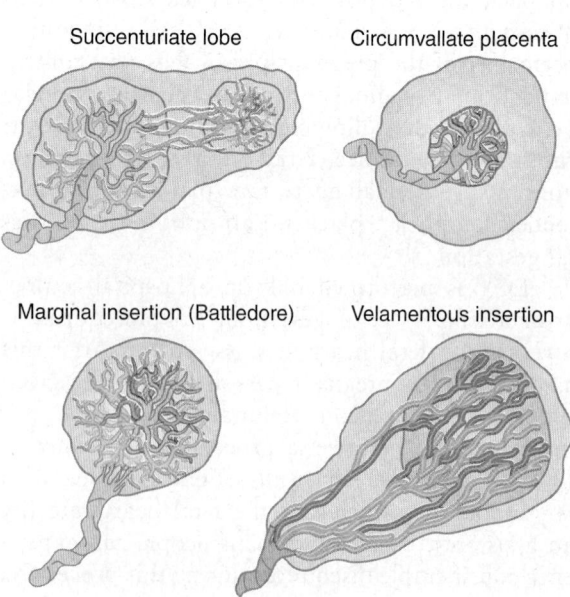

**Figure 23-3** Abnormal placental configurations.

circumvallate placenta and increased incidence of second trimester bleeding, preterm birth, and preterm premature rupture of membranes.[37]

A circummarginate placenta has a ring of membrane that is flat and close to the edge of the placental disc. Circummarginate placentas are not associated with adverse outcomes.

### Succenturiate Lobe

A placenta with a succenturiate lobe has an accessory lobe or cotyledon separate from the primary placental mass. The succenturiate lobe, which is connected to the primary mass by a fetal artery and vein, functions normally. Succenturiate lobes are often clinically insignificant but may be associated with placental abnormalities such as velamentous cord insertion. The most common problem associated with this placental variation is retention of the succenturiate lobe after birth. This is one of the reasons why the midwife should examine the placental edge after birth to look for torn vessels that extend beyond the placental margin.

### Placenta Previa

When the placenta implants over the internal cervical os, the condition is referred to as placenta previa. Approximately 2% of pregnancies will have placenta previa identified during the second trimester anatomy ultrasound.[36,38] However, 90% of these placentas will no longer be located over the cervical os later in pregnancy, as the placenta grows toward the fundus. At the time of birth, placenta previa has an incidence of approximately 1 in 200 births.

Historically, placenta previa was classified as complete, partial, marginal, or low-lying, based on abdominal ultrasound assessment of the degree to which the internal cervical os was covered. However, the availability of transvaginal ultrasound has allowed for a high degree of accuracy in measuring the distance between the placental edge and the cervix. This accuracy gave rise to a change in terminology (Figure 23-4), in which all placentas covering the os to any degree are now called *placenta previa*, with the distance between the placental edge and internal cervical os being noted in the ultrasound report. Placentas close to but not covering the os (within 2 cm) are referred to as *low-lying placenta*.[38]

The primary risk factor for development of placenta previa is previous uterine scarring secondary to cesarean birth or uterine surgery.[39] This risk increases with additional cesarean births. Other risk

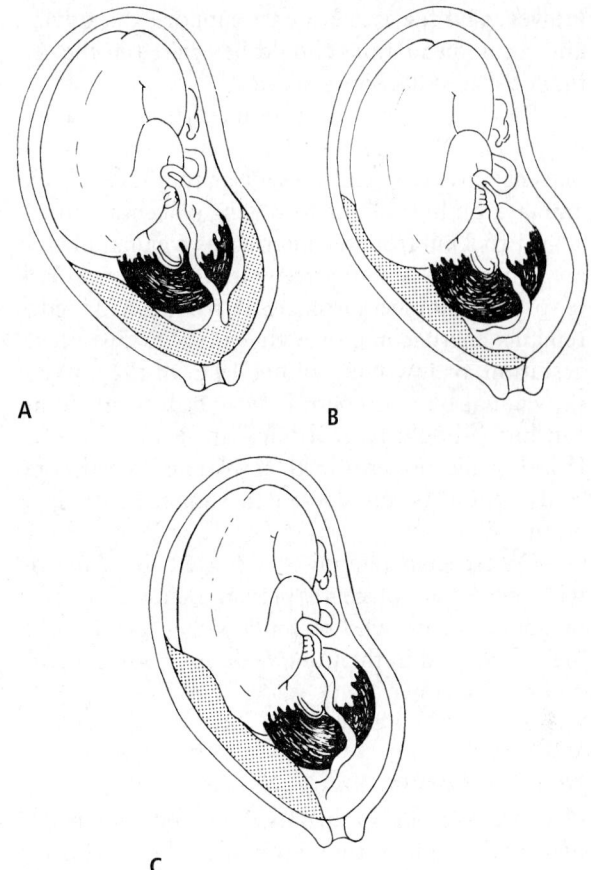

**Figure 23-4 A.** and **B.** Placenta previa. **C.** Low-lying placenta.

factors include age, parity, multifetal gestation, male fetus, smoking, cocaine usage, multiple prior pregnancy terminations, and use of assisted reproductive technology.[38]

The primary complication associated with placenta previa is hemorrhage from the uterus. When the cervix starts to remodel in preparation for labor and birth (i.e., effacement and dilation), the portion of the placenta resting over the cervix separates, which causes bleeding. The gestational age at which vaginal bleeding first occurs is unpredictable. In the majority of cases, the initial bleeding episode presents as a painless gush of blood prior to 36 weeks' gestation. The amount of bleeding is unpredictable.

Once placenta previa is diagnosed, pregnant persons are instructed to call or come to the hospital if vaginal bleeding occurs. There is no further evidence-based counseling for persons with placenta previa. By convention, many midwives and physicians advise avoidance of sexual activity with orgasm or vaginal penetration, so as to avoid uterine contractions or direct trauma to the cervix.

However, no research evidence supports this advice, and recommendations should be offered in the setting of shared decision making.[40,41]

Repeat placenta location ultrasound is recommended at 32 weeks, and then again at 36 weeks (if placenta previa is still present at the 32-week examination). In case of a low-lying placenta with an edge 1 to 2 cm from the internal os, vaginal birth is an option but is associated with an increased risk of postpartum hemorrhage. If the placenta edge remains encroaching over the cervix at 36 weeks' gestation, or low-lying within 1 cm of the internal os, vaginal birth is contraindicated. Instead, cesarean birth should be scheduled at 36 to 37 weeks. If iatrogenic preterm birth is planned, corticosteroids should be considered to enhance fetal lung maturity.

Obstetrician referral is indicated for a person with persistent placenta previa. Acute care of a pregnant person who presents with vaginal bleeding is reviewed in the *Complications During Labor and Birth* chapter.

### Placenta Accreta

Placenta accreta spectrum is an abnormality of placental implantation in which the anchoring placental villi attach to the myometrium instead of to the decidua in the endometrium. Historically, placenta accreta spectrum was subdivided based on how deeply placental villi were anchored. *Placenta accreta* was diagnosed when the

cytotrophoblasts attached to the myometrium, *placenta increta* was diagnosed when the cytotrophoblasts invaded the myometrium, and *placenta percreta* was diagnosed when the cytotrophoblasts extended through the myometrium and serosa, attaching to adjacent pelvic organs (Figure 23-5).[39] In current practice, the term "placenta accreta spectrum" is used for any degree of placenta accreta, to reinforce the understanding that the level of perinatal care needed for management is similar for all presentations.

Placenta accreta occurs when the placenta implants over an area of the uterus that is scarred or damaged. The incidence of placenta accreta has increased dramatically as a result of the rising rate of cesarean birth, as well as uterine procedures associated with assisted reproductive technology (such as myomectomy or resection of a uterine septum). This condition is also more common in people who have placenta previa. Among people with a history of one prior cesarean birth who develop placenta previa in a subsequent pregnancy, 3% will develop placenta accreta. The incidence of accreta increases to 11% in people with placenta previa who had two prior cesarean births, and to 40% in people with placenta previa who had three prior cesarean births.[39]

Hemorrhage at birth is anticipated in all cases of placenta accreta, and most cases require hysterectomy to control the extent of bleeding. With advance planning and specialty center care, fertility-preserving surgical birth may be an

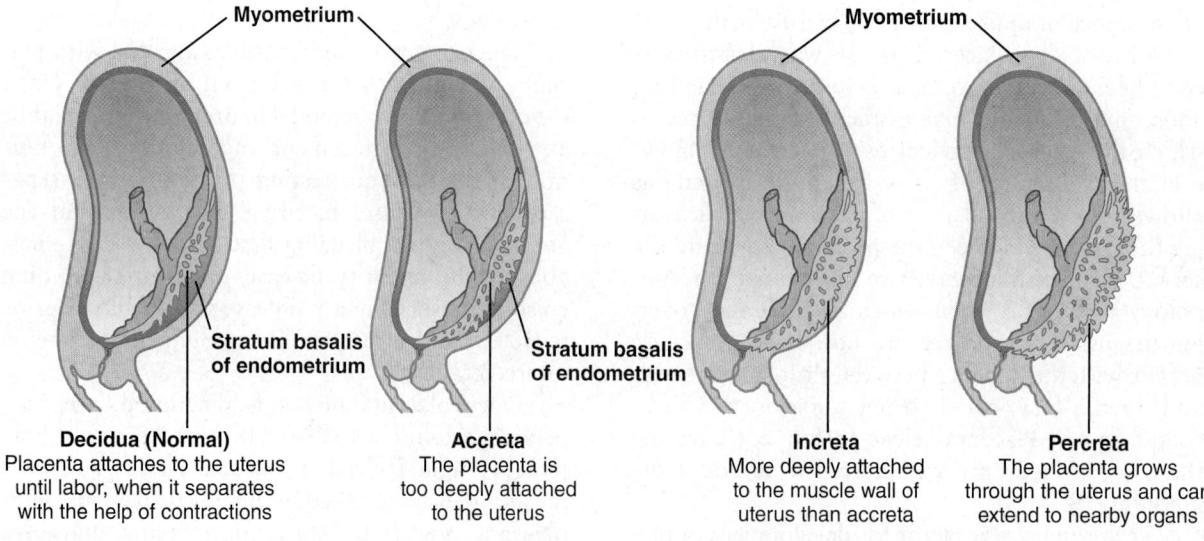

**Decidua (Normal)**
Placenta attaches to the uterus until labor, when it separates with the help of contractions

**Accreta**
The placenta is too deeply attached to the uterus

**Increta**
More deeply attached to the muscle wall of uterus than accreta

**Percreta**
The placenta grows through the uterus and can extend to nearby organs

**Figure 23-5** Placenta accreta spectrum.

option.[40] However, in such cases families need to be prepared for the possibility of cesarean hysterectomy as a life-saving measure for the pregnant person. Midwives can assist families with emotional processing related to this anticipated high-risk birth experience.

Although placenta accreta has characteristic findings on ultrasound, the condition is not always detected during routine ultrasound examination. The role of a midwife is to be alert to risk factors, such as an anterior low-lying placenta in a person who had a previous cesarean birth. Consultation with an MFM is indicated in such cases. Specialized ultrasound and magnetic resonance imaging (MRI) can aid in determining the diagnosis. If placenta accreta is diagnosed, planned cesarean birth in a Level III or Level IV center is needed.[40] Massive transfusion protocols and subspecialist resources are essential to manage this serious and often life-threatening complication of pregnancy.

## Abnormal Amniotic Fluid Volume

Amniotic fluid is primarily composed of fetal urine and lung fluid. The amount of amniotic fluid increases throughout pregnancy until it reaches approximately 1000 milliliters by the beginning of the third trimester; it then gradually decreases to approximately 800 milliliters at term. Amniotic fluid volume can be measured on ultrasound in two ways: by reporting the single deepest vertical pocket of amniotic fluid (DVP) or by calculating the amniotic fluid index (AFI). The AFI is the sum of the deepest vertical pocket in each quadrant of the uterus. Using DVP to diagnose abnormal volume is associated with fewer interventions without an increase in poor pregnancy outcomes. Therefore, DVP is the preferred method for assessing amniotic fluid volume.[42,43]

### *Polyhydramnios*

Polyhydramnios is an excessive amount of amniotic fluid. It is defined as a DVP $\geq$ 8 cm, or an AFI $\geq$ 24 cm or more. This condition is idiopathic in 50% to 60% of cases and most likely to become evident in the third trimester. Several conditions are associated with a higher incidence of polyhydramnios, including fetal structural anomalies, multifetal gestation (especially monozygotic twins with TTTS), diabetes, fetal infection, and fetal

chromosomal abnormalities. Severe polyhydramnios (AFI $\geq$ 35 cm) is more likely to be associated with fetal structural anomalies, such as tracheoesophageal fistula, anencephaly, and meningomyelocele, whereas milder forms are more likely to be idiopathic.[43] Complications of polyhydramnios include preterm labor secondary to uterine distention, premature rupture of membranes, malpresentation of the fetus, umbilical cord prolapse, abruptio placenta, dysfunctional labor, and postpartum hemorrhage.

Polyhydramnios is initially suspected when uterine enlargement, approximated by fundal height, is larger than expected for the gestational age. In such a case, it may be difficult to auscultate fetal heart tones and to palpate the fetal outline and fetal parts. The fetus may have an unstable lie, and a change in lie may be detected during Leopold's maneuvers. In severe cases of polyhydramnios, the pregnant person may experience dyspnea, heartburn, nausea and vomiting, pressure in the abdomen and back, and edema in the vulva or lower extremities.

An ultrasound will confirm the diagnosis and identify any coexisting fetal or placental abnormalities. At this point, consultation with an MFM or obstetrician is needed. Depending on the degree of polyhydramnios and other findings, additional laboratory testing may include rescreening for gestational diabetes, antibody titers to detect isoimmunization, or TORCH (toxoplasmosis, other, rubella, cytomegalovirus, and herpes) titers to assess for infection. Of note, polyhydramnios alone is not an indication for aneuploidy screening by karyotyping.[44] Likewise, uncomplicated polyhydramnios is not an indication for scheduled birth. However, the diagnosis may warrant increased fetal surveillance and attention to difficulties of dyspnea and edema for the pregnant person. On rare occasions, the polyhydramnios is so severe that fluid must be removed via controlled amniocentesis to relieve a pregnant person's respiratory distress.

### *Oligohydramnios*

Oligohydramnios is an abnormally low volume of amniotic fluid, adjusted for the gestational age of the pregnancy. This condition may be suspected on clinical examination but needs to be confirmed via ultrasound. Clinical signs include a fetus that is easily outlined during abdominal palpation, a fetus that is not ballotable, and lagging fundal height measurements. The diagnosis of oligohydramnios is made when the DVP in the third trimester is less than 2 cm, or the AFI is less than 5 cm.

A number of fetal conditions are associated with oligohydramnios, including congenital anomalies (e.g., renal agenesis, Potter's syndrome), viral diseases, fetal growth restriction, uteroplacental insufficiency, preterm prelabor rupture of membranes, response to indomethacin as a tocolytic, and post-term pregnancy.

Oligohydramnios can develop at any time in pregnancy, but its clinical significance in the first trimester is not clear. The fetus normally begins to urinate and swallow fluid in the second trimester, so disorders of the fetal renal/urinary system become apparent at this time. If oligohydramnios is present between 17 and 26 weeks' gestation, the fetus is at risk for developing hypoplastic lungs. In this condition, the fetal lungs do not develop to full size because the fetus is unable to breathe amniotic fluid, a process that normally causes chest expansion and growth.

Oligohydramnios that appears in the third trimester, but preterm, is often associated with uteroplacental insufficiency or preterm prelabor rupture of membranes. Oligohydramnios that appears at full term or late term is often associated with increased resistance in the aging placenta. Management differs depending on the cause and the gestational age, so evaluation of third trimester oligohydramnios focuses on physical, ultrasound, and laboratory examinations to determine the underlying etiology. Physician consultation is also indicated to establish a plan of care.

Oligohydramnios without ruptured membranes and in the absence of other complications is an indication for frequent surveillance of fetal well-being, including fetal movement counts, nonstress tests or biophysical profile (BPP), and possibly umbilical Doppler studies. The timing of birth depends on the evidence for fetal well-being during fetal surveillance. When uncomplicated oligohydramnios occurs in a late-term pregnancy, and tests of fetal well-being are reassuring, evidence supports induction over expectant management.[45]

## Uterine Abnormalities

Uterine anomalies (e.g., bicornuate uterus, septate uterus, uterus didelphys) are congenital variants of the female reproductive tract reviewed in the *Anatomy and Physiology of the Reproductive System* chapter. Uterine anomalies are more common among people seeking fertility care or perinatal care. However, there is not a reliable estimate of the prevalence of uterine anomalies in the general population.[46]

Only some uterine anomalies (e.g. septate, unicornuate) are associated with infertility. Once pregnancy is achieved, however, all uterine anomalies are associated with one or more pregnancy complications. These complications range from miscarriage to fetal growth restriction, preterm labor/birth, malposition, and placental abruption.[46] There is also an increased risk of uterine rupture if the pregnancy occurs in the rare anomaly of rudimentary uterine horn. A rudimentary horn has an underdeveloped myometrium that limits the horn's ability to expand, and it may rupture either catastrophically or silently. Catastrophic rupture has symptoms similar to those of ruptured tubal pregnancy; silent rupture can lead to a secondary abdominal pregnancy.

Uterine anomalies may be identified for the first time during pregnancy, such as during a first trimester ultrasound, or on clinical examination when the uterine outline is displaced to one side of the abdomen. Depending on the gestational age of the fetus and the type of anomaly suspected, three-dimensional ultrasound or MRI may be needed to confirm the diagnosis.

Management of pregnancy in a person with a uterine anomaly requires consultation with an MFM or obstetrician. Depending on the anomaly and the related risk for preterm labor or growth restriction, the plan of care may include cervical length screening or growth ultrasounds. Timing of birth will depend on indicators of fetal well-being. Mode of birth will depend on fetal position. Midwives can continue to act as the primary antepartum care provider, in consultation with a specialist physician.

## Preterm Birth

Preterm birth is defined as birth that occurs before 37 weeks and 0 days gestational age. In the United States, approximately 10% of births occur preterm.[47] Table 23-7 identifies subcategories of preterm gestation based on a combination of the definitions used by the World Health Organization[48] and the National Institute of Child Health and Human Development.[49]

Preterm birth in the United States is more common in non-Hispanic Black persons, compared

| Table 23-7 | Subcategories for Preterm Birth |
|---|---|
| **Category** | **Definition** |
| Periviable gestation | 20 0/7–25 6/7 gestational weeks |
| Extremely preterm | 26 0/7–27 6/7 gestational weeks |
| Very preterm | 28 0/7–31 6/7 gestational weeks |
| Moderate preterm | 32 0/7–33 6/7 gestational weeks |
| Late preterm | 34 0/7–36 6/7 gestational weeks |

to persons from all other racial and ethnic backgrounds.[50] This racial disparity persists even after accounting for risk factors such as smoking, socioeconomic status, and educational level. Although the reasons for the racial disparity in the incidence of preterm birth are not fully understood, cumulative lifetime stress and exposure to racism are implicated.

Globally, preterm birth is the leading cause of neonatal death, accounting for 35% of all neonatal deaths. In the United States, the combination of preterm birth and low birth weight is the leading cause of neonatal death (25%),[51] and the second most common cause of infant death.[52]

For infants who survive preterm birth, short-term adverse outcomes include respiratory distress syndrome, intraventricular hemorrhage, and infection. Long-term adverse outcomes include neurodevelopmental disabilities, altered pulmonary function, and increased risk for adult metabolic and cardiovascular disorders. Morbidity and mortality rates are inversely related to the gestational age at the time of birth. Infants born in the periviable period have the lowest survival rate and highest incidence of long-term morbidities, whereas infants born in the moderate or late preterm gestational age categories have a high chance of surviving without long-term complications.

This chapter presents an overview of preterm birth, including pathophysiology, risk factors, prenatal care for a person with a history of spontaneous preterm birth, and diagnostic criteria for suspected preterm labor. Some of the initial evaluation for preterm labor can be completed in the outpatient setting, but the definitive diagnosis requires assessment in a hospital setting. For this reason, steps involved in the thorough evaluation of a pregnant person with suspected preterm labor are presented in the *Complications During Labor and Birth* chapter.

## Pathophysiology of Spontaneous Preterm Birth

Spontaneous preterm birth can occur following painless dilation and effacement of the cervix, early onset of labor contractions leading to dilation of the cervix, or early rupture of membranes that eventually leads to labor contractions and dilation of the cervix. Painless dilation and effacement can be caused by structural variations in the cervix (discussed in the Cervical Insufficiency section later in this chapter), or by biochemical changes similar to those causing preterm labor or early rupture of membranes. At least five discrete mechanisms have been identified that initiate premature changes in the uterus, cervix, and membranes:

- *Premature activation of the hypothalamic–pituitary–adrenal (HPA) axis.* Physical or psychological stress activates the pregnant person's HPA axis and leads to subsequent release of high levels of corticotropin-releasing hormone (CRH), which in turn increases prostaglandin production and directly stimulates the uterus. Preterm activation of the pregnant person's HPA axis can be caused by emotional-mental stress (depression, post-traumatic stress disorder, anxiety) or physical stress.[53,54] Activation of the fetal HPA axis contributes to release of CRH at term. Preterm activation of the fetal HPA axis can occur secondary to genetic factors, an inhospitable uterine environment, or inflammation (e.g., intra-amniotic infection).[55]

- *Inflammation/infection.* Microorganisms in the genital tract may cause inflammation at the choriodecidual interface, which in turn stimulates contractions.[55]

- *Decidual hemorrhage (placenta abruption or subchorionic hemorrhage).* Localized uteroplacental ischemia can cause necrosis of the decidua. This necrosis is a type of oxidative stress that releases thrombin. Thrombin, in turn, stimulates uterine contractility.[56]

- *Overdistention of the uterus (e.g., polyhydramnios, multifetal gestation).* Overstretching of the myometrium induces formation of gap junctions and upregulation of oxytocin receptors.

- *Genetics.* Genetic factors have long been suspected as an etiology in preterm birth, but the relationship is an area of ongoing research. Four genetic loci have been associated with length of gestation, and variants in three of those loci are associated with preterm birth: *EBF1, EEFSEC*, and *AGTR2*.[57]

| Table 23-8 | Risk Factors for Spontaneous Preterm Birth | |
|---|---|---|
| **Demographic and Related Factors of the Pregnant Person** | | **Fetal Factors** |
| Age < 17 years or > 35 years | | Hydrops fetalis |
| Chronic stress | | Congenital anomalies |
| Exposure to systemic racism[a] | | Fetal growth restriction |
| Genetic variants | | Infection |
| Low pre-pregnancy body weight (BMI < 19.8) | | |
| Low socioeconomic status | | |
| **Medical and Reproductive History of the Pregnant Person** | | **Current Pregnancy Factors** |
| Alloimmunization | | Hypertensive disorders of pregnancy |
| Cervical insufficiency | | Infections during pregnancy |
| Depression and associated disorders (anxiety, post-traumatic stress disorder) | | Intrauterine infection |
| Müllerian tract abnormalities | | Multifetal gestation |
| Pregnant person born preterm | | Placenta previa |
| Previous preterm birth | | Polyhydramnios |
| Prior cervical surgery (cone, dilation and curettage) | | Pyelonephritis |
| Short interpregnancy interval (< 18 months) | | Short cervical length measured on TVUS |
| Substance use (cocaine, methamphetamine, opioids, tobacco) | | Vaginal bleeding during more than one trimester |
| **Factors with Conflicting Evidence Regarding Risk for Preterm Birth** | | **Preventable Iatrogenic Factors** |
| Asymptomatic bacteriuria, cystitis | | Elective induction of labor before term |
| Genital tract infections | | Unknown gestational age |
| Periodontal disease | | |
| Vaginal bleeding | | |

[a] People of Black race living in the United States for multiple generations have increased risk of preterm birth, compared to people of Black race living in continental Africa, England, Canada, the Caribbean, or other parts of the African diaspora.[48,62,63] See the discussion in American College of Obstetricians and Gynecologists. Practice Bulletin No. 234: prediction and prevention of spontaneous preterm birth. *Obstet Gynecol.* 2021;138(2):e65-e90.[64]

Abbreviations: BMI, body mass index; TVUS, transvaginal ultrasound.

Based on Adams MM, Elam-Evans LD, Wilson HG, Gilbertz DA. Rates and factors associated with recurrence of preterm delivery. *JAMA.* 2000;283:1591-1996; Muglia LJ. The enigma of spontaneous preterm birth. *N Engl J Med.* 2010;362:529-535; Zhang G, Feenstra B, Bacelis J, et al. Genetic associations with gestational duration and spontaneous preterm birth. *N Engl J Med.* 2017; 377(12):1156-1167.

## Risk Factors for Preterm Birth

Known risk factors are listed in Table 23-8.[48,57–59] However, approximately 50% of pregnant people who give birth prematurely do not have an identified risk factor for preterm birth[60]; with a few exceptions, risk factors do not reliably predict preterm birth. The most significant risk factor for preterm birth is a history of preterm birth. Persons with such a history are significantly more likely to experience a subsequent preterm birth.[58,61]

## Midwifery Strategies for Prevention of Preterm Birth

A holistic approach to prevention of preterm birth requires attention to modifiable risk factors, as well as the mechanisms involved in each of the possible causes of preterm birth (iatrogenic, short cervix, cervical insufficiency, preterm labor, or premature prelabor rupture of membranes [PPROM]). Preconception care is an opportunity to work toward general health goals such as smoking cessation, stabilization of blood pressure within the normal range, and optimizing weight and nutrition status. It is also an opportunity to support mental health and wellness, and to help patients facing socioeconomic stressors connect with community resources. For more discussion, see the *Preconception Care* appendix and *Health Promotion Across the Lifespan* chapter.

Once the person is pregnant, the midwife's discussion of modifiable risk factors can shift slightly. A conversation about weight should focus on access to nutrition, safe exercise opportunities, and weight gain goals for pregnancy. Discussion about smoking and other substance use becomes time-sensitive, with improved outcomes becoming more likely the earlier a person stops using substances or obtains treatment. Access to mental health care and social resources becomes an immediate need, with the midwife sometimes providing this care directly. See the *Prenatal Care* and *Mental Health Conditions* chapters for further discussion.

Urinary tract infections, periodontal disease, and several urogenital infections—group B *Streptococcus* (GBS), *Chlamydia trachomatis*, bacterial vaginosis, *Neisseria gonorrhea*, syphilis, and *Trichomonas vaginalis*—are associated with preterm labor and PPROM. Even so, a causal relationship between these infections and preterm labor has not been established, and treatment is not associated with lower incidence of preterm labor.[65-68] Therefore, treatment of urogenital infections and periodontal disease is recommended per standard protocols for general health promotion, but it is not considered an intervention for prevention of preterm birth.

## Medical Strategies for Prevention of Preterm Birth

Medical strategies for prevention of preterm birth differ for persons with no history of spontaneous preterm birth versus those with a history of preterm birth, as depicted in Figure 23-6.[64,69] Interventions may include cervical length screening, vaginal progesterone, 17-alpha hydroxyprogesterone caproate (17-OHPC), or cerclage, based on the specific circumstances of a pregnant person's history and current status.

### Screening for Short Cervix

There is a strong positive association between mid-pregnancy cervical length and risk of preterm labor.[70] To ensure accurate results, cervical length measurements should be performed using transvaginal ultrasound. Abdominal ultrasound

measurements of cervical length are not consistent with transvaginal measurements, because of the difficulty maintaining the appropriate angle as the ultrasound is performed. A transvaginal approach allows assessment of the distance between inner and outer os, the shape of the canal (such as "funneling"), and the presence of membranes bulging into the canal. Using a transvaginal approach, 25 mm is the definition of "short cervix" through 24 weeks' gestation. If short cervix is identified, the person should be offered MFM consultation.

For pregnant persons who have a history of spontaneous preterm birth, screening cervical length ultrasound (every 1 to 4 weeks, depending on individual factors) is highly recommended between 16 and 24 weeks' gestation.[71] Prior to 16 weeks' gestation, the lower uterine segment is not well developed, and measurements are not reliable. After 24 weeks' gestation, there is no evidence that medical or surgical intervention for short cervix would significantly improve outcomes. Therefore, a screening cervical length ultrasound outside this time window would have little impact on management.[71]

The routine transvaginal ultrasound measurement of cervical length in people who do not have a history of preterm birth is not universally recommended at this time, because it has not been demonstrated to be a cost-effective screening strategy.[64] However, if the cervix is assessed by abdominal ultrasound, such as during the standard anatomy scan, measurements less than 35 mm should be followed with a transvaginal approach to verify whether the person does, in fact, have a short cervix.[64]

### Progesterone for History of Spontaneous Preterm Birth

For pregnant persons with a history of spontaneous preterm birth, vaginal progesterone or intramuscular progesterone therapy (17-OHPC) should be offered, beginning near 16 weeks' gestation for best outcomes.[64] Vaginal progesterone is administered as suppositories (200 mg) or gel (90 mg), inserted once daily from 16 to 36 weeks' gestation. Intramuscular progesterone is administered as weekly injections of 17-OHPC (250 mg) from 16 to 36 weeks' gestation. Although the mechanism of action is not well understood, progesterone is thought to have an anti-inflammatory effect that curtails inflammatory processes associated with preterm cervical remodeling, contraction onset, and rupture of membranes. Another theory suggests that exogenous progesterone prevents the decrease in progesterone level typically associated with the onset of labor. The data

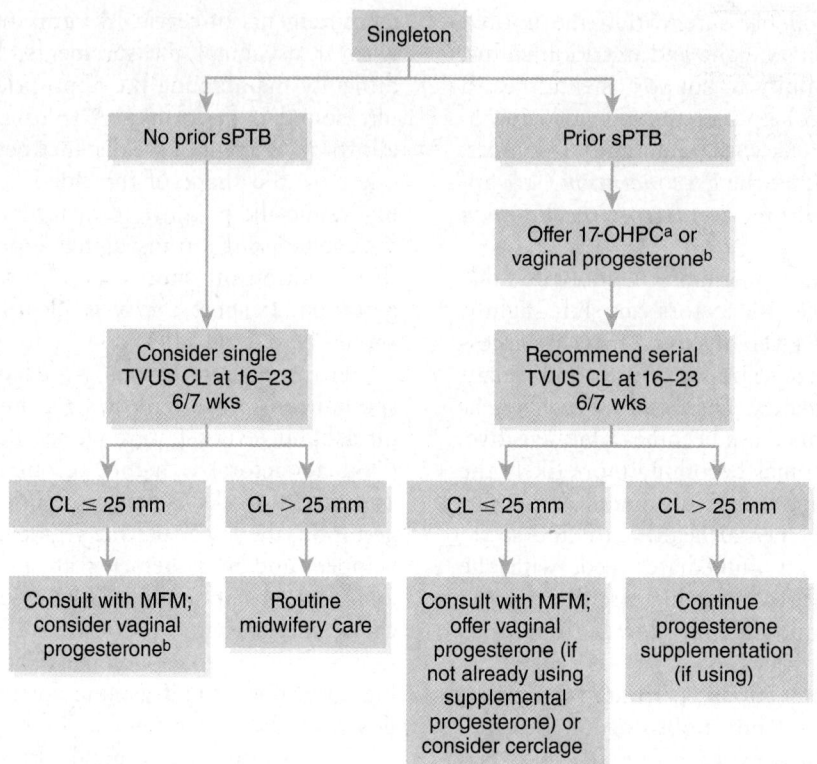

Abbreviations: CL, cervical length; MFM, maternal-fetal medicine specialist; TVUS, transvaginal ultrasound; 17-OHPC, 17-hydroxyprogesterone; sPTB, spontaneous preterm birth.

ᵃ 17-OHPC 250 mg intramuscularly given weekly

ᵇ Daily 200-mg suppository or 90-mg gel

Based on American College of Obstetricians and Gynecologists. ACOG Practice Bulletin No. 234: prediction and prevention of spontaneous preterm birth. *Obstet Gynecol.* 2021;138(2):e65-e90; Society for Maternal-Fetal Medicine. SMFM Statement: response to EPPPIC and considerations for the use of progestogens for the prevention of preterm birth.

**Figure 23-6** Medical strategies for prevention of spontaneous preterm birth.

from randomized controlled trials demonstrating the efficacy of the varied progesterone treatments are conflicting. Ideally, progesterone treatment to reduce the risk of recurrent preterm birth is offered in consultation with maternal fetal medicine specialists.

The safety of progesterone for the developing fetus has been studied in children exposed to progesterone in utero. The studies conducted to date indicate that children 2 to 4 years old have no difference in health status or cognitive skills when compared to a similar cohort of children who were not exposed to this drug in utero.[72] Longer follow-up is needed, however, before safety can

be fully assured. Nonetheless, the balance of unknown long-term risks to the child versus benefits of avoiding preterm birth is such that progesterone is recommended for selected persons at risk for preterm labor.

### Treatment of Short Cervix

Persons with a short cervix but no history of spontaneous preterm birth should be offered timely MFM consultation. In cases of extremely short cervix (< 10 mm), the person may be a candidate for placement of a suture around the cervix, called *cervical cerclage*, that holds the cervix closed.

However, the typical treatment recommendation is vaginal progesterone,[64] which has consistently been shown to reduce the risk of preterm birth prior to 34 weeks.[73] If the decision is made to initiate vaginal progesterone for a person with a short cervix, therapy consists of suppositories (200 mg) or gel (90 mg) inserted once daily from diagnosis of short cervix through 36 completed weeks of gestation.

If a pregnant person with a history of spontaneous preterm birth is found to have a short cervix, management options include beginning vaginal progesterone therapy (if not already taking supplemental progesterone due to preterm birth history) or placing a cerclage. If a person is already taking supplemental progesterone and develops a short cervix, cerclage can be considered as an additional treatment. However, there is no evidence that switching between forms of progesterone, or adding a second form of progesterone, is effective treatment of short cervix.[64]

Use of progesterone therapy outside the indications described here is not advised. Progesterone therapy, whether vaginal or intramuscular, is not effective for prevention of preterm birth in multifetal gestations. Likewise, it is not effective for persons who have current preterm rupture of membranes, or as a tocolytic for persons in active preterm labor.

## Evaluation and Diagnosis of Cervical Insufficiency

Cervical insufficiency (CI) is defined as the painless effacement and dilation of the cervix in the second trimester, leading to birth of a previable fetus or extremely premature neonate. Historically, CI was diagnosed on the basis of one or more second trimester losses and/or early preterm births. This diagnosis can also be used if a short cervix is identified prior to 24 weeks' gestation in a person with a history of spontaneous preterm birth, or if painless shortening and dilation is diagnosed by physical exam, regardless of preterm birth history.[74]

CI is caused by premature remodeling of the cervical matrix. Why this remodeling occurs is poorly understood. Well-established risk factors are structural in nature, such as autoimmune collagen vascular disease, previous mechanical dilation of the cervix, and previous cervical surgery (see Table 23-9 for a full list of risk factors). However,

| Table 23-9 | Risk Factors for Cervical Insufficiency |
|---|---|
| **Congenital Factors** | |
| Müllerian duct anomalies | |
| In utero exposure to diethylstilbestrol (DES) | |
| Collagen vascular disease | |
| **Pregnancy History Factors** | |
| Cervical laceration following vaginal or cesarean birth | |
| Multiple pregnancy terminations | |
| Dilation and evacuation | |
| Dilation and curettage | |
| **Gynecologic History Factors** | |
| Mechanical dilation to allow procedures such as hysterosalpingogram | |
| Cervical loop electrosurgical excision procedure (LEEP) or cold knife cone biopsy | |

Based on Roman A, Suhag A, Berghella V. Overview of cervical insufficiency: diagnosis, etiologies, and risk factors. *Clin Obstet Gynecol.* 2016;59(2):237–240.

some cases of CI are attributed to early-onset biochemical changes in the cervix that could also lead to preterm labor. It is unclear why these cases instead present as CI.

A pregnant person with a history of second trimester losses following painless dilation should be referred to an MFM for evaluation for cervical insufficiency. Depending on the person's current clinical situation and reproductive history, a history-indicated cerclage may be recommended; it is typically placed between 13 and 14 weeks' gestation. A pregnant person with CI may also be a candidate for cervical length monitoring and expectant management. If expectant management is chosen, a cerclage would be considered only if the person develops a short cervix before 24 weeks' gestation. In addition, vaginal progesterone could be considered in a case of CI with a short cervix. The shift away from history-indicated cerclage is due to recognition that cerclage has significant risks that can result in pregnancy loss and maternal morbidity, including rupture of membranes and infection.[64]

If a pregnant person presents with signs or symptoms that suggest possible cervical insufficiency in the early second trimester, such as increased discharge, watery discharge, or vaginal bleeding, an initial speculum examination is indicated. This exam will rule out common causes of symptoms, such as vaginitis. Visible cervical dilation, with or without bulging membranes, indicates a need for immediate MFM consultation. Bimanual and digital examination should be avoided by the midwife in cases of suspected cervical insufficiency. These exams may be performed by the consulting physician, but their occurrence should be minimized to avoid potentially rupturing membranes and introducing infection. If a thorough assessment shows the membranes are intact and the cervix is amenable, emergency placement of a cervical cerclage may be recommended.

Whether a cerclage is indicated by history, ultrasound findings, or physical exam, the cerclage is expected to remain in place throughout the pregnancy. Removal occurs either at the onset of active labor or at 36 to 37 weeks' gestation. Removal of the cerclage suture is within the scope of an obstetrician or experienced midwife.[75]

## Evaluation and Diagnosis of Preterm Labor

The site for assessment of possible preterm labor will depend on the institution, the role of the midwife in that setting, the severity of the pregnant person's symptoms, and the fetus's gestational age. Rapid referral to obstetrician-gynecologist or MFM care is indicated for a person with significant symptoms or whose fetus is at an early gestation. In all settings, the primary role of the midwife is to recognize significant risks for preterm labor and signs of preterm labor.

The diagnosis of preterm labor can be challenging. Most people with symptoms of preterm labor (listed in Table 23-10) do not go on to have a preterm birth,[76,77] and unnecessary intervention is a concern. However, delays in treatment have the potential to increase the risk of adverse perinatal outcomes. For this reason, it is important to evaluate a pregnant person with any symptoms of preterm labor carefully by reviewing the person's history for risks for preterm labor, asking about any additional symptoms from the list in Table 23-11, and observing the person over time if needed.

Diagnostic criteria for active preterm labor include regular uterine contractions ($\geq 6$ contractions in an hour), plus a change in cervical effacement and/or cervical dilation. Some institutions use specific criteria to define this change in cervical

| Table 23-10 | Signs and Symptoms of Preterm Labor[a] |
|---|---|
| **Symptoms** | **Signs** |
| Abdominal tightness or "menstrual-like cramps" | Short cervical length measured on TVUS |
| Diarrhea | Change in cervical effacement or dilation, assessed by digital vaginal exam |
| Fetus dropping low into the pelvis before 36 weeks | |
| Increased vaginal discharge (clear or pink mucus) | Positive fetal fibronectin test |
| Lower back pain | Ruptured membranes |
| Pelvic pressure | |
| Vaginal bleeding | |
| Uterine contractions that are increasing in frequency, duration and intensity | |

[a] Clinical signs and symptoms of preterm labor are not highly predictive of preterm birth.

effacement or dilation, such as cervical dilatation $\geq 3$ centimeters or cervical length $\leq 20$ millimeters. Rupture of membranes or vaginal bleeding increases the diagnostic certainty. If active preterm labor is suspected, inpatient obstetric triage/emergency department assessment is warranted. Further discussion of preterm labor management is found in the *Complications During Labor and Birth* chapter.

## Evaluation and Diagnosis of Preterm Prelabor Rupture of Membranes

Spontaneous rupture of membranes prior to the onset of labor is called prelabor rupture of membranes (PROM). If the rupture occurs before 37 weeks' gestation, it is called *preterm prelabor rupture of membranes* (PPROM). In the United States, PPROM occurs in approximately 3% of all pregnancies.[78] Risk factors for PPROM are the same as the risk factors for preterm labor. Infection can be both a cause of PPROM and a consequence of PPROM. Confirmed PPROM is an indication for obstetrician consultation, and possibly referral.

Ruptured membranes may present as a "gush" that the pregnant person notices or as "a trickle" or constant wetness. In rare cases, a small tear may seal over during the course of a few days or weeks. In that situation, pregnancy is expected to progress normally, although careful monitoring for any additional significant fluid loss is needed. A pregnant person who reports possible PPROM is best evaluated in an inpatient setting. The procedure for assessment and diagnosis is reviewed in the *First Stage of Labor* chapter, and discussion of management can be found in the *Complications During Labor and Birth* chapter.

### Post-Term Pregnancy

A post-term pregnancy is one that has reached or continues beyond 42 0/7 weeks (294 days) of gestation.[79] Historically, "term pregnancy" was defined as a gestation of 37 0/7 weeks to 41 6/7 weeks. In an effort to address the variation in perinatal outcomes in the period between 37 0/7 and 41 6/7 weeks, the following terminology was introduced[80]:

- Early term: 37 0/7 weeks through 38 6/7 weeks
- Full term: 39 0/7 weeks through 40 6/7 weeks
- Late term: 41 0/7 weeks through 41 6/7 weeks
- Post term: 42 0/7 weeks or more

The term "postdates" refers simply to being past one's estimated due date. Because it does not relate to evidence regarding perinatal outcomes or management decisions, it should be avoided when discussing late-term or post-term pregnancy.

In the United States, births during the 41st week of gestation account for 5.2% of all births; births at 42 weeks' gestation and beyond account for 0.25%.[27] The incidence of post-term pregnancy is higher among pregnant people who are older, who are nulliparous, and who have a history of a prior post-term birth. Beyond an error in the dating, the cause of post-term pregnancy is often unknown. In many cases, genetic influences (from either the pregnant person or the fetus) may play a role in initiation of labor. Rare causes of prolonged pregnancy include placental sulfatase deficiency, fetal adrenal insufficiency, and fetal anencephaly.[81]

Pregnancy extending beyond 41 weeks' gestation is associated with increased incidence of adverse outcomes for both the birthing person and the fetus, most of which are the result of excessive fetal growth or placental insufficiency. Risks for the birthing person include severe perineal lacerations, infection, postpartum hemorrhage, operative vaginal birth, and cesarean birth.[81] Reported fetal risks vary somewhat among studies, but include an increased fetal risk of oligohydramnios, meconium aspiration syndrome, macrosomia, and shoulder dystocia.[82] There is also a clear, increased risk of stillbirth and early neonatal death for pregnancies with a late-term or post-term gestation. A large meta-analysis involving more than 15 million pregnancies found that the risk of stillbirth was 0.11 per 1000 pregnancies at 37 weeks, compared to 1.78 per 1000 pregnancies at 41 weeks, and 3.18 per 1000 pregnancies at 42 weeks.[83]

The term *fetal postmaturity syndrome* is used to describe the approximately 10% to 20% of post-term fetuses that are exposed to malnutrition in late pregnancy. Such a fetus has little remaining body fat and is at increased risk for oligohydramnios, umbilical cord compression, and abnormal fetal heart rate patterns. A newborn with postmaturity syndrome is also at greater risk for hypoglycemia, polycythemia, meconium aspiration, and perinatal asphyxia.

Shared decision making about the timing of birth should focus on balancing these perinatal risks for the pregnant person and fetus with the psychosocial and physical benefits of physiologic birth, as well as the availability of local resources for induction of labor. Pregnant persons without complications, who are in the full term period, can be offered the options of induction of labor or expectant management. Induction of labor is associated with decreased risks of both cesarean birth and hypertensive disorders of pregnancy.[84,85] During the full term period, no statistically significant differences in perinatal mortality have been identified for induction of labor versus expectant management.

Beginning at 41 0/7 weeks, it remains advisable to offer pregnant persons without complications the choice of induction of labor or expectant management with fetal surveillance (typically twice weekly). Fetal surveillance is recommended due to the increasing risk of perinatal mortality in the late term and post-term periods.[86] After 42 0/7 weeks, due to the increasing risk of stillbirth and perinatal complications, the recommendation is to induce labor.[79]

### Prevention of Post-Term Pregnancy: Membrane Sweeping

Membrane sweeping is a common intervention performed by both midwives and physicians in the outpatient setting to hasten the onset of labor. Historically called stripping of the membranes, membrane sweeping involves gently dislodging the membranes from where they lay over the cervix; this process releases prostaglandins, which help prepare the cervix for labor. Numerous studies have demonstrated that membrane sweeping increases the likelihood of spontaneous labor before 41 weeks.[87] Evidence also shows membrane sweeping to be safe with no increased risk of infection for either the fetus or the pregnant person, including in the case of GBS carriers.[88-89] Most pregnant persons find this procedure uncomfortable but say they would choose to do it again in a subsequent pregnancy.[87]

Membrane sweeps are typically begun between 38 and 40 weeks, and have greater effectiveness as gestational age advances. However, it may be appropriate to offer a membrane sweep earlier in certain cases, such as to a patient anticipating induction of labor at 39 weeks. Membrane sweeping can be repeated, but clear evidence is lacking that serial sweeps are more effective than a one-time sweep after 38 weeks.

This elective procedure is done only after the pregnant person is informed of the risks and benefits and gives consent for the procedure. The technique for performing membrane sweeping is as follows: The examining fingers of the practitioner's sterile gloved hand are introduced into the vagina, enter the cervical os, and swing circumferentially around the internal os, separating the membranes from the uterine wall. Pregnant persons may experience slight vaginal bleeding and irregular contractions after membrane sweeping. Prelabor rupture of the membranes could occur either during or following the procedure, but this outcome is rare; it is more common when the cervix is already more than 1 cm dilated.[90]

## Dermatoses of Pregnancy

Pruritus is a common problem for pregnant persons. Skin conditions related to or caused by the unique physiologic aspects of pregnancy are classified into four categories: (1) atopic eruption of pregnancy, (2) intrahepatic cholestasis of pregnancy, (3) pemphigoid gestationis, and (4) polymorphic eruption of pregnancy.[91,92] Because both intrahepatic cholestasis and pemphigoid gestationis are associated with serious adverse fetal outcomes, early recognition and differentiation is important to minimize potential fetal risks and provide adequate relief to the pregnant person. These four dermatoses can be differentiated by appearance, location on the body, and time of onset during pregnancy (Table 23-11).[91-95]

### Atopic Eruption of Pregnancy

Atopic eruption of pregnancy is a benign dermatosis of pregnancy characterized by intense itching. This term includes eczema, prurigo of pregnancy, and pruritic folliculitis of pregnancy. It is considered the most common skin disorder during pregnancy, accounting for almost 50% of all rashes experienced by persons who are pregnant.[91] This condition resolves early in the postpartum period, but recurrence in subsequent pregnancies is possible.[93] There are no known adverse effects of atopic eruption of pregnancy on perinatal outcomes.

The presentation of atopic eruption of pregnancy includes intense pruritus with papular, eczematous lesions primarily appearing in the first or second trimester. The rash usually involves the face, neck, and antecubital and popliteal fossae, but can occur on all parts of the body, including the palms and soles. Approximately one-third of cases develop on the trunk and the abdomen.[91,93]

Treatment involves topical corticosteroids and topical or oral antihistamines for relief. Moisturizers and lukewarm showers with mild soap can also provide symptom relief.[93]

### Polymorphic Eruption in Pregnancy

Polymorphic eruption in pregnancy (PEP) is also known as pruritic urticarial papules and plaques of pregnancy (PUPPP). This condition occurs in 0.5% to 1% of pregnancies and typically presents in the third trimester. It is most common during a first pregnancy or multifetal-gestation pregnancy. The pathophysiology of PEP is unclear; theories range from a nonspecific inflammatory reaction to excessive skin stretching, to immunoglobulin E (IgE) release in individuals with atopic disease, to immunoglobulin M (IgM) deposition as would be seen in autoimmune disease. The rash resolves spontaneously after birth. Recurrence in subsequent pregnancies is rare.[91,94]

Except for discomfort, PEP is a benign condition with no adverse effects on the pregnant person or fetus. Its clinical presentation begins with red, itchy, urticarial papules located in the striae. Lesions then spread to cover the trunk. When lesions extend to the extremities, the abdomen and proximal thighs are the most common sites of involvement. The face, palms and soles, and periumbilical area are rarely involved.[94]

Diagnosis of PEP does not require consultation or referral to specialty care, unless there is a need to rule out a rarer dermatosis such as pemphigoid gestationis. Low-potency topical steroids and antihistamines can be used to treat the discomfort. Severe cases may require systemic corticosteroids.

### Intrahepatic Cholestasis of Pregnancy

Intrahepatic cholestasis of pregnancy (ICP) is a hepatic condition specific to pregnancy that features intense itching without rash, elevated serum bile acids, and increased liver enzymes.[96]

| Table 23-11 | **Common Dermatoses in Pregnancy** | | | |
|---|---|---|---|---|
| **Characteristics** | **Atopic Eruption of Pregnancy** | **Polymorphic Eruption of Pregnancy** | **Intrahepatic Cholestasis of Pregnancy** | **Pemphigoid Gestationis** |
| **Historical term** | Eczema in pregnancy[a]<br>Pruritic folliculitis of pregnancy[a]<br>Papular dermatitis of pregnancy | PUPPP[a]<br>Erythema multiforme of pregnancy | Obstetric cholestasis<br>Icterus gravidarum<br>Pruritus gravidarum | Herpes gestationis |
| **Associated conditions** | | | Hepatitis C | Multiparity, hydatidiform mole (rare) |
| **Trimester(s) of onset** | First and second | Third and postpartum | Late second or third | Second and third |
| **Symptoms** | Eczematous rash | Urticarial papules, plaques | Pruritus without rash, jaundice | Urticarial papules, plaques, bullae |
| **Location** | Entire body, including palms/soles | Abdominal striae, then body; spares the face, palms, soles, and periumbilical area | Entire body; may be most intense on palms/soles | Begins on abdomen, then body; spares the face |
| **Diagnosis** | Clinical symptoms and appearance | Clinical symptoms and appearance | Clinical symptoms and elevated bile acids | Skin biopsy |
| **Complications for the pregnant person** | No known risks | No known risks | Steatorrhea, gestational diabetes, preeclampsia | Increased risk for Graves' disease |
| **Complications for the fetus** | No known risks | No known risks | Meconium, preterm birth, stillbirth | Fetal growth restriction, preterm birth, neonatal lesions |
| **Management** | Topical corticosteroids, antihistamines | Topical corticosteroids, antihistamines, emollients | Ursodeoxycholic acid<br>Antenatal fetal testing, fetal movement counts, planned birth at 36–37 weeks | Topical and systemic corticosteroids, antihistamines<br>Antenatal fetal testing, fetal movement counts |
| **Resolution after birth** | Soon after | Weeks | Weeks | Weeks or months |
| **Recurrence in future pregnancies** | Possible | Low | Possible | Frequent |

Abbreviation: PUPPP, pruritic urticarial papules and plaques of pregnancy.

[a] Acceptable term for this condition.

Based on Warshauer E, Mercurio M. Update on dermatoses of pregnancy. *Int J Dermatol*. 2013;52(1):6-13; Bechtel MA, Plotner A. Dermatoses of pregnancy. *Clin Obstet Gynecol*. 2015;58(1):104-111; Mehta N, Chen KK, Kroumpouzos G. Skin disease in pregnancy: the approach of the obstetric medicine physician. *Clin Derm*. 2016;34:320-326; Taylor D, Pappo E, Aronson IK. Polymorphic eruption of pregnancy. *Clin Dermatol*. 2016;34(3):383-391; Lee RH, Greenberg M, Metz TD, Pettker CM. SMFM Consult Series No. 53: intrahepatic cholestasis of pregnancy. *Am J Obstet Gynecol*. 2021;224(2):B2-B9.

The pathophysiology of this condition relates to slow movement of bile acids from hepatocytes into and through the biliary tree. This movement is slowed due to the influence of reproductive hormones (especially estrogen), as well as altered function of bile acid transport molecules in genetically susceptible individuals.[97]

Multifetal gestation, a personal history of hepatitis C, cholelithiasis, and dyslipidemia are associated with increased risk for this disorder.[91] Environmental, dietary, and genetic influences may also contribute to the relative risk of developing ICP. There is wide variation in the incidence of this dermatosis, with rates ranging from 1.5% or less in Europe, to 5.6% or less in the United States (highest in Latinx populations), to as high as 27.6% in indigenous populations in Chile.[96] The recurrence rate of ICP in subsequent pregnancies is as high as 90%, and some affected persons also experience recurrence with use of combined hormonal contraception between pregnancies.[95]

A pregnant person with ICP also has an increased risk of gestational diabetes and preeclampsia.[96] Fetal and neonatal complications include increased incidence of meconium-stained fluid, spontaneous preterm birth, stillbirth, and neonatal respiratory distress. Stillbirth attributed to ICP impacts 1% to 2% of affected pregnancies that proceed past 37 weeks, and it occurs suddenly. The underlying etiology of stillbirth appears to be bile acid–induced fetal arrhythmia and/or vasospasm of placental veins secondary to damage from toxic bile acids.[97]

Symptoms of ICP develop in the second and third trimesters. Intense itching, without rash, occurs all over the body; it may be most severe on the palms and soles, and intensifies at night. In addition, some patients report diarrhea or steatorrhea, and jaundice develops in 10% to 25% of people with ICP. The diagnosis of ICP is based on pruritis without rash, accompanied by laboratory tests that indicate liver dysfunction: aminotransferase levels rise dramatically, and bile acids become elevated to more than 10 mmol/L. Differential diagnoses include preeclampsia (including hemolysis, elevated liver enzymes, and low platelet syndrome), hepatitis, cholelithiasis, and other liver disorders.[95]

Because of the high risk of stillbirth associated with ICP, severe pruritus without rash is sufficient to make a presumptive diagnosis and start treatment, even before laboratory values are available. Treatment with ursodeoxycholic acid (Ursodiol, Actigall) is primarily for the purpose of symptom relief. Data are inconclusive regarding whether treatment improves fetal/neonatal outcomes. The starting dose of ursodeoxycholic acid is 10 to 15 mg/kg body weight daily, divided into 2 to 3 daily doses.

After diagnosing a pregnant person with ICP, a midwife should seek obstetrician or MFM consultation. Serial bile acid testing is not necessary, as it rarely changes the plan of care. Antepartum fetal surveillance is usually recommended as the standard of care, though its value is uncertain, as stillbirth with ICP is not related to chronic uteroplacental insufficiency. Induction of labor is planned at 36 to 37 weeks' gestation, to balance the risks of prematurity with the risk of stillbirth.[95]

## Pemphigoid Gestationis

Pemphigoid gestationis is a rare autoimmune disorder that occurs in approximately 1 in 50,000 pregnancies. Due to the blister-type appearance of lesions, pemphigoid gestationis was originally called herpes gestationis, but it is not related to the herpes viruses. This dermatosis is most common in the third trimester. It usually recurs and worsens in subsequent pregnancies.[93]

Implications of developing this disorder for the pregnant person include a long-term increase in the risk of Graves' disease. Implications for the fetus include an increased risk of fetal growth restriction and spontaneous preterm birth.[93] In addition, there is an estimated 5% to 10% risk of vertical transmission of lesions, due to immunoglobulin G (IgG) crossing the placenta.[98]

Pruritus begins initially with urticarial and annular plaques that make it difficult to distinguish pemphigoid gestationis from other dermatoses. The initial symptoms are followed by vesico-bullous eruptions that begin on the abdomen and spread to the extremities. Skin biopsy by a dermatologist is required for definitive diagnosis.

If pemphigoid gestationis is confirmed, MFM consultation is appropriate. Treatment of pemphigoid gestationis includes potent topical and systemic steroids, as well as topical or oral antihistamines. Antenatal fetal testing is initiated in the third trimester, due to the risk of placental insufficiency. Infants born with the disease do not require treatment, and the condition typically resolves spontaneously.[91]

## Peripartum Cardiomyopathy

Peripartum cardiomyopathy (PPCM) is a rare form of left ventricular systolic heart failure that develops toward the end of pregnancy or during the first year postpartum. This diagnosis is made only in the absence of heart disease or any other identifiable cause for failure. In the United States, the diagnosis is restricted to 1 month before birth and 5 months postpartum[99]; however, the European definition was broadened in 2010 to account for cases of heart failure occurring earlier in pregnancy or later in the postpartum year that cannot be attributed to any cause other than pregnancy.[100] The majority of persons who develop PPCM do so in the postpartum period; thus, this disorder is reviewed in more detail in the *Postpartum Complications* chapter.

People most at risk for PPCM are those with obesity, age older than 30 years, multiparity, and chronic hypertension/preeclampsia. Disparity in the prevalence of this condition is dramatic. Worldwide, PPCM has an incidence of approximately 1/1000 pregnancies, but the incidence in certain geographies climbs to as high as 1/300 (Haiti) and 1/100 (Nigeria), and falls to as low as 1/20,000 (Japan). In the United States, incidence is estimated between 1/1000 and 1/4000, with 40% of those cases occurring in Black individuals.[100] Reasons for the disparity vary, ranging from specific cultural practices (e.g., ritual salt ingestion) to the effects of chronic stress and systemic racism (leading to increased incidence of hypertension/preeclampsia). There is also significant disparity in outcomes in the United States, with increased long-term morbidity and mortality for Black individuals and people of low socioeconomic status. This disparity in outcomes stems directly from delays in diagnosis, which result from systemic barriers to high-quality, nonbiased health care.[100]

There is limited understanding of the pathophysiology of PPCM. Based on animal models, it is understood to be primarily a vascular disease, influenced by the hormonal milieu of late pregnancy and postpartum.[100] Genetics also plays a role, given reports of family clustering of PPCM with heart disease such as dilated cardiomyopathy. However, genetic variants of concern account for only approximately 15% of cases of PPCM, and many people with these variants of concern do not develop PPCM.[100]

Outcomes of PPCM for the pregnant or postpartum person range from rapid decompensation and death, to need for mechanical cardiopulmonary support, to chronic heart failure or complete recovery. Associated complications include thromboembolism and pulmonary edema. Fetal/neonatal outcomes relate specifically to the timing of birth, other pregnancy complications, and PPCM-associated emergencies.

Signs and symptoms of PPCM include all the signs and symptoms of pulmonary edema: shortness

| Table 23-12 | Signs and Symptoms of Heart Failure |
|---|---|
| **Signs of Heart Failure** | **Symptoms of Heart Failure** |
| Cough | Chest pain |
| Tachycardia | Dyspnea (especially with exertion or at night) |
| Peripheral edema | Orthopnea |
| Bilateral basilar crackles | Palpitations |

of breath that is particularly noticeable when the person reclines, cough, tachycardia, palpitations, and chest pain (Table 23-12). Findings may be inaccurately attributed to normal physiologic changes in pregnancy and postpartum, and affected individuals frequently report being given an incorrect diagnosis initially.[101] The role of the midwife is to maintain a high index of suspicion. A person with signs and symptoms should be seen immediately, so that a complete history and physical examination can be performed. Care of a person with PPCM requires a multidisciplinary team of cardiologists, intensive care physicians, MFMs, and respiratory specialists.

## Red Blood Cell Alloimmunization

Alloimmunization (also referred to as isoimmunization) is the process by which a person develops antibodies against human tissue antigens not present in their own body. Events that can lead to red blood cell (RBC) alloimmunization include pregnancy and birth (wherein the pregnant person is exposed to fetal red blood cells), blood transfusion, and tissue/organ transplant. After exposure, the person's immune system develops antibodies against the foreign antigen that has entered circulation. The topic of alloimmunization is introduced in the *Prenatal Care* chapter, and interventions to prevent Rh (D) sensitization are addressed there.

Complications of alloimmunization develop in a subsequent pregnancy, when previously developed antibodies cross the placenta. If the fetus in that subsequent pregnancy is incompatible with antibodies crossing the placenta, the antibodies attach to fetal RBCs and mark them for destruction.[102] The resulting hemolytic disease of the fetus can lead to mild to severe fetal anemia, as well as anemia and hyperbilirubinemia in the newborn. If severe fetal anemia develops, the fetus may develop hydrops fetalis, a condition associated with hepatosplenomegaly, accumulation of fluid in the abdomen, and heart failure.

| Table 23-13 | Red Cell Antibodies and Relationship to Hemolytic Disease of the Fetus and Newborn |
|---|---|
| **Red Cell Antigen** | **Association with Hemolytic Disease of the Fetus and Newborn** |
| Diego D1ª, Diᵇ | Mild to severe |
| Duffy Fyª | Mild to severe |
| Duffy Fyᵇ | Not associated |
| Duffy By³ | Mild |
| Kell K | Mild to severe |
| Kell k, Ko, Kpª, Kpᵇ, Jsª, Jsᵇ | Mild |
| Kidd Jkª | Mild to severe |
| Kidd Jkᵇ, Jk³ | Mild |
| Lewis | Not associated |
| Lutheran Luª, Luᵇ | Mild |
| MSS Mtª | Moderate |
| MSS Vw, Mur, Hil, Hut | Mild |
| Rh D | Mild to severe |
| Rh E, C | Mild to severe |

Note: This list is not an exhaustive list of atypical antibodies that can cause hemolytic disease of the fetus and newborn. Any pregnant person with an atypical antibody should be referred for maternal–fetal medicine specialist consultation and possibly management.

Based on De Haas M, Thurik FF, Koelewijn JM, van der School CE. Haemolytic disease of the fetus and newborn. *VOX Sanguinis.* 2015;109:99-103; ACOG. Practice Bulletin No. 192: management of alloimmunization during pregnancy. *Obstet Gynecol.* 2018;131:e82-e90.

RBC alloimmunization affects approximately 1.15% of pregnancies in the United States.[103] In addition to the Rh (D) antigen, the non-Rh (D) antigens most likely to cause hemolytic disease of the fetus and newborn are Kell and Duffy (Table 23-13).[102,104] The Lewis antigen is commonly encountered, but is not associated with hemolytic disease of the fetus and newborn because it is an IgM antibody and, therefore, too large to cross the placenta.

RBC alloimmunization is diagnosed via antibody screen (indirect Coombs test), one of the routine tests offered to all pregnant persons. Results from antibody screens are reported as positive or negative, and positive screens should be followed with a report of antibody identification and titers.

Titers measure how much antibody-positive serum from the pregnant person is required to agglutinate a standardized sample of antigen-positive RBCs. Titers are reported as dilutions; that is, 1:1 means one full quantity of serum agglutinates a sample of antigen-positive RBCs, whereas 1:16 means 1/16 of the standard quantity of serum agglutinates a sample of antigen-positive RBCs. The higher the titer level, the higher the risk of hemolytic disease of the fetus and newborn. Titer levels associated with pregnancy complications vary between 1:8 and 1:32, depending on the antibody–antigen complex in question.[102]

Persons who have a positive antibody screen in pregnancy should be offered MFM consultation. The MFM may recommend testing the sperm-producing partner (or donor) for the RBC antigen of concern, to determine whether the fetus is genetically at risk. Then, depending on the antibody type and initial titer, titers may be repeated every 4 weeks until 28 weeks, at which time screening frequency increases to every 2 weeks.[102,105] If a person's titers reach critical levels for the antibody in question, the MFM will recommend Doppler studies to assess for fetal anemia. In addition, ultrasound monitoring for hydrops fetalis may be initiated. Identification of anemia or hydrops is an indication for referral to MFM care. At this time, invasive treatments may be considered, such as intrauterine transfusion.[104]

## Population-Specific Special Considerations During Pregnancy

### Adolescent Pregnancy and Advanced Maternal Age

Pregnancy at both ends of the age spectrum—younger and older—is associated with increased risks of adverse outcomes. Adolescent pregnancy is defined as pregnancy before age 20, with pregnancy before age 15 defined as *young adolescent childbearing*.[106] Advanced maternal age (AMA) describes a person who will be 35 years or older at the time of birth. In the United States, approximately 5% of all births are to adolescent individuals.[107] By comparison, approximately 9% of pregnant people in the United States are 35 years or older when they give birth.[108]

### *Adolescent Pregnancy*

The adolescent pregnancy rate in the United States varies significantly by age: 2.2 per 1000 for teens younger than 15 years, 13.6 per 1000 for teens aged 15–17 years, and 56.9 per 1000 for teens aged 18–19 years.[109] Recognizing that some of these pregnancies end in miscarriage and abortion, the composite live birth rate is approximately 15.3 pregnancies per 1000 females aged 15–19 years.[47] Although these rates have declined significantly in recent years, the United States has one of the highest rates of adolescent birth among all industrialized nations.[110]

Adolescent pregnancy is associated with increased rates of adverse outcomes for the pregnant person and fetus. Pregnant adolescents face increased risks for sexually transmitted infections, substance use disorder, anemia, preterm birth, low birth weight, preeclampsia, stillbirth, obstructed labor, postpartum hemorrhage, and endometritis.[111] Worldwide, complications related to pregnancy and birth are the leading cause of death in women between ages 15 and 19 years.[112]

Social implications of adolescent pregnancy include increased risk of stigma, low educational attainment, employment discrimination, and risk of violence (especially from parents or intimate partners).[112] Physical, mental-emotional, and social health complications associated with adolescent pregnancy are highly related to age of the pregnant person, degree of family support, education level already attained, financial status, geographic setting, and cultural perceptions of early parenting. It is important to view a young pregnant individual within the framework of their environment and support structure.

Prenatal care for adolescents in the United States requires increased screening for social risks such as tobacco or other substance use, physical or sexual abuse, food insecurity, and housing instability. Depending on state regulations, mandatory reporting laws may require reporting the pregnancy as evidence of potential sexual abuse, especially if there is a significant age difference between partners. In addition, many adolescents are minors and subject to different regulations regarding parental consent for health care.[113]

Adolescents are less likely to receive adequate prenatal care, as compared to older pregnant persons. Therefore, it is important to create welcoming and accessible prenatal care services for adolescent individuals. In addition to routine prenatal care and social risk screening (as just mentioned), services should include detailed education regarding nutrition, mental-emotional health, reproductive life planning, and preparing for labor, birth, and parenting.[114]

The skills needed to care for adolescents during pregnancy, as well as provide postpartum gynecologic care, are within the scope of independent midwifery practice. However, in many settings, an interdisciplinary team involving midwifery, pediatrics, behavioral health, and social work can provide the best care for this population. The benefits of a CenteringPregnancy prenatal care model are also particularly promising for adolescents.[115] The Resources section at the end of this chapter includes reviews and guidelines that address the specific prenatal needs of adolescents.

### Advanced Maternal Age

Persons who are older than 35 years when they give birth have increased risks for miscarriage, aneuploidy, gestational diabetes, hypertensive disorders of pregnancy, placenta previa, preterm labor/birth, and stillbirth. There are also age-related increases in morbidity and mortality once pregnancy complications arise, particularly regarding the severity of cardiovascular complications.[116]

The association between AMA and these conditions is widely recognized, but little evidence exists regarding their causal mechanisms. A key question emerging from the available data is how much of the association between AMA and pregnancy complications can be accounted for by parity, comorbid conditions, use of assisted reproductive technology, and socioeconomic status, all of which commonly change as a person ages. Another question is whether risks for pregnancy complications apply to all pregnant persons older than 35 years, or whether these risks increase at specific age increments, as is the case for younger versus older adolescents.

In general, screening and interventions for conditions associated with AMA should follow the guidelines for each of the specific conditions. For example, AMA is considered a moderate risk factor for preeclampsia, so low-dose aspirin therapy should be considered for prevention of preeclampsia in pregnant persons who have at least one additional risk factor.[117] See the *Assessment for Genetic and Fetal Abnormalities, Prenatal Care,* and *Medical Complications in Pregnancy* chapters for discussion of screening and interventions for conditions associated with AMA.

Given the increased risk of term stillbirth for pregnant persons with AMA, an ongoing question is whether antenatal fetal surveillance should be recommended for this indication. After pregnant persons with medical comorbidities and pregnant persons giving birth for the first time are excluded from the analysis, individuals ages 35–39 have a 1.28-fold increased relative risk of stillbirth compared with individuals less than 35 years, and individuals 40 years and older have a 1.79-fold increased relative risk.

While notable, this risk is lower than the threshold recommended by the American College of Obstetricians and Gynecologists (ACOG) and Society for Maternal–Fetal Medicine (SMFM) for initiating antenatal fetal surveillance (two-times increased risk).[86] In addition, the pathophysiology by which AMA increases stillbirth risk remains unclear. Some evidence suggests that placental pathology increases in persons aged 40 years and older,[118] but research on the topic is limited. Antenatal fetal surveillance for pregnant persons older than 35 years should be considered and customized on a holistic assessment of risk factors and patient preference.

There are no evidence-based guidelines regarding the timing of birth for pregnant persons with AMA. Birth at 39 weeks' gestation is suggested by some providers as an intervention to decrease the risk of stillbirth due to AMA. However, this recommendation has not been evaluated in large clinical trials, and trials such as ARRIVE were not sufficiently powered to allow subgroup analysis of pregnant persons aged 35 years and older. What can be discussed with pregnant persons with AMA is that, if they choose induction of labor at 39 weeks, they have no increased risk of cesarean birth above the background, age-related risk.[119]

### Pregnancy After Assisted Reproductive Technology

Pregnancy resulting from assisted reproductive technology (ART) is associated with many pregnancy complications, including miscarriage, ectopic pregnancy, congenital anomaly, preterm birth, low birth weight, preeclampsia, placenta previa, placental abruption, stillbirth, and cesarean birth.[120] Even after controlling for parity, age, and multifetal gestation, all of these complications are still independently associated with ART.[121] What remains unclear is whether the process of ART or the underlying infertility is the etiologic factor that explains these associations. Preliminary data indicate that same-sex couples who use ART do not have the same increase in perinatal complications following use of these technologies, compared to couples who use ART due to a history of infertility.[122]

As with pregnancies impacted by AMA, screening and interventions for conditions associated with ART should follow the guidelines established for each of the specific conditions. For example, if a pregnant person has two or more moderate risk factors for preeclampsia, the midwife should recommend low-dose aspirin therapy for prevention of preeclampsia.[117]

Pregnancy after ART is an indication for detailed fetal anatomy ultrasound, as are all pregnancies.[123] All pregnancies conceived through ART have an increased risk of congenital anomaly, with the risk being greatest in multifetal gestations and in pregnancies resulting from intra-cytoplasmic sperm injection (ICSI).[121]

The increased risk of stillbirth in pregnancies resulting from ART is most marked in pregnancies conceived via in vitro fertilization, reaching a peak at 37 to 40 weeks' gestation (2 to 3 times the background risk).[86] Although no studies have evaluated the ability of antenatal fetal surveillance to reduce this risk, antenatal surveillance can be considered beginning at 36 weeks as a precaution.

There is no research evaluating optimal birth timing for pregnancies resulting from ART. As with AMA, birth at 39 weeks' gestation is sometimes suggested as an intervention to decrease the risk of stillbirth. However, in the absence of other medical indications for birth, this cannot be presented as an evidence-based recommendation. Rather, planned birth at 39 weeks should be discussed as an elective intervention.

### Female Genital Mutilation

In Western medical practice, female circumcision is called female genital mutilation (FGM) or female genital cutting (see the *Pelvic Examination* appendix for a discussion of types). This procedure is practiced in parts of Africa, Asia, and the Middle East, and affects more than 90% of women in some countries.[124] As people from these regions have immigrated to Europe and the United States, practitioners in areas previously unfamiliar with this practice have found themselves caring for pregnant persons with FGM.

Although a pregnant person with type I and type II FGM does not usually experience obstetric complications, type III FGM can cause obstruction from the resulting anatomy and scar tissue, necessitating the need for deinfibulation or "anterior episiotomy" prior to birth.[125] Deinfibulation generally does not injure underlying structures, as the scar tissue that forms following infibulation does not fuse with female genital tissue. Discussion of deinfibulation is best initiated early in pregnancy. As much as possible, counseling should occur using the language patients use for the original procedure and their own body parts. Counseling includes information about the medical and obstetric risks associated with birth, as well as the options for deinfibulation. Counseling about deinfibulation may need to proceed over several visits, as the cultural implications of medical deinfibulation can be significant. Obstetrician consultation and involvement early in pregnancy will allow this process to take place over time. Deinfibulation may occur prenatally or during labor.[126]

### Labor After Cesarean

Cesarean birth rates have been increasing for three decades in the United States, with repeat cesarean birth as the leading cause. Both repeat cesarean birth and vaginal birth after cesarean (VBAC) have health benefits and health risks, as evidenced by the composite statistics in Table 23-14.[127–129] However, it is often necessary to consider nuances that impact the benefit–risk balance for a given individual, such as a person's total number of prior cesarean births, history of prior vaginal birth, type of scar(s) from prior cesarean birth(s), whether induction of labor is planned, the experience of the attending provider, and health system capacity and resources where the birth is planned. The decision of whether to perform a repeat cesarean birth or labor after cesarean (LAC) involves balancing several considerations, including (1) the chance of success, (2) the risks for the pregnant person, and (3) the risks for the fetus/newborn.

Compared to repeat cesarean, the primary benefits of LAC include lower risk of intrapartum complication, faster recovery, lower overall healthcare costs, and decreased risk of placenta previa and placenta accreta in future pregnancies. For people who desire multiple future pregnancies, access to LAC is a significant opportunity to reduce morbidity and mortality in those future pregnancies.

The primary risks associated with LAC include unplanned repeat cesarean, which is associated with more morbidity than a planned repeat cesarean, and uterine rupture. Uterine rupture is a complication unique to VBAC, with adverse sequelae including hemorrhage and neonatal morbidity/mortality.[127–129]

Pregnant persons approaching this decision require a detailed review of the benefits and risks of each option, as part of a shared decision-making process.[127–130] Counseling begins with the midwife and often includes other members of the care team, such as a consultant obstetrician or MFM. In many settings, "calculator" tools have been introduced to support this counseling process.

VBAC calculators aim to predict the chance of LAC leading to vaginal birth. The most widely used calculator was developed from data in the Maternal–Fetal Medicine Units (MFMU) Network Cesarean Registry, examining LAC outcomes for pregnant persons with one prior cesarean birth, who were now at term with a single live fetus. The MFMU calculator requires input of age, height, pre-pregnancy weight, history of previous vaginal birth, history of prior labor arrest disorder, and history of chronic hypertension. Until 2021, the calculator also included information about race/ethnicity.[131] This information was originally included to improve the predictive capacity of the calculator, given that persons who identify as Black or Hispanic have higher rates of cesarean birth than persons who identify as non-Hispanic white. However, to many users of the calculator, including race/ethnicity implied that race was a biologic determinant of vaginal birth. Removing race/ethnicity from the calculator allows providers to reframe racial/ethnic disparities in cesarean birth rates in terms of social determinants of health.[131]

One challenge with the use of calculators is that institutions often deny or discourage the option of LAC when pregnant people have a calculated score below a certain threshold.[132] This is not an evidence-based use of calculators; there is no low score cutoff at which the risks for the pregnant person or fetus/neonate clearly outweigh the benefits. In fact, there is minimal correlation between overall VBAC success and risks associated with LAC. For more information on VBAC calculators, see the Resources section at the end of this chapter.

One important point for people considering LAC is that LAC in a hospital setting is associated with better neonatal outcomes than LAC in a birth center or home setting.[133,134] On the basis of these findings, the American College of Nurse-Midwives (ACNM) acknowledges hospital LAC to be the "safest" option but does not specifically recommend against community LAC.[135] The American Association of Birth Centers stresses the importance of shared decision making and careful candidate selection, such as whether a pregnant person has previously given birth vaginally.[136] ACOG specifically recommends against LAC in a community setting.[137] However, ACOG does support the ACNM recommendations that persons considering LAC should be informed about all available hospital and provider resources in their area, including resources in neighboring cities if LAC is not available at a local facility.[137]

### Previous Birth Trauma

Trauma specifically related to childbirth is a recognized cause of perinatal mood disorders and post-traumatic stress disorder (PTSD). Perinatal mood disorders include depression, anxiety, and

| Table 23-14 | Risks Associated with Labor After Cesarean Versus Elective Repeat Cesarean | | |
|---|---|---|---|
| Outcome | Labor After Cesarean | Elective Repeat Cesarean | Analysis |
| **Short-Term Effects for the Birthing Person** | | | |
| Risk of uterine rupture | 4.7 per 1000 women (7 per 1000 women if limited to term pregnancies) | 0.3 per 1000 women | 4–5/1000 fewer uterine ruptures in persons choosing ERCD |
| Maternal mortality | 3.8 per 100,000 women at term | 13.4 per 100,000 women at term | Approximately 9/100,000 fewer maternal deaths in persons undergoing LAC |
| Hysterectomy | 1.57 per 1000 women | 2.8 per 1000 women | No significant difference |
| Blood transfusion | 6.6 per 1000 women at term | 4.6 per 1000 women at term | No significant difference |
| Operative injury | 4.0–5.1 per 1000 women | 2.5–4.4 per 1000 women | Differing study methodologies make this comparison difficult. |
| Infection | 46 per 1000 women | 32 per 1000 women | Differing study methodologies make this comparison difficult. No significant difference |
| Hospital stay | 2.5 days | 3.92 days | Longer for ERCD but longest for a person with LAC that results in repeat cesarean |
| Urinary incontinence | No data | No data | |
| Pelvic floor disorders | No data | No data | |
| **Short-Term and Long-Term Effects: Infant** | | | |
| Perinatal mortality | 13 per 10,000 | 5 per 10,000 | Approximately 1 more death per 1000 LAC |
| Hypoxic ischemic encephalopathy if uterus ruptures[a] | 8.9 per 1000 | 3.2 per 1000 | Strength of evidence is low secondary to methodologic differences in studies |
| Respiratory problem in the first days after birth | 5.4 per 100 | 2.5 per 100 | Insufficient studies to assess differences |
| **Effects on Subsequent Pregnancy Following Cesarean Birth** | | | |
| Placenta previa in subsequent pregnancy | 1% in women with 1 prior cesarean 1.7% in women with 2 prior cesareans 2.8% in women with ≥ 3 prior cesareans | | |
| Placenta accreta in subsequent pregnancy with placenta previa[b] | 5% in women with 1 prior cesarean 24% in women with 2 prior cesareans 47% in women with 3 prior cesareans | | |

Abbreviations: ERCD, elective repeat cesarean delivery; LAC, labor after cesarean.

[a] Rate of hypoxic ischemic injury among all uterine ruptures.

[b] Rate of placenta accreta in subsequent pregnancies that are also affected by placenta previa.

Based on Guise JM, Eden K, Emeis C, et al. Vaginal birth after cesarean: new insights. *Evid ReportTechnology Assess.* 2010;(191):1-397.

psychosis, as well as exacerbation of mental health conditions such as bipolar disorder. Screening and treatment of perinatal mood disorders are reviewed in the *Mental Health Conditions* chapter. Interdisciplinary care can be very helpful for these persons, as midwives work in collaboration with mental health specialists during the preconception, prenatal, and postpartum periods.

Any experience threatening the health or life of the pregnant person, fetus, or neonate may be perceived as traumatic. Screening for birth trauma begins with a compassionate question: "How did your birth go for you?" Referral to behavioral health care is indicated based on the severity of symptoms, the extent to which symptoms interrupt the pregnant or postpartum person's daily life, and the person's previous mental health history. Timely intervention can help prevent the progression of birth trauma into PTSD. Factors that increase the risk of PTSD after a traumatic experience include history of mental health disorders, sexual abuse, family violence, loss of a child or spouse, or other emotional/physical trauma.

Just as midwives take special care during examinations for persons who have experienced sexual abuse, so the same caution applies to persons who have had a previous traumatic birth. Time needs to be provided during prenatal care to gently discuss the traumatic experience. Together with their care team, the pregnant person and family need to articulate plans to avoid and manage trauma reminders ("triggers") during the current pregnancy, birth, and postpartum. These plans should be very individualized. For example, a person who did not consent to emergency procedures in a previous birth may want to avoid epidural anesthesia, to limit any feeling of being controlled or restrained. However, a different person, whose previous birth triggered memories of sexual abuse, may specifically *need* epidural anesthesia to avoid sensations of pelvic touch.

### Stillbirth

After 20 weeks' gestation (or a fetal weight greater than or equal to 350 grams if gestational age is uncertain), fetal death is classified as a stillbirth. This term, rather than "fetal death" or "demise," is preferred. The overall stillbirth rate in the United States is approximately 5.7 per 1000 fetal deaths and live births.[138] Half of all stillbirths occur between 20 and 27 weeks' gestation, and the other half occur at 28 weeks or later. Of particular concern is the racial disparity in the rate of stillbirths, which is twice as high in pregnancies where the pregnant person is non-Hispanic Black (10.3 stillbirths per 1000

fetal deaths and live births), compared to pregnancies where the pregnant person is non-Hispanic white (4.7 stillbirths per 1000 fetal deaths and live births).[138] Factors contributing to this disparity include stress, exposure to racism, limited access to health care, and increased prevalence among Black persons of health conditions such as hypertension and diabetes.[139] However, the full picture of why non-Hispanic Black persons are at increased risk for stillbirth compared to non-Hispanic white persons is not fully understood.

The determination of the cause of the stillbirth is extremely difficult. In the United States, more than half of all stillbirths have no identifiable cause, and approximately 20% are related to infection (which causes preterm labor and/or preterm premature rupture of membranes). In low-resource countries, infection accounts for more than half of all stillbirths. Other causes of stillbirth include congenital or genetic anomalies, fetal growth restriction, fetomaternal hemorrhage, hydrops fetalis secondary to alloimmunization, umbilical cord abnormalities, chronic health conditions of the pregnant person (such as diabetes or hypertension), and exposure to substance use or other toxins. It is best to refrain from discussing any possible cause for the loss until objective facts are clear and post-birth studies are completed.

Often the first sign of a stillbirth is the pregnant person's perception of loss of fetal movement. Inability to detect the fetal heart tones with a Doppler fetal monitor indicates the need for immediate ultrasound to confirm the diagnosis. The midwife should be sensitive to the pregnant person's emotional needs during this uncertainty. It can be beneficial to help the pregnant person connect with a support person and notify the ultrasound staff ahead of time that fetal heart tones could not be found. Once the diagnosis is made, physician consultation is recommended.

The decision to induce labor or wait for labor to occur spontaneously will depend on the pregnant person's choice, the gestational age at which the death occurred, past pregnancy history, current cervical status, and any concomitant medical issues that need to be addressed.[138] Although most pregnant persons choose immediate induction, expectant management is a viable option for a short period of time. The majority of pregnant persons (80% to 90%) will go into labor spontaneously within 2 weeks following a fetal demise. An unusual chronic form of disseminated intravascular coagulation (DIC) can occur if the fetus is retained in utero for more than 4 to 5 weeks; this DIC occurs secondary to slow release of tissue factor from the fetal tissue. If expectant management continues beyond a week or two, coagulation studies measuring prothrombin, partial prothrombin, fibrinogen, and platelets can be performed to screen for DIC prior to induction and at intervals.

The essential components of a stillbirth evaluation should include fetal autopsy; gross and histologic examination of the placenta, umbilical cord, and membranes; and genetic evaluation.[139] Ideally, discussions about testing of the fetal remains should begin prior to labor. See the *Complications During Labor and Birth* chapter for further discussion.

### Pregnancy After Prior Stillbirth

When a person has a history of stillbirth, increased surveillance is indicated in a subsequent pregnancy. Compared with persons who have no history of stillbirth, pregnant individuals who have a previous stillborn infant are 4.83 times more likely to have a subsequent stillbirth.[138] Prior to pregnancy or at the first prenatal visit, a detailed history should be obtained to review all information available about the prior stillbirth and the person's medical and obstetric history. Medical records can be ordered if needed, and obstetrician or MFM consultation is recommended to determine a management plan. Plans can be made to mitigate any modifiable factors, such as smoking, cocaine use, or glycemic control for persons with diabetes. Genetic counseling, as well as thrombophilia and antiphospholipid antibody assessment, can be considered. A detailed anatomic ultrasound at 18 to 20 weeks' gestation should be ordered to screen for fetal anomalies and provide reassurance to the pregnant person and family if the ultrasound findings are normal.

In pregnancy after stillbirth, the gestational age of the prior loss is often a time of grief for the pregnant person, family, and providers. Anxiety can also be heightened throughout the third trimester. It is common for a pregnant person to request additional prenatal appointments or fetal surveillance during this time period.

Evidence regarding the ability of weekly fetal surveillance to reduce recurrent stillbirth risk relates directly to the cause of the previous stillbirth. Therefore, in a 2020 consensus statement,[138] ACOG and SMFM recommended that for prior stillbirths associated with specific conditions, such as hypertension or diabetes, fetal surveillance follow the guidelines established for those conditions. For a pregnant person with a previous unexplained stillbirth, because it is unclear whether uteroplacental insufficiency played a role, once- or twice-weekly antenatal surveillance can be offered at 32 0/7 weeks' gestation, or starting 1 to 2 weeks before the gestational age of the previous stillbirth. For a prior stillbirth that occurred before 32 0/7 weeks' gestation, individualized timing of antenatal surveillance can be considered. A shared decision-making model is useful for helping the pregnant person and their family weigh the risk of recurrent stillbirth versus the risk of neonatal morbidity and mortality due to iatrogenic preterm birth when antepartum testing is abnormal.

Shared decision making should also guide conversations about the optimal gestational age for birth. Birth prior to 39 weeks' gestation is associated with increased neonatal morbidity. However, anxiety for the pregnant person may be extreme in the last weeks of pregnancy. In such cases, early term birth (37 to 38 weeks' gestation) can be considered.[138] Shared decision making on the timing of birth can be conducted with the larger perinatal healthcare team, including MFM.

## Techniques for Fetal Surveillance

The terms "fetal surveillance" and "antenatal testing" refer to tests that assess fetal well-being in the late second or early third trimester. The goals of antenatal fetal testing include (1) prevention of stillbirth, (2) identification of the fetus whose oxygen status is compromised so as to allow intervention before irreversible metabolic acidosis ensues, and (3) avoidance of unnecessary interventions when other clinical parameters are equivocal. This section reviews the theory, indications, methodology, and normal versus abnormal findings for the following tests: fetal movement counting, nonstress test (NST), biophysical profile (BPP), contraction stress test (CST), and Doppler indices.

Antenatal testing is a classic "screening test," in that if the results are normal, fetal well-being is assured. In contrast, if results are abnormal, further assessment is indicated to determine fetal well-being or fetal compromise. Antenatal testing can occur as a scheduled screening (discussed later) or as part of an evaluation of an acute concern, such as decreased fetal movement.

Tests for fetal well-being are clinically useful because their negative predictive value is 99% or higher,[140,141] which means that fetal compromise is rare following a normal test result. However, the positive predictive value of tests for fetal well-being is low, meaning that fetal compromise is not proven following an abnormal test result. The incidence of false-positive tests varies between 30% and 60%, depending on the test. Because the tests have such a high false-positive rate, clinical management of abnormal fetal surveillance tests will vary, determined by the overall clinical scenario (see the *Interpreting Published Research Data with a Clinical Midwifery Lens* Appendix).[142] The interpretation of each test is summarized in Table 23-15.

## Fetal Physiologic Indices and Factors That Affect Fetal Behavior

Prenatal surveillance of fetal well-being is based on the observation that specific fetal behavior states reflect adequate oxygenation. The fetal heart rate pattern, level of fetal activity, and degree of muscle tone are sensitive to hypoxemia and acidosis. Therefore, fetal oxygenation can be indirectly evaluated by assessing biophysical parameters, just as vital signs are used to assess well-being in an adult or child. Fetal biophysical behavior that is assessed in the various prenatal fetal tests includes fetal heart rate parameters, fetal movement, fetal tone, fetal breathing, and quantification of amniotic fluid (because the amount of amniotic fluid is an indication of fetal renal function and renal perfusion). Each of these parameters can be affected by a multitude of factors.

| Table 23-15 | Interpretation of Fetal Surveillance Tests | |
|---|---|---|
| **Name** | **Result** | **Criteria** |
| Contraction stress test (CST) or breast stimulation test (BST)[a] | Negative | Normal FHR without late or significant variable decelerations |
| | Equivocal suspicious | Intermittent late decelerations (occurring with < 50% of contractions) or significant variable decelerations |
| | Equivocal | Decelerations that occur in the presence of contractions more frequent than every 2 minutes or lasting longer than 90 seconds |
| | Unsatisfactory | Fewer than 3 contractions in 10 minutes or an uninterpretable tracing |
| | Positive | Recurrent late decelerations following 50% or more of contractions even if fewer than 3 contractions in 10 minutes |
| Nonstress test (NST)[b] | Reactive | ≥ 2 accelerations meeting gestational age criteria within 20 minutes (some settings extend to 40 minutes)[b] |
| | | Can include variable decelerations that are nonrepetitive and brief (less than 30 seconds) |
| | Nonreactive | < 2 accelerations meeting gestational age criteria within 40 minutes |
| Auscultated acceleration test (AAT) | Reactive | An acceleration is present when the FHR is up by two grid points (2 beats/min) in a 5-second period |
| | | A single FHR acceleration indicates reactivity |
| | Unsatisfactory | No accelerations and no fetal movements after fetal stimulation are noted |
| | Nonreactive | No accelerations are noted, even in the presence of fetal movement |
| Biophysical profile (BPP) | Normal | ≥ 8/10 or 8/8 if NST excluded |
| | Equivocal | 6/10 |
| | Abnormal | ≤ 4/10 and/or DVP ≤ 2 cm |
| Modified NST | Normal | Reactive NST and DVP > 2 cm |
| | Abnormal | Nonreactive NST and/or DVP ≤ 2 cm |

Abbreviations: DVP, deepest vertical pocket of amniotic fluid; FHR, fetal heart rate.

[a] This test is interpreted once the pregnant person has at least 3 contractions within 10 minutes.

[b] An acceleration must be 15 beats per minute above the baseline, and must last 15 seconds or more from onset to resolution, after 32 weeks' gestation. The acceleration must be 10 beats per minute above baseline and last 10 seconds in a preterm fetus between 28 and 32 weeks' gestation.

A pregnant person's awareness of fetal movement begins in the second trimester; parous persons usually start feeling the fetus between 16 and 18 weeks, whereas nulliparous persons usually start feeling the fetus between 18 and 22 weeks. Persons who have an anterior placenta may begin detecting fetal movement somewhat later than those with a posterior placenta. Fetal movement is initially slight and irregular, gradually becoming stronger and more frequent. Fetal movement maximizes around 34 weeks, and then appears to become less frequent. This pattern occurs because, as the central nervous system matures, the fetus begins to exhibit longer and cyclic sleep or quiet alert states wherein movement is minimal. Thus, the pregnant person's perception can be one of decreased movement toward the end of the pregnancy. A pregnant person usually perceives approximately 50% of isolated limb movements and 80% of movements that involve both the trunk and the limb.[143] Table 23-16 lists factors that affect perception of fetal behavior.

| Table 23-16 | Factors That Influence Perception of Fetal Movement |
|---|---|

**Decreased Fetal Movement**

Obesity

Sitting or standing position (fetal movement is perceived best in a recumbent position)

Anterior placenta

Amniotic fluid volume (polyhydramnios and oligohydramnios)

Drugs:
- Corticosteroids
- Sedatives and alcohol prolong quiet sleep states
- Tobacco (short period of time after smoking a cigarette)

Hypoglycemia

Fetal spine in an anterior position (occiput anterior)

**No Difference in Perception of Fetal Movement**

Parity

Anxiety

**Increased Fetal Movement**

Recent meal or increase in blood glucose levels

Evening hours: fetal movement is the least evident in the morning

Based on Hijazi ZR, East CE. Factors affecting maternal perception of fetal movement. *Obstet Gynecol Surv.* 2009;64:489-494.

Fetal behavior—including fetal tone, movement, breathing, and fetal heart rate characteristics—changes as the fetus becomes hypoxic. The functions that appear first in gestation disappear last as hypoxia and acidosis increase. In general, loss of fetal heart rate reactivity, fetal heart rate decelerations, and reduced fetal activity are fetal responses to acute hypoxia, whereas oligohydramnios, fetal growth restriction, and altered umbilical artery blood flow are findings indicative of chronic hypoxia. Additional information on the fetal heart rate responses to acute hypoxia can be found in the *Fetal Assessment During Labor* chapter.

## Indications for Antenatal Testing

Although indications for antenatal testing vary between institutions, Table 23-17 lists those tests that are most common across practice settings. It is important to remember that some pregnant persons will choose not to participate in antenatal testing, even if such tests are indicated. This may be due to the burden of additional appointments (time, travel, cost), anxiety regarding the condition indicating testing, or concerns about a cascade of interventions if antepartum testing is abnormal. A shared decision-making model is useful for helping the pregnant person and their family decide whether to accept recommendations for antenatal testing.

Scheduled antenatal testing generally begins at 32 weeks. However, when to start testing varies by condition; current recommendations are to start testing at the gestational age at which stillbirth risk associated with the condition increases to more than 2 times the general population risk.[86] For early-onset conditions with a very high risk of stillbirth (such as severe fetal growth restriction), the age at which testing starts should also reflect when birth and neonatal resuscitation would be considered for abnormal testing results.

Antenatal testing is conducted 1 or 2 times weekly.[86] If the antenatal testing is reassuring (reactive NST, normal BPP) and the pregnant person has only one, moderate-risk condition indicating surveillance (e.g., obesity, pregnancy conceived through in vitro fertilization), testing can be conducted once per week. However, testing should be conducted 2 times per week or in the inpatient setting if previous testing is not reassuring (nonreactive NST, abnormal BPP), surveillance is indicated due to certain high-risk conditions (e.g., growth restriction with abnormal Doppler results, gestational hypertension/preeclampsia, poorly controlled diabetes, antiphospholipid syndrome), or there are signs of deteriorating status for the pregnant person.

| Table 23-17 | Selected Indications for Antenatal Testing[a,b] | |
|---|---|---|
| **Health History of the Pregnant Person** | **Pregnancy Related** | **Fetal–Placental** |
| Age > 35 years | Abnormal first or second trimester serum screening (one or two abnormal values, unexplained) | Chronic placental abruption |
| Current substance use | | Congenital abnormalities |
| Antiphospholipid antibody syndrome | Assisted reproductive technology | Decreased fetal movement |
| Cyanotic heart disease | Cholestasis of pregnancy | Fetal growth restriction |
| Chronic hypertension | Gestational diabetes requiring medications | Oligohydramnios |
| Diabetes (pregestational) | | Polyhydramnios |
| Hemoglobinopathies | Gestational diabetes poorly controlled | Umbilical cord abnormalities (vasa previa, velamentous cord insertion, single umbilical artery) |
| Pre-pregnancy BMI 35 or greater | Gestational hypertension | |
| Previous fetal growth restriction requiring preterm delivery | Late-term or post-term pregnancy | |
| Renal disease | Multifetal gestation | |
| Stillbirth in previous pregnancy | Preeclampsia | |
| Seizure disorder, poorly controlled | | |
| Sickle cell disease | | |
| Systemic lupus erythematosus | | |
| Thyroid disorder poorly controlled | | |

[a] This table presents a representative list of common indications. Individual practices will have indications for prenatal testing identified in collaboration with consulting physicians that may include additional conditions and that may not include some conditions that appear in this table.

[b] Additional indications include conditions such as preterm premature rupture of membranes, Rh isoimmunization, and fetal surgery.

Based on ACOG. Committee Opinion No. 828: indications for outpatient antenatal fetal surveillance. *Obstet Gynecol.* 2021;137:e177-e197.

## Fetal Movement Counting (Kick Counts)

The rationale for formal fetal movement counting is that 30% to 50% of stillbirths occur in low-risk pregnancies with structurally normal fetuses, in which there were no indications for antenatal testing. In addition, fetal movement starts to decrease several days prior to stillbirth, and pregnant persons who report decreased fetal movement have a higher incidence of fetal growth restriction and stillbirth. These observations became the basis for introducing fetal movement counting for the purpose of preventing stillbirth.

More than 40 years of literature and research now exists on the relationship between fetal movement and adverse pregnancy outcomes. The clinical question has long been, "Should all pregnant persons perform formal fetal movement counts during the third trimester, or just persons who are at high risk for stillbirth?" This question has not been definitively answered due to the scarcity of high-quality randomized trials,[144] but a recent meta-analysis suggests routine fetal movement counting may actually increase the risk for intervention and iatrogenic preterm delivery.[142] Therefore, ACOG does not recommend formal fetal movement counting for patients who are not at risk for chronic fetal hypoxia.[141]

The specific fetal movement count that is the best "alarm" or trigger for additional evaluation has not been determined. The method most commonly used is the "count to 10" method, whereby a pregnant person focuses attention on fetal movement and records how long it takes to document 10 fetal movements. If it takes longer than 2 hours, the person should call their midwife. Appropriate follow-up is for the person to come in for an NST (Figure 23-7).

Pregnant persons close to term often call their midwives to report decreased fetal movement. If the person has no risks for uteroplacental insufficiency, it is reasonable to recommend that they eat something, rest in a semi-recumbent position, and then count fetal movement. If the person notes 10 movements in 2 hours, the person and the midwife can be reassured of normalcy. However, if the pregnant person notes fewer than 10 movements, the midwife should arrange a formal nonstress test. The midwife should have a low threshold for recommending

Name _____

At the same time each day, count the baby's movements. When you have felt 10 movements, record the length of time it took. All movements, even small ones, count toward the total. If you have not felt 10 movements in the usual amount of time, please call your midwife.

Week of_____

Hours taken to feel
10 movements of the baby

| Day | Start Time | 1 | 2 | 3 | 4 | 5 | 6 | 7 | 8 | 9 | 10 |
|-----|-----------|---|---|---|---|---|---|---|---|---|----|
| M | | | | | | | | | | | |
| T | | | | | | | | | | | |
| W | | | | | | | | | | | |
| T | | | | | | | | | | | |
| F | | | | | | | | | | | |
| S | | | | | | | | | | | |
| S | | | | | | | | | | | |

**Figure 23-7** Fetal movement counting chart.

that a pregnant person come in for additional testing, even if a person's recent fetal assessment was normal.

### Contraction Stress Test

The CST was the first antenatal fetal test employed in clinical practice. It is based on the observation that uterine contractions transiently restrict blood flow to the intervillous space, thereby lowering oxygen availability to the fetus. The compromised fetus will respond with a late deceleration. (For more description of the pathophysiology of the fetal heart rate response to contractions, see the *Fetal Assessment During Labor* chapter.) The CST entails intravenous administration of oxytocin to initiate uterine contractions and continuous electronic fetal monitoring. A breast stimulation test (BST) may also be performed to initiate contractions, as an alternative to administering intravenous oxytocin.[145] In the BST, the pregnant person massages one nipple through clothing for 2 minutes, followed by a rest for 5 minutes and then a repeat of the procedure on the other nipple. The person should not stimulate the breast during a contraction. The BST and CST are performed in similar fashion, but the BST is associated with more uterine hyperstimulation.[146] Interpretation of results is the same, however.

The fetal response to 3 contractions in a 10-minute window is measured during the test. The CST has the lowest false-negative rate of all antenatal fetal tests (0.04%), but like other tests it has a high false-positive rate (more than 30%). Because the CST is expensive to perform, it is primarily used in inpatient settings, in situations where it is important to establish the fetus's ability to tolerate uterine contractions prior to induction of labor.

### Nonstress Test

The NST is the most common method of antenatal testing used in practice today. Its false-negative rate ranges from 0.3% to 0.65%, and the false-positive rate is approximately 55%.[147] External fetal monitoring is initiated when the pregnant person is in a semi-recumbent or sitting position. The test is concluded when 2 fetal heart rate accelerations appear within a 20-minute window in a fetal heart rate tracing (Figure 23-8). Accelerations are defined by a rise in fetal heart rate of at least 15 beats per minute above baseline lasting at least 15 seconds for fetuses at least 32 weeks' gestation. For fetuses less than 32 weeks' gestation, accelerations are defined by a rise in fetal heart rate of at least 10 beats per minute above baseline lasting at least 10 seconds. If accelerations do not appear in the first 20 minutes, vibroacoustic stimulation may be applied in an effort to stimulate accelerations, and monitoring may continue another 20 minutes. The generation of accelerations via vibroacoustic stimulation does not cause harm to the fetus, and NSTs that become reactive after vibroacoustic stimulation are as valid

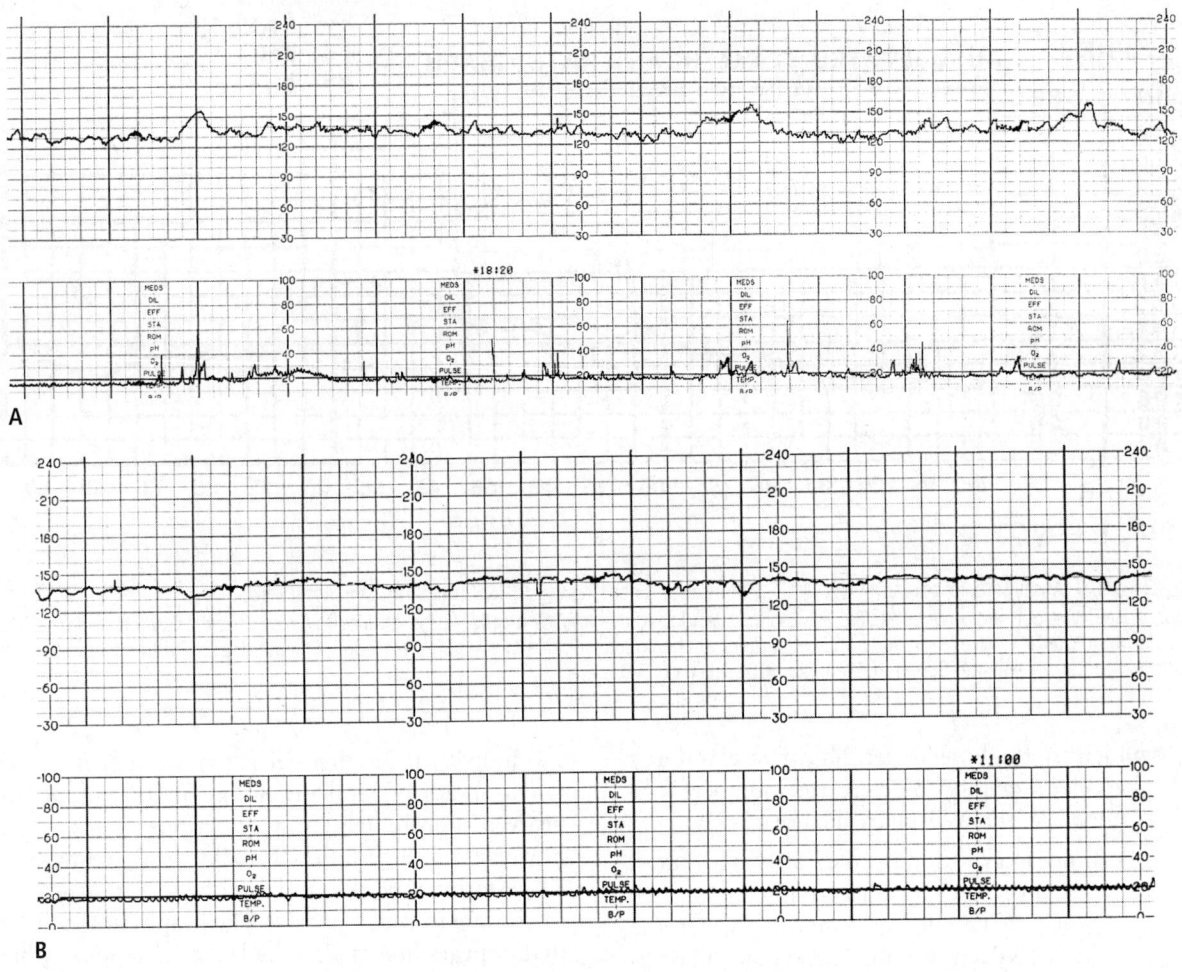

**Figure 23-8 A.** Reactive nonstress test. **B.** Nonreactive nonstress test.

in predicting fetal well-being as NSTs with spontaneous accelerations. The interpretive criteria for NST results are listed in Table 23-16. Management of nonreactive NSTs varies by practice and by the condition for which the NST was performed.

Because a rise in blood glucose can initiate fetal movement, clinicians have traditionally believed that a sudden infusion of glucose via juice or candy would stimulate fetal accelerations. Studies of this practice, however, have found that glucose does not improve the results of antenatal fetal testing.[148]

### Auscultated Acceleration Test

During the 1980s, researchers investigated the use of fetal heart rate auscultation as a means of predicting fetal well-being prenatally.[149] From this work, a method of auscultation was devised as an alternative to the nonstress test. The auscultated acceleration test (AAT) has been validated as a predictor of both reactive and nonreactive NST results

(Figure 23-9).[150] In settings where electronic fetal monitoring is not available or not chosen for use, the AAT is a reliable and valid method of detecting fetal accelerations.

The formal procedure for an AAT requires two clinicians—one auscultating the fetal heart rate and another recording the count on a standard AAT graph. The procedure has the following steps:

- Place the pregnant person in a semi-recumbent, comfortable position.
- Auscultate the fetal heart rate for a maximum of 6 minutes.
- Count every other 5-second interval.
- Record each 5-second count on the AAT graph (Figure 23-9).
- If an acceleration of 2 beats per minute in a 5-second counting interval is noted in conjunction with fetal movement, the test can be stopped.

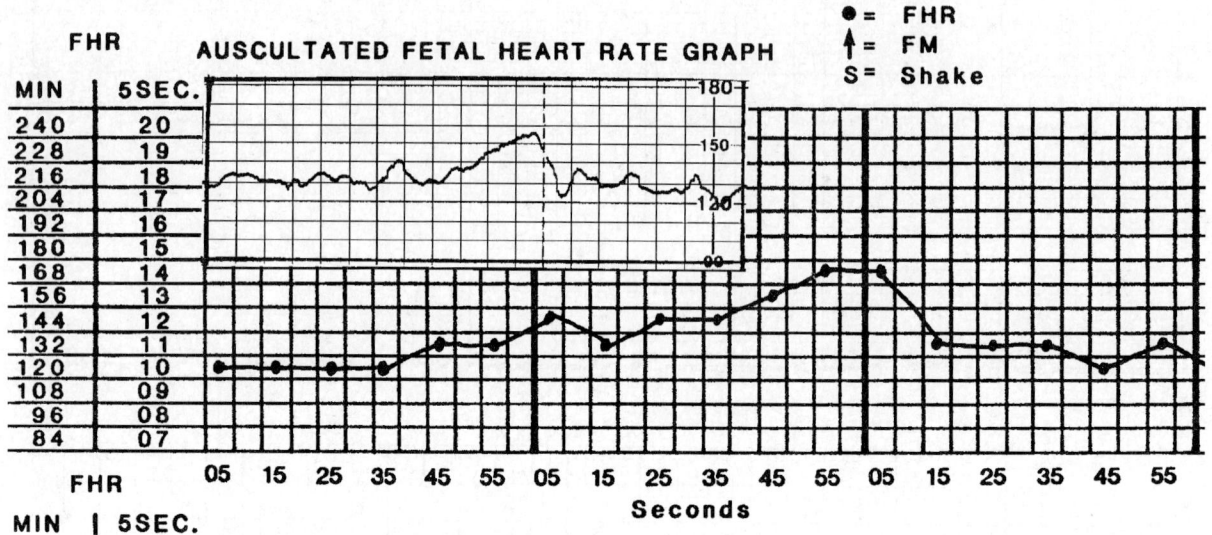

**Figure 23-9** Ausculated acceleration test (AAT) with inset of a nonstress test (NST) completed simultaneously.
Reproduced with permission of Lisa L. Paine, who first developed the AAT with colleagues at Malcolm Grow Medical Center, Andrews AFB, Maryland, and later studied its validity and refinement at the Johns Hopkins Hospital in Baltimore, Maryland, with funding from the NIH National Center for Nursing Research Grant No. R-01-NR-01705-01.

- Identify the baseline fetal heart rate and any accelerations by plotting the numbers obtained on the AAT chart (Figure 23-9).
  - If no acceleration is noted after 3 minutes, the pregnant person's abdomen can be gently shaken in an attempt to awaken the fetus or elicit a more active state. The clinician grasps the fetal head and buttocks and slowly moves the fetus slightly from side to side in a gentle shaking motion for 5 seconds.
  - The fetal heart rate auscultation procedure is repeated for a maximum of 2 to 3 minutes.

### Biophysical Profile

The BPP employs both ultrasound and NST. The ultrasound portion includes observation of amniotic fluid volume, fetal breathing, fetal tone, and fetal movement. The NST provides the fifth component of the test. Each examined factor has a possible score of 2, for a maximum total score of 10 (Table 23-18). The BPP has a lower false-negative rate (0.08%) than the NST. The false-positive rate depends on the specific BPP score, with higher false-positive rates for BPP scores of 6 or 8, compared to scores of 0, 2, or 4.

If all the ultrasound components of the BPP are reassuring, performing the NST is not necessary for confirmation of fetal well-being.

Individual biophysical activities appear at different stages of fetal development. Fetal tone appears at approximately 8 gestational weeks, fetal movement at 9 gestational weeks, fetal breathing at 21 gestational weeks, and fetal heart rate reactivity by the late second trimester. The biophysical activity that appears first is also the last to disappear when acidemia is present. Thus, fetal heart rate variability is first to disappear; conversely, the absence of fetal tone predicts fetal acidemia 100% of the time.

The relationship between the BPP score and fetal acidemia has been studied extensively. A full-term fetus with a score of 8 to 10 has a risk of fetal asphyxia occurring within a week after the test of approximately 1 per 1300 tests, whereas the risk of fetal asphyxia for a fetus with a score of 4 or less is between 91/1000 and 600/1000, respectively.[147]

### Modified Biophysical Profile

The full BPP can take some time to perform. The modified BPP, composed of an NST and AFI, has a similar false-negative rate as the full BPP, though its false-positive rate is 60%. In some clinical settings, it is the most commonly conducted test for fetal surveillance. Nonstress testing can identify acute hypoxia, and decreased amniotic fluid is considered to reflect the presence of chronic hypoxia. The modified BPP has a predictive value similar to that of a full BPP when the NST is reactive and the DVP is higher than 2.0 cm. If the NST is nonreactive or if

| Table 23-18 | The Biophysical Profile | |
|---|---|---|
| **Variable** | **Adequate Score = 2** | **Inadequate Score = 0** |
| Fetal breathing movement | ≥ 1 episode of fetal breathing movements of ≥ 30 seconds in duration | < 30 seconds of sustained fetal breathing movements |
| Fetal movement | ≥ 3 discrete body/limb movements (simultaneous limb and trunk movements are counted as a single movement) | ≤ 2 movements |
| Fetal tone | ≥ 1 episode of active extension with rapid return | Either slow extension with return to partial flexion or movement of limb in full trunk, or hand extension, or absent fetal movement |
| Amniotic fluid volume[a] | DVP > 2 cm that does not include umbilical cord or fetal extremities *or* AFI 5.0–24.0 cm | No pocket of fluid that is > 2 cm *or* AFI < 5.0 cm, oligohydramnios |
| Nonstress test | ≥ 2 accelerations of ≥ 15 beats/min, peak amplitude lasting ≥ 15 seconds from the baseline in 20 minutes | < 2 accelerations or accelerations < 15 beats/min peak amplitude or accelerations < 15 seconds duration in 20 minutes |

Abbreviations: AFI, amniotic fluid index; DVP, deepest vertical pocket.

[a] Either DVP or AFI can be used to assess amniotic fluid volume, though DVP is preferred. Evidence from randomized controlled trials has found that diagnosing oligohydramnios with a DVP < 2 cm is associated with fewer obstetric interventions, when compared to a diagnosis based on AFI.[142]

the DVP is less than 2.0 cm, a complete BPP should be performed.

### Doppler Indices

Doppler ultrasound uses the waveform properties of blood moving through arteries or veins to analyze the rate at which blood passes through those vessels. Evaluation of Doppler velocimetry within the umbilical arteries is an antenatal test used to assess placental resistance in a person who has a growth-restricted fetus.[142]

The umbilical artery velocimetry waveform of normally growing fetuses is characterized by high-velocity diastolic flow. End-diastolic flow in the uterine artery normally increases with advancing gestation, secondary to decreased resistance in the placenta. As more tertiary vessels develop, the pressure within the umbilical artery drops slightly. Thus, the systolic/diastolic ratio of the umbilical artery normally decreases as gestational age increases.[151]

In pregnancies impacted by placental insufficiency, there is increased placental resistance and, therefore, *decreased* umbilical artery end-diastolic flow. In some cases, diastolic flow is absent or even reversed. It is estimated that absent diastolic flow reflects a loss of 60% to 70% of placental function.[152]

Assessment of umbilical artery Doppler velocimetry is a standard component of care for a fetus with growth restriction. Doppler studies should be performed by an experienced ultrasonographer or MFM physician, and they should be interpreted by radiology or MFM. The risk of perinatal death is decreased when uterine artery Doppler studies are added to standard antepartum testing in the setting of fetal growth restriction.

It has been proposed that additional fetal Doppler studies—most notably of the middle cerebral artery and ductus venosus—could improve clinicians' ability to identify a compromised fetus. However, these measurements have not been shown to improve perinatal outcomes for most fetuses with growth restriction.[141] Their use should be directed by MFM and reserved for assessing specific cases, such as a fetus with suspected anemia or cardiac dysfunction.

## Conclusion

Midwives have a long history of caring for persons with complicated pregnancies. Midwives' ability to listen carefully to a pregnant person is an essential component of risk screening and early detection of complications. A midwife who understands the pathophysiology associated with a pregnancy-related condition, as well as the potential impacts of that condition on the pregnant person and fetus/newborn, is well positioned to provide information and continuity of care. Despite complications, midwives can assist persons and families in achieving the best outcomes possible in their current pregnancy, any future pregnancy, and ongoing health. Every person deserves the personalized care of a midwife during pregnancy and birth.

## Resources

| Organization | Description |
| --- | --- |
| **Adolescent Pregnancy** | |
| Geneva Foundation for Medical Education and Research (GFMER) | Guidelines for care of adolescents during pregnancy worldwide. |
| Global Library of Women's Medicine (GLOWM) | Dopkins, Broecker, and Hillard's chapter about pregnancy in adolescence. |
| **Preterm Labor** | |
| Society for Maternal–Fetal Medicine (SMFM) | Preterm Birth Toolkit: SMFM guidelines for risk assessment, prevention, diagnosis, and treatment of spontaneous preterm labor and birth. |
| March of Dimes | The March of Dimes has multiple resources for clinicians and pregnant persons. |
| **Vaginal Birth After Cesarean (VBAC) Calculator** | |
| Maternal–Fetal Medicine Network | Calculator that predicts the chance of VBAC using data available at entry to care or during labor. |

## References

1. American College of Nurse-Midwives, American College of Obstetricians and Gynecologists. Statement of Policy: joint statement of practice relations between Obstetrician-Gynecologists and Certified Nurse-Midwives/Certified Midwives. 2018. http://midwife.org/ACNM/files/ACNMLibraryData/UPLOADFILENAME/000000000224/ACNM-College-Policy-Statement-(June-2018).pdf. Accessed August 19, 2022.

2. American College of Obstetricians and Gynecologists. Obstetric Care Consensus No. 2: levels of maternal care. *Obstet Gynecol*. 2015;2015(125): 502-515.

3. McParlin C, O'Donnell A, Robson SC. Treatments for hyperemesis gravidarum and nausea and vomiting in pregnancy: a systematic review. *JAMA*. 2016;316(13):1392-1401.

4. Boelig RC, Barton SJ, Saccone G, et al. Interventions for treating hyperemesis gravidarum: a Cochrane systematic review and meta-analysis. *J Matern Fetal Neonatal Med*. 2018;31(18):2492-2505. doi:10.1080/14767058.2017.1342805.

5. Fejzo MS, Macgibbon K. Hyperemesis gravidarum: it is time to put an end to the misguided theory of a psychiatric etiology. *Gen Hosp Psychiat*. 2012;34: 699-700.

6. Mitchell-Jones N, Gallos I, Farren J, et al. Psychological morbidity associated with hyperemesis gravidarum: a systematic review and meta-analysis. *BJOG*. 2017;124(1):20-30.

7. Groleau D, Benady-Chorney J, Panaitoiu A, Jimenez V. Hyperemesis gravidarum in the context of migration: when the absence of cultural meaning gives rise to "blaming the victim." *BMC Pregnancy Childbirth*. 2019;19:197. doi:10.1186/s12884-019-2344-1.

8. Lacasse A, Rey E, Ferreira AE, et al. Validity of a modified Pregnancy-Unique Quantification of Emesis and Nausea (PUQE) scoring index to assess severity of nausea and vomiting of pregnancy. *Am J Obstet Gynecol*. 2008;198(1):71.e1-7.

9. King TL, Murphy PA. Evidence-based approaches to managing nausea and vomiting in early pregnancy. *J Midwifery Womens Health*. 2009;54(6):430-444. doi:10.1016/j.jmwh.2009.08.005.

10. Bustos M, Venkataramanan R, Caritis S. Nausea and vomiting of pregnancy: what's new? *Auton Neurosci*. 2017;202:62-72.

11. American College of Obstetricians and Gynecologists. Practice Bulletin No. 189: nausea and vomiting of pregnancy. *Obstet Gynecol*. 2018;131(1):e15-e30. doi:10.1097/AOG.0000000000002456.

12. Oudman E, Wijnia JW, Oey M, et al. Wernicke's encephalopathy in hyperemesis gravidarum: a systematic review. *Eur J Obstet Gynecol Reprod Biol*. 2019;236:84-93. doi:10.1016/j.ejogrb.2019.03.006.

13. Carstairs SD. Ondansetron use in pregnancy and birth defects: a systematic review. *Obstet Gynecol*. 2016;127(5):878-883.

14. Gesterling L, Bradford H. State of the science review: cannabis use in pregnancy. *J Midwifery Womens Health*. November 28, 2021. doi:10.1111/jmwh.13293.

15. Foeller ME, Lyell D. Marijuana use in pregnancy: concerns in an evolving era. *J Midwifery Womens Health*. 2017;62(3):363-367.

16. Alaniz L, Liss J, Metz T, Stickrath E. Cannabinoid hyperemesis syndrome: a cause of refractory nausea

and vomiting in pregnancy. *Obstet Gynecol.* 2015; 125(6):1484-1486.

17. Peter R, Ho J, Valliapan J, Sivasangari S. Symphysial fundal height (SFH) measurement in pregnancy for detecting abnormal fetal growth. *Cochrane Database Syst Rev.* 2015;9:CD008136. doi:10.1002/14651858.

18. American College of Obstetricians and Gynecologists. Practice Bulletin No. 216: macrosomia. *Obstet Gynecol.* 2020;135(1):e18-e35. doi:10.1097 /AOG.0000000000003606.

19. Romero R, Tarca AL. Fetal size standards to diagnose a small- or a large-for-gestational-age fetus. *Am J Obstet Gynecol.* 2018;218(2):S605-S607. doi:10.1016/j.ajog.2017.12.217.

20. World Health Organization. Fetal growth calculator. https://srhr.org/fetalgrowthcalculator/#/. Accessed December 11, 2021.

21. National Institute of Child Health and Human Development. Fetal growth calculator. https://www.nichd .nih.gov/fetalgrowthcalculator. Accessed December 11, 2021.

22. Martins JG, Biggio JR, Abuhamad A. SMFM Consult Series No. 52: diagnosis and management of fetal growth restriction. *Am J Obstet Gynecol.* 2020;223(4):B2-B17. doi:10.1016/j.ajog.2020.05.010.

23. American College of Obstetricians and Gynecologists. Practice Bulletin Number 227: fetal growth restriction. *Obstet Gynecol.* 2021;137(2):e16-e28. doi:10.1097/AOG.0000000000004251.

24. Nardozza LMM, Caetano ACR, Zamarian ACP, et al. Fetal growth restriction: current knowledge. *Arch Gynecol Obstet.* 2017;295(5):1061-1077. doi:10.1007/s00404-017-4341-9.

25. American College of Obstetricians and Gynecologists. Committee Opinion No. 831: medically indicated late-preterm and early-term deliveries. *Obstet Gynecol.* 2021;138(1):e35-e39.

26. Martin JA, Hamilton BE, Osterman MJK. Three decades of twin births in the United States, 1980–2009. *NCHS Data Brief.* 2012;80:1-8. PMID: 22617378.

27. Martin J, Hamilton B, Osterman M, Driscoll A. Births: final data for 2019. *Natl Vital Stat Rep.* 2021;70(2). doi:10.15620/cdc:112078.

28. American College of Obstetricians and Gynecologists. Practice Bulletin No. 231: multifetal gestations: twin, triplet, and higher-order multifetal pregnancies. *Obstet Gynecol.* 2021;137(6):e145-e162. doi:10.1097/AOG.0000000000004397.

29. Goodnight R, Newman W. Optimal nutrition for improved twin pregnancy outcome. *Obstet Gynecol.* 2009;114:1121-1134.

30. Hunter LA. Vaginal breech birth: can we move beyond the term breech trial? *J Midwifery Womens Health.* 2014;59(3):320-327. doi:10.1111/jmwh.12198.

31. Glezerman M. Planned vaginal breech delivery: current status and the need to reconsider. *Expert Rev Obstet Gynecol.* 2012;7:159-166.

32. American College of Obstetricians and Gynecologists. Practice Bulletin No. 221: external cephalic version. *Obstet Gynecol.* 2020;135(5):e203-e212. doi:10.1097/AOG.0000000000003837.

33. Hofmeyr GJ, Kulier R. Cephalic version by postural management for breech presentation. *Cochrane Database Syst Rev.* 2012;10:CD000051. doi:10.1002/14651858.

34. Schlaeger JM, Stoffel CL, Bussell JL, et al. Moxibustion for cephalic version of breech presentation. *J Midwifery Womens Health.* 2018;63(3):309-322. doi:10.1111/jmwh.12752.

35. Asoglu MR, Crimmins S, Kopelman JN, et al. Marginal placental cord insertion: the need for follow up? *J Matern Fetal Neonatal Med.* 2020:1-7. doi:10.1080 /14767058.2020.1763297.

36. Wiedaseck S, Monchek R. Placental and cord insertion pathologies: screening, diagnosis, and management. *J Midwifery Womens Health.* 2014;59:328-335.

37. Taniguchi H, Aoki S, Sakamaki K. Circumvallate placenta: associated clinical manifestations and complications: a retrospective study. *Obstet Gynecol Int.* 2014;2014(986230). doi:10.1155/2014/986230.

38. Reddy UM, Abuhamad AZ, Levine D, Saade GR. Fetal imaging: executive summary of a joint Eunice Kennedy Shriver National Institute of Child Health and Human Development, Society for Maternal–Fetal Medicine, American Institute of Ultrasound in Medicine, American College of Obstetricians and Gynecologists, American College of Radiology, Society for Pediatric Radiology, and Society of Radiologists in Ultrasound Fetal Imaging workshop. *Obstet Gynecol.* 2014;123(5):1070-1082.

39. Silver RM. Abnormal placentation: placenta previa, vasa previa, and placenta accreta. *Obstet Gynecol.* 2015;126:654-668.

40. American College of Obstetricians and Gynecologists, Society for Maternal–Fetal Medicine. Obstetric Care Consensus No. 7: placenta accreta spectrum. *Obstet Gynecol.* 2018;132(6):e259-e275. doi:10.1097/AOG.0000000000002983.

41. MacPhedran SE. Sexual activity recommendations in high-risk pregnancies: what is the evidence? *Sex Med Rev.* 2018;6(3):343-357. doi:10.1016/j .sxmr.2018.01.004.

42. Lim KI, Butt K, Naud K, Smithies M. Amniotic fluid: technical update on physiology and measurement. *J Obstet Gynaecol Can.* 2017;39(1):52-58.

43. Dashe JS, Pressman EK, Hibbard JU. SMFM Consult Series No. 46: evaluation and management of polyhydramnios. *Am J Obstet Gynecol.* 2018;219(4):B2-B8. doi:10.1016/j.ajog.2018.07.016.

44. Sagi-Dain L, Sagi S. Chromosomal aberrations in idiopathic polyhydramnios: a systematic review and meta-analysis. *Eur J Med Genet.* 2015;58(8):409-415.

45. Rossi AC, Prefumo F. Perinatal outcomes of isolated oligohydramnios at term and post-term pregnancy: a systematic review of literature with meta-analysis. *Eur J Obstet Gynecol Reprod Biol.* 2013;169(2):149-154.

46. Kim MA, Kim HS, Kim YH. Reproductive, obstetric and neonatal outcomes in women with congenital uterine anomalies: a systematic review and meta-analysis. *J Clin Med.* 2021;10(21):4797. doi:10.3390/jcm10214797.

47. Hamilton B, Martin J, Osterman M. Births: provisional data for 2020. *Natl Vital Stat Rapid Release.* 2021;12. doi:org/10.15620/cdc:104993.

48. World Health Organization. Born too soon: the global action report on preterm birth. 2012. http://apps.who.int/iris/bitstream/handle/10665/44864/9789241503433_eng.pdf;jsessionid=584814B91A12D6558569844FB1513D6A?sequence=1. Accessed November 26, 2021.

49. American College of Obstetricians and Gynecologists, Society for Maternal–Fetal Medicine. Obstetric Care Consensus No. 6: periviable birth. *Obstet Gynecol.* 2017;130(4):e187-e199. doi:10.1097/AOG.0000000000002352.

50. Manuck TA. Racial and ethnic differences in preterm birth: a complex, multifactorial problem. *Semin Perinatol.* 2017;41(8):511-518.

51. March of Dimes. Neonatal death. 2017. https://www.marchofdimes.org/complications/neonatal-death.aspx. Accessed December 16, 2021.

52. Heron M. Deaths: leading causes for 2019. *Natl Vital Stat Rep.* 2021;70(9). doi:10.15620/cdc:104186.

53. Ding XX, Wu YL, Xu SJ et al. Maternal anxiety during pregnancy and adverse birth outcomes: a systematic review and meta-analysis of prospective cohort studies. *J Affect Disord.* 2014;159:103-110. doi:10.1016/j.jad.2014.02.027.

54. Yonkers KA, Smith MV, Forray A. Pregnant women with posttraumatic stress disorder and risk of preterm birth. *JAMA Psych.* 2014;71(8):897-904.

55. Goldenberg RL, Hauth JC, Andrews WW. Intrauterine infection and preterm delivery. *N Engl J Med.* 2000;342:1500-1509.

56. Han CS, Schatz F, Lockwood CJ. Abruption-associated prematurity. *Clin Perinatol.* 2011;38(3):407-421.

57. Zhang G, Feenstra B, Bacelis JL. Genetic associations with gestational duration and preterm birth. *N Engl J Med.* 2017;377(12):1156-1167.

58. Adams MM, Elam-Evans LD, Wilson HG, Gilbertz DA. Rates and factors associated with recurrence of preterm delivery. *JAMA.* 2000;283:1591-1596.

59. Muglia LJ. The enigma of spontaneous preterm birth. *N Engl J Med.* 2010;362:529-535.

60. Iams JD, Goldenberg RL, Mercer BM. The Preterm Prediction Study: can low risk women destined for spontaneous preterm birth be identified? *Am J Obstet Gynecol.* 2001;184:652-655.

61. McManemy J, Cooke E, Amon E, Leet T. Recurrence risk for preterm delivery. *Am J Obstet Gynecol.* 2007;196(576):1-6.

62. McKinnon B, Yang S, Kramer MS, et al. Comparison of black–white disparities in preterm birth between Canada and the United States. *Can Med Assoc J.* 2016;188(1):E19-E26. doi:10.1503/cmaj.150464.

63. Li Y, Quigley MA, Macfarlane A, et al. Ethnic differences in singleton preterm birth in England and Wales, 2006–12: analysis of national routinely collected data. *Paediatr Perinat Epidemiol.* 2019;33(6):449-458. doi:10.1111/ppe.12585.

64. American College of Obstetricians and Gynecologists. Practice Bulletin No. 234: prediction and prevention of spontaneous preterm birth. *Obstet Gynecol.* 2021;138(2):e65-e90. doi:10.1097/AOG.0000000000004479.

65. Klebanoff MA, Carey JC, Hauth JC. Failure of metronidazole to prevent preterm delivery among pregnant women with asymptomatic *Trichomonas vaginalis* infection. *N Engl J Med.* 2001;345(487):487-493.

66. Manns-James L. Bacterial vaginosis and preterm birth. *J Midwifery Womens Health.* 2011;56(6):575-583.

67. Cunnington M, Korsalioudaki C, Heath P. Genitourinary pathogens and preterm birth. *Curr Opin Infect Dis.* 2013;26:219-230.

68. Schwendicke F, Karimbux N, Allareddy V, Gluud C. Periodontal treatment for preventing adverse pregnancy outcomes: a meta- and trial sequential analysis. *PLoS One.* 2015;10:e0129060.

69. Society for Maternal–Fetal Medicine. SMFM statement: response to EPPPIC and considerations of the use of progestogens for the prevention of preterm birth. 2021. https://www.smfm.org/publications/383-smfm-statement-response-to-epppic-and-considerations-of-the-use-of-progestogens-for-the-prevention-of-preterm-birth. Accessed December 15, 2021.

70. Facco FL, Simhan HN. Short ultrasonographic cervical length in women with low-risk obstetric history. *Obstet Gynecol.* 2013;122(4):858-862. doi:10.1097/AOG.0b013e3182a2dccd.

71. McIntosh J, Feltovich H, Berghella V, Manuck T. SMFM Consult Series No. 40: the role of routine cervical length screening in selected high- and low-risk women for preterm birth prevention. *Am J Obstet Gynecol.* 2016;2016;15(3):B2-B7.

72. Norman JE, Marlow N, Messow CM. Vaginal progesterone prophylaxis for preterm birth

(the OPPTIMUM study): a multicentre, randomised, double-blind trial. *Lancet.* 2016;387(10033): 2106-2116.

73. Romero R, Conde-Agudelo A, Da Fonseca E, et al. Vaginal progesterone for preventing preterm birth and adverse perinatal outcomes in singleton gestations with a short cervix: a meta-analysis of individual patient data. *Am J Obstet Gynecol.* 2018;218(2):161-180. doi:10.1016/j.ajog .2017.11.576.

74. Roman A, Suhag A, Berghella V. Overview of cervical insufficiency: diagnosis, etiologies, and risk factors. *Clin Obstet Gynecol.* 2016;59(2):237-240. doi:10.1097/GRF.0000000000000184.

75. American College of Obstetricians and Gynecologists. Practice Bulletin No. 142: cerclage for the management of cervical insufficiency. *Obstet Gynecol.* 2014;123:372-379.

76. Iams JD, Newman RB, Thom EA. Frequency of uterine contractions and the risk of spontaneous preterm delivery. *N Engl J Med.* 2002;346:250-255.

77. Chao TT, Bloom SL, Mitchell JS, et al. The diagnosis and natural history of false preterm labor. *Obstet Gynecol.* 2011;118:1301-1308.

78. Waters TP, Mercer B. Preterm PROM: prediction, prevention, principles. *Clin Obstet Gynecol.* 2011;54:307-312.

79. American College of Obstetricians and Gynecologists. Practice Bulletin No. 146: management of late term and postterm pregnancies. *Obstet Gynecol.* 2014;124:182-192.

80. American College of Obstetricians and Gynecologists, Society for Maternal–Fetal Medicine. Committee Opinion No. 579: definition of term pregnancy. *Obstet Gynecol.* 2013;122(5):1139-1140.

81. Norwitz ER, Snegovskikh VV, Caughey AB. Prolonged pregnancy: when should we intervene? *Clin Obstet Gynecol.* 2007;50:547-557. doi:10.1097 /GRF.0b013e31804c9b11.

82. Caughey AB, Stotland NE, Washington E, Escobar GJ. Maternal and obstetrical complications of pregnancy are associated with increasing gestational age at term. *Am J Obstet Gynecol.* 2007; 196(155):1-6.

83. Muglu J, Rather H, Arroyo-Manzano D, et al. Risks of stillbirth and neonatal death with advancing gestation at term: a systematic review and meta-analysis of cohort studies of 15 million pregnancies. *PLoS Med.* 2019;16(7):e1002838. doi:10.1371/journal .pmed.1002838.

84. Society for Maternal–Fetal Medicine. SMFM statement: elective induction of labor in low-risk nulliparous women at term: the ARRIVE trial. *Am J Obstet Gynecol.* 2019;221(1):B2-B4. doi:10.1016 /j.ajog.2018.08.009.

85. Middleton P, Shepherd E, Morris J, et al. Induction of labour at or beyond 37 weeks' gestation. *Cochrane Database Syst Rev.* 2020;7. doi:10.1002/14651858 .CD004945.pub5.

86. American College of Obstetricians and Gynecologists. Committee Opinion No. 828: indications for outpatient antenatal fetal surveillance. *Obstet Gynecol.* 2021;137(6):e177-e197. doi:10.1097/AOG .0000000000004408.

87. Finucane EM, Murphy DJ, Biesty LM, et al. Membrane sweeping for induction of labour. *Cochrane Database Syst Rev.* 2020;2. doi:10.1002/14651858 .CD000451.pub3.

88. Kabiri D, Hants Y, Yarkoni TR, et al. Antepartum membrane stripping in GBS carriers, is it safe? (STRIP-G Study). *PLoS One.* 2015;10(12):e0145905. doi:10.1371/journal.pone.0145905.

89. Carlson N, Ellis J, Page K, et al. Review of evidence-based methods for successful labor induction. *J Midwifery Womens Health.* 2021;66(4): 459-469. doi:10.1111/jmwh.13238.

90. Hill MJ, McWilliams GD, Garcia-Sur D, et al. The effect of membrane sweeping on prelabor rupture of membranes: a randomized controlled trial. *Obstet Gynecol.* 2008;111(6):1313-1319. doi:10.1097/AOG .0b013e31816fdcf3.

91. Warshauer E, Mercurio M. Update on dermatoses of pregnancy. *Int J Dermatol.* 2013;52(1):6-13.

92. Mehta N, Chen KK, Kroumpouzos G. Skin disease in pregnancy: the approach of the obstetric medicine physician. *Clin Derm.* 2016;34:320-326.

93. Bechtel MA, Plotner A. Dermatoses of pregnancy. *Clin Obstet Gynecol.* 2015;58(1):104-111.

94. Taylor D, Pappo E, Aronson IK. Polymorphic eruption of pregnancy. *Clin Dermatol.* 2016;34(3):383-391. doi:10.1016/j.clindermatol.2016.02.011.

95. Lee RH, Greenberg M, Metz TD, Pettker CM. SMFM Consult Series No. 53: intrahepatic cholestasis of pregnancy. *Am J Obstet Gynecol.* 2021;224(2):B2-B9. doi:10.1016/j.ajog.2020.11.002.

96. Smith DD, Rood KM. Intrahepatic cholestasis of pregnancy. *Clin Obstet Gynecol.* 2020;63(1):134-151. doi:10.1097/GRF.0000000000000495.

97. Dixon PH, Williamson C. The pathophysiology of intrahepatic cholestasis of pregnancy. *Clin Res Hepatol Gastroenterol.* 2016;40(2):141-153. doi:10.1016/j .clinre.2015.12.008.

98. Sadik CD, Lima AL, Zillikens D. Pemphigoid gestationis: toward a better understanding of the etiopathogenesis. *Clin Dermatol.* 2016;34(3):378-382. doi:10.1016/j.clindermatol.2016.02.010.

99. Cunningham FG, Byrne JJ, Nelson DB. Peripartum cardiomyopathy. *Obstet Gynecol.* 2019;133(1):167-179. doi:10.1097/AOG.0000000000003011.

100. Davis MB, Arany Z, McNamara DM, et al. JACC state-of-the-art review: peripartum cardiomyopathy. *J Am Coll Cardiol*. 2020;75(2):207-221. doi:10.1016/j.jacc.2019.11.014.

101. Dekker RL, Morton CH, Singleton P, Lyndon A. Women's experiences being diagnosed with peripartum cardiomyopathy: a qualitative study. *J Midwifery Womens Health*. 2016;61:467-473.

102. De Haas M, Thurik FF, Koelewijn JM, van der Schoot CE. Haemolytic disease of the fetus and newborn. *VOX Sang*. 2015;109:99-103.

103. Webb J, Delaney M. Red blood cell alloimmunization in the pregnant patient. *Transfus Med Rev*. 2018;32(4):213-219. doi:10.1016/j.tmrv.2018.07.002.

104. American College of Obstetricians and Gynecologists. Practice Bulletin No. 192: management of alloimmunization during pregnancy. *Obstet Gynecol*. 2018;131(3):e82-e90. doi:10.1097/AOG.0000000000002528.

105. American College of Obstetricians and Gynecologists. Practice Bulletin No. 181: prevention of RH D alloimmunization. *Pract Bull*. 2017;130.

106. Mathews TJ. Declines in births to females aged 10–14 in the United States, 2000–2016. *NCHS Data Brief*. 2018;308:1-8.

107. U.S. Department of Health and Human Services, Office of Population Affairs. Trends in teen pregnancy and childbearing. 2021. https://opa.hhs.gov/adolescent-health/reproductive-health-and-teen-pregnancy/trends-teen-pregnancy-and-childbearing. Accessed December 1, 2021.

108. Mathews TJ. Mean age of mothers is on the rise: United States 2000–2014. *NCH Data Brief*. 2016;232:1-8.

109. Maddow-Zimet I, Kost K. *Pregnancies, Births and Abortions in the United States, 1973–2017: National and State Trends by Age*. 2021. https://www.guttmacher.org/report/pregnancies-births-abortions-in-united-states-1973-2017. Accessed December 1, 2021.

110. World Bank. Adolescent fertility rate (births per 1,000 women ages 15–19), 1960–2019. 2021. https://data.worldbank.org/indicator/SP.ADO.TFRT. Accessed February 19, 2022.

111. Leftwich HK, Alves MV. Adolescent pregnancy. *Pediatr Clin North Am*. 2017;64(2):381-388.

112. World Health Organization. Adolescent pregnancy. 2020. https://www.who.int/news-room/fact-sheets/detail/adolescent-pregnancy. Accessed December 1, 2021.

113. American College of Obstetricians and Gynecologists. Committee Opinion No. 803: confidentiality in adolescent health care. *Obstet Gynecol*. 2020;135(4):7.

114. Marvin-Dowle K, Burley VJ, Soltani H. Nutrient intakes and nutritional biomarkers in pregnant adolescents: a systematic review of studies in developed countries. *BMC Pregn Childbirth*. 2016;16(268). doi:10.1186/s12884-016-1059-9. PMID: 27629406; PMCID: PMC5024513.

115. Felder JN, Epel E, Lewis JB. Depressive symptoms and gestational length among pregnant adolescents: cluster randomized control trial of CenteringPregnancy plus group prenatal care. *J Consult Clin Psychol*. 2017;85(6):574-584.

116. Mills TA, Lavender T. Advanced maternal age. *Obstet Gynaecol Reprod Med*. 2014;24(3):85-90.

117. American College of Obstetricians and Gynecologists. Committee Opinion No. 743: low-dose aspirin use during pregnancy. *Obstet Gynecol*. 2018;132(1):9.

118. Lean SC, Derricott H, Jones RL, Heazell AEP. Advanced maternal age and adverse pregnancy outcomes: a systematic review and meta-analysis. *PLoS One*. 2017;12(10):e0186287. doi:10.1371/journal.pone.0186287.

119. Fonseca MJ, Santos F, Afreixo V, et al. Does induction of labor at term increase the risk of cesarean section in advanced maternal age? A systematic review and meta-analysis. *Eur J Obstet Gynecol Reprod Biol*. 2020;253:213-219. doi:10.1016/j.ejogrb.2020.08.022.

120. Stern JE, Luke B, Tobias M, et al. Adverse pregnancy and birth outcomes associated with underlying diagnosis with and without assisted reproductive technology treatment. *Fertil Steril*. 2015;103(6):1438-1445.

121. American College of Obstetricians and Gynecologists. Committee Opinion No. 671: perinatal risks associated with assisted reproductive technology. *Obstet Gynecol*. 2016;128:e61-e68.

122. Downing J, Everett B, Snowden JM. Differences in perinatal outcomes of birthing people in same-sex and different-sex marriages. *Am J Epidemiol*. 2021;190(11):2350-2359. doi:10.1093/aje/kwab148.

123. Wax J, Minkoff H, Johnson A, et al. Consensus report on the detailed fetal anatomic ultrasound examination: indications, components, and qualifications. *J Ultrasound Med*. 2014;33(2):189-195. doi:10.7863/ultra.33.2.189.

124. Goodman D, Danel I. Female genital mutilation/cutting in the United States: updated estimates of women and girls at risk, 2012. *Public Health Rep*. 2016;131(2):340-347.

125. Jacoby SD, Smith A. Increasing certified nurse-midwives' confidence in managing the obstetric care of women with female genital mutilation/cutting. *J Midwifery Womens Health*. 2013;58(4):451-456.

126. Johansen REB. Virility, pleasure and female genital mutilation/cutting: a qualitative study of perceptions

and experiences of medicalized defibulation among Somali and Sudanese migrants in Norway. *Reprod Health*. 2017;14(1):25. doi:10.1186/s12978-017-0287-4.

127. Guise JM, Eden K, Emeis C, et al. Vaginal birth after cesarean: new insights. *Evid Report Technology Assess*. 2010;191:1-397.

128. National Institutes of Health. NIH Consensus Development Conference: vaginal birth after cesarean: new insights. *NIH Consens State Sci Statements*. 2010;27(3). https://consensus.nih.gov/2010/images/vbac/vbac_statement.pdf. Accessed August 19, 2022.

129. American College of Nurse-Midwives. Clinical Bulletin No. 12: care for women desiring a vaginal birth after cesarean. *J Midwifery Womens Health*. 2011;56:517-525.

130. Cox K. Counseling women with a previous cesarean birth: toward a shared-decision making partnership. *J Midwifery Womens Health*. 2014;59:237-245.

131. Grobman WA, Sandoval G, Rice MM, et al. Prediction of vaginal birth after cesarean delivery in term gestations: a calculator without race and ethnicity. *Am J Obstet Gynecol*. 2021;225(6):664.e1-664.e7. doi:10.1016/j.ajog.2021.05.021.

132. Thornton PD, Liese K, Adlam K, et al. Calculators estimating the likelihood of vaginal birth after cesarean: uses and perceptions. *J Midwifery Womens Health*. 2020;65(5):621-626. doi:10.1111/jmwh.13141.

133. Bovbjerg ML, Cheyney M, Brown J, et al. Perspectives on risk: assessment of risk profiles and outcomes among women planning community birth in the United States. *Birth*. 2017;44(3):209-221.

134. Tilden EL, Cheyney M, Guise JM. Vaginal birth after cesarean: neonatal outcomes and United States birth setting. *Am J Obstet Gynecol*. 2017;216(4):403.e1-403.e8.

135. American College of Nurse-Midwives. Share with women: birth options after having a cesarean. *J Midwifery Womens Health*. 2016;61(6):799-800. doi:10.1111/jmwh.12583.

136. American Association of Birth Centers. Clinical bulletin: VBAC: labor and birth after cesarean in the birth center setting. May 10, 2019. https://cdn.ymaws.com/www.birthcenters.org/resource/resmgr/about_aabc_-_documents/AABC_Clinical_Bulletin_-_VBA.pdf. Accessed February 19, 2022.

137. American College of Obstetricians and Gynecologists. Practice Bulletin No. 205: vaginal birth after cesarean delivery. 2019;133(2):18. doi:10.1097/AOG.0000000000003078. PMID: 30681543.

138. Gregory ECW, Valenzuela CP, Hoyert DL. Fetal mortality: United States, 2020. *National Vital Statistics Reports*. 2020; 71(4). doi:10.15620/cdc:118420.

139. American College of Obstetricians and Gynecologists, Society for Maternal–Fetal Medicine. Obstetric Care Consensus No. 10: management of stillbirth. *Obstet Gynecol*. 2020;135(3):e110-e132. doi:10.1097/AOG.0000000000003719.

140. Manning FA. Antepartum fetal testing: a critical appraisal. *Curr Opin Obstet Gynecol*. 2009; 21:348-352.

141. Oyelese Y, Vintzileos AM. The use and limitations of the fetal biophysical profile. *Clin Perinatol*. 2011;38:47-64.

142. American College of Obstetricians and Gynecologists. Practice Bulletin No. 229: antepartum fetal surveillance. *Obstet Gynecol*. 2021;137(6):e116-e127. doi:10.1097/AOG.0000000000004410.

143. Hijazi ZR, East CE. Factors affecting maternal perception of fetal movement. *Obstet Gynecol Surv*. 2009;64:489-494.

144. Mangesi L, Hofmeyr GJ, Smith V, Smyth RMD. Fetal movement counting for assessment of fetal wellbeing. *Cochrane Database Syst Rev*. 2015;10:CD004909. doi:10.1002/14651858.CD004909.pub3.

145. Huddleston JF, Sutliff G, Robinson D. Contraction stress test by intermittent nipple stimulation. *Obstet Gynecol*. 1984;63(5):669-673.

146. Hill WC, Moenning RK, Katz M, Kitzmiller JL. Characteristics of uterine activity during the breast stimulation stress test. *Obstet Gynecol*. 1984;64(4):489-492.

147. Signore C, Freeman RK, Spong CY. Executive summary of a Eunice Kennedy Shriver National Institute of Child Health and Human Development Workshop: antenatal testing: a reevaluation. *Obstet Gynecol*. 2009;113(3):687-701.

148. Tan KH, Sabapathy A. Maternal glucose administration for facilitating tests of fetal wellbeing. *Cochrane Database Syst Rev*. 2012;9:CD003397. doi:10.1002/14651858.CD003397.pub2.

149. Paine LL, Johnson TR, Turner MH, Payton RG. Auscultated fetal heart rate accelerations part II: an alternative to the nonstress test. *J Nurse-Midwifery*. 1989;31(2):73-77.

150. Paine LL, Zanardi LR, Johnson TR, et al. A comparison of two time intervals for the auscultated acceleration test. *J Midwifery Womens Health*. 2001;46(2):98-102. doi:10.1016/s1526-9523(01)00102-7.

151. Kennedy AM, Woodward PJ. A radiologist's guide to the performance and interpretation of obstetric Doppler ultrasound. *RadioGraphics*. 2019;39(3):893-910. doi:10.1148/rg.2019180152.

152. Alfirevic Z, Stampalija T, Dowswell T. Fetal and umbilical Doppler ultrasound in high-risk pregnancies. *Cochrane Database Syst Rev*. 2017;(6). doi:10.1002/14651858.CD007529.pub4.

CHAPTER

# 24

# Medical Complications in Pregnancy

JULIE KNUTSON, ANA SOFIA BARBER DE BRITO, AND LINDA HUNTER

*The editors acknowledge Tekoa L. King, Mayri Sagady Leslie, and Jan M. Kriebs, who were authors of this chapter in previous editions.*

## Introduction

This chapter reviews medical complications that may occur during pregnancy or exist prior to conception. Many chronic illnesses and diseases are affected by the normal physiologic changes that occur during the perinatal period. Conditions may worsen, improve, or exhibit variable trajectories. Common pregnancy symptoms can also impact timely diagnosis, management, and prognosis of newly acquired infections and illnesses. Medical complications during pregnancy may require consultation with the appropriate specialists to develop a comprehensive interdisciplinary plan of care. Ideally, care models should be flexible, dynamic, and responsive to the unique needs of the pregnant person and their family. In all circumstances, the optimal care of the individual and their fetus will drive care decisions, which may necessitate physician referral.

Midwives may be the first healthcare provider to see a person who has increased risks for adverse perinatal outcomes secondary to a medical disorder, including individuals who present for preconception counseling. Identification of risks and consultation, when indicated, is an essential component of midwifery care. Thus, midwives need the knowledge necessary to identify perinatal risks so that they can obtain a thorough history, consult with appropriate specialists, and initiate evaluations when required.

Midwives also often identify social determinants of care and provide ancillary and supportive care for people with increased risks of poor outcomes. For those with complex medical disorders, prenatal visits can involve many tests and discussions of possible adverse outcomes. Midwifery visits can help a person who has a high-risk pregnancy in several ways. For example, a visit may focus on the "normal" aspects of the pregnancy, thereby helping the person preserve their sense of well-being. The midwife may also participate in education and support for the extra care required to treat a medical complication.

This chapter does not provide a comprehensive review of all possible medical conditions that can adversely impact the course of pregnancy. Instead, commonly encountered problems are discussed as exemplars of the approach midwives take in caring for a person with a preexisting medical disorder or when a medical disorder arises during pregnancy. For the convenience of the readers, these conditions are generally presented in an alphabetical order rather than frequency of occurrence.

## Autoimmune Disorders

Autoimmune disorders are a broad classification of disorders in which aberrations in the immune response result in the immune system attacking the individual's healthy body tissue. Examples include systemic lupus erythematosus (SLE), multiple sclerosis, rheumatoid arthritis, and irritable bowel syndrome. During pregnancy, the immune system changes under the influence of various hormonal

963

changes. Because of pregnancy, some autoimmune disorders (e.g., rheumatoid arthritis, multiple sclerosis) can improve. For others, pregnancy has no effect on the progress of the disorder, but the disorder or treatment can have adverse effects on the course of pregnancy (e.g., SLE). Treatment of autoimmune disorders focuses on suppressing abnormal immune function, and a similar group of medications is used to treat many of these disorders. SLE is presented as an example of the topics of import involved in caring for a person with an autoimmune disorder during pregnancy.

## Systemic Lupus Erythematosus

Systemic lupus erythematosus (SLE) is an autoimmune connective tissue disorder involving multiple body systems. The pathogenesis of SLE occurs secondary to an immune dysregulation of B cells that results in abnormally increased production of antibodies to nuclear antigens and other self-antigens not usually identified by the immune system as "foreign." Multiple immune pathways contribute to the inflammation associated with this disorder.[1] SLE is more common among people with two X chromosomes and appears primarily during the reproductive years.[2] The nature of the disease is highly variable, characterized by multiple symptoms, periodic remissions and flare-ups, and differing patterns of progression and prognosis. The genetic and environmental contributions are each approximately 50%.[1]

There are no generally accepted diagnostic criteria for lupus.[1] More than 90% of patients, however, have skin manifestations. Signs and symptoms of flares in pregnancy may include antinuclear antibodies, lupus antibodies, hemolytic anemia or thrombocytopenia, persistent proteinuria, lymphadenopathy, inflammatory arthritis, oral or nasal ulceration, and photosensitive rash.[3] Some symptoms mimic findings associated with normal pregnancy changes, such as facial flushing, fatigue, mild dyspnea, palmar erythema, anemia, and mild thrombocytopenia, which makes detection of an SLE flare challenging.[3]

Several medications from different drug classes are used to help people manage SLE. Some are safe for the pregnant person and the fetus, whereas others are contraindicated.[3] Thus, a thorough review of current medications is one of the initial assessments when caring for a person with SLE or another autoimmune disorder.

SLE does not significantly affect fertility, but pregnancy may increase disease activity and, depending on the systems affected, can lead to serious complications for both the pregnant person and fetus. One meta-analysis of 37 studies on SLE in pregnancy reported increased risks of lupus flare (25%), hypertension (16%), nephritis (16%), preeclampsia (7.6%), and eclampsia (0.8%).[3] People with SLE are at increased risk for thrombotic events during pregnancy and postpartum.[3] Presence of lupus anticoagulant (an antiphospholipid antibody) or autoimmune thyroid antibodies are associated with adverse pregnancy outcomes.[2]

Potential fetal complications of SLE include miscarriage, preterm birth (33%), fetal growth restriction, stillbirth, and neonatal death.[3] Neonatal lupus is an autoimmune disorder acquired by the fetus secondary to passive transfer across the placenta of maternal autoantibodies; these autoantibodies primarily attack the fetus's skin and heart. Fetal/neonatal congenital heart block occurs in approximately 2% of pregnancies affected by SLE and may be identified by Doppler auscultation of the fetal heart; bradycardia warrants urgent referral to a maternal–fetal medicine (MFM) specialist. Risks for all complications increase if the pregnant person has lupus nephritis and antiphospholipid, anti-SS-A(Ro) and anti-SS-B(La) antibodies.[3]

### Management of Lupus Erythematosus

Monitoring of persons with SLE during pregnancy includes baseline and serial laboratory tests to assess for SLE flare, serial ultrasonography with Doppler, weekly biophysical profile in the third trimester, and fetal echocardiography for people who have anti-SS-A(Ro) antibodies or whose fetus has a dysrhythmia.[3] Clients are followed closely for disease exacerbation, thrombotic events, and hypertensive disorders. When a person with SLE is seen for a prenatal visit by a midwife, accurate assessment of blood pressure and urinalysis are essential, as these tests will help detect the onset of a lupus flare. Individuals with a lupus flare are best managed by a team including high-risk obstetric care providers and subspecialists. The best pregnancy outcomes occur among people who have not had a lupus flare for 6 or more months preceding pregnancy.[2]

Risks of preeclampsia and fetal growth restriction can be reduced by initiating low-dose aspirin (LDA) after 12 weeks' gestation and prior to 16 weeks' gestation; LDA is especially important for those individuals with SLE complicated by renal disease, hypertension or a history of preeclampsia, and antiphospholipid syndrome.[3] Daily LDA should continue until shortly before birth and then resume postpartum. Treatment with hydroxychloroquine

(Plaquenil) is considered safe throughout pregnancy and reduces lupus symptoms, risk for thrombosis, and congenital heart block.[2] Low-molecular-weight heparin is indicated to prevent fetal loss and thrombosis in those persons with antiphospholipid syndrome.[2] Nonfluorinated glucocorticoids (i.e., prednisone and prednisolone) can be used for lupus flares throughout pregnancy.[3] Calcium supplementation may reduce risk of preeclampsia and preterm birth. People with lupus are more likely to be vitamin D deficient and may need supplementation.[3] Breastfeeding/chestfeeding is not contraindicated in people with SLE or who are taking the medications used for its treatment; thus, it should be discussed as usual prenatally.[3]

SLE provides an example of how the midwife can collaborate in the care of a person with a high-risk medical condition during pregnancy. The first step is to conduct a thorough history and identify any immediate concerning symptoms. Next, review the individual's current medications to determine whether any are contraindicated or of concern for use in pregnancy. People with significant risks are referred to physician care for urgent evaluation. For people who have SLE but no immediate risks, physician consultation is obtained to identify tests or laboratory evaluations that need to be scheduled and the appropriate timing for a physician visit. Once the person has a plan of care developed with the appropriate obstetric specialist, the midwife can conduct subsequent prenatal visits as indicated.

# Cancer

The incidence of a new cancer diagnosis during pregnancy is approximately 1 in 1000.[4] This incidence is increasing as pregnancy is often delayed until after age 30. Breast cancer accounts for the majority of cases, followed in decreasing incidence by cervical cancer, lymphoma, ovarian cancer, colorectal cancer, and melanoma.[5] Although cancer is a rare event during pregnancy, it is a devastating complication laden with decisional conflict between minimizing fetal risks and optimizing survival for the pregnant person. Diagnosis is often delayed due to overlapping symptoms commonly seen during pregnancy. Fatigue, nausea, breast changes, bowel symptoms, and anemia are a few examples of symptoms that may be overlooked in a developing malignancy.[4] In addition, more recent evidence suggests an association between abnormal noninvasive prenatal testing (NIPT) results and an underlying malignancy in the pregnant person.[6] In situations where a cell-free DNA screening suggests multiple fetal aneuploidies, referral to genetics counseling and/or MFM is warranted.[6]

## Diagnosis and Treatment

The type of diagnostic testing used for suspected cancer is often determined in consultation with specialists. Ultrasound is the preferred diagnostic imaging modality when symptoms of cancer are encountered. Magnetic resonance imaging (MRI) without contrast can also be utilized in situations where ultrasound is inadequate or has questionable value. Due to the increased fetal risks associated with radiation exposure, computed tomography (CT) is not recommended during pregnancy. Chest x-ray and mammography emit lower radiation doses and can be performed with appropriate abdominal shielding. Pregnancy is not a contraindication for other diagnostic tests such as biopsies, endoscopies, bone marrow aspiration, or lumbar puncture.[4]

Any diagnosis of cancer during pregnancy will require a multidisciplinary approach, preferably undertaken at a tertiary center.[5] This will include referral to MFM and the appropriate oncology specialist for coordination of care. Midwives are important members of this team and can provide considerable emotional support and anticipatory guidance with some of the difficult decisions facing the patient and their family.

Pregnant persons with cancer will need detailed counseling regarding treatment options and how the pregnancy might affect the best plan of care. Treatment recommendations and prognosis are similar for pregnant and nonpregnant individuals and will depend on the type of cancer, staging, and gestational age.[4] Most chemotherapy agents are considered safe in the second and third trimesters, but are discontinued during the last 3 weeks of pregnancy to avoid hematologic complications during delivery. Radiation carries significant fetal risks and is generally avoided until after pregnancy.[4] Registries such as the International Network on Cancer, Infertility and Pregnancy (INCIP) can provide updated clinical recommendations based on the best available evidence.[5]

Balancing fetal risks while optimizing the perinatal outcome is paramount. Pregnancy termination options are an essential part of these discussions, especially in previable gestations.[4] Midwives should be aware of the legal status of pregnancy termination and available resources within their respective states, including gestational age limits when the pregnant individual's life is in jeopardy. See the *Early Pregnancy Loss and Abortion* chapter for in-depth discussion of these issues.

## Pregnancy After Cancer

It is well known that most cancer therapies will negatively affect ovarian function and limit the potential for future conception.[7] Over the past several years, however, advances in cancer treatment have improved survivorship, especially for those persons diagnosed during childhood, adolescence, and early adulthood. Recent evidence suggests these subgroups have an overall 80% survival rate, especially for those previously treated for non-Hodgkin lymphoma, melanoma, or thyroid cancer.[8] Given these statistics, younger individuals diagnosed with cancer have likely been counseled on fertility preservation strategies prior to initiating treatment. Details of these options and their implications for cancer treatment can be found elsewhere.[7]

Cancer survivors who desire pregnancy will need multidisciplinary preconception counseling and may conceive via assisted reproductive procedures such as in vitro fertilization (IVF). In general, pregnancy has not been associated with recurrence of cancer; however, research suggests survivors have increased risks of complications such as gestational diabetes and preterm birth.[7] Individuals who achieve pregnancy after cancer treatment are best managed in collaboration with MFM specialists and may give birth at a tertiary center.[7]

## Breastfeeding After Cancer

In those cancer survivors who achieve pregnancy, discussions and support for breastfeeding are vital. Breast cancer survivors in particular may face several challenges, especially after mastectomy. Prior cancer therapies are not known to affect breast milk supply in the remaining (untreated) breast, and contralateral breastfeeding can be encouraged. In contrast, decreased milk supply has been reported in breasts previously treated with radiation.[9]

Despite the benefits of breastfeeding for both infants and survivors, barriers such as negative family and medical advice exist. Fear of breast cancer recurrence in the lactating breast has also been cited as a deterrent, although there is no evidence to support this fear. Strategies to encourage breastfeeding in this unique population include early lactation consultation and evidence-based education to the patient, family, and care team to dispel fears and challenges.[9]

## Cardiovascular Disease

Cardiovascular disease, defined as dysfunction of the heart and vascular system, affects approximately 1% to 4% of pregnant people annually, and accounts for 26.5% of pregnancy-related deaths in the United States.[10] Non-Hispanic Black individuals are disproportionately affected.[10] Disparities in cardiovascular-related disease complications can be explained in part by racial and ethnic bias in health care.[11] Systemic factors contributing to perinatal mortality from cardiac disease include inaccurate diagnosis, underestimation of condition severity, and lack of early referral to cardiac specialists.[12] Additional risk factors for mortality include age older than 40, hypertensive disorders, and pre-pregnancy obesity.[11]

The physiologic changes of pregnancy place increased demands on the cardiovascular system, including an increase in cardiac output and blood volume, a decrease in systemic vascular resistance, and an increase in blood pressure in the third trimester. In healthy people, hemodynamic changes related to pregnancy return to a pre-pregnancy state by 3 to 6 months postpartum.[11] However, people with heart conditions may have greater difficulty adjusting to pregnancy-related cardiovascular changes and can experience a decline in function that may not return after birth. Fetal risks are greater when compared to pregnancies not affected by cardiovascular disease and include miscarriage, preterm birth, and perinatal mortality.[13] Pulmonary edema and arrhythmias are the most common intrapartum cardiac complications.[14] The California Improving Health Care Response to Cardiovascular Disease in Pregnancy and Postpartum toolkit algorithm can be used to screen all people for heart disease during pregnancy and postpartum.[11]

## Management of Cardiovascular Disease

People with cardiovascular disease should be seen by a cardiologist prior to or as early as possible during pregnancy. Multidisciplinary care by a : "pregnancy heart team," including providers with specialty training in managing heart conditions in pregnancy, is essential for achieving optimal outcomes.[11,15] Midwives may contribute to optimal team-based care as part of a multidisciplinary team.[15]

Midwives must be familiar with the signs and symptoms of heart disease to ensure appropriate referral and cardiac evaluation. The type of testing and timing of evaluation depend on the underlying condition and the presenting symptoms. Symptoms of cardiac disease can mimic normal physiologic changes of pregnancy, but individuals with shortness of breath at rest or while sleeping, marked fluid retention, extreme fatigue, chest pain at rest or with little exertion, palpitations, or arrhythmias should undergo prompt evaluation for heart disease. An echocardiogram is indicated for people with these symptoms to assess for cardiomyopathy.[11] Pregnant and postpartum people presenting with chest pain should undergo immediate troponin testing and an electrocardiogram to evaluate for acute coronary syndrome.[11]

A modified World Health Organization (WHO) classification of cardiovascular risk in pregnancy helps providers determine the appropriate frequency for cardiology evaluation.[11] High-risk conditions include pulmonary hypertension, congenital heart disease, noncongenital valvular disease, dilated hypertrophic or peripartum cardiomyopathy, aortic disorders, and coronary artery disease.[11] Pregnancy is strongly discouraged for those people considered to be at very high risk; pregnant individuals falling into this category require close follow-up with cardiac specialists. Lower-risk conditions include uncomplicated or mild pulmonary stenosis, patent ductus arteriosus, mitral valve prolapse, successfully repaired simple lesions, and isolated ectopic beats.[11] Clients with cardiac conditions often require medications in pregnancy; several classes of medications, such as warfarin, angiotensin-converting enzyme inhibitors, angiotensin receptor blockers, and aldosterone antagonists, should be avoided when possible due to potential fetal effects.[11] For the fetus, a history of congenital heart disease in a genetic parent warrants an echocardiogram to screen for defects.

Labor and birth lead to changes in plasma volume, blood pressure, heart rate, and cardiac output, making the early postpartum period an important time for follow-up to screen for complications of cardiac disease. Risks are compounded by birth-related complications such as hypertension, hemorrhage, and infection.[11] Cardiac disease is associated with pregnancy-related death up to 1 year postpartum.[11]

Most medications for cardiac conditions are compatible with breastfeeding/chestfeeding.[16] Intrauterine devices and implants are effective and safe postpartum contraceptive methods for most clients with cardiovascular disease. Combined hormonal contraceptives may increase risks and are typically not appropriate for use in individuals with prothrombogenic states, uncontrolled hypertension, ischemic heart disease, and complicated valvular disease.[11]

## Diabetes

Diabetes is a disease resulting in elevated blood glucose levels that impact numerous body systems. Three general categories of diabetes are distinguished: type 1, type 2, and gestational diabetes

mellitus (GDM). Type 1 and type 2 diabetes are collectively termed *pregestational diabetes mellitus* (PGDM).[17,18,24] A fourth syndrome, *prediabetes*, is defined as high blood glucose levels in a person who does not meet all the criteria for the diagnosis of diabetes, but is at increased risk for developing diabetes.

Gestational diabetes and type 2 diabetes are diseases of insulin resistance, whereas type 1 diabetes is characterized by beta cells in the pancreas producing little or no insulin. GDM is further categorized A1GDM, in which diet and exercise result in euglycemia, and A2GDM, in which medication is needed to maintain euglycemia.[17,24] Although GDM has historically been considered a pregnancy-related complication, today it is evident that the outcomes and treatments of individuals with all types of diabetes are directly related to the severity of glucose dysregulation. Therefore, it is useful to consider this group of diseases together.

In the United States, 1% to 2% of people have type 1 or 2 diabetes in pregnancy and 6% to 9% develop GDM.[19] Alternative diagnostic criteria proposed by the International Association of Diabetes in Pregnancy Summary Groups (IADPSG) would increase the prevalence of GDM to 15% to 20%.[20] The incidences of prediabetes, type 2 diabetes, and GDM are increasing in parallel with rising rates of obesity.[17]

### Pathophysiology of Diabetes in Pregnancy

The dynamics of glucose metabolism evolve from early to late pregnancy as physiologic insulin resistance gradually increases and peaks in the late second to third trimester. As the placenta grows, levels of human placental lactogen (hPL) and other diabetogenic hormones increase. These hormones increase cellular resistance to insulin, which results in higher blood glucose levels. In most people, the pancreas can increase the production of insulin to counterbalance the insulin resistance effect of placental hormones. Overt hyperglycemia occurs when the pancreas is unable to produce adequate amounts of insulin. The peak effect of hPL occurs around 26 to 28 weeks' gestation, which coincides with the recommended window for GDM screening. Pre-pregnant insulin sensitivity returns in the postpartum period. Optimal treatment of diabetes in pregnancy is responsive to these dynamic changes.[21]

If hyperglycemia and hyperinsulinemia remain unchecked during pregnancy, this can stimulate hypergrowth in both the placenta and the fetus. As increasing amounts of glucose cross the placenta, the fetus must increase production of insulin to metabolize the increased glucose.[17] Increased glucose can also cause dramatic growth in the fetus, which has been shown to predispose these infants to childhood obesity, type 2 diabetes, and metabolic syndrome.[22,23]

Gestational diabetes is associated with an increased risk of pregnancy complications, including preeclampsia, preterm birth, macrosomia, shoulder dystocia, neonatal jaundice and hypoglycemia, and neonatal intensive care unit (NICU) admission.[20] The Hyperglycemia and Pregnancy Outcomes trial placed pregnant people ($n = 23,316$) into three categories based on their degree of hyperglycemia and identified a significant increase in adverse pregnancy outcomes as glucose levels rose.[22] Subsequent studies have also shown that people with GDM are 10 times more likely compared to people who had normoglycemic pregnancies to develop type 2 diabetes, with 70% developing type 2 diabetes within 22 to 28 years after pregnancy.[17,23] People with PGDM have increased risks for the same pregnancy complications as those with GDM according to the degree of hyperglycemia experienced throughout pregnancy. Additional risks associated with PGDM include chronic hypertension, retinopathy, nephropathy, acute myocardial infarction, diabetic ketoacidosis, miscarriage, and stillbirth.[24]

Treatment of GDM and PGDM reduces the risk of adverse outcomes in conjunction with improved glucose control.[23–25] Studies suggest that as many as 85% of people with GDM can control their glucose levels with lifestyle changes alone.[21] Individuals with PGDM typically require medication in addition to nutrition and exercise interventions, as described later in this section.

### Diagnosis of Diabetes

The diagnosis of diabetes in nonpregnant adults is reviewed in the *Common Conditions in Primary Care* chapter. However, some people who are given the diagnosis of GDM actually have undiagnosed PGDM. To clarify the distinction between pregestational diabetes and GDM, the American Diabetes Association (ADA) defines GDM as "diabetes diagnosed in the second or third trimester of pregnancy that is not clearly type 1 or 2 diabetes." Diabetes initially detected in the first or early second trimester by HbA1c, fasting plasma glucose greater than 126 mg/dL, or a 2-hour glucose of 200 mg/dL or greater on a 75-gram glucose tolerance test (GTT) is given the diagnosis of PGDM.[18,24] Screening for diabetes during pregnancy is reviewed in the *Prenatal Care* chapter. Diagnosis and prenatal care for people with all types of diabetes are presented in this chapter.

To review, testing for diabetes in pregnancy includes an early assessment for PGDM and a later assessment for GDM:

- *First trimester test for PGDM in people with risk factors.* A hemoglobin A1c level (HbA1c) of 6.5% or higher is diagnostic for diabetes in nonpregnant individuals, and this value is also used for diagnosis of PGDM during pregnancy. However, HbA1c levels are physiologically lower in pregnancy due to increased red blood cell turnover, and mild elevations (5.7% to 6.4%) are associated with an increased risk for developing GDM (27.3% versus 8.7%; odds ratio [OR], 3.9; 95% confidence interval [CI], 2.0–7.7).[26] Therefore, the specific HbA1c value used to indicate a need for further testing or closer surveillance during pregnancy is based on institutional guidelines and population-specific parameters. HbA1c is an indirect measure of glucose level, and a fasting glucose or 2-hour postprandial glucose value following a 75-gram glucose load may be recommended for direct measurement.

- *Screening for GDM between 24 and 28 weeks via a one- or two-step process.* Diagnostic criteria are presented in Table 24-1.[17,18] Choice of the screening method is primarily based on local or regional guidelines. The American Diabetes Association, World Health Organization, and International Federation of Gynecology and Obstetrics (FIGO) recommend the one-step strategy to optimize pregnancy-related outcomes,[18,20] whereas ACOG supports the two-step strategy given the paucity of research demonstrating improved outcomes with the one-step approach.[17]

### Management of Gestational Diabetes Mellitus

Clients diagnosed with GDM should develop a personalized nutrition plan with the help of a registered dietician.[17] Individuals with GDM can often attain euglycemia via lifestyle modifications, primarily diet, and exercise (A1GDM). Dietary changes include consuming complex rather than simple carbohydrates and distributing meals and snacks throughout the day to reduce blood glucose fluctuations, though little evidence supports specific dietary approaches for GDM.[27,28] Exercise should include 30 minutes of moderate-intensity aerobics at least 5 days per week.[17] Treating GDM with nutrition and exercise has been shown to reduce associated risks for preeclampsia, shoulder dystocia, and cesarean birth.[17]

| Table 24-1 | Diagnostic Criteria for Gestational Diabetes in Pregnancy | | | | | |
|---|---|---|---|---|---|---|
| Test Strategy | Glucose Load | Fasting (mg/dL) | 1-Hour Postprandial (mg/dL) | 2-Hour Postprandial (mg/dL) | 3-Hour Postprandial (mg/dL) | Diagnostic Criteria |
| *One-step* | 75 gm | ≥ 92 | ≥ 180 | ≥ 153 | NA | ≥ 1 abnormal value |
| *Two-step* | | | | | | |
| a. Screening | 50 g | NA | ≥ 140 | NA | NA | NA |
| b. GTT | | | | | | |
| NDDG criteria | 100 g | ≥ 105 | ≥ 190 | ≥ 165 | ≥ 145 | ≥ 2 abnormal values |
| Carpenter-Coustan criteria | 100 g | ≥ 95 | ≥ 180 | ≥ 155 | ≥ 140 | ≥ 2 abnormal values |

Abbreviations: GTT, glucose tolerance test; NDDG, National Diabetes Data Group.

Note: Some institutions use a cut-off value of 130–135 mg/dL for the screening step. Either the NDDG or the Carpenter-Coustan cut-off values may be used.

Based on American College of Obstetricians and Gynecologists. Practice Bulletin No. 190: gestational diabetes mellitus. *Obstet Gynecol.* 2018;131:e49-e6419; American Diabetes Association. 2: Classification and diagnosis of diabetes: standards of medical care in diabetes-2020. *Diabetes Care.* 2020;43(Suppl 1):S14-S31.

| Table 24-2 | Target Blood Glucose Values During Pregnancy |
|---|---|
| Time of Test | Target Value (mg/dL) |
| Fasting | ≤ 95 |
| 1-hour postprandial | ≤ 140 |
| 2-hour postprandial | ≤ 120 |
| HbA1c | ≤ 6% |

Abbreviation: HbA1c, hemoglobin A1c.

Based on American Diabetes Association. 14: Management of diabetes in pregnancy: standards of medical care in diabetes-2020. *Diabetes Care.* 2020;43(Suppl 1):S183-S192. doi: 10.2337/dc20-S014.

Glucose monitoring is generally recommended once after fasting and either 1 or 2 hours after each meal. When glucose levels are well controlled by lifestyle recommendations, monitoring may be modified, albeit generally to no less frequently than twice daily. Individuals with A1GDM who are able to maintain euglycemia via diet and exercise alone do not appear to be at risk for stillbirth and are not usually referred for antenatal testing, although induction of labor is usually recommended between 39 6/7 to 40 6/7 weeks.[17]

Medication is indicated when adequate glycemic control is not achieved through lifestyle changes (A2GDM). There is no conclusive evidence for a specific threshold at which medication should be initiated, and practice may vary; recommendations vary from when one or two values exceed target values over 1 or 2 weeks, to when values are "consistently" above target values.[17,29]

Insulin is the preferred medication for individuals with A2GDM; treatment should begin when fasting glucose levels are greater than 95 mg/dL, 1-hour postprandial levels are greater than 140, or 2-hour levels are greater than 120. Insulin doses typically start at 0.7–1.0 unit/kg daily, divided into a regimen combining long- or intermediate-acting doses with short-acting doses throughout the day. Close monitoring is needed initially, and adjustments in doses may be necessary, due to the increased dynamic changes in insulin sensitivity throughout pregnancy.[17] Insulin does not cross the placenta, whereas oral agents do; additionally, the long-term safety of oral medications has not been established.[28]

Metformin, and rarely glyburide, are acceptable alternatives for people who decline or are unable to use insulin.[17] Dosing of metformin for GDM typically starts at 500 mg nightly for the first week, followed by an increase to 500 mg twice daily.[17]

Midwives may participate in care of clients with A2GDM or PGDM, although physicians or other specialists typically manage diabetes medications in pregnancy.[30] Antenatal testing for those persons with A2GDM typically begins at 32 weeks' gestation, and induction of labor is recommended between 39 0/7 and 39 6/7 weeks.[17]

People with GDM should be encouraged to breastfeed/chestfeed. Information on management of individuals with diabetes intrapartum and postpartum is provided in the *Complications During Labor and Birth*, *Postpartum Care*, and *Postpartum Complications* chapters. Postpartum care includes follow-up to assess for type 2 diabetes at 4 to 12 weeks after birth. Lifelong screening for diabetes is recommended at least every 3 years.[18]

## Management of Pregestational Diabetes Mellitus

Table 24-3 presents an overview of prenatal care for individuals with diabetes. Those persons with PGDM, especially type 1 diabetes, may be referred to a physician for pregnancy care. Depending on the type of diabetes, health status, and the healthcare setting, midwives may participate in a multidisciplinary

| Table 24-3 | Overview of Management of Pregestational and Gestational Diabetes | | |
|---|---|---|---|
| **Management** | **PGDM** | **GDM** | **Clinical Considerations** |
| Eye examination | X | | First trimester; monitor each trimester, then every 3 months to 1 year |
| Assessment of renal function | X | | First trimester |
| Four-chamber view of fetal heart including outflow tracts (fetal ultrasound and possible fetal echocardiography) | X | | Increased risk for congenital heart defects |
| Ultrasound for fetal growth, amniotic fluid volume | X | | 28, 32, and 36 weeks depending on clinical situation to assess for fetal growth restriction, polyhydramnios, and macrosomia |
| Nutrition therapy | X | X | All people with diabetes manage blood glucose levels via diet; many with GDM achieve euglycemia with diet changes alone |
| Glucose monitoring: fasting and postprandial | X | X | Some people with PGDM may benefit from preprandial testing |
| Glucose monitoring: measure HbA1c | X | | Target HbA1c is less than 6% |
| Medication: Insulin, metformin, or rarely glyburide | X | X | Insulin is the preferred medication due to placental drug transfer of oral medications and lack of data on long-term outcomes |
| Antenatal fetal testing starting at 32 weeks | X | X | For those with poorly controlled diabetes or A2GDM |
| If chronic hypertension coexists with diabetes | X | X | Target blood pressure is 120–160 mm Hg systolic and 80–105 mm Hg diastolic; blood pressure exceeding the target range may require modifications to antihypertensive medications and preeclampsia screening |
| If EFW ≥ 4500 g, counseling regarding option of cesarean birth | X | X | |
| Postpartum oral GTT 4–12 weeks after birth | | X | |
| Lifelong screening every 1–3 years for diabetes and prediabetes | | X | |

Abbreviations: EFW, estimated fetal weight; GDM, gestational diabetes mellitus; GTT, glucose tolerance test; HbA1c, hemoglobin A1c; PGDM, pregestational diabetes mellitus.

team including diabetes educators and other specialists in diabetes during pregnancy.[30]

Individuals with PGDM receive a first trimester evaluation of HbA1c, thyroid function, electrocardiogram, eye examination to assess for retinopathy, and 24-hour urine.[24] The goal of care in the first trimester is to maintain euglycemia and avoid hypoglycemia. Pregnancies complicated by PGDM have an increased risk for neural tube defects, so supplementing at least 400 micrograms of folic acid daily starting before conception is prudent. Individuals with PGDM also have an increased risk for developing preeclampsia; for these clients, low-dose aspirin (81 mg) daily is recommended after 12 weeks' gestation until birth.[24]

Care during the second and third trimesters additionally focuses on monitoring fetal growth and preventing stillbirth.[30] Second trimester testing typically includes a detailed anatomy ultrasound and fetal echocardiogram. Ultrasounds for fetal growth are generally performed at 28 to 32 weeks. Those pregnant persons who require medication to maintain euglycemia are usually offered antenatal testing twice weekly starting at approximately 32 weeks and asked to perform daily fetal movement counts.

People with PGDM will be seen more frequently during pregnancy and blood glucose values monitored intensively via daily self-monitoring of preprandial and postprandial blood glucose values. Target blood glucose values and target HbA1c values are listed in Table 24-2. The lowest risk for congenital malformations, preeclampsia, and other complications exists when diabetes is well controlled and HbA1c is less than 6.5%.[21]

Insulin is the treatment of choice throughout pregnancy for people with type 1 diabetes, who are especially vulnerable to hypoglycemia in the first trimester. Insulin requirements are often lower in the first trimester, gradually increase in the second trimester, and decrease again in the late third trimester and immediate postpartum period, paralleling plasma levels of placental hormones that induce insulin resistance. Ketoacidosis can occur at lower glucose levels than it would outside of pregnancy.[30]

Individuals with type 2 diabetes may benefit from transitioning from oral agents used before pregnancy to insulin so as to more closely control blood glucose values. Glycemic control in type 2 diabetes often requires higher doses of insulin than are required for type 1 diabetes. Combination therapy with an oral agent and insulin is also an option when diet, exercise, and oral agents do not provide sufficient control of glucose levels.[17,30]

Fetuses of people with diabetes develop respiratory maturity later than do fetuses of those without diabetes, so early birth poses increased risks for respiratory distress. Nevertheless, the presence of comorbidities, fetal growth restriction, or poorly controlled glucose values may indicate a need for preterm induction of labor. If no complications are present, glucose values are stable, and fetal growth is normal, induction of labor is usually recommended by 39 0/7 to 39 6/7 weeks gestation.[24] During labor, patients on insulin typically receive their intermediate- or long-acting evening dose in addition to dextrose and insulin infusions during active labor to keep their blood glucose levels at approximately 100 mg/dL.[24]

## Gastrointestinal Conditions

Many gastrointestinal (GI) conditions commonly arise during pregnancy. In particular, constipation, heartburn, gastroesophageal reflux, abdominal discomfort, nausea, and vomiting frequently occur due to normal physiologic changes in pregnancy and are discussed in the *Pregnancy-Related Conditions* chapter. More serious GI disorders are less common and often difficult to diagnose because of these overlapping symptoms. This section reviews GI disorders that increase the risks of pregnancy complications and those that are adversely affected by pregnancy.

### Acute Abdomen

In general, the definition of acute abdomen encompasses intra-abdominal conditions that will typically require surgical intervention.[31] Classic symptoms of an acute abdomen include severe abdominal pain, tenderness, and rigidity. Differential diagnoses of acute abdominal pain during pregnancy will be the same as for nonpregnant individuals. Additionally, life-threatening pregnancy conditions such as ectopic pregnancy, placental abruption, acute fatty liver, HELLP (hemolysis, elevated liver enzymes, and low platelet count) syndrome, or uterine rupture must be considered.

Identifying a nonpregnancy etiology of acute abdominal pain in pregnancy is further hampered by common pregnancy symptoms and shifts in the normal range of laboratory parameters. Performing a thorough abdominal examination in the presence of a gravid uterus can be difficult. Moreover, standard diagnostic radiologic modalities such as x-ray and CT scan are not recommended during pregnancy.[31] An acute abdomen, however, is a medical emergency that requires urgent evaluation.

The presence of vaginal bleeding along with gestational age may help differentiate pregnancy-related from non-pregnancy-related causes of acute abdominal pain. Initial laboratory tests will further aid in narrowing down the likely etiologies. This evaluation should include a complete blood count (CBC) with differential, urinalysis, and a comprehensive metabolic profile that includes electrolytes, renal, liver, and pancreatic biochemical tests such as aminotransferases, bilirubin, and lipase. Individuals who are hemodynamically unstable, with signs of bleeding or shock, should have coagulation studies and a type and cross-match. In early unlocated gestations, serum human chorionic gonadotropin levels can guide the timing of ultrasound studies to rule out ectopic pregnancy. Abdominal and pelvic ultrasound are the most useful imaging techniques for evaluating abdominal pain in pregnancy and remain first-line modalities for both pregnancy and nonpregnancy causes.[31]

## Appendicitis

The incidence of appendicitis during pregnancy has been reported to range from 1 in 800 to 1 in 1500, with this condition most often appearing during the second trimester.[31] Right lower quadrant pain is the most common presenting symptom in pregnancy. Diagnosis is often delayed in pregnant individuals, because other typical symptoms—such as anorexia, nausea, and vomiting—can also be attributed to a wide range of disorders that frequently occur during pregnancy. In addition, in pregnancy, peritoneal inflammatory signs such as fever, leukocytosis, and right lower quadrant rebound tenderness may be absent. Physiologic leukocytosis is a common finding during pregnancy and is unreliable as a marker for acute appendicitis. Furthermore, the enlarging pregnant uterus displaces the appendix farther away from the right lower quadrant (Figure 24-1), affecting the findings during an abdominal exam and imaging.[31]

The diagnostic work-up for suspected appendicitis includes a CBC with differential, urinalysis, and a comprehensive metabolic panel to rule out renal, liver, and other abdominal organ etiologies. In pregnancy, abdominal or pelvic ultrasound is the first-line imaging modality. In many cases, though, ultrasound will be unable to visualize the appendix, and MRI without contrast will be needed to confirm or rule out the diagnosis.

Once appendicitis is confirmed, surgical referral is warranted. Although conservative therapy for uncomplicated appendicitis in the nonpregnant person may be appropriate, immediate surgical intervention is the preferred treatment during pregnancy due to the increased risks of perforation.[31] A perforated appendix during pregnancy significantly

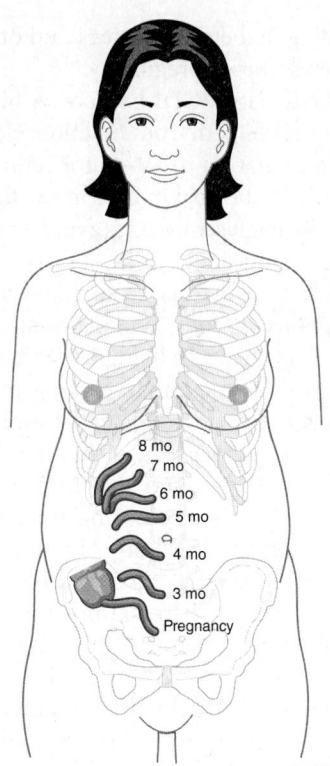

**Figure 24-1** Potential position of the appendix during pregnancy.

increases morbidity and mortality for both the pregnant individual and the fetus.[31]

## Gallbladder: Cholecystitis

Cholecystitis is the second most common etiology of acute abdomen in pregnancy, after appendicitis.[31] During pregnancy, increased estrogen, serum cholesterol, and lipid levels can lead to the accumulation of biliary sludge and the development of gallstones (cholelithiasis). While most pregnant individuals will be asymptomatic or experience manageable episodic symptoms, acute cholecystitis can occur secondary to obstruction and inflammation of the gallbladder. Cholecystitis can lead to serious complications such as jaundice, sepsis, gallstone pancreatitis, abscess, and perforation.[31,32]

Pregnant people with gallbladder disorders often present with the classic symptoms of biliary colic, anorexia, nausea, and bloating. Pain can be mild to severe in the epigastric or right upper quadrant area and may radiate to the back or shoulder.[31,32] Symptoms usually occur 2 to 3 hours after eating a high-fat meal; avoidance of high-fat, low-fiber foods and inclusion of vegetables and whole grains in the individual's diet may reduce symptoms. In persons with mild disease, symptoms typically resolve with supportive treatments such as dietary changes, intravenous fluids, antiemetics, and pain management. Pregnant individuals with acute cholecystitis, however, will present with worsening or unresolved symptoms, fever, nausea, and vomiting. A positive Murphy's sign will be noted, characterized by severe pain on inspiration when directly palpating the lower edge of the liver.[32] In such a case, a complete blood count with differential and liver function tests should be ordered. The differential diagnosis will include other serious liver disorders seen in pregnancy, such as HELLP syndrome, acute fatty liver, and hepatitis.

Diagnosis of cholecystitis is confirmed with ultrasound imaging and generally will require admission to the hospital for bowel rest, pain management, intravenous fluids, and antibiotics.[32] Care in this situation should be managed collaboratively and may include an obstetrician and a GI specialist. Decisions regarding the necessity and timing of cholecystectomy will be individualized based on disease severity. Continued conservative treatment can lead to recurrence and relapse with increased fetal risks.[31]

### Gastroesophageal Reflux Disease

Gastroesophageal reflux disease (GERD) is a common disorder seen in the general population. Pregnancy changes such as slower GI motility and relaxation of the lower esophageal sphincter may contribute to exacerbation of preexisting disease; alternatively, GERD may initially appear during pregnancy, usually in the second or third trimester.[32] Symptoms are similar to those observed in nonpregnant people and include heartburn, epigastric burning, and hypersalivation. Atypical symptoms that indicate increasing severity and a need for medical consultation include dysphagia, noncardiac chest pain, dyspepsia, abdominal pain, hoarseness, sore throat, weight loss, and dental erosions.[32]

The goal of treatment for GERD is to minimize the amount of acid reflux into the esophageal mucosa.[32] Lifestyle modifications are a crucial first step and should be continued regardless of pharmacologic management. Recommendations include avoiding overeating or lying down immediately after a meal, elevating the head of the bed, and not eating for 2 to 3 hours before bedtime. Smoking and high-acid foods should be avoided. Other specific foods known to trigger GERD symptoms include alcohol, carbonated beverages, caffeine, chocolate, and peppermint.

When pharmaceutical methods are needed to control symptoms, antacids are the first-line medications. Antacids promptly reduce acidity by neutralizing stomach contents and can be safely used on demand throughout pregnancy.[33] These medications come in a variety of oral formulations, and those containing calcium, aluminum, and magnesium are considered safe in pregnancy. In contrast, antacids containing sodium bicarbonate should be avoided.[33]

Histamine 2 receptor antagonists ($H_2RA$) reduce gastric acid secretion and are typically the next step if previous measures do not improve symptoms. Famotidine (Pepcid) is an $H_2RA$ commonly prescribed for GERD that has moderate success in controlling symptoms.[33] Proton pump inhibitors (PPI) are more effective than $H_2$-receptor antagonists in inhibiting gastrointestinal acid secretion but should be reserved for those individuals whose symptoms are not controlled by $H_2RAs$.[32] Lansoprazole (Prevacid), rabeprazole (Aciphex), esomeprazole (Nexium), and pantoprazole (Protonix) are all considered safe for use during pregnancy. Omeprazole (Prilosec) has been associated with dose-related teratogenic effects in animals, although more recent data have not supported this finding.[32,33] Antacids, $H_2RAs$, and PPIs can all interfere with iron absorption and should be used with caution when supplemental iron is needed during pregnancy.[32,33] If GERD symptoms persist after birth, antacids and $H_2Ras$ are safe to continue while breastfeeding/chestfeeding, but PPIs are contraindicated.[32,33]

### Inflammatory Bowel Disease

Ulcerative colitis and Crohn's disease are chronic GI disorders collectively known as inflammatory bowel disease (IBD). These conditions commonly affect individuals during their reproductive years and are associated with adverse pregnancy outcomes.[33] Both ulcerative colitis and Crohn's disease are characterized by periods of active symptomatic disease (flares) and quiescent states in which disease remission occurs.[33] Disease flares can cause debilitating symptoms depending on the severity and location of inflammation in the GI tract. The effect of IBD on the course of pregnancy depends on the activity and severity of the disease. Active disease at conception or exacerbation during pregnancy is associated with increased risks for miscarriage, low birth weight, and preterm birth.[33] Crohn's disease also increases risks for cesarean birth, especially in the presence of perianal disease.[33]

Management of IBD is best done by a GI specialist in collaboration with the usual prenatal care provider. Pregnancy has not been shown to affect IBD symptoms and remissions, but the biomarkers used to assess disease activity are often unreliable in pregnant persons due to normal physiologic changes that occur during pregnancy.[33] Most medications used to treat IBD, except for methotrexate, are safe to use in pregnancy and should be continued with close monitoring. Discontinuation of medications could lead to active disease with much higher risks to the fetus.[33] Individuals in remission can be safely managed by midwives during pregnancy with ongoing physician consultation and referral should their IBD worsen.

### Pancreatitis

Pancreatitis is a rare but serious condition that occurs in approximately 1 in 10,000 pregnancies, typically in the third trimester.[31] In the general population, alcohol use and gallbladder disease are the most common causes; however, acute pancreatitis can also result from hypertriglyceridemia.[31,32] In pregnancy, 70% of cases are caused by gallstone blockage of the pancreatic duct, leading to acute inflammation, damage, and leakage of pancreatic enzymes into the systemic circulation.[31,32]

Most individuals with pancreatitis will present with sudden onset of nausea, vomiting, and severe periumbilical pain radiating to the back. Pain improvement associated with leaning forward is a classic sign. Elevated serum pancreatic amylase and lipase twice the normal levels confirm the diagnosis. The precipitating cause of the pancreatitis should be determined. Ultrasound is useful in detecting the presence of gallstones. Other potential causes, including alcohol use, should not be overlooked and require a thorough history.

Pancreatitis increases the risk of preterm birth by 20% and requires careful monitoring for signs of preterm labor.[31] In rare cases, pancreatitis has been associated with preeclampsia and HELLP syndrome.[31] Pregnant persons with acute pancreatitis require admission to the hospital and physician referral.

Pancreatitis often resolves with supportive treatment consisting of intravenous fluids, pain management, bowel rest, and antiemetics. Cholecystectomy may be necessary in severe cases unresponsive to conservative therapies.

## Hematologic Disorders

The hematologic disorders that are the most likely to affect pregnant people include anemias, hemoglobinopathies, and coagulation disorders. A midwife's ability to diagnose and collaborate in managing these disorders can improve outcomes and help prevent morbidity and mortality for both the pregnant individual and their fetus/infant.

### Anemia: An Overview

Anemia is the most common nutritional deficiency worldwide.[34] Anemia in pregnancy is defined as hemoglobin less than 11 g/dL and hematocrit less than 33% in the first and third trimesters.[35] In the second trimester, the criteria for anemia are hemoglobin less than 10.5 g/dL and hematocrit less than 32% (Table 24-4).[36–38] Limited data are available to estimate the current prevalence of iron-deficiency anemia in pregnant individuals in the United States. In North America, anemia rates during pregnancy vary between 5%-20% with prevalence of anemia higher among racial and ethnic minorities, especially non-Hispanic Black or African American identifying people, and economically disenfranchised groups.[39] The prevalence of anemia in pregnant individuals globally is approximately 35% to 56%.[37] In low-resource nations, anemia is also frequently a comorbidity of infection (e.g., malaria) or a hemoglobinopathy.

Consequences of anemia during pregnancy include increased vulnerability to infection, increased

| Table 24-4 | Diagnostic Values for the Diagnosis of Anemia in Pregnancy | |
|---|---|---|
| | Hemoglobin (mg/dL) | Hematocrit (%) |
| **Trimester** | | |
| First trimester | < 11 | < 33 |
| Second trimester | < 10.5 | < 32 |
| Third trimester | < 11 | 33 |
| **Adjustment for Living at High Altitude** | | |
| First trimester | < 11.2–13.0 | < 33.5–39.0 |
| Second trimester | < 10.7–12.5 | < 32.0–38.0 |
| Third trimester | < 11.2–13.0 | < 33.5–39.0 |
| **Adjustment for Smoking** | | |
| 0.5–0.9 pack/day | + 0.3 | + 1.0 |
| 1.0–1.9 pack/day | + 0.5 | + 1.5 |
| 2.0 or more pack/day | + 0.7 | + 2.0 |

Based on American College of Obstetricians and Gynecologists. ACOG Practice Bulletin No. 233: anemia in pregnancy. *Obstet Gynecol.* 2021;138:e55-6441; Mei Z, Cogswell ME, Looker AC, et al. Assessment of iron status in US pregnant women from the National Health and Nutrition Examination Survey (NHANES), 1999-2006. *Am J Clin Nutr.* 2011;93:1312-1320; Chao C, O'Brien KO. Pregnancy and iron homeostasis: an update. *Nutr Rev.* 2013;71(1):35-51.

cardiovascular burden, reduced peripartum blood loss reserves, and increased risk for transfusion. Anemia is also associated with an increase in maternal mortality—an association that is strongly influenced by postpartum hemorrhage. Moreover, individuals who are anemic are at increased risk for preterm birth, fetal growth restriction, low birth weight and prematurity, fetal/infant infection, and infant mortality.[34,36] In addition, fetal iron stores may be compromised when a pregnant person is anemic, and suboptimal iron stores in the neonate are associated with cognitive impairments in the child after birth.[38] Supplementation with iron during pregnancy reduces risks of anemia and iron deficiency in pregnancy.[40,41]

### Differential Diagnosis and Initial Treatment of Anemia

Normocytic anemia is diagnosed when the hemoglobin and hematocrit levels are low, but the mean corpuscular volume (MCV) is in the normal range of 80 to 100 femtoliters (fL; a metric unit of volume equal to $10^{-15}$ liters); microcytic anemia refers to small red blood cells wherein MCV is less than 80 fL; and macrocytic anemia refers to large pale red blood cells wherein the MCV is larger than 100 fL. These definitions, and the causes of the various types of anemia, are summarized in Table 24-5.[36]

Anemia is a symptom of many different disorders, and multiple algorithms for evaluation of patients for anemia are available based on the particular population and the most likely possible diagnoses. However, because most pregnant individuals with anemia have iron-deficiency anemia, the usual practice is to presumptively treat them with iron and then reassess the hemoglobin and hematocrit levels before performing a detailed evaluation of iron status. If iron supplementation is not successful, further evaluation is indicated. One algorithm for evaluating essentially healthy pregnant people who have anemia is presented in **Figure 24-2**.

### Microcytic Anemias

The most common anemia in pregnancy is iron-deficiency anemia. However, thalassemias and sickle cell disease are also associated with microcytic anemia.

### Iron-Deficiency Anemia

In the United States, approximately 18% of pregnant people are anemic overall, but this rate varies by trimester from 6.9% to 14.3% to 29.5% in the first, second, and third trimesters, respectively.[34]

| Table 24-5 | Causes of Anemia by Mean Corpuscular Volume | | |
|---|---|---|---|
| | **Normocytic Anemia: MCV 80–100 fL** | **Microcytic Anemia: MCV < 80 fL** | **Macrocytic Anemia: MCV ≤100 fL** |
| | Chronic disease | Chronic disease | Folic acid deficiency |
| | Early iron deficiency | Iron-deficiency anemia | Drug-induced hemolytic anemia |
| | Hemorrhage | Lead poisoning | Liver disease and/or alcohol abuse disorder |
| | Hemolytic anemia | Thalassemias | Vitamin $B_{12}$ deficiency |
| | Hypothyroidism | | |

Abbreviations: fL, femtoliter (= $10^{-15}$ liters); MCV, mean corpuscular volume.

Note: This table is not comprehensive; rather, these are the most common differential diagnoses for anemia that are likely to occur in people seen for primary care services or prenatal care.

Based on American College of Obstetricians and Gynecologists. ACOG Practice Bulletin No. 233: anemia in pregnancy. *Obstet Gynecol.* 2021;138:e55-64.

Worldwide, the prevalence of iron-deficiency anemia is much higher. Approximately 40% of people begin pregnancy with low or absent iron stores.[37] Increased risks for iron-deficiency anemia include multifetal gestation, multiparity, short interval between pregnancies, anemia prior to pregnancy, lack of access to adequate nutrition, and lower socioeconomic status.

The American College of Obstetricians and Gynecologists (ACOG) and the Centers for Disease Control and Prevention (CDC) endorse the standardized practice of screening for iron deficiency anemia at the initial prenatal visit, at the start of the third trimester, and on admission for labor and birth. To identify iron deficiency anemia, newer evidence recommends in addition to CBC, a serum ferritin or transferrin saturation (TSAT) to evaluate iron storage and risk for developing anemia later in pregnancy.[39] As a preventive measure, research supports offering iron supplementation to all individuals in pregnancy.[40] Intermittent supplementation (1 to 3 times per week) has been shown to be as effective as daily supplementation and has fewer side effects. This may be secondary to the regulation of iron absorption in the duodenum.

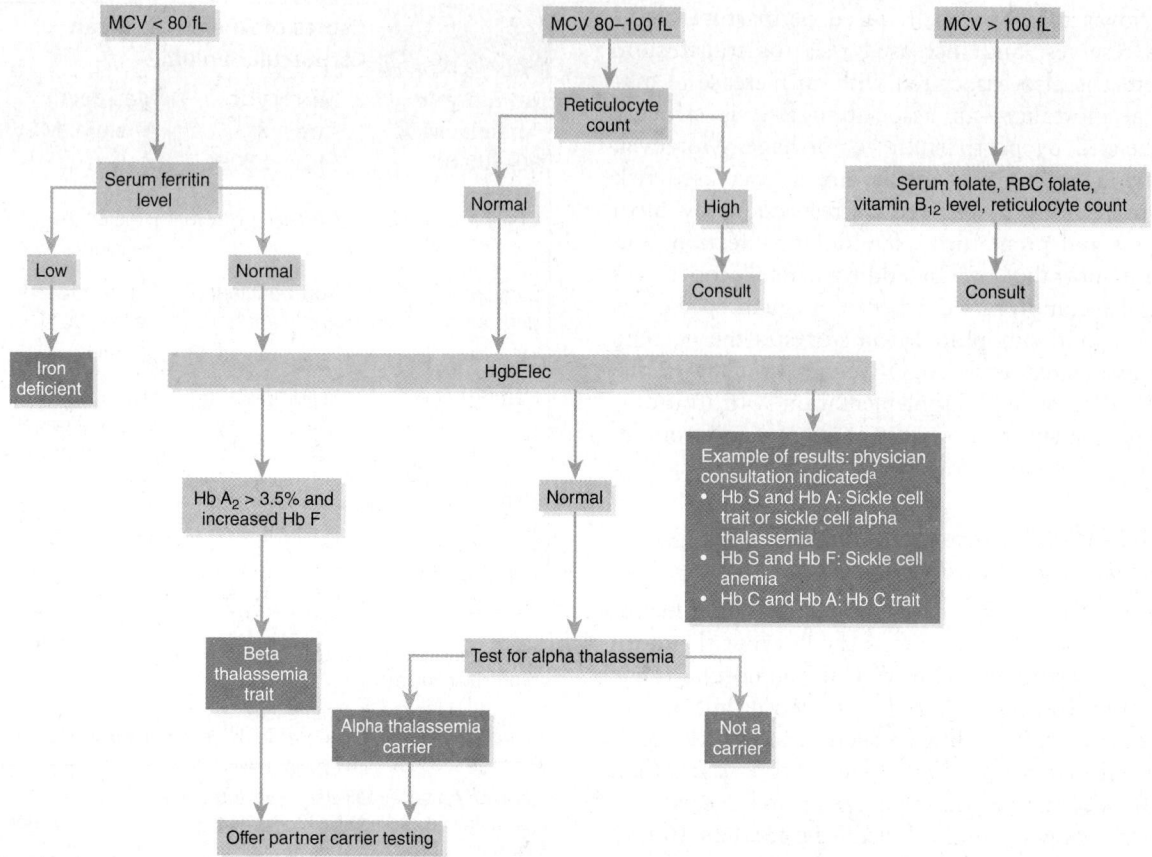

**Figure 24-2** Morphologic evaluation of anemia.

Abbreviations: Hb A, hemoglobin A; Hb A$_2$, hemoglobin A$_2$; Hb C, hemoglobin C; Hb F, hemoglobin F; Hb S, hemoglobin S; Hb SC, hemoglobin SC; HgbElec, hemoglobin electrophoresis; MCV, mean corpuscular volume; RBC, red blood cell.

Note: The hemoglobin electrophoresis reports the type and percentage of different types of hemoglobin. Possible interpretations include sickle cell trait, sickle cell disease, sickle beta-thalassemia, and Hb SC disease, among others.

[a] This figure is an example of an algorithm for a population of essentially healthy pregnant patients who are not at risk for other comorbid conditions or infections.

Iron deficiency is a continuum that ranges from depletion of iron stores to overt anemia. Hemoglobin and hematocrit levels do not begin to decrease until stored iron is depleted, so a pregnant person may have normal hemoglobin and hematocrit values yet also be iron depleted. For this reason, iron supplementation is recommended for all pregnant people.

Serum ferritin levels are the most sensitive measure for diagnosis of iron-deficiency anemia, as ferritin is the storage form of iron. Serum iron levels and total iron-binding capacity can also be measured, but both are subject to diurnal variations, with higher concentrations noted later in the day. Values for hemoglobin, MCV, serum iron, and total iron-binding capacity (TIBC) indicative of iron deficiency are listed in Table 24-6.[35,42]

When iron-deficiency anemia is present, it is important for the midwife to address food insecurity and nutritional deficiencies in the pregnant individual's diet as dietary sources of heme are more readily available for placental transfer than artificial supplementation. If the nutritional gap cannot be resolved, the recommendation is to supplement with 60 to 120 mg per day of elemental iron. The amount of elemental iron in supplements varies, as described in the *Nutrition* chapter. The most common side effects of oral iron preparations include nausea, bloating, constipation, and black stools. In individuals with malabsorption or adverse gastrointestinal effects, recommending alternate-day dosing (every other day) reduces GI side effects and has been shown to result in equivalent outcomes, better tolerance, and increased patient adherence to treatment. A follow-up CBC is performed at the 24–28 weeks venipuncture if tolerating oral supplementation well or 14 days after supplementation is initiated if not tolerating oral iron. Reticulocytosis—that is, an increase in young red blood cells on the CBC—should

| Table 24-6 | Laboratory Tests Indicative of Iron Deficiency, by Degree of Severity | | | |
|---|---|---|---|---|
| | Normal Values | Iron Deficient Without Anemia | Iron Deficient with Anemia | Iron Deficient with Severe Anemia |
| Hemoglobin (Hgb), g/dL | 12–13 | Normal (> 12) | 9–12 | 6–7 |
| Mean corpuscular volume (MCV), fL | 80–100 | 80–100 | < 80 | < 80 |
| Red blood cell (RBC) morphology | Normal | Normal | Normal or slight hypochromia | Hypochromic, microcytic |
| Serum ferritin (ng/dL) | 10–150 | < 40 | < 20 | < 10 |
| Serum iron (SI), mcg/dL | 40–175 | 60–150 | < 60 | < 40 |
| Total iron-binding capacity (TIBC), mcg/dL | 216–400 | 300–390 | 350–400 | > 410 |
| Transferrin saturation (TSAT), % | 16–60 | 30 | < 15 | < 10 |
| Free erythrocyte protoporphyrin (FEP), mcg/dL | < 3 | 30–70 | > 100 | 100–200 |

Based on American College of Obstetricians and Gynecologists. ACOG Practice Bulletin No. 233: anemia in pregnancy. *Obstet Gynecol.* 2021;138:e55–e64; Haider BA, Olofin I, Wang M, Spiegelman D, Ezzati M, Fawzi WW; Nutrition Impact Model Study Group (Anaemia). Anaemia, prenatal iron use, and risk of adverse pregnancy outcomes: systematic review and meta-analysis. *BMJ.* 2013;346:f3443.

be apparent by 7 to 10 days, and the hemoglobin and hematocrit levels should rise within a few weeks.[35]

Intravenous (IV) iron may be preferable to oral supplementation, especially when treating severe iron deficiency anemia as defined by World Health Organization of a hemoglobin < 8 mg/dL. Intravenous iron may also benefit those who do not respond to oral supplementation and/or people who have comorbid conditions associated with hemolysis or malabsorption. For example, people who have undergone bariatric surgery have diminished capacity to absorb oral formulations. Current preparations of intravenous iron, such as low-molecular-weight iron dextran and ferric carboxymaltose (Injectafer), have been shown to increase the pregnant person's hemoglobin at birth, with fewer medication reactions noted in recipients compared to oral iron.[41] Currently, IV iron is not recommended in the first trimester because of lack of data available on fetal development,[39] and oral supplementation should be used unless severe anemia is present. Intravenous administration of iron occurs in a hospital setting or outpatient infusion clinics. Several formulations with different doses and protocols are available. Recheck CBC (ferritin) 2-4 weeks after iron transfusion.

### Hemoglobinopathies

When a person has microcytic anemia and normal iron indices, the next step is to screen for hemoglobinopathies. Normal hemoglobin consists of two pairs of polypeptide chains (two alpha and two beta), each of which has a heme–iron complex attached. More than 100 variant forms of hemoglobin exist.[43] Hemoglobinopathies are genetic synthesis disorders of hemoglobin, which are classified into two types: thalassemias and sickle cell disease. Thalassemias are disorders of reduced synthesis of alpha- or beta-globin chains, whereas structural abnormalities of hemoglobin cause sickle cell disease. Both thalassemias and sickle cell disease cause microcytic anemia. Depending on their genetic inheritance, the individual may be homozygous or heterozygous for one of these disorders, as described in the *Assessment for Genetic and Fetal Abnormalities* chapter. The resulting phenotypes vary and are based on the percentage of different hemoglobin variants, and in the case of thalassemias, which globin genes are affected and how many are affected. Diagnosis and treatments for hemoglobinopathies are determined by hemoglobin electrophoresis. Implications for pregnancy and care for affected individuals during pregnancy are presented in this chapter.

### Sickle Cell Disease and Trait

Sickle cell disease (SCD) is characterized by intermittent, painful "sickle cell crises," especially during viral infections. Sickle cell disease and trait are prevalent in individuals who live in or have ancestry from India, the Mediterranean, the territory known as the Middle East, and sub-Saharan Africa, as this hemoglobin variant is protective against malaria.[45]

978    PART IV Antepartum

People who inherit one sickle cell gene and one normal beta-globin chain gene have sickle cell trait (SCT). People with SCT do not usually manifest symptoms of SCD, but the trait can be inherited by their children.

The exact number of people living with SCD in the United States is unknown, but most studies show that the prevalence rate of sickle cell trait in the United States is 9% among people with African ancestry and 0.2% among people with European ancestry. It is estimated that SCD affects approximately 100,000 individuals in the United States. SCD occurs in approximately 1 out of every 365 people with African ancestry, and about 1 in 13 babies with African ancestry is born with SCT.[44]

SCD is a multiple-organ disorder associated with hemolytic anemia and microvascular obstruction by red blood cell agglutination. Persons who have SCD can experience intensely painful crises, particularly due to interference with oxygenation of vessels and organs. In addition, they can accumulate iron in the spleen from microvascular occlusion, erythrocyte sequestration, and splenic infarction, leading to iron overload despite the presence of microcytic anemia. People with SCD have an increased risk for miscarriage, preterm labor, preeclampsia, stillbirth, fetal growth restriction, prematurity, and low birth weight.[45] These individuals need specialized care during pregnancy, including collaboration with MFM specialists and hematologists.

If a pregnant individual has SCD or SCT, screening of the other biologic parent of the fetus is offered, along with genetic counseling, to determine inheritance patterns and the chance that the fetus will have the trait or disease. SCT follows a Mendelian autosomal recessive inheritance pattern, as described in the *Assessment for Genetic and Fetal Abnormalities* chapter.

### Alpha-Thalassemia

Alpha-thalassemia is one of the most common autosomal recessive disorders in the world, with some studies estimating that as much as 5% of the world's population carries an alpha-thalassemia variant. Alpha-thalassemia is found in most populations worldwide but is most common in populations that live in or have genetic heritage from sub-Saharan Africa through the Middle East and Mediterranean, the Indian subcontinent, and East and Southeast Asia.[46]

Alpha-thalassemia is classified based on how many of the four alpha globin genes are affected, as described in Table 24-7.[46] Individuals with alpha-thalassemia trait have microcytic anemia and a normal hemoglobin electrophoresis. Further DNA

| Table 24-7 | Classification of Alpha-Thalassemias | |
|---|---|---|
| Number of Normal Alpha Globin Genes | Genotype | Clinical Implications |
| 0 | – –/– – | Hemoglobin Bart's hydrops fetalis: incompatible with life. The fetus develops hydrops. |
| 1 | α–/– – | Hemoglobin H disease. Mild to moderate hemolytic anemia. |
| 2 | α –/α – or α α /– – | Homozygous: alpha-thalassemia trait. Mild microcytic anemia that is asymptomatic. This person is a carrier. |
| 3 | α –/ α α | Heterozygous: silent carrier state; not clinically detectable. |
| 4 | α α / α α | Normal: no thalassemia present. |

testing is needed to detect which alpha-globin genes are present, absent, or damaged. The primary purpose of detecting alpha-thalassemia carrier status is to identify couples who are at risk for having a fetus with hemoglobin Bart's hydrops fetalis. Prenatal counseling is of value for these individuals.[46]

### Beta-Thalassemia

Worldwide, approximately 1.5% of people are beta-thalassemia carriers; indeed, beta-thalassemia is one of the most common autosomal recessive disorders in the world, though it is relatively rare in the United States. Historically, the prevalence of beta-thalassemia has been highest in the Mediterranean region, the territory known as the Middle East, and Southeast Asia. Due to migration patterns and increasing numbers in refugees, beta-thalassemia is increasingly more common in non-endemic regions, including Northern Europe and North America.[46]

Beta-thalassemia is the result of insufficient or absent production of the beta-globin chains.[46] This disorder is subclassified as minor, intermediate, or major depending on the number of beta-globin chains produced. People with beta-thalassemia major (Cooley's anemia) or beta-thalassemia intermedia have an increased risk of diabetes and cardiovascular disease during pregnancy. People with beta-thalassemia minor usually have uncomplicated pregnancies and are generally asymptomatic. However, this hemoglobinopathy may be first diagnosed in pregnancy.

Beta-thalassemia trait is diagnosed by hemoglobin electrophoresis, which will reveal increased levels of hemoglobin $A_2$ and hemoglobin F. Once a person is diagnosed as having the trait, partner or sperm source testing can be offered. As of 2017, the American College of Obstetricians and Gynecologists (ACOG) recommended offering carrier screening to people of southeast Asian, African, or Mediterranean descent, as well as to individuals from Middle Eastern and Caribbean territories, as they are considered at higher risk of being carriers of hemoglobinopathies.[45] However, ethnicity is not always a good predictor of genetic risk. See the *Assessment for Genetic and Fetal Abnormalities* chapter for more information on carrier screening.

## Macrocytic Anemia

Macrocytic anemia can occur secondary to glucose-6-phosphate dehydrogenase (G6PD) deficiency, vitamin $B_{12}$ deficiency, alcohol use disorder, folate deficiency, or medications such as those used to treat human immunodeficiency virus (HIV). Macrocytic anemia is not common in pregnant individuals.

### *Glucose-6-Phosphate Dehydrogenase Deficiency*

G6PD deficiency is an inherited defect in a red blood cell enzyme that protects the red blood cell from oxidative injury. Deficiency in G6PD is the most common enzymopathy worldwide, affecting an estimated 400 million people. It is most often found in individuals of African descent.[48] This disorder can range in severity from severe hemolytic anemia to being asymptomatic. Individuals with a G6PD deficiency rarely manifest symptoms, and it is unusual for G6PD deficiency to adversely affect the course of pregnancy. The primary gestational risk for a pregnant person with G6PD deficiency is severe hemolysis as the result of use of medications such as nitrofurantoin and sulfa derivatives, infection or surgery, and ingestion of certain foods such as fava beans.

Infants born with G6PD deficiency may present with severe jaundice and kernicterus. If a pregnant person has G6PD deficiency or a family history of this condition, the pediatric providers for the newborn will need to be aware that the fetus may have this disorder to treat the newborn appropriately.[43]

Neonatal screening for G6PD is not widespread in the United States.

## Thrombocytopenia

Most pregnant individuals receive screening through routine prenatal lab tests that evaluate the platelet count and the white blood cell count. A physiologic reduction in the platelet count occurs during pregnancy, especially in the third trimester. Thrombocytopenia is defined as a platelet count less than 150,000 cells/mL. In practice, platelet counts are often listed in thousands—for example, 100K.

Pregnancy-related thrombocytopenia includes gestational thrombocytopenia and thrombocytopenia related to severe preeclampsia or HELLP syndrome. Types that evolve from causes unrelated to pregnancy, but may first manifest during pregnancy, include immune thrombocytopenia, antiphospholipid syndrome, and thrombotic thrombocytopenia. Due to the serious clinical consequences associated with different forms of thrombocytopenia, an early response to abnormal platelet counts that includes diagnosis, treatment, and/or referral is extremely important.[49] A sudden onset of significant thrombocytopenia in a pregnant person in the third trimester or postpartum period should also lead to consideration of and evaluation for preeclampsia, thrombotic thrombocytopenic purpura, hemolytic uremic syndrome, acute fatty liver, or disseminated intravascular coagulation.

Gestational thrombocytopenia, defined as a platelet level less than 150K cells/mL, is the most common diagnosis of thrombocytopenia made during pregnancy, affecting 5% to 11% of pregnant individuals. There is no specific diagnostic test for gestational thrombocytopenia; rather, it is a diagnosis of exclusion. Midwives can order a CBC and a peripheral blood smear to exclude pseudothrombocytopenia in the evaluation for thrombocytopenia. In general, gestational thrombocytopenia is diagnosed once drugs and other medical disorders are excluded and the pregnant individual has platelet levels between 100K cells/mL and 149K cells/mL without a history of bleeding problems.

Gestational thrombocytopenia can occur at any point in pregnancy, although it typically develops in the mid-second to third trimester; the platelet count is rarely less than 70K cells/mL. This disorder is not associated with increased risk of maternal bleeding complications, fetal hemorrhage, or fetal thrombocytopenia, and generally resolves within days to a few months in the postpartum period. Individuals with gestational thrombocytopenia do not typically require any additional testing or specialized care, except follow-up platelet counts 1 to 3 months after birth. There is currently no evidence available to guide the frequency of platelet counts, so follow-up should be based on clinical reasoning.

Primary immune thrombocytopenia, or idiopathic thrombocytopenic purpura (ITP), is an acquired immune-mediated disorder characterized by isolated thrombocytopenia (a platelet count of less than 100K cells/mL) in the absence of other etiologies. Immune thrombocytopenia can occur at any time during pregnancy, and platelet counts can be less than 50K cells/mL in individuals with severe ITP. Maternal immunoglobulin G (IgG) antiplatelet antibodies can cross the placenta, causing the fetus and neonate to be at risk for thrombocytopenia. Individuals with immune thrombocytopenia are usually referred to hematologists. Expert opinion suggests that serial assessment of the gestational platelet count should be done every trimester in asymptomatic individuals in remission and more frequently in individuals with thrombocytopenia.

Pregnant individuals with ITP should be instructed to avoid nonsteroidal anti-inflammatory drugs (NSAIDs), salicylates, and possible trauma. The goal of medical therapy during pregnancy is to minimize the risk of bleeding complications that can occur with regional anesthesia and birth associated with thrombocytopenia. Corticosteroids and intravenous immunoglobulin (IVIG) are the first-line treatments for ITP. Treatment should be initiated to increase platelet counts to a level considered safe for procedures when the patient has symptomatic bleeding, when platelets fall below 30K cells/mL, or to increase platelet counts to a level considered safe for procedures. Intrapartum management of ITP is based on assessment of maternal bleeding risks associated with giving birth and epidural anesthesia; the minimum platelet counts recommended are 70K cells/mL for epidural placement are and 50K cells/mL for cesarean birth.[50] The mode of delivery in pregnancies complicated with ITP should be determined based on obstetric considerations at the time of birth.

### Venous Thromboembolism and Stroke

Thromboembolic events are one of the leading causes of maternal mortality. Pregnancy is a hypercoagulable state. Although the absolute incidence is low, a person's risk of developing a venous thromboembolic event (VTE)—either deep vein thrombosis (DVT) or pulmonary embolism (PE)—is four-fold higher during pregnancy. A systematic review and meta-analysis of stroke in pregnancy reported an incidence of 30 per 100,000 pregnancies, which is three times the incidence outside of pregnancy in individuals aged 15 to 44, with most strokes

(90%) occurring in the 6 weeks following birth.[51] Additional risk factors for coagulopathy include previous VTE, family history of VTE, inherited thrombophilia, diabetes, autoimmune inflammatory disorders, age greater than 35 years, body mass index (BMI) greater than 30 kg/m$^2$, varicose veins, multifetal gestation, and hospitalization.[52]

A DVT is a blood clot that forms within the deep veins, usually in the leg, although it can also occur in other areas such as the lungs or brain. Symptoms of DVT of extremities include pain, tenderness, unilateral extremity swelling, a palpable "cord" where the DVT is located, and changes in the color and/or circumference of the affected limb. Calf pain may also be present if the clot is located within the lower leg. Most DVTs that develop in pregnant people occur in the left lower extremity, perhaps due to compression of the left iliac artery by the gravid uterus. A DVT is diagnosed via compression ultrasound. Antepartum management includes increased surveillance and anticoagulant treatment with low-molecular-weight heparin.[52]

Individuals with a PE may present with dyspnea, tachypnea, tachycardia, cough, pleuritic chest pain, fever, anxiety, cyanosis, and hemoptysis. The diagnosis of PE in the pregnant population is difficult, however, due to the nature of the invasive testing. PE can be ruled out in the nonpregnant population based on a negative D-dimer result, but D-dimer levels increase during pregnancy. Currently, due to the low specificity and sensitivity of the D-dimer test, all pregnant people with suspected PE undergo CT pulmonary angiography or ventilation/perfusion scanning, both of which involve radiation exposure to the pregnant person and fetus.

People with symptoms of a thromboembolic event require physician evaluation, as VTE has a strong association with stroke. Stroke is defined as a neurologic deficit attributed to acute injury of the central nervous system from a vascular cause, such as cerebral infarction, cerebral vein thrombosis (CVT), intracranial hemorrhage (ICH), or subarachnoid hemorrhage.[51] Although it is not within the scope of practice for midwives to treat strokes, it is imperative that midwives know how to rule out a stroke or promptly recognize symptoms in time to get the individual the care that they require.

Symptoms of stroke include, but are not limited to, unilateral numbness or weakness of the face, arm, or leg; dysphasia; hemianopia (or visual loss in half a visual field); and cerebellar features such as dysarthria and ataxia. Other symptomatic associations include a headache, drowsiness, or confusion. The FAST campaign was created to outline how to

**Box 24-1 FAST Campaign: How to Recognize Stroke**

F: Face drooping

A: Arm weakness

S: Speech difficulty

T: Time to call

Adapted from the Centers for Disease Control and Prevention. Pregnancy and stroke: are you at risk? https://www.cdc.gov/stroke/pregnancy.htm. Published May 6, 2021. Accessed December 10, 2021.

recognize symptoms of stroke (Box 24-1).[53] When a pregnant or recently pregnant individual presents with a suspected stroke, imaging should be done appropriately, with reassurance about fetal safety.[52] MRI is the most accurate and well-tolerated diagnostic option in the pregnant population, but low-dose CT of the head is a valid alternative.

Care during pregnancy for a person with a history of a VTE depends on several factors. VTEs are classified as provoked or unprovoked. A provoked VTE occurs in persons who have a clinical risk factor such as surgery, bone fracture, or bedrest. A VTE is unprovoked if no risk factor is identified. If a pregnant person has a history of a VTE, anticoagulant prophylaxis may be indicated depending on whether the VTE was provoked or unprovoked:

- Individuals with a history of an unprovoked VTE prior to pregnancy are tested for inherited thrombophilias,[54] and it is recommended they receive anticoagulant therapy prophylactically during pregnancy.
- Individuals with a history of provoked VTE are generally not at increased risk for recurrence. However, if the person has an underlying thrombophilia, risk for developing a VTE in pregnancy is significant. Therefore, those with a history of provoked VTE and a first-degree relative with a history of high-risk thrombophilia should be screened for thrombophilia and offered prophylactic anticoagulant therapy if a thrombophilia is diagnosed.[54]

## Disorders of Coagulation

### Clotting Disorders with an Increased Risk of Bleeding

Von Willebrand's disease (VWD) is the most frequent autosomal inherited bleeding disorder. It is caused by quantitative or qualitative defects of von Willebrand factor (VWF),[55] an adhesive protein that binds platelets to exposed sub-endothelium and carries factor VIII (FVII) in circulation. VWD is classified into three types: type 1, the most frequent, caused by a quantitative reduction of a normal VWF; type 2, characterized by qualitative abnormalities of VWF and divided in four subtypes (A, B, M, and N); and type 3, the least frequent but clinically most severe type caused by a virtual absence of VWF. Clinically, VWD is manifested mainly by heavy menstrual bleeding or muco-cutaneous and soft tissue bleeding, with the severity of bleeding being dependent on the degree of VWF and FVIII reduction. Individuals with VWD are treated medically via factor replacement therapy, both VWF and FVIII, or with the antidiuretic hormone vasopressin.

In pregnancy, VWF and FVIII increase significantly in individuals without VWD, reaching their greatest levels during the third trimester. The increased levels of estrogen may assist in bringing clotting capability closer to normal levels during pregnancy in individuals with VWD compared with prior to pregnancy. However, mode of birth, epidural management, operative delivery techniques, and postpartum hemorrhage present risks for those with VWD. Invasive management of labor, such as fetal scalp electrodes, and operative vaginal deliveries should be avoided because of the risk of bleeding in the potentially affected neonate, who may inherit either the autosomal dominant or recessive trait. The third stage of labor should be actively managed to reduce risks of postpartum hemorrhage (as discussed in the *Third Stage of Labor* chapter), and postpartum bleeding closely monitored as lochia is increased by 50% in individuals with VWD.[54,55] These individuals may benefit from postpartum contraception to reduce menstrual flow.

### Thrombophilias and Risk for Venous Thromboembolism

Inherited thrombophilias are genetic conditions that increase the risk for thromboembolism. Approximately 50% to 60% of individuals who develop a VTE during pregnancy have an inherited thrombophilia,[56] such as factor V Leiden (FVL) deficiency, prothrombin G20210A gene mutation, protein S deficiency, or protein C deficiency. Most people with thrombophilias are asymptomatic and undiagnosed; thus, one of these disorders may be first identified in a person who develops a VTE during pregnancy.

Routine screening of pregnant people for inherited thrombophilias is not recommended. However, testing for thrombophilias is offered to pregnant people who have either a history of an unprovoked VTE or a first-degree relative who has a known history of a high-risk thrombophilia or a history of VTE that occurred before the age of 50 years.[54]

***Thrombophilias and Risk for Adverse Pregnancy Outcomes.*** The risk for adverse pregnancy outcomes associated with thrombophilias is controversial. Some thrombophilias, such as FVL, are associated with increased risks of preeclampsia, whereas others do not appear to adversely affect the course of pregnancy. Furthermore, some thrombophilias are associated with a higher frequency of VTE than are others. Care of people who have an inherited thrombophilia depends on the type of thrombophilia as well as their personal and family history of VTE; thus, individuals with a known inherited thrombophilia are referred for physician consultation to establish a plan of care.[54] Although routine screening for thrombophilias is not recommended at this time, current research on pregnancy outcomes associated with specific thrombophilias may identify risks that will change this recommendation.[54]

## Hepatic Disorders

When pregnant individuals present with a constellation of symptoms that includes fatigue, nausea, vomiting, diarrhea, abdominal pain, fever, and jaundice, differential diagnoses will include a variety of hepatic etiologies. Hepatic disorders encompass those that are specific to pregnancy as well as chronic conditions that exist coincidentally.[57] Liver diseases exclusive to pregnancy include hyperemesis gravidarum, preeclampsia/eclampsia, HELLP syndrome, intrahepatic cholestasis of pregnancy, and acute fatty liver of pregnancy. Primary liver diseases that may adversely affect the course of pregnancy include viral hepatitis, autoimmune hepatitis, nonalcoholic fatty liver disease and cirrhosis. Conditions such as preeclampsia, eclampsia, and HELLP syndrome are part of the spectrum of hypertensive disorders seen in pregnancy and are discussed elsewhere in this chapter. Hyperemesis gravidarum and intrahepatic cholestasis of pregnancy are reviewed in the *Pregnancy-Related Conditions* chapter.

The prevalence of liver disease among individuals of childbearing age has risen over the last several years, increasing risks for significant morbidity and mortality among this population.[57] In particular, cases of hepatitis C and nonalcoholic fatty liver disease have increased in this age group and are thought to increase the risks of pregnancy complications such as gestational diabetes.[57]

When hepatic disorders are suspected, differential diagnoses are best assessed with serum analysis of liver function and ultrasound. Liver function tests (LFT) include aspartate aminotransferase (AST), alanine aminotransferase (ALT), alkaline phosphatase (ALP), gamma-glutamyl transferase (GGT), total and indirect bilirubin, and International Normalized Ratio (INR).[57] Abnormal liver tests are seen in 3% to 5% of pregnancies and require careful interpretation and correlation with presenting symptomology.[57,58] Other helpful laboratory tests may include a CBC with differential, a comprehensive metabolic profile that includes renal function (creatinine, blood urea nitrogen [BUN]), electrolytes, and a full hepatitis panel. When hepatic disorders are suspected, physician consultation is indicated with referral to the appropriate specialists once a diagnosis is confirmed.

### Viral Hepatitis

The most common causes of viral hepatitis are hepatitis A, B, and C. Presenting symptoms are similar for each virus, and all result in inflammation of the liver. During pregnancy, clinical manifestations, disease trajectories, and treatment are similar to those for nonpregnant persons.

Hepatitis A is a highly contagious disease that is transmitted via the fecal–oral route from individuals exposed to contaminated food or water. This self-limiting infection is rare in pregnancy and does not cause chronic illness or pose a danger to the fetus. Treatment is supportive and hospitalization is rarely needed. Hepatitis A vaccine is the best ways to prevent this disease and is safe for use during pregnancy.[59]

More commonly, midwives will encounter individuals who are chronic carriers of hepatitis B or C. These bloodborne infections readily cross the placenta and can cause serious risks to the fetus, including chronic disease and death. Screening for hepatitis B and C is recommended during each pregnancy.[59-61] Those persons identified as carriers will require additional testing to determine their viral load and may require antiviral treatment to reduce the risks of transmission to the fetus. Postexposure prophylaxis with hepatitis B immune globulin is available for both adults and newborns, followed by completion of a hepatitis B vaccine series.[60] There is no vaccine or postexposure prophylaxis available for hepatitis C. Additional information regarding diagnosis and treatment of hepatitis can be found in the *Reproductive Tract and Sexually Transmitted Infections* chapter.

### Autoimmune Hepatitis

Autoimmune hepatitis (AIH) is a rare, chronic inflammation of the liver. Its cause is unknown, but the disease can progress to cirrhosis and death if left untreated. It is extremely rare for AIH to initially present during pregnancy, but it should be suspected if the individual develops unexplained acute hepatitis symptoms, such as extreme fatigue, jaundice, poor appetite, or liver pain.[57] Disease presentation is highly variable and characterized by acute disease flares and asymptomatic remission. Flares occur in 20% of people with AIH during pregnancy and 30% to 40% in the postpartum period.[57] The presence of acute disease flares during and in the 12 months preceding pregnancy is associated with adverse fetal outcomes such as prematurity, low birth weight, and neonatal intensive care.[57] First-line treatment with corticosteroids (prednisone) and immunotherapy agents (azathioprine) can be safely continued during pregnancy with physician management.

### Nonalcoholic Fatty Liver Disease

Nonalcoholic fatty liver disease (NAFLD) affects approximately 10% of childbearing-age individuals and is thought to be, at least in part, a hepatic manifestation of metabolic syndrome.[57] Diagnosis is often made during routine screening of liver function. Liver transaminases (AST, ALT, ALP) are elevated, and fatty deposits are seen via ultrasound in the liver, confirming NAFLD. Most nonpregnant people with NAFLD are asymptomatic and are managed expectantly with lifestyle modifications (i.e., losing weight, improving lipid and glucose control). During pregnancy, normal changes in lipid metabolism and increases in insulin resistance can lead to NAFLD or exacerbate existing disease. This increases the risks for gestational diabetes, preeclampsia, cesarean birth, and preterm birth.[57] Therefore, individuals considering pregnancy or those currently pregnant with a history of metabolic syndrome should be carefully screened and monitored for signs of NAFLD and these comorbid conditions.[57]

## Hypertension

Hypertensive disorders are the most common medical disorder occurring during pregnancy, complicating 5% to 10% of all pregnancies.[62] An analysis by the World Health Organization found that 14% of maternal deaths worldwide were attributable to hypertension, second only to deaths from hemorrhage (27.1%).[63] The risks for developing hypertension in pregnancy include age greater than 40, pre-pregnancy obesity, excess gestational weight gain, and pregestational and gestational diabetes.

The prevalence of hypertensive disorders of pregnancy and associated mortalities varies by race and ethnicity. Structural racism has adversely affected health and health care as manifested by higher infant and maternal mortality rates, especially among Black and Hispanic or Latinx individuals.[64] A study of the 2014 and 2015 U.S. birth cohort data noted significant racial disparities in the prevalence of hypertension during pregnancy, with the highest burden in non-Hispanic Black individuals (9.8%) followed by American Indians/Alaska Natives (AIAN) (8.9%).[65]

Hypertensive disorders of pregnancy are classified into four conditions: (1) chronic hypertension, (2) gestational hypertension, (3) preeclampsia–eclampsia, and (4) chronic hypertension with superimposed preeclampsia–eclampsia.[66] Preeclampsia is further subcategorized as preeclampsia with or without severe features.[66] A severe constellation of hemolysis, elevated liver enzymes, and low platelets (HELLP syndrome) is a variant of preeclampsia that occurs in a small subset of people who develop preeclampsia.

The nomenclature for hypertensive disorders of pregnancy has a long history and has changed several times in the past. The 2013 American College of Obstetricians and Gynecologists (ACOG) Task Force on Hypertension in Pregnancy Report provides an important perspective on the current nomenclature for clinical management.[66] Preeclampsia and eclampsia are not distinct pathologies, but rather disorders that exist on a continuum.[66] Preeclampsia was once thought to be a unique pregnancy-related condition that resolved postpartum. However, hypertension is the leading cause of postpartum readmission in the United States. More than one-half of pregnancy-related maternal deaths occur in the fourth trimester.[67] It is now evident that hypertensive disorders during pregnancy span a continuum and are linked to long-term adverse cardiovascular outcomes.

People who have a hypertensive disorder of pregnancy are at increased risk for subsequent cardiovascular disease and mortality as well as for future hypertension and diabetes.[68] The American Heart Association guideline for the prevention of cardiovascular disease in people who identify as women recognizes preeclampsia, eclampsia, and pregnancy-induced hypertension (gestational hypertension) as independent risk factors for cardiovascular disease, such that assessment of pregnancy history is a critical component in determining cardiovascular risk.[68]

Hypertension in pregnant individuals is defined as a clinical systolic blood pressure (SBP) greater than or equal to 140 mm Hg and/or diastolic blood pressure (DBP) greater than or equal to 90 mm Hg on two or more occasions at least 4 hours apart.[66] Blood pressure should always be obtained after the pregnant individual has been at rest for at least 10 minutes and seated with an appropriately sized cuff positioned at the level of their heart.

Severe-range hypertension is defined as sustained SBP greater than or equal to 160 mm Hg and/or DBP greater than or equal to 110 mm Hg. Do not delay treatment with antihypertensives in clients with severe hypertension that is sustained over 15 minutes with a repeat blood pressure reading, as this is a medical emergency.[66]

Differentiating between the types of hypertensive disorders of pregnancy is not always straightforward and requires a clear understanding of specific diagnostic components. Table 24-8 provides an overview of the diagnostic criteria for each condition.

The Hypertension in Pregnancy Task Force Report (2013), released by ACOG and supported by the Society for Maternal–Fetal Medicine, recommends low-dose aspirin (81 mg/day) prophylaxis in individuals at high risk of preeclampsia.[69] Table 24-10 (later in the chapter) outlines the risk factors for developing preeclampsia for pregnant individuals.

Because of the potential for lifelong adverse effects following hypertensive disorders of pregnancy, educating people during the perinatal period is essential. This health education includes discussing the importance of informing all subsequent healthcare providers of the disorder during pregnancy, addressing the importance of health behaviors to ameliorate modifiable risks, and providing ongoing clinical follow-up and, in some cases, specialty referral.[66] For the midwife, it is important to recognize that much of the evidence that associated hypertensive disorders of pregnancy with future health is relatively new. Additional clinical implications of these findings will become evident as research continues.

## Chronic Hypertension

Chronic hypertension affects between 1% and 5% of all pregnant individuals, and the incidence is expected to rise as the incidence of obesity increases. This condition disproportionality affects Black pregnant individuals. Most chronic hypertension is of primary etiology, but in as many as 10% of individuals, it occurs secondary to underlying renal or endocrine disease.[65] Complications associated with chronic hypertension include preterm birth, fetal growth restriction, placental abruption, and superimposed preeclampsia. Approximately 20% to 50% of individuals who have chronic hypertension will develop preeclampsia, although this risk is higher among those individuals with more severe hypertension.[68] Factors that increase an individual's risk for superimposed preeclampsia include having secondary hypertension and cardiovascular disease, diabetes, obesity, maternal age greater than or equal to 40, and preeclampsia in a previous pregnancy. Individuals who have chronic hypertension are often referred to a physician for a management plan for prenatal care. Midwives may be involved in team-based prenatal care visits once a plan of care is established.

When an individual with chronic hypertension first presents for prenatal care, an initial history, physical examination, assessment of current medications, and baseline testing of renal function are performed. Specific tests include serum creatinine, electrolytes, uric acid, liver enzymes, platelet count, and a quantitative measure of urine protein.

Assessing the possibility of secondary hypertension is important because individuals with secondary hypertension may require additional management. Chronic renal disease is the most common etiology of secondary chronic hypertension. Resistant hypertension, hypokalemia, elevated serum creatinine, and a family history of renal disease should raise the index of suspicion for secondary hypertension, and providers may consider a referral to a kidney specialist if this diagnosis is suspected.

Proteinuria is often present in individuals with renal complications of hypertension, and it is particularly important to establish a baseline for this condition at onset of prenatal care. Baseline renal function assessment includes serum creatinine, a urine protein-to-creatinine ratio, and, if needed, a 24-hour urinary collection for total protein and creatinine clearance. A spot urine protein-to-creatinine ratio can be used effectively as a screening test to rule out new-onset proteinuria, or worsening proteinuria as an indicator of the development of superimposed preeclampsia, if there are baseline values with which to compare this measure. Early diabetes screening should also be considered for individuals with chronic hypertension. An echocardiogram may be recommended for pregnant people who have a history of prolonged severe chronic hypertension (more than 4 years). Additional guidelines on baseline evaluation for chronic hypertension in pregnancy can be found in the 2019 ACOG Practice Bulletin.[68]

| Table 24-8 | Diagnostic Criteria for Hypertensive Disorders in Pregnancy | |
|---|---|---|
| **Condition** | **Onset of Hypertension** | **Diagnostic Criteria** |
| Chronic hypertension | Prior to pregnancy or < 20 weeks of pregnancy<br><br>or<br><br>> 12 weeks postpartum | SBP ≥ 140 mm Hg and/or DBP ≥ 90 mm Hg before pregnancy or 20 weeks' gestation<br>or<br>Use of antihypertensive medication before pregnancy<br>or<br>Persistence of hypertension >12 weeks after delivery |
| Chronic hypertension with superimposed preeclampsia/ eclampsia | Prior to pregnancy or < 20 weeks of pregnancy | SBP ≥ 140 mm Hg and/or DBP ≥ 90 mm Hg before pregnancy or 20 weeks' gestation<br>or<br>Use of antihypertensive medication before pregnancy<br>or<br>Persistence of hypertension 12 weeks after delivery<br>AND<br>New development of any of the following: proteinuria, elevated liver enzymes, thrombocytopenia, pulmonary edema, cerebral or visual disturbances, renal insufficiency |
| Gestational hypertension | ≥ 20 weeks of pregnancy | SBP ≥ 140 mm Hg and/or DBP ≥ 90 mm Hg in a previously normotensive person without proteinuria or diagnostic features of preeclampsia on 2 or more occasions 4 hours apart |
| Preeclampsia[a] | ≥ 20 weeks of pregnancy | New-onset hypertension on 2 or more occasions 4 hours apart plus proteinuria (≥ 300 mg per 24-hour urine collection, or > 2+ dipstick if other quantitative methods are not available, or protein/creatinine ratio > 0.3 mg/dL)<br>If no proteinuria, new-onset hypertension with any of the following target organ involvement:<br>• Thrombocytopenia (platelet count < 100,000 cells/mL)<br>• Impaired liver function (elevated liver transaminases to twice normal)<br>• Renal insufficiency (serum creatinine > 1.1 mg/dL or doubling of serum creatinine in the absence of other renal disease)<br>• Pulmonary edema<br>• Cerebral or visual disturbances |
| Preeclampsia with severe features | ≥ 20 weeks of pregnancy | Same diagnostic criteria as for preeclampsia but with the addition of at least one of the following:<br>• SBP ≥ 160 mm Hg and/or DBP ≥ 110 mm Hg measured twice at least 15 minutes apart<br>• Thrombocytopenia (platelet count < 100,000 cells/mL)<br>• Impaired liver function: transaminases 2 times the normal level; severe right upper quadrant or epigastric pain<br>• Renal insufficiency: in the absence of other renal disease, serum creatinine > 1.1 mg/dL or twice the baseline level<br>• Pulmonary edema<br>• New-onset cerebral or visual disturbances |

*(continues)*

| Table 24-8 | Diagnostic Criteria for Hypertensive Disorders in Pregnancy (*continued*) | |
|---|---|---|
| **Condition** | **Onset of Hypertension** | **Diagnostic Criteria** |
| Eclampsia | ≥ 20 weeks of pregnancy | Preeclampsia plus new-onset grand mal seizures<br>or<br>Can present with seizures as the first manifestation |
| Postpartum hypertension, preeclampsia, or eclampsia | After delivery and up to 12 weeks postpartum | Persistence of gestational hypertension–preeclampsia: preexisting condition antepartum/in labor<br>or<br>SBP ≥ 140 mm Hg and/or DBP ≥ 90 mm Hg in a previously normotensive person up to 12 weeks postpartum on 2 or more occasions 4 hours apart<br>New onset hypertension/preeclampsia: onset 3–6 days postpartum<br>Preeclampsia: Same criteria for diagnosis of preeclampsia in antepartum<br>Late-onset eclampsia: headaches, visual changes, seizures, absent neurologic deficits |

Abbreviations: DBP, diastolic blood pressure; SBP, systolic blood pressure.

ᵃ An atypical form of preeclampsia that occurs before 20 weeks' gestation and is associated with hydatidiform mole and antiphospholipid syndrome.

Based on American College of Obstetricians and Gynecologists. ACOG Practice Bulletin No. 222: gestational hypertension and preeclampsia. *Obstet Gynecol.* 2020;135(6):e237-e260.

## Management of Individuals with Chronic Hypertension

A complete assessment of the individual at the initial prenatal visit or preconception visit is vital. Several different classes of medications can be used to treat chronic hypertension, but not all are acceptable for use in pregnancy. Because of these contraindications, a review of current medications can be a critical assessment at a preconception or initial prenatal visit. All antihypertensive medications cross the placenta. Angiotensin-converting enzyme (ACE) inhibitors, angiotensin II receptor blockers (ARBs), mineralocorticoid receptor antagonists (e.g., spironolactone [Aldactone]), and direct renin inhibitors are contraindicated in pregnancy because they are associated with fetal malformations and renal abnormalities.[68,70] Individuals may also be using statins pre-pregnancy that are contraindicated during pregnancy, as these agents may have teratogenic effects.[68] An urgent physician consultation is indicated if a pregnant person presents for prenatal care and is using one of these classes of medications.

Current data do not support an exact algorithm to treat individuals with chronic hypertension, as few randomized controlled trials have been conducted in this population. Treatment of chronic hypertension depends on the severity of the hypertension and the presence or absence of comorbidities. Home blood pressure monitoring can be helpful for some people. "White coat hypertension" refers to elevated blood pressure readings when in the presence of a healthcare provider compared with those readings obtained outside of a clinical setting at home.[71] Home monitoring allows for comparing measurements in different environments to ensure accurate diagnosis. Because preeclampsia typically develops after 20 weeks' gestation, increased frequency of blood pressure checks in the second half of the pregnancy is recommended. For pregnant individuals who are accustomed to engaging in exercise and have well-controlled blood pressure, moderate exercise is recommended during pregnancy. Salt-restricted diets and weight loss are not recommended for management of chronic hypertension in pregnancy.

In 2022, SMFM and ACOG released statements and clinical guidance on treatment for chronic hypertension based on the Chronic Hypertension and Pregnancy (CHAP) study. These organizations recommend utilizing 140/90 as the threshold for initiation or titration of medical therapy for chronic hypertension in pregnancy, as opposed to the previously-recommended threshold of 160/110.[72] The CHAP study demonstrated that a strategy of targeting blood pressure to be less than 140/90 mm Hg was associated with better pregnancy outcomes for pregnant people with chronic hypertension than a strategy of reserving treatment for only severe hypertension, without increasing the risk of small-for-gestational-age birth weight. Pregnant individuals who received active treatment (nifedipine, labetalol, methyldopa, or amlodipine) had a lower risk of preeclampsia with severe features, medically indicated preterm birth at less than 35 weeks' gestation, placental abruption, and fetal or neonatal death.[72] Individuals with severe hypertension should be offered antihypertensive medication.[69]

Antenatal fetal testing is recommended beginning at 32 0/7 weeks' gestation for individuals with chronic hypertension controlled with medication. Serial fetal growth ultrasounds help to monitor for fetal growth restriction when pregnant people have chronic hypertension. Depending on the severity of the maternal disease, weekly or biweekly antenatal fetal testing and amniotic fluid assessment may be recommended starting in the early third trimester or at the time of diagnosis of poorly controlled chronic hypertension or in persons with associated medical conditions.

Timing of birth is based on maternal and fetal indications. For the pregnant individual who has chronic hypertension and is not on medications, birth is recommended between 38 0/7 and 39 0/7 weeks. Expectant management after 39 0/7 weeks should occur only after careful consideration of the risks and benefits and with appropriate surveillance.[68]

## Gestational Hypertension

The distinguishing characteristics of gestational hypertension are two-fold. First, the person does not have proteinuria or meet the other diagnostic criteria for preeclampsia/eclampsia. Second, gestational hypertension resolves by 12 weeks after birth. If there is a continuation of the hypertension beyond this period, the diagnosis is reclassified as chronic hypertension. Approximately 46% of those persons with gestational hypertension will develop preeclampsia.[66] Often, what initially appears to be gestational hypertension is, in fact, evolving preeclampsia. The likelihood of developing preeclampsia increases in those individuals who develop gestational hypertension before 30 weeks' gestation. If diagnostic criteria arise that are consistent with preeclampsia/eclampsia, the diagnosis is reclassified to preeclampsia.

Before confirming the gestational diagnosis, management recommendations include evaluation for signs or symptoms of preeclampsia (e.g., urinary protein excretion; liver enzyme levels; fetal well-being via nonstress test or ultrasound, or both). If preeclampsia is ruled out, weekly in-office blood pressure monitoring and urine protein excretion, as well as twice-weekly home blood pressure measurements, and nonpharmacologic interventions such as 30 minutes of moderate exercise several days a week are appropriate for management.[68] The Society for Maternal–Fetal Medicine recommends twice-weekly antenatal fetal surveillance beginning at diagnosis.[72] The fetus is monitored via fetal movement counts and weekly fetal surveillance testing. An ultrasound for fetal growth may be obtained.

As part of prenatal care, pregnant people are informed of potential warning signs of preeclampsia (Box 24-2) and should have a plan for whom to call and when to call.[66] Pregnant individuals with blood pressures in the severe range should start antihypertensive therapy, and the diagnosis should be reclassified as preeclampsia with severe features. The optimal gestational age for birth depends on the severity of the condition and the status of the fetus. In those persons with uncomplicated gestational hypertension, induction of labor is generally recommended at 37 0/7 weeks.[66]

## Preeclampsia and Eclampsia

Worldwide, approximately 2% to 8% of pregnant people experience preeclampsia.[67] The rate of preeclampsia and eclampsia in the United States

---

**Box 24-2 Preeclampsia Warning Signs**

- Persistent and/or severe headache
- Visual abnormalities (blurred vision, seeing spots, or other changes)
- New onset of swelling of face or sudden weight gain
- New nausea and vomiting in the second half of pregnancy
- Unrelenting pain in the epigastric or right upper quadrant/abdominal area
- New onset of dyspnea, orthopnea

Data from American College of Obstetricians and Gynecologists. ACOG Practice Bulletin No. 222: gestational hypertension and preeclampsia. *Obstet Gynecol*. 2020;135(6):e237-e260.ACOG. Preeclampsia and Pregnancy Infographic. The American College of Obstetric and Gynecology. https://www.acog.org/womens-health/infographics/preeclampsia-and-pregnancy. December 2021. Accessed September 15, 2022.

increased by an estimated 21% from 2005 to 2014, consistent with increases in preeclampsia risk factors of obesity, gestating person's age, and diabetes.[66,73]

## Pathophysiology of Preeclampsia

The primary feature of preeclampsia is hypertension that appears in the second half of pregnancy and is often associated with proteinuria. Although previously believed to be a disorder of late pregnancy, preeclampsia is actually a multisystem disorder that begins early in pregnancy. As a placental disease, preeclampsia progresses in two stages: (1) abnormal placentation earlier in the first trimester, followed by (2) a syndrome in the later second and third trimesters characterized by an excess of antiangiogenic factors.[74] Placental tissue is key to this disorder; that is, placental tissue must be present, but the presence of a fetus is not required. Individuals with a hydatidiform mole pregnancy have a risk for developing signs of preeclampsia early in pregnancy. Furthermore, the only consensus treatment is expediting birth. The disease often resolves spontaneously only after placental tissue is expelled and circulating placental hormones decrease, resulting in preeclampsia being one of the leading causes of nonspontaneous preterm birth. Although placental birth can resolve most signs and symptoms, preeclampsia can persist after birth and, in some cases, people can begin to develop de novo preeclampsia in the postpartum period.

The underlying pathophysiology of preeclampsia is not completely understood. Recent evidence has suggested an imbalance of angiogenic factors as a component of the pathogenesis of preeclampsia.[66] In a normally developing placenta, cytotrophoblast cells extend into the endothelial lining of the decidual segment of the spiral arteries first; later, cytotrophoblast cells invade the myometrial portion of the arteries. This process causes the spiral arteries to be remodeled so they become large, low-resistance vessels that can accommodate increased blood flow. A characteristic feature of preeclampsia, which initiates a cascade of events, is the inappropriate vascular remodeling and a hypoperfused placenta from the shallow cytotrophoblast migration toward the uterine spiral arterioles.[74] The placenta then becomes ischemic, which leads to the release of factors associated with vascular endothelial dysfunction—specifically, endothelin-1 (ET-1), anti-angiogenic factor sFlt-1, agonistic autoantibodies to the angiotensin II type I receptor (ATI-AA), and decreased nitric oxide (NO).[74] The mechanisms responsible for systemic gestational vascular dysfunction are not fully understood, but a continuing cycle of repeated ischemia–reperfusion injury related to immune cells and inflammatory cytokines that cause systemic inflammation, vascular endothelial dysfunction, and a prothrombotic condition is proposed to lead to hypertension during pregnancy and end-organ dysfunction such as damage to the kidneys, liver, and brain.[74]

Early-onset preeclampsia is defined as onset of symptoms after 20 weeks but before 34 weeks' gestation. It poses a high risk to the birthing person for neurologic, cardiorespiratory, and hematologic complications as well as adverse fetoplacental conditions and complications. Pregnant individuals with early-onset preeclampsia often will have abnormal uterine artery Doppler waveforms and fetal growth restriction, and they are more likely to experience adverse perinatal outcomes, including preterm birth.[75] The higher rates of fetal growth restriction and vascular flow disturbances in individuals with early forms of preeclampsia indicate that impaired placentation makes a significant contribution to the etiopathogenesis of early preeclampsia.[75] Late-onset preeclampsia, defined as preeclampsia after 34 weeks' gestation, is associated with more favorable outcomes for the birthing person and fetus.[75] The pathophysiology of preeclampsia and clinical findings are described in Table 24-9.[66,74]

Preeclampsia is associated with placental abruption, as well as stroke, organ failure, and death for the pregnant person. For the fetus, adverse effects of this disorder include preterm birth, fetal growth restriction, stillbirth, and neonatal death. Individuals who develop preeclampsia have a two-fold increase in the risk for cardiovascular disease throughout life and mortality from ischemic heart disease, heart failure, or stroke.[76,77] The likelihood of having hypertension after the perinatal period is increased more than three-fold when a pregnant individual develops preeclampsia. Factors that affect the increased risk for cardiovascular disease include multiparity, prematurity, and severity of the hypertensive disorder.[76,77]

### Risk Factors for Preeclampsia

Risk factors for preeclampsia are listed in Table 24-10. A history of preeclampsia in a prior pregnancy increases the risk of preeclampsia by seven-fold compared to individuals without a history of preeclampsia. The U.S. Preventive Services Task Force and other professional associations recommend that people with high risk factors for preeclampsia take low-dose aspirin (81 mg) daily, starting after 12 weeks' gestation, in subsequent pregnancies.[66,77] Low-dose aspirin in this population significantly reduces the risk for preeclampsia (relative risk [RR], 0.85; 95% confidence interval [CI], 0.75–0.95).[77] A discussion with the patient

| Table 24-9 | Abnormal Findings in Preeclampsia/Eclampsia |
|---|---|
| **Pathophysiology** | **Organ System Findings** |
| **Renal** | |
| Release of placental factors leads to endothelial edema and hypertrophy, reducing the glomerular filtration rate and increasing tubular reabsorption | Proteinuria (urine protein creatinine ratio > 0.30 or 300 mg/24-hour urine collection) <br> ↑ Serum creatinine <br> ↑ Serum uric acid <br> ↑ Blood urea nitrogen (BUN) <br> ↓ Creatinine clearance <br> Oliguria |
| **Cardiovascular** | |
| Inflammation and endothelial dysfunction cause hyperreactivity of vessels | Hypertension |
| Fluid shifts from intravascular to extracellular spaces, causing edema | Peripheral edema |
| Endothelial blood vessel damage leads to fluid leakage into alveoli; most frequently occurs postpartum | Pulmonary edema |
| **Hepatic** | |
| Damage to lining of small blood vessels leads to hemolysis, elevated liver enzymes, and increased fibrin deposits | ↑ Aspartate transaminase (AST) <br> ↑ Alanine transaminase (ALT) |
| The preceding effects can lead to tissue necrosis and infarction; pain is caused by vasospasm | ↑ Right upper quadrant or epigastric pain |
| **Central Nervous System** | |
| Endothelial damage allows fluid to leak into brain tissue, leading to cerebral edema <br> Vasospasm can result in ischemia | Headaches, visual disturbances <br> Seizures <br> Stroke <br> Hyperreflexia |
| **Hematologic** | |
| Fluid shifts from intravascular to extracellular spaces, decreasing serum levels and causing edema <br> Reduction in plasma volume results in hemoconcentration | ↑ Hemoglobin and hematocrit |
| Inappropriate activation of leukocytes, complement, and clotting factors depletes platelets and increases clotting time, leading to hemolysis | Thrombocytopenia <br> ↓ Fibrinogen <br> Fibrin split products <br> Prolonged prothrombin time (PT) <br> Prolonged partial prothrombin time (PPT) |
| **Placental Function** | |
| Inadequate remodeling of spiral arteries leads to vasoconstriction and reduced placental perfusion | Fetal growth restriction <br> ↓ Amniotic fluid index <br> Nonreactive nonstress test <br> Placental abruption |

Based on American College of Obstetricians and Gynecologists. ACOG Practice Bulletin No. 222: gestational hypertension and preeclampsia. *Obstet Gynecol.* 2020;135(6):e237-e260. doi:10.1097/AOG.0000000000003891; Granger JP, Spradley FT, Bakrania BA. The endothelin system: a critical player in the pathophysiology of preeclampsia. *Curr Hypertens Rep.* 2018;20(4):32. doi:10.1007/s11906-018-0828-4.

| Table 24-10 | Risk Assessment for Preeclampsia Based on Medical History | |
|---|---|---|
| **Risk Level** | **Risk Factors** | **Recommendation** |
| High[a] | Autoimmune disease (SLE, APA) | Recommend low-dose aspirin if the pregnant individual has one or more of these high-risk factors |
| | Chronic hypertension | |
| | History of preeclampsia, especially if accompanied by an adverse outcome | |
| | Multifetal gestation | |
| | Renal disease | |
| | Type 1 or 2 diabetes | |
| Moderate[b] | Age ≥ 35 years | Consider low-dose aspirin if the pregnant individual has two or more of these moderate-risk factors |
| | BMI ≥ 30 kg/m$^2$ | |
| | Family history of preeclampsia in mother or sister | |
| | Nulliparity | |
| | In vitro conception | |
| | Personal history risk factors (e.g., history of low fetal birth weight, small for gestational age, previous adverse pregnancy outcome, > 10-year pregnancy interval) | |
| | Sociodemographic characteristics (e.g., exposure to structural racism such as experienced by Black individuals, low socioeconomic status) | |

Abbreviations: APA, antiphospholipid antibody; SLE, systemic lupus erythematosus.

[a] Single risk factors that are consistently associated with the greatest risk for preeclampsia. The incidence of preeclampsia in pregnant people with one or more of these risk factors is approximately ≥ 8%.

[b] A combination of multiple moderate-risk factors (two or more) may be used to identify those persons at high risk for preeclampsia. These risk factors are independently associated with preeclampsia, some more consistently than others. These risk factors vary in their association with an increased risk for preeclampsia.

Modified from the U.S. Preventive Services Task Force. *Final Recommendation Statement: Low-Dose Aspirin Use for the Prevention of Morbidity and Mortality from Preeclampsia: Preventive Medication.* September 28, 2021. https://www.uspreventiveservicestaskforce.org/uspstf /recommendation/low-dose-aspirin-use-for-the-prevention-of-morbidity-and-mortality-from-preeclampsia-preventive-medication. Accessed October 4, 2021.

about their individual risk factors can help with decision making.

### Diagnosis of Preeclampsia

Preeclampsia may slowly progress over a period of weeks, or it may develop in a fulminant manner over a few hours. Recent research has investigated the use of certain biomarkers and uterine artery Doppler studies to help predict preeclampsia. At this time, no screening method for the disorder is recommended, other than taking a complete medical history to assess for known risk factors.[66]

Historically, edema, proteinuria, and hypertension were the classic triad of symptoms that defined preeclampsia. Edema is relatively common in pregnancy, however, so it is no longer considered a diagnostic criterion. Proteinuria, detected via a urine protein creatinine ratio or 24-hour collection for total protein and creatinine clearance, is a common manifestation of reduced renal function, but preeclampsia can manifest in the absence of proteinuria. Today, when hypertension exists but proteinuria is absent, other factors are used to confirm diagnosis, as noted in Table 24-8. When an individual with hypertension develops systemic organ involvement (refer to Box 24-2 for symptoms) or severe hypertension (blood pressure ≥ 160 mm Hg systolic and/ or 110 mm Hg diastolic on two occasions), the diagnosis becomes preeclampsia with severe features.

Although preeclampsia is the most common cause of hypertension and end-organ dysfunction in pregnant people, it is important to remember the differential diagnoses that can mimic preeclampsia:

* Acute fatty liver of pregnancy: In addition to having hypertension and other symptoms of preeclampsia, pregnant persons with acute

fatty liver of pregnancy present with an-orexia, nausea and vomiting, and low-grade fever. Liver dysfunction is more severe, and the individual may develop disseminated in-travascular coagulation.

- Thrombotic thrombocytopenic purpura or hemolytic uremic syndrome: People with this syndrome have microangiopathic hemolytic anemia, thrombocytopenia, neurologic and renal abnormalities, and fever.

- HELLP syndrome (discussed later in this sec-tion): Thought to be a severe form of pre-eclampsia, HELLP syndrome may not present with hypertension or proteinuria. Thus, in-dividuals may have a variable presentation, although the most common symptoms are abdominal pain and mid-epigastric or right upper quadrant tenderness. Nausea and vom-iting and malaise may be present, causing this condition to be mistaken for hepatitis. Jaun-dice, visual changes, and ascites can develop.

These disorders are severe illnesses associated with a high incidence of morbidity for the pregnant person and fetus. Prompt assessment by a physician or MFM specialist is indicated for pregnant patients who have symptoms that suggest a disorder other than preeclampsia.

### Treatment of Individuals with Preeclampsia

The role of the midwife in caring for people who develop hypertension during pregnancy focuses on meticulous screening, early identification, referral or consultation, ongoing assessment, and participation in a collaborative model of care as appropriate. In-patient care is reviewed in more detail in the *Com-plications During Labor and Birth* chapter.

Treatment of preeclampsia often includes expe-diting birth of the fetus and the placenta. Expectant management requires consideration of the health of the pregnant individual and their fetus. Expectant management of and induction of labor in patients with preeclampsia without severe features should be done within a shared decision-making model, which takes into consideration the pregnant person, the fetal risks and benefits, appropriate resources, and ongoing vigilant antenatal surveillance.

No randomized trials have been conducted in this population, but data from retrospective stud-ies recommend that pregnant individuals without severe features continue with antenatal fetal moni-toring until birth at 37 0/7 weeks' gestation for neonatal benefit.[66] Antenatal monitoring of indi-viduals with preeclampsia without severe features

consists of serial ultrasonography to determine fetal growth, weekly antepartum testing, close monitor-ing of blood pressure, and weekly laboratory tests for preeclampsia, although additional proteinuria quantifications are not necessary. Antihyperten-sive medication is not recommended for pregnant individuals with preeclampsia unless they have severe-range blood pressures. Risks associated with expectant management include development of pre-eclampsia with severe features, eclampsia, HELLP syndrome, placental abruption, fetal growth restric-tion, and fetal or maternal death.[67]

### Management of Individuals with Severe Hypertension

Severe hypertension (SBP ≥ 160 mm Hg and/or DBP ≥ 110 mm Hg) is an emergency and can result in acute and long-term complications for both the pregnant individual and the newborn. Evidence-based guidelines for treating severe hyper-tension produced by the National Partnership for Maternal Safety,[78] and endorsed by other profes-sional associations, state that pregnant people with severe hypertension should be evaluated within 15 minutes and treated within 30 minutes. Treat-ment of severe hypertension is reviewed in the *Com-plications During Labor and Birth* chapter.

Potential complications of severe hypertension in pregnancy include pulmonary edema, myocar-dial infarction, stroke, acute respiratory distress syndrome, coagulopathy, renal failure, and retinal injury.[66,67] Birth is recommended when preeclamp-sia with severe features is diagnosed at or beyond 34 0/7 weeks' gestation. ACOG recommends not delaying birth for the administration of steroids in the late preterm period. If a patient is diagnosed with preeclampsia with severe features at less than 34 0/7 weeks' gestation and the fetus and pregnant person are stable, expectant management may be considered until 34 0/7 weeks' gestation. Expectant management is not advised when neonatal survival is not anticipated. Birth is recommended at any time when there is deterioration of the pregnant person or fetus during expectant management. If birth is strongly indicated before 34 0/7 weeks' gestation, administration of corticosteroids for fetal lung mat-uration is recommended.[66,67]

The evaluation of the person with a hypertensive disorder in the postpartum period up to 12 weeks, or the fourth trimester, has not been extensively stud-ied. Based on the scarce data that do exist regarding evaluation and management of blood pressure in the fourth trimester, ACOG recommends that pregnant people with severe hypertension should have a blood pressure evaluation within 72 hours after birth and again no more than 7 to 10 days postpartum.[66,68]

## Eclampsia

Eclampsia is a serious acute complication of pregnancy, which carries high morbidity and mortality for both the pregnant person and the fetus. Eclampsia is defined as the occurrence of one or more generalized, tonic–clonic convulsions unrelated to other medical conditions in the pregnant individual with hypertensive disorder. The reported incidence of eclampsia is 1.6 to 10 per 10,000 deliveries in developed countries, and 50 to 151 per 10,000 deliveries in developing countries. Although 10% of pregnancies are complicated by hypertensive disorders, eclampsia occurs in 0.8% of pregnancies in which the birthing person has a hypertensive disorder.[79]

Risk factors for eclampsia are similar to those associated with preeclampsia or gestational hypertension. Implementing protocols for magnesium sulfate prophylaxis for pregnant individuals presenting with severe hypertension has decreased the incidence of eclampsia. The rate of seizures in pregnant individuals with severe preeclampsia not receiving magnesium sulfate is 2.0%, but only 0.6% in those receiving magnesium sulfate.[79]

Several signs and symptoms can precede eclampsia, such as visual disturbances, epigastric pain, and severe persistent headaches, but none has accurately predicted eclampsia. The most common finding during the neurologic examination following a seizure is altered mental status and deficits of memory or visual perception. Eclamptic convulsions can occur in the antepartum (59% to 70%), intrapartum (20% to 30%), or postpartum period. Most cases of eclampsia occur after 28 weeks' gestation; those that occur before 20 weeks' gestation are usually associated with a molar pregnancy.[79]

Beyond risk of mortality, eclampsia is associated with other significant complications, including increased risk of placental abruption, HELLP, disseminated intravascular coagulation, pulmonary edema, aspiration pneumonia, cardiopulmonary arrest, and acute renal failure. These risks have a higher reported incidence in pregnant individuals who develop eclampsia before 32 weeks' gestation.[79] Treatment of eclampsia is reviewed in the *Complications During Labor and Birth* chapter.

## Chronic Hypertension with Superimposed Preeclampsia

Initial management of pregnant individuals with chronic hypertension and superimposed preeclampsia follows the same guidelines recommended for pregnant people with preeclampsia, including assessment of severity, baseline laboratory values, fetal well-being, and gestational age. When the superimposed preeclampsia has severe features, administration of parenteral magnesium sulfate is indicated during the intrapartum and postpartum periods. Decisions about the timing of birth are driven by consideration of disease severity, the rate at which the disease is progressing, and close assessment of the gestating person and fetal well-being.[80]

## Hemolysis, Elevated Liver Enzymes, and Low Platelets (HELLP) Syndrome

HELLP syndrome is a pregnancy-associated liver disease characterized by the presence of hemolysis (H), elevated liver (EL) enzymes, and a low platelet (LP) count. It is a potentially life-threatening condition manifesting in the context of preeclampsia. This syndrome was initially believed to be a severe form of preeclampsia, as 5% to 20% of pregnant individuals with severe preeclampsia have been reported to develop HELLP syndrome; however, as many as 15% to 20% of pregnant patients with HELLP syndrome do not have preeclampsia prior to developing the syndrome. Furthermore, as many as 30% of people with HELLP syndrome are diagnosed in the postpartum period.[80]

The pathophysiology of HELLP syndrome is similar to that of preeclampsia. Individuals who develop this condition have abnormal placentation that can cause release of inflammatory cytokines and endothelial injury, along with release of other toxic substances that may aid in the development and clinical manifestations of HELLP in the late trimesters. Risk factors include previous hypertensive disorder of pregnancy, previous HELLP syndrome, previous high-risk pregnancy, nulliparity, and multiple gestation.[81,82]

Clinical manifestations of HELLP syndrome include elevated blood pressure, right upper quadrant abdominal or epigastric pain, persistent headaches, visual disturbances, significant weight gain, malaise, dyspnea, nausea, and vomiting. A report of severe pain in the right upper quadrant can also be indicative of a hepatic rupture.[81,82] HELLP syndrome has a peak incidence between 27 and 37 weeks' gestation, but, as mentioned earlier, some cases do not develop until the immediate postpartum period.

The University of Mississippi has developed a classification system to describe the HELLP syndrome based on the nadir platelet count of the pregnant individual: severe or class I (< 50K cells/mL), moderate or class II (50K–100K cells/mL), and mild or class III (100K–150K cells/mL).[83] This system also takes into consideration the diagnosis of partial HELLP syndrome, which is evidence of severe preeclampsia or eclampsia along with two or three laboratory criteria for HELLP syndrome. The Tennessee Classification system categorizes HELLP based on a set of laboratory values rather than disease severity (platelets < 100K cells/mL, LDH ≥ 600 IU/L, AST or ALT ≥ 70 IU/L).[81,83]

There is no definitive cure for HELLP syndrome. Its emergence increases a pregnant person's risk for eclampsia, disseminated intravascular coagulation, acute renal failure, liver hematoma, placental abruption, fetal growth restriction, preterm birth, neonatal respiratory distress syndrome, and perinatal death. Therefore, the standard of care and management of HELLP syndrome focuses on stabilization of the fetus and of the pregnant person's blood pressure. Typically, birth is recommended at 34 weeks' gestation, or earlier in the case of nonreassuring status of the pregnant individual or fetus.[83] If both patient and fetus are stable, administration of antenatal corticosteroids after viability and less than 34 weeks' gestation, magnesium sulfate therapy, and birth are recommended to decrease neonatal morbidity and mortality.[81]

### Fourth Trimester Management of Hypertension

Hypertensive disorders in pregnancy are associated with an increased risk of postpartum readmission and hospitalization and have become a leading cause of postpartum readmission in the United States.[84] More than half of all maternal deaths occur in the fourth trimester,[85] and hypertension is one of the main causes of these deaths. Individuals in the fourth trimester can also develop de novo postpartum preeclampsia, with approximately one-third of eclampsia occurring in the postpartum period. The exact prevalence of de novo postpartum hypertension or preeclampsia is not presently known, but is estimated to be approximately 2% of pregnancies. Only limited data are available regarding the risk factors, pathogenesis, and pathophysiology of postpartum hypertensive disorders.[80] Midwives are essential in early identification and management in individuals with de novo postpartum preeclampsia, as these individuals are at an increased risk of stroke, seizures, pulmonary edema, renal failure, congestive heart failure, and death.

Management of postpartum hypertensive disorders follows the same guidelines as during pregnancy, except regarding antenatal fetal surveillance and testing. Individuals with severe hypertension are treated with intravenous injections of either labetalol or hydralazine in addition to magnesium sulfate

for seizure prophylaxis. Oral antihypertensives are recommended if SBP remains persistently greater than 150 mm Hg and/or if DBP remains persistently greater than 100 mm Hg. These patients with postpartum hypertension must be closely monitored, including follow-up within 1 week after discharge once blood pressure is controlled in the hospital. Daily blood pressure measurements by the patient or visiting nurse and reporting of symptoms should be performed. Antihypertensive medications are discontinued if the patient's blood pressure remains below hypertensive levels for at least 48 hours. This condition may take several weeks to resolve, and those individuals who continue to have persistent hypertension despite antihypertensive therapy need to be further evaluated for other medical concerns.[86,87]

Significant racial disparities exist in postpartum complication and readmission rates. Currently, most hospitals discharge postpartum patients within 24 to 48 hours and many individuals do not return for a blood pressure check until the standard 6-week postpartum visit, which can lead to missed blood pressure measurements and adjustment of treatment.[86] Black individuals with cardiovascular risk factors are more likely to be readmitted postpartum, to have severe morbidity, and to have life-threatening complications including pulmonary edema and acute heart failure compared to white individuals; these increased rates of complications are due to a variety of factors, including systemic societal inequities and racism.[86] More studies are needed to examine hypertensive disorders in the postpartum period and develop management guidelines and a better system to address the fourth trimester and the effects of systemic racism on health.

## Infectious Diseases

Several infectious diseases are known to cause congenital anomalies, fetal harm, or fetal death. Midwives are often involved in screening, diagnosis, counseling about prevention, and obtaining physician consultation as needed for these infections. In adults, symptoms may be mild or difficult to differentiate. Acute or past infection often goes undetected without routine screening. Intrauterine exposure results in various clinical syndromes that are not easily differentiated. For example, neonates born with many of these congenital infections will have a rash, microcephaly, growth restriction, hearing loss, and hepatosplenomegaly. In the past, the acronym TORCH was used to denote the most common of these infections: T for toxoplasmosis, O for syphilis, R for rubella, C for cytomegalovirus, and H for herpes. Although a testing panel for TORCH antibodies is still available in some locations, specific tests for individual infections based on risks, exposure, or maternal/fetal signs have become more widely used, as knowledge and testing modalities have expanded. Nevertheless, the TORCH acronym still provides useful insights into potential differential diagnoses of suspected congenital infections and their sequelae.

In most cases, perinatal diagnosis will include serologic testing for disease-specific immunoglobulins G and M (IgG and IgM). The presence of IgG antibodies usually indicates past infection or immunity, as these antibodies remain present in the body for life. In an acute infection, IgG can take several weeks to appear in the blood. IgM antibodies indicate acute infection; their levels will begin to rise within a much shorter time period, usually 2 to 3 weeks after exposure. IgM antibody production eventually peaks, and the antibodies disappear as infection resolves and IgG levels rise. The exact timing of these changing antibody levels varies depending on the specific disease.

Antibodies can also be measured quantitatively as a titer reported as a ratio (e.g., 1:4). The higher the second number, the higher the antibody level in the blood. Such antibody titers can be followed to detect a rise that could indicate new or worsening infection. Typically, a four-fold or greater rise (e.g., 1:4 to 1:16) is a worrisome finding.

Specialized reference laboratories can conduct antibody avidity testing, which measures the strength of the IgG antibody response over time. Low avidity indicates a recent infection, whereas high avidity suggests infection greater than 3 months prior and immunity in some cases. Pregnant individuals or neonates with findings suggestive of infection warrant prompt consultation with the appropriate specialist(s).

The *Reproductive Tract and Sexually Transmitted Infections* and *Prenatal Care* chapters review prenatal considerations for people who are exposed to or develop syphilis, hepatitis B, herpes, HIV (including treatment in pregnancy and timing of birth), human papillomavirus (HPV), and Zika virus. This section reviews other clinically significant infections that are associated with adverse perinatal outcomes. Many of these infections are considered communicable diseases and, therefore, are reportable to the local public health department. Midwives should be aware of the mandatory reporting laws within their respective states.

## Cytomegalovirus

Cytomegalovirus (CMV) is the most common congenital infection in the United States, affecting 20,000 to 30,000 neonates each year.[89] Transmission of CMV occurs through direct contact with body fluids such as saliva, tears, urine, semen, or vaginal secretions.[87] Symptoms of CMV infection are mild and can include fever, sore throat, swollen glands, and fatigue.

Between 50% and 80% of adults have previously experienced a primary CMV infection, which is typically asymptomatic. Although previously infected individuals have antibodies that can protect them against recurrence, a secondary reinfection can still occur if they are exposed to a newer strain of CMV or reactivation of a latent infection occurs.[88] In addition, asymptomatic viral shedding can occur for months after symptoms have resolved. Children in daycare facilities are frequent sources of infection through continued viral shedding in their saliva. Prevention of CMV centers on behaviors that may mitigate risks, including careful hand washing after exposure to bodly fluids and avoidance of direct contact such as kissing on the mouth or sharing food, cups, and utensils.[88]

When primary CMV infection occurs during pregnancy, the risks of vertical transmission to the fetus increase as gestation advances, from 14% in the first trimester to 68% in the third trimester.[88] Vertical transmission can also occur during a secondary reactivation, albeit at a much lower rate of 1%.[89]

CMV poses many risks to the fetus, including fetal growth restriction, microcephaly, hepatosplenomegaly, thrombocytopenia, hearing loss, vision impairment, and learning disabilities.[88] Among those with primary infection in pregnancy, approximately 10% to 15% of infants will have visible signs at birth (petechial "blueberry muffin" rash, small for gestational age, microcephaly, hepatosplenomegaly, or hyperbilirubinemia).[88] Infected neonates born without these obvious markers have a 10% to 15% risk of progressive hearing loss with a later onset in childhood.[88] The risk of hearing loss also applies to neonates born after a secondary CMV reactivation.[88]

Routine prenatal screening for this virus is not recommended because point-of-care IgG and IgM antibody testing for CMV is not specific and difficult to interpret.[88] Diagnosis of CMV infection in symptomatic pregnant individuals can be confirmed via polymerase chain reaction (PCR) analysis of blood, urine, or saliva, or by monitoring serum IgM and IgG antibodies. IgM alone is not a reliable indicator of primary CMV.[89] Serial monitoring of IgG at least 4 weeks apart and after 18 weeks' gestation provides the most accurate diagnostic information. A four-fold increase in IgG levels or seroconversion from negative to positive during pregnancy confirms the diagnosis of a primary CMV infection.[88]

Antibody avidity testing of IgG can further help determine when the infection occurred in cases where the IgM antibody test is also positive.[89]

Fetal CMV infection should be suspected when specific ultrasound findings such as microcephaly, hydrops fetalis, echogenic bowel, cerebral calcifications, and fetal growth restriction are seen.[88] These signs are also present in many other congenital infections, confounding the diagnosis. The patient should be referred to a MFM specialist for further evaluation. Infection can be confirmed by detecting CMV DNA in the amniotic fluid or testing the neonate after birth.[88] Amniocentesis is more accurate if performed more than 6 weeks after infection and at least 20 weeks' gestation.[89]

### Listeriosis

*Listeria monocytogenes* is a gram-positive bacillus that is readily found in the environment. It can be isolated in soil, water, and decaying vegetation. People acquire infection after ingesting foods contaminated with *Listeria*, such as undercooked meat, dairy products, and cheese.[90] More recently, ready-to-eat foods such as hummus, deli meals, frozen vegetables, unwashed fruits, and salads have also been linked to infections. Although *Listeria* outbreaks are uncommon in the United States, the rate of infection in pregnant persons is 13 times higher than that in the general population.[90] *Listeria* is vertically transmitted to the fetus and is associated with increased rates of miscarriage, preterm labor, stillbirth, and sepsis or meningitis in the neonate.[90] These outcomes are more common when infection occurs earlier in the gestation.[90]

Suspected exposure to listeriosis occurs during known community outbreaks or after ingestion of a recalled food. Symptoms appear within 10 days after exposure, with most infections presenting as mild gastrointestinal complaints followed by flu-like symptoms.[90] There is no PCR test available that can detect *Listeria* in body fluids, and antibody testing is not reliable.[90]

Diagnosis and treatment are based on presumptive exposure, symptoms, and the presence or absence of fever. Asymptomatic individuals and those who are afebrile with mild symptoms can be managed expectantly, and no testing or treatment is recommended.[90] Blood cultures can be offered to confirm the diagnosis but are typically reserved for pregnant persons exposed to *Listeria* and presenting with fever greater than 38.1°C (100.6°F).[90] When blood cultures are ordered, the laboratory should be notified of the clinical suspicion for listeriosis. Once confirmed, treatment with intravenous ampicillin is recommended.[90] Placental cultures should be obtained after delivery.

Midwives should be vigilant for signs and symptoms of listeriosis, and all individuals seeking preconception and prenatal care should receive education on prevention strategies. Washing fruits and vegetables, proper storage of leftovers, and avoiding foods considered to have a high risk of *Listeria* contamination will help mitigate exposure. Foods with a high risk of being contaminated with this pathogen are listed in the *Prenatal Care* chapter. Patients suspected to have listeriosis should be referred to a physician for ongoing management and prompt initiation of antibiotics. Early treatment with antibiotics improves fetal and neonatal outcomes.

### Parvovirus B19

Parvovirus B19, also known as "fifth disease," is a highly contagious virus; outbreaks occur quite frequently among school-age children during the winter months. The virus is transmitted primarily through respiratory droplet and hand-to-mouth exposure.[91] Once someone is exposed, prodromal symptoms will appear within 5 to 10 days and last for about a week. As with other viral illnesses, infected individuals will be contagious prior to the onset of any symptoms. In children, prodromal symptoms include fever, sore throat, and headache followed by a characteristic bright red facial rash resembling "slapped cheeks." Adults typically experience mild prodromal symptoms that are followed by development of a pruritic maculopapular rash on the trunk and extremities along with generalized arthralgias; adults rarely exhibit the facial rash.[92]

Once someone has been infected with parvovirus B19, they have lifelong immunity against future infection. In fact, by age 30, 60% of adults will be fully protected from the virus.[92] For nonimmune individuals, risks of infection are highest for those working with young children (e.g., teachers, daycare workers) or living with an infected child.[91,92]

During pregnancy, nonimmune individuals who acquire a parvovirus B19 infection have a fetal transmission rate of 17% to 33%, with a 1% to 2% risk of acute fetal infection.[91,92] The virus is attracted to red blood cells in the fetal liver, causing lysis, cell death, and severe anemia. When the fetus is infected in the first trimester, the risk of fetal loss is approximately 13%.[92] Parvovirus B19 infection in the second trimester can cause hepatic inflammation, severe anemia, cardiac failure, nonimmune fetal hydrops, and fetal death.[92] Vertical transmission in the third trimester is rare due to normal changes in placental morphology that block the virus from entering the fetal circulation.

Parvovirus B19 infection in a pregnant individual is confirmed through virus-specific serum antibody testing (IgG and IgM titers). A positive IgG antibody titer typically indicates past infection and immunity to parvovirus B19. In this case, there is no risk to the fetus, and further testing is unnecessary. Any positive IgM titer indicates acute infection and referral to an MFM specialist is advised. However, serum IgM antibodies may not appear until 10 to 12 days following exposure. There is also a small window of time in which the IgG titer could start to rise prior to a positive IgM titer in a new exposure.[92] Therefore, if exposure occurred within the previous 2 weeks, a negative IgM should prompt a repeat IgM titer in 2 to 3 weeks regardless of the IgG titer results. If the repeat IgM titer returns positive, this confirms an acute infection.

Once referred to a specialist, pregnant individuals with confirmed parvovirus B19 infections will undergo serial ultrasound examinations to screen for impaired fetal growth, amniotic fluid abnormalities, placentomegaly, and signs of nonimmune fetal hydrops.[91,92] Additionally, Doppler assessment of middle cerebral artery (MCA) peak systolic velocity is performed to detect fetal anemia, a precursor to fetal hydrops.[91] Fetal surveillance continues for 8 to 12 weeks, after which time the risks to the fetus are thought to be rare. If severe anemia and/or nonimmune fetal hydrops is detected, the next steps will likely be fetal transfusion via fetal umbilical cord blood sampling at a specialized center.[92] Figure 24-3 outlines the specific management steps once parvovirus B19 infection is detected during pregnancy.

Universal screening for parvovirus B19 is not currently recommended as a routine part of prenatal care. Any pregnant individual presenting with symptoms suggestive of parvovirus B19 or with a history of a direct exposure (e.g., a household member with confirmed infection) however, should have viral IgG and IgM titers drawn.[91] Screening of pregnant individuals working in high-risk settings (e.g., teachers, daycare workers) is controversial and work restrictions to reduce potential risks of exposure are not necessary. During seasonal parvovirus B19 outbreaks, exposure risks are increased, and testing can be reconsidered. Although pregnant individuals with parvovirus B19 will require referral for fetal surveillance, midwives can resume prenatal, intrapartum, and postpartum care if ultrasound and Doppler evaluation is normal.

### Rubella

Rubella, formerly known as "German measles," is an infection caused by the rubella virus. Also referred to as the 3-day measles, rubella is often confused with the more serious rubeola (measles) virus. In contrast to rubeola, rubella is considered a mild illness with few sequelae unless acquired during pregnancy. Population-level immunization has virtually eliminated perinatal rubella infection and congenital rubella syndrome in the United States, but this risk persists in populations where the vaccine is not in wide use, and outbreaks still occur in other parts of the world.[93]

Rubella is transmitted via contact with respiratory droplets from infected people. The incubation period is approximately 12 to 23 days.[93,94] Prodromal symptoms include low-grade fever, malaise, congestion, and postauricular lymphadenopathy.[94] The characteristic maculopapular rash begins on the face and spreads rapidly down the body. This rash can be mildly pruritic and persists for 1 to 3 days. Peak infectivity exists when symptoms are present; however, viral shedding occurs 7 days before and 7 days after the rash appears, during which time the individual is infectious to others.[93] Up to 50% of children with rubella have a subclinical or asymptomatic course.[93] In adults, the disease is more symptomatic, with 70% of those assigned female gender at birth experiencing arthralgia or arthritis in addition to the other symptoms.[94]

Fetal infection rates vary over the course of pregnancy, and are highest in the first and third trimesters (90% and 100%, respectively) and somewhat lower in the second trimester (25%).[94] Deafness, cataracts, and cardiac defects are the classic triad of congenital anomalies referred to as congenital rubella syndrome.[93,94] Congenital rubella infection is a systemic illness, and can affect almost all fetal organs; thus, miscarriage, preterm birth, fetal growth restriction, and stillbirth are possible.[94] The severity of congenital rubella syndrome depends on the timing of infection, with the highest risks occurring before 18 weeks' gestation.[94]

A pregnant person who is nonimmune and presents with symptoms suggestive of rubella or a history of exposure should be tested immediately. Clinical diagnosis alone is unreliable due to the overlap of symptoms seen in other viral syndromes. PCR testing of specimens from the nasopharynx, urine, or cerebrospinal fluid can detect the presence of rubella virus up to 10 days after the rash appears.[93] As soon as possible after the onset of symptoms, rubella-specific IgG serology should also be obtained. Although often ordered together, serology for IgM is not recommended or helpful in confirming an acute rubella infection. False-positive results can occur depending on when the

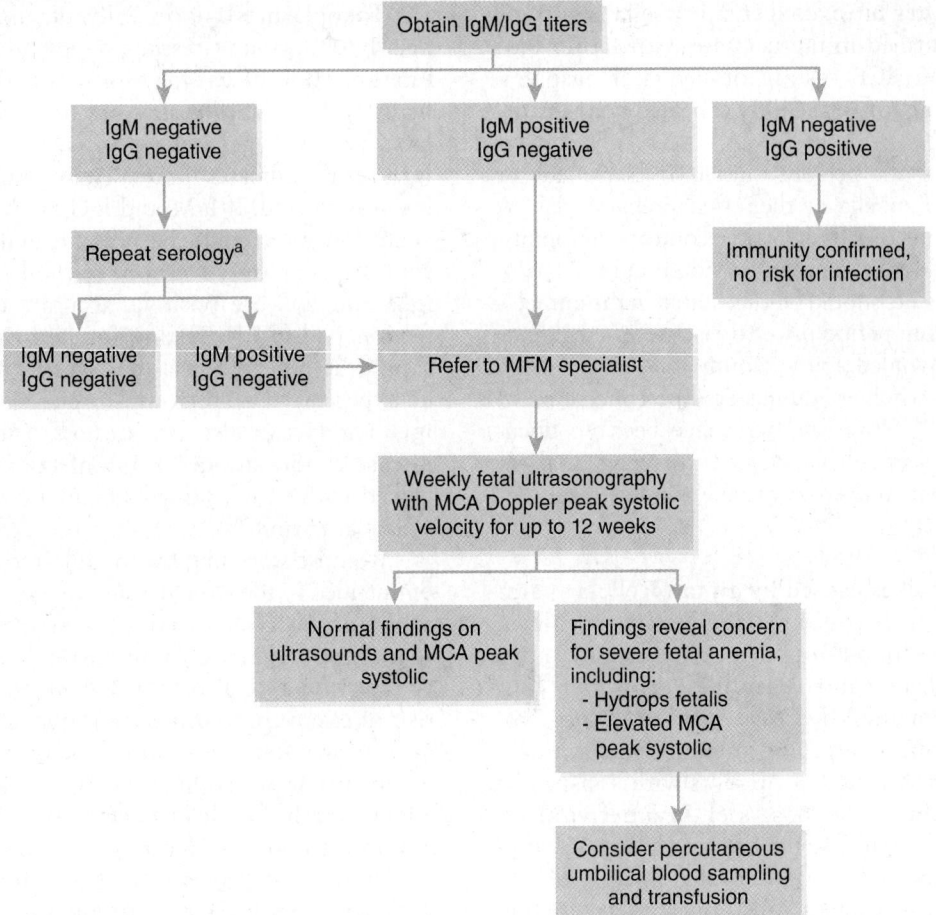

**Figure 24-3** Management algorithm for parvovirus B19 infection during pregnancy.
Abbreviations: IgG, immunoglobulin G; IgM, immunoglobulin M; MCA, middle cerebral artery; MFM, maternal–fetal medicine.
[a] Timing of repeat antibody testing is dependent on timing of exposure and/or symptom onset.
Reproduced with permission from Hunter LA, Ayala NK. Parvovirus B19 in pregnancy: a case review. *J Midwifery Womens Health.* 2021;66(3):385-390. doi:10.1111/jmwh.13254.

specimen was collected.[93] IgG titers can be interpreted as follows:

- A single negative IgG titer indicates a susceptibility to infection and should be repeated in 2 to 3 weeks. Even in cases of known nonimmunity, this baseline titer should be checked when symptoms suggestive of rubella are present. A four-fold increase in IgG titer levels is diagnostic for rubella infection.[94]

- In a symptomatic individual, a single positive IgG does not confirm recent infection versus possible immunity. Subsequent avidity testing, however, can determine the timing of when the infection occurred. Lower avidity testing would indicate a more recent infection. These results can aid in establishing the timing of

infection, especially if symptoms present in the first trimester when the risk of congenital defects from rubella is the highest.[94]

Any pregnant person with a confirmed case of rubella should be isolated from contact with others and referred to MFM for fetal testing and surveillance. Fetal rubella infection can be confirmed via PCR testing of amniotic fluid if timed correctly. The specificity and sensitivity of such testing are highest (100% and 90%, respectively) when amniocentesis is done at least 6 weeks after maternal infection, ideally after 20 weeks' gestation.[94] Amniocentesis should also be offered in case of ultrasound findings such as early-onset fetal growth restriction, microcephaly, intracerebral calcifications, and other signs that are suggestive of fetal infection. After birth, congenital rubella syndrome can be confirmed in the neonate with serum IgM testing. Viral PCR testing of neonatal nasopharyngeal, urine, or oral fluids can also confirm the diagnosis.

All pregnant persons should be screened for immunity to rubella at their first prenatal visit. A positive serum rubella IgG titer confirms immunity. Those individuals identified as nonimmune or with equivocal results should be vaccinated in the immediate postpartum period prior to discharge. Pregnancy should be avoided for a month following rubella vaccination, whether administered preconception or postpartum.[94] However, there have been no documented cases of rubella infection or congenital rubella syndrome related to vaccine administration.[93]

## Toxoplasmosis

Toxoplasmosis is caused by an intracellular parasite known as *Toxoplasma gondii*. This organism is commonly found in undercooked or raw meat, unwashed fruits and vegetables grown in contaminated soil, and the feces of infected cats.[95] In persons with a competent immune system, infection is rarely detected or presents with nonspecific symptoms similar to those seen in other viral illnesses (fever, chills, night sweats, headache, myalgias, pharyngitis, hepatosplenomegaly).[95] A primary toxoplasmosis infection confers lifelong immunity to the pathogen, although certain forms of the parasite can lay dormant in muscle and neural cells indefinitely. The recurrence of infection would only be a risk for immunocompromised individuals.

*T. gondii* is spread to people through ingestion of contaminated foods, improper hand washing after exposure to contaminated soil (i.e., gardening) or cat feces, and transplacental transfer to a fetus during pregnancy.[95] Once a pregnant person has been infected with *T. gondii* during pregnancy, the overall fetal risk of congenital toxoplasmosis is 20% to 50%.[96] The transmission rate increases from 10% in the first trimester to 25% in the second trimester, and then to 60% in the third trimester.[96] Most newborns will be asymptomatic at birth. Unfortunately, 90% of children infected with *T. gondii* in utero will subsequently develop visual impairment, hearing loss, and developmental delay.[96] Fetal ultrasound findings such as intracranial calcifications, microcephaly, ventriculomegaly, ascites, and fetal growth restriction should raise suspicion for congenital infections including toxoplasmosis.[96] Referral to an MFM and/or an infectious disease specialist is warranted when toxoplasmosis is suspected.

Toxoplasmosis is initially diagnosed via IgG and IgM antibody testing, keeping in mind that interpretation of serology for toxoplasmosis is difficult and standard assays are not available in all laboratories. In general, a positive IgG and negative IgM result indicates immunity, and no further testing is indicated. If IgM and IgG are both negative, acute infection could be present, and seroconversion may not yet have occurred. Likewise, if both IgM and IgG are positive, accurate timing of infection is difficult. Testing for both IgM and IgG should be repeated in 2 to 3 weeks, if possible, at an experienced toxoplasmosis reference laboratory. IgG avidity can also be assessed to further aid in disease confirmation.[96] Fetal infection can be confirmed with PCR testing of amniotic fluid after 18 weeks' gestation.[96]

Routine screening for toxoplasmosis is not recommended in the United States due to the low prevalence of this disease and the limited availability of specialized reference laboratories.[96] Primary prevention counseling to help individuals reduce their risk of exposure to *T. gondii* is a standard component of prenatal care. Those persons contemplating pregnancy or presenting for prenatal care should be advised wash their hands before and after handling any raw foods, avoid eating undercooked or raw meats, thoroughly wash all fruits and vegetables, and wear gloves when gardening or handling soil.[95] Cats and kittens can become infected with *T. gondii* and will shed the parasite in their feces, so pregnant individuals should avoid emptying their cat's litter boxes. If this isn't an option, gloves must be worn, with thorough hand washing occurring immediately after handling the litter box. In addition, cat litter should be changed daily, as the parasite is not immediately infectious once shed in the feces.

## Varicella

The varicella zoster virus (VZV) is a DNA virus in the herpesvirus family that can cause both primary (chickenpox) and latent (shingles) infection. Primary infection confers lifelong immunity to chickenpox; however, similar to other herpes viruses, VZV can remain dormant in the sensory nerve ganglia after a primary infection has resolved.[96] It can then be reactivated as a latent infection (shingles). Most adults born prior to 1980 have had a primary VZV infection and are considered immune to chickenpox. In addition, a varicella vaccine has been widely used in the United States since 1995 and has been shown to confer 99% immunity to primary infection.[96] Although this has significantly reduced the incidence of VZV among people of childbearing age, VZV infections still occur and can cause significant perinatal and neonatal morbidity. This section reviews primary and latent VZV infections separately.

### Primary Infection (Chickenpox)

Primary VZV is highly contagious, with an infection rate of 60% to 100% in nonimmune household contacts.[97] Transmission occurs via respiratory droplets or direct contact with vesicular fluid. Following exposure, prodromal signs of infection (fever, malaise, myalgia) will appear within 10 to 21 days. Diagnosis is made clinically from the characteristic appearance of a diffuse pruritic rash that rapidly progresses from macules to papules to vesicles.[97] All stages of the rash can be seen simultaneously. Infectivity begins 2 to 3 days prior to the rash and lasts until all vesicles have crusted over.[96,97] Viral PCR testing can be done on vesicular fluid to confirm the diagnosis but is not necessary in most cases. Any individual (infant, child, or adult) diagnosed with chickenpox should be isolated from all other susceptible persons, especially those known to be immunocompromised. Suspected cases should also be discouraged from coming inside healthcare facilities. Presumptive diagnosis can often be made remotely by symptom description or rash visualization.

At the onset of pregnancy, varicella immunity should be confirmed through either a known history of previous illness, vaccination, or positive varicella IgG titer. Nonimmunity should be documented in the prenatal record and varicella vaccine offered immediately postpartum. Those persons contemplating pregnancy should also have their immunity confirmed and can be offered the vaccine 1 month prior to conception.[96]

A primary VZV infection during pregnancy poses a 20% risk of varicella pneumonia to the pregnant person; this disease has a reported mortality rate of 40%.[96] Varicella-zoster immune globulin (VZIG) should be given as soon as an exposure has been confirmed, ideally within 96 hours and up to 10 days after the exposure, to prevent or diminish symptoms.[96] If symptoms are present, treatment with oral acyclovir can also reduce the risks of serious perinatal illness. Neither VZIG nor acyclovir has been shown to reduce vertical transmission to the fetus.[96]

Congenital varicella syndrome is extremely rare (incidence is 0.4% to 2%) and can occur after a primary infection during the first 20 weeks of gestation.[96,97] Fetal and neonatal consequences include low birth weight, microcephaly, hydrocephaly, limb abnormalities, and cognitive impairment.[96]

Likewise, if a primary VZV infection occurs within 5 days of birth or 48 hours postpartum, the infant can develop neonatal varicella, which carries a neonatal mortality rate of 30% if untreated. Prompt administration of VZIG and intravenous acyclovir has been shown to reduce this risk to 7%.[96,97] If possible, it may be prudent to delay a planned birth until viremia has resolved to reduce neonatal transmission.

### Latent Infection (Shingles)

Reactivation of VZV results in a painful erythematous vesicular eruption known as herpes zoster or shingles. This infection is more commonly seen in older adults and typically presents with erythema and clusters of painful vesicular lesions unilaterally along a sensory dermatome.[97] Rarely does the rash cross the midline. Transmission occurs solely through direct contact with the vesicular fluid. Shingles cannot be transmitted to another person; however, exposure could cause a primary VZV (chickenpox) infection in someone who is not immune to VZV.[97]

Even during pregnancy, a latent VZV infection should be treated with acyclovir to lessen the symptoms and disease severity. There are no known fetal risks from shingles, but infant exposure to open lesions after birth could cause neonatal varicella. Covering of herpes zoster lesions and careful hand washing can greatly reduce the rate of newborn transmission.

## Mental/Behavioral Health Conditions

Mental and emotional health is vital to prenatal and postpartum health and care. Refer to the *Mental Health Conditions* chapter for detailed information on specific conditions.

### Neurologic Conditions

Primary care is within the scope of practice of the midwife; thus, midwives should be equipped to care for pregnant individuals who may have or develop neurologic conditions during pregnancy. Midwifery care of pregnant individuals can include, but is not limited to, diagnosing and treating various neuropathies such as carpal tunnel syndrome, Bell's palsy, migraines, and early detection of stroke or ruling out stroke. A neurologic examination and interpretation of findings are within the midwifery scope of practice. Individuals who have complex neurologic illnesses such as multiple sclerosis or seizure disorders require specialist care during pregnancy.

## Migraine Headache

Headaches are common and can be a symptom of a wide range of disorders, some of which are benign and some of which can be life threatening. As a first consideration, whenever a patient presents with a headache in pregnancy, preeclampsia should be ruled out. Individuals with headaches that are atypical or concerning warrant prompt neurology evaluation (Table 24-11). The most common secondary headache etiologies include stroke, cerebral venous thrombosis, subarachnoid hemorrhage, pituitary tumor, choriocarcinoma, eclampsia, preeclampsia, idiopathic intracranial hypertension, and reversible cerebral vasoconstriction syndrome.[98]

Migraines are a complex neurovascular brain disorder and are estimated to affect 959 million people worldwide. The International Headache Society[99] defines migraines by the criteria shown in Table 24-12.

Migraines are most common during childbearing age (24%) and more common in individuals assigned female at birth (3:1).[100] Many nonpregnant individuals experience an increase in migraine symptoms in conjunction with their menstrual cycle. The physiologic state of pregnancy with its sustained hormone levels—versus the variability in hormone levels seen during the menstrual cycle—can reduce the frequency of migraines. Indeed, migraines often improve or cease during pregnancy, with improvement noted by the end of the third trimester in 67% to 89% of pregnant individuals.[100] Unfortunately, some do not notice a benefit as the pregnancy progresses; others may see an exacerbation of their symptoms, often those with a history of migraine with aura. It is also common for individuals in the postpartum period to experience an exacerbation of migraines within the first few days, which is compounded by sleep disturbances, irregular mealtimes, and stress.[100,101]

Migraine headaches are usually unilateral and may be associated with photophobia or phonophobia, nausea, and vomiting. These headaches are often induced by triggers such as sleep deprivation, stress, or certain foods.[101,102] Migraines do not adversely affect the course of pregnancy, although some studies suggest pregnant individuals who have migraines may have an increased risk for hypertensive disorders in pregnancy and low-birth-weight infants.[101]

Care of people with migraines during pregnancy starts with preconception counseling, particularly if migraine-preventive medications are used that will need to be discontinued prior to conception, such as valproate and topiramate. Other preventive measures start with avoidance of migraine triggers, adequate fluid and rest, and regular meals. Individuals with more frequent or severe migraines may require treatment with migraine-preventive medications, and these treatments should be carried out under the guidance of a neurologist. Evidence is sparse, but certain dietary supplements such as magnesium may have a beneficial effect in preventing migraines. Use of acetaminophen is considered safe during all trimesters of pregnancy and can be used to treat headaches and migraines. Formulations that include butalbital, acetaminophen, and caffeine are considered safe for short-term use (4 to 5 days per month).

NSAIDs are often the first line of treatment in migraine. However, during pregnancy, NSAIDs have been associated with increased risks of miscarriage in the first trimester and premature closure of the ductus arteriosus and pulmonary hypertension after 32 weeks' gestation. Studies have shown that it is reasonable to use ibuprofen or naproxen in the second and early third trimesters.[100] Triptans have vasoconstrictive effects that could theoretically cause vasoconstriction in the placenta, but sumatriptan (Imitrex) has been studied in pregnant women and not found to be associated with adverse effects. The antiemetic metoclopramide (Reglan) is generally thought to be safe in pregnancy; it is useful in migraine treatment and has the added benefit of having an antiemetic effect.[100,102] Ergotamine (Cafergot) is contraindicated during pregnancy due

| Table 24-11 | Red Flags for Headache in Pregnancy That Require Further Investigation |
|---|---|

1. Headache that peaks in severity in under 5 minutes
2. New headache type versus a worsening of a previous headache
3. Change in a previously stable headache
4. Headache that changes with posture (e.g., standing up), physical activity or Valsalva
5. Headache with awakening
6. Neurologic symptoms or seizures
7. Trauma
8. Fever or active infections
9. History of malignancy, pituitary disorders, or thrombophilia
10. Elevated blood pressure (≥ 140/90)

Based on Negro et al., 2017 and Mitsikostas et al., 2015 (European Headache Federation consensus on technical investigation for primary headache disorders).

| Table 24-12 | Migraine Types | |
|---|---|
| **Migraine Without Aura** | **Migraine with Aura** |
| A. At least five attacks fulfilling criteria B–D<br><br>B. Headache attacks lasting 4–72 hours (untreated or unsuccessfully treated)<br><br>C. Headache has at least two of the following characteristics:<br>  1. Unilateral location<br>  2. Pulsating quality<br>  3. Moderate or severe pain intensity<br>  4. Aggravation by or causing avoidance of routine physical activity<br><br>D. During headache at least one of the following:<br>  1. Nausea and/or vomiting<br>  2. Photophobia and phonophobia | A. At least two attacks fulfilling criteria B and C<br><br>B. One or more of the following fully reversible aura symptoms:<br>  1. Visual<br>  2. Sensory<br>  3. Speech and/or language<br>  4. Motor<br>  5. Brainstem<br>  6. Retinal<br><br>C. At least three of the following characteristics:<br>  1. At least one aura symptom spreads gradually over ≥ 5 minutes<br>  2. Two or more symptoms occur in succession<br>  3. Each individual aura symptom lasts 5–60 minutes<br>  4. At least one aura symptom is unilateral<br>  5. At least one aura symptom is positive (adding something to the vision)<br>  6. The aura is accompanied, or followed within 60 minutes, by headache |

Data from Headache Classification Committee of the International Headache Society. The international classification of headache disorders, 3rd edition. *Cephalalgia*. 2018;38(1):1-211.

to fetal hypoxia and potential oxytocic type effects. Pregnant individuals who need other medications or additional therapy are best cared for by a specialist.

## Peripheral Neuropathies

Pathology of the nerve roots may be acquired or inherited. Incidence of peripheral neuropathies during pregnancy is infrequent, especially in individuals without diabetes. The most common neuropathies that occur in pregnancy include Bell's palsy, carpal tunnel syndrome, and sciatica.

### Bell's Palsy

Bell's palsy is defined as an idiopathic, commonly unilateral, lower-motor-neuron facial nerve palsy that may lead to partial or complete facial paralysis. This facial nerve disorder is more common in individuals assigned female at birth and is three times more common during pregnancy. Pregnancy, hypertensive disorders, gestational diabetes, and obesity are independent risk factors for the development of Bell's palsy.[103] This condition is most likely to occur in the third trimester or the first week following birth.

Bell's palsy remains a diagnosis of exclusion, and midwives should be aware of key aspects of the history, examination, and follow-up to differentiate between typical and atypical causes of Bell's palsy (i.e., Guillain-Barré syndrome, infections, central nervous system lesions). Atypical features, such as a more insidious and painful onset or gradual progression over more than 2 weeks, can be a sign of a more serious underlying disease requiring further investigation.[103] Symptoms of Bell's palsy may include pain behind the ear, increased perception of loudness, altered or lost sense of taste, drooling, and difficulty with smiling or eye movement. The condition is painful; reports of dry eye (because the eyelid does not completely close), oversensitive hearing, changes in taste, and headache are common. On examination, the face is smooth and the affected side of the mouth droops. One test is to ask the individual to wrinkle their forehead, which they cannot do if Bell's palsy is present. Compared to nonpregnant population, pregnant individuals with Bell's palsy may be more likely to progress to a complete palsy, wherein both sides of the face can be affected, and to have subsequent poor recovery. Therefore, it is important to continue follow-up and initiate appropriate treatment.

Management in pregnancy ranges from conservative management including patient education, observation, and emotional support, to medical and surgical treatment to encourage recovery and prevent progression. The majority of patients, if left untreated, will show at least partial recovery within 3 weeks of onset. The eyelid may not close, so keeping it moist and protected is important. Corticosteroid treatment can decrease eye irritation and dry eye but must be administered within days of onset of the condition to be of benefit; therefore, rapid referral or consultation with a neurologist is warranted.[103]

### Carpal Tunnel Syndrome

Carpal tunnel syndrome (CTS) is a common medical condition that is one of the most frequently reported forms of median nerve compression. The syndrome is characterized by pain in the hand, numbness, and tingling in the distribution of the median nerve. Risk factors for CTS include obesity, monotonous wrist activity, pregnancy, genetic heredity, and rheumatoid inflammation.[104] CTS can occur at any stage of pregnancy, as well as in the postpartum period, and is more likely to be bilateral in pregnant individuals compared to nonpregnant individuals. Local edema and fluid retention caused by hormonal changes are implicated. Symptoms typically include episodic, recurrent numbness and tingling in the fingertips of the first three digits, often becoming more noticeable at night. Nocturnal awakening that triggers hand shaking is highly characteristic of CTS.[105]

Conservative nonsurgical treatments including wrist splinting or local steroid injections are often sufficient. Neuropathic pain medication is generally avoided during pregnancy. Severe or refractory cases can be considered for carpal tunnel release surgery.[105]

### Meralgia Paresthetica

Meralgia paresthetica is caused by compression of the lateral cutaneous femoral nerve, which produces sensory loss or paresthesia in the lateral thigh. In pregnancy, it is associated with weight gain, obesity, diabetes, or a large fetus.[105] This neuropathy produces purely sensory symptoms and no objective weakness. Affected pregnant individuals may complain of burning, uncomfortable pain, tingling, and numbness over the lateral thigh. Weight change, compressive bands, low belts, and constrictive garments are recognized risk factors. Protective measures include frequent position changes, along with avoidance of prolonged hip flexion or rotation and thigh abduction, especially during labor and birth. Symptom relief may be accomplished by abdominal binders and avoiding tight clothing. Symptoms are typically self-limiting and resolve postpartum. Meralgia paresthesia is not a contraindication for regional anesthesia.[105]

### Pelvic Girdle Pain: Sciatica and Symphyseal Separation

Low back pain, symphyseal pain, and sacroiliac joint pain are all common in pregnancy, with half of all pregnant people experiencing low back pain.[106] Sciatica is much less common, occurring in approximately 1%. These conditions are related to musculoskeletal changes of pregnancy and pressure on pregnancy-involved joints, although peripheral nerves can be entrapped and cause pain that radiates down the back of the buttocks or legs. Pelvic girdle pain can include low back pain, or it may present as isolated pain over one of the pelvic joints. Exaggerated lumbar lordosis, direct uterine pressure, and hormonally induced ligamentous laxity are possible factors in the development of pelvic girdle pain.[105] Sciatic pain may occur secondary to hormonal influences during pregnancy or, rarely, secondary to a herniated disc.[107]

Pelvic girdle pain may be experienced as stabbing, shooting, burning, or dull pain in the low back, sacral or gluteal region or pubis symphysis.[108] Symptoms are typically self-limiting and resolve by 3 months postpartum, but may be disabling in pregnancy and early postpartum.[108] Back pain may be exacerbated by separation, or diastasis, of the rectus abdominis muscles, defined as a gap greater than 25 mm just above the umbilicus; this condition occurs in as many as half of pregnancies.[108]

Treatment is mostly conservative, unless overt root injury develops. Most musculoskeletal pain related to pregnancy responds to activity and postural modifications, which can be taught via exercise therapy or physical therapy.[108] Muscle relaxation, rest with legs flexed using pillows, avoiding prolonged standing, and utilization of kinesio taping may provide some relief for back and pelvic pain.[106] Support binders, acupuncture, and yoga may also improve symptoms.[109] Management of diastasis rectus typically includes abdominal strengthening exercises.[109] Physical therapy is indicated when symptoms impact mobility or activities of daily living. People with severe pain or other neurologic symptoms should be referred to a specialist for consultation. Overt root injury, such as cauda equina syndrome, involves compression of spinal nerve roots and presents as low back pain with bowel or bladder dysfunction, saddle anesthesia, and lower limb sensory and motor deficits; surgery may be indicated for debilitating symptoms.[107]

### Epilepsy

Seizure disorders have a range of manifestations and causes, but are collectively called epilepsy.[110] Epilepsy is one of the most common neurologic conditions encountered during prenatal care.[111] In the United States, epilepsy affects more than 1 million people capable of becoming pregnant annually.[113] In this disorder, abnormal electrical activity in the brain causes altered sensation, lapses in attention, or seizures. Seizure activity may be stimulated by brain trauma, infection, tumors, or specific triggers such as bright lighting. Although epilepsy is most often treated with medications, other treatments include surgical excision of the brain seizure foci, ketogenic diets, and implantable brain neurostimulators.[110] Midwives will encounter patients with epilepsy and must understand this disorder, counsel patients before conception, and collaborate with physicians during pregnancy.

The risks associated with use of antiepileptic drugs during pregnancy are a major concern for individuals with epilepsy who are of reproductive age. Ideally, individuals with epilepsy would seek preconception counseling that focuses on medication optimization. Some clinicians may recommend daily folic acid of 4 mg orally, starting 1 month before conception, when patients use antiepileptic drugs associated with neural tube defects, including valproic acid (Depakote, Convulex) and carbamazepine (Tegretol).[112]

Estrogen and progesterone affect neuronal excitability, thereby changing seizure thresholds. Approximately 15% to 32% of pregnant patients with epilepsy will have changes in seizure type, frequency, or severity during pregnancy, although at least half of pregnant patients experience no change in seizure activity.[112] The best predictor of remaining seizure free during pregnancy is having been seizure free for 9 months prior to pregnancy.[111] Compared to individuals without epilepsy, individuals with epilepsy during pregnancy are at higher risk for spontaneous miscarriage, preterm labor, preeclampsia, small-for-gestational-age newborns, fetal growth restriction, induction of labor, cesarean birth with prolonged hospital stay, and excessive postpartum bleeding.[111,113,114]

Infants born to pregnant individuals with epilepsy have a 4% to 14% risk of having a major congenital malformation. Epilepsy-associated malformations include cleft lip and palate, ventricular septal defect, neural tube defects, hypospadias, club foot, and facial abnormalities such as flattened nasal bridge.[112,113] This increased risk of congenital anomalies is likely secondary to the effects of antiepileptic drugs, but the disorder itself may account for some of the increased risk.

Although some antiepileptic drugs are teratogens, more than 90% of people with epilepsy give birth to healthy newborns. Valproate and phenobarbital, which are known to increase the risk of congenital malformations and cognitive impairments, should be avoided when possible during pregnancy.[113,114] Lamotrigine (Lamictal) and levetiracetam (Keppra) have not been associated with congenital malformations.[114] Adjustment of preconception medication to monotherapy (instead of polytherapy) is preferred, because polytherapy is associated with a higher risk of congenital malformations and long-term cognitive deficits in offspring.[110,111,113] Antiepileptic drugs are cleared more quickly during the second and third trimesters, so serum levels of these agents are monitored regularly during pregnancy.[111] Midwives are encouraged to add data to the Antiepileptic Drug Pregnancy Registry.

## Obesity

Obesity is the most common medical condition in people of reproductive age. In the United States, 29% of people who became pregnant in 2019 met the diagnostic criteria for obesity.[115] Midwives should be equipped to recognize the implications of obesity relative to pregnancy that are often overlooked or ignored due to lack of specific evidence-based treatment options. Midwives should also evaluate their own biases and the effect of those biases on their management of pregnant individuals who have obesity. Information on how to approach conversations about weight can be found in the *Skillful Communication to Mitigate Clinician Bias* appendix. In addition, examination of clinical facilities and equipment to ensure they can accommodate persons of size is important to support safe care. For example, large-size blood pressure cuffs are essential to ensure accurate measurement in individuals with obesity, and chairs and exam tables should be appropriately sized.[116] Health changes related to obesity require

| Table 24-13 | Recommended Pregnancy Weight Gain and Screening According to Body Mass Index | | |
|---|---|---|---|
| **BMI** | **Categorization** | **Suggested Weight Gain (per National Academy of Medicine[a])** | **Suggested Additional Screening or Treatment** |
| 30 or greater | Class I | 11–20 lb<br>(0.5 lb/week in second and third trimesters) | Aspirin after 12 weeks' gestation<br>Early glucose screen<br>Screening for obstructive sleep apnea |
| 35.0–39.9 | Class II | 11–20 lb | All of the above<br>AND<br>Antepartum fetal testing beginning at 37 0/7 weeks |
| 40 or greater | Class III | 11–20 lb | All of the above<br>AND<br>Antepartum fetal testing beginning at 34 0/7 weeks |

[a] The Institute of Medicine was renamed the National Academy of Medicine in 2015.

Based on American College of Obstetricians and Gynecologists. ACOG Practice Bulletin No. 230: obesity in pregnancy. *Obstet Gynecol.* 2021;137(6):e128-e144. doi:10.1097/AOG.0000000000004395.

long-term approaches that range from population-based public health to individual nutritional, behavioral, and surgical interventions.[117]

Obesity is defined most commonly based on body mass index (BMI), a measurement that is used to estimate relative risks for disease compared with normal weight. BMI is calculated by dividing weight in kilograms by height in meters squared. The World Health Organization defines the BMI categories as follows (Table 24-13): A BMI less than 18.5 kg/m$^2$ is underweight; a BMI of 18.5 to 24.9 kg/m$^2$ is considered normal weight; a BMI of 25–29.9 kg/m$^2$ is overweight; and a BMI greater than 30 kg/m$^2$ is classified as obese. Within the obesity category, a BMI of 30–34. is class I, a BMI of 35–39.9 is class II, and a BMI greater than 40 is class III obesity.[116] The degree of obesity may factor into the midwife's decision to transfer a person to a higher level of care; however, there are no well-established BMI cut-offs for recommending transfer of care.[118]

The health implications of pregnancy with obesity can be organized into two categories: (1) comorbidities the person had prior to pregnancy (e.g., chronic hypertension, type 2 diabetes, or heart disease) and (2) complications specific to pregnancy that occur more frequently in people with obesity. Pregnant individuals with obesity have a higher incidence of hypertensive disorders of pregnancy and gestational diabetes compared with individuals who are not obese, as well as increased risks for longer duration of labor, spontaneous abortion, preterm birth, fetal death, congenital anomalies, anesthetic complications, induction of labor, and operative birth.[116,117] Even small pre-pregnancy weight reductions may improve pregnancy outcomes, so midwives should support weight loss prior to pregnancy when possible.[116] However, it is also important to recognize that obesity alone may not indicate an individual's health status or accurately predict pregnancy complications. Emerging evidence suggests that people with obesity who are physically active and have no metabolic indicators of disease have a decreased risk for complications, compared to people with obesity who enter pregnancy in a metabolically unhealthy state.[117]

Care of pregnant individuals with obesity should begin with a BMI calculation at the first prenatal visit, with the midwife then providing diet and exercise counseling guided by the National Academy of Medicine (formerly the Institute of Medicine) recommendations for gestational weight gain during pregnancy and person-centered principles focused on improving health. People with a BMI greater than 30 should aim to gain between 11 and 20 pounds during pregnancy.[116] Midwives should encourage behavioral interventions focused on both nutrition and exercise, which have been shown to reduce excessive gestational weight gain and improve pregnancy-related outcomes.[119]

Obesity can affect testing and diagnostic tools that are frequently used in prenatal care. Cell-free DNA failures are more common in pregnancies with obesity related to a decreased fetal fraction of DNA in the blood. Individuals should be informed that uninterpretable results are associated with a greater risk for abnormalities and should be offered ultrasound screening and diagnostic testing such as amniocentesis. Repeat screening is not recommended in these patients because it is associated with lower success compared to in individuals without obesity.[116] The effect of obesity in pregnancy on ultrasound-estimated fetal weight determination remains unclear, with some studies demonstrating patients with a higher BMI had significantly less accurate estimated fetal weight determination, and other studies suggesting obesity does not affect the accuracy of sonographically predicted fetal weight. Fetal measurements rely on bony markers, which are bright and echogenic and can usually be seen through adipose tissue. While more research is needed, obesity in pregnancy does not appear to create a limitation with regard to the assessment of fetal size.

During the antepartum period, early pregnancy screening for glucose intolerance for gestational diabetes or overt diabetes should be based on risk factors, including BMI of 30 or greater, known impaired glucose metabolism, or previous gestational diabetes. Individuals with obesity should also be screened for obstructive sleep apnea by asking about unexplained shortness of breath, excessive daytime sleepiness, or snoring and referred for sleep evaluation as needed.[116] Midwives can consider weekly antenatal fetal surveillance beginning by 37 0/7 weeks' gestation for patients with a pre-pregnancy BMI of 35.0–39.9. For patients with a pre-pregnancy BMI of 40 or greater, weekly antenatal fetal surveillance may be considered beginning at 34 0/7 weeks' gestation.[116]

Some specialty centers for obesity in pregnancy exist that offer advanced ambulatory and intrapartum care, provide prenatal consultation for intrapartum care, or accept the transfer of intrapartum patients with obesity-related needs. These facilities have specialized equipment and interdisciplinary perinatal teams (MFM specialists, obstetricians, and nurse-midwives) who can work with other specialists (anesthesia, internal medicine/intensive care, physical therapy) to provide individualized care.

During the intrapartum period, midwives should allow for a longer first stage of labor in individuals with obesity prior to declaring labor arrest and considering a cesarean delivery.[116] Anesthesia consultation may be indicated due to increased risk for anesthesia-related complications. In the postpartum period, patients with obesity are at increased risk for thromboembolism and cesarean wound infection.[116] Unfortunately, people in higher obesity classes are less likely to initiate breastfeeding/chestfeeding and should be counseled on the benefits of providing human milk.[120,121] Postpartum considerations for people with obesity are discussed in the *Postpartum Care* chapter.

## Pregnancy After Bariatric Surgery

Bariatric surgery may be recommended for persons living with obesity when lifestyle, diet, and medication therapies have failed and BMI exceeds 35 kg/mm$^2$, or when the individual has comorbid medical conditions (e.g., diabetes or hypertension) and BMI exceeds 30 kg/mm$^2$.[122] Midwives are increasingly providing care for pregnant persons after bariatric surgery, working collaboratively with a network of clinicians, including MFM specialists, nutritionists, and ultrasonographers. Team-based care optimizes a pregnant person's chance for a safe and satisfying pregnancy and birth.

There are two categories of bariatric surgery procedures: (1) restrictive (sleeve gastrectomy, laparoscopic gastric banding) and (2) restrictive/malabsorptive (Roux-en-Y gastric bypass, biliopancreatic diversion/duodenal switch). Knowing the type of bariatric procedure performed is important for ensuring the patient receives appropriate nutritional advice and risk screening.[123,124] Malabsorptive surgeries reduce food, micronutrient, and medication absorption. Deficiencies in iron, vitamin B$_{12}$, folate, vitamin D, calcium, and protein can be common. Baseline vitamin and mineral status should be evaluated at the first prenatal visit, with supplements recommended as needed. A CBC and measurement of vitamin B$_{12}$, iron, ferritin, calcium, and vitamin D levels every trimester should be considered. When at least 12 months has passed between bariatric surgery and pregnancy, these individuals have a reduced risk for gestational diabetes, hypertensive disorders of pregnancy, and large-for-gestational-age neonates.[123] However, if pregnancy occurs soon after surgery, there is a risk of malnutrition and fetal growth restriction.[123]

Persons with a history of bariatric surgery are prone to dumping syndrome, which is aggravated by rapid ingestion of carbohydrates. Therefore, diabetes screening using glucose tolerance tests is not recommended. Instead, gestational diabetes testing can be done by following fasting and postprandial blood glucose levels for 1 week.[124]

## Respiratory Conditions

### Asthma

Asthma affects as many as 8% of pregnant people in the United States and is often undertreated in adults. The course of asthma during pregnancy is variable, with approximately one-third of individuals with this condition experiencing exacerbations, one-third having fewer episodes, and one-third not experiencing any difference in asthma symptoms or frequency.[125] Approximately 10% have severe exacerbations requiring hospitalization and steroids.[126] The more severe or poorly controlled asthma is in the year prior to pregnancy, the higher the risk of worsening disease and hospital admission is during pregnancy.[127]

The effect of asthma on pregnancy is not fully established. However, it appears to be associated with a small increase in various pregnancy complications, including low birth weight, preeclampsia, and preterm birth. It is not clear if these risks occur secondary to asthma, an underlying condition that affects both asthma and pregnancy, or the effects of medications used to treat asthma.[126]

Research consistently demonstrates undertreatment of asthma by providers as well as underutilization of asthma medications during pregnancy. In addition, pregnant people with asthma who visit emergency departments for this disease are less likely to have appropriate medications prescribed than are nonpregnant individuals. Effective management of asthma during pregnancy requires vigilance, and multidisciplinary collaborative care is the optimal model of care for achieving this goal.[128]

When initially evaluating asthma in pregnancy, it is important to determine the asthma classification (see the *Common Conditions in Primary Care* chapter) based on current National Asthma Education and Prevention Program guidelines.[127] Assessment includes obtaining data about the severity, number of episodes, hospitalizations, and medications used in the prior year. Management goals are to (1) prevent chronic symptoms, (2) maintain optimal pulmonary function to support normal levels of activity, (3) prevent exacerbation, (4) maintain fetal oxygenation by preventing prenatal hypoxic episodes, and (5) use treatment with no or minimal side effects.[126,127]

Evaluation of asthma during pregnancy is based on clinical evaluation and peak expiratory flow measurements. A stepwise approach is recommended for treatment, as described in Table 24-14.[127] Treatment

| Table 24-14 | Management of Asthma During Pregnancy |
|---|---|
| Asthma Classification | Step Therapy for Treating Asthma During Pregnancy |
| Mild intermittent | No daily medications<br>Albuterol inhaler as needed |
| Mild persistent | Low-dose inhaled corticosteroid |
| Moderate persistent | Low-dose inhaled corticosteroid and salmeterol (Advair) or medium-dose inhaled corticosteroid is preferred |
| Severe persistent | High-dose inhaled corticosteroid and salmeterol (Advair); oral corticosteroid if needed |

Note: Alternative therapies are available for each step. If an alternative medication is needed, physician consultation should be obtained.

Based on National Asthma Education and Prevention Program. Working group report on managing asthma during pregnancy: recommendations for pharmacologic treatment. https://www.nhlbi.nih.gov/files/docs/astpreg_qr.pdf. Accessed November 11, 2022.

should be stepped up when control is not achieved and stepped down if symptoms have resolved for 3 months or more.

While some people may be concerned about using asthma medications for fear of fetal harm, a fetus needs oxygen. Therefore, it is safer for the birthing person to be treated for asthma in pregnancy than to have asthma symptoms and related complications. There are no documented adverse fetal side effects from the medications for asthma, although only limited data are available on the use of antihistamines in pregnancy.[126,127] People with asthma in pregnancy will benefit from health education and preventive health strategies, including information on how to avoid triggers, how to take medications, importance of smoking cessation, the value of immunization against the flu and COVID-19, and danger signs of worsening disease. Later in pregnancy, teaching includes how to perform fetal movement counts.

### Tuberculosis

The case rate of active tuberculosis (TB) in the United States is approximately 2.8 per 100,000, with two-thirds of infections occurring in people born in other countries.[128] Approximately 5% to 10% of individuals with latent tuberculosis will develop active disease if untreated.[128] Pregnancy does not appear to increase susceptibility to tuberculosis infection or progression from latent to active disease; however, there is an increase in incidence from the level that would otherwise be expected postpartum.[129]

Risk factors for TB include HIV infection, intravenous drug use, being unhoused/homeless, being a close contact of someone with known TB, and recently immigrating from an area of the world with high rates of TB. Individuals with active infection may be asymptomatic. Symptoms include a prolonged, productive cough, fatigue, fever, chills, and night sweats.[130] People suspected to have active TB infection should take measures to reduce spread, including airborne precautions.[129]

Compared to pregnant people without TB, those with active disease have an increased risk of morbidity, anemia, preterm birth, cesarean birth, low-birth-weight infants, birth asphyxia, and perinatal death.[130] Coinfection with HIV is a risk factor for mortality. Infants born from people with tuberculosis can contract congenital tuberculosis, which can cause significant neonatal morbidity.[130]

Individuals at high risk for tuberculosis should be screened during pregnancy. This screening may be done with either the intradermal tuberculin screening test (TST; also referred to as purified protein derivative [PPD]) or the interferon-gamma release assay (IGRA), which uses a serum sample. Both the TST and the IGRA are recommended by the CDC, measure the body's response to tuberculin, and are used in pregnancy. When either test is positive, the diagnosis must be differentiated as either latent or active tuberculosis.[131] An important confounder in diagnosis is the tuberculosis vaccine used in other countries, called bacillus Calmette-Guérin (BCG), which can confer a positive response to the TST but not the IGRA. People who have received BCG can still acquire tuberculosis, so a positive TST result requires follow-up to confirm the diagnosis.[131]

When a tuberculosis screening test is positive, a posterior–anterior chest X-ray using shielding should be performed to detect tuberculosis lesions in the lung. A negative finding rules out active pulmonary disease, and a presumptive diagnosis of latent tuberculosis is then made.[131] If the chest X-ray shows signs of active tuberculosis, a sputum culture positive for *Mycobacterium tuberculosis* confirms the diagnosis.[131]

People with tuberculosis are best cared for by specialists. All tuberculosis diagnoses must be reported to the local health department according to state regulations, and treatment includes directly observed therapy.[128] Treatment for latent tuberculosis should generally be initiated at the time of diagnosis when the risk for active disease is moderate to high.[132] Treatment of latent infection in pregnancy includes 6 to 9 months of isoniazid with supplemental vitamin $B_6$. Treatment of active disease begins at diagnosis and generally consists of 9 months of combination therapy with isoniazid, rifampin, and ethambutol.[129,132] Use of pyrazinamide in pregnancy is controversial in the United States, but this medication is generally administered in cases of immunocompromise, such as HIV coinfection.[132] Individuals who are noninfectious but undergoing treatment should be encouraged to breastfeed/chestfeed.[132]

## Upper Respiratory Infections

In general, symptoms and the course of care for individuals with upper respiratory infections (URIs) are the same for pregnant people as for those who are not pregnant. The hormonal shifts and changing body mechanics of pregnancy can affect respiratory function, reducing lung volume and increasing activity in mucosal membranes. Thus, pregnant people may experience more intense symptoms or have a longer delay before health is restored. Although pregnancy may cause mild dyspnea, tachypnea is never a normal sign of pregnancy. Most importantly, pregnant individuals with a URI are more likely to progress from a cold, bronchitis, or influenza to pneumonia. The differential diagnoses for URI symptoms include the common cold, influenza, bronchitis, sinusitis, SARS-CoV-2, asthma, pertussis, and pneumonia.

Common cold symptoms include rhinitis, sore throat, cough, and malaise, but adults rarely have a fever. Cough may take several days longer to resolve in pregnant people compared to nonpregnant individuals. Acute bronchitis, an inflammation of the bronchi, may follow a common cold and should be considered if a cough persists more than 5 days. People with bronchitis will have clear lungs during auscultation but may have purulent sputum. The color of the sputum does not indicate the presence of bacteria. Most acute respiratory tract infections, including the common cold, bronchitis, pharyngitis, and sinusitis, are caused by viruses and thus do not warrant treatment with antibiotics.[133] Physical preventive measures such as hand washing, use of alcohol-based disinfectants, and masking can reduce transmission of respiratory infections.[134]

Humidified air and acetaminophen for sore throat and headache are safe and effective. Saline nasal spray or nasal irrigation may relieve nasal congestion. Risks of other medications for mitigating common cold symptoms have not been evaluated in randomized trials conducted during pregnancy. Generally, pregnant people should avoid combination over-the-counter medications for treating URI symptoms. Clients who choose drug treatment may use ipratropium bromide nasal spray or intranasal cromolyn sodium for nasal congestion and dextromethorphan or guaifenesin for cough suppression,[133] though these have been found ineffective in the setting of cough from the common cold.[134] Severe cough in pregnancy may cause temporary urinary incontinence.

Pregnancy-related hormonal effects on the nasal passages increase the risk for developing sinusitis following a common cold. Symptoms include nasal congestion, headache, and facial pain or pressure that is worse when bending forward. During pregnancy, these symptoms may be atypical but often appear as worsening of a common cold that was resolving. Sinusitis is generally self-limiting and will resolve in 7 to 10 days. Antibiotic therapy can be initiated if symptoms worsen or do not resolve. The first-line agent is amoxicillin–clavulanate (Augmentin) 875 mg/125 mg administered twice daily, assuming the individual is not allergic to penicillin.[133] A higher-dose formulation is available for those persons with severe infection or risk factors for developing pneumonia.

## COVID-19

SARS-CoV-2 viral infection, also known as coronavirus disease 2019 (COVID-19), is transmitted through person-to-person respiratory contact, causing asymptomatic to severe illness. The most common symptoms in pregnant people include cough, sore throat, body aches, and fever, with one-fourth experiencing symptoms that last for 8 weeks or more.[135] Compared to their nonpregnant peers, symptomatic COVID-19 infection in pregnant individuals is associated with increased risk for intensive care unit admission, mechanical ventilation, and death.[135,136] Severe illness is associated with increased risk for adverse perinatal outcomes including hypertensive disorders of pregnancy, coagulopathy, preterm birth, and stillbirth.[136,137] Those persons with preexisting conditions such as

obesity, asthma, hypertension, and diabetes may be at greater risk for moderate to severe illness.[136]

Individuals who have not been previously vaccinated should be offered vaccination in pregnancy, as COVID-19 infection can be dangerous for pregnant people and their fetuses.[136] Research on the safety and efficacy of vaccination in pregnancy is ongoing; however, there is no evidence of adverse perinatal or infant effects related to COVID-19 vaccination in pregnancy.[138] COVID-19 vaccines may be administered along with other vaccinations routinely given in pregnancy. Those experiencing fever following vaccination may take acetaminophen. Individuals declining vaccination should be counseled on the importance of risk mitigation through mask wearing and social distancing.[138] Vaccination against COVID-19 provides antibody protection to the fetus through the placenta.[139] Human milk provides immune protection to infants, and infected individuals are no more likely to transmit COVID-19 to their infant through breastfeeding/chestfeeding compared to those using human milk alternatives.[137]

As of 2022, there was no cure for COVID-19 infection. Thus, treatments are supportive in nature and, depending on disease severity, may include acetaminophen for fever reduction, monoclonal antibodies, and supplemental oxygen or intubation for people unable to maintain oxygen saturation.[135] Pregnant persons with COVID-19 should discuss the pros and cons of investigational or newly approved treatments such as antiviral agents or immunomodulator medications with their care providers.[137,139] This area of health care is changing rapidly as new research is released; consult current national guidelines when creating a plan of care.

## Influenza

Influenza can be a serious respiratory disease in pregnancy and is associated with increased risk of morbidity and mortality for both the pregnant person and the fetus.[140] The symptoms of influenza are similar to the symptoms of the common cold, but are more severe and include a fever. Hyperthermia that occurs with flu is a well-established risk factor for some congenital anomalies, and first trimester influenza exposure is associated with multiple nonchromosomal congenital anomalies.[141] Although the diagnosis of influenza is usually made on the basis of clinical findings, laboratory tests, including rapid swabs, are also available.

Annual influenza vaccination is recommended for all adults, including in pregnancy.

The injectable inactivated vaccine does not cause harm to pregnant people or their fetuses.[141] In addition, maternal vaccination reduces the incidence of infection among one of the highest-risk populations—infants younger than 6 months who cannot be vaccinated.

Treatment with antivirals should begin as quickly as possible when influenza is suspected, regardless of vaccination status. Oral oseltamivir (Tamiflu) can be safely used during pregnancy.[142] Acetaminophen to reduce fever is an important component of care. Adjunct medications to treat symptoms such as rhinitis are safe and can be used concomitantly with oseltamivir.

### Pneumonia

The symptoms of community-acquired pneumonia in pregnancy are similar to those experienced by nonpregnant people and include cough, shortness of breath, sputum production, chest pain, fever, and malaise. Tachypnea and tachycardia may be present. On examination, lung consolidation, elevated temperature, and signs of respiratory distress including hypoxia may be evident. People with suspected pneumonia should have a shielded chest X ray, CBC, metabolic panel (electrolytes, blood urea nitrogen, creatinine, glucose), and blood gases analysis. Because of the likelihood of rapid disease progression and fetal compromise from decreased oxygenation, hospitalization is often necessary when pneumonia occurs during pregnancy, especially during the third trimester.[143]

In addition to the morbidity directly related to infection, pregnant people with pneumonia have an increased risk of developing preeclampsia. Fetal risks include preterm premature rupture of membranes, fetal growth restriction, prematurity, low birth weight, and small-for-gestational-age infants, as well as morbidity from hypoxemia. People who have symptoms of pneumonia during pregnancy are referred for physician evaluation and consideration for hospitalization. Antimicrobial therapy is chosen based on the microorganism, although empirical treatment with azithromycin and possible addition of a beta-lactam is recommended.[133] Fluoroquinolones should be avoided.[134,143]

### Skeletal Abnormalities

An estimated 7% of pregnant people sustain trauma, most commonly related to motor vehicle accidents.[144] Primary initial concerns after trauma in pregnancy include evaluating vital signs and treating airway or circulation issues as needed as well as monitoring fetal status.[144] Once the patient is stable, imaging may be indicated; in the case of trauma, the test that yields the most accurate diagnosis outweighs the risks of radiation to the fetus.[144] Radiography may be indicated to evaluate for fractures, although femoral and pelvic radiographs should be avoided if possible to limit fetal exposure; MRI can assess trauma in the spinal cord and ligaments, and ultrasound is effective for pelvic images.[145] If surgery is indicated, placing the pregnant person in the left lateral decubitus position prevents aortic compression and decreased oxygenation to the fetus during procedures.[144]

Risk for thromboembolism increases five-fold in pregnancy, and immobilization after an injury greatly increases the risk for thrombosis.[144] Individuals who sustain a break or fracture may be placed on low-molecular-weight heparin.[144] Casts or immobilization devices may sometimes interfere with comfort measures in labor, and alternative support measures may be indicated.

Although back pain in pregnancy is common, certain skeletal abnormalities may cause complications. Pregnancy- and lactation-associated osteoporosis is rare but may result in spinal compression fractures, which present as pronounced back pain.[145] Individuals with scoliosis or a history of spinal surgery may face a longer procedure time for spinal anesthesia placement in labor and would benefit from anesthesia consultation during pregnancy or in early labor.

## Substance Use in Pregnancy

Substance use disorders, especially those that involve opioids, have become a major public health issue in the United States. Substance use plays a role in pregnancy-associated deaths (deaths of individuals who are pregnant or within 365 days of pregnancy) and is a leading cause of maternal death in many states. Tobacco, alcohol, and illicit and/or prescription medications all have fetotoxic properties, as summarized in Table 24-15.[146,147] A midwife's role in caring for a pregnant individual with substance use disorder includes identification of the substance(s) being used at the earliest opportunity, provision of counseling resources, accessing treatment, and referral to social services to address housing, employment, parenting, and transportation issues.

Universal verbal screening for substance use is recommended for all individuals early in pregnancy.

| Table 24-15 | Substances and Associated Harm During Pregnancy | | | | | | | |
|---|---|---|---|---|---|---|---|---|
| Pregnancy-Related Complication | Opioids | Cocaine | Amphetamines | Cannabis | Tobacco | Alcohol | Marijuana |
| Miscarriage | X | X | | X | X | | |
| Placental disruption | | X | | | X | | |
| Preterm birth | X | X | X | X | X | | X |
| Fetal growth restriction | | X | | X | X | X | |
| Low birth weight | X | X | X | X | X | X | X |
| Fetal death | | X | X | X | | | |
| Respiratory disorders/failure | X | | | | X | | |
| Fetal alcohol spectrum | | | | | | X | |
| Neonatal abstinence syndrome | X | | | | X | X | |
| Behavioral and cognitive dysfunction in childhood | | | | | | | X |

Based on Foeller ME, Lyell D. Marijuana use in pregnancy: concerns in an evolving era. *J Midwifery Womens Health*. 2017;62(3): 363-367; Finnegan L. *Licit and illicit drug use during pregnancy: maternal, neonatal and early childhood consequences.* Canadian Centre on Substance Abuse. https://www.ccsa.ca/sites/default/files/2019-04/CCSA-Drug-Use-during-Pregnancy-Report-2013-en.pdf. Published 2013. Accessed October 4, 2021.

Screening based only on factors such as late entry into prenatal care or prior adverse pregnancy outcome can lead to missed cases and adds to stereotyping and stigma.[149] Provider suspicions are subject to conscious and unconscious biases that can overburden some groups and leave other groups undiagnosed.

Despite data showing that usage rates of substances is relatively equal across races and socioeconomic groups, the inequalities seen in a structurally racist society have made it so Black individuals are penalized more often than white individuals for such use. In a recent demographic study on discrepancies in prenatal urine drug screening for cannabis use, results showed Black individuals had 2.8 times higher odds than Latinx individuals of being tested, 2.1 times higher odds than Asian people of being tested, and 1.7 times higher odds than white individuals of being tested.[150] Criminalization of substance use in pregnancy or other methods of penalizing pregnant individuals following disclosure may prevent people from seeking prenatal care and other preventive healthcare services.[151] Patients should be informed that the purpose of verbal screening is to allow treatment of the individual's substance use and not to punish or prosecute them. However, patients should also be informed of the potential ramifications of a positive verbal or laboratory screen result, including mandatory reporting requirements. Providing a positive, compassionate, and nonjudgmental prenatal setting can encourage disclosure, although it may take time to build a trusting relationship.

The recommended process of screening, brief intervention, and referral to treatment (SBIRT) has been validated by the U.S. Preventive Services Task Force and other professional organizations.[148] Screening should occur for all pregnant individuals via use of a validated questionnaire such as the 4 Ps (Table 24-16), NIDA Quick Screen (Table 24-17), and CRAFFT (for individuals younger than 21 years old; Table 24-18). The goal of the screening portion of SBIRT is to identify people at low, moderate, or high risk for substance use disorder and appropriately provide a brief behavioral intervention. Brief intervention is a patient-centered form of counseling that uses the principles of motivational interviewing. The purpose is to identify the person's desire to change behavior. Individuals who are at high risk are referred to specialty treatment.[148] Training in SBIRT is available and resources are listed at the end of this chapter.

A positive response to a self-report screening questionnaire may lead midwives to offer a biologic

| Table 24-16 | 4 Ps Screening Tool: Parents, Partner, Past, and Present |
|---|---|

1.  Have you ever used drugs or alcohol during Pregnancy?
2.  Have you had a problem with drugs or alcohol in the Past?
3.  Does your Partner have a problem with drugs or alcohol?
4.  Do you consider one of your Parents to be an addict or alcoholic?

    5 Ps screening tool adds:

5.  Do any of your Peers have problems with alcohol or drug use?

Use at any time in pregnancy.

Scoring: Any "yes" should be used for further discussion about drug or alcohol use. Persons who answer "yes" to two or more questions should be considered for referral for further assessment.

Adapted from Ewing H. Medical Director, Born Free Project. Contra Costa County, 111 Allen Street, Martinez, CA 94553. Phone: (510) 646-1165. The 5Ps was adapted by the Massachusetts Institute for Health and Recovery in 1999 from Dr. Hope Ewing's 4Ps (1990).

| Table 24-17 | NIDA Quick Screen |
|---|---|

In the past year, how often have you:

1.  Had four drinks a day?
2.  Used tobacco products?
3.  Used prescription drugs for nonmedical reasons?
4.  Used illegal drugs?

Use in patients 18 years and older.

Scoring: If the patient says "never" for all questions, screening is complete. If the patient indicates one or more days of heavy drinking, the patient is an at-risk drinker and needs a brief intervention/referral. If the patient indicates use of tobacco, the patient is at risk and should be advised to quit and given information on smoking cessation. If the patient indicates "yes" for use of illegal or prescription drugs for nonmedical reasons, proceed to NIDA-Modified ASSIST and determine the patient's risk level for referral reasons.

Adapted from National Institute on Drug Abuse. Screening and assessment tools chart. National Institute on Drug Abuse. https://www.drugabuse.gov/nidamed-medical-health-professionals/screening-tools-resources/chart-screening-tools. Published May 6, 2021. Accessed December 10, 2021.

test. After informed consent is obtained and patient confidentiality is discussed, biologic testing can be used to detect or confirm suspected substance use. Drug testing is not recommended for universal

| Table 24-18 | CRAFFT 2.1: Car, Relax, Alone, Forget, Friends, Trouble |
|---|---|

**Part A**

During the PAST 12 MONTHS, on how many days did you:

1.  Drink more than a few sips of beer, wine, or any drink containing alcohol? Put "0" if none.
2.  Use any marijuana (weed, oil, or hash, by smoking, vaping, or in food) or "synthetic marijuana" (like "K2" or "Spice") or "vaping" THC oil? Put "0" if none.
3.  Use anything else to get high (like other illegal drugs, prescription or over-the-counter medications, and things that you sniff, huff, or vape)? Put "0" if none.

If you responded "0" to ALL of these items, answer question 4 and then stop. If you responded "1" or higher to ANY of the items, answer questions 4–9.

**Part B**

4.  C—Have you ever ridden in a car driven by someone (including yourself) who was "high" or had been using drugs or alcohol?
5.  R—Do you ever use alcohol or drugs to relax, feel better about yourself, or fit in?
6.  A—Do you ever use alcohol or drugs while you are by yourself, alone?
7.  F—Do you ever forget things that you did while using alcohol or drugs?
8.  F—Does your family or friends ever tell you that you should cut down on your drinking or drug use?
9.  T—Have you ever gotten into trouble while you were using alcohol or drugs?

Use in adolescents ages 12–21 years.

Scoring: Give each "yes" response in Part B a score of 1 point. A total score of 2 or higher is a positive screen, indicating a need for additional assessment.

Adapted from National Institute on Drug Abuse. Screening and assessment tools chart. National Institute on Drug Abuse. https://www.drugabuse.gov/nidamed-medical-health-professionals/screening-tools-resources/chart-screening-tools. Published May 6, 2021. Accessed December 10, 2021.

screening.[148] Opioid biomarkers may be assayed from blood, saliva, hair, or urine samples; breath testing can be used for other substances, such as alcohol. The short half-lives of most substances and their related metabolites limit detection via biologic testing to recent use only. Urine drug screening is commonly used as a testing mechanism due to its specificity and positive predictive value. A urine drug test assesses only current or recent substance use; thus, a negative test does not rule out sporadic drug use, nor does a positive test diagnose an opioid use disorder or its severity.[151] Its important to be aware of legal mandates, as some states require reporting of substance abuse in pregnancy and in the hospital if a drug screen is positive on admission and/or neonatal samples are positive for drugs. Each practice or hospital should have explicit criteria for drug testing to avoid demographic profiling and discrimination.

Substance use disorder is considered a chronic disease that can be managed and treated successfully. As with other chronic diseases, its treatment will be most effective if it involves a multidisciplinary group of professionals, social support, and treatment availability. Social workers, psychologists, substance abuse counselors, and medical addiction specialists are all needed. Referral to a structured program for pregnant individuals is ideal if locally available. Individuals with substance use disorders have an increased risk for sexually transmitted infections (STIs), hepatitis, and HIV. Rescreening for STIs in the second and/or third trimester may be indicated and should be considered on an individual basis.

## Opioids

Opioid use in pregnancy has increased dramatically in recent years, resulting in a sharp rise in neonatal opioid withdrawal syndrome (NOWS), also known as neonatal abstinence syndrome (NAS). Evidence for higher rate of opioid dependence in pregnancy can be noted from the increased incidence of NOWS, which is characterized by central nervous system irritability, GI effects, and poor weight gain.[151] Care of infants with NOWS is described in the *Neonatal Care* chapter. If a pregnant individual has used opioids during pregnancy for any reason, the pediatric team should be notified.

Opioid withdrawal in pregnancy is not recommended due to associations with decreased neonatal birth weight, illicit drug use relapse, and resumption of high-risk behaviors such as intravenous drug use, criminal activity, or unsafe sex work.[150] Stabilizing patients on medication for opioid use disorder (MOUD) can help reduce acquisition and transmission of infectious diseases such as hepatitis C and HIV. The standard of care for pregnant individuals with opioid use disorder (OUD) is to treat their condition with either methadone or buprenorphine. Because MOUD reduces or eliminates risks associated with dramatic changes in blood opioid levels,

perinatal outcomes are improved for both the patient and the fetus/newborn.

Therapy with methadone initiation occurs in inpatient settings, given that this medication is a full opioid receptor agonist and carries the risks of respiratory depression and overdose. Once dosing is stabilized, patients can receive their therapeutic medication at a federally regulated outpatient methadone treatment facility for supervised dose administration.

Buprenorphine is a Schedule III drug and is associated with less risky withdrawal symptoms than methadone. Therefore, buprenorphine initiation can occur in office-based settings and patients can self-administer their medication by filling a prescription.[150] This agent has also demonstrated shorter treatment duration for NOWS for infants exposed to this medication as compared to methadone. Midwives and nurse practitioners can apply for a buprenorphine waiver application and become a MOUD provider via practitioner training through the Substance Abuse and Mental Health Services Administration, a department within the U.S. Department of Health and Human Services. This is an important tool in helping to eliminate barriers to treatment of this chronic disease.

Even though studies have shown promising findings with MOUD, access to care for pregnant individuals is complicated by transportation difficulties, childcare needs, housing insecurity, and comorbid mental illness. Office-based administration can liberate patients from the stigma associated with methadone treatment facilities as well as help decrease barriers for patients with work or childcare responsibilities. Integrating prenatal care with MOUD is essential.[151,152]

Individuals with opiate use disorder need customized plans of care to manage their postpartum pain. National guidelines recommend encouraging rooming-in and breastfeeding/chestfeeding in patients who are stable on their opioid agonists, are not using illicit drugs, and have no other contraindications. In the event of a relapse, individuals should be counseled about the need to suspend breastfeeding/chestfeeding.

Prescription opiate overdose is a leading cause of pregnancy-related death in many states.[150] For all individuals, providers should be cautious in prescribing excessive amounts of opioids to prevent later OUD. Postpartum pain management is discussed in the *Postpartum Care* chapter. Clinicians should provide naloxone (Narcan) prescriptions and instructions to patients, family members, and friends for potential overdoses. If an opioid prescription is required, such as after a surgical birth, prescribe only the quantity likely to be used. For chronic pain, practitioners should avoid or minimize use of opioids for pain management and instead encourage alternative therapies such as non-pharmacologic (i.e. exercise, physical therapy) and nonopioid pharmacologic treatments.[151] Coordination of controlled prescriptions within a practice group, reviewing the state prescription registry of controlled substances, counseling on the benefits of NSAIDs for pain relief, and referral to pain management specialists may help reduce the rate of prescription misuse.

### Cannabis

Cannabis is widely used in developed and developing countries, with 2.5% to 4.9% of the world's population age 15 to 64 years using this substance. Regionally, about 12.2% of the population in North America engages in cannabis use, although self-reported rates in pregnancy are much lower and likely underestimate of the actual prevalence.[153]

Although medical and social use of cannabis has become more acceptable in the United States, not much is known about the effects of cannabis on fetal growth and development or its effects on pregnant individuals. Studies have demonstrated that cannabinoids readily cross the placenta and appear in human milk. About 34% to 60% of cannabis users continue their use of this substance during pregnancy, with many people believing that it is a "safe and natural herb" that can be safely used for nausea. Some may use cannabis to treat nausea and vomiting in pregnancy.[154] Unfortunately, chronic cannabis use can result in cannabinoid hyperemesis syndrome, which leads to episodic abdominal pain, nausea, and vomiting.[155]

A systematic review/meta-analysis demonstrated that pregnant individuals who used cannabis during pregnancy had an increased odds ratio of anemia compared to those who did not use cannabis. Furthermore, infants exposed to cannabis in utero had lower birth weights and were more likely to need care in the NICU.[153] Some studies have found neurologic sequelae for infants exposed to cannabis in utero. Further research is needed, however, as these studies were limited in their ability to control for environmental and socioeconomic factors.

ACOG recommends that individuals wishing to become pregnant or who are already pregnant should be encouraged to discontinue use of cannabis for medicinal purposes in favor of other evidence-based therapies.[154] Treatment for cannabis use has not been standardized, and treatment

programs are limited. Breastfeeding/chestfeeding by individuals who use cannabis is controversial due to the absence of data on its effects on infants during lactation.

## Thyroid Disorders

As outlined in the *Common Conditions in Primary Care* chapter, thyroid disorders are common in persons of childbearing age. Midwives will both encounter individuals with preexisting thyroid disease and diagnose the condition for the first time during pregnancy. It is estimated that 0.2% to 1% of pregnancies are complicated by hypothyroidism and 0.2% to 0.7% by hyperthyroidism.[156] Both hypothyroidism and hyperthyroidism can be present in a subclinical state and progress to overt disease due to the thyroid changes that occur during pregnancy. Individuals with a new diagnosis may benefit from specialist consultation to optimize perinatal and neonatal outcomes. Careful attention to presenting symptoms and physical examination findings as well as an understanding of thyroid function are essential for prompt recognition of abnormalities. This section reviews pregnancy-related changes in thyroid function and the most common thyroid disorders in pregnancy: hypothyroidism, hyperthyroidism, and thyroid nodules.

### Pregnancy Considerations

During pregnancy, significant changes to the structure and function of the thyroid gland occur, as detailed in the *Anatomy and Physiology of Pregnancy* chapter. Increases in estrogen lead to a two-fold increase in thyroid-binding hormones, which in turn causes increases in thyroid hormone production.[157] In addition, iodine requirements can result in a 30% increase in the size of the thyroid gland to meet this demand. Human chorionic gonadotropin (hCG) secreted early in pregnancy directly stimulates the pituitary to release thyroid-stimulating hormone (TSH). TSH then stimulates the release of higher amounts of free thyroid hormone thyroxine ($T_4$) from the thyroid gland. Free $T_4$ crosses the placenta and is vital for fetal survival. Overall, these normal physiologic changes can increase production of the two primary thyroid hormones, thyroxine ($T_4$) and triiodothyronine ($T_3$), by 20% to 50%.[157]

Since the fetal thyroid does not produce $T_4$ until after 12 weeks' gestation, transplacental passage of $T_4$ is critical for early brain development, fetal growth, and bone maturation.[157] Adequate fetal $T_4$ production does not begin until after 18 weeks'

| Table 24-19 | Overview of Thyroid Hormone Values During Pregnancy in People with Thyroid Dysfunction | | |
|---|---|---|---|
| **Thyroid Hormone** | **Normal Pregnancy** | **Overt Hypothyroidism in Pregnancy** | **Overt Hyperthyroidism in Pregnancy** |
| Thyroid-stimulating hormone (TSH) | Normal | High | Severely decreased or undetectable |
| Free thyroxine ($T_4$) | Normal | Low | Increased |
| Total thyroxine ($T_4$) | Increased | Low | Increased |
| Free triiodothyronine ($FT_3$) | Normal | Low | Increased |
| Total triiodothyronine ($T_3$) | Increased | Low | Increased |
| Thyroid-binding globulin (TBG) | Increased | Normal | Increased |

Based on Alexander EK, Pearce EN, Brent GA, et al. 2017 guidelines of the American Thyroid Association for the diagnosis and management of thyroid disease during pregnancy and the postpartum. *Thyroid.* 2017;27(3):315-389; American College of Obstetricians and Gynecologists. Practice Bulletin No. 148: thyroid disease in pregnancy. *Obstet Gynecol.* 2015 (reaffirmed 2020);125(4):996-1005.

gestation. Careful perinatal assessment for any signs or symptoms suggestive of thyroid dysfunction are especially important during this period.

The reference ranges for TSH and $T_4$ are trimester specific and population based. If local reference ranges are not available, the American Thyroid Association (ATA) has set upper and lower limits that can be used to assess thyroid function.[158] More recently, ACOG published an updated Practice Bulletin containing several divergent approaches and recommendations compared to the ATA, highlighting the need for more-frequent evaluations of the evidence regarding the diagnosis and treatment of thyroid disease in pregnancy.[159] In general, TSH levels decrease slightly in response to hCG activity in the first trimester and begin to normalize to nonpregnant values in the second trimester.[158] Levels of both $T_3$ and $T_4$ increase slowly in the first trimester and can be 50% higher than nonpregnant ranges after 16 weeks' gestation.[156] It may be necessary to inform the lab that an individual is pregnant to correctly discern normal from abnormal thyroid function test results (Table 24-19).

Another necessary component of optimal thyroid function is ensuring newly pregnant individuals have an adequate dietary intake of iodine. Iodine is essential in the production of $T_4$, and during pregnancy, this requirement increases significantly.[156,158] The recommended iodine intake during pregnancy is 220 mcg per day. Iodine deficiency is a known cause of mental impairment worldwide, but can also lead to other neonatal complications, such as goiter, thyroid dysfunction,

congenital iodine-deficiency syndrome (profound intellectual development, motor rigidity, congenital deafness), and stillbirth.[158] Pregnant individuals who are iodine deficient can also develop goiter, and in severe cases, a 30% increase in thyroid nodules has been seen.[158]

In the United States, most people achieve sufficient iodine intake through food sources. Because adequate iodine intake can vary across regions, the ATA recommends a daily supplement of 150 mcg of potassium iodide during pregnancy and lactation.[158] In the United States, most (but not all) prenatal vitamins contain the recommended amount of potassium iodine.[156,158] In addition to iodized salt, other food sources of iodine include certain fish, shellfish, and dairy products.

### Evaluation of Thyroid Nodules

Individuals may present with concerns about thyroid nodules, or such growths may be discovered during routine examination. Thorough examination of the thyroid gland should be included as part of any routine physical exam, but especially in the preconception evaluation and the initial prenatal visit. Pregnancy can cause progression of subclinical thyroid disease, causing changes in the size and structure of the thyroid gland.[158] Both enlargement of the gland and detection of one or more thyroid nodules require further evaluation and consultation. Careful inquiry regarding symptoms and any family history of benign or malignant thyroid disease is key. Examination of the neck for cervical lymphadenopathy is also included in the initial assessment. A serum TSH level (with reflex free $T_4$) should be obtained, and an ultrasound of the thyroid gland ordered.[158]

Ultrasound of the thyroid is the most accurate imaging modality for evaluating thyroid nodules. Specific sonographic patterns can determine risks for malignancy and the need for fine-needle aspiration.[158] Any laboratory or sonographic abnormalities require prompt referral to the appropriate specialists.

### Hypothyroidism

Hypothyroidism during pregnancy can occur as a subclinical state or present as overt hypothyroidism. Causes include autoimmune disease, previous thyroidectomy or radiation treatment, overtreatment of hyperthyroid disorders, and certain medications such as lithium. Subclinical hypothyroidism occurs more frequently (2% to 5%), while overt hypothyroidism complicates fewer than 1% of pregnancies.[156–158]

Screening for hypothyroid disease with a TSH level is recommended for pregnant individuals with a family history of thyroid dysfunction, type 1 diabetes mellitus, or clinical suspicion based on physical exam or symptoms.[156] Universal screening is not recommended; however, other circumstances, such as severe iodine deficiency or multiple pregnancy losses, may warrant consideration for testing. Individuals currently taking lithium, amiodarone, or those who recently received a radiologic contrast agent may also be candidates for TSH screening.[156] Screening is also advised at the onset of pregnancy for those individuals with a personal history of hypothyroid disease regardless of their current treatment with thyroid replacement medications.[159]

An elevated TSH is the hallmark of underactive thyroid function. In the absence of specific regional reference levels, the ATA endorses a range of 0.4 to 4 mIU/L,[158] whereas ACOG identifies a normal TSH level as between 0.1 and 2.5 mIU/L[156] in the first trimester. Reference limits for the second and third trimesters are 0.2 to 3 mIU/L and 0.3 to 3 mIU/L, respectively.[156] A TSH result outside of these parameters requires an evaluation of serum free $T_4$. Note that checking the *total* $T_4$ level is not recommended due to the increased protein binding that occurs during pregnancy. Subclinical hypothyroidism is defined as an elevated TSH level above the upper limits of normal and a normal free $T_4$.[156-158] A free $T_4$ level below the lower limit of normal (with elevated TSH) would then indicate overt hypothyroidism.[156,158]

The most common cause of overt hypothyroidism in pregnancy is Hashimoto thyroiditis, an autoimmune disease in which thyroperoxidase antibodies (TPOAb) destroy the thyroid gland.[156,158] In previously undiagnosed or subclinical cases, the first sign of Hashimoto thyroiditis is typically enlargement of the thyroid gland (goiter). Underactive thyroid function can cause fatigue, cold intolerance, weight gain, constipation, and depression—symptoms commonly seen in pregnancy. In addition, as many as 18% of euthyroid pregnant persons are positive for antithyroid antibodies such as TPOAb and thyroglobulin antibody (TGAb).[156,159] Some studies have shown an association between the presence of antithyroid antibodies and spontaneous pregnancy loss, preterm birth, and the development of Hashimoto's disease during pregnancy.[156,158] For pregnant individuals known to be positive for TPOAb or TGAb antibodies from a previous work-up, monitoring of monthly TSH levels may be prudent.[158]

### Treatment of Hypothyroidism

Daily oral levothyroxine (Synthroid) taken on an empty stomach remains the mainstay of treatment for hypothyroid disease.[156,158] Treatment with levothyroxine is not recommended for subclinical hypothyroidism, as studies have not shown improvement in perinatal or fetal outcomes.[156,158] Treatment could be considered in certain subgroups, however—namely, those TBOAb positive with normal or slightly elevated TSH levels to reduce the risks of early pregnancy loss.[158] Medications containing $T_3$ (desiccated thyroid extract or synthetic $T_3$) are not recommended in pregnancy.

Overt hypothyroidism, if left untreated, can lead to spontaneous abortion, preeclampsia, preterm birth, placental abruption, and stillbirth.[156] In the neonate, low birth weight and impaired neuropsychologic development can occur, especially if severe perinatal iodine deficiency exists.[156] The goals of treatment are to achieve and maintain a TSH level of less than 2.5 mIU/L.[156,158] Additional levothyroxine dosing and monitoring considerations for pregnancy will depend on either the pregnant person's past or current thyroid status. For example, individuals who were previously euthyroid, but are now presenting with an elevated TSH in pregnancy, can be safely started at 1 to 2 micrograms/kg or 100 micrograms daily. Those currently taking levothyroxine should have their dose increased by 25% as soon as pregnancy is confirmed. If the individual has a history of thyroidectomy or previous radiation, higher doses may be required.

TSH levels should be monitored every 4 to 6 weeks and dosing adjusted as needed to maintain a level between the lower reference range limit and 2.5 mIU/L. Individuals who were being treated for hypothyroidism prior to pregnancy can resume their pre-pregnant dosing immediately postpartum. Discontinuation of levothyroxine postpartum can be considered for individuals whose treatment was initiated during pregnancy, especially if the current dose is less than 50 micrograms daily.[158] In either case, a TSH level is recommended in 6 weeks.

### Hyperthyroidism

The presence of excess thyroid hormones in the body can result in a hypermetabolic state known as thyrotoxicosis.[158] Graves' disease is the most common cause of overactive thyroid function (hyperthyroidism), accounting for 95% of cases.[158] Hyperthyroidism with resultant thyrotoxicosis is characterized by suppressed or undetectable TSH and inappropriately elevated $T_4$ and $T_3$.[158] Other causes of thyrotoxicosis include toxic multinodular goiter and toxic adenoma, underscoring the importance of evaluating palpable thyroid nodules.[158] Another cause to consider would be overtreatment of hypothyroidism with levothyroxine ($T_4$ hormone).

The pre-pregnancy incidence of Graves' disease among persons assigned female gender at birth is 0.4% to 1% and approximately 0.2% during pregnancy.[158] In early pregnancy, TSH is commonly suppressed by elevated hCG levels. This transient physiologic process will result in low TSH (less than 0.1 mUI/L) with normal $T_4$. In some cases, excessively high hCG levels (as seen in hyperemesis gravidarum, multiple gestation, hydatidiform mole, and choriocarcinoma) can cause gestational transient thyrotoxicosis.[158] Both new-onset Graves' disease and gestational transient thyrotoxicosis present similarly to overt hyperthyroidism in the first trimester. Symptoms such as palpitations, anxiety, tremors, tachycardia, heat intolerance, weight loss, and hypertension will be present.[156] In Graves' disease, however, additional physical findings of goiter or orbitopathy may be seen. In contrast, serum hCG levels are typically much higher in persons with transient gestational thyrotoxicosis, and are often accompanied by nausea and vomiting. As pregnancy progresses and hCG levels fall, gestational thyrotoxicosis typically resolves without treatment.[156] Regardless of the suspected cause, pregnant individuals presenting with overt hyperthyroidism require referral to a physician.[156]

Normalization of thyroid hormones before and during pregnancy is critical for reducing adverse fetal and maternal outcomes. Thyroid-stimulating antibodies cross the placenta and can stimulate or inhibit the fetal thyroid.[156] Any pregnant person with Graves' disease should be monitored for fetal tachycardia and poor fetal growth—both are signs of fetal thyrotoxicosis. After birth, approximately 1% to 5% of these newborns will develop neonatal Graves' disease and will require close pediatric follow-up.[156]

Treatment of hyperthyroidism focuses on reducing the amount of circulating thyroid hormones in the body through the use of antithyroid medications—that is, propylthiouracil (PTU) or methimazole (Tapazole).[156,159] As both of these medications can cause adverse effects, the choice of treatment will depend, in part, on the trimester. In general, methimazole is avoided in the first trimester due to its association with major fetal malformations—namely, choanal atresia, tracheo-esophageal fistula, and omphalocele.[156] While PTU is preferred in the first trimester, there is an increased risk of perinatal hepatoxicity with use of this medication, and some sources recommend switching to methimazole for the remainder of the pregnancy.[156,158] Ultimately, the choice and monitoring of these medications is best managed by an endocrinologist in collaboration with an MFM specialist (Figure 24-4).

In rare cases of uncontrolled hyperthyroidism, circulating $T_4$ can reach critical levels and cause acute thyroid storm. In most cases, the affected individual will have a history of Graves' disease or presenting symptoms such as fever, tachycardia, cardiac arrhythmias, and/or altered mental status.[156] Patients can rapidly decompensate, especially if a precipitating condition such as preeclampsia, anemia, or sepsis is present. Midwives caring for any pregnant person with hyperthyroidism must be alert for these signs and immediately refer or transfer pregnant individuals with thyroid storm to the nearest appropriate hospital for aggressive critical care management.[156]

## Urinary Disorders

Urinary tract infections (UTIs) are the most common bacterial infection in pregnancy.[160] Such infections include asymptomatic bacteriuria, cystitis, recurrent UTI, and pyelonephritis. In addition to pregnancy itself, other risk factors for UTIs include sexual activity, anatomic or functional urinary tract abnormalities, previous urinary surgeries, low socioeconomic status, previous UTI, and pregestational diabetes.[161] Pregnancy-related changes to the urinary tract predispose individuals to pyelonephritis once a UTI is present.[162] Diagnostic criteria for urinary disorders are presented in the *Common Conditions in Primary Care* chapter.

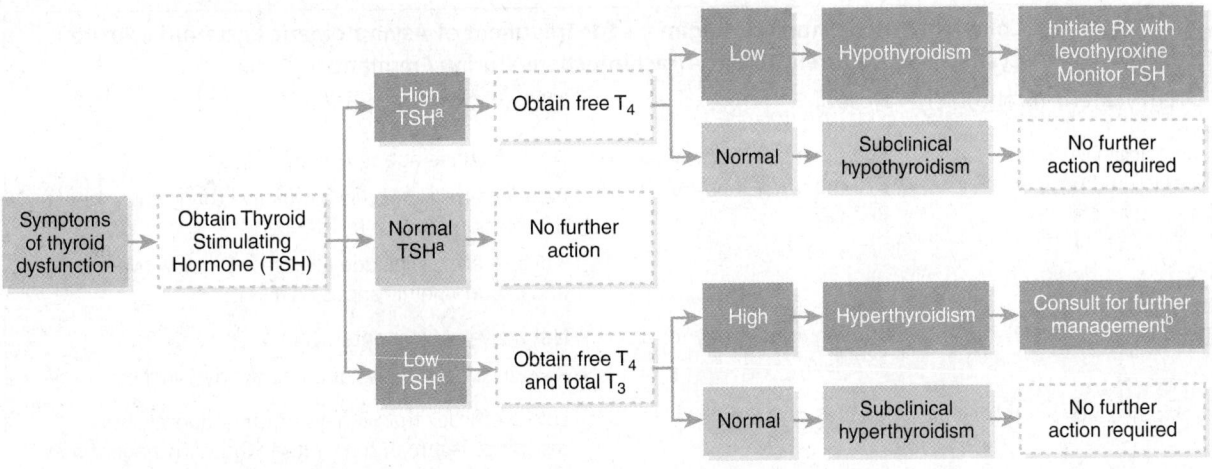

**Figure 24-4** Overview of treatment of thyroid disorders in pregnancy.
Abbreviations: T3, triiodothyronine; T4, thyroxineaTSH.
Based on American College of Obstetricians and Gynecologists: Thyroid disease in pregnancy. *Obstet Gynecol.* 2020;135:e261-e274.
doi: 10.1097/AOG.0000000000003893.

## Asymptomatic Bacteriuria

The incidence of asymptomatic bacteriuria is similar in pregnant and nonpregnant people, with prevalence rates ranging from 2% to 15%.[160] All pregnant people should be screened for asymptomatic bacteriuria upon entry into care via a urine culture. Dipstick analysis and microscopy have poor predictive value. If screening for asymptomatic bacteriuria is negative, routine reculture is neither indicated nor cost-effective in pregnancy. The pathogen most likely to cause this infection is *Escherichia coli*, which accounts for 70% to 80% of such infections.[161] The combination of a lack of overt symptoms associated with a UTI and a clean-catch urine culture that has isolated 100,000 ($10^5$) colonies or more of one bacterium suffices to diagnose asymptomatic bacteriuria.[161] Untreated asymptomatic bacteriuria in pregnancy is associated with up to 40% risk for later symptomatic UTI, including pyelonephritis. Treatment of asymptomatic bacteriuria reduces these risks significantly.[161]

The selection of an antibiotic to treat asymptomatic bacteriuria is guided by resistance patterns, local costs, availability, and allergy history. Nitrofurantoin has bactericidal activity against common urinary pathogens; however, it should be avoided after 36 weeks' gestation due to concern for neonatal hemolysis.[161] Safety data on teratogenicity of nitrofurantoin in the first trimester are conflicting, therefore it is typically only used in the first trimester when suitable alternatives are not available.[161,162]

Sulfonamides and nitrofurantoin are contraindicated for individuals with G6PD deficiency. Some authors recommend avoiding trimethoprim–sulfamethoxazole in the first and third trimesters because trimethoprim is a folic acid antagonist and sulfonamides displace bilirubin from plasma-binding sites in the newborn, which theoretically increases the risk for newborn jaundice. Fluoroquinolones, tetracycline, and doxycycline are contraindicated in pregnancy. Commonly used antibiotic regimens for asymptomatic bacteriuria and other UTIs are presented in Table 24-20.

A urine culture positive for group B *Streptococcus* (GBS) indicates heavy colonization of the vaginal–rectal area; these individuals should be offered prophylactic antibiotics during labor to prevent neonatal GBS infection. Repeat GBS screening at 35 to 37 weeks' gestation is not indicated. Treatment at the time of urine culture is appropriate if the patient is symptomatic, or if the colony count is greater than $10^5$ per milliliter.[163]

A test of cure culture is recommended 1 to 2 weeks after antibiotic treatment is complete, as a significant portion of people with asymptomatic bacteriuria do not clear the infection. Those treated for GBS do not require a test of cure. If an individual experiences a second recurrence of asymptomatic bacteriuria or develops a symptomatic UTI, continuous suppressive therapy should be initiated after treatment of the infection.[161]

| Table 24-20 | Commonly Used Antibiotic Regimens for Treatment of Asymptomatic Bacteriuria, Acute Cystitis, and Recurrent Urinary Tract Infections During Pregnancy | |
|---|---|---|
| **Drug: Generic (Brand)** | **Dose** | **Clinical Considerations** |
| Amoxicillin (Amoxil), ampicillin (Principen) | 500 mg orally 3 times/day or 875 mg orally 2 times/day for 3–7 days | Not a first-line agent, except with GBS. Beta-lactams may be less effective than other agents due to high rates of resistance. Adverse effects include allergies, *Candida* overgrowth, and pseudomembranous colitis. |
| Cephalexin (Keflex) | 500 mg 4 times/day for 3–7 days | Not active against enterococci. Risks include allergies and hepatic dysfunction. |
| Fosfomycin (Monurol) | Single 3-g oral dose | Lower efficacy than 3 days of other agents, but resistance is rare in the United States. This agent may be an option for people with multiple allergies. Does not reach a therapeutic dose in the kidney, so it should not be used if pyelonephritis is suspected. |
| Nitrofurantoin (Macrobid) | 100 mg orally twice daily for 5–7 days | First-choice for uncomplicated UTI. Controversial teratogenic risk; acceptable in first trimester if there are no suitable alternatives. Contraindicated with G6PD deficiency. Resistance is unlikely, but the drug is bactericidal in urine only; poor penetration into tissues. Does not reach a therapeutic dose in the kidney, so it should not be used if pyelonephritis is suspected. Administer with meals to improve absorption. Side effects include gastrointestinal upset, peripheral neuropathy, and pneumonitis. |
| Trimethoprim–sulfamethoxazole (Bactrim, Septra, Septra DS) | 800 mg/160 mg (one double-strength tablet) orally twice daily for 3 days | First-choice agent if resistance in the local area is less than 20%. **Avoid** during the first and third trimesters unless it is the only or best choice. Contraindicated with G6PD deficiency. Allergic reactions are common; serious skin reactions and blood dyscrasias may occur. |
| **Suppressive Therapy** | | |
| Nitrofurantoin (Macrobid) | 50–100 mg orally once daily at bedtime | May be used daily or postcoital if UTI is sexually related. |
| Cephalexin (Keflex) | 250–500 mg orally once daily at bedtime | May be used daily or postcoital if UTI is sexually related. |

Abbreviations: G6PD, glucose-6-phosphate dehydrogenase; GBS, group B *Streptococcus;* UTI, urinary tract infection.

Updated from previous edition based on Glaser AP, Schaeffer AJ. Urinary tract infection and bacteriuria in pregnancy. *Urol Clin North Am.* 2015;42(4):547-560. doi:10.1016/j.ucl.2015.05.004; Kalinderi K, Delkos D, Kalinderis M, Athanasiadis A, Kalogiannidis I. Urinary tract infection during pregnancy: current concepts on a common multifaceted problem. *J Obstet Gynaecol.* 2018;38(4):448-453. doi:10.1080/01443615.2017.1370579; White J, Ory J, Lantz Powers AG, et al. Urological issues in pregnancy: a review for urologists. *Can Urol Assoc J.* 2020;14(10):352-357. doi:10.5489/cuaj.6526.

## Acute Cystitis

Acute cystitis is an infection in the bladder that develops in approximately 1% to 2% of pregnancies.[161] In addition to an increased risk for pyelonephritis, studies have found an increase in both preterm birth and low-birth-weight infants from birthing individuals who have acute cystitis during pregnancy. Symptoms include urgency, frequency, dysuria, hematuria, and suprapubic pressure. Fever, chills, flank pain, and costovertebral angle tenderness suggest possible pyelonephritis.

The diagnosis of a symptomatic UTI is based on urine culture results, but people may be treated presumptively before culture results are available.[161] Nitrites, leukocyte esterase, and white blood cells on a dipstick urinalysis suggest uncomplicated cystitis in symptomatic individuals.[160] Presence of more than 15 to 20 squamous epithelial cells suggests a contaminated sample; in such a case, a new sample should be collected, if possible.[160]

If treatment is initiated prior to availability of culture results, the midwife should check the final report for sensitivities to assure the antibiotic was appropriate. A 3- to 7-day course is initially prescribed, whereas regimens for recurrent infections are 10 to 14 days.[160,162] A repeat urine culture or test of cure is recommended once therapy is completed.[161] If dysuria without bacteriuria persists, testing for STIs is indicated.

## Recurrent Urinary Tract Infections

Recurrent UTI is distinguished from relapse or reinfection.

- *Recurrent UTI* indicates two or more infections within 1 year.
- A *relapse* (persistent infection) occurs when subsequent infections are found to be caused by the same organism as the original infection and the infections occur within 2 weeks of completion of treatment.
- *Reinfection* is defined as a UTI caused by a new organism more than 2 weeks after a negative test of cure.

Individuals who have recurrent UTIs in pregnancy are offered continuous daily suppressive therapy (Table 24-20).

## Pyelonephritis

Pyelonephritis, or infection of the upper urinary tract, typically manifests in the second or third trimester and is often the consequence of undiagnosed or inadequate treatment of a UTI. Age, nulliparity, sickle cell anemia, diabetes, nephrolithiasis, illicit drug use, and a history of pyelonephritis are all risk factors.

Signs and symptoms of pyelonephritis include low back pain, flank pain, fever, chills, nausea, vomiting, costovertebral angle tenderness, and pyuria (white blood cells in the urine). Dysuria is less common. Pyelonephritis carries a risk for sepsis, septic shock, adult respiratory distress syndrome, anemia, renal insufficiency, preterm birth (20% to 50%), and low-birth-weight infant.[161,162] The differential diagnoses for these symptoms are kidney stones, intra-amniotic infection, preterm labor, and placental abruption. Pyuria and bacteriuria will be present with pyelonephritis but do not occur with kidney stones, intra-amniotic infection, or abruption.

Inpatient management is usually recommended for pyelonephritis during pregnancy due to the risk for sepsis. Antibiotics are administered parenterally until the person is afebrile for 24 to 48 hours. These agents are initiated empirically and changed as needed when urine culture results are available. Nitrofurantoin does not reach therapeutic levels in the kidneys, thus other antibiotics including ampicillin plus gentamicin or a single-agent cephalosporin such as ceftriaxone are commonly used to treat pyelonephritis.[161] Once the acute symptoms have resolved, oral medications can be instituted on an outpatient basis. Antibiotics are administered for 7 to 14 days and suppressive therapy is recommended thereafter. Outpatient management may be appropriate when medical follow-up is available. Candidates for outpatient management include those at less than 24 weeks' gestation who do not have severe symptoms and are otherwise healthy or without comorbid conditions.

## Urolithiasis

Urolithiasis, otherwise known as renal calculi or kidney stones, is the most common indication for urologic surgery in pregnancy.[164] Approximately 0.2% of people are affected by symptomatic stones in pregnancy.[164] Kidney stones are associated with increased risk of preterm birth, low birth weight, premature rupture of membranes, preeclampsia, and cesarean section.[165]

Flank pain, microscopic hematuria, and prior history of stones are associated with diagnosis.[164] Ultrasound is not especially sensitive for detecting stones in pregnancy; radiology reports typically note the presence or absence of ureteric jet, with absence supporting obstruction.[164] Initial management of urolithiasis includes intravenous fluids and analgesia.[165] Additional interventions such as surgery may be indicated in patients with refractory pain, bilateral obstruction, or obstruction with infection or sepsis.[164] Physician management is typically indicated beyond initial supportive measures.

## Conclusion

Midwifery care can be of great benefit for individuals whose pregnancy is medically complicated. Listening to patient concerns, meticulous history taking, thorough physical examination, and an understanding of differential diagnoses and danger signs are crucial steps in mitigating adverse effects of these disorders, some of which can have lifelong or fetal effects. The decision to consult, collaborate, or refer to a specialist for ongoing care will be based on the severity of the condition, practice policies, and available resources. A multidisciplinary, team-based approach provides the best possible outcomes when complications are experienced during pregnancy, birth, postpartum, and beyond.

## References

1. Petri M. Systemic lupus erythematosus: clinical updates in women's health care primary and preventive care review. *Obstet Gynecol.* 2020;136(1):226. doi:10.1097/AOG.0000000000003942.

2. Petri M. Pregnancy and systemic lupus erythematosus. *Best Pract Res Clin Obstet Gynaecol.* 2020;64:24-30. doi:10.1016/j.bpobgyn.2019.09.002.

3. Fischer-Betz R, Specker C. Pregnancy in systemic lupus erythematosus and antiphospholipid syndrome. *Best Pract Res Clin Rheumatol.* 2017;31(3):397-414. doi:10.1016/j.berh.2017.09.011.

4. Silverstein J, Post AL, Jo Chien A, et al. Multidisciplinary management of cancer during pregnancy. *JCO Oncol Pract.* 2021;16:545-557.

5. Maggen C, Wolters VE, Cardonick E, et al. Pregnancy and cancer: the INCIP project. *Curr Oncol Rep.* 2020;22:17. doi.org/10.1007/s11912-020-0862-7.

6. Carlson LM, Hardisty E, Coombs CC, Vora NL. Maternal malignancy after discordant cell-free DNA results. *Obstet Gynecol.* 2018;131(3):464-468.

7. Tang M, Webber K. Fertility and pregnancy in cancer survivors. *Obstet Med.* 2018;11(3):110-115.

8. Busnelli A, Vitagliano A. Mensi L. Fertility in female cancer survivors: a systematic review and meta-analysis. *RBMO.* 2020;41(1):96-112.

9. Bhurosy T, Niu Z, Heckman CJ. Breastfeeding is possible: a systematic review on the feasibility and challenges of breastfeeding among breast cancer survivors of reproductive age. *Ann Surg Oncol.* 2021;28:3723-3735.

10. Creanga AA, Syverson C, Seed K, Callaghan WM. Pregnancy-related mortality in the United States, 2011–2013. *Obstet Gynecol.* 2017;130(2):366-373. doi:10.1097/AOG.0000000000002114.

11. American College of Obstetricians and Gynecologists. ACOG Practice Bulletin No. 212: pregnancy and heart disease. *Obstet Gynecol.* 2019;133(5):e320-e356. doi:10.1097/AOG.0000000000003243.

12. Millington S, Magarey J, Dekker GA, Clark RA. Cardiac conditions in pregnancy and the role of midwives: a discussion paper. *Nurs Open.* 2019;6(3):722-732. doi:10.1002/nop2.269.

13. Canobbio MM, Warnes CA, Aboulhosn J, et al. Management of pregnancy in patients with complex congenital heart disease: a scientific statement for healthcare professionals from the American Heart Association. *Circulation.* 2017;135(8):e50-e87. doi:10.1161/CIR.0000000000000458.

14. Silversides CK, Grewal J, Mason J, et al. Pregnancy outcomes in women with heart disease: the CARPREG II Study. *J Am Coll Cardiol.* 2018;71(21):2419-2430. doi:10.1016/j.jacc.2018.02.076.

15. Sharma G, Ying W, Silversides CK. The importance of cardiovascular risk assessment and pregnancy heart team in the management of cardiovascular disease in pregnancy. *Cardiol Clin.* 2021;39(1):7-19. doi:10.1016/j.ccl.2020.09.002.

16. Kearney L, Wright P, Fhadil S, Thomas M. Postpartum cardiomyopathy and considerations for breastfeeding. *Card Fail Rev.* 2018;4(2):112-118. doi:10.15420/cfr.2018.21.2.

17. American College of Obstetricians and Gynecologists. Practice Bulletin No. 190: gestational diabetes mellitus. *Obstet Gynecol.* 2018;131:e49-e64. doi:10.1097/AOG.0000000000002501.

18. American Diabetes Association. 2: Classification and diagnosis of diabetes: standards of medical care in diabetes—2020. *Diab Care.* 2020;43(suppl 1):S14-S31. doi:10.2337/dc20-S002.

19. Centers for Disease Control and Prevention. Diabetes during pregnancy. https://www.cdc.gov/reproductivehealth/maternalinfanthealth/diabetes-during-pregnancy.htm. Updated June 12, 2018. Accessed August 15, 2021.

20. Hod M, Kapur A, McIntyre HD, FIGO Working Group on Hyperglycemia in Pregnancy, FIGO Pregnancy and Prevention of Early NCD Committee. Evidence in support of the International Association of Diabetes in Pregnancy study groups' criteria for diagnosing gestational diabetes mellitus worldwide in 2019. *Am J Obstet Gynecol.* 2019;221(2):109-116. doi:10.1016/j.ajog.2019.01.206.

21. American Diabetes Association. 14: Management of diabetes in pregnancy: standards of medical care in diabetes—2020. *Diab Care.* 2020;43(suppl 1):S183-S192. doi:10.2337/dc20-S014.

22. Lowe WL Jr, Lowe LP, Kuang A, et al. Maternal glucose levels during pregnancy and childhood adiposity in the Hyperglycemia and Adverse Pregnancy Outcome Follow-up Study. *Diabetologia*. 2019;62(4):598-610. doi:10.1007/s00125-018-4809-6.

23. Vounzoulaki E, Khunti K, Abner SC, et al. Progression to type 2 diabetes in women with a known history of gestational diabetes: systematic review and meta-analysis. *BMJ*. 2020;369:m1361. doi:10.1136/bmj.m1361.

24. American College of Obstetricians and Gynecologists. ACOG Practice Bulletin No. 201: pregestational diabetes mellitus. *Obstet Gynecol*. 2018;132(6):e228-e248. doi:10.1097/AOG.0000000000002960.

25. Brown J, Grzeskowiak L, Williamson K, et al. Insulin for the treatment of women with gestational diabetes. *Cochrane Database Syst Rev*. 2017;11(11):CD012037. doi:10.1002/14651858.CD012037.pub2.

26. Fong A, Serra AE, Gabby L, et al. Use of hemoglobin A1c as an early predictor of gestational diabetes mellitus. *Am J Obstet Gynecol*. 2014;211(6):641.e1-641.e7.

27. Han S, Middleton P, Shepherd E, et al. Different types of dietary advice for women with gestational diabetes mellitus. *Cochrane Database Syst Rev*. 2017;(2):CD009275. doi:10.1002/14651858.CD009275.pub3.

28. Martis R, Crowther CA, Shepherd E, et al. Treatments for women with gestational diabetes mellitus: an overview of Cochrane systematic reviews. *Cochrane Database Syst Rev*. 2018;8(8):CD012327. doi:10.1002/14651858.CD012327.pub2.

29. Caissutti C, Saccone G, Khalifeh A, et al. Which criteria should be used for starting pharmacologic therapy for management of gestational diabetes in pregnancy? Evidence from randomized controlled trials. *J Matern Fetal Neonatal Med*. 2019;32(17):2905-2914. doi:10.1080/14767058.2018.1449203.

30. Avery M. Diabetes in pregnancy: the midwifery role in management. *J Midwifery Womens Health*. 2000;45:472-480.

31. Zachariah SK, Fenn M, Jacob K, Arthungal SA, Zachariah SA. Management of acute abdomen in pregnancy: current perspectives. *Int J Womens Health*. 2019;11:119-134. doi:10.2147/IJWH.S151501.

32. Abushamma S, Early DS. A guide to upper gastrointestinal tract, biliary, and pancreatic disorders: clinical updates in women's health care primary and preventive care review. *Obstet Gynecol*. 2021;137(6):1152. doi:10.1097/AOG.0000000000004366.

33. Gomes CF, Sousa M, Lourenço I, et al. Gastrointestinal diseases during pregnancy: what does the gastroenterologist need to know? *Ann Gastroenterol*. 2018;31(4):385-394. doi:10.20524/aog.2018.0264.

34. McLean E, Cogswell M, Egli I, et al. Worldwide prevalence of anaemia: WHO Vitamin and Mineral Nutrition Information System, 1993–2005. *Public Health Nutr*. 2009;12:444-454.

35. Centers for Disease Control and Prevention. Recommendations to prevent and control iron deficiency in the United States. *MMWR Recomm Rep*. 1998;47(RR-3):1-29.

36. American College of Obstetricians and Gynecologists. ACOG Practice Bulletin No. 233: anemia in pregnancy. *Obstet Gynecol*. 2021;138(2):e55-e64. doi:10.1097/AOG.0000000000004477.

37. Mei Z, Cogswell ME, Looker AC, et al. Assessment of iron status in US pregnant women from the National Health and Nutrition Examination Survey (NHANES), 1999–2006. *Am J Clin Nutr*. 2011;93:1312-1320. https://doi.org/10.3945/ajcn.110.007195.

38. Chao C, O'Brien KO. Pregnancy and iron homeostasis: an update. *Nutr Rev*. 2013;71(1):35-51. https://doi.org/10.1111/j.1753-4887.2012.00550.x.

39. Elmore, C., & Ellis, J. (2022). Screening, treatment, and monitoring of iron deficiency anemia in pregnancy and postpartum. *Journal of Midwifery & Women's Health*. https://doi.org/10.1111/jmwh.13370

40. Peña-Rosas JP, De-Regil LM, Garcia-Casal MN, Dowswell T. Daily oral iron supplementation during pregnancy. *Cochrane Database Syst Rev*. 2015;(7):CD004736. doi:10.1002/14651858.CD004736.pub5.

41. Lewkowitz AK, Gupta A, Simon L, et al. Intravenous compared with oral iron for the treatment of iron-deficiency anemia in pregnancy: a systematic review and meta-analysis. *J Perinatol*. 2019;39:519-532. doi:10.1038/s41372-019-0320-2.

42. Haider BA, Olofin I, Wang M, et al. Anaemia, prenatal iron use, and risk of adverse pregnancy outcomes: systematic review and meta-analysis. *BMJ*. 2013;346:f3443. doi:10.1136/bmj.f3443.

43. Thom CS, Dickson CF, Gell DA, Weiss MJ. Hemoglobin variants: biochemical properties and clinical correlates. *Cold Spring Harbor Perspect Med*. 2013;3(3):a011858.

44. Centers for Disease Control and Prevention. Data and statistics on sickle cell disease. https://www.cdc.gov/ncbddd/sicklecell/data.html. Updated December 16, 2020. Accessed September 24, 2021.

45. Howard J, Oteng-Ntim E. The obstetric management of sickle cell disease. *Best Pract Res Clin Obstet Gynecol*. 2012;26:25-36.

46. Petrakos G, Andriopoulos P, Tsironi M. Pregnancy in women with thalassemia: challenges and solutions. *Int J Womens Health*. 2016;8:441-451. doi:10.2147/IJWH.S89308.

47. Kattamis A, Forni GL, Aydinok Y, Viprakasit V. Changing patterns in the epidemiology of β-thalassemia. *Eur J Haematol*. 2020;105(6):692-703. doi:10.1111/ejh.13512.

48. Nkhoma ET, Poole C, Vannappagari V, et al. The global prevalence of glucose-6-phosphate dehydrogenase

deficiency: a systematic review and meta-analysis. *Blood Cells Mol Dis.* 2009;42(3):267-278.

49. Ciobanu AM, Colibab S, Cimpoca B, et al. Thrombocytopenia in pregnancy. *Maedica (Bucur).* 2016;11(1):55-60.

50. American College of Obstetricians and Gynecologists. ACOG Practice Bulletin No. 207: thrombocytopenia in pregnancy. *Obstet Gynecol.* 2019;133(3):e181-e193. doi:10.1097/AOG.0000000000003100.

51. Khalid A, Hadbavna A, Williams D, Byrne B. A review of stroke in pregnancy: incidence, investigations and management. *Obstet Gynaecol.* 2020;22(1):21-33. doi:10.1111/tog.12624.

52. American College of Obstetricians and Gynecologists. ACOG Practice Bulletin No. 196: thromboembolism in pregnancy. *Obstet Gynecol.* 2018;132(1):e1-e17. doi:10.1097/AOG.0000000000002706.

53. Centers for Disease Control and Prevention. Pregnancy and stroke: are you at risk? https://www.cdc.gov/stroke/pregnancy.htm. Published May 6, 2021. Accessed December 10, 2021.

54. American College of Obstetricians and Gynecologists. ACOG Practice Bulletin No. 197: inherited thrombophilias in pregnancy. *Obstet Gynecol.* 2018;132(1):e18-e34. doi:10.1097/AOG.0000000000002703.

55. American College of Obstetricians and Gynecologists. Committee Opinion No. 580: von Willebrand disease in women. *Obstet Gynecol.* 2013 (reaffirmed 2021);122(6):1368-1373. doi:10.1097/01.AOG.0000438961.38979.19.

56. Simcox LE, Ormesher L, Tower C, Greer IA. Pulmonary thrombo-embolism in pregnancy: diagnosis and management. *Breathe (Sheff).* 2015;11(4):282-289. doi:10.1183/20734735.008815.

57. Brady CW. Liver disease in pregnancy: what's new. *Hepatol Comm.* 2020;4(2):145-156. doi:10.1002/hep4.1470.

58. Guarino M, Cossiga V, Morisco F. The interpretation of liver function tests in pregnancy. *Best Pract Res Clin Gastroentero.* 2020;44-45:101667. https://doi.org/10.1016/j.bpg.2020.101667.

59. Nelson NP, Weng MK, Hofmeister MG, et al. Prevention of hepatitis A virus infection in the United States: recommendations of the Advisory Committee on Immunization Practices, 2020. *MMWR Recomm Rep.* 2020;69(RR-5):1-38. http://dx.doi.org/10.15585/mmwr.rr6905a1.

60. Schillie S, Velozzi C, Reingold A, et al. Prevention of hepatitis B virus infection in the United States: recommendations of the Advisory Committee on Immunization Practices. *MMWR Recomm Rep.* 2018;67(RR-1):1-31. https://dx.doi.org/10.15585/mmwr.rr6701a1.

61. Schillie S, Wester C, Osborne M, et al. CDC recommendations for hepatitis C screening among adults—United States 2020. *MMWR Recomm Rep* 2020;69(RR-2):1-17. https://dx.doi.org?10.15585/mmwr.rr6902a1.

62. Folk DM. Hypertensive disorders of pregnancy: overview and current recommendations. *J Midwifery Womens Health.* 2018;63(3):289-300. doi:10.1111/jmwh.12725.

63. Say L, Chou D, Gemmill A, et al. Global causes of maternal death: a WHO systematic analysis. *Lancet Glob Health.* 2014;2(6):e323-e333.

64. Zhang M, Wan P, Ng K, et al. Preeclampsia among African American pregnant women: an update on prevalence, complications, etiology, and biomarkers. *Obstet Gynecol Surv.* 2020;75(2):111-120. doi:10.1097/OGX.0000000000000747.

65. Singh GK, Siahpush M, Liu L, et al. Racial/ethnic, nativity, and sociodemographic disparities in maternal hypertension in the United States, 2014–2015. *Int J Hypertens.* 2018;2018:7897189.

66. American College of Obstetricians and Gynecologists. ACOG Practice Bulletin No. 222: gestational hypertension and preeclampsia. *Obstet Gynecol.* 2020;135(6):e237-e260. doi:10.1097/AOG.0000000000003891.

67. Khedagi A, Bello N. Hypertensive disorders of pregnancy. *Cardiol Clin.* 2021;39:77-90. https://doi.org/10.1016/j.ccl.2020.09.005.

68. American College of Obstetricians and Gynecologists. ACOG Practice Bulletin No. 203: chronic hypertension in pregnancy. *Obstet Gynecol* 2019;133:e26-e50.

69. American College of Obstetricians and Gynecology. ACOG Committee Opinion No. 743: low dose aspirin use during pregnancy. *Obstet Gynecol.* 2018;132:e44–52. doi:10.1097/AOG.0000000000002708.

70. Lu Y, Chen R, Cai J, et al. The management of hypertension in women planning for pregnancy. *Br Med Bull.* 2018;128(1):75-84. doi:10.1093/bmb/ldy035.

71. Tita AT, Szychowski JM, Boggess K, et al. Treatment for mild chronic hypertension during pregnancy. *N Engl J Med.* 2022;386(19):1781-1792. doi:10.1056/NEJMoa220129.

72. Society for Maternal-Fetal Medicine; Publications Committee. Society for Maternal-Fetal Medicine Statement: Antihypertensive therapy for mild chronic hypertension in pregnancy-The Chronic Hypertension and Pregnancy trial. *Am J Obstet Gynecol.* 2022;227(2):B24-B27. doi:10.1016/j.ajog.2022.04.011.

73. Johnson S, Liu B, Kalafat E, et al. Maternal and perinatal outcomes of white coat hypertension during pregnancy: a systematic review and meta-analysis. *Hypertension.* 2020;76(1):157-166. doi:10.1161/HYPERTENSIONAHA.119.14627.

74. Granger JP, Spradley FT, Bakrania BA. The endothelin system: a critical player in the pathophysiology of preeclampsia. *Curr Hypertens Rep.* 2018;20(4):32. doi:10.1007/s11906-018-0828-4.

75. Wójtowicz A, Zembala-Szczerba M, Babczyk D, et al. Early- and late-onset preeclampsia: a

comprehensive cohort study of laboratory and clinical findings according to the New ISHHP Criteria. *Int J Hypertens.* 2019;2019:4108271. doi:10.1155/2019/4108271.

76. Leslie MS, Briggs LA. Preeclampsia and the risk of future vascular disease and mortality: a review. *J Midwifery Womens Health.* 2016;61(3):315-324.

77. U.S. Preventive Services Task Force. *Final Recommendation Statement: Low-Dose Aspirin Use for the Prevention of Morbidity and Mortality from Preeclampsia: Preventive Medication.* September 28, 2021. https://www.uspreventiveservicestaskforce.org/uspstf/recommendation/low-dose-aspirin-use-for-the-prevention-of-morbidity-and-mortality-from-preeclampsia-preventive-medication. Accessed October 4, 2021.

78. Bernstein PS, Martin JN Jr, Barton JR, et al. National Partnership for Maternal Safety: consensus bundle on severe hypertension during pregnancy and the postpartum period. *Obstet Gynecol.* 2017;130(2):347-357.

79. Fishel Bartal M, Sibai BM. Eclampsia in the 21st century. *Am J Obstet Gynecol.* 2020;S0002-9378(20)31128-5. doi:10.1016/j.ajog.2020.09.037.

80. Sharma KJ, Kilpatrick SJ. Postpartum hypertension: etiology, diagnosis, and management. *Obstet Gynecol Surv.* 2017;72(4):248-252. doi:10.1097/OGX.0000000000000424.

81. Wallace K, Harris S, Addison A, Bean C. HELLP syndrome: pathophysiology and current therapies. *Curr Pharma Biotechnol.* 2018;19:816-826. doi:10.2174/1389201019666180712115215.

82. Olutayo Alese M, Moodley J, Naicker T. Preeclampsia and HELLP syndrome, the role of the liver. *J Matern Fetal Neonatal Med.* 2021;34(1):117-123.

83. Kamble RC, Gupte N. Maternal and perinatal outcome in patients with HELLP syndrome. *MVP J Med Sci.* 2018:5(2),198-203. https://doi.org/10.18311/mvpjms/2018/v5i2/18721.

84. Mogos MF, Salemi JL, Spooner KK, et al. Hypertensive disorders of pregnancy and postpartum readmission in the United States: national surveillance of the revolving door. *J Hypertension.* 2018;36(3):608-618.

85. Creanga AA, Syverson C, Seed K, et al. Pregnancy related mortality in the United States. 2011–2013. *Obstet Gynecol.* 2017;130(2):366-373.

86. American College of Obstetricians and Gynecologists. ACOG Committee Opinion No. 736: optimizing postpartum care. *Obstet Gynecol.* 2018;131(5):e140-e150.

87. Aziz A, Gyamfi-Bannerman C, Siddiq Z, et al. Maternal outcomes by race during postpartum readmissions. *Am J Obstet Gynecol.* 2019;220(5):484.e1-e10.

88. Pesch MH, Saunders NA, Abdelnabi S. Cytomegalovirus infection in pregnancy: prevention, presentation, management, and neonatal outcomes. *J Midwifery Womens Health.* 2021;66(3):397-402.

89. Dunkerton SE. Brewster J. Infections in pregnancy. *Obstet Gynaecol Reprod Med.* https://doi.org/10.1016/jogrm.2021.09.002.

90. Craig AM, Dotters-Katz S, Kuller JA, Thompson JL. Listeriosis in pregnancy: a review. *Obstet Gynecol Surv.* 2019;74(6):362-368. doi:10.1097/OGX.0000000000000683.

91. Hunter LA, Ayala NK. Parvovirus B19 in pregnancy: a case review. *J Midwifery Womens Health.* 2021;66(3):385-390. doi:10.1111/jmwh.13254.

92. Attwood LO, Holmes NE, Hui L. Identification and management of congenital parvovirus B19 infection. *Prenatal Diagn.* 2020;40(13):1172-1731.

93. Lanzieri T, Haber P, Icenogle JP, Patel M. Chapter 14: rubella. In: Centers for Disease Control and Prevention. *Epidemiology and Prevention of Vaccine-Preventable Diseases.* 14th ed. Hall E, Wodi AP, Hamborsky J, et al, eds. Washington, DC: Public Health Foundation; 2021.

94. Singh C. Rubella in pregnancy. *J Fetal Med.* 2020;7(1):37-41. doi:10.1007/s40556-019-00238-2.

95. Ratha C. Toxoplasmosis in pregnancy. *J Fetal Med.* 2020;7(1):31-35.

96. American College of Obstetricians and Gynecologists. Practice Bulletin No. 151: cytomegalovirus, parvovirus B19, varicella zoster, and toxoplasmosis in pregnancy. *Obstet Gynecol.* 2015;125(6):1510-1525. doi:10.1097/01.AOG.0000466430.19823.53.

97. Lopez A, Harrington T, Marin M. Chapter 22: varicella. In: Centers for Disease Control and Prevention. *Epidemiology and Prevention of Vaccine-Preventable Diseases.* 14th ed. Hall E, Wodi AP, Hamborsky J, et al, eds. Washington, DC: Public Health Foundation; 2021.

98. Negro A, Delaruelle Z, Ivanova TA, et al. Headache and pregnancy: a systematic review. *J Headache Pain.* 2017;18(1):106. doi:10.1186/s10194-017-0816-0.

99. Headache Classification Committee of the International Headache Society. The international classification of headache disorders, 3rd edition. *Cephalalgia.* 2018;38(1):1-211. https://doi.org/10.1177/0333102417738202.

100. Afridi SK. Current concepts in migraine and their relevance to pregnancy. *Obstet Med.* 2018;11(4):154-159. doi:10.1177/1753495X18769170.

101. Elgendy IY, Nadeau S, Merz CNB, Pepine CJ. Migraine headache: an under-appreciated risk factor for cardiovascular disease in women. *J Am Heart Assoc.* 2019;8(22):e014546.

102. Deneris A, Rosati Allen P, Hart Hayes E, Latendresse G. Migraines in women: current evidence for management of episodic and chronic migraines. *J Midwifery Womens Health.* 2017;62(3):270-285.

103. Hussain A, Nduka C, Moth P, Malhotra R. Bell's facial nerve palsy in pregnancy: a clinical review. *J Obstet Gynaecol.* 2017;37(4):409-415. doi.org/10.1080/01443615.2016.1256973.

104. Genova A, Dix O, Saefan A, et al. Carpal tunnel syndrome: a review of literature. *Cureus.* 2020;12(3):e7333. doi:10.7759/cureus.7333.

105. Weimer L. Neuromuscular disorders in pregnancy. *Handb Clin Neurol.* 2020;172:201-218. doi:10.1016/B978-0-444-64240-0.00012-X.

106. Xue X, Chen Y, Mao X, et al. Effect of kinesio taping on low back pain during pregnancy: a systematic review and meta-analysis. *BMC Pregnancy Childbirth.* 2021;21(1):712. doi:10.1186/s12884-021-04197-3.

107. Ahern DP, Gibbons D, Johnson GP, et al. Management of herniated lumbar disk disease and cauda equina syndrome in pregnancy. *Clin Spine Surg.* 2019;32(10):412-416. doi:10.1097/BSD.0000000000000886.

108. Thabah M, Ravindran V. Musculoskeletal problems in pregnancy. *Rheumatol Int.* 2015;35(4):581-587. doi:10.1007/s00296-014-3135-7.

109. Kinser PA, Pauli J, Jallo N, et al. Physical activity and yoga-based approaches for pregnancy-related low back and pelvic pain. *J Obstet Gynecol Neonatal Nurs.* 2017;46(3):334-346. doi:10.1016/j.jogn.2016.12.006.

110. Liu G, Slater N, Perkins A. Epilepsy: treatment options. *Am Fam Physician.* 2017;96(2):87-96.

111. Chen D, Hou L, Duan X, et al. Effect of epilepsy in pregnancy on fetal growth restriction: a systematic review and meta-analysis. *Arch Gynecol Obstet.* 2017;296(3):421-427.

112. Borgelt L, Hart F, Bainbridge J. Epilepsy during pregnancy: focus on management strategies. *Int J Womens Health.* 2016;8:505-517.

113. Veroniki AA, Rios P, Cogo E, et al. Comparative safety of antiepileptic drugs for neurological development in children exposed during pregnancy and breast feeding: a systematic review and network meta-analysis. *BMJ Open.* 2017;7(7):e017248. doi:10.1136/bmjopen-2017-017248.

114. Danielsson KC, Gilhus NE, Borthen I, et al. Maternal complications in pregnancy and childbirth for women with epilepsy: time trends in a nationwide cohort. *PLoS One.* 2019;14(11):e0225334. doi:10.1371/journal.pone.0225334.

115. Driscoll AK, Gregory ECW. Increases in prepregnancy obesity: United States, 2016–2019. NCHS Data Brief, no 392. Hyattsville, MD: National Center for Health Statistics; 2020. https://www.cdc.gov/nchs/data/databriefs/db392-H.pdf. Accessed September 8, 2021.

116. American College of Obstetricians and Gynecologists. ACOG Practice Bulletin No. 230: obesity in pregnancy. *Obstet Gynecol.* 2021;137(6):e128-e144. doi:10.1097/AOG.0000000000004395.

117. Pétursdóttir Maack H, Larsson A, Axelsson O, et al. Pregnancy in metabolic healthy and unhealthy obese women. *Acta Obstet Gynecol Scand.* 2020;99(12):1640-1648. doi:10.1111/aogs.13929.

118. American College of Obstetricians and Gynecologists. Obstetric Care Consensus #9: Levels of maternal care. *Am J Obstet Gynecol.* 2019;221(6):B19-B30. doi:10.1016/j.ajog.2019.05.046.

119. Reither M, Germano E, DeGrazia M. Midwifery management of pregnant women who are obese. *J Midwifery Womens Health.* 2018;63:273-282. https://doi.org/10.1111/jmwh.12760.

120. Ramji N, Challa S, Murphy PA, et al. A comparison of breastfeeding rates by obesity class. *J Matern Fetal Neonatal Med.* 2018;31(22):3021-3026. doi:10.1080/14767058.2017.1362552.

121. Muktabhant B, Lawrie TA, Lumbiganon P, Laopaiboon M. Diet or exercise, or both, for preventing excessive weight gain in pregnancy. *Cochrane Database Syst Rev.* 2015;6:CD007145. doi:10.1002/14651858.CD007145.pub3.

122. Carreau AM, Nadeau M, Marceau S, et al. Pregnancy after bariatric surgery: balancing risks and benefits. *Can J Diab.* 2017;41(4):432-438.

123. Lindsay NS, Ellsworth Bowers ER. Care of pregnant women with a history of bariatric surgery. *Nurs Womens Health.* 2021;25(5):384-394. doi:10.1016/j.nwh.2021.08.003.

124. Adam S, Ammori B, Soran H, Syed AA. Pregnancy after bariatric surgery: screening for gestational diabetes. *BMJ.* 2017;356:j533. doi:10.1136/bmj.j533.

125. Robijn AL, Murphy VE, Gibson PG. Recent developments in asthma in pregnancy. *Curr Opin Pulm Med.* 2019;25(1):11-17. doi:10.1097/MCP.0000000000000538.

126. Murphy VE, Jensen ME, Gibson PG. Asthma during pregnancy: exacerbations, management, and health outcomes for mother and infant. *Semin Respir Crit Care Med.* 2017;38(2):160-173. doi:10.1055/s-0037-1600906.

127. National Asthma Education and Prevention Program. Working group report on managing asthma during pregnancy: recommendations for pharmacologic treatment. https://www.nhlbi.nih.gov/files/docs/astpreg_qr.pdf. Accessed November 4, 2017.

128. Talwar A, Tsang CA, Price SF, et al. Tuberculosis—United States, 2018. *MMWR.* 2019;68:257-262.

129. Miele K, Bamrah Morris S, Tepper NK. Tuberculosis in pregnancy. *Obstet Gynecol.* 2020;135(6):1444-1453. doi:10.1097/AOG.0000000000003890.

130. Sobhy S, Babiker Z, Zamora J, et al. Maternal and perinatal mortality and morbidity associated with tuberculosis during pregnancy and the postpartum period: a systematic review and meta-analysis. *BJOG.* 2017;124(5):727-733. doi:10.1111/1471-0528.14408.

131. Lewinsohn DM, Leonard MK, LoBue PA, et al. Official American Thoracic Society/Infectious Diseases Society of America/Centers for Disease Control and Prevention clinical practice guidelines: diagnosis of tuberculosis in adults and children. *Clin Infect Dis.* 2017;64(2):111-115.

132. Nahid P, Dorman SE, Alipanah N, et al. Official American Thoracic Society/Centers for Disease Control and Prevention/Infectious Diseases Society of America Clinical Practice Guidelines: treatment of drug-susceptible tuberculosis. *Clin Infect Dis.* 2016;63(7):e147-e195. doi:10.1093/cid/ciw376.

133. Rac H, Gould AP, Eiland LS, et al. Common bacterial and viral infections: review of management in the pregnant patient. *Ann Pharmacother.* 2019;53(6): 639-651. doi:10.1177/1060028018817935.

134. Allan GM, Arroll B. Prevention and treatment of the common cold: making sense of the evidence. *CMAJ.* 2014;186(3):190-199. doi:10.1503/cmaj.121442.

135. Afshar Y, Gaw SL, Flaherman VJ, et al. Clinical presentation of coronavirus disease 2019 (COVID-19) in pregnant and recently pregnant people. *Obstet Gynecol.* 2020;136(6):1117-1125. doi:10.1097/AOG.0000000000004178.

136. Metz TD, Clifton RG, Hughes BL, et al. Disease severity and perinatal outcomes of pregnant patients with coronavirus disease 2019 (COVID-19). *Obstet Gynecol.* 2021;137(4):571-580. doi:10.1097/AOG.0000000000004339.

137. American College of Obstetricians and Gynecologists. *COVID-19 FAQs for obstetricians-gynecologists, obstetrics.* Washington, DC: American College of Obstetricians and Gynecologists; 2021. https://www.acog.org/clinical-information/physician-faqs/covid-19-faqs-for-ob-gyns-obstetrics. Accessed February 15, 2022.

138. Rasmussen SA, Kelley CF, Horton JP, Jamieson DJ. Coronavirus disease 2019 (COVID-19) vaccines and pregnancy: what obstetricians need to know. *Obstet Gynecol.* 2021;137(3):408-414. doi:10.1097/AOG.0000000000004290.

139. Gray KJ, Bordt EA, Atyeo C, et al. Coronavirus disease 2019 vaccine response in pregnant and lactating women: a cohort study. *Am J Obstet Gynecol.* 2021;225(3):303.e1-303.e17. doi:10.1016/j.ajog.2021.03.023.

140. American College of Obstetricians and Gynecologists. ACOG Committee Opinion No. 732: influenza vaccination during pregnancy. *Obstet Gynecol.* 2018;131(4):e109-e114. doi:10.1097/AOG.0000000000002588.

141. Luteijn JM, Brown MJ, Dolk H. Influenza and congenital anomalies: a systematic review and meta-analysis. *Hum Reprod.* 2014;29:809-823.

142. Chambers CD, Johnson D, Xu R, Luo Y, Jones KL; OTIS Collaborative Research Group. Oseltamivir use in pregnancy: risk of birth defects, preterm delivery, and small for gestational age infants. *Birth Defects Res.* 2019;111(19):1487-1493. doi:10.1002/bdr2.1566.

143. Mehta N, Chen K, Hardy E, Powrie R. Respiratory disease in pregnancy. *Best Pract Res Clin Obstet Gynaecol.* 2015;29(5):598-611. doi:10.1016/j.bpobgyn.2015.04.005.

144. Tejwani N, Klifto K, Looze C, Klifto CS. Treatment of pregnant patients with orthopaedic trauma. *J Am Acad Orthop Surg.* 2017;25(5):e90-e101. doi:10.5435/JAAOS-D-16-00289.

145. Hardcastle SA, Yahya F, Bhalla AK. Pregnancy-associated osteoporosis: a UK case series and literature review. *Osteoporos Int.* 2019;30(5):939-948. doi:10.1007/s00198-019-04842-w.

146. Finnegan L. *Licit and Illicit Drug Use During Pregnancy: Maternal, Neonatal, and Early Childhood Consequences.* Canadian Centre on Substance Abuse; 2013. https://www.ccsa.ca/sites/default/files/2019-04/CCSA-Drug-Use-during-Pregnancy-Report-2013-en.pdf. Accessed October 6, 2021.

147. Foeller ME, Lyell D. Marijuana use in pregnancy: concerns in an evolving era. *J Midwifery Womens Health.* 2017;62(3): 363-367.

148. Wright TE, Terplan M, Ondersma SJ, et al. The role of screening, brief intervention, and referral to treatment in the perinatal period. *Am J Obstet Gynecol.* 2016;215(5):539-547.

149. Pflugeisen BM, Mou J, Drennan KJ, Straub HL. Demographic discrepancies in prenatal urine drug screening in Washington State surrounding recreational marijuana legalization and accessibility. *Matern Child Health J.* 2020;24(12):1505-1514. doi:10.1007/s10995-020-03010-5.

150. Krans E, Patrick S. Opioid use disorder in pregnancy: health policy and practice in the midst of an epidemic. *Obstet Gynecol.* 2016;128(1):4-10. doi:10.1097/AOG.000000000001446.

151. American College of Obstetricians and Gynecologists. Committee Opinion No. 711: opioid use and opioid use disorder in pregnancy. *Obstet Gynecol.* 2017 (reaffirmed 2021);130(2):e81-e94. doi:10.1097/AOG.0000000000002235.

152. Sutter MB, Watson H, Bauers A, et al. Group prenatal care for women receiving medication-assisted treatment for opioid use disorder in pregnancy:

an interprofessional approach. *J Midwifery Womens Health*. 2019;64(2):217-224. doi:10.1111/jmwh.12960.

153. Gunn JK, Rosales CB, Center KE, et al. Prenatal exposure to cannabis and maternal and child health outcomes: a systematic review and meta-analysis. *BMJ Open*. 2016;6(4):e009986. doi:10.1136/bmjopen-2015-009986.

154. American College of Obstetricians and Gynecologists. Committee Opinion No. 722: marijuana use during pregnancy and lactation. *Obstet Gynecol*. 2017;130(4):e205-e209. doi:10.1097/AOG.0000000000002354.

155. Badowski S, Smith G. Cannabis use during pregnancy and postpartum. *Can Fam Physician*. 2020;66(2):98-103.

156. American College of Obstetricians and Gynecologists. Practice Bulletin No. 148: thyroid disease in pregnancy. *Obstet Gynecol*. 2015 (reaffirmed 2020);125(4):996-1005. doi:10.1097/01.AOG.0000462945.27539.93.

157. Huget-Penner S, Feig DS. Maternal thyroid disease and its effects on the fetus and perinatal outcomes. *Prenatal Diag*. 2020;40:1077-1084.

158. Alexander EK, Pearce EN, Brent GA, et al. 2017 guidelines of the American Thyroid Association for the diagnosis and management of thyroid disease during pregnancy and the postpartum. *Thyroid*. 2017;27(3):315-389.

159. Pearce EN. A comparison of ATA and updated ACOG guidelines for thyroid disease in pregnancy. *Clin Thyroidol*. 2020;32(7):317-320.

160. Kalinderi K, Delkos D, Kalinderis M, et al. Urinary tract infection during pregnancy: current concepts on a common multifaceted problem. *J Obstet Gynaecol*. 2018;38(4):448-453. doi:10.1080/01443615.2017.1370579.

161. Glaser AP, Schaeffer AJ. Urinary tract infection and bacteriuria in pregnancy. *Urol Clin North Am*. 2015;42(4):547-560. doi:10.1016/j.ucl.2015.05.004.

162. White J, Ory J, Lantz Powers AG, et al. Urological issues in pregnancy: a review for urologists. *Can Urol Assoc J*. 2020;14(10):352-357. doi:10.5489/cuaj.6526.

163. American College of Obstetricians and Gynecologists. ACOG Committee Opinion No. 797: prevention of group B streptococcal early-onset disease in newborns. *Obstet Gynecol*. 2020;135(2):e51-e72. doi:10.1097/AOG.0000000000003668.

164. Ordon M, Dirk J, Slater J, et al. Incidence, treatment, and implications of kidney stones during pregnancy: a matched population-based cohort study. *J Endourol*. 2020;34(2):215-221. doi:10.1089/end.2019.0557.

165. Assimos D, Krambeck A, Miller NL, et al. Surgical management of stones: American Urological Association/Endourological Society Guideline, part I. *J Urol*. 2016;196(4):1153-1160. doi:10.1016/j.juro.2016.05.090.

V

PART

# Intrapartum

**Section Editors**

TEKOA KING

NICOLE CARLSON

CHAPTER

# 25

# Anatomy and Physiology of Labor and Birth

TEKOA L. KING AND ANDREA ZENGION

## Introduction

Heath care that supports the pregnant person during labor and birth requires an understanding of the physiology that underlies this unique event. The anatomy and physiology of the utero-ovarian reproductive system and the changes the body undergoes during pregnancy are described in the *Anatomy and Physiology of the Reproductive System* and *Anatomy and Physiology of Pregnancy* chapters, respectively. This chapter addresses the anatomic and physiologic changes that occur during parturition (i.e., labor and birth) in the pregnant person and the fetus. Particular emphasis is placed on the theories that describe the physiology that changes the uterus from quiescent to actively contracting. A review of maternal physiology during labor and the anatomic relationships between the fetus and the parental pelvis during the process of birth follows.

Traditionally, the processes involved in labor and birth have been conceptualized as affecting three "Ps": the power (uterus), the passenger (fetus), and the passage (pelvis). A fourth "P"—the psyche—is often included in this rubric and will not be addressed in this chapter. However, many complex physiologic processes occur during labor and birth that are often best supported without intervention or via addressing the holistic needs of the laboring person.[1,2] During spontaneous uncomplicated labor and birth, interventions that are common supportive techniques used in medical care (i.e., routine use of intravenous fluids) may potentially disrupt the complex hormonal regulation governing the process.[3–5] Thus, an understanding of the physiology of labor and birth and the ways in which it can be influenced or disrupted is a critical basis for midwifery practice.

The onset of labor is traditionally defined as the occurrence of regular painful contractions that dilate the cervix. Contractions that occur at regular intervals with increasing frequency, duration, and intensity, and that lead to cervical change, are a classic sign of labor.[6,7] Labor is often initiated over a period of several days as multiple interrelated physiologic changes occur in the uterus, decidua, and cervix.

The mechanism underlying onset of labor has not been definitively determined. Many variables, both internal and external, influence this timing. Genetic factors, the health and hormonal status of the pregnant person, placental metabolism, and fetal hormones all play a major role.[2] In addition, environmental influences, stress, and healthcare interventions can affect the onset of labor. Systemic and structural determinants of health are increasingly being recognized as playing roles as well. For example, in the United States, there is marked disparity in the rates of preterm birth for Black, Hispanic, and white persons. While some studies have sought to establish an inherent physiologic cause for this disparity, recent evidence suggests chronic stress and structural inequities can have a biologic effect that increases the risk for and incidence of adverse pregnancy outcomes including preterm birth.[8–11]

Extensive research, including laboratory, animal, epidemiologic, and clinical studies, has identified many of the factors that are associated with the onset of labor.[7,12–14] However, this physiologic transition is complex, and is subject to multiple physiologic cascades that operate in concert with one another. Thus, no specific or individual trigger that initiates the transition from pregnancy to labor has been identified.

## Prelabor Changes: Cervical Remodeling and Uterine Activity

Prior to the onset of progressive labor, cervical remodeling, cervical dilation, and uterine contractions begin to occur. During this period, the fetal presenting part (usually the fetal head) may engage in the pelvis, which is often noted by the pregnant person as increased pressure on the bladder or lower abdomen, with a concomitant decrease in shortness of breath. As the cervix changes in preparation for labor, the pregnant person may also note an increase in cervical discharge, passage of the cervical mucus plug, and/or slight vaginal spotting.

### Cervical Remodeling

Over the full course of pregnancy, labor, birth, and postpartum, the cervix undergoes four phases of remodeling, which are referred to as softening, ripening, dilation, and repair.[15] The cervix gradually softens over the course of pregnancy. The ripening stage occurs just prior to labor and/or during the first hours of labor. During this process, the cervix changes from being relatively firm and measuring approximately 3 to 4 centimeters in length, to being much softer and shorter. The process of thinning, referred to as cervical *effacement*, can be measured when the cervix is palpated clinically. Cervical effacement is evaluated in terms of the cervical length in centimeters or by reporting a percentage of the original length, where no effacement is described as 0% and complete effacement is described as 100%.

The primary physiologic change that occurs during cervical ripening is an increase in hydrophilic noncollagenous proteins, which cause the collagen in the cervix to become soluble and disorganized.[15,16] The process of reducing collagen structure and integrity is furthered by an inflammatory process. Macrophages infiltrate the cervix and generate chemicals and hormones such as pro-inflammatory cytokines and prostaglandins, which also weaken the cervical connective tissue.[17,18] Cervical effacement in a term gestation is likely due to a sterile inflammatory process, while preterm cervical changes are more likely due to pathologic inflammation secondary to infection.[18]

*Dilation* is the opening and widening of the cervical os. During labor, the os expands from an opening that is a few millimeters to being wide enough to allow passage of the fetus during birth. Some cervical dilation may occur prior to labor along with effacement; alternatively, dilation may start after the cervix is significantly effaced (softened and shortened). In nulliparous individuals, effacement typically precedes dilation. In contrast, in parous individuals, some effacement and dilation has taken place prior to the onset of labor, and these two cervical changes continue to occur in tandem as labor progresses. In a multiparous person, some cervical effacement and dilation may be noted days or weeks prior to the onset of labor. Cervical dilation or effacement in the absence of contractions is not a reliable indicator that labor is imminent.

Dilation occurs secondary to the force of uterine contractions, coupled with the hydrostatic action of the amniotic sac and fetal presenting part on the cervix. Dilation is clinically evaluated by measuring the diameter of the cervical opening in centimeters, with 0 centimeters describing a closed external cervical os and 10 centimeters defining complete dilation. Complete dilation is described as 10 centimeters because this degree of cervical dilation is sufficient to accommodate the flexed fetal head.

### Prelabor Uterine Contractions

Uterine contractions may begin to occur irregularly and increase in frequency in the days preceding labor. Historically referred to as Braxton-Hicks contractions, this phenomenon is today known as "prelabor" or "prodromal labor." These contractions do not occur in a regular pattern, nor do they cause the progressive cervical dilation and effacement seen during labor. This prelabor uterine activity likely reflects changes within the uterine musculature that occur with advancing gestation and preparation for labor.

## Clinical Stages of Labor

Labor and birth are divided clinically into four stages.

- The *first stage of labor* includes two to three phases. The *latent phase* is the initial period wherein contractions become regular, more painful, and more frequent but cervical dilation occurs at a slower and highly variable rate. In the *active phase* of labor, the cervix dilates over a period of hours to complete dilation (i.e., 10 centimeters). Historically, it was believed that the active phase of labor includes a *transition phase* in which the cervix dilates rapidly from 8 to 10 centimeters. Contemporary studies of labor progress have not demonstrated that this late transition phase of more rapid dilation occurs consistently in all laboring persons.[19]

- The *second stage of labor* refers to the time from complete cervical dilation to birth of the newborn. During the second stage of labor, the laboring person often actively pushes in concert with uterine contractions. When regional analgesia has not been administered to the individual, the urge to push or bear down is involuntary and thought to occur secondary to pressure of the fetal head on the vaginal floor and rectum.

- The *third stage of labor* is defined as the time between birth of the newborn and placental expulsion.
- The *fourth stage of labor* is the first hour after birth. This stage is not always described in textbooks but is clinically important because it is the time during which the postpartum person is at highest risk for postpartum hemorrhage. This period is discussed in more detail in the *Anatomy and Physiology of Postpartum* chapter.

Significant interindividual variability exists in the normal progress of spontaneous labor.[19,20] Nonetheless, defining standard parameters or average durations for these stages is clinically valuable because sufficient deviance from the anticipated norm is an indication of labor dysfunction. The typical durations and clinical management of each stage of labor are reviewed in the *First Stage of Labor*, *Second Stage of Labor and Birth*, and *Third Stage of Labor* chapters.

## Physiologic Mechanisms That Influence the Onset of Labor

Most of the knowledge of the physiology underlying the onset of labor is based on animal studies, which are not easily translatable to human biology. Although highly informative, some steps in these processes must be acknowledged as theories when applied to human birth. Two initial theories, the progesterone withdrawal theory and the placental–fetal–decidual clock theory, provide partial insights into potential physiologic cascades in the pregnant individual, placenta, and fetus. More recent research on the role of inflammation appears closer to providing an overarching understanding.[21] The primary hormones involved in the mechanisms that initiate and propagate physiologic labor are summarized in Table 25-1.

### Functional Progesterone Withdrawal Theory

In most mammals, labor begins when progesterone levels fall.[22] In humans, however, circulating progesterone levels do not fall; rather, progesterone's actions in the maternal myometrium change prior to the onset of labor.[23–25] Progesterone is synthesized in the placenta. The uterus has several forms of progesterone receptors that initiate different cellular functions. During pregnancy, progesterone primarily binds to progesterone receptor B (PR-B), which causes suppression of the formation of contractile proteins and inhibits upregulation of the prostaglandin and oxytocin receptors that initiate myometrial contractions.[26] During the onset of labor, the myometrium expresses more progesterone receptor A (PR-A) than PR-B. When progesterone binds to PR-A, the result is promotion of the pro-inflammatory effects associated with labor.[27] The increased concentration of PR-A relative to PR-B results in a *functional progesterone withdrawal* without alteration of the circulating progesterone concentrations.[23–25]

### Proposed Roles of the Placenta and Fetus in Labor Initiation

The placenta and fetus help initiate labor in several ways.[7,22,26] Placental production of corticotropin-releasing hormone (CRH) increases over the course of pregnancy and peaks at the time of birth, which has led many researchers to consider a "placental clock" as the inciting mechanism for labor.[7,26] CRH is intimately involved in the positive feedback cascading physiologic mechanisms that initiate and propagate labor. As occurs with progesterone, as the body prepares for labor, the type of CRH receptors present in the uterine myometrium shifts from those that suppress uterine contraction to those that promote contractile activity.[7,22,27,28] The placenta also decreases production of the proteins that bind to CRH in the circulation, thereby making CRH more biologically available to cells, which further potentiates the effects of CRH.[29] This hormone also enhances the uterine response to oxytocin and prostaglandins and promotes a pro-inflammatory response. In addition, placentally produced CRH induces maturation of the fetal hypothalamic–pituitary–adrenal (HPA) axis and has direct effects on the fetal adrenal gland; this is the mechanism by which the fetus is involved in initiation of labor.

In response to placental CRH, the fetal HPA axis stimulates the fetal adrenal gland to synthesize and excrete the chemical precursor the placenta must have to synthesize estrogen. The resultant placental synthesis of estrogen increases such that more estrogen than progesterone is available. Estrogen then initiates multiple changes in the uterine myometrium that facilitate myometrial contraction.[7]

| Table 25-1 | Major Hormones and Functions During Labor | |
|---|---|---|
| **Hormone** | **Source** | **Function During Labor** |
| Corticotropin-releasing hormone | Placenta and fetus | Facilitates maturation of the fetal hypothalamic–pituitary–adrenal axis, which in turn initiates production of cortisol and estrogen precursors from the fetal adrenal gland<br>Induces production of cytokines and other factors that are pro-inflammatory<br>Enhances the uterine response to oxytocin and prostaglandins |
| Estrogen | Fetus, decidua, fetal membranes, placenta | Estrogen does not induce contractions but does cause myometrial cells to become contractile and promotes cellular changes that support coordination of contractions across cells:<br>• Increases expression of oxytocin receptors and prostaglandin receptors on myometrial cells<br>• Promotes synthesis of intracellular enzymes needed in the myometrial contraction sequence<br>• Induces formation of gap junctions<br>• Stimulates local production of oxytocin by the decidua and fetal membranes |
| Oxytocin | Hypothalamus, fetus, fetal membranes, placenta | Upregulates production of prostaglandins<br>When bound to the oxytocin receptors on myometrial cell membranes, induces myometrial contractions by releasing intracellular sequestered calcium |
| Prostaglandins | Fetal membranes | Paracrine and autocrine agents that act locally near their site of production to:<br>• Promote cervical ripening<br>• Increase myometrial sensitivity to oxytocin<br>• Promote formation of gap junctions |

The fetal adrenal gland also produces cortisol, which has multiple critical functions. Cortisol stimulates the placenta to produce more CRH, resulting in the positive feedback mechanism that advances the transition to labor. In addition, cortisol facilitates maturation of the fetal lungs and upregulates catecholamine (epinephrine and norepinephrine) receptors in the fetal lung and heart. Many of the fetal effects of this prelabor cortisol surge support the physiologic maturation the fetus needs to adapt to labor and birth.[3]

## Potential Role of Inflammation in Labor Initiation

Labor is characterized by a heightened state of inflammation. Indeed, multiple inflammatory processes that trigger labor begin days or weeks prior to the onset of labor.[21] Markers of the inflammatory mechanisms involved in the shift from quiescence to labor have been detected in groups of people who experienced either term or preterm labor, and this shift appears to occur approximately 2 to 4 weeks prior to birth.[30]

It has long been known that mechanical stretch of the uterus plays a role in initiation of labor. As the uterus becomes increasingly distended, the mechanical distension causes an inflammatory response within the myometrial cells.[29] Increased myometrial distension also triggers upregulation of oxytocin receptors that induce myometrial contraction.[12] This effect of uterine distension may partially explain why persons pregnant with more than one fetus simultaneously usually experience labor earlier than persons pregnant with a singleton fetus.

Thus, prior to the onset of labor and then extensively during labor, leukocytes invade the myometrium, cervix, chorio-decidua, and amnion.[31,32] Neutrophils release enzymes that further degrade extracellular matrix proteins, including fetal fibronectin and collagen, to allow for progressive cervical effacement and dilation. Inflammatory cytokines and the amount of degrading matrix metalloproteinase enzymes are likewise increased in the fetal membranes, which contributes to weakening and eventual rupture of the membranes.

Pro-inflammatory cytokines released by activated leukocytes promote calcium entry into uterine smooth muscle cells and increased prostaglandin production, enhancing uterine contractions.

In addition, as the gestation reaches term, cellular aging and apoptosis occur in cells within the placenta, decidua, fetal membranes, and fetus. Some products of this cellular senescence also cause an inflammatory response that is believed to play a major role in initiating labor.[21] Among the known triggers for the inflammatory process caused by cellular apoptosis are cell-free fetal DNA and damage-associated molecular pattern (DAMP) markers.[12] DAMPs are molecules from damaged cells that elicit an immune response and are released in higher quantities as cells age.[29] These inflammatory processes are instrumental in progressive cervical effacement, production of oxytocin receptors in the uterus, and rupture of membranes.[12]

The inflammatory process involved in physiologic, term, spontaneous onset of labor does not occur secondary to infection, yet this natural inflammatory process generates cytokines and other chemicals in a manner similar to the inflammatory process that results from infection. With infection-associated labor onset, such as occurs in many cases of preterm labor, microorganisms produce molecules called pathogen-associated molecular patterns (PAMPs). Similar to DAMPs, PAMPs trigger the inflammatory events associated with labor onset.[33,34]

The inflammation theory may also explain the positive associations identified between environment, stress, and preterm birth. Chronic stress is associated with adverse short- and long-term health outcomes. To date, several molecular mechanisms by which stress leads to increased inflammation have been identified.[35,36] Epidemiologic studies show that communities exposed to severe or chronic stress such as that caused by structural and interpersonal racism have higher rates of preterm birth, as well as perinatal mortality and morbidity.[10,11] Initial understanding of the experiences of persons at risk for preterm birth and examination of structural inequities experienced by these individuals is foundational for developing clinical interventions that may interrupt the biologic effects of environmental stresses.[2,37,38]

### Genetic Influences

Genetics may play a role in the inflammatory response.[35,39] An increased risk for preterm birth has been observed among persons who were born preterm, suggesting a genetic predisposition to preterm labor.[35] It is important to remember, however, that hundreds of genes are newly expressed or up-regulated in the placenta, cervix, uterus, and fetal membranes as labor starts. Although research in this area is just beginning, genome-wide association studies have identified genetic loci associated with preterm birth in both the maternal and fetal genomes.[40,41] The genes identified may be related to different pathways that facilitate accelerated cell aging, which in turn may be induced by environmental influences.[35,41,42]

## The Four Phases of Parturition

The overall process of parturition proceeds through four phases (Figure 25-1).[6,43,44]

- *Phase 0: Quiescence.* Period in late pregnancy of uterine quiescence. Inhibitors of uterine

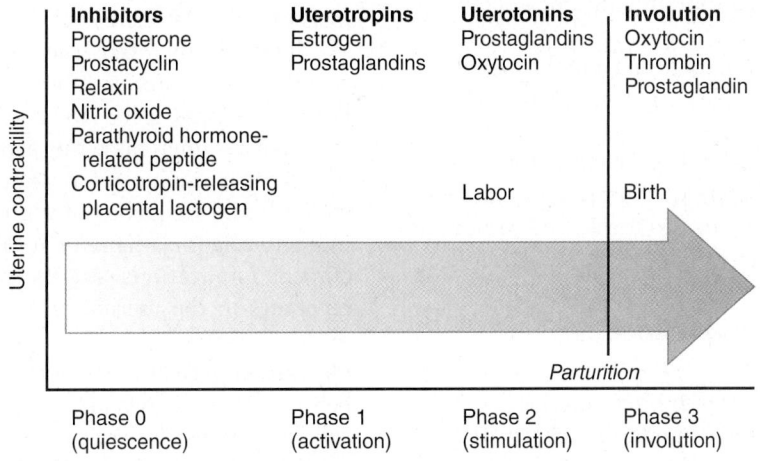

**Figure 25-1** Phases of parturition.

contractions include progesterone, prostacyclin, relaxin, nitric oxide, and other hormones.

- *Phase 1: Activation.* Hormones that prepare the uterus to contract (uterotropins; e.g., estrogen) stimulate upregulation of myometrial receptors for oxytocin and prostaglandins, and activation of gap junctions between myometrial cells.
- *Phase 2: Stimulation.* Hormones that cause uterine contractions (uterotonins; e.g., oxytocin and prostaglandins) promote labor progression.
- *Phase 3: Involution.* Uterine involution after birth is mediated by oxytocin and possibly thrombin.

### Phase 0: Inhibition

Prior to the onset of labor, the uterine myometrium is minimally contractile and essentially quiescent. Progesterone is a potent inhibitor of uterine muscle contraction. Other hormones such as nitric oxide and relaxin increase intracellular concentrations of substances (cyclic adenosine monophosphate [cAMP] and cyclic guanosine monophosphate [cGMP]) that inhibit the intracellular release of calcium, which is essential for myometrial contraction.[28] During this period, the form of progesterone receptor that predominates in the uterus changes, and initial inflammatory processes begin to develop.[7,24]

### Phase 1: Activation

Under the influence of estrogen and the effects of inflammatory cascades,[21] uterine myometrial cells express receptors for prostaglandins and oxytocin and develop gap junctions between myometrial cells that allow direct communication between muscle fibers. *Gap junctions* are transmembrane proteins that create a pore used for communication between two adjacent myocytes. The action potentials that initiate contraction activity propagate through these gap junctions, which results in synchronous uterine contractions characterized by generation of force along a short distance at low velocity. Prostaglandins also facilitate uterine contractions, increase myometrial sensitivity to oxytocin, and stimulate formation of gap junctions.[45]

### Phase 2: Stimulation of Uterine Myometrial Activity

The onset of regular, progressive uterine contractions characterizes the stimulation phase of parturition. During this phase, prostaglandins, in conjunction with oxytocin, increasingly influence myometrial activity. Prostaglandins are produced by the amnion, chorion, and decidua, in part due to upregulation of COX-2 enzymes; they work in a paracrine fashion, affecting nearby tissues to promote uterine contractile activity.[26] Prostaglandin production is also stimulated by inflammatory cytokines and the presence of oxytocin.

### Role of Oxytocin

Oxytocin, a potent uterotonic, is a small, nine-amino acid peptide. The word *oxytocin* is derived from the Greek *oxys*, which means "quick," and *tokos*, which means "birth." Many organs have oxytocin receptors, including the uterus, breast, kidney, and brain. Although oxytocin is not a major player in initiating labor, it has a prominent role in propagating active labor, during birth, and in uterine contraction in the immediate postpartum period.

Oxytocin is produced in the hypothalamus and secreted via the posterior pituitary, in a pulsatile fashion, reaching peak levels during fetal expulsion.[14,45] This hormone is also produced locally by the decidua and fetal membranes.[14] During spontaneous labor, oxytocin pulses occur approximately 4 times per 30 minutes in the first stage of labor and 7 times per 30 minutes in the second stage. The biologic half-life of this molecule is approximately 3 to 4 minutes. Binding of oxytocin to myometrial oxytocin receptors stimulates the smooth muscle contractions that characterize active labor through a calcium-dependent pathway. The interaction between prostaglandins produced in the uterine decidua and oxytocin is an example of the positive feedback mechanisms inherent in labor initiation. Prostaglandins cause an upregulation of oxytocin receptors. Once bound to those receptors, oxytocin promotes production of more prostaglandins, thereby perpetuating the process by which the effects of oxytocin increase.[45,46]

Interestingly, plasma levels of oxytocin do not correlate with uterine contractility or cervical dilation. Changes in oxytocin receptor number and sensitivity, rather than the production and release of oxytocin itself, are the primary influence on the strength and frequency of uterine contractions during active labor.[47] This relationship has important clinical implications. As the number of oxytocin receptors in the uterine fundus increases,[48] the effects of oxytocin are maximized even without an increase in plasma levels of this hormone. The number of oxytocin receptors present on myometrial cell membranes peaks in early labor, reaching as much as 200 times the number of such receptors present prior to the onset of labor.[14] Plasma levels of oxytocin increase and peak in the second stage of labor, possibly enhanced by fetal oxytocin synthesis.[49] Labor and mechanical stretch also increase expression of oxytocin receptors in the uterine myocytes, further enhancing the potential for oxytocin-receptor binding.[46,50]

The oxytocin receptors can, however, become desensitized to oxytocin owing to increased concentrations of oxytocin in the pregnant person's circulation. This can occur as the result of increasing plasma levels of oxytocin or prolonged exposure to oxytocin administered exogenously for induction or augmentation of labor.[51] Prolonged or repeated stimulation of the oxytocin receptors then contributes to downregulation, which reduces the number of receptors available for oxytocin binding. Uterine contractions become less forceful and less frequent because of attenuation of cell signaling and reduced calcium release, potentially leading to impaired labor progress or uterine atony after birth. Thus, elevated risk for postpartum hemorrhage when labor has been prolonged or exogenous oxytocin administered over an extended period may be partially related to oxytocin-receptor desensitization.[52,53]

Oxytocin has obvious and important effects on the uterus. However, the body has receptors for oxytocin in many tissues, and the functions of oxytocin are the subject of current animal research that may inform our understanding of human processes. Oxytocin does not cross the blood–brain barrier well, so the central nervous system's effects of this hormone are caused by oxytocin released from the hypothalamus directly into the adjacent tissues of the brain. In the brain, oxytocin acts as a neuromodulator—it organizes and orchestrates the effects of other hormones. It promotes release of beta-endorphins, whose plasma levels markedly increase during labor, and which may mitigate the effects of pain and stress during labor.[2] It is also postulated that oxytocin plays a critical role in supporting social adaptive behavior, reducing physiologic stress responses, and preparing for parental–infant bonding.[2]

## Mechanism of Uterine Contractions

Located between the decidua and the perimetrium of the uterus, the myometrium consists of four muscle layers, each of which produces a distinct response to substances that promote or inhibit contractions. The inner circular muscle layer runs perpendicular to the long axis of the uterus in a spiral fashion, while the two outer layers run parallel to this axis. In the middle layer, blood vessels pass throughout the interlacing fibers that are located perpendicular to the muscle fibers.[54] The smooth muscle (myometrium) in the uterus is anatomically different from other types of smooth muscle, in that the myometrium fibers have no pacemaker or motor nerve innervation.[7] The uterine myocytes are organized in bundles that generate tension and a shortening of the fibers under local stimulation by uterotonic hormones.

The uterine muscle is thickest in the fundus, which demonstrates the greatest contractile strength. The fundal portion of the uterus becomes the primary contracting portion of the uterus when labor begins (**Figure 25-2**).[55] At the end of pregnancy and

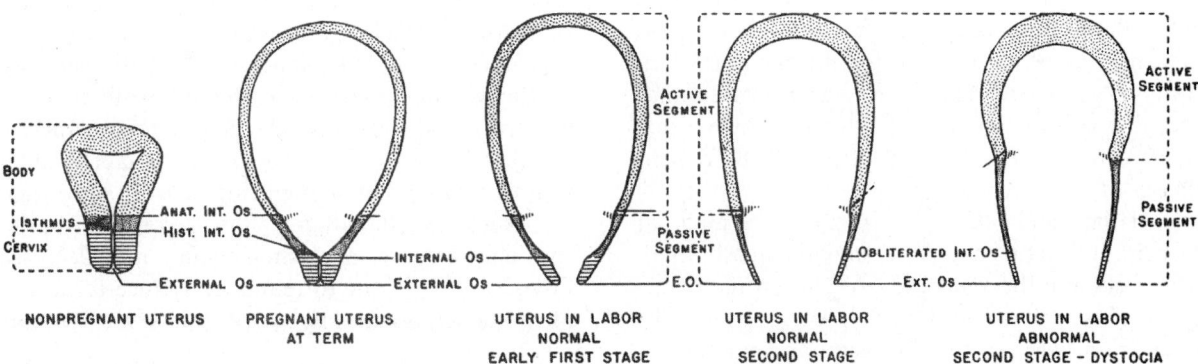

**Figure 25-2** Sequence of development of the segments and rings in the uterus in pregnant people at term and in labor. Note the comparison between the uterus of a nonpregnant person, the uterus at term, and the uterus during labor. The passive lower segment of the uterine body is derived from the isthmus; the physiologic retraction ring develops at the junction of the upper and lower uterine segments. The pathologic retraction ring develops from the physiologic ring.

Abbreviations: Anat. Int. Os = anatomic internal os; E.O. = external os; Hist. Int. Os = histologic internal os.

Reproduced with permission from Cunningham F, Leveno KJ, Bloom SL, et al. Physiology of labor. In: Cunningham F, Leveno KJ, Bloom SL, et al., eds. *Williams Obstetrics*. 25th ed. New York, NY: McGraw-Hill; 2018:408-432.

during labor, the uterine muscle becomes thinner toward the lower uterine segment in the isthmus; this thinner lower uterine segment forms the tube through which the fetus passes. The muscle bundles in the uterine fundus progressively shorten with each contraction, causing the upper portion of the uterus to thicken and gradually become a smaller cavity. This reduced fundal capacity, in turn, promotes descent of the fetus toward the more passive lower uterine segment.

The lower uterine segment muscle bundles become longer in response to contractions in the fundus, creating a distensible structure that is able to accommodate the fetus—a process that promotes fetal descent. The line of demarcation between the active and passive segments is termed the *physiologic retraction ring*. When labor is obstructed, the active segment becomes so much thicker and shorter that the midwife can sometimes see the line between the two uterine segments when observing the abdomen—the so-called *pathologic retraction ring* or *Bandl's ring*.

The propagation of the contraction wave is often called the *triple descending gradient* of fundal dominance, wherein contractions (1) start in the fundus, (2) last longer in the fundus, and (3) progress from the fundus toward the isthmus. This contraction pattern, which is termed *fundal dominance*, appears to be important for effective cervical dilation and progress of labor, though studies offer contradictory evidence regarding the degree to which fundal dominance is important in propagation of the muscle contraction.[56]

Uterine smooth muscle contractions are intermittent, which allows for reperfusion of the uterine muscle and intervillous space between contractions. Each contraction builds in intensity, reaches a peak, and then decreases in intensity until the muscle returns to a state of relaxation, which persists until the next contraction begins. This pattern is often referred to as the increment, acme, and decrement phases of contraction.

At the cellular level, contractile units made of myosin and actin in uterine smooth muscle myocytes promote the generation of tension that leads to synchronous smooth muscle contraction. The interaction between the thin actin and thick myosin filaments is central to the generation of force (**Figure 25-3**).[57] Myosin is arranged in two heavy chains and two light chains, with a globular head attached to a tail that protrudes from the heavy chains at regular intervals. The myosin head also contains a site that binds to actin, which generates the force that is carried along the myosin tails.

Entry of calcium into the myocyte, which occurs in response to specific stimuli such as oxytocin binding and stimulation of gap junctions, prompts intracellular release of calcium from a reservoir in the sarcoplasmic reticulum. Calcium binds to the smooth muscle protein calmodulin, which activates an enzyme called myosin light-chain kinase. In turn, myosin light-chain kinase chemically changes the light chain on the myosin head, allowing a structural link to be established between actin and myosin. Energy is released from the myosin head and the structural cross-bridge shortens the muscle. At this point, the myosin head rotates and pulls on actin, which generates force and shortening. Decreased intracellular calcium concentrations and the action of additional enzyme action reverses the actin–myosin linkages through removal of a phosphate from the myosin light chain, thereby inducing muscle relaxation. The action potentials that pass through gap junctions between myocytes facilitate contraction of adjacent uterine smooth muscle bundles, resulting in a coordinated wave of uterine contraction.

## Systemic Adaptations of the Pregnant Person in Labor

Many of the physiologic adaptations that occur during pregnancy also act as preparation and support for the intrapartum period. Further adaptations occur during labor to support both the pregnant person and the fetus's physiologic needs.

### Cardiovascular System

The pregnant person's blood volume expands by 40% to 50% over the course of pregnancy. Simultaneously, vasodilation in addition to reduction in vascular tone and resistance increase the capacity of the vascular system to accommodate this expanded blood volume.[58] Oxygen-carrying capacity is supplemented by increases in red blood cell (RBC) production, thereby maximizing delivery of oxygen to tissues in both the pregnant person and the fetus. The increase in plasma volume and decrease in viscosity combine to reduce resistance to flow, a phenomenon further supported by lowered vascular resistance.

During labor and birth, additional marked and rapid cardiovascular adaptations occur secondary to uterine contractions, pain, exertion, loss of the placental compartment at birth, and uterine involution.[59] Cardiac output increases by an additional 10% to 15% in first-stage labor and by as much as 50% in second-stage labor, due primarily to

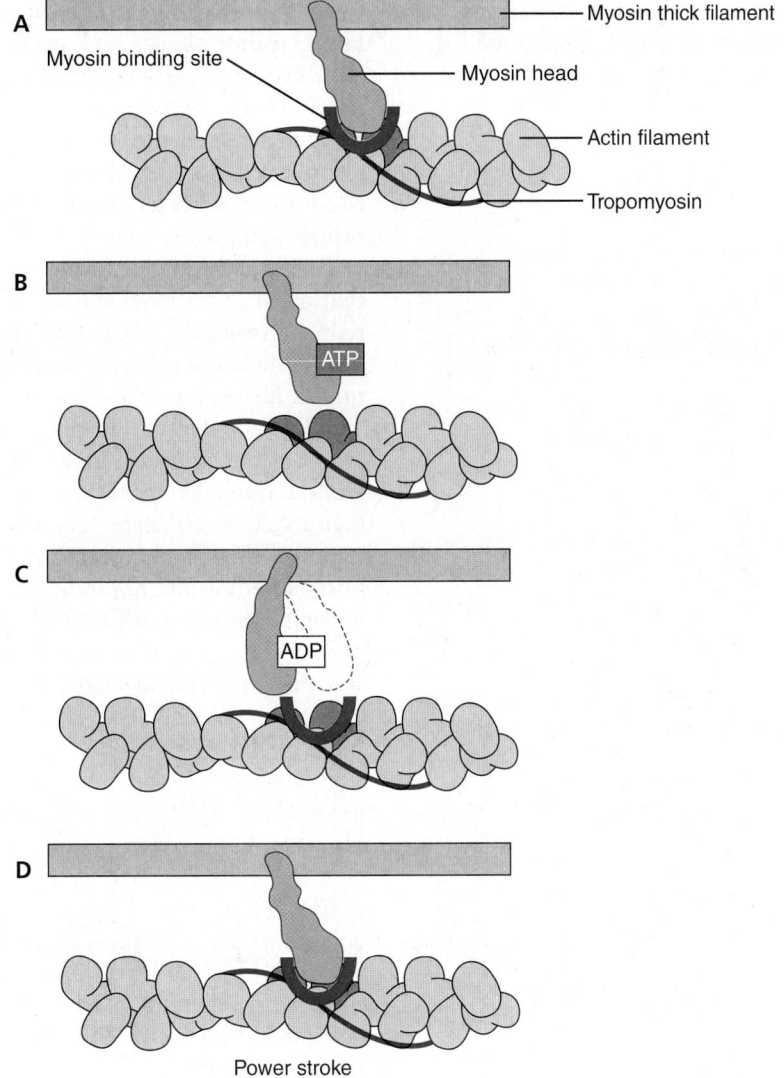

**Figure 25-3** Uterine muscle contraction. **A.** Attached: At the start of the cycle, the myosin head is attached to the myosin binding site on the actin filament. **B.** Recharging: A molecule of ATP binds to a large cleft at the back of the myosin head, which causes a slight change in the conformation of the myosin binding site. This change reduces the affinity the myosin head has for the myosin binding site. **C.** Cocked: The cleft on the myosin head closes around the ATP, which causes a large shape change so that the head is displaced along the actin filament by a distance of approximately 5 nm. **D.** Force-generating: As ATP is hydrolyzed to ADP, the myosin head once again binds tightly to the next myosin binding site on the actin filament. In this process, the myosin head essentially ratchets along the actin filament, creating the muscle contraction.

Abbreviations: ADP, adenosine diphosphate; ATP, adenosine triphosphate.

Reproduced from Lowe NK, Openshaw M, King TL. Labor. In: Brucker MC, King TL, eds. *Pharmacology for Women's Health*. 2nd ed. Burlington, MA: Jones & Bartlett Learning; 2017:1065-1094.

increased stroke volume.[58,60] Cardiac output can also be affected by the laboring person's sensations of pain, anxiety, and any analgesics used. The laboring person's systolic and diastolic blood pressures both rise during uterine contractions, returning to baseline between contractions,[58,59] and may rise in response to pain. Heart rate may either increase or decrease; generally, it rises during contractions and decreases between them, but other variations in heart rate may be observed in response to pain or other factors.

### Blood Flow in the Uterus During Labor

At a term gestation, approximately 500 to 900 mL of the pregnant person's blood flows through the uterine muscle layers into the intervillous space in the placenta each minute.[61,62] An inverse relationship exists between myometrial contractions and placental blood flow. The arteries that supply blood to the uterus and placenta run perpendicular through the uterine muscle, so the arteries become constricted during uterine contractions. Restoration of muscle resting tone between contractions then reestablishes perfusion and refreshes the pool of blood that flows into in the intervillous space from the uterus. Approximately 300 to 500 mL of blood flows back into the maternal venous system from the uterus and intervillous space on the maternal side of the placenta following each uterine contraction.[58]

Circulation is also affected by the posture and position of the pregnant person's body. Supine hypotension secondary to uterine pressure on the inferior vena cava may occur during labor, which is why lateral positions are recommended to ameliorate variant fetal heart rate patterns. Nonetheless, it is not known if asymptomatic supine hypotension has any significant effect on fetal oxygenation. During the second stage of labor, pushing efforts cause an increase in central venous pressure. These shifts in blood pressure can overtax cardiac function in individuals who have significant cardiac disease or structural cardiac abnormalities.[63] In the third stage of labor, the uterus contracts and rapidly reduces its size, which causes a rapid redistribution of a sudden volume of blood into the systemic circulation. This additional circulating blood volume results in an increased central venous pressure, preload, and cardiac output. Because the uteroplacental unit receives such a large proportion of the cardiac output, inadequate uterine contraction and hemostasis at the placental site after placental separation can lead to massive postpartum hemorrhage.

Collectively, the remarkable shifts in blood volume, cardiac output, and systemic venous return during labor and birth can be hazardous for people who have preexisting cardiac disorders. Pregnancy and the intrapartum period can also reveal previously occult cardiovascular disease.

### Hematologic Indices During Labor and Birth

Changes in coagulation factors that initially occur during pregnancy are enhanced during labor, thereby promoting rapid hemostasis after placental separation. Levels of coagulation factors—most notably factor VIII—are markedly increased during labor. Tissue factor release from the placenta and decidua activates the extrinsic coagulation pathway, promoting clot development. The procoagulant condition reaches its maximum after placental separation, with increases in factor V levels, platelet activation, and fibrin clot formation. Clot development that occurs after placental separation contributes to reduced levels of circulating fibrinogen and platelets, as these components are utilized in the production of fibrin clots.

A slight degree of leukocytosis occurs gradually over the course of pregnancy. During labor, the white blood cell (WBC) count peaks and can be as high as $20 \times 10^3/mm^3$. The etiology of this rise in the number of leukocytes is not known, but it is a normal finding and not indicative of infection. Thus, normal ranges for WBC count vary between pregnant and nonpregnant people, and mild leukocytosis cannot reliably identify infection during labor.

## Respiratory System

The pregnant person has a higher requirement for oxygen during labor as well as a reduced total lung capacity. The need for additional oxygen to support the fetus is generally met by normal adaptations during pregnancy, including reduced residual volume and functional residual capacity, as well as increased tidal volume.[64] However, increased muscular work, metabolic rate, and oxygen consumption can be major challenges to the laboring person's respiratory system.

Oxygen consumption increases with the laboring person's muscular activity during uterine contractions. Inter-contraction periods of relaxation allow for reperfusion and restoration of oxygen content to the uterine myometrium. Failure to restore oxygenation to uterine muscle cells over time results in anaerobic metabolism, production of lactic acid, and subsequent ischemic pain that is theorized to contribute to the uterine pain felt during labor.

Pain can also lead to an increased respiratory rate and hyperventilation in the laboring person, promoting respiratory alkalosis. During pushing efforts, voluntary muscle activity further contributes to the increased parental $PCO_2$ (partial pressure of carbon dioxide) and base deficit, leading to a slight lowering of the laboring person's arterial pH. The acid–base balance typically normalizes within 24 hours of delivery as the individual's respiratory rate returns to normal after birth.

## Gastrointestinal System

Some women experience loose stools in the days immediately prior labor; this condition is theorized to occur secondary to prostaglandin release, although the physiologic mechanism has not been clearly established. During labor, the gastrointestinal system exhibits delayed motility. The combined effects of decreased gastric motility, relaxation of the gastroesophageal sphincter, and increased intra-abdominal pressure contribute to an increased risk for emesis and aspiration if a laboring person is sedated or intubated.[64] Transient nausea and vomiting may occur during active labor, particularly during the final stages of cervical dilation; this may also be linked with the person's experience of severe pain. Active pushing and pressure on rectal tissues from the fetal presenting part that occurs during the second stage of labor can also contribute to formation and/or exacerbation of hemorrhoids.

### Nutritional and Hydration Needs During Labor

Energy demands during the first stage of labor are related to increased cardiac output and work of the respiratory and uterine muscles.[65] The additional work required of voluntary muscles in pushing efforts during the second stage of labor further increases the demand for energy. Thus, laboring individuals require calories and hydration but are frequently not comfortable eating food secondary to decreased gastric motility. The natural decreased consumption of nutrients during labor (and/or fasting based on institutional protocols) leads to use of alternative metabolic pathways that result in an accumulation of lactate and ketones.[66] There is a paucity of research on the effects of ketosis during labor, however, so it is unknown if treatment would be beneficial.[66] Intake of isotonic sports drinks and consumption of a light diet by laboring individuals has not been associated with adverse outcomes.[67-69]

Similarly, the effects of dehydration are not fully established. Dehydration is known to adversely affect muscle function in studies of athletes.[70] Studies of laboring women have found increased hydration and light intake of calories may be associated with shorter labor.[71]

### Kidney and Urinary Bladder

Increased uterine size limits bladder capacity. Thus, the average bladder pressure increases during labor, which can contribute to urinary incontinence. When the fetal head is engaged in the pelvis, the bladder may be displaced superiorly and anteriorly. Impingement of the fetal presenting part on the urethra can prevent complete emptying of the bladder; conversely, a full bladder can inhibit descent of the fetal presenting part. The urethra may sustain some trauma from compression during the birth. Oxytocin has a diuretic action, which results in a diuresis in the first days following birth. These factors combine to increase the risk for urinary retention, urinary incontinence, and urinary tract infections (including pyelonephritis) following birth.

## Pain and Psychobiologic Responses in Labor

Laboring people's experiences of pain during labor and methods for mitigating labor pain are reviewed in more detail in the *Support During Labor* chapter and introduced briefly here. Physically, mechanical pressure on anatomic structures (especially in the pelvis and abdomen), uterine contractions, and cervical dilation are the primary physiologic and anatomic mediators of pain during labor.[72] Pain associated with contractions is conducted from pain receptors (nociceptors) to afferent type A delta and C neurons extending from the uterus to the dorsal spinal cord. The afferent neurons enter the spinal cord via segments of the 10–12 thoracic spinal nerves. Fetal descent induces mechanical pressure on the pelvic floor, vagina, and perineum during the second stage of labor, mediating sensory pain impulses via the pudendal nerve to the 2–4 sacral spinal nerves. Interpretation of pain is achieved when the pain impulse ascends the spinal cord to higher cortical brain centers.[72]

The experience of labor pain is, however, a complex dynamic process that is influenced by multiple factors. For example, anxiety and fear of labor appear to increase the pain of labor.[73,74] Previous traumatic birth experience, post-traumatic stress disorder, a history of sexual or other abuse, or other psychoemotional disturbances can also worsen the perception of pain during labor.[75-79]

Modulation of pain can be achieved through interruption of the pain pathway (i.e., entry of pain signals into the spinal cord, spinal neurons, and higher brain centers). This knowledge forms the basis for many pain relief strategies.[79,80] For example, transmission of the pain impulse may be decreased through stimulation of inhibitory afferent type A beta pain fibers using interventions such as massage.

Cognitive strategies such as distraction and relaxation techniques can also reduce pain by targeting the laboring person's higher cortical brain centers. Attenuation of fear, stress, and anxiety via provision of continuous labor support reduces the perception of pain in labor. Other strategies to promote an optimal psychobiologic response to labor include education and anticipatory guidance, support for decision making, and both nonpharmacologic and pharmacologic methods of pain relief.

### Fetal Response to Labor

The fetal cardiovascular and respiratory responses to labor are reviewed in detail in the *Fetal Assessment During Labor* chapter. In brief, a primary clinical focus of the fetal experience of labor is maintenance of gas and nutrient exchange across the placenta as the uterus contracts and the fetus descends and rotates.

The fetus maximizes oxygen-carrying capacity via several physiologic parameters, including fetal hemoglobin, which has a higher affinity for oxygen than does adult hemoglobin; increased amounts of hemoglobin (compared to adult values); a high cardiac output; and a fast heart rate. During labor, approximately 40% of fetal blood volume is located in the fetal–placental circulation.

Uterine contractions interrupt delivery of the pregnant person's blood flow in the intervillous space, which briefly creates a more placid lake of maternal blood in the intervillous space that is actively involved in transfer of gases and nutrients to and from the fetus. Blood flow into and out of the intervillous space resumes between uterine contractions. If the contraction-induced interruption in blood flow to the intervillous space occurs too frequently or for too long, the transfer of these substances to and from the fetal circulation can become impaired. When this occurs, the fetus responds with several compensatory mechanisms, including shunting of blood preferentially to vital organs such as the brain, myocardium, and adrenal glands. In addition, the fetus demonstrates a bradycardic response to hypoxia that lowers the metabolic needs of the fetal heart.[81] The degree to which the fetus is able to tolerate transient episodes of reduced oxygen supply is clinically described as the fetus's "reserve." However, there is no actual reserve; instead, this concept expresses how long the fetus can continue to use compensatory mechanisms to maintain homeostasis and perfusion. If interruptions in delivery of oxygen to the fetus are sustained or too frequent, compensatory mechanisms that might otherwise ensure fetal oxygen delivery can become exhausted and the fetus may develop lactic acidemia, acidosis, and ultimately cardiac dysfunction or central nervous system damage. While the amount and intensity of uterine activity may adversely affect fetal oxygenation, the extent to which it does so is not easy to predict.[82]

Following birth, the newborn must quickly take over several functions that were not needed in utero, including respiration, thermoregulation, independent production of glucose, and oral feeding. Most of these changes occur in the immediate newborn period and are discussed in the *Anatomy and Physiology of the Newborn* chapter. However, the prelabor and intrapartum period prepares the fetus for several of the physiologic changes needed at birth. For example, the cortisol surge that occurs prior to birth induces fetal production of biologically active thyroid hormone. This hormone is involved in initiating metabolism of brown fat, which is needed to maintain thermoregulation in the early neonatal period.[83] Cortisol and marked surges in the release of norepinephrine and epinephrine at birth also have significant effects on the fetal respiratory and cardiovascular system.[2] Infants who are born via cesarean delivery without labor have a higher incidence of transient respiratory distress, an outcome presumed to occur because they did not experience the hormonal surges during labor and vaginal birth that prepare the fetus for extrauterine life.

## The Fetopelvic Relationship During Labor

Basic fetopelvic relationships are reviewed in the *Anatomy and Physiology of Pregnancy* chapter. Because cephalic presentations are by far the most common at the onset of labor, this section will refer to fetopelvic relationships in cephalic (i.e., vertex) presentations. The denominator for a vertex presentation is the occiput. As the fetus descends and rotates during labor, assessments of fetopelvic relationships such as position, station, engagement, synclitism, caput succedaneum, and molding are noted. A full discussion of the vaginal and cervical examination can be found in the appendix *Fetal–Pelvic Relationships*.

### Position

The relationship of the fetal occiput to the laboring person's pelvis is referred to as the fetal *position*. The position is determined by palpating and identifying the posterior and/or anterior fontanel during a vaginal examination and determining where the occiput is in relation to the front, back, and sides of the laboring person's pelvis. The fetal denominator may be on the right or left side and in an anterior, transverse, or posterior section of the laboring person's pelvis.

### Station and Engagement

*Station* describes the position of the fetal head in relation to an imaginary line drawn between the ischial

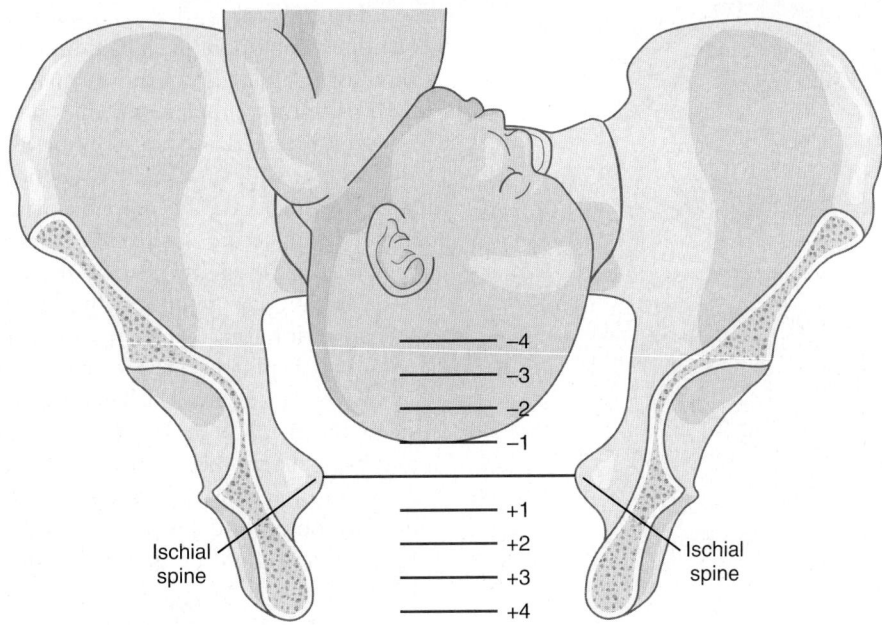

**Figure 25-4** Station, or level of descent of the fetal skull through the pelvis. The location of the forward leading edge (lowest part of the head) is designated in centimeters above or below the plane of the interspinous line. While not shown here, the full scale is from −5 to +5.

spines of the laboring person's pelvis (**Figure 25-4**). When the fetal skull is at the level of the line between the ischial spines, the position is called 0 station. Station of the fetal skull is measured in terms of the number of centimeters above or below this line. When the skull is above the spines, station is designated as −1, −2, −3, −4, or −5. This is stated as minus 1, minus 2, etc. In other words, the lower the number, the farther the fetal skull is from the introitus. When the lowermost part of the fetal skull (the bony structures, not swelling or soft tissue) is lower than the level of the ischial spines, the vertex is at +1, +2, +3, +4, or +5 station. This is stated as plus 1, plus two, etc. When the fetus is at 0 station, the biparietal diameter is descended through the inlet and is considered *engaged*.

*Engagement* occurs when the widest part of the fetal presenting part passes below the plane of the pelvic inlet. In a vertex presentation, this is the biparietal diameter. Engagement may occur prior to labor (most common in nulliparous individuals) or during labor. The fetal head is considered to be "floating" when it can move freely superior to the pelvic inlet. This can have relevance for clinical decision making; for instance, amniotomy is not performed when the head is floating to avoid prolapse of the umbilical cord in front of the head. When the vertex is at +5 station, the fetal head will be visible at the vaginal introitus.

## Synclitism and Asynclitism

*Synclitism* and *asynclitism* are terms that describe the position of the fetal head—specifically, the sagittal suture—in relation to the planes of the pregnant person's pelvis. "Synclitism" is derived from two Greek words, one of which, *klinein*, means "to lean." The fetal head may tilt laterally toward the left or right shoulder to accommodate the various diameters of the pregnant person's pelvis. The fetal head tends to enter the pelvis with the sagittal suture parallel to the transverse diameter of the pelvic inlet and in the middle of the pelvis so that the suture is equidistant from the sacrum and symphysis. This alignment is referred to as *synclitism*. However, the fetus's head may be laterally flexed in relationship to the fetal neck. When such a tilt is present, this is called *asynclitism*.[84]

It is common for the fetal head to enter the pelvis with some degree of asynclitism. When this occurs, the sagittal suture is no longer centered in the middle of the pelvic plane or parallel to the plane of the inlet. In this situation, the region of the fetal head that is lowermost (i.e., presenting) is one of the two parietal bones, and the sagittal suture is shifted either posteriorly toward the sacrum or anteriorly toward the symphysis. Thus, asynclitism is described as either *anterior* or *posterior asynclitism*. Anterior asynclitism occurs when the parietal bone closest to the symphysis pubis is the lowermost or

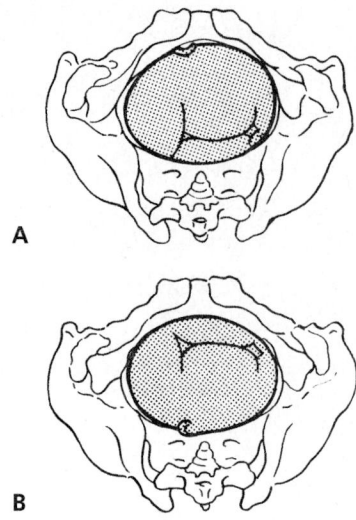

**Figure 25-5** Asynclitism. **A.** Anterior. **B.** Posterior.

leading part of the presenting part. Posterior asynclitism occurs when the parietal bone closest to the sacral promontory is the lowermost part of the presenting part (**Figure 25-5**).

The fetal head often enters the pelvic inlet with a moderate degree of posterior asynclitism, which then changes to anterior asynclitism as the fetus descends farther into the pelvis but before the mechanism of internal rotation occurs. This sequential change, from posterior to anterior asynclitism, facilitates engagement as an accommodation to take advantage of the roomiest portions of the true pelvis. Asynclitism often resolves spontaneously as the fetal head rotates so the sagittal suture is in the anterior-posterior diameter of the midplane but if it does not resolve, it can be associated with labor dystocia and failure of descent.[84] Asynclitism is also seen more often in fetuses in an occiput posterior (OP) position versus an occiput anterior (OA) position.

## Molding and Caput Succedaneum

Molding and caput succedaneum are both conditions that result from pressure exerted on the fetal head by the structures of the birth canal during labor and birth. *Molding* refers to a temporary change to the fetal head structure or shape. The sutures of the fetal skull are not fused, allowing them to overlap, or override, each other as the head conforms to the pressures exerted on it by the pelvis. A minor degree of molding is common as the fetal head negotiates the laboring person's pelvis and is considered a normal finding.

The position and attitude of the fetal head determine which part of the skull presents first and is therefore subjected to the most pressure. OA and OP positions are the most common fetal positions in a vertex presentation, so molding usually occurs as the occiput slides under or over the parietal bones. A bony ridge may be palpable where the parietal bones override the occiput. Parietal bones overlapping across the sagittal suture are uncommon.

Molding can temporarily obscure or minimize the posterior fontanel. It involves the entire skull, with overlapping in one area being counterbalanced by movement elsewhere. This mitigates mechanical stress on the skull and prevents destructive tension and possible rupture of the cranial membrane (i.e., the dura mater). Minor degrees of molding are frequently noted and not associated with adverse effects. Severe molding can occur during prolonged labor or obstructed labor and may cause complications such as injury to the dural membranes and intracranial hypertension.

*Caput succedaneum* (commonly referred to as "caput") is the formation of an edematous swelling superficial to the fetal skull over the most dependent portion of the presenting fetal head. The pressure of the head against the cervix reduces circulation in that area of the head, leading to circulatory congestion and edema of the fetal scalp. If the fetal membranes are ruptured and the fetal head (rather than the membranes) is functioning as the dilating wedge against the cervical opening, a greater amount of caput succedaneum will likely form. As with molding, a few millimeters of caput is a normal finding. Larger degrees of caput succedaneum may develop during prolonged labor. Extensive caput succedaneum can obscure fetal sutures and fontanels, making identification of these landmarks difficult. After birth, caput succedaneum can be differentiated from cephalohematoma (bleeding beneath the periosteum), a more serious condition, by the fact that caput succedaneum crosses suture lines as a generalized swelling, whereas a cephalohematoma may occur over more than one cranial bone but is limited to each individual bone and does not cross any sutures.

Caput succedaneum and molding can be clinically quite important. If the fetal head is significantly molded or a large amount of caput succedaneum develops, the leading edge of the head may be palpable at the level of the ischial spines and appear to be engaged, even though the fetal head (i.e., the biparietal diameters) is not engaged in the pelvis at all. Both molding and caput succedaneum elongate the shape of the fetal skull so that the distance between the leading part of the head and the biparietal diameters is farther than expected with the biparietal diameter not yet through the pelvic inlet.[85] Similarly, as caput succedaneum increases in size, it may appear that the fetus is descending, even if the fetal head is not actually descending through the pelvis. Significant molding and caput are associated with prolonged labor and may result from cephalopelvic disproportion.

## Cardinal Movements of Labor

The *cardinal movements of labor*, also called the mechanisms of labor, describe the movements made by the fetus during labor (Figure 25-6) and immediately before birth that allow the fetal head and shoulders to negotiate the anteroposterior and transverse diameters of the three planes of the pregnant person's pelvis (Table 25-2). Although most fetuses enter labor in a cephalic presentation, knowledge of the cardinal movements for each fetal presentation, position, and denominator is needed to effectively assess fetal descent and rotation.

The cardinal movements are a series of rotations that align the longest anterior-posterior and transverse diameters of the fetal head and the fetal shoulders with the widest diameters of each of the three planes of the pelvis. The pelvic inlet has a larger transverse diameter than anteroposterior diameter; the midplane and the outlet have larger anteroposterior diameters than transverse diameters. In addition, the bony pelvic cavity resembles a curved cylinder, such that the direction of the fetus through it is first downward from the axis of the inlet to just above the tip of the sacrum, and then forward, upward, and outward to the vaginal opening. This curve is called the *curve of Carus* (Figure 25-7).

The cardinal movements include both descent and rotational steps and have been described in a number of ways. Some obstetric textbooks describe the four rotational movements of flexion, internal rotation, extension, and external rotation.[86] Others name the movements of descent as well, thereby listing six or seven steps in the cardinal movements: engagement, descent, flexion, internal rotation, extension, restitution and external rotation, then expulsion.[55,86]

*Engagement* occurs when the biparietal diameter of the fetal head has passed through the pelvic inlet. The fetus typically enters the true pelvis facing transverse or oblique, as the pelvic inlet is widest in the transverse dimension. The biparietal diameter of the fetal skull is in the anteroposterior diameter of the pelvic inlet. It is at this stage that asynclitism may occur if the fetal neck is tilted laterally such that one parietal bone descends before the other to become the denominator. When this occurs, the sagittal suture will still be in the transverse diameter of the pelvis, but will be displaced from the middle to appear more posteriorly or anteriorly.

*Descent* occurs throughout labor and is sometimes omitted from being listed as a step of cardinal movements as it is not a movement performed by the fetal head and shoulders.[86]

*Flexion* of the fetal head (chin toward chest) begins to occur once the vertex is engaged. To understand the importance of flexion, consider the diameters of the fetal head. If the head is unflexed, the occipitofrontal diameter (approximately 11.5 to 12 centimeters) must pass through the pelvis. If flexion occurs, the smaller suboccipitobregmatic diameter (approximately 9.5 centimeters) becomes the largest fetal diameter that moves through the bony pelvis and pelvic planes (Figure 25-8) Flexion occurs as the fetal head meets resistance from maternal tissue and pelvic bones during uterine contractions.

*Internal rotation* brings the now shorter anteroposterior diameter of the fetal head into alignment with the anteroposterior diameter of the midplane of the pregnant person's pelvis. Most commonly, the occiput, which is the lowest descending part of the fetus, rotates anteriorly in the pelvis to a position beneath the symphysis pubis. If internal rotation has not occurred by the time the fetal head has reached the pelvic floor, it takes place shortly thereafter. This motion is encouraged by the dimensions of the pelvis and the V-shape of the levator ani muscles of the pelvic floor. Internal rotation is essential for vaginal birth to occur, except in unusually small fetuses, as it allows the smallest anteroposterior and transverse diameters of the fetal head to pass through the smallest midplane of the pregnant person's pelvis. Internal rotation is expressed in degrees, as it describes the arc that the head must travel from its original position on entering the pelvis to the OA or OP position that precedes birth. When the fetal occiput rotates, the fetal shoulders usually enter the pelvic inlet in one of the oblique diameters (the left oblique diameter for a left occiput anterior and the right oblique diameter for a right occiput anterior).

When the fetus is in an OA position, birth of the head occurs by *extension* of the fetal neck (the fetal chin lifts up from the thorax). Extension occurs as a consequence of the forces exerted by uterine contractions and resistance from the pubic symphysis and pelvic floor. These forces direct the fetal head up toward the vaginal introitus of the laboring person.

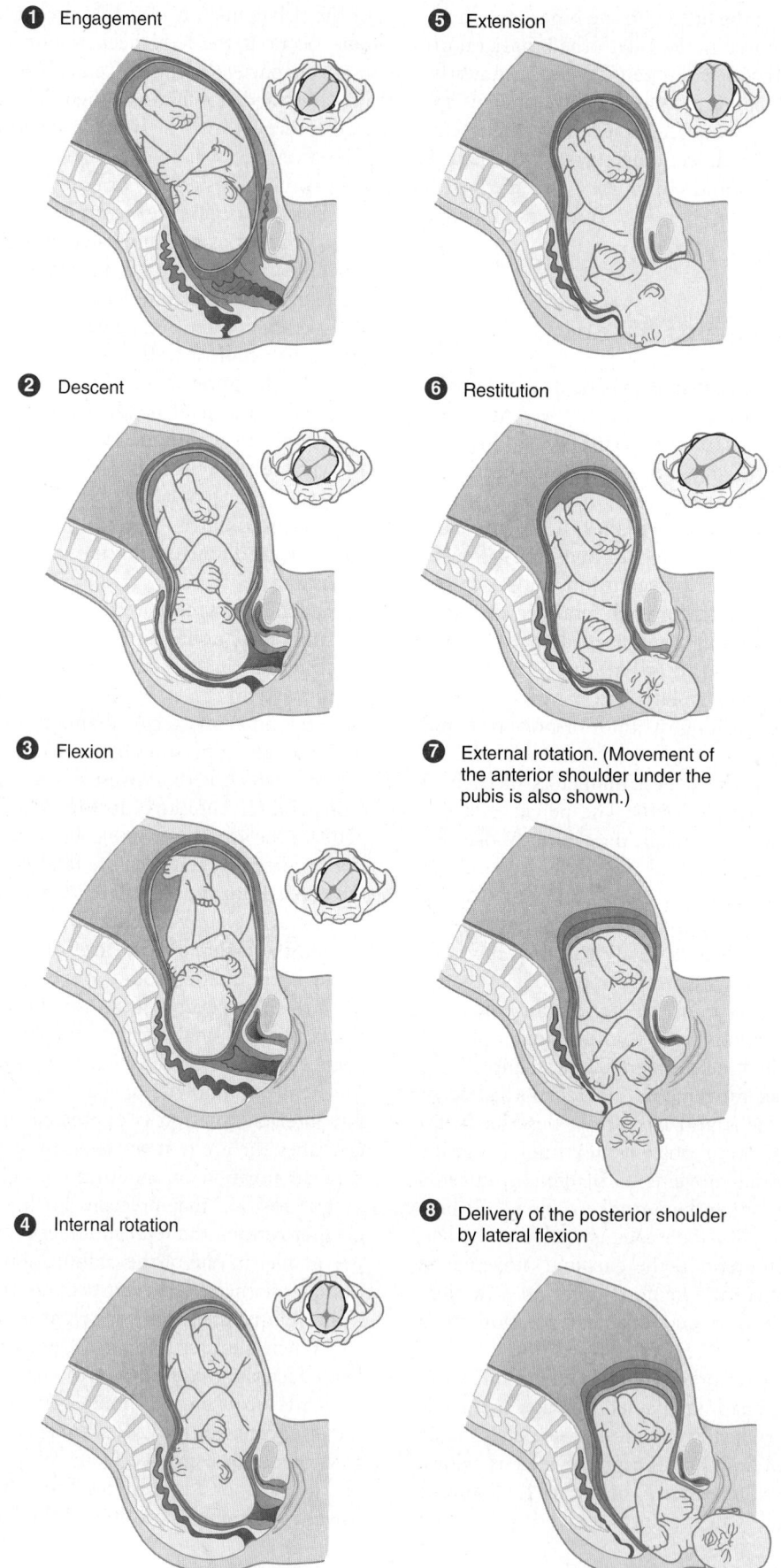

**1** Engagement

**2** Descent

**3** Flexion

**4** Internal rotation

**5** Extension

**6** Restitution

**7** External rotation. (Movement of the anterior shoulder under the pubis is also shown.)

**8** Delivery of the posterior shoulder by lateral flexion

**Figure 25-6** Cardinal movements of labor for a fetus in an occiput anterior position.

| Table 25-2 | Cardinal Movements of Labor for Occiput Anterior and Occiput Posterior Positions | |
|---|---|---|
| Cardinal Movement | Position If Fetus Is Occiput Anterior | Position If Fetus Is Occiput Posterior |
| Engagement | ROT or LOT position | Right or left oblique diameter |
| Descent | Occurs throughout labor | Occurs throughout labor |
| Flexion | Fetal neck flexes chin toward chest | Usually less completely flexed initially, then becomes markedly flexed during internal rotation as the occiput presses against the sacrum during contractions |
| Internal rotation | Undergoes the following degrees of rotation:<br>• 45° for LOA or ROA<br>• 90° for LOT or ROT | 45° for LOP or ROP to OP<br>135° for LOP or ROP to OA |
| Extension | Birth of head by extension of neck | Birth of head by first full flexion of neck (chin to chest) and then extension as the head passes through the introitus |
| Restitution | Undergoes the following degrees of rotation:<br>• 45° to LOA or ROA | Undergoes the following degrees of rotation:<br>• 45° to LOP or ROP |
| External rotation | Undergoes the following degrees of rotation:<br>• 45° to LOT or ROT | Undergoes the following degrees of rotation:<br>• 45° to LOT or ROT |
| Lateral flexion and expulsion | Birth of shoulders by lateral flexion | Birth of shoulders by lateral flexion |

Abbreviations: LOA, left occiput anterior; LOP, left occiput posterior; LOT, left occiput transverse; OA, occiput anterior; OP, occiput posterior; ROA, right occiput anterior; ROP, right occiput posterior; ROT, right occiput transverse.

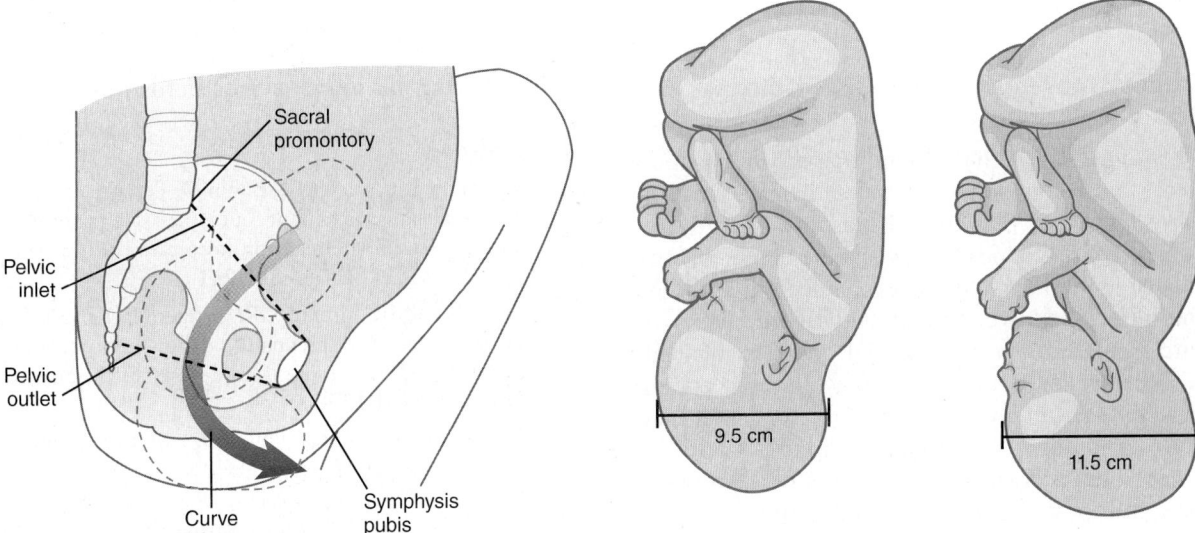

**Figure 25-7** Curve of Carus.

**Figure 25-8** Anterior-posterior fetal skull diameter with and without flexion of the fetal head during labor.

Extension of the head allows it to navigate the curve of Carus. In an OA position, the fetal head is pushed against the symphysis pubis, which acts as a fulcrum, directing the head to extend up underneath it toward the vaginal introitus. Clinically, the head is now visible; it is referred to as "crowning" once it stays visible without the force of a uterine contraction. Thus, the head is born by extension as the occiput, sagittal suture, anterior fontanel, brow, orbits, nose, mouth, and chin sequentially appear over the perineum.

Once the head is born, it will spontaneously rotate 45 degrees to either the left or the right. This movement is called *restitution*. In effect, the neck rotates so that the head is again aligned with the shoulders. The sagittal suture is now in one of the oblique diameters of the pelvis, and the bisacromial diameter of the fetal shoulder is in the other oblique diameter of the pelvis. Restitution may occur either immediately before, during, or immediately after the birth of the head.

*External rotation* occurs as the fetus's shoulders rotate 45 degrees, bringing the bisacromial diameter into alignment with the anteroposterior diameter of the pelvic outlet. This causes the head to rotate externally another 45 degrees into the left occiput transverse or right occiput transverse position, depending on the direction of restitution.

Birth of the shoulders and body occurs by *lateral flexion* to accommodate the curve of Carus. The anterior shoulder comes into view at the vaginal opening, where it impinges under the symphysis pubis; the posterior shoulder then distends the perineum and is born by lateral flexion. Once the shoulders are born, the remainder of the body follows the curve of Carus, completing the birth.

### Cardinal Movements for Persistent Occiput Posterior Position

Ultrasound studies have found that the OP position is the most common position of the fetal head in early labor, but that the OP position typically resolves to an OA position when the cervix is fully dilated and the vertex is descended through the mid-pelvis.[87] However, some fetuses internally rotate from transverse to the OP position through a short arc of 45 degrees with the occiput ending near the sacrum, instead of the more common long arc rotation of 135 degrees to a direct OA position wherein the occiput is near the symphysis. Once the occiput is posterior, the fetal head must traverse the longer posterior portion of the curve of Carus prior to birth. This must occur without the fulcrum and pivot mechanism that happens in an OA position, in which the downward uterine pressure applied to

the occiput, which is resting at the inferior portion of the symphysis pubis, results in extension of the fetal chin toward the introitus. Thus, for the fetus in an OP position, the sinciput eventually impinges beneath the symphysis pubis and becomes the pivotal point for delivery of the head. The head stays flexed as the occiput distends the perineum and is born to the nape of the neck. The remainder of the head is then born by extension, starting with the anterior fontanel and ending with the chin, as the head falls back toward the rectum, with the face looking upward. This process is often slower than when the head is born in an OA position, as the fetal head has less possibility for motion as it descends through the pelvis—the head cannot extend unless and until the occiput is pushed out of the introitus.

Persistent posterior position is considered a variation of normal labor. This position may sometimes be maintained for the entire second stage of labor, or it may resolve to an OA presentation. Diagnosis of a posterior position is made by abdominal examination and confirmed by vaginal examination or ultrasound.

## Conclusion

The physiology of labor is complex, involving hormonal, mechanical, and biochemical events that lead to birth. Endocrine, paracrine, and autocrine feedback cascades in the laboring individual and the fetus contribute to the onset and evolution of labor. Knowledge of the physiology that underlies labor and birth, including an understanding of normal variations and variability between individuals, assures that midwives can best support childbearing people during this unique period in their lives.

### References

1. Mayberry LJ, Avery MD, Budin W, Perry S. Improving maternal and infant outcomes by promoting normal physiologic birth on hospital birthing units. *Nurs Outlook*. 2017;65:240-241.

2. McLemore MR, Altman MR, Cooper N, et al. Health care experiences of pregnant, birthing and postnatal women of color at risk for preterm birth. *Soc Sci Med*. 2018;201:127-135.

3. Buckley SJ. *Hormonal Physiology of Childbearing: Evidence and Implications for Women, Babies, and Maternity Care*. Washington, DC: Childbirth Connection Programs, National Partnership for Women and Families; January 2015. http://www.national partnership.org/research-library/maternal-health /hormonal-physiology-of-childbearing.pdf. Accessed July 31, 2017.

4. American College of Obstetricians and Gynecologists. Committee Opinion No. 687: summary: approaches to limit intervention during labor and birth. *Obstet Gynecol.* 2017;129(2):403-404.

5. American College of Obstetricians and Gynecologists, Society for Maternal–Fetal Medicine, Caughey AB, et al. Safe prevention of the primary cesarean delivery. *Am J Obstet Gynecol.* 2014;210(3):179-193.

6. Liao JB, Buhimschi CS, Norwitz ER. Normal labor: mechanism and duration. *Obstet Gynecol Clin North Am.* 2005;32(2):145-164.

7. Smith R. Parturition. *N Engl J Med.* 2007;356:271-283.

8. York TP, Eaves LI, Neale MC, Straus JF. The contribution of genetic and environmental factors to the duration of pregnancy. *Am J Obstet Gynecol.* 2014;210(5):398-405.

9. York TP, Strauss JF, Neale MC, Eaves LJ. Racial differences in genetic and environmental risk to preterm birth. Lucia A, ed. *PLoS One.* 2010;5(8):e12.

10. Braveman PA, Heck K, Egerter S, et al. The role of socioeconomic factors in Black–White disparities in preterm birth. *Am J Public Health.* 2015;105(4): 694-702.

11. Slaughter-Acey JC, Sealy-Jefferson S, Helmkamp L, et al. Racism in the form of micro aggressions and the risk of preterm birth among black women. *Ann Epidemiol.* 2016;26(1):7-13.

12. Phillippe M. Cell-free fetal DNA, telomeres, and the spontaneous onset of parturition. *Reprod Sci.* 2015; 22(10):1186-1201.

13. Stelzer IA, Ghaemi MS, Han X, et al. Integrated trajectories of the maternal metabolome, proteome, and immunome predict labor onset. *Sci Transl Med.* 2021; 13:eabd9898. doi:10.1126/scitranslmed.abd9898.

14. Walter MH, Abele H, Plappert CF. The role of oxytocin and the effect of stress during childbirth: neurobiological basics and implications for mother and child. *Front Endocrinol (Lausanne).* 2021;12:742236.

15. Word RA, Li XH, Hnat M, Carrick K. Dynamics of cervical remodeling during pregnancy and parturition: mechanisms and current concepts. *Semin Reprod Med.* 2007;25(1):69-79.

16. Baños A, Wolf M, Grawe C, et al. Frequency domain near-infrared spectroscopy of the uterine cervix during cervical ripening. *Laser Surg Med.* 2007;39(8): 641-646.

17. Timmons B, Akins M, Mahendroo M. Cervical remodeling during pregnancy and parturition. *Trends Endocrinol Metab.* 2010;21(6):353-361.

18. Yellon SM. Contributions to the dynamics of cervix remodeling prior to term and preterm birth. *Biol Reprod.* 2017;96(1):13-23. doi:10.1095/biolreprod. 116.142844.

19. Neal JL, Lowe NK. Physiologic partograph to improve birth safety and outcomes among low-risk, nulliparous women with spontaneous labor onset. *Med Hypotheses.* 2012;78(2):319-326.

20. Weckend M, Davison C, Bayes S. Physiological plateaus during normal labor and birth: a scoping review of contemporary concepts and definitions. *Birth.* January 5, 2022. doi: 10.1111/birt.12607.

21. Leimert KB, Xu W, Princ MM, et al. Inflammatory amplification: a central tenet of uterine transition for labor. *Front Cell Infect Microbiol.* 2021;11:660983. doi:10.3389/fcimb.2021.660983.

22. Norwitz ER, Bonney EA, Snegovskikh VV, et al. Molecular regulation of parturition: the role of the decidual clock. *Cold Spring Harb Perspect Med.* 2015;5(11):a023143.

23. Kamel RM. The onset of human parturition. *Arch Gynecol Obstet.* 2010;281(6):975-982.

24. Zakar T, Hertelendy F. Progesterone withdrawal: key to parturition. *Am J Obstet Gynecol.* 2007; 196(4):289-296.

25. Chai SY, Smith R, Zakar T, et al. Term myometrium is characterized by increased activating epigenetic modifications at the progesterone receptor-A promoter. *Molec Hum Reprod.* 2012;18(8):401-409.

26. Ravanos K, Dagklis T, Petousis S, et al. Factors implicated in the initiation of human parturition in term and preterm labor: a review. *Gynecol Endocrinol.* 2015;31(9):679-683.

27. Tan H, Yi L, Rote NS, et al. Progesterone receptor-A and -B have opposite effects on proinflammatory gene expression in human myometrial cells: implications for progesterone actions in human pregnancy and parturition. *J Clin Endocrinol Metab.* 2012;97(5):E719-E730.

28. Vannuccini S, Bocchi C, Severi FM, et al. Endocrinology of human parturition. *Ann Endocrinol (Paris).* 2016;77(2):105-113.

29. Menon R, Bonney EA, Condon J, et al. Novel concepts on pregnancy clocks and alarms: redundancy and synergy in human parturition. *Hum Reprod Update.* 2016;22(5):535-560.

30. Stelzer IA, Ghaemi MS, Han X, et al. Integrated trajectories of the maternal metabolome, proteome, and immunome predict labor onset. *Sci Transl Med.* 2021;13(592):eabd9898.

31. Yulia A, Johnson MR. Myometrial oxytocin receptor expression and intracellular pathways. *Minerva Ginecol.* 2014;66(3):267-280.

32. Osman I, Young A, Ledingham MA, et al. Leukocyte density and pro-inflammatory cytokine expression in human fetal membranes, decidua, cervix and myometrium before and during labour at term. *Molec Hum Reprod.* 2003;9(1):41-45.

33. Behnia F, Taylor BD, Woodson M, et al. Chorioamniotic membrane senescence: a signal for parturition? *Am J Obstet Gynecol.* 2015;213(3):359.e1-359.e16.

34. Romero R, Miranda J, Chaiworapongsa T, et al. Prevalence and clinical significance of sterile intra-amniotic inflammation in patients with preterm labor and intact membranes. *Am J Reprod Immunol.* 2014;72(5):458-474.

35. Jones CW, Gambala C, Esteves KC, et al. Differences in placental telomere length suggest a link between racial disparities in birth outcomes and cellular aging. *Am J Obstet Gynecol.* 2017;216(3):294.e1-294.e8.

36. Miller MW, Lin AP, Wolf EJ, Miller DR. Oxidative stress, inflammation, and neuroprogression in chronic PTSD. *Harv Rev Psychiatry.* 2018;26(2):57-69.

37. Altman MR, Oseguera T, McLemore MR, et al. Information and power: women of color's experiences interacting with health care providers in pregnancy and birth. *Soc Sci Med.* 2019;238:112491.

38. Altman MR, Eagen-Torkko MK, Mohammed SA, et al. The impact of COVID-19 visitor policy restrictions on birthing communities of colour. *J Adv Nurs.* 2021;77(12):4827-4835.

39. Ding W, Chim SSC, Wang CC, et al. Molecular mechanism and pathways of normal human parturition in different gestational tissues: a systematic review of transcriptome studies. *Front Physiol.* 2021;12:730030.

40. Zhang G, Feenstra B, Bacelis J, et al. Genetic associations with gestational duration and spontaneous preterm birth. *N Engl J Med.* 2017;377(12):1156-1167.

41. Wadon M, Modi N, Wong HS, et al. Recent advances in the genetics of preterm birth. *Ann Hum Genet.* 2020;84(3):205-213.

42. Latendresse G. Perinatal genomics: current research on genetic contributions to preterm birth and placental phenotype. *Annu Rev Nurs Res.* 2011;29:331-351.

43. Sfakianaki AK, Norwitz ER. Mechanisms of progesterone action in inhibiting prematurity. *J Matern Fetal Neonatal Med.* 2006;19(12):763-772.

44. Challis RJG, Gibb W. Control of parturition. *Prenat Neonat Med.* 1996;1;238.

45. Blanks AM, Thornton S. The role of oxytocin in parturition. *BJOG.* 2003;110(suppl 20):46-51.

46. Terzidou V, Blanks AM, Kim SH, et al. Labor and inflammation increase the expression of oxytocin receptor in human amnion. *Biol Reprod.* 2011;84(3):546-552.

47. Weiss G. Endocrinology of parturition. *J Clin Endocrinol Metab.* 2000;85(12):4421-4425.

48. Kim SH, Bennett PR, Terzidou V. Advances in the role of oxytocin receptors in human parturition. *Molec Cell Endocrinol.* 2017;449:56-63.

49. Dawood MY, Raghavan KS, Pociask C, Fuchs F. Oxytocin in human pregnancy and parturition. *Obstet Gynecol.* 1978;51(2):138-143.

50. Terzidou V, Sooranna SR, Kim LU, et al. Mechanical stretch up-regulates the human oxytocin receptor in primary human uterine myocytes. *J Clin Endocrinol Metab.* 2005;90(1):237-246.

51. Phaneuf S, Rodriguez Linares B, TambyRaja RL, et al. Loss of myometrial oxytocin receptors during oxytocin-induced and oxytocin-augmented labour. *J Reprod Fertil.* 2000;120(1):91-97.

52. Terzidou V. Biochemical and endocrinological preparation for parturition. *Best Pract Res Clin Obstet Gynecol.* 2007;21(5):729-757.

53. Page K, McCool WF, Guidera M. Examination of the pharmacology of oxytocin and clinical guidelines for use in labor. *J Midwifery Womens Health.* 2017;62(4):425-433.

54. Young RC. Myocytes, myometrium, and uterine contractions. *Ann NY Acad Sci.* 2007;1101:72-84.

55. Cunningham F, Leveno KJ, Bloom SL, et al. Physiology of labor. In: Cunningham F, Leveno KJ, Bloom SL, et al., eds. *Williams Obstetrics.* 25th ed. New York, NY: McGraw-Hill; 2018:408-432.

56. Kissler KJ, Lowe NK, Hernandez TL. An integrated review of uterine activity monitoring for evaluating labor dystocia. *J Midwifery Womens Health.* 2020;65(3):323-334.

57. Lowe N, Openshaw M, King TL. Labor. In: Brucker MC, King TL, eds. *Pharmacology for Women's Health.* 2nd ed. Burlington, MA: Jones & Bartlett Learning; 2017:1065-1094.

58. Ozuounian JG, Elkayam U. Physiologic changes during normal pregnancy and delivery. *Cardiol Clin.* 2012;30:317-332.

59. Fujitani S, Baldisseri MR. Hemodynamic assessment in a pregnant and peripartum patient. *Crit Care Med.* 2005;33(10 suppl):S354-S361.

60. Soma-Pillay P, Nelson-Piercy C, Tolppanen H, Mebazaa A. Physiological changes in pregnancy. *Cardiovasc J Afr.* 2016;27(2):89-94.

61. Konje JC, Howarth ES, Kaufmann P, Taylor DJ. Longitudinal quantification of uterine artery blood volume flow changes during gestation in pregnancies complicated by intrauterine growth restriction. *BJOG.* 2003;100:301-305.

62. Flo K, Wolsgaard T, Vartun A, Acharya G. A longitudinal study of the relationship between maternal cardiac output measured by impedance cardiography and uterine artery blood flow in the second half of pregnancy. *BJOG.* 2010;117:837-844.

63. Earing MG, Webb GD. Congenital heart disease and pregnancy: maternal and fetal risks. *Clin Perinatol.* 2005;32(4):913-919.

64. Chang J, Streitman D. Physiologic adaptations to pregnancy. *Neurol Clin.* 2012;30(3):781-789.

65. Kardel KR, Henriksen T, Iversen PO. No effect of energy supply during childbirth on delivery outcomes in nulliparous women: a randomised, double-blind, placebo-controlled trial. *J Obstet Gynaecol.* 2010; 30(3):248-252.

66. Toohill J, Soong B, Flenady V. Interventions for ketosis during labour. *Cochrane Database Syst Rev.* 2008;3: CD004230. doi:10.1002/14651858.CD004230.pub2.

67. Singata M, Tranmer J, Gyte GM. Restricting oral fluid and food intake during labour. *Cochrane Database Syst Rev.* 2013;8:CD003930.

68. American College of Nurse-Midwives. Providing oral nutrition to women in labor. *J Midwifery Womens Health.* 2016;61(4):528-334.

69. ACOG Committee Opinion No. 766: approaches to limit intervention during labor and birth. *Obstet Gynecol.* 2019;133(2):e164-e173.

70. Casa DJ, Clarkson PM, Roberts WO. American College of Sports Medicine roundtable on hydration and physical activity: consensus statements. *Curr Sports Med Rep.* 2005;4(3):115-127.

71. Ciardulli A, Saccone G, Anastasio H, Berghella V. Less restrictive food intake during labor in low-risk singleton pregnancies: a systematic review and meta-analysis. *Obstet Gynecol.* 2017;129(3):473-478.

72. Lowe NK. The nature of labor pain. *Am J Obstet Gynecol.* 2002;186(5 suppl):S16-S24.

73. Alder J, Breitinger G, Granado C, et al. Antenatal psychobiological predictors of psychological response to childbirth. *J Am Psychiatr Nurs Assoc.* 2011;17(6): 417-425.

74. Hodnett ED. Pain and women's satisfaction with the experience of childbirth: a systematic review. *Am J Obstet Gynecol.* 2002;186(5 suppl):S160-S172.

75. Lally JE, Murtagh MJ, Macphail S, Thomson R. More in hope than expectation: a systematic review of women's expectations and experience of pain relief in labour. *BMC Med.* 2008;6:7. doi:10.1186/1741-7015-6-7.

76. Choi KR, Seng JS. Predisposing and precipitating factors for dissociation during labor in a cohort study of posttraumatic stress disorder and childbearing outcomes. *J Midwifery Womens Health.* 2016;61(1): 68-76.

77. Leeners B, Görres G, Block E, Hengartner MP. Birth experiences in adult women with a history of childhood sexual abuse. *J Psychosom Res.* 2016;83:27-32.

78. LoGiudice JA. A systematic literature review of the childbearing cycle as experienced by survivors of sexual abuse. *Nurs Womens Health.* 2016-2017;20(6): 582-594.

79. Bohren MA, Hofmeyr G, Sakala C, et al. Continuous support for women during childbirth. *Cochrane Database Syst Rev.* 2017;7:CD003766. doi:10.1002/14651858.CD003766.pub6.

80. Smith CA, Levett KM, Collins CT, et al. Relaxation techniques for pain management in labour. *Cochrane Database Syst Rev.* 2018;3:CD009514. doi:10.1002/14651858.CD009514.pub2.

81. Turner JM, Mitchell MD, Kumar SS. The physiology of intrapartum fetal compromise at term. *Am J Obstet Gynecol.* 2020;222(1):17-26.

82. Reynolds AJ, Geary MP, Hayes BC. Intrapartum uterine activity and neonatal outcomes: a systematic review. *BMC Pregnancy Childbirth.* 2020;20(1):532.

83. Nathanielsz PW, Berghorn KA, Derks JB, et al. Life before birth: effects of cortisol on future cardiovascular and metabolic function. *Acta Paediatr.* 2003;92(7):766-772.

84. Malvasi A, Barbera A, Di Vagno G, et al. Asynclitism: a literature review of an often forgotten clinical condition. *J Matern Fetal Neonatal Med.* 2015;28(16): 1890-1894.

85. Iversen JK, Kahrs BH, Torkildsen EA, Eggebø TM. Fetal molding examined with transperineal ultrasound and associations with position and delivery mode. *Am J Obstet Gynecol.* 2020;223(6):909 .e1-909.e8.

86. Iversen JK, Kahrs BH, Eggebø TM. There are 4, not 7, cardinal movements in labor. *Am J Obstet Gynecol MFM.* 2021;3(6):100436.

87. Hjartardóttir H, Lund SH, Benediktsdóttir S, et al. When does fetal head rotation occur in spontaneous labor at term: results of an ultrasound-based longitudinal study in nulliparous women. *Am J Obstet Gynecol.* 2021;224(5):514.e1-514.e9.

C H A P T E R

# 26

# First Stage of Labor

JEREMY L. NEAL, HEATHER M. BRADFORD, AND JULIA C. PHILLIPPI

*The editors acknowledge Nancy K. Lowe, Sharon L. Ryan, and Linda A. Hunter for contributions to this chapter in the previous edition.*

## Introduction

A physiologic labor and birth are powered by the innate human capacity of the birthing person and fetus. Midwifery care of laboring people is a cyclic process that is responsive to the dynamic nature of individual and fetal responses to labor. Continual reassessment, with ongoing evaluation and modification of the care plan throughout labor, is the basis of safe and responsive midwifery care. The science of physiologic childbirth has been examined closely in the last three decades and is supported by a consensus statement defined by leading midwifery organizations (Table 26-1).[1] Care provided in labor to low-risk individuals should be person-centered and focus on the physiologic needs and personal preferences of the individual. In addition, the midwife should compassionately assess all important factors and make suggestions for changes and interventions as needed, according to the individual's wishes and medical needs.

This chapter focuses on the midwifery care of laboring individuals who are at low risk of perinatal complications. Despite consensus among perinatal care clinicians on the importance of factors that promote physiologic birth, 98% of birthing individuals in the United States experience childbirth in hospital settings,[2] where interventions that have limited or uncertain benefits are commonly used.[3] In 2017, the American College of Obstetricians and Gynecologists (ACOG) Committee on Obstetrical Practice released *Approaches to Limit Intervention During Labor and Birth*,[4] which was endorsed by the ACNM and reaffirmed in 2021; this document calls for expansion of evidence-based means to support physiologic birth for low-risk individuals.[5] Similar documents and resources from other professional associations can be found in the Resources section at the end of this chapter. As the U.S. perinatal care system examines the overuse of intrapartum interventions, midwifery skills and techniques are valuable components for supporting healthy individuals to have physiologic births.

This chapter reviews care for essentially healthy individuals during spontaneous labor and provides information about the promotion of optimal care during labor and birth. Care for individuals who require induction of labor and those who have labor complications is presented in the *Complications During Labor and Birth* chapter. Even if complications arise, midwives can promote physiologic labor care where possible in the birth process.

## Choice of Birth Setting and Birth Attendant

Ideally, all birthing persons would have the opportunity to give birth in their setting of choice, whether that be the home, birth center, or hospital. They would also have the freedom to choose a birth attendant whose training and background are congruent with their wishes. However, in the United States, birthing people's options for their preferred birth setting or type of birth attendant are often limited due to health complications, insurance or financial limitations, workforce insufficiencies, and political restrictions. For example, a facility may not accept all insurance types, or restrictions on scope of practice in a state may decrease the availability of midwives. Alternatively, pregnancy risk factors such as a multiple gestation may necessitate physician consultation, collaboration, and/or referral (more information on levels of care in pregnancy and birth

| Table 26-1 | Physiologic Birth |
|---|---|
| **Characteristics of Physiologic Birth** | |
| Labor begins and progresses spontaneously | |
| Includes biologic and psychological conditions that promote effective labor | |
| Promotes vaginal birth | |
| Facilitates immediate and ongoing skin-to-skin contact between the birthing person and infant during the postpartum period and keeps the new dyad together in the same room throughout the facility stay | |
| Encourages breastfeeding soon after birth using newborn cues to guide feeding | |
| **Factors That Influence Physiologic Birth** | |
| *For the Birthing Person* | |
| Individual health status and physical fitness | |
| Autonomy and self-determination in childbirth | |
| Personal knowledge and confidence about birth, including cultural beliefs, norms, and practices and education about the value of normal physiologic birth | |
| Fully-informed, shared decision making | |
| Access to healthcare systems, settings, and clinicians supportive of and skilled in normal physiologic birth | |
| *For the Clinician* | |
| Education, knowledge, competence, skill, and confidence in supporting physiologic labor and birth, including helping birthing persons cope with pain | |
| Commitment to working with birthing persons through education to enhance their confidence in birth and diminish their fear of the process | |
| Commitment to shared decision making | |
| Working within an infrastructure supportive of normal physiologic birth | |
| **Factors That Disrupt Physiologic Birth** | |
| Situations in which the individual feels unsupported, threatened, or unsafe | |
| Facility factors that increase fear or decrease comfort (e.g., lack of privacy, multiple clinicians, lack of supportive companions, lack of trusted providers, characteristics of the birth room) | |
| Routine induction without a medical indication | |
| Routine augmentation of labor without an indication | |
| Use of rigid time constraints for labor based on policy and/or staffing in lieu of parameters based on research evidence | |
| Requirements surrounding fluids and foods | |
| Opioids, regional analgesia, or general anesthesia | |
| Routine episiotomy | |
| Operative vaginal (vacuum, forceps) or cesarean birth | |
| Immediate umbilical cord-clamping | |
| Manual removal of the placenta | |

Based on Supporting healthy and normal physiologic childbirth: a consensus statement by ACNM, MANA, and NACPM. *J Perinat Educ.* 2013;22(1):14-18. doi:10.1891/1058-1243.22.1.14; Saftner MA, Neerland C, Avery MD. Enhancing women's confidence for physiologic birth: maternity care providers' perspectives. *Midwifery.* 2017;53:28-34; Zielinski RE, Brody MG, Low LK. The value of the maternity care team in the promotion of physiologic birth. *J Obstet Gynecol Neonatal Nurs.* 2016;45(2):276-284.

is found in Table 23-2 (Chapter 23), which focuses on levels of perinatal care). Midwives attend births in homes, birth centers, and hospitals, and they partner with birthing persons to provide care that is individualized to their health status and desires whenever possible.

## Person-Centered and Culturally Centered Care

All people deserve reproductive care that promotes not only their physical health, but also the social, cultural, and environmental factors that support them. This consideration is especially important for individuals who are marginalized due to their race, ethnicity, religion, gender identity, sexual orientation, financial resources, body shape and size, intellectual ability, or any other characteristic. Labor and birth are important life transitions that often provoke feelings of vulnerability, fear, and loss of control in birthing people and their families.[6] By centering their care in respect for the whole person, midwives can not only promote optimal birth outcomes, but also provide a calm, safe place where birthing people can thrive.

## Prelabor

Many pregnant individuals experience premonitory signs or symptoms of impending labor. Common signs and symptoms suggestive of physiologic progress toward labor include descent of the fetus, cervical changes, an increase in uncoordinated uterine contractions, bloody show or increased mucus-like vaginal discharge, perception of increased energy, and gastrointestinal distress. Anticipatory guidance for individuals in late pregnancy includes reassurance that these signs and symptoms are normal, promotion of comfort measures, and support for watchful waiting.

"False labor" and "prodromal contractions" are terms historically used to describe the experience of uterine contractions of varying intensity not associated with progressive cervical change. Use of the term "prelabor contractions" is now preferred, as it better affirms a pregnant person's discomfort. Prelabor contractions are an intensification of the usually painless contractions that may occur in the third trimester or even earlier. Prelabor contractions do not intensify over time and are often relieved by rest, walking, or position changes, whereas labor contractions will become longer, stronger, and closer together over time and are associated with progressive cervical change. Labor contractions sometimes intensify with walking and are not relieved by position changes.

If a pregnant individual is preterm and experiencing prelabor contractions, thorough assessment of signs and symptoms of preterm labor is warranted, but at term these feelings are physiologic. Prelabor contractions may occur for days or weeks before the onset of labor. A pregnant person experiencing persistent or recurrent prelabor contractions may become fatigued over time and have difficulty coping, as these contractions can be painful and distressing. The clinician can assure the individual they will be able to identify a change in the labor pattern when labor begins. Comfort measures for prelabor contractions are the same as those used in latent-phase labor.

### Descent of the Fetus

Notable descent of the fetus prior to labor, or "lightening," occurs following the gradual softening of the uterine isthmus (lower uterine segment). The fetal presenting part, most commonly the head, descends to or through the inlet of the pelvis (**Figure 26-1**). Pregnant persons often subjectively refer to the physical experience and appearance of lightening as "the baby has dropped." Although lightening is not synonymous with engagement of the fetal presenting part (i.e., when the widest diameter of the fetal presenting part is at or below the pelvic inlet), engagement may result from lightening. A small reduction in fundal height is common following this prelabor fetal descent. After lightening, a cervical examination (if needed for other reasons) may reveal that the presenting part is "fixed" and not ballotable.

Among many—but not all—nulliparous individuals, prelabor descent of the fetus may occur 2 or more weeks in advance of labor. When this happens at term, it is reassuring that the fetus fits through the pelvis at the plane of the inlet. For those persons who have previously given birth, notable descent may not occur until labor is advanced. When this sign and the resulting increase in pelvic pressure happen before 37 weeks' gestation, additional assessment of the risk of preterm birth is warranted.

Fetal descent associated with lightening can result in the pregnant person having more room in the upper abdomen, allowing for better lung expansion and increased stomach capacity. However, lightening often causes new discomforts because of pressure of the presenting part on other pelvic

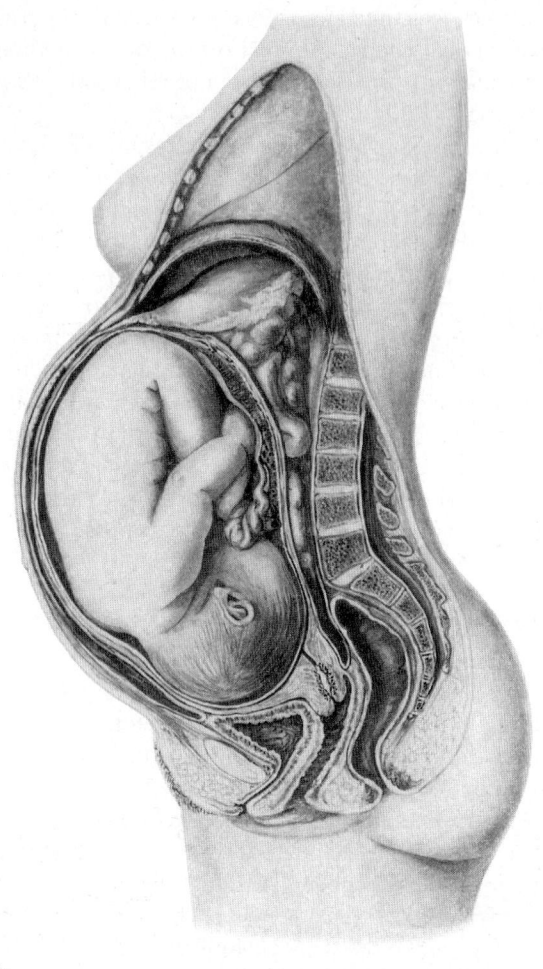

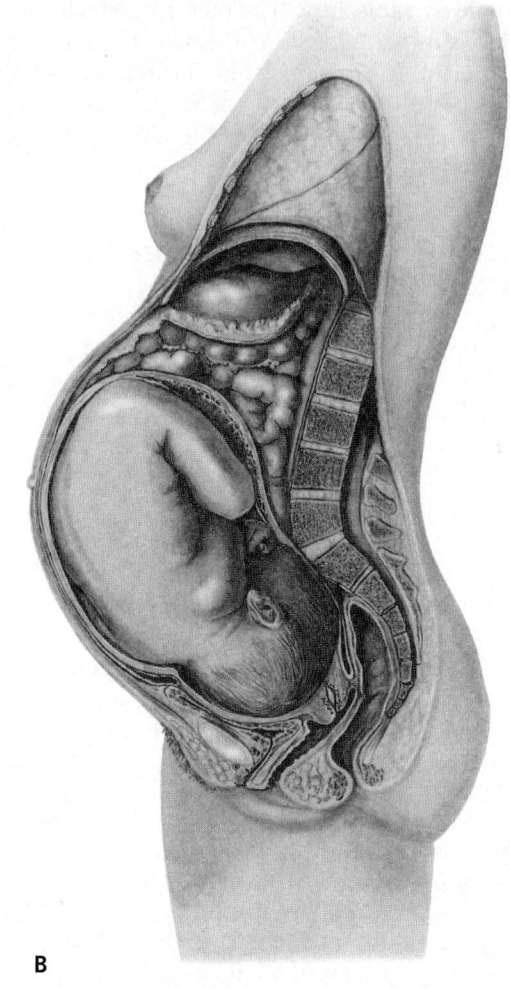

A

B

**Figure 26-1** **A.** Prelightening. **B.** Postlightening.
© Childbirth Connection 2013. Used with permission.

structures. For example, compression of the bladder can cause urinary frequency. Pregnant persons may describe a constant feeling of pelvic pressure, which contributes to the straddling walk of late pregnancy. Increased pelvic congestion and venous insufficiency can cause more dependent edema, development of hemorrhoids, and vulvar or lower-extremity varicosities.

Finally, sciatic nerve pain, characterized by unilateral shooting pain radiating from the buttocks down the back of the leg, can be aggravated or initiated by the fetal descent. Sciatic pain may be relieved by massage, application of heat/cold, gentle stretching exercises, or specialized applications of tape. Sciatic nerve pain that is debilitating or persists into the postpartum period warrants a referral for evaluation, as it can indicate vertebral disc herniation or other complications.

## Cervical Ripening

The process of cervical change preparatory to labor is referred to as "ripening." The cervix, which is typically long, closed, and semi-firm throughout pregnancy, becomes soft and malleable though a process described in the *Anatomy and Physiology of Labor and Birth* chapter. Cervical ripening may occur with or without uterine contractions.

Cervical ripening can be objectively assessed via digital cervical examination. Changes that occur in preparation for labor may include effacement, dilation, softening, and anterior positioning of the cervix. At term, cervical exam findings are often associated with parity. For example, during the final weeks of pregnancy, a nulliparous person's cervix may remain firm and closed until the onset of labor, whereas a multiparous person's cervix may be soft and dilated several centimeters. Therefore, while ripening is suggestive of progress toward labor, it is not a reliable predictor of actual labor onset. For this reason, unless cervical evaluation is needed to inform clinical decision making, routine assessment via digital examination in late pregnancy should not be performed. Quantification of cervical ripening as part of induction-related decision making is explored in the *Complications During Labor and Birth* chapter.

## Bloody Show

The mucus plug that sits in the cervix throughout pregnancy is often released as the cervix thins and opens. It may consist of clear mucus, or it may be tinged with red or brown blood. Bloody show can be a premonitory sign of labor and may be accompanied by other signs of labor, including cramping, pelvic pressure, and contractions. Spontaneous bloody show usually signals the onset of labor within the next few days. However, bloody show can also result from recent vaginal examination or sexual intercourse due to minor trauma to the cervix or disruption of the mucus plug. A thorough patient history and examination can help differentiate benign bloody show from frank bleeding.

## Energy Spurt

Some pregnant persons perceive an energy spurt in the days preceding labor onset, the cause of which is unknown. Many may focus their energy on cooking, baking, cleaning, or organizing closets or baby care items—activities that are sometimes known as "nesting." They may benefit from anticipatory guidance cautioning them against over-exerting themselves.

## Gastrointestinal Distress

In the absence of any other causative factors, a brief occurrence of diarrhea, indigestion, nausea, and vomiting can be indicative of impending labor. These gastrointestinal distress symptoms are likely associated with the increased production of prostaglandins and estrogen and the decrease in progesterone levels that occur with the approach of labor.

## Prelabor Rupture of Membranes

Rupture of the fetal membranes with associated loss of amniotic fluid prior to the onset of labor is called prelabor rupture of membranes (PROM). PROM occurs in approximately 8% of term pregnancies and is generally followed by a spontaneous onset of labor.[7,8] Accurate diagnosis of PROM can sometimes be difficult. The pregnant person's perceptions of the event, careful physical examination, and laboratory testing contribute to confirming an accurate diagnosis. The steps for assessment and diagnosis of PROM are described in the *Assessment and Diagnosis of Rupture of Membranes* appendix. Differential diagnoses that need to be excluded include urinary incontinence, vaginal or cervical discharge, leakage of semen following vaginal intercourse, and rupture of the chorion alone. Midwifery care for confirmed PROM is described briefly later in this chapter and in more detail in the *Complications During Labor and Birth* chapter.

## Definitions of Labor

Labor is the process leading to childbirth, requiring uterine contractions of sufficient frequency, duration, and intensity to cause effacement and dilation of the cervix. Determining the time of labor onset can be difficult, because individuals perceive contractions differently and for varying durations of time before recognizing the feelings as labor. Complicating the prospective diagnosis of labor even more is that the mechanisms underlying the onset and progress of spontaneous labor remain largely unknown, and cervical examinations are performed episodically, if at all, in early labor. Most often, the onset of labor is a diagnosis made retrospectively, based on cervical changes that have already occurred.

Physical changes such as cervical dilation and fetal descent can be used to evaluate labor progress. The word *dilation* is used to describes the process of the cervix becoming wider and more open, whereas *dilatation* is the noun that describes the estimate of the cervical opening. Cervical dilation in active labor, expressed in centimeters per hour (cm/hr), has long been a key aspect of decision making for clinicians providing care to laboring individuals. Accuracy in determining cervical dilation depends on the skill of the examiner. Even between experienced clinicians, the assessment may vary slightly. In addition, cervical dilatation can change rapidly. Nevertheless, because cervical dilation rates are highly related to labor duration, this facet of assessment is the most commonly used indicator of labor progress.

While descriptions of labor often divide the labor process into stages such as first stage and second stage and phases such as latent phase and active phase based on cervical dilatation, individuals experience labor as a continuous process. Each stage and phase of labor is characterized by physical changes and behavioral responses. The birthing person's behaviors may be used to estimate labor progress without a cervical examination, although individual and cultural responses to labor vary, and the clinician's implicit biases can result in misinterpretation. Thus, understanding the individual's goals, expectations, and concerns as well as their cultural framework may assist in assessment of labor progress. In addition, a midwife's interpretation of nonverbal behaviors should always be verified with the individual. Understanding normal first-stage labor allows clinicians to support birthing people by providing sufficient time for the events of physiologic labor to unfold without unnecessary interventions, while simultaneously evaluating whether interventions may be indicated.

The *first stage of labor*, also known as the cervical dilation stage, begins with labor contractions that cause progressive cervical changes and ends when the cervix is completely dilated (approximately 10 cm for term births) and ready for passage of the fetal presenting part. Traditionally, the first stage of labor has been divided into two sequential phases: latent and active. The *latent phase* begins with the onset of regular uterine labor contractions; the *active phase* begins when the rate of cervical dilation increases or in clinical practice is sometimes defined by a dilatation. While the exact dilatation at which cervical change increases varies between individuals, there is a current presumption that most individuals are in active labor by the time their cervix is dilated 6 cm.[9,10] As the cervix nears 10 cm dilation, laboring persons may experience contractions that are stronger and closer together, a phenomenon termed *transitional labor*.

Following the first stage, the *second stage of labor*, known as the expulsive stage, begins with complete cervical dilatation and ends with the birth of the infant. The *third stage of labor* is the time between birth of the infant and expulsion of the placenta. The second and third stages of labor are discussed in detail in separate chapters.

Abnormalities in expected durations of the latent, active, and second stages of labor are associated with maternal fatigue and perinatal morbidities such as intra-amniotic infection, cephalopelvic disproportion, cesarean birth, and postpartum hemorrhage. Definitions and management of these conditions are discussed in later chapters and appendices.

## Stages of Physiologic First Stage of Labor

### Latent Phase of Labor

The *latent phase of labor* encompasses the period of time from the beginning of regular uterine contractions to the point when cervical dilation begins to accelerate. The onset of the latent phase is difficult to determine objectively, as individuals typically do not seek labor care until after the onset of labor. Thus, identification of latent-phase onset often depends on memory of the pregnant person and discernment of prelabor versus labor contractions. The end of the latent phase is also difficult to determine due to the wide variability in when cervical dilation becomes more rapid. In multiparous individuals, the rate of cervical dilation commonly accelerates after 6 cm dilation; however, the average labor curve for nulliparous individuals does not always have a clear inflection point of dilation acceleration that marks the end of the latent phase.[10]

Uterine contractions become established during the latent phase as they increase in frequency, duration, and intensity. It is common for contractions during latent labor to initially be of mild intensity, occurring every 10 to 20 minutes and lasting 15 to 20 seconds. As latent labor advances, contractions typically increase to moderate intensity, occurring approximately every 5 to 7 minutes and lasting 30 to 40 seconds. These parameters alone do not define latent labor, however, as the experience of contractions may vary greatly among individuals at similar points of the labor process. Only demonstrable effacement and/or dilation of the cervix in combination with regular uterine contractions defines labor. For most individuals, little to no descent of the presenting part occurs during the latent phase.

### Active Phase of Labor

The *active phase of labor* is the period of time that starts with an increase in the rate of cervical dilation (the end of the latent phase of labor) and ends with complete cervical dilatation (the beginning of the second stage of labor). Progressive descent of the fetal presenting part also typically occurs during the latter part of the active phase. Accurate diagnosis of active labor is important because the rate of cervical dilation in this phase serves as the basis against which labor progress is assessed. It is also useful in deciding about admission to the birth facility, though it is not the only variable used for this decision.

Cervical dilation rates indicative of active labor may begin at varying dilatation points for different individuals. In the presence of regular, painful contractions and complete or near-complete effacement, it is reasonable to consider a laboring person to be in active labor at 4 cm or 5 cm dilatation[11,12] if that state is immediately preceded by active cervical change over time (i.e., 1 cm or more in a 2-hour or shorter window, as determined by two or more

| Table 26-2 | Definition of Active Labor |
| --- | --- |

In the presence of regular, painful contractions and complete or near-complete effacement, an individual can be considered to be in active labor:

- At 4 cm or 5 cm dilation,[11,12] if that dilatation is immediately preceded by active cervical change over time (i.e., 1 cm or more in a 2-hour or shorter window), OR
- At 6 cm or more[13] regardless of the rate of previous cervical change, unless their body mass index (BMI) exceeds 30 kg/m$^2$, in which case active-phase labor may not occur until 7 to 8 cm, with individuals having higher BMIs experiencing the onset of active-phase labor at more advanced dilatations.[15]

Adapted from *Intrapartum care for healthy women and babies.* London: National Institute for Health and Care Excellence (NICE); 2017 Feb. PMID: 32212591. https://www.nice.org.uk/guidance/cg190/resources/intrapartum-care-for-healthy-women-and-babies-pdf-35109866447557; *WHO Labor Care Guide: User's Manual.* Geneva: World Health Organization; 2020. https://www.who.int/publications/i/item/9789240017566#:~:text=The%20WHO%20Labour%20Care%20Guide%20is%20a%20tool,and%20managers%20of%20maternal%20and%20child%20health%20services; Caughey AB, Cahill AG, Guise JM, Rouse DJ. Safe prevention of the primary cesarean delivery. *Am J Obstet Gynecol.* 2014;210(3):179-193; Kominiarek MA, Zhang J, Vanveldhuisen P, Troendle J, Beaver J, Hibbard JU. Contemporary labor patterns: the impact of maternal body mass index. *Am J Obstet Gynecol.* 2011;205(3):244.e241-248.

sequential cervical examinations ideally performed by the same clinician) or at 6 cm or more,[13] regardless of the rate of previous cervical change (Table 26-2).[14] Unless labor is clearly advanced, a single cervical dilation measurement does not reliably differentiate labor phases. For this reason, a period of triage prior to admission to the birth facility and ongoing midwifery care can be helpful to determine whether progressive cervical changes are occurring.

## Initial Evaluation of the Person Presenting with Signs and Symptoms of Labor

Many primary care and pregnancy-related concerns can mimic labor onset. Initial evaluation of an individual presenting with signs and symptoms of labor includes review of their history, physical assessment, and, often, laboratory investigations. The *Assessment for Diagnosis of Labor* appendix provides information on the initial evaluation. The initial assessment should aim to holistically and thoroughly assess the current physical well-being of the laboring person and fetus, and understand and contextualize their health and pregnancy history, social situation, and expectations.

In making a diagnosis of labor, clinicians must carefully differentiate not only between prelabor and labor, but also between labor and any obstetric or non-obstetric pregnancy-related or non-pregnancy-related discomforts or complications, such as urinary tract infections, vaginitis, and placental abruption. Care for non-obstetric pregnancy-related complications is discussed in the *Medical Complications in Pregnancy* chapter.

A comprehensive approach to assessment is necessary to identify actual and potential problems and to create a mutually agreeable and appropriate plan of care. The beginning of labor is a time for reassessment of the individual's personal preferences and health needs for the birth and postpartum period. Thorough assessment and open discussion are important at the beginning of labor and throughout the birthing process.

### History and Current Concerns

Many individuals have signs and symptoms that mimic labor during pregnancy. Listening to the person's concerns is important for a thorough and accurate assessment. Information about the person's history can be obtained from their health record, when possible, but key aspects of their history should be confirmed. See the *Assessment for Diagnosis of Labor* appendix for more information on obtaining a thorough history.

### Physical Examination

A complete chart review, history, and physical examination are important in the first assessment of someone who presents with signs and symptoms of labor. Signs of labor can mimic many other conditions, and individuals may have developed risk factors that need additional care. The examination is presented in the remainder of this section by system, consistent with typical charting. However, the physical exam should happen in an organized manner that minimizes disruption to the individual. The *Assessment for Diagnosis of Labor* appendix presents the essential components of the physical and pelvic examinations performed at the initial labor evaluation.

### Fetal Heart Rate

Assessment of the fetus is an essential component of care for individuals with signs of labor. The

*Fetal Assessment During Labor* chapter provides details regarding obtaining and interpreting fetal heart rate (FHR). National guidelines are silent on the preferred method of evaluating FHR for those pregnant individuals presenting for evaluation with labor signs and symptoms. In institutions that have continuous electronic fetal monitoring capability, it is common practice to obtain a baseline FHR recording (e.g., 20 minutes) as part of the initial evaluation of fetal well-being. This practice, when applied to individuals who do not have a prenatal or health risk for fetal acidemia, does not improve perinatal outcomes and, when compared to initial assessment by intermittent monitoring, may be associated with an increase in intrapartum interventions, including continuous electronic fetal monitoring (relative risk [RR] = 1.30; 95% confidence interval [CI] = 1.14–1.48) and cesarean birth (RR = 1.20; 95% CI = 1.00–1.44).[16] National guidelines are clear regarding the appropriateness of intermittent auscultation for ongoing evaluation of low-risk individuals in labor.[4,17]

### Laboratory Studies

Available prenatal records can provide valuable information on the birthing person's blood type and Rh status, anemias, glucose tolerance testing, and specific perinatal infections including group B *Streptococcus* (GBS) carrier status, hepatitis B and C infection or carrier status, and prior sexually transmitted infections. If prenatal records are not available, all routine prenatal laboratory tests should be obtained. Clinical judgment and institutional policy will influence the decision to order further laboratory studies when the person presents to the birth facility. If intravenous access is indicated, blood specimens can be obtained concurrently with intravenous catheter placement. The *Assessment for Diagnosis of Labor* appendix identifies laboratory studies commonly performed for evaluation of an individual with labor signs and symptoms.

## Assessment of Individuals Presenting with Signs and Symptoms of Labor and Developing a Plan of Care

After a thorough history and physical exam, an assessment of the status of the individual presenting with signs and symptoms of labor is made. Facets of this assessment include whether the individual is in labor, fetal factors, and whether the individual needs ongoing midwifery care.

Differentiating between latent labor and active labor is one of the important elements of assessment for people presenting with signs of labor. Diagnosis of active labor and timing of labor admission are clinical decision points that influence birth outcomes, specifically cesarean birth. Table 26-2 (Chapter 26) summarizes the criteria for diagnosis of active labor. Admission to the birth facility or midwifery presence for a planned home birth is appropriate for individuals in active labor, but may also be appropriate for individuals not yet in active labor depending on other facets of the assessment.

Fetal heart rate, if assessed by continuous fetal monitoring, is categorized in the assessment portion of the clinical note using standardized terminology. This approach provides a concise summary of the risk of fetal acidemia and is useful in planning clinical care.

Overall maternal status and well-being, GBS status, and pertinent other items are also summarized in the assessment following a comprehensive assessment. Following a comprehensive assessment, a customized plan is made.

### Determination of Need for Ongoing Midwifery Care

Based on the laboring individual's preferences, latent versus active labor status, FHR assessment, a thorough history and physical exam, and health and pregnancy risk factors, a determination can be made regarding whether the individual should be admitted into the birth facility and their level of needed care. For individuals planning a home birth, the midwife makes decisions on the need for midwifery presence and the need for transfer to a birth facility.

#### *In Active Labor*

For low-risk individuals admitted in active labor, ongoing midwifery care and presence has been associated with improved birth outcomes.[18] Some laboring individuals with high-risk conditions, such as hypertensive disorders, infection, obstetric hemorrhage, or preterm gestation, may require team-based care with physician colleagues or transfer to a birth facility with a higher level of resources. To reduce perinatal morbidity and mortality, ensuring the laboring individual is receiving risk-appropriate care specific to their healthcare needs is essential.[19] Local clinical practice guidance, often based on national guidelines, can provide more detail on which facilities are appropriate based on the laboring individual's medical needs and regional facility capabilities.

### Not in Active Labor and Without Risk Factors

Studies support that delaying admission to the birth facility until the individual is in active labor improves outcomes for low-risk individuals. Many low-risk individuals admitted to hospitals for labor are not yet in the active phase.[20,21] Early admission to the birth facility has been associated with increased rates of intervention.[21-23] Following assessment, otherwise well individuals who are not in active labor can be sent home with information on when to return to the clinic or birth facility.

However, many factors can influence admission timing, including other health needs, lack of safe places for the individual to be during early labor, and the preference of the laboring individual. After shared decision making, an individual at term may opt to remain at the hospital in latent labor. If an individual needs or wants to be admitted prior to active labor, best practice includes minimizing unnecessary interventions and using labor progress rather than time from admission to guide decision making. Early labor lounges may be an alternative to facility admission that allow the individual to stay close to the location of birth but not receive intensive monitoring.[24]

### Not in Active Labor but Needing Ongoing Midwifery Care

Individuals who are not in active labor may need to be admitted to the birth facility. For example, some individuals may have developed complications that require ongoing midwifery care. Without intervention, these complications may be associated with poor perinatal outcomes. Some individuals may benefit from additional outpatient monitoring, while others may need inpatient care such as an induction of labor, especially at term gestation. Examples of complications include nonreassuring testing, PROM, intrauterine infection, and hypertensive disorders. Individuals experiencing complications may also need transfer to a facility that can provide a higher level of care for the laboring person or newborn.[19,25] Care of pregnant and laboring individuals with complications is discussed in the *Pregnancy-Related Conditions* and *Complications During Labor and Birth* chapters.

### Care Following Prelabor Rupture of Membranes

Prelabor rupture of membranes is discussed in more detail in the *Complications During Labor and Birth* chapter. If the decision is made to expedite labor and birth, the plan of care should take into consideration the status of the cervix, the presence of uterine contractions, and the status of the fetus. More information on induction of labor is discussed in the *Complications During Labor and Birth* chapter. Cervical ripening with prostaglandins or mechanical methods or immediate induction of labor with oxytocin can be used as appropriate depending on the individual's cervical status. Vaginal methods of cervical ripening can be used for persons with PROM.

## Admission to the Birth Facility

When a person is admitted to a birth facility, orders are placed that outline their perinatal care. This set of orders provides information useful to the team providing the care. Table 26-3 outlines common facets of care addressed in admission orders.

| Table 26-3 | Common Orders on a Birthing Person's Admission to a Birth Facility |
|---|---|
| **Orders** | |
| Admission to the birth facility or transfer of care to a different facility | |
| Medications (home and intrapartum) | |
| • Home medication reconciliation | |
| • Intrapartum medications as indicated (group B *Streptococcus* prophylaxis, hypertension treatment, labor induction as indicated) | |
| • Postpartum medications planned for third stage | |
| Labs: Often include a complete blood count (CBC) with platelets and lab tests as needed based on any medical conditions; in some areas with high rates of sexually transmitted infections, human immunodeficiency virus (HIV) and syphilis testing are repeated on admission | |
| Blood bank orders | |
| Vital signs (temperature, pulse, respirations, blood pressure) | |
| Comfort techniques or medications desired by individual (consult with anesthesia as needed) | |
| Fetal heart rate monitoring | |
| Uterine monitoring | |
| Activity level of the birthing person | |
| Oral fluids and diet | |
| IV access, fluid type, and rate of infusion (if applicable) | |

---

**Sample Intrapartum Admission Note**

---

**Patient Name: [REDACTED] Date: [TODAY] Time: <u>0100</u>**

**Chart Review:**

Prenatal course: Uncomplicated—routine prenatal care with midwives since 8 weeks' gestation. Declined genetic testing. Singleton gestation.

Prenatal labs: A positive, rubella immune, GC/CT/HIV/RPR neg at 8 weeks' gestation HIV/RPR negative at repeat testing at 28 weeks, H/H at 28 weeks = 34.0/13.2, 1-hour GTT at 28 weeks = 90, GBS positive and GC/CT negative at 35 weeks.

Health/surgical/psych/family/social history: No previous surgeries, all first-degree relatives alive and well, mild depression in college resolved with counseling, regular exercise per patient report

Vaccination history: COVID vaccine × 2 plus booster shot; received flu vaccine at 16 weeks' gestation and Tdap at 28 weeks' gestation

Height, 5 ft 6 in; prepregnancy weight, 125 lb; prepregnancy BMI, 20; last weight at 41.3 weeks, 150 lb (total weight gain, 25 lb)

No known drug allergies

Current medications: PNV 1 po qd

**Subjective:**

This is a 25-year-old, G1P0 cisgender woman at 40.6 weeks' gestation by sure LMP who reports spontaneous onset of contractions at 1600, which became strong, q 3 minutes since 2200. Breathing through contractions. Denies rupture of membranes or vaginal bleeding. Reports active fetus. May want epidural for pain. Here with partner and doula. Reviewed birth preferences: Patient desires upright positioning during labor, epidural upon request, mirror at time of crowning, partner to assist with catch, delayed cord-clamping, skin-to-skin contact after birth. Patient consents to vitamin K and hepatitis B vaccination for newborn. Plans to breastfeed and prefers discharge at 24 hours after birth if possible.

**Objective:**

BP (standing), 122/74; temp, 97.0°F; respirations, 15; pulse, 80

Abdomen: Gravid, left occiput (LOA) by palpation, estimated fetal weight 7 lb

Fetal monitoring: Within 20-minute monitoring segment: baseline 130 beats per minute (bpm), three 15 × 15 bpm accelerations, no decelerations, moderate variability of >10 bpm

Contractions: q 3 minutes lasting 60 seconds, moderate to palpation and soft uterine resting tone

Vaginal examination: 6 cm/75% effaced/–1 station/cervix is soft and anterior position, fetus left occiput transverse (LOT) with bag of water palpably intact

**Assessment:**

25-year-old, nulliparous woman in active labor desires unmedicated labor at this time

Fetus Category I

GBS-positive without drug allergy

**Plan:**

1. Admit to birthing unit under midwifery service, OB hospitalist notified of patient admission, anticipate 1-night length of stay from time of birth
2. Labs: Type and screen, complete blood count (CBC) with platelets, and syphilis (due to local prevalence rate)
3. Orders placed for ambulation as desired and consumption of clear liquids and light solids
4. Intermittent fetal monitoring with Doppler every 30 minutes while in active phase without epidural anesthesia
5. IV penicillin G 5 million units now for GBS prophylaxis, then every 4 hours until birth; after initial infusion, change IV access to heplock until needed again
6. Will provide 1-to-1 labor support as needed and if patient requests epidural, will consult anesthesia provider on call

---

An admission order often triggers the provider to input additional information, such as the reason for admission, the preferred hospital unit (such as labor and delivery or postpartum), the provider team, and the anticipated length of stay. In case of a hospital admission, the provider will conduct a medication reconciliation that includes identification of all medications the individual takes at home and information on whether each should be continued during labor. In general, prenatal vitamins do not need to be continued during labor, but other routine medications such as thyroid medication and antidepressants can be administered at their regular intervals or held until postpartum if the birth is expected within the next 24 hours.

Intrapartum medications are also ordered at this time. They may include treatment of hypertension and preeclampsia, or GBS prophylaxis if the birth person has tested positive or has known risk factors for infant infection. (See the *Complications During Labor and Birth* chapter for more information.) Many birthing facilities also require a plan for management of third-stage labor to be entered at the time of the birthing person's admission. The *Third Stage of Labor* chapter provides more detail on medications for management of this phase of labor.

One decision needed on admission orders is which type of laboratory test is indicated regarding holding of blood (i.e., "hold," "screen," or "cross"). All three choices include assessment of blood type and Rh status. A "type and hold" test holds off on further evaluation of a coagulated sample until the need for a blood transfusion is identified. A "type and screen" test evaluates the blood type, Rh status, and antibodies present. The "type and hold" or "type and screen" test is typically chosen for individuals at low to medium risk of postpartum hemorrhage, respectively, although blood bank recommendations should be based on institutional availability and policies. Some institutions no longer hold a specimen in the blood bank, while others request a "type and screen" on all birthing individuals using automated technology (even if they are considered to be at low risk). For individuals at high risk for postpartum hemorrhage, the midwife can order a "type and cross," which determines the same information, but additionally performs a cross-match between the individual's sample and a unit of blood to prepare a product for immediate transfusion.[26]

The exact content and format of orders placed on admission vary by location and facility. Each order represents a decision about intrapartum care, and the plan for care and the orders within the system may change over the course of labor. Where possible, the midwife should discuss the order with the laboring person and used shared decision making to craft the plan of care. More information about the options for each order are discussed in the next section on components of midwifery care for laboring individuals.

## Components of Midwifery Care for Laboring Individuals

Continuing evaluation during labor has three primary foci: (1) well-being of the laboring person (general condition, vital signs, labor support and pain management, laboring person's position and level of activity, hydration and nutrition, intravenous access and infusion, urinary output, membrane status, vaginal mucus discharge and bleeding, infection surveillance, and deep vein thrombosis prophylaxis), (2) fetal assessment, and (3) labor progress (cervical dilation/effacement, fetal presentation and position, fetal adaptation to the maternal pelvis).

### Well-Being of the Laboring Person
#### General Condition of the Laboring Person
Continuing evaluation of the laboring person's well-being includes evaluation of several areas that interrelate and overlap: level of fatigue and physical depletion, behavior and responses to labor, perception of pain, and access to coping strategies/supports.[27] The level of fatigue and depletion of a laboring person is affected by their state at the start of labor, hydration during labor, length of labor, and access to labor coping strategies. This can be a vicious cycle: A lack of access to internal or external coping resources may increase fatigue, and fatigue can decrease the ability to access coping strategies. Occasionally, a laboring person enters labor exhausted and dehydrated from days of the symptoms characteristic of the end of pregnancy or a prolonged latent phase. Labor care should be individualized to the person's needs for rest and hydration to support labor progress.

A laboring person's behavior changes throughout labor, and these changes can be used to evaluate the best ways to support their labor progress. Expressions and behaviors are affected by the person's culture, their degree of labor self-efficacy, anxiety or fear, expectations, social support, and perceived pain. Support for laboring persons during labor is discussed in the *Support During Labor* chapter.

#### Vital Signs
The frequency with which vital signs are assessed in the absence of complications varies among settings and is typically detailed in institutional policies. The frequency of vital signs for low-risk individuals in labor may be based on tradition rather than current evidence. A commonly used pattern of vital signs assessment for low-risk individuals without epidural anesthesia during the first stage of labor is detailed in Table 26-4.

| Table 26-4 | Vital Signs Frequency for Low-Risk Individuals in Labor Without Anesthesia |
|---|---|

Respirations on admission

Heart rate: Every 1 to 4 hours (4 hours for low-risk individuals)

Pulse oximetry may be included with heart rate at some facilities.

Blood pressure: On admission and every 1 to 4 hours for normotensive, low-risk individuals

Temperature: On admission and every 2 to 4 hours when the temperature is normal and the membranes are intact, and every 1 to 2 hours if the temperature is greater than 100.4°F or 38°C and/or after the membranes have been ruptured

As a person's risk status may change over the course of labor, the frequency of vital signs assessment should be adjusted to match their unique situation.

### Labor Support and Pain Management

Labor support and pain management are intertwined. Labor support consists of techniques and interventions that support the physical and emotional experiences of the individual in labor and includes recognizing the therapeutic value of human presence—a hallmark of midwifery. Reviewed in detail in the *Support During Labor* chapter, support and pain management are basic components of midwifery care throughout labor.

### Laboring Person's Position and Level of Activity

The level of physical activity and positions during labor are ideally chosen by the birthing person. It is rare to have a contraindication to a position. When given a choice, many people prefer an upright position or ambulation throughout much of labor, alternating with supported positions for rest. However, the birth environment may affect the level of empowerment the laboring person has to assert their desires. Many hospitals have a culture of laboring in bed, which is often not optimal for either labor progress or the laboring person's comfort. Midwives should advocate on behalf of the rights of laboring people to have autonomy in their positions, movement, and level of activity.

Laboring persons assuming upright positions have shorter labor durations by approximately 1 hour and are less likely to have an epidural or cesarean birth, as compared to those who maintain recumbent positions.[28] Furniture, pillows, birthing balls, or an adjustable bed can be used creatively to support a laboring person in a variety of upright positions, including hands and knees, sitting, standing, and squatting. The midwife can support activity and freedom of choice of positions through routine use of intermittent fetal auscultation and a hand-held Doppler fetoscope.

Individuals who have physical mobility disabilities often require additional modifications to facilitate comfort and labor progression and can work with their team to meet their needs. Finally, individuals who have a history of sexual or physical abuse may find certain labor and birth positions, or having clinicians stand over them, particularly triggering of their previous trauma. For these individuals, if a plan has not been established prenatally for labor care, discussion early in labor to identify preferred positions is recommended. All laboring individuals should receive trauma-informed, respectful care that makes them feel supported during labor and birth.

When resting in bed is desired or necessary, lateral recumbent positions are preferred to supine positions because they reduce the potential for aortic/vena cava compression with resulting hypotension and potential fetal compromise. Lateral positions also facilitate kidney function and do not interfere with coordination and efficiency of uterine contractions.

If the fetus is in a cephalic presentation and the presenting part is engaged in the pelvis or well applied to the cervix, there is no reason to restrict ambulation or upright positions after rupture of membranes. These activities may be desirable to the laboring person, as the intensity of the contractions often increases after rupture of membranes, and upright positions facilitate comfort. Ambulation or upright positions may be contraindicated in case of rupture of membranes with malpresentation or an unengaged fetal head because of the heightened risk of umbilical cord prolapse.

Individuals with an epidural or conditions such as preeclampsia, placental abruption, or acute infection may need to restrict their activity due to their physiologic instability, the effect of medications, or the need for continuous electronic fetal monitoring. Even if walking is not a possibility, the individual can change positions frequently in the bed. While in bed, frequent position changes are encouraged, as well as use of pillows, birth balls, and/or peanut balls between the legs. These supportive measures can increase comfort for the laboring person as well as promote widening of the diameter of the pelvic outlet, fetal repositioning, and fetal descent. Further information on nonpharmacologic support measures in labor can be found in the *Support During Labor* chapter.

### Hydration and Nutrition

Oral consumption of fluids during labor is important for the birthing person's hydration, nutrition, and comfort. Self-regulated oral intake in labor has also been associated with increased feelings of control and lower stress levels.[29,30] Adequate hydration during labor assists in the delivery of oxygen and nutrients as well as facilitates the elimination of waste from the contracting uterus, aiding in uterine efficiency during labor. Clear liquid options include water, fruit juices without pulp, coconut water, carbonated beverages, low-sodium broth, clear tea, black coffee, and sports drinks.[29,31] Isotonic sports drinks have been studied as a means of supplying energy and electrolytes during labor.[32] An important component of selection is for the laboring person to have fluids they enjoy consuming.

Food and fluid consumption in early labor is important to provide nutrients, energy, and hydration for the labor ahead, especially for nulliparous individuals. In a 2017 meta-analysis of 3982 birthing persons, researchers found that less-restrictive food intake was associated with significantly shorter duration of labor and no negative perinatal outcomes.[30] It is common for individuals in active labor to not be hungry or to be mildly nauseous, especially when they are experiencing pain. Gastric emptying rates depend on volume, pH, osmolality, and fat content. Therefore, oral intake in labor should include easily digestible foods and fluids that are low in acid and fat, noncaffeinated, and nonaromatic, and that contain some sugar and salt. For individuals without anesthesia, these foods must be able to be easily consumed in the break between contractions. Suggested food examples include fresh or dried fruit, ice pops, toast or bagel with jam or peanut butter, applesauce, honey sticks, and oatmeal.

Vomiting is common during the period of rapid cervical change. Emesis in active labor necessitates common sense for decreasing intake of fluids and food. Single-episode vomiting in labor does not warrant treatment with antiemetics, but if vomiting is repeated, pharmacologic treatment should be offered. Vomiting may be a pain response, so adjustment of coping strategies should be considered. Rarely, when vomiting is excessive, a bolus of

intravenous fluid hydration (lactated Ringer's solution with or without glucose) may be beneficial.

Despite the known benefits of oral intake in labor, protocols in many U.S. facilities limit food intake due to a 1946 review by Dr. Curtis Mendelson that reported a risk of gastric content aspiration during or after the administration of anesthesia.[31,33] However, prolonged fasting in labor is associated with production of ketones, which may result in ketosis for the birthing person.[29] Consequences of limited fluid or food intake can include a rising pulse and fatigue, as well as dissatisfaction with the birth experience.[34] In 2016, the American Society of Anesthesiologists (ASA) revised its position to recommend that birthing persons in hospital settings whose labors are progressing normally be offered modest amounts of clear liquids.[31] Circumstances that put the individual at increased risk for pulmonary aspiration, such as preoperative poor physical status, hypertension, severe preeclampsia, neurologic disorder, gastritis, previous abdominal surgery, esophageal disease, elevated body mass index (BMI), and increased risk for difficult intubation, provide a basis for risk identification and targeted recommendations.[31] In light of the 2017 meta-analysis noting the benefits of less restrictive food intake, other current evidence,[3,29] and the 2016 ASA revised recommendations,[31] some hospitals have lifted their restrictions on oral intake during labor. Home and birth center settings do not have stipulations around oral intake during labor. Instead, these settings encourage normal food and fluid consumption in early labor and then follow the cues of the laboring person during active labor to support physiologic labor processes.

### Intravenous Access and Infusion

Intravenous (IV) access involves placement of a small catheter within a superficial vein. The needle and tubing can then be hooked up to a continuous infusion, often known as an IV, or can be capped off and used as needed, often known as a saline lock. IV access in labor can be initiated when needed or placed prophylactically.

Routine prophylactic insertion of IV access is unnecessary in the provision of physiologic labor and birth care for those persons with no significant prenatal or health risks. Although found to be safe, this intervention limits freedom of movement and is not necessary. Requiring IV access and/or fluid infusion in the absence of prenatal or health risks is not in alignment with guidance on supporting normal physiologic labor and birth.[4,29]

The decision to initiate IV access during labor should be based on individual risk factors, such as whether the laboring person can tolerate oral fluids and whether they are at risk for postpartum hemorrhage. IV access is also necessary for administration of epidural anesthesia and some medications, such as antibiotics, pain medications, and oxytocin. Placement of the IV in a body location that allows freedom of movement is important. For example, using a ventral or dorsal forearm vein instead of a radial or antecubital vein will allow the laboring person to bend their wrist and arm, which is helpful for laboring and pushing. If initiating IV access is indicated, the clinician should consider use of a saline lock when medications are not infusing to avoid tethering the laboring person to an IV pole.

Appropriate use of IV fluids can decrease the likelihood of adverse events. For example, prior to initiation of epidural anesthesia, establishing IV access allows for administration of isotonic fluid such as lactated Ringer's solution to mitigate epidural-related hypotension. Continuing access after epidural placement allows for ongoing fluid administration and medication administration should complications develop. A saline lock (as a primary or secondary line) may be beneficial for a birthing person at moderate or high risk of postpartum hemorrhage to allow for rapid use of IV uterotonics during and after the third stage of labor.

### Urinary Output

A distended bladder can impede the progress of labor by preventing fetal descent as well as increasing discomfort and pain. A laboring person should be encouraged to empty their bladder at least every 2 hours during the active phase of labor. The individual can walk to the toilet if there are no contraindications to ambulation. Methods to promote voiding include listening to the sound of running water, running warm water over the perineum, applying light suprapubic pressure, and perineal relaxation. If the laboring person is unable to be out of bed, they can be provided with a clean disposable pad or a bedpan on which to void. If these strategies are unsuccessful, catheterization may be indicated. If this intervention is needed, consider whether it will likely be the only catheterization prior to second-stage labor. If multiple catheterizations are likely, placement of an indwelling catheter may decrease the number of catheterizations, improving comfort and decreasing risk of infection.[35]

With deepening descent of the fetal presenting part into the pelvis during labor, the bladder may be compressed to the point at which even small urine volumes cause distension. Bladder distension can occur in any laboring person, but is especially likely in those with epidural anesthesia who received a bolus of fluid prior to initiating the epidural. Once the epidural is active, the urge to urinate is not felt, and the muscle control needed to void is not present. A distended bladder may appear as a bulge above the symphysis pubis. When the fetus is in a posterior position, the contour of the abdomen may look as though there is a full bladder; bladder distension must be ruled out in such a case. In the event of bladder distension, the first step is to facilitate spontaneous voiding. If efforts are not successful, intermittent or indwelling insertion of a urinary catheter to drain the bladder is recommended to minimize the risk of urinary retention or infection, especially if the laboring person is remote from delivery.

### Membrane Status Evaluation

During labor, with increasing strength of contractions and fetal descent, the membranes may spontaneously rupture. Careful attention should be paid to the laboring individual's report of a release of vaginal fluids, or when changing protective pads or sanitary pads, to assess for ruptured membranes. The time of rupture, amount, and color of the fluid provide important assessment information. Depending on institutional policies and birth setting, meconium-stained fluid may require additional staff to assist with the newborn assessment and transition to life. Immediately after the membranes rupture, the fetal heart rate should be assessed as ROM is a risk for prolapsed cord.

### Vaginal Mucus Discharge and Bleeding

It is not uncommon for laboring individuals to have increased small amounts of bloody show and vaginal mucus, which often indicates cervical change. Frank, bright red bleeding in moderate amounts may be indicative of an obstetric emergency such as placenta previa and requires immediate assessment and intervention.

### Infection Surveillance

Vital signs are one part of surveillance for infection during labor. Increased temperature (greater than 100.4°F or 38°C) and pulse (more than 100 beats per minute) are other important signs of infection that should guide further investigation and treatment. Amniotic fluid odor can also be a sign of infection. The laboring person's report of chills, which are normal in the first hour after epidural anesthesia due to the sympathetic nervous system reaction, can also be a symptom of a spiking fever. Prompt treatment of suspected infection can improve perinatal outcomes. For more information about labor care in the presence of infection, as well as GBS prophylaxis, refer to the *Complications During Labor and Birth* chapter.

### Deep Vein Thrombosis Prophylaxis

Pregnancy and the postpartum periods present an increased risk for venous thromboembolism (VTE), including deep vein thrombosis (DVT) and pulmonary embolism. Risk for VTE in the perinatal period is also increased for individuals with inherited thrombophilias, history of a VTE, elevated BMI, and increasing parity (more than three children).[36] Individuals at greater risk for VTE may have been on anticoagulants (e.g., heparin) during pregnancy. However, these medications should be discontinued prior to or at the start of labor and not resumed until after the birth.

To mitigate the risk of VTE during the intrapartum period, the use of sequential (or pneumatic) compression devices can be considered for a nonambulatory laboring person, such as during the use of epidural anesthesia if the person has minimal motor control.[37] These devices are also used when magnesium sulfate is administered. The compression device is placed on the legs and has cuffs that fill with air to squeeze the legs. The squeezing increases blood flow through the veins of the legs in an effort to prevent blood clots.

## Fetal Assessment

Fetal monitoring is important for ongoing FHR evaluation and should be conducted via the method most appropriate to the individual and fetus. The *Fetal Assessment During Labor* chapter details the methods and indications for intermittent auscultation of FHR as well as continuous external and continuous internal FHR assessment.

## Labor Progress

### Uterine Contraction Assessment

Contractions usually increase in frequency and strength over the course of the first stage of labor. Strong, regular contractions are usually needed to cause the necessary cervical changes during physiologic birth at term. Assessment of uterine contractions begins with discussion with and observation of the laboring person. The person's response to contractions provides insights into the frequency, duration, and intensity of contractions, though responses to labor vary widely. The person's external response to a contraction is influenced by environment, culture, and individual coping abilities. Individuals generally sense contractions when the contractions exert approximately 15 mm Hg of intrauterine pressure; this is also the minimum strength of contraction that can be detected by an observer's hand. The rise of the uterus within the abdomen during a contraction can be visualized or palpated with an individual of low or normal BMI. Palpation of the fundus provides information on the strength, frequency, and duration of the contraction, as well as relaxation time between contractions. Contractions are measured as mild, moderate, or strong in intensity. They are presumed to be sufficient to produce labor progression when they are moderate or strong as determined by palpation—that is, when the uterine fundus does not allow indentation on palpation at their acme. Thus, for laboring people at low risk for complications, palpation may be all the assessment needed, especially if labor is progressing well. While progressive cervical changes are the best indicator of contractions that will progress labor, it is generally accepted that three contractions within 10 minutes, as averaged over 30 minutes, is the minimum frequency necessary to achieve progressive cervical changes in active labor, while 5 contractions per 10 minutes is considered the upper limit of normal.[38,39]

If assessment of uterine strength, frequency, and duration is inconclusive via observation and/or palpation and more information is needed, uterine activity can be further evaluated with one or more electronic monitoring methods: an external tocodynamometer, an intrauterine (intra-amniotic) pressure catheter (IUPC), or electrical uterine myography. When considering continuous electronic uterine monitoring, the need for data should be described to the individual and their preferences discussed using shared decision making. Some electronic monitoring devices (external and internal) can assess contractions without tethering the individual to the monitor.

An external electronic tocodynamometer functions by capturing a graphic image of a contraction as the abdomen lifts against the pressure transducer, which is held in place by an abdominal band or adhesive. External tocodynamometry can measure the frequency and duration of uterine contractions; however, it relies on correct placement and calibration and may not work well for individuals with elevated BMIs. In addition, the tocodynamometer is highly sensitive to a person's movement, predisposing the data to artifacts and errors.

Internal monitoring is the most accurate—and most invasive—method of evaluating uterine activity. Introduction of an IUPC may be indicated when labor dystocia is suspected or to treat recurrent FHR variable decelerations with amnioinfusion. See the *Intrauterine Pressure Catheter* appendix for information on placement of this device. When placed correctly, the IUPC provides information about the frequency, duration, and intensity of contractions. Internal uterine monitoring may detect increases in uterine tone slightly sooner than the individual or attendants.[40] The IUPC also allows for instillation of an isotonic fluid, such as a normal saline, into the uterus (amnioinfusion) to treat recurrent variable FHR decelerations associated with fetal umbilical cord compression.[13,41] To use this kind of catheter, the membranes must be ruptured. Placement of an IUPC carries with it a rare risk of uterine perforation, thought to range between 1 in 300 and 1 in 1400 placements, usually due to improper placement in the extramembranous space.[42] Insertion of an IUPC has been associated with some other rare adverse outcomes as well, such as placental abruption, placental vessel perforation, and development of intrauterine infection; in regard to the last possibility, IUPCs are often placed for assessment of prolonged labor, which is also associated with development of intrauterine infection.

When using an IUPC, Montevideo units (MVUs) are used to assess the strength of uterine contractions (see the *Fetal Assessment During Labor* chapter for more information). MVU levels are determined by subtracting the numeric amplitude of each contraction that occurs in a 10-minute window from the baseline uterine tonus amplitude (in millimeters of mercury, mm Hg), and then summing the total calculated rise in amplitude over the 10-minute time period. "Adequate" contractions with an IUPC are defined as greater than 200 MVUs.[43]

To counter the limitations of tocodynamometers, researchers and some hospitals are using electrical uterine myography.[44] This emerging method of electronic uterine monitoring uses electrodes placed on the abdomen to ascertain electrical activity of the uterine muscle, similar to how an electrocardiogram records electrical conduction in the heart. This promising technology provides the same information as a tocodynamometer, but has the advantage of not being as strongly affected by BMI, abdominal wall thickness, or the person's position.

### Vaginal Examinations During Labor

Vaginal examinations are used to assess labor progress. The cervix is usually assessed in labor using

| Table 26-5 | Indications for Vaginal Examination During Labor |
|---|---|
| Determine labor status prior to labor admission (prelabor, latent, or active labor) | |
| Inform care decisions related to management of labor pain | |
| Determine fetal presentation, position, and adaptation to the pelvis | |
| Assess progress in labor (ensure adequate time between exams to note progress) | |
| Assess reasons for fetal heart rate changes (deep or prolonged decelerations) | |
| Check for a suspected prolapsed cord after spontaneous rupture of membranes (e.g., previously ballotable presenting part or fetal heart rate decelerations) | |
| Verify complete dilatation | |

the examiner's fingers, or digits—a process known as digital cervical examination. During normal first-stage labor, a vaginal examination may be indicated for the reasons shown in Table 26-5.

The unique clinical situation of the laboring person and their preferences, along with the clinical judgment and expertise of the clinician, are important when considering the necessity of performing an examination. An examination is needed only if it will provide information useful in providing appropriate labor care. Internal examinations are intrusive and uncomfortable, and they increase the risk of infection; however, they can inform labor management. Frequency of examinations depends on the laboring person's condition, the fetal heart tones, and the midwife's ability to use other parameters for labor progress evaluation. These other parameters include the individual's behavior, contraction pattern, signs and symptoms of transition into second-stage labor, change of location of back pain, change in location of maximum intensity of fetal heart tones, and electronic fetal monitoring (EFM) tracing. Shared decision making between the midwife and the laboring person should be used to decide if and when to perform a vaginal examination. Cervical examinations require explicit, informed, and ongoing consent using trauma-informed language before each time they are performed throughout labor. Because each examination carries a risk of infection, the midwife should maximize the information obtained with each exam. Many important components should be assessed during a vaginal examination, as summarized in Table 26-6.

| Table 26-6 | Intrapartum Vaginal Exam Assessment Components |
|---|---|

Cervical position (posterior, mid-position, anterior)

Cervical consistency (firm, medium, or soft)

Cervical effacement

Cervical dilatation

Membrane status and presence of a forebag
If amniotic fluid is present, color and odor

Fetal presentation, position, and synclitism

Fetal caput succedaneum formation

Fetal station (as measured from the fetal skull, not the caput)

Adaptation of the fetal presenting part to the space available in the pelvis

Presence of show or bleeding, including amount and color

Digital examinations rely on the proprioceptive skill of the clinician. Clinicians who provide labor care accurately determine actual cervical dilatation in only half of all cases, but are accurate to within 1 cm (plus or minus 1 cm) of actual cervical dilatation in approximately 90% of cases.[45–47] Cervical evaluations in laboring persons with advanced dilatation (7 to 10 cm) and low effacement (25%) are more difficult.[48] It is recommended that serial examinations be performed by the same clinician whenever possible to allow for assessment of progress over time.

### Expected Progression of Labor

Clinical expectations of cervical dilation and fetal descent during labor were influenced for decades by the research of Emanuel Friedman, beginning in the 1950s.[49–54] Friedman obtained data for laboring individuals within a fairly demographically homogeneous population and plotted their cervical dilatation to depict the typical progress of labor. He reported that the slowest acceptable rates of cervical dilation in the most progressive part of active labor for nulliparous and multiparous persons were 1.2 cm per hour and 1.5 cm per hour, respectively.[50,51,53,54] Broad but flawed application of these findings in clinical practice culminated in what became known as the "1 cm per hour rule," wherein it became commonplace for clinicians to expect the cervix to dilate at least 1 cm per hour during active labor. Labors that did not progress at this minimal rate were considered too slow. The 1 cm per hour rule was pervasive in clinical settings for more than half a century.

Labor care now differs in many ways from that offered in the era in which Friedman conducted his research. Today, laboring individuals frequently use epidural analgesia to manage labor pain, whereas in the 1950s they used sedatives and morphine. In Friedman's work, if a laboring person had not birthed spontaneously after 2 hours in the second stage of labor, an episiotomy and forceps delivery were performed; today, operative vaginal birth is used much less frequently. Most importantly, demographic and birth-related factors have changed since the time of Friedman's research. Today, birthing people enter labor with significantly higher BMIs and age compared to those in Friedman's studies—both factors are known to slow labor progress.[15,55] Thus, the Friedman estimates are no longer applicable to modern laboring populations.

Much of the current understanding of labor patterns comes from a group of researchers led by Zhang et al., who used modern statistical techniques to provide evidence about both the duration of first-stage labor and the pattern of labor progression with spontaneous labor onset.[10] The Zhang team analyzed observational data of 228,668 birthing persons from different areas of the United States, 87% of whom gave birth from 2005 to 2007.[10] Their labors were typical of contemporary populations in the United States, as many of these individuals received interventions such as amniotomy, oxytocin augmentation, and epidural analgesia. Zhang and colleagues found that the average labor curve for nulliparous persons did not show a clear inflection point when dilation accelerated to indicate the beginning of active labor; in contrast, in multiparous individuals, labor appeared to accelerate after 6 cm.[10,56–58] These researchers also demonstrated that the slope of cervical dilation was not linear; instead, cervical dilation rates progressively accelerated with each passing centimeter for nulliparous, primiparous, and multiparous individuals.[10,57,58] Accordingly, the duration of time needed to dilate from one centimeter to the next was commonly shorter with each passing centimeter after the spontaneous onset of labor. Moreover, as rates of cervical dilation accelerated with advancing labor, the time necessary to dilate from one centimeter to the next was typically less variable.[10,58]

Findings from Zhang and other researchers on labor progress have been adopted by U.S. clinicians in whole or in part and are a central part of the guidelines proposed by ACOG and the Society for

Maternal–Fetal Medicine (SMFM) for the safe prevention of primary cesarean births.[13] As reflected by these guidelines, clinicians can be reassured by the findings of Zhang and colleagues that vaginal birth is frequently the outcome for slow but progressive labor without evidence of compromise in the birthing person or fetus. No longer should cesarean births be recommended to birthing persons for the sole indication of slow labor progression. However, assessment and interventions to speed labor progress should be considered when the duration of the active phase is statistically beyond the normal range (i.e., more than 2 standard deviations slower than the average cervical dilation rate, or beyond the 95th percentile).

In the face of modern evidence that cervical dilation rates typically become faster as active labor advances, the World Health Organization (WHO) now recommends nonlinear assessment of active labor, wherein advancing cervical dilatations have shorter clinical alert time values regardless of the birthing person's parity.[12] The WHO time parameters for normal labor progression are longer than the durations endorsed by ACOG and SMFM. For example, under the WHO labor care guidelines, clinicians would be alerted when cervical dilatation remains at 5 cm during active labor for 6 or more hours, when dilatation remains at 6 cm for 5 or more hours of active labor, when dilatation remains at 7 cm for 3 or more hours, when dilatation remains at 8 cm for 2.5 or more hours, or when dilatation remains at 9 cm for 2 or more hours.[12]

Many midwives provide care for laboring people with physiologic labor that does not involve use of interventions aimed at speeding the laboring process. Albers[59,60] and Jones and Larson[61] studied the duration of spontaneous active labor among low-risk individuals who gave birth vaginally without oxytocin, epidurals, or operative deliveries. In their studies, active labor was defined as the time necessary for the cervix to dilate from 4 cm to 10 cm (Table 26-7). Viewed linearly, active labor dilation rates in these studies averaged 0.8 to 1.0 cm per hour for nulliparous individuals and 1.1 to 1.4 cm per hour for multiparous individuals, whereas the slowest but still normal rate (i.e., mean dilation rate = 2 standard deviations) rates were 0.3 to 0.5 cm per hour and 0.4 to 0.5 cm per hour, respectively. Unfortunately, these studies are decades old, and criteria for active labor determination have appropriately changed based on newer research evidence.

Tilden and colleagues studied the duration of spontaneous labor using a cohort of more than

| Table 26-7 | Duration and Cervical Dilation During Spontaneous Active-Phase Labor in Laboring People with Physiologic Labor and Vaginal Birth | | | | | |
|---|---|---|---|---|---|---|
| Publication | N | Dilation for Active-Phase Onset (cm)[a] | Active-Phase Duration (in hours) | | Rate of Dilation (cm/hr)[b] | |
| | | | Mean (SD) | Mean Multiplied by 2 SD | Mean | Limit |
| **Nulliparous Individuals** | | | | | | |
| Albers et al., 1996 | 949 | 4 | 7.7 (5.9) | 19.4 | 0.8 | 0.3 |
| Albers, 1999 | 2511 | 4 | 7.7 (4.9) | 17.5 | 0.8 | 0.3 |
| Jones et al., 2003 | 240 | 4 | 6.2 (3.6) | 13.4 | 1.0 | 0.5 |
| **Multiparous Individuals** | | | | | | |
| Albers et al., 1996 | 949 | 4 | 5.7 (4.0) | 13.7 | 1.1 | |
| Albers, 1999 | 2511 | 4 | 5.6 (4.1) | 13.8 | 1.1 | |
| Jones et al., 2003 | 240 | 4 | 4.4 (3.4) | 11.6 | 1.4 | |

*Abbreviations:* N, number of individuals within the sample; SD, standard deviation.

[a]Absolute value taken as evidence of active-phase onset (in centimeters).
[b]Calculated based on the assumption that the cervical dilation phase ends at 10 cm, which approximates complete cervical dilation.

Based on Albers LL, Schiff M, Gorwoda JG. The length of active labor in normal pregnancies. *Obstet Gynecol.* 1996;87(3):355-359; Albers LL. The duration of labor in healthy women. *J Perinatol.* 1999;19(2):114-119; Jones M, Larson E. Length of normal labor in women of Hispanic origin. *J Midwifery Womens Health.* 2003;48(1):2-9.

75,000 individuals who had planned a home or birth center birth. The definitions used for data collection in this study differed from those used in other data sets, making comparisons among studies difficult. In the Tilden et al. data set, active labor was defined by the midwife's assessment and did not require a cervical exam, and the end of first stage was defined as the beginning of pushing phase as noted by the midwife attendant. These researchers found that the mean time from when the midwife recorded that the person was in active labor until the "pushing" phase began was 11.9 hours (standard deviation, 15.4 hours); for multiparous individuals, however, the mean time was 4.6 hours (standard deviation, 5.6 hours).[62]

More contemporary studies of physiologic labor are needed. Only by understanding spontaneous labor progression can clinicians decide if and when interventions aimed at speeding labor progress should be presented as appropriate options to laboring persons.[14] Reinforcing the value of using appropriate norms to assess labor progress are research findings that some populations have significantly longer labor durations than those studied by Zhang and colleagues, including people in countries outside the United States,[63–65] as well as those with an elevated BMI,[15] with diabetes,[66] or of older age.[67] Normal progress of induced labor also includes longer durations between each centimeter, particularly before 6 cm.[68] Even fetal gender has been reported to influence labor progress, with male fetuses being associated with longer active phases.[69,70]

### Fetal Presentation, Position, and Station

Assessment of descent and internal rotation of the fetal presenting part is as important as assessment of progressive cervical dilation when monitoring labor progress. Fetuses rotate and descend differently depending on their size, their position, and the birthing person's pelvis. The fetus negotiates the birth canal based on the diameter of the fetal head and the birthing person's pelvis and, with the force of the contractions, naturally takes advantage of the roomiest portions of the pelvis. (See the *Anatomy and Physiology of Labor and Birth* chapter and the *Fetal-Pelvic Relationships* appendix for more information.) Therefore, once the cervix is dilated enough to feel the fetal presenting part, assessment of the fetal presentation and position are important clinical findings. Station can be assessed regardless of the extent of dilatation.

Studies defining normal labor duration and progression are largely based on cohorts of laboring individuals with a singleton fetus in a vertex presentation. Most commonly, the fetus enters the pelvis in an occiput transverse position and then internally rotates to occiput anterior at the level of the pelvic ischial spines. This can happen before labor, during early labor, or in active labor.

By contrast to the slow dilation that occurs as the fetus in an occiput position descends and rotates, prolonged arrest of descent, even in the presence of cervical dilation, may indicate cephalopelvic disproportion or fetal malpositioning. For more on these complications, refer to the *Complications During Labor and Birth* chapter.

Because cephalic presentations are by far the most common, it is important to identify the essential landmarks of the fetal skull (as described in the *Anatomy and Physiology of Labor and Birth* chapter) with each internal examination. In addition to the landmarks, variations in the shape of the fetal head, such as molding and caput succedaneum, can be important assessment findings, as the fetal head is subjected to the pressure of the birth canal, pelvic floor muscles, and surrounding structures. More information is in the *Fetal-Pelvic Relationships* appendix. The formation of a few millimeters of caput succedaneum is not unusual or abnormal. By contrast, formation of extensive caput succedaneum, which makes the identification of fetal sutures and fontanels difficult, combined with molding, occurs when intrauterine pressure has been great and labor prolonged. Cephalopelvic disproportion must be suspected when significant molding or overriding sutures are noted. A sizable caput may also be seen when the fetal position is occipitoposterior.

Recently, point-of-care ultrasound has been explored as a tool for diagnosing malpositions and asynclitism. Ultrasound appears to be a promising modality for this application; however, the data may not be clinically useful given the relative lack of evidence-based treatments for specific fetal malpositions.[71] Use of different positions and movements for treatment of fetal malpositions is reviewed in the *Complications During Labor and Birth* chapter. Care of laboring persons who have a fetus in a persistent occiput posterior position is reviewed in the *Second Stage of Labor and Birth* chapter.

### Influence of Elevated Body Mass Index on Labor Progression

Individuals with an elevated BMI (greater than or equal to 30 kg/m$^2$) have an increased risk for labor, birth, and postpartum complications compared to individuals with a BMI less than 30 kg/m$^2$.[72,73] However, professional guidelines on care of laboring

| Table 26-8 | Median and 95% percentile (hours) for Progression of Cervical Dilation from 4 to 10 cm in Nulliparous and Multiparous People by Body Mass Index (BMI) Category (kg/m²) | | | | |
|---|---|---|---|---|---|
| | **BMI Category (kg/m²)** | | | | |
| | **< 25.0** | **25.0–29.9** | **30.0–34.9** | **35.0–39.9** | **> 40.0** |
| Nulliparous | 5.4(18.2) | 5.7(18.8) | 6.0(19.9) | 6.7(22.2) | 7.7(25.6) |
| Multiparous | 4.6(17.5) | 4.5(17.4) | 4.7(17.9) | 4.0(19.0) | 5.4(20.6) |

Data from Kominiarek MA, Zhang J, Vanveldhuisen P, Troendle J, Beaver J, Hibbard JU. Contemporary labor patterns: the impact of maternal body mass index. *Am J Obstet Gynecol*. 2011;205(3):244.e1-8. doi:10.1016/j.ajog.2011.06.014.

individuals with elevated BMIs are lacking, unclear, or discrepant.[74,75] Current evidence indicates that labor progression slows with each additional BMI point, even when adjusting for confounding variables such as height, age, epidural anesthesia use, gestational weight gain, and fetal size.[15,55,76,77] Several changes in the body caused by excess leptin or cholesterol, and by adipose accumulation in myometrial cells, are theorized to cause functional impairment of uterine contractility.[15,78-80]

In general, augmentation of labor or operative delivery should not be recommended in an otherwise healthy laboring person and fetus until their labor traverse times are as slow or slower than 95% of other people with similar BMIs and parity (Table 26-8). For example, it can take more than 7 hours longer (25.6 − 18.2 = 7.4 hours) for a person with a BMI greater than 40 kg/m² to dilate from 4 cm to 10 cm, as compared to a person whose BMI is less than 25 kg/m².

Given that most clinicians do not individualize their expectations of labor progression based on the birthing person's BMI, interventions such as oxytocin augmentation are more often used with individuals with higher BMIs.[81] When oxytocin is utilized for augmentation, higher doses and a longer duration may be needed to support progression of labor.[78,82] In addition, amniotomy for labor augmentation may not be as effective in laboring people with higher BMIs as it is for individuals with BMIs less than 30 kg/m².[83] Despite these challenges, laboring people with an elevated BMI can be supported to achieve a safe vaginal birth with appropriate encouragement and watchful waiting using evidence-based guidelines.

### Influence of Pain and Anesthesia on Labor Progression

For laboring individuals, the experience of pain can be complex. Decisions about how to manage pain should be based on patient preference, stage of labor, institutional options, and side effects. A thorough informed consent discussion must include the risks, benefits, and alternatives to the pain relief options being considered. While epidural anesthesia is the most effective form of pharmacologic pain relief for laboring individuals planning a vaginal birth and is associated with high patient satisfaction, it is also associated with higher rates of oxytocin augmentation, a longer second stage of labor, and higher rates of operative births.

### Amniotic Membranes

There are limited indications for artificial rupture of membranes (AROM) during labor (amniotomy), and routine use of this procedure with a spontaneous term labor may do more harm than good.[3] Risks associated with AROM include discomfort from the procedure, umbilical cord compression with resultant FHR decelerations, umbilical cord prolapse, increased risk of infection, abrasion of the fetal head and, rarely, rupture of fetal vessels (with vasa previa). AROM has commonly been believed to accelerate the progress of labor and is used frequently in contemporary practice. It can also be used in the late second stage of labor to examine the amniotic fluid and determine whether additional help is needed at the time of birth in case of moderate or thick meconium-stained fluid.

The use of AROM as a routine measure to speed the progress of labor in those persons without labor dystocia has been evaluated in several randomized trials. In a Cochrane meta-analysis of 15 randomized control trials (*n* = 5583), routine AROM in the first stage of normally progressing spontaneous labor was not associated with significant reductions in the length of labor, cesarean delivery, or neonatal outcomes compared with no amniotomy.[84] ACOG concurs, stating that amniotomy should not be performed in individuals with normally progressing labor, unless required to facilitate fetal monitoring—guidance that aligns with long-standing midwifery practice.[4] AROM is also used as an intervention to induce labor either alone or with other agents, or as a treatment for dystocia, as discussed in the *Complications During Labor and Birth* chapter.

If there is a clinical rationale for performing an amniotomy, a cephalic presentation and engagement in the pelvis should be confirmed. Before performing AROM, the midwife should carefully assess fetal station and ensure the fetal head is well applied to the cervix (if the cervix is still present). Keeping the fingers against the cervix, the membranes can be gently disrupted with the amnihook; care should be taken to avoid scratching the fetal head. The clinician's fingers should be left in place during the initial gush of fluid to assess for prolapsed cord. The FHR should be assessed during the procedure and monitored frequently for at least one full contraction cycle afterward.

---

**Sample Labor Progress Note @ 0430**

**Subjective:**

25-year-old, G1P0 cisgender woman is laboring well. Now comfortable in semi-recumbent position after epidural placed at 0400. Has questions about what to expect with pushing. Partner and doula at bedside providing supportive care.

**Objective:**

Vital signs: Blood pressure, 128/68 between contractions; pulse, 76; respirations, 20; temperature, 98.9°F

2.5 mu IV PCN completed for GBS prophylaxis at 0300

Abdomen: Remains LOA by abdominal palpation

Contractions per toco q 3 minutes lasting 80 seconds, strong to palpation and relaxed tone in between contractions

Continuous electronic fetal monitoring: Baseline 135 beats per minute (bpm), positive accelerations, no decelerations, moderate variability of 10 bpm

Vaginal exam deferred at patient request (last cervical exam at 0100: 6 cm/75%/–1 station/intact)

**Assessment:**

Nulliparous woman with contraction pattern suggesting normal active labor per external monitoring

Category I fetal heart rate

GBS-positive status with administration of 1 dose of penicillin G

Membranes intact

**Plan:**

1. Next penicillin dose due at 0700 for adequate GBS prophylaxis
2. Recheck cervix with permission for increased pressure or if indicated by EFM.
3. Continue to provide labor support, encourage rest and frequent position changes every 20–30 minutes. Review what to expect in second stage of labor with respect to urge to push, pushing effort, and typical length of second stage.
4. Anticipate spontaneous vaginal birth

---

# Conclusion

Physiologic labor is an intricate interplay of physiologic and psychological forces within the laboring person and with their care environment. Caring for individuals in labor involves attention to multiple but equally important variables, including the well-being of the laboring person, the well-being of the fetus, and labor progress. Care during the first stage of labor should be based on evidence, but also be personalized for each individual and consider the person's preferences for care as well as their medical needs. Attentive and evidence-based care can greatly improve perinatal outcomes. Supporting physiologic birth is a hallmark of midwifery. Individuals remember the care they received in labor throughout their lives, and compassionate and affirming intrapartum care creates positive memories and a sense of accomplishment.

## Resources

| Organization | Description |
|---|---|
| American College of Nurse-Midwives (ACNM) | *Evidence-Based Practice: Pearls of Midwifery*: PowerPoint presentation and printable checklists on evidence for labor care practices |
| Healthy Birth Initiative | Resources for consumers, midwives, and maternity care institutions |
| American College of Nurse-Midwives (ACNM), Midwives Alliance North America (MANA), National Association of Certified Professional Midwives (NACPM) | *Supporting Healthy and Normal Physiologic Childbirth*: a consensus statement by ACNM, MANA, and NACPM, 2012 |
| American College of Nurse-Midwives (ACNM), Association of Women's Health, Obstetric, and Neonatal Nurses (AWHONN), National Association of Certified Professional Midwives (NCAP), Lamaze | The *Birth Tools* website has tools for clinicians to safely optimize the outcomes of labor. Content includes tools for coping in labor, promoting spontaneous onset of labor, nutrition and hydration, and physiologic second stages. |
| American College of Obstetricians and Gynecologists (ACOG) and Society for Maternal–Fetal Medicine (SMFM) | *Safe Prevention of the Primary Cesarean: Obstetric Consensus #1* reviews recommended labor care practices that can reduce the incidence of cesarean birth. |
| Childbirth Connection | *Transforming Childbirth* provides a blueprint for action, including steps toward a high-quality, high-value maternity care system. |
| National Institute for Health and Care Excellence (NICE) | Based in Britain, this organization provides information about intrapartum care for healthy individuals and their infants. |
| World Health Organization (WHO), Department of Reproductive Health and Research | *WHO Labor Care Guide* provides guidance for supportive care, monitoring, and documentation of labor care around the world. |

## References

1. Supporting healthy and normal physiologic childbirth: a consensus statement by ACNM, MANA, and NACPM. *J Perinat Educ.* 2013;22(1):14-18.

2. Osterman M, Hamilton B, Martin JA, et al. Births: final data for 2020. *Natl Vital Stat Rep.* 2021;70(17): 1-50.

3. Alhafez L, Berghella V. Evidence-based labor management: first stage of labor (part 3). *Am J Obstet Gynecol MFM.* 2020;2(4):100185.

4. American College of Obstetricians and Gynecologists. ACOG Committee Opinion No. 766: approaches to limit intervention during labor and birth. *Obstet Gynecol.* 2019;133(2):e164-e173.

5. American College of Nurse-Midwives. BirthTools. org: tools for optimizing the outcomes for labor safely. http://birthtools.org/MOC-Promoting-Physiological -Pushing. Published 2015. Accessed September 30, 2021.

6. Nilsson C, Hessman E, Sjöblom H, et al. Definitions, measurements and prevalence of fear of childbirth: a systematic review. *BMC Pregnancy Childbirth.* 2018;18(1):28.

7. Middleton P, Shepherd E, Flenady V, et al. Planned early birth versus expectant management (waiting) for prelabour rupture of membranes at term (37 weeks or more). *Cochrane Database Syst Rev.* 2017;1(1):Cd005302.

8. Siegler Y, Weiner Z, Solt I. ACOG Practice Bulletin No. 217: prelabor rupture of membranes. *Obstet Gynecol.* 2020;136(5):1061.

9. Caughey AB. Is Zhang the new Friedman: How should we evaluate the first stage of labor? *Semin Perinatol.* 2020;44(2):151215.

10. Zhang J, Landy HJ, Ware Branch D, et al. Contemporary patterns of spontaneous labor with normal neonatal outcomes. *Obstet Gynecol.* 2010;116(6): 1281-1287.

11. National Institute for Health and Care Excellence. In: *Intrapartum Care for Healthy Women and Babies: Clinical Guideline.* London, UK: National Institute for Health and Care Excellence; 2017. https://www .nice.org.uk/guidance/cg190. Accessed November 21, 2022.

12. World Health Organization. *WHO Labour Care Guide: User's Manual.* Geneva, Switzerland: World Health Organization; 2020.

13. Caughey AB, Cahill AG, Guise JM, Rouse DJ. Safe prevention of the primary cesarean delivery. *Am J Obstet Gynecol.* 2014;210(3):179-193.

14. Neal JL, Lowe NK, Schorn MN, et al. Labor dystocia: a common approach to diagnosis. *J Midwifery Womens Health.* 2015;60(5):499-509.

15. Kominiarek MA, Zhang J, Vanveldhuisen P, et al. Contemporary labor patterns: the impact of

maternal body mass index. *Am J Obstet Gynecol.* 2011;205(3):244.e241-e248.

16. Devane D, Lalor JG, Daly S, et al. Cardiotocography versus intermittent auscultation of fetal heart on admission to labour ward for assessment of fetal wellbeing. *Cochrane Database Syst Rev.* 2017;1(1):Cd005122.

17. Arnold JJ, Gawrys BL. Intrapartum fetal monitoring. *Am Fam Physician.* 2020;102(3):158-167.

18. Neal JL, Carlson NS, Phillippi JC, et al. Midwifery presence in United States medical centers and labor care and birth outcomes among low-risk nulliparous women: a Consortium on Safe Labor study. *Birth.* 2019;46(3):475-486.

19. Levels of maternal care: Obstetric Care Consensus No. 9. *Obstet Gynecol.* 2019;134(2):e41-e55.

20. Neal JL, Lowe NK, Phillippi JC, et al. Likelihood of cesarean birth among parous women after applying leading active labor diagnostic guidelines. *Midwifery.* 2018;67:64-69.

21. Neal JL, Lowe NK, Phillippi JC, et al. Likelihood of cesarean delivery after applying leading active labor diagnostic guidelines. *Birth.* 2017;44(2):128-136.

22. Mikolajczyk RT, Zhang J, Grewal J, et al. Early versus late admission to labor affects labor progression and risk of cesarean section in nulliparous women. *Front Med (Lausanne).* 2016;3:26.

23. McNiven PS, Williams JI, Hodnett E, et al. An early labor assessment program: a randomized, controlled trial. *Birth.* 1998;25(1):5-10.

24. Paul JA, Yount SM, Breman RB, et al. Use of an early labor lounge to promote admission in active labor. *J Midwifery Womens Health.* 2017;62(2):204-209.

25. AAP Committee on Fetus and Newborn, ACOG Committee on Obstetric Practice. *Guidelines for Perinatal Care.* 7th ed. Elk Village, IL: American Academy of Pediatrics Books; 2017. doi.org/10.1542/9781610020886.

26. Lagrew D, McNulty J, Sakowski, C, Cape V, Main E, Morton, CH. *Improving Health Care Response to Obstetric Hemorrhage: A California Maternal Quality Care Collaborative Toolkit.* 2022. https://www.cmqcc.org/resources-tool-kits/toolkits. Accessed September 30, 2021.

27. Howard ED. Promoting maternal confidence, coping, and comfort in latent labor: evidence-based strategies and resources. *J Perinat Neonatal Nurs.* 2018;32(4):291-294.

28. Lawrence A, Lewis L, Hofmeyr GJ, Styles C. Maternal positions and mobility during first stage labour. *Cochrane Database Syst Rev.* 2013;8:Cd003934.

29. Providing oral nutrition to women in labor: American College of Nurse-Midwives. *J Midwifery Womens Health.* 2016;61(4):528-534.

30. Ciardulli A, Saccone G, Anastasio H, Berghella V. Less-restrictive food intake during labor in low-risk singleton pregnancies: a systematic review and meta-analysis. *Obstet Gynecol.* 2017;129(3):473-480.

31. Practice guidelines for obstetric anesthesia: an updated report by the American Society of Anesthesiologists Task Force on Obstetric Anesthesia and the Society for Obstetric Anesthesia and Perinatology. *Anesthesiology.* 2016;124(2):270-300.

32. Kubli M, Scrutton MJ, Seed PT, O'Sullivan G. An evaluation of isotonic "sport drinks" during labor. *Anesth Analg.* 2002;94(2):404-408, table of contents.

33. Mendelson CL. The aspiration of stomach contents into the lungs during obstetric anesthesia. *Am J Obstet Gynecol.* 1946;52:191-205.

34. Bouvet L, Garrigue J, Desgranges FP, et al. Women's view on fasting during labor in a tertiary care obstetric unit: a prospective cohort study. *Eur J Obstet Gynecol Reprod Biol.* 2020;253:25-30.

35. Millet L, Shaha S, Bartholomew ML. Rates of bacteriuria in laboring women with epidural analgesia: continuous vs intermittent bladder catheterization. *Am J Obstet Gynecol.* 2012;206(4):316.e311-317.

36. Alsheef MA, Alabbad AM, Albassam RA, et al. Pregnancy and venous thromboembolism: risk factors, trends, management, and mortality. *Biomed Res Int.* 2020;2020:4071892.

37. Pacheco LD, Saade G, Metz TD. Society for Maternal–Fetal Medicine Consult Series #51: thromboembolism prophylaxis for cesarean delivery. *Am J Obstet Gynecol.* 2020;223(2):B11-B17.

38. ACOG Practice Bulletin No. 107: induction of labor. *Obstet Gynecol.* 2009;114(2 pt 1):386-397.

39. Executive summary: neonatal encephalopathy and neurologic outcome, second edition. Report of the American College of Obstetricians and Gynecologists' Task Force on Neonatal Encephalopathy. *Obstet Gynecol.* 2014;123(4):896-901.

40. Parer J, King T, Ikeda T. *Electronic Fetal Heart Rate Monitoring: The 5-Tier System.* Burlington, MA: Jones & Bartlett Learning; 2018.

41. Caughey AB, Cahill AG, Guise J, Rouse DJ, American College of Obstetricians and Gynecologists. Safe prevention of the primary cesarean delivery. *Am J Obstet Gynecol.* 2014;210(3):179-193.

42. Lind BK. Complications caused by extramembranous placement of intrauterine pressure catheters. *Am J Obstet Gynecol.* 1999;180(4):1034-1035.

43. Krapohl AJ, Myers GG, Caldeyro-Barcia R. Uterine contractions in spontaneous labor: a quantitative study. *Am J Obstet Gynecol.* 1970;106(3):378-387.

44. Huber C, Shazly SA, Ruano R. Potential use of electrohysterography in obstetrics: a review article. *J Matern Fetal Neonatal Med.* 2021;34(10):1666-1672.

45. Buchmann EJ, Libhaber E. Accuracy of cervical assessment in the active phase of labour. *BJOG.* 2007;114(7):833-837.

46. Phelps JY, Higby K, Smyth MH, et al. Accuracy and intraobserver variability of simulated cervical dilatation measurements. *Am J Obstet Gynecol.* 1995;173(3 Pt 1):942-945.

47. Tuffnell DJ, Bryce F, Johnson N, Lilford RJ. Simulation of cervical changes in labour: reproducibility of expert assessment. *Lancet.* 1989;2(8671):1089-1090.

48. Nitsche JF, Goodridge E, Kim SM, et al. Evaluation of the patterns of learning in the labor cervical examination. *Simul Healthc.* 2019;14(6):378-383.

49. Friedman E. The graphic analysis of labor. *Am J Obstet Gynecol.* 1954;68(6):1568-1575.

50. Friedman EA. Primigravid labor: a graphicostatistical analysis. *Obstet Gynecol.* 1955;6(6):567-589.

51. Friedman EA. Labor in multiparas: a graphicostatistical analysis. *Obstet Gynecol.* 1956;8(6):691-703.

52. Friedman EA, Kroll BH. Computer analysis of labour progression. *J Obstet Gynaecol Br Commonw.* 1969;76(12):1075-1079.

53. Friedman EA, Kroll BH. Computer analysis of labor progression. III. Pattern variations by parity. *J Reprod Med.* 1971;6(4):179-183.

54. Friedman E. *Labor: Clinical Evaluation and Management.* 2nd ed. Norwalk CT: Appleton-Century-Crofts; 1978.

55. Norman SM, Tuuli MG, Odibo AO, et al. The effects of obesity on the first stage of labor. *Obstet Gynecol.* 2012;120(1):130-135.

56. Zhang J, Troendle J, Mikolajczyk R, et al. The natural history of the normal first stage of labor. *Obstet Gynecol.* 2010;115(4):705-710.

57. Laughon SK, Branch DW, Beaver J, Zhang J. Changes in labor patterns over 50 years. *Am J Obstet Gynecol.* 2012;206(5):419.e411-e419.

58. Zhang J, Troendle JF, Yancey MK. Reassessing the labor curve in nulliparous women. *Am J Obstet Gynecol.* 2002;187(4):824-828.

59. Albers LL, Schiff M, Gorwoda JG. The length of active labor in normal pregnancies. *Obstet Gynecol.* 1996;87(3):355-359.

60. Albers LL. The duration of labor in healthy women. *J Perinatol.* 1999;19(2):114-119.

61. Jones M, Larson E. Length of normal labor in women of Hispanic origin. *J Midwifery Womens Health.* 2003; 48(1):2-9.

62. Tilden EL, Snowden JM, Bovbjerg ML, et al. The duration of spontaneous active and pushing phases of labour among 75,243 US women when intervention is minimal: a prospective, observational cohort study. *EClin Med.* 2022;48:101447.

63. Lu D, Zhang L, Duan T, Zhang J. Labor patterns in Asian American women with vaginal birth and normal perinatal outcomes. *Birth.* 2019;46(4):608-615.

64. Ashwal E, Livne MY, Benichou JIC, et al. Contemporary patterns of labor in nulliparous and multiparous women. *Am J Obstet Gynecol.* 2020;222(3):267.e261-267.e269.

65. Suzuki R, Horiuchi S, Ohtsu H. Evaluation of the labor curve in nulliparous Japanese women. *Am J Obstet Gynecol.* 2010;203(3):226.e221-226.

66. Timofeev J, Huang CC, Singh J, et al. Spontaneous labor curves in women with pregnancies complicated by diabetes. *J Matern Fetal Neonatal Med.* 2012;25(1):20-26.

67. Zaki MN, Hibbard JU, Kominiarek MA. Contemporary labor patterns and maternal age. *Obstet Gynecol.* 2013;122(5):1018-1024.

68. Harper LM, Caughey AB, Odibo AO, et al. Normal progress of induced labor. *Obstet Gynecol.* 2012;119(6):1113-1118.

69. Cahill AG, Roehl KA, Odibo AO, et al. Impact of fetal gender on the labor curve. *Am J Obstet Gynecol.* 2012;206(4):335.e331-335.e335.

70. Meibodi MR, Mossayebi E, Najmi Z, Moradi Y. Normal labor curve is affected by fetus gender: a cohort study. *Med J Islam Repub Iran.* 2017;31:93.

71. Dall'Asta A, Rizzo G, Masturzo B, et al. Intrapartum sonographic assessment of the fetal head flexion in protracted active phase of labor and association with labor outcome: a multicenter, prospective study. *Am J Obstet Gynecol.* 2021;225(2):171.e171-171.e112.

72. Marchi J, Berg M, Dencker A, et al. Risks associated with obesity in pregnancy, for the mother and baby: a systematic review of reviews. *Obes Rev.* 2015;16(8):621-638.

73. Reither M, Germano E, DeGrazia M. Midwifery management of pregnant women who are obese. *J Midwifery Womens Health.* 2018;63(3):273-282.

74. American College of Obstetricians and Gynecologists. ACOG Practice Bulletin No 156: obesity in pregnancy. *Obstet Gynecol.* 2015;126(6):e112-e126.

75. National Academies of Sciences, Engineering, and Medicine. *Birth Settings in America: Outcomes, Quality, Access, and Choice.* Washington, DC: National Academies Press; 2020.

76. Hilliard AM, Chauhan SP, Zhao Y, Rankins NC. Effect of obesity on length of labor in nulliparous women. *Am J Perinatol.* 2012;29(2):127-132.

77. Carlhall S, Kallen K, Blomberg M. Maternal body mass index and duration of labor. *Eur J Obstet Gynecol Reprod Biol.* 2013;171(1):49-53.

78. Carlson NS, Hernandez TL, Hurt KJ. Parturition dysfunction in obesity: time to target the pathobiology. *Reprod Biol Endocrinol.* 2015;13:135.

79. Muir R, Ballan J, Clifford B, et al. Modelling maternal obesity: the effects of a chronic high-fat,

high-cholesterol diet on uterine expression of contractile-associated proteins and ex vivo contractile activity during labour in the rat. *Clin Sci (Lond)*. 2016;130(3):183-192.

80. Carlson NS, Breman R, Neal JL, Phillippi JC. Preventing cesarean birth in women with obesity: influence of unit-level midwifery presence on use of cesarean among women in the Consortium on Safe Labor data set. *J Midwifery Womens Health*. 2020;65(1):22-32.

81. Carlson N, Lowe N. Intrapartum management associated with obesity in nulliparous women. *J Midwifery Womens Health*. 2014;59(1):43-53.

82. Carlson N, Corwin E, Lowe N. Oxytocin augmentation in spontaneously laboring, nulliparous women: multilevel assessment of maternal BMI and oxytocin dose. *Biol Res Nurs*. 2017;19(4):382-392.

83. Hiersch L, Rosen H, Salzer L, et al. Does artificial rupturing of membranes in the active phase of labor enhance myometrial electrical activity? *J Matern Fetal Neonatal Med*. 2015;28(5):515-518.

84. Smyth RM, Markham C, Dowswell T. Amniotomy for shortening spontaneous labour. *Cochrane Database Syst Rev*. 2013;6:Cd006167.

APPENDIX

# 26A

# Assessment for Diagnosis of Labor

NICOLE S. CARLSON, JEREMY L. NEAL, HEATHER M. BRADFORD, AND JULIA C. PHILLIPPI

Individuals present for midwifery care in late pregnancy with multifaceted concerns, including possible labor. It is often hard to differentiate labor from other sensations of late pregnancy, including increased vaginal discharge, prelabor contractions, and low back pain. A thorough history and examination can provide information valuable in assessment and diagnosis of labor, as well as other pregnancy-related and primary care conditions. Individuals experiencing pain or anxiety can feel very vulnerable when presenting for care; thus, the tone of this assessment visit is crucial, as it can be the basis for the future trust versus wariness with which the laboring person will approach their healthcare providers in the future. As with all assessments, assessment of individuals for possible labor should be sensitive to their needs and allow for the development of a plan of care that is founded on evidence, personalized, and congruent with their culture.

## History

If the prenatal record is available, it can be used as the source of information for much of the history. Specifically, personal information, past pregnancy history, past health and primary healthcare history, and family history should be reviewed. Present pregnancy history should be reviewed to confirm the items in Table 26A-1, such as gestational age and estimated date of birth, significant prenatal events, and presence of a personalized plan for birth. This spares the laboring person from having to reiterate history they provided prenatally and being disturbed at a time when they may be coping with the demands of labor. However, critical items of the history should be double-checked with the individual, including verification of the existence

of drug allergies, blood transfusions and reactions, and major pregnancy or health complications during pregnancy. Documentation that the prenatal record was reviewed should be included in the intrapartum admission note. An interim history that includes any change in health status from the time of the last documented visit, chief concern, and history of present illness, coupled with a brief review of pertinent systems, will complete the history and help guide the physical examination. Table 26A-1 outlines the essential components of the health history when evaluating an individual presenting for labor evaluation.

An individual presenting for labor evaluation without an available prenatal record or no previous perinatal care presents a challenge to the care team. The individual may have received regular prenatal care but simply not have records available for a variety of reasons, such as miscommunication about the expected birth location or travel. In the absence of a prenatal record, the clinician must elicit essential information from the laboring person directly, beginning with those data most relevant to the acuity of the clinical scenario.

## Physical Examination

Essential components of the physical examination performed at the initial labor evaluation are presented in Table 26A-2. When a prenatal record is available, components performed prenatally can be used as a baseline and compared with the current physical examination. The review of the previous examination should be documented in the health record.

The exam is usually conducted by doing noninvasive assessment first, moving from head to toe, and then getting specific consent before conducting a speculum or pelvic exam. The physical exam

| Table 26A-1 | Essential Components of the Health History When Evaluating an Individual Presenting in Labor |
|---|---|
| **Component** | **Clinical Implications** |
| Presenting concern(s) | Allows the individual to disclose their concerns and needs and provides important details needed for differentiation of labor from other concerns and diagnoses |
| History of present concern(s) | It is useful to organize the history of the present concern using the OLD CARTS mnemonic: Onset, Location, Duration, Character, Aggravating factors, Relieving factors, Timing, Severity. For example, if the presenting concern is contractions, include the time of contraction onset, location of contractions (e.g., back, lower abdomen), duration/character of contractions from onset to the present (including frequency, duration, and intensity), aggravating and relieving factors, and coping strategies. |
| Age | Birth at the extremes of the reproductive life span is associated with an increased risk for adverse perinatal outcomes. |
| Parity | Influences labor progress and labor duration (e.g., progress is typically slower in nulliparous individuals compared to multiparous individuals) |
| Estimated date of birth (EDD) and estimated weeks of gestational age | Identifies the potential for newborn complications related to prematurity or postmaturity; establishes a baseline for evaluating fetal size as related to gestational age |
| Gestational weight gain and body mass index (BMI) based on latest prenatal weight | Excess gestational weight gain and BMIs greater than 30 kg/m$^2$ in late pregnancy are associated with larger fetal size and glucose intolerance. It is normal for labor to last longer with each increase above 25 kg/m$^2$ in the BMI. |
| Fetal testing, including ultrasound findings (note the placental location if known), noninvasive prenatal genetic screening, maternal-serum alpha feto-protein results | Identifies potential fetal concerns or need for additional staff at the time of birth. Placental placement affects many aspects of care. For example, individuals with low-lying placental placement presenting with frank vaginal bleeding should not receive any internal examinations and should be assessed for placenta previa. |
| Laboratory results including group B *Streptococcus* (GBS) status, hemoglobin/hematocrit, glucose tolerance testing results, human immunodeficiency virus (HIV) testing and dates, other sexually transmitted infection (STI) testing such as syphilis | Can be used to prevent vertical transmission of infections, guide decisions about current testing, and/or inform labor care |
| Complications of current pregnancy | Identifies existing or potential problems that may influence midwifery care of the current labor and birth |
| Current medications and vitamins | Current medications and supplements provide insight into the person's health status and valuable information needed to avoid drug interactions. |
| | Most medications can be continued during labor. A few, such as insulin, require more intensive titration during labor. Some medications, such as those used to treat HIV, can interact with commonly used intrapartum medications. |
| | Medications that should be discontinued before or during labor include anticoagulants such as heparin. Low-dose aspirin does not need to be administered in labor but is not associated with peripartum complications. |

*(continues)*

| Table 26A-1 | Essential Components of the Health History When Evaluating an Individual Presenting in Labor (*continued*) |
|---|---|
| **Component** | **Clinical Implications** |
| Major complications of previous pregnancies, including prenatal, intrapartum, and postpartum periods. Key items to assess are history of postpartum hemorrhage, shoulder dystocia, and/or history of an infant with GBS early-onset disease. | Identifies potential recurring problems that may affect the current labor and birth |
| Previous labor experience, including mode of labor onset, labor duration, and previous coping strategies | Provides information about potential labor progress and labor coping strategies |
| Mode of previous births | Identifies previous operative vaginal deliveries or cesarean birth, which may influence midwifery care of the current labor and birth |
| Size of previous infants | Provides estimates of fetal weight and prior vaginal birth of infants similar to the current size of the fetus; suggests ability to allow fetal passage through pelvis |
| Recent fetal movement pattern | Reflects fetal status |
| Vaginal discharge including fluid, show, and bleeding | Differentiated from bloody show, frank vaginal bleeding is abnormal and typically contraindicates performance of a vaginal exam. Frank bleeding requires further evaluation for placenta previa or abruption. Duration of ruptured membranes and characteristics of amniotic fluid will influence care decisions. |
| Activities of the past 24 hours and since beginning of labor signs and symptoms | Can provide insight into other causes of labor-like symptoms such as recent increase in physical activity; also provides more details on the individual's well-being and level of fatigue |
| Recent food and fluids | Provides a baseline from which to assess energy reserves and hydration; also useful in anesthesia care during labor and may be helpful in determining if the individual experiences food insecurity |
| Review of pertinent systems based on history; examples include respiratory, urinary, or neurologic symptoms, and changes in extremities | Provides additional details to assist in a thorough assessment |
| Labor care and coping preferences | Plans for labor care and coping allow for the perinatal team to meet the needs and preferences of the individual. Reviewing a previously submitted birth plan is helpful, but the individual's preferences may have changed and should be solicited anew. |
| History of trauma | History of past trauma and sexual abuse can inform optimal perinatal care. |
| Social determinants of health, including problems with housing, food, utilities, and personal safety | The conditions in which people live profoundly affect their health, and are major contributors to maternal/infant health outcome inequities. Violence is a major cause of maternal death, and resources can be provided to promote safety. Food, housing, and utility insecurity are major barriers to pregnancy health. Short screening tools are available from multiple sources.[1,2] |

| Table 26A-2 | Physical Examination for an Individual Presenting with Labor Signs and Symptoms |
|---|---|
| **Component** | **Significance** |
| **General Health and Abdominal Assessment** | |
| Observation | Person-centered observation throughout the visit is useful in assessing overall physical and emotional state, developmental stage, coping with current sensations, and interactions with support people |
| Vital signs: blood pressure, temperature, pulse, respirations | Elevated blood pressure may indicate a hypertensive disorder; in the presence of a normal diastolic measurement, elevation in systolic blood pressure may indicate anxiety or pain |
| | Elevated temperature indicates an infectious process or dehydration |
| | Elevated pulse and/or respirations may indicate infection, shock, dehydration, or anxiety |
| Auscultation of heart and lungs | Screens for and identifies acute or previously unrecognized conditions that could adversely affect the current labor and birth, including heart murmur or asthma |
| Assessment for costovertebral angle tenderness | Provides information useful in the diagnosis of urinary tract infections, including pyelonephritis |
| Assessment of contractions though observation and palpation | The contraction pattern helps determine labor status and should be assessed by observing the individual and palpating the uterus to determine contraction strength and length as well as resting tone between the contractions. Individuals presenting with signs of preterm labor will benefit from external contraction monitoring as well as observation and palpation. |
| Visual inspection of the abdomen | Identification of dermatoses or bruises could indicate possible dermatologic conditions or history of interpersonal violence needing further assessment; identification of surgical scars confirms surgical history or identifies previously unidentified surgical procedures, including cesarean births |
| Abdominal and uterine palpation for tenderness | Abdominal tenderness can be useful in determining whether gastrointestinal conditions may be causing pain. Examples of conditions that have abdominal tenderness as a symptom include appendicitis, acute fatty liver, cholecystitis, HELLP (hemolysis, elevated liver enzymes, and low platelet count) syndrome, and pancreatitis. See the *Medical Complications in Pregnancy* chapter. |
| | Uterine tenderness can indicate intrauterine infection and/or placental abruption. |
| Abdominal palpation to determine fetal lie, presentation, position, engagement, and estimated fetal weight | Fetal lie, presentation, position, and engagement influence the course of labor and guide decisions regarding positioning in labor, mode of birth, and necessity for consultation, collaboration, or referral. |
| | In relation to gestational age, fetal size identifies the possibility of inaccurate dating, growth that is greater or less than expected, multifetal gestation, oligohydramnios or polyhydramnios, or other abnormalities and their associated complicating factors. Estimated fetal weight via palpation in pregnant individuals with a normal weight body mass index (BMI) can also help guide planning for the birth of a large fetus (i.e., shoulder dystocia).[3] |
| Assessment of fetal heart tones including baseline, variability, accelerations, and decelerations before, during, and after contractions | Provides information on fetal well-being and risk of hypoxia. See the *Fetal Assessment During Labor* chapter. |
| Visual assessment of extremities for rashes, bruises, varicosities, and signs of deep vein thrombosis | Assists in diagnosis of venous thromboembolism disorders. Edema, especially if severe and developing rapidly, can occur during preeclampsia. Bruises can indicate physical trauma. |

*(continues)*

| Table 26A-2 | Physical Examination for an Individual Presenting with Labor Signs and Symptoms (*continued*) |
|---|---|
| **Speculum Examination if Indicated** | |
| Visualization of the vagina, cervix, and vaginal vault | Inspection of the vaginal walls can reveal lesions such as occur with syphilis or herpes, and provides information useful in assessment and diagnosis of vaginitis. See the *Reproductive Tract and Sexually Transmitted Infections* chapter. |
| | Allows visualization of the cervix and vaginal vault to confirm rupture of membranes, collect laboratory specimens, and estimate cervical dilatation and effacement if a digital vaginal exam is too risky, such as in case of prelabor rupture of membranes (PROM). See the *Assessment and Diagnosis of Rupture of Membranes* appendix. |
| Assessment of rupture of membranes | See the *Assessment and Diagnosis of Rupture of Membranes* appendix for more information |
| Collection of fetal fibronectin if indicated | For individuals with signs of preterm labor, a fetal fibronectin test can provide information useful in management. See the *Complications During Labor and Birth* chapter. |
| Collection of a swab of vaginal discharge for assessment of vaginitis if indicated | Allows for microscopy and pH testing of vaginal discharge for diagnosis of candidiasis, bacterial vaginosis, or trichomoniasis. See the *Collecting Laboratory Specimens* appendix. |
| **Pelvic and Cervical Examination if Indicated** | |
| Visual inspection of perineum | Identification of lesions (especially herpetic lesions), vulvar varicosities, and/ or vaginal discharge including amniotic fluid and frank bleeding will impact midwifery care. If there is frank bleeding, consider the placental location before performing a vaginal exam. |
| Cervical examination including position and consistency of the cervix, effacement, and dilatation | Location of the cervix in an anterior or middle position is associated with greater readiness for labor compared to a posterior cervix |
| | Consistency of the cervix (soft, medium, or firm) is an indicator of cervical readiness for change |
| | Progressive cervical effacement and dilation are the diagnostic criteria for labor |
| Membrane status | Palpation of intact fetal membranes or amniotic fluid expulsion on cervical examination is suggestive of membrane status |
| Fetal presentation, position, attitude, and synclitism/asynclitism Station of fetal presenting part Presence of molding or caput succedaneum | Digital examination findings confirm those found abdominally and provide additional detail; if unable to determine cephalic position digitally, ultrasound is indicated |
| | Progressive fetal descent is indicative of active labor |
| | Molding and/or caput can indicate fetal adaptation to the pelvis |
| Relationship of fetus and pelvis | The interaction of the fetal presenting part with the bony pelvis changes over the course of labor and is part of assessment of labor status and progression. See the *Fetal-Pelvic Relationships* appendix. |
| **Optional or Supplemental Examinations** | |
| Measurement of weight | Although rarely measured in labor, the most recent prenatal weight is relevant as a predictor of labor duration (e.g., BMI > 24.99 kg/m² in late pregnancy is associated with longer labor duration, compared to lower BMIs);[4] rapid weight gain may be an indirect measure of edema |

components can be truncated if an individual is clearly in advanced labor and about to give birth, or can be expanded if the individual is experiencing nonlabor distress. For example, individuals presenting with constant pain may need more in-depth assessment for gallbladder-, liver-, and kidney-related disorders.

For some individuals, the initial examination may be insufficient for making clinical decisions. The diagnosis of labor and many other conditions often requires repeat examination over a period of time. Subsequent assessments should include interval history from the individual and needed physical exam components. Ideally, reassessment of the cervix will be performed by the same examiner to improve detection of changes.

The time frame for repeat examination depends on the component or measurement needing reassessment. For example, blood pressure measurements need to be reassessed in accordance with current evaluation for pregnancy-induced hypertension; severe range blood pressures (greater than 160 mm Hg systolic or greater than 110 mm Hg diastolic) should be reassessed in 15 minutes and treatment begun within 30 to 60 minutes.[5] The time frame for reassessment of cervical dilatation should be determined based on the individual's parity, previous labor history, current dilatation, and plans for coping and pain relief. The spacing of cervical exams should allow for enough change to occur for meaningful decision making; for most nulliparous individuals, this interval will likely be at least 2 hours.

If an individual is otherwise considered to be at low risk with no concerning findings in the initial history and examination (i.e., fetal heart rate abnormalities), walking or being upright and active can be encouraged between assessments. Depending on their personal needs and facility guidance, the individual may want to walk around the building, go to a local park, or return home for a few hours prior to reassessment.

## Laboratory Studies

Available prenatal records should be reviewed. Important information to review includes hemoglobin, glucose tolerance testing, and perinatal infections with risk for vertical transmission including group B *Streptococcus* (GBS), hepatitis B and C, syphilis, and human immunodeficiency virus (HIV). Repeat testing may be indicated if these tests were

not obtained in the third trimester or need to be repeated at the time of birth per Centers for Disease Control and Prevention guidelines (e.g., tests for HIV, syphilis, and hepatitis B).[6] Clinical judgment and institutional policy will influence the decision to order further laboratory studies when the person presents to the birth facility. If there are no prenatal records, all routine prenatal laboratory tests should be obtained. If intravenous access is indicated, blood specimens can be obtained concurrently with intravenous catheter placement. Table 26A-3 identifies laboratory studies commonly performed for evaluation of an individual with labor signs and symptoms.

Physical exam findings should be conveyed to the individual. Following the physical exam, further discussion with the individual about their symptoms, concerns, and needs is important. For example, if the person is afebrile, in extreme pain, has a large amount of blood in their urine, and shows no uterine contractions on the monitor, more information about urinary symptoms and family history of renal calculi is indicated. Another example is a pregnant person with anxiety symptoms caused by traumatic life events, such as recent violence or loss, who requires validation of their feelings and resources for support. For all pregnant people presenting for care in late pregnancy, a trauma-informed approach is essential to encourage shared decision making and trust with the client.

## Assessment

Information obtained from the history and physical exam are essential when addressing the pregnant person's concerns and partnering with them to plan for their care. More information about assessment for labor-related concerns at term can be found in the *First Stage of Labor* chapter. Information on nonlabor but pregnancy-related diagnoses can be found in the *Medical Complications in Pregnancy* chapter.

Individuals who present for assessment frequently may need in-depth assessment of their physical concerns by specialists and could benefit from discussion about their larger needs as well. For some pregnant people, triage assessments provide them with relief from anxiety, a safe place to rest, or a warm meal that they are not able to obtain on their own. A holistic and interprofessional approach to care that engages local resources can meet the person's emotional and health needs and improve perinatal outcomes.

| Table 26A-3 | Potential Laboratory Investigations for an Individual Presenting with Labor Signs and Symptoms |
|---|---|
| **Laboratory Test** | **Significance** |
| Complete blood count (CBC) with platelets | Provides baseline measures of hemoglobin and hematocrit, thereby evaluating for anemia (a risk factor for postpartum hemorrhage) |
| | Provides a baseline for the white blood cell (WBC) count, which can indicate infection—although transiently high values (< 15,000/mL) are common in late pregnancy, and normal WBC counts can be as high as 23,000/mL on day 1 postpartum[7] |
| | Provides a baseline platelet count, which may be used by anesthesia personnel when determining eligibility for neuraxial procedures |
| ABO blood type, Rh status, and antibody | Most valuable for individuals being admitted to hospital in labor |
| | Confirms prenatal blood group and Rh status |
| | Facility blood banks may want to screen and/or hold blood in the event that a transfusion is needed later |
| Urinalysis | Most useful for individuals who are not in active labor |
| | Identifies abnormal components in the urine, such as blood, nitrites, and leukocytes, consistent with urinary tract infection |
| | Identifies the presence of ketones, a reflection of fat metabolism and a lack of recent food intake compared to energy expended |
| | Indicates hydration status (i.e., specific gravity measurement) |
| | Identifies protein, a marker for preeclampsia (however, clean-catch urine is not a reliable indicator of proteinuria) |
| **Supplemental Labs as Indicated** | |
| Group B *Streptococcus* | Individuals with unknown GBS status can be tested for GBS using nucleic acid amplification test (NAAT) techniques, be offered GBS treatment if they had a positive GBS test in a previous pregnancy, or be treated if they develop risk factors for neonatal GBS disease[8] |
| Infectious disease screening: HIV, syphilis, others as locally indicated | Initial or repeat labs for infections with the potential for vertical transmission per Centers for Disease Control and Prevention (CDC) guidelines and considering local prevalence rates[6] |
| | Offer opt-out rapid testing in labor for individuals without previous HIV testing in pregnancy and in the third trimester |
| | A test for syphilis should be performed at the initial prenatal visit and at 28 weeks and at the time of labor/birth if in a geographic area with high syphilis rates or with personal risk factors for syphilis acquisition |
| | Hepatitis B virus (HBV) testing is needed for individuals not screened during pregnancy, or who are at high risk or have signs and symptoms of infection |
| Testing for gestational hypertension and preeclampsia | If indicated due to blood pressure (systolic > 140 mm Hg, diastolic > 90 mm Hg), or clinical symptoms (e.g., headache, visual changes, right upper quadrant pain, or signs of pulmonary edema), labs to diagnose hypertensive-related disorders in pregnancy include CBC with platelets, serum creatinine, uric acid, lactate dehydrogenase (LDH), aspartate aminotransferase (AST), alanine aminotransferase (ALT), and urine protein (protein to creatinine ratio or 24-hour urine collection may be appropriate).[5] See the *Medical Complications in Pregnancy* chapter. |
| Ultrasound for presentation and cervical length (if preterm) | Determination of fetal presentation if unable to be confirmed through examination (i.e., fetal skull landmarks palpated digitally during vaginal exam) |
| | Cervical length is indicated for signs of preterm labor in the absence of an indication for birth; transvaginal ultrasound of cervical length may provide information useful in clinical management[9] |
| If no prior prenatal care or records are unavailable | If not already available, order prenatal labs including blood type (plus Rh), red blood cell (RBC) antibody screen, rubella titer, hepatitis B surface antigen (HBsAg), HIV, Venereal Disease Research Laboratory (VDRL)/rapid plasma reagin (RPR), gonorrhea/chlamydia (via urine or vaginal sample), and hemoglobin A1c (although HgbA1c is not a substitute for antenatal glucose tolerance testing, values less than 6.5% are associated with reduced rates of complications)[10] |

## Conclusion

Midwifery assessment of individuals with potential signs of labor should be holistic and person-centered. Individuals presenting with concerns about labor should be assessed carefully in a manner that validates their concerns, is trauma-informed, and includes appropriate history, physical exam, and laboratory components to assess for relevant physiologic and pathologic processes and diagnoses. During labor triage visits, individuals bring with them hope, excitement, and their fears. Midwifery care that fosters trust can form the basis of later affirming and evidence-based health care.

## References

1. O'Gurek DT, Henke C. A practical approach to screening for social determinants of health. *Fam Pract Manag.* 2018;25(3):7-12.

2. Billioux A, Verlander K, Anthony S, Alley D. Standardized screening for health-related social needs in clinical settings: the accountable health communities screening tool. Discussion Paper. *NAM Perspectives.* 2017. https://nam.edu/wp-content/uploads/2017/05/Standardized-Screening-for-Health-Related-Social-Needsin-Clinical-Settings.pdf. Accessed November 11, 2022.

3. Preyer O, Husslein H, Concin N, et al. Fetal weight estimation at term: ultrasound versus clinical examination with Leopold's manoeuvres: a prospective blinded observational study. *BMC Pregnancy Childbirth.* 2019;19(1):122.

4. Kominiarek MA, Zhang J, Vanveldhuisen P, et al. Contemporary labor patterns: the impact of maternal body mass index. *Am J Obstet Gynecol.* 2011;205(3):244.e241-244.248.

5. American College of Obstetricians and Gynecologists' Committee on Practice Bulletins. Gestational hypertension and preeclampsia: ACOG Practice Bulletin, Number 222. *Obstet Gynecol.* 2020;135(6):e237-e260.

6. Workowski KA, Bachmann LH, Chan PA, et al. Sexually transmitted infections treatment guidelines, 2021. *MMWR Recom Rep.* 2021;70(4):1.

7. Dockree S, Shine B, Pavord S, Impey L, Vatish M. White blood cells in pregnancy: reference intervals for before and after delivery. *EBioMedicine.* 2021;74:103715.

8. American College of Obstetricians and Gynecologists. Committee Opinion No. 782: prevention of group B streptococcal early-onset disease in newborns. *Obstet Gynecol.* 2019;134(1):e19-e40.

9. Society for Maternal–Fetal Medicine. When to use fetal fibronectin. https://www.smfm.org/publications/117-when-to-use-fetal-fibronectin. Published 2016. Accessed May 3, 2022.

10. Finneran MM, Kiefer MK, Ware CA, et al. The use of longitudinal hemoglobin A1c values to predict adverse obstetric and neonatal outcomes in pregnancies complicated by pregestational diabetes. *Am J Obstet Gynecol MFM.* 2020;2(1):100069.

APPENDIX

# 26B

# Assessment and Diagnosis of Rupture of Membranes

HEATHER M. BRADFORD AND JEREMY L. NEAL

*The editors acknowledge Nancy Lowe, Sharon Ryan, Linda Hunter, and Amy Marowitz for contributions to this appendix in the previous edition.*

Spontaneous rupture of membranes (SROM) most often occurs during labor, unless an artificial rupture of membranes (AROM) is performed by the clinician. However, prelabor rupture of membranes (PROM) occurs in approximately 8% of individuals with term pregnancies, while preterm (i.e., less than 37 weeks' gestation) prelabor rupture of membranes (PPROM) complicates 2% to 3% of pregnancies.[1] Accurate diagnosis of rupture of membranes (ROM) is essential for determining subsequent assessment strategies and care provision. False-positive diagnoses contribute to misallocation of resources and unnecessary interventions, whereas false-negative diagnoses may lead to adverse birth outcomes. The physiologic basis for spontaneous rupture of membranes is described in the *Anatomy and Physiology of Labor and Birth* chapter. This appendix covers assessment and diagnosis of SROM, PROM, and PPROM. For management steps for individuals not in labor, refer to the *Complications During Labor and Birth* chapter.

Most cases of ROM can be diagnosed through collection of the pregnant person's history and a four-point clinical assessment, including two laboratory tests performed on samples of fluid obtained during the physical examination: the arborization test (fern test) and pH testing (nitrazine test). When findings are equivocal, additional testing for amniotic fluid proteins (e.g., placental alpha microglobulin-1), fetal fibronectin in vaginal secretions, and ultrasound assessment of amniotic fluid volume may be of value.[1,2] When evaluating for SROM, PROM, and PPROM, differential diagnoses include urinary incontinence, normal vaginal or cervical discharge, vaginitis, sexually transmitted infections, and semen or lubricant leakage.

A comprehensive assessment of ROM is presented next. This assessment may be truncated based on results from the beginning steps of the assessment. For example, during active labor at term gestation, visualization of amniotic fluid from the introitus is all that is needed to diagnose ROM, but nitrazine testing of fluid can also prove helpful in differentiating urine from amniotic fluid.

## Chart Evaluation

1. Confirm pregnancy dating (especially if less than 37 weeks' gestation).
2. Review the prenatal record for past pregnancy history, prenatal issues, or current health problems.
3. Review prenatal labs including group B *Streptococcus* (GBS) testing and other infections with the potential for vertical transmission including gonorrhea, chlamydia, human immunodeficiency virus (HIV), syphilis, and herpes.

## History

1. Inquire about the time, amount, color (e.g. clear, pink, bloody, light green, yellow), consistency (i.e., liquid, mucus-like, mixed with particulate meconium), odor, and pattern of

reported fluid leakage (e.g., large gush, continued leaking, single incident of moistness).

a. These data are especially important for development of a management plan because the length of time from ROM to birth is directly correlated with the risk of infection in both the pregnant person and the fetus. The characteristics of the fluid can reveal clues to fetal well-being and be used to determine neonatal care decisions.

b. PROM will often cause a large gush of fluid, followed by a continuous watery discharge that soaks through the person's underwear, necessitating use of sanitary pads or even towels. However, PROM may also present as repeated leaking of small volumes of fluid. In some instances of ruptured membranes, the only symptom the individual may notice is a feeling of moistness on their undergarments from a small, continuous discharge. Pregnant individuals may be able to differentiate between leaking of urine or semen versus PROM by putting on a dry pair of underwear and evaluating for further leaking with ambulation over a period of time.

c. In contrast to PROM, ROM during active labor may not be noticed, especially in cases where the fetal head is low. Presence of a "forebag," or bag of fluid present in front of the fetal head, does not always indicate an intact bag of waters. This is because a laboring person can have ROM from a tear higher in the amniotic sac, then develop a forebag when the fetus descends in labor.

2. Inquire about any recent fever, abdominal trauma or pain, vaginal bleeding, abnormal discharge, bloody show, or urinary symptoms. Ask the individual when they last underwent a vaginal exam or had vaginal intercourse. Examination of the cervix can increase uterine cramping, and the lubricant can cause vaginal discharge or persistent moistness. Increased vaginal discharge may be noted after sexual activity. If present, semen expelled from the vagina can be mistaken for amniotic fluid by the pregnant person. Semen in the vagina can also make diagnosis of ROM difficult, as it has the same pH as amniotic fluid. In these cases,

it is sometimes necessary to use additional testing for amniotic fluid protein.

3. Inquire about signs of labor such as back pain, contractions, and bloody show.

4. Ask about recent fetal movement patterns as part of fetal assessment.

## Physical Examination

A full examination for labor may be appropriate when ROM is reported, and the *Assessment for Diagnosis of Labor* appendix details a full physical examination appropriate for individuals presenting with signs of labor. The earlier an examination is performed after ROM occurs, the easier it is to diagnose this condition. When more than 6 to 12 hours passes, many of the diagnostic observations become unreliable because of decreased fluid leakage. Not all components of the physical exam detailed here are warranted if the initial assessment reveals obvious ROM.

1. Assess the fetal heart rate as described in the *Fetal Assessment During Labor* chapter.

2. Inspect the vulva and vaginal introitus.

a. Observe for copious amniotic fluid from the vagina, which is diagnostic for ROM.

b. Note the color, consistency, and amount of any fluid leaking from the introitus.

c. Ask the person to cough and look for fluid release from the urethra and/or introitus.

d. Inspect the vulva for lesions, if indicated by history and presenting concerns.

3. Perform a sterile speculum exam.

a. Be alert for any evidence of prolapsed cord, bulging forebag, or protruding fetal parts.

b. Observe the vaginal walls for discharge (clear, thin white, or curd-like) and the vaginal vault for pooling of fluid.

c. Visualize the cervical os and note any fluid leaking directly from the os.

If there is no visible fluid from the os, have the individual perform a Valsalva maneuver or cough and observe for fluid from the os. Alternatively, consider having an assistant apply gentle fundal pressure or gently elevate the presenting part abdominally to allow fluid to pass by the presenting part and flow through the cervical os. Another option is to have the individual remain semi-reclining for

30 to 60 minutes to allow for further leaking of fluid and then repeat the sterile speculum examination.

If fluid is present, observe:

  i. Color: Normal amniotic fluid can be clear, straw colored, or cloudy. Flecks of white or creamy vernix may be noted in the amniotic fluid of preterm or near-term infants. Dark yellow or green fluid indicates the presence of meconium in the amniotic fluid. Meconium-stained fluid increases the risk for chorioamnionitis, and thick meconium can be an indication of fetal compromise. Undiluted meconium may be indicative of breech presentation. Bacterial vaginosis often presents with thin, white or gray discharge, whereas candidiasis often presents with thick, white or curd-like discharge.

  ii. Odor: Amniotic fluid has a distinct musty odor, which differentiates it from urine. Foul-smelling fluid can indicate infection.

  iii. Bleeding: Blood or bloody show may be present in the vaginal vault or at the cervical os.

d. Note any visible cervical dilatation and length/effacement as well as whether there is a bulging forebag.

e. Do not perform a digital vaginal/cervical examination unless the information is required for clinical decision making, as vaginal exams increase the risk of infection.

4. During the sterile speculum exam, samples can be collected as indicated.

   a. If indicated by signs of preterm labor, collect the fetal fibronectin test prior to performing a vaginal exam or ultrasonography, as manipulation of the cervix may release fetal fibronectin. After collection, ROM should be ruled out prior to sending this sample to the lab since fetal fibronectin is found in amniotic fluid and the fetal membranes. Follow the manufacturer's directions; sample collection usually involves placing the swab in the posterior fornix and gently rotating for 10 seconds.[3]

   b. Collect samples of fluid by placing two sterile swabs in the vaginal fluid in the posterior fornix or along the vaginal wall for 10 to 15 seconds. Care must be taken not to touch the cervical os to avoid collecting cervical mucus.

   i. If nitrazine paper is being used, touch the tip of one swab to the pH paper. A well-saturated cotton swab can be used to prepare both a slide for the fern test and the nitrazine paper. Alternatively, the paper can be dabbed in the fluid collected at the tip of the sterile speculum after the exam. (Interpretation of results is discussed later in this appendix).

   ii. Immediately after touching the swab to the nitrazine paper, roll the swab across a dry, clean slide to create a thin film. Thick specimens may obscure ferning. Set the slide aside to dry for 10 minutes without a coverslip. Once it is dry, inspect the slide using a microscope at 10× power. Ferning occurs as the liquid on the slide evaporates, so false-negative results are possible if the slide is examined before it is completely dry.

   iii. Use the second swab for a wet mount for assessment of candidiasis, bacterial vaginosis, and/or trichomoniasis.

5. Other specimens may be obtained as indicated:

   a. GBS testing is appropriate for individuals without known GBS status who have ROM. The sample should be obtained without a speculum. The swab is inserted into the lower vagina and then into the rectum, passing through the anal sphincter. Treatment for GBS should be based on risk factors until the results of testing are known.[4]

   b. Testing for other infections with the potential for vertical transmission may be indicated based on history and physical exam findings, or may not have been performed (or repeated in the third trimester) per the Centers for Disease Control and Prevention (CDC) guidelines. Examples include gonorrhea, chlamydia, HIV, herpes, and syphilis.

## Interpretation of Tests

The *fern test* may be indicative of ROM but must be considered within the context of a comprehensive clinical assessment (**Figure 26B-1**). An observed

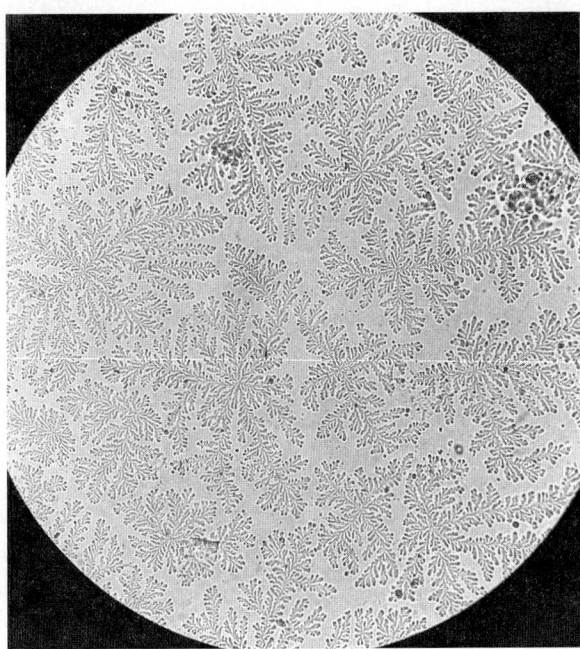

**Figure 26B-1** Fern pattern of amniotic fluid.
© Karnnara/Shutterstock.

fern-like pattern (arborization) is caused by crystallization due to the high sodium chloride and protein concentrations in amniotic fluid. The sensitivity and specificity of the fern test among nonlaboring individuals are 51.4% and 70.8%, respectively; for those in labor, these results improve to 98% and 88.2%, respectively.[5] Cervical mucus and semen can also show fern-like patterns, which may cause a false-positive result. Ferning is not affected by meconium at any concentration, nor is it influenced by small amounts of blood or by changes in vaginal pH.[6]

The *nitrazine test* uses limited-range pH paper or a commercially prepared swab to detect the increase in pH of vaginal discharge associated with the presence of amniotic fluid. The normal pH of the vagina in most individuals is acidic (approximately 4.5), whereas amniotic fluid is neutral to slightly alkaline (7.0–7.5). In the presence of alkaline material such as amniotic fluid, the mustard-gold nitrazine will turn dark blue. The sensitivity and specificity of the nitrazine method in confirming ROM are approximately 87% and 81%, respectively.[7] False-positive results can occur in the presence of vaginal infections (e.g., trichomoniasis and bacterial vaginosis), lubricants, blood, semen, or other alkaline substances, while false-negative results can occur with minimal leaking of amniotic fluid.

Other tests may be useful for determining the reason for increased vaginal discharge. A *wet prep* can be used to determine the presence of candidiasis, bacterial vaginosis, and trichomoniasis. These diagnoses can coexist with rupture of membranes, so even in the presence of one or more of these disorders, it is important to rule out ruptured membranes. For more information on the interpretation of wet prep, refer to the *Reproductive Tract and Sexually Transmitted Infections* chapter.

When the results of the initial testing and clinical assessment are equivocal, several commercially available *laboratory tests for amniotic fluid proteins* (e.g., placental alpha microglobulin-1 [PAMG-1], placental protein 12 [PP12], alpha-fetoprotein) can be considered as supplemental testing options. For these tests, a speculum exam is not required, as the swab is inserted vaginally to collect cervicovaginal fluid. The PAMG-1 test (marketed as AmniSure, Qiagen Sciences, Germantown, MD) was the first commercially available test for ROM to be approved by the U.S. Food and Drug Administration (FDA). Many manufacturer-sponsored studies and meta-analyses have been published regarding the accuracy of amniotic fluid protein tests, and research findings have demonstrated that they have high sensitivity and specificity.[8–11] However, a 2018 U.S. FDA letter recommended that healthcare providers use these tests only in conjunction with other clinical assessments because of concerns about "misuse, overreliance, and inaccurate interpretation of lab test results," which "can lead to serious adverse events, including fetal death, infection, and other health complications in pregnant women."[12] In addition, these tests usually cost more than nitrazine and wet prep testing.

A *test for fetal fibronectin* is a sensitive but nonspecific test for ROM. A positive test result does not confirm ROM, but a negative test result suggests intact membranes. It may be difficult to interpret the results in the presence of active vaginal bleeding or if a vaginal examination or ultrasound was performed prior to sample collection. In addition, use of vaginal lubricants, disinfectants, soaps, or creams, or vaginal intercourse within 24 hours, may contribute to false-positive results.

*Ultrasound quantification of amniotic fluid* may also be used to test for ROM, although a person can have ruptured membranes and still have a normal amount of amniotic fluid, especially if there was not a moderate gush of fluid. Ultrasound documentation of oligohydramnios does not confirm ROM but may be helpful in developing a management plan.

## Diagnosis of Rupture of Membranes

The diagnosis of ruptured membranes provides useful information for labor management and infection prevention. During labor, copious amniotic fluid from the introitus is enough to diagnose rupture; additional assessment and testing can be used if needed. Diagnosis of PROM is typically made via the constellation of history and a four-point clinical assessment—that is, (1) pooling of fluid in the posterior vaginal vault, (2) visualizing of fluid from the cervix, (3) positive fern test, and (4) positive nitrazine test. The results of a fern and/or nitrazine test must be viewed within the context of the history and sterile speculum examination, and these tests may best be viewed as supportive rather than conclusive if active leaking from the cervical os or pooling is not visible. If the results are equivocal, other testing options can be considered. Physician consultation may be needed if the diagnosis is inconclusive, especially for an individual at preterm gestation.

### References

1. Siegler Y, Weiner Z, Solt I. ACOG Practice Bulletin No. 217: prelabor rupture of membranes. *Obstet Gynecol*. 2020;136(5):1061. doi:10.1097/aog.0000 000000004142.

2. Esplin SM, Hoffman MK, Theilen L, Kupchak P. Prospective evaluation of the efficacy of immunoassays in the diagnosis of rupture of the membranes. *J Matern Fetal Neonatal Med*. 2020;33(15):2594-2600. doi:10.1080/14767058.2018.1555809.

3. Hologic. *Rapid fFN for the TLiIQ System Specimen Collection Kit*. https://www.hologic.com/file/43496/download?token=6K-f96uH. Published August 2020. Accessed November 13, 2022.

4. American College of Obstetricians and Gynecologists. Committee Opinion No. 797: prevention of group B streptococcal early-onset disease in newborns: correction. *Obstet Gynecol*. 2020;135(4):978-979. doi:10.1097/aog.0000000000003824.

5. de Haan HH, Offermans PM, Smits F, et al. Value of the fern test to confirm or reject the diagnosis of ruptured membranes is modest in nonlaboring women presenting with nonspecific vaginal fluid loss. *Am J Perinatol*. 1994;11(1):46-50. doi:10.1055/s-2007-994535.

6. Bennett SL, Cullen JB, Sherer DM, Woods JR Jr. The ferning and nitrazine tests of amniotic fluid between 12 and 41 weeks gestation. *Am J Perinatol*. 1993;10(2):101-104. doi:10.1055/s-2007-994637.

7. Abdelazim IA, Makhlouf HH. Placental alpha microglobulin-1 (AmniSure® test) for detection of premature rupture of fetal membranes. *Arch Gynecol Obstet*. 2012;285(4):985-989. doi:10.1007/s00404-011-2106-4.

8. Thumm B, Walsh G, Heyborne KD. Diagnosis of rupture of membranes: AmniSure, clinical assessment, and the Food and Drug Administration warning. *Am J Obstet Gynecol MFM*. 2020;2(4):100200. doi:10.1016/j.ajogmf.2020.100200.

9. Ramsauer B, Vidaeff AC, Hösli I, et al. The diagnosis of rupture of fetal membranes (ROM): a meta-analysis. *J Perinat Med*. 2013;41(3):233-240. doi:10.1515/jpm-2012-0247.

10. Palacio M, Kühnert M, Berger R, et al. Meta-analysis of studies on biochemical marker tests for the diagnosis of premature rupture of membranes: comparison of performance indexes. *BMC Pregnancy Childbirth*. 2014;14:183. doi:10.1186/1471-2393-14-183.

11. Committee on Practice Bulletins – Obstetrics. ACOG practice bulletin No. 217: prelabor rupture of membranes. *Obstet & Gynecol*. 2020 Nov 1;135(3):e80-97.

12. Food and Drug Administration. FDA alerts healthcare providers, women about risks associated with improper use of rupture of membranes tests. 2018. https://www.fda.gov/news-events/press-announcements/fda-alerts-healthcare-providers-women-about-risks-associated-improper-use-rupture-membranes-tests. Accessed November 23, 2022.

APPENDIX

# 26C

# Fetal–Pelvic Assessment

KATHLEEN DANHAUSEN AND JULIA C. PHILLIPPI

*The editors acknowledge Jennifer M. Demma, Karen Trister Grace, and
Tekoa L. King for their contributions to this appendix in the last edition*

## Introduction

Clinical pelvimetry measures the length and shape of pelvic structures to assess the dimensions of the pelvic inlet, the mid-pelvis, and the pelvic outlet. The pelvic planes cannot be measured directly, but rather are estimated during pelvimetry and assessed in relationship to the presentation, position, and size of a fetus. The size and shape of the interior of the pelvis are important because during birth the fetus must navigate the pelvic inlet, then move through the mid-pelvis, and then out of the pelvic outlet. Pelvic diameters are most accurately measured by X ray, computed tomography (CT), or magnetic resonance imaging (MRI). However, there is a lack of research supporting the value of these measurements except in rare cases or for some nulliparous individuals planning vaginal breech birth.[1]

While pelvimetry can be performed at any time, the information it provides is most valuable in labor, when the dimensions of the pelvis can be assessed in relation to a specific fetus. The fetal presentation, position, and flexion, as well as the estimated fetal weight, are important facets in assessing how and if a fetus will negotiate the pelvic diameters (Figure 26C-1). Assessment of a pelvis as adequate or borderline is also not clinically meaningful unless it is in relationship to a particular fetus. For example, a person who had a prior cesarean delivery in the second stage of labor with a 9-pound fetus in an occiput-posterior position might have a rapid second stage with a preterm fetus in an occiput-anterior position.

In the past, clinical pelvimetry was used to categorize the pelvis into types. However, the Caldwell-Malloy typing system uses a racialized nomenclature and does not provide clinically meaningful information. A more comprehensive assessment of the planes of the pelvis in relationship to a presenting fetus provides information specific to the birthing person and fetus that is useful in clinical decision making.

Clinical pelvimetry has also been used to assess a pelvis as "adequate," "borderline," or "contracted" for the birth of an average-size fetus by numerically estimating the shape and size of the pelvic inlet, midplane, and outlet. In the past, the higher prevalence of rickets and other nutritional

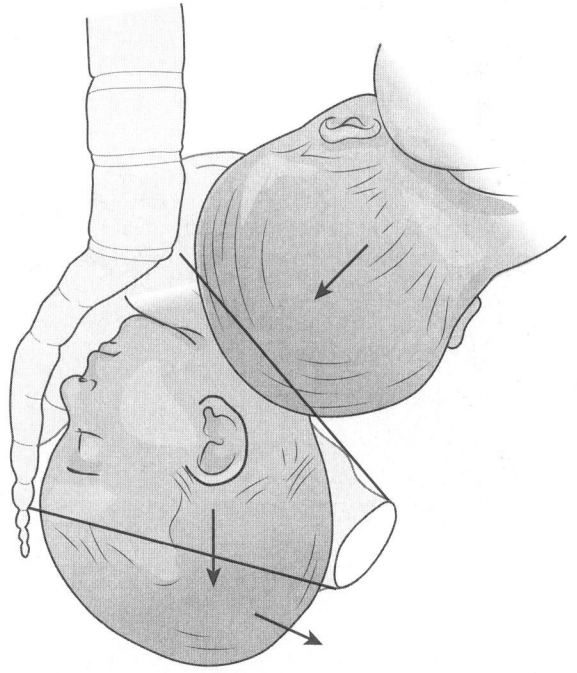

**Figure 26C-1** Typical Movement of the fetal head through the pelvis.

disorders and diseases meant more individuals had pelvic architecture that precluded safe vaginal birth.[2] In the United States and Canada, gross abnormalities of the pelvis are rare, and there is no need to routinely assess a person's pelvis for contracture ahead of labor.[3] However, if an individual has a comorbidity affecting the pelvis or has had fractures of the pelvic bones or coccyx, pelvimetry might provide information useful in labor planning.

Accurate assessment of the pelvic structures prior to late pregnancy can be difficult, as the pelvic muscles and ligaments have not softened under the effects of relaxin and other hormones. Fetal–pelvic assessment should be ongoing throughout labor, as the pelvic dimensions can change slightly as the birthing person changes position and the joints of the pelvis also have some give to them. Moreover, the dimensions of the fetal vertex change during labor (Figure 26C-2). Since the fetal position and cranial dimensions as well as the birth person's pelvic dimensions are dynamic in labor, clinical pelvimetry should not be used to exclude people from laboring and vaginal birth. Nearly all individuals without a history of disease or trauma that affects the pelvis should not need pelvic assessment prior to labor. During labor, assessment should include the pelvis as well as fetal position, presentation, and adaptation to the pelvis as part of a comprehensive assessment.

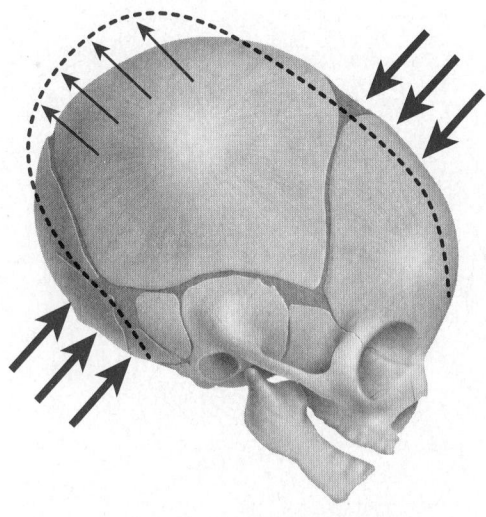

**Figure 26C-2** Typical skull molding from vaginal birth in a well-flexed, vertex presentation. As pressure is applied to the fetal skull in one dimension (shown with darker arrows), the skull expands in another dimension (shown with lighter arrows and the dotted line.

## Foundational Knowledge for Pelvimetry

1. The midwife should have an understanding of:

   a. Pelvic anatomy and the typical dimensions of the pelvic planes, as described in the *Anatomy and Physiology of the Reproductive System* chapter.

   b. Basic dimensions of the fetal skull, as outlined in the *Anatomy and Physiology of Pregnancy* chapter. The examiner should understand how to determine the presentation and position of the fetus from palpation of the presenting part. It is important to know the presenting diameters of all cephalic presentations and the dimensions of breech presentations if assessing the pelvis for breech birth.

   c. Cardinal movements of the fetus through the pelvis during labor and birth, as described in the *Anatomy and Physiology of Labor and Birth* chapter.

2. If a numeric estimate of the pelvis is desired, the size of the examiner's fingers and hand should be measured.

   a. The length of the reach of the examining fingers is measured from the tip of the longest finger to the juncture of the first finger and thumb.

   b. The fist is measured from the lateral (ulnar) aspect to the medial (radial) aspect of the tops of the knuckles of the fingers where they attach to the hand. If this does not measure at least 8 cm, then position the thumb in the way that it will be positioned each time and add the joint or knuckle of the thumb into the measurement.

3. Knowledge of the pregnant or birthing person's history serves as the foundation for clinically relevant fetal–pelvic assessment, including the following information:

   a. Number of vaginal births and the fetal presentation and position and birth weight

   b. Prior cesarean births and their indications, including length of labor, fetal presentation/position, and birth weight

   c. History of pelvic surgery or injury

   d. Number of fetuses in the uterus

e. Estimated presentation, position, and weight of the fetus from abdominal or ultrasound examination

f. Membrane status (intact or ruptured)

## Preparation of the Individual

Discuss with the individual the benefits and potential risk of the exam. Explain that pelvic assessment includes additional pressure compared with exams that solely assess cervical dilation and fetal position. The steps of pelvimetry add time to the exam, as well as the potential for additional discomfort, so if the laboring person is uncomfortable and planning an epidural, it is reasonable to postpone pelvimetry until they are comfortable. After obtaining consent, use a trauma-informed approach to the exam itself.

The person should be offered the opportunity to empty their bladder. The midwife should wash their hands with soap and water and don gloves (sterile gloves if the person's amniotic membranes are ruptured or per facility protocol). Apply lubricant to the gloves prior to initiating the examination. Explain to the individual that the exam can be paused or stopped at any point.

## Assessment of Fetal Presentation, Position, and Attitude

An assessment of the presentation, position, and attitude of the fetus is important in understanding how a particular fetus may move through a particular pelvis. Refer to the *Anatomy and Physiology of Labor and Birth* chapter and the *Assessment for Diagnosis of Labor* appendix for foundational information. Figure 26C-3 depicts what is palpable when an individual is in active labor with a fetus in the most common fetal position at zero station (occiput anterior, well flexed). While many images depict the anterior fontanel of the fetal head when it is within the pelvis, during a vaginal exam it is rare for an examiner to easily palpate both the anterior and the posterior fontanels, especially prior to complete cervical dilatation.

## Steps of Pelvimetry

### Assessment of the Pelvic Inlet

The pelvic inlet is the upper brim of the pelvis and is defined by the anterior aspect of the symphysis pubis and the sacral promontory (**Figure 26C-4**). The

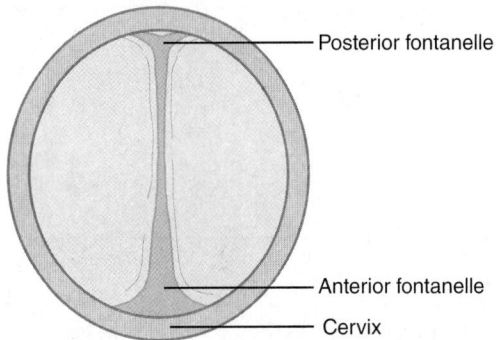

**Figure 26C-3** Fetal vertex in occiput-anterior position as palpated during a vaginal exam in active labor.

line between these two areas is referred to as the obstetric conjugate.

1. Using your dominant hand for the vaginal exam, reach posteriorly in the pelvis with your examining fingers to locate the sacral promontory. As your fingers slide up the center of the sacrum, lower your wrist and elbow to direct your fingers toward the upper sacrum. Use gentle downward pressure on the perineum to avoid undue pressure on the urethra or clitoris.

   The *diagonal conjugate*, the clinical measurement that best approximates the obstetric conjugate, is assessed by locating the most prominent sacral bone, the *sacral promontory*. With your middle finger touching the sacral promontory (if it is palpable), lift your wrist until your hand contacts the lower border of the symphysis pubis (**Figure 26C-5**). The average length of the diagonal conjugate is 12 to 12.5 cm, and many midwives will not be able to reach the sacral promontory with their fingers. A narrow diagonal conjugate can impact the ability of the fetus to engage into the pelvis. If the fetal head has descended into the pelvis and past the sacral promontory, assessment of the pelvic inlet is not needed, as it is adequate for the presenting part of the fetus.

2. From the sacral promontory, sweep your fingers from side to side and estimate the distance between the side walls of the pelvis. A pelvic inlet diameter of more than 10 cm is normal. If the fetal head is within the pelvis, the upper side walls will not be easily palpable, and assessment of this diameter is not necessary as it accommodates the fetus.

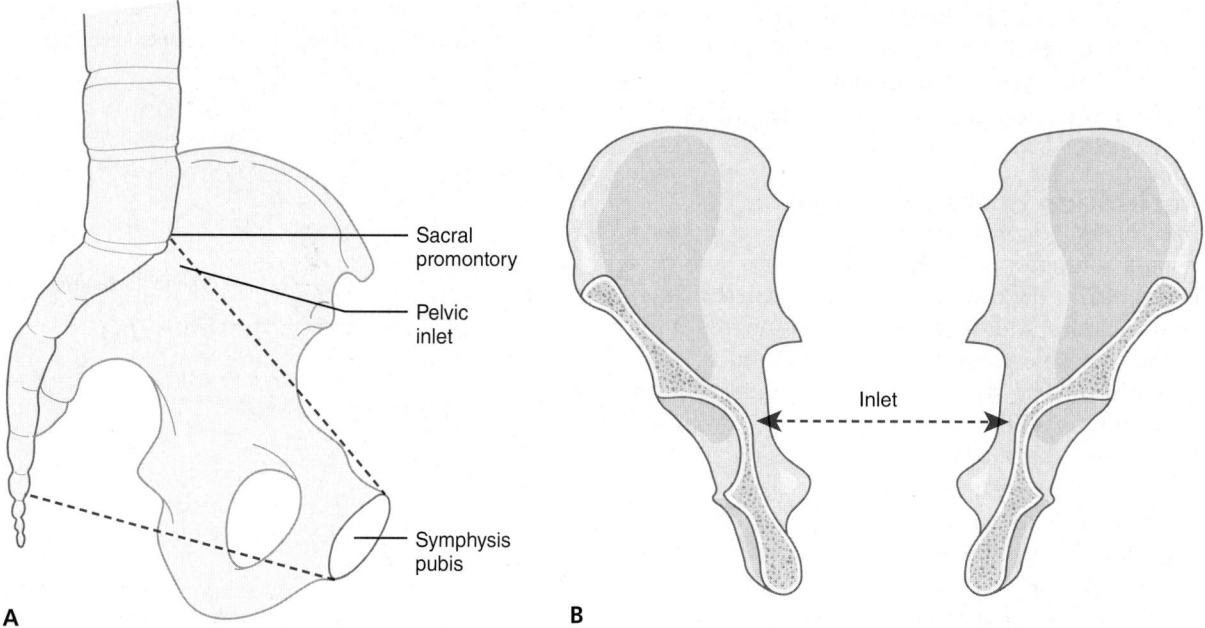

**A**

**B**

**Figure 26C-4  A.** Sagittal section of the pelvis noting the pelvic inlet. **B.** Coronal section of the pelvis noting the pelvic inlet.

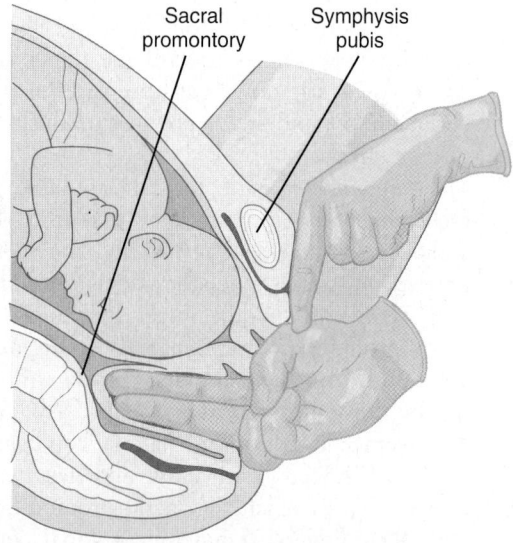

**Figure 26C-5** Measurement of the diagonal conjugate.

## Assessment of the Mid-Pelvis

The mid-pelvis, also known as the pelvic cavity, encompasses the area within the pelvis between the symphysis pubis and the sacrum below the sacral promontory and above the coccyx (**Figure 26C-6**). Important aspects of the mid-pelvis to assess include the angle of pelvic sidewalls, the prominence of the ischial spines, the interspinous diameter, and the curvature of the sacrum.

1. Sweep the fingers down the sidewalls of the pelvis (**Figure 26C-7**), and note how the sidewalls

are angled. Most sidewalls are *parallel*. *Convergent sidewalls* narrow as they approach the outlet. *Divergent sidewalls* flare outward toward the outlet (**Figure 26C-8**).

2. There are several techniques for locating the ischial spines, which feel like small bony prominences and are located next to the pudendal nerve. Depending on the pelvic anatomy, the ischial spines may be difficult or impossible to palpate. Spines that are blunt and not easily palpated are a normal finding and do not interfere with fetal descent.

   First, exert gentle lateral pressure as you sweep your fingers around the sidewall to locate the ischial spine (**Figure 26C-9**). If unable to locate the spine in this manner, move your fingers medially to the sacrum and locate the sacrospinous ligament, which will feel like a firm, band-like ligament that attaches at the tip of the sacrum. Follow the sacrospinous ligament laterally until you reach the ischial spine. If still unable to locate the spine, sweep the sidewalls of the pelvis with your examining fingers and ask the birthing person to tell you when it feels like you have hit a nerve (the pudendal nerve). Once you have found the nerve, feel in all directions until you palpate a bony prominence. Ischial spines are described as *blunt* when they are not easily palpated and/or are flattened against the pelvic sidewalls, *prominent* when they are easily palpable, and *encroaching* when they are long, sharp, or encroach into the pelvic cavity. Ischial spines are typically blunt.

3. To measure the interspinous diameter between the ischial spines, rotate your palm

down, sweeping your fingers across the sacrum and ending when your palm is facing in the opposite direction to locate the other spine; then sweep your finger back to the first position. Do not flex your fingers as you sweep from side to side. Estimate how much space is available between the two spines. A typical interspinous diameter is 10 cm or greater. A pelvis that is narrow in the mid-plane will restrict your side-to-side motion and may impair fetal rotation and/or descent.

4. As you sweep your fingers from side to side, note the curvature and inclination of the sacrum, which can affect how the fetus navigates the mid-pelvis. Bring your fingers to midline. Angle your fingers upward and make contact with the sacrum. Sweep your fingers down the sacrum and note the sacral curvature and the length. The sacrum is described as *hollow*, *flat*, or *forward/J-shaped* (Figure 26C-10).

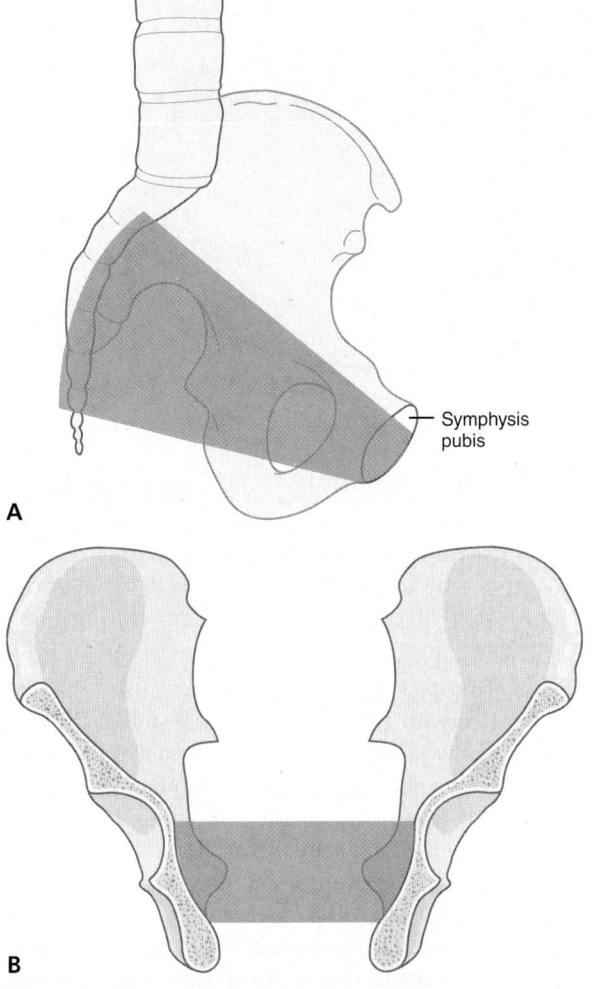

**Figure 26C-6 A.** Sagittal section noting the mid-pelvis. **B.** Coronal section of the pelvis noting the mid-pelvis.

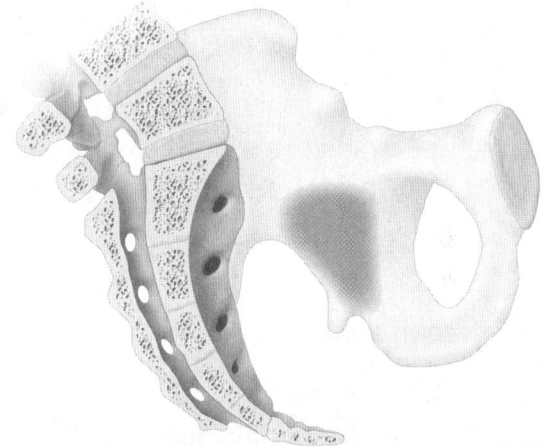

**Figure 26C-7** Location of pelvic sidewalls.

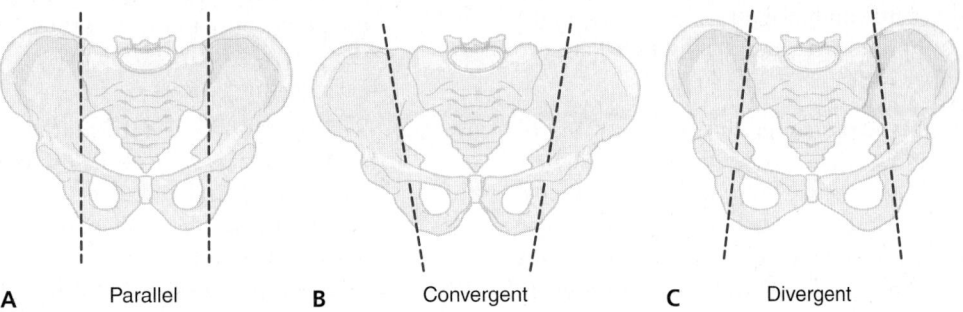

**Figure 26C-8** Inclination of pelvic sidewalls. **A.** Parallel. **B.** Convergent. **C.** Divergent.

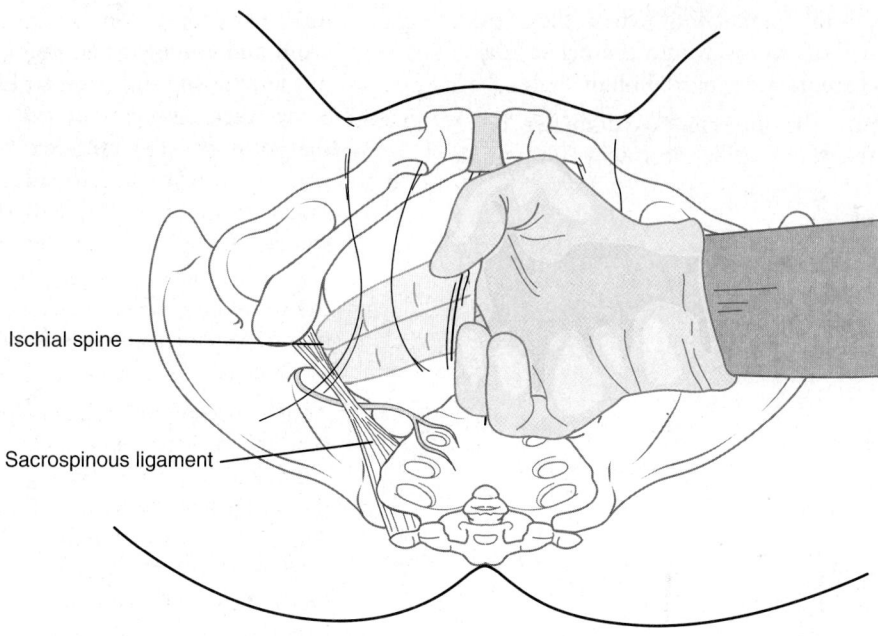

Ischial spine

Sacrospinous ligament

**Figure 26C-9** Assessment of an ischial spine.

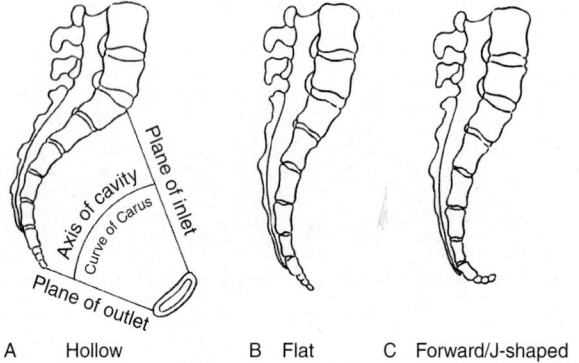

A   Hollow    B   Flat    C   Forward/J-shaped

**Figure 26C-10** Sacral shapes. **A.** Hollow. **B.** Flat.
**C.** Forward/J-shaped.

## Assessment of the Pelvic Outlet

The pelvic outlet boundaries include the symphysis pubis, tip of the coccyx (tailbone), ischial tuberosities, and sacrospinous ligaments. The outlet is assessed for the shape and mobility of the coccyx, the angle of the subpubic arch, and the distance between the ischial tuberosities.

1. To estimate the shape and mobility of the coccyx, locate the base of the sacrum, where it joins the coccyx. Press firmly on the coccyx to determine its shape and mobility. You may need to place your thumb, or the middle finger of your other hand, externally against the coccyx to assess the rigidity of the sacrococcygeal joint. The coccyx is described as J-shaped or flat, and immobile or fixed. A coccyx that is J-shaped or immobile may break during childbirth. Labor may or may not be impeded, but significant pain in the area of the coccyx can occur during birth and postpartum if it breaks.

2. To assess the angle of the subpubic arch, rotate your fingers to touch the side of the pelvis as you begin to remove your hand from the vagina. Just prior to removing your hand and when your fingers are within the vagina to the second set of finger joints, rotate your examining hand so the palmar surface is up (**Figure 26C-11**). Evaluate how easily your two examining fingers fit under the arch. If two fingers fit comfortably, the angle is approximately 90 degrees. If the fingers must overlap to fit in the subpubic arch, the angle is less than 90 degrees. If the pubic arch is narrow, the fetal head must use the space of the pelvic outlet closer to the sacrum to exit the pelvis, which can increase the chance of perineal lacerations.

3. Remove your hand from the vagina. The transverse diameter of the outlet is the space between the ischial tuberosities. Place your fist between the tuberosities and assess whether the space is greater, equal to, or less than the premeasured width of your fist. A typical measurement is approximately 8 cm (**Figure 26C-12**).

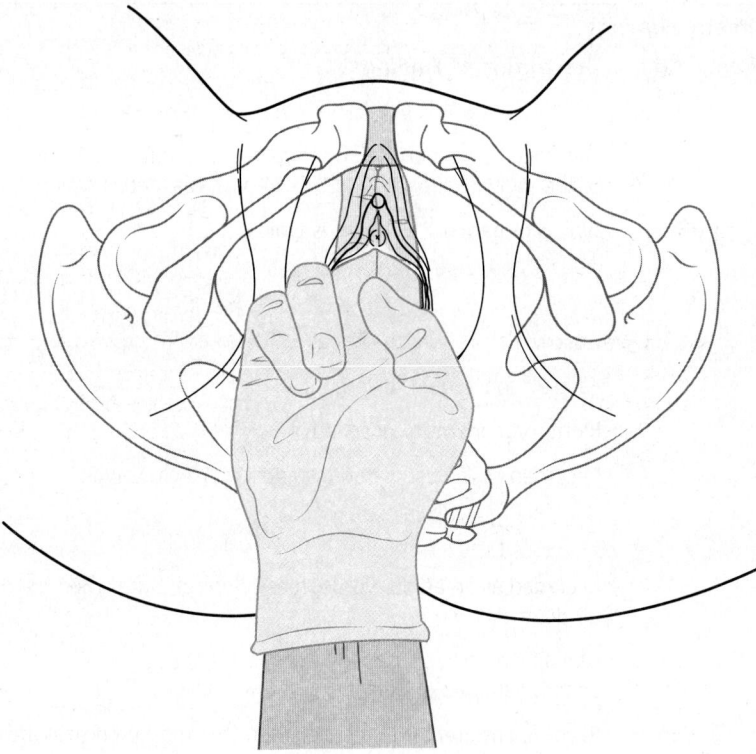

**Figure 26C-11** Assessment of the subpubic arch.

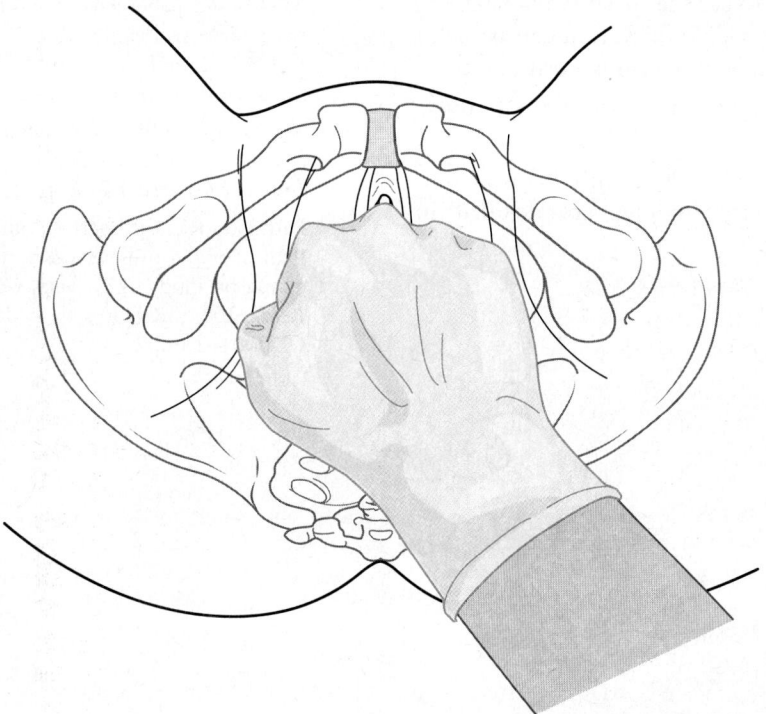

**Figure 26C-12** Assessment of the intertuberous diameter.

| Table 26C-1 | Pelvimetry Findings |
|---|---|
| **Pelvic Plane and Anatomic Area** | **Description of Findings** |
| **Pelvic Inlet** | |
| Diagonal conjugate | Recorded as greater than or equal to the measured distance of the midwife's reach; > 11.5 cm or unreached is typical |
| Transverse diameter of pelvic inlet | Typical or narrow; ≥ 10 cm is typical |
| **Mid-Pelvis** | |
| Sacral shape | Hollow, flat, forward/J-shaped |
| Sidewalls | Parallel, convergent, divergent |
| Ischial spines | Blunt, prominent, or encroaching |
| Interspinous diameter | Recorded as the estimated distance; ≥ 10 cm is typical |
| **Pelvic Outlet** | |
| Subpubic arch | Recorded as an angle; 90 degrees is typical, but can be greater than or less than 90 degrees |
| Coccyx | Mobility: mobile or fixed<br>Shape: J-shaped or flat |
| Intertuberous diameter | Recorded as greater than or equal to the measured size of the midwife's fist; 8 cm is typical |

4. After you have assessed the fetus and the pelvis, consider how this fetus will likely rotate and descend to use the space available in the pelvic cavity. This information can be helpful in assisting with laboring positioning.

5. Wash your hands and describe the findings to the pregnant person.

6. Record findings in the health record. Common pelvimetry findings are detailed in Table 26C-1.

### References

1. Klemt AS, Schulze S, Brüggmann D, Louwen F. MRI-based pelvimetric measurements as predictors for a successful vaginal breech delivery in the Frankfurt Breech at Term cohort (FRABAT). *Eur J Obstet Gynecol Reprod Bio.* 2019;232:10-17.

2. MacLennan HR. Contracted pelvis in childbirth: a study of its morbid effects on mother and child. *J Obstet Gynaecol Br Emp.* 1944;51:293-317.

3. Pattinson RC, Cuthbert A, Vannevel V. Pelvimetry for fetal cephalic presentations at or near term for deciding on mode of delivery. *Cochrane Database Syst Rev.* 2017;3:CD000161. doi:10.1002/14651858.CD000161.pub2.

CHAPTER

# 27

# Fetal Assessment During Labor

JENIFER O. FAHEY

*The editors acknowledge Tekoa L. King who was the author of this chapter in the previous edition*

## Introduction

Fetal assessment during labor is intended to identify the fetus experiencing acute impairment of gas exchange to allow for timely intervention. When the fetus is exposed to decreased oxygen, it responds by modulating its heart rate in a way to help reduce oxygen consumption. Similarly, when a fetus is experiencing profound oxygen deprivation, the fetal heart rate (FHR) is affected. These predictable and visually identifiable physiologic responses of the FHR to oxygenation provide the theoretical underpinnings that have led to the use of electronic fetal monitoring (EFM) as the primary means to assess fetal well-being in labor in the United States and other high-income countries. Unfortunately, even with the use of adjunct assessment modalities, EFM has not been demonstrated to reliably perform better than intermittent FHR auscultation in terms of neonatal and maternal outcomes.[1]

The seeming failure of EFM to improve outcomes has been due to its premature adoption into clinical practice, which preceded research that has since helped providers gain an improved, albeit still incomplete, understanding of existing associations between the fetal response to compromised oxygenation and the FHR patterns observed via EFM. To optimize outcomes without unnecessarily increasing intervention requires an approach that (1) is grounded in the most current understanding of the physiology of fetal oxygenation and FHR patterns, (2) considers the capacity and limitations of each fetal assessment modality, and (3) appropriately utilizes existing FHR pattern classification and categorization tools to guide the interpretation and management of FHR variations.

This chapter reviews current understanding of the physiology of fetal oxygenation and acid–base balance as well as the pathophysiology of fetal asphyxia and how these physiologic and pathologic states are reflected in FHR patterns. The methods used for assessment of fetal well-being in labor, including EFM, intermittent auscultation, and umbilical cord gas assessment, are presented. Finally, classification and categorization frameworks for FHR patterns are introduced, along with some guidance on how these can be used to support the interpretation and management of FHR patterns in labor.

## Physiology of Fetal Oxygenation

Fetal survival and growth are dependent on effective transfer of nutrients and oxygen to the fetus and removal of the waste products of fetal metabolism, including carbon dioxide, from fetal circulation. Optimal maternal–fetal gas exchange can occur only when the following five components function well: (1) adequate flow of well-oxygenated maternal blood into the intervillous space, (2) a large enough placental area for gas exchange, (3) efficient diffusion of gases across the placental tissues that separate the maternal and fetal circulations, (4) unimpaired umbilical vein circulation into the fetus, and (5) adequate oxygen transport capacity in the fetus.

Maternal adaptations during pregnancy promote optimal gas exchange with the fetus. As gestation progresses, there is increased blood flow to the uterus. At the beginning of pregnancy, blood flow to the uterus is estimated to be 20 to 50 mL per minute[2]; by comparison, at term, approximately 500 to

900 mL of maternal blood flows to the uterus each minute.[3,4] The majority of this blood (70% to 90%) enters the maternal spiral arteries. As reviewed in the *Anatomy and Physiology of Pregnancy* chapter, the uterine spiral arteries become deinnervated during pregnancy as their endothelial linings are replaced with trophoblastic tissue. Consequently, the arteries become maximally dilated to facilitate blood flow into the intervillous space at the placenta, where substances are transferred between the maternal and fetal circulations.[5,6] In individuals without preexisting medical disorders, placental growth is usually sufficient to provide the necessary surface area for gas and nutrient exchange. An increase in maternal minute ventilation promotes a lowering of the partial pressure of carbon dioxide ($PCO_2$) in the maternal arterial blood, helping to create a $CO_2$ gradient that facilitates the transfer of $CO_2$ from the fetal circulation to the maternal circulation for elimination via the maternal lungs and kidneys. At term, maternal $PCO_2$ is approximately 34 mm Hg, whereas fetal $PCO_2$ is approximately 40 mm Hg. This maternal state of compensated respiratory alkalosis also creates a greater potential for oxygen–hemoglobin dissociation during pregnancy, thereby facilitating oxygen delivery across the placenta.

Fetal anatomic and physiologic adaptations also promote optimal gas exchange. In the fetal circulation, deoxygenated blood flows from fetal tissues through the two umbilical arteries to the placenta and to the capillary beds at the end of the fetal villi, where gas exchange happens via diffusion across the four tissue layers that separate the maternal and fetal circulations (see Figure 19-8). Oxygen and carbon dioxide are highly permeable across the placental tissues, which facilitates gas exchange. Furthermore, the fetus resides in an environment of comparatively low oxygen. The fetal arterial $PO_2$ is approximately 35 mm Hg, similar to the $PO_2$ in the maternal venous system, while the maternal arterial $PO_2$ is in the range of 80 to 100 mm Hg. This gradient facilitates oxygen transfer to the fetus.

Additional aspects of fetal physiology that promote oxygenation include fetal hemoglobin type and concentration as well as adaptations of the fetal circulation. The hemoglobin concentration in fetal blood (43% to 63%) is higher than that in the pregnant adult's circulation at term (28% to 40%). Fetal hemoglobin also has a higher affinity for oxygen than does adult hemoglobin. From the placenta, oxygenated blood travels back to the fetus via the umbilical vein. Fetal circulation, which is discussed in more detail in the *Anatomy and Physiology of Pregnancy* chapter, includes shunts that allow the

fetal heart and brain to be preferentially perfused with well-oxygenated blood while blood with lower oxygen content is circulated to the lower body.

## Pathophysiology of Intrapartum Fetal Hypoxia, Acidosis, and Asphyxial Injury

During active labor, uterine contractions cause intermittent increases in uterine venous pressure and constriction of maternal spiral arteries, temporarily interrupting blood flow in and out of the intervillous space (Figure 27-1). This leads to intermittent decreases in $PO_2$ and increases in $CO_2$ in fetal circulation. Uterine contractions and/or maternal expulsive efforts can also lead to compression of the umbilical cord, resulting in a decrease or interruption of fetal blood flow.

In a healthy fetus and pregnant individual, the uterine contractions that are characteristic of a normal labor typically do not significantly alter fetal oxygenation overall. The adaptations that allow a fetus to survive and grow in a comparatively low-oxygen environment also serve as a buffer to the intermittent decreases in blood flow that occur during labor and birth. When the amount of available oxygen is not sufficient to meet the oxygen requirements of fetal tissue despite these adaptive mechanisms, fetal *hypoxia* occurs. Definitions related to hypoxia are listed in Table 27-1.[7,8]

A fetus usually becomes hypoxic through three potential mechanisms: (1) a decrease in oxygen content in maternal blood, (2) insufficient uterine/placental blood flow, or (3) insufficient umbilical blood blow. Less common causes of fetal hypoxia include fetal anemia, which decreases oxygen-carrying capacity, and pyrexia, which results in increased oxygen consumption.

In a healthy, term fetus, a common cause of acute intrapartum hypoxia is an abnormal uterine contraction pattern. Studies of fetal oxygenation have found that an interval of approximately 60 seconds between contractions is associated with stable fetal cerebral oxygenation, whereas intervals between contractions that are less than 60 seconds are associated with lower umbilical artery pH levels.[9-11] Simpson et al. measured fetal oxygenation ($FSpO_2$) via pulse oximetry among pregnant individuals who were being induced at term.[9] These researchers found that when fewer than five contractions occurred in a 10-minute window, fetal oxygen saturation was unaffected; when five or more contractions occurred in a 10-minute window, fetal $FSpO_2$ dropped 20% in 30 minutes; and when more than six contractions occurred in 10 minutes, fetal

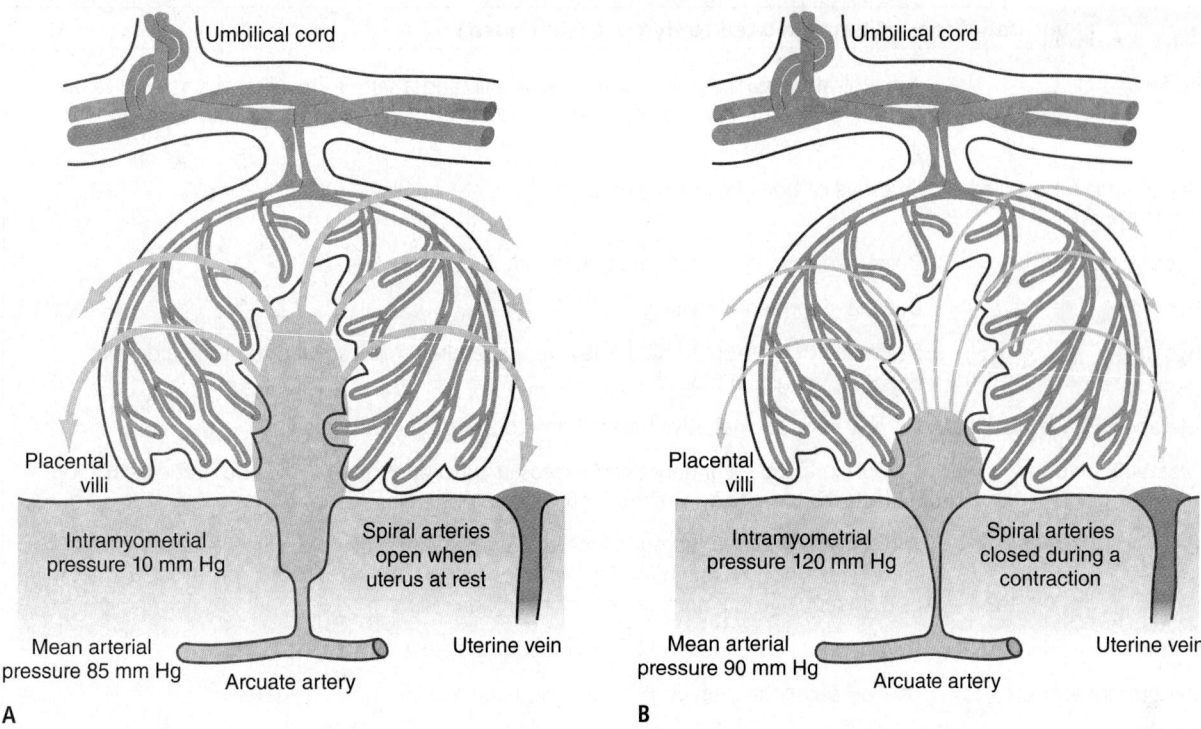

**Figure 27-1** Effect of uterine contraction on blood flow into the intervillous space in the placenta. **A.** Blood flow into the intervillous space between uterine contractions. **B.** Blood flow into the intervillous space stops or is reduced during myometrial contractions.

| Table 27-1 | Definitions of Terms Related to Hypoxia |
|---|---|
| **Term** | **Definition** |
| Acidemia | Increased concentration of hydrogen ions in the blood, which is measured as pH. Acidemia refers to low pH in blood. |
| Acidosis | Increased concentration of hydrogen ions in the tissues of the body, which is measured as pH. Acidosis refers to low pH in both blood and tissues. Acidosis is not directly measurable, as pH in tissues cannot be sampled. |
| Aerobic metabolism | Metabolism of glucose using oxygen. The end products of aerobic metabolism are ATP and carbon dioxide. |
| Anaerobic metabolism | Metabolism of glucose without the use of oxygen. The end products of anaerobic metabolism are ATP and lactic acid. |
| Asphyxia | Any decrease in $O_2$ and increase in $CO_2$ secondary to impairment of gas exchange. Asphyxia is a continuum described by degrees of acidosis. Clinically, this term is typically used only when tissue damage or death occurs. |
| Base | A substance that is capable of accepting hydrogen ions, thereby decreasing acidity. Bases such as bicarbonate ($HCO_3^-$) and hemoglobin act as acid–base buffers in blood. |
| Base excess (BE) | The amount of base or $HCO_3^-$ that is available for buffering hydrogen ions. As metabolic acidosis increases, the base excess decreases. |
| Bicarbonate (bicarb) | $HCO_3^-$ is the base or hydrogen acceptor that is part of the primary buffering system within the blood. |

*(continues)*

| Table 27-1 | Definitions of Terms Related to Hypoxia (*continued*) |
|---|---|
| Buffer | A chemical substance that is both a weak acid and a salt. Buffers can absorb or give up hydrogen ions, thereby maintaining a constant pH value. The primary buffer involved in fetal oxygenation is $HCO_3^-$. |
| Hypercarbia (also called hypercapnia) | Excessive carbon dioxide in blood. |
| Hypoxemia | Decreased oxygen concentration in blood. |
| Hypoxia | Decreased oxygen in tissues. |
| Ischemia | Decreased or interrupted blood flow to tissues. Ischemia can lead to hypoxia despite adequate oxygen in blood. |
| Metabolic academia | Low bicarbonate (negative base excess) concentration in blood. |
| Metabolic acidosis | Low pH in tissue secondary to an increased concentration of lactic acid in the circulation. Reflects the severity of asphyxia and hypoxia–ischemia. |
| pH | The concentration of hydrogen ions in blood. The term pH refers to *puissance hydrogen*, which is French for "strength (or power) of hydrogen." A pH of 7.0 is the same as 0.0000001 ($10^{-7}$) mole per liter of hydrogen ions. |
| Respiratory acidemia | Low pH secondary to high $PCO_2$ in blood and tissues. |
| Respiratory acidosis | Low pH secondary to high $PCO_2$ in blood and tissues. |

Abbreviations: ATP, adenosine triphosphate; $CO_2$, carbon dioxide; $HCO_3^-$, bicarbonate; $PCO_2$, partial pressure of carbon dioxide.

Adapted from Parer JT, King TL, Ikeda T. *Electronic Fetal Heart Rate Monitoring: The 5-Tier System*. 3rd ed. Burlington, MA: Jones & Bartlett Learning; 2018.

$FSpO_2$ dropped 29% in 30 minutes. Contraction patterns of more than five contractions in 10 minutes can occur in spontaneous labor,[12] but are more common when induction or augmentation agents such as oxytocin are administered.[13–15]

### Fetal Response to Hypoxia

In response to hypoxia, the fetus can mount a complex, coordinated cardiovascular response to maintain adequate oxygen delivery to the vital organs. This response includes (1) a transient decrease in heart rate; (2) redistribution of blood to vital organs including the heart, brain, and adrenal glands; and (3) use of anaerobic metabolism.

A slowing of the FHR and decrease in fetal body movements lowers oxygen consumption during periods of hypoxia. This compensatory slowing of the FHR is believed to occur when the peripheral chemoreceptor reflex is triggered. The cardioregulatory center in the medulla oblongata receives input from the central nervous system (CNS), peripheral chemoreceptors, baroreceptors, and circulating catecholamines, and it sends out acceleratory or inhibitory signals to the heart via the sympathetic and parasympathetic nervous systems. Parasympathetic control of the FHR occurs via the 10th cranial nerve, the vagus nerve. Vagal stimulation results in a slowing of the FHR. There appears to be a gradient of chemoreflex activation that is dependent on fetal oxygenation. This gradient is reflected in the amount of slowing (deceleration) of the FHR, such that with more profound degrees of impairment of fetal oxygenation, there will be more profound decelerations of the FHR.[16–18]

In addition to decreasing the amount of oxygen consumption by the myocardium, a slowing of the FHR prolongs the period of cardiac filling. This allows more time for the fetal heart to extract oxygen and to maintain adequate cardiac output despite the lower heart rate by increasing the filling time and, by extension, the amount of blood pumped out of the heart during each systolic heart contraction (stroke volume).[19] With prolonged or recurrent hypoxic insults, a progressive oxygen debt occurs with a loss of buffering capacity. Eventually, fetal decompensation occurs, and the intermittent slowing of the FHR may reflect not only the chemoreceptor-mediated compensatory reflex, but also depressed myocardial function.[18]

During episodes of hypoxia, vasodilation in the fetal coronary and cerebral vascular beds, in combination with peripheral vasoconstriction, contributes to a redistribution of fetal blood flow so that essential organs such as the brain, heart, and adrenal gland are preferentially perfused.[19] In the presence of hypoxemia sufficient to trigger fetal redistribution of blood flow, there is also, initially, an increase in arterial blood pressure and a decrease in cerebral vascular resistance that promotes an increase in cerebral blood flow. In addition to this "brain sparing" effect, a reduction in blood flow to the intestines, spleen, kidney, and musculoskeletal system decreases overall oxygen consumption.

Under normal circumstances, most of the body's cellular energy is produced via aerobic metabolism, the oxygen-dependent process by which carbohydrates, protein, and fats are used to produce adenosine triphosphate (ATP). This process generates carbon dioxide ($CO_2$) as a waste product, which in extrauterine life is eliminated via the lungs. In the fetus, waste products of metabolism, including $CO_2$, must be transported across the placenta for elimination by the maternal lungs and kidneys. As described earlier, $CO_2$ diffuses across the placental membranes from the fetal circulation to the maternal circulation very easily, so if there is adequate uteroplacental circulation, the $CO_2$ produced by fetal metabolism is eliminated without significant changes in fetal blood pH. If maternal–fetal gas exchange is compromised and the concentration of $CO_2$ in the fetal circulation increases, the condition is referred to as *respiratory acidosis*.

When oxygen is not available for aerobic metabolism despite compensatory mechanisms to preserve oxygen, *anaerobic metabolism* occurs. Anaerobic metabolism utilizes glucose and glycogen to produce energy (i.e., ATP), a process that generates lactic acid ($C_3H_6O_3$) as the final dissociation product. Unlike water and $CO_2$, lactic acid does not diffuse across the placenta quickly. While anaerobic metabolism allows cells to survive and function during short periods of oxygen insufficiency, when this metabolic process persists for a longer period, accumulating lactic acid in the fetal compartment can lead to a drop in pH. The lower pH then can cause cellular metabolism to fail, eventually resulting in cellular and tissue death with ensuing organ and system failure.

The fetus, like the adult, has a buffering capacity to maintain pH at normal levels. The major buffers utilized by the fetus for neutralizing hydrogen ion and lactic acid production are plasma bicarbonate and hemoglobin. If hypoxia is unrelieved, these buffering substances are depleted, fetal buffering capacity is overwhelmed, and the pH in fetal circulation falls, resulting in a state of *metabolic acidosis*. When metabolic and respiratory acidosis become severe, normal metabolic processes begin to fail.

## Fetal Asphyxia and Asphyxial Injury

If unabated, hypoxia and metabolic acidosis will eventually overwhelm the fetal compensatory mechanisms and tissue damage and organ failure will ensue. This state of extreme deficiency of oxygen and carbon dioxide excess is referred to as *asphyxia*. However, this term is imprecise and not used clinically or in written medical documentation. Asphyxia is a continuum that cannot be directly measured. Although metabolic acidemia can be measured in umbilical or neonatal blood, due to individual variations in the response to profound oxygen deprivation, the measured metabolic acidemia may not be an exact reflection of the degree of acidosis in tissues. Thus, there is no clear threshold at which one can say metabolic acidemia reflects the presence of asphyxia. This explains why, as a single measure, the presence of metabolic acidemia is not a strong predictor of long-term adverse effects in the fetus and newborn.[7(p69)]

When the arterial $O_2$ falls below a critical threshold, the cardiovascular adaptive mechanisms that preserve cerebral perfusion become overwhelmed. In the profoundly hypoxic fetus, autoregulation of cerebral blood flow fails, and cerebral perfusion becomes pressure dependent. Neurons have a high metabolic rate, and the brain does not store glucose, so the fetal brain is particularly vulnerable to asphyxial damage. If myocardial function becomes depressed to a degree that cardiac output is not sufficient to maintain adequate blood pressure, the brain also becomes hypotensive and ischemic.[7(p65),20] Cellular metabolism in the brain is quickly compromised (Figure 27-2) secondary to both loss of oxygen and ischemia. Thus, the final pathway to cell death and brain injury is termed "hypoxic–ischemic."

## Neonatal Hypoxic–Ischemic Brain Injury and Neonatal Encephalopathy

Although the terms *hypoxic–ischemic encephalopathy* (HIE) and *neonatal encephalopathy* are often used interchangeably, neither hypoxia nor ischemia can be assumed to have been the unique initiating causal mechanism for a specific newborn with neurologic impairment. The term "hypoxic–ischemic encephalopathy," therefore, is not used clinically and has been replaced by "neonatal encephalopathy."[21]

Neonatal encephalopathy (NE) is a complex disease of the newborn associated with multi-organ dysfunction that occurs in approximately 3 per 1000 live births in high-income nations. It is defined as "a clinically defined syndrome of disturbed neurologic function in the earliest days of life in the infant born at or beyond 35 weeks of gestation manifested by

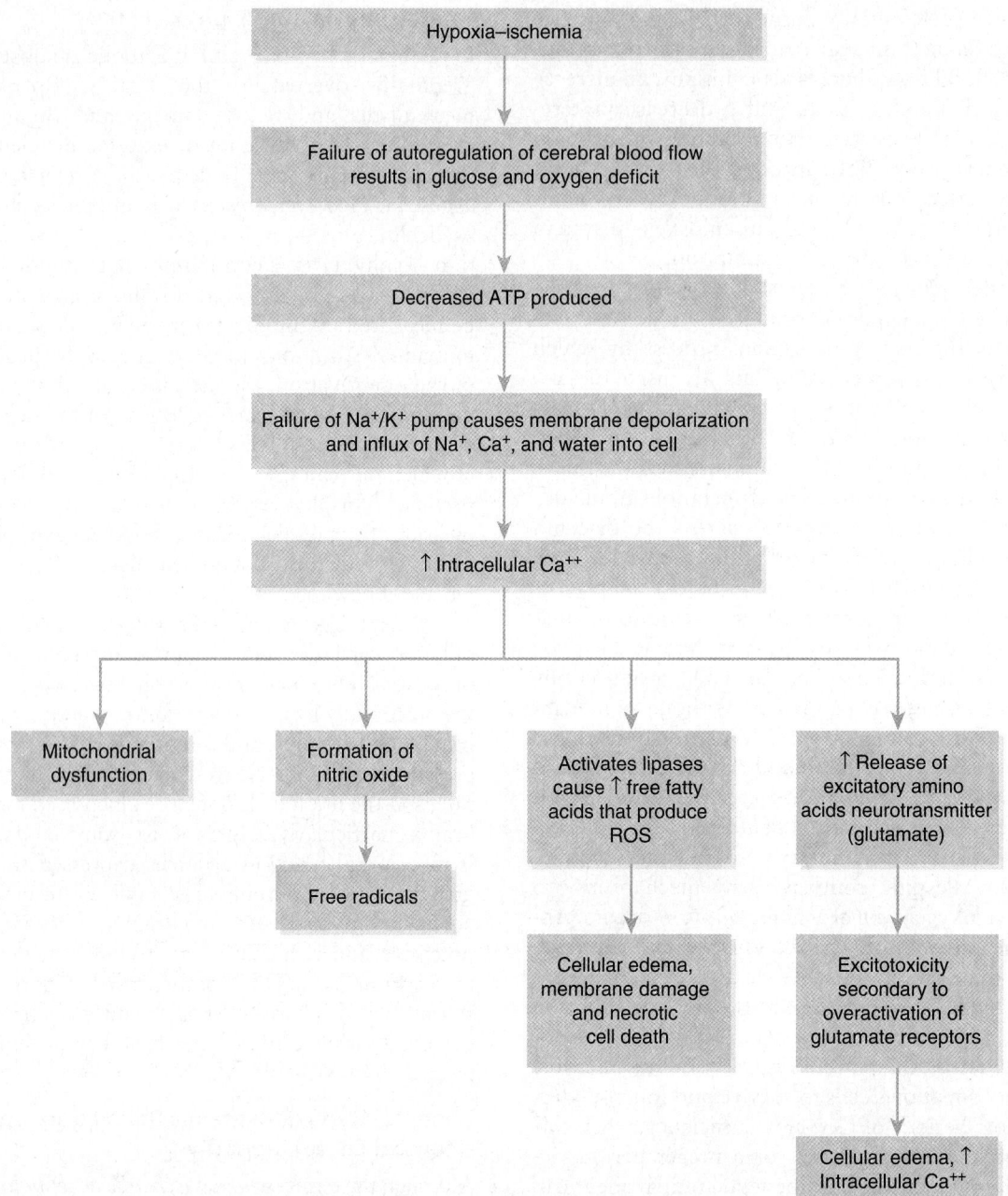

**Figure 27-2** Primary energy failure: the mechanism of hypoxic–ischemic injury.
Abbreviations: ATP, adenosine triphosphate; ROS, reactive oxygen species.
Reproduced from Parer JT, King TL, Ikeda T. *Electronic Fetal Heart Rate Monitoring: The 5-Tier System.* 3rd ed. Burlington, MA: Jones & Bartlett Learning; 2018.

subnormal level of consciousness or seizures, and often accompanied by difficulty with initiating and maintaining respiration and depression of tone and reflexes."[21] Hypoxic–ischemic brain injury is one of many etiologies of NE. Notably, perinatal infections, placental abnormalities, metabolic disorders, coagulopathies, and neonatal vascular stroke can also result in NE. Often, the cause of NE remains unidentified.[22]

The criteria necessary to assign the etiology of NE to intrapartum asphyxia are listed in Table 27-2.[21]

Neonatal encephalopathy due to hypoxic–ischemic injury occurs in approximately 1.5 per 1000 term births.[21,23] Approximately 66% of newborns with severe HIE will die or experience long-term sequelae. Conversely, the majority of infants with mild HIE have no adverse effects.[24]

| Table 27-2 | Acute Peripartum or Intrapartum Events Sufficient to Cause Neonatal Encephalopathy |
|---|---|
| **Neonatal Characteristic** | **Description** |
| Apgar score | < 5 at 5 and 10 minutes after birth. |
| Umbilical artery acidemia | pH < 7.0 and/or base deficit ≥ 12 mmol/L. |
| Magnetic resonance imaging | MRI abnormalities that appear after 24 hours of life. MRI obtained between 24 and 96 hours after birth is the most sensitive for determining the timing of cerebral injury. Conventional qualitative MRI findings of diffusion abnormalities, deep nuclear gray matter, or watershed cortical injury are most likely to indicate hypoxic–ischemic injury. |
| Multisystem organ failure | Can include renal injury, hepatic injury, hematologic abnormalities, gastrointestinal injury, cardiac dysfunction, metabolic derangements, or a combination of these abnormalities. |
| Sentinel hypoxic or ischemic event | A hypoxic or ischemic event that occurred immediately before or during labor and delivery (e.g., ruptured uterus, placental abruption, vasa previa, amniotic fluid embolism, or maternal cardiovascular collapse). |
| Fetal heart rate patterns | Category II pattern identified on presentation or for longer than 60 minutes that includes minimal/absent variability and no accelerations; suggests a previously compromised fetus. Category I FHR pattern that develops into a Category III pattern over the course of labor. Additional FHR patterns consistent with hypoxic ischemic events: tachycardia with recurrent decelerations and persistent minimal variability with recurrent decelerations. |
| Other proximal or distal factors | No evidence of other proximal or distal factors that could contribute to neonatal encephalopathy. |

Abbreviations: FHR, fetal heart rate; MRI, magnetic resonance imaging.

Based on American College of Obstetricians and Gynecologists Task Force on Neonatal Encephalopathy. *Neonatal Encephalopathy and Neurologic Outcome.* 2nd ed. Washington, DC: American College of Obstetricians and Gynecologists; 2014 (Reaffirmed 2019).

Therapeutic hypothermia, the purposeful cooling of a neonate's head or full body, can improve the probability of survival without severe disability of infants with signs of hypoxic–ischemic brain injury.[25] This treatment is thought to prevent the second stage of neuronal death that can occur following a severe episode of asphyxia. The latent period between the primary and delayed stages of neuronal death is approximately 6 hours.[26] Thus, this is the therapeutic window of opportunity for the initiation of therapeutic hypothermia. Infants more than 36 weeks' gestation who have either (1) a cord pH ≤ 7.0 or base deficit ≥ −16 or (2) a pH of 7.01 to 7.15 or base deficit of −10 to −15.9 on cord gas or blood gas within 1 hour of birth, with a history of an acute perinatal event (e.g., cord prolapse, placental abruption, or uterine rupture) and an Apgar score ≤ 5 at 10 minutes or at least 10 minutes of positive-pressure ventilation, are candidates for therapeutic hypothermia if their clinical exam reveals seizures or other evidence of moderate-to-severe encephalopathy.[27,28]

### Neonatal Encephalopathy and Cerebral Palsy

Cerebral palsy is a permanent disorder of movement and posture that is caused by damage to the fetal or neonatal brain. Historically, it was believed that cerebral palsy was always caused by asphyxia during the birth process. However, the relationship between NE, hypoxic–ischemic injury related to oxygen deprivation during labor, and cerebral palsy is complex. NE is the typical initial presentation of cerebral palsy in the neonate. Due to the timing of its presentation, it is now understood that NE is the result of a common final pathologic pathway that can be initiated by different inciting events (sometimes in combination), but does not always involve fetal asphyxia. Placental lesions, intrauterine infection, and intrauterine stroke may—either on their own or in combination with other factors—also result in fetal brain damage that eventually manifests as NE and subsequent cerebral palsy.[21,29]

## Techniques for FHR Assessment During Labor

Monitoring of the FHR, either intermittently or continuously, is the mainstay of fetal assessment in labor. The goal is to use what is known both about the FHR compensatory response to hypoxemia and signs of fetal decompensation that are detectable via observation of the FHR to determine whether intervention is needed before hypoxic injury occurs.

Assessment of the fetal heart can be conducted via intermittent auscultation or via intermittent or continuous electronic fetal monitoring (EFM). Electronic FHR monitoring can be conducted using either external or internal monitors. Assessment of fetal well-being during labor relies on assessment of the response to the fetal heart to contractions, so monitoring of contractions is also necessary. Like the FHR, uterine contractions can be monitored either externally or internally. Graphing of continuous EFM (FHR tracing) together with graphing of continuous electronic monitoring of contractions is sometimes referred to as cardiotocography (CTG). Often, the term EFM is used synonymously with CTG.

## Intermittent Auscultation

Noncontinuous, or intermittent, auscultation of the FHR may be performed with a fetoscope, a Doppler device, or even the external ultrasound transducer of the electronic fetal monitor. Because fetoscopes that do not use Doppler sonography (such as the DeLee-Hillis and Allen devices) rely on bone conduction of sound, and therefore require proximity of the examiner's head to the pregnant abdomen, factors such as maternal position, habitus, and activity can limit assessment of the FHR with a fetoscope.

Intermittent FHR assessment is most often conducted using handheld Doppler devices. Doppler ultrasound technology projects an ultrasound wave into the uterus. This wave is reflected off the moving fetal ventricle, and the waveform changes as it is reflected to the Doppler transducer. The transducer detects the heart movement of each heartbeat and emits an electronically created sound that can be counted or displayed digitally. Doppler devices can detect the fetal heart movement when the parturient is in most positions. In addition, some models can be safely used underwater, allowing for their use during hydrotherapy in labor and birth. The technique for performing and interpreting intermittent auscultation is presented in the *Intermittent Auscultation During Labor* appendix.

Use of the EFM Doppler transducer for intermittent auscultation of the FHR is somewhat controversial. Advocates find use of the EFM ultrasound transducer to be convenient, and a printout of the FHR pattern can be made. When a graphic or paper FHR tracing is obtained, data including the FHR variability, accelerations, and types of decelerations must be identified and interpreted according to continuous EFM guidelines. Caution is warranted, as no standard exists for this technique; each institution and individual clinician must consider the pros and cons of relying on these data. The American College of Obstetricians and Gynecologists (ACOG) recommends use of either intermittent auscultation or EFM for persons who are at low risk for fetal acidemia at the onset of labor.[30] Professional association guidelines from Canada and the United Kingdom recommend intermittent auscultation for persons who are not at risk for fetal acidemia at the onset of labor.[31,32]

## Electronic Fetal Heart Rate Monitoring

EFM devices are placed externally on the maternal abdomen or internally into the uterus through the vagina. The fetal monitor graphic display has both upper and lower display areas. The upper portion displays the FHR pattern, with increments of 10 beats per minute (bpm) graphed on the vertical axis. The lower portion displays the uterine contractions, with gradations for 0 to 100 units on the vertical axis. The horizontal axis is divided into 10-second and 1-minute segments. Therefore, the FHR pattern, the contraction pattern, and the timing and relationship between the two are displayed on the device. EFM has become nearly ubiquitous for fetal assessment in certain birth settings, utilized at some point in approximately 90% of individuals who labor in U.S. hospitals.[33]

EFM devices were introduced as instruments for monitoring individuals with high-risk pregnancies in the 1960s and were rapidly adopted in clinical practice before adequate research assessing the relationship between FHR characteristics and newborn outcomes had been conducted. The first observational studies of FHR monitoring compared newborn outcomes in settings before the introduction of FHR monitoring to outcomes after widespread adoption of FHR monitoring. Those before-and-after studies documented a significant decrease in the incidence of intrapartum stillbirth in individuals who were continuously monitored during labor—an outcome that remains one of the key benefits of EFM.[34]

No randomized controlled trials (RCTs) have compared continuous EFM during labor to no fetal monitoring during labor. Several RCTs, performed in the 1980s and 1990s, compared continuous EFM to intermittent auscultation of the fetal heart with a Pinard stethoscope or a handheld Doppler device. Most of these trials included one-to-one nursing, and several included individuals at high risk for adverse outcomes. Neither the RCTs nor the subsequent meta-analyses found that EFM improved outcomes when compared to intermittent auscultation with regard to Apgar scores, incidence of cerebral palsy, or perinatal mortality.[1,35] However, continuous EFM was associated with an approximately 50% increase in rates of cesarean birth (relative risk [RR], 1.63; 95% confidence interval [CI], 1.29–2.07) and a slight increase in operative vaginal birth (RR, 1.15; 95% CI, 1.01–1.33).[35]

Newborn seizures were used as an indicator of long-term neurologic dysfunction and perinatal mortality in these trials. The largest RCT, which was performed in Dublin, Ireland, found EFM resulted in a 50% decrease in neonatal seizures (1.8% in the EFM group versus 4.1% in the intermittent auscultation group). When the cohort of newborns in this trial who had seizures and survived were reexamined at age 4 years, those in the EFM group and those in the intermittent auscultation group had equal proportions of cerebral palsy—a finding that suggests EFM was not effective in decreasing the rate of cerebral palsy.[36,37] It is not possible to draw clinically relevant conclusions about the effect of EFM from these data and the small number of affected children. Nonetheless, EFM may have a protective effect in decreasing the incidence of early newborn seizures, although the long-term implications are unclear.

The negative findings of the meta-analysis of the RCTs evaluating EFM resulted in many clinicians concluding that EFM has no clinical value. However, the RCTs' failure to detect a benefit of EFM occurred secondary to several methodologic problems; thus, the results are not considered conclusive or reliable for practice today.[38] In short, the RCTs did not answer the question of whether EFM improves neonatal outcomes because they had the wrong outcome measures, they did not monitor for FHR patterns that are known today to indicate fetal compromise, cerebral palsy is not always the result of intrapartum hypoxia, and the studies were not large enough to detect meaningful changes in perinatal mortality. Thus, it is as inappropriate to claim EFM has no value as it is to advocate for universal use of EFM. Studies conducted in the last decade have identified some FHR patterns that are indicative of developing acidemia.[39–41] While more data are needed, it is possible that this refined understanding of when intervention for variant FHR patterns is warranted will help reduce both the incidence of newborn acidemia and the rate of operative births performed secondary to abnormal FHR patterns.[42]

### External Monitoring

External FHR monitoring is accomplished via the placement of a Doppler device that has a transducer and a receiver that is secured onto the maternal abdomen, over the area of the fetal heart. The Doppler transducer transmits a high-frequency ultrasound pulse of approximately 2.5 MHz. The receiver detects the change in the ultrasound wave length as it is reflected by the fetal heart as it moves during each heartbeat. In brief, the monitor counts the time interval between each detected fetal heartbeat and calculates a beats per minute (bpm) rate based on that interval. The monitor then plots the bpm rate on a graph, which scrolls continuously so that the individual plot points are merged into a jagged line. This line is jagged because the time interval between each fetal heartbeat typically varies slightly.[43]

External fetal monitoring is appropriate for most laboring individuals for whom continuous EFM during labor is indicated. In most situations, with careful placement of the abdominal transducer and tocodynamometer, the FHR and uterine contractions will be visually displayed adequately for interpretation. In some cases, such as with individuals who have a high body mass index (BMI) or persons using frequent position changes, the FHR can be difficult to obtain or may require frequent repositioning of the transducer. The equipment and electrical cords of most EFM units limit their mobility unless a telemetry unit is available that allows transmission across long distance, thus allowing for ambulation of the pregnant person. Some of these units can work in a shower or submerged in a tub.

### Sources of Artifact and Error in External Electronic Fetal Monitoring

EFM has some limitations secondary to the Doppler technique itself. The Doppler signal can fail to detect the FHR as the fetus moves or the laboring person changes position. Periodic "drop-out" of the signal can then result in misinterpretation of the FHR pattern. If the FHR has minimal variability, and the clinician has a concern that the fetus is experiencing hypoxia, use of an internal fetal scalp electrode will record an accurate fetal electrocardiogram (ECG) and can aid clinical decision making.

Maternal heart rate artifact is also an important source of signal processing errors in EFM. This kind of artifact is generated when the Doppler device detects movement of maternal vessels, which are then recorded as the FHR. The second stage of labor is a time of increased risk for maternal heart rate artifact, as the Doppler device is often placed lower on the maternal abdomen, where it is more likely to detect the movement of large maternal vessels.

This can lead to a failure to recognize an abnormal FHR or a fetal demise. Irrespective of the type of monitoring unit used, the midwife must be sure to disambiguate the maternal and fetal signals. When doubt arises regarding whether the monitor is recording the FHR, the provider should verify the maternal rate by checking maternal radial pulse and, if a clear difference cannot be detected this way, by placing a maternal ECG monitor or using a finger pulse oximeter to provide a continuous pulse reading. Adjusting the Doppler transducer position or placing an internal fetal monitor may be necessary if continuous monitoring is needed and a repeated loss of the fetal heart signal allows for the maternal heart rate to mask the FHR.

### Internal Fetal Heart Rate Monitoring

Internal monitoring is used when the fetal heart rate needs to be monitored continuously and obtaining an adequate tracing via external monitoring is difficult. Internal monitoring requires ruptured membranes. A fetal scalp electrode (FSE) is placed a few millimeters into the fetal scalp. The FSE transmits the fetal electrocardiogram to the monitor, which displays a digital signal of the FHR as well as a continuous graph of the heart rate. The procedure for placing an FSE is described in the *Fetal Scalp Electrode* appendix.

### Uterine Activity Monitoring

Uterine contractions can be monitored via maternal perception, manual palpation, external tocodynamometer attached to an electronic fetal monitor, or internal placement of an intrauterine pressure catheter (IUPC). A uterine contraction is first detectable via manual palpation when the intrauterine pressure exceeds 10 mm Hg; by comparison, maternal perception of a painful contraction usually occurs when the intrauterine pressure reaches a minimum of 15 mm Hg.[44] This amount of pressure is required to distend the lower uterine segment and create pressure on the cervix. Assessment of uterine contraction by palpation should be conducted over the uterine fundus, which should be easy to indent in between contractions. During a contraction, fetal parts become unpalpable and the uterus difficult to indent. While manual palpation can be used to assess for the presence of contractions,[45] assessment of contraction strength by manual palpation correlates poorly to contraction strength assessed via pressure catheter.[46]

For external electronic monitoring of uterine activity, a uterine pressure tocodynamometer is placed on the maternal fundus and secured with a belt around the laboring person's abdomen. The tocodynamometer records the changes in pressure that occur when the fundus tightens during a contraction and shows the continuous pressure changes on a graphic display. Although this device records contraction duration and frequency, it does not accurately record contraction intensity. Tightening the monitor straps or changing the position of the tocodynamometer can alter the appearance of contraction intensity. Internal uterine monitoring is needed to detect and measure contraction intensity.

If the progress of labor is slower than expected, an IUPC may be inserted through the cervix into the uterine cavity to provide a quantitative measurement of uterine contraction intensity. The procedure for placing an IUPC and interpretation of its data output are described in the *Intrauterine Pressure Catheter* appendix. The IUPC has the advantage of providing specific information about the resting tone of the uterus, the actual pressure generated by the contractions, and accurate timing of the onset, peak, and completion of a contraction. If amnioinfusion is needed, it can be done through the same catheter used to perform internal uterine monitoring. Disadvantages of this technology include an increased risk of infection if the IUPC is left in place for an extended period and the requirement that the individual in labor remain tethered to a bed.

### Adjunct Surveillance Methods

Adjunct fetal surveillance methods have been studied to determine if they can increase the accuracy of EFM. These included FHR electrocardiogram ST-segment analysis (STAN) via an electrode that is passed through the cervix and attached to the fetal head; analysis of fetal scalp blood for lactate or pH, with the sample being retrieved by making a small incision in the fetal scalp and collecting blood with a capillary tube; and pulse oximetry, which uses a noninvasive probe that sits along the fetal head and records both pulse rate and arterial oxygen saturation to derive an estimate of fetal peripheral perfusion. None of these methods has been associated with a reduced risk of neonatal acidemia, neonatal intensive care unit (NICU) admission, Apgar scores, or perinatal death compared to EFM alone or intermittent auscultation.[1] Currently research is being conducted on the use of noninvasive sensors placed on the maternal abdomen that detect the fetal ECG and on use of computerized interpretation of FHR characteristics.

## Fetal Heart Rate Characteristics and Patterns: Terminology, Etiology, and Clinical Significance

In the decades following the introduction of EFM, a barrier to the useful application of this technology in both research and clinical practice was the lack of a standardized lexicon to describe the visually distinct characteristics and patterns in an FHR tracing. In the late 1960s, Edward Hon first described FHR decelerations as early versus late based on their appearance and timing in relation to uterine contractions.

It was not until 1997, however, that the National Institute of Child Health and Human Development (NICHD) convened an expert panel charged with developing a standard terminology for interpreting FHR patterns. This panel created mutually exclusive definitions for each distinct FHR characteristic that have been widely adopted for research and clinical use (Table 27-3).[47] These FHR characteristics are classified as baseline, periodic, or episodic.[47] The baseline features, which include the heart rate, variability, and accelerations, are assessed between uterine contractions. *Periodic changes*, which include early and late decelerations, occur in association with uterine contractions. *Episodic changes*, including variable and prolonged decelerations, are not clearly associated with uterine contractions.

This standard nomenclature was later reaffirmed in a second NICHD expert panel in 2008.[48] This nomenclature is used in the United States and most high-income nations to describe FHR characteristics during labor. Familiarity with the NICHD definitions and FHR categorization system is thus an essential component of intrapartum care. However, it is important to note that the NICHD terminology is essentially a description of visual characteristics, and that our understanding of the clinical significance of the FHR patterns described by these terms is based on incomplete and evolving knowledge of the pathophysiology of fetal asphyxia.

### Baseline Fetal Heart Rate

The baseline fetal heart rate at term ranges from 110 to 160 bpm. The average baseline heart rate in the normal term fetus before labor is 140 bpm. Early in pregnancy, the average FHR is higher, albeit not significantly higher. Because parasympathetic (vagal) tone does not predominate until the third trimester, heart rates of 140 to 160 bpm are normal baseline rates in a preterm fetus.

### Tachycardia

Fetal tachycardia is defined as a baseline rate of more than 160 bpm. Short periods of tachycardia are a normal compensatory response to transient hypoxia, and in the absence of other FHR abnormalities, are not usually associated with poor outcomes in the term fetus. Mild tachycardia is common in the fetus of less than 28 weeks' gestation.

Nonhypoxic causes of tachycardia include administration of beta-mimetic drugs or ephedrine given to correct maternal hypotension. Tachycardia in a term fetus may also be due to developing hypoxia when it is part of a constellation of characteristics that include recurrent decelerations of the FHR and decreasing variability, along with maternal or fetal infection.[49] Other conditions associated with tachycardia include cardiac arrhythmias[50] and, rarely, fetal anemia (Rh isoimmunization), acute fetal blood loss (placental abruption), an abnormal fetal conduction system (fetal arrhythmia), or poorly controlled maternal hyperthyroidism. Sustained fetal tachycardia should not be dismissed as a benign finding without consideration of the full clinical picture and other FHR characteristics.[39,51,52]

### Bradycardia

Both hypoxic and nonhypoxic causes of fetal bradycardia are possible. Nonhypoxic causes include fetal heart block and maternal hypothermia. A mild bradycardia in the 100 to 120 bpm range can be idiopathic and is often seen in the postmature fetus, as the heart rate progressively slows over the course of gestation and early childhood. Bradycardia can also develop during rapid descent of the fetal presenting part or at the end of the second stage of labor when fetal head compression causes increased intracranial pressure, which then initiates a vagal response and bradycardia. In such a case, the fetus will maintain cerebral oxygenation if the FHR remains higher than 80 bpm and variability will be retained. A mild drop in FHR, which presents as a prolonged deceleration, can also can occur after administration of intrathecal opioids or local anesthetics for epidural analgesia. This etiology is usually attributed to maternal hypotension secondary to the sympathetic block leading to decreased uteroplacental blood flow. These transient bradycardias usually retain normal FHR variability and are rarely associated with adverse outcomes. In short, fetal bradycardia that is accompanied by moderate variability is not associated with fetal acidemia.[53]

Hypoxic causes of bradycardia include acute emergency events such as prolapsed cord,

| Table 27-3 | Terminology for Fetal Heart Rate Characteristics |
|---|---|
| **Term** | **Definition** |
| Baseline rate | Mean FHR rounded to increments of 5 bpm during a 10-minute segment excluding periodic or episodic changes, periods of marked variability, and segments of baseline that differ by > 25 bpm. Duration must be ≥ 2 minutes. |
| Bradycardia | Baseline rate < 110 bpm. |
| Tachycardia | Baseline rate > 160 bpm. |
| Variability | Fluctuations in the baseline FHR ≥ 2 cycles/min. |
| Absent variability | Amplitude from peak to trough undetectable. |
| Minimal variability | Amplitude from peak to trough > undetectable and ≤ 5 bpm. |
| Moderate variability | Amplitude from peak to trough 6–25 bpm. |
| Marked variability | Amplitude from peak to trough > 25 bpm. |
| Acceleration | Visually apparent abrupt increase (onset to peak < 30 seconds) of FHR above baseline. Peak ≥ 15 bpm. Duration ≥ 15 bpm and < 2 minutes. In gestations < 32 weeks, peak ≥ 10 bpm above baseline and duration ≥ 10 seconds is an acceleration. |
| Prolonged acceleration | Acceleration ≥ 2 minutes and < 10 minutes' duration. An acceleration ≥ 10 minutes is a baseline change. |
| Early deceleration | Visually apparent *gradual* decrease (onset of deceleration to nadir ≥ 30 seconds) of FHR below baseline. Return to baseline associated with a uterine contraction. Generally, the onset, nadir, and recovery of the deceleration occur at the same time as the onset, peak, and recovery of the contraction, respectively. |
| Late deceleration | Visually apparent *gradual* decrease (onset of deceleration to nadir ≥ 30 seconds) of FHR below baseline. Return to baseline associated with a uterine contraction. The nadir of the deceleration occurs *after* the peak of the contraction. Generally, the onset, nadir, and recovery of the deceleration occur after the onset, peak, and recovery of the contraction, respectively. |
| Variable deceleration | Visually apparent *abrupt* decrease (onset of deceleration to nadir < 30 seconds) in FHR below baseline. Decrease ≥ 15 bpm below baseline. Duration ≥ 15 seconds and < 2 minutes from onset to return to baseline. |
| Prolonged deceleration | Visually apparent decrease in FHR below baseline. Decrease ≥ 15 bpm below baseline. Duration ≥ 2 minutes but < 10 minutes from onset to return to baseline. |

Abbreviations: bpm, beats per minute; FHR, fetal heart rate.

Based on National Institute of Child Health and Human Development Research Planning Workshop. Electronic fetal heart rate monitoring: research guidelines for interpretation. *Am J Obstet Gynecol.* 1997;17:1385-1390; *JOGNN.* 1997;26:635-64047; and Macones GA, Hankins GD, Spong CY, Hauth J, Moore T. The 2008 National Institute of Child Health and Human Development Research Workshop report on electronic fetal heart rate monitoring. *Obstet Gynecol.* 2008;112:661-666; *JOGNN.* 2008;37:510-515.

placental abruption, uterine rupture, and vasa previa,[54] though bradycardia can also be the result of progressive hypoxia that overwhelms the fetal compensatory mechanisms, leading to direct myocardial depression. When an acute bradycardia occurs, the depth and duration of the bradycardia and the presence or absence of variability are key factors associated with subsequent neonatal morbidity. In general, if the FHR remains greater than 80 bpm, both coronary and cerebral oxygenation will be preserved, and variability is often retained.[55] In contrast, when the FHR is persistently less than 80 bpm, the variability will diminish rapidly as a metabolic acidemia develops. An FHR baseline of less than 60 bpm is an emergency. At this heart rate, the fetus is unable to sustain adequate circulation through the heart to supply the coronary arteries and brain. If this condition is unrelieved, it will result in brain injury, cardiac failure, and fetal death.

The presence of a pattern of FHR decelerations preceding the bradycardia signals the presence of lower fetal reserves. In a retrospective analysis of cases of uterine rupture, Leung et al. found that none of the newborns without decelerations preceding the bradycardia had significant metabolic acidemia when the bradycardia-to-birth time was less than 18 minutes.[56] By comparison, when the bradycardia was preceded by recurrent decelerations, metabolic acidemia occurred as early as 10 minutes after the bradycardia started.

### Fetal Heart Rate Variability

The vagus nerve controls the baseline FHR. Because the vagus nerve is responsive to input from the CNS, it stimulates frequent changes in the timing between each heartbeat. This variability in FHR can be seen on EFM tracings as unidirectional, short-term fluctuations in the line that records the FHR. This variability reflects CNS function and well-being. Variability is described as absent, minimal, moderate, or marked based on the amplitude of the fluctuations. The presence of moderate FHR variability signifies that the fetus has an intact cerebral cortex, midbrain, vagus nerve, and cardiac conduction system, and is one of the best indicators that the fetus does not have cerebral tissue hypoxia or ischemia.[53] Approximately 98% of all fetuses with moderate variability will not have clinically significant acidemia at the time the variability is observed, even if recurrent FHR decelerations are present (Figure 27-3).[53]

Minimal variability is interpreted based on the presence or absence of accelerations or recurrent decelerations. If the variability is minimal and FHR decelerations are not present, this condition has no correlation with fetal acidemia.[53] Fetal rest cycles are associated with periods of uncomplicated minimal variability typically lasting 20 to 40 minutes, but sometimes persisting for as long as 75 to 80 minutes.[57] Administration of opioids (e.g., morphine, butorphanol, fentanyl), promethazine (Phenergan), or beta-adrenergic agents such as terbutaline to the pregnant person will also decrease the amplitude of FHR variability.

Absent variability, like minimal variability, should be interpreted based on the presence or absence of decelerations. Absent variability without decelerations is rare but can be idiopathic and is not consistently associated with fetal acidemia. In contrast, minimal or absent variability in the presence of recurrent late or variable decelerations is one of the FHR patterns most consistently associated with fetal acidemia and requires urgent assessment and intervention.[30,38–40,42,48] The evolution of moderate to minimal to absent variability in the presence of recurrent decelerations that become progressively deeper is the classic pattern evolution that reflects developing fetal acidemia over time.[30,38–40,42,48]

Marked variability is relatively rare. While it is not associated with adverse long-term newborn outcomes, it has been associated with abnormal arterial cord gases and neonatal respiratory distress and, therefore, may warrant intervention to optimize fetal oxygenation.[58] Marked variability in FHR patterns may represent an increased sympathetic response in the neonate due to short periods of hypoxia that are of neither a frequency nor an intensity to cause overt acidemia.

### Accelerations

Accelerations are visually abrupt, transient increases of the FHR above the baseline (Figure 27-4), often occurring with fetal movement and, sometimes, with uterine contractions. They are thought to be due to sympathetic activity. Accelerations are associated with a normal pH at the time they occur, so they are considered a reassuring indicator of fetal well-being.[59]

### Early Decelerations

Early decelerations are periodic decreases in the FHR that "mirror" uterine contractions. Their onset, nadir, and resolution coincide with the onset, peak, and resolution of the contraction, respectively (Figure 27-5). The precise mechanism underlying early decelerations has not been determined. A commonly referenced theory suggests that early decelerations are caused by head compression, though this theory has never been substantiated.[7(p5)] Studies of FHR response to head compression have demonstrated either no response or a vagal response resulting in variable decelerations.

Despite the lack of knowledge about the underlying physiologic mechanism, clinical observation has been useful in determining how to interpret this deceleration pattern. Early decelerations that are not recurrent and present with moderate variability are not associated with fetal acidemia and can be considered a benign finding not requiring intervention.[7(p5)] However, early decelerations that are recurrent have been observed to evolve into a pattern of late decelerations, suggesting that they may also be an initial

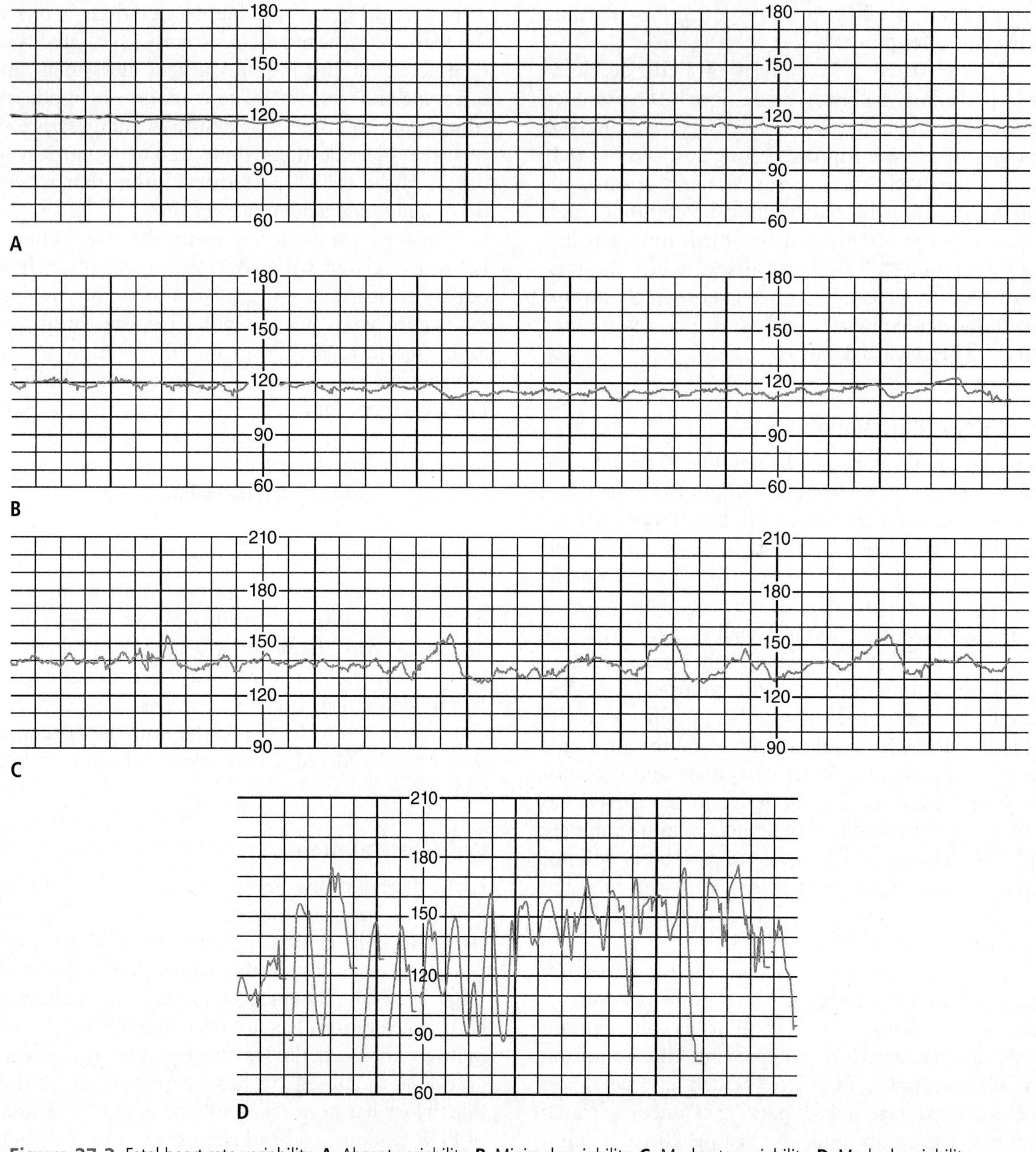

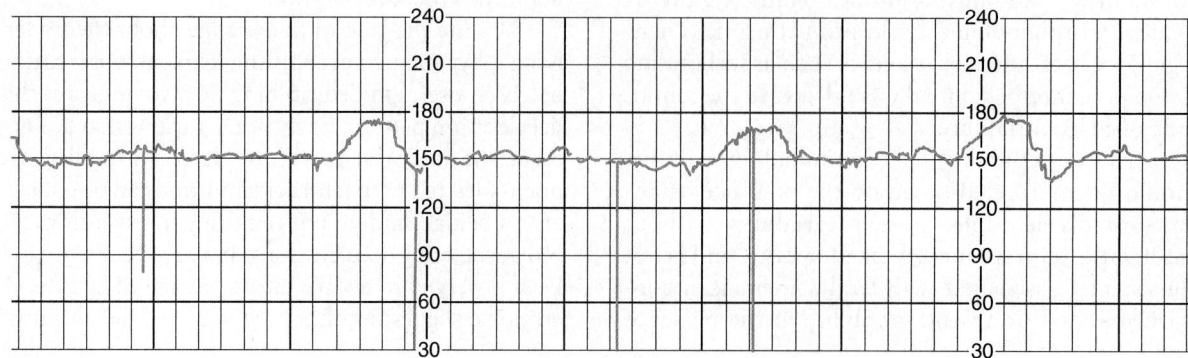

**Figure 27-3** Fetal heart rate variability. **A.** Absent variability. **B.** Minimal variability. **C.** Moderate variability. **D.** Marked variability.

**Figure 27-4** Accelerations of the fetal heart rate.

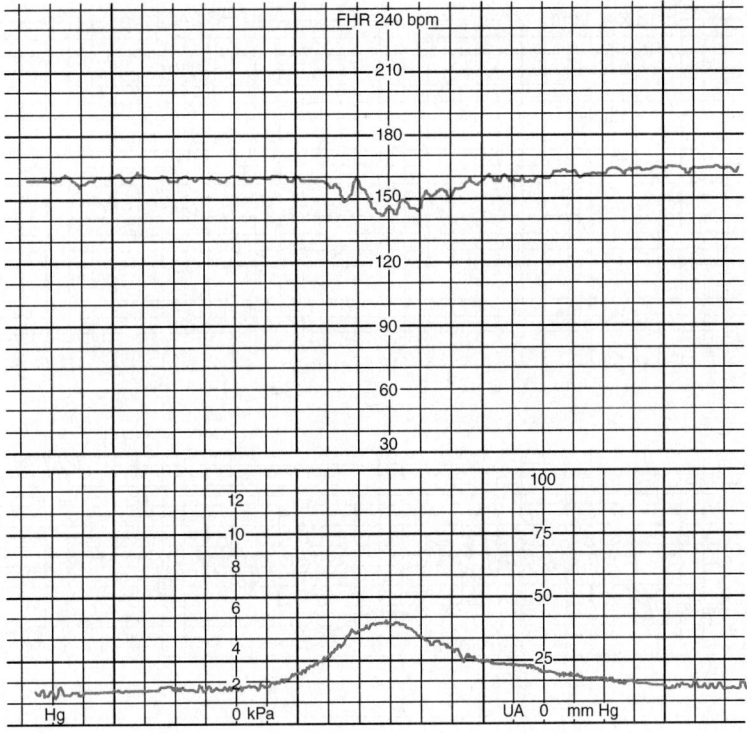

**Figure 27-5** Early decelerations.
Abbreviations: bpm, beats per minute; FHR, fetal heart rate; UA, uterine activity.

response to decreased fetal oxygenation. Recurrent and deepening decelerations, particularly with an accompanying decrease in FHR variability, should not be dismissed as benign, as they may signal a developing fetal acidemia regardless of the timing of the onset of the deceleration.

### Late Decelerations

Unlike for early decelerations, the underlying mechanism that causes late decelerations has been established. These decelerations occur in response to transient decreases in oxygen tension. This compensatory mechanism starts with a uterine contraction that causes a decrease in uteroplacental perfusion, which is followed by lower oxygen levels in the blood returning from the placenta to fetal circulation. The hypoxemia is detected by chemoreceptors in the fetal carotid artery, carotid sinus, and aortic arch. Chemoreceptor activation signals a vagally mediated drop in the FHR. The nadir of the fetal bradycardia is "late" relative to the peak of the uterine contraction because the CNS needs time to first detect the physiologic pathway that results in chemoreceptor stimulation and then generate a response via the vagus nerve (Figure 27-6).

Recurrent late decelerations (occurring with more than 50% of contractions in a 20-minute period)

are associated with uteroplacental insufficiency. *Uteroplacental insufficiency* refers to any condition in which the placenta is not able to supply sufficient oxygen or nutrients to the fetus. It can be either chronic or acute. Causes of chronic uteroplacental insufficiency include maternal hypertensive disorders, diabetes, hyperthyroidism, autoimmune disorders such as lupus, and abnormal placentation. All of these disorders are associated with narrowed spiral arteries, small placentas, and/or placental infarcts that decrease the placental area available for transfer of oxygen and nutrients. In addition, uteroplacental insufficiency is associated with postmaturity. Acute uteroplacental insufficiency can develop in the setting of uterine tachysystole or maternal hypotension. Finally, fetal anemia secondary to fetal–maternal hemorrhage, Rh sensitization, and nonimmune hydrops will effectively lower the oxygen-carrying capacity of the fetus so that the transient decreases in oxygen present in the intervillous spaces associated with uterine contractions result in significant declines in fetal oxygen tension and resultant late decelerations.

In the presence of moderate heart rate variability, late decelerations usually indicate a fetus with normal CNS status having an expected, compensatory response to decreased oxygenation related to labor contractions, rather than the presence of

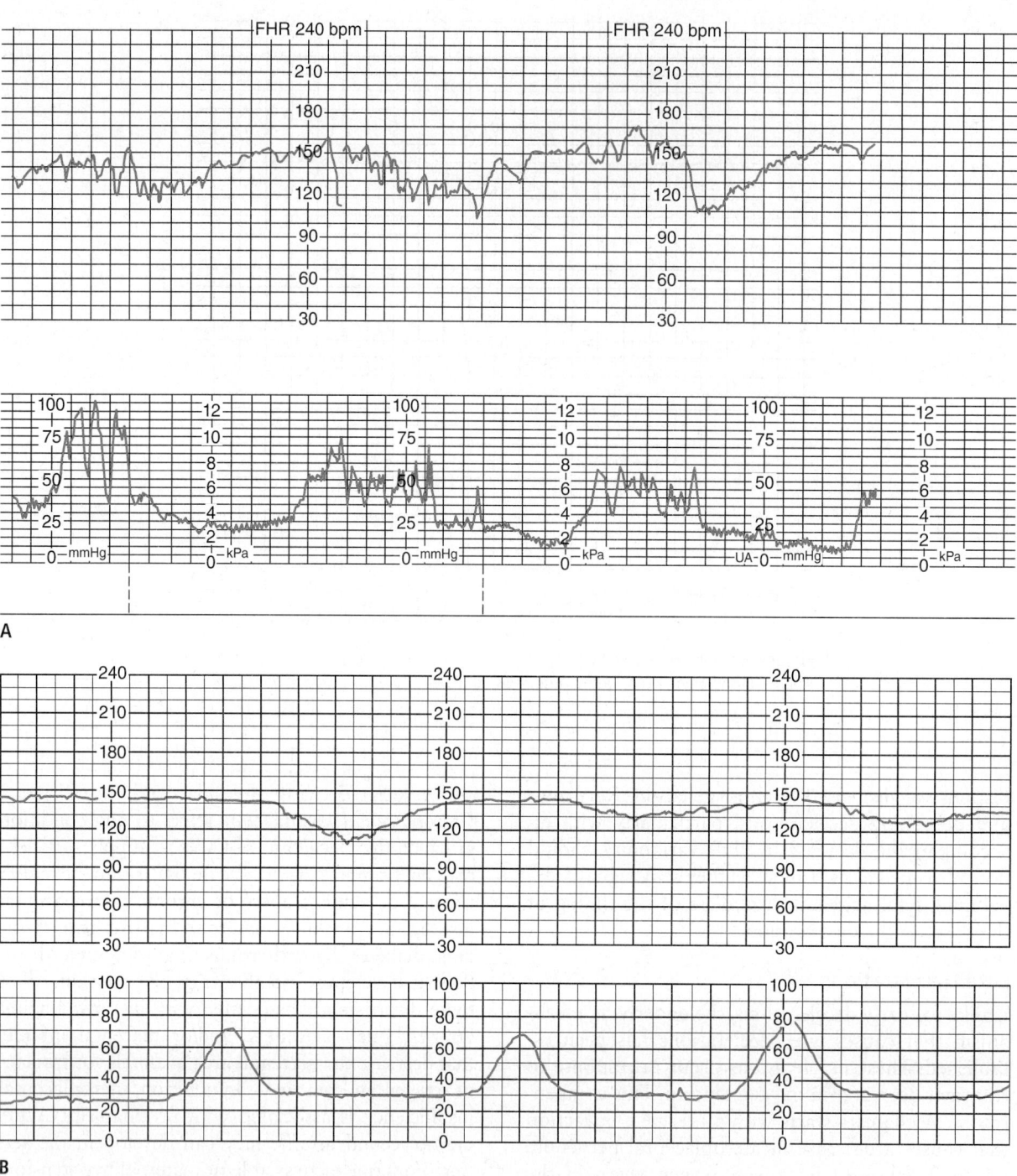

**Figure 27-6** Late decelerations. **A.** Late deceleration with moderate variability. **B.** Late deceleration with absent variability.
Abbreviations: bpm, beats per minute; FHR, fetal heart rate.

acidemia.[53] Conversely, recurrent late decelerations in the presence of minimal or absent variability is one of the FHR patterns most closely associated with fetal acidemia.[48,53]

Late decelerations can be classified as mild (≤ 15 bpm drop from baseline to nadir), moderate (15 to 45 bpm drop from baseline to nadir), or severe (≥ 45 bpm drop from baseline to nadir). Although these classifications are not part of the NICHD nomenclature, good evidence supports the observation that late decelerations become progressively deeper as fetal acidemia worsens.[53,60,61] These deep, late decelerations are usually accompanied by minimal or absent variability and are thought to be due to direct myocardial depression that occurs when fetal compensatory mechanisms are insufficient to maintain adequate cerebral and myocardial oxygenation.[18]

### Variable Decelerations

Variable decelerations are the most common variant FHR pattern, seen in approximately 45% to 75% of all labors.[62,63] These abrupt decreases in FHR can be either episodic (occurring at random times) or periodic (occurring with each uterine contraction). A common theory on the cause of variable decelerations is that umbilical cord occlusion causes an increase in fetal peripheral resistance and hypertension, which then triggers baroreflex-mediated decelerations in an effort to restore normal arterial pressure. While baroreceptor activation may contribute to this finding, recent evidence suggests that variable decelerations, like late decelerations, are mediated primarily by peripheral chemoreceptors in response to abrupt reductions in fetal oxygenation often related to interruptions in umbilical blood flow related to cord compression.[18,64]

Numerous causes of umbilical cord compression have been identified. These etiologies include cord occlusion secondary to the cord around the fetus's neck or body, true knots in the cord, frank and occult prolapse of the cord, and compression due to decreased amniotic fluid (this fluid cushions the cord). Variable decelerations are also common in the second stage of labor, in which case they are presumed to occur secondary to either head compression and the direct effect of increased intracranial pressure on the vagus nerve, or interruptions in the uteroplacental flow that occur when maternal pushing efforts are superimposed on contractions.

Variable decelerations that return to baseline in less than 60 seconds with concomitant normal baseline and moderate variability are not associated with fetal acidemia. In contrast, similar to recurrent late decelerations, recurrent variable decelerations with minimal or absent variability are associated with fetal acidemia and require urgent evaluation and consideration of intervention (Figure 27-7).

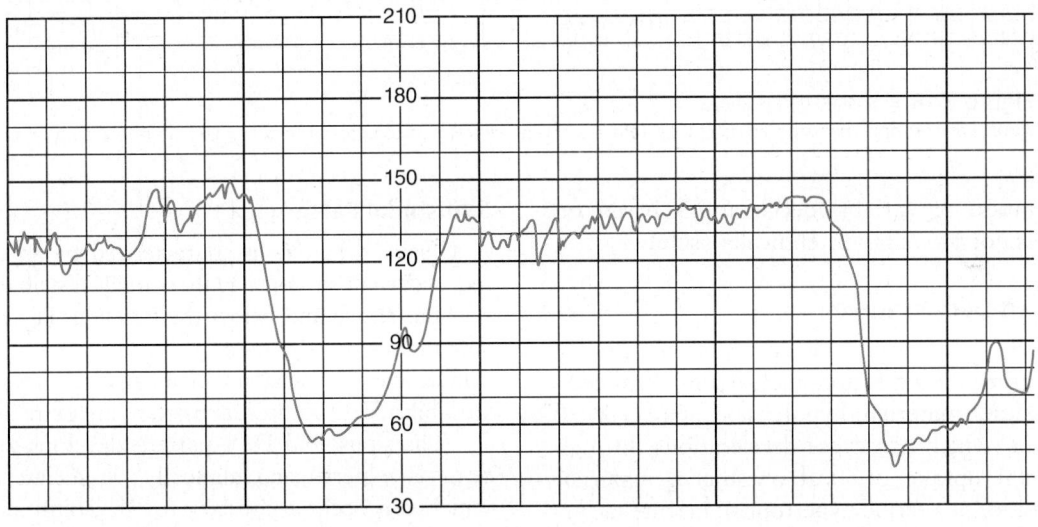

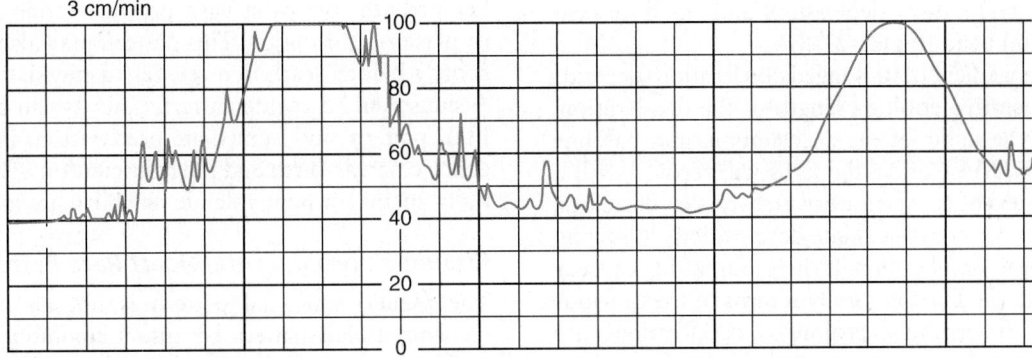

**Figure 27-7** Variable decelerations.

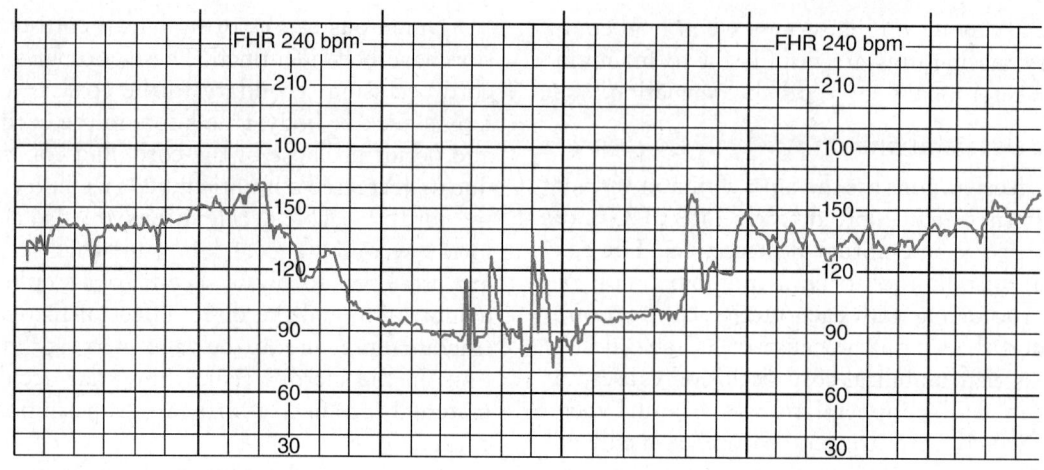

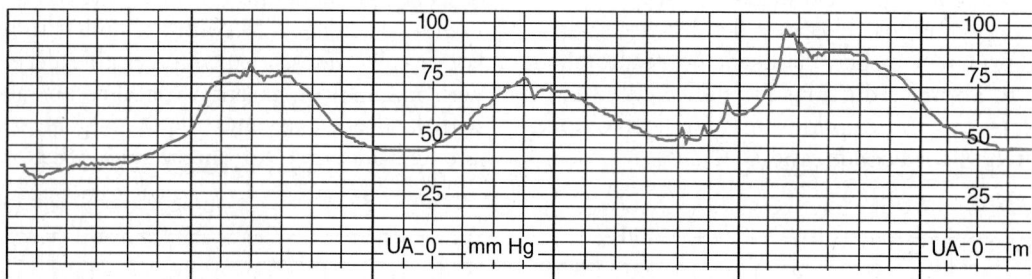

**Figure 27-8** Prolonged decelerations.
Abbreviations: bpm, beats per minute; FHR, fetal heart rate; mm Hg, millimeters of mercury; UA, uterine activity.

Interpretation of variable decelerations based on shape has not proved to be clinically useful.

## Prolonged Decelerations

Prolonged decelerations have multiple causes. Known precipitating factors include umbilical cord compression, maternal hypotension, paracervical anesthesia (which can cause decelerations through direct fetal uptake of local anesthetic, maternal hypotension, or uterine hypertonus), uterine tachysystole, maternal hypoxia associated with seizures or acute respiratory depression, and rapid descent of the fetal head (Figure 27-8).

Management of prolonged decelerations depends on the putative etiology, length of the deceleration, FHR at the nadir of the deceleration, and baseline variability. Most often, the fetus will recover with a short period of compensatory tachycardia, decreased variability, or occasional late decelerations following a prolonged deceleration. If the precipitating cause is alleviated, the FHR generally returns to the previous baseline. Intermittent prolonged decelerations are not associated with an increased risk for fetal acidemia in the presence of moderate variability.

## Sinusoidal Pattern

A sinusoidal pattern is characterized by an undulating, recurrent uniform FHR equally distributed 5 to 15 bpm above and below the baseline (Figure 27-9). The undulation occurs at a rate of 2 to 6 cycles per minute and is associated with an absence of short-term variability. True sinusoidal patterns are extremely rare.

The sinusoidal FHR pattern develops when the fetus is experiencing clinically significant anemia, which can occur secondary to Rh isoimmunization or, more commonly today, during a maternal–fetal hemorrhage following vasa previa, uterine rupture, or placental abruption. This pattern may also appear shortly before death in a severely asphyxiated fetus. A sinusoidal heart rate pattern is always an ominous FHR pattern, and immediate preparations for emergency cesarean birth and the resuscitation of a potentially anemic or hypovolemic newborn are indicated.

### Pseudo-sinusoidal Fetal Heart Rate Pattern

The pseudo-sinusoidal pattern is not an NICHD-recognized FHR pattern because it commonly results from opioid administration, rather than being an intrinsic FHR characteristic. This clinically insignificant

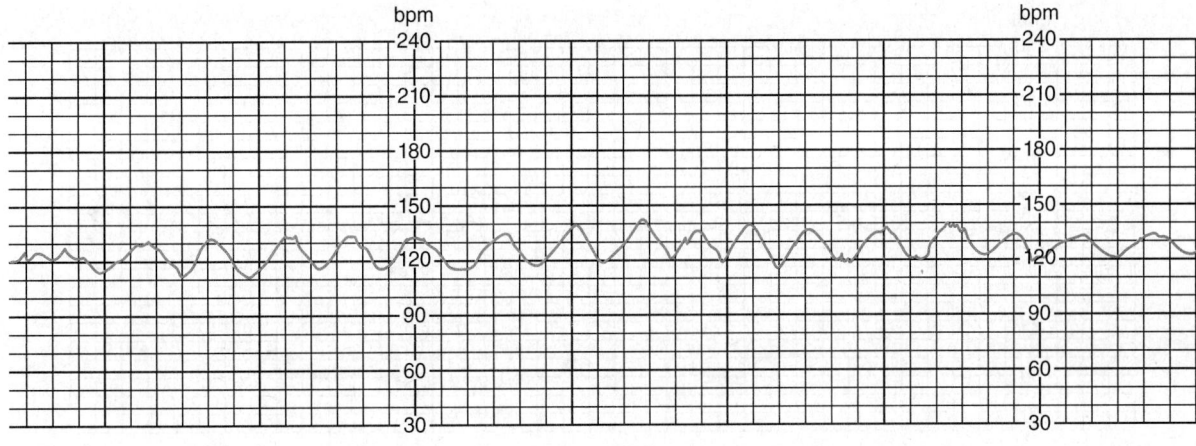

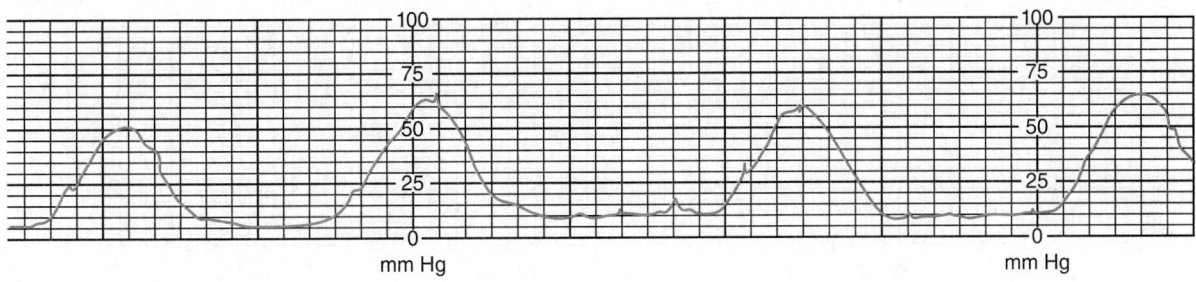

**Figure 27-9** Sinusoidal pattern.
Abbreviation: bpm, beats per minute; mm Hg, millimeters of mercury.

pattern is intermittent and associated with moderate variability. A pseudo-sinusoidal FHR pattern differs from a real sinusoidal pattern in two ways—namely, variability is retained and there are more than 2 to 6 cycles per minute (Figure 27-10). In addition, pseudo-sinusoidal patterns are not persistent, whereas sinusoidal patterns may initially be intermittent but will eventually become persistent and continuous.

### Wandering Baseline

*Wandering baseline* is not part of the official NICHD FHR nomenclature, but this term continues to be used in clinical practice and, therefore, deserves mention. A wandering baseline is a very late development in the progression of fetal deterioration. It is often within the normal baseline parameters of 110 to 160 bpm and is identifiable by absent variability. This pattern is an ominous indicator of fetal acidemia and requires preparation for emergency operative birth if vaginal birth is not imminent.

### Fetal Arrhythmias

Fetal arrhythmias occur among approximately 1% to 3% of fetuses at term.[65,66] Approximately 90% of

fetal arrhythmias are transient and benign in nature. A consulting physician should evaluate any fetus with an arrhythmia, and a plan should be made for ongoing collaboration as long as the arrhythmia is present. Arrhythmias can be heard on audible Doppler devices and seen on FHR tracings, but cannot be accurately diagnosed via EFM. Thus, neonatal/pediatric attendance at birth may be recommended depending on the rate and persistence of the arrhythmia.

## Classification of Fetal Heart Rate Patterns

Despite increasing knowledge of FHR characteristics that are associated with hypoxemia and acidemia, the poor sensitivity and high false-positive rates found in studies that sought to correlate FHR patterns with newborn outcomes present a clinical conundrum that has not yet been solved. In an effort to improve the predictive value of these data and to facilitate their use to help guide clinical practice, various professional organizations and groups have created classification systems for FHR patterns based on the risk of fetal acidemia.[48,67,68]

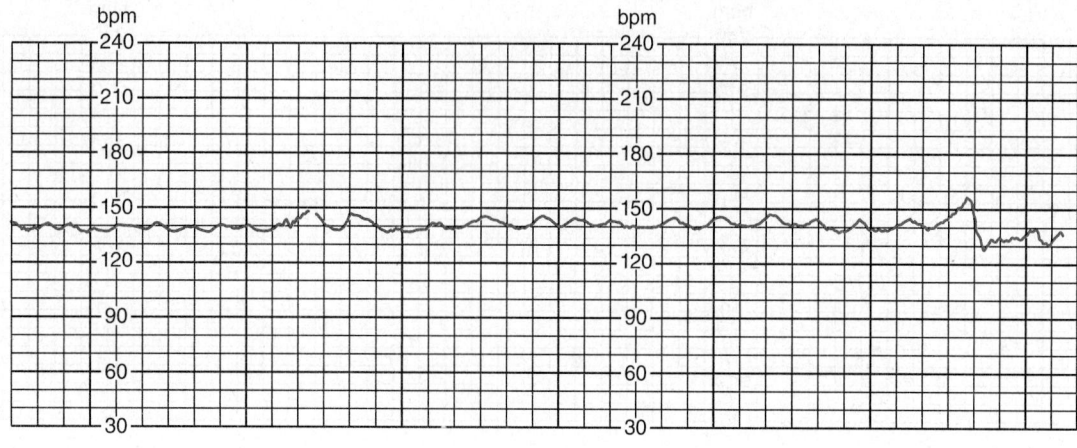

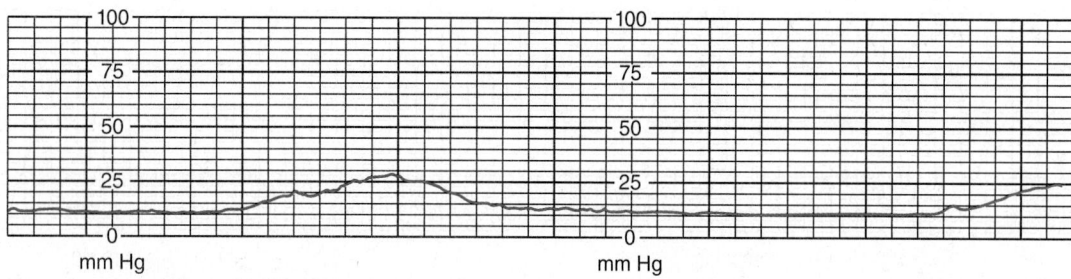

**Figure 27-10** Pseudo-sinusoidal FHR pattern that appeared shortly after intravenous administration of fentanyl given for pain relief. The irregularity of the sine wave distinguishes this pattern from a true sinusoidal pattern.

## National Institute of Child Health and Human Development's Three-Tier System

In 2008, the NICHD convened an expert panel on FHR monitoring to evaluate the research since the 1995 meeting and to address the interpretation and clinical management of FHR patterns in labor. The report from this workshop reaffirmed the 1997 FHR characteristics terminology, provided a new definition for uterine tachysystole, and recommended a three-tier system for interpreting FHR patterns (**Table 27-4**) that has been adopted in many labor and birth settings in the United States.[48]

The interpretation guidelines from the NICHD expert panels apply to intrapartum FHR tracings for term fetuses. Although the same terminology is often used for preterm fetuses, there is a paucity of research on the relationship between FHR patterns and neonatal outcomes in preterm births.

The NICHD system is built around two extremes: patterns that have reliably been demonstrated to predict a well-oxygenated fetus (Category I) and those patterns that have been most reliably associated with a fetus with significant acidemia or one at high risk of acidemia (Category III).[48] Between these two extremes fall a wide range of patterns exhibited at some point in labor by most fetuses. Category II FHR patterns constitute a heterogenous group with differing risks for fetal acidemia. All fetuses with pH of 7.1 or less, as well as 97.6% of fetuses with pH greater than 7.1, demonstrate a Category II pattern in the 30 minutes preceding birth.[69] This high prevalence of Category II patterns significantly limits the utility of this system in clinical practice.

The NICHD system has been widely adopted in birth settings across the United States and is recommended for use by ACOG.[30] However, this system has not been demonstrated to be superior to other classification systems, nor has it been shown to lead to improved neonatal outcomes.

## Parer-Ikeda Five-Tier System

The Parer-Ikeda five-tier FHR classifications system was devised using a grid of all 134 possible FHR patterns based on baseline FHR and type of decelerations, stratified by variability, and including sinusoidal and marked variability as distinct

| Table 27-4 | Fetal Heart Rate Interpretive Categories |
|---|---|
| **Category** | **FHR Patterns Assigned to This Category** |
| **Category I (Normal)** | |
| Baseline rate 110–160 bpm, moderate variability, and absence of late or variable decelerations must *all* be present. | Baseline rate: 110–160 bpm<br>Baseline FHR variability: moderate<br>Late or variable decelerations: absent<br>Early decelerations: present or absent<br>Accelerations: present or absent |
| **Category II (Indeterminate)** | |
| All FHR patterns not categorized as Category I or Category III. Includes *any* of these patterns. | Baseline rate:<br>• Bradycardia not accompanied by absent baseline variability<br>• Tachycardia<br>Baseline FHR variability:<br>• Minimal baseline variability<br>• Absent baseline variability<br>• Marked baseline variability<br>Accelerations:<br>• Absence of induced accelerations after fetal stimulations<br>Periodic or episodic decelerations:<br>• Recurrent[a] variable decelerations accompanied by minimal or moderate baseline variability<br>• Prolonged deceleration > 2 minutes but < 10 minutes<br>• Recurrent[a] late decelerations with moderate baseline variability<br>• Variable decelerations with other characteristics, such as slow return to baseline, "overshoots," or "shoulders" |
| **Category III (Abnormal)** | |
| Includes *either* pattern. | Absent baseline FHR variability and any of the following:<br>• Recurrent[a] late decelerations<br>• Recurrent[a] variable decelerations<br>• Bradycardia<br>Sinusoidal pattern |

Abbreviations: bpm, beats per minute; FHR, fetal heart rate.

[a] Decelerations are defined as recurring if they occur with 50% or more of uterine contractions in any 20-minute segment.

Based on Macones GA, Hankins GD, Spong CY, Hauth J, Moore T. The 2008 National Institute of Child Health and Human Development Research Workshop report on electronic fetal heart rate monitoring. *Obstet Gynecol.* 2008;112:661-666; *JOGNN.* 2008;37:510-515.

patterns (Table 27-5). These patterns were categorized into five color-coded levels of risk for fetal acidemia based on a review that evaluated all studies published between the 1960s and 2005 that examined the relationship between FHR patterns and newborn outcomes in term gestations.[53,67]

Research suggests that five-tier systems have the best accuracy of the currently available FHR categorization systems in correlating FHR patterns to newborn acidemia.[40,42,70–74] However, this interpretation framework has been criticized for being too complicated to implement clinically, a factor that has affected its adoption.[40,71,72] Computer-assisted algorithms and a mobile application have been developed to facilitate the clinical use of this system of interpretation. Additionally, modifications to align the

| Table 27-5 | Risk Categories for Fetal Acidemia Related to Fetal Heart Rate Variability, Baseline Rate, and Presence of Recurrent Decelerations |

**Moderate (Normal) Variability**

| | No | Early | Mild VD | Mod VD | Sev VD | Mild LD | Mod LD | Sev LD | Mild PD | Mod PD | Sev PD |
|---|---|---|---|---|---|---|---|---|---|---|---|
| Tachy | B | B | B | Y | O | Y | Y | O | Y | Y | O |
| Normal | G | G | G | B | Y | B | Y | Y | Y | Y | O |
| Mild Brd | Y | Y | Y | Y | O | Y | Y | O | Y | Y | O |
| Mod Brd | Y | Y | | | O | | O | O | | | O |
| Sev Brd | O | O | | | O | | | O | | | O |

**Minimal Variability**

| | No | Early | Mild VD | Mod VD | Sev VD | Mild LD | Mod LD | Sev LD | Mild PD | Mod PD | Sev PD |
|---|---|---|---|---|---|---|---|---|---|---|---|
| Tachy | B | Y | Y | O | O | O | O | R | O | O | R |
| Normal | B | B | Y | O | O | O | O | R | O | O | R |
| Mild Brd | O | O | R | R | R | R | R | R | R | R | R |
| Mod Brd | O | O | | | R | | R | R | | R | R |
| Sev Brd | R | R | | | R | | | R | | | R |

**Absent Variability**

| | No | Early | Mild VD | Mod VD | Sev VD | Mild LD | Mod LD | Sev LD | Mild PD | Mod PD | Sev PD |
|---|---|---|---|---|---|---|---|---|---|---|---|
| Tachy | R | R | R | R | R | R | R | R | R | R | R |
| Normal | O | R | R | R | R | R | R | R | R | R | R |
| Mild Brd | R | R | R | R | R | R | R | R | R | R | R |
| Mod Brd | R | R | | | R | | R | R | | R | R |
| Sev Brd | R | R | | | R | | | R | | | R |

**Other Patterns**

| | | |
|---|---|---|
| Sinusoidal | R | |
| Marked Variability | Y | |

Abbreviations: B, blue; Brd, bradycardia; G, green; LD, late decelerations; Mod, moderate; O, orange; PD, prolonged decelerations; R, Red; Sev, severe; Tachy, tachycardia; VD, variable decelerations.; Y, yellow.

Reproduced with permission from Parer JT. Standardization of fetal heart rate pattern management: is international consensus possible? *Hypertens Pregnancy.* 2014;29(20):51-58.

| Table 27-6 | Aligned 5- and 3-Tier FHR Classification Systems with Interpretation and Management Recommendations | |
| --- | --- | --- |
| 5-Tier Category | Modified NICHD Category | Interpretation and Management Overview |
| Green | I | No action needed, not associated with acidemia and unlikely to progress to higher-risk FHR category. |
| Blue | II(A) | Not associated with acidemia and low probability of progression to higher risk FHR category. Monitor more closely and, if not self-resolving, implement techniques to improve fetal oxygenation.[a] |
| Yellow | II(B) | Not associated with fetal acidemia, but moderate risk of progression to higher-risk FHR category. Implement measures to improve fetal oxygenation and consider preparations for expedited birth.[b] |
| Orange | II(C) | Rarely associated with existing fetal acidemia, but high risk of progression to Category III/Red FHR category. Implement measures to improve fetal oxygenation and prepare for expedited birth. |
| Red | III | Represents increased risk for development of fetal acidemia or, rarely, presence of existing fetal acidemia. Expedited birth is indicated (by cesarean or assisted vaginal birth if spontaneous vaginal birth not imminent). Measures to improve fetal oxygenation should be implemented while necessary steps toward expedited birth are occurring. |

[a] Measures to improve fetal oxygenation include maternal position changes, intravenous fluid bolus, discontinuation of oxytocic agents, and administration of tocolytics if tachysystole present or if decision has been made to proceed with operative birth. Maternal oxygen administration should be considered if there is compromised maternal oxygenation.

[b] Preparations for expedited birth may need to begin sooner and/or at a lower risk FHR category (e.g., Blue/Category IIA vs Yellow/Category IIB) in situations where there is increased risk of progression to higher category (e.g., fetus with growth restriction) or in settings where longer time may be required to prepare for operative birth (e.g., sites where providers needed for operative birth are not immediately available).

Based on Parer JT, Ikeda T. A framework for standardized management of intrapartum fetal heart rate patterns. *Am J Obstet Gynecol.* 2007;197:26e.1-26.e6.

five-tier system categories with the NICHD three-tier system allow for the concurrent application of these two systems. This may allow providers in sites that have adopted the NICHD system to better interpret and manage Category II patterns by incorporating the increasing risk of acidemia and evolution represented by FHR pattern in the blue, yellow, and orange categories of the 5-tier system.[30] The five tiers, classified by color and adapted to the NICHD three-tier system, as well as the corresponding recommended management actions are shown in Table 27-6.

### International FHR Classification Systems

Professional associations in countries such as the United Kingdom and Canada as well as the International Federation of Gynaecology and Obstetrics (FIGO) have established FHR classification systems similar to those used in the United States. These systems are aligned regarding the FHR patterns that are known to be associated with or without fetal acidemia

and differ only in how the FHR patterns that inconsistently reflect acidemia are subdivided.[31,32,68]

## Interpretation and Management of FHR Patterns: A Physiologic Approach

Categorization frameworks can help reduce variability in the interpretation and management of FHR patterns. There are risks, however, when providers become overly focused on the terminology defining specific decelerations and categorization of patterns. Misclassification can result in unwarranted intervention to expedite the birth of a fetus who is successfully compensating during intermittent fetal hypoxia or, alternatively, in a failure to intervene when a fetus is experiencing loss of compensatory reserve and developing acidemia. These errors can also happen when the FHR pattern is correctly identified but falls into a category (such as NICHD Category II) for which there are no clear management

| Table 27-7 | FHR Pattern Interpretation: General Physiologic Principles |
|---|---|

1. Moderate variability is strongly predictive of neo-natal vigor independent of the presence of variant patterns. Moderate FHR variability has a negative predictive value of 98% to 99% in a term fetus.

2. Minimal and absent variability in the presence of late or severe variable decelerations are the FHR patterns most likely to be associated with fetal acidemia, although the positive predictive value is only in the range of 10% to 30%.

3. An increasing FHR baseline and sustained tachycardia in the presence of or following a period of recurrent decelerations may be a sign of developing acidemia.

4. The frequency, duration, and severity of decelerations is more important than the type of deceleration in determining risk of fetal acidemia. A positive relationship can be found between the total depth and duration of decelerations or bradycardia ("area under the curve" or "total deceleration area") and the degree of acidemia.

5. Newborn acidemia with decreasing FHR variability in combination with decelerations develops over a period of approximately 1 hour in a previously healthy term fetus.

Abbreviation: FHR, fetal heart rate.

Sources: Parer JT et al. 2018; Macones et al. 2008; Parer JT et al. 2006; Jia YJ. 2021; Furukawa A et al. 2021; Cahill AG. 2018; Giannubilo SR. 2007; Tranquilli AL. 2014.

recommendations. A physiologic approach to FHR pattern interpretation that complements the standardized categorization system will optimize the likelihood of identifying the fetus with acidemia requiring expedited birth. General principles that help guide such a physiologic approach are presented in **Table 27-7**.[7,48,52,53,61,69,75,76]

A normal FHR baseline with moderate variability and the absence of FHR decelerations is a reliable sign that there is no acute fetal acidemia and can continue to be monitored. All other patterns warrant assessment of the clinical situation for the presence of factors that increase the risk of progressive fetal hypoxia. In the presence of moderate variability, the fetus can reliably be assumed to not be acidotic, even when recurrent decelerations are observed. The presence of accelerations reliably indicates the absence of acidemia at the time the accelerations are evident. Thus, prior to initiating interventions for variant FHR patterns, stimulation of fetal accelerations may be employed to assess for fetal acidemia.

## Fetal Scalp Stimulation and Vibroacoustic Stimulation

The goal of fetal scalp stimulation (FSS) and vibroacoustic stimulation (VAS) is to indirectly assess fetal pH to help guide management by attempting to elicit an FHR acceleration with an amplitude of at least 15 bpm lasting at least 15 seconds. FSS or VAS that elicits an acceleration provides reassurance that the fetal pH is higher than 7.2 at that time.[59] These adjunct assessment techniques are most useful in the setting of minimal variability and decelerations, or in case of minimal variability without decelerations. For example, if an individual has been given opioids, the FHR variability may be iatrogenically decreased. If this individual's fetus has an FHR pattern that includes late or variable decelerations, FSS may be of value to differentiate this iatrogenic decrease in variability from a decrease that may be related to fetal hypoxia.

FSS is performed between contractions and usually conducted by exerting digital pressure (often with a rubbing motion) on the fetal scalp, but can also be performed with a gentle pinch of the fetal scalp with an atraumatic clamp (e.g., Allis clamp). VAS is performed using a handheld vibroacoustic stimulator (artificial larynx), which is applied to the maternal abdomen over the region of the fetal head, where it delivers a sound stimulus for 3 to 5 seconds. FSS and VAS should not be performed during a deceleration and are not interventions to improve fetal oxygenation.

Approximately 50% of fetuses who do not respond to scalp stimulation or VAS with an acceleration will have a normal pH.[59] Thus, this test is useful only if, when performed between contractions, it results in an FHR acceleration. If an acceleration occurs, the clinician can be assured that the fetus is not acidemic at that moment. Conversely, when an acceleration does not occur, no conclusion can be made about the presence or absence of fetal acidemia; thus, management must be based on other clinical factors. If an acceleration occurs in response to FSS or VAS but no improvement is seen in the FHR pattern and no intervening events take place that change the clinical picture, a repeat assessment should be conducted.

## Pattern Evolution Suggestive of Progressive Fetal Hypoxia

Midwives, nurses, and physicians interpreting EFM results should recognize the typical pattern evolution that occurs as acidemia is developing (**Figure 27-11**). In all cases, this pattern starts with recurrent decelerations and ends with a terminal bradycardia that heralds fetal demise if the problem is not remedied before the fetus is born.

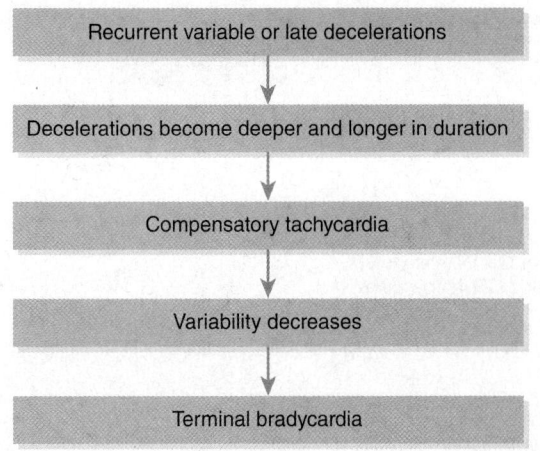

**Figure 27-11** Fetal heart rate pattern evolution from normal to fetal acidemia.
Reproduced from Parer JT, King TL, Ikeda T. *Electronic Fetal Heart Rate Monitoring: The 5-Tier System.* 3rd ed. Burlington, MA: Jones & Bartlett Learning; 2018.

A rise in baseline FHR, an increase in the depth and duration of recurrent decelerations, and a decrease is variability indicate the fetus is using compensatory mechanisms to maintain oxygenation to vital organs. When these findings are all present, the fetus may no longer be compensating adequately. However, the onset of deeper decelerations, tachycardia, and diminution of variability can appear in any order. For example, tachycardia may develop before or after the variability starts to decrease. Similarly, the decelerations may not become visibly deeper and of longer duration until after the variability begins decreasing. Sustained tachycardia, especially if accompanied by minimal variability and recurrent decelerations, appears to indicate that the fetus's ability to compensate for hypoxia is limited.[39,53] This pattern can appear after recurrent decelerations are present for some period, but before a terminal bradycardia becomes evident, and is characteristic of FHR pattern evolution when acidemia is increasing.

In a term, healthy fetus, it takes approximately 1 hour for clinically significant metabolic acidemia to develop once a pattern of recurrent late or variable decelerations and diminishing variability begins during labor.[53] However, variant FHR patterns must be considered in conjunction with other factors in the clinical scenario that can independently reduce the fetus's ability to tolerate repeated hypoxic events, as the reserves that individual fetuses have can vary considerably. The midwife needs to be vigilant for signs of progression of fetal acidemia to anticipate the need for operative birth. The amount of time needed for preparation of the operating room and anticipatory notification of the consultant physician is site dependent and must be considered in the development of any FHR management protocols.

## Management of FHR Patterns Suggestive of Developing Fetal Acidemia

Management of FHR patterns in the normal baseline range should be based first on the degree of FHR variability and then on the presence or absence of recurrent decelerations. **Figure 27-12** presents a template for managing variant FHR patterns that is based on current evidence and most professional organizations' guidelines. In the face of a pattern of recurrent decelerations with decreasing variability, the midwife should assume the presence of fetal hypoxia. The midwife should then try to identify its likely source and whether it is modifiable (e.g., tachysystole) or not (e.g., uteroplacental insufficiency secondary to hypertension).

In the case of incremental and potentially modifiable reductions in fetal oxygenation, several corrective measures (also referred to as *intrauterine resuscitation techniques*), such as position changes, amnioinfusion, intravenous fluid bolus, judicious oxygen administration, and administration of tocolytics, can be implemented. When implemented in response to a Category II FHR pattern, these measures, collectively, are associated with an improvement to Category I within 60 minutes.[77] Individually, some of these measures have been shown to improve fetal oxygenation, neonatal outcomes, or both, whereas others, such as administration of oxygen, have uncertain benefit.

### Reduction in Contraction Frequency

Interventions to decrease the frequency of uterine contractions, including intravenous bolus of fluids, reduction or discontinuation of oxytocin, and administration of tocolytics (usually beta-adrenergic agents such as 0.25 mg of terbutaline), can improve Category II FHR patterns and mitigate the development of acidemia, particularly in the presence of uterine tachysystole. In the Simpson et al. study, discontinuation of oxytocin infusion resulted in resolution of tachysystole in approximately 14.2 minutes.[78] Discontinuing oxytocin and administering an intravenous bolus (at least 500 mL) resulted in resolution in approximately 9.8 minutes. Discontinuing oxytocin, administering an intravenous bolus, and ensuring lateral positioning together resolved tachysystole in approximately 6 minutes.[78]

Administration of a tocolytic will also reliably resolve tachysystole. There are insufficient data to

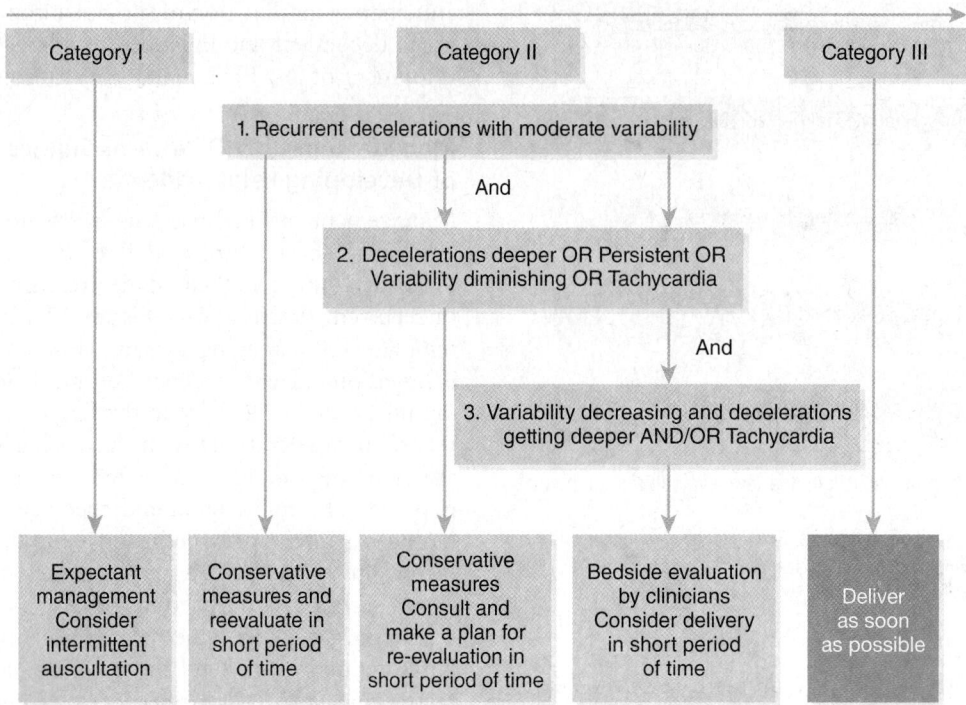

**Figure 27-12** Management of fetal heart rate patterns during labor.

support the use of tocolytics in cases involving an abnormal FHR pattern without concomitant tachysystole.[79] Maternal pushing with every other contraction can mitigate the negative effect of uterine contractions on fetal oxygenation and may decrease the severity or frequency of decelerations during second-stage pushing.

### Position Changes, Amnioinfusion, and Bolus of Intravenous Fluids

During pregnancy, the uterine vasculature is maximally dilated and the uterine spinal arteries are deinnervated, so that placental flow is pressure-dependent. As a result, very little can be done physiologically to increase blood flow to the placenta to compensate for decreases in maternal perfusion. Nonetheless, maximal arterial flow to the spiral arteries can be supported via use of a side-lying position to prevent compression of the inferior vena cava combined with the administration of intravenous fluids. Position changes may also relieve pressure on the umbilical cord. Position changes and lateral positioning are associated with improvements in the FHR pattern in observational studies.[77,80] Randomized controlled trials have demonstrated a clear benefit from amnioinfusion for patterns suggesting recurrent cord compression (e.g., recurrent variable decelerations or prolonged decelerations), including a reduction in cesarean birth, fewer

infants with Apgar scores less than 7 at 5 minutes or meconium below the neonatal vocal cords, and higher mean cord umbilical artery pH.[81] The technique for amnioinfusion is reviewed in the *Intrauterine Pressure Catheter* appendix.

Intravenous bolus of crystalloid fluids, such as lactated Ringer's solution, appears to work in two ways. First, an intravenous bolus of fluids appears to dilute the concentration of circulating oxytocin, which can in turn reduce the frequency of uterine contractions.[82] A bolus of fluid can also optimize placental perfusion through an increase in maternal intravascular volume. Administration of intravenous fluid bolus has been demonstrated to improve fetal oxygen saturation, even in the absence of maternal hypovolemia or hypotension.[82] A 1000 mL bolus has been shown to have a greater effect than 500 mL, and the positive effect is maintained for more than 30 minutes post-infusion.[82] Caution should be exercised to avoid fluid overload in individuals at risk for pulmonary edema, such as those with preeclampsia.

### Administration of Maternal Supplemental Oxygen

Although administration of oxygen to laboring individuals with variant FHR patterns is common, evidence of this intervention's effectiveness is lacking.[83–85] Furthermore, this practice has been the source of debate given concerns regarding the potential risk of fetal harm following exposure to free radicals associated with administration of supplemental oxygen.[86,87] Both hyperoxia and re-oxygenation following periods of hypoxia have been demonstrated to lead to tissue damage, such as retinopathy of prematurity, in both animal models and human neonates. While there is currently no evidence that maternal administration of oxygen leads to this type of damage in a fetus, there is also no clear evidence that maternal oxygen administration improves outcomes even in situations where the FHR patterns improve.[77] Recent studies have demonstrated no additional benefit of supplemental oxygen over room air in terms of neonatal outcomes[83–85,88] or rates of operative birth.[84] Given the concerns regarding the potential dangers of hyperoxia related to supplemental oxygenation and the lack of evidence to support its use for variant FHR patterns, a judicious approach to the administration of supplemental oxygen is warranted.

### Relationship Between Fetal Heart Rate Patterns and Newborn Outcomes

Several different newborn variables have been used in studies to identify the relationship between FHR patterns and neonatal outcomes, including Apgar scores, newborn seizures, umbilical cord blood gases, and—more recently—magnetic resonance imaging (MRI) findings in newborns with signs of neonatal encephalopathy.

Umbilical artery cord pH and base deficit are the most useful measurements for determining the presence or absence of fetal acidemia at the time of birth. When umbilical cord blood gases are in the normal range, intrapartum development of acidemia can be ruled out as the etiology of neonatal encephalopathy in a depressed or compromised newborn.[21] A description of the technique to obtain cord gases and guidelines for interpretation of the results are included in the *Umbilical Cord Gas Technique and Interpretation* appendix.

## Special Populations

The fetal response to hypoxic stress can be significantly affected by fetal and maternal medical or obstetric disorders, gestational age, and in utero exposures to fetotoxic substances. For example, although the pathophysiologic pathways differ, both preterm and post-term fetuses are more vulnerable to asphyxial stress than are term fetuses. Furthermore,

the fetus responds differently to chronic hypoxia, which is more likely to develop during the prenatal period, than to acute hypoxia, which is more likely to occur in the intrapartum period. Although a detailed discussion of these modifying factors is beyond the scope of this chapter, a brief review of the most common clinical scenarios—that is, preterm gestation, infection, fetal growth restriction, and hypertensive disorders—is presented here. Persons with these conditions during pregnancy are at increased risk for adverse maternal and fetal outcomes, are not candidates for intermittent monitoring during labor, and often need consultation with a physician for their care.

### Preterm Fetus

The preterm fetus has different inherent FHR characteristics as compared to the term fetus. These characteristics include a higher baseline heart rate, smaller-amplitude heart rate accelerations (especially prior to 32 weeks' gestation), and decreased baseline variability.[89] Short, shallow variable decelerations appear more frequently in FHR tracings of preterm fetuses. The preterm fetus is also more vulnerable to cerebral injury from a hypoxic event and more likely to be exposed to hypoxic stress via preterm rupture of membranes, preterm labor, or infection. Thus, tachycardia should be evaluated as a possible sign of infection, even though the baseline rate in a preterm fetus may be only slightly elevated above the normal baseline rates seen in term fetuses. Pattern evolution that reflects developing acidemia, characterized by diminishing variability, deeper decelerations, and tachycardia, progresses more rapidly than the expected 1-hour duration that has been reported in term fetuses.

### Infection

Infection may reduce the threshold at which hypoxia causes cerebral damage, thereby increasing the fetus's risk for subsequent cerebral palsy. Infection also increases the fetal metabolic rate, such that the fetus requires more oxygen. The fetal inflammatory response to infection, in addition to the direct effects of the bacterial toxins, causes dysregulation of cerebral blood flow and subsequent hypoxic–ischemic injury.[90,91] Preterm birth is closely linked to this inflammatory process, as infection also initiates release of prostaglandins, which cause preterm labor. Indeed, intra-amniotic infection is often the cause of preterm labor. The cardinal FHR characteristic associated with intra-amniotic infection is tachycardia. Treatment is reviewed in the *Complications During Labor and Birth* chapter.

## Fetal Growth Restriction

The term *fetal growth restriction* (FGR) is applied when a fetus fails to reach the genetic growth potential—that is, when the fetus's estimated weight is less than 10% of the predicted weight based on gestational age. Most commonly, the etiology of FGR is placental dysfunction. *Uteroplacental insufficiency* (UPI) refers to any condition in which the placenta is not able to supply sufficient oxygen or nutrients to the fetus. In addition to FGR, uteroplacental insufficiency is most often associated with preeclampsia, diabetes, maternal vascular disorders, and postdates. In the setting of uteroplacental insufficiency, the fetus can be exposed to chronic hypoxia and must balance reduced oxygen delivery with oxygen consumption. The result is a diminution of metabolic function and growth restriction.

Baseline FHR variability is generally diminished in fetuses with FGR compared to the FHR variability commonly seen in fetuses with appropriate growth.[92,93] During labor, fetuses with FGR are more likely to develop late decelerations than are fetuses without FGR.

## Conclusion

The assessment of fetal well-being is a critical component of midwifery management of the maternal–fetal dyad during labor. All midwives can use the methodologies that promote normal labor and birth while screening for and managing deviations from normal. The midwife may be the primary supporter of intermittent auscultation and the educator of other professionals in the birthing environment. Use of intermittent auscultation is a clear opportunity to blend the art and science of midwifery in a way that can make substantive positive change in clinical practice. Similarly, by applying a thoughtful, physiologic approach to the interpretation and management of EFM patterns, the midwife can identify the fetus for whom expedited birth may be indicated. Just as importantly, the midwife can advocate for increased surveillance and the judicious use of intrauterine resuscitation methods, and against operative birth, when there are variant FHR patterns such as recurrent decelerations with moderate variability that, while suggestive of hypoxia, also contain signs of fetal compensatory reserves. Regardless of the use of intermittent auscultation, EFM, or a combination of the two, the focus of fetal monitoring in labor must be on the full clinical scenario encompassing both the birthing person and the fetus, not just the information generated by FHR assessment technologies.

## References

1. Al Wattar BH, Honess E, Bunnewell S, et al. Effectiveness of intrapartum fetal surveillance to improve maternal and neonatal outcomes: a systematic review and network meta-analysis. *CMAJ.* 2021;193(14):E468-E477.

2. Thaler I, Manor D, Itskovitz J, et al. Changes in uterine blood flow during human pregnancy. *Am J Obstet Gynecol.* 1990;162(1):121-125.

3. Graham EM, Petersen SM, Christo DK, Fox HE. Intrapartum electronic fetal heart rate monitoring and the prevention of perinatal brain injury. *Obstet Gynecol.* 2006;108(3 pt 1):656-666.

4. Kurinczuk JJ, White-Koning M, Badawi N. Epidemiology of neonatal encephalopathy and hypoxic–ischaemic encephalopathy. *Early Hum Dev.* 2010;86(6):329-338.

5. Brosens I, Puttemans P, Benagiano G. Placental bed research: I. The placental bed: from spiral arteries remodeling to the great obstetrical syndromes. *Am J Obstet Gynecol.* 2019;221(5):437-456.

6. Turco MY, Moffett A. Development of the human placenta. *Development.* 2019;146(22):dev163428.

7. Parer JT, King TL, Ikeda T. *Electronic Fetal Heart Rate Monitoring: The 5-Tier System.* 3rd ed. Burlington, MA: Jones & Bartlett Learning; 2018.

8. Fahey J, King TL. Intrauterine asphyxia: clinical implications for providers of intrapartum care. *J Midwifery Womens Health.* 2005;50:498-506.

9. Simpson KR, James DC. Effects of oxytocin-induced uterine hyperstimulation during labor on fetal oxygen status and fetal heart rate patterns. *Am J Obstet Gynecol.* 2008;199:34.e1-34.e5.

10. Simpson KR. Clinician's guide to the use of oxytocin for labor induction and augmentation. *J Midwifery Womens Health.* 2011;56:214-221.

11. Bakker PCAM, Kurver PHJ, Kuik DJ, Van Geijn HP. Elevated uterine activity increases the risk of fetal acidosis at birth. *Am J Obstet Gynecol.* 2007;196:313.e1-313.e6.

12. Ahmed AI, Zhu L, Aldhaheri S, et al. Uterine tachysystole in spontaneous labor at term. *J Matern Fetal Neonatal Med.* 2016;29(20):3335-3339.

13. Tsakiridis I, Mamopoulos A, Athanasiadis A, Dagklis T. Induction of labor: an overview of guidelines. *Obstet Gynecol Surv.* 2020;75(1):61-72.

14. Kunz MK, Loftus RJ, Nichols AA. Incidence of uterine tachysystole in women induced with oxytocin. *J Obstet Gynecol Neonatal Nurs.* 2013;42(1):12-18.

15. Page K, McCool WF, Guidera M. Examination of the pharmacology of oxytocin and clinical guidelines for use in labor. *J Midwifery Womens Health.* 2017;62(4):425-433.

16. Itskovitz J, LaGamma EF, Rudolph AM. Heart rate and blood pressure responses to umbilical cord

compression in fetal lambs with special reference to the mechanism of variable deceleration. *Am J Obstet Gynecol.* 1983;147(4):451-457.

17. Baan J Jr, Boekkooi PF, Teitel DF, Rudolph AM. Heart rate fall during acute hypoxemia: a measure of chemoreceptor response in fetal sheep. *J Develop Physiol.* 1993;19(3):105-111.

18. Lear CA, Galinsky R, Wassink G, et al. Sympathetic neural activation does not mediate heart rate variability during repeated brief umbilical cord occlusions in near-term fetal sheep. *J Physiol.* 2016;594(5):1265-1277.

19. Giussani DA. The fetal brain sparing response to hypoxia: physiological mechanisms. *J Physiol.* 2016;594(5):1215-1230.

20. Greco P, Nencini G, Piva I, et al. Pathophysiology of hypoxic–ischemic encephalopathy: a review of the past and a view on the future. *Acta Neurol Belg.* 2020;120(2):277-288.

21. American College of Obstetricians and Gynecologists Task Force on Neonatal Encephalopathy. *Neonatal Encephalopathy and Neurologic Outcome.* 2nd ed. Washington, DC: American College of Obstetricians and Gynecologists; 2014, reaffirmed 2019.

22. Nelson KB, Bingham P, Edwards EM, et al. Antecedents of neonatal encephalopathy in the Vermont Oxford Network Encephalopathy Registry. *Pediatrics.* 2012;130:878-886. doi:10.1542/peds.2012-0714.

23. Graham EM, Ruis KA, Hartman AL, et al. A systematic review of the role of intrapartum hypoxia–ischemia in the causation of neonatal encephalopathy. *Am J Obstet Gynecol.* 2008;199(6):587-595.

24. Shah PS, Beyene J, To T, et al. Postasphyxial hypoxic–ischemic encephalopathy in neonates: outcome prediction rule within 4 hours of birth. *Arch Pediatr Adolesc Med.* 2006;160:729-736.

25. Jacobs SE, Berg M, Hunt R, et al. Cooling for newborns with hypoxic ischaemic encephalopathy. *Cochrane Database Syst Rev.* 2013;1:CD003311.

26. Chiang MC, Lien R, Chu SM, et al. Serum lactate, brain magnetic resonance imaging and outcome of neonatal hypoxic ischemic encephalopathy after therapeutic hypothermia. *Pediatr Neonatol.* 2016;57(1):35-40.

27. McAdams RM, Juul SE. Neonatal encephalopathy: update on therapeutic hypothermia and other novel therapeutics. *Clin Perinatol.* 2016;43(3):485-500.

28. Committee on Fetus and Newborn; Papile LA, Baley JE, Benitz W, et al. Hypothermia and neonatal encephalopathy. *Pediatrics.* 2014;133(6):1146-1150.

29. Hankins GD, Speer M. Defining the pathogenesis and pathophysiology of neonatal encephalopathy and cerebral palsy. *Obstet Gynecol.* 2003;102(3):628-636.

30. American College of Obstetricians and Gynecologists. Practice Bulletin No. 106: Intrapartum fetal heart rate monitoring: nomenclature, interpretation, and general management principles. *Obstet Gynecol.* 2009 Jul;114(1):192-202.

31. National Institute for Health and Care Excellence. Intrapartum care for healthy women and babies. https://www.nice.org.uk/guidance/cg190/chapter/Recommendations#monitoring-during-labour. Published 2017. Accessed January 22, 2022.

32. Liston R, Sawchuck D, Young D. Fetal health surveillance: antepartum and intrapartum consensus guideline: fetal health surveillance in labour. *J Obstet Gynaecol Can.* 2007;29(9):S27.

33. Declercq ER, Sakala C, Corry MP, et al. Major survey findings of Listening to Mothers III: new mothers speak out: report of national surveys of women's childbearing experiences conducted October–December 2012 and January–April 2013. *J Perinat Educ.* 2014;23(1):17-24.

34. Yeh SY, Diaz F, Paul RH. Ten year experience of intrapartum fetal monitoring in Los Angeles County/University of Southern California Medical Center. *Am J Obstet Gynecol.* 1982;143:496-500.

35. Alfirevic Z, Devane D, Gyte GML, Cuthbert A. Continuous cardiotocography (CTG) as a form of electronic fetal monitoring (EFM) for fetal assessment during labour. *Cochrane Database Syst Rev.* 2017;2:CD006066. doi:10.1002/14651858.CD006066.pub3.

36. MacDonald D, Grant A, Sheridan-Periera M, Chalmers I. The Dublin randomized controlled trial of intrapartum fetal heart rate monitoring. *Am J Obstet Gynecol.* 1985;152:524-539.

37. Grant S, O'Brien N, Joy MT, et al. Cerebral palsy among children born during the Dublin randomized trial of intrapartum monitoring. *Lancet.* 1989;2:1233-1235.

38. Parer JT, King T. Fetal heart rate monitoring: is it salvageable? *Am J Obstet Gynecol.* 2000;182(4):982-987.

39. Vintzileos AM, Smulian JC. Decelerations, tachycardia, and decreased variability: have we overlooked the significance of longitudinal fetal heart rate changes for detecting intrapartum fetal hypoxia? *Am J Obstet Gynecol.* 2016;215(3):261-264.

40. Coletta J, Murphy E, Rubeo Z, Gyamfi-Bannerman C. The 5-tier system of assessing fetal heart rate tracings is superior to the 3-tier system in identifying fetal acidemia. *Am J Obstet Gynecol.* 2010;206:226.e1-226.e5.

41. Ogunyemi D, Jovanovski A, Friedman P, et al. Temporal and quantitative associations of electronic fetal heart rate monitoring patterns and neonatal outcomes. *J Matern Fetal Neonatal Med.* 2019;32(18):3115-3124.

42. Katsuragi S, Parer JT, Noda S, et al. Mechanism of reduction of newborn metabolic acidemia following application of a rule-based 5-category color coded fetal heart rate management framework. *J Matern Fetal Neonatal Med.* 2015;28(13):1608-1613.

43. Ayers-de-Campo D, Nogueira-Reis Z. Technical characteristics of current cardiotocograph monitors. *Best Pract Res Clin Obstet Gynecol.* 2016;30:22-32.

44. Bakker PCAM. Uterine activity monitoring during labor. *J Perinat Med.* 2007;35:468-477.

45. Cohen WR. Clinical assessment of uterine contractions. *Int J Gynaecol Obstet.* 2017;139(2):137-142.

46. Arrabal PP, Nagey DA. Is manual palpation of uterine contractions accurate? *Am J Obstet Gynecol.* 1996;174(1 pt 1):217-219.

47. National Institute of Child Health and Human Development Research Planning Workshop. Electronic fetal heart rate monitoring: research guidelines for interpretation. *Am J Obstet Gynecol.* 1997;17:1385-1390; *JOGNN.* 1997;26:635-640.

48. Macones GA, Hankins GD, Spong CY, et al. The 2008 National Institute of Child Health and Human Development Research Workshop report on electronic fetal heart rate monitoring. *Obstet Gynecol.* 2008;112:661-666; *JOGNN.* 2008;37:510-515.

49. Aina-Mumuney AJ, Althaus JE, Henderson JL, et al. Intrapartum electronic fetal monitoring and the identification of systemic fetal inflammation. *J Reprod Med.* 2007;52(9):762-768.

50. Zoeller BB. Treatment of fetal supraventricular tachycardia. *Curr Treat Options Cardiovasc Med.* 2017;19(1):7.

51. Liu L, Tuuli MG, Roehl KA, et al. Electronic fetal monitoring patterns associated with respiratory morbidity in term neonates. *Am J Obstet Gynecol.* 2015;213(5):681.e1-681.e6.

52. Jia YJ, Chen X, Cui HY, et al. Physiological CTG interpretation: the significance of baseline fetal heart rate changes after the onset of decelerations and associated perinatal outcomes. *J Matern Fetal Neonatal Med.* 2021;34(14):2349-2354.

53. Parer JT, King TL, Flanders S, et al. Fetal acidemia and electronic fetal heart rate patterns: is there evidence of an association? *J Matern Fetal Neonatal Med.* 2006;19:289-294.

54. Fahey JO. The recognition and management of intrapartum fetal heart rate emergencies: beyond definitions and classification. *J Midwifery Womens Health.* 2014;59(6):616-623.

55. Takano Y, Furukawa S, Ohashi M, et al. Fetal heart rate patterns related to neonatal brain damage and neonatal death in placental abruption. *J Obstet Gynecol.* 2013;39(1):61-66.

56. Leung TY, Chung PW, Rogers MS, et al. Urgent cesarean delivery for fetal bradycardia. *Obstet Gynecol.* 2009;114(5):1023-1038.

57. Mirmiran M, Maas YG, Ariagno RL. Development of fetal and neonatal sleep and circadian rhythms. *Sleep Med Rev.* 2003;7(4):321-334.

58. Polnaszek B, López JD, Clark R, et al. Marked variability in intrapartum electronic fetal heart rate patterns: association with neonatal morbidity and abnormal arterial cord gas. *J Perinatol.* 2020;40(1):56-62.

59. Clark SL, Gimovsky ML, Miller FC. The scalp stimulation test: a clinical alternative to fetal scalp blood sampling. *Am J Obstet Gynecol.* 1984;148:274-277.

60. Sameshima H, Ikenoue T. Predictive value of late decelerations for fetal acidemia in unselective low-risk pregnancies. *Am J Perinatol.* 2005;22:19-23.

61. Furukawa A, Neilson D, Hamilton E. Cumulative deceleration area: a simplified predictor of metabolic acidemia. *J Matern Fetal Neonatal Med.* 2021;34(19):3104-3111.

62. Sameshima H, Ikenoue T, Ikeda T, et al. Unselected low-risk pregnancies and the effect of continuous intrapartum fetal heart rate monitoring on umbilical blood gases and cerebral palsy. *Am J Obstet Gynecol.* 2004;190:118-123.

63. Hader A, Sheiner E, Hallak M, et al. Abnormal fetal heart rate tracing patterns during the first stage of labor: effect on perinatal outcome. *Am J Obstet Gynecol.* 2001;185:863-868.

64. Lear CA, Kasai M, Booth LC, et al. Peripheral chemoreflex control of fetal heart rate decelerations overwhelms the baroreflex during brief umbilical cord occlusions in fetal sheep. *J Physiol.* 2020;598(20):4523-4536.

65. Jaeggi ET, Masalo M. Fetal brady- and tachyarrhythmias: new and accepted diagnostic and treatment methods. *Semin Fetal Neonatal Med.* 2005;10:504-511.

66. Donofrio MT, Moon-Grady AJ, Hornberger, et al., for American Heart Association Adults with Congenital Heart Disease Joint Committee of the Council on Cardiovascular Disease in the Young and Council on Clinical Cardiology, Council on Cardiovascular Surgery and Anesthesia, and Council on Cardiovascular and Stroke Nursing. Diagnosis and treatment of fetal cardiac disease: a scientific statement from the American Heart Association. *Circulation.* 2014;129(21):2183-2242.

67. Parer JT, Ikeda T. A framework for standardized management of intrapartum fetal heart rate patterns. *Am J Obstet Gynecol.* 2007;197:26.e1-26.e6.

68. Ayres-de-Campos D, Spong CY, Chandraharan E; FIGO Intrapartum Fetal Monitoring Expert Consensus Panel. FIGO consensus guidelines on intrapartum fetal monitoring: cardiotocography. *Int J Gynaecol Obstet.* 2015;131(1):13-24.

69. Cahill AG, Tuuli MG, Stout MJ, et al. A prospective cohort study of fetal heart rate monitoring: deceleration area is predictive of fetal acidemia. *Am J Obstet Gynecol.* 2018;218(5):523.e1-523.e12.

70. Soncini E, Paganelli S, Vezzani C, et al. Intrapartum fetal heart rate monitoring: evaluation of a standardized system of interpretation for prediction of metabolic acidosis at delivery and neonatal neurological morbidity. *J Matern Fetal Neonatal Med.* 2014;27(14):1465-1469.

71. Ikeda S, Okazaki A, Miyazaki K, et al. Fetal heart rate pattern interpretation in the second stage of labor using the five-tier classification: impact of the degree and duration on severe fetal acidosis. *J Obstet Gynaecol Res.* 2014;40(5):1274-1280.

72. Di Tommaso M, Seravalli V, Cordisco A, et al. Comparison of five classification systems for interpreting electronic fetal monitoring in predicting neonatal status at birth. *J Matern Fetal Neonatal Med.* 2013;26(5):487-490.

73. Sadaka A, Furuhashi M, Minami H, et al. Observation on validity of the five-tier system for fetal heart rate pattern interpretation proposed by Japan Society of Obstetricians and Gynecologists. *J Matern Fetal Neonatal Med.* 2011;24(12):1465-1469.

74. Penfield CA, Hong C, Ibrahim Sel H, et al. Easy as ABC: a system to stratify Category II fetal heart rate tracings. *Am J Perinatol.* 2016;33(7):688-695.

75. Giannubilo SR, Buscicchio G, Gentilucci L, et al. Deceleration area of fetal heart rate trace and fetal acidemia at delivery: a case-control study. *J Matern Fetal Neonatal Med.* 2007;20(2):141-144.

76. Tranquilli AL, Biagini A, Greco P, et al. The correlation between fetal bradycardia area in the second stage of labor and acidemia at birth. *J Matern Fetal Neonatal Med.* 2013;26(14):1425-1429.

77. Reddy UM, Weiner SJ, Saade GR, et al.; Eunice Kennedy Shriver National Institute of Child Health and Human Development (NICHD) Maternal–Fetal Medicine Units (MFMU) Network. Intrapartum resuscitation interventions for Category II fetal heart rate tracings and improvement to Category I. *Obstet Gynecol.* 2021;138(3):409-416.

78. Simpson KR. Intrauterine resuscitation during labor: should maternal oxygen administration be a first-line measure? *Semin Fetal Neonatal Med.* 2008;13(6):362-367.

79. Eller AG. Interventions for intrapartum fetal heart rate abnormalities. *Clin Obstet Gynecol.* 2020;63(3):635-644.

80. Raghuraman N, López JD, Carter EB, et al. The effect of intrapartum oxygen supplementation on Category II fetal monitoring. *Am J Obstet Gynecol.* 2020;223(6):905.e1-905.e7.

81. Hofmeyr GJ, Lawrie TA. Amnioinfusion for potential or suspected umbilical cord compression in labour. *Cochrane Database Syst Rev.* 2012;1:CD000013. doi:10.1002/14651858.CD000013.pub2.

82. Simpson KR. Clinicians' guide to the use of oxytocin for labor induction and augmentation. *J Midwifery Womens Health.* 2011;56(3):214-221.

83. Raghuraman N, López JD, Carter EB, et al. The effect of intrapartum oxygen supplementation on Category II fetal monitoring. *Am J Obstet Gynecol.* 2020;223(6):905.e1-905.e7.

84. Burd J, Quist-Nelson J, Moors S, et al. Effect of intrapartum oxygen on the rate of cesarean delivery: a meta-analysis. *Am J Obstet Gynecol MFM.* 2021;3(4):100374.

85. Raghuraman N, Temming LA, Doering MM, et al. Maternal oxygen supplementation compared with room air for intrauterine resuscitation: a systematic review and meta-analysis. *JAMA Pediatr.* 2021;175(4):368-376.

86. Garite TJ, Nageotte MP, Parer JT. Should we really avoid giving oxygen to mothers with concerning fetal heart rate patterns? *Am J Obstet Gynecol.* 2015;212(4):459-460, 459.e1.

87. Hamel MS, Anderson BL, Rouse DJ. Oxygen for intrauterine resuscitation: of unproved benefit and potentially harmful. *Am J Obstet Gynecol.* 2014;211(2):124-127.

88. Moors S, Bullens LM, van Runnard Heimel PJ, et al. The effect of intrauterine resuscitation by maternal hyperoxygenation on perinatal and maternal outcome: a randomized controlled trial. *Am J Obstet Gynecol MFM.* 2020;2(2):100102.

89. Hurtado-Sánchez MF, Pérez-Melero D, Pinto-Ibáñez A, et al. Characteristics of heart rate tracings in preterm fetus. *Medicina (Kaunas).* 2021;57(6):528.

90. Kim CJ, Romero R, Chaemsaithong P, et al. Acute chorioamnionitis and funisitis: definition, pathologic features, and clinical significance. *Am J Obstet Gynecol.* 2015;213(4 suppl):S29-S52.

91. Ugwumadu A. Infection and fetal neurologic injury. *Curr Opin Obstet Gynecol.* 2006;18:106-111.

92. Stampalija T, Casati D, Monasta L, et al. Brain sparing effect in growth-restricted fetuses is associated with decreased cardiac acceleration and deceleration capacities: a case-control study. *BJOG.* 2015;123(12):1947-1954.

93. Nijhuis IJ, ten Hof J, Mulder EJ, et al. Fetal heart rate in relation to its variation in normal and growth retarded fetuses. *Eur J Obstet Gynecol Reprod Biol.* 2000;89(1):27-33.

# APPENDIX

# 27A

# Intermittent Auscultation During Labor

TEKOA L. KING

The purpose of intrapartum assessment of the fetal heart rate (FHR) is to monitor this rate over the course of labor so as to identify the fetus who is developing clinically significant acidemia. Effective methods of evaluation and accurate interpretation of the FHR during labor have long been the subjects of debate. Continuous electronic fetal monitoring (EFM) is the most commonly used method of intrapartum fetal surveillance, but has not been found to be more effective than intermittent auscultation (IA) in women who are at low risk for acidemia at the onset of labor.[1,2] National and international professional organizations recommend use of IA for individuals with term gestations who do not have a known a priori risk for developing fetal acidemia during labor.[3–10] This appendix presents the technique for IA, interpretation of findings from IA, and management recommendations.

When comparing IA to continuous EFM, there are both advantages and disadvantages associated with this technique for fetal surveillance. IA is performed frequently, so it ensures recurrent and regular close physical contact between the midwife or nurse and the laboring individual. This contact increases interactions that facilitate emotional and clinical support. IA also allows the pregnant person to assume any position of comfort, thereby promoting upright postures and mobility. IA is labor intensive, in that it requires more provider time at the bedside when compared to continuous EFM. Learning the technique and interpretation of FHR characteristics identified using IA requires training.[4]

## Fetal Heart Rate Characteristics Detectable on Intermittent Auscultation

A handheld Doppler device can effectively detect the baseline FHR as well as the occurrence of accelerations or decelerations if the technique is performed correctly.[3–7] Conversely, IA can fail to detect significant FHR decelerations if this rate is not auscultated during the latter half and immediately after a uterine contraction. Table 27A-1 lists the FHR characteristics that can be detected via IA and EFM. Auscultation can determine the baseline FHR, changes in the rhythm of the heart rate, and accelerations.[3–7] IA cannot determine FHR variability.[3–7] Decelerations can be identified as a decrease in the heart rate, but the specific timing of the decelerations in relation to uterine contractions cannot be determined reliably, nor can the degree of decline of the heart rate, such as "sudden" or "gradual," be confirmed. Thus, decelerations cannot be categorized as early, variable, or late in character when using IA. Instead, detection of decreases in the FHR are categorized as "brief" or "prolonged" based on the auscultated duration and the slowest rate that is counted or registered on the Doppler device.

## Indications and Contraindications for Intermittent Auscultation

There is no standard or uniform list of indications or contraindications for use of IA, although it is recommended that institutional protocols and

| Table 27A-1 | Fetal Heart Rate Characteristics Detectable via Handheld Doppler and Electronic Monitoring Devices | |
|---|---|---|
| **FHR Characteristic** | **Handheld Doppler** | **Electronic FHR Monitor** |
| Variability | Not quantifiable | Can be quantified<br><br>Categorized as absent, minimal, moderate, or marked |
| Baseline rate | Quantifiable<br><br>Categorized as brady-cardia, normal rate, or tachycardia | Quantifiable<br><br>Categorized as bradycardia, normal rate, or tachycardia |
| Accelerations | Detects brief increases in FHR above the baseline that occur between uter-ine contraction activity<br><br>Not reliably quantifiable | Detects brief increases in FHR above the baseline rate that occur between uterine contraction activity<br><br>Categorized by the maximum increase above baseline (number of bpm) and the duration (seconds) |
| Decelerations | Detects decreases in FHR and duration of decrease but not quantifiable in bpm<br><br>Categorized as brief or prolonged | Detects decreases in FHR and duration of decrease and records duration and depth in bpm<br><br>Categorized as early, late, variable, or prolonged decelerations |
| Rhythm[a] | Arrhythmia will be audible | Arrhythmia can be detected audibly and will be identified as an arrhythmia in the graphic representation of the FHR that is displayed and/or printed if a paper recording is obtained.<br><br>The type of arrhythmia cannot be determined. May double or halve the count and report an inaccurate FHR if arrhythmia is present. |
| Differentiation of maternal and fetal heart rates | May detect maternal heart rate instead of FHR | May detect and record maternal heart rate instead of FHR |

Abbreviations: bpm, beats per minute; FHR, fetal heart rate.

[a] The FHR is identified as regular or irregular. None of these devices can diagnose the type of fetal arrhythmia.

Data from American College of Nurse-Midwives. Intermittent auscultation for intrapartum fetal heart rate surveillance. *J Midwifery Womens Health*. 2015;60(5):626-632. [Erratum, *J Midwifery Womens Health*. 2016;61(1):134]; Lyndon A, Wisner K. *Fetal Heart Monitoring Principles and Practices*. 6th ed. Washington, DC: Association of Women's Health, Obstetric and Neonatal Nurses; 2021. Dubuque, IA: Kendall Hunt Publishing; 2021;83-89.

standard procedures include such a list. The underlying concept is that IA is appropriate for individuals who (1) have no identifiable risks for developing fetal acidemia or adverse perinatal outcomes during labor and birth, (2) are at a term gestation with a singleton fetus, and (3) have a fetus in the vertex presentation. Table 27A-2 lists examples of indications for electronic FHR monitoring based on risks for adverse outcomes that are present in the laboring individual, in the fetus, or during labor progress.

## Equipment: Doppler Fetoscopes

Intermittent auscultation is typically conducted using a handheld Doppler fetoscope. Pinard-type fetoscopes may be used prenatally, but they have limitations for intrapartum use and are not commonly used in the United States.[11]

Doppler devices use ultrasound to detect the movement—that is, opening and closing—of the ventricular valves by noting the change in ultrasound wavelength caused by the heart movement. The device converts the wavelength change into an audible sound and visual digital recording. Doppler devices require use of a gel that is placed between the face of the transducer and the maternal skin to ensure transmission of sound without air interference. Some handheld devices will generate a printout record. Many Doppler fetoscopes are waterproof and can be used to record the FHR when a person is in water.

| Table 27A-2 | Examples of Indications for Electronic Fetal Heart Rate Monitoring |
|---|---|
| **Risks for Fetal Acidemia During Labor** | **Selected Conditions** |
| Maternal risks | Maternal disorders that indicate decreased uteroplacental function, such as hypertension, diabetes, preeclampsia, prior cesarean birth, or uterine scar |
| Fetal risks | Abnormal antenatal nonstress test or biophysical profile |
| | Fetal heart rate decelerations, bradycardia, or tachycardia |
| | Intrauterine growth restriction |
| | Known fetal chromosomal abnormality compatible with life and a desire to intervene if needed |
| | Multiple gestation |
| | Nonvertex presentation |
| | Oligohydramnios |
| | Preterm gestation |
| | Post-term gestation ($\geq$ 42 weeks) |
| | Rh isoimmunization |
| Intrapartum risks | Abnormal vaginal bleeding |
| | Regional analgesia |
| | Induction or augmentation of labor with oxytocin |
| | Intra-amniotic infection or maternal fever |
| | Meconium (thick) |
| | Prolonged first or second stage of labor |
| | Anticipated operative vaginal birth or cesarean birth |
| | Tachysystole |

## Technique for Performing Intermittent Auscultation

The method for performing IA described in this appendix is concordant with the American College of Nurse-Midwives (ACNM) guidelines.[3] Individual institutions or practices may develop protocols specific to their settings and populations.[3] ACNM recommends auscultating the FHR through a contraction and for 30 to 60 seconds after the contraction every 15 to 30 minutes in the active phase of labor and every 5 minutes in the second stage of labor.[3] However, as labor progresses, uterine contractions increase in intensity and fetal position changes, so auscultation may be indicated more frequently because vents that can affect fetal oxygenation also change over the course of labor. Strict adherence to a designated time–minute interval for assessing the FHR fails to account for changes in labor status that could potentially affect fetal tolerance of the labor process. More frequent auscultation may be appropriate based on labor characteristics such as the frequency of contractions, clinical signs of fetal descent (e.g., rupture of membranes, bloody show, urge to push, nonrecurrent decelerations), and institution of hydrotherapy or other interventions that may affect the FHR.

The original randomized controlled trials recommended auscultating between contractions, and for many years professional organizations' guidelines maintained this recommendation. However, listening between contractions can result in missing clinically significant variable decelerations that occur during a contraction and resolve as the contraction ends. For this reason, the current guidelines recommend listening through a contraction and for a period of time after the contraction ends.[3–7] If no decreases in the FHR are noted, the midwife may begin auscultation at the peak of a contraction and continue listening for 30 to 60 seconds after the contraction is over. Listening between contractions is not effective and should not be part of the technique.

Only a few studies have been conducted that assessed the reliability and accuracy of IA using

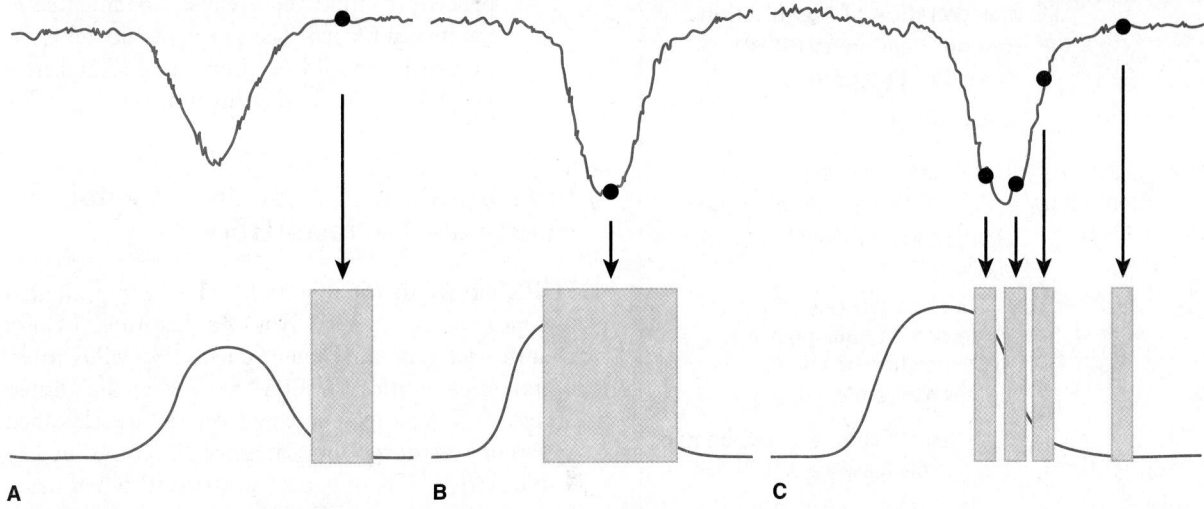

**Figure 27A-1** Multicount strategy for assessing the fetal heart rate via intermittent auscultation. **A.** A single count strategy for less than 1 minute between contractions may miss a deceleration. **B.** A single count strategy for 30 to 60 seconds that starts after the peak of the contraction will detect the presence of a deceleration qualitatively. **C.** A multicount strategy for 10 seconds with a 5- to 10-second break between counts allows the clinician to graphically sketch the deceleration.

differing techniques.[11] In general, these studies have found significant interindividual variability in accuracy of recognizing decelerations, which suggests training and practice are needed to attain and maintain proficiency with the technique.[11] Determination of the FHR rate is less accurate when the fetus has tachycardia or bradycardia.[11]

To quantify the FHR baseline in beats per minute (bpm), a multicount technique has been shown to be more reliable than counting once throughout the period of assessment.[12] When using a multicount strategy, the listener counts the FHR for a period of 6, 10, or 15 seconds several times over the course of the listening period. A defined rest period of 5 or 10 seconds occurs between each count. Each count is then multiplied by the appropriate number to obtain a bpm rate. In a study conducted by Shiffrin et al., the multicount strategy identified approximately 93% of FHR decelerations; by comparison, a single-count strategy identified 74% of the FHR decelerations.[12] The counts can be plotted to diagram the FHR changes over the course of the auscultation period, as shown in Figure 27A-1. Some anecdotal evidence suggests that this technique will reveal FHR variability, but this relationship has not been evaluated scientifically.

1. Discuss options for fetal surveillance with the laboring individual. IA should be chosen as part of a shared decision-making process.[13]

2. Conduct abdominal palpation (Leopold's maneuver) to determine the fetal lie. Listening through the fetal back provides the clearest sound.

3. Assist the person into a position that allows the midwife to listen to the FHR while preserving comfort.

4. Determine the duration and frequency of uterine contractions.

5. Count and record the maternal heart rate.

6. Count and record the baseline FHR:

   a. Check the maternal radial pulse at the same time to confirm that the Doppler fetoscope is detecting the FHR.

   b. Place the Doppler transducer on the maternal abdomen over the fetal thorax or back. Perform the initial auscultation for a minimum of 60 seconds, between contractions, to determine the baseline FHR and to listen for regularity of the rate.

   c. Listen between contractions for several intervals within a 10-minute period to confirm consistency of the FHR and to identify the baseline.

   d. Count for 6 to 10 seconds several times, with a 5- or 10-second pause between counts; then multiply each count by 10 or 6, respectively, to obtain the bpm numeric value.

7. Listen for the presence of FHR accelerations. Accelerations can be detected qualitatively as short, irregular increases in the FHR

| Table 27A-3 | Interpretation of Auscultation Findings Relative to NICHD Three-Tier Categories |
|---|---|
| **Category** | **Description** |
| Category I FHR characteristics by auscultation | FHR baseline between 110 and 160 bpm with regular rhythm |
| | No decreases of the FHR from the baseline |
| | FHR increases (accelerations) of 15 seconds in duration and amplitude from the baseline may or may not be present |
| Category II FHR characteristics by auscultation | Tachycardia (baseline > 160 bpm) or bradycardia (baseline < 110 bpm) |
| | Audible irregular rhythm |
| | Presence of FHR decreases or decelerations from the baseline |

Abbreviations: bpm, beats per minute; FHR, fetal heart rate; NICHD, National Institute of Child Health and Human Development.

baseline that occur when a uterine contraction is not present. Accelerations do not need to be present to identify the FHR as Category I if the FHR has a normal baseline and no decelerations are present. However, FHR accelerations are a sign of fetal well-being and should be assessed for and documented as present if auscultated.

8. Determine the presence of FHR decelerations. Begin listening at the peak of the contraction and continue for at least 30 to 60 seconds after the contraction is over.

   a. If a deceleration is heard, listen through successive contractions or several contractions in a 10-minute window to determine whether they are recurrent or nonrecurrent.

   b. A multicount method to document the drop in FHR baseline and depth of the decrease may be used.

9. Document the bpm rate for each assessment and inform the laboring person and their support team of the findings. Documentation of the FHR following use of IA should define the method of conducting IA, the frequency and duration of IA, the indications for IA, and the indications for transfer to EFM if appropriate. The type of Doppler technology used and the multicount

procedure employed are also documented in the health record. The graph for documentation of IA should be simple and straightforward, to facilitate documentation.

## Interpretation of Auscultated Fetal Heart Rate Characteristics

FHR changes identifiable on IA have been evaluated in concert with the 2008 National Institute of Child Health and Human Development (NICHD) interpretative categories for EFM for use in the United States. FHR changes detected on IA are classified as either Category I or Category II, as outlined in Table 27A-3.[2] There is no Category III when using IA, because Category III FHR patterns have no variability and the degree of FHR variability cannot be detected via IA.

## Management of Category II Fetal Heart Rate Changes Detected Via Intermittent Auscultation

Category I FHR patterns reliably suggest the fetus is well oxygenated and intervention is not indicated. Category II FHR changes require increased surveillance. A longer listening period may be initiated, the frequency of auscultation increased, or transfer to EFM undertaken. If recurrent decelerations are noted, the parturient can be asked to assume a different position (e.g., side-lying) and the FHR immediately reevaluated. If the decelerations do not resolve with position changes, intravenous fluids, oxygen therapy, or tocolysis may be initiated depending on the depth and duration of the decelerations. If the Category II FHR pattern does not resolve in a short period of time, frequent auscultation and documentation of results should continue while transferring the person to a setting where continuous EFM and operative delivery are available.

## Discussion

Both continuous EFM and IA have limitations. The FHR is affected by multiple physiologic signals, and some of the FHR characteristics associated with acidemia are not strongly predictive.[14] The presence of FHR minimal or moderate variability is one of the key variables used to assess for developing acidemia. Therefore, the inability of IA to reliably detect FHR variability or to discriminate between types of FHR decelerations must be addressed.

Despite the fact that IA cannot differentiate between absent, minimal, and moderate FHR variability, and despite the lack of direct scientific studies of this technique, IA is considered a viable option for persons at low risk for adverse perinatal outcomes at term for two reasons. First, the incidence of adverse outcomes in this population is very low. Second, when metabolic acidemia develops de novo during labor, the FHR pattern will reflect the developing acidemia with recurrent decelerations that are detectable via properly conducted IA. However, obstetric emergencies that result in a sudden bradycardia and fetal decompensation (e.g., umbilical cord prolapse or vasa previa compression) are very rare but may not be detected as quickly with IA as it would be with continuous EFM. These facts can be shared with pregnant persons considering the type of fetal surveillance they prefer during labor.

- IA is recommended only for those pregnant persons who do not have an a priori risk (known risk) for developing fetal acidemia during labor. The incidence of clinically significant metabolic acidemia in newborns in a healthy population of parturients is approximately 3 per 1000 births.[15,16] Of these infants, a small proportion (approximately 4%) have no risk factors that could be identified antenatally.[15] Screening for a priori risks is a critical step in identifying individuals who are candidates for this method of fetal surveillance.

- A very low incidence of adverse perinatal outcomes has been found in large population-based studies of out-of-hospital birth.[17-22] Individuals who are low risk, are at a term gestation with a singleton fetus, and experience spontaneous labor that is monitored with IA during labor have a low incidence of adverse perinatal outcomes, particularly when they are cared for by trained clinicians and in an integrated setting that facilitates transfer to higher-level care when indicated.[17-22]

- When significant fetal acidemia does develop during the intrapartum period in a previously healthy fetus, it occurs over a period of time, during which the fetus will develop recurrent FHR decelerations that are detectable on IA or as an acute unremitting bradycardia.[23]

- Randomized controlled trials of IA included one-to-one nursing care, which is associated with a positive effect on labor outcomes. Thus, the continuous or very frequent presence of a healthcare provider necessary to conduct IA may also independently increase the chance of a positive birth outcome.

- Although the incidence of acute bradycardia in a rigorously screened low-risk population is quite low, this important fact needs to be included in shared decision making when a pregnant individual is choosing a mode of fetal surveillance.

- IA will not detect a sinusoidal FHR pattern if decelerations are not also present. This rare FHR pattern is associated with placental abruption, Rh isoimmunization, and maternal–fetal hemorrhage. A person with symptoms of one of these conditions is not a candidate for IA.

## References

1. Alfirevic Z, Devane D, Gyte GML, Cuthbert A. Continuous cardiotocography (CTG) as a form of electronic fetal monitoring (EFM) for fetal assessment during labour. *Cochrane Database Syst Rev.* 2017;2:CD006066. doi:10.1002/14651858.CD006066.pub3.

2. Martis R, Emilia O, Nurdiati DS, Brown J. Intermittent auscultation (IA) of fetal heart rate in labour for fetal well-being. *Cochrane Database Syst Rev.* 2017;2:CD008680.

3. American College of Nurse-Midwives. Intermittent auscultation for intrapartum fetal heart rate surveillance. *J Midwifery Womens Health.* 2015;60(5):626-632. [Erratum: *J Midwifery Womens Health.* 2016;61(1):134.]

4. Lewis D, Downe S; FIGO Intrapartum Fetal Monitoring Expert Consensus Panel. FIGO consensus guidelines on intrapartum fetal monitoring: intermittent auscultation. *Int J Gynaecol Obstet.* 2015;131(1):13-24.

5. Lyndon A, Wisner K. *Fetal Heart Monitoring Principles and Practices.* 6th ed. Washington, DC: Association of Women's Health, Obstetric and Neonatal Nurses; 2021. Dubuque, IA: Kendall Hunt Publishing; 2021.

6. World Health Organization. *Intrapartum Care for a Positive Childbirth Experience.* Geneva, Switzerland: World Health Organization; 2018. http://apps.who.int/iris/bitstream/handle/10665/260178/9789241550215-eng.pdf;jsessionid=FFFEDA8EB7DFB4F0309AEF5B74A9672C?sequence=1. Accessed September 15, 2021.

7. National Institute for Health and Care Excellence. Intrapartum care for health women and babies [Clinical guideline]. December 2014. https://www.nice.org.uk/guidance/cg190/resources/intrapartum-care-for-healthy-women-and-babies-pdf-35109866447557. Accessed September 15, 2021.

8. American College of Obstetricians and Gynecologists. Practice Bulletin No. 116: management of

intrapartum fetal heart rate tracings. *Obstet Gynecol.* 2010;116:1232-1240.

9. Dore S, Ehman W. Society of Obstetricians and Gynaecologists of Canada No. 396: fetal health surveillance: intrapartum consensus guideline. *J Obstet Gynaecol Can.* 2020;42(3):316-348.e9. [Erratum: *J Obstet Gynaecol Can.* 2021;43(9):1118.]

10. International Confederation of Midwives. Use of intermittent auscultation for assessment of foetal well-being during labour [Position statement]. https://www.internationalmidwives.org/assets/files/statement-files/2018/04/eng-use_intermittend_auscultation.pdf. Accessed September 16, 2021

11. Blix E, Maude R, Hals E, et al. Intermittent auscultation fetal monitoring during labour: a systematic scoping review to identify methods, effects, and accuracy. *PLoS One.* 2019;14(7):e0219573.

12. Shiffrin BS. The accuracy of auscultatory detection of fetal cardiac decelerations: a computer simulation. *Am J Obstet Gynecol.* 1992;166(2):566-576.

13. Hersh S, Megregian M, Emeis C. Intermittent auscultation of the fetal threat rate during labor: an opportunity for shared decision-making. *J Midwifery Womens Health.* 2014;59:334-339.

14. Graham EM, Adami RR, McKenney SL, et al. Diagnostic accuracy of fetal heart rate monitoring in the identification of neonatal encephalopathy. *Obstet Gynecol.* 2014;124:507-513.

15. Task Force on Neonatal Encephalopathy. *Neonatal Encephalopathy and Neurologic Outcome.* 2nd ed. Washington, DC: American College of Obstetricians and Gynecologists; 2014, reaffirmed 2019.

16. Morgan JL, Casey BM, Bloom SL, et al. Metabolic acidemia in live births at 35 weeks of gestation or greater. *Obstet Gynecol.* 2015;126(2):279-283.

17. de Jonge A, van der Goes BY, Ravelli ACJ, et al. Perinatal mortality and morbidity in a nationwide cohort of 529,688 low-risk planned home and hospital births. *BJOG.* 2009;116(9):1177-1184.

18. Stapleton SR, Osborne C, Illuzzi J. Outcomes of care in birth centers: demonstration of a durable model. *J Midwifery Womens Health.* 2013;58(1):1-12.

19. Olsen O, Clausen JA. Planned hospital birth versus planned home birth. *Cochrane Database Syst Rev.* 2012;9:CD000352. doi:10.1002/14651858.CD000352.pub2.

20. Cheng Y, Snowden JM, King TL, et al. Selected perinatal outcomes associated with planned home births in the United States. *Am J Obstet Gynecol.* 2013;209(4):325.e1-e8.

21. Birthplace in England Collaborative Group, Brocklehurst P, Hardy P, et al. Perinatal and maternal outcomes by planned place of birth for healthy women with low risk pregnancies: the Birthplace in England national prospective cohort study. *BMJ.* 2011;343:d7400.

22. Rossi AC, Prefumo F. Planned home versus planned hospital births in women at low-risk pregnancy: a systematic review with meta-analysis. *Eur J Obstet Gynecol Reprod Biol.* 2018;222:102-108.

23. Parer JT, King TL, Flanders S, et al. Fetal acidemia and electronic fetal heart rate patterns: is there evidence of an association? *J Matern Fetal Neonatal Med.* 2006;19:289-294.

# 27B

# Fetal Scalp Electrode

EMILY S. SLOCUM

*The editors acknowledge Tekoa L. King who was the author
of this appendix in the previous edition*

A fetal scalp electrode (FSE) is a small, thin, spiral wire that, when attached to the fetal scalp or buttocks, detects the fetal electrocardiogram (ECG). The FSE is attached via a cord to an electronic fetal heart rate (FHR) monitor. The monitor can convert the ECG into an audible sound and a continuous electronic recording. Placement of an FSE requires that the laboring person has ruptured membranes, and a cervix dilated at least 1 to 2 centimeters.

An FSE is not recommended for routine fetal monitoring during labor. Instead, an FSE is used *only* when a continuous legible recording is considered necessary to inform clinical management and an externally placed Doppler or fetoscope is *not* able to supply such a record.

Although there are no specific indications for use of an FSE in the United States, this technology is commonly used when continuous FHR monitoring is indicated and an external Doppler device is unable to continuously detect the FHR. The inability to monitor may be secondary to artifact interference.

In the past, first-generation electronic monitors exaggerated FHR variability when the abdominal Doppler device was used, so an FSE would be applied to provide a more accurate rendition of FHR variability. Today, electronic FHR monitors use an autocorrelation technique that counts the FHR multiple times during the Doppler signal so that FHR variability is portrayed more accurately when an external Doppler is used.[1] Thus, the need to better assess variability is rarely an indication for use of an FSE if a continuous legible tracing is present.

Nevertheless, it is important to note that the external Doppler device is subject to interference from various artifacts, such as signal drop-out from changes in maternal position. The Doppler device can also erroneously detect a maternal heart rate or double or halve the signal, which can, in rare situations, confound interpretation of its output.[1,2] Therefore, difficulty in monitoring the FHR when there is a risk of fetal metabolic acidemia or fetal death can be an indication for use of an FSE. One common scenario in which this occurs is when caring for a person with a high body mass index (BMI).[2] The FSE can assure accurate data are gathered, and it provides reassurance in the context of an illegible or uninterpretable FHR pattern.[3]

Complications following FSE use may include scalp laceration, localized infection, and (rarely) abscess. Some case reports describe facial injury, or insertion in the eye or ear when the FSE is placed without accurate diagnosis of fetal presentation and position. In 2022, Philips recalled its FSE because of case reports of the spiral tip breaking off in the scalp due to over rotation during insertion or after pulling the tip during removal. An FSE also provides a potential pathway for ascending infection. Early studies found a correlation between prolonged use of an FSE (more than 12 hours) and neonatal sepsis, but subsequent retrospective analyses determined that FSE alone is not associated with an increased risk for neonatal sepsis.[4-7] To date, none of the studies conducted has been sufficiently powered to definitely answer this question. When attachment of an FSE is done in a fetus with known vertex presentation and the procedure is performed under aseptic conditions, complications are very rare.

## Mechanism of Action

The FSE spiral electrode contains two electrodes in close proximity. One penetrates the fetal scalp to the depth of approximately 2 millimeters, with vaginal secretions providing electrical conduction between the two wires; the difference in voltage between the two electrodes is then measured and recorded. A third reference electrode that helps eliminate electrical interference is placed on the maternal thigh.

## Contraindications to Use of Fetal Scalp Electrode

- Active infection that might be vertically transmitted to the fetus such as human immunodeficiency virus (HIV), herpes, or hepatitis B or C
- Placenta previa
- Unknown fetal presentation or position
- Face presentation
- Do not place on genitalia or a fontanel.

## Equipment

- Sterile fetal spiral electrode
- Sterile gloves
- Electronic FHR monitor
- Leg plate with Velcro strap or adhesive patches and cable to fetal monitor
- Water-based lubricant

## Procedure for Attaching a Fetal Scalp Electrode

1. Explain to the laboring person the indication for use of an FSE, and review the procedure, along with its benefits and risks. Answer any questions. Obtain informed consent prior to placement.
2. Perform hand hygiene.
3. Attach the leg plate to the laboring person's thigh.
4. Prepare a clean site, often on the bed, for the material needed.
5. Open the FSE packaging.
6. Put on sterile gloves.
7. Remove the wires from between the drive tube and the guide tube, keeping the materials sterile.
8. Perform a vaginal examination; confirm the fetal lie, presentation, and position. Keep the examining hand on the area of the presenting part where the FSE will be applied.

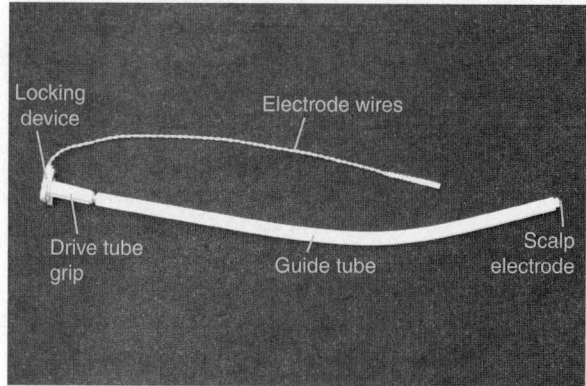

**Figure 27B-1** Fetal monitoring spiral electrode assembly.

9. Select the FSE with the non-examining hand. Verify that the spiral end of the electrode is withdrawn so it is completely within the guide tube. This assures that the device will not inadvertently injure any tissues of the laboring person or the examiner (Figure 27B-1).
10. Advance the guide tube between the examining fingers, and position it firmly against the fetal presenting part, avoiding sutures, fontanels, or genitalia. If uncertain about the exact presentation, do not attach the FSE.
11. Advance the drive tube until it touches the fetal presenting part.
12. Maintain pressure on the guide tube so that it remains touching the fetal presenting part, and rotate the drive tube clockwise approximately 1.5 rotations until mild resistance is felt and the drive tube recoils. Rotating the drive tube causes the tip of the spiral electrode to penetrate the fetal skin and become attached.[1]
13. Release the end of the electrode wires from the locking device at the end of the drive tube grip.
14. Carefully retract the guide tube a few inches, and check the placement and security of the scalp electrode with the examining hand.
15. Remove the guide tube from the vagina and dispose of it per institutional policy.
16. Remove and discard gloves.
17. Attach the electrode wires to the leg plate and the cable from the leg plate to the fetal monitor.
18. Evaluate the FSE recording of FHR to determine if the recording is legible and to assess

the FHR pattern for at least 5 to 10 minutes before leaving the room.

19. Explain the FHR findings to the laboring person and the support team.

20. Document the procedure and FHR pattern in the health record.

## Procedure for Removing a Fetal Scalp Electrode

1. Discuss the removal procedure with the laboring individual and get consent for removal.

2. Perform hand hygiene.

3. Put on sterile gloves and perform a vaginal examination if the presenting part is not visible.

4. With the examining hand on the electrode, rotate it counterclockwise until it is free of the fetal presenting part. Do not pull the electrode directly before rotating the electrode out of the fetal scalp, as this could cause a scalp laceration.

5. Guard the sharp portion of the FSE to protect the vaginal tissues during removal.

6. Safely discard the sharp portion of the FSE in an approved sharps container.

7. Discard gloves and perform hand hygiene.

## References

1. Parer JT, King TL, Ikeda T. *Electronic Fetal Heart Rate Monitoring: The 5-Tier System.* 3rd ed. Burlington, MA: Jones & Bartlett Learning; 2018.

2. Frolova AI, Stout MJ, Carter EB, et al. Internal fetal and uterine monitoring in obese patients and maternal obstetrical outcomes. *Am J Obstet Gynecol MFM.* 2021;3(1):100282.

3. Fairbairn S, McParlin C. The lived experience of staff caring for women in labour who have a BMI ≥ 40 kg/m². *Br J Midwifery.* 2021;29(7):376-385.

4. Bernardes J, Ayres-de-Campos D. The persistent challenge of foetal heart rate monitoring. *Curr Opin Obstet Gynecol.* 2010;22(2):104-109.

5. Nakatsuka N, Jain V, Aziz K, et al. Is there an association between fetal scalp electrode application and early-onset neonatal sepsis in term and late preterm pregnancies? A case-control study. *J Obstet Gynaecol Can.* 2012;34(1):29-33.

6. Harper LM, Shanks AL, Tuuli MG, et al. The risks and benefits of internal monitors in laboring patients. *Am J Obstet Gynecol.* 2013;209(1):38.e1-38.e6.

7. Kawakita T, Reddy UM, Landy HJ, et al. Neonatal complications associated with use of fetal scalp electrode: a retrospective study. *BJOG.* 2016;123(11):1797-1803.

# 27C

# Intrauterine Pressure Catheter

EMILY S. SLOCUM

An intrauterine pressure catheter (IUPC) is a device used to generate quantified information about the frequency, duration, and intensity of uterine contractions as well as baseline uterine tone. Since it requires placement in the uterus, use of an IUPC requires ruptured membranes and adequate cervical dilation for insertion (usually at least 1 to 2 centimeters). The IUPC consists of double-lumen tubing with a pressure transducer (sensor) at the tip (Figure 27C-1). The catheter is introduced into the uterus and amniotic cavity through a curved plastic "introducer" guide that is inserted through the vagina. The external end of the IUPC is attached to a reusable cable connected to an electronic fetal heart rate (EFM) monitor. The changes in pressure detected by the transducer tip are translated into electronic signals that display the intrauterine pressure in units of millimeters of mercury (mm Hg). The first lumen is closed at the external end and transmits the pressure reading from the transducer catheter tip to the cable. The second lumen is open and allows fluid to be instilled into the amniotic cavity when an amnioinfusion is performed.

An IUPC is not recommended for routine care of persons in labor, as it has not been shown to improve maternal or fetal outcomes as compared to external tocodynamometry.[1] Thus, an IUPC is used when detailed assessment of the uterine contraction pattern is needed to make decisions about labor management. A common indication for IUPC use is when a tocodynamometer placed on the abdomen is unable to provide a consistent or clear recording. This can be due to many reasons, including maternal obesity or frequent position changes/movements.[2,3] Internal contraction monitoring can also add valuable information when evaluating for protracted labor, titrating oxytocin (Pitocin), or assessing if tachysystole

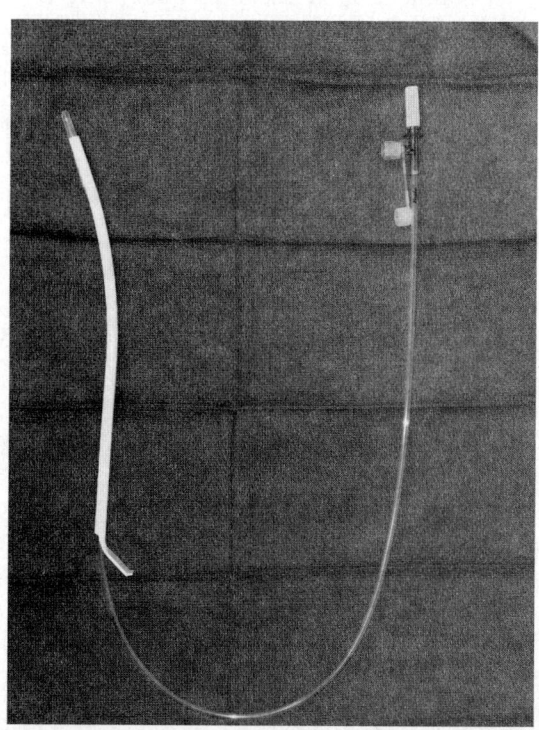

**Figure 27C-1** Intrauterine pressure catheter.

may be contributing to fetal heart abnormalities. An IUPC is also used for amnioinfusion.[4]

The use of an IUPC does have potential risks—notably, increased incidence of maternal infection.[5,6] Though rare, other adverse effects, such as placental abruption or uterine perforation, and even perforation of fetal vessels, have been described.[4-7] Extramembranous insertion rather than intra-amniotic placement of the IUPC increases these risks. In addition, at the time of insertion, there is a risk of displacing the fetal presenting part, which could result in cord prolapse. Care must be taken at time of IUPC insertion to minimize these risks.[7]

## Contraindications to Use of Intrauterine Pressure Catheter

### Absolute Contraindications

- Diagnosed or suspected placenta previa or vasa previa
- Contraindication to rupture of membranes
- Insufficient cervical dilation

### Relative Contraindications

- Excessive bleeding of unknown origin
- Chorioamnionitis
- Some guidelines discourage use with infections with a risk of vertical transmission.

## Equipment

- Sterile IUPC (Figure 27C-1)
- Sterile gloves
- Electronic fetal monitor
- Proper cable to attach the IUPC to the fetal monitor

## Procedure for Attaching an Intrauterine Pressure Catheter

1. Verify that the person does not have placenta previa.
2. Explain to the laboring person the recommendation and indication for use of the IUPC. Review the procedure, along with its benefits and risks. Answer any questions. Obtain informed consent prior to placement.
3. Perform hand hygiene.
4. Prepare a clean, level site, often on the bed, for the material needed.
5. Open the IUPC packaging.
6. Put on sterile gloves.
7. Perform a vaginal examination; confirm cervical dilatation, fetal presentation, and rupture of the membranes. Artificial rupture of the membranes can be performed prior to insertion of an IUPC if indicated. Place the internal fingers of the examining hand between the cervix and the presenting part. This placement helps protect the presenting part from trauma from the IUPC as it is being placed in the uterus next to the fetus.

8. Remove the IUPC from its packaging with the non-examining sterile hand. Keeping the IUPC introducer sterile, thread the introducer and catheter between the examining hand and the presenting part, to just beyond the examining fingers. Do not continue to advance the introducer beyond the tips of the examining fingers or place the introducer into the uterus.
9. Advance the IUPC catheter, threading it with the non-examining hand beyond the introducer and into the uterine cavity (Figure 27C-2). Thread the catheter up to the first mark that is visible on the tubing, or about 10 to 14 centimeters. If resistance is met at any time, retract the catheter back to the level of the introducer and change the angle, or reposition the introducer. The presence of amniotic fluid in the catheter tubing indicates that the catheter is correctly placed in the amniotic space.[8] Advance the IUPC catheter until the second guide mark on tubing is at the introitus, or to about 45 centimeters. This should ensure correct placement near the fundus of the uterus.
10. Gently remove the introducer, taking care not to injure the patient's genitalia. The introducer can be placed on a site on the bed for disposal later, along with sterile gloves, which can be removed now.
11. The IUPC tubing should be secured to the inner thigh of the laboring person; this can be done with nonsterile gloves or by assisting personnel.
12. The IUPC sensor should be attached via cable to the fetal monitor. For correct interpretation, the IUPC may need to be "zeroed" at

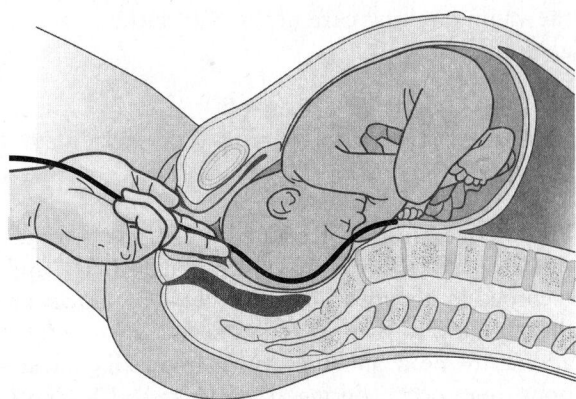

**Figure 27C-2** Technique for placing an intrauterine pressure catheter transcervically.

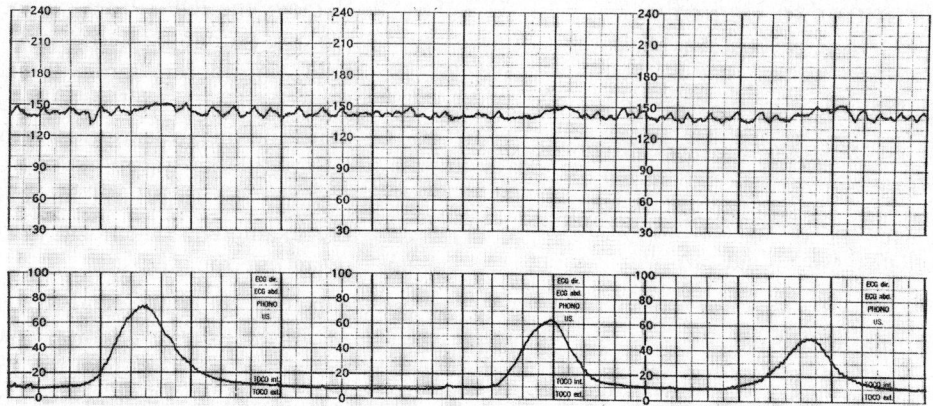

**Figure 27C-3** The calculation of Montevideo units. In this 10-minute period, there are three uterine contractions of 73, 63, and 50 mm Hg peak intensity. Subtracting 10 mm baseline tone from each contraction results in 156 Montevideo units.

this time, ensuring that the baseline pressure is accurately read. This is usually done by depressing a button on the cable before attaching the proximal end of the IUPC to the cable.

13. Ask the patient to cough. The contraction monitor should trace a sharp increase from baseline, indicating the IUPC and monitor are functioning and recording well.

14. Dispose of materials per protocol, and share impressions and the plan of care with the laboring person and the support team.

15. Assess the baseline tone, uterine activity, fetal heart rate, and any complications from the procedure. Document in the health record.

## Removing an IUPC

With sterile or nonsterile gloves, gently grasp the catheter tubing near the introitus and retract slowly until the catheter is fully removed from the vagina, taking care not to injure the patient's genitalia.

## Interpretation of Uterine Activity with IUPC

Intrauterine pressure generated by uterine contractions is measured in Montevideo units (MVUs) and recorded by the area under the curve as shown on the monitor.[9,10] The MVU value is calculated by adding the peak pressures (mm Hg) of all contractions that occur during a designated 10-minute period. The baseline uterine tone (mm Hg) is subtracted from the peak pressure of each contraction

(Figure 27C-3). Traditionally, "adequate" contractions—that is, those associated with successful vaginal birth—have been defined as between 200 to 250 MVUs in a 10-minute time period.

## Documentation

After insertion of an IUPC, the following items should be assessed and then documented in the individual's health record:

- Indications for IUPC placement
- Resting baseline tone following insertion
- Color of amniotic fluid
- Uterine activity: frequency, duration, and intensity (in either mm Hg or MVU)
- Tachysystole: present or absent
- FHR pattern
- Complications from the procedure

### References

1. Bakker JJ, Janssen PF, van Halem K, et al. Internal versus external tocodynamometry during induced or augmented labour. *Cochrane Database Syst Rev.* 2013;8:CD006947. doi:10.1002/14651858. CD006947.pub3. PMID:23913521.

2. Frolova AI, Stout MJ, Carter EB, et al. Internal fetal and uterine monitoring in obese patients and maternal obstetrical outcomes. *Am J Obstet Gynecol MFM.* 2021;3(1):100282. doi:10.1016/j.ajogmf .2020.100282. Epub 2020 Nov 27. PMID: 33451595; PMCID: PMC8087154.

3. American College of Obstetrics and Gynecology Committee on Practice Bulletins—Obstetrics. ACOG Practice Bulletin Number 49, December 2003:

dystocia and augmentation of labor. *Obstet Gynecol.* 2003;102(6):1445-1454.

4. Gee SE, Frey HA. Contractions: traditional concepts and their role in modern obstetrics. *Semin Perinatol.* 2020;44(2):151218.

5. Harper LM, Shanks AL, Tuuli MG, et al. The risks and benefits of internal monitors in laboring patients. *Am J Obstet Gynecol.* 2013;209(1):38.e1-38.e6.

6. Gee SE, Ma'ayeh M, Ward C, et al. Intrauterine pressure catheter use is associated with an increased risk of postcesarean surgical site infections. *Am J Perinatol.* 2020;37(6):557-561.

7. Wilmink FA, Wilms FF, Heydanus R, et al. Fetal complications after placement of an intrauterine pressure catheter: a report of two cases and review of the literature. *J Matern Fetal Neonatal Med.* 2008;21(12):880-883.

8. Koala. Instructions for use [Online brochure]. Clinical Innovations. https://clinicalinnovations.com/wp-content/uploads/2018/07/054-0044.pdf. Accessed September 2, 2021.

9. Caldeyro-Barcia R, Poseiro J. Physiology of the uterine contraction. *Clin Obstet Gynecol.* 1960;3(2):386-410.

10. Bakker PC, Van Rijswijk S, van Geijn HP. Uterine activity monitoring during labor. *J Perinat Med.* 2007;35(6):468-77. [Erratum: *J Perinat Med.* 2008;36(2):184. Van Rijsiwijk, Suzanne corrected to Van Rijswijk, Suzanne.]

APPENDIX

# 27D

# Umbilical Cord Gas Technique and Interpretation

TEKOA L. KING

Umbilical cord gases should be obtained in situations in which an adverse newborn outcome may occur. Normal umbilical cord gases virtually rule out intrapartum acidemia as a contributing factor affecting the newborn's health status.[1] Umbilical cord blood gases are obtained from a section of umbilical cord that has been clamped at both ends. First a sample of umbilical arterial blood and then a sample of umbilical venous blood are collected in heparinized syringes and transported to a laboratory for blood gas analysis. The fetal vessels on the surface of the placenta may be used if a length of umbilical cord is not available.

The blood gases in the umbilical artery (UA) reflect the status of the fetus, whereas the blood gases in the umbilical vein (UV) reflect the status of the intervillous space. Thus, the values of import with regard to acidemia in the fetus immediately before and during birth are those obtained from the UA. However, both UA and UV samples are needed so the results can be correctly interpreted. When only one sample is obtained or when the samples yield the same results, one cannot be certain if the values are from the UA or the UV.

## Selected Indications for Umbilical Cord Blood Gas Analysis

There are no national or international guidelines that recommend when to obtain umbilical cord blood gases. Individual institutions may or may not have a protocol that lists indications for umbilical cord gas analysis. In general, umbilical cord blood should be collected from one UA and the UV following any birth in which a concern arises that the fetus/newborn may have been developing clinically significant acidemia (Table 27D-1).[1] Umbilical cord gas analysis may be performed if needed or the collected blood discarded if the newborn is transitioning to extrauterine life without difficulty.

## Equipment

- Sterile gloves
- Two heparinized syringes
- Section of umbilical cord that is double-clamped. If a section of umbilical cord is not available, vessels that are visible on the fetal side of placenta may be used. Umbilical arteries cross over the umbilical veins.

## Procedure for Obtaining Umbilical Cord Blood Gases

1. Put on sterile gloves.
2. Prior to cutting the umbilical cord to separate the newborn from the placenta, four clamps are placed on the cord in two sets of two, with a distance of 10 to 20 centimeters between each of pair of two clamps. The cord is cut in two places between each set of two clamps. The result will be a clamp on the cord attached to the newborn, a clamp on the cord attached to the placenta, and a cut section of umbilical cord that is clamped at both ends (Figure 27D-1).[2]

| Table 27D-1 | Indications for Collection of Umbilical Cord Gases |
|---|---|

**Antepartum**

Diabetes (requiring medications)

Fetal growth restriction or low birth weight

Hypertension/preeclampsia

Maternal thyroid disease (uncontrolled)

Multifetal gestations

Substance use disorder

**Intrapartum**

Low Apgar score at 5 minutes[a]

Assisted vaginal birth performed for nonreassuring fetal status

Breech presentation

Category II or III fetal heart rate pattern prior to birth

Cesarean birth performed for nonreassuring fetal status or other intrapartum emergency

Intrapartum fever (intrapartum amniotic infection)

Meconium-stained amniotic fluid

Preterm birth

Shoulder dystocia

True knot in cord

[a] Definitions vary (Apgar score < 4 or < 7).

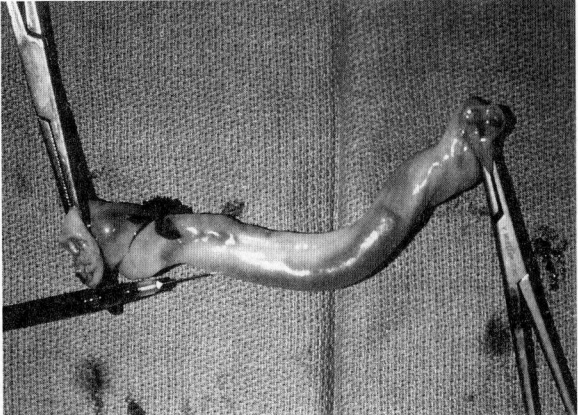

**Figure 27D-1** Section of umbilical cord clamped at both ends.
Reproduced from Parer JT, King TL, Ikeda TL. *Electronic Fetal Heart Rate Monitoring: The 5-Tier System.* 3rd ed. Burlington, MA: Jones & Bartlett Learning; 2018.

3. Using a heparinized syringe, draw blood from the umbilical vein in one syringe and then from an umbilical artery in the other syringe. The vein is larger and more distended. Aspirate anaerobically.

4. Draw approximately 0.5 mL in each syringe.

5. Remove all residual air from the syringe and cap it.

6. Transport the syringes to the laboratory. The syringes are generally placed on ice for transport, but the sample can be kept at room temperature for up to a maximum of 20 minutes.[3]

## Interpretation of Umbilical Cord Blood Gases

Umbilical cord gases report values for (1) pH, (2) partial pressure of carbon dioxide ($PCO_2$), (3) partial pressure of oxygen ($PO_2$), and (4) base deficit (positive number) or base excess (negative number). These indices are evaluated together to determine if the acid–base status of the fetal circulation just prior to birth was normal, indicated a respiratory acidemia, or indicated the presence of metabolic acidemia (Table 27D-2).[1,4]

The pH reflects the degree of acidemia. The $PCO_2$ is used to help determine whether the pH value is related to a respiratory acidosis. For example, acute cord compression during the last phase of birth may result in a sudden rise in $PCO_2$ and a corresponding drop in pH; because the insult is short term, however, the fetus will not need to use anaerobic metabolism and so will not generate lactic acid, which otherwise accumulates as a metabolic acidemia.

The base deficit reflects the concentration of bicarbonate in the newborn circulation that is available to buffer lactic acid and is the primary indicator of metabolic acidemia. A low pH and a high base deficit are the primary umbilical cord gas values that suggest the presence of metabolic acidemia, which is associated with newborn morbidity. A UA pH of less than 7.0 and a base deficit higher than 12 mmol/L are the threshold values most reliably associated with newborn morbidity and mortality.[1] These pH and base deficit values have consistently been identified as the inflection point at which the risk for neonatal encephalopathy becomes significant statistically.[5-7] Infants with a UA pH between 7.0 and 7.1 have an increased risk for short-term neonatal problems such as transient tachypnea, need for supplemental oxygen, or hypothermia. A clinically significant metabolic acidemia is highly unlikely in newborns with a UA pH greater than 7.1.

| Table 27D-2 | Guidelines for Interpretation of Umbilical Arterial Cord Gases in Term Newborns | | | |
|---|---|---|---|---|
| **Diagnosis** | **pH** | **PCO$_2$ (mm Hg)** | **Bicarbonate (HCO$_3^-$)** | **Base Deficit$^a$ (mEq/L)** |
| Normal,$^b$ mean (SD) | 7.26 (± 0.07) | 53 (± 10) | 22.0 (± 3.6) | 4 (± 3) |
| Respiratory acidemia | Normal or low | High | Normal | Normal |
| Metabolic acidemia$^c$ | Low | Normal | Low | High |
| Mixed (metabolic–respiratory) acidemia$^c$ | Low | High | Low | High |

$^a$ May be reported as base excess (negative values) or base deficit (positive value); however, the numeric value is the same.

$^b$ Data from term infants with an Apgar score ≥ 7 at 5 minutes.

$^c$ Clinical association exists with adverse neonatal outcomes when pH < 7 and base deficit > 12 mEq/L.

Based on Helwig JT, Parer JT, Kilpatrick SJ, Laros RK Jr. Umbilical cord blood acid–base state: what is normal? *Am J Obstet Gynecol.* 1996;174(6):1807-1814; American College of Obstetricians and Gynecologists, American Academy of Pediatrics. *Neonatal Encephalopathy and Neurologic Outcome.* 2nd ed. Washington, DC: American College of Obstetricians and Gynecologists; 2014, reaffirmed 2020.

## Limitations of Umbilical Cord Blood Gas Analysis

The risk of neonatal morbidity is inversely related to newborn UA cord blood pH, although the precise level of acidemia that is pathologic for an individual newborn remains unknown. The effects of fetal acidemia reflect an interaction between the magnitude of the stress and the responsiveness of the fetus, with the latter being subject to a great deal of individual variation. In addition, although one might expect a small amount of asphyxia to cause a small amount of damage and larger amounts of asphyxia to have more adverse consequences, the concept of a "continuum of causality" may not be an accurate description of the fetal response to hypoxia. Instead, the fetal response to hypoxia is more likely a threshold effect—that is, damage becomes evident only after a certain threshold has been exceeded.

Umbilical cord blood gases have additional important limitations. Measurements of the UA pH and base deficit suggest the severity of the asphyxial insult but do not provide any information about the duration, whether the insult was continuous or intermittent, or the ability of the individual fetus to compensate for the insult. Although cord blood gases are positively associated with neonatal morbidity, they are only one of many factors that can affect long-term outcomes and neurodevelopment. For example, comorbidities such as anemia or prior infarction may potentiate the effects of fetal acidemia. In addition, greater duration of acidemia likely worsens outcomes, but duration of metabolic acidemia cannot be determined from a single post-birth sample obtained from the umbilical cord.

## Effect of Delayed Cord Clamping

The effect of delaying clamping until after newborn breathing is established may alter the respiratory components of the blood gases (i.e., carbon dioxide and oxygen). In addition, over time, delayed cord clamping may alter the metabolic components secondary to gaseous diffusion and ongoing metabolism. The respiratory components are less important than the metabolic components, so a short delay has not been determined to alter the blood gases significantly.

In term infants born vaginally who appear healthy at birth, delayed cord clamping may be performed for up to 120 seconds prior to obtaining umbilical cord blood gases before there is a clinically significant effect on the cord blood acid–base balance.[8] A recent before-and-after study compared umbilical cord blood gases following immediate cord clamping versus a delay of up to 3 minutes in pregnant individuals who were at increased risk for fetal metabolic acidemia (*n* = 6884).[9] This study did not find significant differences in the blood gases between the two groups.

If delayed cord clamping is performed and umbilical cord gas analysis is indicated, samples can be obtained from the pulsating unclamped cord immediately after the birth. The midwife then places a finger over the puncture sites to stop bleeding for the duration of the period of delayed cord clamping.

## References

1. American College of Obstetricians and Gynecologists, American Academy of Pediatrics. *Neonatal Encephalopathy and Neurologic Outcome.* 2nd ed. Washington, DC: American College of Obstetricians and Gynecologists; 2014, reaffirmed 2020.

2. Parer JT, King TL, Ikeda TL. *Electronic Fetal Heart Rate Monitoring: The 5-Tier System.* 3rd ed. Burlington, MA: Jones & Bartlett Learning; 2018.

3. Valero J, Desantes D, Perales-Puchalt A, et al. Effect of delayed umbilical cord clamping on blood gas analysis. *Eur J Obstet Gynecol Reprod Biol.* 2012;162(1):21-23.

4. Helwig JT, Parer JT, Kilpatrick SJ, Laros RK Jr. Umbilical cord blood acid–base state: what is normal? *Am J Obstet Gynecol.* 1996;174(6):1807-1814.

5. Yeh P, Emary K, Impey L. The relationship between umbilical cord arterial pH and serious adverse neonatal outcome: analysis of 51,519 consecutive validated samples. *BJOG.* 2012;119(7):824-831.

6. Victory R, Penava D, da Silva O, et al. Umbilical cord pH and base excess values in relation to adverse outcome events for infants delivering at term. *Am J Obstet Gynecol.* 2004;191:2021-2028.

7. Malin GL, Morris RK, Khan KS. Strength of association between umbilical cord pH and perinatal and long term outcomes: systematic review and meta-analysis. *BMJ.* 2010;340:c1471.

8. Nudelman MJR, Belogolovsky E, Jegatheesan P, et al. Effect of delayed cord clamping on umbilical blood gas values in term newborns: a systematic review. *Obstet Gynecol.* 2020;135(3):576-582.

9. Colciago E, Fumagalli S, Ciarmoli E, et al. The effect of clamped and unclamped umbilical cord samples on blood gas analysis. *Arch Gynecol Obstet.* 2021;304(6):1493-1499

CHAPTER

# 28

# Support During Labor

LEISSA ROBERTS, JULIA S. SENG, AND KATE WOEBER

*The editors acknowledge Elizabeth Nutter, who was the author of this chapter in the previous edition.*

## Introduction

Every labor and birth are unique, and interpretation of labor pain is highly individual. The actions of care providers can have a strong effect on how a person copes with labor pain and views their experience of labor.[1] A parent's memory of each labor and birth persists for many years, and likely for their lifetime. Provision of person-centered and culturally safe support in labor is an essential component of midwifery care.[2]

Labor is an area of perinatal care where substantial disparities have occurred in the care of marginalized and racialized individuals. People from these groups have been less likely to have their wishes heard or respected in labor, including the provision of desired comfort measures. Midwives need to work to identify and alleviate personal, systemic, and societal biases that may affect support in labor.

The World Health Organization (WHO) states in their 2014 report The Prevention and Elimination of Disrespect and Abuse during Facility-based Childbirth, "Every woman has the right to the highest attainable standard of health, which includes the right to dignified, respectful health care."[3] This includes facility-based obstetric care. The Organic Law on Women's Right to a Violence-Free Life defines "obstetric violence" in Article 15(13) as

> the appropriation of a woman's body and reproductive processes by health personnel, in the form of dehumanizing treatment, abusive medicalization and pathologization of natural processes, involving a woman's loss of autonomy and of the capacity to freely make her own decisions about her body and her sexuality, which has negative consequences for a woman's quality of life.[3]

An implication of this policy statement is that the desires of the pregnant person should be assessed, documented, and fulfilled to the extent possible; and that regular practices or limitations of the birth environment that are not subject to change and that go against these wishes should be disclosed prenatally so the individual can decide if the facility meets their needs.

In a 2019 study, WHO researchers reported that mistreatment occurred during 42% of childbirths in the four nations studied (Ghana, Guinea, Nigeria, and Myanmar), but that evidence suggests it occurs worldwide, including in developed countries.[4] Mistreatment during childbirth, including physical and verbal abuse and discrimination, is characterized as "negligent, reckless, discriminatory and disrespectful acts by health professionals . . . legitimized by the symbolic relations of power that naturalize and trivialize their occurrence."[5] Examples include doing vaginal examinations without consent and cutting episiotomies without informed consent or anesthesia.[5] Within the United States, patterns of obstetric violence are characterized by large disparities according to race and ethnicity.[6]

Severe, unwanted labor pain and traumatic birth experiences, whether due to the pain or perceptions of poor care, are associated with the development of chronic pain and birth-related post-traumatic stress symptoms in the postpartum period. A review of data from the Listening to Mothers II survey found that the rate of post-traumatic stress disorder (PTSD) after childbirth in people who gave birth in the United States was approximately 9%.[7] Approximately 2% of these individuals were still symptomatic 6 months postpartum.[8] Across nations, the rates of birth-related PTSD in the postpartum period are similar, approximately 6%, but are higher among those who experienced high-risk situations such as having an infant in intensive care or experiencing life-threatening complications. Subdiagnostic levels of PTSD symptoms are associated with similar levels of distress and impairment. Of the 6% of birthing persons who develop PTSD symptoms postpartum, approximately 1.5% experience new-onset PTSD. Another 4.5% with PTSD after birth had PTSD at some point before the birth; although these people's postpartum symptoms (e.g., nightmares, intrusive memories) are related to the birth experience, their condition is considered a "retraumatization."[9,10] That is, the birth experience seems to have caused a recurrence of their extant PTSD.

Severe pain is also associated with postpartum depression.[11] Consistent intrapartum predictors of PTSD after birth include unwelcome or intrusive or painful procedures, negative patient–staff interactions, and feelings of loss of control over the birth. These intrapartum risk events likely interact with natal and prepregnancy predictors of traumatic birth—namely, past trauma and mental health conditions.

Empowering laboring people to trust their bodies, having a deeper understanding of how labor works, and providing a positive environment with social, emotional, and, if desired, comfort and pharmacologic support can affect labor and birth outcomes. Support in labor that focuses on the birthing individual's needs and affirms that person's desires for coping, comfort, and support is a foundation of midwifery care. This chapter divides coverage of support during labor into three sections: (1) a review of the physiology of labor pain and factors that influence the experience of labor and birth, (2) nonpharmacologic techniques for providing support in labor, and (3) pharmacologic techniques used to provide support during labor.

## Physiology of Pain

Pain is the result of a complex interplay between physical, biologic, psychologic, and sociocultural factors, each of which contributes to the overall perception of the experience.[12,13] The formal definition of pain used in health care today comes from the International Association for the Study of Pain (IASP):

> [Pain is] an unpleasant sensory and emotional experience associated with . . . actual or potential tissue damage . . . Pain is always a personal experience that is influenced to varying degrees by biological, psychological, and social factors. . . . Through their life experiences, individuals learn the concept of pain.[14]

Pain is generally characterized as either acute or chronic, and is further characterized as somatic (deep or superficial) or visceral. Deep somatic pain is dull, aching, and poorly localized, whereas superficial somatic pain is sharp and well localized. Visceral pain is caused by ischemia or inflammation in visceral structures (internal organs). Over the course of labor, visceral, deep somatic, and superficial somatic pain can all be experienced.

Pain is caused by stimulation of nociceptors—that is, sensory neurons that detect noxious substances. The pain impulse is transmitted from nociceptors in the periphery or viscera via fast, lightly myelinated A-delta fibers and slower, unmyelinated C fibers (**Figure 28-1**). Pain traveling along the A-delta fibers is perceived within 0.1 second, whereas pain transmitted along the C fibers takes longer—approximately 1 second or more—to be perceived by the individual. Numerous types of stimuli, such as mechanical, thermal (temperature related), inflammatory mediators, and chemical agents, can stimulate nociceptors. For example, uterine stretching

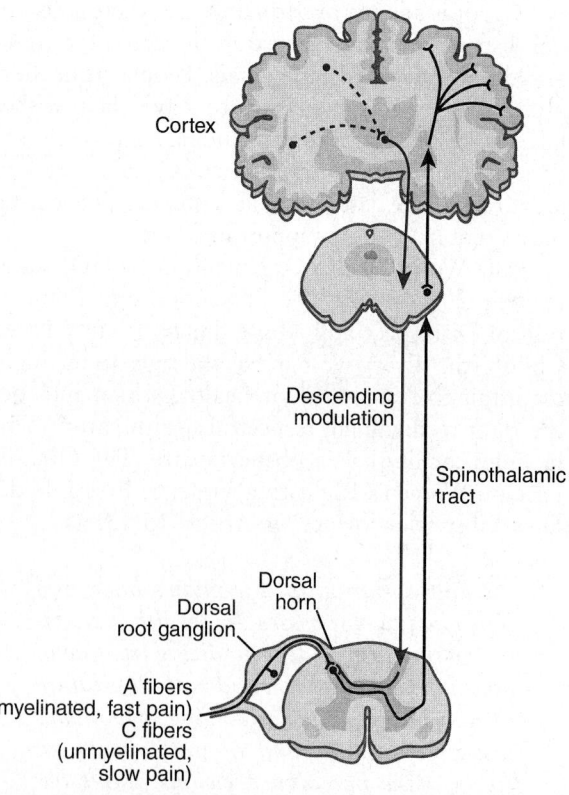

Cortex

Descending modulation

Spinothalamic tract

Dorsal horn

Dorsal root ganglion

A fibers (myelinated, fast pain)
C fibers (unmyelinated, slow pain)

**Figure 28-1** Transmission of pain between periphery and central nervous system.

during labor causes mechanical pain, but lactic acid in uterine muscle can also stimulate uterine pain. Chemical mediators of pain include substance P, glutamate, bradykinin, acetylcholine, serotonin, and histamine. Pain management during labor is aimed at minimizing or allaying the effects of both mechanical and chemical mediators.[15]

Once pain is transmitted from the nociceptors at the anatomic source of the pain, the impulse is transmitted via A-delta and C fibers to the dorsal column of the spinal cord, where these fibers synapse with other neurons in the cord. During the first stage of labor, the pain fibers from the contracting uterus enter the spinal cord at the T10 to L1 levels; in contrast, during the second stage of labor, the pain fibers enter the spinal cord at the S2 to S4 level.[16] Nerves within the dorsal horn of the spinal cord transfer the impulse to the contralateral spinothalamic tract, where nerves ascend to the cerebral cortex.

Prior to ascending to the central nervous system (CNS), the pain impulse crosses from one side of the dorsal horn to the other. The impulse can be modulated by several different mechanisms in the dorsal horn. The gate-control theory of pain modulation is the hypothesis that stimulation of A-delta fibers via massage, sterile water injections, or transcutaneous electric nerve stimulation (TENS) results in impulses rapidly traversing to the dorsal horn, where they effectively close a "gate" that blocks impulses from the slower C fibers that transmit deeper pain signals.[12,13] This theory, which was proposed in 1965 by Melzack and Walls, is not exactly correct in its details: Notably, the mechanism for how the small and larger fibers interact is more complex.[17] Nonetheless, the gate-control theory of pain correctly identified the general process and sparked subsequent research that has greatly expanded knowledge of pain pathways and the factors that influence them. The contemporary IASP definition of pain given earlier builds upon founding member Melzack's 1968 work, stating that pain is a multidimensional complex with numerous sensory, affective, cognitive, and evaluative components.

The pain impulse travels to the brain via two pathways: the neospinothalamic tract and the paleospinothalamic tract. Most of the fibers of the neospinothalamic tract terminate in brain areas such as the brain stem and the thalamus, where the pain signal is transmitted to basal areas of the brain as well as the somatosensory cortex, causing the parturient to "feel" pain. The paleospinothalamic tract fibers terminate in the brain stem, in the areas of the medulla, pons, mesencephalon, and periaqueductal

gray region. These lower regions of the CNS also play a role in the perception of pain. Thus, the perception of pain is the result of CNS integration of pain impulses in the thalamus, lower brain areas, and the cortex.

The pathways of pain perception are bidirectional. The CNS also has the capability of modifying the perception of pain. First, inhibitory neurons in the CNS can dampen the pain sensation via activation of an endogenous opiate system. The brain includes an analgesic system that varies from person to person, which partially explains some of the individual differences in pain perception. In addition, the periaqueductal gray and the periventricular areas (the areas around the third and fourth ventricles of the brain) possess neurons that transmit anti-nociceptive impulses to the dorsal horns of the spinal cord. The impulses from these fibers block the ascending pain impulse before it is relayed to the brain, via release of neurotransmitters such as enkephalin and serotonin at their terminus in the dorsal horn of the spinal cord.

Serotonin promotes release of enkephalin, which is known to inhibit both presynaptic and postsynaptic type C and A-delta pain fibers at the dorsal horns. Several other naturally occurring physiologic opiates, such as beta-endorphin and dynorphin, also play roles similar to that of enkephalin. Although these opioid-like substances can make people feel a "natural high," they do not cause addiction. In contrast, exogenous opioids, whether natural or synthetic, can cause dependence and addiction. Most of the naturally occurring opioids now used exogenously to treat pain are derived from opium. These opium-derived opioids, which are referred to as "opiates," include heroin, morphine, and codeine. Opioids can also be created synthetically, such as fentanyl.

Over the past decade, additional avenues for understanding internal sensations—not only pain—have been integrated to create the new science of "interoception." This field of science seeks to explain how we sense, integrate, interpret, and regulate signals within ourselves.[18] Interoceptive information can be transmitted and interpreted by the brain via non-neural signals that are biologic, mechanical, or electromagnetic and thermal. Although much interoception likely remains entirely below the level of conscious awareness, perception of interoceptive states and conscious processing may come to greatly expand the possibilities for assessments and interventions in labor. Theoretically, our current, rather singular focus on treating pain could expand to shared patient–provider attention to numerous other sensations. Although very little clinically applicable research has emerged so far, studies of interoception have the potential to advance options for facilitation of physiologic labor tailored to the individual's interoception of relevant body processes.

## Labor Pain

Labor pain is felt in three general physical locations. Virtually all people in labor experience lower abdominal pain. In addition, approximately 74% experience contraction-related back pain, and 33% experience continuous low back pain.[11] In Melzack's classic study of 42 nulliparous and 37 multiparous women who completed hourly pain assessments throughout labor, there was a wide variability between individuals in the spatial distribution of where pain was felt.[19]

In addition to spatial variation, variation in intensity of labor pain is apparent. Generally, compared to multiparous people, nulliparous people report higher average intensity levels of pain on the McGill Pain Questionnaire, a tool developed by Melzack. This is especially true for nulliparous people who have had no preparation for childbirth.[19] However, there is variability in the pain reported at hourly intervals by individuals, just as there is a great deal of variability among different laboring people. Although for most birthing persons, the average intensity of pain increases as labor progresses, nulliparous people often report more pain in early labor, whereas multiparous people tend to report more pain in active labor. In addition, many people report periods during active labor where pain does not increase or actually decreases for a short time. In summary, despite the general observation that labor pain increases as cervical dilation increases, labor pain can be independent of cervical dilation for both nulliparous and multiparous people, and there is interindividual variability in the location, intensity, and progression of pain during labor.[11,18-20]

### Physiologic Response to Labor Pain

Pain during the first stage of labor is generally believed to be caused by mechanical distension of the lower uterine segment, cervical dilation, and perhaps acidemia in uterine muscles that develops as a result of recurrent uterine contractions. A number of physiologic systems are affected by pain. One of the first responses comes from the sympathetic nervous system, which releases stress-related hormones such as cortisol, catecholamines (norepinephrine

and epinephrine), and cytokines. Concomitantly, the levels of angiotensin II, antidiuretic hormone, growth hormone, and glucagon increase. The effects of these changes include heightened alertness, increased cardiac output, increased heart rate, increased respiratory rate, elevated blood pressure, higher serum glucose levels, and more extracellular fluid in the periphery and lungs. Increased levels of catecholamines also slow gastrointestinal and genitourinary motility and alter coagulation and immune responses.

The relationship between catecholamine release and uterine contractility during labor is poorly understood. It has long been theorized and noted in observational studies of small numbers of laboring people that the uterus does not contract well when catecholamine levels are very high.[21] Levels of epinephrine, a known tocolytic, increase proportionately more than levels of norepinephrine during labor, albeit with a great deal of interindividual variability. Poorly controlled pain can cause anxiety and fear, which in turn further stimulate the hypothalamic–pituitary–adrenal (HPA) axis and exacerbate the stress response, leading to the release of even more catecholamines and cytokines. Despite the identification of some physiologic mechanisms, the exact effects of stress and fear on uterine contractility during labor have not yet been clearly delineated.[21] However, contemporary understandings of the oxytocin system's roles in stress reduction and stress recovery, as well as its importance to feeling connected to others and protected, have implications for support in labor.[22]

It may be helpful to those managing and supporting labor to understand that oxytocin is *both* a paracrine and pituitary hormone *and* a neurotransmitter.[23] As a paracrine and pituitary hormone, it is secreted from and acts on smooth muscle tissue, including that found in the heart, airway, bowel and bladder, breast, and uterus. Oxytocin also acts centrally to affect stress regulation and behavioral functions such as face and voice recognition and prosocial activity. As a neurotransmitter, oxytocin has a key role in the parasympathetic nervous system, down-regulating cortisol and facilitating recovery from stress.[24] It stimulates feelings of connectedness, including affiliation for protection, as well as bonding and caregiving behavior. Reciprocally, oxytocin is stimulated by social interaction that offers closeness and support, such as caregiving in labor.[25]

Currently, research in the field of stress, labor, contractility, and bonding is challenging, complex, and still evolving. However, the current knowledge base suggests that labor practices supporting the parasympathetic facilitation of oxytocin while decreasing disruptions of the sympathetic nerve system could have important implications for both the birthing person's peripheral and central nervous systems.

## Factors Affecting the Perception of Labor Pain

To help account for the significant interindividual variability in the perception and response to pain, Melzack expanded the gate-control theory into the neuromatrix theory of pain.[12,13,26] According to this theory, the perception of pain by any individual, including during labor, is a dynamic process with physical, psychological, and behavioral components.

The interplay of psychological preparation, expectations, past experience of pain, fear of childbirth, and emotional support during labor are just a few of the factors that affect the degree of pain perceived during labor. Expectations appear to play a large role in perception and ability to cope with the pain of labor.[26] In a review of this body of work, Lally et al. found that, in general, there is a significant gap between expectations and experience, with most people who give birth reporting more pain than anticipated and expectations that were not met.[27]

The effects of genetics and culture on pain perception are complex.[15] Culture does not appear to influence perception of pain, but it does affect behavioral responses to pain.[15] Genetic variability in opioid receptors can affect pain sensation, with specific polymorphisms in opioid receptors occurring more frequently in some genetic groups.[28,29] For example, genetic differences in the microsomal enzymes involved in metabolizing drugs can play a clinically important role in the body's ability to metabolize the opioids used for pain management during labor.[30] In addition, several polymorphisms in the cytochrome CYP2D6 system have been identified that adversely affect the metabolism of codeine in affected individuals.[30]

Unfortunately, systemic bias has often resulted in differentially poor management of pain for race- and ethnic-minority people,[31] including pain in labor.[32] This health disparity can be redressed by consistently attending to individual differences in pain experience and expression rather than applying false generalizations about race or ethnicity. Current international understandings of pain underscore the importance of prioritizing the pain experience of the individual.

One of the key aspects of the IASP's definition of pain is the understanding that pain is learned through lifetime experience.[14] This suggests that "history" is among the physical, psychological, and behavioral aspects operating in pain. One in five adults is a survivor of childhood maltreatment. For people who experience early life pain in the form of abuse or neglect, pain can also include both interpersonal and emotional components. Many people are resilient despite maltreatment, but others develop depression or PTSD marked by "reexperiencing" of any and all aspects of the trauma.[33] These responses can include somatic memory, automatic and potentially maladaptive coping, fear, hypervigilance for betrayal, and strong efforts to avoid any reminders—including efforts to avoid being in pain or needing help.

Healthcare providers frequently encounter patients whose responses to pain may be complicated by childhood maltreatment. Other traumatic life experiences may similarly affect pain response; for example, survivors of life-threatening illness or medical or reproductive experiences that were traumatic may also experience pain complicated by post-traumatic stress reactions. A trauma-informed approach to pain assessment and management is critical for all healthcare providers. This approach allows care providers to address the physical, psychological, and behavioral domains, while also providing the patient with an uplifting experience of being treated optimally and with respect by a caregiver during a time when they experienced pain.

Multiple antecedents may affect labor pain, and knowledge of these factors can inform the therapeutic approach. It is usually possible to assess for these factors and discuss needs ahead of labor. For example, those individuals who have a history of severe dysmenorrhea are more likely to have severe labor pain. This outcome may be related to increased prostaglandin synthesis, which results in intense uterine contractions.[15] Pain also tends to be worse at night than in the daytime. Laboring in an unfamiliar setting can increase self-reports of pain intensity. Likewise, fear of labor and lack of self-efficacy are associated with severe labor pain. A person's ability to use mental strategies to cope with labor pain appears to be related to their self-confidence in being able to use those strategies, although this is a simplification that does not fully account for the many factors involved.[15] As explained earlier, trauma survivors' experiences may be affected by their history of pain in the context of violence or betrayals in caregiving relationships. For all these reasons, it is critical that the midwife provide each laboring person with an individualized pain management assessment, including sensitive and appropriate assessment of trauma-related needs, followed by tailored pain management and individualized support during labor.

### Childbirth Fear or Anxiety

Fear of childbirth affects 6.3% to 14.8% of people giving birth.[34] It can range from mild anxiety to avoidance of childbearing because the fear is so great; the latter extreme is labeled *tokophobia*. Most of the research on fear of childbirth has been conducted in Northern Europe. Although there is a paucity of data on this topic from the United States, significant fear appears to be more common than previously thought.[35,36] Studies of pregnant people's fear of childbirth have found increased fear is associated with nulliparity, young maternal age, preexisting psychological conditions, low self-esteem, and a history of abuse.[35-37] Fear of childbirth is also associated with increased severity of labor pain.[37,38] Such a fear can overshadow the experience of pregnancy, though interventions during this period can improve outcomes. Brief instruments for assessing fear of childbirth are available that can be useful for quantifying tokophobia and facilitating treatment.[35]

### Trauma History

As explained earlier, a personal history of trauma can affect an individual's experience of pain in labor. It also can affect other aspects of the childbearing year, ranging from somatic discomforts to nightmares and trouble sleeping, to labor, to lactation, to postpartum mental health status, and on into parenting.[39] For all of these reasons, universal screening and prenatal practices and programs to address trauma-related needs are important.[40]

A trauma-informed approach in prenatal care[41] follows the public health norm of using a tiered system of responses, as detailed in the *Mental Health Conditions* chapter. At the "universal" tier, screening and incorporating attention to trauma into the whole team's habits of mind is vital. At the "targeted" tier, providers enact practices and implement evidence-based programs that address individual or group unmet needs. At the "specialist" or intensive tier, referral to mental health services must be available to address diagnostic-level problems. Screening or assessing needs only upon admission to labor is awkward and eliminates opportunities to address trauma-related needs holistically and with the whole perinatal team.[41]

### Childbirth Education

Starting with the first edition of Grantly Dick-Read's classic *Childbirth Without Fear*, which was published in the 1930s, various childbirth preparation programs have assisted people in preparing to give birth. By the 1970s, childbirth education classes had become a common means of preparing for labor and birth. The initial focus of these classes was on reducing the fear–pain–tension cycle by providing people with knowledge about the labor process so pain medications could be avoided during labor. Dick-Read postulated that fear generates physical tension, which in turn increases pain; he also suggested that fear could be alleviated with knowledge and skills. Subsequently introduced natural psychoprophylactic methods of childbearing have varied in the emphasis they place on preparatory muscular and breathing exercises, but all educate the birthing person about the process of labor and various means of coping with pain, thereby reducing fear.

A Cochrane review of the effects of childbirth preparation classes was not able to identify how childbirth classes affect labor pain, self-efficacy, or knowledge acquisition, with the researchers citing multiple methodologic flaws in the trials that made up their systematic review of this topic.[42] A subsequent large randomized trial that involved an intention-to-treat analysis found some significant benefits of childbirth education. In this study, participants were randomly assigned to a group that received 9 hours of formal childbirth education versus a group that received usual care. The researchers found that participants in the intervention group— that is, those receiving childbirth education—were more likely to be admitted in active labor (relative risk [RR], 1.45; 95% confidence interval [CI], 1.26–1.65) and less likely to use epidural analgesia for labor (RR, 0.84; 95% CI, 0.73–0.97).[43]

### General Principles for Assessment of Labor Coping and Provision of Labor Support

In 2002, Hodnett performed a systematic review that analyzed results from 137 studies (both qualitative and quantitative) involving more than 14,000 birthing people to determine the major factors that influence birth satisfaction.[26] This analysis identified four major components of birth satisfaction: (1) prenatal expectations, (2) support from caregivers, (3) quality of the caregiver–birthing person relationship, and (4) involvement in decision making. These results have been validated and replicated in multiple studies since the publication of this seminal analysis. Surprisingly, adequate pain relief is not one of the four factors that affect birth satisfaction. Hodnett concluded:

> *The influences of pain, pain relief, and intrapartum medical interventions on subsequent*

| Table 28-1 | General Principles for Supporting Coping and Mitigating Pain During Labor |
|---|---|

**General Principles**

Listen to, respect, and support individuals' informed preferences for comfort and pain management

Facilitate the presence of chosen support persons

Ensure privacy and prevent exposure

Promote an optimal laboring environment

Use calm, quiet, purposeful communication

Offer labor support and pain relief strategies

**Physical Care Activities**

Support relaxation to prevent fatigue

Encourage an empty bladder

Keep the perineum clean and dry

Offer liquids and lip moisteners for oral care

Encourage regular changes in position and support the extremities with pillows

*satisfaction are neither as obvious, as direct, nor as powerful as the influence of the attitude and behaviors of the caregivers.*[26(pS160)]

This suggests that other factors, which go beyond the narrow focus on pain management, are highly significant and could be addressed prior to the acute episode of labor. Table 28-1 shows general principles for supporting coping and mitigating labor pain.

### Promote an Optimal Laboring Environment

Any midwife can take several key steps to create an optimal laboring environment (these steps are adapted from the Samueli Institute's Optimal Healing Environment).[44] An optimal environment includes four components: internal, interpersonal, behavioral, and external. Optimal internal and interpersonal environments support a person's expectations and intentions through open communication, compassion, social support, and empathy. A key component of interpersonal communication and an optimal laboring environment is ensuring that the laboring person feels heard. Birthing plans are a popular method for the birthing person (and their partner) to communicate their desires for labor to the midwife and care team. An optimal

behavioral environment supports integrative team-based care with use of complementary therapies as desired by the individual. Another optimal component supports the use of color, light, aroma, music, and sound therapies.[44]

An additional critical part of an optimal laboring environment is the healing skills of the midwife. In their qualitative review of complementary and alternative care providers, Churchill and Schenk identified several core healing skills that mirror the philosophy of midwifery care: take time, be open and listen, do the little things, be committed, let the patient explain, remove barriers, and share authority.[45]

### Assure Privacy and Prevent Exposure

Assurance of privacy and prevention of exposure are of particular importance in a hospital.[46] Ideas of modesty vary widely, often according to one's past experiences and culture. Some people may not feel the need to be draped to prevent exposure, whereas others will be uncomfortable exposing their body. Walburg et al. found that feelings of embarrassment could be minimized during exposure of genitalia by limits on the number of personnel present, a professional and kind attitude from providers, and explanation of procedures.[47]

### Promote Comfort

Mitigation of pain is a key strategy for supporting individuals in labor, but it is not the only one. Kolcaba[48] and Schuiling[49] advanced theories of comfort, including comfort in labor. The concept of comfort is broader than just relief of pain in labor. Pain is only one aspect of the labor experience, which also includes social, spiritual, physical, and psychological dimensions. Provision of comfort care during labor encompasses all of these dimensions of the experience. Comfort during labor is increased by ensuring continuity of care and continuous emotional support, as well as attention to pain management.

### Support Coping During Labor

The work of Hodnett and others expanded our knowledge of the experience of labor, including clarifying the point that the mitigation or diminution of labor pain and coping with labor are not the same thing.[18,26] In physiologic labor, increasing pain or discomfort generally signifies progress toward birth, not pathology. Each individual's expectations and interpretation of pain play a critical role in their ability to cope in labor. Labor pain can be welcomed and embraced as productive and purposeful.[50,51]

Research suggests that the ability to cope in labor is more important to birth satisfaction than relief of pain.[52]

Adequate pain relief is considered an important patient right by The Joint Commission. In most acute care settings in the United States, a numeric rating scale (NRS), where 0 is no pain and 10 is the worst possible pain, is used to assess pain, plan interventions, and evaluate the effect of those interventions. However, this numeric rating scale does not capture how a person is coping with their labor.[52-54] The NRS also medicalizes labor pain, presuming that like other pain experiences, labor pain creates suffering and must be eradicated.[54,55]

The mindset that labor is a medicalized state where pain needs to be managed may be slowly shifting in the United States. In 2019, the American College of Obstetricians and Gynecologist (ACOG) released a revised bulletin (No. 209) regarding obstetric analgesia and anesthesia, which acknowledged that nonpharmacologic options may be useful alternatives in labor.[56] Moreover, The Joint Commission does not dictate that the NRS must be used for all populations, but rather encourages the use of more appropriate tools for specialized populations.

Roberts et al. developed the Coping with Labor Algorithm (Figure 28-2) to capture the variable of coping in laboring, while complying with The Joint Commission standards.[53,54] Simply asking "How are you coping?", instead of asking the laboring person to rate their pain, can generate important information, allowing the midwife and other care team members to offer appropriate support.

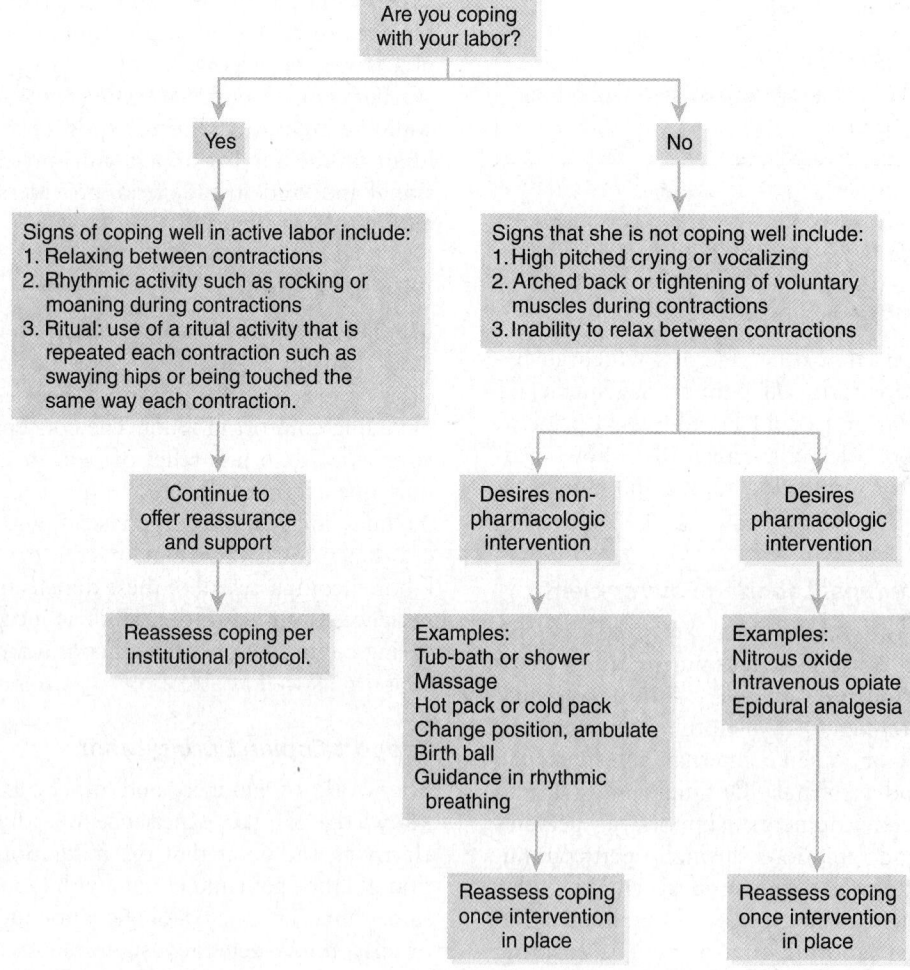

**Figure 28-2** Coping with labor algorithm.
Modified with permission from Leissa Roberts, CNM, DNP, FACNM. The coping with labor algorithm: an alternate pain assessment tool for the laboring woman. *J Midwifery Womens Health*. 2010;55(2): 107-116.

Simkin analyzed the behaviors of individuals who were coping well in labor and found three consistent behaviors that may serve as cues, in addition to self-reports: (1) the ability to relax during or between contractions, (2) use of a ritual, and (3) a rhythmic activity (breathing, rocking, swaying).[55] If a person is coping well with labor, it is likely the individual is not suffering or experiencing acute emotional distress. Simkin and Bolding stated:

> Although pain and suffering often occur together, one may suffer without pain or have pain without suffering . . . one can have pain coexisting with satisfaction, enjoyment and empowerment. Loneliness, ignorance, unkind or insensitive treatment during labor, along with unresolved past psychological or physical distress, increase the chance that the woman will suffer.[1(p489)]

Bergstrom et al. observed four broad categories of behavior during the second stage of labor: (1) not expressing pain or distress, (2) low-level pain, (3) focused working, and (4) severe pain.[57] In all but the last category, the laboring persons were able to maintain their sense of self-control. An effective technique identified by the researchers for caregivers to use when laboring people's pain is severe enough that they are unable to maintain a sense of self-control is to position oneself very close to the person's face (en face position) to gain their attention and talk in a low tone of voice. The researchers found when this method was used, pain intensity was lowered and the person in labor was able to maintain their sense of control.[57]

### Accurately Assess Coping

Care providers are not very accurate in their assessment of a person's coping or pain during labor. Studies that have compared providers' assessments to laboring persons' assessments have found that the provider's estimate of the person's degree of pain is consistent with the individual's report only approximately 50% of the time.[58] The remaining 50% was split evenly, with 25% of providers overestimating pain and 25% underestimating labor pain.[58]

Two factors contributing to providers' underestimation of birthing people's labor pain are multiparity and cultural differences with the laborer.[59] There is a recognized problem of racial bias in pain assessment and treatment recommendations in the United States, which results in Black people being systematically undertreated for their pain compared to white people.[31] In addition, minimal expression of pain experienced by a laboring person can lead to inaccuracy in pain assessment. For example, in one study, midwives estimated mild or moderate labor pain fairly well, but underestimated a reported experience of severe pain.[60] Another study found that midwives' personal experiences influenced their estimation of the degree of pain in labor.[61] Although these investigations were small studies conducted in different countries, they are still quite valuable. Clearly, the laboring persons' self-report is the most critical piece of data for assessing and mitigating labor pain.

### Offer Labor Support and Pain Relief Strategies

In the United States, there are a vast array of options for mitigation of labor pain and promotion of coping. These can be split into two major categories: pharmacologic and nonpharmacologic. The goal of pharmacologic interventions is to eliminate or minimize pain in labor, whereas the nonpharmacologic model offers resources for effective coping during the labor and birth experience.[54]

When advising birthing people about their options for labor pain relief, it is important that the midwife has a clear understanding of how research, or evidence, is graded for quality, as detailed in the *Interpreting Published Research Data with a Clinical Midwifery Lens* appendix. Choices about pain management in labor should be informed by evidence-based practice, meaning practice based on solid, relevant information from research, combined with an individual's medical needs, desires, values, and preferences. It *is* evidence-based practice to arrive at treatment choices collaboratively, through the provider giving full information for informed consent,[62] with discussion of risks and benefits during prenatal discussions as well as in the moment of labor. By interpreting the strength of the evidence, healthcare providers can present an accurate picture of both the benefits and the potential harms of interventions to the birthing people in their care.

As midwives, we have a primary responsibility to help our patients make decisions about appropriate treatments, care measures, and interventions. Ethics is an important attribute that is inseparable from the art and science of midwifery. Midwives have an obligation to provide care that will benefit those persons receiving that care, and to respect their social and cultural values and principles, while ensuring that they do no harm.

The ethical principles of beneficence and nonmaleficence were first stated by Hippocrates and incorporated as tenets of the Hippocratic oath, which all healthcare providers abide by. Beneficence is the principle that one should act for the benefit of the patient. Nonmaleficence is the obligation to do no harm.[63] Many of the nonpharmacologic methods of pain relief that midwives offer have insufficient data, limited evidence, or low evidence for their use—yet they do not cause harm or have a clear mechanism by which they could cause harm. Knowing an intervention does not cause harm is an important distinction when presenting options and ensuring informed consent of patients. The principles of beneficence and nonmaleficence help midwives negotiate this point of tension created by the lack of supporting evidence for interventions by emphasizing the simple fact that most of the nonpharmacologic care measures that midwives employ cause no harm. Put simply, if a patient feels a particular intervention is helping them to cope with labor and there is no evidence of harm, the midwife should support its use.

# Nonpharmacologic Methods of Mitigating Labor Pain

A variety on nonpharmacologic methods can be used to support labor comfort and coping. Not all methods are available in all settings, but the midwife should be knowledgeable about their potential value and application. Providing options and supporting individuals in use of methods they find helpful is an important consideration in person-centered care. The following sections describe some of these methods and are organized in alphabetical order. Table 28-2 provides information on the mechanism of action of nonpharmacologic methods commonly used to mitigate labor pain.[1]

## Acupressure or Acupuncture

Traditional Chinese medicine recognizes acupuncture as a means to correct imbalances in the vital

| Table 28-2 | Mechanism of Action for Reducing Pain via Selected Nonpharmacologic Methods | | | | |
|---|---|---|---|---|---|
| | Affects Nerve Conduction of Pain Stimuli | Changes Pressure Sensations | Decreases Tension and Anxiety | Distracts Away from Pain Sensation | Increases Sense of Control to Aid in Coping |
| Acupuncture/acupressure | | | • | | |
| Ambulation and position changes | | • | • | • | • |
| Aromatherapy | • | | • | • | |
| Audioanalgesia | • | | • | • | • |
| Breathing/relaxation | | | • | • | • |
| Education about labor and birth | | | • | | • |
| Heat and cold therapies | • | | • | • | |
| Hydrotherapy/water immersion | • | • | • | • | |
| Hypnotherapy | | | • | • | • |
| Spirituality and religious expression | | | • | • | • |
| Sterile water injections | • | | | • | |
| Support (physical and emotional) from other people | | | • | | • |
| Touch and massage | • | • | • | • | |
| Transcutaneous electrical nerve simulation | • | | | • | • |

Based on: Bohren MA, Hofmeyr GJ, Sakala C, et al. Continuous support for women during childbirth. *Cochrane Database Syst Rev.* 2017;7:Cd003766; Lawrence A, Lewis L, Hofmeyr GJ, Styles C. Maternal positions and mobility during first stage labour. *Cochrane Database Syst Rev.* 2013;10:Cd003934; Simkin P, Bolding A. Update on nonpharmacologic approaches to relieve labor pain and prevent suffering. *J Midwifery Womens Health.* 2004;49(6):489-504; Smith CA, Levett KM, Collins CT, et al. Relaxation techniques for pain management in labour. *Cochrane Database Syst Rev.* 2018;3:Cd009514.

energy known as Qi (pronounced "chee"). Acupuncture involves the needling of specific points along meridian pathways, thereby promoting the circulation of blood and stimulating the flow of Qi to promote harmony of yin and yang. Acupuncture is thought to stimulate the body to produce endogenous opioids (endorphins), and to secrete neurotransmitters that maintain the normal physiology and provide comfort. Minimizing the stress response may be another mechanism of action underlying acupuncture's efficacy.[64-66] Acupuncture should be performed only by a qualified practitioner, and most states require a diploma from the National Certification Commission for Acupuncture and Oriental Medicine for licensing to practice acupuncture.

An alternative to acupuncture is acupressure, in which firm steady pressure is applied to acupoints with a thumb or finger instead of needles (Figure 28-3). Commonly cited acupoints utilized to help difficult or slowed labor progress and/or labor pain are Sanyinjiao/spleen 6 (SP6), Hoku or Hegu/large intestine 4 (LI4), bladder 67 (BL67), and gallbladder 21 (GB21).[64] Although no license is required to administer acupressure, training and education in these techniques are recommended.[66]

Although there is some heterogeneity in the published studies of acupuncture and acupressure, results consistently show that these techniques reduce labor pain when compared to no intervention or placebo acupuncture/acupressure.[64-66] A theoretical risk of acupuncture is possible infection if sterile needles are not used. Licensed practitioners, however, would be expected to use sterile needles (usually disposable).

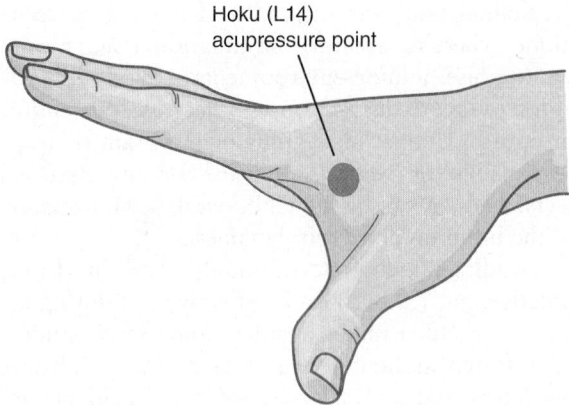

Hoku (L14)
acupressure point

**Figure 28-3** Correct positioning of small ice bag for massage stimulation of LI4.

Reproduced with permission from Waters BL, Raisler J. Ice massage for the reduction of labor pain. *J Midwifery Womens Health.* 2003;48:317-321.

Acupuncture/acupressure has also been evaluated for effectiveness in improving uterine contractility and labor induction. These studies have found a modest increase in cervical ripening (as measured by Bishop's score) with use of acupuncture, but have not adequately assessed other clinically important variables such as time to onset of labor. Nonetheless, contraindications to use of acupressure during labor may include fetal intolerance of labor, uterine tachysystole, tetanic contractions, preterm gestation, or any other clinical condition in which uterine contractions are contraindicated (e.g., placenta previa).[64]

The most current Cochrane meta-analysis of 28 randomized controlled trials (RCTs; 13 on acupuncture and 15 on acupressure) reported on 3960 individuals who received these pain management interventions in labor.[67] This review highlighted the following points and the need for additional research. Acupuncture may reduce the use of pharmacologic pain relief and increase satisfaction with pain relief, but the evidence has very low certainty. Acupuncture may help with pain relief. Both methods appear to have little to no effect on the likelihood of assisted vaginal birth; however, acupuncture may reduce the risk of cesarean birth. Midwives with appropriate training can incorporate acupressure into their labor care.

## Ambulation and Position Changes

When laboring people are not confined to bed or acculturated to believe they should be in bed during labor, they frequently change positions throughout the intrapartum course. As labor progresses, people tend to gradually limit how often they change positions, using less ambulation and sitting during active-phase labor compared to latent-phase labor.[68]

Upright positions are likely to improve maternal comfort during labor via several mechanisms. First, pelvic dimensions are wider in the upright or squatting position, and movement is thought to facilitate optimal fetal positioning.[68,69] Second, optimal feto-pelvic relationships may decrease the pain associated with malpositions.[1] Third, uterine contractility may be improved with upright positions, which could shorten the duration of labor.[69] Finally, upright positions may enhance the individual's sense of control and self-efficacy, which may make coping with labor easier. Contraindications to movement in labor are rare, but may include ruptured membranes with high fetal station when the presenting part is not well applied to the cervix, or any other condition for which reduction in movement is necessary.

Lawrence et al. conducted a Cochrane meta-analysis ($n = 5218$; 25 RCTs) of studies involving first-stage labor in an upright position as opposed to recumbent position. Upright positions were associated with a shorter labor by approximately 1 hour and 22 minutes (average MD, −1.36; 95% CI, −2.22 to −0.51).[70] Study participants who were upright were more likely to experience a vaginal birth, and were less likely to have a cesarean birth, epidural analgesia, or admission of their neonate to the neonatal intensive care unit (NICU). There were no significant differences between groups in terms of duration of second-stage labor, nor were there any differences in other outcomes between the groups who were upright versus those who were recumbent during the first stage of labor.[70]

A Cochrane meta-analysis of studies involving participants (primigravida and multigravida) who did not have epidural analgesia and who assumed upright positions in the second stage of labor, when compared with individuals who assumed supine positions ($n = 9015$; 32 RCTs), revealed fewer operative vaginal deliveries, fewer abnormal fetal heart rate patterns, fewer episiotomies, no change in cesarean section rates, and an increased risk of an estimated blood loss of more than 500 mL for the former group.[71] The analysis found a possible increase in second-degree perineal lacerations among those using upright positions (RR, 1.20; 95% CI, 1.00–1.44; low-quality evidence), but no difference in third- or fourth-degree perineal tears (RR, 0.72; 95% CI, 0.32–1.65; very low-quality evidence).[71] The difference in estimated blood loss may be related to discrepancies in estimating rather than changes in actual blood lost. Another Cochrane meta-analysis assessed studies of epidural analgesia use in the second stage of labor ($n = 879$; 5 RCTs) and revealed no statistically significant difference between upright and recumbent positions in regard to mode of birth, duration of the second stage of labor, lacerations requiring suturing, operative birth for fetal distress, low cord pH, or admission to a NICU.[72] Although this body of work is limited by heterogeneity in study designs and small numbers of participants, the findings suggest that upright positions may benefit persons who do not receive an epidural, but may decrease laboring individuals' likelihood of having an intact perineum.

## Aromatherapy

Aromatherapy refers to the medicinal or therapeutic use of essential oils that are absorbed through the skin or olfactory system. Essential oils are derived from plants and are utilized to enhance physical and psychological well-being. Clinical aromatherapy is the controlled use of pure essential oils to achieve a desired measurable outcome based on the chemical constituents of an oil. Every essential oil has a variety of chemical constituents (e.g., esters, alcohols, phenols, aldehydes, ketones, terpenes, sesquiterpenes) that may have therapeutic effects.

Research into the effectiveness of aromatherapy in reducing pain during childbirth has yielded inconsistent results. In a Cochrane review of two RCTs ($n = 535$), researchers found no difference between groups in terms of pain intensity, assisted vaginal birth, cesarean section, use of pharmacologic pain relief, spontaneous vaginal birth, duration of labor, or augmentation using clary sage, chamomile, lavender, ginger oil, or lemongrass essential oils compared to those participants receiving standard care.[73] In contrast, a combined systematic review and meta-analysis identified a significant positive effect of aromatherapy (compared to placebo or usual treatment controls) in reducing pain reported on a visual analog scale. This study found that aromatherapy was effective in treating nociceptive, acute, postoperative, and obstetric and gynecologic pain ($p < 0.0001$).[74]

Essential oils are generally considered safe for use in childbirth. Midwives wanting to integrate essential oils into their clinical practice should seek additional training on the clinical application of essential oils prior to their utilization in practice. Midwives using essential oils need to understand relevant essential oil physiology, chemistry, and pharmacology, and know how to blend and administer the oils safely and appropriately.[75]

## Audioanalgesia

Audioanalgesia was originally defined as a technique whereby auditory stimulation (e.g., music, white noise, and/or environmental sounds) is provided to create distraction and decrease perception of pain by activating regions of the brain that are responsible for mediating reward and anxiolytic effects. These areas of the CNS overlap with regions of the brain involved with analgesia.[76]

Audioanalgesia is commonly used in dental practice, but research on its effectiveness during labor has yielded mixed results. Some small studies have found audioanalgesia may be beneficial during latent and active labor and may positively affect pain perception via elevation of mood and an increase in pain tolerance.[77,78] However, Cochrane systematic reviews of these studies have found insufficient evidence to support the effectiveness of audioanalgesia for labor pain management.[79] The wide variation in personal choices may account for the lack of sufficient evidence to make recommendations for the use of music for labor pain management, but being allowed to play their favorite music may be pleasant for the birthing person and family.

### Birthing Balls

Birthing balls were introduced in the 1980s and can help with control and empowerment in labor. Birth balls come in several shapes and sizes, and the best choice is one that fits the size of the person laboring. When sitting on the ball, the individual's legs should be bent at a 90-degree angle. They should sit on the birthing ball with their feet approximately 2 feet apart and flat on the floor. This creates an upright position from which the hips can be rotated in ways that relieve back pain and encourage fetal descent. Another position of comfort can be to sit on the ball and lean forward, or to lean against the birthing ball while in either a kneeling (ball on floor) or standing (ball on a bed or table) position (Figure 28-4). These positions support the birthing person's body and provide a position that can promote rest. They also align the long axis of the uterus and the fetus with the laboring person's pelvis and facilitate occiput anterior positions. The hypothesized mechanism of action with regard to mitigating pain is similar to the purported mechanisms for upright positions.

In a 2019 systematic review and meta-analysis of four randomized trials and an aggregated sample of 220 pregnant women, Delgado et al. concluded that a moderate level of evidence supports reductions in pain after 20 to 90 minutes of using a birthing ball in the first stage of labor. The meta-analysis also determined there was no difference in labor length, use of oxytocin or analgesia, laceration, episiotomy, or type of delivery between those using the birthing ball and those receiving usual care.[80] Grenvik et al. reviewed seven trials ($N = 533$) with laboring persons randomized to an intervention group (use of the birthing ball) or a control group (no birthing ball). The results indicated that the birthing ball can be an effective tool for nonpharmacologic pain relief in the active phase of first-stage labor.[81]

Another type of birthing ball is known as the "peanut ball." As the name implies, it is shaped like a peanut shell, with the middle circumference being smaller than the circumference at the ends. The peanut ball can be placed between or under the person's legs while they are in the bed. This positioning widens the diameter of the pelvic outlet, allowing more room for fetal descent or repositioning of the fetus. One RCT evaluated the impact of the peanut ball on the duration of the first and second stages of labor for individuals who were planning elective induction at 39 weeks' gestation or more and epidural anesthesia for pain management. The researchers found that use of a peanut ball reduced the duration of the first stage of labor for primiparous participants ($p = 0.018$), but did not lead to any significant difference (reduction) in the length of first-stage labor for multiparous participants ($p = 0.057$). Since the authors did not report actual differences in time, the clinical relevance of their findings is not clear. Use of the peanut ball did not alter the duration of second-stage labor in either group undergoing induction of labor.[82]

A second RCT evaluated use of the peanut ball in laboring persons who received epidural analgesia, compared to laboring persons who received standard care with epidural analgesia and no peanut ball. Those researchers found that the peanut ball decreased both the duration of labor (first stage, 29 minutes; $P = 0.053$ and second stage, 11 minutes; $P < 0.001$) and the incidence of cesarean deliveries (10.3% versus 21.1%, respectively, $P = 0.011$).[83]

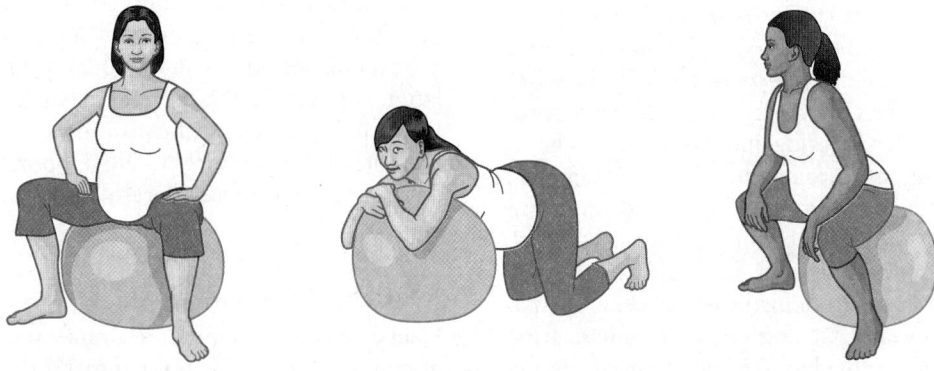

**Figure 28-4** Possible positions when using a birthing ball.

Although these studies suggest that both the birthing ball and the peanut ball have positive effects on labor outcomes, their results are considered low-level evidence. More research is needed to determine the effectiveness of these techniques. However, as neither type of ball has been associated with harm, they can be a helpful option to offer laboring people.

### Breathing

Breathing and relaxation exercises can be useful in labor by decreasing anxiety and fear, and increasing a sense of control or self-efficacy.[1] Use of these techniques is directly related to childbirth satisfaction, and they are essential components of most childbirth education programs.[1] Approximately 48% of persons giving birth in the United States use breathing and relaxation methods during labor, and 77% of them report that these techniques were either somewhat helpful or very helpful.[7] Practice may play a large role in how well these techniques work. Specific breathing techniques work best in early labor but do not help coping with labor when introduced for the first time during active labor.

Breathing techniques that focus on progressive relaxation may be more effective than those that focus on specific types of breathing patterns. Progressive relaxation can be practiced prenatally, to facilitate rapid relaxation between contractions during labor. A knowledgeable caregiver can also teach some relaxation techniques during labor. Breathing techniques used for relaxation, yoga, or mindfulness may help a person feel more in control of their labor, thereby increasing satisfaction and reducing anxiety or pain. The wide variation of techniques makes study comparisons difficult and most trials have not reported on safety or birth outcomes.[84]

### Continuous Labor Support/Doula Care

Multiple RCTs have shown that continuous labor support improves labor outcomes and has a positive influence on the childbirth experience.[85,86] The word "continuous" refers to one support person who provides care to the laboring individual and who is physically present throughout labor. Doulas are trained nonmedical persons who provide continuous nonmedical care, including physical comfort, emotional support (reassurance and encouragement), information (nonmedical advice, anticipatory guidance), and facilitation of communication with healthcare providers. The word *doula* is derived from the Greek word *doulē*, meaning "one

who serves." Doulas can provide many of the comfort measures during labor that are detailed in this chapter.

The effects of continuous labor support were evaluated in a systematic review of 27 RCTs that included 15,858 subjects from high- and middle-income countries.[85] In this review, continuous labor support during labor was associated with the following outcomes:

- Increased likelihood of spontaneous vaginal birth (RR, 1.08; 95% CI, 1.04 to 1.12)
- Lower risk of cesarean births (RR, 0.75; 95% CI, 0.64 to 0.88)
- Shorter duration of labor (mean duration: −0.69 hour; 95% CI, −1.04 to −0.34)
- Reduced need for pharmacologic pain relief (RR, 0.90; 95% CI, 0.84 to 0.96)
- Decreased negative perceptions of childbirth experiences (RR, 0.69; 95% CI, 0.59 to 0.79).
- Reduced risk for low 5-minute Apgar scores (RR, 0.62; 95% CI, 0.46 to 0.85)

No significant differences were found with continuous labor support in the use of synthetic oxytocin, newborn admission to a special care nursery, or breastfeeding at 1 to 2 months postpartum.[85]

In RCTs, researchers have found that continuous labor support is most effective when provided by doulas, rather than by partners, other relatives, nurses, or midwives.[85–87] Nevertheless, in smaller nonrandomized studies where continuous labor support was provided by midwifery students, nursing students, or trained relatives (following some training), positive birth outcomes were also found.[88]

Hodnett[89] and Hofmeyr et al.[90] have offered two theoretical explanations for the effectiveness of labor support, both of which posit that labor support increases the laboring individual's sense of being in control and self-efficacy. Hofmeyr et al. hypothesized that continuous companionship serves as a buffer to the stressors of labor, particularly in a hospital environment.[90] Hodnett suggested that labor support enhances fetal passage by promoting mobility and upright positions, with improved comfort of the mother.[89] Labor support may also reduce anxiety and fear, thereby decreasing the stress response.[90]

### Heat or Cold Therapies

Heat and cold therapies are simple and inexpensive nonpharmacologic pain relief methods. Application of cold for minimizing pain is based on gate-control theory; cold therapy effectively blocks neural transmission via sensory fibers, thereby elevating the pain threshold. Cold therapy can also lead to a reduction in pain by inducing numbness, decreasing muscle tension, and offering distraction. Heat therapy, in addition to utilizing the same mechanisms of action related to application of cold, stimulates heat receptors in the derma and deeper tissues, which purportedly leads to closure of the gate, thereby subsequently impeding neural impulses from reaching the brain. Topical application of heat increases circulation to the area, thereby combating pain from tissue anoxia.

Most studies of heat or cold therapy published to date have been small and hindered by differing methodologies. In general, these studies have found some benefits from heat or cold therapy with regard to decreasing labor pain.[91,92] Caution is warranted when using heat packs, as burns can be caused by using too high a temperature or by putting heat on an area to which creams, oils, or ointments have already been applied. Using a microwave to heat hot packs can be particularly dangerous, as microwaves heat elements at different temperatures; thus, the hot pack can be differentially heated in various places within the pack. It is recommended that at least one layer of cloth be placed between the skin and hot or cold pack. The pack should be tested prior to placement on the skin. Use of heat or cold should also be avoided in the dermatomes anesthetized by an epidural due to concerns that individual may not be able to perceive if the temperature is too hot or cold. Fever is a contraindication to using heat. Contraindications to use of cold include sickle cell anemia, cold hypersensitivities, cryoglobulinemia, Raynaud's phenomenon, and cultural proscriptions.[1]

### Hydrotherapy and Water Immersion

Intrapartum hydrotherapy is the therapeutic use of water for pain relief and relaxation during childbirth. This practice may reduce a laboring person's perception of pain by transmitting a therapeutic temperature into targeted tissues, changing the state of irritant receptors.[93,94] Intrapartum hydrotherapy can be provided in a shower, bathtub, pool, or any body of water available.

Intrapartum immersion is hydrotherapy that involves submersion in a pool or tub that is deep enough for the water to cover the abdomen. More specifically, intrapartum immersion can be divided into water immersion during labor and water immersion during birth. Water labor is defined as use of immersion during some portion of labor, but where the actual birth does not take place in the tub. Water birth is defined as birth of the neonate underwater.[93] Water immersion causes an increase in hydrostatic pressure and a shift of extracellular fluid into the circulation, which provides a central blood volume bolus, increases cardiac output, and subsequently decreases circulating catecholamine levels. It is postulated that the improved blood flow results in improved uteroplacental perfusion and increased uterine efficiency.[94,95]

In 2017, Shaw-Battista[96] performed a systematic review of RCTs in which standard care was compared to immersion hydrotherapy in labor. The review, which included seven studies with 2615 participants, found that hydrotherapy promoted physiologic labor and did not cause maternal, fetal, or neonatal harm.[96] In addition, intrapartum immersion was associated with increased mobility, lower episiotomy rates, decreased likelihood of third- and fourth-degree perineal lacerations, and increased patient satisfaction in several small studies; these findings are not yet considered conclusive.[97]

In 2018, the Cochrane Collaboration completed a systematic review of the effects of intrapartum immersion on labor and birth by examining 15 clinical trials involving more than 3663 people.[98] Water immersion during the first stage of labor was associated with a small reduction in the use of epidural/spinal analgesia from 43% to 39% (RR, 0.91; 95% CI, 0.83–0.99). There was little to no difference in spontaneous vaginal birth (83% versus 82%). The researchers did not find sufficient evidence to determine the effects on blood loss, third- or fourth-degree lacerations, neonatal infections, or NICU admissions. No evidence was found of increased adverse events during first- or second-stage labor for either the laboring person or the infant.[99]

The timing of intrapartum immersion warrants consideration. Immersion is recommended after active labor is established.[97] Immersion in water during latent labor may result in longer labors that can require pharmacologic intervention and oxytocin augmentation.[99,100] The American College of Nurse-Midwives has developed a model template for hydrotherapy in labor that describes eligibility for this therapy, techniques, and recommended policies.[97] Water immersion for birth is discussed in the *Second Stage of Labor and Birth* chapter.

### Hypnotherapy

Hypnosis employs specific mind–body techniques that are used to induce profound relaxation. The goal of using hypnosis during labor is to help achieve a state of deep relaxation within a state of focused attention, thereby reducing perception of external stimuli and increasing receptivity to specific suggestions. The ability to experience hypnosis varies, but hypnotic susceptibility has generally been found to increase during pregnancy.[101] Hypnosis can involve a hypnotist, or it can be self-administered (i.e., self-hypnosis).

Studies evaluating hypnosis during childbirth have yielded conflicting findings. Individuals who practice self-hypnotic techniques during the prenatal period may reduce their need for analgesia during labor and may have shorter labors when compared to those who use other childbirth preparation techniques.[102–104] A systematic analysis using a mixed-methods appraisal tool found that hypnosis-based interventions improved the childbirth experience. Hypnosis-based interventions led to increased confidence and less fear about one's ability to go through labor, improved feelings of empowerment, and increased self-reported ability to control emotions during childbirth.[105] The beneficial effects of introducing hypnosis for the first time when a person is in labor, however, have not been confirmed.[104] Further research is needed to assess the value of hypnosis during labor and birth and its effect on the use of pharmacologic pain relief, labor, delivery, neonatal outcomes, and postnatal well-being. Notably, this technique is contraindicated for persons with a history of psychosis or a severe mental health condition.

## Spirituality and Religious Expression

Individuals have unique conceptual frameworks for existential meaning during labor and birth, which can generally be classified as spirituality, religion, prayer fellowship, ceremony, and other. Care providers should welcome and support religious or spiritual ceremonies such as praying, blessings, mantras, smudging, and use of talismans, blessed items, or other artifacts to bring meaning and fulfillment to the birthing family. Aziato et al. conducted a descriptive phenomenologic study of 13 Ghanaian women to explore religious practices and identify religious artifacts used in pregnancy and labor.[106] Practices included prayers, singing, anointing, laying of hands, tribal rituals, fellowship, and food and water restrictions. Artifacts included items such as anointing oil, blessed water, stickers of pastors or churches, blessed white handkerchiefs, blessed sand, bibles, and rosaries.[106] A 2016 study of Danish mothers found that 65% of them responded affirmatively when asked if they had prayed or meditated in labor.[107] The Navajo have traditionally used a blessing ceremony during pregnancy to prepare for birth. In 1988, when Maureen Hartle-Schutte

conducted an ethnographic study to investigate the frequency of use of the blessingway, she found that 14% of Navajo women at the hospital had undergone a blessingway.[108] Across cultures, spiritual expressions can be a source of comfort throughout labor and birth, and individuals' religious and spiritual practices should be supported by all involved in perinatal care.

## Sterile Water Injections

Sterile water injections, or sterile water papules, involve intradermal injections of sterile water administered in four places in the lower lumbosacral area of the back to form papules. The therapeutic goal is to relieve back pain in labor. Since the cutaneous afferent nerves from the lower back converge to the dorsal horns in the same segments, pain may be referred to the lower back. It is speculated that sterile water injections work through the mechanism described by the gate-control theory, whereby stimulation of specific areas can relieve this referred pain. The hypotonic nature of sterile water injections is thought to cause increased osmotic pressure in the surrounding cells, and subsequently tissue distension, which stimulates nociceptors and mechanoreceptors, thereby providing noxious stimulation of nociceptors. This effect results in a subsequent release of endorphins and stimulation of A-delta fibers, which overwhelm the visceral sensations transmitted to the brain by the slower C fibers.[109]

A 25-gauge needle containing 0.6 to 1.0 mL of sterile water (not saline) is used to inject 0.1 to 0.3 mL of sterile water intradermally at each of four sites, where referred pain from uterine contractions is usually felt. An intense stinging sensation is felt for approximately 20 to 40 seconds during (and immediately following) the injection, with pain relief then lasting for approximately 1 to 3 hours.[110] The *Sterile Water Injections for the of Low Back Pain in Labor* appendix reviews this procedure.

Sterile water injections have been found to significantly reduce severe back pain. However, the overall need for additional pain medication is not reduced. This may be related to the fact that water injections given for back pain have no effect on abdominal pain, and that back pain appears to occur more commonly in the latent or early active phase of labor. When Derry et al. performed a meta-analysis of seven RCTs, they concluded that the evidence is insufficient to recommend this practice, due to perceived limitations of the studies involved.[109] In contrast, the meta-analysis of eight RCTs performed by Hutton et al. found sterile water papules were associated with a significant reduction in visual analog scores for pain and a decreased rate of cesarean births in the sterile water group (4.6%) versus the comparison groups (9.9%) (RR, 0.51; 95% CI, 0.30–0.87).[110] Investigators in a 2020 multisite, placebo-controlled RCT ($N = 1166$ laboring people) supported the use of water injections to relieve back pain in labor, finding that 60.8% of participants reported a 30% reduction in pain 30 minutes after receiving the injections.[111]

### Touch and Massage

Massage, defined as purposeful manipulation of soft tissues for therapeutic purposes, is widely utilized during labor. Massage is applied to a specific body part, such as the hands, feet, scalp, shoulders, or back. Touch can be firm or light and repeated in a specific pattern (e.g., effleurage), or it can consist of still pressure or kneading. A specific form of touch often used to aid with back pain is firm, steady counterpressure applied to the center of the sacroiliac portion of the back during a contraction. With counterpressure, the amount of pressure increases during the contraction and decreases as the contraction wanes. Massage can be performed through use of the hands or with massage devices, and with or without lotions, oils, and powders.[112]

Touching and massage will be effective only if the person is comfortable being touched, as cultural views of touch appropriateness vary. This technique's probable mechanism of action in reducing pain is an increase in the endogenous release of endorphins and oxytocin. In 2018, a Cochrane review found low-quality evidence that massage in the first stage of labor reduces intensity of pain (self-reported) more than usual care. This review also indicated there was no clear benefit of massage over usual care regarding length of labor or use of pharmacologic pain relief.[113] By contrast, in a 2017 trial that compared a specific form of massage/counterpressure over the sacrum and lower back, applied for 30 minutes at three different times during labor, researchers found a significant decrease in reported lower back pain and increased satisfaction with the birth experience among the massage group compared to the non-massage group.[114]

While these studies demonstrate that massage may have a role in pain reduction and help to increase laboring individuals' sense of control and birth satisfaction, the quality of the evidence supporting its improvement of birth outcomes varies from low to very low. Further research is needed to address the possible positive impact that touch, massage, and specific types of massage may have on labor. However, targeted massage may be helpful to some laboring people, and does not have evidence of harm.

### Transcutaneous Electrical Nerve Stimulation

Transcutaneous electrical nerve stimulation (TENS) units are handheld, battery-operated devices that use low-voltage electric current to reduce pain. TENS has been used in childbirth to help reduce labor pain since the 1970s. With this technique, stimulation electrode pads are placed on the skin over the low back on the paraspinal muscles, on either side of the spine, at the vertebral positions of T10 and S2, which correspond to the nerve pathways through which the pain signal from the uterus enters the spinal cord. With the pads in place, the TENS unit emits low-voltage impulses. The frequency and intensity of the nerve stimulation can be controlled by the individual. The low-voltage sensation is not painful, but rather is experienced as a tingling or buzzing feeling at the site of the electrodes.[115]

The mechanism of action for TENS is based on the gate-control theory of pain, as well as the theory that painful stimulation results in the release of neurotransmitters. TENS units are believed to induce the release of endorphins. Endorphins' primary function is to inhibit the transmission of pain signs, similar to the effect produced by opioids. A Cochrane meta-analysis ($n = 1466$; 17 trials) of subjects who used TENS units in labor was unable to find consistent evidence that TENS units have any impact on interventions or labor outcomes.[115]

Table 28-3 identifies various methods of pain relief and support for labor. This table presents the pros, cons, pertinent notes, and strength of the evidence for each method. For the purposes of the table, "sufficient evidence" meets the high or moderate level according to the Agency for Healthcare Research and Quality (AHRQ) definitions. Keep in mind that each person who labors is an individual, and each labor is unique. Therefore, if a method has insufficient evidence to support it, yet is working for an individual, the care team should be supportive so long as it will not create harm. Some nonpharmacologic care measures and coping techniques are quite simple, whereas others require specialized training to perform.

## Pharmacologic Methods of Mitigating Labor Pain

Pregnant individuals can be knowledgeable and prepared for labor, desire active participation in the natural, normal process of childbearing, and still

| Table 28-3 | Methods of Labor Support and Pain Relief | | |
|---|---|---|---|
| **Technique** | **Pros** | **Cons/Cautions** | **Level of Evidence on Effectiveness/Notes** |
| **Nonpharmacologic** | | | |
| Acupressure and acupuncture | May reduce intensity of pain<br><br>May increase sense of satisfaction with birth<br><br>Fewer operative vaginal births (low evidence) | Avoid use in preterm gestation<br><br>Not readily available<br><br>Facility may not allow<br><br>No consensus on forbidden points in pregnancy[116] | Insufficient evidence[65]<br><br>Benefits likely outweigh theoretical risks[67] |
| Ambulation and upright positions (first stage) | Benefits physiologic birth<br><br>Reduces duration of labor, risk of cesarean birth, and need for epidural | Not always possible with certain interventions<br><br>Ensure fetal head is engaged if membranes are ruptured | Sufficient evidence to encourage use in first-stage labor[70] |
| Aromatherapy | May decrease anxiety<br><br>Easy to use<br><br>Scents can evoke positive emotions<br><br>Theory for mechanism of action: stimulation of the limbic system—decrease cortisol and increase serotonin[117]<br><br>Some research supports use of lavender in labor[118] | Do not use with patients who have allergies to the ingredients of the essential oils, sensitive skin, or uncontrolled asthma<br><br>Requires expertise and understanding[75]<br><br>Some fragrances are contraindicated during labor<br><br>May be expensive<br><br>May be hard to find<br><br>Lack of availability or support in birth facility | Insufficient evidence[73,119] |
| Audioanalgesia | Decreases perception of pain[76] | None | Insufficient evidence[1,79] |
| Birthing ball | Reduces pain after 20–90 minutes of use[80]<br><br>Reduces anxiety<br><br>Improves fetal head descent and rotation<br><br>Widens the pelvis<br><br>Shortens duration of first-stage labor<br><br>Enhances satisfaction and well-being | Must have ability to balance to use safely<br><br>Limited availability<br><br>Facility may not support use<br><br>Body confidence is better if the individual practices antepartum | Insufficient/low evidence[80,81,120]<br><br>No evidence of harm |
| Breathing | May assist in coping with labor<br><br>May increase satisfaction<br><br>Different patterns work for individuals | Some breathing patterns are complicated<br><br>Hyperventilation | Insufficient evidence[84]<br><br>No evidence of harm |
| Continuous labor support or doula care | May improve outcomes: increased spontaneous vaginal births, shorter labor times, decreased cesarean birth, and less use of analgesia[85]<br><br>Meets emotional and physical needs | Not always available<br><br>Can be difficult for support person if labor is long | Low evidence[85]<br><br>No evidence of harm<br><br>Most effective with a labor companion or doula |

| Technique | Pros | Cons/Cautions | Level of Evidence on Effectiveness/Notes |
|---|---|---|---|
| Heat and cold | May decrease muscle tension and reduce perception of pain<br><br>Inexpensive<br><br>May increase joint mobility | Only use in persons with normal sensation<br><br>Avoid use with fevers<br><br>Avoid use with open sores or rash | Insufficient evidence<br><br>No evidence of harm |
| Hydrotherapy intrapartum | Easy to use<br><br>Promotes normal physiologic birth<br><br>Increased relaxation<br><br>Increased pain relief<br><br>Decreases anxiety<br><br>Increased maternal ease of movement<br><br>Decreased use of analgesia<br><br>No effect on neonatal outcomes | Entry timing, duration, and water temperature are important<br><br>Not always available<br><br>Policy may not allow<br><br>Contraindications:<br>• Pathophysiologic vaginal bleeding<br>• Infection risk to fetus or birth attendants<br>• Decreased maternal mobility<br>• Epidural anesthesia | Sufficient evidence[96,121]<br><br>Limited evidence[98]<br><br>Candidates should be healthy with an uncomplicated pregnancy from 37 to 41 6/7 weeks' gestation, with a singleton, vertex fetus |
| Hypnotherapy or care based on the philosophy of hypnosis and birthing | Person directed<br><br>Incorporates other pain relief methods<br><br>Life skill<br><br>May reduce fear and increases satisfaction<br><br>May shorten the duration of labor<br><br>Embraces physiologic birth | Must be learned and practiced by the laboring person<br><br>Lack of support or understanding in birth facility | Limited low-level evidence[103,105,122,123]<br><br>Recommend that individuals start classes prior to third trimester<br><br>No evidence of harm |
| Massage or touch | Decreases perception of pain and anxiety[124]<br><br>Increases sense of control and satisfaction with labor<br><br>May reduce length of labor | Lack of availability or support in birth facility | Insufficient evidence[113]<br><br>No evidence of harm |
| Sterile water injections | May reduce back pain in labor<br><br>May decrease risk of cesarean birth[111] | Pain with administration<br><br>Facilities may not have a person with knowledge to administer the injections | Limited evidence[109,110,125] |
| Transcutaneous electrical nerve stimulation (TENS) | Use at any stage of labor<br><br>May reduce perception of pain in labor<br><br>May shorten active-phase labor[126,127] | Availability may be limited<br><br>Skin irritation under the pad<br><br>Do not use with hydrotherapy, heat, or epidural. | Limited evidence[128]<br><br>No evidence of harm |
| Upright positions: second stage—without epidural[62] | Reduces duration of second stage slightly<br><br>Reduces episiotomy and assisted delivery rates | Increased risk of blood loss > 500 mL.<br><br>Possible increased risk of second-degree lacerations | Encourage birth in a position of comfort.[71] |

*(continues)*

| Table 28-3 | Methods of Labor Support and Pain Relief (*continued*) | | |
|---|---|---|---|
| **Technique** | **Pros** | **Cons/Cautions** | **Level of Evidence on Effectiveness/Notes** |
| **Pharmacologic** | | | |
| Intravenous or intramuscular opioid pain medication | Short acting<br><br>Fast acting<br><br>Sedates between contractions | Crosses the placental barrier<br><br>Effects for fetus or newborn may be loss of variability in fetal heart rate (FHR), reduction in FHR baseline, neonatal respiratory depression, or neurobehavioral changes[56]<br><br>Monitor for side effects of nausea, vomiting, excessive sedation, and respiratory depression | Low- to very-low-quality evidence[129] |
| Nitrous oxide | Minimal effect on fetus<br><br>Commonly used in other countries<br><br>Less expensive than epidural medication<br><br>Allows individual control<br><br>High satisfaction | Requires equipment not always available<br><br>Eases the intensity of pain, but does not eliminate pain<br><br>Limits ability to move<br><br>Maternal side effects of nausea, dizziness, and lethargy | Insufficient evidence[130,131] |
| Regional anesthesia | Provides effective pain relief<br><br>High satisfaction<br><br>Permits rest and sleep<br><br>Associated with potential for reduced postpartum depression risks—more study needed | Limits mobility<br><br>Oral intake may be limited<br><br>Maternal adverse effects may include:<br>• Pruritus<br>• Shivering<br>• Hypotension<br>• Fever<br>• Urinary retention<br>• Reactivation of oral herpes<br>• Postdural puncture headache<br>Can affect the FHR tracing[56] | Sufficient evidence[132,133]<br><br>Factors associated with failed epidurals: prolonged duration of anesthesia, higher body mass index, placement in early labor[134] |

choose to use medication to mitigate pain. Medications may be used during labor to relieve pain, allow rest, decrease anxiety, provide sedation, or control nausea and vomiting. All medications used during labor should be evaluated for (1) effectiveness, (2) safety for the laboring person, (3) safety for the fetus and newborn, and (4) effects on labor progress. It is important to note that "effectiveness" does not always correlate with reduction of pain; individuals rating their satisfaction with labor pain management may be evaluating a more global impression of coping assistance that might include manageability of pain and anxiety, degree of sedation, and sense of control.

Two types pain relief are used during labor and birth: analgesia and anesthesia. Analgesia aims to reduce pain, whereas anesthesia aims to block or remove the sensation of pain. Depending on the method, this difference reflects the type and/or the amount of medication administered, in addition to the method by which medication is delivered. Both analgesia and anesthesia may be systemic or regional in their effects on pain receptors. The most commonly used systemic analgesics for labor include intravenous medications and inhaled nitrous oxide, and the most commonly employed strategies for regional analgesia include neuraxial analgesia (spinal, epidural, or combined) and pudendal blocks. For cesarean birth, pain is most often managed using neuraxial anesthesia, but general anesthesia may be necessary if other methods are not available, not effective, or contraindicated. Beyond its effects on coping and pain perception, the choice of pharmacologic strategy may affect patients' mental status and mobility, as well as a variety of outcomes.

Providing patients with information about the benefits and risks of available options contributes to patient autonomy, empowerment, and satisfaction. Beyond counseling patients about their pain management options, midwives work interprofessionally to implement chosen strategies and manage any persistent discomforts and complications. Prior to administering any medication during labor, a careful assessment of the patient's vital signs, fetal heart rate pattern, allergies, indications and contraindications, concurrent medications, and stage of labor is made. Those data, plus details about patient counseling and the chosen plan of care, are documented clearly in the health record.

### Systemic Analgesic Medications

Systemic medications were the mainstay agents used to reduce labor pain for most of the first half of the twentieth century. Today, they are used by those who prefer to reduce, but not eliminate sensation, and by those for whom neuraxial techniques are undesirable, contraindicated, ineffective, or unavailable.[135] These methods do not limit the laboring person's mobility, although mobility precautions are advisable for those experiencing sedation or dizziness. Sedating effects on the fetus and newborn vary, and influence the optimal timing of administration. Systemic medications are given by the intravenous, intramuscular, or inhalation route, and they act on the entire nervous system, rather than a specified area. The most popular of these agents are opioids, mixed opioid agonist–antagonists, and nitrous oxide.

### Opioids

Opioid analgesics act by binding to one or more of the three main types of opioid receptors: mu opioid receptors (MOR), kappa opioid receptors (KOR), and delta opioid receptors (DOR). These receptors are all found in the central and peripheral nervous systems, with MOR also found in the gastrointestinal tract. When opioids bind to their receptors, nerve transmission by norepinephrine, acetylcholine, neuropeptide, and substance P is inhibited, thereby blocking ascending pain impulses through the spinal cord to the brain.[136] In addition, binding of opioid analgesics to MOR inhibits descending pain signals from the brain stem.[137] The type of receptor activated influences the more specific effects of the medication. MOR stimulation causes spinal (ascending neural pathway) and supraspinal (descending neural pathway) analgesia, euphoria, sedation, slowed gastrointestinal motility, nausea and vomiting, respiratory depression, urinary retention, and pruritus. KOR stimulation causes spinal analgesia, sedation, dyspnea, dysphoria, miosis (pupil constriction), and dependence. DOR stimulation is not as well studied, but is associated with both spinal and supraspinal analgesia and has dysphoric and psychomimetic effects.[136,138] Generally, opioid medications bind to MOR, but have variable binding to KOR and DOR.

Specific drugs may function as agonist, antagonist, or mixed agonist–antagonist at different receptors. Agonists trigger the expected opioid effects, antagonists bind to receptors without eliciting effects while blocking agonists from binding, and agonist–antagonists act as agonists at one type of receptor but antagonists at another. For example, fentanyl is a pure agonist at all types of receptors, morphine is a pure agonist at both MORs and KORs, and butorphanol and nalbuphine are KOR agonists and MOR antagonists.[138] Most agonist–antagonists have a "ceiling effect," meaning that above a particular dosage, side effects may increase but analgesia and respiratory depression do not.[138] As an opioid antagonist with a strong affinity for all types of opioid receptors, naloxone (Narcan) is able to displace medications bound to opioid receptors when used to reverse overdose symptoms.[137]

An individual's biologic response to opioids also depends on factors such as age, sex, renal function, use of concurrent medications, and pharmacogenetics. In some people, a genetic polymorphism causing inactivation of the CYP2D6 gene will prevent metabolization of the prodrug codeine to morphine, resulting in inadequate pain relief. In others, excessive CYP2D6 activation may result in rapid metabolism of codeine, potentially leading to a strong, brief response. Especially for people with rapid drug metabolism, it is important to remember that some opiates, such as morphine and meperidine, have active metabolites that can build up and cause harm if the drug is used repeatedly.[138] For perinatal patients, it is important to consider that drugs and their metabolites usually pass through the placenta and to breast milk. Since effects on the birthing person and the fetus or neonate may differ, monitoring each for signs of excessive sedation and respiratory depression is indicated, especially after extended use or administration of multiple high doses.

For intrapartum pain management, opioids are administered by the intramuscular (IM) or intravenous (IV) routes or through regional anesthesia (discussed later in this chapter); if opioids are used for postpartum analgesia, the oral route is preferred. Compared with IM injections, IV administration produces a faster onset of action, more predictable plasma levels of medication, and less variability of peak concentrations. While IM injections involve the pain of being stuck by a needle with each dose, this route often results in a longer duration of action. IV administration involves only one needle stick, but the presence of an IV access port can be bothersome for many patients, and the duration of action of the medication may be shorter.[135,136]

Patient-controlled analgesia (PCA) pumps, which are often used to allow patients to self-administer a programmed dose of medication through an epidural catheter (see the later section on regional anesthesia), may also be used for patient titration of IV opioids, with minimum intervals between doses. Intravenous PCA pumps provide for a rapid onset of action, greater reduction of pain compared to intermittent parenteral opioid injection, and a sense of control for the patient without adversely affecting the mode of delivery.[135,136,139] Although IV PCA administration is widely used internationally, it is not used as commonly in the United States due to adverse effects and their practical implications. For example, fentanyl IV PCA is associated with lower Apgar scores in neonates, an increased need for neonatal resuscitation, and increased use of neonatal naloxone. This method of pain relief may also result in a longer labor with a higher rate of augmentation and operative vaginal delivery. Due to these potential adverse effects, IV PCA analgesia during labor requires continuous one-to-one care, continuous oxygen-saturation monitoring, and a dedicated IV catheter. Midwives should consider reserving this method for patients with a nonviable fetus, or be prepared for a newborn needing pediatric physician assistance after birth.[136,140] If IV PCA administration is being considered, consultation with anesthesia personnel is indicated.[141]

Systemic opioids are readily available, easy to administer, fast acting, and less invasive than neuraxial analgesia. They have no apparent effect on labor progress when administered during the active phase of labor.[138] In systematic reviews of parenteral opioids, researchers found that data on opioids' effectiveness for pain relief during labor are limited, but that birthing people generally rate their satisfaction with analgesia provided by this method

as moderate.[129] Two-thirds of laboring patients receiving opioids report moderate or severe pain and/or poor or moderate pain relief 1 to 2 hours after parenteral opioid administration.[129] The effectiveness of opioids may be reduced if they are administered near the end of the first stage of labor, from 7 to 9 centimeters dilation.[138]

Although some patients feel an unwelcome loss of control after being given an opioid, that experience is not common. The more common side effects of such therapy include euphoria and sedation. Other dose-dependent, potential side effects include nausea and vomiting, dizziness, pruritis, and urinary retention. Some opiates, such as morphine, are associated with hyperthermia.[136] All opioids are associated with the adverse effect of respiratory depression, but this complication is rare with the IV and IM doses typically used to treat labor pain.

All of the opioids have some drug–drug interactions that can be clinically significant in some populations.[136] For pregnant patients with opioid use disorder, use of opioid antagonists (i.e., naloxone) and mixed agonist–antagonists (i.e., butorphanol, nalbuphine) can precipitate acute withdrawal symptoms when administered to either the adult or the neonate. In general, midwives should avoid administering opioids to persons with opioid use disorder during labor, focusing instead on strategies such as neuraxial analgesia, nitrous oxide, and nonpharmacologic strategies.[142]

Systemic opioids are lipid soluble, so they cross the placenta freely and enter into the fetal circulation.[136] As a result, a common effect of IV and IM opioid use during labor is a temporary decrease in variability of the fetal heartbeat, lasting up to 30 minutes.[138] With administration of some medications—primarily butorphanol (Stadol), but also nalbuphine (Nubain), fentanyl (Sublimaze), and meperidine (Demerol)—a transient pseudosinusoidal fetal heart rate pattern may be noted.[136] After birth, neonatal effects of recent or long-acting opioid exposure include respiratory depression, decreased muscle tone and reflexes, and impaired early breastfeeding.[135,136]

Opioids also transfer into breast milk and can be harmful to the newborn, especially in the presence of reduced drug clearance or reduced function of the blood–brain barrier. However, short-term use by breastfeeding parents (2 to 3 days) is considered safe for their newborns.[143] Individuals receiving buprenorphine for treatment of opioid use disorder may provide breast milk to their infants.

The opioids most commonly used to treat labor pain in the United States are listed in

| Table 28-4 | Pharmacokinetic Profiles of Selected Systemic Opioids | | | | |
|---|---|---|---|---|---|
| Drug (Brand) | Opioid Receptor Binding | Usual Intrapartum Dose | Onset/Peak Effect | Labor Implications | Neonatal and Breastfeeding Implications[138,145] |
| Morphine | MOR and KOR agonist | Labor:<br>• IV: 2–5 mg every 4 hr<br>• IM: 10 mg every 4 hr<br>Therapeutic rest: 10–15 mg SC/IM × 1 dose | IV: 5 min/20 min<br>IM: 10–20 min/30–45 min | Faster absorption when administered in deltoid muscle compared to gluteal muscle<br>Use lower doses for people with impaired ventilation or asthma | Half-life:<br>• Morphine: 6.5 ± 2.8 hr<br>• Active (potent) metabolite: 13.9 hr |
| Fentanyl (Sublimaze) | MOR, KOR, and DOR agonist | IV: 50–100 mcg every hr<br>IM: 50–100 mcg every hr | IV: 1 min/5 min<br>IM: 7–15 min/ 10–20 min | Maximum cumulative labor dose is usually 500–600 mcg when given IV or IM | Half-life: 75 min–7.3 hr<br>Associated with fewer newborn effects than morphine |
| Butorphanol (Stadol) | MOR antagonist KOR agonist | IV: 1–2 mg every 3–4 hr<br>IM: 1–2 mg every 3–4 hr | IV: 2–3 min/ 5–10 min<br>IM: 10–20 min/30–60 min | Maternal ceiling effect<br>May trigger withdrawal symptoms in individuals with OUD<br>Transient fetal pseudo-sinusoidal FHR pattern | May increase serum prolactin<br>Brief (10-min) delay in breastfeeding |
| Nalbuphine (Nubain) | MOR antagonist KOR partial agonist | IV or IM: 10 mg every 3 hr | IV: 2–3 min/ 30 min<br>IM: <15 min/ 30–60 min | Maternal ceiling effect<br>May trigger withdrawal symptoms with OUD | May increase serum prolactin<br>Brief (10-min) delay in breastfeeding |

Abbreviations: DOR, delta opioid receptor; FHR, fetal heart rate; IM, intramuscular; IV, intravenous; KOR, kappa opioid receptor; MOR, mu opioid receptor; OUD, opioid use disorder; SC, subcutaneous.

*Based on Lexicomp Online.* UpToDate, Inc.; 2021. https://online-lexi-com.frontier.idm.oclc.org/lco/action/home. Accessed September 30, 2021.

Table 28-4.[138,144] Comparative effectiveness studies have not found one opioid to be superior to the others for balancing pain management with side effects. The choice of medication will depend on the timing during labor and the medication's half-life. Drugs with longer half-lives or that have active metabolites with longer half-lives, such as morphine, should be used only during latent labor and for therapeutic rest. For instance, the active metabolite of morphine is morphine-6-glucuronide, which has a half-life of 2 to 4 hours in the adult patient but 13.9 hours in the neonate; its administration during active labor or near the time of birth could cause respiratory depression in the transitioning neonate.[136,138]

Newborns with respiratory depression should receive care according to the most recent Neonatal Resuscitation Program (NRP) guidelines. Although naloxone (Narcan) is an opiate/opioid agonist used in the United States and internationally to treat respiratory depression due to opiates administered during labor, the 2021 NRP guidelines state that there is insufficient evidence to support the use of naloxone in neonates; the benefits are unclear and the long-term effects of newborn exposure to naloxone are unknown. A Cochrane review concluded that use of naloxone in neonates should be reserved for RCTs aimed at building evidence about risks and benefits.[146] Its use is contraindicated in newborns of mothers with opioid use disorder, as its use in opioid-habituated newborns can result in opioid withdrawal and seizures.[147,148]

Morphine and fentanyl are the two MOR agonists most frequently used for labor pain in the United States. Morphine is most often used to treat prolonged latent labor, as it decreases uterine activity prior to active labor but does not inhibit active labor contractions.[138,149] A common combination for treating prolonged latent-phase labor is 10 to 15 mg of morphine sulfate and 25 to 50 mg of promethazine (Phenergan) given intramuscularly. Because morphine has active metabolites that can cause maternal or newborn depression, it is generally contraindicated for use in the later stages of labor.

Fentanyl has a short half-life, and has not been associated with neonatal respiratory depression. Repeated doses may be used during active labor, and due to its short duration of action, fentanyl may be used even toward the end of the first stage of labor. It can also be helpful for pain relief during intrapartum procedures such as intracervical balloon catheter insertion, or in the third stage when local or regional analgesia is ineffective, undesired, contraindicated, or unavailable.

Butorphanol and nalbuphine are KOR agonists and MOR antagonists. They have a longer half-life and, anecdotally, have been reported to provide better pain relief than fentanyl. As MOR antagonists, both are contraindicated for use in patients with opioid use disorder.

Historically, meperidine (Demerol) was the most frequently used opioid for treating labor pain worldwide; however, it has largely fallen out of favor in the United States. Meperidine has limited effectiveness for pain relief. It has a long half-life and active metabolites; therefore, its use is associated with a high risk of neonatal respiratory depression.[135,150]

## Opioid Adjuncts

Several medications are used as adjuncts to opioids during labor. Medications such as promethazine and hydroxyzine (Vistaril) may be used concomitantly with opioids to potentiate pain relief; used alone, these sedatives are less effective for pain relief.[151] Some patients may benefit from the anxiolytic or antipruritic effects of medications such as hydroxyzine or prochlorperazine. Opiate adjuncts may also treat the nausea and vomiting that are common side effects of opioids, although nonsedating choices, such as ondansetron (Zofran), may be used for this purpose as well. The sedating effect may be useful for stopping contractions during prolonged latent labors as part of therapeutic rest.[149] Non-opioid agents frequently utilized in combination with opioids during labor are listed in Table 28-5.

Few guidelines are available to describe the optimal use of opioid adjuncts to manage labor pain and opioid side effects. As adjuncts, sedatives and antihistamines are associated with increased patient satisfaction with labor pain management without an increase in assisted births or low 5-minute Apgar scores.[151] Ideally, use of non-opioid adjuvants may reduce the amount of opioids administered. Without high-quality research exploring relevant effects and outcomes for those and other medications, specific guidance is lacking on how to best consider the strength and timing of these medications during labor.

### Inhaled Analgesia: 50:50 Nitrous Oxide/Oxygen

First used to manage labor pain in the 1880s, nitrous oxide inhalation analgesia is currently used by the majority of laboring people in many developed countries, including Canada, Australia, Scandinavia, and the United Kingdom.[135] In the United States, use of this therapy has been growing since the U.S. Food and Drug Administration (FDA) approved a delivery system in 2012.[131,152] The mixture of 50% nitrous oxide ($N_2O$) and 50% oxygen ($O_2$)—$N_2O/O_2$—is widely considered both safe and effective, especially in the absence of additional sedating medications.[131,153] Lagging uptake of inhaled nitrous oxide for labor pain in the United States may be related to challenges with the logistics of introducing a new technology, reimbursement questions, safety concerns based on animal studies (using different concentrations and combinations of gas), or perceived lack of need. Those challenges must be weighed against the value of having an additional safe and effective option that leaves patients with lasting higher positive perceptions of labor pain management.[131,152,154]

Nitrous oxide is a weak anesthetic when used in high doses, and has analgesic and anxiolytic effects at low doses.[155] Its biologic effects are thought to result from its action of increasing the release of natural opioids and dopamine in the brain and neuromodulators in the spinal cord. In addition, it reduces the hormonal response to stress by increasing prolactin release and decreasing cortisol release.[155] Otherwise, nitrous oxide has minimal effects on the hemodynamic and respiratory systems, and no effect on uterine contractions or on the fetal heart rate.[131,155] Less than 1% of inhaled nitrous oxide is metabolized by the body; 99% is exhaled.[155] The half-life in the neonate is approximately 3 minutes,

| Table 28-5 | Opioid Adjuncts for Potentiation and Side-Effect Relief | | | |
|---|---|---|---|---|
| Generic (Brand) | Drug Class | Dosing | Effects of Short-Term Use on Newborns and Breastfeeding[145] | Comments |
| Promethazine (Phenergan) | Phenothiazine | Opioid potentiation or relief of nausea/vomiting: 12.5–25 mg PO/IM/PR/IV every 4–6 hr prn  Therapeutic rest: 50 mg PO/IM or 25 mg IV × 1 dose | Generally little effect. Repeated doses can be sedating.  Can lower basal prolactin secretion and may delay onset of lactogenesis. | Potentiates opioid analgesia  Relieves nausea and vomiting  Sedating, may cause dizziness  IM administration preferred; IV infiltration may cause severe tissue injury |
| Hydroxyzine (Vistaril) | Antihistamine | Opioid potentiation: 25–50 mg IM/ PO × 1 dose or every 6–8 hr prn  Relief of pruritis: 25–50 mg PO × 1 dose or every 4 hr prn | Generally little effect. Repeated doses can be sedating. Can lower basal prolactin secretion. | Potentiates opioid analgesia  Relieves nausea and vomiting, urticaria, anxiety  Sedating |
| Diphenhydramine (Benadryl) | Antihistamine | 25–50 mg IV/IM/PO × 1 dose or every 4–6 hr prn | Generally little effect. Repeated doses can be sedating. Can lower basal prolactin secretion. | Relieves allergic symptoms |
| Prochlorperazine | Antiemetic | 5–10 mg PO every 6–8 hr  5–10 mg IM/IV × 1 dose or every 3–4 hr prn | No published data on newborns. May cause galactorrhea in adults by increasing prolactin. | Relieves nausea and vomiting, anxiety |
| Ondansetron (Zofran) | Antiemetic | 4–8 mg IV/PO × 1 dose or every 4–8 hr prn  Oral tablets and film dissolve | No published data on newborn effects after use during pregnancy, but this medication is used in newborns. No published data on lactation effects. | May cause headache, fatigue, constipation or diarrhea, fever |

Abbreviations: IM, intramuscular; IV, intravenous; PO, by mouth; PR, by rectum; prn, as needed.
Based on *Lexicomp Online.* UpToDate, Inc.; 2021. https://online-lexi-com.frontier.idm.oclc.org/lco/action/home. Accessed September 30, 2021.

and no neonatal adverse effects on fetal heart rate, umbilical cord gases, or Apgar scores have been found following maternal use during labor.[131,155] One study found that those persons who used nitrous oxide during labor had significantly higher breastfeeding rates at 1 month and 3 months postpartum.[154] Nitrous oxide can be used safely during any part of labor,[130,131,135] and no concomitant IV access is needed.[153] It may also be used to enhance postpartum comfort during procedures.

Patients have generally reported high degrees of satisfaction with the use of N$_2$O/O$_2$ in labor, even when they experience only mild or moderate degrees of pain relief following its use.[135,154,156] One study that compared the effectiveness of epidural analgesia to that of N$_2$O/O$_2$ found that patients who relied on N$_2$O/O$_2$ without later choosing neuraxial analgesia reported higher satisfaction scores compared to those who later used epidural analgesia, despite lower scores on actual pain diminution.[157] This finding may relate to patient feelings of control; relaxation, distraction, and decreased anxiety; and/or to the high level of mobility maintained with this method.[156] As discussed previously, direct analgesia is not the only factor associated with birth satisfaction.

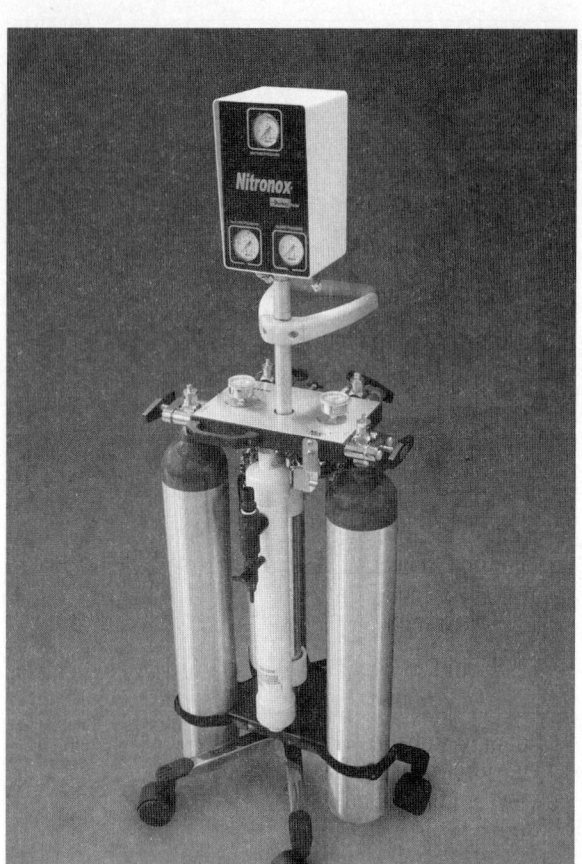

**Figure 28-5** A nitrous oxide machine.
Courtesy of Porter Instrument Division, Parker Hannifin Corp.

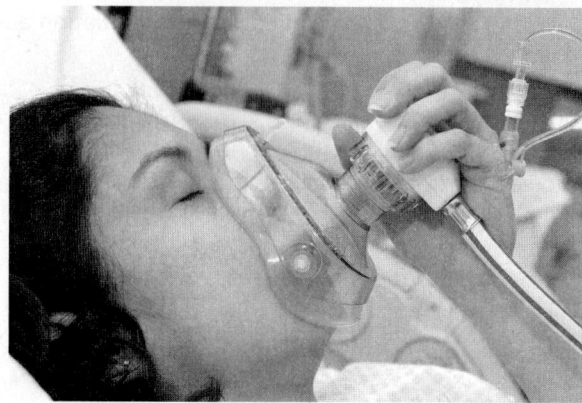

**Figure 28-6** Use of 50:50 nitrous oxide/oxygen for pain relief during labor.
© dblight/E+/Getty Images

The American Society of Anesthesiologists describes $N_2O/O_2$ as analgesia, not anesthesia, so midwives and registered nurses may be responsible for management.[153] The gas mixture is blended in a machine attached to nitrous oxide and oxygen tanks, or attached to piped nitrous oxide and oxygen sources (Figure 28-5). It is then self-administered by the patient via a handheld face mask that covers the nose and mouth or via a mouthpiece (Figure 28-6). A demand valve opens with inhalation and closes with exhalation. Self-administration is not only empowering for the patient, but also allows patients to titrate safe amounts of the gas—because patients experiencing sedation drop the mask from their face. Guidelines for use of this agent are listed in Table 28-6.[153,155]

Potential side effects of $N_2O/O_2$ include nausea in 5% to 40% of patients, vomiting in as many as 15%, and rarer side effects such as dizziness and dysphoria.[135] Approximately 40% to 70% of those who start using $N_2O/O_2$ switch, or "convert," to another type of analgesia later in labor.[131,157] The likelihood of converting is higher with nulliparity

or with labor challenges such as induction, oxytocin augmentation, or prior cesarean.[131,157]

To protect individuals in the room from $N_2O/O_2$ exposure, scavenging equipment to collect the exhaled gas is essential.[135,152] Use of scavenging equipment, inspiratory demand valves, and a 50:50 $N_2O/O_2$ mixture results in environmental levels well below strict safety standards set by the U.S. National Institute for Occupational Safety and Health.[135]

As with all medications, it is important to assess patients for contraindications and to ensure informed consent prior to administration of nitrous oxide. General contraindications to the use of this intervention during labor include inability of the patient to hold the mask, excessive sedation, impaired oxygenation, hemodynamic instability, and a Category III fetal heart rate pattern.[153] Relative contraindications include extreme vitamin $B_{12}$ deficiency and methylenetetrahydrofolate reductase (MTHFR) gene polymorphisms, although robust data on the relationships between $N_2O/O_2$ used during labor, vitamin $B_{12}$ deficiency, MTHFR polymorphisms, and possible adverse outcomes are lacking.[158,159]

Overall, $N_2O/O_2$ is very safe, and can be considered for use by most patients in a variety of situations.[135,153] For example, it can provide effective analgesia for several painful or anxiety-provoking procedures: labor, IV placement, placement of a balloon catheter for labor induction, postpartum suturing, or manual removal of the placenta.[135,153] Limited studies have found no improvement from $N_2O/O_2$ use during external cephalic version on pain scores or satisfaction, although the rate of success may be increased for multiparous patients.[160] As a non-opioid analgesic with beneficial effects on anxiety, nitrous oxide is an excellent choice for

| Table 28-6 | Use of Nitrous Oxide During Labor: Patient Instructions and Rationale |
|---|---|
| **Patient Instructions** | **Rationale** |
| Using nitrous oxide can reduce pain and anxiety, and people who use it during labor report that they are more satisfied with their labor. You will still feel contractions, but the medication may help make them more manageable. | Informed consent is fundamental to practice. Patient satisfaction with this intervention may be higher if correct expectations are shared. |
| If you experience side effects like nausea, dizziness, or drowsiness, you can use the mask less and/or switch to a different strategy for pain management. A separate medication is available to treat nausea. | |
| You can use the mask either all the time or just surrounding contractions. | Continuous inhalation is easier to initiate but may be more likely to result in central nervous system effects of dizziness or dysphoria. |
| If you are using the gas only during contractions, place the mask over the nose and mouth about 30 seconds before the contraction. Then take several breaths. | Intermittent inhalation 30 seconds prior to the onset of contraction maximizes the peak effect of $N_2O/O_2$ so the peak analgesic effect occurs during the peak of the uterine contraction. |
| Be sure the mask has a tight seal on the face. | A tight seal with inhalation allows the $N_2O/O_2$ to pass through a second-stage regulator. |
| Hold the mask on without anyone else's assistance. If you are too drowsy to hold the mask in place, leave the mask off until you feel ready to hold it again. This will keep you from becoming too sedated from the gas. | Excessive sedation from $N_2O/O_2$ is possible if the patient continues to inhale the gas after they can no longer hold the mask tightly to their face. |
| | Self-administration gives the patient personal control of management of pain, and this control may potentiate the analgesic effect. |
| Breathe out into the mask. | To protect others nearby from inhaling the gas and to prevent the $N_2O$ from going into the environment, a scavenging system is connected to the mask. |

Modified from Migliaccio L, Lawton R, Leeman L, Holbrook A. Initiating intrapartum nitrous oxide in an academic hospital: considerations and challenges. *J Midwifery Womens Health.* 2017;62(3):358-362; Rooks JP. Safety and risks of nitrous oxide labor analgesia: a review. *J Midwifery Womens Health.* 2011;56(6):557-565.

individuals with opioid use disorder who have co-morbid PTSD, and whose pain may not be effectively or safely managed with opioids.[153] For those at high altitudes, there are no statistically significant differences by elevation in neonatal outcomes or in the rate of patient conversion to another analgesic.[161]

## Regional Analgesia

Regional analgesia and anesthesia provide pain relief within a defined area of the body. Many regional analgesia techniques are only available within hospitals where they are administered by specially-trained providers such as nurse-anesthetists or anesthesiologists. Individuals receiving regional anesthesia often have impaired mobility and need additional assistance with activities such as urination or changing positions.

### Neuraxial Analgesia

Neuraxial analgesic techniques include spinal (intrathecal injection), epidural, and combined spinal/epidural injections. In the United States, 71% of laboring patients choose neuraxial analgesia to manage labor pain, and almost 90% of those undergoing cesarean delivery have neuraxial anesthesia.[162] This intervention provides high levels of patient satisfaction, and compared to IV/IM opioids and inhalation anesthetics, it provides the most effective relief of labor pain.[133] Over the past three decades, the use of neuraxial methods has increased dramatically, reflecting improvements in administration, greater access to the procedure, and consumer demand.

#### Effectiveness and Indications

When deciding whether to use neuraxial analgesia for labor, individuals must weigh a variety of considerations. A choice for neuraxial analgesia may be made out of empowerment, because of fear of labor pain, or depending on labor progression and intensity. Many patients desire to feel as little of the labor sensations as possible, and choose epidurals to be alert for their birth. Some perceive that they will have greater control over decision making without systemic medications. Many wish to avoid passing systemic medications to the fetus.

Conversely, many people approach labor with some level of commitment to avoiding neuraxial analgesics. For many, that intent or commitment is tied to their trust in the normalcy of physiologic birth, as well as to a sense of adequate personal agency, social support, and clinical resources. Others may be planning in response to incomplete or misinformation about the procedure's risks and benefits, or in the face of pressure from significant others. Individuals in some cultures may be more likely to believe that pain is important for labor, or to avoid neuraxial procedures due to distrust of the medical establishment—a distrust that may be legitimately based on biases and disparities in existing and historical U.S. medical practice.[163] For the midwife providing respectful counseling about available, safe pain management options, it is important to gain a full understanding of the patient's priorities, and to include in the discussion those persons whose support is needed by the patient. Ultimately, midwives aim to further empower patients in their decision making while ensuring that well-informed choices are made autonomously by the patient.

Beyond those personal reasons for choosing neuraxial analgesia, this intervention has benefits for some specific populations. For individuals who have a history of sexual abuse, labor can induce anxiety about painful stimuli in the vaginal/rectal area or flashbacks of abusive events. Thus, the "numbing" effect of epidural analgesia can mitigate some aspects of the post-traumatic stress caused by labor and birth. For people with opioid use disorder, neuraxial analgesia can provide more effective control of pain while avoiding the use of systemic opioids.[164] For people with a medical need to diminish maternal expulsive efforts (e.g., maternal cardiac or ophthalmologic disease), neuraxial analgesia can allow for greater patient control over the pushing efforts during the second stage of labor. If a patient's medical or obstetric condition places them at increased risk for needing an emergent cesarean section, early placement of an epidural catheter may be recommended to expedite action if the emergency occurs. This "double setup" is sometimes done, for example, if membranes are to be ruptured when the fetal presenting part is not in the pelvis, for a vaginal breech birth, or for a patient with a multifetal gestation.

Not everyone is a good candidate for neuraxial analgesia or anesthesia. Indications for consultation with an anesthesiologist during the antepartum and/or intrapartum periods are listed in **Table 28-7**.[56,165]

| Table 28-7 | Indications for Anesthesiology Consultation for Midwifery Patients | |
|---|---|---|
| **Category** | **Examples** | **Rationale** |
| **Cardiac risk factors or disease** | Current or past heart disease, birth defects, or surgeries; rhythm abnormalities | The stress and hemodynamic shifts of labor, birth, and cesarean surgery may require intensive management |
| **Hematologic abnormalities** | Thrombocytopenia, anticoagulant medications, coagulopathies | Epidural or spinal analgesia could lead to bleeding into the spinal or epidural spaces |
| **Spinal, muscular, and neurologic risk factors or disease** | Structural abnormalities in the spinal column, scoliosis, prior spinal surgeries, spinal cord injury | Surgical scarring and bone fusion could interfere with placement of regional analgesia/anesthesia |
| **Risk factors for anesthesia complications including difficult intubation** | Obstructive sleep apnea, anatomic or functional defects of the head or neck, obesity impacting the neck, difficult-to-visualize uvula, previous difficulties with epidural, spinal, or general anesthesia; allergy to local anesthetics | Facilitates appropriate choices of analgesia/anesthesia agents or techniques, planning for the possibility of general anesthesia |

Based on American College of Obstetrician and Gynecologists Practice Bulletin No. 209: obstetric analgesia and anesthesia. *Obstet Gynecol.* 2019;133(3):e208-e225; Kollmeier BR, Boyette LC, Beecham GB, et al. Difficult airway. In: *StatPearls.* Treasure Island, FL: StatPearls Publishing; 2022. https://www.ncbi.nlm.nih.gov/books/NBK470224/. Accessed December 12, 2022.

In many cases, a telephone consultation and access to previous medical records may be sufficient; in other cases, a face-to-face consultation with a physical exam is appropriate.

Absolute contraindications to neuraxial analgesia and anesthesia include the patient's refusal of these interventions, skin or soft-tissue infection at the site of needle placement, frank coagulopathy, untreated sepsis, increased intracranial pressure, and hemodynamic instability. Relative contraindications include inability to maintain safe positioning for insertion, neurologic disease of the spinal cord, and heparin therapy or thrombocytopenia.[56] Depending on the criteria set by anesthesia specialists, a stable platelet count of at least 70,000 to 100,000 cells per microliter without additional diagnoses or use of anticoagulants is required before administration of the medication.[56,134] Contrary to popular belief, a tattoo over the insertion area is not a contraindication to epidural analgesia.[166]

Determination of whether to use a spinal, an epidural, or a combined spinal–epidural (CSE) depends on the situational needs and timing, and is guided by the anesthesia specialist. In general, CSE is associated with faster relief, lower pain scores, less need for rescue analgesia, and fewer side effects than traditional epidurals; however, there is conflicting evidence as to whether it reduces operative vaginal births, and consistent evidence that other outcomes for the patient and the newborn are similar.[167] For routine labor, epidurals or CSEs are used most often because they are effective, and a continuous infusion of medication can be used for prolonged periods as needed. For emergent or time-limited situations requiring fast onset of action without the need for an extended block or ongoing infusion (i.e., scheduled cesarean delivery or rapidly progressing labors), spinal anesthesia may be used. Spinal analgesia does not affect motor ability, so this therapy is often called "the walking epidural" despite the fact that it does not deliver analgesia into the epidural space. The major drawback of spinal analgesia is that it requires a dural puncture, which is not safe to do multiple times. Because it is not easy to predict how long laboring patients will need analgesia, spinal analgesia is not used as often as is epidural or CSE analgesia.

### Placement and Mechanism of Action

The process for initiating neuraxial analgesia is similar from the patient's standpoint regardless of whether spinal, epidural, or CSE analgesia is being used. In settings with experienced and available anesthesia specialists, pain relief takes approximately 10 to 20 minutes after informed consent is obtained by the anesthesia provider. The patient either sits on the side of the bed or rests in a lateral position with the spine curved. After a local anesthetic is used to numb the area of insertion, the anesthesia provider places the epidural or spinal needle between the spinal processes and into the desired space. When correct placement is assured for an epidural, a catheter is passed into the space and secured. The needle is removed and the epidural catheter is injected with medication and attached to a pump for a continuous infusion and/or patient-controlled dosing of the medication. For initiation of spinal analgesia, a catheter is not usually placed; thus, while onset of action is rapid, the length of pain management is limited to the duration of the specific opioid used. For CSE, both spaces are injected and an epidural catheter is left in place for ongoing infusion. Throughout the analgesia process, there is close monitoring of the patient's oxygenation saturation and blood pressure as well as the fetal heartbeat. Transient changes in the patient's blood pressure and the fetal heartbeat are common and discussed in more detail later in this section.

The effects of neuraxial analgesia depend on where the medication is placed, which medications are used (and their dosages), and how dosing is administered. To block sensory input from the uterus and perineum, neuraxial analgesia must block T10 to L1 during the first stage of labor and extend to S2 to S4 during the late first and second stages of labor. For spinal anesthesia, a single injection of opioid is administered in the intrathecal (subarachnoid) space that contains cerebrospinal fluid, spinal nerves, and blood vessels, all of which are enclosed by the membrane of the dura mater. For epidural anesthesia, an injection of a local anesthetic, with or without the addition of an opioid, is placed into the epidural space (Figure 28-7). Located exterior to the dura mater and interior to the ligamentum flavum, this area contains nerve roots, fat, lymphatics, and blood vessels. For CSE, anesthetic and opioid medications are injected into both the intrathecal and epidural spaces. When an anesthetic or opioid medication is placed in either space, impulses traveling in the sensory and motor nerves in contact with the drug are blocked.[150] The effect occurs more quickly (several minutes) after spinal and CSE injections compared with epidural placements (10 to 15 minutes).[167]

The anesthetic agents most commonly used to produce a sensory block are bupivacaine (Marcaine) and ropivacaine (Naropin). Fentanyl or remifentanyl can be added to potentiate the analgesic

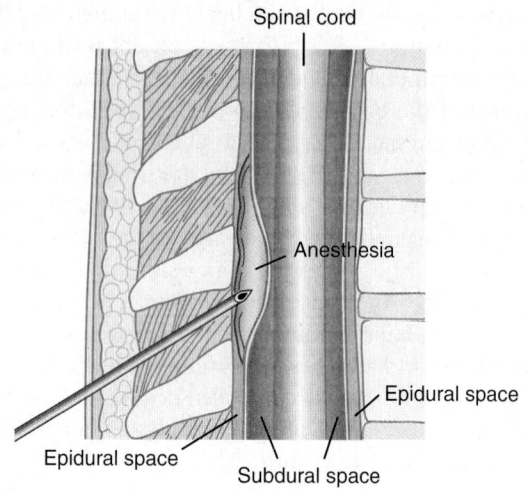

**Figure 28-7** Placement of anesthesia in the epidural space.

| Table 28-8 | Signs of Intrathecal or Systemic Toxicity Following Misplaced Epidural Injection |
|---|---|
| **Placement of Anesthetic** | **Signs and Symptoms of Toxicity** |
| Intrathecal | Rapid cephalad spread of anesthesia<br>Symptomatic hypotension (maternal or fetal)<br>Respiratory depression<br>Loss of consciousness |
| Intravascular | Seizures<br>Cardiac dysrhythmias<br>Cardiac arrest |

effect, and the combination of medications allows for smaller doses of each drug, along with fewer adverse effects. Often epinephrine is added to the local anesthetic solution because it prolongs the duration of action; sodium bicarbonate may added either alone or with epinephrine because alkalinization can speed and intensify the effect.[132] CSE placement leads to a 2- to 5-minute faster onset of action compared to placement of a traditional epidural, along with more even analgesia and fewer supplemental doses.[132] Ongoing delivery of epidural medication is by intermittent, continuous, or patient-controlled infusion, or with a combination of these dosing methods. When a continuous background infusion is added to patient-controlled epidural analgesia, pain control appears to be maximized.[132,150]

Some of the individual differences noted in the quality of neuraxial blocks, despite use of a consistent technique, may reflect individual anatomic variations that occur in the epidural space. For example, differences in nerve root size or the presence of membranes in the epidural space that prevent equal spread of the medication to all nerves passing through the epidural space may lead to variable effects. When the patient's block is uneven from side to side, changing position may allow for a more even distribution of the anesthetic. If the pain is persistent, the anesthesia provider should be alerted so they can adjust the epidural dose, change the position of the catheter, or replace the epidural altogether.[150]

### Side Effects and Adverse Effects

The anesthesia provider will remain involved to ensure desired effectiveness of the analgesia or anesthesia, as well as to manage severe or persistent adverse effects. Midwives need to anticipate the effects of the procedure, be prepared to manage routine side effects and complications, and collaborate with anesthesia specialists when patient conditions demand.

Adverse effects that are immediately related to implementation of the epidural analgesia procedure are rare. The incidence of epidural abscess is fewer than 1 in 60,000, epidural hematoma approximately 1 in 250,000, and serious neurologic injury approximately 1 in 36,000; postpartum changes in sensation, weakness, and loss of bladder or bowel control require evaluation.[134] Inadvertent intrathecal (subarachnoid) or intravascular placement can result in toxicity because the high dose of anesthetic can cause high spinal block, leading to respiratory compromise. Inadvertent intravenous placement can lead to to seizures and cardiac arrest (Table 28-8). Total spinal anesthesia occurs in 0.03% of people; in this condition, the level of the anesthesia rises dangerously high, resulting in paralysis of the respiratory muscles including the diaphragm (1 in 4000).[134] When this effect occurs, the patient will experience numbness of the hands and fingers, as well as dyspnea. Treatment includes assisted respiration until the anesthesia resolves.

Another complication related to neuraxial insertion is postdural puncture headache, commonly known as a "spinal headache." Its incidence is 1% to 2% after uncomplicated epidural or spinal procedures, but rises to more than 50% in those persons with accidental dural puncture.[162,168] If excessive cerebrospinal fluid leaks into the epidural space, the drop in intrathecal pressure can cause a positional headache, which increases in severity when the patient is in the sitting or standing position. Resolution of the headache occurs spontaneously within 4 to 5 days. If not severe, this headache may be treated with oral hydration, caffeine, and simple analgesics such as acetaminophen (Tylenol) or ibuprofen (Motrin, Advil). If the headache is severe or prolonged, it can be treated per anesthesia with other medications or a blood patch, which is an epidural injection of the patient's blood to seal the leaking membrane.[162] Postpartum headaches are common, and postdural puncture headaches account for approximately 16% of these outcomes.[168] Thus, midwives must evaluate birthing persons thoroughly for other possible causes of headache, and consult anesthesia specialists appropriately as indicated.

Hypotension, defined as a systolic blood pressure of less than 100 mm Hg or 80% of baseline, is a common occurrence with neuraxial pain management strategies and can be accompanied by signs and symptoms in the pregnant patient and the fetus.[133,169] Local anesthetics cause a sympathetic blockade that leads to decreased vascular tone, peripheral vasodilation, and a subsequent drop in blood pressure. Significant complications are uncommon, but symptomatic patients may report nausea or dizziness. Blood flow to the uterus diminishes with hypotension, and fetal heart rate decelerations (e.g., prolonged deceleration or late decelerations) frequently appear for a short time within 10 to 20 minutes after the epidural placement. When changes in fetal heart rate patterns are associated with moderate fetal heart rate variability and resolve spontaneously or following a bolus of IV fluids within a few minutes, they are not associated with adverse newborn outcomes. However, sustained hypotension resulting in nonreassuring fetal heart rate patterns and requiring treatment with vasopressors such as phenylephrine or epinephrine has been associated with fetal acidemia and neurobehavioral changes at 4 to 7 days of life.[169] An anesthesia provider should be consulted for management of symptomatic hypotension that persists after a change in position and a bolus of IV fluids. Evidence-based efforts to prevent hypotension include lateral or tilted positioning for supine patients, a 1000 mL co-load (i.e., IV fluids infuse while insertion is occurring—a technique superior to preloading before insertion) of crystalloid IV fluids such as lactated Ringer's solution, or a 500 mL preload of colloid IV fluids such as 6% hydroxyl-ethyl starch or albumin.[169]

Pruritus, of varying degrees of severity, occurs in 60% to 100% of patients receiving opioids in neuraxial analgesia/anesthesia.[170] Antihistamines such as diphenhydramine (25 mg given intravenously) or hydroxyzine (25 mg by mouth or intramuscularly) can be of value in this situation; in severe cases, naloxone can be administered with caution. If naloxone is needed, be aware that the anesthetic effect of the spinal analgesia will also be reversed.[171]

Urinary retention can occur when the patient experiences loss of the sensation to void, relaxation of overall bladder tone, and loss of control of the urinary sphincter. If many hours will elapse between initiation of an epidural and birth, and the patient is unable to void independently, an indwelling catheter or intermittent catheterization may be indicated. The catheter should be discontinued during the second stage of labor.[172]

An increase in the incidence of intrapartum fever, defined as a body temperature of at least 38°C (100.4°F), occurs in approximately 20% of people who labor with neuraxial analgesia.[173] Temperature elevations tend to increase immediately after the epidural is initiated and average 0.18°C (0.33°F) per hour. The occurrence of fever equal to or higher than 38°C (100.4°F) is apparent after approximately 4 hours.[174,175] Most likely, epidural-related fever is attributable to inflammation from labor and from the neuraxial method, as well as to thermoregulatory alterations such as a decrease in heat dissipation secondary to sympathetic block of sweating.[173] Some individuals who develop a fever after epidural initiation have intra-amniotic infection. Unfortunately, it is not possible to reliably distinguish fever of benign versus infectious origin, so all patients who develop a fever in labor should be treated for intra-amniotic infection.[176] A meta-analysis demonstrated no increased rate of neonatal bacteremia or antibiotic treatment in such cases, but newborns of those who develop a fever during labor are more likely to be evaluated for sepsis.[176]

A secondary analysis of data from a large study that followed patients in labor to determine fetal position confirmed the increased incidence of a rise in temperature in patients who have an epidural.[177] This analysis found that a rise in temperature was positively associated with occiput posterior position at birth despite the groups having a nonsignificant difference in the incidence of occiput posterior position at the onset of labor. Furthermore, the incidence of occiput posterior position at birth and cesarean section increased proportionately as the maternal temperature increased (17.2% versus 9.2% in people with and without fever respectively; odds ratio [OR], 2.0; 95% CI, 1.5–2.8).[177] This finding remained significant after controlling for confounding factors such as body mass index, gestational age, birth weight, and length of labor (OR, 1.5; 95% CI, 1.1–2.1).[177]

Back pain is a common side effect of labor and birth, with or without an epidural. When lower back pain occurs following regional analgesia, the back pain may be attributed to the epidural. However, robust evidence of a correlation between postpartum back pain and neuraxial strategies is lacking.[133] To prevent back pain from labor, midwives can ensure that recumbent patients frequently change their position and have proper body alignment supported by pillows. Before and after birth, back pain may be alleviated by measures such as analgesics, pelvic belts, acupuncture, core-strengthening exercises, and physical therapy.[178]

### Effect of Neuraxial Analgesia on Labor Progress and Outcomes

Neuraxial analgesia is an excellent method for reducing labor pain, and patient satisfaction is high for those who choose this method. However, it is associated with several adverse effects that frequently require attention—namely, hypotension, pruritis, headache, urinary retention, and fever. Relatively consistent data showing a reassuring absence of effect from epidurals in terms of the rate of cesarean section, long-term postpartum backache, and neonatal outcomes.[133] In regard to how neuraxial analgesia affects labor progress and the mode of delivery, data are inconsistent. While these inconsistencies reflect the many confounding variables involved, they also illustrate the improvements in neuraxial methods over time. Ethical care requires midwives to provide accurate counseling about available options, as well as to show deference to patients' decisions about their preferred comfort strategies.

*Length of Labor.* In general, labor progress is slower when neuraxial analgesia is used. According to a 2018 Cochrane review of RCTs, the use of epidurals results in longer first and second stages of labor, as well as an increased likelihood of having oxytocin augmentation.[133] Separate, retrospective studies add nuance to these findings.[179] For instance, one retrospective study determined that without induction, the average labor (50th percentile of labor duration, first and second stages combined) was 76 minutes longer for nulliparous patients and 7 minutes longer for multiparous patients using an epidural.[180] A retrospective study of only nulliparous patients found that patients using CSE analgesia had latent phases of labor that were relatively faster, and active phases that were relatively slower, than those of the comparison group without CSE analgesia.[181] A retrospective study of only multiparous patients who did and did not receive epidurals demonstrated that those receiving epidurals at 4 centimeters dilation or more did not have prolonged labors, but

those receiving early epidurals at 2 to 3 centimeters had labors that were 50 minutes longer.[182] It is unclear whether the laboring persons receiving earlier epidurals were experiencing more dysfunctional labors before the epidural was placed, or whether the slowing of the labor occurred afterward.

Thus, parity, use of induction or augmentation, and timing of epidural/CSE placement confound attempts to decipher the exact effects of neuraxial analgesia on labor progress. Additional variables include whether an epidural or CSE is used and which medication is included in the analgesia. A Cochrane review conducted in 2012 determined that although CSE takes effect more quickly than a traditional epidural, the rate of augmentation does not differ with the two methods.[167] Retrospective cohort studies suggest that for CSE, labor is lengthened when the medications used include an opioid and an anesthetic versus only an anesthetic.[183] For epidurals, length of labor is comparable to when nonepidural analgesia is used if lower-concentration anesthetics are used instead of higher-concentration anesthetics—a change in practice that has become increasingly popular.[184]

Perhaps most importantly, individual anatomy, physiology, and psychology influence the effects of neuraxial analgesia on labor progress. Most patients may experience a longer labor with neuraxial analgesia; this extended duration is presumed to occur secondary to the lack of sensation for bearing down and perhaps the relaxation of the levator ani muscles that make up the pelvic floor. However, some patients experience an accelerated course of labor after epidural analgesia is initiated. This effect may be due to improved uterine contractility after previous inhibition from markedly elevated catecholamine levels in people experiencing severe pain. Alternatively, the higher level of pain that inspired the request for epidural analgesia might have reflected rapid dilation that occurred spontaneously. Given these offsetting reasons for responding differently to pain relief, it can be difficult to draw clinically meaningful conclusions from these data.

*Mode of Delivery.* Epidural and CSE analgesia are not associated with an increase in cesarean births.[133,185] They are associated with operative vaginal birth (RR, 1.44; 95% CI, 1.29–1.60), but this rate has declined over the past decades due to the evolution of the low-dose epidural, which allows for less motor block and a shorter second stage of labor compared to higher concentrations; implementation of CSE; and use of patient-controlled neuraxial analgesia.[133,185] However, a 2012 Cochrane review indicated that operative vaginal delivery is less likely for laboring persons who receive a CSE than for those who receive an epidural (RR, 0.81; 95% CI, 0.67–0.97),[167] and a 2018 Cochrane review found that after eliminating trials performed prior to 2005, the higher rate of operative vaginal birth with CSE versus no neuraxial analgesia was eliminated (RR, 1.19; 95% CI, 0.97–1.46).[133]

A variety of practices are, or have been, used to optimize the outcomes of people using neuraxial analgesia during labor. Frequent position changes—at least hourly, if not every 20 to 30 minutes—shorten both the first and second stages of labor, and reduce the rate of cesarean delivery.[186] Use of peanut balls between side-lying patients' legs has been implemented to maintain the pelvis in an open position; however, while these balls may be used for their contribution to patient comfort, the practice does not seem to affect the length of labor or the rates of occiput posterior position or cesarean delivery (studies did not report the rate of operative vaginal birth).[186,187] "Laboring down"—that is, delaying second-stage pushing until the presenting part is low in the pelvis—reduces active pushing time, but does not increase the rate of spontaneous vaginal birth; moreover, it increases the rates of intra-amniotic infection and postpartum hemorrhage.[188] Two Cochrane reviews comparing upright and recumbent positioning during the second stage with epidurals suggest that upright positioning either does not increase the rate of spontaneous birth[72] or is associated with an increase in cesarean delivery without a decrease in operative vaginal birth.[189] Some practitioners have advocated cessation of epidural analgesia during second-stage labor to enable the laboring person to experience the urge to push and to be able to actively participate in expulsive efforts. However, evidence suggests that the reoccurrence of severe pain following discontinuation of an epidural in second-stage labor may interfere with the laboring person's ability to push, thereby lengthening the second stage's progress and increasing interventions.[190] Discontinuing the epidural infusion during labor is not recommended.

### Effects of Neuraxial Analgesia on the Fetus and Neonate

Anesthetics and opioids are both highly lipid soluble and can cross into the fetal circulation in small amounts, depending on the quantity found in the maternal circulation. Nevertheless, neonatal outcomes such as low 5-minute Apgar scores, cord pH, and NICU admissions have not been shown to be significantly different between patients using neuraxial analgesia and those using IV opioids or no medications.[133,191] Robust studies of long-term developmental sequelae are generally lacking.

The effects of epidural analgesia on breastfeeding outcomes have also been controversial. Patients cannot be randomized prospectively to epidural analgesia or no-epidural analgesia groups, and because those with epidural analgesia tend to have longer second stages, more fevers, and a higher rate of operative birth, it is not clear if lower rates of breastfeeding initiation occur secondary to the epidural analgesia or to the labor course. Overall, rates of breastfeeding initiation and continuation through 6 weeks postpartum appear to be unchanged regardless of the method of analgesia.[192,193]

### Pudendal Block

A pudendal block is used to alleviate pain stemming from the perineum and vagina during the second stage of labor.[194] Before the widespread adoption of epidural analgesia for mitigating labor pain, pudendal blocks were the preferred analgesic technique for birth. A pudendal block can be an effective form of analgesia for a low vaginal or perineal procedure if a patient has a contraindication to neuraxial anesthesia. The lower vagina, perineum, and vulva obtain most of their sensory and motor innervation from sacral nerve roots 2, 3, and 4 via the pudendal nerve. Infiltration of a local anesthetic around the pudendal nerve at the level of the ischial spine results in analgesia of these areas. Pudendal nerve blocks do not decrease the pain associated with uterine contractions or cervical dilation. The *Pudendal Nerve Block* appendix describes the procedure in detail.[194]

Pudendal blocks are simple to perform and provide satisfactory analgesia for many individuals. However, 10% to 50% of bilateral pudendal blocks are ineffective on one or both sides. Pudendal blocks do not interfere with uterine contractions, so they have no adverse effects on labor progress or maternal or fetal well-being. Neonatal local anesthetic toxicity after maternal pudendal block is extremely rare. A report described three cases of neonatal lidocaine intoxication, which manifested as transient hypotonia, apnea, seizures, mydriasis, cyanosis, and need for mechanical ventilation; all of the neonates recovered completely.[195] Potential maternal complications are also rare, but may include post-block fetal bradycardia, systematic toxicity after intravascular administration, lower-extremity paresthesia, vaginal hematoma, and infection.[194,195] Postpartum urinary retention is not increased after pudendal block.[196]

## General Anesthesia

General anesthesia refers to the use of an inhaled anesthetic agent to induce unconsciousness. During perinatal care, this intervention is used primarily for emergency cesarean birth. Induction of anesthesia is accomplished with short-acting agents that render the patient unconscious, such as thiopental or propofol. After the induction agent is administered, a muscle relaxant such as succinylcholine is typically administered to facilitate intubation.[197] Although general anesthesia is rarely used in elective cesareans in the United States, it is used in as many as 19% of emergency cases.[168]

Complications such as "failed" intubation and pulmonary aspiration are rare, but they occur more often for pregnant people. The risk of intubation difficulty is increased during pregnancy because of increased vascularity and edema of the oral and nasal mucosa and decreased functional residual capacity and increased oxygen consumption.[168] Pulmonary aspiration risk is increased especially for those persons with labor, neuraxial analgesia, obesity, diabetes, hypertension, embolism, hemorrhage, gastroesophageal reflux, or emergent procedures.[168,198] Because of these risks and those for fetuses exposed to anesthetics, general anesthesia is avoided when possible.

Concern about potential complications associated with unplanned use of general anesthesia affects labor decision making. Fasting, preoperative antacids, and advances in intubation technique have greatly decreased rates of complications associated with general anesthesia during pregnancy below what they were in past decades. Some argue that even the low incidence of pulmonary aspiration justifies policies restricting oral intake during labor—especially because several RCTs comparing groups with restricted versus liberal oral intake found no difference in duration of labor, neonatal outcomes, or mode of delivery.[168] Others note that since fasting has been found to increase acid secretion (possibly even increasing gastric volume) and since there is a lack of evidence that fasting reduces the odds of death due to aspiration, withholding oral energy intake is unnecessary and potentially harmful.[198]

In general, community birth settings are unlikely to restrict oral intake of laboring persons. U.S. hospitals often restrict intake to clear liquids during latent labor and ice chips during active labor, with a significant minority of hospitals allowing nothing by mouth during latent and/or active labor. Notably, people birthing in several other countries—that is, Britain, Australia, and the Netherlands—have greater or full autonomy over oral intake without an increased rate

of fatal aspiration.[198] Respectful care requires midwives and other clinical personnel to help individuals weigh personal risks, benefits, and preferences regarding oral intake. When patient risks for anesthesia complications are high and/or clinical conditions indicate a risk for an urgent cesarean delivery, shared decision making can be used to consider limiting oral intake, administration of antacids, early consultation with anesthesia, and early placement of intrathecal catheters.[198] In many clinical situations where a surgical birth becomes necessary, there is adequate time for placement of spinal anesthesia, which has less potential for maternal–fetal complications.

## Conclusion

Each person's labor is unique, and each person has a variety of options to consider as they decide how to manage their labor. As advocates for informed choice, shared decision making, and the right to self-determination, midwives provide laboring people with the knowledge and support they need to make safe, empowering choices about their comfort during labor. By supporting a range of pharmacologic and nonpharmacologic options and effectively leading a team centered on the needs and preferences of the laboring person, midwives foster patient- and family-centered care as standards for all birth settings. Memories of childbirth are powerful and last a lifetime, and it is a midwife's honor to ensure that those memories capture the dignity and empowerment of each experience.

## References

1. Simkin P, Bolding A. Update on nonpharmacologic approaches to relieve labor pain and prevent suffering. *J Midwifery Womens Health*. 2004;49(6):489-504.
2. Simkin P. Just another day in a woman's life? Part II: nature and consistency of women's long-term memories of their first birth experiences. *Birth*. 1992;19(2):64-81.
3. *The Prevention and Elimination of Disrespect and Abuse During Facility-Based Childbirth*. Geneva, Switzerland: World Health Organization; 2015.
4. Bohren MA, Mehrtash H, Fawole B, et al. How women are treated during facility-based childbirth in four countries: a cross-sectional study with labour observations and community-based surveys. *Lancet*. 2019;394(10210):1750-1763.
5. van Brunnersum S. Women around the world face widespread abuse during childbirth. *Deutche Welle*. https://www.dw.com/en/women-around-the-world-face-widespread-abuse-during-childbirth/a-51393868. Published November 11, 2019.

6. Campbell C. Medical violence, obstetric racism, and the limits of informed consent for Black women. *Mich J Race Law.* 2021;26(Special Issue).

7. Declercq E, Sakala C, Corry M, Applebaum S. *Listening to Mothers II: Pregnancy and Birth.* New York, NY: Childbirth Connection; 2006.

8. Beck CT, Gable RK, Sakala C, Declercq ER. Posttraumatic stress disorder in new mothers: results from a two-stage U.S. national survey. *Birth.* 2011;38(3): 216-227.

9. Yildiz PD, Ayers S, Phillips L. The prevalence of post-traumatic stress disorder in pregnancy and after birth: a systematic review and meta-analysis. *J Affect Disord.* 2017;208:634-645.

10. Seng JS, Sperlich M, Low LK, et al. Childhood abuse history, posttraumatic stress disorder, post-partum mental health, and bonding: a prospective cohort study. *J Midwifery Womens Health.* 2013; 58(1):57-68.

11. Melzack R, Schaffelberg D. Low-back pain during labor. *Am J Obstet Gynecol.* 1987;156(4):901-905.

12. Melzack R. From the gate to the neuromatrix. *Pain.* 1999;Suppl 6:S121-S126.

13. Trout KK. The neuromatrix theory of pain: implications for selected nonpharmacologic methods of pain relief for labor. *J Midwifery Womens Health.* 2004;49(6):482-488.

14. Raja SN, Carr DB, Cohen M, et al. The revised International Association for the Study of Pain definition of pain: concepts, challenges, and compromises. *Pain.* 2020;161(9):1976-1982.

15. Lowe NK. The nature of labor pain. *Am J Obstet Gynecol.* 2002;186(5 suppl Nature):S16-S24.

16. Eltzschig HK, Lieberman ES, Camann WR. Regional anesthesia and analgesia for labor and delivery. *N Engl J Med.* 2003;348(4):319-332.

17. Mendell LM. Constructing and deconstructing the gate theory of pain. *Pain.* 2014;155(2):210-216.

18. Chen WG, Schloesser D, Arensdorf AM, et al. The emerging science of interoception: sensing, integrating, interpreting, and regulating signals within the self. *Trends Neurosci.* 2021;44(1):3-16.

19. Melzack R. The myth of painless childbirth (the John J. Bonica lecture). *Pain.* 1984;19(4):321-337.

20. Melzack R, Kinch R, Dobkin P, et al. Severity of labour pain: influence of physical as well as psychologic variables. *Can Med Assoc J.* 1984;130(5):579-584.

21. Lowe NK, Corwin EJ. Proposed biological linkages between obesity, stress, and inefficient uterine contractility during labor in humans. *Med Hypotheses.* 2011;76(5):755-760.

22. Olza I, Uvnas-Moberg K, Ekström-Bergström A, et al. Birth as a neuro-psycho-social event: an integrative model of maternal experiences and their relation to neurohormonal events during childbirth. *PLoS One.* 2020;15(7):e0230992.

23. Mitchell BF, Fang X, Wong S. Oxytocin: a paracrine hormone in the regulation of parturition? *Rev Reprod.* 1998;3(2):113-122.

24. Engert V, Koester AM, Riepenhausen A, Singer T. Boosting recovery rather than buffering reactivity: higher stress-induced oxytocin secretion is associated with increased cortisol reactivity and faster vagal recovery after acute psychosocial stress. *Psychoneuroendocrinology.* 2016;74:111-120.

25. Uvnas-Moberg K. The inner guide to motherhood. In: *Oxytocin: The Biological Guide to Motherhood.* Amarillo, TX: Praeclarus Press; 2014.

26. Hodnett ED. Pain and women's satisfaction with the experience of childbirth: a systematic review. *Am J Obstet Gynecol.* 2002;186(5 suppl Nature): S160-S172.

27. Lally JE, Murtagh MJ, Macphail S, Thomson R. More in hope than expectation: a systematic review of women's expectations and experience of pain relief in labour. *BMC Med.* 2008;6:7.

28. Mogil JS. Pain genetics: past, present and future. *Trends Genet.* 2012;28(6):258-266.

29. Landau R. Genetic contributions to labor pain and progress. *Clin Perinatol.* 2013;40(3):575-587.

30. Landau R, Smiley R. Pharmacogenetics in obstetric anesthesia. *Best Pract Res Clin Anaesthesiol.* 2017; 31(1):23-34.

31. Hoffman KM, Trawalter S, Axt JR, Oliver MN. Racial bias in pain assessment and treatment recommendations, and false beliefs about biological differences between Blacks and whites. *Proc Natl Acad Sci U S A.* 2016;113(16):4296-4301.

32. Morris T, Schulman M. Race inequality in epidural use and regional anesthesia failure in labor and birth: an examination of women's experience. *Sex Reprod Healthc.* 2014;5(4):188-194.

33. *Diagnostic and Statistical Manual of Mental Disorders.* 5th ed. Washington, DC: American Psychiatric Association; 2013.

34. Nilsson C, Hessman E, Sjöblom H, et al. Definitions, measurements and prevalence of fear of childbirth: a systematic review. *BMC Pregnancy Childbirth.* 2018; 18(1):28.

35. Roosevelt L, Low LK. Exploring fear of childbirth in the United States through a qualitative assessment of the Wijma Delivery Expectancy Questionnaire. *J Obstet Gynecol Neonatal Nurs.* 2016;45(1): 28-38.

36. Lowe NK. Self-efficacy for labor and childbirth fears in nulliparous pregnant women. *J Psychosom Obstet Gynaecol.* 2000;21(4):219-224.

37. Laursen M, Johansen C, Hedegaard M. Fear of childbirth and risk for birth complications in nulliparous

women in the Danish National Birth Cohort. *BJOG.* 2009;116(10):1350-1355.

38. Haines HM, Rubertsson C, Pallant JF, Hildingsson I. The influence of women's fear, attitudes and beliefs of childbirth on mode and experience of birth. *BMC Pregnancy Childbirth.* 2012;12:55.

39. Sperlich M, Seng J, Rowe H, et al. A cycles-breaking framework to disrupt intergenerational patterns of maltreatment and vulnerability during the childbearing year. *J Obstet Gynecol Neonatal Nurs.* 2017; 46(3):378-389.

40. Granner JR, Seng JS. Using theories of posttraumatic stress to inform perinatal care clinician responses to trauma reactions. *J Midwifery Womens Health.* 2021;66(5):567-578.

41. Seng J, Taylor J. *Trauma-Informed Care in the Perinatal Period.* Edinburgh, UK: Dunedin Academic Press; 2015.

42. Gagnon AJ, Sandall J. Individual or group antenatal education for childbirth or parenthood, or both. *Cochrane Database Syst Rev.* 2007;3:Cd002869.

43. Maimburg RD, Vaeth M, Dürr J, et al. Randomised trial of structured antenatal training sessions to improve the birth process. *BJOG.* 2010;117(8):921-928.

44. Sakallaris BR, MacAllister L, Voss M, et al. Optimal healing environments. *Glob Adv Health Med.* 2015; 4(3):40-45.

45. Churchill LR, Schenck D. Healing skills for medical practice. *Ann Intern Med.* 2008;149(10):720-724.

46. Hodnett ED, Stremler R, Weston JA, McKeever P. Re-conceptualizing the hospital labor room: the PLACE (Pregnant and Laboring in an Ambient Clinical Environment) pilot trial. *Birth.* 2009;36(2):159-166.

47. Walburg V, Friederich F, Callahan S. Embarrassment and modesty feelings during pregnancy, childbirth and follow-up care: a qualitative approach. *J Reprod Infant Psychol.* 2014;32(2):126-136.

48. Kolcaba KY. A theory of holistic comfort for nursing. *J Adv Nurs.* 1994;19(6):1178-1184.

49. Schuiling KD, Sampselle CM. Comfort in labor and midwifery art. *Image J Nurs Sch.* 1999;31(1):77-81.

50. Whitburn LY, Jones LE, Davey MA, Small R. Women's experiences of labour pain and the role of the mind: an exploratory study. *Midwifery.* 2014;30(9): 1029-1035.

51. Whitburn LY, Jones LE, Davey MA, Small R. The meaning of labour pain: how the social environment and other contextual factors shape women's experiences. *BMC Pregnancy Childbirth.* 2017;17(1):157.

52. Lowe NK. Context and process of informed consent for pharmacologic strategies in labor pain care. *J Midwifery Womens Health.* 2004;49(3):250-259.

53. Gulliver BG, Fisher J, Roberts L. A new way to assess pain in laboring women: replacing the rating scale with a "coping" algorithm. *Nurs Womens Health.* 2008;12(5):404-408.

54. Roberts L, Gulliver B, Fisher J, Cloyes KG. The Coping with Labor Algorithm: an alternate pain assessment tool for the laboring woman. *J Midwifery Womens Health.* 2010;55(2):107-116.

55. Simkin P, Rohls K. The three R's in childbirth preparation: relaxation, rhythm and ritual. https://www.pennysimkin.com/the-3-rs-in-childbirth-preparation-relaxation-rhythm-and-ritual. Published June 14, 2016. Accessed December 12, 2022.

56. ACOG Practice Bulletin No. 209 summary: obstetric analgesia and anesthesia. *Obstet Gynecol.* 2019; 133(3):595-597.

57. Bergstrom L, Richards L, Morse JM, Roberts J. How caregivers manage pain and distress in second-stage labor. *J Midwifery Womens Health.* 2010;55(1): 38-45.

58. Sheiner E, Sheiner EK, Hershkovitz R, et al. Overestimation and underestimation of labor pain. *Eur J Obstet Gynecol Reprod Biol.* 2000;91(1):37-40.

59. Sheiner EK, Sheiner E, Shoham-Vardi I, et al. Ethnic differences influence care giver's estimates of pain during labour. *Pain.* 1999;81(3):299-305.

60. Baker A, Ferguson SA, Roach GD, Dawson D. Perceptions of labour pain by mothers and their attending midwives. *J Adv Nurs.* 2001;35(2):171-179.

61. Williams AC, Morris J, Stevens K, et al. What influences midwives in estimating labour pain? *Eur J Pain.* 2013;17(1):86-93.

62. Rice MJ. Evidence-based practice principles: using the highest level when evidence is limited. *J Am Psychiatr Nurses Assoc.* 2011;17(6):445-448.

63. Varkey B. Principles of clinical ethics and their application to practice. *Med Princ Pract.* 2021;30(1): 17-28.

64. Schlaeger JM, Gabzdyl EM, Bussell JL, et al. Acupuncture and acupressure in labor. *J Midwifery Womens Health.* 2017;62(1):12-28.

65. Smith CA, Armour M, Dahlen HG. Acupuncture or acupressure for induction of labour. *Cochrane Database Syst Rev.* 2017;10:Cd002962.

66. Waters BL, Raisler J. Ice massage for the reduction of labor pain. *J Midwifery Womens Health.* 2003;48(5):317-321.

67. Smith CA, Collins CT, Levett KM, et al. Acupuncture or acupressure for pain management during labour. *Cochrane Database Syst Rev.* 2020;2:Cd009232.

68. Carlson JM, Diehl JA, Sachtleben-Murray M, et al. Maternal position during parturition in normal labor. *Obstet Gynecol.* 1986;68(4):443-447.

69. Fenwick L, Simkin P. Maternal positioning to prevent or alleviate dystocia in labor. *Clin Obstet Gynecol.* 1987;30(1):83-89.

70. Lawrence A, Lewis L, Hofmeyr GJ, Styles C. Maternal positions and mobility during first stage labour. *Cochrane Database Syst Rev.* 2013;10:Cd003934.

71. Gupta JK, Sood A, Hofmeyr GJ, Vogel JP. Position in the second stage of labour for women without epidural anaesthesia. *Cochrane Database Syst Rev.* 2017;5:Cd002006.

72. Kibuka M, Thornton JG. Position in the second stage of labour for women with epidural anaesthesia. *Cochrane Database Syst Rev.* 2017;2:Cd008070.

73. Smith CA, Collins CT, Crowther CA. Aromatherapy for pain management in labour. *Cochrane Database Syst Rev.* 2011;7:Cd009215.

74. Lakhan SE, Sheafer H, Tepper D. The effectiveness of aromatherapy in reducing pain: a systematic review and meta-analysis. *Pain Res Treat.* 2016;2016:8158693.

75. Sheppard-Hanger S, Hanger N. The importance of safety when using aromatherapy. *Int J Childbirth Educ.* 2015;30(1):42-47.

76. Hsieh C, Kong J, Kirsch I, et al. Well-loved music robustly relieves pain: a randomized, controlled trial. *PLoS One.* 2014;9(9):e107390.

77. Phumdoung S, Good M. Music reduces sensation and distress of labor pain. *Pain Manag Nurs.* 2003;4(2):54-61.

78. Dehcheshmeh FS, Rafiei H. Complementary and alternative therapies to relieve labor pain: a comparative study between music therapy and Hoku point ice massage. *Complement Ther Clin Pract.* 2015;21(4):229-232.

79. Smith CA, Collins CT, Cyna AM, Crowther CA. Complementary and alternative therapies for pain management in labour. *Cochrane Database Syst Rev.* 2006;4:Cd003521.

80. Delgado A, Maia T, Melo RS, Lemos A. Birth ball use for women in labor: a systematic review and meta-analysis. *Complement Ther Clin Pract.* 2019;35:92-101.

81. Grenvik JM, Rosenthal E, Wey S, et al. Birthing ball for reducing labor pain: a systematic review and meta-analysis of randomized controlled trials. *J Matern Fetal Neonatal Med.* 2021:1-10.

82. Roth C, Dent SA, Parfitt SE, et al. Randomized controlled trial of use of the peanut ball during labor. *MCN Am J Matern Child Nurs.* 2016;41(3):140-146.

83. Tussey CM, Botsios E, Gerkin RD, et al. Reducing length of labor and cesarean surgery rate using a peanut ball for women laboring with an epidural. *J Perinat Educ.* 2015;24(1):16-24.

84. Smith CA, Levett KM, Collins CT, et al. Relaxation techniques for pain management in labour. *Cochrane Database Syst Rev.* 2018;3:Cd009514.

85. Bohren MA, Hofmeyr GJ, Sakala C, et al. Continuous support for women during childbirth. *Cochrane Database Syst Rev.* 2017;7:Cd003766.

86. Fortier JH, Godwin M. Doula support compared with standard care: meta-analysis of the effects on the rate of medical interventions during labour for low-risk women delivering at term. *Can Fam Physician.* 2015;61(6):e284-e292.

87. Hodnett ED, Lowe NK, Hannah ME, et al. Effectiveness of nurses as providers of birth labor support in North American hospitals: a randomized controlled trial. *J Am Med Assoc.* 2002;288(11):1373-1381.

88. Paterno MT, Van Zandt SE, Murphy J, Jordan ET. Evaluation of a student-nurse doula program: an analysis of doula interventions and their impact on labor analgesia and cesarean birth. *J Midwifery Womens Health.* 2012;57(1):28-34.

89. Hodnett ED. Caregiver support for women during childbirth. *Cochrane Database Syst Rev.* 2002;1:Cd000199.

90. Hofmeyr GJ, Nikodem VC, Wolman WL, et al. Companionship to modify the clinical birth environment: effects on progress and perceptions of labour, and breastfeeding. *Br J Obstet Gynaecol.* 1991;98(8):756-764.

91. Taavoni S, Abdolahian S, Haghani H. Effect of sacrum–perineum heat therapy on active phase labor pain and client satisfaction: a randomized, controlled trial study. *Pain Med.* 2013;14(9):1301-1306.

92. Shirvani MA, Ganji Z. The influence of cold pack on labour pain relief and birth outcomes: a randomised controlled trial. *J Clin Nurs.* 2014;23(17-18):2473-2479.

93. Nutter E, Meyer S, Shaw-Battista J, Marowitz A. Waterbirth: an integrative analysis of peer-reviewed literature. *J Midwifery Womens Health.* 2014;59(3):286-319.

94. Benfield RD, Hortobágyi T, Tanner CJ, et al. The effects of hydrotherapy on anxiety, pain, neuroendocrine responses, and contraction dynamics during labor. *Biol Res Nurs.* 2010;12(1):28-36.

95. Benfield RD. Hydrotherapy in labor. *J Nurs Scholarsh.* 2002;34(4):347-352.

96. Shaw-Battista J. Systematic review of hydrotherapy research: does a warm bath in labor promote normal physiologic childbirth? *J Perinat Neonatal Nurs.* 2017;31(4):303-316.

97. Kane Low L, Nutter E. A model practice template for hydrotherapy in labor and birth. *J Midwifery Womens Health.* 2017;62(1):120-126.

98. Cluett ER, Burns E, Cuthbert A. Immersion in water during labour and birth. *Cochrane Database Syst Rev.* 2018;5:Cd000111.

99. Cluett ER, Burns E. Immersion in water in labour and birth. *Cochrane Database Syst Rev.* 2009;2:Cd000111.

100. Eriksson M, Ladfors L, Mattsson LA, Fall O. Warm tub bath during labor: a study of 1385 women with prelabor rupture of the membranes after 34 weeks of gestation. *Acta Obstet Gynecol Scand.* 1996;75(7):642-644.

101. Alexander B, Turnbull D, Cyna A. The effect of pregnancy on hypnotizability. *Am J Clin Hypn.* 2009; 52(1):13-22.

102. Werner A, Uldbjerg N, Zachariae R, et al. Antenatal hypnosis training and childbirth experience: a randomized controlled trial. *Birth.* 2013;40(4):272-280.

103. Madden K, Middleton P, Cyna AM, et al. Hypnosis for pain management during labour and childbirth. *Cochrane Database Syst Rev.* 2016;5:Cd009356.

104. Landolt AS, Milling LS. The efficacy of hypnosis as an intervention for labor and delivery pain: a comprehensive methodological review. *Clin Psychol Rev.* 2011;31(6):1022-1031.

105. Catsaros S, Wendland J. Hypnosis-based interventions during pregnancy and childbirth and their impact on women's childbirth experience: a systematic review. *Midwifery.* 2020;84:102666.

106. Aziato L, Odai PN, Omenyo CN. Religious beliefs and practices in pregnancy and labour: an inductive qualitative study among post-partum women in Ghana. *BMC Pregnancy Childbirth.* 2016;16(1):138.

107. Prinds C, Hvidtjørn D, Skytthe A, et al. Prayer and meditation among Danish first time mothers: a questionnaire study. *BMC Pregnancy Childbirth.* 2016; 16:8.

108. Hartle-Schutte M. *Contemporary Usage of the Blessingway Ceremony for Navajo Births.* Tucson, AZ: University of Arizona; 1988.

109. Derry S, Straube S, Moore RA, et al. Intracutaneous or subcutaneous sterile water injection compared with blinded controls for pain management in labour. *Cochrane Database Syst Rev.* 2012;1: Cd009107.

110. Hutton EK, Kasperink M, Rutten M, et al. Sterile water injection for labour pain: a systematic review and meta-analysis of randomised controlled trials. *BJOG.* 2009;116(9):1158-1166.

111. Lee N, Gao Y, Collins SL, et al. Caesarean delivery rates and analgesia effectiveness following injections of sterile water for back pain in labour: a multicentre, randomised placebo controlled trial. *EClin Med.* 2020;25:100447.

112. Simkin P, Ancheta R, Hanson L. *The Labor Progress Handbook: Early Interventions to Prevent and Treat Dystocia.* 3rd ed. Hoboken, NJ: Wiley-BLackwell; 2011.

113. Smith CA, Levett KM, Collins CT, et al. Massage, reflexology and other manual methods for pain management in labour. *Cochrane Database Syst Rev.* 2018;3:Cd009290.

114. Unalmis Erdogan S, Yanikkerem E, Goker A. Effects of low back massage on perceived birth pain and satisfaction. *Complement Ther Clin Pract.* 2017; 28:169-175.

115. Dowswell T, Bedwell C, Lavender T, Neilson JP. Transcutaneous electrical nerve stimulation (TENS) for pain relief in labour. *Cochrane Database Syst Rev.* 2009;2:Cd007214.

116. Carr DJ. The safety of obstetric acupuncture: forbidden points revisited. *Acupunct Med.* 2015;33(5): 413-419.

117. Dekker R. Aromatherapy during labor for pain relief. Evidence Based Birth website. https://evidencebased birth.com/aromatherapy-for-pain-relief-during -labor/. Published 2018. Accessed November 8, 2021.

118. Kazeminia M, Abdi A, Vaisi-Raygani A, et al. The effect of lavender (*Lavandula stoechas L.*) on reducing labor pain: a systematic review and meta-analysis. *Evid Based Complement Alternat Med.* 2020;2020:4384350.

119. Jones L, Othman M, Dowswell T, et al. Pain management for women in labour: an overview of systematic reviews. *Cochrane Database Syst Rev.* 2012;3: Cd009234.

120. Makvandi S, Latifnejad Roudsari R, Sadeghi R, Karimi L. Effect of birth ball on labor pain relief: a systematic review and meta-analysis. *J Obstet Gynaecol Res.* 2015;41(11):1679-1686.

121. Dykes H, Johnson J, Frazer C, Hussey L. Overview of hydrotherapy during labor. *Int J Childbirth Educ.* 2017;32(4):45-47.

122. Uludağ E, Mete S. The effect of nursing care provided based on the philosophy of hypnobirthing on fear, pain, duration, satisfaction and cost of labor: a single-blind randomized controlled study. *Health Care Women Int.* 2021;42(4-6):678-690.

123. Imannura P, Budhiastuti UR, Poncorini, E. The effectiveness of hypnobirthing in reducing anxiety level during delivery. *J Matern Child Health.* 2016;1(3):200-204.

124. Pachtman Shetty SL, Fogarty S. Massage during pregnancy and postpartum. *Clin Obstet Gynecol.* 2021; 64(3):648-660.

125. Stulz V, Liang X, Burns E. Midwives and women's experiences of sterile water injections for back pain during labour: an integrative review. *Midwifery.* 2021;103:103164.

126. Njogu A, Qin S, Chen Y, et al. The effects of transcutaneous electrical nerve stimulation during the first stage of labor: a randomized controlled trial. *BMC Pregnancy Childbirth.* 2021;21(1):164.

127. Shahoei R, Shahghebi S, Rezaei M, Naqshbandi S. The effect of transcutaneous electrical nerve stimulation on the severity of labor pain among

nulliparous women: a clinical trial. *Complement Ther Clin Pract.* 2017;28:176-180.

128. Bedwell C, Dowswell T, Neilson JP, Lavender T. The use of transcutaneous electrical nerve stimulation (TENS) for pain relief in labour: a review of the evidence. *Midwifery.* 2011;27(5):e141-e148.

129. Smith LA, Burns E, Cuthbert A. Parenteral opioids for maternal pain management in labour. *Cochrane Database Syst Rev.* 2018;6:Cd007396.

130. Likis FE, Andrews JC, Collins MR, et al. Nitrous oxide for the management of labor pain: a systematic review. *Anesth Analg.* 2014;118(1):153-167.

131. Nodine PM, Collins MR, Wood CL, et al. Nitrous oxide use during labor: satisfaction, adverse effects, and predictors of conversion to neuraxial analgesia. *J Midwifery Womens Health.* 2020;65(3):335-341.

132. Lim G, Facco FL, Nathan N, et al. A review of the impact of obstetric anesthesia on maternal and neonatal outcomes. *Anesthesiology.* 2018;129(1):192-215.

133. Anim-Somuah M, Smyth RM, Cyna AM, Cuthbert A. Epidural versus non-epidural or no analgesia for pain management in labour. *Cochrane Database Syst Rev.* 2018;5:Cd000331.

134. Toledano RD, Leffert L. What's new in neuraxial labor analgesia. *Curr Anesthesiol Rep.* 2021:1-8.

135. Markley JC, Rollins MD. Non-neuraxial labor analgesia: options. *Clin Obstet Gynecol.* 2017;60(2):350-364.

136. Phillips SN, Fernando R, Girard T. Parenteral opioid analgesia: does it still have a role? *Best Pract Res Clin Anaesthesiol.* 2017;31(1):3-14.

137. Ghelardini C, Di Cesare Mannelli L, Bianchi E. The pharmacological basis of opioids. *Clin Cases Miner Bone Metab.* 2015;12(3):219-221.

138. Anderson D. A review of systemic opioids commonly used for labor pain relief. *J Midwifery Womens Health.* 2011;56(3):222-239.

139. Weibel S, Jelting Y, Afshari A, et al. Patient-controlled analgesia with remifentanil versus alternative parenteral methods for pain management in labour. *Cochrane Database Syst Rev.* 2017;4:Cd011989.

140. Karol D, Weiniger CF. Update on non-neuraxial labor analgesia. *Curr Anesthesiol Rep.* 2021:1-7.

141. Practice guidelines for moderate procedural sedation and analgesia 2018: a report by the American Society of Anesthesiologists Task Force on Moderate Procedural Sedation and Analgesia, the American Association of Oral and Maxillofacial Surgeons, American College of Radiology, American Dental Association, American Society of Dentist Anesthesiologists, and Society of Interventional Radiology. *Anesthesiology.* 2018;128(3):437-479.

142. Rizk AH, Simonsen SE, Roberts L, et al. Maternity care for pregnant women with opioid use disorder: a review. *J Midwifery Womens Health.* 2019;64(5):532-544.

143. Ito S. Opioids in breast milk: pharmacokinetic principles and clinical implications. *J Clin Pharmacol.* 2018;58(suppl 10):S151-S163.

144. *Lexicomp Online.* UpToDate, Inc.; 2021. https://online-lexi-com.frontier.idm.oclc.org/lco/action/home. Accessed September 30, 2021.

145. *Drugs and Lactation Database (LactMed).* U.S. National Library of Medicine; 2021. https://www.ncbi.nlm.nih.gov/books/NBK501922/.

146. Moe-Byrne T, Brown JVE, McGuire W. Naloxone for opioid-exposed newborn infants. *Cochrane Database Syst Rev.* 2018;10:Cd003483.

147. Gibbs J, Newson T, Williams J, Davidson DC. Naloxone hazard in infant of opioid abuser. *Lancet.* 1989;2(8655):159-160.

148. Neonatal drug withdrawal. American Academy of Pediatrics Committee on Drugs. *Pediatrics.* 1998;101(6):1079-1088.

149. Maykin MM, Ukoha EP, Tilp V, et al. Impact of therapeutic rest in early labor on perinatal outcomes: a prospective study. *Am J Obstet Gynecol MFM.* 2021;3(3):100325.

150. Nanji JA, Carvalho B. Pain management during labor and vaginal birth. *Best Pract Res Clin Obstet Gynaecol.* 2020;67:100-112.

151. Othman M, Jones L, Neilson JP. Non-opioid drugs for pain management in labour. *Cochrane Database Syst Rev.* 2012;7:Cd009223.

152. Vallejo MC, Zakowski MI. Pro–con debate: nitrous oxide for labor analgesia. *Biomed Res Int.* 2019;2019:4618798.

153. Migliaccio L, Lawton R, Leeman L, Holbrook A. Initiating intrapartum nitrous oxide in an academic hospital: considerations and challenges. *J Midwifery Womens Health.* 2017;62(3):358-362.

154. Zanardo V, Volpe F, Parotto M, et al. Nitrous oxide labor analgesia and pain relief memory in breastfeeding women. *J Matern Fetal Neonatal Med.* 2018;31(24):3243-3248.

155. Rooks JP. Safety and risks of nitrous oxide labor analgesia: a review. *J Midwifery Womens Health.* 2011;56(6):557-565.

156. Richardson MG, Raymond BL, Baysinger CL, et al. A qualitative analysis of parturients' experiences using nitrous oxide for labor analgesia: it is not just about pain relief. *Birth.* 2019;46(1):97-104.

157. Sutton CD, Butwick AJ, Riley ET, Carvalho B. Nitrous oxide for labor analgesia: utilization and predictors of conversion to neuraxial analgesia. *J Clin Anesth.* 2017;40:40-45.

158. Nagele P, Zeugswetter B, Wiener C, et al. Influence of methylenetetrahydrofolate reductase gene

polymorphisms on homocysteine concentrations after nitrous oxide anesthesia. *Anesthesiology.* 2008; 109(1):36-43.

159. Nagele P, Brown F, Francis A, et al. Influence of nitrous oxide anesthesia, B-vitamins, and MTHFR gene polymorphisms on perioperative cardiac events: the Vitamins in Nitrous Oxide (VINO) randomized trial. *Anesthesiology.* 2013;119(1):19-28.

160. Dochez V, Esbelin J, Misbert E, et al. Effectiveness of nitrous oxide in external cephalic version on success rate: a randomized controlled trial. *Acta Obstet Gynecol Scand.* 2020;99(3):391-398.

161. Wood C, Arbet J, Amura CR, et al. Multicenter study evaluating nitrous oxide use for labor analgesia at high- and low-altitude institutions. *Anesth Analg.* 2021;134(2):294-302.

162. Delgado C, Bollag L, Van Cleve W. Neuraxial labor analgesia utilization, incidence of postdural puncture headache, and epidural blood patch placement for privately insured parturients in the United States (2008–2015). *Anesth Analg.* 2020;131(3):850-856.

163. Roberson MC. Refusal of epidural anesthesia for labor pain management by African American parturients: an examination of factors. *AANA J.* 2019; 87(4):299-304.

164. Hoyt MR, Shah U, Cooley J, Temple M. Use of epidural clonidine for the management of analgesia in the opioid addicted parturient on buprenorphine maintenance therapy: an observational study. *Int J Obstet Anesth.* 2018;34:67-72.

165. Kollmeier BR, Boyette LC, Beecham GB, et al. Difficult airway. In: *StatPearls.* Treasure Island, FL: StatPearls Publishing; 2022. https://www.ncbi.nlm.nih.gov/books/NBK470224/. Accessed December 12, 2022.

166. Zipori Y, Jakobi P, Solt I, Abecassis P. The need for an epidural "window of opportunity" in pregnant women with a lumbar tattoo. *Int J Obstet Anesth.* 2018;33:53-56.

167. Simmons SW, Taghizadeh N, Dennis AT, et al. Combined spinal–epidural versus epidural analgesia in labour. *Cochrane Database Syst Rev.* 2012; 10:Cd003401.

168. McQuaid E, Leffert LR, Bateman BT. The role of the anesthesiologist in preventing severe maternal morbidity and mortality. *Clin Obstet Gynecol.* 2018;61(2):372-386.

169. Kinsella SM, Carvalho B, Dyer RA, et al. International consensus statement on the management of hypotension with vasopressors during caesarean section under spinal anaesthesia. *Anaesthesia.* 2018;73(1):71-92.

170. Yurashevich M, Carvalho B, Butwick AJ, et al. Determinants of women's dissatisfaction with anaesthesia care in labour and delivery. *Anaesthesia.* 2019;74(9):1112-1120.

171. Kumar K, Singh SI. Neuraxial opioid-induced pruritus: an update. *J Anaesthesiol Clin Pharmacol.* 2013;29(3):303-307.

172. Wilson BL, Passante T, Rauschenbach D, et al. Bladder management with epidural anesthesia during labor: a randomized controlled trial. *MCN Am J Matern Child Nurs.* 2015;40(4):234-242; quiz E217-E238.

173. Sharpe EE, Arendt KW. Epidural labor analgesia and maternal fever. *Clin Obstet Gynecol.* 2017; 60(2):365-374.

174. Shatken S, Greenough K, McPherson C. Epidural fever and its implications for mothers and neonates: taking the heat. *J Midwifery Womens Health.* 2012;57(1):82-85.

175. Osborne C, Ecker JL, Gauvreau K, et al. Maternal temperature elevation and occiput posterior position at birth among low-risk women receiving epidural analgesia. *J Midwifery Womens Health.* 2011;56(5):446-451.

176. Jansen S, Lopriore E, Naaktgeboren C, et al. Epidural-related fever and maternal and neonatal morbidity: a systematic review and meta-analysis. *Neonatology.* 2020;117(3):259-270.

177. Lieberman E, O'Donoghue C. Unintended effects of epidural analgesia during labor: a systematic review. *Am J Obstet Gynecol.* 2002;186(5 suppl Nature):S31-S68.

178. Vermani E, Mittal R, Weeks A. Pelvic girdle pain and low back pain in pregnancy: a review. *Pain Pract.* 2010;10(1):60-71.

179. Hung TH, Hsieh TT, Liu HP. Differential effects of epidural analgesia on modes of delivery and perinatal outcomes between nulliparous and multiparous women: a retrospective cohort study. *PLoS One.* 2015;10(3):e0120907.

180. Shmueli A, Salman L, Orbach-Zinger S, et al. The impact of epidural analgesia on the duration of the second stage of labor. *Birth.* 2018;45(4):377-384.

181. Ando H, Makino S, Takeda J, et al. Comparison of the labor curves with and without combined spinal–epidural analgesia in nulliparous women: a retrospective study. *BMC Pregnancy Childbirth.* 2020;20(1):467.

182. Luo S, Chen Z, Wang X, et al. Labor epidural analgesia versus without labor epidural analgesia for multiparous women: a retrospective case control study. *BMC Anesthesiol.* 2021;21(1):133.

183. Zhang L, Xu C, Li Y. Impact of epidural labor analgesia using sufentanil combined with low-concentration ropivacaine on maternal and neonatal outcomes: a retrospective cohort study. *BMC Anesthesiol.* 2021;21(1):229.

184. Wang TT, Sun S, Huang SQ. Effects of epidural labor analgesia with low concentrations of local

anesthetics on obstetric outcomes: a systematic review and meta-analysis of randomized controlled trials. *Anesth Analg.* 2017;124(5):1571-1580.

185. Sultan P, Murphy C, Halpern S, Carvalho B. The effect of low concentrations versus high concentrations of local anesthetics for labour analgesia on obstetric and anesthetic outcomes: a meta-analysis. *Can J Anaesth.* 2013;60(9):840-854.

186. Hickey L, Savage J. Effect of peanut ball and position changes in women laboring with an epidural. *Nurs Womens Health.* 2019;23(3):245-252.

187. Mercier RJ, Kwan M. Impact of peanut ball device on the duration of active labor: a randomized control trial. *Am J Perinatol.* 2018;35(10):1006-1011.

188. Cahill AG, Srinivas SK, Tita ATN, et al. Effect of immediate vs delayed pushing on rates of spontaneous vaginal delivery among nulliparous women receiving neuraxial analgesia: a randomized clinical trial. *J Am Med Assoc.* 2018;320(14):1444-1454.

189. Walker KF, Kibuka M, Thornton JG, Jones NW. Maternal position in the second stage of labour for women with epidural anaesthesia. *Cochrane Database Syst Rev.* 2018;11:Cd008070.

190. Zheng S, Zheng W, Zhu T, et al. Continuing epidural analgesia during the second stage and ACOG definition of arrest of labor on maternal–fetal outcomes. *Acta Anaesthesiol Scand.* 2020;64(8):1187-1193.

191. Wang K, Cao L, Deng Q, et al. The effects of epidural/spinal opioids in labour analgesia on neonatal outcomes: a meta-analysis of randomized controlled trials. *Can J Anaesth.* 2014;61(8):695-709.

192. Bai DL, Wu KM, Tarrant M. Association between intrapartum interventions and breastfeeding duration. *J Midwifery Womens Health.* 2013;58(1):25-32.

193. Orbach-Zinger S, Landau R, Davis A, et al. The effect of labor epidural analgesia on breastfeeding outcomes: a prospective observational cohort study in a mixed-parity cohort. *Anesth Analg.* 2019; 129(3):784-791.

194. Anderson D. Pudendal nerve block for vaginal birth. *J Midwifery Womens Health.* 2014;59(6):651-659.

195. Pagès H, de la Gastine B, Quedru-Aboane J, et al. [Lidocaine intoxication in newborn following maternal pudendal anesthesia: report of three cases]. *J Gynecol Obstet Biol Reprod (Paris).* 2008;37(4):415-418.

196. Waldum ÅH, Staff AC, Lukasse M, et al. Intrapartum pudendal nerve block analgesia and risk of postpartum urinary retention: a cohort study. *Int Urogynecol J.* 2021;32(9):2383-2391.

197. Lim MJ, Tan HS, Tan CW, et al. The effects of labor on airway outcomes with Supreme™ laryngeal mask in women undergoing cesarean delivery under general anesthesia: a cohort study. *BMC Anesthesiol.* 2020;20(1):213.

198. American College of Nurse-Midwives. Providing oral nutrition to women in labor. *J Midwifery Womens Health.* 2016;61(4):528-534.

APPENDIX

# 28A

# Sterile Water Injections for the Relief of Low Back Pain in Labor

LENA B. MÅRTENSSON AND NIGEL LEE

Approximately 30% of individuals in labor experience severe continuous low back pain.[1] Back pain in labor is often associated by intrapartum providers with a fetal occipito-posterior position;[2] however, it is equally prevalent with occipito-anterior fetal positions.[3,4] The tension caused by low back pain has been associated with an increased need for pain medication.[5] Several techniques have been reported to be helpful in managing this pain, including massage, counterpressure, applied heat or ice, transcutaneous electrical nerve stimulation (TENS), and hydrotherapy. However, only the use of sterile water injections is specific to the management of back pain in labor.

While earlier reviews suggested sterile water injections were effective in providing pain relief in labor,[5-7] a Cochrane review published in 2012 reported that there was insufficient evidence to support the analgesic effect of water injections from placebo-controlled trials.[8] However, evidence published in 2020 confirmed the findings of previous systematic reviews and meta-analyses[5-7] that intradermal sterile water injections provide pain relief for back pain during labor.[4] In that large ($N = 1166$), placebo-controlled trial, sterile water injections resulted in an immediate 30% to 50% reduction in pain for as long as 2 hours.[4]

Sterile water injections offer the advantage of requiring minimal, readily available equipment; moreover, they are adaptable to any birth setting and are easy to administer. There are no systemic side effects for the person or the fetus. Birthing people who use this method of pain relief are able to ambulate and move freely afterward. There is no need for additional fetal heart rate monitoring or other supplemental interventions.[9]

The main disadvantage of sterile water injections is the sensation of intense burning or stinging at time of application—an effect that lasts 20 to 40 seconds. This pain can discourage laboring people from initial use or reapplication of the injections. In a study conducted with female persons who were not pregnant, researchers found that subcutaneous injections were less painful than intradermal injections.[10] However, this experience of lower pain during subcutaneous sterile water injections was not noted in another study with laboring participants, although their pain relief was the same, regardless of injection method.[11]

## Method to Place Sterile Water Injections

1. Prior to beginning the procedure:
   - Prepare two 1-cc syringes (one for two midwives) with 0.6 mL of sterile water each (do not use normal saline) and a 25-gauge needle. It is preferable for two midwives, or a midwife and a nurse, to give the injections simultaneously.
   - Gather alcohol swabs, pen(s) for marking the skin, and gloves to avoid introduction of pathogens and to protect the provider from exposure to the woman's blood.

2. Explain the procedure to the laboring person and their support people.
   - Benefits include relief of back pain, lack of systemic maternal or fetal side effects, and continued ability to ambulate or move as desired.

- Risks include intense burning pain at the injection sites for 30 to 90 seconds and less effective pain relief than desired.
- Relief occurs by 2 minutes of completion of injections. Prepare the laboring person and their support persons with methods of maintaining a stable position and coping with discomfort during the procedure.

3. Place the person in a sitting, kneeling, lying, or standing position where they can stabilize themselves with their arms and hands as they lean forward slightly. The injection sites in the sacral area will be more visible when the person leans forward and flattens their back.

4. Expose their lower back enough to visualize the sacral dimples, which correspond to the superior iliac spines. The iliac spines are connected to the skin by a ligament; in some people this ligament is shortened, forming the sacral dimple. If the sacral dimple is not evident, place your hands on the person's waist and move your thumbs down to the sacral area at approximately a 30-degree angle. In this position, your thumbs will rest approximately on the iliac spines. Mark these landmarks with a pen.

5. Place the index finger at these pen marks and move the thumbs about 3 to 4 cm down and 1 to 2 cm inward to form a trapezoid (Figure 28A-1); mark these points as well. Alternatively, ask the person to indicate the most painful area of their back pain and plot four injection points surrounding that local area. The positions of the injection points are not integral to the pain relief experienced, provided the injection points surround the localized area of pain.

6. Clean the sites with an alcohol swab, taking care not to erase the marks indicating the area to be injected. Put on sterile gloves. Remind the person that they will feel temporary burning and stinging as the injections are placed.

7. Plan to do the injections quickly during a contraction.
- The intradermal injections are very shallow in depth. Position the syringe almost parallel with the skin, with the bevel end of the needle facing up. Insert the needle into the skin just beyond the depth of the bevel.
- Inject 0.1 to 0.3 mL intradermally in each of the four points until the distended skin forms a small (0.3 to 0.5 cm) blanched bleb or papule. The papule or bleb should start to appear as soon as you start to inject the sterile water.
- The amount you inject will depend on your visual estimation of the resulting bleb, which should be 3 to 5 mm in diameter.
- If the intradermal injection is too deep, you will not see a bleb. In that case, you need to reposition your needle and injected more fluid.
- If using the subcutaneous method, insert the needle vertically into the anterior subcutaneous tissue and inject 0.5 mL for each injection. The resulting bleb will be less obvious.

8. The onset of relief should occur within 2 minutes.

9. Once the effects have worn off (in 1 to 3 hours), the injections may be repeated with the laboring person's consent.

10. Document the person's consent for the procedure. Also, document the time of injections and patient pain scores both before and after the procedure.

## References

1. Melzack R, Schaffeberg D. Low-back pain during labour. *Am J Obstet Gynecol*. 1987;158:901-905. https://doi.org/10.1016/0002-9378(87)90349-8.

2. Lee N, Kildea S, Stapleton H. "Facing the wrong way": exploring the occipito posterior position/back pain discourse from women's and midwives' perspectives. *Midwifery*. 2015;31(10):1008-1014. https://doi.org/10.1016/j.midw.2015.06.003.

3. Lieberman E, Davidson K, Lee-Parritz A, Shearer E. Changes in fetal position during labor and their association with epidural analgesia. *Obstet Gynecol*. 2005;105(5 pt 1):974-982. doi:10.1097/01.AOG.0000158861.43593.49.

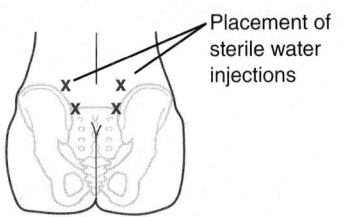

**Figure 28A-1** Placement of sterile water injections.

4. Lee N, Gao Y, Collins SL, et al. Caesarean delivery rates and analgesia effectiveness following injections of sterile water for back pain in labour: a multicentre, randomised placebo controlled trial. *EClin Med.* 2020;25:100447. https://doi.org/10.1016/j.eclinm.2020.100447.

5. Hutton EK, Kasperink M, Rutten M, et al. Sterile water injection for labour pain: a systematic review and meta-analysis of randomised controlled trials. *BJOG.* 2009;116(9):1158-1166. https://doi.org/10.1111/j.1471-0528.2009.02221.x.

6. Fogarty V. Intradermal sterile water injections for the relief of low back pain in labour: a systematic review of the literature. *Women Birth.* 2008;21(4):157-163. https://doi.org/10.1016/j.wombi.2008.08.003.

7. Martensson L, Wallin G. Sterile water injections as treatment for low-back pain during labour: a review. *Austral NZ J Obstet Gynaecol.* 2008;48(4):369-374. doi:AJO856. pii:10.1111/j.1479-828X.2008.00856.x.

8. Derry S, Straube S, Moore RA, et al. Intracutaneous or subcutaneous sterile water injection compared with blinded controls for pain management in labour. *Cochrane Database Syst Rev.* 2012;1. doi:10.1002/14651858.CD009107.pub2.

9. Mårtensson LB, Hutton EK, Lee N, et al. Sterile water injections for childbirth pain: an evidenced based guide to practice. *Women Birth.* 2018;31(5):380-385. https://doi.org/10.1016/j.wombi.2017.12.001.

10. Martensson L, Nyberg K, Wallin G. Subcutaneous versus intracutaneous injections of sterile water for labour analgesia: a comparison of perceived pain during administration. *BJOG.* 2000;107(10):1248-1251. https://doi.org/10.1111/j.1471-0528.2000.tb11615.x.

11. Martensson L, Wallin G. Labour pain treated with cutaneous injections of sterile water: a randomised controlled trial. *Br J Obstet Gynaecol.* 1999;106(7):633-637.https://doi.org/10.1111/j.1471-0528.1999.tb08359.x.

CHAPTER

# 29

# Second Stage of Labor and Birth

HEATHER BRADFORD

*The editors acknowledge Lisa Kane Low and Kathryn Osborne for their contributions to this chapter in the previous edition. Julia Phillippi contributed information on management of perineal lacerations to this version of the chapter.*

## Introduction

The second stage of labor is a vulnerable and transformational phase of the birth experience for most people. Birth is a developmental and societal milestone, during which the birthing person transitions to the role of parent. By providing a continuous, supportive, and therapeutic presence during the second stage, midwives can not only support physiologic labor and birth, but also encourage optimal outcomes for the family. During pregnancy and labor, the role of the midwife has best been described as watchful waiting or "the art of doing 'nothing' well."[1] The midwife anticipates needs and is vigilant in assessment of birthing persons during labor and birth, while remaining cognizant of the wide range of what constitutes normal and where the boundaries of abnormal begin. All persons involved participate in shared decision making, with the midwife being responsive, rather than reactive, and supportive, rather than directive during physiologic birth. This chapter reviews midwifery management during the second stage of labor and birth.

## Definition and Phases of Second-Stage Labor

Second-stage labor is defined as beginning with complete dilation of the cervix (10 cm) and ending with birth of the neonate.[2] In birthing persons without epidural analgesia who are not coached to push, three distinct phases are typically experienced within the second stage of labor.[3,4]

The first phase, called the latent phase, is experienced if the fetus is above 0 station when the cervix becomes completely dilated. A subtle indicator of the latent phase is a lull in the frequency and intensity of contractions.

In the second phase, called the active expulsive phase, the physiologic urge to push is typically activated when the fetal presenting part reaches +1 station. Bearing-down efforts become progressively stronger, promoting fetal rotation and descent. Many people experience the beginning of the active expulsive phase as a need to have a bowel movement. Signs of the active expulsive phase also include location of the fetal heart rate (FHR) in progressively lower parts of the abdomen, rectal bulging, perineal bulging, and progressive visibility of the presenting part at the vaginal introitus. In addition, there may be an increase in bloody show, and the FHR pattern may demonstrate variable decelerations secondary to the presenting part descending with spontaneous bearing-down efforts. In rare cases, some birthing persons not using epidural analgesia do not feel the urge to bear down.

The final phase of second-stage labor occurs when the fetal head is visible at the introitus. During this last phase, a strong sense of pressure combined with a sensation of stretching often results in pushing efforts even between contractions.[2,5]

### Fetal Descent During Second-Stage Labor

During the second stage of labor, the fetus descends. Internal rotation often takes place during the late first stage or in the second stage. Birth of the head occurs first with flexion of the fetal neck, followed by extension and external rotation. This process can occur very quickly, especially for an individual who has given birth before, or it can occur over a period of time, as is more common for a nulliparous individual. A detailed description of the cardinal movements that describe fetal passage through the birth canal during labor and birth is found in the *Anatomy and Physiology of Labor and Birth* chapter.

### Duration of Second-Stage Labor

For several decades, the norms used to define the duration of second-stage labor were based on investigations conducted in the 1950s and early 1960s by Emanuel A. Friedman using a small sample of 500 participants from one geographic location.[4,6] According to Freidman, the average length of the second stage was 46 minutes for nulliparous individuals and 14 minutes for multiparous individuals.[4] During this era, labor management strategies differed from those employed in contemporary practice. For example, approximately 55% of participants in Friedman's observations had their second stage expedited by application of low or mid-forceps. In addition, widespread use of epidural analgesia for pain management in the past few decades has slowed the pace of fetal descent during bearing-down efforts compared to this time period. Thus, Friedman's analysis of second-stage duration was more an observation of practice patterns at the time rather than an investigation of the natural course of the second stage that would be applicable to modern individuals.

New definitions of second-stage labor were provided in 2010 by Zhang et al. in their study of 62,414 term, spontaneous vaginal deliveries. Those researchers reported a wider range of "normal" second-stage labor duration, with the 95th percentile of nulliparous study participants progressing to a spontaneous vaginal birth after as long as 2.8 and 3.6 hours without and with an epidural, respectively.[7] More recently, a systematic review reported that among nulliparous birthing persons with an epidural ($n = 4081$) and prolonged (more than 3 hours) second stage, the primary cesarean and operative vaginal birth rates were low (19.8% and 21.6%, respectively), and the spontaneous vaginal birth rate was high (58.9%).[8] This suggests that the 3-hour time limit is too stringent in nulliparous birthing persons who receive epidural analgesia. This study did not report adverse perinatal outcomes, but other studies of prolonged second-stage labor have not reported higher rates of severe morbidity or mortality.[9]

It is difficult to precisely define the outer bounds of safe second-stage labor duration for every person due to the multiple short- and long-term perinatal outcomes that must be considered. However, in 2014, the American College of Obstetricians and Gynecologists (ACOG) and Society for Maternal–Fetal Medicine (SMFM) published guidelines that defined a prolonged second stage for nulliparous individuals as more than 3 hours without epidural analgesia or 4 hours with epidural analgesia, and for multiparous people, 2 hours without or 3 hours with epidural analgesia (Table 29-1).[10] Outcomes research examining the perinatal complications associated with a prolonged second-stage is discussed in the *Complications During Labor and Birth* chapter.

Factors associated with the duration of the second stage of labor are listed in Table 29-2.[2,10–14] For birthing persons who have no health or antenatal conditions at the onset of labor, the three factors that have the strongest association with the duration of the second stage are parity, fetal position, and the presence or absence of epidural analgesia. More information on assessment of labor progress can be found in the *Fetal–Pelvic Relationships* appendix.

| Table 29-1 | Average Length of Second Stage of Labor in Hours | | | |
|---|---|---|---|---|
| | **Nulliparous** | | **Multiparous** | |
| | **Without Epidural** | **With Epidural** | **Without Epidural** | **With Epidural** |
| Median length[*] | 0.6 | 1.1 | 0.1–0.2 | 0.3–0.4 |
| Prolonged labor (95%)[†] | > 3 | > 4 | > 2 | > 3 |

[*] Based on Consortium on Safe Labor data ($n = 62,415$).[7]

[†] Based on American College of Obstetricians and Gynecologists and Society for Maternal–Fetal Medicine guidelines.[10]

| Table 29-2 | Factors Associated with Length of Second Stage of Labor |
|---|---|
| Passage factors | Parity |
| | Position of birthing person |
| | Soft-tissue resistance |
| | Pelvic architecture |
| | Body habitus and height of the birthing person |
| Passenger factors | Occiput position and degree of flexion |
| | Station at complete dilation |
| | Fetal weight |
| Power factors | Uterine contraction activity (strength and frequency) |
| | Spontaneous onset versus induction of labor |
| | Pain or discomfort |
| | Infection status |
| | Pushing effort, effectiveness, and fatigue |
| Other factors | Epidural analgesia |
| | "Laboring down" approach prior to active pushing |
| | Length of first stage |
| | Fear or anxiety |
| | History of sexual abuse or trauma |
| | Health/antenatal conditions such as hypertensive disorders and gestational diabetes |
| | Age of the birthing person |
| | Level of engagement and support from nurses and clinicians |

Sources: Caughey AB, Cahill AG, Guise JM, Rouse DJ. Safe prevention of the primary cesarean delivery. *Am J Obstet Gynecol.* 2014;210(3):179-193. doi:10.1016/j.ajog.2014.01.026; Obstetric Care Consensus No. 1: safe prevention of the primary cesarean delivery. *Obstet Gynecol.* 2014;123(3):693-711. doi:10.1097/01.AOG.0000444441.04111.1d; Morcos C, Caughey AB. Passive descent in the second stage: evaluation of variation in practice patterns. *J Matern Fetal Neonatal Med.* 2018;31(17):2271-2275. doi:10.1080/14767058.2017.1340448; Cheng YW, Caughey AB. Defining and managing normal and abnormal second stage of labor. *Obstet Gynecol Clin North Am.* 2017;44(4):547-566. doi:10.1016/j.ogc.2017.08.009; Myers ER, Sanders GD, Coeytaux RR, et al. *AHRQ Comparative Effectiveness Reviews: Labor Dystocia.* Rockville, MD: Agency for Healthcare Research and Quality; 2020; National Academies of Sciences, Engineering, and Medicine. *Birth Settings in America: Outcomes, Quality, Access, and Choice.* 2020. https://doi.org/10.17226/25636.

## Assessment of Well-Being in Second Stage of Labor

Assessment during the second stage of labor includes evaluation of the birthing person's well-being, fetal well-being, and progress of labor, as described in Table 29-3.[15,16] In general, the midwife stays with the birthing person during the second stage. Critical elements of a second-stage labor note are presented in the following subsections.

### Vital Signs

The birthing person's blood pressure is taken between contractions and is, on average, 10 mm Hg higher in the second stage than the values obtained during the first stage of labor if the person has been pushing. Similarly, an increase in the birthing person's pulse is often seen during contractions. However, immediate action is required when any Maternal Early Warning Signs (MEWS) criteria for blood pressure, heart rate, respiratory rate, oxygen saturation, and oliguria are met. See the *Complications During Labor and Birth* chapter for more information.

Among birthing persons who have an epidural, approximately 30% will experience a temperature higher than 99.5°F, and this rate increases with the duration of the epidural and in nulliparous individuals. It is not associated with infection, and the etiology remains unknown.[17] Fever (temperature greater than or equal to 100.4°F orally that persists after 30 minutes) requires intervention. See the *Medical Complications in Pregnancy* chapter for information on management of intrauterine infection.

### Bladder

With an unmedicated birth, birthing persons should be encouraged to empty their bladder frequently, especially if they are receiving intravenous fluids. An empty bladder allows more space for the fetal descent, and the ambulation and position changes needed to get to the toilet also promote progress of the second stage.

Epidural analgesia reduces the ability to void, so it increases the laboring person's risk for urinary retention and distension.[18] In those persons who receive epidural analgesia, the bladder often contains larger volumes of residual urine compared to those individuals who have not had an epidural. If an indwelling catheter is in place at the onset of the second stage, it should be removed when pushing

| Table 29-3 | Overview of Midwifery Care and Charting During the Second Stage of Labor | |
|---|---|---|
| **Category** | **Component** | **Charting Section** |
| Foundational background | Gravida, para | Presenting concern and background |
| | Gestational age | |
| | Spontaneous/inducted/augmented labor and indication if applicable | |
| | Length of first and second stages, including active pushing time | |
| | Membrane status and rupture time/duration and fluid color if applicable | |
| | Current coping strategies, including medications and position | |
| | Support people present and their engagement | |
| Birthing person's subjective report | Comments about well-being, comfort/pressure/pain, anxiety, fear, and needs | Subjective |
| | Plans/desires for birth, postpartum, and parenting as relevant | |
| Birthing person's overall well-being | Coping/pain response | Objective |
| | Current comfort measures and their effectiveness | |
| | Level of fatigue | |
| | Hydration and nutrition | |
| Birthing person's vital signs | Blood pressure is taken between contractions every 15 minutes unless more frequent evaluation is indicated. | Objective |
| | Temperature and pulse are measured hourly, unless more frequent evaluations are indicated. Assessment of respirations is facility dependent. | |
| | Bladder distension (and urinary output as needed) is assessed hourly.<br>• Individuals in second-stage labor may need to be reminded to void, as their feeling of bladder pressure is altered.<br>• Intermittent catheterization may be needed if the individual is unable to void spontaneously.<br>• If an indwelling catheter is in place at the onset of the second stage, it should be removed when pushing is initiated and fetal descent is noted. | |
| Labor progress | Contraction pattern (frequency, duration, intensity, resting tone) and method of assessment (palpation, tocodynamometer, intrauterine pressure catheter). Note if the birthing person's sensations of contractions are not reflected by monitors. | Objective |
| | If applicable, current rate of Pitocin administration and total hours of use | |
| | Pushing effort | |
| | Fetal descent | |
| | Fetal position including synclitism or asynclitism, and any notable changes from the last exam | |
| | Fetal station (molding or caput succedaneum obscuring assessment) and change from last exam or with pushing effort | |
| | See the *Fetal–Pelvic Relationships* appendix. | |
| Fetal well-being[a] | Assess fetal heart rate every 5–15 minutes, noting the type of monitoring performed (intermittent, external monitor, fetal scalp electrode).[15,16] Increase frequency of assessment as the presenting part descends, or with longer second-stage labor durations. | Objective |
| | Describe the fetal heart rate using standard terminology. | |
| | See the *Fetal Assessment During Labor* chapter. | |

| Category | Component | Charting Section |
|---|---|---|
| Assessment and summary | Present concise summary of foundation information | Assessment |
| | Gravida, para at gestational age in (spontaneous/inducted/augmented) labor | |
| | Total time in second-stage labor and total time actively pushing | |
| | Progress (descent and rotation) made during second-stage labor | |
| | Pertinent diagnoses of the birthing person (e.g., preeclampsia) | |
| | Assessment of the birthing person's well-being | |
| | Categorize fetal status using standard terminology | |
| Planning for future care | Planned midwifery management (e.g., continued pushing or plans for rest, position changes every *x* minutes, hydration) | Plan |
| | Address any nonreassuring information provided in the assessment | |
| | Anticipated time to reevaluate progress and dyadic health, or plan to consult with a physician and the indication | |
| | Anticipated mode of birth if applicable (physiologic birth, assisted birth, cesarean) | |

is initiated and fetal descent is noted to minimize trauma to the urethra with fetal head compression.

If the individual has a distended bladder and is unable to void, intermittent catheterization may be indicated to facilitate fetal descent and minimize risk of postpartum hemorrhage. If the fetal head is in the true pelvis, it may be necessary to direct the catheter upward and over the fetal head to guide it into the bladder due to displacement of the urethra.

## Hydration and Nutrition in Second Stage

Oral consumption of fluids and food during labor is important for hydration, nutrition, and comfort. Self-regulated oral intake in labor has also been associated with increased feelings of control and lower stress levels.[19] The second stage of labor requires active physical work. However, historically, laboring people had their oral intake of fluids and food limited in hospital settings due to the care team's concerns about aspiration during or after the administration of general anesthesia, especially among birthing persons with epidural anesthesia. However, prolonged fasting in labor is associated with increased production of ketones, which may result in ketosis for the birthing person. Consequences of limited fluid or nutritional intake can include a rising pulse rate and limited energy or fatigue, as well as dissatisfaction with the birth experience. Theoretically, ketosis can cause dysfunctional uterine contractions, although this has not been definitively shown.

In a 2017 meta-analysis of 3982 birthing persons, researchers found that less-restrictive food intake was associated with significantly shorter duration of labor and no negative perinatal outcomes.[19] In 2016, the American Society of Anesthesiologists revised its position to recommend that birthing persons in hospital settings whose labors are progressing normally be offered modest amounts of clear liquids.[20] Clear liquid options include water, fruit juices without pulp, carbonated beverages, clear tea, black coffee, and electrolyte-enhanced drinks.[20,21] In the wake of this research and updated recommendations, some hospitals lifted their restrictions on oral intake during labor. By contrast, in community birth settings, oral hydration and nutrition during labor is encouraged.

The midwife can promote self-determination of appropriate oral intake, considering the health status of the individual, their preferences, the risk of surgical intervention, and the policies of the birth setting. Birthing persons should be encouraged to take oral hydration by offering clear liquids or ice chips between pushing efforts. After the intensity of the labor transition, encouragement of sips of fluids with calories and electrolytes during the second stage may be beneficial. If the individual is unable to maintain oral hydration, intravenous fluids may be indicated. The presence of an epidural should not alter the recommendation to maintain oral hydration during labor if the individual desires it.[21]

## Assessment of Pain and Coping

During the second stage of labor, new physical sensations occur as the birthing person nears the time of birth. Anticipatory guidance as the second stage progresses can help the individual cope with pressure sensations, perineal stretching, and potentially, an uncontrollable urge to bear down.

If a birthing person is crying out rather than grunting and bearing down, or is unable to sustain any position of comfort, they may be suffering distress instead of coping. Some individuals will experience sudden fear and anxiety with the sensations of vaginal stretching. Birthing persons who have experienced past sexual abuse or assault may be at particular risk for fear or panic, which may escalate when the presenting part induces new sensations in the pelvic floor or perineum.[22] Orienting the person to typical sensations, providing close support, and assisting the person in finding a location in the room or position that promotes their sense of control may be helpful. Some individuals find that perineal support (provided with their own hand or by the midwife) can be helpful, as can the application of warm washcloths. If those measures are not helpful, pain relief that ameliorates this perineal sensation may be necessary for the birthing person to push. A pudendal block can be used if an epidural is not available or desired[23] (see the *Pudendal Nerve Block* appendix). Nitrous oxide may also be used to support coping in second stage of labor.

### Fatigue

Some individuals begin the active process of pushing with renewed energy and excitement. Others enter the second stage of labor with exhaustion, especially if their first stage was tiring. Since fatigue can contribute to a prolonged second stage, it is important to monitor the energy level of the birthing person, provide appropriate support, and encourage periods of rest between bearing-down efforts. Suggestions to offer the birthing person to promote the burst of energy often needed in the second stage include increasing the lighting in the room, consuming a popsicle or sips of fluids with calories and electrolytes, washing the neck or forehead with a cold cloth, listening to different music, and/or brushing the teeth. The amount of added energy a birthing person requires for the process of pushing varies greatly depending on their previous birth history and the factors identified in Table 29-2. The labor support team often becomes more engaged as birth nears and provides encouragement to the birthing person.

### Evaluation of Fetal Well-Being

The assessment of the FHR or fetal heart tones during the second stage of labor is reviewed in more detail in the *Fetal Assessment During Labor* chapter. Variant FHR patterns are more common in the second stage than in the first stage, especially variable decelerations, prolonged decelerations, and bradycardias. Thus, the FHR is evaluated more frequently in second-stage labor. Current standards recommend assessment every 15 minutes in the absence of risk for fetal acidemia and every 5 minutes when an increased risk for acidemia is present.[15,16] In practice, the FHR is evaluated more frequently as the second stage progresses and is often checked every two to three contractions in the final phases of the second stage. This information is used to guide the midwife in determining the optimal position of the laboring person, planning for the location of birth, and determining whether additional personnel should be present or nearby at the moment of birth.

## Midwifery Management of the Second Stage of Labor

A hallmark of midwifery care is the empowerment of individuals as partners in their care, which is of utmost importance during the second stage of labor.[24] The midwife can promote a quiet, calm, client-centered atmosphere and encourage a birthing person to listen to their body, trust their body, and engage in pushing efforts in ways that feel most comfortable to them. Incorporating a clinical assessment of fetal position is also of value when the birthing person asks for specific suggestions.[25] In addition, the midwife can facilitate the efforts of everyone in the birthing room to provide additional support. Suggestions can be offered without the intent to coach or provide directive instructions and within the context of what has occurred thus far in labor and/or prior labor and birth experiences. Collectively, support and implementation of physiologic birth tools can promote spontaneous vaginal birth and prevent adverse perinatal outcomes.[26-28]

### The Family-Centered Birth Environment

The decision of who to include in the birth room is important. Community birth settings generally have few or no restrictions on the number of persons present. By contrast, most hospitals allow only a limited number of support persons in the labor room, with additional restrictions on the number of support people in the operating room for cesarean birth. Birthing facilities often allow children/siblings to be present during labor and birth, although they may require the presence of a designated adult whose primary responsibility is care of the children. Children may want or need to leave the birth environment, so the designated adult should be prepared to leave the birth room as necessary.

It can be helpful to orient the birth person's support team regarding what to expect during the second stage, including normal responses of the birthing person and the potential length of the second stage based on the birthing person's history and labor course. Midwives should also consider the hydration, nutrition, and energy status of the support team and encourage their self-care based on the expected length of the second stage.

## Pushing Efforts

Several management approaches may facilitate fetal descent, including passive descent, open versus closed glottis technique, and spontaneous versus directed pushing. An initial consideration is whether a period of passive descent (often termed "laboring down") would be beneficial for the birthing person who has an epidural or is without the urge to push. Once active pushing begins, pushing efforts can be open glottis or closed glottis (Valsalva maneuver) and spontaneous or directive. In addition, pushing efforts and fetal descent among individuals with epidural anesthesia may be improved by turning down (but not off) the infusion rate of the epidural.

### Delayed Pushing: Passive Descent Versus Immediate Maternal Pushing Efforts

Passive descent, also called "laboring down," was initially introduced as a management approach to reduce the incidence of instrumental birth in individuals with epidural analgesia. Its implementation was based on the theory that in response to force generated from contractions alone, the fetus would descend and begin to internally rotate, once the presenting part reached the pelvic floor. Moreover, passive descent was thought to increase the efficiency of pushing efforts by allowing the birthing person to rest and conserve energy until there was a physical stimulus to actively push. Then, once active pushing started, efforts would be more effective in the presence of physical cues from pressure of the presenting part on the pelvic floor.[29]

Over the past 25 years, investigators in multiple randomized, controlled trials (RCTs) and meta-analyses have compared perinatal outcomes for birthing persons assigned to immediate versus delayed pushing, finding conflicting results.[11,30–33] In most of these studies, passive descent was defined as no active pushing for a minimum of 1 hour unless an uncontrollable urge to push developed, or the fetal head was visible at the introitus. Perinatal outcomes were compared among groups who used passive descent and groups who started pushing at the beginning of the second stage. A 2008 meta-analysis of seven RCTs found delayed pushing was associated with a modest increase in the incidence of spontaneous birth (risk ratio [RR], 1.08; 95% confidence interval [CI], 1.01–1.15; $P = 0.025$), and fewer operative births (RR, 0.77; 95% CI, 0.77–0.85; $P \leq 0.0001$), less maternal exhaustion, and no increase in adverse maternal or neonatal outcomes.[31] However, investigators in more recent, high-quality RCTs reported no improvement in spontaneous vaginal births and many adverse perinatal outcomes with passive descent, including an increase in cesarean births, operative vaginal births, maternal fever, chorioamnionitis, postpartum hemorrhage, neonatal acidemia, and confirmed or suspected sepsis, compared to immediate pushing.[30,32–35]

In light of this evidence, it is prudent to encourage active pushing when the presenting part reaches +1 station in all people, so as to avoid possible short-term and long-term adverse effects. In people whose fetus is above 0 station, allowing time for rest with passive descent may be beneficial if the initial pushing efforts do not result in any fetal movement. For example, delayed pushing may be especially useful for nulliparous individuals with an epidural in place who have no urge to push after complete dilation. Identification of how long to wait and when to transition to active pushing efforts requires careful consideration. Intra-amniotic infection, FHR patterns that indicate a risk for fetal acidemia, vaginal bleeding, or other clinical indications for expediting birth are likely contraindications to delayed pushing.

### Open-Glottis Versus Closed-Glottis (Valsalva) Pushing

Open-glottis pushing is similar to the semi-voluntary grunting and pushing associated with defecation. Because the glottis is not closed, this form of pushing effort does not greatly increase intrathoracic pressure and, therefore, does not affect cardiac output. Beginning in the 1950s, birthing persons were counseled to use closed-glottis (also known as Valsalva) pushing to hasten the birth and address the challenges of the lithotomy position.[36] This approach involves taking a deep breath, holding it, and pushing forcefully throughout the duration of a uterine contraction. The use of breath holding combined with prolonged bearing down can decrease cardiac output and subsequent blood flow to the uterus.

Studies comparing Valsalva-type, closed-glottis pushing to open-glottis pushing have found conflicting results regarding the effectiveness of each method and associated perinatal outcomes. In a 2017 Cochrane review of 21 RCTs (n = 884 birthing persons), investigators found no significant differences by pushing technique in the duration of the second stage, perineal lacerations, mode of birth, or adverse neonatal outcomes.[32] In a 2020 RCT (n = 250), French investigators also saw no statistically significant differences in the effectiveness of one method over the other in terms of adverse outcomes including perineal lacerations, episiotomies, postpartum hemorrhage, and umbilical cord pH.[37] Further studies are warranted in this area; however, birthing persons should be encouraged to use their preferred and most effective method of pushing.[38]

### Spontaneous Versus Directed Pushing

Spontaneous pushing occurs when a birthing person responds to the strong sensations of vaginal/rectal pressure and an urge to push with bearing-down efforts and open-glottis pushing. In contrast, directed or coached pushing occurs when the clinician instructs the birthing person to push in a specific manner, such as to take a deep breath and hold it for a sustained period, typically "to the count of 10." Directed pushing may also include suggestions for the person to push before the urge to do so and to hold the push beyond the spontaneous urge. By contrast, verbal support for spontaneous bearing-down efforts often includes words of encouragement in a natural speaking voice, such as "Your body knows what to do," "There is plenty of room for this baby," or "You are moving your baby with every push."[39]

Table 29-4 summarizes the differences between spontaneous pushing and directed pushing. While there are gaps in the literature regarding the benefits of spontaneous pushing, its use has not been shown to cause harm to either the birthing person or the neonate.[37]

### Turning Down the Epidural

Some authors have suggested reducing the concentration of anesthetic in the epidural infusion during the second stage so that the sensory block is less strong and the birthing person feels a stronger urge to push.[40] This strategy can be effective if the birthing person wants to have more sensation, the epidural is able to be titrated, and consent has been given. Nevertheless, total discontinuation of the epidural is not recommended because it results in more pain and no increase in the spontaneous vaginal birth rate.[41] As research on epidural infusion reduction during second stage is inconclusive, decisions should be considered on an individual basis depending on the pace of labor progression using shared decision making.[40]

### Positioning During the Second Stage of Labor

Birthing persons benefit from autonomy in choosing the positions that feel best for them. Principles to consider when recommending positions to promote labor progress in the second stage are reviewed in Table 29-5. An individual can push in any position—on their side, hands and knees, kneeling, standing, or squatting. The positions assumed during second-stage labor depend on the birthing person's preferences, as well as on the health status of the laboring person and fetus. Authors of several RCTs have examined upright versus supine positions during the second stage of labor.[42-44] In a 2017 meta-analysis (N = 30 RCTs, 9015 individuals)

| Table 29-4 | Comparison of Spontaneous to Directed Approaches to Pushing During Second-Stage Labor |
|---|---|
| **Spontaneous** | **Directed** |
| Also referred to as physiologic and supportive pushing. | Also referred to as Valsalva and authoritative pushing. |
| Bearing-down efforts begin when a clinician assesses that the individual is fully dilated (10 cm) and when the birthing person feels an overwhelming urge to push. | Bearing-down efforts begin when a clinician assesses that the individual is fully dilated (10 cm) and ready to push. |
| Pushing is spontaneous—in response to natural urges and sensations. Usually results in 5–6 bearing-down efforts per contraction of 3–10 seconds each. | Pushing is directed—with instructions from a nurse or clinician about when and how long to bear down. Usually results in 3 pushes per contraction of 8–10 seconds each. |
| Pushing often occurs during exhalation, with open mouth and open glottis. Usually results in grunting and low groaning. | Pushing occurs while holding the breath. Silence is encouraged. Often results in a Valsalva maneuver. |

comparing the outcomes of laboring people without an epidural who pushed in upright positions versus supine or lithotomy positions, the authors identified several potential benefits of pushing in upright positions—namely, a small reduction in duration of second-stage labor, fewer episiotomies and assisted deliveries, and fewer abnormal FHR patterns. However, pushing in upright positions was also associated with an increase in second-degree perineal tears and blood loss greater than 500 mL. The researchers concluded that without a specific indication to adopt a particular position, birthing persons should be encouraged to use the position that is most comfortable and that supports ongoing progress of the second stage.[42] In a more recent 2020 systematic review (N = 7 RCTs, 1219 individuals), researchers found no difference in length of second stage, rate of spontaneous delivery, or perinatal outcomes with pushing in squatting position versus any supine position.[45] Thus, the choice of birthing position should be individualized, facilitated by sharing information, inquiring about preferences, and using supportive direction.[25]

| Table 29-5 | Principles to Consider When Recommending Positions in Second-Stage Labor |
|---|---|

1. Supine and lithotomy positions are associated with uterine pressure on the vena cava, maternal hypotension, decreased uterine perfusion, and variant fetal heart rate patterns.
2. When the back is rounded rather than arched, the uterus and fetal presenting part are better aligned with the pelvis.
3. Leaning forward in an upright position increases the angle between the uterus and the spine, thereby directing the fetal presenting part toward the larger posterior segment of the pelvis.
4. Changing positions frequently promotes changes in pelvic diameters, which could aid the fetus finding the "best fit" while moving through the pelvis.
5. Regardless of position, the legs should not be abducted laterally in an exaggerated manner (lithotomy position) because these positions put increased stress and tension on the perineum.

Sources: Simkin P, Hanson L, Ancheta R. *The Labor Progress Handbook*. 4th ed. Hoboken, NJ: John Wiley & Sons; 2017; Gupta JK, Sood A, Hofmeyr GJ, Vogel JP. Position in the second stage of labour for women without epidural anaesthesia. *Cochrane Database Syst Rev*. 2017;5(5):Cd002006. doi:10.1002/14651858.CD002006.pub4.

## Preparing for the Birth

The midwife should be aware of the institutional/practice birth protocols. For example, the presence of thick meconium-stained fluid may require transfer to another facility or added personnel to be in attendance. General preparations are outlined in Table 29-6.

During and immediately following birth, both the birthing person and the neonate may need care simultaneously. Thus, at least two healthcare professionals trained in care at birth, neonatal resuscitation, and management of third-stage labor should always be present. Additional personnel may also be needed, depending on any risk factors that may be present. It is the responsibility of the midwife to consider the unique risk factors of the dyad, to request the necessary resources in anticipation of the birth, and to know how to activate emergency support should an unexpected complication occur.

In general, if labor is progressing normally, it is best to begin preparations for birth before complete dilation if the birthing person is multiparous and at the beginning of second-stage labor if the individual is nulliparous. The midwife will need to decide when to don protective wear, including a waterproof gown or clothing, a mask, and eye protection per birth setting protocol. If a water birth is

| Table 29-6 | Preparation for Birth |
|---|---|

1. Encourage the birthing person to empty their bladder as indicated.
2. Determine the most appropriate place for the birth to occur and move as indicated (e.g., from the shower to the birthing stool).
3. Inform the labor support team, including nursing staff, that birth is imminent and review roles and what to expect.
4. Consider securing supplies that may be needed for a shoulder dystocia or postpartum hemorrhage.
5. Confirm that neonatal resuscitation equipment and supplies are present and in proper working condition.
6. Confirm that necessary birth instruments and supplies are accessible and maintain a sterile field.
7. Don protective clothing and gloves using sterile technique.
8. Set the tone for the room using a calm, positive approach, placing the birthing person and their support team at the forefront of all care.

planned, the midwife will need to don longer gloves or a gown that is fully waterproof to maintain universal precautions.

## Midwifery Care During Birth

Midwifery care during birth includes standard hand maneuvers to support the birth and immediate assessment of the neonate and birthing person afterward. Hand maneuvers are reviewed in the *Hand Maneuvers for Birth* appendix. In managing the birth, the midwife makes quick sequential decisions about the following: (1) providing supportive direction to the birthing person through the final perineal phase of the second stage of labor; (2) using techniques to maintain perineal integrity while supporting birth of the fetal head; (3) deciding where to place the neonate immediately after birth based on risk factors and immediate neonatal assessment; and (4) timing of when to clamp and cut the umbilical cord.

### *Perineal Integrity*

One area of focus prior to crowning should be use of techniques to promote perineal integrity and prevent perineal lacerations. Studies have produced conflicting findings regarding the association of specific birth positions (e.g., squatting, upright, lying down) and rates of perineal trauma.[42,44,46] Squatting may be associated with more second-degree lacerations because it is a position in which the midwife has less control of the fetal head. The position associated with the highest incidence of genital tract trauma is lithotomy. In that position, marked abduction of the thighs stretches the perineum transversely so that it becomes a tight band without significant ability to flex around the emerging head.

Perineal support techniques that are purported to decrease the incidence of genital tract trauma include warm compresses and a "hands on" technique (versus "hands off").[46–49] In a 2019 meta-analysis of RCTs (*n* = 2103), researchers found that compared to usual perineal care, placing warm, wet compresses on the perineum during and between contractions prior to crowning was associated with a higher rate of intact perineums (22.4% versus 15.4%; RR, 1.46; 95% CI, 1.22–1.74), lower rates of third-degree tears (1.9% versus 5.0%; RR, 0.38; 95% CI, 0.22–0.64), fourth-degree tears (0.0% versus 0.9%; RR, 0.11; 95% CI, 0.01–0.86), third- and fourth-degree tears combined (1.9% versus 5.8%; RR, 0.34; 95% CI, 0.20–0.56), and episiotomy (10.4% versus 17.1%; RR, 0.61; 95% CI, 0.51–0.74).[48] Although more

| Table 29-7 | Strategies to Promote an Intact Perineum |
|---|---|

Make certain the individual's thighs and legs are not abducted laterally.

All body jewelry should be removed from the vulva and perineum.

Use of warm compresses during the perineal phase may increase the incidence of intact perineum and decrease the incidence of third- and fourth-degree lacerations.

Avoid vigorous or sustained perineal massage during the second stage, as it may cause perineal edema and tearing.

Facilitate birth of the fetus slowly between contractions, controlling extension of the fetal head using a "hands on" technique so pressure on the perineum and vulva is not suddenly forceful.

If blanching of the perineum is observed, encourage the individual to breathe instead of push, to support slower birth of the fetal head.

Based on Aasheim V, Nilsen ABV, Reinar LM, Lukasse M. Perineal techniques during the second stage of labour for reducing perineal trauma: updated review. *Cochrane Database Syst Rev.* 2017;6. doi:10.1002/14651858.CD006672.pub3; Magoga G, Saccone G, Al-Kouatly HB, et al. Warm perineal compresses during the second stage of labor for reducing perineal trauma: a meta-analysis. *Eur J Obstet Gynecol Reprod Biol.* 2019;240: 93-98. doi:10.1016/j.ejogrb.2019.06.011; Van Hoover C, Rademayer CA, Farley CL. Body piercing: motivations and implications for health. *J Midwifery Womens Health.* 2017;62(5): 521-530. doi:10.1111/jmwh.12630.

research is needed, the potential for benefit and absence of harm from warm (not hot) compresses supports use of this technique by midwives. The "hands on" technique entails using one hand to maintain flexion of the fetal occiput and the other hand to guard the perineal body by placing fingers on both sides of the perineum. "Hands off" means not touching the fetal head or perineum until the fetal head is crowning (i.e., the biparietal diameter of the fetal head is through the vulva). In a 2015 meta-analysis of nonrandomized studies (*N* = 3 studies; 74,744 individuals) the "hands on" technique was associated with lower rates of perineal and sphincter tears.[50] Table 29-7 summarizes these strategies to reduce the risk of perineal tearing.

### Birth of the Fetal Head

The ideal time for birth of the fetal head is between contractions. The combination of the uterine contraction and the birthing person's pushing effort exerts a double force on the perineum at the moment of birth, which makes birth of the head more rapid and the release of restraining pressure more abrupt. However, each birth has unique factors and midwives should adjust their management in response to the needs of the birthing person and fetus. Close communication between the midwife and the birthing person facilitates a team approach to help them gently give birth while making every effort to protect perineal integrity.

### Head-to-Body Interval During Birth

Once the head is born and the midwife assesses for a nuchal cord, the midwife can move immediately to guide the birth of the fetal body or wait for the next contraction and spontaneous restitution and birth of the shoulders before guiding the neonate's body out of the vagina. In the *one-step approach*, the midwife attempts to keep the head-to-body interval shorter, thereby decreasing the duration of the expulsive phase and (in theory) mitigating neonatal acidemia. By contrast, in the more physiologic *two-step approach*, the midwife allows a longer head-to-body interval. Although it is common practice in the United States to effect birth of the neonate quickly once the head is born, no evidence supports the contention that rapid birth is safer than a two-step birth in terms of clinical outcomes.[51]

The choice of performing a one-step or two-step method for facilitating birth is based on the individual circumstance. The one-step procedure may be better if the FHR pattern indicates that acidemia may be developing or if other clinical factors place the fetus at increased risk for adverse effects of acidemia. Another factor to consider when making the decision about a longer expulsive stage is the risk for shoulder dystocia. Although clinical risk factors for shoulder dystocia are not strongly predictive, some authors have proposed that a rapid birth will prevent the anterior shoulder from becoming impacted behind the symphysis. However, little evidence supports this claim, and other authors argue that utilizing the two-step approach might actually reduce rates of shoulder dystocia by allowing the shoulders to rotate into an ideal position for birth.[52,53] The birth of the shoulders may also occur spontaneously, without any guidance from the midwife.

### Water Immersion for Birth

Water immersion for birth refers to birth of the neonate completely underwater. The neonate's face is gently and directly brought to the surface within 5 to 10 seconds, while attention is paid to the length of the umbilical cord so cord avulsion does not occur.[54] Midwives should offer evidence-based information with respect to water birth.

Access to water immersion for birth in hospital settings is limited in the United States. Consequently, there are limited data on associated outcomes. However, several recent studies have identified an association between water immersion for birth and lower rates of first- and second-degree lacerations. as well as lower rates of neonatal intensive care unit (NICU) admissions.[55,56] A 2018 systematic review and meta-analysis ($N = 39$ studies, 12,592 births under water) examined whether water immersion was associated with one of 12 adverse neonatal outcomes; no evidence was found to support this linkage when compared to land deliveries.[57] A 2021 retrospective cohort study that matched 17,530 water births to similar land births found water birth was not associated with an increased risk of neonatal death or hospitalization, but was associated with uterine infection and umbilical cord avulsion.[58]

An American College of Nurse-Midwives (ACNM) position statement recommends that birthing persons with uncomplicated pregnancies and labors can be safely offered water birth, especially those people who would like to avoid pharmacologic pain relief.[59] However, ACOG does not support birth in the water. Midwives may need to work at the health-system level to facilitate access to water birth. Logistical considerations are multi-level and include ensuring the floor can hold the weight of a full tub, setting up the birthing pool to have quick access to the laboring person and newborn, providing adequate protective equipment for birth attendants, and maintaining water temperature and cleanliness. For midwives planning to facilitate water birth in a new location, ACNM has published guidelines for water birth that include indications, contraindications, protocols, and requirements for quality control.[54]

Contraindications to water immersion for birth include conditions that are indicative of perinatal compromise or that pose an infection risk to the birthing person, fetus, or birth attendants. Preparation for water birth includes balancing support and realistic expectations. A birthing person will need to be open about their comfort and medical needs in the moment.

## Immediately Following the Birth

### Placing the Neonate in Skin-to-Skin Contact

Following birth, the ideal placement for the neonate is on the birthing person's abdomen, with skin-to-skin contact, promoting a positive transition

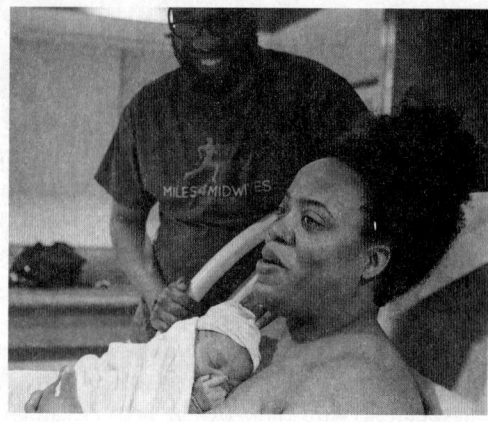

**Figure 29-1** Skin-to-skin care.
Reproduced with permission from Ebony Marcelle.

from intrauterine to extrauterine life (**Figure 29-1**). Skin-to-skin contact promotes thermoregulation of the neonate, reduces physiologic stress, enhances successful breastfeeding both initially and at 3 months postpartum, and results in improved bonding between the birthing person and their baby. Evaluation of the neonate, the assignment of Apgar scores, and initial vital signs can be completed while maintaining this skin-to-skin contact.[60]

### Cord-Clamping

Delayed cord-clamping is an evidence-based practice and standard of care across all gestational ages that promotes the transition from intrauterine to extrauterine life and offers numerous other health benefits without any adverse effects.[61-66] It allows the blood that was circulating in the umbilical vessels and the placenta to return to the neonate's circulation after birth. This process, known as placental transfusion, increases blood volume in the neonate by approximately 30% and red blood cell volume by 50%.[67] In the past, many newborns had their cords clamped and cut nearly immediately after birth, but this routine should be discontinued. Delayed cord-clamping involves waiting at least 1 minute, and as long as 5 minutes, after the birth before the umbilical cord is clamped and cut.[64]

The increased volume of red blood cells, stem cells, and other blood components received by the neonate during delayed cord-clamping has significant health benefits. For the term neonate, this practice results in higher ferritin levels, reduces the risk of iron-deficiency anemia, and can increase stores of brain myelin, which is important for more rapid and efficient brain communication.[63,68] Neonates at all gestational ages have better neurodevelopmental outcomes when cutting of the umbilical cord is delayed.[69,70,71] The procedure for clamping the umbilical cord in different clinical situations is presented in the *Umbilical Cord-Clamping at Birth* appendix.

Most birthing individuals/families desire to separate the baby from the placenta; however, some prefer to keep the two attached until the cord separates from the baby naturally, referred to as a lotus birth. Research is conflicting regarding the safety of this practice and the risk of neonatal infection.

### Umbilical-Cord-Blood Banking

Cord-blood banking involves collecting and storing umbilical cord blood after birth, whereas tissue banking involves storing the umbilical cord or placenta. Cord blood is a source of stem cells for treatment of hematologic malignancies, hemoglobinopathies, severe forms of T-lymphocyte and other immunodeficiencies, and metabolic diseases. A public bank stores blood or tissue at no cost to parents, but they give up ownership of the cells and the stem cells can go to any person who qualifies for them. A private bank requires fees for storage, but the stem cells are "saved" for use by that family. The American Academy of Pediatricians and ACOG both encourage donation to and use of cord blood in public banks.[72] ACOG suggests stem cells should be stored in public banks because generally these banks distribute more stem cells for transplant. However, public cord-blood donation should not alter the routine practice of delayed umbilical cord-clamping, except in the rare circumstance of directed donation.[72,73]

### Inspection of the Perineum and Laceration Repair

The third stage of labor begins as soon as the neonate is born. Management of this phase of labor is described in detail in the *Third Stage of Labor* chapter, and care of the newborn is discussed in the *Neonatal Care* chapter. Once the neonate is safely being observed/cared for by another healthcare professional, the midwife checks for vaginal bleeding while inspecting the vagina and perineum for lacerations and arterial bleeding. Most vaginal births are associated with some degree of perineal trauma.[46] The types of perineal lacerations are described in Table 29-8.[47,74] Third- and fourth-degree lacerations are sometimes termed "obstetric anal sphincter injuries" (OASIS). Perineal lacerations can result in both short-term and long-term morbidity and pain, especially with OASIS.[46] The systematic inspection process, technique for initiating local or pudendal

| Table 29-8 | Types of Perineal Lacerations |
|---|---|
| **Classification** | **Location of Injury** |
| First degree | Vulvar and/or perineal epithelium |
| Second degree | Perineal muscles (perineal body) |
| Third degree | Perineal muscles and the anal sphincter complex<br>3a: < 50% of the external anal sphincter<br>3b: > 50% of the external anal sphincter<br>3c: Both the external and internal anal sphincter torn |
| Fourth degree | Perineal muscles, anal sphincter complex, and anal epithelium |
| Sulcus tears | Vaginal mucosa and underlying tissue along one or both sides of the posterior column of the vagina instead of the middle inferior part of the vagina |
| Labial | Fourchette anteriorly in one or both of the labia majora bodies |
| Periurethral | Labia minora near the urethra |
| Clitoral | Periurethral extending into or near the clitoral body |
| Cervical | Any part of the cervix, usually on one or both of the lateral sides at 3 o'clock and/or 9 o'clock where the anterior and posterior aspects join |

Based on American College of Obstetricians and Gynecologists. reVITALize: obstetrics data definitions. https://www.acog.org/practice-management/health-it-and-clinical-informatics/revitalize-obstetrics-data-definitions?utm_source=vanity&utm_medium=web&utm_campaign=pm. Accessed September 25, 2021; Ducarme G, Pizzoferrato AC, de Tayrac R, et al. Perineal prevention and protection in obstetrics: CNGOF clinical practice guidelines. *J Gynecol Obstet Hum Reprod.* 2019;48(7):455-460. doi:10.1016/j.jogoh.2018.12.002.

anesthesia, and laceration repair are summarized in the following appendices: *Genital Tract Injury: Immediate Postpartum Inspection of the Vulva, Perineum, Vagina, and Cervix*; *Local Infiltration for the Genital Tract Repair*; and *Repair of Genital Tract Lacerations and Episiotomy*. Usually the perineum is repaired after the birth of the placenta and an initial period of parental–newborn bonding.

After a thorough inspection, the midwife should decide whether lacerations require intervention. Lacerations with active bleeding need immediate attention to decrease overall blood loss and hematoma risk. For example, vaginal sulcus tears often bleed heavily, requiring suturing immediately following the birth of the neonate. Larger bleeding vessels may require a stitch to hold them closed. Smaller bleeding vessels may be treated with sustained manual pressure for 1 to 2 minutes; the pressure stops active bleeding and approximates vessel walls, allowing for clot formation.

After care of bleeding vessels, the midwife assesses if the laceration would benefit from intervention to promote closure and discusses the need for repair with the birthing person. The goals when caring for a perineal laceration include promotion of immediate healing and long-term sexual and pelvic floor function as well as prevention of infection and perineal pain.

In case of a first-degree laceration that approximates well when the individual's legs are not abducted, repair may not be needed. Leaving the superficial skin layer unrepaired has been shown to decrease postpartum perineal pain and is not associated with poor healing or anatomic dysfunction.[75,76] First-degree interior vaginal tears and lacerations to the hymenal ring that are not bleeding also do not require repair, as suturing in these areas is associated with increased postpartum perineal pain.

Labial, periurethral, and periclitoral lacerations can be left to heal if they are hemostatic and the overall appearance of the area is unaffected, but repair should be offered if spontaneous healing would result in anatomic distortion.[77] If there are bilateral labial lacerations and the wound edges touch, the two labia could potentially heal together; to prevent fusion, the person can separate their labia each time they void, petroleum jelly can be applied to the wound surfaces, or one or both labial lacerations can be sutured.

There is no clear evidence on the value of repair for second-degree lacerations that are well approximated and hemostatic. Research on perineal pain in the first 8 to 12 weeks postpartum for these patients demonstrates that suturing may increase perineal pain, compared to nonsuturing.[75,76] In addition, in comparison of outcomes up to 12 weeks postpartum, researchers did not find any differences based on suture use in rates of infection, incontinence, or sexual activity and function.[76,78] However, high-quality research assessing longer-term adverse outcomes like incontinence is lacking. Thus, clinical judgment about the value of wound approximation for muscle healing and function should be incorporated into shared decision making surrounding perineal repair.

If the laceration does not approximate, or if muscle or anatomic function will likely be affected if it is not repaired, closure of the laceration should be offered to the individual. Third- and fourth-degree lacerations should be repaired, and usually these procedures involve consultation with collaborating physicians.

Multiple methods of repair are available, including suturing with a variety of materials and application of surgical glues. In selecting the type of suture, synthetic materials (i.e., polyglactin) are preferred over natural materials (i.e., catgut and chromic), as use of synthetic sutures is associated with less tissue inflammation and pain.[77] However, natural suture materials are less expensive and may be more readily available in lower-resource settings. Continuous stitches are preferred for perineal repair compared with interrupted stitches, as they are associated with lower rates of perineal pain in the immediate postpartum period and require less time to perform.[77,78]

Compared to use of sutures for perineal repair, surgical glues have similar functional outcomes and are associated with less postpartum perineal pain. In addition, glues require less time to apply than sutures and are more cost-effective than sutures in most settings. Techniques for use of glues during perineal repair are not standardized, but usually involve drying the wound surface, approximating the tissue manually or with forceps, and applying the adhesive per the manufacturer's instructions from the interior portion of the laceration moving toward the introitus.[75,79,80]

---

### Sample Birth Note

**Labor:**

This 30-year-old, G2P1001 cisgender woman at 40.2 weeks' gestation by LMP and second-trimester ultrasound, GBS negative, had an onset of uterine contractions at 3 P.M. and presented to the Midwifery Birth Center in active labor 5 hours later with contractions every 3 minutes lasting 60 seconds. FHR pattern demonstrated a baseline of 135 in a Category 1 pattern with accelerations and no decelerations on admission. The cervical assessment was 6/90/0 with the fetus in left occiput anterior (LOA) position. Maternal preferences were to labor and birth in the tub, skin-to-skin contact immediately after the birth, with delayed cord-clamping. Maternal coping was characterized by controlled breathing. Various comfort measures and interventions were employed, including partner support, position changes, and hydrotherapy. Following spontaneous urge to push, cervical assessment 10/100/+1 station in fetus in OA position at 2225. Spontaneous rupture of membranes (SROM) at 2235 in birthing tub and appeared to be clear.

**Birth:**

At 2245, after 20-minute second stage, normal spontaneous vaginal birth (NSVB) of live female (8 lb 1 oz; 3657 grams). Nuchal cord not present. Shoulders birthed with ease. The newborn was immediately placed on the maternal abdomen and dried. She was vigorous with Apgar scores 9/9. Using active management of the third stage, 10 IU of IM Pitocin was given. After 5 minutes, the umbilical cord was clamped and cut by the father of baby. Cord blood was not obtained (mother's blood type A+).

**Third stage:**

Mother moved to the bed. After 10-minute third stage, the placenta delivered via Schultz mechanism spontaneously with trailing membranes. Fundus massaged to firm. Placenta, membranes, and cord were examined and found to be morphologically normal and intact, with a 3-vessel cord. Quantified blood loss 375 cc.

**Fourth stage:**

The perineum, vagina, and cervix were inspected and second-degree perineal laceration noted and repaired without complication using 3-0 polyglactin (Vicryl) under local anesthetic and sterile conditions. Perineum well approximated with no further bleeding noted.

**Newborn:**

Skin-to-skin immediately after birth. No birth injuries evident. Newborn breastfeeding at 25 minutes old. Latch achieved with rhythmic sucking. Mother and newborn bonding and in satisfactory condition. Plan discharge home at 24 hours of age.

## Conclusion

Throughout all stages of the birthing process, the midwife maintains a safe, secure, respectful environment that supports an optimal labor and birth. To do so, the midwife must have full awareness of the desires and expectations of the individuals involved in the labor and birth. This will allow the midwife to support a birth experience within the boundaries of the individual circumstances, birth environment, and clinical factors that influence the care provided to the laboring family.

## References

1. Kennedy HP. A model of exemplary midwifery practice: results of a Delphi study. *J Midwifery Womens Health*. 2000;45(1):4-19. doi:10.1016/s1526-9523 (99)00018-5.

2. Caughey AB, Cahill AG, Guise JM, Rouse DJ. Safe prevention of the primary cesarean delivery. *Am J Obstet Gynecol*. 2014;210(3):179-193. doi:10.1016/j .ajog.2014.01.026.

3. Roberts JE. A new understanding of the second stage of labor: implications for nursing care. *J Obstet Gynecol Neonatal Nurs*. 2003;32(6):794-801. doi: 10.1177/0884217503258497.

4. Friedman A. *Labor: Clinical Evaluation and Management*. 2nd ed. New York, NY: Appleton-Century-Crofts; 1978.

5. Roberts J, Hanson L. Best practices in second stage labor care: maternal bearing down and positioning. *J Midwifery Womens Health*. 2007;52(3):238-245. doi:10.1016/j.jmwh.2006.12.011.

6. Friedman EA. Primigravid labor: a graphicostatistical analysis. *Obstet Gynecol*. 1955;6(6):567-589. doi:10.1097/00006250-195512000-00001.

7. Zhang J, Troendle J, Reddy UM, et al. Contemporary cesarean delivery practice in the United States. *Am J Obstet Gynecol*. 2010;203(4):326.e1-326.e10. doi:10.1016/j.ajog.2010.06.058.

8. Gimovsky AC, Guarente J, Berghella V. Prolonged second stage in nulliparous with epidurals: a systematic review. *J Matern Fetal Neonatal Med*. 2017;30(4): 461-465. doi:10.1080/14767058.2016.1174999.

9. Laughon SK, Berghella V, Reddy UM, et al. Neonatal and maternal outcomes with prolonged second stage of labor. *Obstet Gynecol*. 2014;124(1):57-67. doi:10.1097/aog.0000000000000278.

10. Obstetric Care Consensus No. 1: safe prevention of the primary cesarean delivery. *Obstet Gynecol*. 2014;123(3):693-711. doi:10.1097/01.AOG.000044 4441.04111.1d.

11. Morcos C, Caughey AB. Passive descent in the second stage: evaluation of variation in practice patterns. *J Matern Fetal Neonatal Med*. 2018;31(17): 2271-2275. doi:10.1080/14767058.2017.1340448.

12. Cheng YW, Caughey AB. Defining and managing normal and abnormal second stage of labor. *Obstet Gynecol Clin North Am*. 2017;44(4):547-566. doi:10.1016/j.ogc.2017.08.009.

13. Myers ER, Sanders GD, Coeytaux RR, et al. *AHRQ Comparative Effectiveness Reviews: Labor Dystocia*. Rockville, MD: Agency for Healthcare Research and Quality; 2020.

14. National Academies of Sciences, Engineering, and Medicine. *Birth Settings in America: Outcomes, Quality, Access, and Choice*. 2020. https://doi.org /10.17226/25636.

15. Intermittent auscultation for intrapartum fetal heart rate surveillance: American College of Nurse-Midwives. *J Midwifery Womens Health*. 2015;60(5):626-632. doi:10.1111/jmwh.12372.

16. Fetal heart monitoring. *J Obstet Gynecol Neonatal Nurs*. 2018;47(6):874-877. doi:10.1016/j.jogn.2018 .09.007.

17. ACOG Practice Bulletin No. 209: obstetric analgesia and anesthesia. *Obstet Gynecol*. 2019;133(3): e208-e225. doi:10.1097/aog.0000000000003132.

18. Mulder FE, Oude Rengerink K, van der Post JA, et al. Delivery-related risk factors for covert postpartum urinary retention after vaginal delivery. *Int Urogynecol J*. 2016;27(1):55-60. doi:10.1007 /s00192-015-2768-8.

19. Ciardulli A, Saccone G, Anastasio H, Berghella V. Less-restrictive food intake during labor in low-risk singleton pregnancies: a systematic review and meta-analysis. *Obstet Gynecol*. 2017;129(3):473-480. doi: 10.1097/aog.0000000000001898.

20. Practice guidelines for obstetric anesthesia: an updated report by the American Society of Anesthesiologists Task Force on Obstetric Anesthesia and the Society for Obstetric Anesthesia and Perinatology. *Anesthesiology*. 2016;124(2):270-300. doi:10.1097 /aln.0000000000000935.

21. Providing oral nutrition to women in labor: American College of Nurse-Midwives. *J Midwifery Womens Health*. 2016;61(4):528-534. doi:10.1111/jmwh .12515.

22. Leeners B, Görres G, Block E, Hengartner MP. Birth experiences in adult women with a history of childhood sexual abuse. *J Psychosom Res*. 2016;83:27-32. doi:10.1016/j.jpsychores.2016.02.006.

23. Smith A, Laflamme E, Komanecky C. Pain management in labor. *Am Fam Physician*. 2021;103(6):355-364.

24. American College of Nurse-Midwives. *ACNM Core Competencies for Basic Midwifery Practice*. Silver Spring, MD: ACNM; 2020.

25. Nieuwenhuijze MJ, Low LK, Korstjens I, Lagro-Janssen T. The role of maternity care providers

in promoting shared decision making regarding birthing positions during the second stage of labor. *J Midwifery Womens Health*. 2014;59(3):277-285. doi:10.1111/jmwh.12187.

26. Garpiel SJ. Effects of an interdisciplinary practice bundle for second-stage labor on clinical outcomes. *MCN Am J Matern Child Nurs*. 2018;43(4):184-194. doi:10.1097/nmc.0000000000000438.

27. American College of Nurse-Midwives. BirthTools.org: tools for optimizing the outcomes for labor safely. http://birthtools.org/MOC-Promoting-Physiological-Pushing. Accessed September 30, 2021.

28. *Nursing Care and Management of the Second Stage of Labor: Evidence-Based Clinical Practice Guideline*. 3rd ed. Washington, DC: Association of Women's Health, Obstetric and Neonatal Nurses; 2019.

29. Spong CY, Berghella V, Wenstrom KD, et al. Preventing the first cesarean delivery: summary of a joint Eunice Kennedy Shriver National Institute of Child Health and Human Development, Society for Maternal–Fetal Medicine, and American College of Obstetricians and Gynecologists workshop. *Obstet Gynecol*. 2012;120(5):1181-1193. doi:10.1097/aog.0b013e3182704880.

30. Tuuli MG, Frey HA, Odibo AO, et al. Immediate compared with delayed pushing in the second stage of labor: a systematic review and meta-analysis. *Obstet Gynecol*. 2012;120(3):660-668. doi:10.1097/AOG.0b013e3182639fae.

31. Brancato RM, Church S, Stone PW. A meta-analysis of passive descent versus immediate pushing in nulliparous women with epidural analgesia in the second stage of labor. *J Obstet Gynecol Neonatal Nurs*. 2008;37(1):4-12. doi:10.1111/j.1552-6909.2007.00205.x.

32. Lemos A, Amorim MM, Dornelas de Andrade A, et al. Pushing/bearing down methods for the second stage of labour. *Cochrane Database Syst Rev*. 2017;3(3):Cd009124. doi:10.1002/14651858.CD009124.pub3.

33. Yee LM, Sandoval G, Bailit J, et al. Maternal and neonatal outcomes with early compared with delayed pushing among nulliparous women. *Obstet Gynecol*. 2016;128(5):1039-1047. doi:10.1097/aog.0000000000001683.

34. Cahill AG, Srinivas SK, Tita ATN, et al. Effect of immediate vs delayed pushing on rates of spontaneous vaginal delivery among nulliparous women receiving neuraxial analgesia: a randomized clinical trial. *JAMA*. 2018;320(14):1444-1454. doi:10.1001/jama.2018.13986.

35. Di Mascio D, Saccone G, Bellussi F, et al. Delayed versus immediate pushing in the second stage of labor in women with neuraxial analgesia: a systematic review and meta-analysis of randomized controlled trials. *Am J Obstet Gynecol*. 2020;223(2):189-203. doi:10.1016/j.ajog.2020.02.002.

36. Simkin P, Hanson L, Ancheta R. *The Labor Progress Handbook*. 4th ed. Hoboken, NJ: John Wiley & Sons; 2017.

37. Barasinski C, Debost-Legrand A, Vendittelli F. Is directed open-glottis pushing more effective than directed closed-glottis pushing during the second stage of labor? A pragmatic randomized trial: the EOLE study. *Midwifery*. 2020;91:102843. doi:10.1016/j.midw.2020.102843.

38. American College of Obstetricians and Gynecologists. ACOG Committee Opinion No. 766: approaches to limit intervention during labor and birth. *Obstet Gynecol*. 2019;133(2):e164-e173. doi:10.1097/aog.0000000000003074.

39. Hanson L. Low-technology clinical interventions to promote labor progress. In: Simkin P, Hanson L, Ancheta R, eds. *The Labor Progress Handbook*. 4th ed. Hoboken, NJ: John Wiley & Sons; 2017:231-259.

40. Polnaszek BE, Cahill AG. Evidence-based management of the second stage of labor. *Semin Perinatol*. 2020;44(2):151213. doi:10.1016/j.semperi.2019.151213.

41. Mhyre JM. What's new in obstetric anesthesia? *Int J Obstet Anesth*. 2011;20(2):149-159. doi:10.1016/j.ijoa.2010.10.008.

42. Gupta JK, Sood A, Hofmeyr GJ, Vogel JP. Position in the second stage of labour for women without epidural anaesthesia. *Cochrane Database Syst Rev*. 2017;5(5):Cd002006. doi:10.1002/14651858.CD002006.pub4.

43. Walker KF, Kibuka M, Thornton JG, Jones NW. Maternal position in the second stage of labour for women with epidural anaesthesia. *Cochrane Database Syst Rev*. 2018;11(11):Cd008070. doi:10.1002/14651858.CD008070.pub4.

44. Upright versus lying down position in second stage of labour in nulliparous women with low dose epidural: BUMPES randomised controlled trial. *BMJ*. 2017;359:j4471. doi:10.1136/bmj.j4471.

45. Dokmak F, Michalek IM, Boulvain M, Desseauve D. Squatting position in the second stage of labor: a systematic review and meta-analysis. *Eur J Obstet Gynecol Reprod Biol*. 2020;254:147-152. doi:10.1016/j.ejogrb.2020.09.015.

46. Aasheim V, Nilsen ABV, Reinar LM, Lukasse M. Perineal techniques during the second stage of labour for reducing perineal trauma. *Cochrane Database Syst Rev*. 2017;6(6):Cd006672. doi:10.1002/14651858.CD006672.pub3.

47. Ducarme G, Pizzoferrato AC, de Tayrac R, et al. Perineal prevention and protection in obstetrics: CNGOF clinical practice guidelines. *J Gynecol Obstet Hum Reprod*. 2019;48(7):455-460. doi:10.1016/j.jogoh.2018.12.002.

48. Magoga G, Saccone G, Al-Kouatly HB, et al. Warm perineal compresses during the second stage of labor

for reducing perineal trauma: a meta-analysis. *Eur J Obstet Gynecol Reprod Biol.* 2019;240:93-98. doi:10.1016/j.ejogrb.2019.06.011.

49. Ma DM, Hu W, Wang YH, Luo Q. A multicentre study on the effect of moderate perineal protection technique: a new technique for perineal management in labour. *J Obstet Gynaecol.* 2020;40(1):25-29. doi:10.1080/01443615.2019.1587605.

50. Bulchandani S, Watts E, Sucharitha A, et al. Manual perineal support at the time of childbirth: a systematic review and meta-analysis. *BJOG.* 2015;122(9):1157-1165. doi:10.1111/1471-0528.13431.

51. Locatelli A, Incerti M, Ghidini A, et al. Head-to-body delivery interval using "two-step" approach in vaginal deliveries: effect on umbilical artery pH. *J Matern Fetal Neonatal Med.* 2011;24(6):799-803. doi:10.3109/14767058.2010.531307.

52. Kotaska A, Campbell K. Two-step delivery may avoid shoulder dystocia: head-to-body delivery interval is less important than we think. *J Obstet Gynaecol Can.* 2014;36(8):716-720. doi:10.1016/s1701-2163(15)30514-4.

53. Menticoglou S. Delivering shoulders and dealing with shoulder dystocia: should the standard of care change? *J Obstet Gynaecol Can.* 2016;38(7):655-658. doi:10.1016/j.jogc.2016.03.012.

54. A model practice template for hydrotherapy in labor and birth. *J Midwifery Womens Health.* 2017;62(1):120-126. doi:10.1111/jmwh.12587.

55. Bailey JM, Zielinski RE, Emeis CL, Kane Low L. A retrospective comparison of waterbirth outcomes in two United States hospital settings. *Birth.* 2020;47(1):98-104. doi:10.1111/birt.12473.

56. Sidebottom AC, Vacquier M, Simon K, et al. Maternal and neonatal outcomes in hospital-based deliveries with water immersion. *Obstet Gynecol.* 2020;136(4):707-715. doi:10.1097/aog.0000000000003956.

57. Vanderlaan J, Hall PJ, Lewitt M. Neonatal outcomes with water birth: a systematic review and meta-analysis. *Midwifery.* 2018;59:27-38. doi:10.1016/j.midw.2017.12.023.

58. Bovbjerg ML, Cheyney M, Caughey AB. Maternal and neonatal outcomes following waterbirth: a cohort study of 17,530 waterbirths and 17,530 propensity score-matched land births. *BJOG.* 2021; doi:10.1111/1471-0528.17009.

59. American College of Nurse-Midwives. Position statement: hydrotherapy during labor and birth. 2014. https://www.midwife.org/ACNM/files/ACNMLibraryData/UPLOADFILENAME/000000000286/Hydrotherapy-During-Labor-and-Birth-April-2014.pdf. Accessed February 10, 2023.

60. Moore ER, Bergman N, Anderson GC, Medley N. Early skin-to-skin contact for mothers and their healthy newborn infants. *Cochrane Database Syst Rev.* 2016;11(11):Cd003519. doi:10.1002/14651858.CD003519.pub4.

61. Gomersall J, Berber S, Middleton P, et al. Umbilical cord management at term and late preterm birth: a meta-analysis. *Pediatrics.* 2021;147(3). doi:10.1542/peds.2020-015404.

62. World Health Organization. WHO recommendation on delyaed umbilical cord clamping. https://srhr.org/rhl/article/who-recommendation-on-delayed-umbilical-cord-clamping#:~:text=Delayed%20umbilical%20cord%20clamping%20(not,infant%20health%20and%20nutrition%20outcomes. Accessed February 18, 2023.

63. Mercer JS, Erickson-Owens DA, Deoni SCL, et al. The effects of delayed cord clamping on 12-month brain myelin content and neurodevelopment: a randomized controlled trial. *Am J Perinatol.* 2020. doi:10.1055/s-0040-1714258.

64. American College of Nurse-Midwives. Position statement: delayed umbilical cord clamping. https://www.midwife.org/ACNM/files/ACNMLibraryData/UPLOADFILENAME/000000000290/Delayed-Umbilical-Cord-Clamping-May-2014.pdf. Accessed October 5, 2021.

65. American College of Obstetricians and Gynecologists. Delayed umbilical cord clamping after birth: ACOG Committee Opinion, Number 814. *Obstet Gynecol.* 2020;136(6):e100-e106. doi:10.1097/aog.0000000000004167.

66. Rabe H, Gyte GM, Díaz-Rossello JL, Duley L. Effect of timing of umbilical cord clamping and other strategies to influence placental transfusion at preterm birth on maternal and infant outcomes. *Cochrane Database Syst Rev.* 2019;9(9):Cd003248. doi:10.1002/14651858.CD003248.pub4.

67. Yao AC, Moinian M, Lind J. Distribution of blood between infant and placenta after birth. *Lancet.* 1969;2(7626):871-873. doi:10.1016/s0140-6736(69)92328-9.

68. Bayer K. Delayed umbilical cord clamping in the 21st century: indications for practice. *Adv Neonatal Care.* 2016;16(1):68-73. doi:10.1097/anc.0000000000000247.

69. Fogarty M, Osborn DA, Askie L, et al. Delayed vs early umbilical cord clamping for preterm infants: a systematic review and meta-analysis. *Am J Obstet Gynecol.* 2018;218(1):1-18. doi:10.1016/j.ajog.2017.10.231.

70. Aziz K, Lee CHC, Escobedo MB, et al. Part 5: neonatal resuscitation. 2020 American Heart Association guidelines for cardiopulmonary resuscitation and emergency cardiovascular care. *Pediatrics.* 2021;147(suppl 1). doi:10.1542/peds.2020-038505E.

71. Rana N, Kc A, Målqvist M, et al. Effect of delayed cord clamping of term babies on neurodevelopment at 12 months: a randomized controlled trial. *Neonatology.* 2019;115(1):36-42. doi:10.1159/000491994.

72. Shearer WT, Lubin BH, Cairo MS, Notarangelo LD. Cord blood banking for potential future transplantation. *Pediatrics*. 2017;140(5). doi:10.1542/peds.2017-2695.

73. ACOG Committee Opinion No. 771: umbilical cord blood banking. *Obstet Gynecol*. 2019;133(3):e249-e253. doi:10.1097/aog.0000000000003128.

74. American College of Obstetricians and Gynecologists. reVITALize: obstetrics data definitions. https://www.acog.org/practice-management/health-it-and-clinical-informatics/revitalize-obstetrics-data-definitions. Accessed September 25, 2021.

75. Swenson CW, Low LK, Kowalk KM, Fenner DE. Randomized trial of 3 techniques of perineal skin closure during second-degree perineal laceration repair. *J Midwifery Womens Health*. 2019;64(5):567-577.

76. Elharmeel SM, Chaudhary Y, Tan S, et al. Surgical repair of spontaneous perineal tears that occur during childbirth versus no intervention. *Cochrane Database Syst Rev*. 2011;8. doi: 10.1002/14651858.CD008534.pub2.

77. American College of Obstetricians and Gynecologists' Committee on Practice Bulletins–Obstetrics, Cichowski S, Rogers R. Committee Opinion 198: prevention and management of obstetric lacerations at vaginal delivery. *Obstet Gynecol*. 2018;132(3):E87-E102.

78. Leeman LM, Rogers RG, Greulich B, Albers LL. Do unsutured second-degree perineal lacerations affect postpartum functional outcomes? *J Am Board Fam Med*. 2007;20(5):451-457.

79. Mota R, Costa F, Amaral A, et al. Skin adhesive versus subcuticular suture for perineal skin repair after episiotomy: a randomized controlled trial. *Acta Obstet Gynecol Scand*. 2009;88(6):660-666.

80. Ochiai AM, Araújo NM, Moraes S, et al. The use of non-surgical glue to repair perineal first-degree lacerations in normal birth: a non-inferiority randomised trial. *Women Birth*. 2021;34(5):e514-e519.

APPENDIX

# 29A

# Pudendal Nerve Block

AMY KAYLER

*The editors acknowledge Deborah Anderson, who contributed to this appendix in the previous edition.*

## Introduction

Pudendal nerve block is a regional nerve anesthetic that is administered by a midwife or other birth provider, rather than by an anesthesiologist. It involves a one-time injection of local anesthetic near the pudendal nerve that results in the elimination of pain perception in the muscles and tissue innervated by that nerve, including the lower vagina, labia, perineum, and rectum. It does not provide pain relief to the upper vagina or cervix.[1]

## Indications

This technique is primarily used to achieve analgesia for the following situations:

- Operative vaginal birth
- Repair of genital tract lacerations
- Minor surgical procedures involving the perineum
- Late second-stage pain relief related to introital distension with spontaneous vaginal birth
- Birthing people who do not have adequate or satisfactory pain relief during perineal repair following instillation of local anesthesia to the perineum[2]

## Advantages

- Provides anesthesia to the vulva, clitoris, labia majora, labia minora, perineal body and rectum, thereby offering broader anesthesia coverage than is accomplished with local infiltration

- Does not alter the strength or frequency of uterine contractions or the pain of cervical dilation, but may decrease the urge to push during the second stage of labor[1]
- Confers minimal risk to the parturient, fetus, or newborn when administered correctly, using the appropriate medication within the safe dosage range
- Does not require an anesthesiologist

## Equipment for Pudendal Block

The equipment needed to perform a pudendal block is listed in **Table 29A-1**. The needle guide, procedure needle, and syringe used for this technique are shown in **Figure 29A-1**.

## Anesthetic Agent for Pudendal Block

The most commonly used local anesthetic for pudendal nerve block is 1% (10 mg/mL) lidocaine hydrochloride (Xylocaine) without added epinephrine.[1] Lidocaine is rapidly absorbed, crosses the placenta, and is detectable in maternal venous and fetal scalp blood within 5 minutes after injection, with peak levels attained between 10 and 20 minutes after the injection.[3] A maximum block may take up to 20 minutes to achieve because the pudendal nerve is a large peripheral nerve with a smaller surface area to volume ratio, and a myelin sheath. Hence, the time to maximum block takes longer to achieve than the usual 5 minutes for subcutaneous infiltration of the perineum.[4]

The duration of anesthesia depends on the success of the pudendal block and on the medication

1209

| Table 29A-1 | Equipment for Pudendal Block |
|---|---|

Sterile gloves

Local anesthetic: lidocaine (Xylocaine) 1% without added epinephrine

Prepackaged pudendal nerve block set, which includes:
- Needle guide (e.g., Iowa trumpet)
- 12- to 15-cm (5- to 6-inch) 20- or 22-gauge procedure sterile needle
- 10-mL sterile syringe
- 18- to 20-gauge sterile needle for drawing up the anesthetic

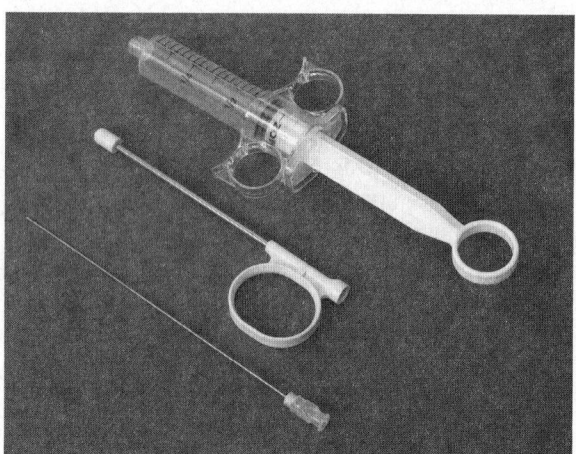

**Figure 29A-1** Pudendal nerve block set: needle, guide, and syringe.
Reproduced with permission from Anderson D. Pudendal nerve block for vaginal birth. *J Midwifery Womens Health*. 2014;59(6): 651-659. © 2014, with permission from Wiley.

used. The average duration of action of lidocaine is 30 to 60 minutes. Safe dosing of 1% lidocaine is 3 to 4.5 mg/kg, with the maximum recommended dose being 300 mg or 30 mL.[4,5]

## Pudendal Block

### Anatomic Location of Pudendal Nerve

A successful pudendal block requires an understanding of the anatomy of the nerve. The pudendal nerve derives from sacral roots S2–S4. It lies between the piriformis and the coccygeus muscle, and exits the pelvis through the greater sciatic foramen. It then courses on the posterolateral surface of the sacrospinous ligament, medial to the internal pudendal vessels that lie on the posterior aspect of the ischial spine. Inferior to the ischial spine, the nerve travels along the lateral pelvic wall through the pudendal

canal (also known as Alcock's canal) and divides into three branches (inferior rectal nerve, perineal nerve, and dorsal nerve of the clitoris).[6]

### Key Principles for Achieving an Effective Pudendal Nerve Block

1. To target the pudendal nerve effectively and safely, an understanding of the locations of the pudendal nerve and internal pudendal artery is essential.

2. Understand the key anatomic landmarks used to locate the optimal point of lidocaine infiltration to most effectively target the pudendal nerve.

3. Allow for a sufficient amount of time to effect adequate analgesia.

### Contraindications to Pudendal Nerve Block

Contraindications to pudendal nerve block include coagulation disorders, infection in the vagina, allergy to local anesthetic, and a parturient who is unable to cope with the procedure, or who declines pudendal nerve block.

## Procedure for Pudendal Nerve Block: Multiple-Injection Method

The procedure can be performed using either the transvaginal or transperineal approach.[1] However, because the transvaginal approach is almost universally employed intrapartum, we will focus on this technique in the following procedure notes. Readers may also refer to a video of this procedure at https://drive.google.com/file/d/1ySj-BFOog8A25Q_LnFqdKuEJ3PMM0n9X/view.

1. Before beginning the procedure, explain the risks and benefits of pudendal nerve block to the patient and **obtain informed consent**. Risks of the procedure are rare, but include hematoma, localized infection, inadvertent injection of anesthetic into the fetal scalp or the mother's vasculature, and temporary nerve issues. Benefits were highlighted earlier in this appendix.

2. Ask the person to move into "butterfly" or lithotomy position.

3. Draw up 10 mL of 1% lidocaine into the syringe, attach the pudendal needle, and clear the air from the syringe and needle.

4. Palpate the ischial spine along the vaginal sidewall. If the location of the ischial spine is

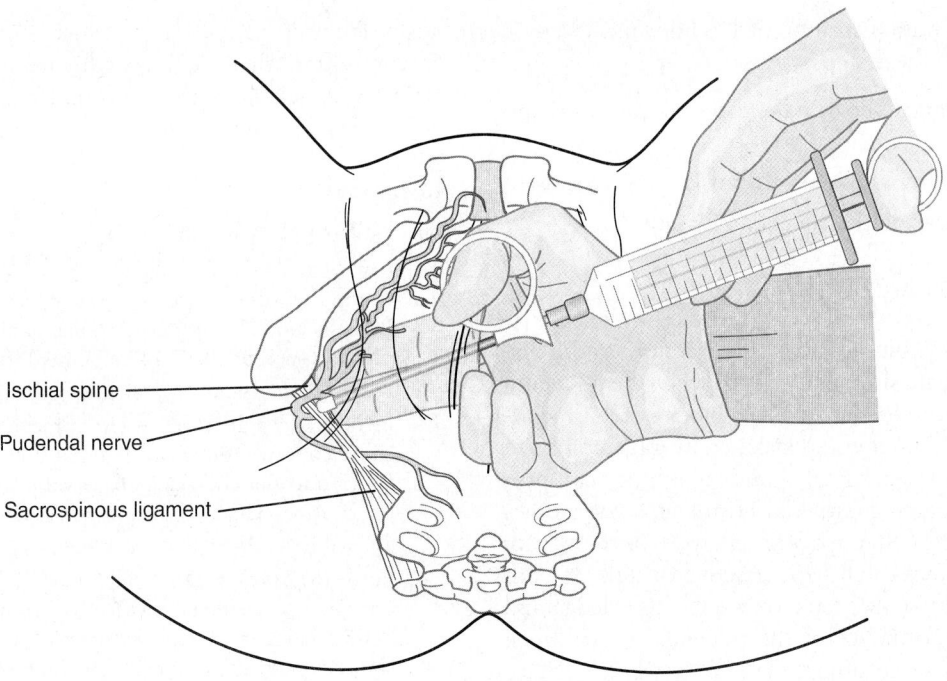

Ischial spine

Pudendal nerve

Sacrospinous ligament

**Figure 29A-2** Pudendal block procedure.

unclear, palpate the sacrospinous ligament, and follow it laterally to its attachment point on the ischial spine.

5. Introduce the needle guide into the vagina and place the tip of the guide on the sacrospinous ligament, 1 cm medial and inferior to the ischial spine (**Figure 29A-2**). To perform a right-sided block, place the right index finger on the ischial spine. Place the middle finger on the adjacent sacrospinous ligament, stabilizing the guide between the two fingers. This is reversed for the opposite side.

6. Holding the guide against the vaginal mucosa, insert the needle and syringe into the guide taking care to avoid an inadvertent needle stick. Advance the needle through the vaginal mucosa approximately 1 cm deep.

7. **Aspirate** to confirm that the needle is not in a vessel, and then inject 3 mL of local anesthetic into the ligament.

8. Advance the needle slightly until the resistance of the ligament is lost. The needle should now be in the tissue behind the ligament where the pudendal nerve is located.

9. **Aspirate again** to confirm the absence of a vessel, and then inject the remaining 7 mL of anesthetic.

10. Repeat the procedure on the contralateral side to achieve a bilateral block. This may require waiting for a contraction to pass.

Placing the pudendal nerve block while the fetal head is deep in the pelvis can be challenging, as this procedure often stimulates an urge to push. Timing the injections between contractions and encouraging the parturient to breathe deeply between contractions may help them to overcome the urge to bear down during the procedure.

The maximum analgesic effect is achieved after 10 to 20 minutes. To test for an effective block, the midwife can stroke the skin adjacent to the anus. An effective block will prevent the reflexive constriction of the anal sphincter. Repeat on the opposite side.[3]

If the block is ineffective or unilateral, an additional 5 mL of 1% lidocaine may be administered on one or both sides, but the total dose administered should not exceed a total of 30 mL (300 mg) 1% lidocaine.[1]

## Variation of Pudendal Block Procedure: Single-Injection Approach

Variations of the standard procedure have been described by several authors.[1,5,7] While the multiple-injection approach may decrease the chance of inadequate block, the single-injection approach may minimize the risks of pudendal nerve block complications. However, no studies have been conducted comparing the safety or efficacy of the single- and multiple-injection techniques. For the single-injection pudendal block,[1,5] the midwife should follow the procedure outlined earlier until the point of administration of 1% lidocaine (Step 7). Then follow these steps:

1. Advance the needle through the sacrospinous ligament.
2. Aspirate and inject 10 mL of 1% lidocaine.
3. Repeat on the contralateral side.

## Outcomes and Efficacy

Within 4 to 5 minutes after the injection is administered, little pain should be elicited when the perineum is pinched. The full effect of the block is achieved after 10 to 20 minutes and lasts, on average, for 30 to 60 minutes. If successful, a pudendal block can provide satisfactory anesthesia. However, some studies have estimated that approximately 10% to 50% of pudendal blocks will be ineffective on one or both sides.[3] Ford has suggested that poor knowledge and variable performance of the pudendal nerve block may contribute to suboptimal effectiveness.[4]

In a small double-blind trial ($N = 72$) conducted at a single medical center in China in 2020, investigators used ultrasound guidance to improve the accuracy of pudendal nerve blocks. They found that nulliparous people who had epidural anesthesia had a shorter second-stage duration (33.8 minute shorter; 95% confidence interval, 15.6–52.0, $p < 0.001$) when they received a pudendal at 9 cm cervical dilation compared to similar laboring people with only an epidural.[8] These researchers theorized that pushing efforts were more effective when participants avoided epidural bolus dosing in second-stage labor due to the superior perineal pain relief offered by pudendal nerve block.

A pudendal block can also be an excellent analgesia choice for the repair of perineal lacerations. In a trial comparing single-shot spinal anesthesia with pudendal block pain relief in the active phase of labor, the two were reported to be equivalent for episiotomy repair.[9] However, the single-shot spinal analgesia provided better general pain relief than the pudendal block.

## Complications

Complications of pudendal nerve block are rare, but can be serious. They include hematoma with or without infection, localized infection (retropsoas and subgluteal abscess), infection at the site of injection, systemic toxicity from inadvertent intravascular administration or excessive doses of anesthetic, temporary ischial paresthesia, sacral neuropathy, and inadvertent needle injection of anesthetic into the fetal scalp, laboring person, or provider.[7,10–12] It is therefore important that providers who are new to pudendal nerve blocks have the opportunity to train with a skilled provider, and follow recommended procedures.

## References

1. Anderson D. Pudendal nerve block for vaginal birth. *J Midwifery Womens Health*. 2014;59(6):651-659.

2. Committee on Practice Bulletins—Obstetrics. Practice Bulletin No. 177: obstetric analgesia and anesthesia. *Obstet Gynecol*. 2017;129:e73. Reaffirmed 2019.

3. Zador G, Lindmark G, Nilsson BA. Pudendal block in normal vaginal deliveries: clinical efficacy, lidocaine concentrations in maternal and foetal blood, foetal and maternal acid–base values and influence on uterine activity. *Acta Obstet Gynecol Scand*. 1974;34(suppl):51-64.

4. Ford JM, Owen DJ, Coughlin LB, Byrd LM. A critique of current practice of transvaginal pudendal nerve blocks: a prospective audit of understanding and clinical practice. *J Obstet Gynaecol*. 2013;33(5):463-465.

5. Cunningham FG. Obstetrical anesthesia. In: Cunningham FG, ed. *William's Obstetrics*. 24th ed. New York, NY: McGraw-Hill; 2014:504-522.

6. Standring S, ed. Gray's *Anatomy: The Anatomical Basis of Clinical Practice*. 39th ed. Edinburgh, UK: Elsevier Churchill Livingstone; 2005.

7. Kurzel RB, Au AH, Rooholamini SA. Retroperitoneal hematoma as a complication of pudendal block: diagnosis made by computed tomography. *West J Med*. 1996;164(6):523-525.

8. Xu J, Zhou R, Su W, et al Ultrasound-guided bilateral pudendal nerve blocks of nulliparous women with epidural labour analgesia in the second stage of labour: a randomised, double-blind, controlled trial. *BMJ Open*. 2020;10:e035887. doi:10.1136/bmjopen-2019-035887.

9. Pace MC, Aurilio C, Bulletti C, et al. Subarachnoid analgesia in advanced labor: a comparison of subarachnoid analgesia and pudendal block in advanced labor: analgesic quality and obstetric outcome. *Ann NY Acad Sci*. 2004;1034:356.

10. Svancarek W, Chirino O, Schaefer G Jr, Blythe JG. Retropsoas and subgluteal abscesses following paracervical and pudendal anesthesia. *JAMA*. 1977;237(9):892-894.

11. Langhoff-Roos J, Lindmark G. Analgesia and maternal side effects of pudendal block at delivery: a comparison of three local anesthetics. *Acta Obstet Gynecol Scand*. 1985;64(3):269-272.

12. Pages H, de la Gastine B, Quedru-Aboane J, et al. Lidocaine intoxication in newborn following maternal pudendal anesthesia: report of three cases. *J Gynecol Obstet Biol Reprod (Paris)*. 2008;37(4):415-418.

# 29B

# Hand Maneuvers for Birth

HEATHER BRADFORD

*The editors acknowledge Barbara Reale, who was the author of this appendix in the previous edition.*

## Introduction

Hand placement during pushing is directed toward preserving perineal integrity as the fetus emerges. Techniques to promote perineal integrity are discussed in the *Second Stage of Labor and Birth* chapter. Once the head emerges, placement of the second hand, as described in this appendix, is critical, as it will allow the midwife to maintain two secure grips on the neonate throughout and immediately after the birth. Neonates are slippery, and sometimes the combination of pushing and uterine contractions results in a rapid, forceful birth. It is imperative that the midwife is able to hold the neonate securely throughout the process. The hand maneuvers presented in this appendix can be used in any setting.

## Hand Maneuvers When the Fetus Is in an Occiput Anterior Positioning While in a Semi-Sitting, Lateral, or Dorsal Position

1. Ensure both access to the perineum and visibility of the vulvar–perineal area.

   a. The midwife stands or sits in a position that allows for a clear visual field and comfortable access to the birthing person's perineum. Many birthing persons appreciate a warm, moist washcloth or compress on the rectal area during the final stages of pushing. Use a clean technique when applying warm compresses and ensure the compress is not too hot prior to application.

   b. A sterile field is made on a surface within easy reach, on which instruments and a bowl for the placenta are arranged. While the instruments used at a birth are sterile, the birth itself is not sterile. Therefore, consider protecting instruments needed for a possible repair by covering them with a sterile towel. Some midwives double-glove or request a second set of sterile gloves to use for perineal repair.

   c. If stool is expelled during pushing, the midwife should cover the anus with a towel to prevent it from touching the fetus. Repeated stools may be removed using sterile gauze, a washcloth, or toilet paper to decrease unpleasant smells from distracting the birthing person. During a water birth, stool should be removed using a net.

2. Control extension of fetal head to minimize the likelihood of perineal laceration.

   a. The hands-on technique refers to placement of one hand on the fetal head to control extension. Using the hand that is not controlling the pace of extension of the fetal head, a thumb and one finger are placed on the perineum near the ischial tuberosities below the fourchette, so that the midline area of the perineum, which is likely to tear, is between the thumb and the finger. Applying pressure with the thumb and fingers inward toward each other and the middle of the perineum (perineal body) reduces the transverse pressure created as the fetal head extends.

b. During extension of the head, the anterior–posterior diameter of the fetal vertex gradually changes from the suboccipitobregmatic diameter (9.5 cm) to the occipitofrontal diameter (11.5 cm), and then to the occipitomental diameter (12.5 cm). Gradual extension prevents perineal trauma as these increasing anterior–posterior diameters stretch the perineum during the birth.

c. To control extension of the fetal head during crowning, the midwife places the palmar side of one hand, with fingers held straight, on the portion of the occiput of the fetal vertex visible at the vaginal introitus. This should be done as the vulva begins to stretch around the presenting part, with crowning imminent (Figure 29B-1). Control of extension is maintained best when the *fingers are kept in a straight plane with the hand.* This finger positioning allows the midwife to control extension of the head. When just the fingertips are placed on the head, the midwife does not have as much control. If sudden extension occurs with a contraction or pushing, the fingertips are likely to slide along the curve of the fetal head, or touch or hurt the sensitive clitoral area, and the head will pop into the midwife's palm, placing rapid pressure on the perineum. The use of one hand to control extension leaves the other hand free to check for a nuchal cord and handle any equipment or supplies that may be needed. Given that midwives' hands vary in size and that people give birth

in many different positions, the actual placement may be less important than identifying how the midwife can comfortably provide the needed control and simultaneously visualize the perineum. Good body mechanics are important to prevent injury to the midwife.

i. Sometimes the fetal head emerges with a nuchal hand. If this is the case, the hand maneuvers do not change. The fetal arm should not be pulled, as this practice is associated with brachial plexus injury.

ii. If the birthing person is **lateral** (side-lying), their legs should be bent at the knee, and when open, remain parallel to each other. Pillows or a peanut ball between the knees can increase comfort in this position. If the upper leg is pushed toward the birthing person's head and flexed more dramatically than the lower leg, the pelvis is forced out of alignment and the perineum becomes tightly stretched. When given the opportunity to raise and position the upper leg spontaneously, many individuals will not do so until birth is imminent. Visualization of the perineum and maintaining flexion of the fetal head is easiest if the midwife stands behind the birthing person's back. If facing their abdomen, visualization of the perineum is impaired, but guiding the rest of the birth can be easier. In either position, the midwife's fingers can be placed on the occiput, exerting pressure with the palmar surfaces, toward the perineum as needed to control extension of the head during the birth.

3. Check for a nuchal cord. As soon as the head has emerged, place the pad side of the fingertips of one hand on the neonate's neck, sweeping the fingers along the neck in both directions, to determine if the umbilical cord is looped around the neck. If a nuchal cord is present, ascertain how tight the cord is. There are four options for proceeding with the birth if a nuchal cord is present:

a. *Cord reduction:* If the cord is loose, slip it forward over the fetal head before delivery of the shoulders (referred to as reducing the cord over the head).

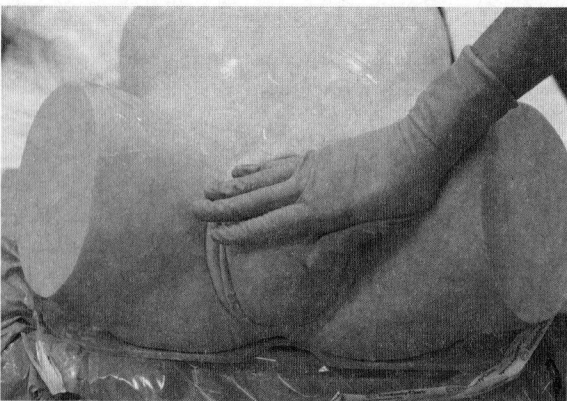

**Figure 29B-1** The midwife's fingers are in a flat plane with the palm of the hand to allow maximum control of extension of the fetal head.

b. *Birth through the cord:* If the cord is too tight to reduce but still has some mobility, slip it back over the fetal shoulders as the neonate is born, allowing the neonate to be born through the cord.

c. *Somersault maneuver:* If the cord is too tight to slip over the shoulders but loose enough to permit some movement, use one hand to keep the fetal head close to the birthing person's thigh throughout the birth of the body and the other hand to "somersault" the body over the perineum, which will limit the traction placed on the cord. The somersault maneuver is depicted in **Figure 29B-2**.

d. *Clamp and cut:* If the cord is too tight to accomplish the other preferred steps, double-clamp and cut the cord between the clamps at the neck before the neonate's body is born, while protecting the infant's skin from the scissors.

4. If planning a two-step, head-to-body birthing process (assuming the cord has not been clamped and cut): While waiting for restitution, external rotation, and the next contraction, the midwife or staff member may wipe fluid from the neonate's face, nose, and mouth with a soft, absorbent cloth. It is not necessary to stimulate the neonate at this moment. Suctioning with a bulb syringe

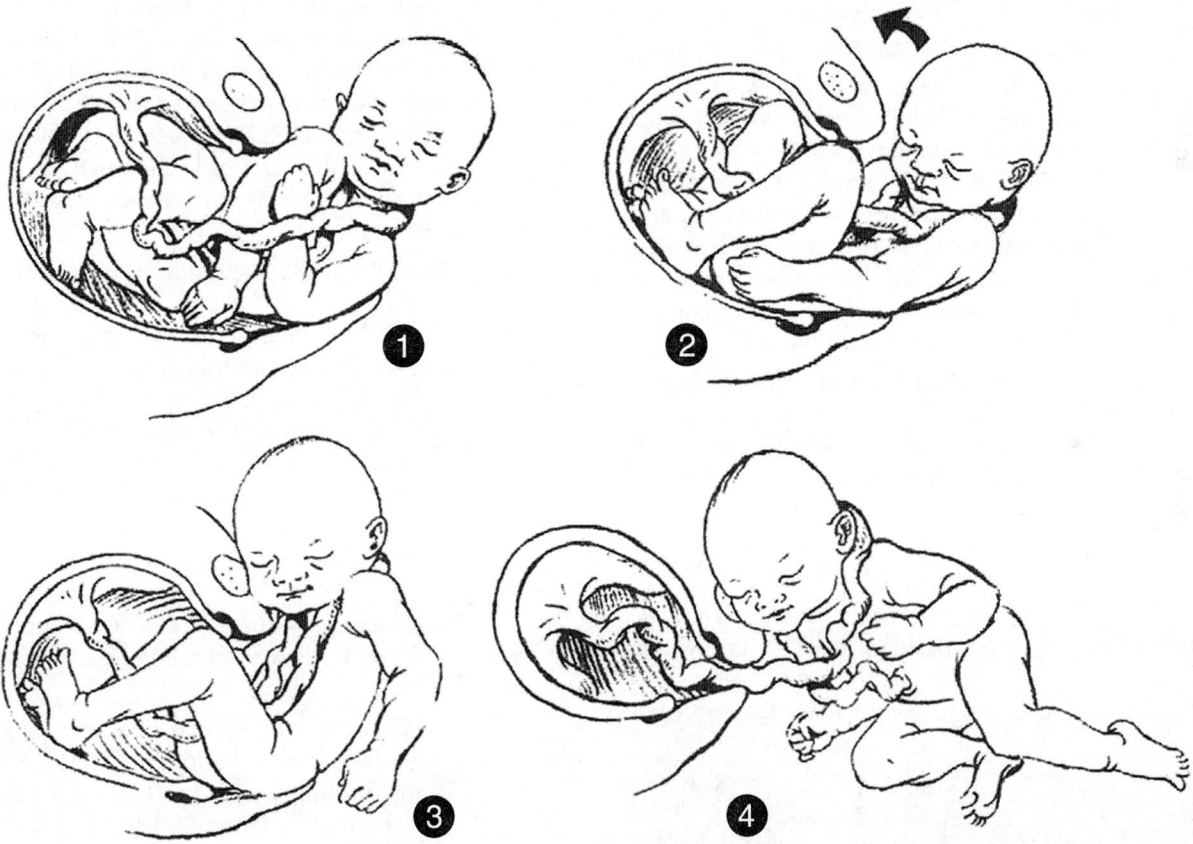

**Figure 29B-2** The somersault maneuver involves holding the neonate's head flexed and guiding it upward or sideways toward the pubic bone or thigh, so the neonate does a "somersault," ending with the neonate's feet toward the birthing person's knees and the head still at the perineum.

1. Once the nuchal cord is discovered, the anterior and posterior shoulders are slowly delivered under control without manipulating the cord.
2. As the shoulders are delivered, the head is flexed so that the face of the neonate is pushed toward the birthing person's thigh.
3. The neonate's head is kept next to the perineum while the body is delivered and "somersaults" out.
4. The umbilical cord is then unwrapped, and the usual management ensues.

Reprinted with permission of Judith Mercer. Copyright © Judith Mercer.

of the fetal nasal and oral passages is not recommended.

a. Wait for the next contraction and for restitution and external rotation to occur, which will be evident when the occiput rotates 90 degrees.

b. If there is a need to expedite the birth (e.g., the cord has been clamped and cut or there is evidence of fetal distress), rotation of the fetal shoulders into the anterior–posterior position to facilitate restitution and external rotation can be facilitated by using a modified Rubin's maneuver if needed. Insert and place two fingers over the scapula of the anterior shoulder, and two fingers against the clavicle of the posterior shoulder.

5. Facilitate birth of the shoulders.

a. Place one hand on each side of the head over the parietal and cheek bones so that the midwife's *fingers point toward the fetal face* and nose, as depicted in Figure 29B-3. The midwife's little fingers are closest to the perineum and the thumb is farthest away. This step ensures that all subsequent maneuvers will result in maintaining a secure hold on the neonate. Remember: *"Pinkies to the perineum."*

   i. A fetus in the left occiput transverse (LOT) position will be facing the birthing person's right leg. The midwife's left hand will be the bottom hand underneath the fetal head, and the midwife's right hand will be the hand on top of the fetal head.

   ii. A fetus in the right occiput transverse (ROT) position will be facing the

birthing person's left leg. The midwife's right hand will be the bottom hand underneath the head, and the midwife's left hand will be the hand on top of the head.

   iii. Remember: *"Fetus faces the birthing person's right; the midwife's right hand is on top"* (Figure 29B-3).

b. Assist with the birth of the anterior shoulder. Avoid gripping the fetus's neck by keeping the fingers straight so the hands are flat on the sides of the head. During the next contraction, while the individual pushes, exert **gentle**, downward pressure on the head until the top of the anterior shoulder and axilla can be seen beneath the symphysis pubis. Maintain parallel alignment between the head and the fetal spine during this process. Pulling down on the head alone laterally flexes the fetal head toward the posterior shoulder. This widens the angle between the neck and anterior shoulder, which can cause undue stretch and injure the neonate's brachial plexus.

c. Once the anterior shoulder and axilla are visible, apply gentle upward pressure on the fetal head with both hands, lifting the neonate's head and following the natural arc of the curve of the pelvis toward the birthing person's abdomen. Avoid laterally flexing the neonate's neck during this maneuver. Some midwives suggest that the perineum can be protected during the birth of the posterior shoulder by sliding the bottom hand over the neonate's shoulder and keeping the neonate's arms and hands close to the body during the birth.

d. As the posterior shoulder is emerging, pivot the bottom hand under the fetal head, forming a C-shape cup with that hand facing the fetus, so that the palmar side of the hand is facing the perineum. Loosely grasp the neonate's chest and back between the thumb and fingers. The head will be supported by the midwife's forearm in this position. If the midwife's hands have been placed properly during birth of the head, the midwife's thumb will come to rest near the scapula and the fingers will lay across the neonate's thorax, with the neck and head resting

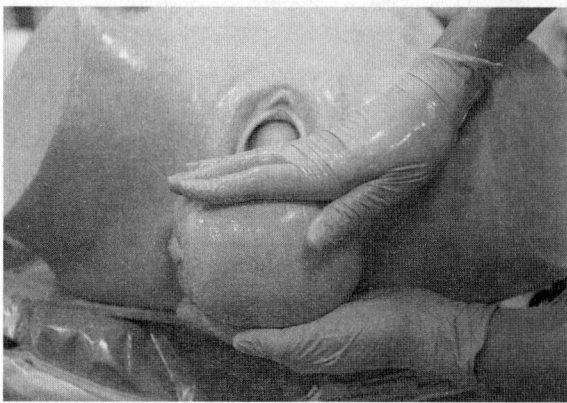

**Figure 29B-3** Placement of hands for birth of the body.

gently between the thumb and fingers in the webbing between the thumb and fingers of the bottom hand. This is the first secure grip that will be maintained. With the bottom hand in this position, a forceful push will not result in the midwife losing a secure grip on the neonate's body. This bottom hand positioning also stabilizes the neonate's neck and head. The thumb and fingers are directed down toward the center of the neonate's body, which prevents circling the neck.

    e. Slide the hand that was on the top of the fetal head down the neonate's back; grasp one or both thighs, using this hand. This is the second secure grip that will be maintained.

6. As the body of the neonate emerges, the healthy neonate can be placed immediately onto the birthing person's abdomen, pivoted to rest on the midwife's forearm facing the midwife, or handed to another clinician for assessment.

    a. To place the neonate immediately on the birthing person's abdomen: Using the bottom hand that is supporting the head by cupping the chest and scapula, move the neonate in a smooth arc from over the perineum onto the abdomen. Position the neonate laterally on the abdomen with the head and face slightly lower than the body to facilitate drainage of oral and nasal fluids.

        i. While moving the neonate onto the abdomen, confirm that there is no tension on the umbilical cord.

        ii. Maintain both secure grips on the neonate until the birthing person is safely holding the neonate.

    b. To hand the neonate to another clinician: Pivot the hand cupping the neonate's chest and scapula in one of two ways:

        i. Keeping the thumb and fingers around the neonate's shoulders, extend a finger to support the occiput and stabilize the neck. The neonate's shoulders are in the palm of the hand, and the thumb and remaining fingers are *resting*—not pressing—against the sides of the neck. The top hand continues its grasp around legs during this maneuver.

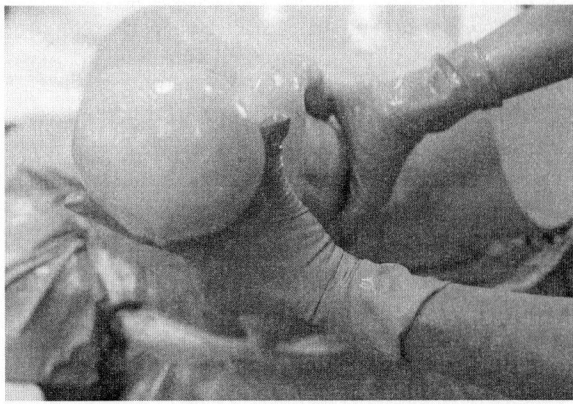

**Figure 29B-4** Stabilize the neck of the baby with one hand.

        ii. Alternatively, the bottom hand can slide up toward the head and grasp the two parietal bones between the thumb and fingers, with the occiput resting in the palm of the hand. With this maneuver, the neck is stabilized because the scapula rests on the bottom of the midwife's palm (Figure 29B-4).

        iii. The neonate's hips and legs are then tucked securely between the midwife's bottom arm and body at waist level. The neonate's back is supported on the midwife's lower arm. The neonate's head is held firmly, in a slightly dependent and lateral position to encourage postural drainage. This is the third secure grip that can be maintained regardless of the birthing person's position. An initial assessment should be conducted at this time. The midwife now has one hand (the original top hand) free to clamp and cut the umbilical cord when necessary.

## Hand Maneuvers for a Fetus in the Occiput Posterior Position

The same hand maneuvers used to facilitate birth when the fetus is in the occiput anterior (OA) position are applicable for the fetus in the occiput posterior (OP) position, with one exception: The direction of pressure exerted to maintain flexion of the head is maintained by upward pressure instead of downward pressure because the occiput is closer to the rectum than it is to the symphysis. Once the biparietal diameters are visible, releasing the upward pressure on the occiput, in a controlled manner, controls extension.

This technique is also used for the fetus in a face presentation. In a face presentation, the mentum (chin) will be under the symphysis and the rest of the head will be born by flexion of the neck. A face presentation that rotates so the mentum is posterior is not compatible with vaginal birth because the neck is too short. Once the head is out, the remaining hand maneuvers are the same as described previously.

## Hand Maneuvers When the Birthing Person Is in a Hands-and-Knees Position or Standing Position

While the mechanisms of labor are not changed by the hands-and-knees position, the way the neonate emerges appears reversed and requires variations in the direction of support and positioning of hands as a result. Visibility and access to effect maneuvers are enhanced in this position. However, in this position, while the birthing person can hear the midwife, they are not able to see the midwife. As a result, anticipatory guidance about what to expect, and where to position themselves to receive the neonate, should be communicated prior to birth if possible. In addition, there may be increased stress on the anterior labia and on the periurethral area when the birthing person assumes a hands-and-knees position for birth.

Figure 29B-5 shows a birth in a hands-and-knees position, with the neonate in an occiput anterior position. Typically, when a birthing person is standing, they are leaning forward, so the same hand maneuvers for the hands-and-knees position applies with the clinician standing behind them.

1. As the head emerges, maintain flexion by directing pressure on the occiput in the direction of the anus.

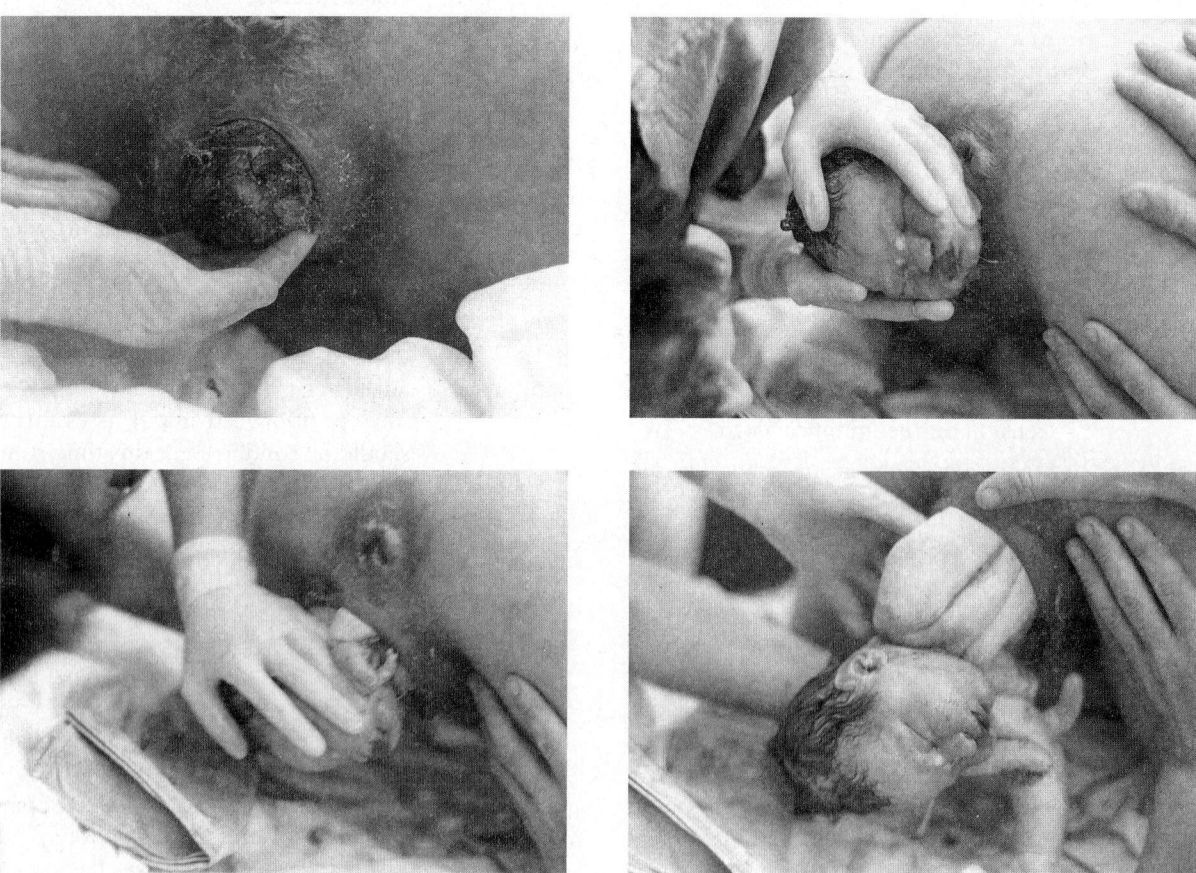

**Figure 29B-5** Birth of a neonate with a compound anterior arm in a hands-and-knees position.
Photograph courtesy of Tekoa L. King.

2. Allow the head to extend gradually, maintaining a steady but gentle counterpressure on the vertex. Maintaining flexion until the occiput passes under the symphysis pubis and extension begins will reduce the possibility of perineal trauma.

3. It is possible to support the perineum with the other hand alone or with a warm, moist towel.

4. The hand maneuvers involved in checking for a nuchal cord and watching for restitution and external rotation are the same as the maneuvers for birth when the birthing person is in any other position. In the hands-and-knees position, the hand checking for the presence of a nuchal cord will be palm up and sliding back under the neonate's head.

5. To effect birth of the shoulders: Some clinicians guide the anterior shoulder past the symphysis first, just as though the birthing person were in a dorsal position; others reverse the order and deliver the shoulder nearest the birthing person's sacrum first.

6. As the upper half of the neonate is born, follow the curve of the pelvis and, using the same hand that checked for a nuchal cord, hold the arms close against the neonate's body to protect the perineum and anterior structures.

7. The neonate can then be passed to the birthing person through the legs, keeping a secure hold until the birth person has a firm grasp on them. The midwife then moves to face the birthing person and helps them sit down. It is important to observe for tension on the umbilical cord if this maneuver is selected.

8. Alternatively, the birthing person can carefully lift one leg, with the neonate and cord being passed under that leg as they complete a turn to sit down facing the midwife. The neonate can then be placed on their abdomen.

9. Immediately after birth, many birthing persons will naturally start to sit back. If the individual sits before passage of the neonate to their arms, they may sit on the cord or neonate. To prevent this problem, the midwife instructs the birthing person and the support team on what to expect both prior to and during the birth process.

## Hand Maneuvers When the Birthing Person Is in a Deep Squatting or Supported Squat Position

To facilitate visibility, access, and control when the birthing person is in a squatting position, the midwife sits on a low stool or the floor in front of them. In a deep squat, the birthing person's legs are bent and abducted, with weight bearing distributed between the legs and feet. This position brings the perineum close to the surface they are squatting on, so the neonate emerges just inches above the surface. Moreover, the curve of the pelvis is such that the natural arc of the neonate's path is into the birthing person's arms as an extension of the arc.

In the supported squatting position, the buttocks can be partially supported by the edge of a birthing bed, a birthing chair, or a stool. The birthing person may use a squatting bar or handles on the stool, which then distributes weight bearing between their hands, buttocks, legs, and feet. The birthing person may also be supported in a semi-squat position by another person. This person may stand against a wall for back support, holding the birthing person under their arms and across their chest. Both people bend their legs and squat gently, while the birthing person bears down with support from behind. It is helpful to place a pillow on the floor between the pair's legs so that there is a place to slide down onto and sit after the birth. There is usually ample space between the perineum and floor for assisting with birth in a supported squat. The perineum may be less taut when the birthing person is in a supported squatting position compared to the deep squatting position.

The following hand maneuvers are performed to support giving birth in a squatting position:

1. As the vertex appears at the vaginal introitus, flexion of the crowning vertex should be maintained with the palmar side of the fingers and hand. Perineal support can be provided in the same manner described previously for other positions, but is done by feel, not sight, in this position.

2. It is important to watch the introitus while the head extends and is born, paying attention to the labial borders. When the presenting part emerges with the birthing person in a squatting position, the pressure exerted on the introitus is distributed equally between the labia and the perineum. Lacerations along the labial borders are more common

but tend to be shallow if extension of the head is controlled.

3. Using the maneuvers described previously, the neonate may be brought to the birthing person's abdomen, where they can easily grasp and hold the neonate if supported.

4. The hand maneuvers involved in checking for a nuchal cord, wiping the neonate's head, watching for restitution and external rotation, and delivering the anterior and posterior shoulders and body are the same as described previously.

APPENDIX

# 29C

# Umbilical Cord-Clamping at Birth

DEBRA A. ERICKSON-OWENS AND JUDITH S. MERCER

## Introduction

Following birth, neonates are separated from their placentas by the simple procedure of clamping and cutting the umbilical cord. Although a relatively straightforward procedure, it is important that the midwife understand the optimal timing and steps of cord-clamping/cutting. In this appendix, we review basic steps of clamping/cutting the umbilical cord, including how to adapt the clamping technique if neonatal resuscitation is required and how to assist a family member to cut the cord. We begin by discussing the timing of cord-clamping.

## Overview

A delay in clamping the umbilical cord results in a placental transfusion that supplies the newborn with a major source of red blood cells, stem cells, plasma, large amounts of progesterone, growth factors, and important messengers directing cellular function.[1,2] Placental transfusion continues for several minutes after birth if the umbilical cord is not clamped, and results in approximately 30% more blood volume and 50% more iron-rich red blood cells being delivered to the newborn, as compared to immediate clamping of the umbilical cord.[3] Recent randomized controlled trials have demonstrated both short- and long-term benefits of delaying cord-clamping for term and preterm newborns, without any adverse effects.[4-7] The focus of this appendix is the practice of delayed cord-clamping (DCC) for term newborns.

The definition of DCC varies, but is often described as clamping that occurs 1 to 3 minutes after birth.[4,8-11] By contrast, immediate cord-clamping (ICC) in term infants is usually defined as clamping and cutting the umbilical cord within 30 seconds after birth.[10] The World Health Organization recommends not clamping the cord immediately and suggests instead waiting for at least 1 to 3 minutes.[8] However, a delay of 5 minutes or more is encouraged when the infant is held skin-to-skin (above the level of the placenta) to ensure greatest benefit.[10] Reflecting this evidence, the most recent American College of Nurse-Midwives (ACNM) position statement on optimal management of the umbilical cord at birth recommends waiting 3 to 5 minutes before clamping.[9]

Benefits of DCC for preterm infants include reduced death rates during neonatal intensive care unit (NICU) stay, improved hemodynamic stability resulting in less intraventricular hemorrhage, reduced rates of neonatal transfusion in the NICU, higher blood volume, and blood pressure compared to ICC.[6,12] Benefits of DCC for term infants, as compared to ICC, include higher birth weights and increased early hematocrit levels, better iron stores in infancy along with less anemia, more myelin volume in early-developing areas in the brain, and better social and motor skills at 4 years of age, especially for boys.[5,7,10,13]

## Key Points

- DCC substantively increases iron stores in early infancy. Inadequate iron stores in infancy may have an irreversible impact on the developing brain despite oral iron supplementation.

- Gravity influences the amount of placental transfusion that the newborn receives. Placing the newborn in skin-to-skin contact with the birthing person immediately after birth requires a longer delay in cord-clamping.

- Uterotonics can be safely administered before clamping the umbilical cord.

- Cord milking is a safe alternative to DCC for neonates with a gestational age greater than 28 weeks, when waiting is not clinically feasible.

- The concern that DCC can cause hyperbilirubinemia or symptomatic polycythemia is unsupported by the available research.

- A change in cord-clamping practice requires collaboration between all types of providers who attend births.

## Management Steps

Briefly review the benefits of placental transfusion with the laboring person and their support person(s). Explain that DCC at the time of birth is standard practice, unless the laboring person requests otherwise.

Several issues must be considered in regard to the management of umbilical cord-clamping/cutting: timing, position of the newborn, use of uterotonics, the influence of the birth setting, and complex clinical situations (including cord milking).

A step-by-step guide for clamping/cutting the cord is provided in this appendix. It offers guidance to assist a family member in clamping/cutting the cord, if the birthing person so desires.

### Timing

- Gravity affects the amount of placental transfusion that the newborn receives. Holding the newborn below the level of the placenta accelerates the transfusion, while holding the newborn above the level of the placental slows the transfusion. Holding the baby skin-to-skin requires a little longer delay.[10,14]

- Once the transfusion is complete, the umbilical cord will become pale, white, and flat, and will look obviously emptied; at that point, the umbilical cord can be clamped and cut.[9,15] "Wait for white" is a mnemonic that is used to signal when the transfusion is complete (Figure 29C-1).

- Cessation of palpable pulsations of the umbilical cord vessels means only that the umbilical arteries have constricted; it does not indicate that it is time to clamp the cord. There is still more blood left behind in the placenta that will be transferred via the umbilical vein to the newborn during the third-stage uterine contractions.[16]

### Position of the Newborn

- Assess the newborn. Only newborns with good tone and respiratory effort should go immediately onto the birthing person's abdomen. Place the stable newborn skin-to-skin. Dry and cover the newborn with a warm blanket, and leave the umbilical cord intact for 5 minutes or until the placenta is ready to emerge.[16]

- For any person who does not want skin-to-skin placement of their newborn, place the newborn on a clean pad between the birthing person's legs, keep the neonate warm, and wait for the placental transfusion to complete.[16]

### Use of Uterotonics

- Uterotonics can be safely administered before clamping the umbilical cord.[4,17]

- The use of uterotonics may speed the rate of placental transfusion by increasing the strength and frequency of uterine contractions. A widely held misconception is that the

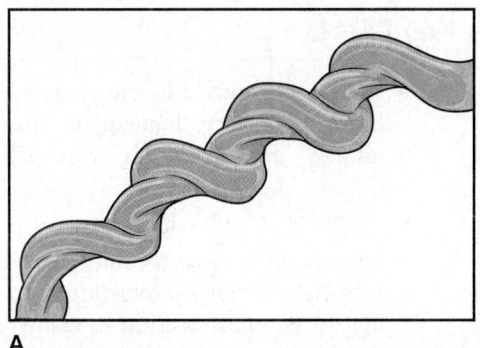
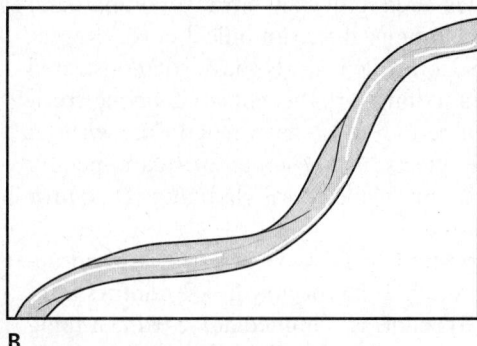

A                                                                B

**Figure 29C-1** Umbilical cord before **(A)** and after **(B)** placental transfusion.

newborn will be over-transfused; however, the evidence is clear that over-transfusion does not occur.[15]

## Complex Clinical Situations

### Tight Nuchal Cord

Approximately one-third of all newborns are born with a nuchal cord. Usually this is a nonemergent event. A tight nuchal cord is less common but can be associated with hypovolemia in the newborn. Keeping the cord intact is strongly encouraged and can be supported by performing the somersault maneuver (see Figure 29B-2 in the *Hand Maneuvers for Birth* appendix).[18] This can be followed by transitioning (or resuscitation) with an intact cord.[19]

### Shoulder Dystocia

Hypovolemia frequently accompanies a shoulder dystocia. After a birth complicated by a shoulder dystocia, assess the newborn and use techniques such as DCC or cord milking to restore blood volume before clamping. If the shoulder dystocia is accompanied by a tight nuchal cord, avoid clamping the cord before birth of the newborn's shoulders.[10]

### Slow-to-Start Newborn Requiring Neonatal Resuscitation

If the newborn has poor tone or is "slow to start," a plan of action is needed to support a safe neonatal transition.[15,19] Providers in out-of-hospital settings usually resuscitate the newborn at the perineum while maintaining an intact cord.[20] The newborn should be kept warm during the resuscitation (using warmed blankets or towels) to avoid cold stress. The hospital setting is more challenging in this respect, and the provider may not be able to resuscitate the newborn with an intact cord, without prior planning. When a neonatal resuscitation is required and the clinical situation does not allow for resuscitation with an intact cord, the cord should be clamped using two hemostats, leaving a longer section of cord (4 to 5 cm) between the neonate and the first clamp. This will allow venous or arterial access, if needed. Later, the cord can be clamped and cut closer to the neonate.

### Resuscitation with an Intact Cord

The newborn can be placed on a clean pad at the perineum or held below the level of the placenta to accelerate placental transfusion. According to the Neonatal Resuscitation Program (NRP) guidelines, breathing, heart rate, and tone need to be assessed. Heart rate can be assessed by lightly feeling the stump of the umbilical cord or by an assistant listening with a Doppler device placed on the newborn's chest, which allows all involved to hear the heart rate.[21] The heart rate is often normal even when the newborn is not initially breathing. Resuscitation, as recommended by NRP, can then proceed. The midwife should check the heart rate again; if it has not improved, all the usual resuscitation maneuvers can be instituted at the perineum without detaching the newborn. Once the newborn is breathing and tone is regained, the newborn can be placed skin-to-skin. This method of resuscitation has been practiced safely for many years in out-of-hospital settings.[10]

### Resuscitation and Umbilical Cord Milking

For infants greater than 28 weeks' gestation, and when it is necessary to transfer the newborn to a warmer for resuscitation, an alternative is to milk the umbilical cord.[10,15,16,22] While milking the cord does not provide as much blood to the newborn as DCC does, it does provide the newborn with some additional blood and red blood cell volume.[8,9] If the heart rate is low, the cord can be milked 3 to 5 times toward the newborn to accelerate transfer of blood volume before clamping.[19] To milk (or strip) the cord, a portion of the cord nearest the introitus is grasped between the thumb and the forefinger, and the cord is then compressed (milked) down the length of cord toward the newborn's umbilicus 3 to 5 times. Following a vaginal birth, start at the introitus; at the time of cesarean birth, start near the insertion site on the placenta. Take about 2 seconds to move over the length of the cord; wait about 2 seconds for cord to refill after milking, and then milk again.[15,23]

## Umbilical Cord Blood Gas Sampling

Within the hospital setting, a cord blood gas sample may be required or be a component of a standard protocol. To collect a sample, the provider double-clamps and cuts the cord near the neonate's abdomen using both a plastic cord clamp and a hemostat. A second hemostat is placed approximately 10 to 20 cm away from the first hemostat and cut (Figure 29C-2).[24] This procedure creates a section of the cord that can be used to obtain blood samples to assess acid–base balance. For more information on how to collect umbilical cord blood gases, refer to the *Third Stage of Labor* chapter and the *Umbilical Cord Gas Technique and Interpretation* appendix.

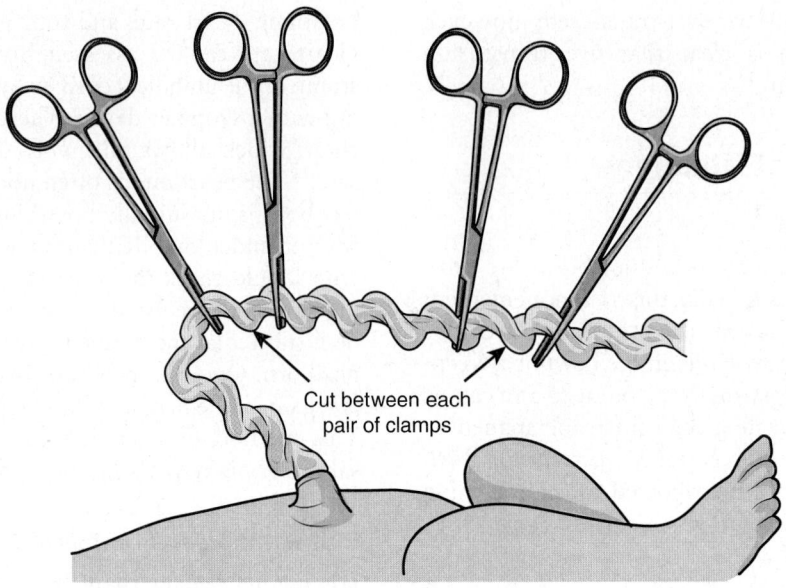

Cut between each
pair of clamps

**Figure 29C-2** Correct placement of clamps for collection of umbilical cord blood. Cut between each set of clamps, as shown by the arrows.

A delay in cord-clamping can safely be used in situations of where umbilical cord blood gas sampling is desired. In a recent systematic review, it was reported that a 2-minute delay in clamping did not significantly affect cord gas results.[25] An alternative technique supports cord gas sampling while maintaining an intact cord.[26] With this procedure, an assistant holds the newborn immediately after birth. The midwife then uses both hands to collect the umbilical cord blood gas samples. Using a tuberculin syringe with a very small-gauge needle (25 or 27 gauge), the sample is collected first from an umbilical artery and then from the umbilical vein. A small, 2 × 2 gauze pad is placed over the insertion site and very gentle pressure applied to stop the oozing. DCC is maintained and, if appropriate, the newborn is placed skin-to-skin.

## Steps of Umbilical Cord-Clamping/Cutting

1. Before birth, have the instruments needed for cord-clamping/cutting readily available. This equipment includes scissors, two hemostats, and a plastic (often yellow) cord clamp or sterile cloth tie. Instruments are sterile, and are placed on a sterile surface until used for cord-clamping/cutting.

2. After birth and when it is time to clamp the cord, place a plastic cord clamp or sterile cloth tie approximately 3 cm from the newborn's abdomen. Verify that the umbilical cord is visually normal (without evidence of bowel) before placing the clamp.

3. Grasping the cord above the cord clamp between your fingers, gently milk blood out of this section of the cord and away from the neonate for a distance of 2 to 3 cm. Hold your finger at this position while you grasp a hemostat with your other hand. This ensures that blood is not trapped between the cord clamp and hemostat, and avoids blood spray during cord-cutting. However, if the midwife "waits for white," this step will not be necessary, as blood will have transfused out of the cord.

4. Place the hemostat between your fingers and the yellow cord clamp. Now, use the scissors to cut the cord between the hemostat and the yellow cord clamp. Figure 29C-3 depicts the correct placement of instruments during cord-cutting.

5. Alternatively, if the birthing person desires, assist the family member (or birthing person) to cut the cord. Carefully pass the family member (or birthing person) a pair of scissors, handle first. Instruct them to cut between the cord clamp and hemostat, while placing the blunt end of the scissors (if applicable) toward the newborn.

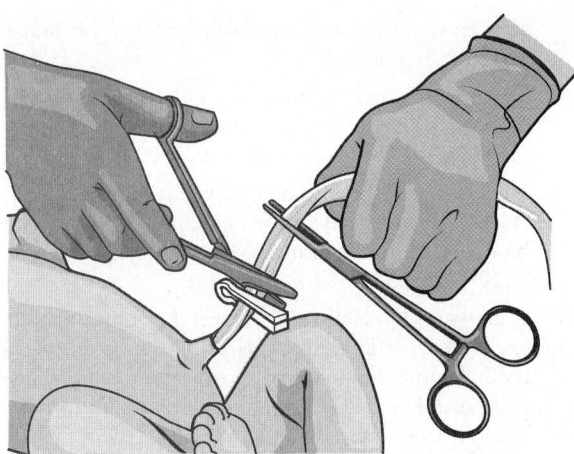

**Figure 29C-3** Correct positioning of two cord clamps prior to cutting of the umbilical cord.

6. Protect the baby during the cutting procedure. Keep moving legs and/or the penis out of the path of the scissors.

7. Once the cord is cut, take the scissors back from the helper without getting your sterile gloves contaminated. This is easiest if you grasp the scissors by their closed tips. Place the dirty scissors on the edge of the instrument table to avoid contaminating sterile instruments.

## References

1. Chaudhury S, Saqibuddin J, Birkett JR, et al. Variations in umbilical cord hematopoietic and mesenchymal stem cells with bronchopulmonary dysplasia. *Front Pediatr.* 2019;7:475. https://doi.org/10.3389/fped.2019.00475.

2. Mercer JS, Erickson-Owens DA, Rabe H. Placental transfusion: may the "force" be with the baby. *J Perinatol.* 2021;41(6):1495-1504. doi:10.1038/s41372-021-01055-0.

3. Yao AC, Moinian M, Lind J. Distribution of blood between infant and placenta after birth. *Lancet.* 1969;2(7626):871-873.

4. McDonald SJ, Middleton P, Dowswell T, Morris PS. Effect of timing of umbilical cord clamping of term infants on maternal and neonatal outcomes. *Cochrane Database Syst Rev.* 2013;7:CD004074. doi:10.1002/14651858.CD004074.pub3.

5. Andersson O, Lindquist B, Lindgren M, et al. Effect of delayed cord clamping on neurodevelopment at 4 years of age: a randomized clinical trial. *JAMA Pediatr.* 2015;169(7):631-638.

6. Rabe H, Gyte GML, Díaz-Rossello JL, Duley L. Effect of timing of umbilical cord clamping and other strategies to influence placental transfusion at preterm birth on maternal and infant outcomes. *Cochrane Database Syst Rev.* 2019;9:CD003248. doi:10.1002/14651858.CD003248.pub4.

7. Mercer JS, Erickson-Owens DA, Deoni SCL, et al. The effects of delayed cord clamping on 12-month brain myelin content and neurodevelopment: a randomized controlled trial. *Am J Perinatol.* 2022 Jan;39(1):37-44. doi:10.1055/s-0040-1714258.

8. World Health Organization. WHO recommendation on delayed umbilical cord clamping. https://srhr.org/rhl/article/who-recommendation-on-delayed-umbilical-cord-clamping. Accessed February 18, 2023.

9. American College of Nurse Midwives. Position statement: optimal management of the umbilical cord at the time of birth. http://midwife.org/acnm/files/acnmlibrarydata/uploadfilename/000000000290/optimal%20management%202021_final.pdf. Published May 2014. Updated July 2021. Accessed March 24, 2023.

10. Andersson O, Mercer J. Cord management of the term newborn. *Clin Perinatol.* 2021;48:447-470.

11. ACOG Committee Opinion: delayed umbilical cord clamping at birth (#814). *Obstet Gynecol.* 2020; 136(6):e100-e106.

12. Fogarty M, Osborn DA, Askie L, et al. Delayed vs early umbilical cord clamping for preterm infants: a systematic review and meta-analysis. *Am J Obstet Gynecol.* 2018;218(1):1-18. https://doi.org/10.1016/j.ajog.2017.10.231.

13. Mercer J, Erickson-Owens D, Deoni S, et al. Effects of delayed cord clamping on four-month ferritin levels, brain myelin content and neurodevelopment: a randomized controlled trial. *J Pediatr.* 2018;203:266-272.e2.

14. Yao AC, Lind J. Effect of gravity on placental transfusion. *Lancet.* 1969;2(7619):505-508.

15. Katheria AC, Lakshminrusimha S, Rabe H, et al. Placental transfusion: a review. *J Perinatol.* 2017;37(2):105-111.

16. Mercer JS, Erickson-Owens DA, Collins J, et al. Effects of delayed cord clamping on residual placental blood volume, hemoglobin and bilirubin levels in term infants: a randomized controlled trial. *J Perinatol.* 2017;37(3):260-264.

17. Vain NE, Satragno DS, Gordillo JE, et al. Postpartum use of oxytocin and volume of placental transfusion: a randomised controlled trial. *Arch Dis Child Fetal Neonatal Ed.* 2020;150(1):14-17. doi:10.1136/archdischild-2018-316649.

18. Mercer JS, Skovgaard RL, Peareara-Eaves J, Bowman TA. Nuchal cord management and nurse-midwifery practice. *J Midwifery Womens Health.* 2005;50(5):373-379.

19. Katheria AC, Brown MK, Rich W, Arnell K. Providing a placental transfusion in newborns who need resuscitation. *Front Pediatr.* 2017;5:1.

20. Fulton C, Stoll K, Thordarson D. Bedside resuscitation of newborns with an intact umbilical cord: experiences of midwives from British Columbia. *Midwifery*. 2016;34:42-46.

21. Hutchon D. A practical approach to measuring and documenting the heart rate at birth [Unpublished manuscript]. 2021.

22. Katheria A, Reister F, Essers J, et al. Association of umbilical cord milking vs delayed umbilical cord clamping with death or severe intraventricular hemorrhage among preterm infants. *JAMA*. 2019;322(19):1877-1886. doi:10.1001/jama.2019.16004.

23. Erickson-Owens DA, Mercer JS, Oh W. Umbilical cord milking in term infants delivered by cesarean section: a randomized controlled trial. *J Perinatol*. 2012;32(8):580-584.

24. Saneh H, Mendez D, Srinivasan VN. Cord blood gas. *StatPearls*. 2021. https://pubmed.ncbi.nlm.nih.gov/31424874/. Accessed January 20, 2022.

25. Nudelman MJR, Belogolovsky E, Jegatheesan P, et al. Effect of delayed cord clamping on umbilical blood gas values in term newborns. *Obstet Gynecol*. 2020;135(3):576-582.

26. Andersson O, Hellstrom-Westas L, Andersson D, et al. Effects of delayed compared with early umbilical cord clamping on maternal postpartum hemorrhage and cord blood gas sampling: a randomized trial. *Acta Obstet Gynecol Scand*. 2013;92(5):567-574.

APPENDIX

# 29D

# Genital Tract Injury: Immediate Postpartum Inspection of the Vulva, Perineum, Vagina, and Cervix

BARBARA J. REALE AND NICOLE S. CARLSON

*The editors acknowledge Lisa Kane Low, who contributed to this appendix in the previous edition.*

## Introduction

After birth, the midwife explains to the client the need to inspect, examine, and repair any injuries. Consent should be obtained from the birthing person for each of these stages. Comfort and pain relief measures are offered. Inspection of the vulva, perineum, vagina, and cervix for the presence of tissue trauma, lacerations, or hematomas takes place immediately after the birth to prevent unnecessary blood loss. During this inspection, the midwife identifies:

- The presence of any arterial bleeding that needs immediate ligation
- The location, severity, and type of lacerations
- Whether the lacerations require repair[1,2]
- The presence or absence of signs of a hematoma

While many repairs can be performed by the midwife alone, an assistant is often helpful or necessary. Another midwife, a nurse, scrub tech, physician, or trained birth assistant can fulfill this role.

## Key Points

### Pain Relief

Inspection of the vagina and cervix can be uncomfortable or painful for the postpartum person. The first step is to obtain consent, and then determine whether the individual is bleeding heavily from a laceration. If so, hemostasis must be achieved prior to or simultaneously with analgesic considerations. Hemostasis may be achieved initially with a combination of manual pressure, placement of hemostats, and suture ligation.

Once hemostasis is achieved, the midwife must determine whether the person needs an analgesic for the remaining components of the inspection. Before proceeding with analgesia, the midwife should obtain the birthing person's consent. The decision of which type of analgesia to offer will depend on both how extensive the inspection is likely to be and what the person's pain level is. If an extensive inspection or repair is likely, the postpartum person may need an intravenous dose of an opiate such as fentanyl or morphine. Nitrous oxide may be offered if available. If the patient has an epidural, the anesthesiologist should be consulted to determine if the epidural can be used to provide the necessary pain relief. If the patient has a patient-controlled epidural analgesia pump, they should be asked to press the button for another dose. A pudendal or local injection of anesthetic may be given as needed.

### Adequate Lighting

Ensure that an adequate, directional lighting source is available. Inadequate lighting can result in misidentification of anatomy, a laceration, or a prolonged inspection and repair. It may be necessary to move the person to a different place or different room to ensure adequate visualization.

### Positions for the Patient and the Provider

Position the person in a manner that will maximize their comfort and also allow the midwife to conduct an adequate examination. For most inspections, having the person assume a modified lithotomy position by reclining and flexing their knees and placing their feet on the bed or other surface is sufficient. However, if an upper vaginal vault or cervical laceration is suspected, positioning the person with feet in foot rests or stirrups may be preferable if available.

### Visualization

The midwife will need to insert three or four fingers into the vagina to provide adequate space to visualize the cervix and possibly the apex of a vaginal tear. Alternatively, a single-blade speculum or vaginal retractor may be inserted to apply pressure against the anterior vaginal wall for better visualization of the vagina. An assistant can gently and firmly hold the instrument in place. Actions to be taken include:

- Assess whether the laceration is hemostatic or bleeding.
- Identify the margins and anatomic location of the laceration so that a suturing plan can be formulated.
- Determine which type of laceration is present, whether repair is indicated, and which materials will be needed for the repair.[3] Table 29-8 in the *Second Stage of Labor and Birth* chapter provides descriptions of different types of perineal lacerations, and Figure 29D-1 demonstrates the appearance of common first- and second-degree genital tract lacerations following birth. Repair techniques, including selection of materials for repair, are reviewed in the *Repair of Genital Tract Lacerations and Episiotomy* appendix.

## Equipment

- Sterile gloves
- Sterile gauze pads (or lap sponge pads detectable by X ray)
- Tissue forceps
- Vaginal retractor or single-blade speculum
- Two ring forceps
- Antiseptic solution

## Procedure for Examination of the Vulva and Perineum

1. Inspection of the vulva and the perineum is achieved by using sterile, gloved fingers to gently separate the labia. A sterile cloth or gauze may be used to gently clean away blood or clots that obscure a laceration.

2. The periurethral, periclitoral, labial, fourchette, perineal, and rectal areas are completely visualized.

3. The edges of irregular lacerations may be visually approximated best if a tissue forceps is used to carry one side of the laceration to the other. This helps the midwife begin a plan for repair of the laceration.

4. If a third- or fourth-degree laceration is suspected, don an additional glove and insert the index finger into the rectum to assess the integrity of the rectal sphincter and epithelium. With palmar side up, gently lift upward to expose the full extent of the laceration. Remove this glove and discard it after the rectal examination.

## Procedure for Thorough Examination of the Vaginal Vault

For the purpose of this procedure, the vaginal vault is divided into four sections: posterior, anterior, and two lateral walls. Each section is visualized separately to identify lacerations in the vaginal mucosa. A systematic approach to this examination ensures that all areas are quickly, yet thoroughly, inspected. Gauze sponges should be counted both prior to use and after the repair is complete.

1. A 4 × 4 gauze sponge folded in fourths and clamped with a long-length ring forceps can be used to clean away blood. If the cervix is prolapsed or the anterior vaginal wall is lowered and preventing visualization, a second ring forceps, a vaginal retractor, or single-blade speculum can be used to gently lift the cervix and elevate the anterior wall, allowing for an unobstructed view of the lateral, posterior, and anterior fornices of the vaginal vault.

2. To examine each section of vaginal wall, insert the full length of several fingers of one sterile, gloved hand palmar side down and exert pressure away from the area being examined. Once one area has been inspected, release the pressure and reposition the

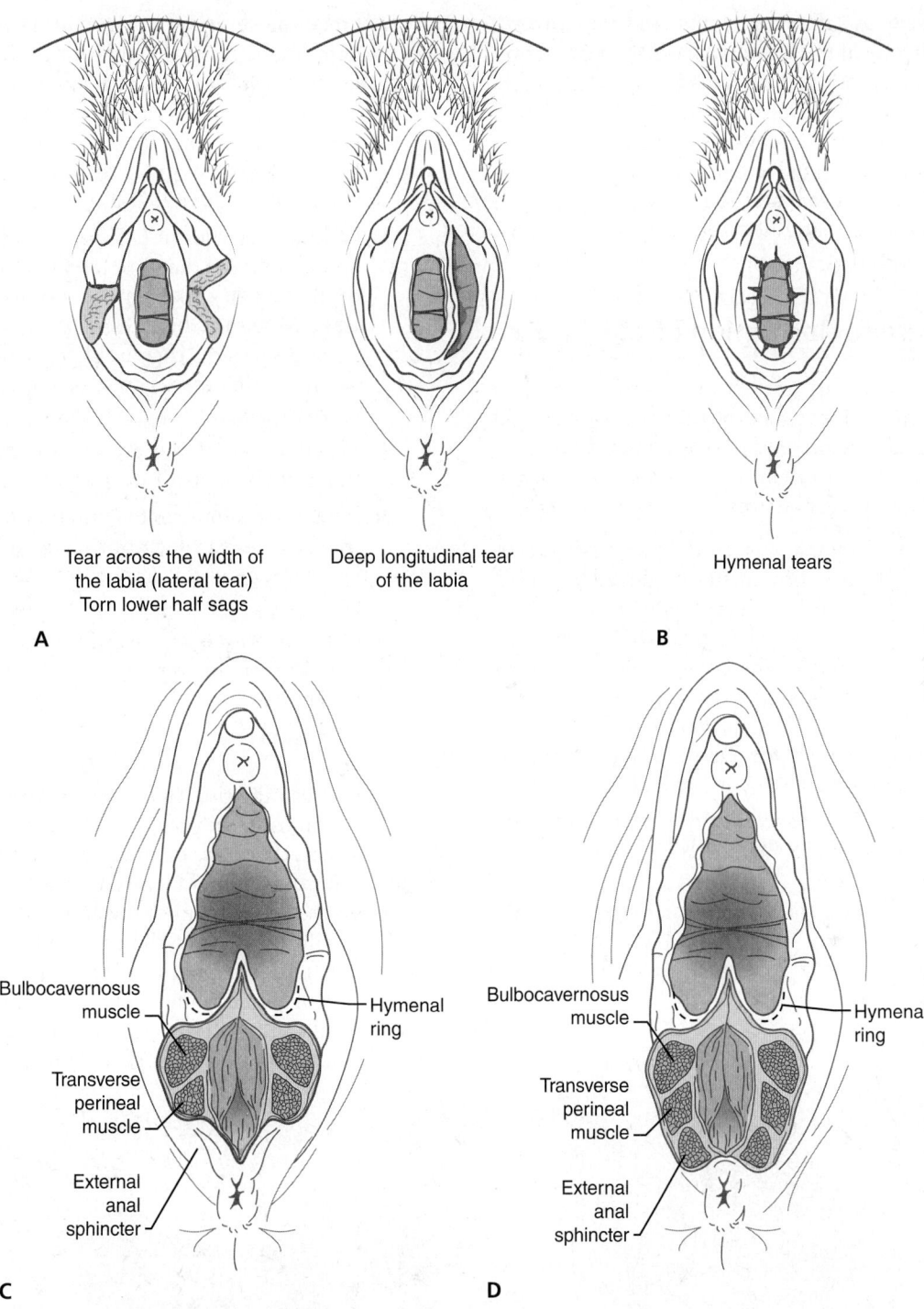

Tear across the width of
the labia (lateral tear)
Torn lower half sags

Deep longitudinal tear
of the labia

Hymenal tears

**A**

**B**

Bulbocavernosus
muscle

Hymenal
ring

Transverse
perineal
muscle

External
anal
sphincter

**C**

Bulbocavernosus
muscle

Hymenal
ring

Transverse
perineal
muscle

External
anal
sphincter

**D**

**Figure 29D-1** Common lacerations of the genital tract following birth. The images show lacerations of the **(A)** labia, **(B)** hymen, and **(C)** perineum, as well as **(D)** a laceration involving the anal sphincter.

vaginal hand in the new area to be inspected before force is applied again.

3. Insert the ring forceps with the gauze sponge on it by sliding it down the top of the vaginal fingers. This maneuver minimizes the

amount of gauze touching the vaginal walls, as the gauze is abrasive to these tissues. The gauze serves as a sponge to blot blood and other fluids from the exposed area, thereby facilitating visualization. If the gauze sponge becomes saturated, remove the ring forceps, dispose of the saturated gauze sponge, clamp on a clean one, and reinsert the ring forceps. During this procedure, the midwife should be careful to monitor use of gauze sponges so none is inadvertently left in the vagina. Dedicating an area on a delivery table or drape for saturated sponges to be counted is essential.

## Procedure for Inspection of the Cervix

Although not a part of the routine genital tract inspection following vaginal birth, the cervix should be thoroughly inspected for lacerations if the midwife notices greater than usual vaginal bleeding in the presence of a firm uterus.

1. Insert a vaginal retractor, single-blade speculum, or three or four sterile, gloved fingers of the nondominant hand, palmar side down, along the posterior vaginal wall to the area just in front of the cervix. The instrument or hand is used to exert pressure to expose the posterior vaginal wall and facilitate visualization of the cervix (Figure 29D-2). An assistant using a vaginal retractor or single-blade speculum will make this procedure easier and more efficient.

2. Once the cervix is in view, using the dominant hand, grasp the anterior lip of the cervix with one of the ring forceps. The first ring forceps is used to help bring the anterior part of the cervix into view. The second ring forceps is used to grasp the posterior part of the cervix (Figure 29D-3).

3. Hold the handles of *both* ring forceps in the dominant hand. Pull on the ring forceps gently, if necessary, to bring the cervix more into view. Move the handles of the instruments toward one side, thereby slightly pulling the cervix so the lateral apex of the cervix can be visualized.

4. Visually inspect the area of the cervix between the two ring forceps on one side.

5. If necessary, confirm the visual inspection by using the index finger of the vaginal hand to feel the edge of the cervix.

6. Repeat the procedure, moving the handles of the instruments toward the other side to visualize and inspect the other lateral side of the cervix.

7. If the cervix is very patulous, all of the cervix may be difficult to visualize adequately between the ring forceps placed on the anterior and posterior lips of the cervix. In such a case, the entire circumference of the cervix can be visualized by placing one ring forceps on the anterior lip of the cervix and the second forceps to the right of the first. Release the first forceps and place it on the other side of the second. Continue to leap-frog or "walk" the ring forceps around the cervix clockwise, clamping at 12 and 3, 3 and 6,

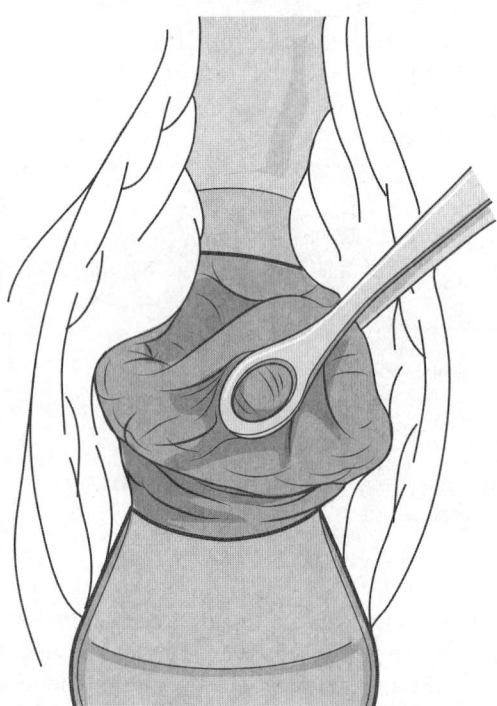

**Figure 29D-2** Visualization of the posterior fornix and cervix.

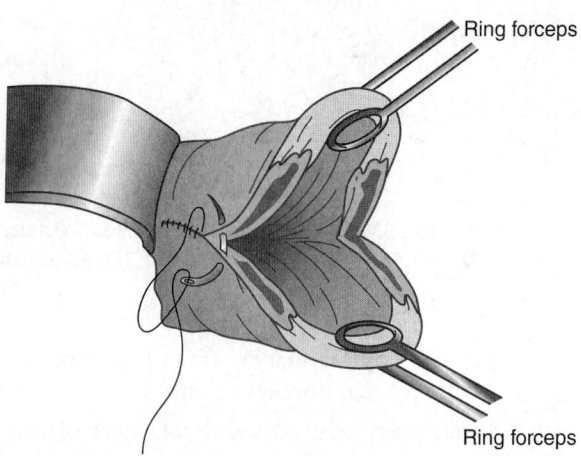

Ring forceps

Ring forceps

**Figure 29D-3** Visualization and repair of the cervix.

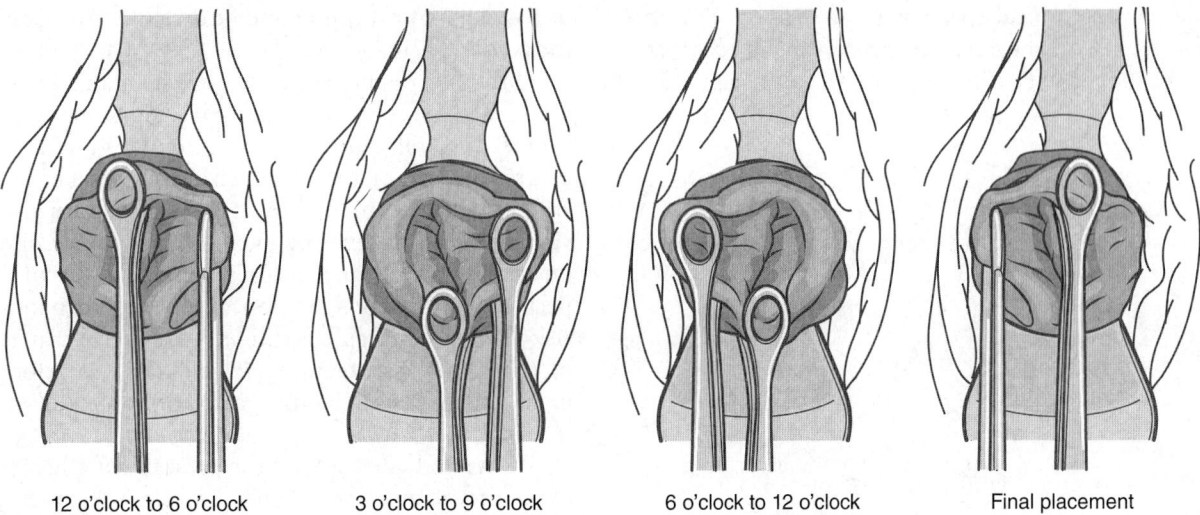

12 o'clock to 6 o'clock     3 o'clock to 9 o'clock     6 o'clock to 12 o'clock     Final placement

**Figure 29D-4** Inspection of the cervix.

6 and 9, and 9 and 12 o'clock sequentially (Figure 29D-4). This technique can also be used when the posterior lip of the cervix cannot be located easily.

8. If there are no cervical lacerations, remove the instruments or hand used for visualization.

9. If a cervical laceration is identified, it is crucial to identify the apex of the laceration, so as to rule out the possibility of an extension into the lower uterine segment. An extension would require transfer of the patient to a physician, and use of the operating room for visualization, anesthesia, and sterile technique. If the apex is difficult to visualize, place one or more sutures into the proximal aspect of the laceration and apply traction to the long ends, to bring more of the cervix into view.

10. If the cervix is bleeding from a cervical laceration, position the ring forceps to apply direct pressure on each side of the laceration to decrease or stop the bleeding, prior to repair. This method can help to significantly reduce the amount of blood lost. Cervical lacerations that continue to bleed require repair, whereas small hemostatic lacerations less than 2 cm do not need repair.

## Procedure for Identification of Hematomas

Hematomas can develop rapidly, and can be extremely painful for those birthing persons who do not have regional anesthesia.[4] They can also involve significant blood loss, causing the patient to rapidly develop signs of shock. A classic presentation is pain that is unrelieved or worsens despite administration of pain medication, typically 2 to 6 hours following birth. The most common symptom in birthing people who have epidural anesthesia is rectal pressure or rectal pain.

The most common puerperal hematomas can be classified anatomically as vulvar, vulvovaginal, or paravaginal.[4] Both vulvar and vulvovaginal hematomas can be visualized, as reviewed in the following section, whereas paravaginal hematomas may be silent until signs of hypovolemia present.[4] Hematomas are reviewed in more detail in the *Third Stage of Labor* and *Postpartum Complications* chapters.

Vulvar and vulvovaginal hematomas typically develop secondary to damage affecting one of the branches of the pudendal artery, and are the easiest of the genital tract hematomas to identify on examination. These hematomas grow superficially toward the skin and loose subcutaneous tissue. They present as swellings in the labia majora that can extend into the vagina (Figure 29D-5).[5]

Paravaginal hematomas are the typically the result of injury to the descending branch of the uterine artery.[4] These vessels are not surrounded by fascia, so bleeding can extend into the upper or lower vaginal areas, causing the walls of the vagina to push inward (Figure 29D-6).[5] Often, paravaginal hematomas are not immediately observable on exam, but if large enough, they can be palpated via careful vaginal exam. However, paravaginal hematomas can sometimes extend away from the vagina into the retroperitoneal space, making them more difficult to detect on exam. For this reason, any postpartum patient with symptoms of worsening perineal or rectal pain/pressure should be carefully evaluated for possible hematoma.

Midwifery management of hematomas is performed in collaboration with a physician colleague. For all patients, the midwife should be aware of risk factors for hematoma formation, which include proximal factors such as operative vaginal birth, presence of a genital tract injury, and injection of local anesthesia during a repair of a perineal or vaginal laceration, as well as pregnancy risk factors such as coagulopathy. The full range of pregnancy risk factors for hematoma development are reviewed in the *Postpartum Complications* chapter.

If the midwife suspects the presence of a hematoma, they should immediately evaluate the patient, including assessment of the person's pain, review of vital signs trends, and examination of the vulvovaginal area using inspection and gentle palpation. A complete blood count should be obtained so the care team can track any trends indicating blood loss. An intravenous line should be started, if not already present. Obstetric management may include interventions to identify the location and extent of the hematoma, such as ultrasonography, computed tomography scan, or magnetic resonance imaging.[6] Depending on the location and stability of the hematoma, the obstetrician and the midwife may manage it using observation, surgery, and/or referral to intervention radiology for endovascular management.[7]

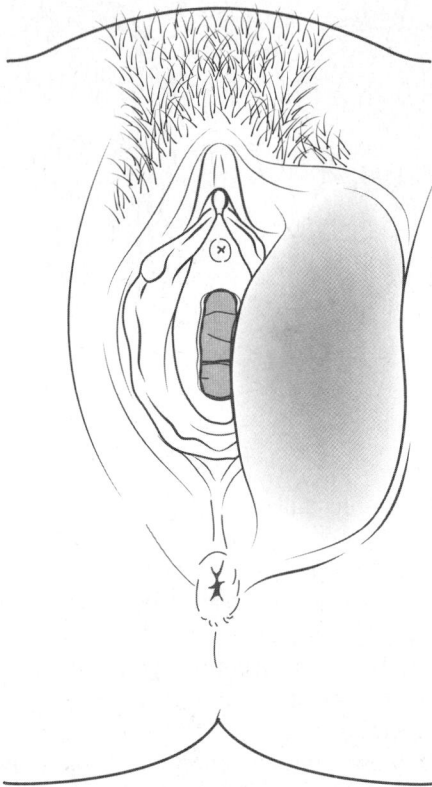

**Figure 29D-5** Vulvar hematoma causing labial bulge.

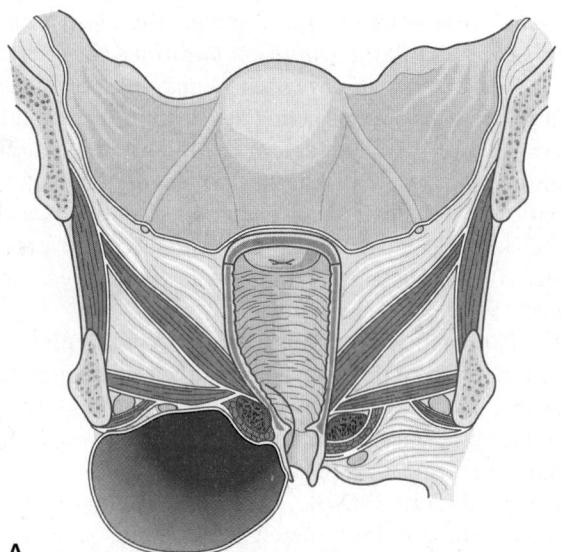

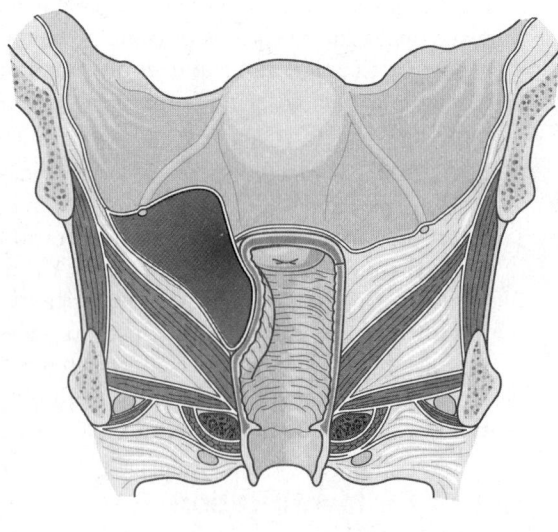

A

B

**Figure 29D-6** Paravaginal hematoma causing **(A)** posterior wall bulge (infralevator hematoma) and **(B)** lateral wall vaginal bulge (supralevator hematoma).

## References

1. Cioffi JM, Swain J, Arundell F. The decision to suture after childbirth: cues, related factors, knowledge and experience used by midwives. *Midwifery*. 2010;26(2):246-255.

2. Cioffi JM, Arundell F, Swain J. Clinical decision-making for repair of spontaneous childbirth trauma: validation of cues and related factors. *J Midwifery Womens Health*. 2009;54(1):65-72.

3. Swenson CW, Low LK, Kowalk KM, Fenner DE. Randomized trial of 3 techniques of perineal skin closure during second-degree perineal laceration repair. *J Midwifery Womens Health*. 2019;64(5):567-577. doi:10.1111/jmwh.13020.

4. Genital tract lacerations and hematomas. In: Yeomans ER, Hoffman BL, Gilstrap LC III, Cunningham F., eds. *Cunningham and Gilstrap's Operative Obstetrics*. 3rd ed. New York, NY: McGraw-Hill; 2017: 482-492.

5. Mirza FG, Gaddipati S. Obstetric emergencies. *Semin Perinatol*. 2009;33:97-103.

6. Youssef A, Margarito E, Cappelli A, et al. Two- and three-dimensional transperineal ultrasound as complementary tool in management of vaginal hematoma. *Ultrasound Obstet Gynecol*. 2019;53(2):272-273. doi:10.1002/uog.19043.

7. Gentric JC, Koch G, Lesoeur M, et al. Diagnosis and management of puerperal hematomas: two cases. *Cardiovasc Intervent Radiol*. 2013;36:1174-1176. https://doi-org.proxy1.lib.tju.edu/10.1007/s00270 -012-0504-z.

# A P P E N D I X

# 29E

# Local Infiltration for Genital Tract Repair

BARBARA J. REALE AND NICOLE S. CARLSON

*The editors acknowledge Lisa Kane Low, who contributed to this appendix in the previous edition.*

## Introduction

Local infiltration of an anesthetic solution in the genital tract area can occur just prior to birth (e.g., when performing an episiotomy or pudendal block) or following birth in the areas or structures that need to be sutured. This appendix focuses on the use of local infiltration for episiotomy or during the postpartum period for genital tract injury. The *Pudendal Nerve Block* appendix reviews pudendal nerve blocks.

## Anesthetic Agent for Local Injection

The medication recommended for local infiltration of genital tract tissue injuries is 1% lidocaine hydrochloride (Xylocaine) 10 mg/mL.[1] Lidocaine is available either with or without added epinephrine. Epinephrine produces vasoconstriction—an action that helps retain the drug in the tissue being sutured longer, thereby extending the period of anesthesia. Limited evidence suggests that lidocaine *with* added epinephrine has a longer anesthetic effect compared to lidocaine *without* epinephrine for local infiltration after birth.[2] However, lidocaine with epinephrine should *not* be used prior to birth, as epinephrine can have significant negative effects on uterine blood flow and the fetus.[3] Currently, most providers use lidocaine *without* added epinephrine for genital tract anesthesia, regardless of when they are infiltrating.

Topical anesthetic has benefits over lidocaine infiltration because it does not distort the tissue needing repair. For this reason, some providers use topical anesthetics such as lidocaine-prilocaine (EMLA) cream in addition to, or in place of, lidocaine infiltration for genital tract repair. In clinical trials, these two methods led to similar levels of pain control for repair of spontaneous lacerations or episiotomy.[4]

## Lidocaine Toxicity

Lidocaine toxicity is usually the result of accidental intravenous injection, rapid absorption from a very vascular area such as mucous membranes, or overdose. Lidocaine toxicity can cause light-headedness, dizziness, tinnitus, abnormal taste, facial tingling, circumoral numbness, and confusion.[1,5] Severe toxicity results in loss of consciousness and respiratory arrest. If lidocaine without epinephrine is injected intravascularly, the first signs may be hypotension and bradycardia.

Because lidocaine toxicity has serious side effects, a maximum dose that is safe to use is specified for this drug. It is important that the midwife carefully monitor the total volume of lidocaine injected, and not exceed the maximum recommended dose (Table 29E-1). In addition, aspiration to check for blood return is a crucial step when injecting lidocaine to avoid accidental intravenous injection (see the discussion of the procedure for local infiltration for repair after birth later in this appendix).

| Table 29E-1 | Local Anesthetic Dose and Durations for the Genital Tract | | | | |
|---|---|---|---|---|---|
| Lidocaine Type | Recommended Dose | Maximum Recommended Dose | Time Until Onset of Action and Peak Plasma Concentration | Duration of Action |
| Lidocaine 1% without epinephrine (10 mg lidocaine hydrochloride per mL) | For episiotomy: 5–10 mL (50–100 mg) infiltrated prior to episiotomy, then 10–15 mL (100–150 mg) for repair. For spontaneous genital tract injury: 10–20 mL (100–200 mg) divided between sites being repaired | 30 mL (300 mg) | Onset: 3 min. Peak: 3–15 minutes | 30–60 minutes |

Sources: Lidocaine hydrochloride: drug summary. *Prescribers Digital Reference*. http://www.pdr.net/drug-summary/Lidocaine-Viscous-Solution-lidocaine-hydrochloride-2696. Accessed June 10, 2022; Drugs.com. Lidocaine and epinephrine injection prescribing information. https://www.drugs.com/pro/lidocaine-and-epinephrine-injection.html#:~:text=The%20elimination%20half%2Dlife%20of,may%20alter%20lidocaine%20HCl%20kinetics. Accessed June 10, 2022; Phillipson EH, Kuhnert BR, Syracuse CD. Maternal, fetal, and neonatal lidocaine levels following local perineal infiltration. *Am J Obstet Gynecol*. 1984;149(4):403-407.

## Equipment for Local Infiltration

Equipment used to perform local infiltration is listed in Table 29E-2.

Lidocaine toxicity can also affect the fetus. Case reports of toxic levels of lidocaine in the fetus have been described secondary to direct injection into the fetal scalp. The risk of this unanticipated event is more likely if the fetus is in an occiput posterior (OP) position or if large amounts of lidocaine are injected more than 4 minutes prior to the birth.

## Lidocaine Dose and Pharmacokinetics

Lidocaine doses and pharmacokinetics are described in Table 29E-1. Note that this medication's onset of action occurs 3 minutes after injection. Thus, it is crucial that the midwife pause between infiltration and starting the genital tract repair to allow time for the drug to take effect. Occasionally, multiple infiltrations may be necessary if the first attempt does not provide sufficient pain relief. After each infiltration, a 3-minute pause prior to repair should again be observed.

## Local Infiltration Prior to Cutting an Episiotomy

Local infiltration prior to cutting an episiotomy is done when the perineal body has been thinned and flattened considerably by the crowning of the fetal head or pressure from the presenting fetal part. At this point, there is typically little anteroposterior tissue and only one plane that requires anesthesia.

| Table 29E-2 | Equipment Necessary for Local Infiltration of Anesthetic Solution |
|---|---|

Sterile gloves

1% lidocaine without epinephrine (10 mg/mL)

A 10- to 20-mL syringe

Needles:
- 18-gauge, 1½-inch needle to draw up the anesthetic from its original container
- 22-gauge, 1½-inch needle for episiotomy, perineal or vaginal laceration, or vaginal sulcus tear
- 25-gauge, 1-inch needle for periurethral or clitoral lacerations

While the thin and flattened perineal body allows for easier administration of anesthetic and ready identification of the area where infiltration has occurred, it also presents the challenge of potentially piercing the posterior perineal wall and inserting local anesthetic uselessly into the vagina or dangerously into the fetus. To avoid this risk, the following principles and procedure are recommended.

### General Principles
1. Always inject slowly.
2. Aspirate regularly during the injection to check for blood return and to avoid intravascular injection.
3. Keep track of the total amount infiltrated, making sure it is less than the 30 mL (300 mg) maximum recommended dose.

## Procedure

1. Place two fingers of the nondominant hand 3 to 4 cm into the vagina between the fetal presenting part and the flattened perineal body. Bring a small amount of pressure onto the posterior perineal surface to create a space between the area where the local infiltration will occur and the presenting fetal part.

2. Either of two techniques for local infiltration of the perineal body may be used. *If the plan is to cut a mediolateral episiotomy, the direction of the needle and resultant wheal(s) should not be placed centrally but instead directed to the side, following the intended path of the mediolateral cut that will be made.*

a. Technique 1: Insert the needle at the center of the fourchette and direct the needle in the mediolateral direction (infiltration for mediolateral episiotomy; Figure 29E-1) or toward the rectum (infiltration for midline episiotomy; Figure 29E-2). After aspirating, inject 5 to 10 mL (50 to 10 mg) of lidocaine slowly as the needle is withdrawn. The desired effect is to create a large, visible, and palpable perpendicular wheal approximately 2 to 2.5 cm wide and extending from top to bottom in a mediolateral or midline wedge of the perineal body.

b. Technique 2: Insert the needle point at the center of the fourchette and aspirate. Inject a maximum of 2 to 3 mL (20 to 30 mg) while steadily inserting the needle toward the perineum, making a raised line-shaped wheal from the anesthetic. Withdraw the needle up to the insertion point and redirect it to inject 2 to 3 mL again, approximately 30 degrees to the left, using the same technique. Repeat on the right side. The wheals raised by the anesthetic create an upside-down fan shape in the perineum body. This technique provides more anesthesia in a wider section of the perineum. Its goal is to avoid multiple sticks by not removing the needle before re-angling it (Figure 29E-3). **For a mediolateral episiotomy, the middle wheal of anesthetic should be centered on the line of intended incision.**

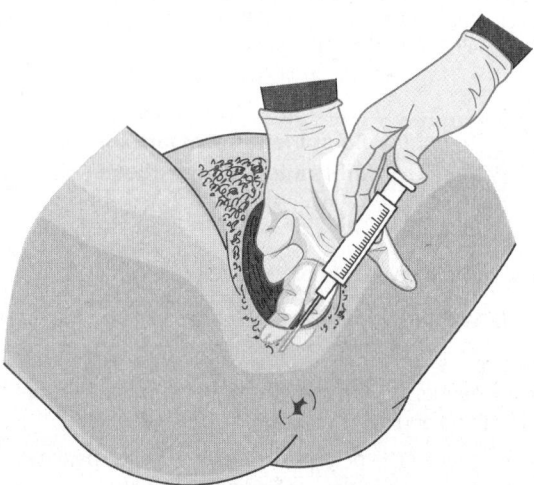

**Figure 29E-1** Technique 1 for local infiltration for a mediolateral episiotomy.

**Figure 29E-2** Technique 1 for local infiltration for a midline episiotomy.

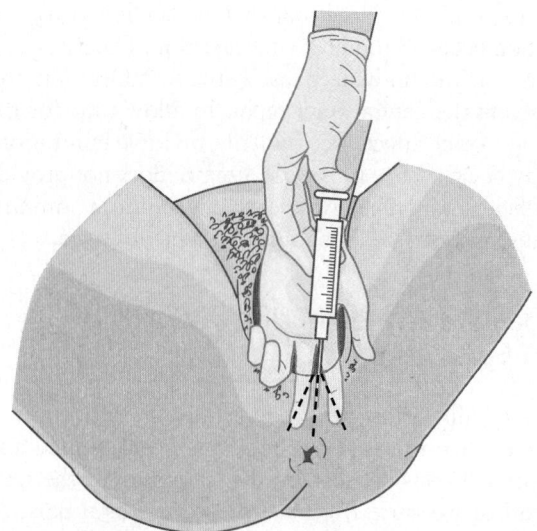

**Figure 29E-3** Technique 2 for local infiltration for a midline episiotomy.

## Local Infiltration for Repair After Birth

Local infiltration for repair of a laceration after birth may be needed if pre-birth anesthesia has dissipated, a post-birth pudendal block has failed, or local infiltration is the mode of choice. The primary disadvantage of local infiltration for repair is that it can distort the tissue, thereby making identification of landmarks and tissue approximation potentially more challenging. For this reason, the midwife should use the smallest amount of lidocaine that provides adequate pain relief according to the birthing person.

The equipment listed in Table 29E-2 can also be used for post-birth local infiltration.

### Procedure

1. Identify all tissue that requires anesthesia and repair.
2. Place the needle tip at the end or corner of the laceration nearest the posterior fourchette, and insert it for the length of the wound, reaching the areas where the suture needle will be either entering or exiting the tissue.
3. Aspirate to confirm that the needle is not in a vessel.
4. Inject the anesthetic as the needle is withdrawn along the line of the wound edge.
5. Without fully withdrawing the needle, continue injecting medication as the needle is withdrawn to just under where it entered the wound. The needle should not exit the skin.
6. Redirect the needle along the open wound into any additional tissue just under the wound that requires suturing.
7. Inject anesthetic as the needle is withdrawn back to the point of entrance.
8. Repeat this process until the area that needs suturing has been anesthetized.
9. Once the area requiring anesthesia is fully infiltrated, withdraw the needle. Another, noncontiguous area can then be anesthetized by following the same process, paying attention to ensure that the total amount of lidocaine infiltrated does not exceed the maximum suggested dose.

### References

1. Lidocaine hydrochloride: drug summary. *Prescribers Digital Reference*. http://www.pdr.net/drug-summary /Lidocaine-Viscous-Solution-lidocaine-hydrochloride -2696. Accessed June 10, 2022.
2. Colacioppo PM, Riesco MLG. Effectiveness of local anaesthetics with and without vasoconstrictors for perineal repair during spontaneous delivery: double blinded randomised controlled trial. *Midwifery*. 2009;25:88-95.
3. Drugs.com. Lidocaine and epinephrine injection prescribing information. https://www.drugs.com/pro /lidocaine-and-epinephrine-injection.html#:~ :text=The%20elimination%20half%2Dlife%20of ,may%20alter%20lidocaine%20HCl%20kinetics. Accessed June 10, 2022.
4. Abbas AM, Mohamed AA, Mattar OM, et al. Lidocaine-prilocaine cream versus local infiltration anesthesia in pain relief during repair of perineal trauma after vaginal delivery: a systematic review and meta-analysis. *J Matern Fetal Neonatal Med*. 2020;33(6):1064-1071.
5. Phillipson EH, Kuhnert BR, Syracuse CD. Maternal, fetal, and neonatal lidocaine levels following local perineal infiltration. *Am J Obstet Gynecol*. 1984;149(4):403-407.

APPENDIX

# 29F

# Repair of Genital Tract Lacerations and Episiotomy

BARBARA J. REALE AND NICOLE S. CARLSON

*The editors acknowledge Lisa Kane Low, Mary C. Brucker, Saraswathi Vedam, and Tekoa L. King, who contributed to this appendix in the previous edition.*

## Introduction

Approximately 85% to 90% of nulliparous individuals and 60% of multiparous individuals sustain some genital tract laceration during vaginal birth.[1,2] These lacerations can be either minor or extensive. Lacerations to the perineum often need repair, whereas lacerations to other parts of the genitalia usually need repair only to control bleeding or prevent later anatomic distortion. More information about decisions regarding the need to repair lacerations appears in the *Second Stage of Labor and Birth* chapter. In addition, an episiotomy—a surgical incision of the posterior perineal body—should always be repaired. (See the *Urgent Maneuvers to Shorten Second Stage* appendix.) Repair of genital tract lacerations is an essential midwifery skill.

This appendix reviews general principles for suturing, different stitches used in repairing genital tract lacerations, and techniques for repairing common genital tract lacerations sustained with birth. Genital tract lacerations are categorized according to the extent of tissue and muscle involvement, as noted in Table 29-8 in the *Second Stage of Labor and Birth* chapter.

A note regarding the directional relationships in this appendix: Step-by-step instructions for stitches are provided from the perspective of a provider who is situated at the postpartum person's perineum, while the postpartum person is positioned on their back. In this appendix, "left" and "right" sides of the wound or suture refer to the patient's left and right sides, respectively. Instructions are provided that are easiest for right-handed providers. For left-handed providers, stitches are typically initiated on the opposite side of the wound from their initiation point for a right-sided provider. Similarly, left-handed stitches are completed on the opposite side of the wound from right-sided stitches. For example, a continuous locked (blanket) stitch is secured or locked along the left side of the wound line in right-handed suturing, but is locked along the right side of the wound in left-handed suturing.

Figure 29F-1 illustrates the general anatomy of a perineal laceration. The anatomy that can be disrupted includes the skin, vaginal mucosa, hymenal ring, fourchette, bulbocavernosus muscle, transverse perineal muscle, and—if the laceration extends into the rectum—the external rectal sphincter, internal rectal sphincter, and rectal mucosa.

## Controversies Regarding Laceration and Episiotomy Repair

Controversy has emerged about when to repair genital lacerations versus when to allow them to heal spontaneously. Because every laceration is unique, meaningful evidence has been difficult to find regarding this question. In general, if the edges of the laceration appear to be well approximated when the tissue is not being handled or when the person's legs are relaxed in a natural position, then the use of suture for repair may be avoided. Today, some professionals question whether even a second-degree

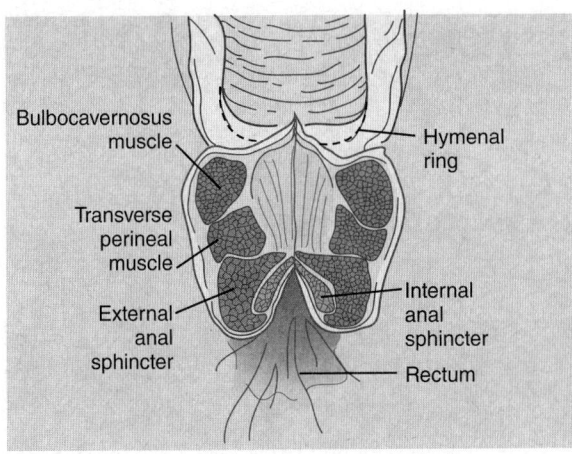

**Figure 29F-1** Anatomy of a third-degree perineal laceration.

laceration might heal in that manner, but available evidence on this topic is scant and inconsistent.[3] More information on this topic can be found in the *Second Stage of Labor and Birth* chapter.

## To Repair Skin Edges or Not to Repair Skin Edges

Some authors have suggested that leaving the skin edges unsutured may result in less pain or dyspareunia, as the sutures themselves can cause irritation. A randomized trial of two-layer versus three-layer repair found that leaving the skin edges unrepaired does result in less pain and dyspareunia at 3 months postpartum, without disadvantages such as infection or repair breakdown.[4] Glue has also been used to approximate skin edges, as reviewed in the *Second Stage of Labor and Birth* chapter.

## Equipment for Repair of Genital Tract Trauma

- Sharp scissors
- Sterile gauze sponges (4 × 4)
- Needle holder (also called a needle driver)
- Tissue forceps with and without teeth
- Suture
- 1% lidocaine without epinephrine (10 mg/mL)
- 10- to 20-mL syringe and 18-gauge needle for filling syringe with lidocaine
- 22-gauge needle for local infiltration of lidocaine

Optional as needed:
- Iowa trumpet and needle for pudendal block
- Single-blade speculum/vaginal retractor

Third- or fourth-degree laceration:
- Vaginal retractors (Gelpi)
- Locking tissue clamps with teeth (Allis)

## General Principles and Suture Technique

Repair of a genital tract laceration or episiotomy accomplishes three goals: (1) hemostasis, (2) return to functional integrity, and (3) cosmetic repair. Multiple sources exist electronically online that demonstrate various aspects of perineal laceration repair for learners who need a visual demonstration. Active practice using models and under the direct supervision of an experienced midwife or physician cannot be underestimated.

### Achieving Hemostasis

Hemostasis must first be achieved before a wound is closed. Blood clots increase the inflammatory reaction and serve as a culture media for bacteria. Large clots can cause tissue necrosis by creating pressure on adjoining tissues.

Hemostasis is accomplished by applying direct and sustained pressure for 2 minutes, or by tying off bleeding vessels. The following techniques also aid in promoting hemostasis:

1. Gently probe the depth of the wound before suturing to identify the true depth that needs repair beneath the mucosal layer.
2. Start any line of suture at least 1 cm beyond the apex of the wound to include any retracted blood vessels.
3. Use stitch types that facilitate hemostasis in the most vascular areas, such as the continuous locked or blanket stitch.
4. Use an atraumatic (tapered) needle instead of a cutting needle.

### Promoting Wound Healing

Wound healing involves three phases: inflammation, proliferation, and maturation.[5] Although healthy tissues tend to heal well, it is critical that aseptic technique is maintained to avoid the risk of infection. Asepsis may require changing gloves following the birth and redraping the area if necessary to create a sterile field; using an extra sterile glove over

| Table 29F-1 | | Suture Gauge and Common Sites for Use of Suture Material | |
|---|---|---|---|
| | **Gauge** | **Common Repair Sites** | **Usual Types of Stitches** |
| *Thinner* | 4-0 | Clitoral lacerations | Continuous, interrupted |
| | | Shallow periurethral lacerations | Continuous, interrupted |
| | | Anterior wall of rectum (repair of fourth-degree laceration) | Continuous, locked |
| | 3-0 | Vaginal mucosa | Continuous locked or unlocked |
| | | Deep periurethral lacerations | Subcutaneous, continuous |
| | | Pelvic muscles that are not extensive | Continuous unlocked, interrupted |
| | 2-0 | External anal sphincter | Continuous, interrupted |
| *Thicker* | | Cervical lacerations | Continuous locked, interrupted |
| | | Lateral wall lacerations | Continuous, interrupted |
| | | Deep pelvic muscles | Interrupted |

the sterile glove(s) already on an examining hand when checking the rectum and discarding the extra glove immediately after use; and careful placement of suture on the sterile field as the process of the repair is conducted.

During the process of wound repair, the following techniques promote wound healing:

- Use the smallest suture, suture gauge, and needle size that are needed.
- Use an atraumatic round needle.
- Align tissues as close to their original positions as possible for optimal functional integrity and good cosmetic results. Tissue forceps can be used to approximate the opposing margins of the wound into alignment, and then sutures may be placed to hold "like" tissues together.
- Carefully choose where sutures are placed the first time. Do not remove and replace sutures to obtain a more perfect result.
- Do not place stitches too close together or make them too tight. Tissue strangulation can result from very tight stitches.
- Avoid repeated unnecessary sponging, prodding, and probing of the wound. Dab—do not wipe—to avoid creating additional trauma to the tissue.
- Avoid use of instruments that crush tissue.
- Remove blood clots and debris before closure.
- Establish visible hemostasis before closure to avoid formation of hematomas.
- Ensure closure obliterates all dead space.

## Selection of Suture Material

Types of sutures used in perineal repair include standard synthetic suture, rapidly absorbing synthetic suture, and chromic catgut suture.[6] Synthetic sutures are preferred, as they are associated with less pain in the immediate postpartum period.[5,7] When compared to catgut, standard synthetic suture is absorbed more slowly; in consequence, it is less likely to require resuturing, but more likely to require removal.[5,7] Catgut has the disadvantage of causing a marked tissue inflammatory reaction that produces edema, which places tension on the sutures and can cause tissue necrosis. Ultimately, more scarring can occur, which results in a weaker functional repair. The two most commonly used types of absorbable synthetic sutures are polyglycolic acid (Dexon) and polyglactin 910 (Vicryl).

## Selection of Suture Gauge and Needle Type

Muscle heals by deposition of scar tissue and requires a stronger suture than does other tissue, which regenerates itself. The larger the gauge number, the finer the suture (e.g., 4-0 is finer than 3-0 or 2-0). The suture gauges used for various conditions are listed in Table 29F-1.

The use of an atraumatic or tapered round needle is recommended instead of a cutting needle, so as to reduce tissue trauma and the risk of increased bleeding (Figure 29F-2). A cutting needle is triangular in shape, and each edge has a sharp surface; in contrast, the atraumatic needle is a round needle with a tapered point. The latter moves through soft tissues more easily than a cutting needle and is less likely to lacerate a blood vessel. The anatomy of a needle is identified in **Figure 29F-3**.

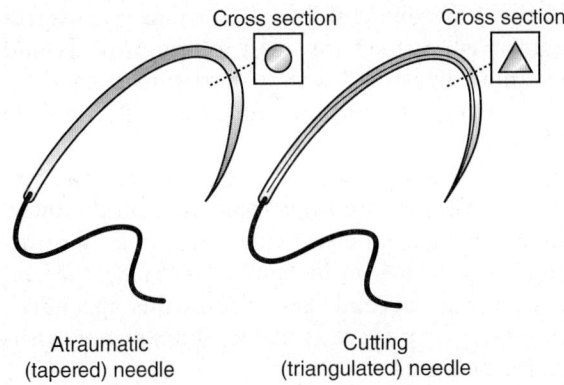

Atraumatic
(tapered) needle

Cutting
(triangulated) needle

**Figure 29F-2** Types of curved needles usually attached to suture material (swaged).

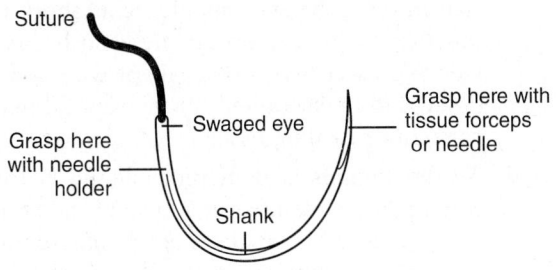

**Figure 29F-3** Anatomy of a needle.

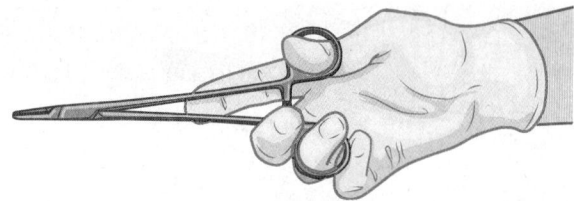

**Figure 29F-4** One method for holding a needle holder.

## Suturing

### Key Points

1. The tissue should be carefully visualized and landmarks identified. A plan should be made for the types of suture, needles, and techniques to be used for the repair.

2. The needle holder is clamped proximal to the swaged end of the needle, but not on the junction of the needle and suture.

3. The needle is clamped by the tip of the needle holder so that the plane of the curve of the needle is perpendicular to the plane of the needle holder.

4. Excess suture can be gathered up in the palm of the hand holding the needle holder, so as to prevent the length of suture from contacting other areas and causing contamination.

5. The needle holder is controlled by wrist action. It can be held so that the thumb holes are in the palm of the hand and secured by the ring and little fingers. With this positioning, the thumb and middle fingers are on either lateral side of the shaft, with the index finger on one side (usually the upper) of the broad side of the shaft (rather than placing fingers through the holes) (**Figure 29F-4**).

6. Suturing is begun by holding the needle with its curved midportion turned so the tissue can be entered with the point of the needle at an angle to the tissue that controls the depth of penetration. The closer to perpendicular to the tissue the needle is, the deeper the stitch will be. The hand holding the shaft of the needle holder is positioned so that the back of the hand is up as the needle point is positioned for entry. As the needle enters the tissue, the wrist is rotated approximately 180 degrees (palm up) so that the needle follows the necessary directional path for exit, completing the stitch.

7. The needle should be guided through tissue along the angle of its curve. When following the circle of the needle, the suture will lie in the smallest space possible, a track left by the needle. If the needle is pulled straight, its arced shape will enlarge the space it creates in the tissue and the suture will lie in a larger track, which may result in a less stable stitch, or collection of blood and fluids. Turning the wrist to follow the same arc as the needle promotes smooth movement.

8. As the point of the needle emerges, it should be grasped either by tissue forceps (without teeth) or by releasing the needle holder from its original position and repositioning the needle holder to grasp the emerging point (**Figure 29F-5**). The needle should never be handled with fingers, as doing so can cause a needle stick.

    Tissue forceps always should be used when suturing deep to moderately deep wounds. In such a case, the amount of tissue is often large enough that it is impossible to release the needle holder and grasp the other end of the needle without losing the needle in the tissue. When shallow stitches are being

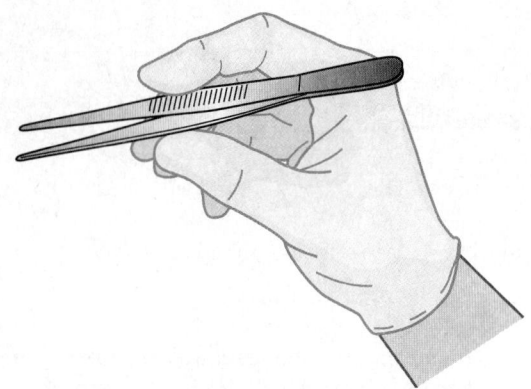

**Figure 29F-5** Tissue forceps without teeth.

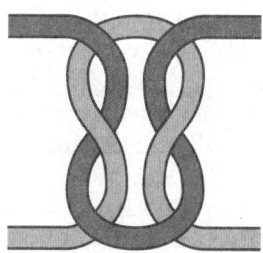

**Figure 29F-6** Square knot.

made, such as subcuticular stitches, the needle holder may be released and reclamped to the other end of the needle to complete the stitch, without concern for the needle being retracted into the tissue.

9. Excessive suture in the wound slows the healing process by causing an inflammatory reaction to foreign material. Unnecessary needle punctures, stitches, and the incorrect placement of stitches should be avoided.

## Knots

A square knot is the basic knot used for repairing an episiotomy or a laceration (Figure 29F-6). A square knot results after a left-handed overhand knot is created, followed by a right-handed knot. Each step is referred to as a "throw." Most experts advocate not only completing the square knot, but also adding one more throw to ensure that the stitch does not come undone. If either the first or third throw were to become loose, or if the suture were to dissolve more rapidly than anticipated, one complete square knot would remain.

A square knot can be tied by hand, by instrument, or by both, as all of these options can ensure that the knot is correctly tied and placed flat against

the tissue. Becoming skillful at instrument ties is recommended, as they are safest for the provider and the knot can be tied with a short suture length. A hand tie requires longer ends of suture to complete the knot.

Attaining skill in tying knots requires practice. Multiple resources on this topic exist on the Internet, including a variety of video recordings illustrating how to tie a knot by hand or instrument in real time (a topic beyond the scope of this appendix). Knot-tying boards are available, although not essential for practice.[8]

### Key Points for Tying Knots

1. The knot should be as small as possible to minimize the use of excessive suture material; in turn, the ends should be as short as possible. Extra ties do not necessarily provide extra security, but they do provide additional and unwarranted suture material that can irritate healing tissue.

2. As the knot is tied, tension should be as equal as possible in each step, and the final tension should be made as nearly horizontal as possible. The midwife may need to change physical orientation to tie the most effective knot.

3. Crimping of the suture should be avoided except when grasping the free end of the suture during an instrument tie.

4. Sutures used simply to approximate skin and subcutaneous tissue should not be tied with excessive tension because this may cause further tissue damage and unnecessary pain.

## Types of Stitches

Challenges in any discussion of the types of stitches used in repairing genital tract lacerations include the existence of many, often minor variations to a basic technique and multiple names for both the same stitch and those variations. The most commonly used stitches—continuous, continuous locked, interrupted, subcuticular, and figure of eight—are illustrated in Figure 29F-7. The description of each of these techniques presented here usually assumes a right-handed practitioner; the direction should be reversed if suturing in a left-handed manner.

### Figure of Eight Stitch

A figure of eight stitch is used to provide hemostasis and tie off actively bleeding vessels (Figure 29F-7). This step should be performed prior to undertaking

| Stitch | Alternative nomenclature | Illustration |
|---|---|---|
| Continuous locked | Blanket | 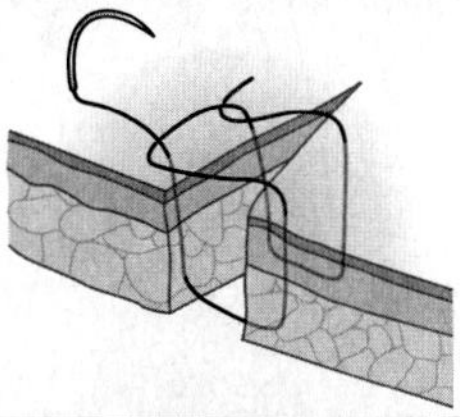 |
| Continuous | Running | 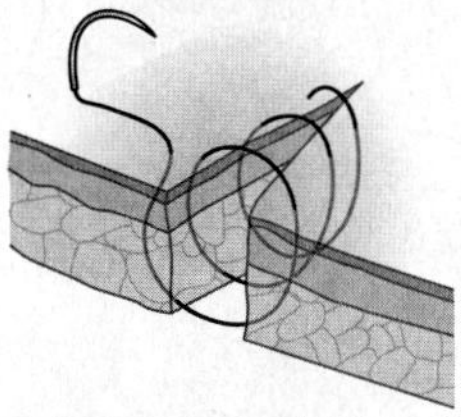 |
| Interrupted | | 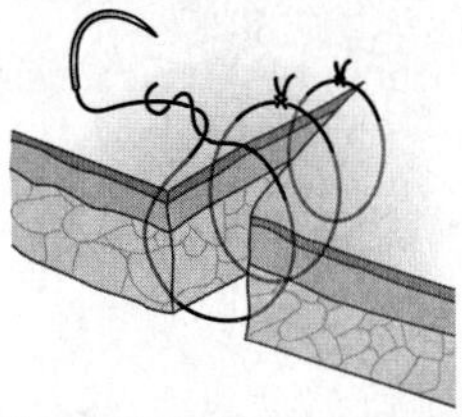 |
| Double interrupted for third-degree laceration | | 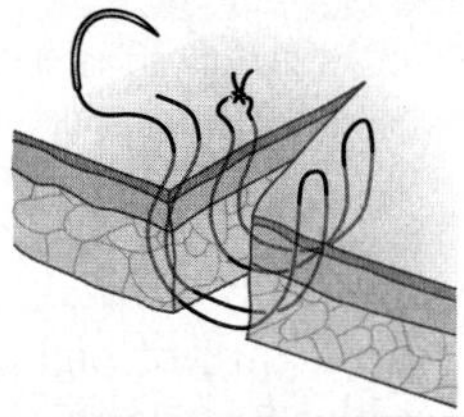 |
| Subcuticular | Mattress | 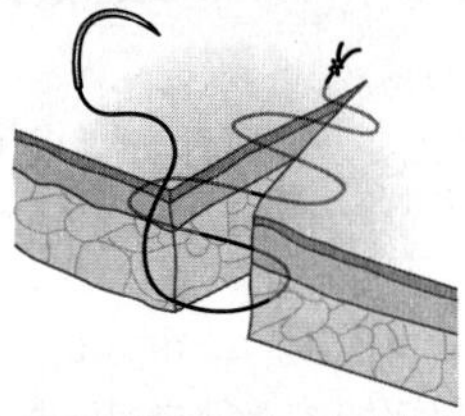 |
| Figure of eight | | 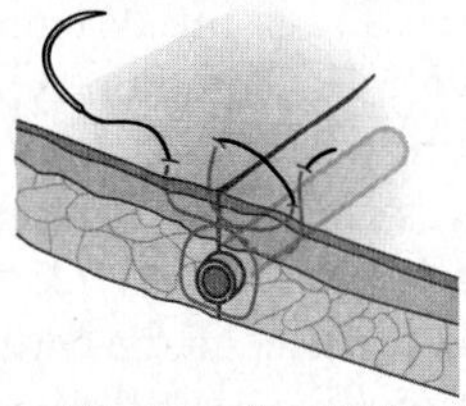 |

**Figure 29F-7** Stitches.

other genital tract repairs so as to prevent unnecessary blood loss.

1. Start the stitch by entering the tissue on one side of the bleeding vessel, moving from deep to shallow. An end for tying should remain loose.

2. Continuing with the same needle and suture, create a second, parallel stitch on the other side of the bleeding vessel, again moving from deep to shallow.

3. Create another end for tying by cutting the needle off from the suture. The two ends of

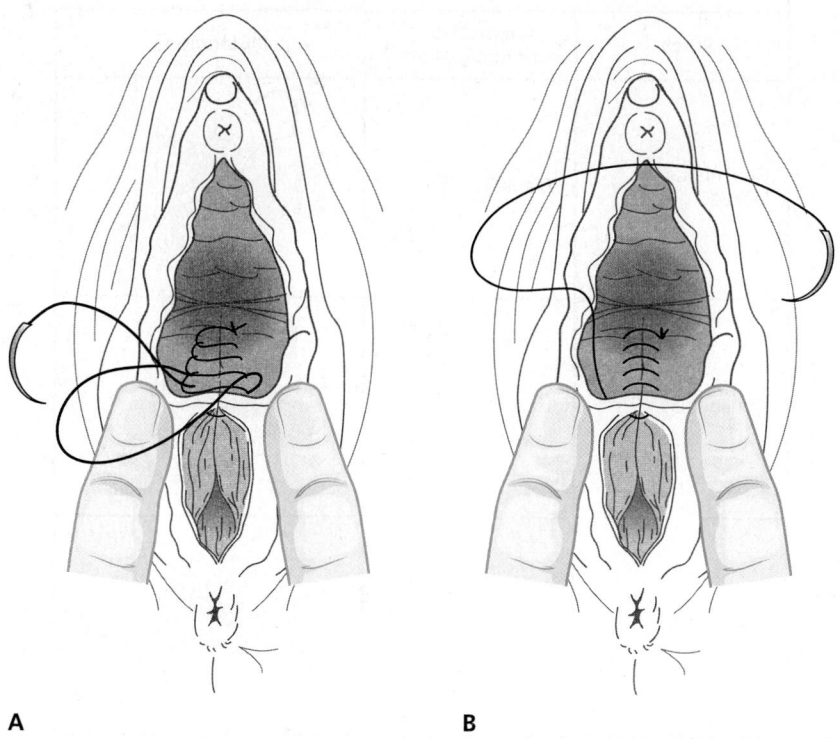

A                                                                                        B

**Figure 29F-8** Repair of vaginal mucosa and recto-vaginal fascia using **(A)** continuous locked (blanket) stitches and **(B)** continuous unlocked stitches.

suture can be tied diagonally across the tissue surface, creating a figure of eight. The suture constricts the bleeding vessel within its configuration.

### Continuous Locked (Blanket) and Continuous (Running) Stitches

A continuous stitch is often called a running stitch. However, each stitch can also be locked to provide additional security. This locking is the differentiating factor between the two most common types of continuous stitches. Steps to perform each of these stitches are presented here, as are figures demonstrating their use in the vagina (Figure 29F-8). Continuous running stitches can also be used in the perineum to repair subcutaneous tissue (Figure 29F-9).

1. For both types of stitches, the needle is inserted into the (patient's) right side of the wound and brought through the incision to emerge on the left side of the wound. The amount of tissue on each side should be approximately the same. Based on the amount of the tissue, it may be advisable to bring the point of the needle out into the midline of the wound to verify positioning before continuing to the left side. In this two-step process,

it is important that the needle enters the left side directly across from where it exited the right side, for correct approximation.

2. An anchoring knot is tied on the left side of the stitch and one end is cut short.

   a. For a continuous locked (blanket) stitch, the long end of the suture is held in front of the stitch, on the opposite side of the needle holder. The needle point emerges in front of the previous stitch but within a loop of the long end of the suture. As the needle exits the tissue, the loop of suture is pulled through until it locks the stitch.

   b. For a continuous (running) stitch, the long end of the suture lies to the outside of the needle holder. The needle point emerges in front of the previous stitch— *not* within a loop of the suture.

3. The needle and suture should be guided through the tissue, following the curve of the needle.

   a. A continuous locked (blanket) stitch is secured or locked along the left side of the wound line in right-handed suturing, and locked along the right side of the wound in left-handed suturing.

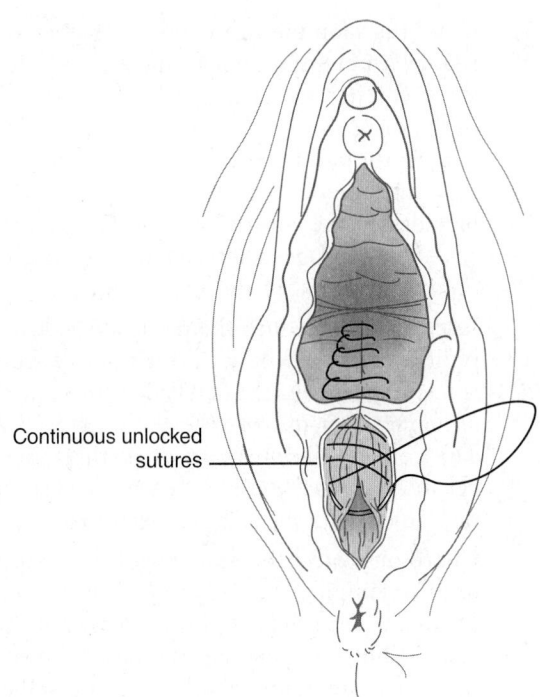

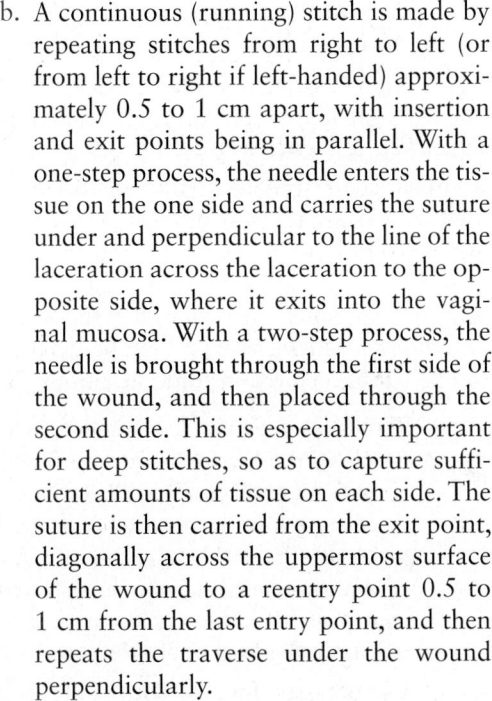

**Figure 29F-9** Repair of perineal subcutaneous fascia using continuous stitches.

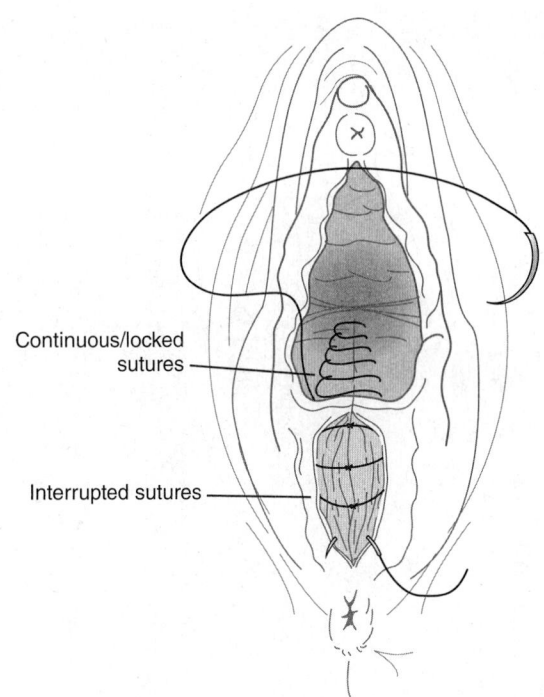

**Figure 29F-10** Repair of muscles using interrupted stitches.

b. A continuous (running) stitch is made by repeating stitches from right to left (or from left to right if left-handed) approximately 0.5 to 1 cm apart, with insertion and exit points being in parallel. With a one-step process, the needle enters the tissue on the one side and carries the suture under and perpendicular to the line of the laceration across the laceration to the opposite side, where it exits into the vaginal mucosa. With a two-step process, the needle is brought through the first side of the wound, and then placed through the second side. This is especially important for deep stitches, so as to capture sufficient amounts of tissue on each side. The suture is then carried from the exit point, diagonally across the uppermost surface of the wound to a reentry point 0.5 to 1 cm from the last entry point, and then repeats the traverse under the wound perpendicularly.

These steps should be repeated until the layer of tissue is closed.

### Interrupted Stitch

An interrupted stitch consists of a single stitch and knot. Both ends of the suture are cut short. These stitches are used to repair deep muscles of the perineum and anus (**Figure 29F-10**).

1. The needle is inserted into the side of the wound and brought through the wound to emerge on the other side of the wound, directly across from the origination, in a one- or two-step process. Sufficient suture length should remain on one end for tying.

2. The amount of tissue picked up by the needle on each side of the laceration should be approximately the same, unless the depths of the sides of the wound are uneven (e.g., in a mediolateral episiotomy). In case of a deep stitch, with a large amount of tissue to bring together, it is advisable to use two steps—first, bring the needle out in the midline of the wound; then, take another stitch into the other side of the wound. This approach will verify positioning and ensure that the needle grasps the appropriate amount of tissue on each side.

3. Tie a square knot to secure the stitch. If the interrupted stitch is used for deep muscle, care should be taken to avoid leaving any unsutured dead space behind the closed wound.

Separate interrupted stitches should be placed as needed by following these steps.

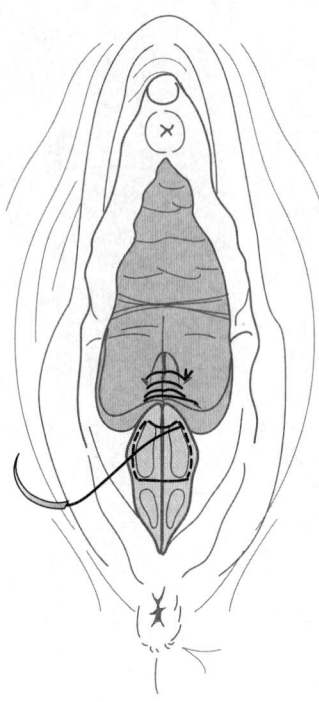

**Figure 29F-11** Crown stitch.

## Crown Stitch

The crown stitch is used to reapproximate the bulbocavernosus muscle (Figure 29F-11), also known as the bulbospongiosus muscle. This step restores the anatomy of the perineum, introitus, and labial junction at the mucocutaneous junction. When the bulbocavernosus muscle is torn, the ends usually retract superiorly and posteriorly. The crown stitch is placed in a manner that securely grasps each end, and brings both ends down and medial, to approximate them.

1. Begin by entering the tissue in an upper diagonal slant at the upper-left side of the wound line near the junction of the perineum and the vagina. Adequate space should be allowed away from the edge of the tear to enable subcutaneous continuous stitches and potentially a subcuticular closure over the completed crown stitch.

2. Direct the needle so that it follows a sequence of moving upward, then laterally, downward, and medially so that it exits in the same plane, but posterior to the original entry site. Leave a length of suture for tying a knot. Experience is essential to perform this technique well because the amount of lateral thrust must be just enough to reach the retracted cut end of the bulbocavernosus muscle. The more lateral tissue obtained, the

more vascular the area and the higher the risk of a potential hematoma will be. After the first stitch is placed, grasp the two ends of the suture a short distance from the tissue and gently pull them to provide verification that the bulbocavernosus muscle has been included in the suture. If the bulbocavernosus muscle has been sutured, the entire labia on that side (ipsilateral) will be pulled.

3. Insert the needle into the tissue at the lower right side of the wound directly across from the exit point on the left side. Direct it in a manner that mirrors the action in Step 2. The correct placement through the bulbocavernosus muscle can be ascertained using the same technique as described in Step 2.

4. Guard or protect the needle while it is not in use by clamping the swaged end in the needle driver with the tip of the needle pointed toward but not touching the needle holder, so you cannot inadvertently stick yourself or someone else. Alternatively, cut the needle off and tie the two ends of suture in a square knot, then cut the ends short. Care must be taken to only closely approximate the muscle when repairing it; pulling and suturing the two sides together too tightly may result in increased scar tissue and dyspareunia.

## Subcuticular (Mattress) Stitch

A subcuticular stitch is a buried horizontal stitch used for closing the subcuticular perineal skin during a laceration or episiotomy repair so that the suture is not visible on the skin. Figure 29F-12 demonstrates this stitch. As reviewed in the *Second Stage of Labor and Birth* chapter, the superficial skin layer can be left unrepaired in some situations.

1. Typically, subcuticular stitches, when used to close the perineum during repair of a second-degree laceration, will follow a series of running continuous stitches using the same piece of suture. However, if this is not the case, the subcuticular stitch is started with a new piece of suture, making sure to secure the suture with an anchoring stitch and knot.

2. Use of tissue forceps with teeth, to hold the skin and adjacent tissue stable while placing a stitch, may be helpful. Pick up the tissue ahead of where the needle will enter and exit.

3. Insert the needle on one side of the incision. Unlike with other stitches, this insertion is shallow. The suture is placed immediately

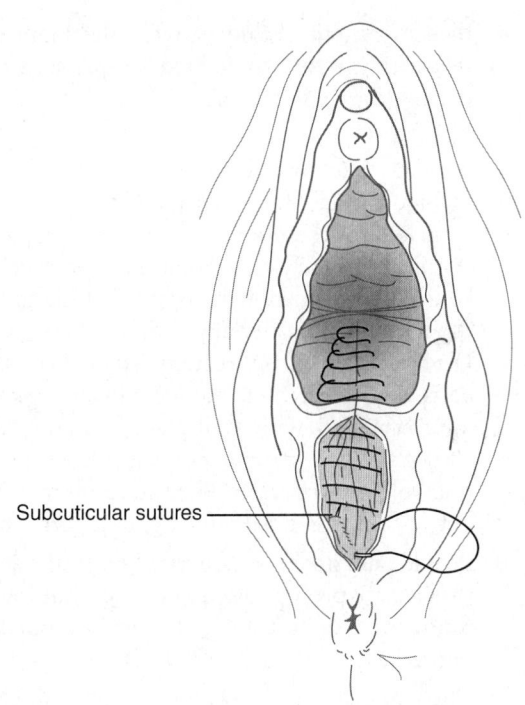

Subcuticular sutures

**Figure 29F-12** Reapproximation of skin using subcuticular (mattress) stitches.

below the skin layer and will run parallel to the line of the wound under the skin.

4. Gently guide the suture through the tissue for approximately 0.5 cm in length. Avoid catching or piercing the skin, as this could result in delayed healing and, possibly, a granuloma.

5. Make the next stitch in the same manner on the opposite side of the wound. The entry point on this side should be directly across from the exit point of the preceding stitch on the opposite side of the wound. If exit and entry points are not directly across from each other, the skin will appear "bunched up." Careful placement will result in smooth, even closure.

These steps are repeated until the wound is closed.

## Repair of First-Degree Lacerations

The majority of first-degree lacerations are small skin disruptions that barely lacerate the vaginal mucosa and will heal spontaneously without suturing. Tears in the hymenal ring do not need repair. Small, hemostatic first-degree lacerations may be repaired with glue or suture if desired by the individual.[9] More-extensive first-degree lacerations can

be repaired using continuous running stitches. In some situations, a single interrupted stitch or two may accomplish closure.

The midwife should assess the area to be repaired, approximate the laceration prior to suturing, and visualize all appropriate landmarks; the midwife should then plan the number of stitches that may be required in advance with the principle of placing the fewest possible to accomplish hemostasis and tissue edge reapproximation. A finer-gauge suture, such as 3-0 or 4-0 polyglactin on a small needle, may provide adequate tensile strength and be less traumatic.

## Repair of Periurethral, Clitoral, and Labial Lacerations

Periurethral and labial lacerations are usually longitudinal lacerations that follow the general contour of the vestibule of the perineum. They vary in depth as well as in length, with some extending superiorly to the glans of clitoris, or inferiorly exposing the crus of the clitoris. At other times, they may be transverse lacerations extending into the labia minora and occasionally across the labia majora so that it is torn into two sections. (See the *Genital Tract Injury: Immediate Postpartum Inspection of the Vulva, Perineum, Vagina, and Cervix* appendix for more information.) It is important to consider underlying tissue when repairing the skin above it.

Repair of periurethral lacerations depends on their depth, bleeding, and the need for a cosmetic repair. Repair of any laceration close to the urethra should be preceded by insertion of a urinary catheter to prevent accidental closure of the urethra. Small, superficial periurethral lacerations that are not bleeding will often heal spontaneously without stitches. Although this complication is rare, bilateral labial lacerations directly across from each other may potentially heal together, fusing the labia. At least one of these lacerations should be closed to prevent this outcome. Application of topical ointments such as petroleum jelly to the inner surfaces of the labia for several days can also help prevent labial adhesion. When significant labial edema is present, bilateral suturing and postpartum treatments such as initial application of cold packs can reduce the extent of labial edema.

When repair is indicated, most periurethral lacerations should be repaired with 4-0 suture using an interrupted technique. Prior to beginning the repair, the midwife should determine the best approach, using the smallest number of stitches possible while accomplishing reapproximation and hemostasis. There is no precise pattern or sequence of stitches to use, as each laceration is unique.

Repair of labial lacerations may also be done with 4-0 gauge suture using an interrupted stitch. Interrupted stitches can be approximately 0.5 to 1 cm apart and should not be tied too tightly, as this tissue can very easily become edematous. Continuous sutures are not recommended for labial lacerations because they can constrict edematous tissue and distort the healing process.

## Repair of a Second-Degree Laceration or Midline Episiotomy

Following are the steps that are used to repair a second-degree laceration or midline episiotomy. Although mediolateral episiotomy is now preferred over the midline procedure due to a lower risk for extension to a third- or fourth-degree laceration, repair of midline episiotomy is presented here first, as the steps are similar to those for a spontaneous second-degree laceration. The steps for a mediolateral episiotomy repair are provided in the following subsection.

As with several other midwifery skills, the steps reviewed here are only one of several possible repair strategies. This method includes both continuous and interrupted stitches. Closures dependent only on interrupted suturing techniques are associated with more pain.[10]

### Key Points Prior to Repair

1. An aseptic field must be established and meticulously maintained. Establish this field by clearing away soiled materials, irrigating or cleansing soiled skin areas, and, if needed, placing clean or sterile drapes under the buttocks.

2. Good visualization of the area of repair is critical. Lighting and positioning may need to be adapted. Uncomplicated repairs can be completed in 15 to 60 minutes, depending on the experience level of the midwife. For repairs of complicated lacerations, the birthing person can be positioned using stirrups. An assistant should be requested, and the time should be limited to less than 90 minutes, to decrease the risk of impaired circulation or thrombophlebitis.

3. Visualize the vulva, labia, vestibule, vaginal walls, cervix, and perineum to identify all sites of bleeding and tissue disruption prior to beginning the repair.

4. Identify and tie off any actively bleeding vessels with a figure of eight stitch prior to repairing the main laceration.

5. Identify the depths of the lacerations in all directions. Shallow lacerations usually do not include muscle, but occasionally the muscle is nicked. In these instances, where a muscle is mostly intact, a well-placed continuous suture can give enough support to the muscle to facilitate well-approximated healing. Deep lacerations bifurcate muscles. The two ends of a bifurcated muscle can be closely approximated with well-placed interrupted sutures. When severed perineal muscles are not well approximated, the end result may be pelvic floor weakness and a gaping introitus.

6. Provide adequate anesthesia. Epidural anesthesia may provide adequate relief, but local infiltration or a pudendal block should be performed as needed.

7. Throughout the procedure, the midwife should continually communicate with the person and family and provide anticipatory guidance.

### Technique for Repair of Second-Degree Perineal Laceration or Midline Episiotomy

1. A sponge or other absorbent material that has a tail, which remains outside the vagina, may be inserted as a tampon if necessary to maintain visualization of the field. Some portion of the internal material should always be visible outside of the vagina.

   a. Insert two fingers along the posterior vaginal wall, apply downward pressure, and slide the rolled gauze against the posterior aspect of the fingers toward the posterior fornix of the vagina.

   b. Secure the tail with a clamp to a drape where it can be seen and will not be forgotten or left in the vagina when the repair is complete.

2. Check the integrity of the anal sphincter. Feel the depth of the defect and ascertain that the anal sphincter is intact. To do this, place a second glove over the examining hand, apply lubricant to the index finger, and insert this finger into the anus. Gently press this finger toward the vagina to visualize and palpate the integrity of the sphincter and rectal mucosa; discard the outer glove immediately after examining the rectum.

3. Before starting the repair, gently support the tissue so that it falls together naturally; identify key landmarks, including the hymenal ring, apex of vaginal mucosa, mucocutaneous junction, and perineal apex. It may be helpful to use a tissue forceps with teeth to pick up one side of the laceration and carry it over to the other side to visualize how it should come together, before beginning suturing.

4. The tissue between the vaginal mucosa and rectum consists of muscle, fascia, and other tissue fibers that are collectively referred to as the recto-vaginal septum. It is repaired in stages, and in different planes. From within the vagina, sutures are placed in the vaginal mucosa with insertion directed down into the septum. On the perineum, sutures are placed below the perineal skin, and directed inward, toward the patient's back.

5. Repair the vaginal mucosa and underlying recto-vaginal fascia: The vaginal mucosa and fascia are repaired with a 3-0 synthetic absorbable suture using an atraumatic, tapered needle with locked or unlocked continuous suturing (Figure 29F-8 and Figure 29F-13A).

   a. Visualize the vaginal apex by placing both fingers along the wound edges and applying gentle downward pressure. The anchoring stitch is placed approximately 1 cm beyond the vaginal apex of the wound. This stitch is tied and one side cut close to the knot, leaving an approximately 0.5-cm tail.

   b. Repair the vaginal mucosa and fascia of the recto-vaginal septum from the posterior aspect of the wound in the vagina to the hymenal ring, using continuous stitches. Traditionally, these are locked to achieve uniform tension across the wound, but unlocked continuous stitches are adequate if bleeding is minimal. Unlocked continuous stitches have been demonstrated to cause less pain than locked continuous stitches in the recovery phase.[11] Stitches should be placed approximately 1 to 1.5 cm apart. The first one or two stitches should be deep enough to include adequate tissue on each side of the wound to close it completely. As the repair approaches the perineal muscles, the stitches should be shallower and include only the vaginal mucosa. The muscle should stay exposed so that it can be visualized and repaired. Avoid placing sutures through or over the hymenal ring, as they may cause discomfort in the healing process.

   c. Use a transition stitch to bring the suture from the vagina down to the perineum (Figure 29F-13B). If using unlocked continuous stitches on the vaginal floor, direct the needle downward into the mucosa and exit in the subcutaneous tissue of the perineum. If using locked continuous stitches, place the needle so that it locks the last vaginal stitch as it is directed downward to bring the suture from the vagina behind the hymenal ring into the perineal plane.

6. Repair of the perineal muscles and subcutaneous fascia: Alternative approaches can be used to complete repair of the perineum. The first approach involves continuous (unlocked) suturing down toward the anus, followed by subcuticular stitches using the same suture back up to the fourchette. The second is a three-layer, multi-suture approach. Both are described in detail in the following section.

   If the perineal wound is shallow and appears to have spared the transverse perineal muscles, continuous suturing is done as described in option (a). In contrast, if the wound appears deep enough to have separated the bulbocavernosus and superficial transverse perineal muscles (generally, deeper than 1 cm when a finger is inserted into the perineal wound, just beneath the repaired vaginal mucosa), deep interrupted stitches as part of a three-layer perineal repair provide better support for a reconstructed perineal body, as described in option (b).

   a. Continuous unlocked suturing of perineum: When the perineal wound is shallow and does not appear to involve the transverse perineal muscles, continuous suturing may be used to repair the wound. Continuous running (unlocked) stitches should be used.

      i. Repair the bulbocavernosus muscle (Figure 29F-10 and Figure 29F-13C). After pulling the suture from the vagina into the perineal plane using a transition stitch, perform a crown stitch to reapproximate the ends of

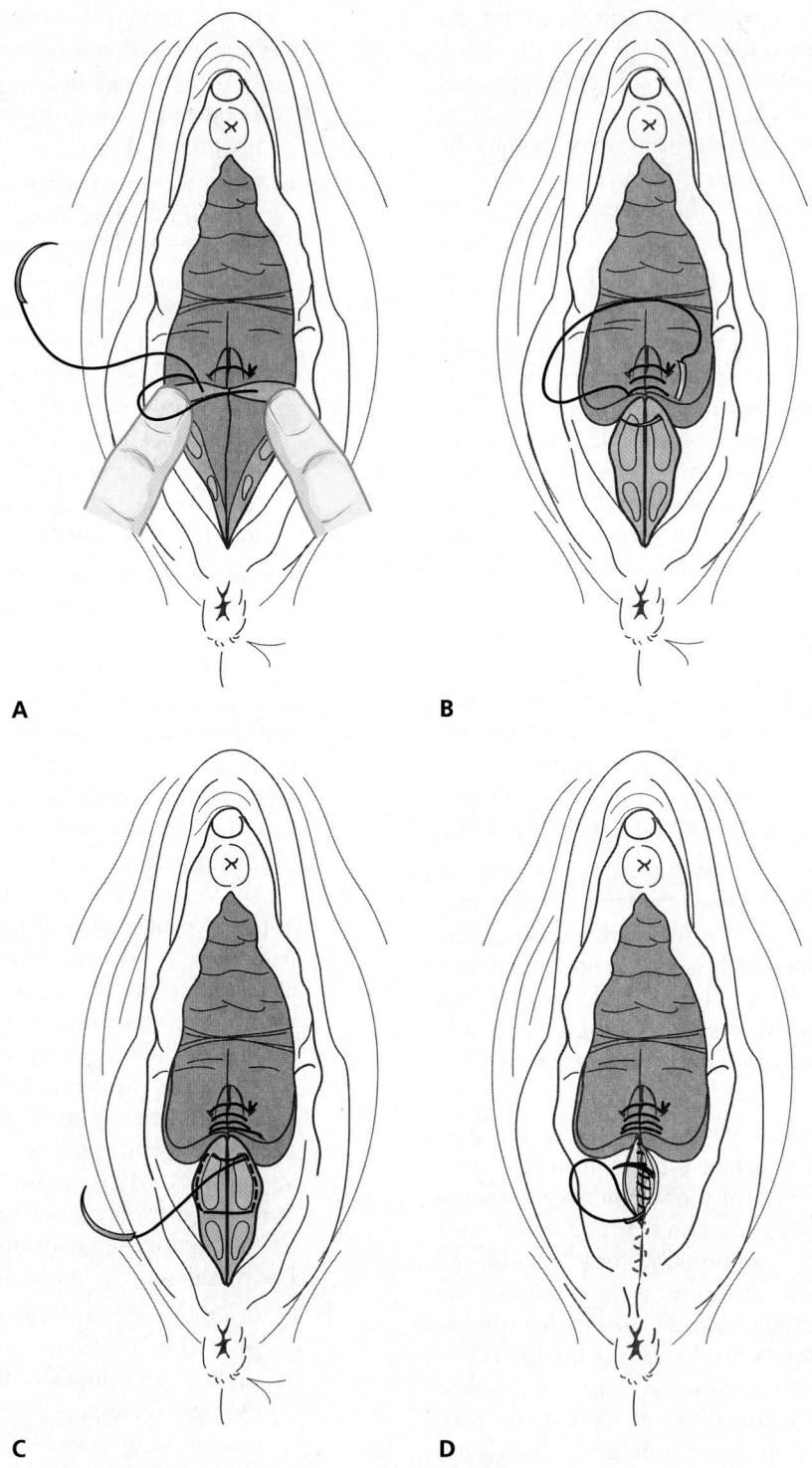

**A**

**B**

**C**

**D**

**Figure 29F-13** Repair of second-degree laceration or midline episiotomy. **(A)** Placement of an anchor stitch above the wound apex, with continuous locked suture of the vaginal epithelium. **(B)** Transition stitch to bring the suture from the vagina to the perineum. **(C)** Reapproximation of the bulbocavernosus muscle using a crown stitch. **(D)** Closure of the perineal skin using a subcuticular stitch from the bottom of the perineal laceration upward. Not shown is the final knot tied inside the hymenal ring.

this muscle (which often retract into the deeper perineal layers when torn).

ii. Repair the perineal subcutaneous fascia. Using the same suture from Step i, run a series of continuous unlocked stitches from below the hymen down to the apex of the perineal laceration. To do this, insert the needle perpendicular to the wound so as to avoid accidentally placing stitches in the rectum. To properly orient the needle into the perineum, hold the needle holder parallel to your body, with the handle near the edge of the bed (in hospital births where the person is on a bed with an edge). In a community birth setting where repairs are often performed in a bed, the needle holder can be oriented with the handle up toward the ceiling. Make sure the needle grasps subcutaneous fascia and deep perineal muscles together on each side of the wound. Place each stitch 0.5 to1.0 cm below the previous one.

iii. Perform a gentle one-finger rectal exam to identify any suture that may have inadvertently entered the rectum. Afterward, discard the glove used to examine the rectal tissue and don a new one. If suture is palpated in the rectum, the repair must be dismantled and the rectally placed suture removed to prevent infection or creation of a sinus tract. (If continuous stitches were used, they must be removed until sufficient length of suture to tie a knot is left; then restart with a new suture.) Proceed to subcuticular closure.

iv. If reapproximating the perineal skin, use subcuticular stitches (Figure 29-F12 and Figure 29F-13D), moving from the apex of the perineal wound (nearest to the anus) toward the fourchette. Skin reapproximation does not have to be tight to allow for swelling during the normal healing process.

v. Reverse the direction of the transition stitch and tie off the suture. Diving below the hymenal ring with the needle,

pull the suture from the perineum back through the vaginal mucosa, behind the hymen. Make one additional stitch in this location. Do not pull the suture through the tissue entirely, but instead leave a loop to create one side of the tie. Cut the needle off of the opposite side and tie the knot across the laceration, posterior to (behind) the hymen. The knot should be made securely, but not tight enough to cause tissue bunching. Placement of the knot behind the hymen decreases the risk of postpartum discomfort. Trim suture ends to 0.5 to 1 cm long.

b. Three-layer, multi-suture repair of perineum: When the perineal wound is deeper and involves both the bulbocavernosus and transverse perineal muscles, correct placement of a layer of deep interrupted stitches will improve approximation and give additional support to the muscles of the perineal body during healing. Afterward, a second layer of continuous unlocked suture repairs subcutaneous tissue, followed by a third layer of subcuticular stitches to reapproximate the skin.

i. Secure the needle and suture from the vaginal repair. For this three-level repair, two different sutures are used: (1) the suture used during repair of the vaginal tissues and (2) a new length of suture to be used for deep interrupted stitches. After using the transition stitch to bring the suture used for vaginal repair down to the perineum, secure the needle for this suture and place on a sterile drape located under the birthing person's bottom. It is important to "guard" the needle not in use with a needle driver.

ii. Prepare suture for repair of the perineal muscles. Load a 2-0 absorbable synthetic suture with an atraumatic needle onto a new needle driver.

iii. Repair the bulbocavernosus muscle (Figure 29F-10 and Figure 29F-13C). Using the new length of 2-0 suture, perform a crown stitch to reapproximate the ends of this muscle (which often retract into the deeper perineal layers when torn). Cut the suture, tie the two ends in a square knot, and then cut the ends to a length of 0.5 to 1 cm.

iv. Repair the transverse perineal muscles. Using the 2-0 suture, place another interrupted stitch to repair the transverse perineal muscles; these muscles retract laterally when torn. Holding the needle holder perpendicular to the floor and the introitus, direct the needle from superficial to deep, so it exits at the back of the perineal wound. The needle is then grasped with forceps and held, while the needle holder is removed and replaced on the other end of the needle to draw it through using a twisting motion of the wrist. Care must be taken to not "lose" the needle in the retracting muscle. Next, direct the needle from deep to superficial, incorporating the other side of the wound. It is important that the needle exit and entry points are directly across from each other.

v. Perform a rectal exam. After the interrupted stitches are placed, put aside the 2-0 suture, and perform a rectal examination to determine whether any of the stitches can be palpated within the rectal mucosa. The risk of a rectal suture is diminished if all interrupted stitches are placed carefully in the horizontal plane.

vi. Repair the perineal subcutaneous fascia. Using the same suture you set aside in Step i (3-0 suture used to repair the vaginal mucosa), run a series of continuous unlocked stitches down the length of the perineal laceration toward the anus. The goal is to obliterate space that would be created by closing the skin edges over a subcutaneous defect.

vii. If reapproximating the perineal skin using suture, place subcuticular stitches (Figure 29-F12 and Figure 29F-13D), moving from the apex of the perineal wound (nearest to the anus) toward the vagina.

viii. Reverse the transition stitch and tie off the suture. Diving below the hymenal ring with the needle, pull the suture from the perineum back through the vaginal mucosa, behind the hymen. Make one additional stitch in this location, tying off the suture. Trim suture ends to a length of 0.5 to 1 cm.

7. After suturing, remove any gauze that may have been inserted in the vagina. Inspect and verify that the suture line is intact and without any hematoma or active bleeding along the suture lines.

8. Conduct a count of gauze pads and needles with the birthing assistant or nurse, assuring safety for all. In general, it is the responsibility of the provider to safely dispose of all needles.

9. Ascertain the firmness of the fundus and remove any vaginal blood clots that may have developed during the repair. Wash the perineal area, thighs, and buttocks as needed. Assist in helping the person assume a comfortable position. Apply ice to the repaired laceration.

## Repair of Sulcus Tears

Sulcus tears are a type of second-degree laceration in which the vaginal mucosa and underlying tissue are lacerated along one (unilateral) or both (bilateral) sides of the posterior column of the vagina, instead of up the middle. The posterior column of the vagina is a longitudinal ridge of the inner surface of the lining extending the length of the vagina. The lateral edges of the column meld into the lateral vaginal walls and create a slight groove (sulcus), from which this type of laceration derives its name.

Due to the depth of the wound and potential difficulty with visualization, extra lighting, vaginal retractors, and a second person to hold the retractors are often needed during assessment and repair of sulcus tears. Significant blood loss can occur with deep sulcus tears, requiring prompt placement of figure of eight stitches to effect hemostasis. Repair of sulcus lacerations is an advanced suturing skill, and many midwives consult with obstetricians for repair of these lacerations.

Repair of sulcus tears differs from the repair of the vaginal mucosa only if the tear is bilateral. In this event, a midline tear will bifurcate in the posterior vagina and the laceration can have a Y shape. Two apices (plural for apex) and two separate lines of continuous locked stitches are needed to close the separate tears in the Y portion of the laceration. At their common base, one line of sutures is tied with a final stitch and a square knot, while the other line of sutures continues to draw the larger base opening together.

Sulcus tears are usually deep lacerations and may require two layers of deep interrupted stitches when the deep muscle layer is repaired. To provide better access for placing the deep interrupted stitches, the vaginal mucosa may be repaired with a few stitches placed in the common base of the bilateral tear for approximation of the tissues, followed by interrupted stitches, followed by the return to the repair of the vaginal mucosa.

## Technique for Repair of Mediolateral Episiotomy

The mediolateral episiotomy differs from the median episiotomy in that the surgical incision is at an angle of approximately 60 degrees off the midline of the perineum (Figure 29F-14). The tissue exposed on the medial side of the incision appears shorter in width than the tissue on the lateral side. A mediolateral episiotomy tends to be deeper and involves a more extensive repair than a midline episiotomy, but has the advantage of less often extending to form a third- or fourth-degree perineal laceration.[10] The following concepts must be understood to succeed with a well-approximated repair.

1. Stitching from side to side of the incision must be done in accordance with the angle of the incision, rather than situating stitches straight across the wound. This is facilitated by holding the needle holder parallel to the perineal edge of the incision, on the same side where the needle will first enter. This concept also applies to stitches placed vaginally.

2. The medial aspect of the wound (closest to the rectum) tends to retract more than the lateral aspect. Therefore, the needle must pick up less tissue on the medial side, and more on the lateral side.

3. Deep perineal muscles are repaired using two steps, allowing the provider to account for medial retraction and uneven widths of tissue on each side of the wound. This also helps the midwife avoid losing the needle within the deep tissue. A two-step technique is done in the following manner:
   a. Hold the needle holder perpendicular to the skin on the lateral side of the

laceration. Have the needle enter the deep tissue on the lateral side of the incision and exit at the middle base of the wound. Use a forceps to secure the needle, bring it completely through, and replace it on the needle holder.
   b. Reposition the needle holder so it is parallel to the medial edge of the incision. Have the needle enter directly across from where it exited the lateral side. Pick up approximately half as much tissue in the medial side, as compared to the lateral side.

Repair the mediolateral episiotomy using the same sequence of stitches as used for the repair of the median episiotomy. As in that repair, if the perineal transverse muscles appear to be intact, a continuous unlocked suture may be used rather than the triple-layer approach with interrupted stitches.

1. Begin on the posterior vaginal floor, placing an anchor stitch behind the apex of the incision (Figure 29F-14A). Bring the vaginal mucosa together using a continuous unlocked stitch (unless locking is preferred for a wound requiring more tension for control of small bleeding vessels). Any larger bleeding vessels created by an episiotomy should be repaired first using interrupted stitches (see the figure of eight stitch instructions). Bring the needle under the hymen and exit in the subcutaneous tissue of the perineum using a transition stitch.

2. Assess the depth of the incision. If the perineal wound is deep and the perineal transverse muscles appear to be injured, use a triple-layer repair with interrupted stitches. To do this, guard the needle used in Step 1 and put aside for the triple-layer approach. Then, prepare a new needle with 2-0 suture. If the perineal wound is not deep (less than 1 cm in depth), prepare to use the original needle for repair of the bulbocavernosus muscle.

3. Reapproximate the bulbocavernosus muscle (Figure 29F-14C). If using the three-layer suture approach, repair this muscle using the new 2-0 suture, then tie the suture off. If using the continuous suture approach, use the needle and suture from Step 1.

4. If they are injured, repair the transverse perineal muscles. Using a new needle with 2-0 suture, repair the deep transverse muscles of

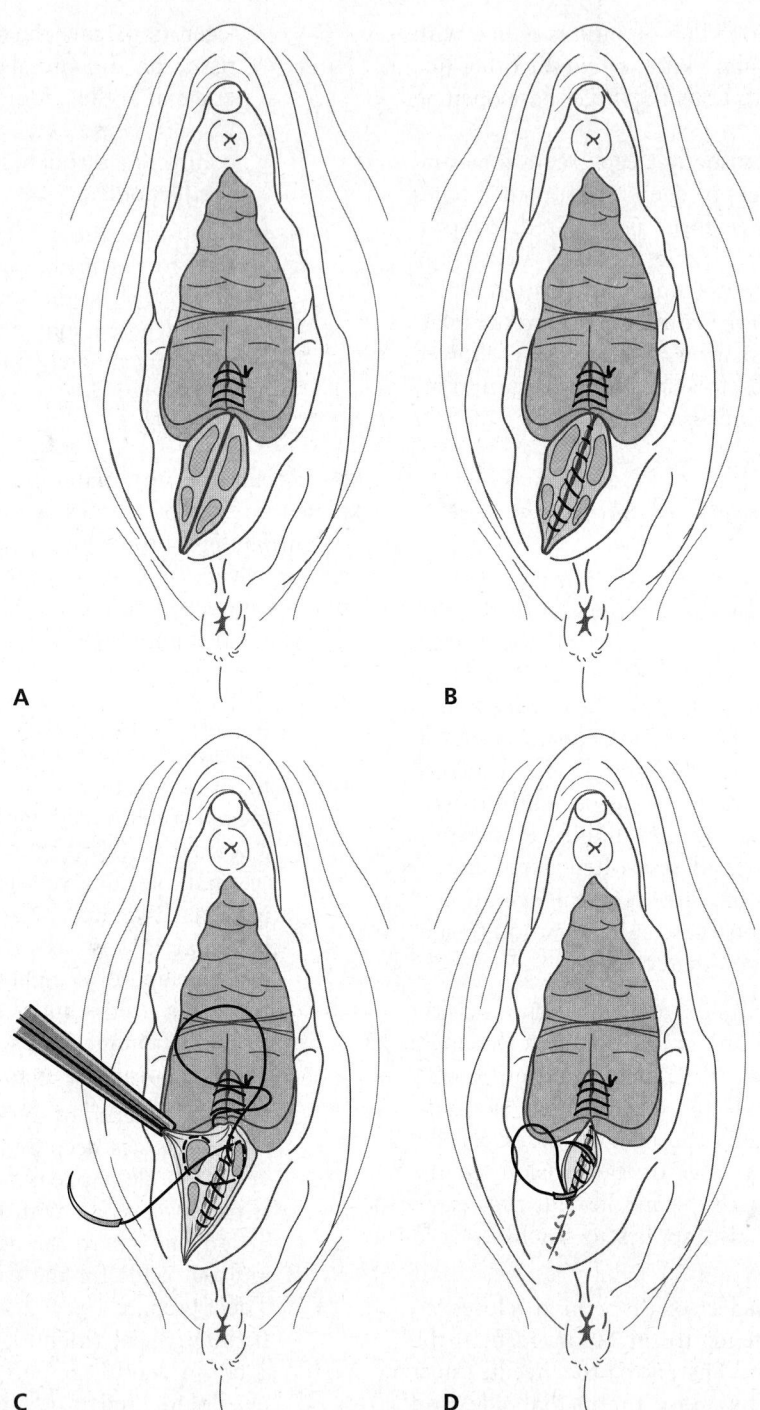

**Figure 29F-14** Repair of a mediolateral episiotomy. **(A)** Repair of vaginal tissues using a single continuous suture. **(B)** Reapproximation of deeper perineal tissues using continuous stitches (may not be necessary if the perineal wound is not deep). **(C)** Reapproximation of the bulbocavernosus muscle using crown stitch. **(D)** Closure of the perineal skin.

the perineum with interrupted stitches; avoid entering the rectum by using the two-step process. These stitches will provide stability to the repair and, if the suture should break prematurely, the other stitches will remain in place.

5. If stitches were placed near the rectum, perform a rectal exam to confirm that no suture has entered the rectum. If suture is found, it must be cut and removed. Don a new glove and repair as needed. (If continuous stitches were used, they must be removed until a sufficient length of suture to tie a knot is left; then restart with a new suture.)

6. The fascia and subcutaneous layers are closed using continuous stitching. Pick up the needle that was used to repair the vagina in Step 1. Bring together the sides of the incision by running continuous unlocked stitches down to the lower apex of the perineal incision, picking up more muscle tissue on the lateral side. Place stitches approximately 0.5 cm apart on both sides of the wound, moving under and away from the vaginal floor (Figure 29F-14B). This layer of stitching should "even up the wound," resulting in close approximation of the skin.

7. Repair the skin by running a subcutaneous stitch from the lower apex to the introitus. Complete the repair in the same manner as the repair of a median episiotomy (Figure 29F-14D).

## Repair of Third- and Fourth-Degree Lacerations

Repair of third- and fourth-degree lacerations is an advanced skill beyond the American College of Nurse-Midwives' Core Competencies for Basic Midwifery Practice. The experienced midwife may be credentialed to perform repairs of third- or fourth-degree lacerations. Appropriate education, experience, and institutional privileges are needed prior to implementing this skill.

### Key Points

1. Good visualization and adequate anesthesia are essential to accurately repair a third- or fourth-degree laceration. Assistance is likely needed to secure the visualization needed and should be requested by the midwife while collaborating team members for the repair are assembled.

2. Third- and fourth-degree lacerations are always repaired before repairing the rest of the perineal laceration, if present.

3. The goal of repair is to reconstruct the muscular cylinder of the rectal sphincter, which is approximately 2 cm thick and 3 cm long.

4. The area may be irrigated with saline prior to being repaired. In contrast to practice years ago, antiseptic solutions generally are no longer employed, as they may irritate this tissue.

### Repair of Fourth-Degree Lacerations

Fourth-degree lacerations involve the external anal sphincter, internal sphincter, and anterior rectal mucosa (Figure 29F-15). The rectal mucosa and the internal anal sphincter are always repaired before the external rectal sphincter is repaired. After identifying the tear in the anterior rectal wall and the torn ends of the anal sphincter, the repair begins by rejoining the anterior rectal mucosa. This area is repaired in two layers with 3-0 or 4-0 polyglactin suture (Vicryl) on an atraumatic needle.

1. The first layer of suturing starts at the internal apex and consists of a row of interrupted stitches placed in the rectal submucosa to approximate the rectal mucosa without placing stitches in the lumen of the bowel. A CT-1 atraumatic curved needle is typically used, taking small amounts of tissue into each stitch.

2. The second layer is the internal anal sphincter; it appears as a shiny pink, thick tissue that surrounds the rectal mucosa. It often

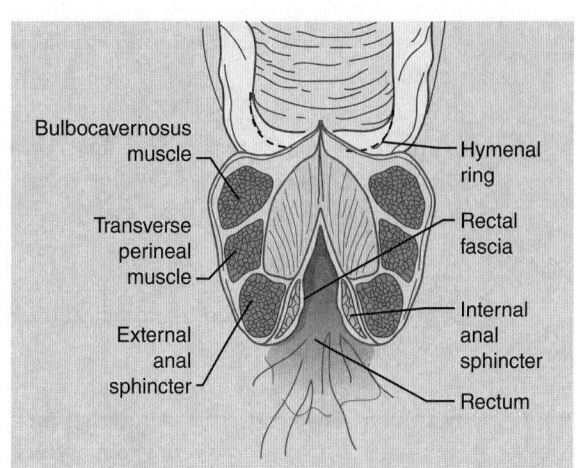

**Figure 29F-15** Fourth-degree perineal laceration.

retracts laterally and superiorly when torn. Repair is made with a continuous technique using 3-0 polyglactin suture. This repair also starts at the internal apex and is brought out to the cutaneous junction, where it is tied off.

3. After verification that no sutures are in the rectal lumen, repair of the external anal sphincter (described in the next section), followed by standard repair of the laceration or episiotomy, is completed.

### Repair of Third-Degree Lacerations

A third-degree laceration differs from a fourth-degree laceration in that it does not include the rectal mucosa. Otherwise, repair of the anal sphincter is the same for both types of lacerations.

1. Identify the torn external anal sphincter. As the torn ends retract, they are found flush with, or as dimples in, the lateral walls at the bottom of the perineal aspect of the wound near the surface. The muscle fibers of the sphincter are visually different from the surrounding fascia. Often one side is dimpled, and the muscle can be visualized emerging from the other side.

2. Grasp both torn ends with a tissue clamp with teeth and pull them toward each other, causing them to meet. The suture of choice is 2-0 synthetic, absorbable suture. Some midwives prefer to first anchor a 3-0 absorbable suture within the inferior apex of the skin extension of the laceration and take a few subcuticular stitches in the posterior anal capsule, then lay this suture aside until the end. This approach is intended to avoid later difficulty in repairing the subcuticular area over the rectal sphincter, as it is sometimes difficult to visualize this apex after repair of the sphincter.

3. Repair a lacerated external anal sphincter with either doubled interrupted stitches or a figure of eight stitch after approximating the torn ends grasped by the tissue clamp with teeth.

   a. Inclusion of the anterior and posterior fascial layers surrounding the sphincter muscle strengthens the repair.

   b. The internal and external sphincters may both be lacerated. The internal anal sphincter appears as a shiny pink, thick tissue that surrounds the rectal mucosa. It often retracts laterally and superiorly

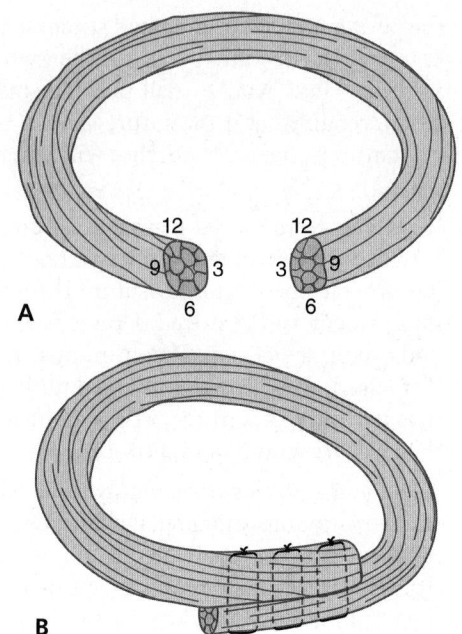

**Figure 29F-16** Repair of anal sphincter. **A.** End-to-end technique. **B.** Overlapping technique.

when torn. Repair of this layer is made with a continuous technique using 3-0 polyglactin suture. This repair also starts at the internal apex and is brought out to the cutaneous junction, where it is tied off. After verification that no sutures are in the rectal lumen, repair of the external anal sphincter (described in the next section), followed by standard repair of the laceration or episiotomy, is completed.

   c. The external sphincter can be repaired by one of two methods: The first places the torn section "end to end" and the second uses an "overlapping" technique (Figure 29F-16). The overlapping technique is superior in that it is associated with less fecal incontinence and pain.[10,12–14] The overlapping method is recommended for a complete tear but cannot be used for an incomplete tear (grade 3a or partial-thickness grade 3b).[10]

   d. Technique for a doubled interrupted stitch:

      i. Put the needle into the right side of the muscle and bring it out in the left side of the muscle.

      ii. Put the needle into the left side of the muscle near where it came out and bring it out in the right side.

iii. The suture now has two strands and will be tied off on the side where it was started.

  e. *End-to-end repair:* Place four doubled interrupted sutures starting at the posterior aspect (Figure 28F-16A), with one in each quadrant at the 6 o'clock, then 9 o'clock, then 12 o'clock, and then 3 o'clock positions.

  f. *Overlapping technique:* Using the tissue clamp with teeth, overlap the ends of the sphincter and place three doubled interrupted sutures in both parts of the muscle where they overlap (Figure 29F-16B).

4. After repairing the sphincter and before continuing with the remainder of the repair, perform a rectal examination to confirm that sutures have not been placed in the rectal mucosa as previously described. If no stitches are palpated, repair of the laceration or episiotomy then continues in standard fashion.

5. When a person has a third- or fourth-degree perineal laceration, it is common practice to order stool softeners, oral analgesics, and sitz baths for their initial postpartum recovery. In addition, a single dose of antibiotics has been shown to decrease wound complications in the postpartum period for OASIS wounds, and was designated as "reasonable" in the 2018 practice guidelines published by the American College of Obstetricians and Gynecologists.[10]

## Repair of Cervical Lacerations

Cervical lacerations can be difficult to identify and can bleed extensively. Availability of an assistant to hold the retractors and good lighting are invaluable in this situation to enable good visualization.

### Key Points

1. Good visualization is necessary, including adequate lighting and effective use of the ring forceps on the cervix to bring the cervix and its laceration into full view (see Figure 29D-3 in the *Genital Tract Injury: Immediate Postpartum Inspection of the Vulva, Perineum, Vagina, and Cervix* appendix). A well-contracted uterus can also be beneficial so potentially obscuring uterine bleeding is minimal.

2. Use of a vaginal retractor helps provide better visualization. In the optimal scenario, an assistant will be available to hold the retractor during the repair. Since cervical lacerations can extend into the lower uterine segment, it is critical to be able to visualize the apex with certainty.

3. Epidural anesthesia will be of benefit and allows relaxation that will promote better visualization. Alternatively, nitrous oxide or intravenous opioids can be used.

4. Cervical lacerations more than approximately 1 cm in length or a laceration of any length that is bleeding should be repaired.

5. Cervical lacerations are repaired with 2-0 absorbable synthetic suture.

### Steps to Repair Cervical Lacerations

1. Approximation of the two sides of the tear is facilitated by the placement of a ring forceps on each side of the laceration. The ring forceps should be placed close enough to the edges to be of use, but far enough away from the edges that the stitches can be taken without sewing through the ring of the forceps.

2. Cervical lacerations are repaired with interrupted stitches, a continuous stitch, or a continuous locked stitch if additional hemostasis is required. Selection of the best stitch is at the discretion of the person placing the sutures.

3. The first stitch should be placed approximately 1 cm above or beyond the apex of the laceration to include any retracted blood vessels.

4. Care should be taken in the placement of each stitch approximating the two sides of the tear so that only the sides of the wound are included in the stitch, thereby maintaining the patency of the cervical canal.

### References

1. Albers L, Garcia J, Renfrew M, et al. Distribution of genital tract trauma in childbirth and related postnatal pain. *Birth.* 1999;26:11-17.

2. Smith LA, Price N, Simonite V, Burns EE. Incidence and risk factors for perineal trauma: a prospective observational study. *BMC Pregnancy Childbirth.* 2013;13:59. doi:10.1186/1471-2393-13-59.

3. Elharmeel SMA, Chaudhary Y, Tan S, et al. Surgical repair of spontaneous perineal tears that occur during childbirth versus no intervention. *Cochrane Database*

*Syst Rev.* 2011;8:CD008534. doi:10.1002/14651858 .CD008534.pub2.

4. Gordon B, Mackrodt C, Fern E, et al. The Ipswich childbirth study: 1. A randomized evaluation of two stage postpartum perineal repair leaving the skin un-sutured. *Br J Obstet Gynecol.* 1998;105:435-440.

5. Leffell DJ, Brown MD. *Manual of Skin Surgery: A Practical Guide to Dermatologic Procedures.* New York, NY: Wiley; 1997.

6. Kettle C, Dowswell T, Ismail KMK. Absorbable suture materials for primary repair of episiotomy and second degree tears. *Cochrane Database Syst Rev.* 2010;6: CD000006. doi:10.1002/14651858.CD000006.pub2.

7. Bharathi A, Reddy DB, Kote GS. A prospective randomized comparative study of Vicryl Rapide versus chromic catgut for episiotomy repair. *J Clin Diagn Res.* 2013;7(2):326-330. doi:10.7860/JCDR/2013 /5185.2758.

8. Ethicon. Knot tying manual. http://surgsoc.org.au /wp-content/uploads/2014/03/Ethicon-Knot-Tying -Manual.pdf. Accessed December 12, 2017.

9. Arnold MJ, Sadler K, Leli K. Obstetric lacerations: prevention and repair. *Am Fam Physician.* 2021; 103(12):745-752.

10. ACOG Practice Bulletin No. 198: prevention and management of obstetric lacerations at vaginal delivery. *Obstet Gynecol.* 2018;132(3):e87-e102. doi: 10.1097/AOG.0000000000002841.

11. Kettle C, Dowswell T, Ismail KM. Continuous and interrupted suturing techniques for repair of episiotomy or second-degree tears. *Cochrane Database Syst Rev.* 2012;11:CD000947.

12. Fernando RJ, Sultan AH, Kettle C, et al. Repair techniques for obstetric anal sphincter injuries. *Obstet Gynecol.* 2006;107(6):1261-1268.

13. Leeman L, Spearman M, Rogers R. Repair of obstetric perineal lacerations. *Am Fam Physician.* 2003; 68(8):1585-1590.

14. Fernando RJ, Sultan AH, Kettle C, Thakar R. Methods of repair for obstetric anal sphincter injury. *Cochrane Database Syst Rev.* 2013;12:CD002866. doi:10.1002/14651858.CD002866.pub3.

15. Jiang H, Qian X, Carroli G, Garner P. Selective versus routine use of episiotomy for vaginal birth. *Cochrane Database Syst Rev.* 2017;2:CD000081. doi:10.1002/14651858.CD000081.pub3.

16. Sooklim R, Thinkhamrop J, Lumbiganon P, et al. The outcomes of midline versus medio-lateral episiotomy. *Reprod Health.* 2007;4:10-16.

17. Ma K, Byrd L. Episiotomy: what angle do you cut to the midline? *Eur J Obstet Gynecol Reprod Biol.* 2017;213:102-106.

CHAPTER

# 30

# Complications During Labor and Birth

AMY MAROWITZ AND SHAUGHANASSEE VINES

*The editors acknowledge Linda A. Hunter, who was the author of this chapter in the previous edition.*

## Introduction

Even under the most normal of circumstances, intrapartum complications can occur. While many of these situations develop gradually or are associated with known risk factors, some will arise without warning. This chapter builds on material reviewed in the *Pregnancy-Related Conditions* and *Medical Complications in Pregnancy* chapters as well as the content on the physiologic first and second stages of labor. An overview of selected complications and conditions during the intrapartum period is presented. Familiarity with intrapartum complications and emergencies is essential to midwifery practice and requires frequent review of current guidelines. Additional resources and study may be necessary to obtain a more thorough exploration of the underlying pathophysiology associated with certain preexisting high-risk conditions.

Team-based care is a type of interprofessional collaborative practice that is ideal for the situations in which intrapartum complications occur. With this approach, a midwife partners with colleagues (e.g., obstetricians, maternal–fetal medicine specialists, and/or pediatricians) to provide care according to the person's preferences and needs and as clinical circumstances dictate. Members of the healthcare team utilize their expertise to the full extent of their scope of practice.[1,2]

Communication and collaboration practices as part of team-based care vary according to the severity of the pregnant person's pregnancy complication(s). There are three main types of team-based care: consultation only, collaborative care, and referral. Each is reviewed here, with the midwife and physician roles being defined for each approach; this subject is also discussed in detail in the *Professional Midwifery Today* chapter. For all types of team-based care, the rationale for consultation, collaboration, or referral as well as the resultant personnel involved in a pregnant person's care should be clearly documented in the health record.

During consultation, the midwife formulates the management plan with input from a physician. This model of team-based care is appropriate for complications that are only slightly outside the midwife's normal range of care. For more intense complications, a collaborative mode of care can be used.

Within a collaborative model of care, the midwife provides continuity of care, advocates for the pregnant person, protects normal labor progress as the clinical situation allows, and keeps the consulting physician and interprofessional team informed of any changes in the pregnant person's condition. On their end, the physician leads the process of formulating the management plan related to the complication in collaboration with the midwife and pregnant person. In cases where a complication is identified antenatally, a collaborative management plan with a physician should already be in place prior to the onset of labor. If not, the development of a new intrapartum complication or deviation from normal labor progress may require the midwife to seek physician consultation or to establish a collaborative plan of care.

When referral of care is indicated, the midwife can maintain an active role in the supportive care of the pregnant person and their family, seeking the most appropriate balance of medicine and midwifery in collaboration with the physician. This supportive role is ongoing throughout the pregnant person's intrapartum clinical course and continues into the postpartum period as needed. Individuals who experience an unanticipated intrapartum complication or emergency will greatly benefit from the continuity and emotional support provided by their midwife.

Shared decision making is an essential component of each type of team-based care. Whether a consultation is being requested for a deviation from normal, or a referral of care is requested for more severe complications, changes in the care plan should include shared decision making with the pregnant person.[3] In a shared decision-making model, the pregnant person is at the center of the team, with their support persons also included when requested.

If an emergency occurs during the intrapartum period, prompt recognition and action are required to avoid serious adverse maternal or fetal outcomes, and shared decision making may not always be possible. In these cases, the midwife should make every effort to maintain communication during the emergency with the pregnant person and their support persons about the need for a change in the plan of care, and a plan should be made to debrief with them after the emergency is resolved. The midwife must also be ready and able to manage acute emergent situations within the appropriate institutional and legal boundaries of midwifery practice until the complication is resolved or the collaborating physician can take over.

## Preterm Labor/Birth

Preterm birth is one of the leading causes of neonatal mortality in the United States.[4] Infants born prior to 37 weeks' gestation also have an increased risk of morbidity, such as neurologic and developmental disabilities.[4] The *Pregnancy-Related Conditions* chapter details risk assessment for preterm birth and the role of prevention strategies. In this chapter, the focus is on the evaluation and management of individuals who have suspected or confirmed active preterm labor with a singleton pregnancy.

### Evaluation for Possible Preterm Labor with a Singleton Pregnancy

Anticipatory guidance about signs and symptoms of possible preterm labor (PTL) should be provided during prenatal care, and pregnant individuals should be encouraged to report any such signs or symptoms. Those who are experiencing persistent uterine contractions with pelvic pressure and/or backache, vaginal bleeding, or any loss of fluid prior to 37 weeks' gestation should be evaluated promptly for possible preterm labor.[5] Other less-specific symptoms, such as cramping, abdominal pain, and watery vaginal discharge, could also indicate preterm labor.

The differential diagnoses for spontaneous PTL include physiologic causes such as contractions without labor (i.e., Braxton Hicks contractions), dehydration, lax vaginal tone, and round ligament pain. Other, more serious etiologies, such as infection (intrauterine, renal, genital tract), abruption, trauma, or appendicitis, must also be considered and assessed for when obtaining a history and conducting a physical examination. The evaluation procedure for preterm labor is outlined in the *Assessment for Diagnosis of Labor* appendix.

Contraction frequency is a poor predictor of subsequent preterm birth. When evaluating individuals for possible preterm labor, diagnostic accuracy may be improved with use of measurement of cervical length by vaginal ultrasound and fetal fibronectin.[5–8]

### Cervical Length Measurement and Fetal Fibronectin

As discussed in the *Pregnancy-Related Conditions* chapter, transvaginal ultrasound cervical length measurement can be used as a screening tool for preterm birth in asymptomatic pregnant persons. A cervical length of 25 mm or less after 16 weeks' gestation and before 24 weeks' gestation is associated with an increased risk of preterm birth.[7–9] In individuals who are more than 24 weeks' gestation with signs or symptoms of possible preterm labor, cervical length assessment by ultrasound can be a helpful adjunct to examination.[7] The cutoff value for short cervical length during this period of pregnancy varies between 20 mm and 30 mm.

*Fetal fibronectin* (fFN) is a biochemical marker whose identification may aid in management of pregnant persons with symptoms of preterm labor. This extracellular glycoprotein, which is found in the amniochorionic membrane, serves as an adhesive binder between the membranes and the decidua. It is normally present in cervicovaginal secretions prior to 20 weeks' gestation and again after 37 weeks' gestation as cervical remodeling takes place in preparation for normal full-term labor. Between 24 and 34 weeks' gestation, the presence of fFN is atypical and could indicate inflammation or uterine activity—both of which are precursors to preterm birth.[10]

Unfortunately, studies have found that fFN has a poor positive predictive value (PPV). (See the *Interpreting Published Research Data with a Clinical Midwifery Lens* appendix for more information on positive predictive value.) The reported PPV among pregnant persons who present with preterm labor symptoms is about 13%.[10] Conversely, fFN has a high negative predictability (97.6%) for indicating that birth will not occur within 7 days.[10,11] In practical terms, this means that fFN should not be used as a screening test.[9] A positive fFN test in symptomatic pregnant persons has limited clinical utility and should not be used alone to determine management. However, a negative fFN test can be helpful in avoiding unnecessary treatment when symptoms are present, especially in equivocal situations such as a pregnant person with contractions who has a negative fFN, and no cervical change over several hours. Pregnant persons with symptoms of preterm labor between 24 and 34 weeks' gestation and a negative fFN culture (or assay) have approximately a 3% chance of giving birth within the next 7 to 14 days.[10,11]

Fetal fibronectin is tested by sampling vaginal secretions; this sample must be collected prior to any other vaginal examinations. The accuracy of fFN testing is decreased in the presence of lubricants, blood, recent intercourse, or cervical manipulation within the previous 24 hours. However, a negative fFN result can prove useful even in these situations; therefore, these conditions are not contraindications to the use of fFN. A sample of vaginal secretions should not be submitted for fFN testing if the cervix is more than 3 cm dilated or 80% effaced, and fFN sampling is contraindicated if there is evidence of ruptured membranes.

Typically, the fFN sample is collected at the beginning of the pelvic examination of a pregnant person presenting with preterm labor symptoms and set aside until the results of a digital cervical examination and possibly a transvaginal ultrasound cervical length measurement are available. The fFN can then be sent or discarded, depending on the clinical situation. The fFN collection technique is outlined in Figure 30-1.

Some researchers and professional organizations suggest combining fFN and cervical length in standardized preterm labor algorithms.[9-11] In these protocols, persons presenting with preterm labor symptoms between 24 and 34 weeks' gestation would have an fFN sample collected during their initial speculum examination, followed by a digital examination. If the cervix is less than 3 cm dilated and 80% effaced, cervical length measurement by ultrasound is performed. The results of the cervical length measurement determine whether the fFN test is needed. The fFN test does not aid in diagnosis if the cervical length is very short (less than 20 mm) or very long (more than 30 mm). For example, a cervical length of 30 mm or more is considered normal and has a negative predictive value—that is, it suggests preterm birth will not occur—that ranges from 96% to 100%.[9] In these circumstances, the fFN sample can be discarded and the pregnant person discharged home pending any other clinical problems that need to be addressed. Alternatively, if the cervical length is between 20 and 29 mm, the fFN is sent for analysis. A negative fFN would again be reassuring and indicates preterm birth is unlikely. In contrast, a positive fFN in this situation or a cervical length of less than 20 mm would warrant admission

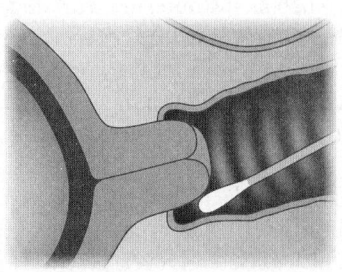 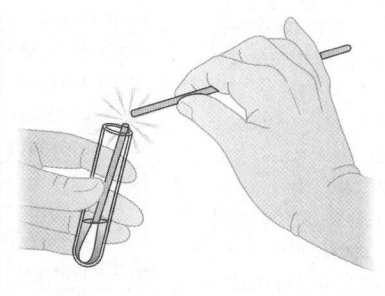 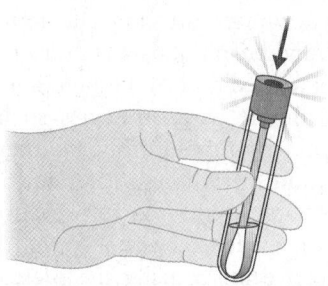

**Step 1**
During speculum examination, lightly rotate swab across posterior fornix of vagina for 10 seconds to absorb cervicovaginal secretions

**Step 2**
Remove swab and immerse polyester tip in buffer; break shaft at score even with top of tube

**Step 3**
Align the shaft with hole inside the tube cap and push down tightly over shaft, sealing tube; ensure shaft is aligned to avoid leakage

**Figure 30-1** Fetal fibronectin specimen collection procedure.
Courtesy of Hologic, Inc., and affiliates.

and initiation of preterm labor treatment. Because the positive predictive value of both fFN and cervical length measurements is inexact, management should not rely on these measurements alone when a pregnant person has preterm labor symptoms.

It can be challenging to formulate a plan for individuals who have some symptoms of preterm labor but no cervical dilation. The Society for Maternal–Fetal Medicine (SMFM) recommends the following: If the cervical length is normal (more than 30 mm), the pregnant person should be discharged.[5] Alternatively, the digital vaginal examination can be repeated after 1 to 2 hours of observation. If no cervical change is noted, discharge is reasonable.[5]

## Treatment of Preterm Labor

For pregnant persons in active preterm labor between 34 and 37 weeks' gestation, the midwife should follow local communication practices regarding physician collaboration for a management plan. If the pregnant person is less than 34 weeks' gestation and the initial cervical examination is more than 3 cm dilated or 80% effaced, preterm labor treatment should be initiated unless contraindicated. Many birth facilities will transfer pregnant persons in preterm labor to a tertiary care center, because these facilities have specialized neonatal care available. Guidelines vary from hospital to hospital in terms of the gestational age at which transfer is recommended, reflecting the facility's ability to care for preterm newborns. Midwives in all practice settings should be aware of the current preterm labor treatment recommendations and initiate these interventions as the clinical situation requires.[12] For example, corticosteroids (described in the next subsection) can be given prior to transfer to a tertiary care facility. Any other abnormalities, such as urinary tract infection, encountered by the midwife during the initial data collection should be managed and treated according to practice guidelines.

In the past, strategies such as bedrest, home contraction monitoring, maintenance tocolysis, hydration, periodontal care, and abstinence from intercourse were used to prevent preterm labor and birth. Evidence has not found these methods to be effective in reducing the preterm birth rate; thus, they are no longer used as specific preventive or treatment therapies.[9]

## Corticosteroids for Fetal Lung Maturity

The administration of corticosteroids to pregnant persons in preterm labor between 24 and 34 weeks' gestation has been conclusively shown to improve fetal lung maturity and decrease other morbidities associated with prematurity.[9] Either betamethasone (Celestone) 12 mg intramuscularly (IM) given in two doses 24 hours apart, or dexamethasone (Decadron) 6 mg IM given in four doses 12 hours apart, can be used.[9] Once the patient has received a complete course of steroids, tocolysis is discontinued. If the pregnant person does not give birth, the full steroid course can be repeated once as a "rescue dose" if more than 2 weeks has passed, the gestational age is less than 33 weeks, and there is a risk of birth within 7 days.[9] Some evidence suggests that a "rescue dose" may also be beneficial when the time since the last course of steroids is 7 to 14 days.[9]

Newer research suggests that administration of steroids in the late preterm period may also be beneficial.[13] Therefore, in pregnant persons with a gestational age of 34 0/7 to 36 6/7 weeks at risk of preterm birth within the next 7 days who have not yet received steroids, a complete course of the treatment should be considered. In addition, administration of steroids from 23 to 24 weeks' gestation may be considered based on the family's wishes for resuscitation during this time.[9]

## Tocolytics

There is extensive evidence regarding the use of tocolytic medications to prolong pregnancy. Although several different agents have been studied over the past 50 years, none appears to effectively reduce the preterm birth rate or decrease neonatal mortality and morbidity (Table 30-1).[9,12] All tocolytic agents slow uterine contractions to some degree, but they generally delay birth for only about 48 hours.[9] It is important to remember that tocolysis is contraindicated if the pregnant person has any condition that requires labor, such as intrauterine fetal demise, nonreassuring fetal status, severe preeclampsia, intra-amniotic infection, lethal fetal anomaly, maternal bleeding with hemodynamic instability, or any maternal contraindication to use of one of the tocolytic agents.[9]

In the past, magnesium sulfate and beta mimetics (terbutaline [Brethine]) were the most widely used tocolytic medications. However, research has shown that calcium-channel blockers (nifedipine [Procardia]) and prostaglandin synthetase inhibitors (indomethacin [Indocin]) have the best clinical efficacy and a lower incidence of toxicity and maternal side effects when compared to magnesium sulfate and terbutaline.[9] As a result, terbutaline is no longer recommended for acute tocolysis, and magnesium sulfate should be reserved for clinical situations in

| Table 30-1 | Tocolytic Medications Used to Treat Preterm Labor | | | |
|---|---|---|---|---|
| **Mechanism of Action** | **Dose** | **Common Maternal Side Effects** | **Fetal Effects** | **Contraindications/ Cautions** |
| **Nifedipine (Procardia)** | | | | |
| Calcium channel blocker that directly blocks calcium ion influx through cell membrane and release of intracellular calcium from sarcoplasmic reticulum. This inhibits myometrial contractions. | Optimal dose has not been established. Common regimen is loading dose of 20–30 mg orally given in divided doses. Then 10–20 mg orally every 3–8 hours. | Peripheral vasodilator; may induce transient nausea, flushing, headache, palpitations, hypotension, dizziness, tachycardia | Secondary to maternal hypotension | Contraindications: preload-dependent cardiac disorder, left ventricular dysfunction, heart failure, or hemodynamic instability. Do not use concurrently with terbutaline or magnesium sulfate. |
| **Indomethacin (Indocin)** | | | | |
| Cyclo-oxygenase (COX) inhibitor reduces prostaglandin production by COX | Loading dose: 50–100 mg orally or 50 mg rectally. Then 25–50 mg orally every 6 hours, for 48 hours. | Gastrointestinal: nausea, vomiting, reflux, gastritis Platelet dysfunction | Premature closure of ductus arteriosus Oligohydramnios | Contraindicated for pregnant persons with platelet dysfunction, bleeding diathesis, hepatic dysfunction, gastrointestinal ulcerative disease, and asthma if sensitive to aspirin. Not recommended for more than 48 hours of continuous use. Not recommended for pregnant persons at $\geq$ 32 weeks' gestation. |
| **Magnesium Sulfate** | | | | |
| Mechanism of action unknown but probably competes with calcium at cell membrane, reducing calcium available for myometrial contraction. | Loading dose: 4–6 g intravenously (IV) over 20–30 minutes. Then 2 g/ hour by continuous IV infusion (pump required). | Flushing, nausea, blurred vision, headache, lethargy, muscle weakness, hypotension Rare effects: pulmonary edema, respiratory or cardiac arrest | Neuroprotective, decreased fetal heart rate variability Decreased neonatal tone | Contraindicated in pregnant persons with impaired renal function, myasthenia gravis, or cardiac conduction defects. Do not use concurrently with nifedipine. Toxicity: loss of patellar reflexes, decreased urine output < 30 mL/hour, respiratory rate < 12/minute. Toxicity risks increase with serum creatinine > 1.0 mg/dL. |

*(continues)*

| Table 30-1 | Tocolytic Medications Used to Treat Preterm Labor (*continued*) |
|---|---|

**Terbutaline (Brethine)**

| | | | | |
|---|---|---|---|---|
| Beta-agonist binds to beta- 2 adrenergic receptors that cause a chain reaction resulting in depletion of intracellular calcium, thereby blocking myometrial receptors.<br><br>Receptors can become desensitized with prolonged use, thereby diminishing effectiveness. | Varying doses used. Common regimen is 0.25 mg subcutaneous (SQ) injection every 20 to 30 minutes up to 4 doses. Then 0.25 mg SQ every 3–4 hours.<br><br>May be administered by continuous IV infusion. | Tachycardia, peripheral vasodilation, hypotension, bronchial relaxation, pulmonary edema, hyperglycemia, myocardial infarction | Tachycardia<br><br>Neonatal hypoglycemia | Contraindications: tachycardia sensitive cardiac disease, poorly controlled hypertension, poorly controlled diabetes.<br><br>Use with caution in individuals with hemorrhage, as tachycardia and hypotension can complicate symptoms of hemorrhage.<br><br>The FDA has mandated a black box warning stating that terbutaline should not be used for tocolysis for more than 72 hours secondary to the risk for maternal cardiac problems and recommends against use of oral terbutaline secondary to lack of effectiveness.<br><br>ACOG states that terbutaline can be used for short-term, inpatient use. |

Abbreviations: ACOG, American College of Obstetricians and Gynecologists; FDA, U.S. Food and Drug Administration.

Based on American College of Obstetricians and Gynecologists' Committee on Practice Bulletins—Obstetrics. Practice Bulletin No. 171: management of preterm labor. Reaffirmed 2020; Nijman TA, Vliet EO, Koullali B, et al. Antepartum and intrapartum interventions to prevent preterm birth. *Semin Fetal Neonatal Med.* 2016;21:121-128. https://www.acog.org/clinical/clinical-guidance/practice-bulletin /articles/2016/10/management-of-preterm-labor.

which nifedipine and indomethacin are contraindicated or fetal/newborn neuroprotection is sought.[9]

Regardless of the agent chosen for tocolysis, the primary goal is to delay birth long enough to administer a full course of corticosteroids to facilitate fetal lung development and arrange for transfer of the pregnant person to a tertiary center if needed. These two interventions have demonstrated significant improvements in neonatal outcomes and are the mainstay of preterm labor management.

### Group B Streptococcus Prophylaxis

Another important intervention in the event of preterm labor is administration of antibiotics to prevent group B *Streptococcus* (GBS) disease. Preterm infants are especially susceptible to GBS sepsis, and pregnant persons experiencing preterm labor will likely have an unknown colonization status because the standard screening culture is not performed until 35 to 36 weeks' gestation. All pregnant persons in preterm labor prior to 37 weeks with unknown GBS status should receive antibiotic prophylaxis.[14]

### Magnesium Sulfate for Neuroprotection

In addition to having some tocolytic properties, magnesium sulfate reduces the risk of cerebral palsy in infants born prior to 32 weeks' gestation.[9] Many institutions now include administration of magnesium sulfate as part of preterm labor management. Although the exact mechanisms of fetal neuroprotection are unknown, it is hypothesized that the magnesium sulfate improves fetal cerebral blood flow and safeguards the fetus against hypoxic stress. Given that prematurity and low birth weight are the most significant risk factors for cerebral palsy, fetal neuroprotection has the potential to greatly improve the neurodevelopmental future of children born prior to 32 weeks' gestation.

Institutions that use magnesium sulfate for fetal neuroprotection should establish written guidelines and dosing protocols for this therapy.[9] These guidelines should also include an informed consent process and shared decision-making discussion with the pregnant person and their family regarding the risks and potential benefits of magnesium sulfate in preventing cerebral palsy.

### Follow-Up

Pregnant persons admitted for treatment for preterm labor will typically remain in the hospital for at least 24 hours. Once the full course of steroids is completed, tocolysis is usually discontinued and expectant management is resumed if the pregnant person has not given birth. Those with advanced cervical dilatation may need prolonged inpatient care and monitoring, especially if the fetus is at a previable, extremely preterm, or very preterm gestational age. The midwife can maintain an active supportive role in the pregnant person's care during hospitalization and discuss the continued management plan with the physician as the clinical scenario changes. Prior to discharge from the hospital, the midwife may be involved in reassessment for preterm birth risk factors and initiation of any necessary treatments or interventions.

Outpatient monitoring will include weekly prenatal visits for the remainder for the pregnancy with either the midwife or the physician, or both, according to the plan of care. The pregnant person should also be counseled about any signs of preterm labor and advised to call if any symptoms are noted. If symptoms do occur, the pregnant person should be reassessed promptly in the hospital and the appropriate treatments repeated if needed.

## Post-Term and Late Term Pregnancy

Late term and post-term gestational age is associated with increased risks of multiple pregnancy complications, including perinatal mortality.[15,16] Researchers have sought to determine whether routine induction improves outcomes and, if so, at what gestational age induction of labor is most protective. Researchers have also sought to identify any associated risks of labor induction, especially the risk of cesarean birth.

### Expectant Management Versus Induction of Labor

The risks of cesarean birth or other complications associated with induction of labor for late term or post-term gestation must be considered separately from the risks of cesarean birth associated with elective induction at earlier gestational ages. Elective labor induction is discussed in the "Induction of Labor" section of this chapter.

For pregnant people at or beyond 41 weeks' gestation, labor induction compared to expectant management resulted in a lower perinatal mortality rate (0.03% or 2/5472 birth versus 0.35% or 19/5437 births, respectively) and a decrease in cesarean births (15.6% or 882/5662 versus 17.4% or 979/5642, respectively) in the largest analysis of data from clinical trials on labor induction to date.[15]

The American College of Obstetricians and Gynecologists (ACOG) supports induction of labor between 41 0/7 and 41 6/7 weeks and recommends induction of labor at 42 0/7 weeks to avoid an increased risk of perinatal mortality and morbidity.[16] In 2018, ACOG extended its recommendations for labor induction based on gestational age to also include low-risk nulliparous people at 39 weeks' gestation (for more on this topic, see the "Induction of Labor" section).[17]

### Midwifery Care of People at Late Term and Post-Term Gestational Ages

When a pregnant person approaches 41 0/7 weeks' gestation, prenatal care must include a discussion of care options for late term and post-term pregnancy. During this discussion, it is important to clearly separate the evidence on (1) risks of late term and post-term pregnancy, and (2) outcomes of people who are induced compared to those who elect for expectant management with fetal surveillance during late term and post-term pregnancy.

Principles of shared decision making can best guide this discussion, which includes an explanation of the evidence showing increased risks for both the pregnant person and the fetus after 41 weeks' gestation, and evidence on pros and cons of the different care options. These principles include the use of absolute risk as opposed to relative risk, and may include use of a visual aid such as a pictograph.[18] Perinatal mortality is a rare outcome, and the absolute risk of stillbirth and early neonatal death in uncomplicated pregnancies is small. The use of relative risk to explain this numeric evidence can introduce unintended bias.[18]

A discussion of the person's values, goals, and preferences as they relate to the options for care is another principle of shared decision making and is a critical component of midwifery care with a person who has a late term and post-term pregnancy. Some pregnant people are anxious to end their pregnancies and will readily request induction of labor at 41 weeks. Some pregnant individuals find any increase in risk of perinatal mortality unacceptable and choose induction to mitigate this risk. Others have a strong preference for avoiding induction and may choose to await spontaneous labor.

Expectant management of pregnant persons with late term and post-term pregnancy includes antepartum fetal surveillance such as a nonstress test and/or a biophysical profile. Fetal surveillance has not been conclusively shown to decrease perinatal morbidity and mortality,[19] as studies in people with post-term pregnancies have not included an unmonitored control group for ethical reasons. Regardless, starting antepartum fetal surveillance, including weekly nonstress tests and a biophysical profile with amniotic fluid measurement, at 41 weeks' gestation provides reassurance and is a commonly accepted practice.

If a pregnant person declines induction at 42 0/7 weeks' gestation, consultation with a physician usually occurs for a continued plan of care. Referral of care may be indicated. Careful fetal surveillance must be recommended, as well as ongoing discussion with the pregnant person regarding the risks and benefits of induction versus awaiting spontaneous labor. Any consultation, results of fetal surveillance, and details of the discussion with the pregnant person are documented in the health record.

## Prelabor Rupture of Membranes

Prelabor rupture of membranes (PROM) is defined as rupture of the membranes prior to onset of labor. This condition is also referred to as premature rupture of the membranes, although the use of the word "premature" may be confusing in this context because it is often used to refer to gestational age. When this event occurs in pregnant persons who are less than 37 weeks' gestation, it is referred to as premature prelabor rupture of membranes (PPROM). PROM at term gestation is a normal process associated with physiologic weakening of the amniotic membrane as labor nears. PPROM, in contrast, is thought to result from some type of underlying pathology, such as infection. The recommended care differs considerably for term and preterm PROM; thus, these conditions are considered separately here.

### Evaluation for Ruptured Membranes

The diagnosis of PROM is clinical and based on a thorough physical exam. Many normal events (e.g., sexual intercourse) and medical conditions can mimic rupture of membranes. Evaluation of the pregnant person with possible ruptured membranes is reviewed in the *Assessment and Diagnosis of Rupture of Membranes* appendix.

#### *Premature Prelabor Rupture of Membranes*

Care of pregnant people with PROM at any gestational age can consist of either expectant management or induction of labor. In contrast, the care of people with PPROM must weigh the risks of prematurity against the risks of infection following prolonged latency and delayed delivery. In general, the latency period with PPROM lasts an average of approximately 1 week with expectant management, but in some cases may last several weeks. In contrast to individuals with PROM at term, subclinical or clinical infection is often present in people with PPROM; approximately 15% to 20% are diagnosed with intra-amniotic infection, and 15% to 20% go on to have postpartum endometritis.[20] Reflecting this reality, clinical intra-amniotic infection with PPROM is an indication for birth. Other indications for birth in the presence of PPROM include abnormal fetal testing or placental abruption. Cervical examination is avoided for individuals with PRROM to decrease the risk of infection.

In the absence of indications for birth following PPROM, the preterm fetus will benefit from a longer period in utero. Care decisions at the time of diagnosis are based on gestational age, presence of other complications such as infection or preterm labor, fetal well-being, fetal lung maturity, and access to a neonatal intensive care unit (NICU). Collaborative care with a physician is typical.

#### *Previable PPROM*

In situations where PPROM occurs between 14 and 24 weeks' gestation, an individualized collaborative approach that includes the neonatal team is necessary to determine the best course of treatment. GBS prophylaxis, tocolysis, corticosteroids, and magnesium sulfate for fetal neuroprotection are not recommended if the fetus is at a previable gestational age.[20] Extensive counseling and shared decision making with the pregnant person and their family should occur. The midwife fills a valuable role by listening and providing assistance to the family in understanding the complex information given in this situation.

### PPROM at 24 to 33 6/7 Weeks

In gestations between 24 and 33 6/7 weeks, expectant management is preferred if there are no clinical signs of infection, fetal compromise, or labor. Transfer to a tertiary center should be arranged if necessary. In addition, a single course of corticosteroids (two doses of 12 mg of betamethasone 12 hours apart or four doses of 6 mg of betamethasone every 12 hours) is administered to improve fetal lung maturity upon diagnosis of PPROM, and GBS testing should also be completed.

If there are no contraindications, antibiotics are administered for neonatal GBS prevention and to prolong the latency period. ACOG's current guidelines for GBS prophylaxis detail the evaluation and care of pregnant persons with PPROM in regard to culturing for GBS, the time period over which to administer antibiotics, and care if the pregnant person does or does not go into labor.[14] ACOG recommends against the use of tocolytics in this situation.[19] Magnesium sulfate for fetal neuroprotection is recommended if the gestational age is less than 32 0/7 weeks.[20] Digital cervical examinations are contraindicated to reduce the risk of chorioamnionitis.

### PPROM at 34 to 36 6/7 Weeks

The gestational age at which the risks of infection outweigh the risks associated with prematurity is not clear. According to ACOG, either expectant management or induction of labor is reasonable for a diagnosis of PPROM at 34 0/7 to 36 6/7 weeks' gestation.[20] A single course of corticosteroids to reduce respiratory morbidity in the newborn is recommended if induction is undertaken and birth is anticipated in 1 to 7 days.[20]

### The Term PROM Controversy

The primary risk associated with term PROM is development of infection, which is termed either intra-amniotic infection or chorioamnionitis. Factors most strongly associated with an increased risk of infection are digital cervical examinations, colonization of the pregnant person with GBS, duration of membrane rupture, duration of labor, and duration of latency period (i.e., the time between rupture of membranes and onset of labor).[21] Neonates born after prolonged rupture of membranes are at increased risk for sepsis and may need additional testing and assessment after birth.[22]

The two options for pregnant persons with term PROM are induction of labor and expectant management. Primary questions of concern are which care option results in lower infection rates, and whether one of these options is associated with more cesarean births. The 1996 TermPROM study is the most relevant contemporary research due to its randomized design and large sample size.[23] In this study, neonatal infection rates and cesarean birth rates were similar in pregnant persons who underwent induction and those who were managed expectantly, but a higher rate of infection was noted in members of the expectant management group. Several study limitations likely affected the risk of infection in the expectant management group, including an atypical diagnosis of chorioamnionitis, more digital cervical examinations in the expectant management group, and no prenatal GBS screening and therefore no antibiotic prophylaxis during labor for those who tested positive for GBS.[22]

ACOG recommends induction of labor as the optimal care approach for individuals with term PROM but recognizes expectant management as an acceptable option for those who decline induction.[20] The American College of Nurse-Midwives' (ACNM) Position Statement on Premature Rupture of Membranes at Term reaffirms the pregnant person's rights to self-determination and supports the option of expectant management for selected persons.[24] Table 30-2 summarizes these recommendations.

Pregnant persons who choose or require induction of labor should be admitted and a plan of care made, including decisions regarding cervical ripening and/or oxytocin infusion. Bedside ultrasounds can be used to confirm cephalic presentation before initiating interventions to initiate labor, rather than performing digital cervical examinations for this purpose. Some evidence indicates that the use of an intracervical balloon catheter for induction/cervical ripening is associated with a higher rate

| Table 30-2 | Criteria for Expectant Management of Prelabor Rupture of Membranes |
|---|---|

Full term (> 37 0/7 weeks)
Singleton, uncomplicated pregnancy
Cephalic presentation
Clear amniotic fluid
No fever or infection
Reassuring fetal status

Based on American College of Nurse-Midwives position statement: premature rupture of membranes at term. ACNM Division of Standards and Practice, Clinical Practice Section. https://www.midwife.org/acnm/files/ACNMLibraryData/UPLOADFILENAME/000000000233/PS-Prelabor-rupture-of-membranes-FINAL-22-MAR-18.pdf. Published 2008; reviewed and updated 2018.

of intra-amniotic infection as compared to oxytocin induction.[20,25] Oral dosing of cervical ripening medications (misoprostol) are attractive options in these clinical situations, as they avoid vaginal application. Physician consultation may be indicated depending on the institutional guidelines and the individual clinical scenario. If induction is chosen, it is important to allow adequate time for the latent phase of labor to avoid cesarean birth for failed induction. Multiple cervical examinations are a primary risk factor for infection, so digital cervical examinations should be minimized during induction, and deferred if possible during early labor.[20,21]

If expectant management is chosen, the care plan should include where the pregnant person will await onset of labor and for how long, and how well-being of both the birthing person and fetus will be monitored during this time. There is little evidence on which to base the decision about the best location for awaiting the onset of labor,[21] and a return to home for a predetermined time may be considered. A pregnant person who returns home for expectant management should be advised to monitor their temperature (with a thermometer) every 2 to 4 hours as well as the contraction frequency and fetal movement. It is important to also counsel the pregnant person to avoid inserting anything into their vagina. The midwife should be contacted immediately if any of the following conditions occur: temperature of 38°C or higher, decreased fetal movement, signs of active labor, and either meconium-stained or foul-smelling amniotic fluid. Plans for follow-up evaluation should also be made.

In the TermPROM study, the median latency duration was 33 hours and 95% of participants gave birth within 95 to 107 hours after rupture of the membraines.[23] The optimal maximum duration of expectant management is not known. The TermPROM study allowed up to 96 hours before induction was performed.[23] Pregnant persons choosing expectant management may elect to have their labor induced at any time

During labor, individuals with ruptured membranes must be monitored for developing infection, regardless of the care option chosen. Fetal or maternal tachycardia, fever, uterine tenderness, and foul-smelling fluid are all signs of possible chorioamnionitis. Any of these signs or symptoms requires admission and prompt initiation of the appropriate treatment interventions. To avoid infection, digital cervical examinations should be minimized during induced or spontaneous labor.

## Intra-amniotic Infection

Intrauterine infection or inflammation refers to infection of the amniotic sac, the amnion, and the chorion.[26,27] *Chorioamnionitis* is the historical term, but refers to a heterogeneous set of conditions characterized by infection and/or inflammation, which have differing degrees of severity. Therefore, the terms *intrauterine infection*, *intrauterine inflammation*, or *intrauterine infection and inflammation* (Triple I) have been proposed as replacements. The term *intra-amniotic infection*, which has also been proposed as a replacement for chorioamnionitis, is used in this chapter.

A common cause of intra-amniotic infection is ascending bacteria from the lower genital tract. Organisms such as group B *Streptococcus*, *Escherichia coli*, *Ureaplasma urealyticum*, *Fusobacterium* species, and *Mycoplasma hominis* have all been implicated as causative pathogens.[27] Because the membranes provide some protection against fetal infection, prolonged rupture of membranes and long labor are risk factors for intra-amniotic infection. Manipulative vaginal or intrauterine procedures and frequent digital cervical examinations are also associated with an increased risk of intra-amniotic infection, especially once the membranes have ruptured.[26,28] Many of these factors are interrelated and, therefore, their independent effects have not been fully established. For example, an increased number of cervical examinations during labor is associated with longer labor and longer duration of membrane rupture, both of which are also associated with an increased risk of infection.[28]

The definitive diagnosis of intra-amniotic infection can be made only after the birth, through histologic examination of the placenta and membranes.[29,30] However, fever in the birthing person during labor is the primary clinical marker of intra-amniotic infection and is associated with 95% of cases.[29]

Noninfectious causes of fever in the birthing person are also possible, such as epidural analgesia, dehydration, overheated room temperature, and possibly prolonged time in the shower or tub. Given these ambiguities, the National Institute of Child Health and Human Development (NICHD) Expert Panel was convened in 2015 to evaluate the research on intra-amniotic infection. It released new guidelines for diagnosis and care of this condition that specified criteria for three different diagnoses: isolated maternal fever, suspected intra-amniotic infection, and confirmed intra-amniotic infection.[30] In cases of isolated maternal fever, NICHD suggested that treatment may not be needed. This recommendation was based on concerns about the adverse effects of unnecessary treatment, including exposure of laboring persons to antibiotics and overuse of diagnostic work-ups and antibiotic treatment of neonates.

In response to NICHD's intra-amniotic infection recommendations, ACOG published a Committee Opinion on the subject.[26] The authors of this opinion expressed concern about the lack of sensitivity of the NICHD criteria for intra-amniotic infection, given the serious implications of untreated infections. As a result, the ACOG recommendations for diagnosis and care are different from the NICHD recommendations. A key difference between the NICHD and ACOG guidelines concerns the diagnosis of a laboring person with a single temperature of 39°C (102.2°F) or higher measured on one occasion. The ACOG authors argued that this temperature is most often the result of an infectious process, so it should not be diagnosed as an isolated maternal fever. Instead, the ACOG guidelines recommend that this temperature be considered diagnostic for intra-amniotic infection. The ACOG authors also recommended antibiotic treatment for isolated maternal fever unless a source other than intra-amniotic infection is confirmed (Table 30-3).

Although no randomized trials have compared the various antibiotic regimens, broad-spectrum antibiotics such as ampicillin or penicillin, used in

| Table 30-3 | Diagnostic Criteria for Intra-amniotic Infection According to NICHD Expert Panel Workshop and ACOG | |
|---|---|---|
| **Diagnosis** | **Diagnostic Criteria According to NICHD Expert Panel Workshop** | **Diagnostic Criteria According to ACOG** |
| Isolated maternal fever (documented fever) | Oral temperature of ≥ 39°C (102.2°F) on one occasion OR Oral temperature of 38–38.9°C (100.4–102.1) that persists when the temperature measurement is repeated after 30 minutes | Oral temperature of 38–38.9°C (100.4–102.1°F) that persists when the temperature measurement is repeated after 30 minutes |
| Suspected intrauterine infection | Isolated maternal fever (see definition above) without a clear source and ONE OR MORE of the following: 1. Fetal tachycardia: FHR > 160 beats/min for 10 minutes or longer excluding accelerations, decelerations, and periods of marked variability 2. Maternal leukocytosis: WBC count > 15,000/mm³ in the absence of corticosteroids 3. Purulent discharge from the cervical os | Isolated maternal fever (see definition above) without a clear source and ONE OR MORE of the following: 1. Fetal tachycardia: FHR > 160 beats/min for 10 minutes or longer excluding accelerations, decelerations, and periods of marked variability 2. Maternal leukocytosis: WBC count > 15,000/mm³ in the absence of corticosteroids 3. Purulent discharge from the cervical os OR Oral temperature of ≥ 39°C (102.2°F) on one occasion |
| Confirmed intra-amniotic infection | All of the above AND: 1. Amniocentesis-proven infection via positive Gram stain 2. Low glucose or positive amniotic fluid culture 3. Placental histopathology with diagnostic features of infection | All of the above AND: 1. Amniocentesis-proven infection via positive Gram stain 2. Low glucose or positive amniotic fluid culture 3. Placental histopathology with diagnostic features of infection |

Abbreviations: ACOG, American College of Obstetricians and Gynecologists; FHR, fetal heart rate; NICHD, National Institute of Child Health and Human Development; WBC, white blood count.

American College of Obstetricians and Gynecologists. Committee Opinion No. 712: intrapartum management of intraamniotic infection. *Obstet Gynecol.* 2017;130:e95-e101; Higgins RD, Saade G, Polin RA, et al. Evaluation and management of women and newborns with a maternal diagnosis of chorioamnionitis: summary of a workshop. *Obstet Gynecol.* 2016;127(3):426-436. doi:10.1097/AOG.0000000000001246.

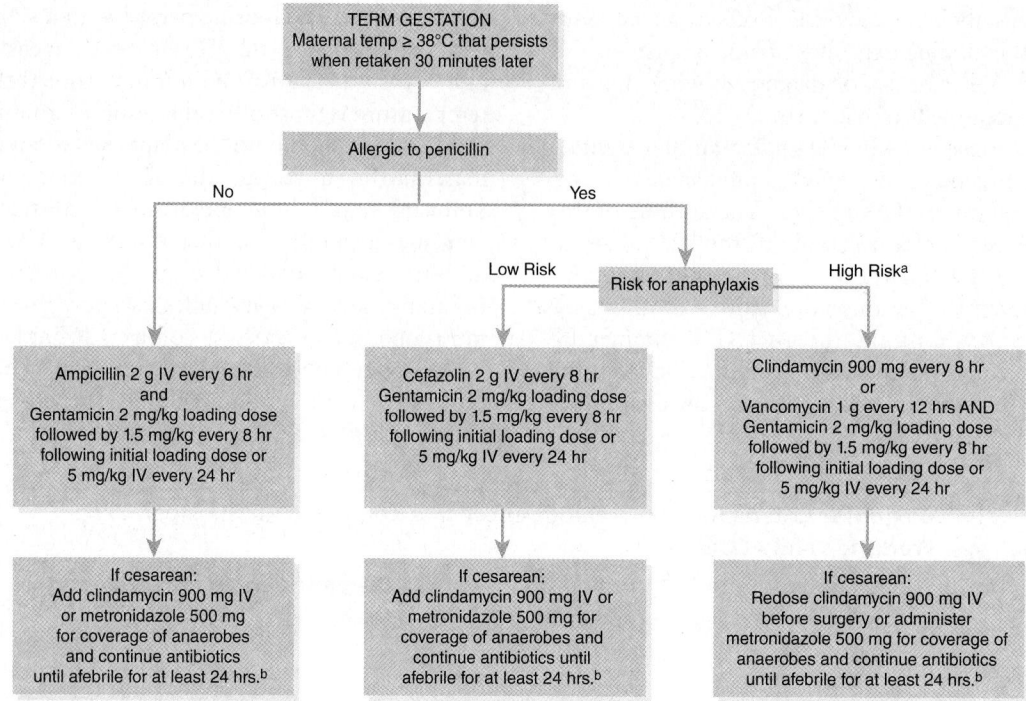

**Figure 30-2** Treatments for isolated maternal fever and suspected intra-amniotic infection based on ACOG guidelines.
[a] High risk for anaphylaxis includes history of angioedema, respiratory distress, anaphylaxis, or urticaria (hives) after exposure to penicillin.
[b] Some authors suggest one dose following birth is sufficient. Thus, the duration of antibiotic administration after birth is based on institutional guidelines.

Based on American College of Obstetricians and Gynecologists. Committee Opinion No. 712: intrapartum management of intraamniotic infection. *Obstet Gynecol.* 2017;130:e95-e101.

combination with gentamicin (Garamycin), are the most commonly recommended treatment for suspected infection. Administered intravenously until birth, these antibiotics have consistently demonstrated the highest efficacy against the two leading causes of neonatal sepsis—namely, GBS and *E. coli*. Figure 30-2 shows the recommended dosing regimens, including alternatives for individuals with penicillin or ampicillin allergy.[26,27,30]

Administration of penicillin or ampicillin for GBS prophylaxis is not sufficient for treatment of intra-amniotic infection. If a pregnant person who is receiving penicillin for GBS prophylaxis develops a fever during labor, a broad-spectrum antibiotic that is effective against anaerobic bacteria must be initiated. Oral acetaminophen (Tylenol) up to 1000 mg may also be given. Some evidence suggests that reducing the pregnant person's temperature can improve labor progress and fetal acid–base balance.[26] The pregnant person's condition and labor progress should be monitored closely. Oxytocin should be used if labor is not progressing normally.

Intra-amniotic infection alone is not an indication for cesarean birth. If a cesarean birth is performed, additional anaerobic antibiotic coverage with clindamycin or metronidazole to prevent postpartum endometritis may be needed. Once birth occurs, the placenta is sent to the pathology laboratory for histologic evaluation and the infant closely monitored for any signs of sepsis or infection. Intravenous antibiotics should not be routinely continued after birth unless fever or other signs of postpartum endometritis occur.[26]

### Induction of Labor

Induction of labor refers to stimulation of cervical ripening and uterine contractions through artificial means. Methods for inducing labor include both hormonal and nonhormonal approaches. The decision to induce labor should be made via shared decision making between the pregnant person and the care provider, and involves assessing the risks associated with continuing pregnancy versus the risks associated with labor induction.

| Table 30-4 | Common Indications for Induction |
|---|---|
| **Pregnancy Indications** | **Fetal Indications** |
| Gestational hypertension | Fetal growth restriction |
| Preeclampsia/eclampsia | Fetal demise |
| Cholestasis of pregnancy | Nonreassuring fetal status |
| Diabetes mellitus | |
| Intra-amniotic infection | |
| Oligohydramnios | |
| Prelabor rupture of membranes | |
| Post-term or late term pregnancy | |

Induction of labor can be elective or medically indicated. Table 30-4 provides examples of evidence-based medical indications for an induction of labor.

Induction of labor often occurs in hospital settings; however, a growing body of evidence supports outpatient cervical ripening prior to stimulating contractions. Induction of labor is contraindicated in any situation that precludes vaginal birth, such as placenta previa, vasa previa, transverse lie, umbilical cord prolapse, previous myomectomy entering the endometrial cavity, previous classical uterine incision, active genital herpes infection, or presence of a Category III fetal heart rate (FHR) tracing.[31]

Elective induction (i.e., no medical indication for induction) is an intervention that has received considerable attention from researchers over the past decade. Factors such as convenience, history of fast labors, distance from the hospital, relief of physiologic pregnancy discomforts, avoidance of certain calendar dates or holidays, institutional staffing concerns, and patient satisfaction have all been cited as reasons for elective induction. In addition, recent research findings that elective induction reduces risks of perinatal death, cesarean birth, maternal hypertensive disease, and NICU admission compared to expectant management have increased interest in labor induction—even among birthing people with no complications.[32] Risks associated with induction of labor include uterine tachysystole, fetal intolerance of labor, and postpartum uterine atony. Adverse outcomes include increased incidence of neonatal morbidity from iatrogenic prematurity if the estimated gestational age is incorrect.[31]

The relationship between cesarean birth and induction of labor remains complex. Induction for certain indications, such as late term and post-term pregnancy[15] and prelabor rupture of membranes at term is not associated with an increased risk of cesarean birth.[23] In the early 2000s, a considerable body of evidence emerged that showed the risk of cesarean birth is substantially increased with induction in nulliparous persons, with most researchers finding the risk to be at least doubled.[31,33] However, these studies compared labor outcomes in pregnant individuals who were induced versus labor outcomes in pregnant individuals who experienced spontaneous labor at the same gestational age. Since that time, researchers have noted that the proper comparison group for pregnant individuals who are induced are actually pregnant individuals at the same gestational age who are managed expectantly.[34] Several recent studies, including a systematic review that used this comparison group, demonstrated a decreased rate of cesarean births in pregnant individuals whose labors were induced as compared to pregnant individuals who were managed expectantly.[35-38]

In 2018, investigators of the ARRIVE[32] (A Randomized Trial of Induction Versus Expectant Management) trial studied the effects of elective induction on low-risk, nulliparous persons at 39 weeks' gestation to determine if elective induction lowered the neonatal mortality and morbidity rate and if elective inductions affected the risk of cesarean births. They concluded that there was no statistical difference in perinatal mortality and severe neonatal morbidity between groups; however, they found a decreased rate of cesarean birth and hypertensive disease in the birthing persons who underwent induction compared to the expectant management group.[32]

The external validity of the ARRIVE trial may be limited by selection bias and induction practice patterns used during the study.[39] It is also possible that the relationship between induction and cesarean birth may be affected by multiple factors not explored in the ARRIVE trial, including differences in labor care practices at non-academic medical centers.[37] However, in the most recent Cochrane review of randomized controlled trials (RCTs) on this subject, induction was associated with reductions in perinatal death, stillbirth, cesarean birth, NICU admission, and 5-minute Apgar scores less than 7.[15] Importantly, in that review of 34 trials ($N > 21,000$ laboring people), investigators did not see differences in these benefits of induction, regardless of the laboring person's parity, gestation, or Bishop's score.

Nonetheless, the ACNM continues to recommend person-centered decision making regarding

| Table 30-5 | Clinical Considerations Prior to Induction of Labor and/or Cervical Ripening |
|---|---|

1.  Physician consultation according to local communication practices and collaboration with the interprofessional team should occur prior to the initiation of labor induction. In some cases, a collaborative plan of care is required.

2.  The indications for induction (if present) should be discussed with the birthing person and support person(s). The risks and benefits of each proposed agent (or technique) should be thoroughly reviewed. The birthing person's preferences should be taken into consideration. This discussion should be documented in the health record.

3.  The labor induction record should include the following information:

    a.  Documentation of the gestational age and criteria used to establish the final estimated due date

    b.  Bishop's score

    c.  Indications for labor induction

    d.  Verification of no contraindications for induction

    e.  Clinical pelvimetry

    f.  Confirmation of a cephalic presentation

    g.  Confirmation of Category I fetal heart rate pattern. Induction may proceed with oxytocin if a Category II fetal heart rate pattern is present, following consultation with a physician.

4.  Communicate with the physician according to local patterns if the birthing person declines a medically indicated induction of labor.

5.  Caution should be exercised when prescribing or recommending alternative methods of labor induction that are not supported in the scientific literature.

6.  During cervical ripening and induction, practices that encourage the normal process of labor (e.g., balloon catheters, ambulation with telemetry, oral hydration, discontinuation of oxytocin infusion in active-phase labor) should be encouraged. Encourage adequate nutrition during induction, especially those of longer duration.

7.  Water immersion in the shower or tub (with waterproof fetal telemetry monitoring) may be considered during induction of labor with oxytocin.

labor induction, including the option of waiting for the onset of spontaneous labor when desired by the birthing person.[40] The authors of the ACNM clinical bulletin on labor induction stress the importance of sharing the risks and benefits of this intervention with the pregnant person, including the induction success rates (citing absolute numbers whenever possible) from not only the research studies but also from the hospital and practice where the induction will take place. To do this, midwives should track rates of failed induction and unplanned cesarean birth in their practice and facility.

Regardless of its possible benefits at 39 weeks or beyond, labor induction prior to 39 weeks' gestation is associated with an increased rate of iatrogenic prematurity. Strict criteria for gestational age dating are now in place, and elective induction prior to 39 weeks' gestation is contraindicated.[41] Most institutions have adopted stringent guidelines for elective induction at term that also require a signed consent form and a pre-induction checklist for providers.[42]

Prior to the initiation of labor induction, the pregnant person should be counseled about the indication for induction as well as the risks and benefits that are associated with both induction and expectant management. In addition, a collaborative plan of care between the midwife and the physician regarding the plan of care for cervical ripening and induction of labor is indicated according to local practice. Table 30-5 summarizes key midwifery considerations when caring for pregnant individuals who require an induction of labor.

## Cervical Ripening Techniques

For most pregnant people, the first intervention in a labor induction involves the use of cervical ripening techniques. As pregnancy approaches full term, the cervix gradually begins to soften, efface, and move anteriorly in the vaginal vault. This process, which is commonly referred to as "ripening," occurs as a result of normal remodeling of the collagen fibers and other glycoprotein connective tissues within the cervix. Cervical ripening occurs more readily in multiparous individuals, and the process may begin in the days to weeks before the onset of labor.

The degree of ripening can be quantified using the modified Bishop's score, which assesses factors associated with cervical remodeling. Bishop's score is a numeric assessment of four different characteristics of the cervix and fetal station; it is used to

| Table 30-6 | The Bishop Scoring System | | | |
|---|---|---|---|---|
| **Point Value** | **0** | **1** | **2** | **3** |
| Cervical position | Posterior | Midline | Anterior | |
| Cervical consistency | Firm | Medium | Soft | |
| Cervical effacement[a] | 0–30% | 40–50% | 60–70% | 80% or greater |
| Cervical dilatation | 0 | 1–2 cm | 3–4 cm | > 5 cm |
| Fetal station[b] | –3 | –2 | –1/0 | +1/+2 |

Abbreviation: ACOG, American College of Obstetricians and Gynecologists.

[a] Either the original percentage effacement or centimeters of cervical length may be used.

[b] Station is based on a –3 to +3 range. This denotes thirds of the level above/below the ischial spines. Although ACOG has redefined station using centimeters (–5 to +5), Bishop's score is still based on the –3/+3 range.

Based on Bishop EH. Pelvic scoring for elective induction. *Obstet Gynecol*. 1964;24:266-2684; Lange AP, Secher NJ, Westergaard JG, Skovgård I. Prelabor evaluation of inducibility. *Obstet Gynecol*. 1982;60(2):137-147; American College of Obstetricians and Gynecologists. Practice Bulletin No. 107: induction of labor. *Obstet Gynecol*. 2009;114:386-397. [Reaffirmed 2016].

predict the success of induction and the need for cervical ripening.[43] The currently used version of Bishop's score is shown in **Table 30-6**.[41,43] This scoring system indicates whether the pregnant person's cervix is "favorable" or "unfavorable" with regard to predicting the success of labor induction and is the best predictor of induction duration known to date.

According to the California Maternal Quality Care Collaborative (CMQCC), a pregnant person's cervix is considered "ripe" at 8 or greater in nulliparous individuals and at 6 or greater for multiparous individuals.[44] Pregnant persons with a Bishop's score less than these values have an unfavorable cervix, and cervical ripening is recommended during their labor induction to decrease their induction duration and the chances they will have a failed induction. Cervical ripening agents can act directly on the glycoproteins within the cervix (hormonal) or through mechanical dilatation of the cervix. Some cervical ripening methods can be used in tandem; for example, balloon catheters can be used with prostaglandins to decrease the duration of labor induction. No cervical ripening method should be employed before 39 weeks' gestation unless there is a medical indication for induction.

Many variables—such as provider preference, availability, cost, and institutional guidelines—will determine which agents or methods are used for cervical ripening. All hormonal agents can cause excessive uterine activity (tachysystole) or induce labor, so assessment of fetal well-being is an important prerequisite before hormonal ripening is initiated. The midwife should monitor the birthing person's response to cervical ripening and remain vigilant for signs of tachysystole or fetal intolerance to uterine activity. Mechanical methods are easier to discontinue than pharmacologic methods.

### Outpatient Cervical Ripening

Outpatient cervical ripening is an option for some pregnant people at term and can be used during labor after prior cesarean birth.[44–48] Most outpatient cervical ripening involves use of a balloon catheter or laminaria (also known as mechanical ripening) although some practices in the United States have administered medications such as oral misoprostol or dinoprostone for outpatient ripening. Due to the length of time that cervical ripening may require, low-risk pregnant people may prefer outpatient cervical ripening. Outpatient cervical ripening may also prove less costly since inpatient resources are not being utilized.

A 2021 systematic review by the Agency for Healthcare Research and Quality (AHRQ) found that, in low-risk birthing people, there was no significant difference in the incidence of cesarean birth, intra-amniotic or neonatal infection, or birth trauma with dinoprostone or single-balloon catheter used for outpatient cervical ripening compared to the inpatient setting.[49] To date, ACOG has not issued a recommendation regarding this practice; however, more research is warranted. The risks, benefits, and expected side effects should be explained to the pregnant individual as a part of informed consent prior to the use of a ripening technique and documented with a procedure note in the medical record.

### Membrane Sweeping

In the intervention known as membrane sweeping, the clinician inserts one or two gloved fingers into the cervical canal and "sweeps" the amniotic membrane away from the lower uterine wall. Sweeping of these membranes releases prostaglandins.[50,51] Membrane sweeping can be performed for two different reasons: to help hasten the onset of spontaneous labor or to decrease the duration of labor induction. When used to hasten labor induction, membranes should be swept at the initiation of the induction, or whenever the cervix has dilated sufficiently to allow passage of a finger through the inner os. The literature shows that serial membrane sweeping is no more efficacious than a single sweep performed after 38 weeks' gestation. Membrane sweeping appears to be safe in birthing persons colonized with GBS and is not associated with perinatal or neonatal adverse effects.[52,53] This procedure is reviewed in detail in the *Pregnancy-Related Conditions* chapter.

### Balloon Catheter

The most common method of mechanical dilation is use of a balloon catheter, although hygroscopic dilators (laminaria) are used in some locations. Two types of balloon devices are used in practice: a single-balloon device and a double-balloon device.[44] Although researchers have not shown differences in effectiveness or adverse perinatal or neonatal outcomes between the two catheter types, single-balloon catheters are often preferred clinically due to their lower cost.[44] The benefits of mechanical dilation using a balloon catheter are that it works directly on the cervix, has few adverse or systemic effects, and can be easily removed.[44]

Balloon catheters are inserted directly into the cervix and advanced beyond the internal os using aseptic technique. Insertion can be done with direct visualization of the cervix using a speculum or during a digital examination. Depending on the type of balloon catheter used, differing amounts of sterile water or saline are then used to inflate the balloon(s). Some evidence suggests that larger fill volumes (50 to 60 mL versus 30 mL) are associated with shorter labor durations.[45] Balloon catheters typically fall out of the cervix when the cervix dilates to 3 to 4 cm, often within 6 to 12 hours. The insertion procedure may cause some discomfort for the pregnant person and lead to persistent lower abdominal cramping. Some birthing people are more comfortable during balloon catheter insertion with the use of nitrous oxide or other pain-relieving agents. Accidental rupture of the membranes or cervical bleeding can occur during balloon insertion.

### Prostaglandin Agents for Cervical Ripening

The two hormonal agents currently used for cervical ripening are prostaglandin $E_2$ (dinoprostone) and the synthetic prostaglandin $E_1$ analogue (misoprostol [Cytotec]). Dinoprostone, the prostaglandin $E_1$ analogue, is approved by the Food and Drug

Administration (FDA) for cervical ripening and is available in two formulations: Prepidil, a vaginal gel, and Cervidil, a vaginal insert. By contrast, misoprostol, the prostaglandin $E_2$ analogue, is not approved by the FDA for cervical ripening or labor induction; therefore, these are off-label uses of this medication.[44]

Prostaglandins work by softening the cervix and stimulating myometrial contractions.[44,49] Side effects include uterine tachysystole, fever, chills, vomiting and diarrhea; however, the frequency of these side effects depends on which prostaglandin is used, the dose, and the route of administration. Contraindications to prostaglandin use include history of a prior cesarean birth or other uterine surgery (e.g., myomectomy) and the presence of regular uterine contractions. The current preparations, dosing regimens, and clinical considerations for these agents are outlined in Table 30-7.[41,54]

### Misoprostol

Misoprostol is available as 100- or 200-microgram (mcg) scored tablets that can be broken to provide 25 or 50 mcg doses.[54] The tablets are not formulated for vaginal use, and misoprostol is not FDA-approved for cervical ripening. Nonetheless, misoprostol is effective for cervical ripening and is commonly used on an off-label basis for this indication. Like all prostaglandins, misoprostol is contraindicated for birthing persons who have had a prior cesarean birth or uterine surgery.

Misoprostol may be administered either orally or vaginally. The uterine response to misoprostol can be somewhat strong, especially with vaginal dosing. As a precaution, the dose is not usually administered if the birthing person experiences more than 3 contractions in a 10-minute period.

Terbutaline should always be readily available to treat uterine tachysystole that is associated with abnormal or indeterminate FHR patterns. Interestingly, although caution is warranted, episodes of FHR decelerations that occur in response to misoprostol-induced tachysystole have not been associated with adverse neonatal outcomes in the studies that assessed the effectiveness of misoprostol for cervical ripening.[54]

### Combination Methods for Cervical Ripening

There is a considerable amount of research on cervical ripening techniques that combine hormonal agents with mechanical dilation.[44] These studies suggest that this is a safe and effective method of cervical ripening, especially for nulliparous people.[44]

| Table 30-7 | Hormonal Cervical Ripening Agents[a] | | | | | |
|---|---|---|---|---|---|---|
| **Drug: Generic (Brand)** | **Dose and Route** | **Onset of Action (min)** | **Peak Plasma Level (min)** | **Duration of Action (hr)** | **Mean Time to Sustained Uterine Activity (min)** | **Clinical Considerations** |
| **Prostaglandin E$_1$** | | | | | | |
| Misoprostol (Cytotec) | 25–50 mcg orally/buccally every 3–6 hours | 12 ± 3 | 20–30 | 2 | 90 | Contraindicated in birthing persons with a scarred uterus<br><br>Consider continuous fetal heart rate monitoring for a period of time to ensure stable maternal and fetal status |
| Misoprostol (Cytotec) | 25 mcg every 3–6 hours in posterior vaginal fornix | 20.9 ± 5.3 | 60–80 | 4.5–5 | 106 | Vaginal doses of 50 mcg are associated with higher incidence of uterine tachysystole and are not recommended<br><br>Oxytocin may be started 4 hours after last dose |
| **Prostaglandin E$_2$** | | | | | | |
| Dinoprostone (Prepidil) | 0.5 mg in 2.5 mL syringe; endocervical gel | Rapid onset | 60–120 | Variable | 127 | Pregnant person must remain supine for 30 minutes after insertion<br><br>May be repeated 6–12 hours after initial application |
| Dinoprostone (Cervidil) | 10 mg 0.3 mg/hour Vaginal insert | Rapid onset | Unknown | Variable | Unknown | Should be removed after 12 hours, or when active labor begins<br><br>Remove insert if more than 5 contractions/10 minutes (tachysystole)<br><br>Oxytocin may be started 30–60 minutes after removal<br><br>Monitor fetal heart rate for 1–2 hours after each dose<br><br>Oxytocin may be started 6–12 hours after last dose |

[a] Cervical ripening agents are contraindicated if there is an abnormal fetal heart rate tracing or more than 3 contractions in a 10-minute window.

Based on American College of Obstetricians and Gynecologists. Practice Bulletin No. 107: induction of labor. *Obstet Gynecol.* 2009;114:386-397. [Reaffirmed 2016]; Yount S, Lassiter N. The pharmacology of prostaglandins for induction of labor. *J Midwifery Womens Health.* 2013;58:133-144.

## Uterine Contraction Stimulation Techniques

Once the cervical ripening stage of labor induction is complete, uterine contraction stimulation is accomplished using a range of interventions, including amniotomy and oxytocin infusion. These interventions can be used sequentially, or—more often—in tandem.

### Amniotomy

Planned artificial rupture of the membranes (AROM) may be used as a method of labor induction either alone or concurrently with oxytocin. Studies have shown amniotomy to be more effective when the cervix is favorable (Bishop's score of at least 5), but individual responses to amniotomy can be unpredictable, which can result in long intervals between AROM and the onset of regular uterine contractions.[41] There is a potential risk of infection from a prolonged labor and cesarean birth if amniotomy is performed when the cervix is unfavorable. In addition, once the membranes have been ruptured, the birthing person is committed to giving birth and no longer has the possibility of reverting to a period of expectant management if a trial of induction fails to initiate labor. For laboring individuals with cervical dilatation of 4 cm or more, one study showed that early amniotomy was not associated with adverse maternal or neonatal outcomes and shortened labor by 2 hours or more.[55] When amniotomy is combined with oxytocin, the induction-to-birth interval is decreased.[41]

The primary risk associated with amniotomy is umbilical cord compression—or, more emergently, a prolapsed umbilical cord. For this reason, amniotomy should be avoided if the fetal vertex is high in the pelvis, or not well applied to the cervix. Variable decelerations are commonly seen when the umbilical cord is compressed; the management of variable decelerations is discussed in the *Fetal Assessment During Labor* chapter. Umbilical cord prolapse is a perinatal emergency regardless of whether the membranes ruptured spontaneously or following amniotomy. It is the primary reason why amniotomy should not be performed if the fetal head is not engaged in the pelvis and firmly applied to the cervix. See the "Intrapartum Emergencies" section of this chapter and the *Emergency Interventions for Umbilical Cord Prolapse* appendix for detailed guidelines for a prolapsed umbilical cord.

### Oxytocin Infusion

Oxytocin is a small, nine-amino-acid peptide hormone produced in the hypothalamus and secreted from the posterior pituitary gland. This hormone is similar to vasopressin and has a direct antidiuretic effect on the kidney. Most importantly, oxytocin is a potent uterotonic agent that causes uterine contractions. Although pituitary secretion appears to be the primary source of oxytocin, this hormone is also synthesized and secreted by the placenta and fetus. Synthetic oxytocin (Pitocin), which is chemically identical to endogenous oxytocin, is one of the most prescribed medications in midwifery practice today.

When this medication is used appropriately, the clinical benefits are undeniable, especially for treating postpartum hemorrhage. However, oxytocin is associated with adverse fetal and maternal outcomes and, therefore, is frequently implicated in intrapartum litigation cases.[56,57] As a result, oxytocin is now considered a "high alert" medication, which mandates compliance with safety measures to reduce the errors that may result in morbidities in either the birthing person or the neonate. Some of the safeguards currently in place include standardized intravenous concentrations, mandatory use of an infusion pump, continuous FHR monitoring, and dosing protocols.[56,57]

Oxytocin exerts its effect via agonist action on oxytocin receptors that are present in the uterine myometrium. These receptors become active or "upregulate" significantly by the end of pregnancy as described in the *Anatomy and Physiology of Labor and Birth* chapter. Oxytocin receptor expression and function are theorized to be the key reasons for the marked interindividual variability in responses to this drug. The oxytocin receptors also downregulate or become desensitized following prolonged exposure to oxytocin, which may partially explain why pregnant persons who are exposed to oxytocin therapy during labor induction are at increased risk for postpartum hemorrhage.[58,59]

The onset of action for synthetic oxytocin is 3 to 4 minutes, and the half-life is approximately 3 to 4 minutes. The uterine response reaches a steady state after 30 to 40 minutes.[59] Individual responses to a particular dose are both variable and dose dependent: As the infusion rate increases, the frequency and intensity of contractions follow if oxytocin receptors are expressed in sufficient quantities on the myometrium. As mentioned in the earlier discussion of cervical ripening in this chapter, oxytocin infusions for labor induction should generally be avoided until the cervix is ripe.

***Oxytocin Dosing Regimens.*** The variability in the individual response to oxytocin requires that the medication be started at a small dose and titrated until the desired contraction response is met. Various dosing regimens have been proposed, including those based on the starting dose and on the frequency at which the dose is increased and the amount of increase. Regimens are generally referred to as "low dose" or "high dose," although these terms are not well defined. Generally, the higher-dose regimens include a starting dose of 6 mU/minute that is increased by 3 to 6 mU/minute every 15 to 40 minutes. In contrast, the low-dose protocols are based on the pharmacokinetics of oxytocin and use a starting dose of 0.4 to 2 mU/minute, which is increased by 1 to 2 mU/minute every 40 minutes. High-dose regimens are associated with more uterine tachysystole, a shorter interval between starting oxytocin and adequate labor, and shorter duration of labor. The evidence regarding cesarean birth rates with high-dose versus low-dose regimens has been inconsistent, but most studies have not found that high-dose protocols increase the cesarean birth rate.[59-61] The influence of provider behavior on cesarean birth rates when oxytocin augmentation is used is not known.

Despite a lack of standard protocols, most clinicians use low-dose regimens that call for waiting at least 30 to 40 minutes before increasing the dose, to allow for evaluation of the full effects of the prior dose. This time frame allows the oxytocin administered to reach a steady-state plasma concentration and reduces the chance of dysfunctional uterine activity or tachysystole. Moreover, during the first stage of labor, a small baseline concentration of endogenous oxytocin may be present in the pregnant person's circulation, which may combine with the intravenous oxytocin infusion to produce a cumulative effect on uterine contractions.[59,62]

***Discontinuation of Oxytocin Infusion in Active-Phase Labor.*** Newer evidence shows that discontinuing oxytocin infusions once active labor has begun reduces the risk of uterine tachysystole and abnormal FHRs.[63] In these studies, active labor is defined as well-defined contractions and cervical dilatation of at least 5 cm.[64] The literature is mixed on the effects on cesarean birth.[63–65] Oxytocin discontinuation during active labor is a promising practice that should be considered in labor induction to allow movement in the birthing person.

***Side Effects and Adverse Effects of Oxytocin.*** Oxytocin has an antidiuretic effect, so it must be used with caution in individuals who need fluid restriction or who are at increased risk for pulmonary edema. Oxytocin can also cause hypotension, tachycardia, and transient myocardial ischemia that results in electrocardiogram (EKG) changes if given as a bolus dose.

The most commonly encountered side effect of oxytocin is uterine tachysystole. Tachysystole is defined as more than 5 contractions in 10 minutes averaged over a 30-minute window.[66] Due to the short half-life of oxytocin, decreasing or stopping an oxytocin infusion will rapidly slow the frequency of contractions. In many cases, uterine tachysystole does not result in obvious fetal compromise, but still requires an oxytocin dose adjustment to allow for adequate fetal oxygenation in between contractions. Titration of the infusion is highly individualized, with some finesse required to find a balance between

the desired effect and avoidance of uterine tachysystole. Birthing persons who are receiving oxytocin also require an assessment of their own and their fetus's status every 15 minutes during the active phase of labor and every 5 minutes during second-stage labor.[57,62] This important safeguard ensures prompt recognition and treatment of tachysystole and abnormal FHR patterns.

Regardless of the contraction pattern, any sign of fetal compromise requires immediate discontinuation of the oxytocin infusion. Additional interventions include lateral repositioning of the pregnant person and up to a 500-mL intravenous fluid bolus of lactated Ringer's solution. A single dose of terbutaline 0.25 mg can be administered subcutaneously if these initial interventions fail to ameliorate the contraction pattern. The midwife should notify the physician and remain at the bedside with the pregnant person until fetal well-being is ensured, in which case the oxytocin infusion can be resumed after 15 to 30 minutes, or when indicated. The *Fetal Assessment During Labor* chapter details the suggested tachysystole care guidelines.

In some cases, induction with oxytocin takes longer than anticipated, especially if cervical ripening was discontinued prematurely (Bishop's score < 6 in a multiparous individual, or < 8 in a nulliparous individual).[44] Desensitization (downregulation) of the oxytocin receptor sites on the uterus may occur following continuous exposure to oxytocin over a prolonged period.[59] Alternatively, inadequate progress in the phases of parturition can result in too few oxytocin receptors being expressed in the first place. When either of these events happens, oxytocin is less effective and increasing the dose merely adds to the risk of tachysystole and inefficient uterine contraction activity, without necessarily dilating the cervix.

Prolonged use of oxytocin can also increase the risk of postpartum hemorrhage from uterine atony from desensitization. Thus, it is important to be alert for this possibility and consider active management of third-stage labor to minimize the risk for postpartum hemorrhage in individuals who have been exposed to exogenous oxytocin for several hours. (For more information, see the *Third Stage of Labor* chapter.)

In addition to carrying an increased risk of postpartum hemorrhage, the use of oxytocin in the first and second stages of labor is associated with an increased risk of uterine rupture. Uterine rupture in a birthing person who does not have a scar on their uterus is a rare event in the United States (fewer than 1 incident per 10,000 pregnant individuals).[67] In developed countries, uterine rupture is almost exclusively associated with laboring individuals attempting labor after cesarean (LAC). Although oxytocin for labor induction or augmentation is not contraindicated for birthing persons who are attempting LAC, higher doses significantly increase the risks of uterine rupture and should be avoided.

If the birthing person's condition is stable and the individual is not yet in active labor, it is reasonable to discontinue the oxytocin infusion after 10 to 12 hours. This conservative approach will correct any receptor downregulation and enable the laboring person to rest. It will also reduce the risk of postpartum uterine atony from a prolonged infusion. Moreover, this approach allows time for additional cervical ripening overnight if needed. The oxytocin can then be restarted the next day and the induction plan will proceed accordingly. For some birthing persons, achieving a vaginal birth through labor induction requires considerable patience on the part of the caregivers. The criteria for a diagnosis of "failed induction" are not clearly defined in the literature, and this possibility should be considered only after the person reaches the active phase of labor.[41]

One last issue with oxytocin is the conflicting goals and miscommunication that sometimes occur between the nurses at the bedside managing the infusion and the ordering providers.[56] Often this conflict revolves around the dosing intervals of the oxytocin infusion. One possible solution is to implement mutually agreed-upon checklist-based protocols for oxytocin administration.[56,57,62] Such checklists focus on the fetal and uterine response to oxytocin instead of specifying a particular dosing regimen, allowing time for normal labor progress rather than automatically calling for more oxytocin. Also included are other safety measures such as appropriate staffing ratios and standard order sets for treating tachysystole. Prompt initiation of interventions without additional orders from the provider is an essential component of best practice recommendations for oxytocin use.[62]

## Other Methods of Induction

The use of more natural techniques to stimulate labor or facilitate cervical ripening is of interest for many birthing individuals. In many cases, these methods are used to help birthing persons avoid an induction of labor with oxytocin.

### Nipple Stimulation

Researchers have evaluated the safety and effectiveness of nipple or breast stimulation as a method to stimulate or induce labor.[68] Stimulation of the nipples is known to induce the release of endogenous oxytocin from the pituitary gland, which in turn causes uterine contractions.[69] In fact, nipple stimulation protocols have been used as an alternative to oxytocin administration for performing a contraction stress test. Various techniques have been employed, such as rolling one or both nipples between the fingers or using a manual or electric breast pump.

The authors of a systematic review of the available studies on nipple stimulation reported that low-risk women ($N = 719$) with a favorable cervix who used this technique were more likely to be in labor within 72 hours, compared to those who did not perform such stimulation.[68] Other significant findings related to nipple stimulation were a decreased incidence of postpartum hemorrhage and no difference in uterine tachysystole or abnormal FHR changes. Although the amount of endogenous oxytocin released by nipple stimulation appears to be minimal, it is not known if uterine contractions caused by nipple stimulation can significantly decrease placental perfusion. Therefore, nipple stimulation should be discouraged for birthing people who are at risk for fetal acidemia.[68]

### Herbal Preparations

Several herbal preparations, such as castor oil, evening primrose oil, raspberry leaf, and blue or black cohosh, have been used for the purpose of stimulating labor. Information regarding herbal methods of labor induction is often shared informally among colleagues and is likely based on anecdotal experiences, folklore, and traditional practices. There is wide variation among midwives in how and when these preparations are prescribed.

Midwives who recommend herbal preparations believe these methods are safe, are inexpensive, and help women avoid medical induction and prolonged pregnancy.[70,71] These preparations can also be self-administered by the birthing person at home or used in a birth center, where intrapartum oxytocin and prostaglandin may not be used.

Reviewers of the literature regarding herbal methods of labor induction reported an overall lack of scientific evidence regarding these treatments' efficacy or clinical benefit.[72] In case reports, blue cohosh has been associated with perinatal stroke and acute myocardial infarction; therefore, it should not be used.[73] Currently, there is no scientific literature that documents the safety or efficacy of black cohosh. Until scientific studies can be conducted to refute these concerns, blue and black cohosh, either together or in combination with other substances, should not be used in clinical practice.

Evening primrose oil and raspberry leaf, in contrast, have demonstrated no evidence of harm over many years of use. Whether they actually cause contractions or promote cervical ripening is not conclusively seen in the evidence, but their use during pregnancy is considered to be safe.[73]

The use of castor oil can be traced back to Egyptian times, and this product is still commonly used today to induce or stimulate labor. Although the exact mechanism of action is not completely understood, ingestion of castor oil produces a powerful gastrointestinal effect that releases endogenous prostaglandins, which in turn induces uterine contractions. Some birthing persons have reported rapid, tumultuous labors after ingesting castor oil, and use of this preparation may be associated with an increased risk of meconium-stained amniotic fluid. The evidence from several studies remains inconclusive regarding the effectiveness of castor oil. Although castor oil ingestion is safe for birthing individuals during pregnancy, midwives who elect to use it for labor induction should be aware of the inconsistent evidence as well as the lack of standard dosing protocols. Also, castor oil may be less effective for labor induction in nulliparous people.

In summary, caution should be exercised when prescribing or recommending alternative methods of cervical ripening or induction of labor not supported in the scientific literature. The midwife should also inform the laboring person of the known risks, benefits, and safety concerns prior to prescribing or endorsing the use of any herbal preparations.

### Acupressure/Acupuncture

Acupuncture/acupressure has also been evaluated for effectiveness in improving uterine contractility and labor induction. These studies have found a modest increase in cervical ripening (as measured by a Bishop's score) in pregnant persons exposed to acupuncture, but have not adequately assessed other clinically important variables such as time to onset of labor. Nonetheless, contraindications to use of acupressure during labor may include fetal intolerance of labor, uterine tachysystole, tetanic contractions, preterm gestation, or any other clinical condition in which uterine contractions are contraindicated (e.g., placenta previa).[54]

## Labor Progress Abnormalities

Evaluation of labor progress is an ongoing intrapartum assessment done to ensure the health of the pregnant person and their baby. However, the relationship between labor duration and maternal and neonatal outcomes is not well understood.[74–76] Obstructed labor resulting from true cephalo-pelvic disproportion is a real phenomenon, and neglected obstructed labor is a significant contributor to maternal and neonatal morbidity and mortality in low-resource countries.[77] Primary contributors to this problem are undernourishment in childhood resulting in a small pelvis and lack of access to needed medical care during abnormal labors. The situation in developed countries is quite different. It is not clear that the frameworks used for diagnosing and treating prolonged labor in the United States improve outcomes.[74,76,78] Nonprogressive labor is the most common reason for primary cesarean births and indirectly for many repeat cesareans. Most agree that this condition is overdiagnosed.[79-81]

Many terms are used to denote abnormally slow labor—for example, *labor dystocia*, *dysfunctional labor*, and *failure to progress*. There is no current consensus on the diagnostic criteria for these terms or on which term should be used.[80] Contemporary research and expert opinions on the parameters of normal labor progress are reviewed in the *First Stage of Labor* chapter. Questions about the appropriate labor progress make this an evolving and complex topic.[82–85]

For many years, assessment of labor progress was based on the work of Friedman, who published original labor curve data in the 1950s.[82] In the Friedman framework, there are two types of abnormally slow labor progress in the first stage: protracted labor (slower than normal progress) or arrested labor (no progress for a designated time frame). Friedman's parameters for abnormal labor progress are as follows:[86]

- Latent phase (criteria for prolonged latent phase diagnosis):
  - Nulliparas: greater than 20 hours
  - Multiparas: greater than 14 hours
- Active phase:
  - Protracted active phase:
    - Nulliparas: less than 1.2 cm per hour dilation
    - Multiparas: less than 1.5 cm per hour dilation
  - Active-phase arrest: no progress in 2 hours

More recent research based on two large data sets, the Collaborative Perinatal Project (CPP) from 1959–1966[83] and the Consortium on Safe Labor (CSL) from 2002–2008,[84] have challenged Friedman's criteria, suggesting that labor progress is much slower for both nulliparous and multiparous individuals. Analysis of the CSL data set found significant individual variability in the time interval to dilate from one centimeter to the next during the active phase of labor.[84] A delay in cervical dilation, also called a physiologic labor plateau, appears to be a normal variation of some labors.[87] No progress for 2 hours, especially before 7 cm dilatation is a common occurrence.[88] Another key finding is that most pregnant individuals are not in the active phase of labor until their cervix is 6 cm dilated.

Currently proposed evidence-based definitions for abnormal labor progress based on the CSL database are as follows:[83,84]

- Latent phase:
  - Nulliparas and multiparas: labor durations can vary greatly prior to 6 cm cervical dilatation
- Active phase:
  - Nulliparas: less than 0.5 to 0.7 cm per hour dilation
  - Multiparas: less than 0.5 to 1.3 cm per hour dilation

Use of these parameters to distinguish normal and slow labor progress in the active phase is supported by ACOG, SMFM, and is consistent with recommendations from the World Health Organization (WHO).[79,89]

## Midwifery Care During Slow First-Stage Labor

### Slow Labor in the Latent Phase

Although Friedman used the 95th percentile threshold to define prolonged latent phase as greater than 20 hours for nulliparas and 14 hours for multiparas,[86] researchers working with contemporary populations have not focused on the duration of latent phase except for consistently identifying that, for most persons, active labor does not begin until cervical dilation has reached about 6 cm.[83,84] Accurate measurement of the latent phase of labor is problematic because it is often difficult to mark the beginning and end of this part of labor with certainty.[90] The relationship between duration of the latent phase and outcomes is unclear.[90]

Delaying admission of the patient to the birth setting until the active phase of labor is optimal, because earlier admission is associated with an increased risk of a variety of interventions, such as oxytocin augmentation, epidural analgesia, and cesarean birth.[86] However, researchers cite qualitative evidence that many pregnant persons find coping with latent labor at home difficult and stressful, and desire admission earlier than recommended.[91] Additionally, individuals in these studies report that their experience of latent labor often did not match what they were told to expect by healthcare providers.[91] This shows the importance of providing accurate anticipatory guidance on latent labor, including potential variations in duration and degree of discomfort. This will help to normalize latent-phase labor and help pregnant persons prepare for the realities of this part of labor.

Long latent phases are particularly challenging for both pregnant persons and their care providers. The use of coping techniques at home will be sufficient for some laboring persons. Among these strategies are the presence of a supportive companion, a warm bath or shower, fluid and food, resting or sleeping when able, comfort measures such as massage, ambulation and rhythmic movement, music, and aromatherapy.[91] Regular phone contact with the midwife, outpatient check-ins, reassurance of normalcy, realistic anticipatory guidance, and emotional support will also help enable some individuals to manage this part of labor at home.

Medications that have a sedative effect are sometimes used to help pregnant persons sleep during latent-phase labor.[91] There is a paucity of research on the effectiveness or safety of these agents during labor. Some, such as diphenhydramine (Benadryl) and hydroxyzine (Vistaril), have a long history of use during pregnancy and appear to be quite safe. Others, such as secobarbital (Seconal), have very long half-lives that could adversely affect the newborn, so they are no longer in common use. Short-acting nonbenzodiazepine sedatives such as zolpidem (Ambien) may be used for this purpose, but no studies that have assessed either their safety or their effectiveness have been published.

If the pregnant person becomes significantly dehydrated or sleep deprived because of a prolonged latent phase, they may need admission to the birth site. The two treatment options in such a case are intravenous fluids plus (1) therapeutic rest to stop contractions and allow a period of rest or (2) uterotonic drugs to encourage organized effective contractions. It is best to base care decisions on maternal and/or fetal status and shared decision making with the pregnant person, rather than on the duration of the latent phase.

Therapeutic rest typically involves a single dose of morphine sulfate administered intramuscularly (or intravenously), which is sometimes combined with promethazine (Phenergan) or hydroxyzine (Vistaril).[91] Nalbuphine (Nubain) and butorphanol (Stadol) are sometimes used instead of morphine sulfate. A variety of dosing strategies are used, all of which have a primary goal of inducing heavy sedation or sleep. Commonly encountered side effects in the pregnant person include respiratory depression, euphoria, sedation, dizziness, and nausea and vomiting. Neonatal respiratory depression is also a potential concern, especially if labor progresses rapidly or if morphine is administered close to the time of birth. In many cases, those persons managed with therapeutic rest will sleep for several hours and awaken in active labor.

### Slow Labor in the Active Phase

Care of persons experiencing slow labor in the active phase requires decisions about when and how to intervene. Current professional organization and expert opinion recommendations focus on the threshold for intervening with oxytocin, amniotomy, or cesarean birth. Midwives generally view the care of individuals with slow labor through a broader lens, understanding that there are other ways to promote labor progress that are low technology, low risk, and supportive of physiologic labor.

To date, no evidence has been published that evaluates the timing and sequencing of various interventions to reverse slow active-phase labor. Starting with less invasive measures and moving toward more invasive interventions as needed is a common-sense approach. However, shared decision making should be used, and the strategy to address slow labor should be chosen in collaboration with the laboring person.

Before initiating interventions for slow active-phase labor progress, the well-being of the birthing person and the fetus must first be confirmed. Next, all factors that might contribute to slow labor progress must be assessed, including physical, psychological, and environmental factors (Table 30-8).

---

| Table 30-8 | Data Collection for Slow Labor Progress |
|---|---|

1. Determine the laboring person's body mass index at the time of labor admission. Active labor proceeds more slowly in people who have BMIs in the overweight or obese range, compared to those whose BMI is in a normal range (up to 7 hours longer in nulliparas and 3 hours longer in multiparas).[92] If elevated BMI is present in the laboring person, reassure them that their slow labor progress may be normal.

2. Observe the pregnant person for signs of exhaustion and/or decreased coping.

3. Assess the adequacy of the pregnant person's labor support.

4. Assess the pregnant person's environment for factors that may impede labor progress.

5. Explore the possibility of fear or anxiety related to labor or the pending birth that might impede labor progress.

6. Assess comfort and need for pain relief.

7. Determine the pregnant person's activity level and movement.

8. Determine if the pregnant person is taking in adequate fluids and calories.

9. Check the pregnant person's vital signs for fever or tachycardia.

10. Determine the frequency and intensity of the contractions and note any trends or changes.

11. Reassess estimated fetal weight and fetal lie, presentation, position and attitude with Leopold's maneuvers.

12. Assess fetal well-being with intermittent auscultation or continuous electronic fetal monitoring.

13. Review the labor progress up until this point.

14. Request permission from the pregnant person to perform a pelvic examination and carefully assess:
    - Dilatation
    - Effacement
    - Station
    - Fetal presentation and position of the fetal head
    - Asynclitism
    - Molding or caput
    - Pelvic cavity including dimensions of the mid-pelvis and outlet
    - Relationship of the fetal head to the space within the pelvis

Abbreviation: BMI, body mass index.

Data from Kominiarek MA, Zhang J, Vanveldhuisen P, et al. Contemporary labor patterns: the impact of maternal body mass index. *Am J Obstet Gynecol.* 2011;205(3):244.e1-244.e2448. doi:10.1016/j.ajog.2011.06.014.

One consideration when caring for individuals with slow labor progress is the hormonal physiology of labor—that is, the neurobiologic processes that result in the onset and progress of labor and birth. Several hormonal systems are involved: oxytocin, beta-endorphins, and stress hormones. These processes are not fully understood, but a growing body of research supports their impacts on labor.[93-95] During labor, a delicate interplay of these hormonal systems occurs. For example, endogenous oxytocin causes contractions and reduces fear, anxiety, and pain.[93-95] Events or stimuli that cause anxiety and increased pain may lead to overproduction of stress hormones such as epinephrine. This, in turn, decreases oxytocin and may mute the protective effects of oxytocin on anxiety, pain, and slow labor progress.

In addition to increasing stress hormones, certain environmental factors are thought to overstimulate the neocortex. These include noise, bright lights, lack of privacy, and practices such as mobility restrictions, restriction of food and fluids, and frequent vaginal examinations. These stimuli are theorized to inhibit the part of the brain that initiates the cascade of hormones required for effective labor.[93-95] Strategies that promote a sense of emotional well-being and safety while reducing environmental stimuli are appropriate in any labor and may be helpful if labor progress is slow. For example, continuous labor support, especially the therapeutic presence of the midwife or a trusted person, and attention to an optimal environment are primary strategies in the care of individuals with slow labor.

Measures to increase coping and comfort, and to relieve pain, are also important factors in decreasing levels of stress hormones and promoting labor progress.[93] These measures include nonpharmacologic methods such hydrotherapy (either a warm shower or warm water immersion in a bath), position changes, touch and massage, application of heat and cold, sterile water injections, and pharmacologic methods such as nitrous oxide, systemic analgesics, and neuraxial analgesia. (See the *Support During Labor* chapter for more detailed information on comfort and pain relief methods.)

### Oxytocin Infusion for Labor Augmentation.
In the past, recommendations for oxytocin were based on the Friedman criteria for protracted and arrested labor. When labor was protracted or arrested according to these criteria, oxytocin augmentation and amniotomy were recommended. There are no currently agreed-upon protocols indicating when such interventions should begin. The authors of the ACOG/SMFM consensus document stated, "when the first stage of labor is protracted or arrested, oxytocin is commonly recommended."[79] Other experts advise "at more than 5 cm dilatation, oxytocin augmentation may be considered any time there is a more than a 4 h delay in cervical change."[76] Though not clearly elucidated, the specific wording of such recommendations for initiation of oxytocin augmentation seems to imply that these thresholds are not absolute.

### Amniotomy.
Amniotomy is commonly performed to stimulate or augment labor when slowed progress is encountered. This procedure is not associated with a shortening of the duration of labor in pregnant persons who start labor spontaneously and progress normally.[96] Evidence is mixed on the use of amniotomy for those experiencing slow labor progress. In one study, pregnant persons with active-phase arrest were randomized to receive either amniotomy with oxytocin or oxytocin alone ($n = 108$).[97] No significant differences in mode of birth or duration of labor were observed between the two groups. In a Cochrane review examining amniotomy and oxytocin augmentation for prevention of or treatment for delays in progress during the first-stage labor, use of oxytocin and amniotomy to prevent dystocia was found to decrease the number of cesarean births.[98] This reduction was not seen in the three studies included in the meta-analysis in which oxytocin and amniotomy were used to treat more significant delays in labor progress.

### Cesarean Birth.
Past recommendations for slow labor treatment, which were based on the Friedman criteria and included short durations of oxytocin augmentation followed by cesarean birth, contributed to an unacceptably high rate of cesarean birth, especially among nulliparous people.[99] More recent recommendations from ACOG and SMFM assert that slow but progressive labor is *not* an indication for a cesarean birth in isolation.[87] They state that before a cesarean birth for arrested active labor is initiated, the pregnant person should be at 6 cm cervical dilatation or more, have ruptured membranes, and have no cervical change over 4 hours in the presence of "adequate" uterine activity, or no cervical change with at least 6 hours of oxytocin with "inadequate" uterine activity.[79] "Adequate" uterine activity is defined as more than 200 Montevideo units (MVUs).[79] Calculation of MVUs requires an intrauterine pressure catheter (IUPC) to measure peak contraction strength and uterine resting tone in millimeters of mercury (mm Hg). The strength

of the contraction is calculated by subtracting the resting pressure from the peak pressure. MVUs are determined by adding together the strength of all contractions in a 10-minute window. (See the *First Stage of Labor* chapter and the *Intrauterine Pressure Catheter* appendix for more information.) There is no consensus on the necessity of using an IUPC during oxytocin augmentation for slow labor progress. A 2013 Cochrane review compared internal and external tocodynamometry and found no differences in rates of cesarean birth or other outcomes.[100]

Some organizations, such as the California Maternity Quality Care Collaborative (CMQCC), encourage intrapartum care providers to use checklists to decrease the rate of unnecessary cesarean birth for labor dystocia. In the CMQCC checklist, IUPC monitoring can be substituted with palpation monitoring by the intrapartum provider, with moderate to strong palpation assumed to be similar to MVUs greater than 200.[101]

*Fetopelvic Factors Causing Slow Labor.* Cephalopelvic disproportion (CPD) as a cause of slow labor progression is often assumed to result from size discrepancies alone. Although this does occur, more often CPD is caused by a misalignment of various aspects of the pregnant person's pelvic architecture and the presentation and position of the fetal head. Malpresentations related to asynclitism or deflexion attitudes of the fetal head, as well as malpositions such as occiput posterior, are common causes of delayed progress during the first and second stages of labor. These factors can occur individually or in combination.

Malpresentations and malpositions alter the presenting fetal head diameter, as well as the biomechanics of labor and birth, and are discussed in the *Fetal–Pelvic Relationships* appendix. Cervical dilation can be slow because of uneven or reduced pressure on the cervix from the head. Descent may also be delayed until the fetal head rotates, flexes, or aligns with the plane of the pelvis, or may simply take longer due to a larger presenting diameter.

Theoretically, diagnosis of malpositions and malpresentations is possible via abdominal palpation or digital vaginal examination. Anecdotally, observations of abdominal shape, location of pain, the contraction pattern, and where the fetal heart rate is most easily heard can help in diagnosing a posterior position. However, studies show that these diagnostic techniques are not reliable.[102–105] For example, researchers in one study found that back pain was as common among pregnant persons with occiput anterior or occiput transverse fetuses as in those

with occiput posterior fetuses.[106] The most accurate way to diagnose a malposition or malpresentation is through ultrasound performed by an experienced operator.[105,107,108]

## Midwifery Care During Slow Second-Stage Labor

There are three clinically significant questions related to prolonged duration of the second stage: (1) What is the time frame during which the laboring person's chance of successful vaginal birth declines? (2) What are the maternal outcomes? and (3) What are the fetal outcomes?

Researchers have shown a positive correlation between the duration of the second stage and spontaneous vaginal birth rates. Furthermore, there is a second-stage labor duration at which the chance of vaginal birth diminishes significantly. In a secondary analysis of an RCT in which 94% of the participants had an epidural, Rouse et al found that 85% of laboring persons who pushed for less than 1 hour had a spontaneous vaginal birth. Among those who pushed between 1 and 2 hours, 78.7% had a spontaneous vaginal birth; among those who pushed between 2 and 3 hours, the rate was 59.1%; and among those who pushed between 3 and 4 hours, the rate was 24.7%. When laboring persons pushed 5 hours or more, the vaginal birth rate was 8.7%.[109] Those authors concluded that duration of second-stage labor could be safely extended for some individuals, but decisions to terminate the second stage should not be made based on duration alone.

To date, no prospective randomized trial has been conducted to address the question of "how long is too long" for the duration of second-stage labor; retrospective cohort studies and secondary analyses, however, support longer durations.[110] This debate is ongoing in the literature, with some investigators advocating caution in regard to extending the duration beyond 2 hours for multiparous individuals and 3 hours for nulliparous individuals because of concerns about increased maternal and neonatal morbidity.[111] Other investigators have identified that the parameters for second-stage labor duration can be safely extended without an increase in adverse maternal–fetal outcomes and recommend a reexamination of the definition of prolonged second-stage labor.

## Maternal Complications Associated with Prolonged Second-Stage Labor

A prolonged duration of second-stage labor is associated with an increased risk of maternal morbidity. The specific complications in such cases are intra-amniotic infection,[110-114] postpartum hemorrhage,[110-117] and third- and fourth-degree lacerations.[110,111,113-120] It is not clear if prolonged duration of the second stage results in intra-amniotic infection or if intra-amniotic infection adversely affects uterine contractility sufficiently to cause a prolonged duration. Thus, intra-amniotic infection may be both a cause and an effect of prolonged labor.

Additionally, interpretation of the body of evidence on this topic is complicated by numerous factors. These include varied outcomes in different studies, inconsistent definitions of prolonged second stage, different outcomes for nulliparous and multiparous individuals, different outcomes with and without epidural use in some studies, and lack of data on delayed versus immediate pushing in some studies. Perhaps most significantly, many studies did not account for increased use of interventions with longer second stages such as operative vaginal birth and cesarean birth. These interventions are clearly associated with a higher incidence of maternal morbidity. It is not clear if the complications are due to the duration of the second stage itself, or the interventions commonly used when the second stage is prolonged.

### Neonatal Complications Associated with Prolonged Second-Stage Labor

The relationship between prolonged second-stage labor and neonatal outcomes is less clear. Some studies have not found any increase in neonatal complications with a prolonged second stage.[117,118,121] Others have observed an increased risk of 5-minute Apgar scores less than 7,[111,112,121,122] NICU admission,[111,112,115-117,122] neonatal sepsis,[115,122] and shoulder dystocia.[115,118] One study found an increased incidence of sepsis in infants born to nulliparous individuals only.[111] In regard to neonatal mortality, most studies found no increase with a prolonged second stage.[111-113,115-118,121-123] In contrast, the study by Laughton et al. found an increased risk of neonatal mortality for both nulliparous and multiparous individuals who did not receive epidurals.[111] Although these are statistically significant increased odds, the absolute risk of adverse neonatal outcomes was quite low for all the newborn outcomes. Nonetheless, as second-stage labor progresses beyond the recommended guidelines, ongoing fetal assessment should be part of the consideration in balancing the risks versus the benefits of a spontaneous vaginal birth.[111]

In summary, the criteria for the diagnosis of prolonged second-stage labor have evolved from the strict limitations described by Freidman to the latest recommendations,[84] to offer greater latitude in evaluation of the ongoing progress of rotation and descent and identification of prolonged second-stage labor. In the absence of maternal exhaustion, other maternal complications, or signs that the fetus is developing acidemia, there are no clear reasons for rigidly adhering to any preset time limit for duration of second-stage labor. Instead, emphasis should be placed on evidence of progress in rotation and descent of the presenting part in response to the laboring person's pushing efforts, their stamina, and fetal well-being.

Ongoing assessment during second-stage labor includes continuous evaluation and documentation of fetal descent, rotation, other aspects of fetal position such as asynclitism, and the degree to which the fetus and the laboring person are tolerating the vigorous work of the second stage. Most people will progress through second-stage labor by following their physiologic urges and sensations without the need for intervention. The point in time at which the midwife first consults the physician for suspected (or anticipated) prolonged second-stage labor varies from practice to practice and is influenced by the circumstances under which the midwife works. For example, a midwife practicing in a rural hospital whose physician colleague is 25 minutes away would likely consult the physician sooner than a midwife whose physician colleague is always available in the hospital. The prudent midwife–physician team has preestablished parameters, relative to prolonged second stage and consultation, that meet the unique needs of the individuals served by that practice.

In general, the midwife stays with the laboring person and continues to offer support when physician consultation becomes necessary. During the consultation, the midwife and the physician establish a plan of care that often involves co-management, such that the midwife provides ongoing care and assessment of the laboring person and gives periodic updates to the physician.

## Descent Abnormalities in Second-Stage Labor

Descent abnormalities in second-stage labor can occur secondary to malpositions such as persistent occiput posterior or asynclitism, uterine hypocontractility, cephalopelvic disproportion, or fatigue of the laboring person. Failure of descent is present if the fetal presenting part makes no descent after 1 to 2 hours of adequate contractions and pushing efforts. Relative cephalopelvic disproportion may also manifest as protracted descent and prolonged second-stage labor. Protracted descent is more common than failure of descent or arrest of descent, and malpositions are a common cause of protracted descent. The process of rotation and descent should be regularly assessed to determine whether progress is ongoing or has stopped.

Assessment of station, fetal position, and presentation at the onset of second-stage labor is critical in determining the amount of progress that has been made over time, particularly if concerns about duration arise. From a clinical standpoint, it is important not to confuse molding or caput with true descent; progress should be measured from the location of the fetal skull. Physician consultation should be obtained when second-stage progress is protracted.

### Protracted Descent and Persistent Occiput Posterior Position

A common reason for delayed fetal descent is persistent occiput posterior (OP) position. Many fetuses are in an OP position during labor, and most rotate to an anterior position spontaneously, often in the late first stage or early second stage.[108] However, when the fetus remains in an OP position during descent in the second stage of labor, the cardinal movements of labor are slightly different, as described in the *Anatomy and Physiology of Labor and Birth* chapter.

Flexion of the fetal head (fetal chin touching fetal chest) may be incomplete, so that the larger occipitofrontal diameter is the anterior–posterior diameter that descends through the pelvis (Figure 30-3). When the fetus is in an occiput anterior (OA) position, the occiput descends and flexes, so the chin is against the chest as the occiput moves down the 5-cm anterior–posterior diameter of the posterior inferior

portion of the symphysis pubis; then, once the occiput is out from under the symphysis, the head is born by extension of the neck. In contrast, when the fetus is in an OP position, the occiput descends along the 10-cm distance between the top of the sacrum to the bottom of the coccyx and the final few centimeters along the floor of the birth canal before the fetal head is born via flexion, with the occiput presenting in the lower portion of the introitus, then extension on the fetal head occurring only as the occiput fully exits the vagina.

### Persistent Occiput Posterior Position

***Epidural Analgesia.*** Several observational studies show a correlation between epidural analgesia and an OP position.[124–126] Other studies show this association only when an epidural is placed before engagement of the head.[127,128] It is not known if this association is the result of the epidurals causing persistent posterior positions, or if those laboring persons experiencing this fetal position are more likely to request epidurals. However, when a persistent OP position results in exhaustion of the laboring person, epidural analgesia can provide an opportunity for that individual to rest in preparation for the work to come.

***Amniotomy.*** There is uncertainty about the role of amniotomy in persistent posterior positions. Amniotomy is commonly performed as a treatment for delayed progress. There is a theoretical concern that rupturing the membranes might decrease the changes of fetal rotation to a more favorable position because intact forewaters may allow for more fetal maneuverability. Only one study has provided evidence on this issue, finding an association between persistent OP position and ruptured membranes.[125]

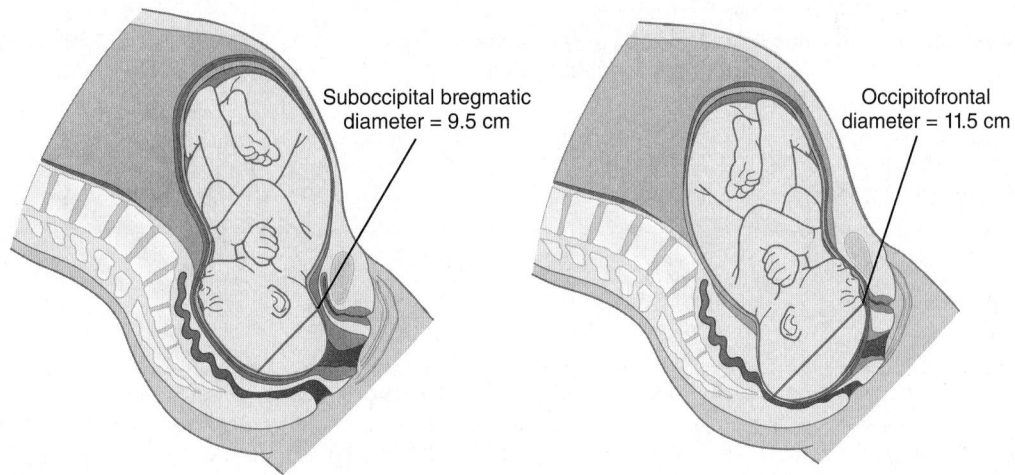

**Figure 30-3** Presenting anterior–posterior fetal skull diameters in occiput anterior and occiput posterior positions.

***Maternal Movement and Position Changes.***
Many midwives recommend movement and position changes of the laboring person to correct a fetal malposition or malpresentation and thereby encourage labor progress. A substantial body of evidence shows that maternal positions and movements result in changes in pelvic dimensions and the forces of gravity.[129–132] In theory, these changing forces and dimensions may improve the biomechanics of labor and promote optimal fetopelvic relationships.

Anecdotal reports of corrections of malpositions and malpresentations with position changes, followed by rapid labor progress, suggest that these measures may sometimes be effective.

Evidence on the use of maternal position changes to optimize fetal pelvic relationships is mixed. Five RCTs have examined specific positions to encourage rotation to OA position, following ultrasound diagnosis of an OP position (Table 30-9).[133–137] However, only in one study did researchers show a statistically

| Table 30-9 | | Positions to Encourage Rotation to Occiput Anterior | | | |
|---|---|---|---|---|---|
| **Study** | ***N*** | **Treatment** | **Epidural Rate** | **Ruptured Membranes at Randomization** | **Rotation to Occiput Anterior** |
| Stremmler et al. (2005)[133] | 147 | Hands and knees for at least 30 minutes | | | 16% versus 7%[a,e] |
| Intervention arm | | | 19% | 43% | |
| Control arm | | | 22% | 48% | |
| Desbriere et al. (2013)[134] | 220 | One of three positions based on fetal station until rotation to OA or birth[c] | | | 78.2% versus 76.4%[b,e] |
| Intervention arm | | | 93.6% | 100% | |
| Control arm | | | 95.5% | 100% | |
| Guittier et al. (2016)[136] | 439 | Hands and knees for at least 10 minutes | | | 17.2% versus 11.5%[a,e] |
| Intervention arm | | | 94.5% | 88.6% | |
| Control arm | | | 93.1% | 93.1% | |
| LeRay et al. (2016)[135] | 322 | Side-lying, opposite side of fetal spine for 1 hour | | | 21.9% versus 21.6%[a,e] |
| Intervention arm | | | 90% | 90% | |
| Control arm | | | 89.5% | 89.5% | |
| Bueno-Lopez et al. (2017)[137] | 120 | Side-lying, same side as fetal spine, 40 minutes per hour until rotation to OA or birth | | | 50.8% versus 21.7%[d] |
| Intervention arm | | | 100% | 100% | |
| Control arm | | | 100% | 100% | |

Abbreviation: OA, occiput anterior.

[a] One hour after randomization.

[b] At birth.

[c] –3 to –5 station: hands and knees; –2 to 0 station: side-lying, same side as fetal spine, inferior leg folded, superior leg extended and within axis of body; > 0 station: side-lying, same side as fetal spine, inferior leg extended, superior leg 90-degree angle with leg support.

[d] Timing of assessment for rotation not specified.

[e] Not statistically significant.

Data from Hanson L. *Simpkin's Labor Progress Handbook: Early Interventions to Prevent and Treat Dystocia*. 5th ed. Hoboken, NJ: Wiley-Blackwell.

significant difference between the control and intervention groups.[137] Interpretation of this body of evidence is complicated by confounding variables such as very high rates of epidural analgesia and amniotomy. In addition, it is not known if a minimum amount of time in certain positions is needed, if position changes are more effective in the first or second stage, or if the sequential use of several different positions is more likely to result in fetal rotation to OA. Frequent changes of position, such as occur during use of the traditional Mexican rebozo technique, may be more useful than any single specific position.[138]

Research examining the activity of all laboring persons has generally shown that those who are upright versus recumbent[139] or active in labor versus not active in labor[140] have fewer cesarean births and shorter labors. Given this evidence, it is reasonable to recommend maternal activity and the use of different positions when labor progress is slow, especially if a malposition or malpresentation is known or suspected. More research on positions for resolving malpositions and malpresentations is needed, especially for persons with intact membranes and no epidural.

***Digital and Manual Rotation of Occiput Posterior Position.*** Both digital and manual rotation reduce the incidence of OP birth.[141] The techniques for digital and manual rotation are described in Table 30-10 and shown in Figure 30-4. Although these interventions carry a theoretical risk of umbilical cord prolapse, fetal injury, fetal intolerance, or cervical lacerations, these complications appear to be rare, and the procedures are considered safe.[141] In fact, manual rotation is encouraged in the ACOG and SMFM guidelines for safe prevention of cesarean birth. Rotation can be performed during the second stage prophylactically (at the beginning of second stage) or therapeutically (after the second stage has become prolonged). There is debate on

| Table 30-10 | Technique for Digital and Manual Rotation of Occiput Posterior Position |
|---|---|
| **For Both Techniques** | |

Using a process of shared decision making, review the risks and benefits of the procedure and obtain informed consent.
Make certain the person's bladder is empty.

Bedside ultrasound can be used to visualize the fetal position precisely to plan which direction to rotate, and which of the provider's hands should be used.

| **Digital Rotation** | **Manual Rotation** |
|---|---|
| Place the tips of the gloved index and middle fingers in the anterior portion of the lambdoidal suture near the posterior fontanel. | Place four gloved fingers behind the posterior parietal bones, with the palm and fingers resting on the occipital bone. |
| Place the thumb of the same hand over the parietal bone. | Place the thumb of the same hand over the anterior parietal bone. |
| Move the fetal head up toward the pelvic brim slightly and flex it with upward pressure from the two fingers. | Flex and rotate the fetal head anteriorly during a contraction and when the laboring person is pushing. Mild upward pressure of the fetal head toward the pelvic brim may facilitate rotation. |
| Rotate the fetal head to the OA position via the shortest arc during a contraction and when the laboring person is pushing (i.e., if the fetus was right OP, then rotate to right OA). | |
| If the fetal head does not rotate with this mechanism, rotation of the fetal head can be attempted when the laboring person is not pushing, again following the short arc. | |

Abbreviation: OA, occiput anterior.

[a] One hour after randomization.

[b] At birth.

[c] −3 to −5 station: hands and knees; −2 to 0 station: side-lying, same side as fetal spine, inferior leg folded, superior leg extended and within axis of body; > 0 station: side-lying, same side as fetal spine, inferior leg extended, superior leg 90-degree angle with leg support.

[d] Timing of assessment for rotation not specified.

[e] Not statistically significant.

Data from Hanson L. *Simpkin's Labor Progress Handbook: Early Interventions to Prevent and Treat Dystocia.* 5th ed. Hoboken, NJ: Wiley-Blackwell.

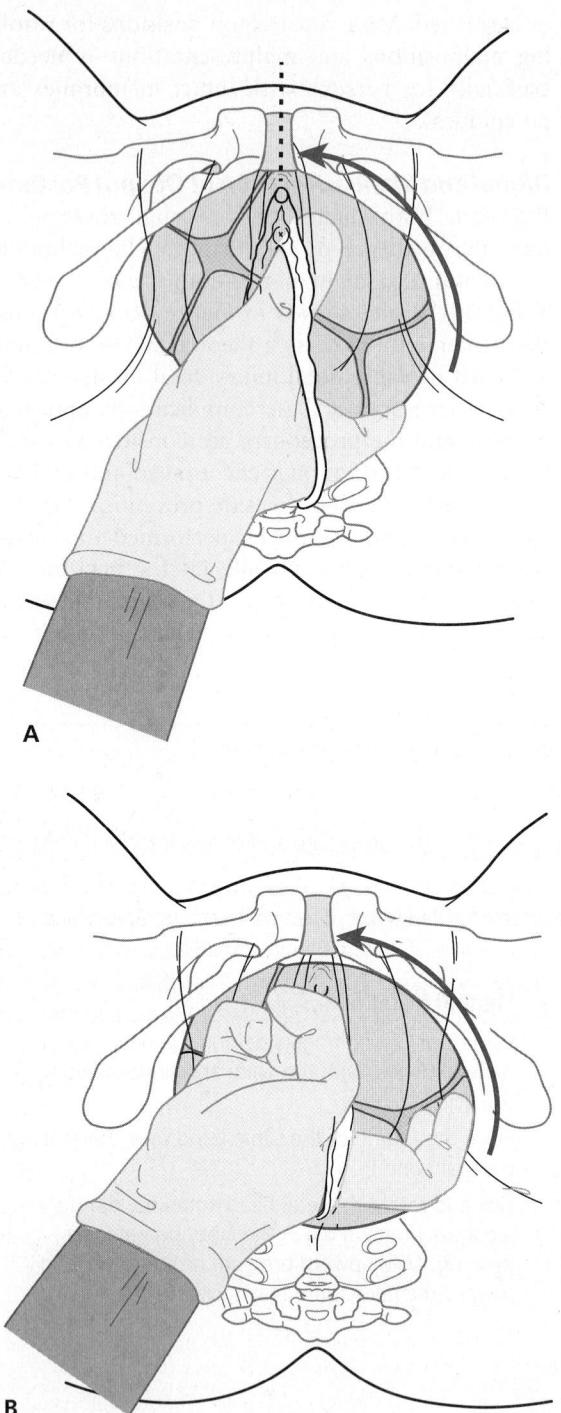

**Figure 30-4** Two techniques for rotation to reduce occiput posterior position. **A.** Manual rotation. **B.** Digital rotation.

the optimal timing of manual or digital rotation, although many providers recommend performing rotation before significant fetal caput develops to increase their ability to palpate the fetal skull.[142,143] Manual rotation should not be performed prior to the second stage of labor. It is not known if it is

best to perform this procedure during or in between contractions, although most providers rotate during a contraction.[141]

## Methods to Expedite Late Second-Stage Labor
### Episiotomy

Routine episiotomy was part of standard obstetric management until the 1990s, as it was historically believed that an episiotomy would decrease the incidence of perineal lacerations and brain damage in the fetus/newborn.[144] The change from routine episiotomy to the rare use of episiotomy occurred over the course of the 1990s, following the release of a 1989 seminal study in which researchers found that episiotomies are more likely to result in third- or fourth-degree lacerations than were spontaneous perineal tears (rectal laceration with episiotomy: 28.4% versus 2.2% without episiotomy (adjusted odds ratio [aOR], 8.9; 95% confidence interval [CI], 6.1–13.0).[145] A large national review of discharge data from hospitals, addressing translation of evidence-based guidelines into the practice of reducing episiotomy use, found that the incidence of episiotomy had decreased from 20.3% in 2002 to 9.4% in 2011.[146]

Today, routine episiotomy is not recommended.[147] The primary reason for an indicated episiotomy is to expedite birth secondary to fetal bradycardia or other FHR patterns suggestive of a significant risk of fetal acidemia when the muscles of the perineum are the likely impediment to birth. An episiotomy can also be beneficial in anticipation of use of forceps or vacuum extractor. However, there is no evidence that an episiotomy is beneficial prophylactically in these situations, and this procedure clearly increases the risk for an extension to or through the anal sphincter.[148]

If an episiotomy is indicated, anesthesia is a prerequisite. Even if the birthing person has an epidural, local anesthesia or a pudendal block may still be needed to provide pain relief during the surgical repair. After anesthesia is in place, one of two types of episiotomy is most often performed: midline or mediolateral. A mediolateral episiotomy is less likely to result in a third- or fourth-degree laceration than is a midline episiotomy. However, a midline episiotomy is less painful than a mediolateral episiotomy during the healing process because there are fewer nerve branches in the locale of a midline episiotomy and its repair. For more information about how to perform an episiotomy, see the *Urgent Maneuvers to Shorten Second Stage* appendix.

## Manual Fetal Head Extension (Ritgen Maneuver)

Manual fetal head extension, previously known as the Ritgen maneuver or modified Ritgen maneuver, is an old technique in which the clinician applies pressure on the fetal chin with one hand and pressure on the occiput with the other hand to control the birth of the head. The fetal chin is palpated behind the laboring person's rectum and pulled forward while the other hand maintains flexion of the occiput. As a result, the fetal head is pulled forward. This maneuver is performed between uterine contractions. The original rationale for using it was to control extension of the fetal head and prevent perineal lacerations. Over time, it became a practice used when the birth needed to be expedited. This maneuver is rarely used today, as vacuum or forceps are chosen when operative vaginal birth is indicated.

The original maneuver for manual fetal head extension involved placing fingers in the laboring person's rectum. The modified version of this maneuver involves placement of the fingers between the rectum and the coccyx.

Manual fetal head extension in any of its forms is not associated with a decrease in perineal lacerations,[149] but may expedite birth by a short period if needed and if other resources are not available. The steps involved in performance of this maneuver are detailed in the *Urgent Maneuvers to Shorten Second Stage* appendix.

## Labor After Cesarean

For the past several decades, pregnant individuals with a history of one or more previous cesarean births have encountered a series of changing professional opinions regarding the optimal mode of birth for subsequent pregnancies. Prior to the early 1980s, the predominant philosophy was "once a cesarean, always a cesarean." However, early reports of successful vaginal birth after cesarean (VBAC) began to challenge this long-standing practice. In 1980, the National Institutes of Health (NIH) published a landmark statement endorsing a trial of labor for pregnant persons who had one previous lower transverse cesarean birth.[150] Over the next 10 years, VBAC continued to grow in popularity, with several large studies reporting a 60% to 80% success rate for pregnant persons who underwent labor after cesarean (LAC).[151] These studies also demonstrated that planned repeat cesarean delivery (PRCD) was associated with more maternal morbidity than a LAC and subsequent VBAC.[150,151]

The NIH had hoped that promoting a trial of labor would reduce the rising cesarean birth rates, along with their associated costs in terms of morbidity and economic expense. This strategy initially appeared to be successful: By 1996, the rate of cesarean births in the United States had reached an all-time contemporary low of 20.7%.[151] However, as more individuals underwent LAC, reports of uterine rupture during a trial of labor emerged, leading to increased safety concerns. In 1996, a large clinical trial was published that examined a composite measure of serious maternal morbidity including uterine rupture, hysterectomy, and operative injury.[152] The absolute risk of this measure was found to be 1.6% in pregnant persons who underwent LAC and 0.8% in pregnant persons who had a PRCD. Moreover, the highest risk of these complications was found in the 40% of pregnant persons in the LAC group who had an unplanned, repeat cesarean birth.

This study, which was widely publicized, reported the relative risk of a doubling of serious perinatal complications with LAC versus PRCD. Almost immediately, enthusiasm for LAC began to wane and VBAC rates steadily fell. Concern about the risk of uterine rupture and its associated liability resulted in ACOG guidelines stipulating that patients seeking to birth by LAC have immediate in-house availability of an obstetrician and an anesthesiologist to perform an emergent cesarean birth if needed.[153] Many hospitals and providers who were unable or unwilling to accommodate this recommendation subsequently stopped offering LAC services, radically altering childbirth choices. By 2007, VBAC rates had plummeted to 8.9% and, in turn, cesarean birth rates rose to 32.8%.[154] While many factors have been cited as drivers of the cesarean epidemic, decreased access to LAC services—particularly in rural areas that do not have immediate in-house anesthesia availability—is a frequently cited cause of this unfortunate trend.

Concerns about the rising primary cesarean birth rates and associated morbidities, particularly placenta previa and placenta accreta in birthing people with prior cesarean births, led the NIH to revisit the comparative safety of having a VBAC versus PRCD. In 2010, the NIH Consensus Development Conference Statement on this topic was published; it concluded that pregnant persons with a previous low transverse cesarean birth can be safely offered labor when no other contraindications to vaginal birth exist.[154] The NIH statement also encouraged perinatal providers to improve access to LAC services and support pregnant individuals' preferences when possible. ACNM published a position statement and an updated clinical practice bulletin that supported the NIH's consensus report; it continues to reaffirm that birthing people have a right to safe and accessible options for LAC, and that certified nurse-midwives/certified midwives are qualified to provide counseling around the mode of birth to people with a uterine scar.[155]

In 2017, ACOG published revised guidelines that recommend pregnant individuals who are candidates for LAC can be safely offered these services in Level 1 hospital settings.[156] These settings are not required to have immediate in-house anesthesia, but should have the ability to initiate an emergency cesarean delivery in life-threatening situations.[156]

### Risks of LAC and PRCD

The comparative risks of LAC versus PRCD are presented in the *Pregnancy-Related Conditions* chapter, reflecting the reality that discussion of these issues begins during prenatal care. The most serious and catastrophic risk for a laboring person who elects LAC is *uterine rupture*, defined as an anatomic separation of the uterine muscle.[157] This outcome can be further differentiated into uterine scar dehiscence versus full separation of all uterine layers. Scar dehiscence does not include the serosa layer and is an incidental, asymptomatic finding with no adverse maternal or fetal consequences. A complete uterine rupture, in contrast, is a symptomatic, life-threatening emergency. Currently, the risk of uterine rupture remains low; however, the risk of rupture is greater in pregnant persons with a scarred uterus (0.47%, or 1 in 200 people with a LAC).[157,158] Uterine rupture is associated with a 14% to 33% rate of immediate hysterectomy and a 6% intrapartum fetal death rate (or 2.9 fetal deaths per 10,000 birthing persons who have a LAC).[154]

PRCD carries risks for both the current pregnancy and any subsequent pregnancies. There is an increased risk of abnormal placentation (placenta previa, accreta, and abruption) with a history of cesarean birth, and this risk increases with each cesarean birth. For example, after one cesarean birth, the risk of placenta previa is 9 per 1000, but this risk increases to 17 per 1000 after two cesareans.[154]

A history of previous classical or "T" uterine incision, previous uterine rupture, or any type of fundal uterine surgery (i.e., myomectomy) significantly increases the risk for uterine rupture.[156,157] Pregnant persons presenting for prenatal care with any of these risk factors are not candidates for LAC; instead, it is recommended that they undergo a PRCD. The optimal gestation age for PRCD is 39 weeks.[147] In addition, these individuals require prompt evaluation in the hospital with continuous fetal monitoring and physician consultation should regular contractions occur before the scheduled date of surgery.

Factors such as a history of two or more previous (low transverse) cesarean births, or previous preterm cesarean birth, increase the risks of uterine rupture to varying degrees.[157] A review of the existing evidence found weak associations for these factors and concluded that evidence for most of the factors is limited.[147] Consequently, pregnant persons with these obstetric histories can now safely be offered a LAC if desired and after a discussion about the individualized risks. These individuals should also receive prenatal counseling explaining that they have conditions that may increase the risk of uterine rupture to some extent.

### Induction or Augmentation of Labor During LAC

Abnormal labor progress is associated with a small increased risk of uterine rupture.[150,156] One study estimated that approximately half of uterine ruptures in people with a LAC could be prevented if abnormal labor progress was treated early with oxytocin augmentation.[159] Some studies have shown a slightly increased risk of uterine rupture when oxytocin is used for augmentation of labor in pregnant persons undergoing LAC, except when the Bishop's score was greater than 6 at the time of oxytocin initiation, or if the person had a prior vaginal birth.[150] The increased risk of uterine rupture associated with oxytocin augmentation is minimal, however, and does not rule out this medication's use when medically indicated.[150,156] Although upper limits for oxytocin dosing in persons with LAC have not been established, a conservative approach is preferred. Some authors recommend limiting oxytocin titrations to a maximum of 8 mU/minute, accompanied by close monitoring of fetal well-being, uterine activity, and labor progress.

Similarly, the risk of uterine rupture is higher in pregnant persons whose labor is induced with oxytocin, but the absolute risks are still low (0.74% risk for uterine rupture without induction versus 1.5% risk with induction).[156] Some evidence indicates that labor induction in a person with a prior uterine scar is more likely to result in a successful VBAC if initiated prior to 41 weeks' gestation, and ideally at 39 weeks' gestation. Similar to the case for people without a uterine scar, induced labor in people with a previous uterine scar is less likely to result in a successful vaginal birth if the cervix is not ripe when the oxytocin infusion is initiated.[156]

Therefore induction of labor should include cervical ripening when indicated and should occur in hospital settings where physician consultation for a cesarean birth is available.

Cervical ripening in people with a prior uterine scar is limited to mechanical methods, due to the association of prostaglandins during labor induction with increased rates of uterine rupture. Prostaglandin $E_1$ (misoprostol) is contraindicated in people with a uterine scar.[156] Due to limited evidence regarding the effects of prostaglandin $E_2$ (dinoprostone) on people with a uterine scar, use of this medication is discouraged.[156] By contrast, mechanical methods (i.e., osmotic dilators, single- or double-balloon cervical catheters) have not been associated with increased risks of uterine rupture and can be used for cervical ripening.[156]

## Intrapartum Care During LAC

Table 30-11 outlines intrapartum care guidelines for pregnant persons attempting LAC. When a person with a history of previous cesarean birth presents for a labor evaluation, the prenatal record should be reviewed, along with any previously discussed labor care options. The person's continued desire for LAC should be reaffirmed and the informed consent documentation reviewed. It is also important to assess the laboring person's desires for LAC, even if they had previously indicated a wish for PRCD. For example, if the cervical dilatation is advanced, some laboring people may wish to proceed with labor. One extenuating circumstance is that if there is a known fetal demise, LAC is the preferred method for stillbirth. The intrapartum assessment should also include a thorough review of the

| **Table 30-11** | **Intrapartum Care Guidelines for Individuals Attempting Labor After Cesarean Birth** |
|---|---|

1. If required by local communication patterns, the consultant physician should be notified when a birthing person desiring LAC is admitted in labor.

2. Intravenous access (i.e., heparin or saline lock) may be required according to institutional policies.

3. Clear liquid intake is not contraindicated; however, some institutional policies may restrict this intake to ice chips or sips of water.

4. More frequent fetal heart rate monitoring is required—either continuous electronic monitoring or intermittent monitoring per high-risk guidelines (i.e., every 15 minutes in active labor and every 5 minutes in second-stage labor). A telemetry monitor can be used to encourage freedom of movement.

5. The birthing person should be monitored closely for indications of uterine rupture. The most common initial sign is either recurrent fetal heart rate decelerations that become progressively deeper or an abrupt fetal heart rate bradycardia. Other signs include changes or cessation of uterine contractions, vaginal bleeding, or a sudden loss of fetal station.

6. Epidural anesthesia is not contraindicated and will not mask the most common signs and symptoms of uterine rupture.

7. Labor progress should be closely monitored for signs of abnormally slow progress, keeping in mind that the laboring person will typically progress according to their previous number of vaginal births, not their parity. Oxytocin should be used with nonpharmacologic methods to promote labor progress. Physician consultation should be obtained prior to initiating labor augmentation with oxytocin.

8. High-dose oxytocin protocols are contraindicated.

9. Intrauterine pressure catheters have not been shown to accurately depict an impending uterine rupture and should not be used solely for that purpose.

10. Hydrotherapy (i.e., tub or shower) is not contraindicated if waterproof fetal monitoring is available, although it is frequently restricted according to institutional policies.

11. There are no contraindications to alternative positions for birth if fetal assessment guidelines are followed.

12. Care during third-stage labor is the same following VBAC as it is following a normal vaginal birth. The midwife and the birthing person can opt for either expectant or active management of the third stage. There is no need to explore the uterine scar for signs of asymptomatic dehiscence after the delivery of the placenta.

13. Birthing persons with a previous uterine scar have an increased risk of abnormal placentation (e.g., placenta accreta). A physician should be consulted for a retained placenta prior to any attempts for manual removal.

Abbreviations: LAC, labor after cesarean; VBAC, vaginal birth after cesarean.

Data from Hanson L. *Simpkin's Labor Progress Handbook: Early Interventions to Prevent and Treat Dystocia*. 5th ed. Hoboken, NJ: Wiley-Blackwell.

obstetric history, paying particular attention to the indications for and circumstances surrounding the previous cesarean birth. Equally important is confirming the type of uterine incision (if known) and ascertaining whether the person has undergone any other uterine surgeries since the last birth. Lastly, the collaborating physician should be notified using local communication preferences if there is any contraindication to VBAC or if the person is opting for PRCD.

Use of a VBAC calculator can help estimate the laboring person's probability of vaginal birth after previous cesarean and may be helpful during intrapartum shared decision-making discussions. However, the clinician should be careful to use the updated VBAC calculator, which does not include race or ethnicity, to avoid structural bias against people of color.[160]

Midwifery care for individuals in labor who desire LAC is similar to the care of any laboring person with a few exceptions, including the recommendation for continuous FHR and uterine contraction monitoring and, possibly, a requirement for intravenous access. In addition, laboring persons who have experienced a previous unplanned cesarean birth often present with intense feelings regarding their past birth. They may have psychological milestones to overcome at the point in labor in which the events leading to the cesarean birth occurred. The midwifery model of care supports practices that promote normal labor and birth and are beneficial for pregnant persons who desire LAC. All interventions, therefore, should be evaluated for safety and interference with normal labor progress and mechanisms within a trauma-informed model of care.

## Intrapartum Care for Pregnant Individuals with Coexisting Medical Conditions

Three common medical conditions that can have adverse effects for a pregnant person and the fetus are obesity, diabetes, and hypertension. When caring for a pregnant person with these conditions during labor, collaboration between the midwife and the consulting physician will greatly depend on institutional policies, the evolving clinical situation, and the midwife's level of experience. It is important for midwives to have knowledge of what to expect for these individuals and to recognize that the intrapartum clinical course could change suddenly, necessitating immediate referral of care to the obstetrician. Ongoing and clear communication between the

physician and the midwife is paramount throughout labor to ensure the best outcome for both the birthing person and the fetus.

When midwives collaborate in the care of birthing people with coexisting medical complications requiring active treatment, they often monitor and manage labor progress, while the physician monitors and manages interventions required to minimize adverse effects of the medical condition. For example, if the birthing person has diabetes, the midwife may provide care during labor and birth, while the physician oversees administration of insulin and other tests to monitor diabetes.

### Elevated Body Mass Index and Labor Progress

The prevalence of obesity in the United States has risen sharply over the past three decades. Currently, 39.7% of people of childbearing age (20 to 39 years) have a body mass index (BMI) in the obese range. Obesity patterns are also characterized by racial disparities, with Latinx and Black birthing people being more likely to have BMIs in the obese range during their pregnancy compared to white birthing people.[161]

During the intrapartum period, the pregnant person's adiposity has profound effects on uterine efficiency,[162,163] is associated with considerable slowing of labor, with each point increase in the birthing person's BMI being associated with longer labor duration.[162] For example, among nulliparous individuals with a BMI of at least 35 kg/m$^2$, labor can take as much as 7 hours longer than in people who have a BMI in the normal range, whereas people with BMIs in the overweight range (25 to 29.9 kg/m$^2$) will labor for only 0.6 hour longer. However, because people with higher BMIs have slower labors, they are more often augmented with oxytocin than people in the normal-weight range.[164] As in birthing people with normal-range BMIs, labor tends to accelerate in people with higher BMIs during late active-phase labor. Thus, the greatest differences in the speed of cervical dilation between birthing people who are obese versus not obese occurs from 0 to 7 cm, while late active-phase labor and second-stage labor tend to proceed similarly, regardless of BMI.[162,163]

People with higher BMIs tend to go into spontaneous labor later in their pregnancies than birthing people with lower BMIs.[165] Thus, labor induction for late term or post-term pregnancy is more likely in people with larger bodies. When labor is induced, it is more likely to fail in people with obesity, largely because providers do not allow adequate time for cervical ripening and latent labor before performing a cesarean.[166] For example, compared to birthing people with BMIs in the normal range, people with BMIs in the obese range had a labor induction that lasted nearly 6 hours longer.[167] Evidence also shows that people with higher BMIs do not complete cervical ripening as easily with dinoprostone, compared to those who receive misoprostol.[168] In addition, the higher a person's BMI, the less likely they are to have a uterine activation following AROM.[169]

As experts in watchful waiting, midwives are ideally suited to care for birthing people with higher BMIs during labor. Midwives should individualize their expectations for labor duration and their choice of intrapartum interventions based on maternal BMI, and focus their care on education about what to expect and labor support. As a higher BMI during pregnancy is associated with a small increased risk of shoulder dystocia, especially with comorbid diabetes, midwives should also be prepared for this eventuality.

## Diabetes in Pregnancy

Approximately 6% to 7% of pregnancies in the United States occur in people with diabetes, with 90% of these affected people having gestational diabetes.[170,171] For pregnant people with well-controlled, pregestational diabetes, induction of labor is recommended between 39 0/7 and 39 6/7 weeks' gestation.[170] For pregnant people with well-controlled gestational diabetes, ACOG and SMFM recommend that birth occur between 39 0/7 and 39 6/7 weeks' gestation.[170] Nonetheless, a plan for fetal surveillance and timing of birth should be developed in collaboration with the birthing person and the perinatal care team physician.

Pregnant individuals with either pregestational or gestational diabetes have an increased risk of shoulder dystocia during birth. This trend reflects the increased risk of macrosomia and a tendency for the infants of birthing people with diabetes to have larger shoulder diameters at a given weight.[172] Prediction of macrosomia is an inexact process, with estimates of fetal weight via ultrasonography being no more accurate than those obtained through clinical palpation.[172] Induction of labor prior to 39 0/7 weeks gestation is not recommended for suspected macrosomia.[172] Nevertheless, the option of cesarean birth is offered to birthing persons with diabetes who have a fetus with an estimated fetal weight of 4500 grams or more.[172] This practice is based on evidence showing a higher risk of brachial plexus injury in the infants born to birthing persons with this risk factor. The *Shoulder Dystocia* appendix reviews the care with shoulder dystocia.

Infant lung maturity may be delayed in the newborns of birthing persons with diabetes. Seemingly full-term newborns can exhibit respiratory distress and other related complications immediately following birth.

Intrapartum considerations include a careful assessment of fetal size by Leopold's maneuvers when the birthing person is admitted, and close monitoring of labor progress. The pediatric team should also be notified, especially if the laboring person has poor glycemic control or fetal lung immaturity is a possibility. Continuous fetal monitoring is required if an insulin infusion is administered. The midwife should be prepared for the possibility of shoulder dystocia at the time of birth and have a low threshold for requesting the presence of the consulting obstetrician during the second stage of labor.

During labor, monitoring the birthing person's blood glucose and maintaining glycemic control have been shown to reduce the incidence of neonatal hypoglycemia.[173] For euglycemic individuals whose diabetes is treated with dietary changes only, it may not be necessary to monitor glucose levels during labor. However, birthing persons who are using insulin or oral glycemic agents will require finger-stick glucometer testing approximately every 2 hours. Any evidence of intrapartum hyperglycemia should be treated promptly with intravenous insulin. Institutional variations on care guidelines may exist; nonetheless, the midwife should develop the most appropriate plan of care with a physician. When a person in labor has an insulin infusion, that individual is best cared for collaboratively by a physician who manages the diabetes and a midwife who manages labor progress.

## Hypertensive Disorders in Pregnancy

The diagnostic criteria for hypertensive disorders in pregnancy are described in the *Medical Complications in Pregnancy* chapter. In all cases, these diagnoses may become indications for birth, but the timing will vary according to the severity of the laboring person's condition and the gestational age of the fetus. Although some fetal risks are associated with these disorders, mortality and morbidity in the birthing person are the primary concern, and treatment focuses on preventing end-organ damage in the pregnant individual. Most importantly, clinicians should recognize that hypertension and preeclampsia exist on a continuum that is often unpredictable. For this reason, pregnant individuals admitted with either of these diagnoses require vigilant monitoring during labor for subtle changes or a sudden worsening of symptoms. The midwife works closely with the collaborating physician to develop the most appropriate plan of care, especially if the individual is diagnosed with preeclampsia.

Intrapartum considerations include an ongoing assessment of the laboring individual for the presence of headache, visual changes, or epigastric pain.[174] Any headache should be taken seriously and reported to the consulting physician, especially if unrelieved with oral acetaminophen. Visual changes such as scotomata (loss of visual field) or scintillating spots and epigastric or right upper quadrant pain are also worrisome symptoms that require prompt evaluation and consultation with the physician.[174] Careful monitoring of fluid balance is essential as well. Although individuals with preeclampsia may have intravascular volume depletion, they are at risk for pulmonary edema following intravenous fluid administration secondary to impairments in their kidney function. Table 30-12 outlines specific assessments that should be included in the plan of care during labor.

Severe hypertension and eclampsia are two of the most serious consequences of preeclampsia. The National Partnership for Maternal Safety has a consensus bundle (set of evidence-based guidelines) of recommendations for recognizing early warning signs (triggers) of these conditions and treating severe hypertension (Table 30-13).[174,175]

Magnesium sulfate remains the standard of care for the prevention and treatment of eclampsia for individuals with preeclampsia with severe features.[174,175] Magnesium sulfate is administered as a bolus of 4 to 6 grams in 100 mL over 20 minutes, followed by an intravenous infusion of 1 to 2 grams per hour throughout labor and for 24 hours post birth. Magnesium sulfate therapy is not recommended when preeclampsia occurs without severe features.[174,175] Nonetheless, progression of

---

| Table 30-12 | Labor Assessment for Individuals with Preeclampsia |
|---|---|

1. Hourly blood pressure monitoring[a]:
   a. Any result higher than or equal to 160 mm Hg systolic or 110 mm Hg diastolic requires immediate physician consultation and administration of an intravenous antihypertensive medication.[174,175]

2. Lung auscultation and/or pulse oximetry:
   a. Any shortness of breath, abnormal breath sounds (crackles, wheezes), or other signs of pulmonary edema require the immediate presence of a physician.
   b. Obtain pulse oximetry if the individual has any shortness of breath.

3. Deep tendon reflexes:
   a. Hyper-reflexive (+4) deep tendon reflexes is an indicator of nervous system involvement. Hypo-reflexive or absent reflexes can be a sign of magnesium toxicity.

4. Laboratory monitoring:
   a. Obtain at admission and per practice/institutional guidelines. Consult with a physician for abnormalities.
   b. Obtain a complete blood count (CBC) with platelets, serum creatinine, uric acid, lactate dehydrogenase (LDH), aspartate aminotransferase (AST), alanine aminotransferase (ALT), and urine protein (protein to creatinine).

5. Strict intake/output:
   a. Measure urine output at least every 2 to 4 hours. If the urine output is averaging 30 mL/hour or less, consult the physician.
   b. Carefully monitor intravenous and oral fluids.

6. If magnesium sulfate is infusing:
   a. Perform hourly assessments of respiratory rate, deep tendon reflexes, and urine output. The infusion should be discontinued and the physician notified immediately for any signs of magnesium toxicity (respiratory rate less than 12 breaths/min, absent or diminished deep tendon reflexes, or urine output less than 30 mL/hour).
   b. The antidote for magnesium toxicity is calcium gluconate 10 mL of a 10% solution administered intravenously over 3 minutes.

[a] Manual blood pressure measurements are preferred, as they are the most accurate.

| Table 30-13 | Treatment of Severe Hypertension | |
|---|---|---|
| **Drug: Generic (Brand)** | **Dose** | **Contraindications[a]** |
| Hydralazine (Apresoline) | 5 mg IV or IM, then 5–10 mg IV every 20–40 minutes<br>Maximum total dose: 20 mg or IV infusion of 0.5–10 mg/hour | Tachycardia |
| Labetalol (Normodyne, Trandate) | 10–20 mg IV bolus, followed by 20–80 mg every 30 minutes if not effective<br>Maximum total dose: 300 mg or IV infusion at 1–2 mg/min | Asthma, heart failure |
| Nifedipine | 10–20 mg orally, can repeat in 20 minutes; then 10–20 mg every 2–6 hours if needed<br>Maximum total daily dose: 180 mg<br>Note: Not to be given sublingually | Tachycardia |
| Magnesium sulfate | Not recommended as an antihypertensive agent but used for seizure prophylaxis and controlling eclamptic seizures<br>4–6 g in 100 mL IV bolus over 20 minutes<br>1–2 g/hour IV infusion throughout labor and for 24 hours after birth<br>Titration based on blood levels and clinical signs of toxicity. | Renal failure; myasthenia gravis |

Abbreviations: IM, intramuscular; IV, intravenous.

[a] Contraindications may be relative contraindications depending on the clinical condition.

Note: If blood pressure is ≥ 160 mm Hg systolic or ≥ 110 mm Hg diastolic, verify within 15 minutes. If confirmed by a second reading, administer an antihypertensive agent within 30–60 minutes.

Based on Bernstein PS, Martin JN Jr, Barton JR, et al. National Partnership for Maternal Safety: consensus bundle on severe hypertension during pregnancy and the postpartum period. *Obstet Gynecol.* 2017;130(2):347-357; Gestational hypertension and preeclampsia: ACOG Practice Bulletin Summary, Number 222. *Obstet Gynecol.* 2020;135(6):1492-1495. doi:10.1097/AOG.0000000000003892.

preeclampsia can occur suddenly, and the individuals must be monitored very closely for any such changes.

Deep tendon reflexes are part of both the initial evaluation and ongoing assessments in people receiving magnesium sulfate. Reflexes are evaluated on a scale of 0 to 4+:

0: absent; no response

1+: decreased; diminished; sluggish

2+: normal; average

3+: brisk

4+: very brisk; hyperactive (usually associated with clonus)

Reflexes designated as 1+ are low-normal reflexes; 3+ reflexes are more brisk than the average reflex response and indicate the possible, but not absolute, presence of disease. 0 and 4+ reflexes are abnormal and indicate disease requiring a minimum of physician consultation. Normally, deep tendon reflexes are evaluated as 1+ or 2+. A sign of magnesium toxicity is absent or depressed deep tendon reflexes. Therefore, when magnesium sulfate is infusing, it is important that deep tendon reflexes are assessed hourly.

## Intrapartum Emergencies

Midwives in clinical practice will inevitably encounter intrapartum emergencies. Fortunately, most intrapartum emergencies are rare occurrences, and in some cases, they can be anticipated. Consideration must be given to the appropriate location of care when risk factors are present, and recruitment of the appropriate care team. Regardless, midwives are responsible for the care of individuals during the intrapartum period, which requires a thorough understanding of how to manage emergent events during labor and birth. Prompt recognition and immediate action are imperative until the situation is resolved or the physician or interprofessional team can assume care.

The following sections review the clinical care for several intrapartum emergencies, including intrapartum hemorrhage, shoulder dystocia, prolapsed umbilical cord, uterine rupture, twin gestation, and breech birth. Appendices also review in detail how these conditions should be handled by the midwife, including how to collect umbilical cord gases to assess the newborn's status following an urgent or emergency intrapartum situation.

| Table 30-14 | **Maternal Early Warning Signs and Triggers** | |
| --- | --- | --- |
| **Sign or Symptom** | **Criteria** | **Trigger** |
| Blood pressure | Systolic: < 90 or > 160 mm Hg | Systolic: < 80 or > 155 mm Hg |
| | Diastolic: > 100 mm Hg | Diastolic: < 45 or > 105 mm Hg |
| Heart rate | < 50 or > 120 beats/min | < 50 or > 110 beats/min |
| Respiratory rate | < 10 or > 30 breaths/min | < 12 or > 24 breaths/min |
| Maternal symptoms | Agitation, confusion, unresponsiveness | Altered mental status |
| | If preeclampsia: nonremitting headache or shortness of breath | |
| Oxygen saturation at room air at sea level | < 95% | ≤ 93% |
| Oliguria | < 35 mL/hour for > 2 hours | — |

Data from Zuckerwise LC, Lipkind HS. Maternal early warning systems: towards reducing preventable maternal mortality and severe maternal morbidity through improved clinical surveillance and responsiveness. *Semin Perinatol.* 2017;41(3):161-165. doi:10.1053/j.semperi.2017.03.005.

Recent studies suggest that nearly two-thirds of pregnancy-related deaths in the United States are preventable.[176] Delays in recognition and treatment have prompted the development of early warning signs and rapid response teams to help clinicians more effectively anticipate and respond to intrapartum emergencies. Each sign also includes "triggers" that identify patients at risk and in need of further evaluation.[177] These early warning signs and triggers requiring immediate attention are listed in Table 30-14. All maternity care providers should know these signs and triggers as well as the plans for intervention. Resources for learning more about maternal early warning systems are listed at the end of this chapter.

### Intrapartum Hemorrhage

The differential diagnoses for vaginal bleeding in the second or third trimester include placenta previa, placental abruption, uterine rupture, and vasa previa. The midwife's role in the care of a laboring individual who is bleeding is to notify the interprofessional team and initiate stabilization measures until the team arrives. An obstetrician or maternal fetal medicine specialist, anesthesia specialist, operating room team, and the neonatal/pediatric team should be mobilized and on standby for fluid resuscitation, emergent birth, and possible neonatal resuscitation. If the person is hemodynamically unstable or the fetus is in jeopardy, birth will be expedited, regardless of gestational age.

Initial evaluation of hemodynamic status includes assessment of vital signs, mental status, and skin color (pallor), as well as a visual evaluation of blood loss. The physician is called for an immediate bedside consultation. If there is evidence of significant blood loss on the person's clothes or body with any signs of hemodynamic compromise, two large-bore intravenous lines should be started; one with normal saline. The person should be given oxygen and placed on continuous electronic fetal monitoring. Laboratory evaluation includes a complete blood count, coagulation studies, blood type, antibody screen, and cross-match for a minimum of 4 units of blood if the person is actively bleeding. In addition, a Kleihauer-Betke test (a quantitative fetal blood screen) should be obtained on all individuals who are Rh negative to quantify the degree of fetomaternal transfusion to guide the dosing of Rh immune globulin (RhoGAM).

No digital examinations should be performed when a person presents with vaginal bleeding until placenta previa has been ruled out. Prenatal ultrasound records should be obtained and reviewed as quickly as possible. If previous ultrasound studies have confirmed a normal placental location, placenta previa can be ruled out, but other possibilities such as placental abruption or vasa previa should still be considered.

### Placenta Previa

Placenta previa can cause a small amount of vaginal bleeding, or it may result in acute hemorrhage. In most cases, individuals with placenta previa will present with an initial episode of painless vaginal bleeding. During this first episode, the bleeding usually stops, the individual and fetus remain stable, and expectant management in the hospital is initiated. During this hospitalization, the person is monitored for signs of labor and, depending on the fetus's gestational age, steroids may be administered to enhance fetal lung maturity and/or magnesium sulfate administered for fetal neuroprotection.

In cases of placenta previa, the individual's care is managed by a physician in expectation of cesarean birth. The midwife may continue in a collaborative role to provide emotional support and anticipatory guidance. Preparation for breastfeeding/chestfeeding and parenting as well as family adjustments to hospitalization are an important midwifery component of the individual's plan of care.

### Placental Abruption (Abruptio Placentae)

One of the leading causes of intrapartum hemorrhage in the second and third trimesters is placental abruption, defined as a premature separation of a normally implanted placenta resulting in decreased oxygen and nutrient exchange to the fetus.[178] Placental abruption occurs in approximately 0.6% to 1% of all pregnancies and is associated with significant perinatal and neonatal mortality and morbidity.[178,179]

In most cases of abruption, bleeding occurs between the membranes and the decidua, and passes through the cervix into the vagina. In severe cases of abruption, significant blood loss, fetal hypoxia, and fetal death can occur rapidly, necessitating an emergency cesarean birth.[178] Less commonly, the abruption is concealed, such that the blood accumulates behind the placenta with no obvious vaginal bleeding. In concealed abruptions, the blood may penetrate through the uterine decidua and escape into the peritoneum via a phenomenon termed a *Couvelaire uterus*.

An abruption can be either total (involving the entire placenta) or partial (involving only a portion of the placenta) (Figure 30-5). A total abruption is a catastrophic intrapartum event, often leading to fetal death and significant morbidity for the birthing person.

Although the specific etiology of abruption is unknown, several factors associated with it have been identified (Table 30-15). The most common of these risk factors is hypertensive disorders, especially chronic hypertension with superimposed preeclampsia.[180,181] A history of previous abruption, smoking, and cocaine use also significantly increase the risks of placental abruption. In addition, any maternal trauma (e.g., fall, abdominal injury, intimate-partner violence, or motor vehicle accident) warrants an evaluation in the hospital to rule out and monitor for an abruption.

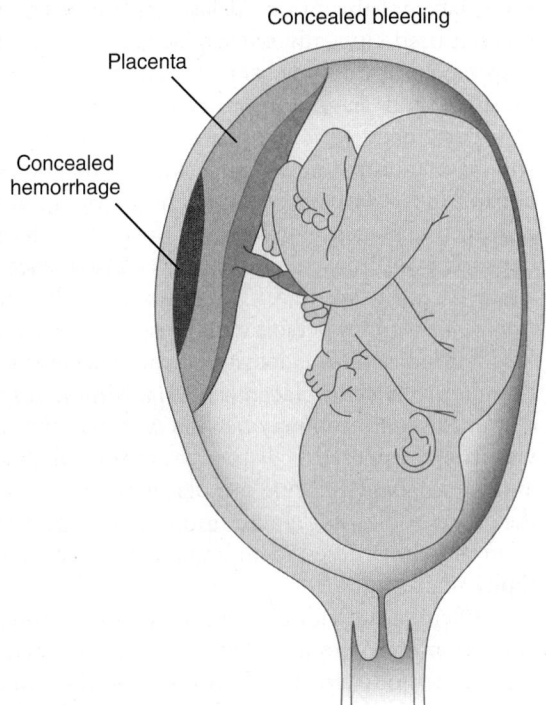
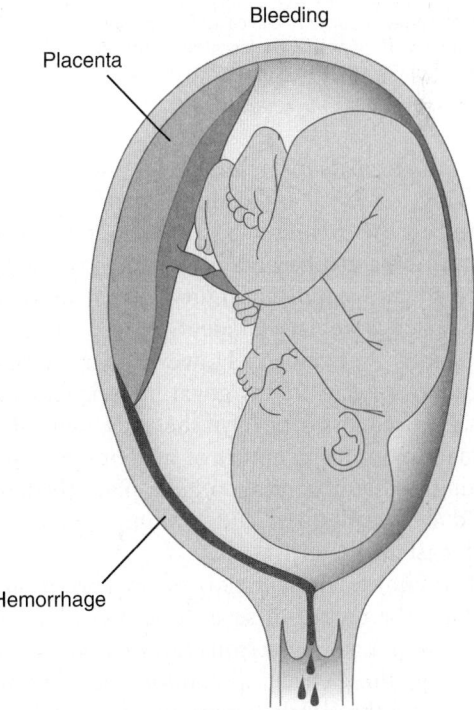

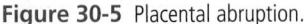

**Figure 30-5** Placental abruption.

| Table 30-15 | Risk Factors for Placental Abruption |
|---|---|
| **Individual Risk Factors** | |
| Advanced birthing person age | |
| Cocaine use | |
| Smoking during pregnancy | |
| **Pregnancy Risk Factors** | |
| Intra-amniotic infection | |
| Fetal growth restriction | |
| History of placental abruption | |
| Hypertensive disorders (chronic, gestational, preeclampsia) | |
| Multifetal gestation | |
| Premature rupture of membranes | |
| Polyhydramnios | |
| Oligohydramnios | |
| Thrombophilias | |
| **Acute Etiology** | |
| Trauma (fall, abdominal injury, motor vehicle accident) | |
| External cephalic version for breech presentation | |

Based on Oyelese Y, Ananth CV. Placental abruption. *Obstet Gynecol.* 2006:108:1005-1016; Hladky K, Yankowitz J, Hansen WF. Placental abruption. *Obstet Gynecol Surv.* 2002;57(5):299-305; Ananth CV, Lavery JA, Vintzileos AM, et al. Severe placental abruption: clinical definition and associations with maternal complications. *Am J Obstet Gynecol.* 2016;214(2):272.e1-272.e9. doi:10.1016/j.ajog.2015.09.069.159.

Pregnant persons who are at more than 24 weeks' gestation should have continuous fetal monitoring for a minimum of 4 hours following minor trauma to the abdomen that is not accompanied by any significant injury to that individual. (This includes vehicle accidents where the person was properly restrained.) However, if more than 4 contractions occur in any given hour, if fetal heart tones are nonreassuring, or if there are signs of serious maternal injury, rupture of membranes, vaginal bleeding, or significant abdominal pain, the person should be hospitalized and monitoring continued for at least 24 hours.

The clinical presentation of an abruption depends on the degree of separation and blood loss. Symptoms in birthing persons can vary widely, from mild generalized back discomfort or abdominal cramping to the classic symptoms of vaginal bleeding, severe abdominal pain, tetanic contractions, and/or abnormal fetal heart tracings.[179] Early signs of an abruption can mimic those of labor, and the birthing person may report periodic mild contractions with what may be perceived as bloody show or bloody amniotic fluid. Low backache may be the only symptom if the placenta is posterior and there is a concealed abruption. The person may also report decreased fetal movement.

On examination, the individual's demeanor or distress may be out of proportion to the objective clinical signs, and vital signs may be normal with no obvious signs of hemodynamic compromise. The abdomen may be mildly tender with palpable contractions, or it may feel firm, rigid, or board-like. Once placenta previa has been ruled out, a pelvic examination may reveal minimal to no bleeding; however, this will not correlate with the amount of blood loss from a concealed hemorrhage. Fetal status will also greatly depend on the degree of separation and blood loss. Thus, a variety of FHR patterns have been associated with a placental abruption, including recurrent late or variable decelerations, loss of FHR variability, bradycardia, and a sinusoidal pattern.[180,182] In most cases, frequent, low-amplitude contractions are seen on the external fetal monitor. Fetal demise is associated with more than a 50% placental separation; however, this degree of abruption rarely occurs without other overt symptoms.[180,182]

There are no definitive procedures used to diagnose placental abruption. Although ultrasonography is often used clinically when placental abruption is suspected, it is rarely helpful in confirming a placental abruption diagnosis or determining the degree of separation.[182] The literature shows that the sensitivity of ultrasound findings for the diagnosis of abruption is relatively low, and the sonographic appearance of placental separation varies considerably depending on how much time has passed since the acute bleeding event.[180,182] An ultrasound evaluation of a pregnant person who presents with vaginal bleeding is useful in identifying the placental location and ruling out placenta previa. Although some degree of separation may be seen with placenta previa, it is considered a distinctly separate diagnosis and would, in effect, rule out placental abruption as the cause of bleeding. In addition, radiologic assessment may be ordered including a computed tomography scan.

When an individual presents with symptoms of abruption, they should be immediately assessed for signs of hemodynamic compromise and the fetus assessed for signs that suggest an increased risk for fetal acidemia. If the individual is Rho(D) negative, they should be given Rho(D) immune globulin (RhoGAM) within 72 hours of the trauma (300 micrograms IM is sufficient to protect against Rh isoimmunization of approximately 30 mL of fetal blood). A Kleihauer-Betke test, also known as a fetal cell screen, may be used to determine if more RhoGAM is indicated. The continued care will depend in part on the gestational age and in part on the conditions of the laboring person and the fetus. The physician should be notified immediately of the midwife's clinical assessment and evaluation and seek to determine the most appropriate plan of care. The midwife should also initiate the maternal–fetal stabilization measures and laboratory assessments discussed in the previous section.

Depending on the severity of the abruption and gestational age, the birthing person may be transferred to a medical center with the capacity for more specialized care. Although care may vary depending on the degree of maternal–fetal compromise, a diagnosis of placental abruption near term will warrant an expedited birth. In many cases, the placental abruption will stimulate vigorous contractions, with labor then rapidly progressing on its own. The midwife can collaboratively manage this situation with a physician and conduct the birth as planned. During labor, the fetus should be monitored continuously, and any signs of fetal compromise promptly reported to the physician. Even with a mild abruption, the situation could deteriorate rapidly, and the individual is at significant risk for coagulopathy and hypovolemic shock. In addition to blood transfusions, the individual may need aggressive replacement of coagulation factors. Many hospitals have a massive transfusion protocol that designates the ratio of blood products administered following large blood losses. After the birth, the placenta should be sent to pathology, and the individual closely monitored collaboratively with a physician until their condition stabilizes.

### Uterine Rupture

Uterine rupture is an anatomic separation of the uterine muscle.[150,151,156] Rupture can be further differentiated between uterine scar dehiscence and full separation of all three uterine layers (i.e., endometrium, myometrium, and perimetrium).[182] Uterine scar dehiscence does not include the perimetrium layer and is an incidental, asymptomatic finding with no adverse consequences to the birthing person or fetus. In contrast, a complete uterine rupture is nearly always symptomatic and a life-threatening emergency. Uterine rupture occurs in an estimated one in every 5000 to 7000 births, and the incidence is increasing worldwide due to more birthing individuals desiring

a trial of labor after cesarean birth (TOLAC). Uterine rupture is more common in birthing individuals with a prior cesarean birth, with the risk being highly dependent on the number and type of cesarean births an individual has had. The rate of uterine rupture is approximately 1% for individuals with one previous cesarean birth, but increases to more than 3% for those with more than one previous cesarean birth.[182] A history of previous classical or "T" uterine incision, previous uterine rupture, or any type of fundal uterine surgery (i.e., myomectomy) significantly increases the risk for uterine rupture.

Midwives must be vigilant for the signs and symptoms of uterine rupture. Fetal bradycardia is the most common abnormality associated with uterine rupture. A more ominous sign is absent fetal heart tones. Initial signs in the birthing person include hemodynamic instability, including hypotension and tachycardia; changes or cessation of uterine contractions; and loss of fetal station. Acute abdominal pain may occur, though this symptom may be masked in an individual with an epidural. If bleeding occurs, it tends to be intra-abdominal and undetectable to the patient.[182]

### Prolapsed Umbilical Cord

There are three types of umbilical cord prolapse: compound cord presentation, funic cord prolapse, and overt cord prolapse.[183] A compound cord presentation occurs when the umbilical cord is compressed alongside the presenting part in the lower uterine segment or inner cervix. The cord may not be palpable during a cervical examination but will often cause variable decelerations or bradycardia like that seen with umbilical cord compression. In a funic umbilical cord prolapse, the cord is palpable in front of the presenting part. In an overt umbilical cord prolapse, the cord slips completely out of the uterus through the cervix and may be protruding at the vaginal introitus. Variant FHR patterns may be present depending on the degree of cord compression from the presenting part.

When an overt umbilical cord prolapse is encountered, the birthing person will need an emergent cesarean birth and immediate interventions to improve fetal oxygenation. Prolapsed umbilical cord statistics, risk factors, and emergency care are outlined in the *Emergency Interventions for Umbilical Cord Prolapse* appendix.

### Amniotic Fluid Embolism

Amniotic fluid embolism (AFE) is a rare and potentially life-threatening perinatal emergency that may occur anytime from the onset of an apparently uncomplicated labor to within 30 minutes of placental expulsion. The incidence in the United States ranges from 1.9 to 6.1 per 100,000 births, but the mortality rate is as high as 60%.[184,185] AFEs are highly unpredictable and can be difficult to prevent; nonetheless, reported risk factors for AFE involve situations where there is an exchange of amniotic fluid or fetal material between the birthing person and the fetus. Such circumstances may include operative vaginal birth, cesarean birth, placenta previa, multiple gestation, trauma, abruption, and uterine rupture.[186] AFE is characterized by sudden cardiorespiratory arrest that might include hypotension, dyspnea, and cyanosis.[187] Its traditional presentation is quite dramatic, including a triad of symptoms: hypoxia, hypotension, and coagulopathy.[186] Blood pressure falls rapidly, and peripheral oxygen saturation is less than 90%. The onset of disseminated intravascular coagulation (DIC) varies, with some people having these symptoms immediately following cardiovascular arrest, whereas others experience DIC later in the symptom triad, ultimately resulting in massive hemorrhage.[186]

Clinically, an individual with an AFE has sudden respiratory distress with simultaneous cardiovascular system deterioration. The cause of AFE was previously thought to be mechanical obstruction of the pulmonary vasculature by fetal cells in the amniotic fluid, caused by sudden inflow of this fluid into the maternal circulation. More recently, the presence of pulmonary vasospasm has been documented during autopsies of individuals with fatal AFE, indicating an anaphylactoid reaction to fetal cells. As a result, AFE is now proposed to be an immune-inflammatory reaction, most likely mediated by factor VII activation.[184,185] Differential diagnoses include occult hemorrhage, septic shock, pulmonary thromboembolism, and anaphylaxis. An anesthetic accident is also a possible etiology if symptoms occur during cesarean birth.[187]

The responsibility of the midwife present when symptoms occur is to summon a team for emergency medical assistance, initiate cardiopulmonary resuscitation, and provide help as part of the response team. The person with an AFE will require intensive care, including cardiopulmonary support and correction of coagulopathy.

The midwife will have an important role in providing support to the individual during recovery and assisting in their transition to parenthood after stabilization.

## Shoulder Dystocia

Shoulder dystocia is defined as a birth in which additional maneuvers are required to release the fetal shoulders after gentle downward traction on the fetal head has failed.[188–191] Shoulder dystocia occurs in 0.2% to 3% of vaginal births with a fetus in a cephalic presentation.[188–191] It is believed to be caused by impaction of the fetal anterior shoulder on the symphysis pubis, or less commonly by the fetal posterior shoulder on the sacral promontory.[188–191] Although there is no standard description of shoulder dystocia, failure to deliver the fetal shoulders by the usual methods, prolonged head-to-body delivery time, and need for ancillary maneuvers are suggested criteria.[188–191] Once the fetal head is born, retraction of the head against the birthing person's perineum (the "turtle sign") is highly suggestive of shoulder dystocia; however, it is not diagnostic.

### Risk Factors for Shoulder Dystocia

Antepartum risk factors for shoulder dystocia include macrosomia, pregestational and gestational diabetes, previous shoulder dystocia, obesity of the pregnant person, excessive weight gain during pregnancy, and multiparity.[188–191] The combination of two or more of these factors significantly increases the risk of shoulder dystocia.[188–191] Macrosomia is an especially significant risk factor. The incidence of shoulder dystocia is thought to rise with increasing fetal size, especially among infants born to persons with diabetes.[190,192] The principal intrapartum risk factors for shoulder dystocia are a precipitous second stage of labor and operative vaginal birth. Rapid descent of the fetus during second-stage labor may not allow enough time for normal internal rotational maneuvers and compression of the shoulders toward the thorax, which results in impaction of the anterior shoulder behind the pubic bone.

### Prediction and Prevention Strategies

Experts caution that although multiple risk factors for shoulder dystocia have been identified, this event cannot be accurately predicted or prevented.[188–191] Known risk factors have a very low positive predictive value, in part due to the lack of an accurate means of diagnosing macrosomia prenatally.[188–191] Additionally, the great majority of macrosomic infants do not have shoulder dystocia, and many shoulder dystocias occur with infants who are not macrosomic. Cesarean birth may help prevent shoulder dystocia and most neonatal morbidity associated with an impacted shoulder. However, planned cesarean birth for suspected macrosomia is recommended only in pregnant persons with diabetes whose fetus has an estimated fetal weight of more than 4500 grams, and in pregnant persons without diabetes whose fetus has an estimated fetal weight of more than 5000 grams.[190,192]

### Complications of Shoulder Dystocia

Even when managed appropriately, shoulder dystocia can result in neonatal injuries, such as a fractured humerus or clavicle and either temporary or permanent damage to the infant's brachial plexus. Prolonged fetal asphyxia during a difficult shoulder dystocia can also result in neonatal encephalopathy, seizures, and infant death. Complications for the birthing person may include excessive blood loss (e.g., from postpartum hemorrhage) and perineal, vaginal, or rectal lacerations. Last-resort maneuvers such as cephalic replacement or abdominal rescue via cesarean birth significantly increase the risks for both perinatal morbidity and neonatal mortality.

The neonatal consequences of shoulder dystocia are at the root of many lawsuits. For this reason, brachial plexus injury, in particular, has received considerable attention in the literature. This injury is thought to occur from forceful stretching or hyperextension of one side of the neck, which then results in avulsion or rupture of one or all of the brachial plexus nerves. Lateral traction applied to the infant's neck while attempting to deliver the anterior shoulder is believed to be the cause in most cases. However, this injury can also occur prior to birth and may be unavoidable in certain circumstances.[188–191,193]

### Management of Shoulder Dystocia

The steps involved in management of shoulder dystocia are detailed in the *Shoulder Dystocia* appendix. There is no evidence on which to base the sequence of release maneuvers for a shoulder dystocia.[190] Professional obstetric organizations in the United States (ACOG), France (French College of Obstetricians and Gynecologists [CNGOF]), Canada (Society of Obstetricians and Gynaecologists of Canada [SOGC]), and the United Kingdom (Royal College of Obstetricians and Gynaecologists [RCOG]) recommend the McRoberts maneuver as a first step, either with or without suprapubic pressure in tandem.[188–191] All professional organization recommendations emphasize that fundal pressure should never be used.

The routine use of episiotomy to assist with shoulder dystocia is no longer recommended due to a lack of scientific evidence proving its efficacy in relieving obstruction from the maternal bony pelvis and concerns that it may unnecessarily increase birthing persons' risk of third- and fourth-degree lacerations.[188–191] Episiotomy can be reserved for cases in which the provider believes that incising the perineum would provide additional room for maneuvers.[191] Detailed guidance on the use of episiotomy can be found in the *Urgent Maneuvers to Shorten Second Stage* appendix.

RCOG recommends against the use of any lateral traction to facilitate delivery of the fetal shoulders, even in the absence of shoulder dystocia, instead recommending axial traction (i.e., in line with the fetal spine).[188] In addition, RCOG and CNGOF recommend no maternal pushing efforts until the impacted shoulder is released.[188,189] However, ACOG and SOCG do not comment on this issue in their Practice Bulletin on shoulder dystocia.[190,191]

Use of the hands-and-knees position is another strategy to resolve a shoulder dystocia. ACOG, RCOG, and SOGC include this position, which is known as the "Gaskin maneuver" (after midwife Ina May Gaskin), in their shoulder dystocia algorithms. However, these professional organizations do not recommend use of hands-and-knees repositioning until after multiple maneuvers have been attempted while the birthing person is on their back, including the McRoberts maneuver, rotational maneuvers, and delivery of the posterior arm.[188,190] Although numerous anecdotal reports cite the person's movement to the hands-and-knees position itself as relieving the impacted shoulder, professional organizations may be concerned that many providers are unfamiliar with assisting birth in this position. However, midwives tend to have a greater familiarity with individuals giving birth on hands and knees. Thus, if the birthing person is mobile, use of this strategy earlier than indicated in the RCOG and SOGC algorithms is reasonable.

Other maneuvers use gentle traction around the posterior shoulder and under the axilla to release an impacted shoulder. The *shoulder shrug* uses the attendant's fingers by circling the thumb and forefinger. The maneuver called *posterior axilla sling traction* uses a neonatal suction tube for traction. (See the *Shoulder Dystocia* appendix for a more detailed description of these techniques.[192,193])

Last-resort rescue maneuvers include intentional fracture of the clavicle, cephalic replacement (Zavanelli maneuver), and abdominal rescue.[194,195] The latter two require a full operating room team and a physician capable of performing a cesarean delivery.

### Shoulder Dystocia Simulation

Simulation is a helpful tool in preparing for shoulder dystocia because it occurs relatively infrequently. ACOG recommends simulation and team training to improve the clinician's skills and confidence in managing a shoulder dystocia.[191]

Another advantage of simulation is the ability to train groups of learners to work together as a multidisciplinary team for resolving a specific clinical emergency, such as shoulder dystocia. At the end of the scenario, participants have an opportunity to debrief on the experience under the guidance of a skilled simulation coordinator. Teaching points are highlighted, and the team is given constructive feedback related to the original learning objectives for the session. Studies have shown improvements in both confidence and skills when simulation is used for shoulder dystocia training.[196,197]

### Twin Gestation

The incidence of twins and higher-order multifetal gestations had previously been on the rise; however, in recent years, these numbers have slowly declined.[198] In 2018, the twin birth rate was 32.6 twins per 1000 total births in the United States.

Approximately 60% of twin gestations are preterm, and the infant mortality rate is nearly five times higher compared to singleton gestations.[198] In addition, higher rates of congenital anomalies and growth restriction are noted with multifetal pregnancies. Complications such as gestational hypertension, preeclampsia, and diabetes are also more frequent among birthing people with multifetal gestations than those with singleton gestations.[198] Lastly, intrapartum complications such as malpresentation, prolapsed umbilical cord, placental separation, and postpartum hemorrhage occur more frequently in twin gestations.[199]

When referring to twin gestations, it is critical to know the chorionicity (one or two placentas) and the amnionicity (one or two amniotic sacs)—that is, whether the twins will be dichorionic–diamniotic (di-di), monochorionic–diamniotic (mono-di), or monochorionic–monoamniotic (mono-mono). Chorionicity is explained further in the *Pregnancy-Related Conditions* chapter.

In many midwifery practice settings, mono-mono twin gestation requires physician referral, as this chorionicity is associated with the highest risks. For either mono-di or di-di twins, a collaborative care plan with a physician can be considered (per local practice guidelines) with criteria for referral of care. The birthing person will need ongoing surveillance for both individual and fetal complications throughout the remainder of the pregnancy. An individualized plan of care regarding the optimal timing and mode of birth with the appropriate informed consent discussion will also be needed.

### Mode of Birth in Twin Gestations

The mode of birth depends on the fetal presentation. Therefore, as the pregnancy progresses, the presentation and lie of each fetus will be carefully assessed and documented in the prenatal record. Birthing persons with diamniotic twins in a vertex–vertex presentation are ideal candidates for a vaginal birth.[198,200] This option should be discussed with the birthing person well before the onset of labor using shared decision making, including consideration of the risks and benefits of vaginal birth versus elective cesarean birth. Current evidence does not show that cesarean birth improves perinatal outcomes in vertex–vertex presentations; thus, vaginal birth should be encouraged for all vertex–vertex presenting twins.[198,200]

Vaginal birth is still a possibility in twin gestations where one twin is not vertex. Birthing persons at or beyond 32 weeks' gestation with diamniotic twins, in which the first twin is in a vertex presentation and the second twin is in a breech or transverse presentation, are candidates for vaginal birth if a provider skilled in internal podalic version and vaginal breech birth is present.[198,200] However, when the presenting fetus is breech, cesarean birth is recommended.[198,200]

Upon admission in labor, the presentation and lie of each fetus should be reassessed with ultrasound. The midwife should notify the physician, and a collaborative care plan should be established if the birthing person desires a trial of labor. Intrapartum management guidelines for individuals with a twin gestation are found in the *Intrapartum Management of Twin Gestation* appendix. Some midwives attend twin births; therefore, these skills should be periodically reviewed as needed.

### Fetal Malpresentations

The three possible fetal presentations are cephalic, shoulder, and breech. Cephalic presentations include vertex, military, brow, and face, based on the degree of the flexion or extension of the fetal head.[201] See the *Anatomy and Physiology of Pregnancy* chapter for more detailed information on fetal presentation. This section reviews variations of each fetal presentation that can complicate labor and birth.

#### Cephalic Presentations

- Vertex presentation
  - Attitude: well-flexed head
  - Presenting part: vertex (posterior part)
  - Denominator: occiput (O)

- Presenting diameter with an occiput anterior (OA) position: suboccipto-bregmatic

Variations with a vertex presentation occur, including occiput posterior (OP) position and asynclitism, both of which can change presenting fetal diameters.

- Military/median presentation
  - Attitude: deflexed head (neither flexed nor extended)
  - Presenting part: vertex (median part)
  - Denominator: occiput (O)
  - Presenting diameter: occipto-frontal
- Brow presentation
  - Attitude: partial extension
  - Presenting part: brow
  - Denominator: forehead/frontum (Fr)
  - Presenting diameter: vertico-mental

This is the largest presenting fetal head diameter. A fetus in a brow presentation may convert to a vertex or face presentation. If this does not occur, vaginal birth is often not possible due to the large presenting diameter.

- Face presentation
  - Attitude: complete extension
  - Presenting part: face
  - Denominator: chin/mentum (M)
  - Presenting diameter: submento-bregmatic

If the fetus is in a mento-anterior position, a vaginal birth is possible. However, if the fetus is in a mento-posterior position, the fetal brow presses against the maternal symphysis pubis and limitations in the length of the fetal neck prohibit the head from extending enough to maneuver past the maternal sacrum pubis. If the head does not rotate to a more favorable position (mentum anterior), a cesarean birth will be needed.

### Shoulder Presentation (Transverse Lie)

A shoulder presentation occurs when a fetus in a transverse lie. A cesarean birth is required if the fetus does not convert to a cephalic or breech presentation by the time labor starts or membranes rupture.

### Breech Presentation

Prior to the late 1990s, vaginal breech birth was a common occurrence and an important component of intrapartum training for both midwives and physicians. The publication of the Term Breech Trial

in 2000 dramatically changed practice patterns regarding vaginal breech births.[202] This multicenter, randomized study originally reported that planned cesarean birth for breech, as compared to planned vaginal breech birth, significantly decreased perinatal mortality and serious short-term neonatal morbidity.[202] Almost immediately, pregnant persons with a breech presentation were restricted from a vaginal birth by their providers. Over the past decades, severe limits on vaginal breech births have limited choices for pregnant persons, while also decreasing expertise in vaginal breech birth among intrapartum providers, as clinical learning opportunities have diminished.[203]

Closer examination of the Term Breech Trial has resulted in several challenges to some of its findings.[202-204] For example, several protocol violations in the trial have been identified, and investigators in subsequent studies reported conflicting results with regard to perinatal mortality and neonatal morbidity in breech presentations with different modes of birth.[202-204] Current evidence suggests that planned vaginal breech birth as compared to planned cesarean breech birth is associated with an increased risk of perinatal mortality and *short-term* neonatal morbidity, with no difference in *long-term* neurologic morbidity.[203-205] The absolute risk of perinatal mortality is small with either option. For example, the perinatal mortality cited by the SOGC in its guidelines on breech presentations is 0.8 to 1.7 deaths per 1000 planned vaginal breech births and 0 to 0.8 deaths per 1000 planned cesarean breech births.[204] Also, maternal morbidity and mortality are higher with cesarean breech birth compared to vaginal breech birth. Several observational studies with strict inclusion criteria and labor care protocols for vaginal breech birth have also reported excellent outcomes with this mode of delivery.[204]

Following these research findings that vaginal breech birth is not as dangerous as once believed, ACOG updated its recommendation on the mode of birth for term singleton breech in 2018, stating that "planned vaginal (birth) of a term singleton breech fetus may be reasonable under hospital-specific protocol guidelines for eligibility and labor care."[205] Prior to a vaginal breech birth, shared decision making with the pregnant person should include a comparison of the risks and benefits of planned cesarean breech birth versus planned vaginal breech birth. Some persons with a breech presentation will seek out a provider who will perform a planned vaginal breech birth. The option for planned vaginal breech birth is based on the availability and willingness of an obstetrician experienced in this mode of birth. Guidelines for these circumstances have been established, and institutions that can safely offer this service are encouraged to develop protocols for intrapartum care.[205] Some sources have outlined selection criteria shown to improve success rates, such as sonographically determined estimated fetal weight between 2500 and 4000 grams, frank or complete breech, absence of fetal anomalies, normal amniotic fluid levels, and flexion of the fetal head as documented by ultrasound.[205,206,207]

Even with careful assessment techniques, some pregnant persons will present in labor with an undiagnosed breech presentation; thus, a breech presentation may first be diagnosed during a vaginal examination. Signs of a breech presentation can include high fetal station, a difference in the feel of the presenting part, and a lack of palpation of sutures and fontanels. Palpation of fetal small parts, usually the feet, or the buttocks may be encountered, although sometimes it is very difficult to distinguish the fleshy part of the breech (especially when the fetus is in frank breech presentation) from the soft-tissue caput on the fetal vertex. In some cases, the breech presentation is not discovered until the individual is well into active labor, when fresh meconium stool is seen. Ultrasound can be helpful in determining the presentation if the midwife cannot confirm the fetus is vertex.

Once a breech presentation is confirmed, the pregnant person should be informed, and the consulting physician notified immediately. If the birth is imminent or a cesarean birth is not immediately available, the midwife should be prepared to perform a safe vaginal breech birth. The need for resuscitation is increased following breech birth, and neonatal team should be notified to be present at the birth.[206] The *Breech Birth* appendix reviews the steps for a vaginal breech birth. All midwives caring for laboring persons should be thoroughly familiar with these techniques.

## Special Clinical Situations

Birth is often thought of as a beginning—but it can also be an end. Although birth is a joyous occasion for most families, stillbirth and the birth of a newborn with a critical illness or lethal anomaly are among the most profound traumas that a family can experience. These clinical scenarios can be traumatic for all involved, including the midwife and other members of the care team.

### Intrapartum Care with an Expected Stillbirth

Before the birthing person who is diagnosed with a stillbirth arrives at the birth facility, staff should be informed of the situation and have a labor room

arranged that will ensure privacy and liberal visitation from support people. Many facilities have mechanisms in place that discreetly communicate a fetal demise or lethal anomaly to the entire staff (e.g., a special door magnet). It is especially important that the birthing person is not accidentally approached by a staff member who is unaware of the diagnosis and assumes they are expecting a healthy newborn.

The midwife's role in the care of an individual with a stillbirth or a fetus with a lethal anomaly will vary according to local practice guidelines and the specific clinical circumstances. A physician should be consulted to establish the most appropriate plan of care, which may in some cases require co-management or referral. The midwife's continued presence and availability, however, can provide emotional support and comfort for the bereaved family, especially in the immediate postpartum period. Midwives caring for individuals in these situations must balance their own emotions, while also prioritizing the birthing person's immediate needs.

Once the birthing person is admitted, the midwife should thoroughly review the prenatal chart and all documentation of previous discussions regarding the proposed plan of care. A thorough patient history should be obtained to assess for known conditions or symptoms associated with stillbirth.[208] Laboratory studies should include a complete blood count with platelets, lupus anticoagulant, rapid plasma reagin (RPR) or Venereal Disease Research Laboratory (VDRL) test for syphilis, immunoglobulin G (IgG) and immunoglobulin M (IgM) for anticardiolipin and β-2 glycoprotein antibodies, and a Kleihauer-Betke test (fetal cell screen) for individuals who are Rh negative. Additional laboratory studies could include an indirect Coombs test, glucose levels, or toxicology screening. All testing requires the permission of the pregnant person, and toxicology testing may have legal implications for the pregnant person.[208]

The method and timing of delivery depend on the gestational age at which fetal death occurred, perinatal history, institutional expertise, and family preference. Depending on the gestational age, either dilation and evacuation (recommended in the second trimester) or induction of labor (recommended in the second and/or third trimester) can be offered to the bereaved family, in combination with a discussion of each option's potential risks, benefits, and alternatives. Shared decision making plays a vital role in determining the optimal method of birth.[208] If an induction of labor is planned, a physician should be consulted to determine the most appropriate method of induction and cervical ripening. The specific agents and protocols used will depend on the person's diagnosis, fetal gestational age, past perinatal history, and current Bishop's score.[208] Evidence supports the use of mifepristone and misoprostol to manage pregnancy loss prior to 20 weeks' gestation, rather than using misoprostol alone. In pregnancies between 20 and 28 weeks, 400 to 600 micrograms of vaginal misoprostol every 3–6 hours is the recommended induction agent, regardless of the Bishop's score.[208] High-dose oxytocin is another acceptable option.[208,209] After 28 weeks' gestation, induction of labor should be managed according to the usual intrapartum protocols. The induction plan should be reviewed with the bereaved family, with clear explanations of what to expect as labor and birth progress. The birthing person may need information repeated and should be given opportunities to openly express feelings and ask questions. Every effort must be made to honor the person's choices and requests.

Most labor and birth units have specific protocols and checklists in place for bereaved parents that include referrals to social services and bereavement counseling, the availability of a chaplain, assistance with burial plans, and collection of photographs, footprints, and other keepsakes (i.e., lock of hair) from the baby following the birth. These services are offered to the bereaved family at the appropriate times over the course of hospitalization. Bereavement care should also include the recognition of parenthood, acknowledgment of partner and family grief, and an understanding that grief is unique to each person.[208] Care must be individualized to respect and support the personal, religious, and cultural choices of the bereaved family.[208] Cost may be an issue as well, but some charitable organizations, such as Now I Lay Me Down to Sleep, provide free services, and some local funeral homes will assist with stillbirths for free or a greatly reduced cost.

The bereaved family will also be informed about the availability of a detailed fetal evaluation after the birth. This evaluation includes a prompt general examination of the stillborn fetus noting dysmorphic features, height, body weight, foot length, and head circumference; a standard autopsy; genetic evaluation; collection of blood or tissue samples; and a gross and histologic evaluation of the placenta, membranes, and umbilical cord for pathology.[208] Test and imaging results should be clearly communicated to the family once they are available. If the family is uncomfortable with a full autopsy, less invasive options may be available, such as photographs, magnetic resonance imaging,

X rays, and ultrasonography.[208] It can be gently emphasized that this information may be useful for subsequent review and consultation with a specialist as well as in planning future pregnancies. Analyzing tissue or amniotic fluid samples for fetal karyotype may allow for diagnosis of a syndrome or chromosomal abnormality even without the results from a full autopsy.[208] Sending the placenta and umbilical cord for pathologic examination after the birth is another option, with permission from the parents. Parents should be informed of the costs of all these options, as they can be considerable.

Parents may have difficulty making firm decisions, especially regarding seeing or holding the infant at birth. If the parents have previously stated that they do not wish to see the infant after the birth, the nursing staff should be prepared to take the infant to another location after the birth. Parents may change their minds, however, and the midwife should remain open to all possibilities.

The birth itself is managed in the same way as any other vaginal birth, except that there may be softening or overriding of the fetal skull bones or anomalies not previously identified that can complicate the labor or birth. In addition, there is an increased risk of shoulder dystocia.[210] Caution should be used when applying even gentle traction to any part of the fetus during the birth, as body parts can easily be dislocated. Instead, it is best to rely mostly on the birthing person's expulsive efforts. The umbilical cord should be clamped and cut as close to the abdomen as possible, and the infant gently wrapped in a blanket or towel. The placenta should be delivered in the usual fashion, with cautions taken to avoid umbilical cord avulsion, and any perineal lacerations should be repaired.

After the birth, the infant, umbilical cord, placenta, and membranes should be carefully examined for any recognizable abnormalities. Any deviations from normal should be shown to the parents. Sometimes seeing an obvious cause of death is reassuring for grieving families who are searching for answers. Unfortunately, most intrauterine deaths cannot be attributed to a known cause; therefore, it is important not to offer a potential diagnosis without clear evidence. During the exam, a clip of hair and a foot or hand print can be obtained for a memory book or box.

The parents can be encouraged to view, touch, and hold the infant and allowed as much time as needed. They can wrap the infant in a blanket of their choice and allow family members to visit and hold the newborn. Specialized cooling beds are available that can allow parents to keep the infant's body in the room with them for a longer amount of time if desired. Once they are ready to say goodbye, the infant can be brought to the morgue per local hospital policy. The infant's blanket can be kept as a remembrance.

The grieving family can guide many of the decisions in this time. Birth facilities sometimes have a place to store mementos from the birth if the parent does not want them at that moment but may at a later date. Compassion shown to families can assist their processing and healing and will be remembered throughout their lives.

### Life-Threatening or Fatal Fetal Diagnosis

Due to improvements in diagnostic technology, more parents have advanced knowledge of a life-threatening fetal diagnosis prior to birth. This early diagnosis may enable prenatal transfer of the birthing person to a tertiary center and consultation with neonatal specialists capable of interventions that will improve the infant's survival. In other cases, the birthing person and partner have the task of deciding whether to continue the pregnancy to term. Depending on the gestational age at the time of diagnosis and individual state laws, elective termination of the pregnancy or a preterm induction of labor may not be an option. This section focuses on pregnant persons with a known fatal fetal anomaly who present at full-term gestations either in spontaneous labor or for a planned induction.

In most cases, the birthing person and family will likely be receiving care from a multidisciplinary team that includes neonatology, maternal–fetal medicine, genetics specialists, and social services. In some settings, a perinatal palliative care plan has been established, and many of the decisions facing grieving parents during labor and birth have been discussed. Perinatal palliative care is an emerging field that moves beyond traditional bereavement support and is initiated at the time of diagnosis rather than during labor and birth.[211] This holistic approach incorporates the principles of bereavement care by integrating the family's choices and understanding with realistic goals for care of the baby after birth, including perinatal hospice care. Ensuring quality of life, reducing pain and suffering, and honoring the infant's life and death are at the core of this framework.[211]

Once the birthing person is admitted to the labor unit, a collaborative plan of care with a consulting physician should be considered in accordance with local practice guidelines. Other care team providers (e.g., neonatology, pediatrics, chaplaincy) are notified of the impending birth. Depending on the type of anomaly, the gestational age, the expected perinatal outcome, and medical conditions of the birthing person, referral for physician care may be necessary.

The intrapartum care in this situation is similar to the care of a person with a stillbirth. Regardless of the amount of prenatal counseling and support, the birthing person may exhibit a wide range of emotional responses during labor. All pain relief options should be available, if requested. Additionally, as second-stage labor nears, the birthing person may experience more difficulty coping and become conflicted about pushing, as the birth represents confirmation that the infant is going to die—"holding on" subconsciously may be seen as preventing this outcome from happening. Providing gentle encouragement, support, and patience will allow the birthing person to work through emotions and facilitate their sense of control over the situation.

If the neonatal team is planning to examine the newborn after birth, it may be less distracting for them to wait outside the room until after the birth occurs. Having a perinatal palliative care plan in place will facilitate the seamless transition from birth to end-of-life care.[211]

## Conclusion

Complications during labor and birth can occur at any time, and knowledge of these conditions is essential for midwifery practice. Understanding the condition, its natural course, the effects on the pregnant person and their fetus, and the degree of interprofessional communication (consultation, collaboration, or referral) required are the basic competencies needed for all intrapartum complications.

Emergencies are unpredictable, and knowledge of how to care for those individuals with the most common intrapartum complications will enable midwives to care for pregnant persons safely. All those who experience an intrapartum complication will greatly benefit from the continuity, education, and support that a midwife provides.

### References

1. American College of Obstetricians and Gynecologists. *Collaboration in Practice: Implementing Team-Based Care*. Washington, DC: American College of Obstetricians and Gynecologists; 2016.

2. American College of Nurse Midwives, American Congress of Obstetricians and Gynecologists. *Joint Statement of Practice Relations Between Obstetrician-Gynecologists and Certified Nurse-Midwives/Certified Midwives*. Washington, DC: American College of Nurse Midwives and American Congress of Obstetricians and Gynecologists; 2018.

3. Megregian M, Emeis C, Nieuwenhuijze M. The impact of shared decision-making in perinatal care: a scoping review. *J Midwifery Womens Health*. 2020;65(6):777-788. doi:10.1111/jmwh.13128.

4. Frey HA, Klebanoff MA. The epidemiology, etiology, and costs of preterm birth. *Semin Fetal Neonatal Med*. 2016;21(2):68-73. doi:10.1016/j.siny.2015.12.011.

5. Society for Maternal–Fetal Medicine Preterm Birth Task Force. SMFM preterm birth toolkit. https://www.smfm.org/publications/231-smfm-preterm-birth-toolkit. Published 2016. Accessed April 25, 2023.

6. Koullali B, Oudijk MA, Nijman TA, et al. Risk assessment and management to prevent preterm birth. *Semin Fetal Neonatal Med*. 2016;21(2):80-88. doi:10.1016/j.siny.2016.01.005.

7. McIntosh J, Feltovich H, Berghella V, Manuck T. The role of routine cervical length screening in selected high- and low-risk women for preterm birth prevention. *Am J Obstet Gynecol*. 2016;215(3):B2-B7. doi:10.1016/j.ajog.2016.04.027.

8. American College of Obstetricians and Gynecologists' Committee on Practice Bulletins—Obstetrics. Prediction and prevention of spontaneous preterm birth: ACOG Practice Bulletin, Number 234. *Obstet Gynecol*. 2021;138(2):e65-e90. doi:10.1097/AOG.0000000000004479.

9. American College of Obstetricians and Gynecologists' Committee on Practice Bulletins—Obstetrics. Practice Bulletin No. 171: management of preterm labor. *Obstet Gynecol*. 2016;128(4):e155-164. [Reaffirmed 2020].

10. Wax JR, Cartin A, Pinette MG. Biophysical and biochemical screening for the risk of preterm labor: an update. *Clin Lab Med*. 2016;36(2):369-383. doi:10.1016/j.cll.2016.01.019.

11. Son M, Miller ES. Predicting preterm birth: cervical length and fetal fibronectin. *Semin Perinatol*. 2017;41(8):445-451. doi:10.1053/j.semperi.2017.08.002.

12. Nijman TA, van Vliet EO, Koullali B, et al. Antepartum and intrapartum interventions to prevent preterm birth and its sequelae. *Semin Fetal Neonatal Med*. 2016;21(2):121-128. doi:10.1016/j.siny.2016.01.004.

13. Gyamfi-Bannerman C, Thom EA, Blackwell SC, et al. Antenatal betamethasone for women at risk for late preterm delivery. *N Engl J Med*. 2016;374(14):1311-1320. doi:10.1056/NEJMoa1516783.

14. Prevention of group B streptococcal early-onset disease in newborns: ACOG Committee Opinion, Number 797. *Obstet Gynecol*. 2020;135(2):e51-e72. [Published correction appears in *Obstet Gynecol*. 2020;135(4):978-979.] doi:10.1097/AOG.0000000000003668.

15. Middleton P, Shepherd E, Morris J, et al. Induction of labour at or beyond 37 weeks' gestation. *Cochrane Database Syst. Rev*. 2020;7:CD004945. https://doi.org/10.1002/14651858.CD004945.pub5.

16. American College of Obstetricians and Gynecologists. Practice Bulletin No. 146: management of late term and postterm pregnancies. *Obstet Gynecol*. 2014;124:182-192. [Reaffirmed 2016].

17. American College of Obstetricians and Gynecologists. Clinical guidance for integration of the findings of the ARRIVE trial: labor induction versus expectant management in low-risk nulliparous women. https://www.acog.org/clinical/clinical-guidance/practice-advisory/articles/2018/08/clinical-guidance-for-integration-of-the-findings-of-the-arrive-trial. Published August 2018. Accessed April 25, 2023.

18. Edwards A, Elwyn G, Mulley AL. Explaining risks: turning numerical data into meaningful pictures. *Br Med J*. 2002;324:827-830.

19. Sanchez-Ramos LF, Oliver F, Delke I, Kaunitz AM. Labor induction versus expectant management for postterm pregnancies: a systematic review with meta-analysis. *Obstet Gynecol*. 2003;101:1312-1318.

20. Prelabor rupture of membranes: ACOG Practice Bulletin Summary, Number 217. *Obstet Gynecol*. 2020;135(3):739-743. doi:10.1097/AOG.0000000000003701A.

21. Marowitz A. Evidence-based management of prelabor rupture of the membranes at term. In: Anderson B, Rooks J, Barroso R, eds. *Best Practices in Midwifery* (2nd ed.). New York, NY: Springer; 2017:411-427.

22. Middleton P, Shepherd E, Flenady V, et al. Planned early birth versus expectant management (waiting) for prelabour rupture of membranes at term (37 weeks or more). *Cochrane Database Syst Rev*. 2017;1:CD005302. doi:10.1002/14651858.CD005302.pub3.

23. Hannah ME, Ohlsson A, Farine D, et al. Induction of labor compared with expectant management for prelabor rupture of the membranes at term. TERMPROM Study Group. *N Engl J Med*. 1996;334(16):1005-1010. doi:10.1056/NEJM199604183341601.

24. American College of Nurse-Midwives position statement: premature rupture of membranes at term. ACNM Division of Standards and Practice, Clinical Practice Section. https://www.midwife.org/acnm/files/ACNMLibraryData/UPLOADFILENAME/000000000233/PS-Prelabor-rupture-of-membranes-FINAL-22-MAR-18.pdf. Published 2008; reviewed and updated 2018. Accessed April 25, 2023.

25. Mackeen AD, Quinn ST, Movva VC, et al. Intracervical balloon catheter for labor induction after rupture of membranes: a systematic review and meta-analysis. *Am J Obstet Gynecol*. 2021;224(6):624-628. doi:10.1016/j.ajog.2021.03.002.

26. American College of Obstetricians and Gynecologists. Committee Opinion No. 712: intrapartum management of intraamniotic infection. *Obstet Gynecol*. 2017; e95-e101. doi:10.1097/AOG.0000000000002236.

27. Conde-Agudelo A, Romero R, Jung EJ, Garcia Sánchez ÁJ. Management of clinical chorioamnionitis: an evidence-based approach. *Am J Obstet Gynecol.* 2020;223(6):848-869. doi:10.1016/j.ajog.2020.09.044.

28. Cahill AG, Duffy CR, Odibo AO, et al. Number of cervical examinations and risk of intrapartum maternal fever. *Obstet Gynecol.* 2012;119(6):1096-1101. doi:10.1097/AOG.0b013e318256ce3f.

29. Jones C, Titus H, Belongilot CG, et al. Evaluating definitions for maternal fever as diagnostic criteria for intraamniotic infection in low-risk pregnancies. *Birth.* 2021;48(3):389-396. doi:10.1111/birt.12548.

30. Higgins RD, Saade G, Polin RA, et al. Evaluation and management of women and newborns with a maternal diagnosis of chorioamnionitis: summary of a workshop. *Obstet Gynecol.* 2016;127(3):426-436. doi:10.1097/AOG.0000000000001246.

31. Bonsack CF, Lathrop A, Blackburn M. Induction of labor: update and review. *J Midwifery Womens Health.* 2014;59:606-615.

32. Grobman WA, Rice MM, Reddy UM, et al. Labor induction versus expectant management in low-risk nulliparous women. *N Engl J Med.* 2018;379:513-523. doi:10.1056/NEJMoa1800566.

33. Glantz J. Elective induction vs. spontaneous labor associations and outcomes. *J Reprod Med.* 2005;50:235-240.

34. Little SE, Caughey AB. Induction of labor and cesarean: what is the true relationship? *Clin Obstet Gynecol.* 2015;58(2):269-281.

35. Caughey AB, Sundaram V, Kaimal AJ, et al. Systematic review: elective induction of labor versus expectant management of pregnancy. *Ann Intern Med.* 2009;151:252-263.

36. Osmundsen S, Ou-Yang R, Grobman W. Elective induction compared with expectant management in nulliparous women with a favorable cervix. *Obstet Gynecol.* 2010;116:601-605.

37. Osmundsen S, Ou-Yang R, Grobman,W. Elective induction compared with expectant management in nulliparous women with an unfavorable cervix. *Obstet Gynecol.* 2011;117:583-587.

38. Wood S, Cooper S, Ross S. Does induction of labour increase the risk of caesarean section? A systematic review and meta-analysis of trials in women with intact membranes. *BJOG.* 2013;121:674-685.

39. Carmichael SL, Snowden JM. The ARRIVE trial: interpretation from an epidemiologic perspective. *J Midwifery Womens Health.* 2019;64(5):657-663. doi:10.1111/jmwh.12996.

40. American College of Nurse-Midwives position statement: induction of labor. ACNM Division of Standards and Practice. https://www.midwife.org/ACNM/files/ACNMLibraryData/UPLOADFILENAME/000000000235/Induction%20of%20Labor%2010.10.pdf. Published 2016.

41. American College of Obstetricians and Gynecologists. Practice Bulletin No. 107: induction of labor. *Obstet Gynecol.* 2009;114:386-397. [Reaffirmed 2016].

42. Fisch JM, English D, Pedaline S, et al. Labor induction process improvement: a patient quality-of-care initiative. *Obstet Gynecol.* 2009;113:797-803.

43. Bishop EH. Pelvic scoring for elective induction. *Obstet Gynecol.* 1964;24:266-268.

44. Carlson N, Ellis J, Page K, et al. Review of evidence-based methods for successful labor induction. *J Midwifery Womens Health.* 2021;66(4):459-469. doi:10.1111/jmwh.13238.

45. Ausbeck EB, Jauk VC, Xue Y, et al. Outpatient Foley catheter for induction of labor in nulliparous women: a randomized controlled trial. *Obstet Gynecol.* 2020;136(3):597-606. doi:10.1097/AOG.0000000000004041.

46. Son SL, Benson AE, Hart Hayes E, et al. Outpatient cervical ripening: a cost-minimization and threshold analysis. *Am J Perinatol.* 2020;37(3):245-251.

47. Katz Eriksen JL, Chandrasekaran S, Delaney SS. Is Foley catheter use during a trial of labor after cesarean associated with uterine rupture? *Am J Perinatol.* 2019;36(14):1431-1436. doi:10.1055/s-0039-1691766.

48. ACOG Practice Bulletin No. 205: vaginal birth after cesarean delivery. *Obstet Gynecol.* 2019;133(2):e110-e127. doi:10.1097/AOG.0000000000003078.

49. McDonagh M, Skelly AC, Tilden E, et al. Outpatient cervical ripening: a systematic review and meta-analysis. *Obstet Gynecol.* 2021;137(6):1091-1101. https://doi.org/10.1097/AOG.0000000000004382.

50. Finucane EM, Murphy DJ, Biesty LM, et al. Membrane sweeping for induction of labour. *Cochrane Database Syst Rev.* 2020;2:CD000451.

51. Avdiyovski H, Haith-Cooper M, Scally A. Membrane sweeping at term to promote spontaneous labour and reduce the likelihood of a formal induction of labour for postmaturity: a systematic review and meta-analysis. *J Obstet Gynaecol.* 2019;39(1):54-62.

52. Kabiri D, Hants Y, Yarkoni TR, et al. Antepartum membrane stripping in GBS carriers, is it safe? (The STRIP-G study). *PLoS One.* 2015;10(12):e0145905.

53. Prevention of group B streptococcal early-onset disease in newborns: ACOG Committee Opinion, Number 782. *Obstet Gynecol.* 2019;134(4):1.

54. Yount S, Lassiter N. The pharmacology of prostaglandins for induction of labor. *J Midwifery Womens Health.* 2013;58:133-144.

55. Macones GA, Cahill A, Stamilio DM, Odibo AO. The efficacy of early amniotomy in nulliparous labor induction: a randomized controlled trial. *Am J Obstet Gynecol.* 2012;207:403.e1-403.e5.

56. Clark SL, Simpson KR, Knox GE, Garite TJ. Oxytocin: new perspectives on an old drug. *Am J Obstet Gynecol.* 2009;200:35.e1-35.e6.

57. Simpson KR. Clinicians guide to the use of oxytocin for labor induction and augmentation. *J Midwifery Womens Health.* 2011;56:214-221.

58. Gimpl G, Fahrenholz F. Oxytocin receptor system: structure, function, and regulation. *Physiol Rev.* 2001;81(2):629-683.

59. Page K, McCool WM, Guidera M. Examination of the pharmacology of oxytocin and clinical guidelines for use in labor. *J Midwifery Womens Health.* 2017;62:425-433.

60. Wei S, Luo Z, Qi H, et al. High-dose vs low-dose oxytocin for labor augmentation: a systematic review. *Am J Obstet Gynecol.* 2010;204:296-304.

61. Budden A, Chen LJY, Henry A. High-dose versus low-dose oxytocin infusion regimens for induction of labour at term. *Cochrane Database Syst Rev.* 2014;10:CD009701. doi:10.1002/14651858.CD009701.pub2.

62. Simpson KR, Miller L. Assessment and optimization of uterine activity during labor. *Clin Obstet Gynecol.* 2011;54:40-49.

63. Saccone G, Ciardulli A, Baxter JK, et al. Discontinuing oxytocin infusion in the active phase of labor: a systematic review and meta-analysis. *Obstet Gynecol.* 2017;130(5):1090-1096. https://doi.org/10.1097/AOG.0000000000002325.

64. Merriam J, Bergen K, Kienzle D, et al. What are the risks and benefits of discontinuing oxytocin after reaching the active phase of labor in patients undergoing labor induction or augmentation? *Evid Based Pract.* 2021;24(10):23-24. doi:10.1097/EBP.0000000000001227.

65. Boie S, Glavind J, Uldbjerg N, et al. Continued versus discontinued oxytocin stimulation in the active phase of labour (CONDISOX): double blind randomised controlled trial. *BMJ Clin Res.* 2021;373:716. https://doi.org/10.1136/bmj.n716.

66. Macones GA, Hankins GD, Spong CY, et al. The 2008 National Institute of Child Health and Human Development workshop report on electronic fetal monitoring: update on definitions, interpretation, and research guidelines. *Obstet Gynecol.* 2008;112:661-666.

67. Dow M, Wax JR, Pinette MG, et al. Third-trimester uterine rupture without previous cesarean: a case series and review of the literature. *Am J Perinatol.* 2009;26:739-744.

68. Kavanagh J, Kelly AJ, Thomas J. Breast stimulation for cervical ripening and induction of labour. *Cochrane Database Syst Rev* 2005;3:CD003392. doi:10.1002/14651858.CD003392.pub2.

69. Levine LD, Valencia CM, Tolosa JE. Induction of labor in continuing pregnancies. *Best Pract Res Clin Obstet Gynaecol.* 2020;67:90-99. doi:10.1016/j.bpobgyn.2020.04.004.

70. McFarlin BL, Gibson MH, O'Rear J, Harman P. A national survey of herbal preparation use by nurse-midwives for labor stimulation. *J Midwifery Womens Health.* 1999;44:205-216.

71. Mollart L, Skinner V, Adams J, Foureur M. Midwives' personal use of complementary and alternative medicine (CAM) influences their recommendations to women experiencing a post-date pregnancy. *Women Birth.* 2018;31(1):44-51. doi:10.1016/j.wombi.2017.06.014.

72. Hall HG, McKenna LG, Griffiths DL. Complementary and alternative medicine for inductions of labor. *Women Birth.* 2012;25:142-148.

73. Dugoua JJ, Perri D, Seely D, et al. Safety and efficacy of blue cohosh (*Caulophyllum thalictroides*) during pregnancy and lactation. *Can J Clin Pharm.* 2008;15:e66-e73.

74. Blankenship SA, Raghuraman N, Delhi A, et al. Association of abnormal first stage of labor duration and maternal and neonatal morbidity. *Am J Obstet Gynecol.* 2020;223(3):445.e1-445.e15. doi:10.1016/j.ajog.2020.06.053.

75. Hamilton EF, Warrick PA, Collins K, et al. Assessing first-stage labor progression and its relationship to complications. *Am J Obstet Gynecol.* 2016;214(3):358.e1-358.e3588. doi:10.1016/j.ajog.2015.10.016.

76. Neal JL, Lowe NK. Physiologic partograph to improve birth safety and outcomes among low-risk, nulliparous women with spontaneous labor onset. *Med Hypotheses.* 2012;78(2):319-326. doi:10.1016/j.mehy.2011.11.012.

77. Neilson JP, Lavender T, Quenby S, Wray S. Obstructed labour. *Br Med Bull.* 2003;67:191-204. doi:10.1093/bmb/ldg018.

78. Oladapo OT, Diaz V, Bonet M, et al. Cervical dilatation patterns of "low-risk" women with spontaneous labour and normal perinatal outcomes: a systematic review. *BJOG.* 2018;125(8):944-954. doi:10.1111/1471-0528.14930.

79. Caughey AB, Cahill AG, Guise JM, Rouse DJ. Safe prevention of the primary cesarean delivery. *Am J Obstet Gynecol.* 2014;210(3):179-193. doi:10.1016/j.ajog.2014.01.026.

80. Neal JL, Ryan SL, Lowe NK, et al. Labor dystocia: uses of related nomenclature. *J Midwifery Womens Health.* 2015;60(5):485-498. doi:10.1111/jmwh.12355.

81. Thuillier C, Roy S, Peyronnet V, et al. Impact of recommended changes in labor management for prevention of the primary cesarean delivery. *Am J Obstet Gynecol.* 2018;218(3):341.e1-341.e9. doi:10.1016/j.ajog.2017.12.228.

82. Friedman EA. Primigravid labor: a graphicostatistical analysis. *Obstet Gynecol*. 1955;6(6):567-589. doi:10.1097/00006250-195512000-00001.

83. Zhang J, Troendle J, Mikolajczyk R, et al. The natural history of the normal first stage of labor. *Obstet Gynecol*. 2010;115(4):705-710. [Published correction appears in *Obstet Gynecol*. 2010;116(1):196.] doi:10.1097/AOG.0b013e3181d55925.

84. Zhang J, Landy HJ, Ware Branch D, et al. Contemporary patterns of spontaneous labor with normal neonatal outcomes. *Obstet Gynecol*. 2010;116(6):1281-1287. doi:10.1097/AOG.0b013e3181fdef6e.

85. Neal JL, Lowe NK, Phillippi JC, et al. Likelihood of cesarean delivery after applying leading active labor diagnostic guidelines. *Birth*. 2017;44(2):128-136. doi:10.1111/birt.12274.

86. Friedman EA. *Labor: Clinical Evaluation and Management* (2nd ed.). New York, NY: Appleton-Century-Crofts; 1978.

87. Weekend MJ, Bayes S, Davison C. Exploring concepts and definitions of plateaus during normal labor and birth: a scoping review protocol. *JBI Evid Synth*. 2021;19(3):644-651. doi:10.11124/JBIES-20-00105.

88. Neal JL, Lowe NK, Ahijevych KL, et al. "Active labor" duration and dilation rates among low-risk, nulliparous women with spontaneous labor onset: a systematic review. *J Midwifery Womens Health*. 2010;55(4):308-318. doi:10.1016/j.jmwh.2009.08.004.

89. *WHO Recommendations: Intrapartum Care for a Positive Childbirth Experience*. Geneva, Switzerland: World Health Organization; 2018.

90. Tilden EL, Phillippi JC, Ahlberg M, et al. Describing latent phase duration and associated characteristics among 1281 low-risk women in spontaneous labor. *Birth*. 2019;46(4):592-601. doi:10.1111/birt.12428.

91. Marowitz A. Assessment and care at the onset of labor. In: Jordan R, Farley C, Grace K, eds. *Prenatal and Postnatal Care: A Woman-Centered Approach*. Hoboken, NJ: Wiley Blackwell; 2019:393-399.

92. Kominiarek MA, Zhang J, Vanveldhuisen P, et al. Contemporary labor patterns: the impact of maternal body mass index. *Am J Obstet Gynecol*. 2011;205(3):244.e1-244.e2448. https://doi.org/10.1016/j.ajog.2011.06.014/.

93. Buckley SJ. *Hormonal Physiology of Childbearing: Evidence and Implications for Women, Babies, and Maternity Care*. Washington, DC: Childbirth Connection Programs, National Partnership for Women & Families; 2015.

94. Olza I, Uvnas-Moberg K, Ekström-Bergström A, et al. Birth as a neuro-psycho-social event: an integrative model of maternal experiences and their relation to neurohormonal events during childbirth. *PLoS One*. 2020;15(7):e0230992. doi:10.1371/journal.pone.0230992.

95. Uvnäs-Moberg K, Ekström-Bergström A, Berg M, et al. Maternal plasma levels of oxytocin during physiological childbirth: a systematic review with implications for uterine contractions and central actions of oxytocin. *BMC Pregn Childbirth*. 2019;19(1):285. doi:10.1186/s12884-019-2365-9.

96. Smyth RM, Alldred SK, Markham C. Amniotomy for shortening spontaneous labour. *Cochrane Database Syst Rev*. 2013;1:CD006167. doi:10.1002/14651858.CD006167.pub3.

97. Rouse DJ, McCullough C, Wren AL, et al. Active-phase labor arrest: a randomized trial of chorioamnion management. *Obstet Gynecol*. 1994;83(6):937-940. https://doi.org/10.1097/00006250-199406000-00007.

98. Wei S, Wo BL, Qi HP, et al. Early amniotomy and early oxytocin for prevention of, or therapy for, delay in first stage spontaneous labour compared with routine care. *Cochrane Database Syst Rev*. 2013;8:CD006794. doi:10.1002/14651858.CD006794.pub4.

99. American College of Obstetrics and Gynecology Committee on Practice Bulletins—Obstetrics. ACOG Practice Bulletin Number 49, December 2003: dystocia and augmentation of labor. *Obstet Gynecol*. 2003;102(6):1445-1454. doi:10.1016/j.obstetgynecol.2003.10.011.

100. Bakker JJ, Janssen PF, van Halem K, et al. Internal versus external tocodynamometry during induced or augmented labour. *Cochrane Database Syst Rev*. 2013;8:CD006947. https://doi.org/10.1002/14651858.CD006947.pub3.

101. Smith H, Peterson N, Lagrew D, Main E. *Toolkit to Support Vaginal Birth and Reduce Primary Cesareans: A Quality Improvement Toolkit*. Stanford, CA: California Maternal Quality Care Collaborative; 2016. https://www.cmqcc.org/BirthToolkitResource.

102. Simkin P. The fetal occiput posterior position: state of the science and a new perspective. *Birth*. 2010;37(1):61-71. doi:10.1111/j.1523-536X.2009.00380.x.

103. Malvasi A, Bochicchio M, Vaira L, et al. The fetal head evaluation during labor in the occiput posterior position: the ESA (evaluation by simulation algorithm) approach. *J Matern Fetal Neonatal Med*. 2014;27(11):1151-1157. doi:10.3109/14767058.2013.851188.

104. Malvasi A, Barbera A, Di Vagno G, et al. Asynclitism: a literature review of an often forgotten clinical condition. *J Matern Fetal Neonatal Med*. 2015;28(16):1890-1894. doi:10.3109/14767058.2014.972925.

105. Malvasi A, Tinelli A, Barbera A, et al. Occiput posterior position diagnosis: vaginal examination or intrapartum sonography? A clinical review. *J Matern Fetal Neonatal Med*. 2014;27(5):520-526. doi:10.3109/14767058.2013.825598.

106. Sherer DM. Can sonographic depiction of fetal head position prior to or at the onset of labor predict mode of delivery? *Ultrasound Obstet Gynecol*. 2012;40(1):1-6. doi:10.1002/uog.11213.

107. Bellussi F, Ghi T, Youssef A, et al. Intrapartum ultrasound to differentiate flexion and deflexion in occipitoposterior rotation. *Fetal Diagn Ther.* 2017;42(4):249-256. doi:10.1159/000457124.

108. Hjartardóttir H, Lund SH, Benediktsdóttir S, et al. When does fetal head rotation occur in spontaneous labor at term: results of an ultrasound-based longitudinal study in nulliparous women? *Am J Obstet Gynecol.* 2021;224(5):514.e1-514.e9. doi:10.1016/j.ajog.2020.10.054.

109. Rouse DJ, Weiner SJ, Bloom SL, et al. Second-stage labor duration in nulliparous women: relationship to maternal and perinatal outcomes. *Am J Obstet Gynecol.* 2009;201(4):357.e1-357.e3577. https://doi.org/10.1016/j.ajog.2009.08.003.

110. Gimovsky AC, Berghella V. Prolonged second stage: what is the optimal length? *Obstet Gynecol Surv.* 2016;71(11):667-674. https://doi.org/10.1097/OGX.0000000000000368.

111. Laughon SK, Berghella V, Reddy UM, et al. Neonatal and maternal outcomes with prolonged second stage of labor. *Obstet Gynecol.* 2014;124(1):57-67. https://doi.org/10.1097/AOG.0000000000000278.

112. Allen VM, Baskett TF, O'Connell CM, et al. Maternal and perinatal outcomes with increasing duration of the second stage of labor. *Obstet Gynecol.* 2009;113(6):1248-1258. doi:10.1097/AOG.0b013e3181a722d6.

113. Altman MR, Lydon-Rochelle MT. Prolonged second stage of labor and risk of adverse maternal and perinatal outcomes: a systematic review. *Birth.* 2006;33(4):315-322. doi:10.1111/j.1523-536X.2006.00129.x.

114. Cheng YW, Hopkins LM, Laros RK Jr, Caughey AB. Duration of the second stage of labor in multiparous women: maternal and neonatal outcomes. *Am J Obstet Gynecol.* 2007;196(6):585.e1-585.e5856. doi:10.1016/j.ajog.2007.03.021.

115. Pergialiotis V, Bellos I, Antsaklis A, et al. Maternal and neonatal outcomes following a prolonged second stage of labor: a meta-analysis of observational studies. *Eur J Obstet Gynecol Reprod Biol.* 2020;252:62-69. doi:10.1016/j.ejogrb.2020.06.018.

116. Rouse DJ, Weiner SJ, Bloom SL, et al. Second-stage labor duration in nulliparous women: relationship to maternal and perinatal outcomes. *Am J Obstet Gynecol.* 2009;201(4):357.e1-357.e3577. doi:10.1016/j.ajog.2009.08.003.

117. Matta P, Turner J, Flatley C, Kumar S. Prolonged second stage of labour increases maternal morbidity but not neonatal morbidity. *Aust N Z J Obstet Gynaecol.* 2019;59(4):555-560. doi:10.1111/ajo.12935.

118. Myles TD, Santolaya J. Maternal and neonatal outcomes in patients with a prolonged second stage of labor. *Obstet Gynecol.* 2003;102(1):52-58. doi:10.1016/s0029-7844(03)00400-9.

119. Naqvi M, Jaffe EF, Goldfarb IT, et al. Prolonged second stage of labor and anal sphincter injury in a contemporary cohort of term nulliparas. *Am J Perinatol.* 2020;10.1055/s-0040-1718878. doi:10.1055/s-0040-1718878.

120. Aiken CE, Aiken AR, Prentice A. Influence of the duration of the second stage of labor on the likelihood of obstetric anal sphincter injury. *Birth.* 2015;42(1):86-93. doi:10.1111/birt.12137.

121. Cheng YW, Hopkins LM, Caughey AB. How long is too long: does a prolonged second stage of labor in nulliparous women affect maternal and neonatal outcomes? *Am J Obstet Gynecol.* 2004;191(3):933-938. doi:10.1016/j.ajog.2004.05.044.

122. Infante-Torres N, Molina-Alarcón M, Arias-Arias A, et al. Relationship between prolonged second stage of labor and short-term neonatal morbidity: a systematic review and meta-analysis. *Int J Environ Res Public Health.* 2020;17(21):7762. doi:10.3390/ijerph17217762.

123. Infante-Torres N, Molina-Alarcón M, Gómez-Salgado J, et al. Relationship between the duration of the second stage of labour and neonatal morbidity. *J Clin Med.* 2019;8(3):376. doi:10.3390/jcm8030376.

124. Lieberman E, Davidson K, Lee-Parritz A, Shearer E. Changes in fetal position during labor and their association with epidural analgesia. *Obstet Gynecol.* 2005;105(5 pt 1):974-982. doi:10.1097/01.AOG.0000158861.43593.49.

125. Cheng YW, Shaffer BL, Caughey AB. Associated factors and outcomes of persistent occiput posterior position: a retrospective cohort study from 1976 to 2001. *J Matern Fetal Neonatal Med.* 2006;19(9):563-568. doi:10.1080/14767050600682487.

126. Menichini D, Mazzaro N, Minniti S, et al. Fetal head malposition and epidural analgesia in labor: a case-control study. *J Matern Fetal Neonatal Med.* 2021;1-10. doi:10.1080/14767058.2021.1890018.

127. Robinson CA, Macones GA, Roth NW, Morgan MA. Does station of the fetal head at epidural placement affect the position of the fetal vertex at delivery? *Am J Obstet Gynecol.* 1996;175(4 pt 1):991-994. doi:10.1016/s0002-9378(96)80039-1.

128. Le Ray C, Carayol M, Jaquemin S, et al. Is epidural analgesia a risk factor for occiput posterior or transverse positions during labour? *Eur J Obstet Gynecol Reprod Biol.* 2005;123(1):22-26. doi:10.1016/j.ejogrb.2005.02.009.

129. Desseauve D, Fradet L, Lacouture P, Pierre F. Position for labor and birth: state of knowledge and biomechanical perspectives. *Eur J Obstet Gynecol Reprod Biol.* 2017;208:46-54. doi:10.1016/j.ejogrb.2016.11.006.

130. Huang J, Zang Y, Ren LH, et al. A review and comparison of common maternal positions during the

second-stage of labor. *Int J Nurs Sci.* 2019;6(4): 460-467. doi:10.1016/j.ijnss.2019.06.007.

131. Hemmerich A, Bandrowska T, Dumas GA. The effects of squatting while pregnant on pelvic dimensions: a computational simulation to understand childbirth. *J Biomech.* 2019;87:64-74. doi:10.1016/j .jbiomech.2019.02.017.

132. Siccardi M, Valle C, Di Matteo F. Dynamic external pelvimetry test in third trimester pregnant women: shifting positions affect pelvic biomechanics and create more room in obstetric diameters. *Cureus.* 2021;13(3):e13631. doi:10.7759/cureus.13631.

133. Stremler R, Hodnett E, Petryshen P, et al. Randomized controlled trial of hands-and-knees positioning for occipitoposterior position in labor. *Birth.* 2005;32(4): 243-251. doi:10.1111/j.0730-7659.2005.00382.x.

134. Desbriere R, Blanc J, Le Dû R, et al. Is maternal posturing during labor efficient in preventing persistent occiput posterior position? A randomized controlled trial. *Am J Obstet Gynecol.* 2013;208(1):60. e1-60.e608. doi:10.1016/j.ajog.2012.10.882.

135. Le Ray C, Lepleux F, De La Calle A, et al. Lateral asymmetric decubitus position for the rotation of occipito-posterior positions: multicenter randomized controlled trial EVADELA. *Am J Obstet Gynecol.* 2016;215(4):511.e1-511.e5117. doi:10.1016/j .ajog.2016.05.033.

136. Guittier MJ, Othenin-Girard V, de Gasquet B, et al. Maternal positioning to correct occiput posterior fetal position during the first stage of labour: a randomised controlled trial. *BJOG.* 2016;123(13):2199-2207. doi:10.1111/1471-0528.13855.

137. Bueno-Lopez V, Fuentelsaz-Gallego C, Casellas-Caro M, et al. Efficiency of the modified Sims maternal position in the rotation of persistent occiput posterior position during labor: a randomized clinical trial. *Birth.* 2018;45(4):385-392. doi:10.1111/birt.12347.

138. Cohen SR, Thomas CR. Rebozo technique for fetal malposition in labor. *J Midwifery Womens Health.* 2015;60(4):445-451. doi:10.1111/jmwh.12352.

139. Lawrence A, Lewis L, Hofmeyr GJ, Styles C. Maternal positions and mobility during first stage labour. *Cochrane Database Syst Rev.* 2013;10:CD003934. doi:10.1002/14651858.CD003934.pub4.

140. Lepleux F, Hue B, Dugué AE, et al. Données obstétricales dans une population bénéficiant de variations posturales en cours de travail et d'accouchement [Obstetric data in a population with postural changes during labor and delivery]. *J Gynecol Obstet Biol Reprod (Paris).* 2014;43(7): 504-513. doi:10.1016/j.jgyn.2013.06.013.

141. Elmore C, McBroom K, Ellis J. Digital and manual rotation of the persistent occiput posterior fetus. *J Midwifery Womens Health.* 2020;65(3):387-394. doi:10.1111/jmwh.13118.

142. de Vries B, Hyett JA, Kuah S, Phipps H. Persistent occiput posterior position-OUTcomes following manual rotation (the POP-OUT trial): a randomized controlled clinical trial. *Am J Obstet Gynecol MFM.* 2021;3(6):100388. doi:10.1016/j .ajogmf.2021.100388.

143. Broberg JC, Caughey AB. A randomized controlled trial of prophylactic early manual rotation of the occiput posterior fetus at the beginning of the second stage vs expectant management. *Am J Obstet Gynecol MFM.* 2021;3(2):100327. doi:10.1016/j .ajogmf.2021.100327.

144. DeLee J. The prophylactic forceps operation. *Am J Obstet Gynecol.* 1920;1(34):34-44.

145. Green JR, Soohoo SL. Factors associated with rectal injury in spontaneous deliveries. *Obstet Gynecol.* 1989;73(5 pt 1):732-738.

146. Kozhimannil KB, Karaca-Mandic P, Blauer-Peterson CJ, et al. Uptake and utilization of practice guidelines in hospitals in the United States: the case of routine episiotomy. *Jt Comm J Qual Patient Saf.* 2017;43(1):41-48. doi:10.1016/j.jcjq.2016.10.002.

147. ACOG Committee on Practice Bulletins—Obstetrics. ACOG Practice Bulletin No. 198: prevention and management of obstetric lacerations at vaginal delivery. *Obstet Gynecol.* 2018;132(3): e87-e102. doi:10.1097/AOG.0000000000002841.

148. Mahgoub S, Piant H, Gaudineau A, et al. Risk factors for obstetric anal sphincter injuries (OASIS) and the role of episiotomy: a retrospective series of 496 cases. *J Gynecol Obstet Hum Reprod.* 2019;48(8):657-662. doi:10.1016/j.jogoh .2019.07.004.

149. Aquino CI, Saccone G, Troisi J, et al. Is Ritgen's maneuver associated with decreased perineal lacerations and pain at delivery? *J Matern Fetal Neonatal Med.* 2020;33(18):3185-3192. doi:10.1080/14767 058.2019.1568984.

150. National Institutes of Health. *Consensus Development Conference on Cesarean Childbirth.* Publication No. 82: 2067. Bethesda, MD: National Institutes of Health, Department of Health and Human Services; 1981.

151. Guise JM, Denman MA, Emeis C, et al. Vaginal birth after cesarean: new insights on maternal and neonatal outcomes. *Obstet Gynecol.* 2010;115(6):1267-1278.

152. McMahon MJ, Luther ER, Bowes WA Jr, Olshan AF. Comparison of a trial of labor with an elective second cesarean section. *N Engl J Med.* 1996;335(10):689-695. doi:10.1056/NEJM199609053351001.

153. American College of Obstetricians and Gynecologists. *ACOG Practice Bulletin No. 5: Vaginal Birth After Previous Cesarean Delivery.* Washington, DC: American College of Obstetricians and Gynecologists; July 1999.

154. National Institutes of Health consensus development conference statement on vaginal birth after cesarean: new insights March 8–10, 2010. *Obstet Gynecol.* 2010;115(6):1279-1295.

155. American College of Nurse-Midwives. Position statement: vaginal birth after cesarean. https://www.midwife.org/acnm/files/ACNMLibraryData/UPLOADFILENAME/000000000090/VBAC-PS-FINAL-10-10-17.pdf. Published September 2017. Accessed November 9, 2021.

156. Committee on Practice Bulletins—Obstetrics. Vaginal birth after previous cesarean delivery: Practice Bulletin No. 184. *Obstet Gynecol.* 2017;130:217-233.

157. Togioka BM, Tonismae T. Uterine rupture. In: *StatPearls [Internet].* Treasure Island, FL: StatPearls Publishing; July 1, 2021. https://www.ncbi.nlm.nih.gov/books/NBK559209/.

158. Al-Zirqi I, Stray-Pedersen B, Forsén L, et al. Uterine rupture: trends over 40 years. *BJOG.* 2016;123(5):780-787.

159. Vachon-Marceau C, Demers S, Goyet M, et al. Labor dystocia and the risk of uterine rupture in women with prior cesarean. *Am J Perinatol.* 2016;33(6):577-583. doi:10.1055/s-0035-1570382.

160. Grobman WA, Sandoval G, Rice MM, et al. Prediction of vaginal birth after cesarean delivery in term gestations: a calculator without race and ethnicity. *Am J Obstet Gynecol.* 2021;225(6):664.e1-664.e7. doi:10.1016/j.ajog.2021.05.021.

161. Hales CM, Carroll MD, Fryar CD, Ogden CL. *Prevalence of Obesity and Severe Obesity Among Adults: United States, 2017–2018. NCHS Data Brief,* No. 360. Hyattsville, MD: National Center for Health Statistics; 2020.

162. Kominiarek MA, Zhang J, Vanveldhuisen P, et al. Contemporary labor patterns: the impact of maternal body mass index. *Am J Obstet Gynecol.* 2011;205(3):244.e1-244.e2448. doi:10.1016/j.ajog.2011.06.014.

163. Norman SM, Tuuli MG, Odibo AO, et al. The effects of obesity on the first stage of labor. *Obstet Gynecol.* 2012;120(1):130-135. doi:10.1097/AOG.0b013e318259589c.

164. Khalifa E, El-Sateh A, Zeeneldin M, et al. Effect of maternal BMI on labor outcomes in primigravida pregnant women. *BMC Pregn Childbirth.* 2021;21:753. https://doi.org/10.1186/s12884-021-04236-z.

165. Slack E, Best KE, Rankin J, Heslehurst N. Maternal obesity classes, preterm and post-term birth: a retrospective analysis of 479,864 births in England. *BMC Pregn Childbirth.* 2019;19(1):434. doi:10.1186/s12884-019-2585-z.

166. Wolfe KB, Rossi RA, Warshak CR. The effect of maternal obesity on the rate of failed induction of labor. *Am J Obstet Gynecol.* 2011;205(2):128.e1-128.e1287. doi:10.1016/j.ajog.2011.03.051.

167. Dammer U, Bogner R, Weiss C, et al. Influence of body mass index on induction of labor: a historical cohort study. *J Obstet Gynaecol Res.* 2018;44(4):697-707.

168. Suidan RS, Rondon KC, Apuzzio JJ, Williams SF. Labor outcomes of obese clients undergoing induction of labor with misoprostol compared to dinoprostone. *Am J Perinatol.* 2015;30(2):187-192.

169. Hiersch L, Rosen H, Salzer L, et al. Does artificial rupturing of membranes in the active phase of labor enhance myometrial electrical activity? *J Matern Fetal Neonatal Med.* 2015;28(5):515-518.

170. Committee on Obstetric Practice, Society for Maternal–Fetal Medicine. ACOG Committee Opinion: medically indicated late-preterm and early-preterm deliveries. *Obstet Gynecol.* 2021;831(1):e35-e39.

171. American College of Obstetricians and Gynecologists' Committee on Practice Bulletins—Obstetrics. ACOG Practice Bulletin No. 201: pregestational diabetes mellitus. *Obstet Gynecol.* 2018;132(6):e228-e248. doi:10.1097/AOG.0000000000002960.

172. Macrosomia: ACOG Practice Bulletin, Number 216. *Obstet Gynecol.* 2020;135(1):e18-e35. doi:10.1097/AOG.0000000000003606.

173. ACOG Practice Bulletin No. 190: gestational diabetes mellitus. *Obstet Gynecol.* 2018;131(2):e49-e64. doi:10.1097/AOG.0000000000002501.

174. Gestational hypertension and preeclampsia: ACOG Practice Bulletin Summary, Number 222. *Obstet Gynecol.* 2020;135(6):1492-1495. doi:10.1097/AOG.0000000000003892.

175. Bernstein PS, Martin JN Jr, Barton JR, et al. National Partnership for Maternal Safety: consensus bundle on severe hypertension during pregnancy and the postpartum period. *Obstet Gynecol.* 2017;130(2):347-357. doi:10.1097/AOG.0000000000002115. Erratum in: *Obstet Gynecol.* 2019;133(6):1288.

176. Pregnancy-related deaths in the United States. Centers for Disease Control and Prevention. https://www.cdc.gov/hearher/pregnancy-related-deaths/index.html. Published September 14, 2021. Accessed April 25, 2023.

177. Zuckerwise LC, Lipkind HS. Maternal early warning systems: towards reducing preventable maternal mortality and severe maternal morbidity through improved clinical surveillance and responsiveness. *Semin Perinatol.* 2017;41(3):161-165. doi:10.1053/j.semperi.2017.03.005.

178. Downes KL, Grantz KL, Shenassa ED. Maternal, labor, delivery, and perinatal outcomes associated with placental abruption: a systematic review. *Am J Perinatol.* 2017;34(10):935-957. doi:10.1055/s-0037-1599149.

179. Ananth CV, Lavery JA, Vintzileos AM, et al. Severe placental abruption: clinical definition and

associations with maternal complications. *Am J Obstet Gynecol.* 2016;214(2):272.e1-272.e9. doi:10.1016/j.ajog.2015.09.069.

180. Oyelese Y, Ananth CV. Placental abruption. *Obstet Gynecol.* 2006;108:1005-1016.

181. Hladky K, Yankowitz J, Hansen WF. Placental abruption. *Obstet Gynecol Surv.* 2002;57(5):299-305.

182. Togioka BM, Tonismae T. Uterine rupture. In: *Stat-Pearls.* Treasure Island, FL: StatPearls Publishing; https://www.ncbi.nlm.nih.gov/books/NBK559209/. Published July 1, 2021.

183. Wong L, Kwan AHW, Lau SL, et al. Umbilical cord prolapse: revisiting its definition and management. *Am J Obstet Gynecol.* 2021;225(4):357-366. doi:10.1016/j.ajog.2021.06.077.

184. Pacheco LD, Clark SL, Klassen M, Hankins GDV. Amniotic fluid embolism: principles of early clinical management. *Am J Obstet Gynecol.* 2020;222(1): 48-52. doi:10.1016/j.ajog.2019.07.036.

185. Tamura N, Farhana M, Oda T, Kanayama N. Amniotic fluid embolism: pathophysiology from the perspective of pathology. *J Obstet Gynaecol Res.* 2017;43(4):627-632.

186. Pacheco LD, Saade G, Hankins GD, Clark SL. Amniotic fluid embolism: diagnosis and management. *Am J Obstet Gynecol.* 2016;215(2):B16-B24. doi:10.1016/j.ajog.2016.03.012.

187. Clark S, Romero R, Dildy G, et al. Proposed diagnostic criteria for the case definition of amniotic fluid embolism in research studies. *Am J Obstet Gynecol.* 2017;217(2):228-229.

188. Royal College of Obstetricians and Gynaecologists. *RCOG Green-Top Guideline No. 42.* London, UK: Royal College of Obstetricians and Gynaecologists; 2012:13.1-13.13.

189. Sentilhes L, Sénat MV, Boulogne AI, et al. Shoulder dystocia: guidelines for clinical practice from the French College of Gynecologists and Obstetricians (CNGOF). *Eur J Obstet Gynecol Reprod Biol.* 2016;203: 156-161. doi:10.1016/j.ejogrb.2016.05.047.

190. Society of Obstetricians and Gynaecologists of Canada. Chapter 13: Shoulder dystocia. In: *Advances in Labour and Risk Management Textbook: ALARM International Program Manual.* 22nd ed. Ottawa, Canada: Society of Obstetricians and Gynaecologists of Canada; 2016.

191. Practice Bulletin No 178: shoulder dystocia. *Obstet Gynecol.* 2017;129(5):e123-e133. doi:10.1097/AOG .0000000000002043.

192. Sancetta R, Khanzada H, Leante R. Shoulder shrug maneuver to facilitate delivery during shoulder dystocia. *Obstet Gynecol.* 2019;133(6):1178-1181. doi:10.1097/AOG.0000000000003278.

193. Hoek J, Verkouteren B, van Hamont D. Posterior axilla sling traction: a new technique for severe shoulder dystocia. *BMJ Case Rep.* 2019;12(3):e226882. doi:10.1136/bcr-2018-226882.

194. Macrosomia: ACOG Practice Bulletin, Number 216. *Obstet Gynecol.* 2020;135(1):e18-e35. doi:10.1097/AOG.0000000000003606.

195. Johnson GJ, Denning S, Clark SL, Davidson C. Pathophysiologic origins of brachial plexus injury. *Obstet Gynecol.* 2020;136(4):725-730. doi:10.1097/AOG.0000000000004013.

196. Andrighetti TP, Knestrick JM, Marowitz A, et al. Shoulder dystocia and postpartum hemorrhage simulations: student confidence in managing these complications. *J Midwifery Womens Health.* 2012;57:55-60.

197. Allen EDG. Simulation of shoulder dystocia for skill acquisition and competency assessment: a systematic review and gap analysis. *Simul Healthc.* 2018;13(4):268-283. doi:10.1097/SIH.0000000000000292.

198. American College of Obstetricians and Gynecologists. Multifetal gestations: twin, triplet, and higher-order multifetal pregnancies. *Obstet Gynecol.* 2021;137(6):e145-e162. doi:10.1097/AOG .0000000000004397.

199. Lee YM. Delivery of twins. *Semin Perinatol.* 2012;36:195-200.

200. Hofmeyr GJ, Barrett JF, Crowther CA. Planned caesarean section for women with a twin pregnancy. *Cochrane Database Syst Rev.* 2015;12:CD006553. doi:10.1002/14651858.CD006553.pub3.

201. Posner G, Dy J, Black A, Jones G. *Oxorn-Foote Human Labor and Birth.* 6th ed. New York, NY: McGraw-Hill Professional; 2013.

202. Hannah ME, Hannah WJ, Hewson SA, et al. Planned caesarean section versus planned vaginal birth for breech presentation at term: a randomised multicentre trial. Term Breech Trial Collaborative Group. *Lancet.* 2000;356(9239):1375-1383. doi:10.1016/s0140-6736(00)02840-3.

203. Impey LWM, Murphy DJ, Griffiths M, Penna LK; Royal College of Obstetricians and Gynaecologists. Management of breech presentation: Green-top Guideline No. 20b. *BJOG.* 2017;124(7):e151-e177. [Published correction appears in *BJOG.* 2017; 124(10):e279.] doi:10.1111/1471-0528.14465.

204. Kotaska A, Menticoglou S. No. 384: management of breech presentation at term. *J Obstet Gynaecol Can.* 2019;41(8):1193-1205. doi:10.1016/j. jogc.2018.12.018.

205. ACOG Committee Opinion No. 745: mode of term singleton breech delivery. *Obstet Gynecol.* 2018;132(2):e60-e63. doi:10.1097/AOG .0000000000002755.

206. Ekéus C, Norman M, Åberg K, et al. Vaginal breech delivery at term and neonatal morbidity and mortality: a population-based cohort study in Sweden.

*J Matern Fetal Neonatal Med.* 2019;32(2):265-270. doi:10.1080/14767058.2017.1378328.

207. Hofmeyr GJ, Hannah M, Lawrie TA. Planned caesarean section for term breech delivery. *Cochrane Database Syst Rev.* 2015;7:CD000166. doi:10.1002/14651858.CD000166.pub2.

208. American College of Obstetricians and Gynecologists; Society for Maternal–Fetal Medicine in collaboration with Metz TD, et al. Obstetric Care Consensus #10: management of stillbirth: (replaces Practice Bulletin Number 102, March 2009). *Am J Obstet Gynecol.* 2020;222(3):B2-B20. doi:10.1016/j.ajog.2020.01.017.

209. Lemmers M, Verschoor MA, Kim BV, et al. Medical treatment for early fetal death (less than 24 weeks). *Cochrane Database Syst Rev.* 2019;6:CD002253. doi:10.1002/14651858.CD002253.pub4.

210. Larsen S, Dobbin J, McCallion O, Eskild A. Intrauterine fetal death and risk of shoulder dystocia at delivery. *Acta Obstet Gynecol Scand.* 2016;95(12):1345-1351. doi:10.1111/aogs.13033.

211. Cortezzo DE, Ellis K, Schlegel A. Perinatal palliative care birth planning as advance care planning. *Front Pediatr.* 2020;8:556. doi:10.3389/fped.2020.00556.

APPENDIX

# 30A

# Urgent Maneuvers to Shorten Second Stage

SHARON L. HOLLEY

Whenever possible, the natural process of second-stage labor should be supported. However, when circumstances arise that indicate a need for a shortened second stage, the midwife can choose among several techniques to expedite birth. In this appendix, episiotomy and manual fetal head extension (Ritgen maneuver) are reviewed.

## Episiotomy

### Definition

An episiotomy is a surgical incision that is performed to enlarge the vaginal opening. The procedure involves incising the posterior aspect of the vagina to the perineum during the last part of the second stage of labor, just prior to a vaginal birth.[1-3]

### Background

Multiple randomized trials and a Cochrane meta-analysis have demonstrated that routine episiotomy is associated with an increased risk for severe perineal lacerations.[4] Routine use of episiotomy is linked to over-medicalization and an increase in severe perineal injury, and is financially driven rather than patient-driven care.[5,6] Consequently, birth providers should not routinely perform an episiotomy, but rather use a restricted policy and consider risk factors.[3,6,7] The one accepted indication for an episiotomy is a need to expedite birth secondary to fetal bradycardia or another fetal heart rate pattern that suggests a significant risk of newborn acidemia. Other suggested but controversial indications include operative birth, suspected shoulder dystocia, and short perineum.[2]

Cutting and repair of an episiotomy is a skill that should be part of the repertoire of a midwife so that, when needed, it can be performed competently. An understanding of perineal anatomy is critical to the discussion of episiotomies and lacerations, and relevant information can be found in the *Anatomy and Physiology of the Reproductive System* chapter.

The midwife should also understand the advantages and disadvantages of each type of episiotomy and share their recommendations based on this understanding with the laboring person as part of informed consent. For example, there is conflicting evidence regarding the risk of obstetric anal sphincter injury (OASIS) in laboring persons who are exposed to a policy of non-episiotomy versus selective episiotomy.[8] Evidence also indicates that a mediolateral episiotomy cut at a crowning angle of 60 degrees decreases the risk of OASIS, particularly when vacuum or forceps are used.[4,9]

Ideally, the potential need for episiotomy should be discussed prior to labor so the person is aware of possible indications and risks, should this procedure become necessary. Even if not discussed before labor, informed consent should always be obtained prior to performing an episiotomy to ensure that the birthing person's human rights are respected.[6] The discussion about the need for an episiotomy to expedite birth may occur under urgent conditions such as prolonged fetal heart rate decelerations. This limits the opportunity to engage in in-depth discussion of the risks and benefits of the procedure. Nevertheless, it is important to get fully informed consent and to avoid coercive communication. If a fully informed birthing person then declines, a respectful discussion of alternative options should be pursued. Individuals have the right for their decisions to be respected. The discussion may continue as conditions change.

## When to Cut an Episiotomy

There is little evidence to guide a midwife regarding when to cut an episiotomy. Performing this procedure too early may result in extra blood loss. Waiting until the perineum is paper thin and the tissue bulging, however, may result in a rapid and perhaps uncontrolled birth of the fetal head, with resulting extension of the episiotomy. Many midwives advocate making the incision when the head is crowning and not retracting between contractions, such that birth is expected within a few contractions. When the head is well applied to the perineum, it also provides a type of tamponade to decrease bleeding.

Sometimes the discussion for consent leads to a change in pushing intensity that expedites birth without the need for future intervention. Similarly, the act of inserting the needle to provide local anesthetic can weaken perineal tissue, resulting in a laceration that expedites birth without an incision.

After the episiotomy is performed, the midwife should continue to apply gentle pressure to the fetal head to control and direct a slow extension of the head. This will help avoid a rapid birth, sudden pressure on the perineum, and extension of the incision. Pressure on the wound to control bleeding may also be required between maternal pushing efforts.

## Preparation

During labor, when it becomes apparent that an episiotomy may be necessary, the midwife should discuss the indication and recommendation with the laboring person and their support persons. Continuous communication as the procedure is performed informs them of events, especially if the patient has regional anesthesia and impaired sensation.

Appropriate equipment should be available, including a pair of sterile gloves and episiotomy scissors have one rounded outer blade to protect the fetal head from injury. Left-handed versions of standard episiotomy scissors and needle drivers are also available but may need to be specifically requested. Include items needed for providing pain relief prior to and after an episiotomy, such as a 10-mL syringe with a 22-gauge needle for administering lidocaine. There should be appropriate lighting to provide visualization of the area prior to cutting the episiotomy. It is also best to have available any equipment that will be needed to repair the episiotomy following the birth of the baby: a needle driver, suture scissors, forceps with teeth, Allis clamps, sterile

sponges, and suture material. A handheld retractor is also helpful for visualizing deep vaginal lacerations, or repairing third- or fourth-degree perineal lacerations.[10–12]

Anesthesia is a prerequisite before an episiotomy is performed, and the level of anesthesia should be appropriate for the extent of surgical repair. Although nitrous oxide or parenteral opioids may be useful as analgesia, the denser pain relief offered by an epidural or a pudendal nerve block will be more effective. Under some circumstances, local infiltration may be performed prior to cutting an episiotomy, although this intervention may distort tissue and cause edema. Descriptions of the techniques for local infiltration and pudendal block can be found in the *Local Infiltration for Genital Tract Repair* and *Pudendal Nerve Block* appendices, respectively.

## Classification of Episiotomy

There are seven classifications of episiotomy: midline (median, medial), modified median, mediolateral, "J"-shaped, lateral, and radical lateral. Currently, there is more evidence about mediolateral and midline episiotomies; therefore, this appendix will focus on these surgical techniques.

### Midline Versus Mediolateral Episiotomy

Two types of episiotomy are the most frequently performed: midline incision and mediolateral incision. The midline episiotomy is used more commonly in the United States and Canada, whereas the mediolateral episiotomy is used more frequently in Europe.[3,5] Evidence indicates that using a mediolateral episiotomy may help to avoid OASIS, particularly when vacuum or forceps are used.[2,9,13,14]

### Midline Episiotomy

The midline (or median) episiotomy has a vaginal apex and proceeds from anterior to posterior along the midline through the central tendon of the perineal body, separating the bulbocavernosus and superficial transverse perineal muscles.[5] Depending on the depth of the cut, the deep transverse perineal muscle may also be cut into two sides. The perineal apex is above the anal sphincter, with the incision extending to roughly half the length of the perineum. The pre-birth incision angle from midline should be between 0 and 25 degrees of the sagittal plane.[5]

***Advantages.*** The primary advantage of a midline episiotomy is ease of repair and a better cosmetic result. Although retrospective studies of postpartum pain have found that midline episiotomies are associated with less pain than mediolateral episiotomies, prospective studies have not found a significant difference. Using this technique also avoids risk of incising the Bartholin's gland and duct.[15]

***Disadvantages.*** Because the inferior apex of the midline episiotomy is directly above the rectal sphincter, extension into a third- or fourth-degree laceration is more likely to occur than with a mediolateral episiotomy.[2,16]

### Mediolateral Episiotomy

A mediolateral episiotomy also begins with a midline vaginal apex at the central tendinous point of the perineum and is then directed laterally and downward away from the rectum.[5] This incision cuts through the bulbocavernosus and the superficial and deep transverse perineal muscles, and into the pubococcygeus (levator ani) muscle. A mediolateral episiotomy is cut on the diagonal (right or left) starting at the midline or up to 3 mm from the posterior fourchette, with the points of the scissors directed right or left toward the ischial tuberosity on the same side as the incision (Figure 30A-1).[2] The pre-birth incision angle should be at 60 degrees away from the midline to achieve a post-birth suture angle of 45 degrees.[3,5,9]

***Advantages.*** The primary advantage of a mediolateral episiotomy is that fewer extensions into a third- or fourth-degree laceration occur, as compared to the outcomes of midline episiotomies. A growing body of evidence has demonstrated that a mediolateral episiotomy is protective of OASIS, particularly with use of forceps or vacuum extraction for nulliparous patients.[13,14]

***Disadvantages.*** Some studies have found mediolateral episiotomies to be associated with more blood loss; others have not. If not done using the correct technique, there is a potential risk of injury to the Bartholin's gland and duct. Compared to midline episiotomies, mediolateral episiotomies can be more challenging to repair. Distortion of the site may occur during repair if suturing is done horizontally, as would occur with repair of a medial episiotomy. Instead, suture of a mediolateral episiotomies should follow a diagonal slant along the line of the incision.[2] Additionally, the superior side of the incision has a larger area of exposed tissue than the inferior side, requiring larger "bites" of tissue superiorly when stitching.

### Angle of Episiotomy

Previous studies have demonstrated that the angle of the episiotomy when it is performed during crowning of the fetal head is greater than the angle of the resulting incision. This is due to the perineal degree of distortion. For example, an episiotomy performed at 40 degrees from the midline of the posterior fourchette would result in an incision

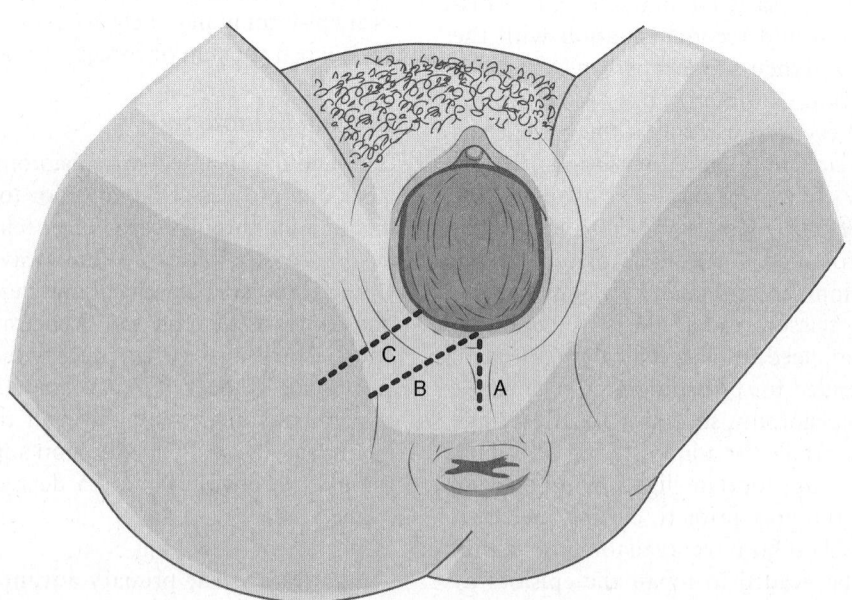

**Figure 30A-1** Types of episiotomies. **A.** Midline. **B.** Mediolateral. **C.** Lateral.

angle of 20 degrees, and an episiotomy performed at a 60-degree angle would result in an incision angle of 45 degrees.[9] Note that the angle of the incision after birth is more important than the pre-birth episiotomy angle; therefore, it is important for each midwife to understand the correct angle to cut with each type of episiotomy.[12,17]

### Technique for Performing an Episiotomy

1. Obtain informed consent for the procedure from the individual.

2. Assess for and ensure adequate pain control. Pain control may be accomplished using (in no particular order): an epidural, pudendal block, or local tissue infiltration with an anesthetic agent.

3. The episiotomy should be performed when the fetal head is at approximately +4 station or with approximately 4 cm of the fetal head showing.[15]

4. Place the index and middle fingers of the nondominant hand into the vagina, palmar side down and facing away from the birthing person. The fingers should be slightly separated and provide gentle outward pressure on the perineal body to create adequate space between the perineum and the head to allow the scissors to slip between the fingers. Thus, the fetal head is protected from being touched by the scissors. The pressure also slightly flattens the perineal area, providing an easier incision.

5. Holding the scissors in the dominant hand, place the blades in the appropriate direction—either straight anterior–posterior or diagonally, depending on the type of episiotomy to be cut. One blade of the scissors should be against the posterior vaginal wall, while the other blade should be against the skin of the perineal body, with the point where the blades cross at the midline of the posterior fourchette.

6. Locate the external anal sphincter by palpation using the fingers in the vagina and the thumb of the same hand placed externally to the perineal body (Figure 30A-2). Knowing the location of the external anal sphincter minimizes hesitation in cutting an adequate episiotomy due to fear of accidentally cutting through the sphincter.

    a. When cutting a **midline** episiotomy, adjust the length of the blades of the scissors on the perineal body to the projected length of the incision and terminate above the anal sphincter. Performing a single incision through both the vagina and the perineum with one cut avoids the need for multiple incisions and increased tissue trauma.

    b. When cutting a **mediolateral** episiotomy, position the blades so that there is

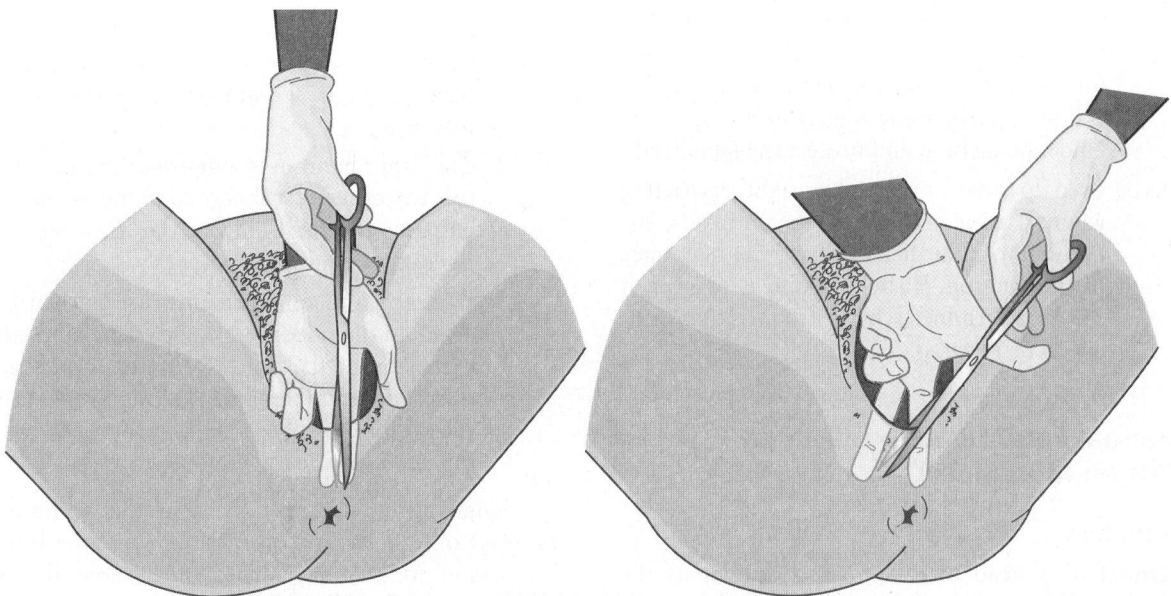

**Figure 30A-2** Hand and finger positions for midline and mediolateral episiotomies.

approximately 1 cm of levator ani muscle between the incision and the sphincter. Another way to visualize this is to cut laterally from the midline at a 40- to 60-degree angle toward the ischial tuberosity.[2,15,18] This directs the incision far enough laterally to avoid the sphincter during the process of cutting the episiotomy and when performing the repair. Some sources advocate starting the incision 3 mm from the midline of the posterior fourchette. If this is done, the midwife should be careful to avoid starting the incision too high laterally. If it is too high up, there is a potential of injuring the Bartholin's gland or not providing the desired relaxation of the median portion of the levator ani muscle.[2]

7. Incise the perineum with a 3- to 4-cm single cut that is sufficient to open the perineal body and extend into the vaginal vault. Incising in this manner opens the vagina and the perineum and avoids making successive small cuts that create distorted edges. If the episiotomy is not large enough, tension remains on the perineal tissue and a weak point is created that may increase the risk of extension, creating an uncontrolled laceration.[2]

8. After the initial incision, observe and evaluate the area to identify any active bleeding. Adequate visualization usually requires gentle use of gauze sponges to blot away blood, excessive and aggressive blotting or wiping can further harm the tissue.

9. If a second incision is necessary, it can be performed at this time. Extension of an incision is best made by using fingers in the vagina to guide the incision and protect the fetal head.

10. By palpating for a band of tight, restricting vaginal tissue just inside the introitus, the midwife can further evaluate the adequacy of the incision. If such a band is present, it can be determined whether the band must be cut to be released.

## Manual Fetal Head Extension (Ritgen Maneuver)

### Definition

Manual fetal head extension, also known as the Ritgen maneuver, is the use of an upward pressure from the coccygeal region to extend the head during actual delivery of the fetal head. It can only be used when the fetus is distending the perineum and in the occiput anterior position.

### Background

The manual fetal head extension technique was first described in 1855 and was originally named after Dr. Ferdinand August Maria Franz von Ritgen. It has long been thought to decrease second-stage labor just prior to birth. However, it is not protective for severe perineal lacerations and is associated with increased postpartum pain. Therefore, this technique should not be used routinely during the second stage of labor.[19]

### Technique

Manual fetal head extension can be used when the fetal head extends approximately 5 cm from the introitus and is not retracting between contractions. To perform manual fetal head extension, the midwife uses the second through fourth fingers of their nondominant hand to provide upward pressure on the posterior perineum between the coccygeal area and the anus. These fingers gently lift the fetal chin (Figure 30A-3). At the same time, the fingers of the dominant hand are placed on the fetal occiput. and gentle pressure is applied to slow birth of the fetal head. This results in the gradual extension of the head.[19,20]

### Technique for Performing Manual Fetal Head Extension Maneuver

1. One hand remains on the occiput as the fetus is crowning to maintain flexion until after the biparietal diameters are visible at the introitus.

2. The other hand uses a gauze or sterile towel to protect against rectal contamination and palpates the fetal chin in the area between the coccyx and rectum.

3. Forward and outward pressure is then exerted on the underneath side of the chin, and extension of the head is controlled between this hand and the hand exerting pressure on the occiput to control the pace of the birth of the neonate's head.

Some have recommended that this technique be used only between contractions with the birthing person not pushing. This creates a slow birth of the fetal forehead but avoids an abrupt emergence, which may increase the risk of lacerations.

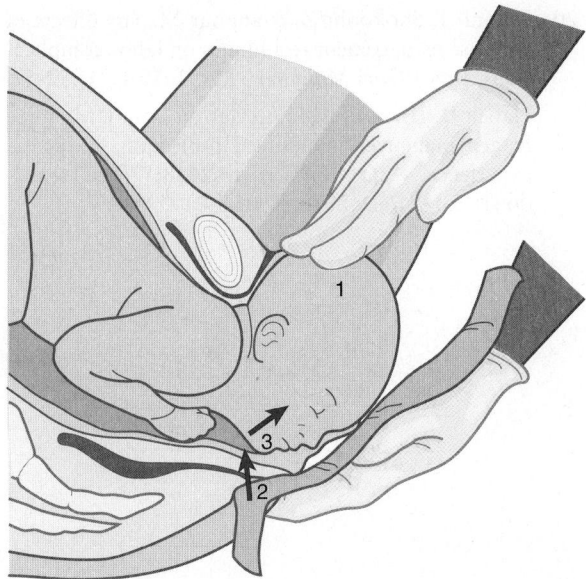

**Figure 30A-3** Manual fetal head extension maneuver (Ritgen maneuver).

An alternative to the traditional maneuver is the modified Scandinavian technique, which aims to provide additional perineal protection. In this technique, the dominant hand is spread on the perineum so that the index finger and thumb pull toward each other or squeeze the perineum as the third finger lifts the fetal chin up. Some evidence indicates that this modified technique, when compared to a hands-off approach, may decrease risk of OASIS, episiotomy, and severe perineal lacerations.[21]

## References

1. Carroli G, Mignini L. Episiotomy for vaginal birth. *Cochrane Database Syst Rev.* 2009;1:CD000081. doi:10.1002/14651858.CD000081.pub2.

2. Hersh SR, Emeis CL. Mediolateral episiotomy: technique, practice, and training. *J Midwifery Womens Health.* 2020;65(3):404-409. doi:10.1111/jmwh.13096.

3. American College of Obstetricians and Gynecologists. Practice Bulletin No. 165: prevention and management of obstetric lacerations at vaginal delivery. *Obstet Gynecol.* 2016;128:e1-e15.

4. Jiang H, Qian X, Carroli G, Garner P. Selective versus routine use of episiotomy for vaginal birth. *Cochrane Database Syst Rev.* 2017;2:CD000081. doi:10.1002/14651858.CD000081.pub3.

5. Kalis V, Laine K, de Leeuw JW, et al. Classification of episiotomy: towards a standardization of terminology. *BJOG.* 2012;119(5):522-526. doi:10.1111/j.1471-0528.2011.03268.x.

6. *WHO Recommendations: Intrapartum Care for a Positive Childbirth Experience.* Geneva, Switzerland: World Health Organization; 2018.

7. Mahgoub S, Piant H, Gaudineau A, et al. Risk factors for obstetric anal sphincter injuries (OASIS) and the role of episiotomy: a retrospective series of 496 cases. *J Gynecol Obstet Hum Reprod.* 2019;48:657-662.

8. Pereira GMV, Hosoume RS, de Castro Monteiro MV, et al. Selective episiotomy versus no episiotomy for severe perineal trauma: a systematic review with meta-analysis. *Int Urogynecol J.* 2020;31(11):2291-2299. doi:10.1007/s00192-020-04308-2.

9. Sultan AH, Thakar R, Ismail KM, et al. The role of mediolateral episiotomy during operative vaginal delivery. *Eur J Obstet Gynecol Reprod Biol.* 2019;240:192-196. doi:10.1016/j.ejogrb.2019.07.005.

10. Leeman L, Spearman M, Rogers R. Repair of obstetric perineal lacerations. *Am Fam Physician.* 2003;68(8):1585-1590.

11. Arnold MJ, Sadler K, Leli K. Obstetric lacerations: prevention and repair. *Am Fam Physician.* 2021;103(12):745-752.

12. Royal College of Obstetricians and Gynaecologists. The management of third- and fourth-degree perineal tears: Green-Top Guideline No. 29. https://www.rcog.org.uk/media/5jeb5hzu/gtg-29.pdf. Published 2015. Accessed July 12, 2021.

13. Kalis V, Landsmanova J, Bednarova B, et. al. Evaluation of the incision angle of mediolateral episiotomy at 60 degrees. *Int J Gynaecol Obstet.* 2011;112:220-224.

14. Sooklim R, Thinkhamrop J, Lumbiganon P, et al. The outcomes of midline versus medio-lateral episiotomy. *Reprod Health.* 2007;4:10. doi:10.1186/1742-4755-4-10.

15. Ankarcrona V, Zhao H, Jacobsson B, et al. Obstetric anal sphincter injury after episiotomy in vacuum extraction: an epidemiological study using an emulated randomised trial approach. *BJOG.* February 4, 2021. doi:10.1111/1471-0528.16663.

16. van Bavel J, Hukkelhoven CWPM, de Vries C, et al. The effectiveness of mediolateral episiotomy in preventing obstetric anal sphincter injuries during operative vaginal delivery: a ten-year analysis of a national registry. *Int Urogynecol J.* 2018;29(3):407-413. doi:10.1007/s00192-017-3422-4.

17. Muhleman MA, Aly I, Walters A, et al. To cut or not to cut, that is the question: a review of the anatomy, the technique, risks, and benefits of an episiotomy. *Clin Anat.* 2017;30(3):362-372. doi:10.1002/ca.22836.

18. Ma K, Byrd L. Episiotomy: what angle do you cut to the midline? *Eur J Obstet Gynecol*

*Reprod Biol.* 2017;213:102-106. doi:10.1016/j.ejogrb .2017.04.006.

19. Aquino CI, Saccone G, Troisi J, et al. Is Ritgen's maneuver associated with decreased perineal lacerations and pain at delivery? *J Matern Fetal Neonatal Med.* 2020;33(18):3185-3192. doi:10.1080/14767058.2019.1568984.

20. Fahami F, Shokoohi Z, Kianpour M. The effects of perineal management techniques on labor complications. *Iran J Nurs Midwifery Res.* 2012;17(1):52-57.

21. Habek D, Tikvica Luetić A, Marton I, et al. Modified Ritgen maneuver in perineal protection: sixty-year experience. *Acta Clin Croat.* 2018;57(1):116-121. doi:10.20471/acc.2018.57.01.14.

# APPENDIX

# 30B

# Shoulder Dystocia

AMY MAROWITZ AND SHAUGHANASSEE VINES

*The editors acknowledge Linda A. Hunter, who was the author of this appendix in the previous edition.*

Shoulder dystocia is an intrapartum emergency that most midwives will inevitably encounter in clinical practice. Care is focused on systematic steps designed to minimize adverse outcomes, especially injury to the infant's brachial plexus. This appendix reviews the key points and steps required for safe intrapartum practice in the event of a shoulder dystocia.

Clinically, signs of an impending shoulder dystocia occur while the birthing person is pushing as the infant's head slowly extends and emerges over the perineum. Instead of fully extending, the vertex partially retracts back into the vagina, a phenomenon commonly referred to as the "turtle sign" (Figure 30B-1). For some birthing individuals with larger bodies, it may appear as if the "turtle sign" is occurring when, in reality, there is simply perineal soft tissue that impedes the extension and rotation of the infant's head.

Following birth of the head, restitution and external rotation do not occur, as the infant's shoulders have not followed the normal cardinal movements through the pelvis and are impacted in an anterior–posterior position. Abducting the person's hips (the McRoberts maneuver) causes the symphysis pubis to shift its inclination, which usually allows enough room for normal birth mechanisms to occur (Figure 30B-2).

During a shoulder dystocia, it is crucial that the midwife accurately diagnose the situation, remain calm, and perform a rapid assessment. After the head is born, some shoulder dystocias may resolve spontaneously if the midwife waits for the next contraction to allow for normal restitution and external rotation, then encourages the laboring person to push. If restitution and external rotation do not occur, it is important to first assess the location of the

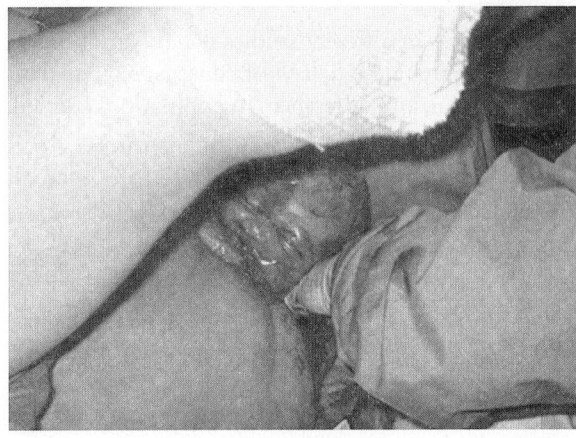

**Figure 30B-1** Turtle sign. Note that (1) the infant's chin cannot be seen because the head has retracted into the vagina and (2) the attendant has rotated the head. The turtle sign appears immediately following the birth of the head when the fetal face is looking toward the birthing person's back.

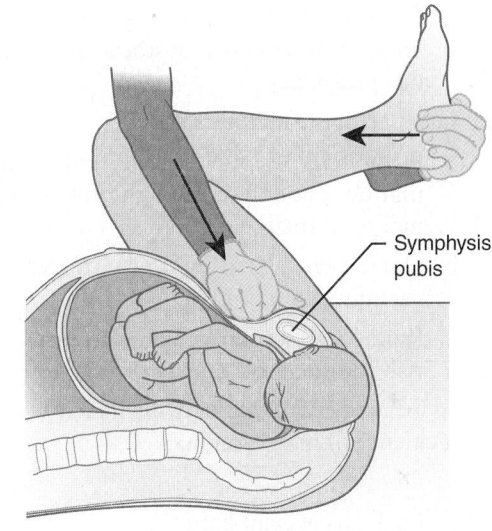

Symphysis pubis

**Figure 30B-2** McRoberts maneuver and suprapubic pressure.

shoulders prior to initiating any maneuvers (other than repositioning the birthing person).

Midwives who are attending births at home or in a birth center may need to enlist the assistance of the birthing person's partner and/or family if a shoulder dystocia is encountered. Even if the dystocia is resolved quickly, resuscitation assistance and ambulance transfer to the nearest hospital may still be needed for both the birthing person and their newborn.

## Definition of Shoulder Dystocia[1–4]

Need for ancillary maneuvers to deliver the shoulders.

## Incidence[1–4]

1. Varies in different studies due to variations in research design, lack of consensus on its definition, and differences in populations studied.
2. Contemporary review of literature: Incidence is approximately 0.2% to 3% of all births.
3. May be under-reported due to variations in study design, definition, and population.
4. Incidence rises with increasing fetal weight.
5. Incidence is highest in birthing persons who have diabetes and a macrosomic fetus.

## Risk Factors[1–4]

1. Prenatal risk factors
   a. Fetal macrosomia (more than 4000 grams)
   b. Maternal diabetes
   c. History of shoulder dystocia in a previous pregnancy
2. Intrapartum risk factors
   a. Precipitous second stage: Rapid descent that does not allow enough time for normal rotational maneuvers
   b. Operative vaginal delivery (forceps or vacuum extraction)
   c. Prolonged second stage (increases the risk for operative delivery)
3. Associated risks (all of which increase the incidence of macrosomia)
   a. Obesity
   b. Excessive weight gain
   c. Late term and post-term gestation

## Key Points

1. Stay calm and clearly communicate to the laboring person and the team.
2. Do not panic and do not rush.
3. Be systematic and deliberate in moving through the procedures.
4. Minimize traction on the fetal head.
5. Although there is no consensus on this issue, several professional organizations recommend that maneuvers be done when the laboring person is *not* pushing.
6. Do *not* let anyone perform suprapubic pressure until asked for by the person attending the birth.
7. Under *no* circumstances should anyone *ever* perform fundal pressure.
8. Try a maneuver once and then move on to another one; spend no more than 30 seconds on each maneuver.
9. Keep the team informed as each maneuver is performed.
10. Cut an episiotomy *only* if unable to get an entire hand into the vagina.
11. Continuously monitor the fetal heart rate if possible.
12. Do not clamp or cut a nuchal cord during a shoulder dystocia; plan to deliver the infant with the somersault maneuver once the dystocia is resolved (see the *Hand Maneuvers for Birth* appendix).
13. Be prepared for a postpartum hemorrhage after the infant is born.
14. Be prepared for a full neonatal resuscitation. Analysis of cord blood gases should be obtained if the shoulder dystocia was prolonged or if there is any sign of neonatal distress after the birth.
15. Neonatal asphyxia becomes a significant risk by 5 minutes. Rescue maneuvers (cephalic replacement or abdominal rescue) should be considered by 4 minutes. These will require transfer to the operating room and the availability of an obstetrician.

## Management Steps

There is no clear superiority in terms of the order in which release maneuvers are attempted. The circumstances and the midwife's judgment should guide the order of maneuvers when a shoulder dystocia occurs.

1. *Diagnose, inform the room, and ask for help.*
   - As soon as a shoulder dystocia is suspected, have the laboring person *stop* pushing and immediately assess the position of the fetal shoulders with a vaginal examination.
   - If the anterior shoulder is impacted, calmly and clearly state, "I have a shoulder dystocia."
   - Request help—additional nurses, the consulting physician, the neonatal team, and anesthesia should be called immediately.

2. *Perform McRoberts maneuver and suprapubic pressure.*
   - Have the laboring person move to the edge of the bed and then into *McRoberts position* (head flat on the bed, and knees and hips hyperflexed toward the abdomen; Figure 30B-3). Hyperflexing the legs does not increase pelvic diameters but causes cephalic rotation of the symphysis, so the symphysis slides up and over the anterior shoulder.
   - Direct another person to perform *suprapubic pressure* at a slight angle in the direction you are trying to rotate the shoulder toward the fetal chest.
   - The combination of McRoberts maneuver and suprapubic pressure will likely relieve

most shoulder dystocias. If it is not working, additional maneuvers are required.

3. *Begin internal maneuvers.* There is no evidence or expert consensus on the optimal order of internal maneuvers, although most clinicians advocate focusing the initial internal maneuvers on release of the posterior arm. Cut an episiotomy *only* if more room is needed to insert your hand. Keep team members, including the birthing person, informed.
   - *Delivery of the posterior arm.* Insert an entire hand in the posterior aspect of the vagina and follow the posterior arm to the infant's elbow. If the arm is extended, try to reach the forearm and bend the arm at the elbow until you can feel the infant's hand. Either grasp the hand or put gentle forward pressure on the elbow to sweep the arm across the chest and out of the vagina. There is an increased risk of humerus or clavicle fracture, but in the majority of cases, delivery of the posterior arm will relieve the dystocia.
   - *Shoulder shrug.* Gently move the fetal head anteriorly with one hand to make room for insertion of the other hand under the posterior shoulder. Using a pincer grasp (making a circle out of the thumb and forefinger) so that these fingers come together in the axillary fossa. Pull toward the vaginal opening to "shrug" the

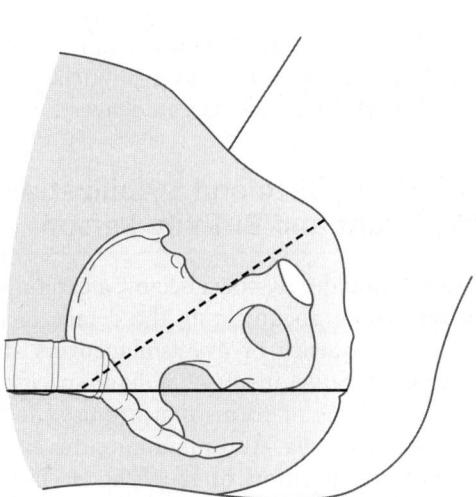 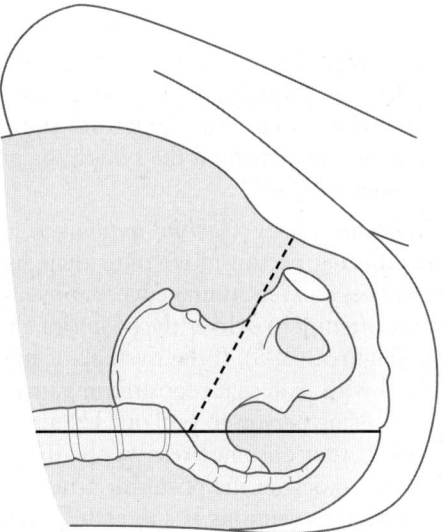

**Figure 30B-3** Effect of McRoberts maneuver on the symphysis. Notice that adduction of the legs toward the laboring person's abdomen moves the symphysis up so it slides over the fetal anterior shoulder.

shoulder. Maintain the grasp of the shoulder and the gentle pressure on the head, and rotate the head and shoulder as a unit toward the front of the fetus. The rotation may be done toward the fetal back if unable to rotate in the opposite direction. Once the fetus is rotated 180 degrees, deliver the anterior shoulder.[5]

- *Posterior axilla sling traction.* This technique uses the same principles as the shoulder shrug to release an impacted shoulder. However, rather than the attendant's finger, a neonatal suction tube is used for traction. This is accomplished by folding the suction tube in half and sliding it under the posterior arm in the axilla. One side of the tube is pulled through with the other hand.[6]

- *Rubin maneuver.* Insert a hand (or as many fingers as possible) behind the anterior shoulder on the fetal back and try to rotate the shoulder forward into an oblique position in the pelvis. This is also referred to as "collapsing the shoulders" and may help reduce the bisacromial shoulder diameter. An assistant can use directed suprapubic pressure at the same time. Use minimal and very gentle lateral traction (on the fetal shoulder—not the fetal head or neck). If this does not easily relieve the dystocia, repeated attempts will increase the force and the risk of brachial plexus injury and should not be continued.

- *Woods' screw maneuver.* Insert a hand (or as many fingers as possible) behind the anterior shoulder and in front of the posterior shoulder, and try to rotate the shoulders until the anterior shoulder emerges from behind the symphysis pubis (Figure 30B-4).

4. *Hands and Knees (Gaskin) maneuver.* Have the laboring person move onto their hands and knees and repeat maneuvers above, such as the attempt to deliver the posterior shoulder (Figure 30B-5). If the dystocia is not resolved with maternal repositioning, instruct the laboring person to pull one leg up into a lunge. If that does not resolve the dystocia, attempt to deliver the posterior arm. If none of these interventions is successful, *internal rotational maneuvers of the fetus* can be attempted in this position.

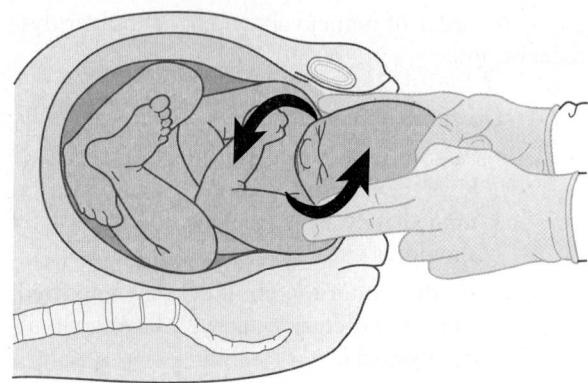

**Figure 30B-4** Woods' screw (rotational) maneuver.

To perform internal rotational maneuvers of the fetus, place a hand firmly against either the posterior or anterior shoulder, and push the shoulder clockwise or counterclockwise in an attempt to rotate it in a 180-degree arc. Continue to rotate the shoulders back and forth in whichever direction they will move until the impaction is dislodged and the infant is born. This maneuver may require both hands (one anterior and one posterior) pushing in opposite directions.

5. When the consulting physician or another provider enters the room, brief them about the steps taken so far and make a joint decision about who should try to facilitate the birth.

6. Intentional fracture of the clavicle may decrease the bisacromial diameter but may be difficult to perform in an emergent situation.

7. Rescue maneuvers include cephalic replacement (Zavanelli maneuver) or abdominal rescue, both of which require a full operating room team and a physician capable of performing a cesarean delivery.

## Following Birth and Stabilization of the Infant and Birthing Person

After a shoulder dystocia occurs, a carefully written delivery note documenting the details of the birth and the sequence of events/maneuvers should be completed. Some institutions have specific delivery note templates or forms that are used following a shoulder dystocia. At a minimum, this note should include the position of the head at birth, which shoulder was anterior, time of the birth of the head, who was present or called, maneuvers that were

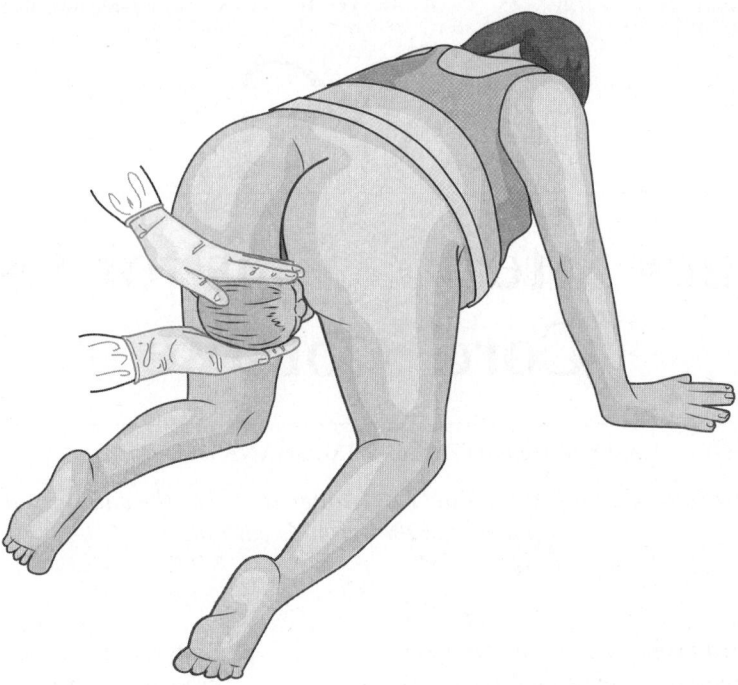

**Figure 30B-5** Hands and knees maneuver with attempt to deliver the posterior shoulder.

done and in which order, time of the delivery of the body, newborn weight and Apgar scores, cord blood gas results if obtained, disposition of the newborn, and any motor deficit in the upper extremities noted on initial newborn examination. In addition, any maternal injuries should be noted. Midwives should avoid using the term "traction" or trying to quantify the amount of force used when documenting their care during a shoulder dystocia. From a medicolegal standpoint, it should be noted that fundal pressure was not used. The events should be explained clearly and simply with no attempts to editorialize or speculate.

Shoulder dystocia is a traumatizing event for all involved. It may be helpful for the midwife to organize a debriefing with the other staff and providers who were present as soon as possible to discuss what happened in a nonthreatening, supportive way. The midwife should also stay in close contact with the laboring person and their support persons. In the event of a serious shoulder dystocia, they may be facing devastating neonatal consequences and need ongoing support and follow-up. It is also essential that the midwife provides honest and accurate information to the laboring person and their support persons regarding what happened during the birth without any blame or judgment.

## References

1. Hansen A, Chauhan SP. Shoulder dystocia: definitions and incidence. *Semin Perinat.* 2014;38:184-188.
2. American College of Obstetricians and Gynecologists. ACOG Practice Bulletin No. 40: shoulder dystocia. *Obstet Gynecol.* 2002;100:1045-1050. [Reaffirmed 2015].
3. Royal College of Obstetricians and Gynaecologists. *RCOG Green-Top Guideline No. 42.* London, UK: Royal College of Obstetricians and Gynaecologists; 2012.
4. Society of Obstetricians and Gynaecologists of Canada. Shoulder dystocia. In: *Advances in Labour and Risk Management Textbook. ALARM International Program Manual.* 22nd ed. Ottawa, Canada: Society of Obstetricians and Gynaecologists of Canada; 2016. https://www.glowm.com/resource-type/resource/textbook/title/advances-in-labor-and-risk-management/resource-doc/15. Accessed October 23, 2017.
5. Sancetta R, Khanzada H, Leante R. Shoulder shrug maneuver to facilitate delivery during shoulder dystocia. *Obstet Gynecol.* 2019;133(6):1178-1181. doi:10.1097/AOG.0000000000003278.
6. Hoek J, Verkouteren B, van Hamont D. Posterior axilla sling traction: a new technique for severe shoulder dystocia. *BMJ Case Rep.* 2019;12(3):e226882. doi:10.1136/bcr-2018-226882.

A P P E N D I X

# 30C

# Emergency Interventions for Umbilical Cord Prolapse

AMY MAROWITZ AND SHAUGHANASSEE VINES

*The editors acknowledge Linda A. Hunter, who was the author of this appendix in the previous edition.*

An overt umbilical cord prolapse is an intrapartum emergency that will require an expedited birth, almost always via cesarean delivery. However, under some circumstances, such as an umbilical cord prolapse with a double footling breech presentation during the second stage of labor, a vaginal birth can occur more quickly and safely than a cesarean birth.

Often the first sign of a cord prolapse is a sudden fetal bradycardia or recurrent variable decelerations that rapidly become more severe. Management of this acute situation requires prompt action on the part of the midwife in recognizing the prolapse and performing the appropriate life-saving interventions while an operating room team and the consulting physician are mobilized. Figure 30C-1 depicts the types of umbilical cord prolapse.

## Definitions[1–3]

1. *Overt cord prolapse:* The cord slips completely out of the cervix and is protruding in the vagina (Figure 30-1, panel A).

2. *Funic cord prolapse (also called cord presentation):* The cord is palpable in front of the presenting part (Figure 30-1, panel B).

   a. A funic presentation requires consultation with the collaborating physician to develop the most appropriate management plan.

3. *Compound cord presentation:* The cord is compressed alongside the presenting part in the lower uterine segment or inner cervix (Figure 30-1, panel C).

   a. Maternal repositioning or gentle upward pressure on the fetal head during a cervical examination can relieve an occult cord prolapse.

   b. If fetal heart rate (FHR) decelerations are present, intrauterine resuscitation measures should be initiated (see the *Fetal Assessment During Labor* chapter).

## Risk Factors[1–3]

1. Prematurity
2. Multifetal gestation
3. Multiparity
4. Polyhydramnios
5. Breech or shoulder presentation
6. Rupture of membranes: intentional or spontaneous with an unengaged head
7. Interventions such as manual rotation of the fetal head, amnioinfusion, insertion of transcervical balloon catheters, insertion of an intrauterine pressure catheter (IUPC), or application of scalp electrode

## Management Steps[1–3]

1. Call for help immediately and do not leave the pregnant person.
2. Clearly state, "I have a prolapsed umbilical cord."

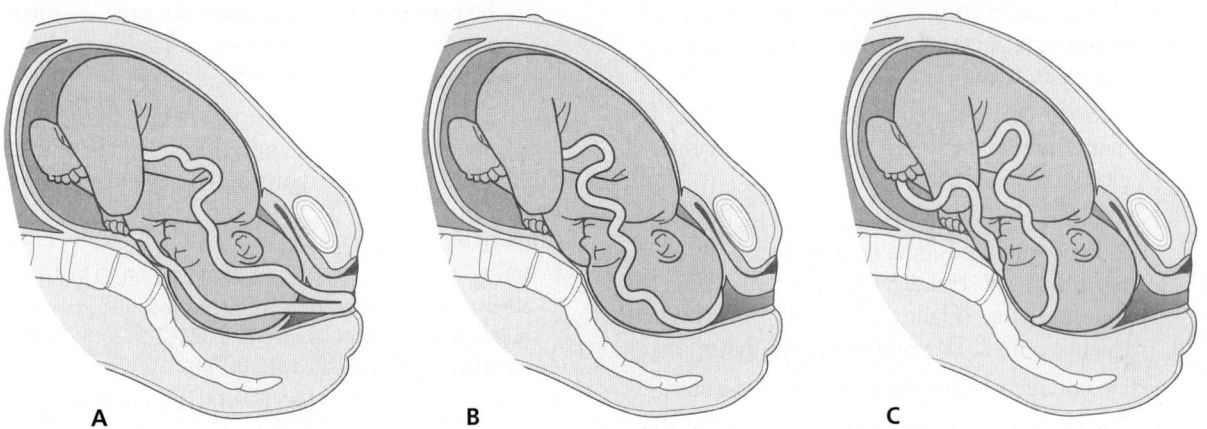

**Figure 30C-1** Umbilical cord prolapse. **A.** Overt cord prolapse. **B.** Funic cord prolapse. **C.** Compound cord presentation.

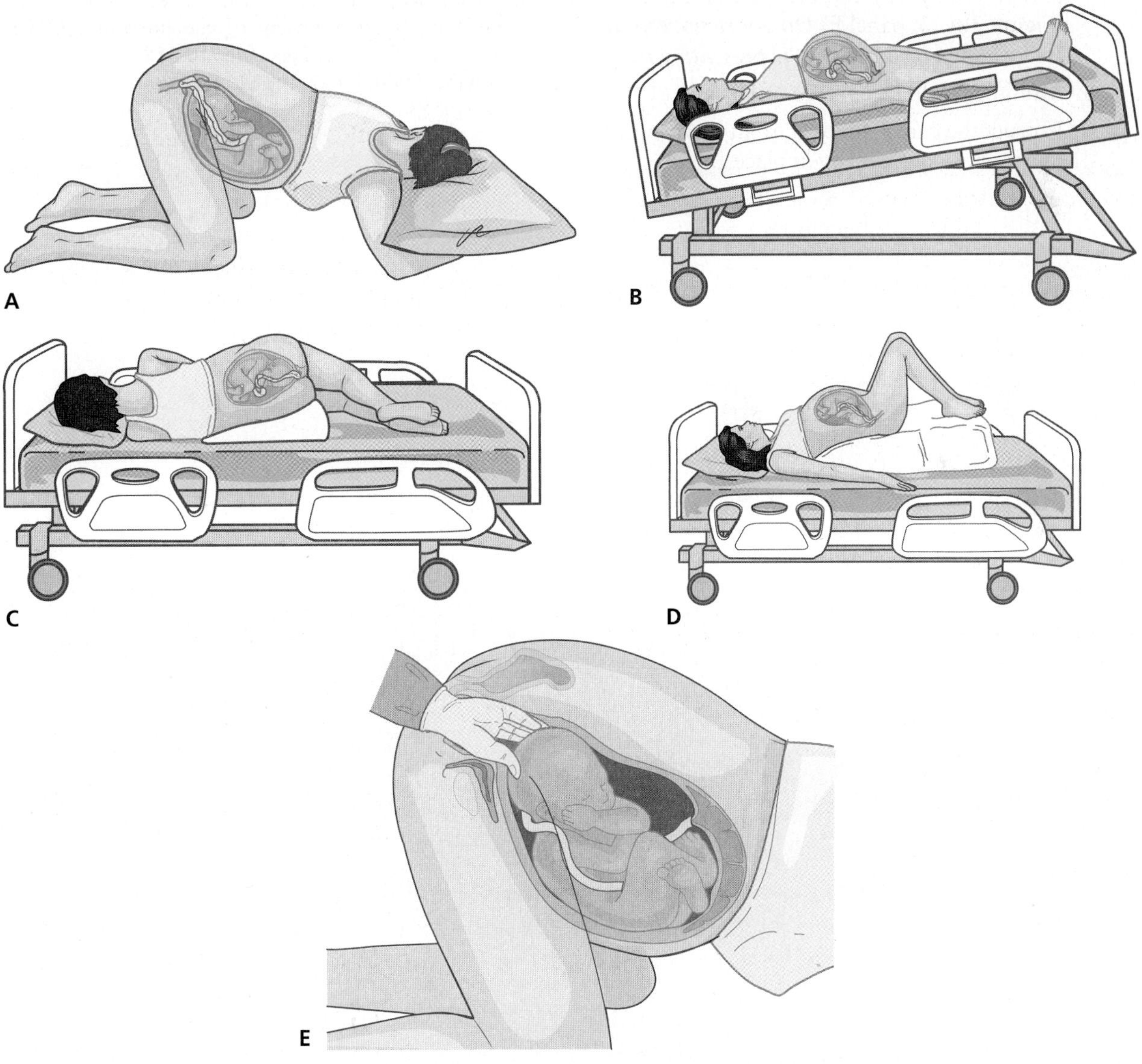

**Figure 30C-2** Repositioning of the birthing person during umbilical cord prolapse. **A.** Knee–chest. **B.** Trendelenburg. **C.** Side-lying with pelvic wedge. **D.** Supine with pelvic wedge. **E.** Hand/fingers pushing up on fetal head while laboring person is in knee–chest position.

3. Direct others to page a physician capable of performing a cesarean and notify the operating room team.

4. Inform the pregnant person of what is happening and explain the need for an emergency cesarean birth.

5. Reposition the pregnant person in the bed. A knee–chest position is best (**Figure 30C-2, A**). However, Trendelenburg (**Figure 30C-2, B**), side-lying (**Figure 30C-2, C**), or supine (**Figure 30C-2, D**) are other position options.

6. Do *not* attempt to replace the cord in the uterus.

7. Put a sterile glove on and get into or on the bed. Insert several fingers or a hand into the vagina and firmly push up on the presenting part to relieve any compression on the cord (**Figure 30C-3, panel E**) *Do not remove your fingers/hand or let up on the presenting part.*

8. Monitor the FHR continuously.

9. Instruct the care team to start an intravenous line if one is not already in place.

10. Be prepared to accompany the pregnant person into the operating room in this position while riding on the bed.

11. The operating room staff will place the sterile drapes over you, and the physician will let you know when you can remove your hand.

## References

1. Wong L, Kwan AHW, Lau SL, et al. Umbilical cord prolapse: revisiting its definition and management. *Am J Obstet Gynecol.* 2021;225(4):357-366. doi:10.1016/j.ajog.2021.06.077.

2. Sayed Ahmed WA, Hamdy MA. Optimal management of umbilical cord prolapse. *Int J Womens Health.* 2018;10:459-465. doi:10.2147/IJWH.S130879.

3. Pagan M, Eads L, Sward L, et al. Umbilical cord prolapse: a review of the literature. *Obstet Gynecol Surv.* 2020;75(8):510-518. doi:10.1097/OGX.0000000000000818.

# 30D

# Intrapartum Management of Twin Gestation

AMY MAROWITZ AND SHAUGHANASSEE VINES

*The editors acknowledge Linda A. Hunter, who was the author of this appendix in a previous edition.*

Midwifery management of a planned twin birth should always occur in a hospital in close collaboration with a physician capable of performing a cesarean birth. Many institutions require vaginal delivery of twins to occur in the operating room with anesthesia and an operating room team on standby. The neonatal (or pediatric) team should also be notified as soon as possible of a twin labor admission to ensure the presence of adequate nursing staff and personnel capable of full neonatal resuscitation of both newborns. Regardless of how the fetuses were identified during pregnancy, the first twin to deliver is referred to as "Baby A" and the second twin is "Baby B."

## Incidence

Approximately 3% of all births are multiple gestations.

## Types of Twins[1]

1. Monochorionic–monoamniotic (mono-mono)
   a. Requires referral for medical management
   b. Delivery by cesarean birth typically at 32 weeks[1]
2. Monochorionic–diamniotic (mono-di)
3. Dichorionic–diamniotic (di-di)

## Risks Associated with Twin Deliveries[1]

- Preterm birth
- Malpresentation
- Prolapsed umbilical cord
- Placental separation (especially between the birth of Twin A and Twin B)
- Postpartum hemorrhage
- Preeclampsia
- Placenta previa

## Intrapartum Care Guidelines for Twin Gestations

1. Upon arrival in labor, the presentation and lie of each fetus should be reassessed with ultrasound.
2. Ultrasound findings should be reviewed with the consulting physician to determine the risks and benefits of planned vaginal birth in light of the findings. This plan should be discussed with the laboring person and their informed consent obtained.
3. The laboring person should have an intravenous line inserted with blood drawn for a blood type, antibody screen, and cross-match.

4. Care related of labor pain is no different for twins, including use of epidural anesthesia if the laboring person desires this intervention. Epidural analgesia is recommended in many institutions because it can provide anesthesia for an emergency cesarean birth if needed, as well as assure comfort of the laboring person during complex internal maneuvers, if necessary.

5. Continuous fetal monitoring of both fetuses is required throughout labor with an electronic fetal monitor that can record both fetuses' heart rates simultaneously. A fetal scalp electrode should be inserted on Baby A only if medically indicated.

6. The consulting physician should be in the hospital and present in the room during the births. It is generally recommended that the births occur in an operating room, as there is a significant risk of needing an emergency cesarean birth for Baby B.

7. The management of Baby A's birth is no different than a singleton gestation. An episiotomy should be done only if medically indicated.

8. The umbilical cord from Baby A should be clamped and marked so that it is clear that this cord is from Baby A. For example, use one clamp for Baby A and two clamps for Baby B.

9. After the birth of Baby A, Baby B's position and presentation should be immediately assessed with ultrasound and the laboring person's cervix checked for dilation and the station of the presenting part determined.

10. Baby B's fetal heart rate should be monitored continuously, as this is the period of risk for umbilical cord prolapse.

11. If Baby B is presenting vertex, care should be taken if rupturing the membranes to avoid a prolapsed umbilical cord. Do not rupture the membranes if Baby B is not engaged in the pelvis.

12. If Baby B is not vertex, the physician should take over care, especially if a breech extraction is anticipated.

13. A postpartum hemorrhage should be anticipated and the appropriate uterotonic medications and/or blood products should be immediately available.

14. The umbilical cords should be carefully marked to differentiate Baby A from Baby B and the placenta(s) sent to pathology if necessary.

## Reference

1. American College of Obstetricians and Gynecologists' Committee on Practice Bulletins—Obstetrics, Society for Maternal-Fetal Medicine. Multifetal gestations: twin, triplet, and higher-order multifetal pregnancies: ACOG Practice Bulletin, Number 231. *Obstet Gynecol.* 2021;137(6):e145-e162. doi:10.1097/AOG.0000000000004397.

APPENDIX

# 30E

# Breech Birth

AMY MAROWITZ AND SHAUGHANASSEE VINES

As discussed in the chapter, there may be circumstances when a pregnant person with a known breech presentation is planning a vaginal birth. Planned vaginal breech births should take place within a hospital setting under the primary care of an obstetrician. Midwives in clinical practice are more likely to encounter a pregnant person in advanced labor with a previously unknown breech presentation. Every attempt should be made to mobilize a team to perform a cesarean birth or have an experienced individual assist with a breech birth. However, if the birth is imminent, it may occur vaginally. This appendix reviews the techniques for a vaginal breech birth. All midwives are encouraged to periodically review these steps so as to be prepared if this situation arises. As with other intrapartum emergencies, participation in simulation drills focused on vaginal breech birth has been shown to improve provider confidence and team communication. Midwives are encouraged to participate in these types of training experiences.

## Incidence of Breech Presentation

Of all pregnancies, 3% to 4% have a breech presentation at term.[1]

## Types of Breech Presentations[1]

There are three types of breech presentations, as shown in Figure 30E-1.

- *Frank breech (50% to 70%)*. The lower extremities are flexed at the hips, with the legs extended and the feet near the infant's head ("pike" position). The presenting part is the infant's buttocks. One buttock may present ahead of the other, making it harder to diagnosis the breech via vaginal exam.

- *Complete breech (5% to 10%)*. Both the hips and knees are flexed, with both feet above the infant's buttocks ("cannonball" position). The presenting part is the infant's buttocks. One buttock may present ahead of the other, making it harder to diagnosis via vaginal exam.

- *Footling (incomplete) breech (10% to 40%)*. One or both feet extend below the infant's buttocks and present in the vagina. This can be either a single or double footling presentation.

## Predisposing Factors[2-4]

- Preterm gestation
- Multifetal gestation
- Multiparity with lax uterine tone
- Polyhydramnios
- Oligohydramnios
- Uterine anomalies (bicornuate uterus)
- Uterine fibroids (especially in the lower uterine segment)
- Placenta previa
- Fetal anomalies (hydrocephaly, aneuploidy, nuchal masses)

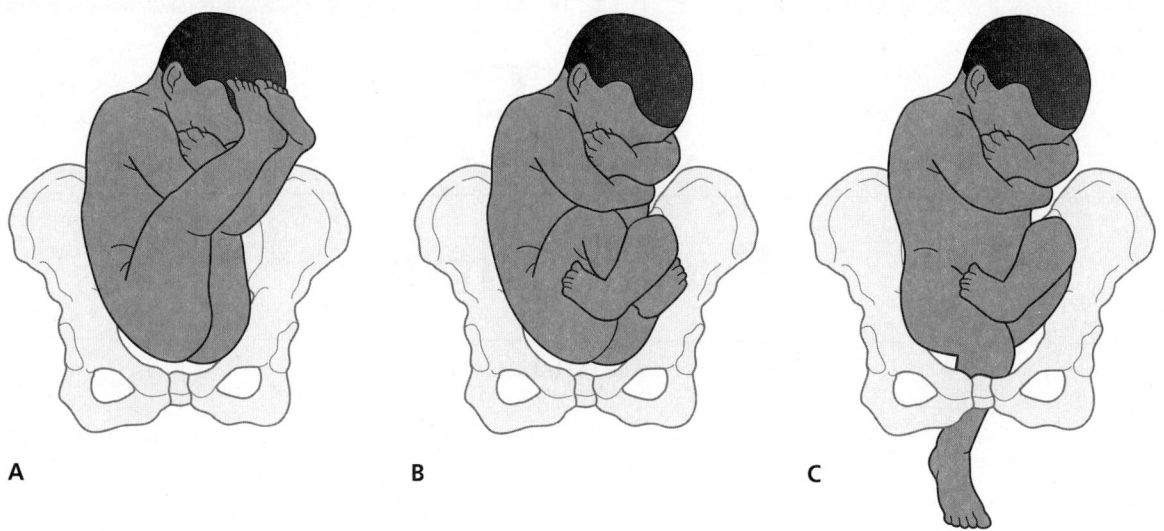

A                                    B                                    C

**Figure 30E-1** Types of breech presentation. **A.** Frank breech. **B.** Complete breech. **C.** Footling (incomplete) breech.

## Factors That May Improve the Success of Vaginal Breech Birth[2-4]

- Average-size fetus (2500–3800 grams) with no known anomalies
- Pelvis of sufficient size to allow for previous vaginal birth of fetus as big as or bigger than in the current pregnancy
- Frank or complete breech
- Documentation of fetal head flexion (by ultrasound)
- Spontaneous labor with normal progress
- Easy, spontaneous delivery of the buttocks and thighs

## Key Points

1. Abdominal palpation for fetal presentation is an important assessment tool but may be unreliable in determining presentation during active labor.

2. When performing a cervical examination on a person in labor, palpation of the fetal skull sutures confirms a vertex presentation.

3. *Any* suspicion for breech presentation should always be confirmed with ultrasound.

4. In out-of-hospital sites, the midwife may have to rely on abdominal palpation and a careful vaginal examination to palpate the fetal skull sutures. There should be no hesitation to transfer the laboring person to a hospital if a breech presentation is suspected. The midwife should also call 911 for additional help and notify the consulting physician, especially if the laboring person declines transfer or the birth is imminent.

5. The infant's sacrum is the denominator (anatomic landmark for determining the position in the pelvis).

6. If the pregnant person has any contraindications to a vaginal breech birth, transfer to a hospital or operating room and preparation for a cesarean birth is indicated. If contraindications are present, the midwife should assist with a vaginal birth only if the birth occurs before a cesarean birth can be facilitated.

7. When a breech birth is imminent, the midwife should request the assistance of any available obstetrician (or a more experienced midwife if a physician is not available). The neonatal or pediatric team should also be called and the staff prepared for full infant resuscitation. Anesthesia and an operating room team should be on standby in the event that surgical intervention is needed.

8. During the birth, the infant may pass thick meconium stool from compression of the abdomen and breech in the vagina. This is

often the first indication during labor of a "missed breech" presentation.

9. The fetal heart rate should be monitored continuously. The laboring person should also have an intravenous line inserted if possible.

10. Vaginal breech birth requires a "hands-off" approach until the breech is delivered to the level of the umbilicus. Considerable patience is required to allow for spontaneous progression of the normal cardinal movements (listed in the next section). The laboring person should be encouraged to push, and their progress monitored closely.

11. Vaginal breech birth in an upright position (hands and knees, kneeling or standing) has been investigated as an alternative to a supine position. One recent study found that an upright position for a vaginal breech birth resulted in shorter second stages, less need for extraction techniques, and fewer neonatal injuries.[5]

## Cardinal Movements and Techniques for a Breech Birth

1. Descent occurs throughout and is facilitated by the laboring person's pushing efforts.

2. Engagement of the hips usually takes place when the infant's bitrochanteric diameter (the distance between the outer points of the hips) enters the oblique diameter of the maternal pelvis. The position will then be either right sacrum anterior (RSA) or left sacrum anterior (LSA).

3. The anterior hip usually descends more rapidly than the posterior hip.

4. As resistance from the pelvic floor is encountered, internal rotation of 45 degrees will occur and the anterior hip will pass under the pubic bone. The bitrochanteric diameter of the hips is now in the anterior–posterior diameter of the laboring person's pelvis in either a right sacrum transverse (RST) or left sacrum transverse (LST) position.

5. As descent continues, the anterior hip provides a pivot for the posterior hip, which usually crosses the perineum first. Delivery of the anterior hip will follow through lateral flexion of the spine.

6. Until this point in time, the laboring person should push as needed, and descent of the breech should be observed closely. The midwife should resist the temptation to pull the buttocks out and allow the pushing efforts to continue as in any normally progressing second stage. If the infant is born too quickly, the head may not have time to flex or the fetal arms may become entrapped.

7. Once the buttocks are born and the umbilicus is visible at the perineum, the legs should birth spontaneously through the vaginal opening, usually one at a time. Sometimes when the infant is in a frank breech presentation, full extension of the legs can hinder descent and birth of the legs.

8. If the fetal legs do not birth after 20-30 seconds, the birth of the legs can be assisted in between pushing efforts by inserting either the right or left hand (depending on the sacrum's position) and following the thigh to the popliteal fossa behind the knee. The midwife's thumb should be on the anterior side of the fetal thigh. Gently press on the popliteal fossa and move the leg laterally away from the midline. This will cause the leg to flex at the knee, thereby bringing the foot down to where it can be grasped. Bring the leg down and out of the vagina by drawing it across the infant's abdomen in its natural range of motion. Repeat the maneuver for the other leg if needed. This procedure, called *Pinard's maneuver*, is used to "break up the breech" (Figure 30E-2).

9. After the trunk, legs, and feet are delivered, external rotation will occur, aligning the

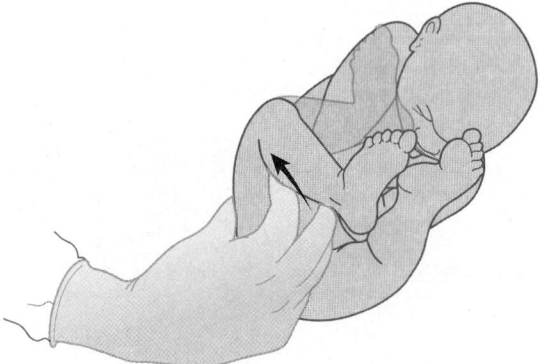

**Figure 30E-2** If there is a delay with the birth of the legs after the breech has been born to the umbilicus, the midwife can apply gentle pressure in the popliteal fossa and move the leg laterally away from the midline to reach the fetal foot (Pinard's maneuver).

infant's back into a sacrum anterior position ("bum to tum"). This will cause the shoulders to rotate internally into the oblique diameter of the maternal pelvis and pass under the pubic bone. It is important for the fetus to be aligned this way

10. The remainder of the birth should occur within the next 3 to 5 minutes to avoid hypoxia from compression of the umbilical cord. A generous loop of the umbilical cord can be pulled down to prevent stress at the umbilical insertion site.

11. Wrap a warm towel around the infant's lower body just below the umbilicus. This will keep the infant warm and provide a hold on the hips that is not slippery.

12. To facilitate birth of the shoulders, gently grasp the hips by placing the thumbs on the sacrum and the fingers on the corresponding iliac crests (**Figure 30E-3**). Avoid any pressure on the soft-tissue areas of the abdomen or flank.

13. Provide downward and outward traction on the body with coordinated pushing from the laboring person, and gently rotate the infant to either an RST or LST position (Figure 30E-4).

14. Continue downward traction with the labor person's pushing efforts until both the scapula and the axilla of the anterior shoulder are visible.

15. *Delivery of shoulders and arms.* There are different techniques for delivery of the shoulders and arms, and it does not matter which shoulder is delivered first. Typically, the anterior shoulder will appear as a result of the downward traction placed on the body. Once the axilla is visible, the arm can then be delivered by reaching in to the elbow and sweeping the arm up across the chest. Once the anterior arm is out, the infant should be rotated 180 degrees, keeping the back up. This will bring the posterior scapula and axilla into view anteriorly, and this arm can be delivered in the same manner.

16. *Delivery of the posterior arm.* If the anterior shoulder does not appear with downward traction, the posterior arm can be delivered first. Grasp the feet securely in one hand and lift the body up and over toward the maternal abdominal side until the scapula and

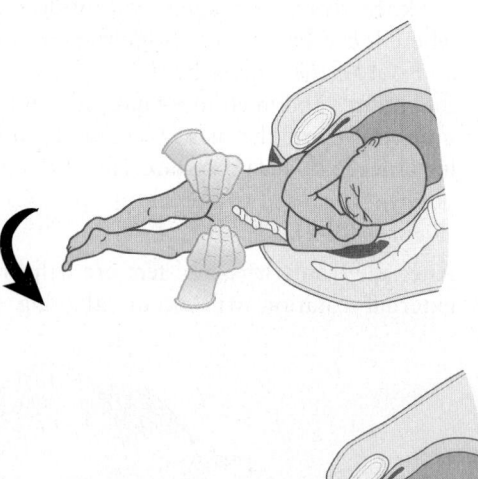

**Figure 30E-3** If rotation is needed, the midwife's hands can be placed on the infant's lower body with thumbs over the sacroiliac joint and gentle rotational pressure applied to the pelvis. Not shown in this figure is a towel, which should be wrapped around the newborn's lower body, just below the umbilicus.

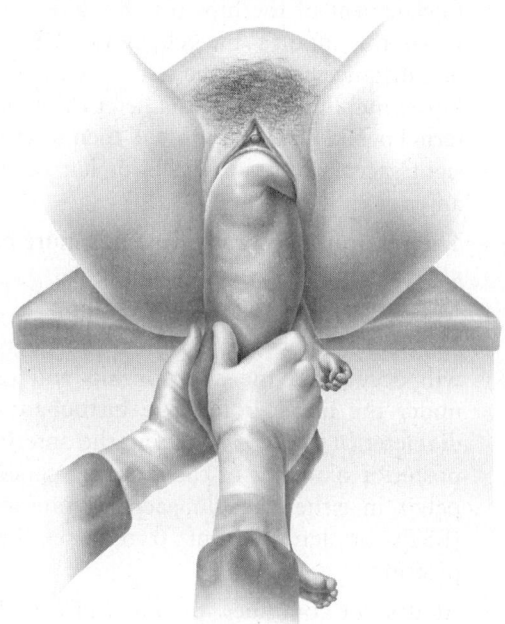

**Figure 30E-4** Birth of the anterior shoulder by downward traction. Note the placement of the midwife's hands on the infant's hips. Not shown: Towel wrapped around newborn's lower body.

axilla are visible posteriorly at the perineum. Insert the other hand along the upper arm to the elbow and sweep the arm across the chest. Now the infant can be either repositioned with gentle downward traction again or rotated until the anterior shoulder and axilla are in view (Figure 30E-5).

17. Engagement of the head usually occurs in one of the oblique pelvic diameters. Internal rotation is facilitated by delivery of the shoulders; once the arms are released, the head is generally in an occiput anterior position, with the back of the neck visible at the vaginal introitus.

18. It is very important *not* to let the head rotate to the occiput posterior position, as any traction on the body will cause extension of the head and increase the chances of entrapment.

19. Delivery of the head is best accomplished by stabilizing the fetal head between both of the provider's hands, maintaining head flexion, and applying gentle directional pressure, known as the *Mauriceau–Smellie–Veit*

*maneuver* (Figure 30E-6). Several variations of this maneuver exist, in which the hand is inserted posteriorly into the vagina and the fingers are positioned carefully around the fetal face to facilitate flexion of the head. Most commonly, the index and middle fingers are placed on either side of the nose on the maxilla and downward pressure is applied to maintain flexion of the head. Extreme care must be taken to avoid any pressure on the lower jaw or accidentally inserting the fingers into the orbit of the eyes. Although insertion of a finger into the infant's mouth is sometimes described as part of this maneuver, this modification could cause serious damage to the tongue, jaw, and surrounding tissues.

20. Once the fingers of the posterior hand are in place on the maxilla, rest the infant's body astride the length of the arm. Place the other hand on top of the infant and hook the index and middle fingers of this hand onto the shoulders on each side of the infant's neck.

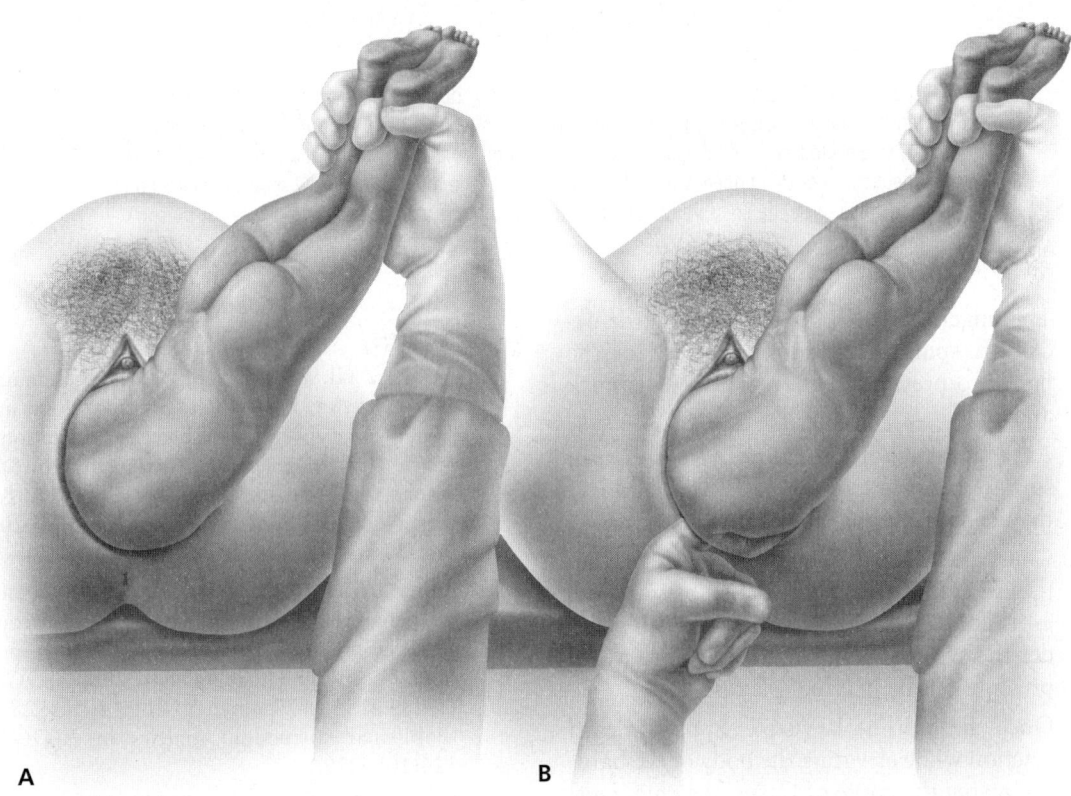

**A**  **B**

**Figure 30E-5** Delivery of the posterior arm. **A.** Birth of the posterior shoulder by upward traction. **B.** Freeing the posterior arm. Not shown: Towel wrapped around the newborn's lower body.

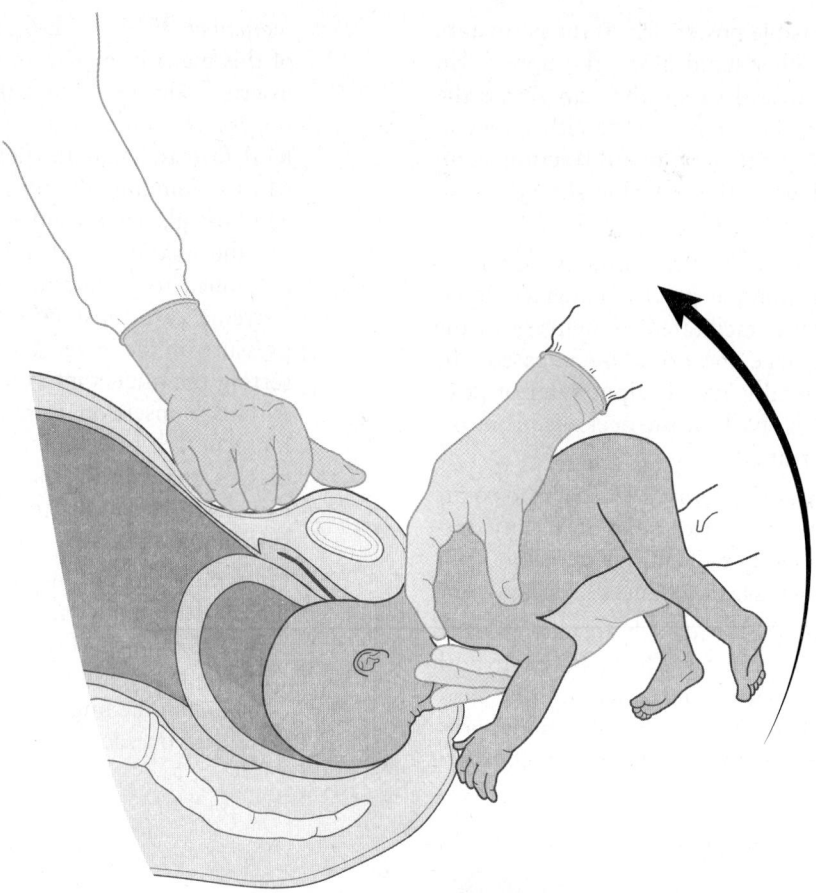

**Figure 30E-6** To assist with the birth of the head, downward traction is applied until the infant's hairline is visible. Then, gentle upward traction (shown here) is applied while the infant's body is elevated and suprapubic pressure is provided by an assistant (Mauriceau–Smellie–Veit maneuver). Note that fingers are on the maxilla, not in the mouth. The arrow shows the direction of the curve of gentle pressure to help birth the head by pivoting it against the birthing person's pelvic bone.

The fingers can also be placed along the occiput to splint the infant's head between the hands to prevent any extension of the neck and head.

21. An assistant should be directed to perform suprapubic pressure to maintain flexion of the head during this part of the birth.

22. Continue to apply gentle downward traction with the infant sandwiched between the arms/hands until the hairline is visible under the symphysis pubis. Take care to avoid pressure on the brachial plexus.

23. Once the hairline is visible, apply upward traction while elevating the body of the baby. Following the curve of Carus, the chin, face, brow, anterior fontanel, and the remainder of the head are delivered in sequence across the perineum.

## References

1. Hofmeyr GJ. Overview of breech presentation. In: *UpToDate*. Lockwood CJ, ed. https://www.uptodate.com/contents/overview-of-breech-presentation?search=overview-of-breech-%20presentation&source=search_result&selectedTitle=1~150&usage_type=default&display_rank=1. Published 2021. Accessed November 10, 2021.

2. Impey LWM, Murphy DJ, Griffiths M, Penna LK, on behalf of Royal College of Obstetricians and Gynaecologists. Management of breech presentation: Green-top Guideline No. 20b. *BJOG*. 2017;124(7):e151-e177. doi:10.1111/1471-0528.14465. [Published correction appears in *BJOG*. 2017;124(10):e279.]

3. Kotaska A, Menticoglou S. No. 384: management of breech presentation at term. *J Obstet Gynaecol Can*. 2019;41(8):1193-1205. doi:10.1016/j.jogc.2018.12.018.

4. ACOG Committee Opinion No. 745: mode of term singleton breech delivery. *Obstet Gynecol.* 2018;132(2):e60-e63. doi:10.1097/AOG.0000000000002755.

5. Louwen F, Daviss BA, Johnson KC, Reitter A. Does breech delivery in an upright position instead of on the back improve outcomes and avoid cesareans? *Int J Gynaecol Obstet.* 2017;136(2):151-161. doi:10.1002/ijgo.12033.

CHAPTER

# 31

# Third Stage of Labor

MAVIS N. SCHORN

## Introduction

The birth of a child is exciting and the pinnacle of an intense and emotional period for the birthing person and family. However, the time immediately following the birth is also a critical one for both the person who gave birth and the newborn. The expulsion of the placenta and physiologic stabilization immediately following this event represent a period of great vulnerability. Postpartum hemorrhage (PPH) is one of the leading causes of childbirth-related perinatal morbidity and mortality, both worldwide and in the United States; when it occurs, it most often does so during the third or fourth stage of labor.[1] Moreover, the first hour after birth is a "sensitive period" both psychologically and physiologically, wherein continuous contact potentially has significant benefits for the person who gave birth as well as the newborn.[2] This chapter reviews the third stage of labor, methods for promoting normal physiologic adaptation, perinatal complications that can occur during this time period, and management strategies for complications of the third stage.

## Definitions

The third stage of labor is defined as the period following the birth of the newborn through the expulsion of the placenta. A duration of longer than 30 minutes without placental expulsion is the conventionally accepted criterion for the diagnosis of *prolonged third stage of labor*, which is also known as *retained placenta*. Retained placenta is associated with an increased risk for hemorrhage and related complications arising from manual removal of the placenta.[3-6]

## Physiology of the Third Stage of Labor

### Duration of the Third Stage

The length of time for the third stage of labor to be completed is usually within 10 minutes.[6,7] Based on a review of more than 12,000 births, only 3% of third stages have a duration that is longer than 30 minutes.[8] The duration of the third stage of labor is commonly longer in preterm gestations compared to term gestations[9] and for individuals with higher body mass index (BMI).[10] Although the outer limit of normalcy has not been conclusively determined for any gestational age or maternal BMI, the risk of complications increases with longer duration of the third stage at all gestations and peripartum weights.[3-6]

In a setting in which uterotonic medications were routinely administered during the third stage of labor, researchers reported that the mean duration of the third stage was 5.6 minutes and the 99th percentile was 28 minutes.[8] In this analysis, the risk for PPH was significantly increased (adjusted odds ratio [aOR] 1.82; 95% confidence interval [CI], 1.43–3.21; 13.2% versus 8.3%) when the duration of the third stage was greater than 20 minutes.[8] Although this finding suggests the diagnosis of retained placenta should be applied when the third stage lasts 20 minutes or more,[8] a period of 30 minutes without placental expulsion continues to be the standard definition for the prolonged third stage or retained placenta in the United States. The World Health Organization (WHO) recommends that, in the absence of bleeding, intervention not be initiated until 60 minutes after birth if the placenta has not been expelled,[11] and European countries have wide variations in practices related to this condition.[5]

## Placental Separation

Contraction frequency and intensity in the third stage of labor are similar to the corresponding measures during the second stage of labor,[9,12] although contractions are often felt only minimally, if at all, by the birthing person, especially compared to the sensations associated with contractions immediately before the birth of the neonate. These post-birth contractions constrict the blood vessels that supply the placenta, resulting in hemostasis. Placental separation is the result of an abrupt decrease in size of the uterine cavity following birth of the neonate. As the uterus contracts, the placental implantation surface area decreases without a corresponding change in the placental size. This sudden disproportion between the area of implantation and the placental size causes the placenta to buckle and separate from the decidua.

After the placenta separates, it descends through the lower uterine segment and into the upper vaginal vault, causing clinical signs of placental separation. Table 31-1 lists the common signs of placental separation. During placental separation, women who do not have analgesia may experience a slight increase in the perception of contraction intensity and pelvic floor discomfort.

## Placental Expulsion

Expulsion of the placenta occurs by one of two mechanisms: Schultze or Duncan.

| Table 31-1 | Signs of Placental Separation |
|---|---|
| **Signs of Placental Separation** | **Physiologic Explanation** |
| A small gush of blood | With separation, some blood escapes from between the placenta and the decidua. |
| Lengthening of the umbilical cord | As the placenta descends into the vagina, the cord lengthens at the vaginal introitus. |
| Rise of the uterus into the abdomen | As the placenta descends into the vagina, the uterus is displaced cephalad. |
| The uterus becomes firm and rounded | Once the placenta is expelled from the uterus, the uterine smooth muscles contract more firmly, altering the shape of the uterus. |

In the *Schultze mechanism*, which is the most common, the placenta separates centrally. The fetal side of the placenta—the side with a smooth, shining membrane continuous with the sheath of the chorion (which also covers the umbilical cord)—drops to the lower portion of the uterus. It then exits, fetal side first, through the cervix into the vagina, onto the birthing person's pelvic floor, and is expelled. The membranes are expelled last, with the uterine side of the placenta inside the amniotic sac. This mechanism, in effect, inverts the placenta and amniotic sac, and causes the membranes to peel off the remainder of the decidua and trail behind the placenta. The majority of bleeding that occurs during this mechanism may remain hidden until the placenta and membranes are expelled, as the blood is captured behind the placenta and inside the amniotic sac (Figure 31-1).

During the *Duncan mechanism*, which occurs less frequently, the placenta separates marginally. The placenta then slides into the cervical opening without inverting, so that the uterine side of the placenta, with dark red cotyledons, is expelled at the same time as the fetal side. Blood escapes between the membranes and uterine wall, and is more likely to be visible externally earlier in the separation process than is seen with the Schultze mechanism. The amniotic sac does not invert, trailing behind the placenta.

The memory aid for correctly identifying the mechanisms of placental expulsion is based on the appearance of the two different sides of the placenta first seen at the vaginal introitus. The fetal side is shiny and glistening from the fetal membranes covering the placenta, whereas the uterine side is dark and beefy—hence the sayings "Shiny Schultze" and "Dirty Duncan." In past years, some sources have suggested that there is a higher risk of postpartum bleeding during the Duncan mechanism, but no evidence has been found to substantiate this belief.

## Management of the Third Stage of Labor

Although more research in the area of third-stage management is being conducted, little is known about how the first and second stages of labor affect the third stage. The primary focus of routine management techniques used during the third stage of labor is to prevent PPH. Evidence-based management of the third stage is controversial and

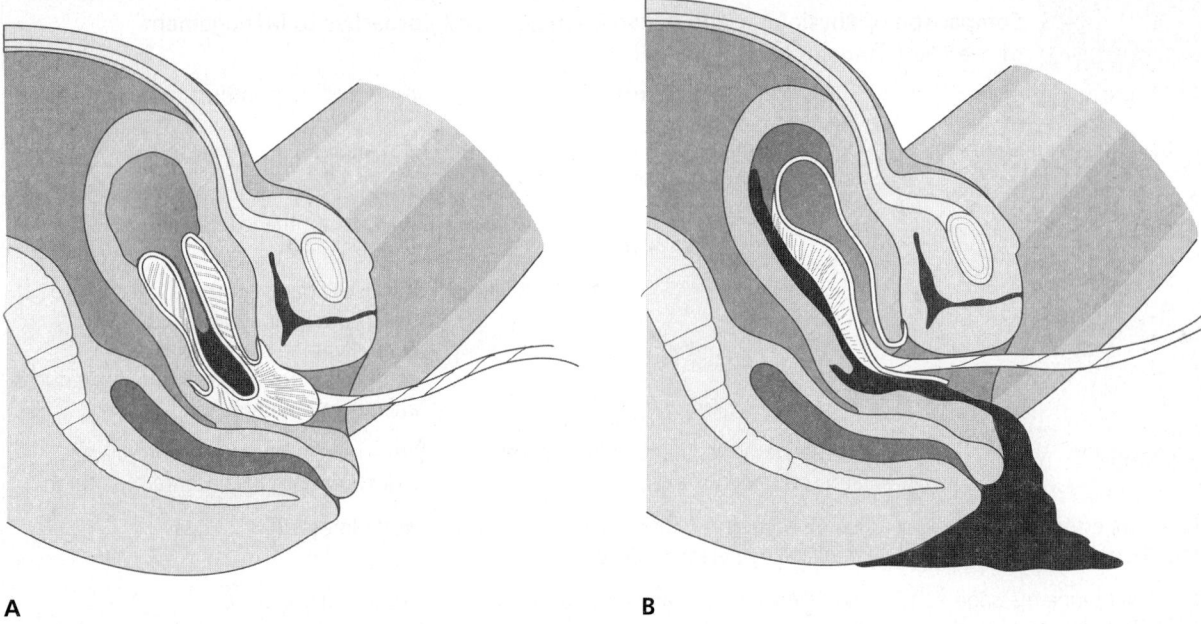

A                                                                        B

**Figure 31-1** Mechanisms of placental expulsion. **A.** Schultze. **B.** Duncan.

practices vary. Best practice is rapidly evolving as research identifies new evidence.

The two standard approaches to third-stage management are commonly described as physiologic management (sometimes referred to as expectant management) and active management.[13,14] The physiologic approach supports normal physiologic processes to enhance optimal outcomes.[13,14] This strategy is more commonly followed by midwives in many parts of the world compared to active management.[15–18] Nevertheless, active management is the approach recommended by the International Confederation of Midwives (ICM), the International Federation of Gynecologists and Obstetricians (FIGO), and WHO based on their interpretation of data reporting decreased PPH with this approach compared to expectant management.[11,19] Table 31-2 compares these two approaches. Studies have shown that birth attendants and birth facilities often use a mixed approach that incorporates portions of each approach, rather than strictly following one or the other.[17,18,20,21]

### Active Management of the Third Stage

Active management of the third stage of labor has been shown to decrease the risk of PPH in a general perinatal population.[13] The most recent meta-analysis of active management protocols compared active management of the third stage of labor

to physiologic management for the Cochrane Collaboration.[13] For individuals who were at mixed levels of bleeding risk, it was not clear whether active management reduced the risk of severe PPH (more than 1000 mL). In that analysis, patients with active management saw a reduced mean blood loss, had a lower rate of blood loss greater than 500 mL, and less often needed therapeutic uterotonic administration, compared to those whose third stage of labor was managed expectantly.[13,22] Other researchers have found that active management of the third stage of labor may not be beneficial to individuals undergoing physiologic birth.[20] In fact, use of active management in the third stage of labor for individuals undergoing physiologic birth has been associated with a higher risk for PPH and prolonged third stage of labor.[20] These findings are of particular importance in low-resource settings where treatment options for PPH are limited and in settings that support physiologic birth.

The active management approach, as initially evaluated in randomized controlled trials (RCTs), included four elements: (1) controlled cord traction to facilitate placental expulsion, (2) early cord-clamping and cutting, (3) routine administration of a prophylactic uterotonic, and (4) fundal massage (in some studies).[13] However, the individual components of active management were not well studied, and each has possible adverse

| Table 31-2 | Comparison of Physiologic and Active Management Approaches to Management of the Third Stage of Labor | |
|---|---|---|
| **Intervention** | **Physiologic Management** | **Active Management** |
| Birthing person positioning | Upright positioning of the birthing person to promote gravity assistance | Not addressed |
| Delayed cord-clamping | Yes | WHO recommends delayed cord-clamping<br><br>ICM/FIGO has a footnote attached to the recommendation for controlled cord-clamping stating that delaying cord-clamping by 1 to 3 minutes reduces anemia in the newborn |
| Cord traction | No—generally a "hands-off" approach and spontaneous expulsion | Yes—continuous gentle cord traction following signs of placenta separation |
| Birthing person efforts to expel the placenta | Expulsion occurs with the aid of gravity or the birthing person's efforts | Not addressed |
| External uterine massage following placental expulsion | No—generally a "hands-off" approach to the uterus | Yes (ICM/FIGO only) |
| Routine administration of a uterotonic agent | No | Yes |
| Early infant suckling | Yes | Not addressed |
| Draining the umbilical cord | Not addressed | Not addressed |

Abbreviations: FIGO, International Federation of Gynecology and Obstetrics; ICM, International Confederation of Midwives; WHO, World Health Organization.
Based on World Health Organization. WHO recommendations for the prevention and treatment of postpartum haemorrhage. 2012. http://apps.who.int/iris/bitstream/10665/75411/1/9789241548502_eng.pdf. Accessed October 1, 2021; Begley CM, Gyte GM, Devane D, McGuire W, Weeks A, Biesty LM. Active versus expectant management for women in the third stage of labour. *Cochrane Database Syst Rev.* 2019 Feb 13;2(2):CD007412. doi: 10.1002/14651858.CD007412.pub513; International Confederation of Midwives; International Federation of Gynaecologists and Obstetricians. Joint statement: management of the third stage of labour to prevent post-partum haemorrhage. *J Midwifery Womens Health.* 2004 Jan-Feb;49(1):76-77. doi:10.1016/j.jmwh.2003.11.005. PMID: 14710151.

consequences when examined independently. In addition, management of the first and second stages of labor may influence third-stage management.[22] Therefore, as protocols for active management of labor and the predictive understanding of labor characteristics have evolved, some individual components have been deleted from the package of care practices.

The ICM/FIGO joint statement recommends three steps: (1) controlled cord traction (once pulsation stops in a healthy newborn), (2) use of a uterotonic agent, and (3) fundal massage after expulsion of the placenta.[19] Early cord-clamping was not included in this recommendation because delayed cord-clamping has known positive benefits for the newborn.[19,20,22] WHO recommends use of a uterotonic agent in all settings, but controlled cord traction only in settings where a skilled birth attendant is present; in support of this recommendation, WHO cites evidence that both controlled cord traction and early cord-clamping can be harmful to the birthing person and the infant, respectively.[11] Sustained fundal massage is not recommended by WHO.[11]

Since the initial active management protocols were published, controlled cord traction, uterotonics, fundal massage, and early versus delayed cord-clamping have all been the subject of considerable research.[23–26] As new information has emerged, the recommended components of active management have further evolved.[13] Current evidence suggests that administration of a uterotonic agent during the third stage of labor is the most effective treatment for prevention of PPH and likely the only component within the active management triad that has consistent clinical utility.[25]

A variety of uterotonic drugs are available, and controversy exists about the best route, dose, and timing for their administration when used as part of an active management of the third stage of labor protocol. The current guidelines from ICM/FIGO and WHO recommend oxytocin (Pitocin) 10 U administered intramuscularly or intravenously after being diluted in solution as the first-choice agent.[11,19] Other studies have found that intravenous oxytocin is more effective than intramuscular injection.[27–30] Although the guidelines refer to administration of oxytocin after the birth of the neonate, this medication can be given as the anterior shoulder is released under the symphysis pubis during the birth, after the birth, or after placental expulsion. The timing of administration does not influence the amount of bleeding or the rate of PPH.[13,31–33] For people who experience physiologic labor, the benefits of prophylactic administration of oxytocin in the third stage of labor are less clear, and this intervention may increase the risk of PPH and a prolonged third stage of labor.[20]

## Physiologic Management

Physiologic management of the third stage of labor includes no routine uterotonic administration, delayed cord-clamping, and gentle—if any—cord traction. Efforts by the birthing person to expel the placenta are encouraged. A Cochrane Collaboration analysis found heterogeneity in how the components of physiologic management were implemented in the studies analyzed.[13] However, the same analysis also found that there were no significant differences in the risk for severe PPH among individuals who did not have an a priori risk for PPH when active management was compared to expectant management.

A secondary analysis of data from RCTs suggests that prophylactic oxytocin for the reduction of PPH (greater than 1000 mL) in individuals who do not receive intrapartum oxytocin for induction or augmentation may not have the same protective effect as for individuals who received intrapartum oxytocin.[22] Therefore, individuals who are at low risk for PPH and successfully complete the first and second stages of labor without oxytocin use may be offered physiologic management in settings that have ready access to treatments for PPH. By contrast, active management may be more beneficial in low-resource settings.

## Mixed Management

Mixed management incorporates components of both active and physiologic management of the third stage of labor, and is a common practice.[13,16] The primary change in practice that has resulted in widespread adoption of a mixed management strategy is the introduction of delayed cord-clamping, which has proven benefits for the newborn.[23–26] In this scenario, the midwife may routinely administer a uterotonic agent after the birth but delay clamping the cord either for an arbitrary period of time or until it stops pulsating; then, after clamping and cutting the cord, the midwife applies gentle, controlled cord traction. In clinical practice, the combination of a midwife's usual practice, the birth site, institutional or practice guidelines, the birthing person's history, the birth situation, and the birthing person's particular preferences likely influence how the third stage of labor is managed, with this management rarely conforming strictly to either expectant or active protocols.

A survey of midwives and physicians reported more than 100 interventions that they or others may use during the third stage of labor.[17,21] However, the myriad techniques used during the third stage were found to cluster into distinct practice patterns, ranging from primarily hands-off care to higher hands-on interventions.[21] The effect of these patterns—that is, these clusters of care practices—on the rate of PPH remains unknown.

## Uterotonics to Prevent Postpartum Hemorrhage

Although oxytocin is the first choice for PPH prophylaxis, it may not be as effective for those individuals who received large doses of oxytocin during labor for induction or augmentation.[21] In this case, a different uterotonic agent may be indicated. Ergot alkaloids (methylergonovine maleate), prostaglandins, and Syntometrine (an oxytocin/ergometrine combination drug not available in the United States) are second-line prophylactic uterotonic agents.[27] Misoprostol is not as effective for prophylaxis but may be used if other uterotonics are not available.[27]

The routine use of oxytocin, or any other uterotonics, with normal saline via umbilical vein injection has not been found to be effective and should not be used for prevention of PPH.[27,28] The effectiveness of complementary treatments such as herbs or homeopathic remedies for PPH reduction is still unclear.[32]

## Cord Traction

Continuous cord traction initially was recommended as part of the active management package, without examining its individual effectiveness. Systematic reviews in 2013 and 2014 found no significant difference with respect to incidence of severe PPH, need for blood transfusion, or administration of therapeutic uterotonics with the use of controlled cord traction, in comparison to hands-off care.[34,35]

Gentle cord traction may be needed to guide the placenta out of the vagina during expulsion. Following signs of placental separation, the midwife applies gentle counter-traction to the lower uterine segment abdominally with one hand, while the other hand applies continuous gentle downward traction on the cord. An instrument such as a hemostat is used to clamp the umbilical cord close to where the cord exits the introitus; alternatively, a piece of gauze can be wrapped around the cord to promote easy traction. The traction should follow the curve of the pelvis. For example, if the person giving birth is in a semi-recumbent position, the cord is guided inferiorly as the placenta descends to the pelvic floor, and as the placenta becomes visible at the introitus, the cord is guided superiorly.

If the birthing person is in a squatting or other upright position, cord traction is likely not necessary and may even be dangerous. Excessive cord traction increases the risk for uterine inversion—a risk that theoretically might be further increased if the birthing person is in an upright position. A birthing person in an upright position will likely feel the pressure of the placenta as it descends to the pelvic floor and spontaneously expel it.

### Umbilical Cord Drainage

Umbilical cord drainage in the third stage of labor involves the removal of the clamp from the previously clamped and cut umbilical cord (after necessary cord blood samples have been obtained), allowing for drainage of any remaining blood from the cord and placenta. In two meta-analyses, one including three RCTs ($N = 1257$)[36] and the other including nine RCTs ($N = 2653$),[37] cord drainage reduced the length of the third stage of labor by 2 to 3 minutes. The investigators in one of these studies found that total blood loss was reduced by less than 80 mL[36] and the other group found no difference in total blood loss when compared to no cord drainage.[37] Corroborating findings of a drainage benefit, Wu et al. found a 3% reduction in the incidence of PPH following spontaneous vaginal births in which blood was drained from the cord when compared to no drainage.[36] It is still unclear if changes to the third stage of labor as a result of cord drainage are clinically significant, but this technique is noninvasive

and does not result in complications. If umbilical cord drainage is incorporated into third-stage management, the blood from this source should not be counted in the estimated or quantified blood loss, as it is fetal blood.

### External Uterine Massage Following Placental Expulsion

Uterine massage following the expulsion of the placenta is a component of active management of the third stage of labor that is recommended by both ICM and FIGO.[19] However, the precise benefit (if there is one) of routine external uterine massage is still undetermined. Assessment of uterine contractility is necessary and should be considered different than sustained uterine massage. If the uterus is not firm when assessed, uterine massage should be initiated.

One RCT ($N = 1170$) compared uterine massage to no uterine massage in individuals who also received 10 units of oxytocin intramuscularly immediately after the neonate's shoulder emerged.[38] The incidence of more than 400 mL blood lost and the incidence of more than 1000 mL blood loss were not statistically different between the groups.[38]

Thus, if a uterotonic agent is administered, external massage may not further increase the protection against an early PPH. Moreover, uterine massage following placental expulsion can cause significant discomfort.[38,39] Uterine massage *before* expulsion of the placenta is not recommended because this practice may cause incomplete separation of the placenta, resulting in iatrogenic hemorrhage.

### Blood Loss Measurement

Previously, the generally accepted definition of PPH was a blood loss of more than 500 mL after a vaginal birth or more than 1000 mL blood loss following a cesarean birth. In 2014, to encourage standardization, a U.S. multidisciplinary collaborative which included member representation from the American College of Nurse-Midwives, defined early PPH as a cumulative blood loss of 1000 mL or more accompanied by signs and symptoms of hypovolemia within 24 hours following a birth.[40] Although most healthy women can tolerate a blood loss of 1000 mL without adverse consequences, cumulative blood loss of 500 to 999 mL should trigger increased supervision and intervention as clinically indicated.

Measurement of blood loss at birth provides objective data that will help inform care of the laboring individual following birth. Visual estimation of blood loss (EBL) has been routine practice for many years, although repeated studies have demonstrated the inaccuracy of this simple method.[41-45] If a large blood loss occurs in the immediate postpartum period, the amount is commonly underestimated visually. Although training improves the accuracy of blood loss estimation, quantitative methods of assessing blood loss are now recommended.[42]

Two quantitative blood loss (QBL) methods that are relatively easy to implement are measuring and weighing. A calibrated under-buttocks drape can be used to measure blood loss. If a calibrated drape is not available or the person gives birth in a position that does not allow for an under-buttocks drape (e.g., supported squat), weighing blood-saturated items can be implemented. Because *1 gram is equivalent to 1 milliliter in volume*, weighing blood-saturated items and subtracting the weight of the item when dry provides a relatively accurate measurement. Either the pads or calibrated drapes should be used immediately after birth to limit additional content such as amniotic fluid or urine from being included in the blood loss measurement. The most effective QBL method to reduce hemorrhage-related morbidity has not been determined.[46]

Some birth sites routinely collect QBL data; however, this step can also be instituted if blood loss is estimated to be higher than normal to improve accuracy and guide management. A worksheet with the weight of commonly used items can be used to expedite the process of calculating a quantitative measure of blood loss.[45,47] Some hospitals have incorporated these calculations into their electronic medical records.

Water birth increases the difficulty of performing blood loss measurement. If the third stage of labor occurs in the water, quantitative measurement of blood loss is not possible.[48] However, several groups have published visual tools for estimating blood loss in a pool that significantly improved the accuracy of blood loss estimation among small groups of midwives. Midwives who care for birthing people whose third stage occurs in water should be familiar with these visual tools to help guide their management in these cases.[49]

## Midwifery Management of the Third Stage of Labor

The sequential steps for midwifery management of the third stage of labor are presented in the *Management of the Third Stage of Labor* appendix.

## Supporting a Birthing Person's Choices

Requests by a birthing person for nonintervention during the natural progress of the third stage are important to address prior to labor. The process of shared decision making will include discussion of ways to support normalcy during the third stage and the evidence for interventions known to minimize the risk for PPH. Prenatal preventive measures such as a healthy diet to prevent anemia will lessen adverse effects of blood loss at birth. Avoiding procedures during labor and birth that may increase postpartum blood loss, such as induction, augmentation, and episiotomy, also decreases the risk of hemorrhage. Conversely, it is important to remember that delaying the use of uterotonics until bleeding is excessive may increase the risk of hemorrhage.

The placenta, umbilical cord, and membranes have special or spiritual significance in many cultures. In turn, additional requests for third-stage management by birthing people reflecting these beliefs may be quite varied. The birthing person or family may want to save the placenta for a variety of purposes.[50] The ritual of burying the placenta may be undertaken for the purpose of protecting the child, protecting the birthing person, or establishing a spiritual or sacred link between the land and the child.[51,52] Parents may also be interested in leaving the placenta attached to the newborn until the cord falls off spontaneously, often referred to as a lotus birth.[52] Some individuals practice placentophagia, consuming the placenta in either raw or cooked form, or encapsulate the placenta in pill form, with hopes of preventing postpartum depression or as a galactogogue.[53-55] Although humans have engaged in placentophagia since ancient times, findings related to these practices generally have been inconclusive or have demonstrated potential harm.[53-56] Safe consumption necessitates proper sanitization, handling, and testing of the placenta.[55]

Rituals also may involve the umbilical cord and even the membranes. The cord may be kept as a charm or used for medicinal purposes. In traditional lore, when a newborn is born in a caul (i.e., with membranes covering the head), it means that the child will never drown; thus, these membranes have been sold to sailors for protection.

When a pregnant person has a special request, the focus should be on safety while also attempting to honor the request. Honoring the variety of beliefs among families is important whenever possible, following a process of shared decision making.

## Examination of the Placenta and Placental Pathology

After the uterus is evaluated and assessed, and the uterine bleeding has slowed, the midwife should perform a methodical inspection of the placenta. Routine inspection of the placenta assists in recognizing abnormal findings and reduces the likelihood of overlooking a significant finding. The steps for inspection of the cord, placenta, and membranes are reviewed in the *Inspection of the Umbilical Cord, Placenta, and Membranes* appendix.

Table 31-3 lists common variations noted with the cord, placenta, and membranes (also refer to the *Pregnancy-Related Conditions* chapter and

| Table 31-3 | Umbilical Cord, Placenta, and Membrane Variations |
|---|---|
| **Variation** | **Significance** |
| **Umbilical Cord** | |
| Two-vessel cord | A two-vessel cord occurs in 0.5% to 1% of neonates. Two-vessel cords are associated with gastrointestinal, genitourinary, and cardiovascular abnormalities. |
| Long cord | A long cord, more than 75 cm, is associated with knots and fetal entanglement, as well as increased amniotic fluid and fetal activity. |
| Short cord | Short cords, less than 32 cm, are associated with disorders that limit fetal movement, such as neuromuscular disorders, fetal limb dysfunction, and Down syndrome. During labor, short cords are also associated with fetal heart rate abnormalities as a result of traction on the cord with fetal descent. |
| Thin cord | Associated with oligohydramnios and poor fetal growth. |
| Thick cord | Associated with polyhydramnios and macrosomia. |
| Marginal (Battledore) insertion | The cord is inserted at or within 1.5 cm of the margin of the placenta. Associated with preterm labor, abnormal fetal heart rate patterns in labor (compression), and bleeding in labor (vessel rupture). |
| Velamentous insertion | The umbilical cord vessels run through the amnion and chorion before entering the placenta, leaving the vessels unprotected (see Figure 31B-3 in the *Inspection of the Umbilical Cord, Placenta, and Membranes* appendix). This type of insertion may lead to rupture and fetal hemorrhage, particularly if associated with vasa previa (transcervical position). This finding is more common in a twin placenta. |
| Knots, loops, torsion, or strictures | These variations are associated with increased fetal mortality and morbidity. |
| **Placenta** | |
| Pale placenta | A pale placenta is associated with immature neonates and anemia. Edematous, pale, and bulky placentas are seen with immune and nonimmune hydrops fetalis, twin-to-twin transfusion syndrome, fetal congestive heart failure, and infection. |
| Green-stained placenta | With extended exposure to meconium, the placenta may be stained green. |
| Calcifications | The uterine surface is usually smooth but may have gritty white areas of calcification. Generally, the quantity of calcifications has no clinical importance. |
| Avulsed cotyledon | Incomplete expulsion of the placenta and retained products of conception. Associated with uterine atony, subinvolution, delayed hemorrhage, and postpartum infection. |
| Small, light placenta | A small placenta, defined as less than the 10% percentile for gestational age, may be associated with intrauterine infections, genetic mutations, or hypertension. |
| Large, heavy placenta | A large placenta, more than the 90% percentile for gestational age, is often due to various pregnancy or fetal conditions such as diabetes, fetal erythroblastosis and fetal hydrops, fetal congestive heart failure, and syphilis. |

| Variation | Significance |
|---|---|
| Infarctions | Usually grossly recognizable placental lesions on the uterine side, central or marginal. Acute infarcts are red and irregular, and have firm consistency. Subacute infarcts are tan-red, and remote infarcts are white-tan. Small infarcts are normal variants. Larger infarcts are associated with fetal growth restriction and stillbirth. Any condition that interferes with uteroplacental circulation can lead to placental infarcts (e.g., hypertensive disorders in pregnancy, post-term pregnancies, retroplacental hemorrhage). |
| Nodules or plaques on the fetal surface | Associated with oligohydramnios and renal agenesis, squamous metaplasia (benign), and infection. |
| Foul odor | Associated with infection. |
| **Placenta** | |
| Circumvallate placenta | The membranes appear to arise a short distance inward toward the umbilical cord, rather than from the edge of the placenta, and fold back upon themselves, creating a dense, gray-white ring that surrounds the outer margin of the placenta. The fetal vessels stop at this ring. Usually this finding is insignificant, but it has been associated with threatened abortion, preterm labor, painless vaginal bleeding after 20 weeks' gestation, placental insufficiency, fetal growth restriction, and intrapartum and postpartum hemorrhage. |
| Marginate or circummarginate placenta | A form of circumvallate placenta in which the fetal membranes do not fold back, creating the white ring. In this variation, placental tissue appears to extend beyond the marginate ring where the membranes arise. Usually this finding is insignificant. |
| Succenturiate placenta | One or more smaller accessory lobes of placenta develop within the membranes and are attached to the main placenta by fetal vessels. This finding is more common in multifetal gestations. The accessory lobes may be retained, leading to postpartum hemorrhage or infection. These placentas can be associated with velamentous insertion of the cord. |
| Bilobate placenta | Also referred to as bipartite or duplex. A placenta with three or more lobes is referred to as multilobate. |
| **Membranes** | |
| Cloudy membranes | Associated with infection. |
| Incomplete membranes | Remnants of membranes are usually spontaneously expelled after the birth; however, they can cause subinvolution of the uterus, uterine atony, or infection if retained. |

*Inspection of the Umbilical Cord, Placenta, and Membranes* appendix). Some variations, such as a true knot in the cord, may be simple incidental findings, yet are also associated with an increased risk for newborn morbidity. When observed, their presence should be noted in the health records of both the birthing person and the newborn. See the *Pregnancy-Related Conditions* chapter and the *Inspection of the Umbilical Cord, Placenta, and Membranes* appendix for more information.

## Placental Pathology

Placental evaluation by a pathologist is not indicated for all placentas. A pathology examination of the placenta can be diagnostic in some situations, however, and the College of American Pathologists has published recommendations, last updated in 1997, for when placental pathology examination should be performed.[57] For example, a pathology examination of the placenta can help establish a diagnosis when stillbirth occurs.[58,59] Indications to send a placenta for a detailed pathology examination commonly fall into four categories:

- Identification of a previously unsuspected disease process in the birthing person or neonate that requires immediate attention (e.g., unusual infection such as *Listeria*)
- Conditions with a high probability of subsequent reoccurrence (e.g., placenta accreta)
- Information that can guide management of future pregnancies or influence long-term care of

the birthing person or neonate (e.g., spontaneous preterm birth with histologic chorioamnionitis)

- Diagnosis that provides an explanation for an adverse outcome such as fetal death or growth restriction[59]

A detailed placental pathology examination may provide valuable information or an explanation for neonatal neurodevelopmental impairment or other adverse pregnancy outcomes.[60,61] Table 31-4 lists some of the clinical scenarios that are commonly cited as indications for requesting a detailed pathology examination of the placenta.[57]

### Postplacental Intrauterine Device Insertion

The use of immediate long-acting reversible contraception has increased in the United States over the past few decades. Postplacental intrauterine device (IUD) insertion is one factor contributing to this increase. Insertion of an IUD within 10 minutes after the placenta is expelled is convenient and cost-effective, with similar risks to insertion at other time points.[62] Specific risks include perforation, infection, vaginal bleeding, and expulsion. Data are inconsistent about expulsion rates; however, cesarean birth, increased provider experience, and

the use of a copper IUD may result in lower rates of expulsion.[62] The benefits of immediate effective contraception often outweigh the risk of expulsion for many birthing people. It is essential that shared decision making be used to determine the appropriateness of postplacental IUD insertion for each birthing person. Given U.S. history of reproductive coercion and the fact that an IUD requires a healthcare visit to discontinue its use, postplacental IUDs should not be considered unless the individual understands how it can be removed. Additional information and sequential steps for inserting a postplacental IUD are presented in the *Postplacental IUD Insertion* appendix.

## Complications of the Third Stage of Labor

Although most births end with an uncomplicated third stage of labor, some of the most severe childbirth complications occur during the third stage, including retained placenta, placenta accreta, and uterine inversion. Early (also called immediate) PPH occurs during the third stage of labor or up to 24 hours postpartum. Excessive blood loss after

| Table 31-4 | Clinical Conditions That May Indicate Need for a Pathology Examination of the Placenta After Birth | | |
|---|---|---|---|
| **Birthing Person Indications** | **Fetal or Neonatal Indications** | **Placental Indications** | |
| Abruption, unexplained third trimester bleeding, or excessive bleeding | Congenital anomalies | Gross placental abnormalities (shape, infarct, mass, amnion nodosum, abnormal coloration, malodor, thrombosis) | |
| Fever or chorioamnionitis | Fetal growth restriction or birth weight less than 10th percentile | | |
| Infection during this pregnancy (e.g., human immunodeficiency virus, syphilis, cytomegalovirus, parvovirus, primary herpes, toxoplasmosis, rubella, Zika) | Gestational age < 34 weeks or > 42 weeks | | |
| | Hydrops fetalis | Morbidly adherent placenta | |
| Invasive procedure with suspected placental trauma | Infection or suspected neonatal sepsis | Placental abruption | |
| Oligohydramnios | Neonatal neurologic problems (e.g., seizures) | Umbilical cord abnormalities (long or short, marginal or velamentous insertion, two-vessel cord) | |
| Polyhydramnios | Newborn with abnormal umbilical cord blood gas values, low Apgar scores, or requiring neonatal intensive care unit admission | | |
| Systemic disorder with clinical concerns for mother or neonate (e.g., autoimmune disease, diabetes, hypertension, collagen disease, seizures, severe anemia, thrombophilia, or thromboembolic disorder) | Multifetal gestation | | |
| | Stillbirth/early neonatal death | | |
| | Thick meconium | | |
| Substance abuse | Vanishing twin first trimester | | |
| Physical trauma | Very-low-birth-weight infant | | |

Based on Langston C, Kaplan C, Macpherson T, et al. Practice guideline for examination of the placenta: developed by the Placental Pathology Practice Guideline Development Task Force of the College of American Pathologists. *Arch Pathol Lab Med.* 1997;121:449-4757; Cypher RL. Placental pathology and liability: a window to fetal health? *J Perinat Neonatal Nurs.* 2020 Oct/Dec;34(4):294-296.

24 hours through 4 weeks postpartum is considered late, delayed, or secondary PPH.

## Retained Placenta

The prevalence of retained placenta has been reported to range from 0.5% to 4.8%.[63] A literature review of original research articles published between 1990 and 2020 found advanced age in the birthing person, previous retained placenta, previous surgical uterine procedures, and labor induction with oxytocin were the most recurrent, independent risk factors.[63] The primary risk associated with retained placenta is hemorrhage.

In birthing people who receive oxytocin prophylaxis in the third stage of labor, only 1 in 200 takes longer than 20 minutes to expel the placenta;[6,64] therefore, in the absence of bleeding, the midwife should start interventions to promote separation and expulsion at the 20-minute mark, and consider manual removal by 30 minutes in these situations. By contrast, in birthing people who have physiologic management of their third stage, 98% will expel their placenta by 60 minutes following birth of the newborn.[65] For these individuals, the midwife should start interventions to promote separation and expulsion at the 30-minute mark, including prophylactic oxytocin administration, and consider manual removal by 60 minutes.[65] This also allows for notification of the interprofessional team and gathering of needed supplies and personnel.

The midwife can implement several conservative interventions when the third stage is prolonged, including encouraging an upright position for the birthing person, nipple stimulation via encouraging the newborn to breastfeed or manual nipple stimulation, and ensuring an empty bladder, by means of catheterization if indicated. If oxytocin has not been administered, provision of oxytocin—via intramuscular injection, through an intravenous line, or intraumbilical—may promote placental expulsion.[66] A consultation should be obtained once a prolonged third stage has been diagnosed, and relocation of the birthing person to an appropriate place to conduct manual removal of the placenta should be considered. Nonemergency manual removal of the placenta should occur in a hospital setting both for reasons of safety and to enable the birthing person to receive anesthesia or deep analgesia for this usually painful procedure.

The *Manual Removal of the Placenta* appendix reviews the procedure for manual removal of the placenta. In a nonemergency situation, the midwife may manually remove the placenta in consultation with a physician or wait for a physician to perform the procedure. If the individual is hemorrhaging, the midwife may need to manually remove the placenta emergently.

## Avulsed Cord

Excessive cord traction before complete placental separation, or normal cord traction with a thin or velamentous umbilical cord insertion into the placenta, can cause the umbilical cord to detach or avulse from the placenta, necessitating manual removal of the placenta—an intervention that exposes the birthing person to unnecessary pain and an increased risk of infection. A sensation of tearing is often felt by the midwife as the cord is detaching. If this is noticed, cord traction should be discontinued immediately and signs of placental separation should be apparent before resuming. Repositioning the birthing person in an upright position may facilitate placental expulsion. Grasping the placental aspect of the torn umbilical cord with ring forceps, or other atraumatic instrument, may allow gentle traction to continue, if needed.

## Uterine Inversion

Uterine inversion occurs when the fundus collapses into the endometrial cavity, which turns the uterus partially or completely inside out. Uterine inversion is a rare event, occurring in approximately 1 in 3448 births; however, as many as 50% of cases occur without precipitating factors.[67] Strong umbilical cord traction and fundal placental implantation are two risk factors associated with this condition, although it may also occur spontaneously.[67,68] The uterine inversion can be incomplete (fundus within the endometrial cavity), complete (fundus protrudes through the cervical os), prolapsed (fundus protrudes to or beyond the vaginal introitus), or total (both the uterus and the vagina are inverted).[67,68] Incomplete or complete inversions feel like a soft tumor that can be felt in the cervical or vaginal orifice, while abdominally a funnel-like depression may be felt instead of a rounded fundus.

Uterine inversion is associated with shock and disseminated intravascular coagulation (DIC). Thus, this complication can be a life-threatening emergency. Uterine inversion should be suspected and a vaginal examination performed if the person, after giving birth, develops symptoms of shock for no obvious reason. Excessive bleeding and severe uterine pain may or may not be present. The *Initial Management of Uterine Inversion* appendix presents the management of uterine inversion and describes the position of the midwife's hands during this maneuver. If the placenta is still attached, the uterus should be replaced *prior* to removing the placenta.

## Placenta Accreta

*Placenta accreta* is the term for a placenta that is abnormally adherent to the uterine wall. Placenta accreta is further subcategorized as *placenta increta*, when the placenta invades the myometrium, and *placenta percreta*, when it has extended through the myometrium and uterine serosa and into adjacent tissue, often the bladder. The range of clinical and pathologic meanings associated with these conditions have resulted in the introduction of a newer term, *placenta accreta spectrum*.

Placenta accreta spectrum most often occurs when the placenta implants over an area where there is a deficiency of decidual formation, such as over a uterine scar or in the lower uterine segment, with the most important risk factor being placenta previa.[69,70] Individuals who experience a cesarean birth are at increased risk for placenta accreta spectrum in subsequent pregnancies. People who have had one or more previous cesarean births and who have a placenta previa in the current pregnancy are particularly at risk for placenta accreta spectrum.[69,71]

The overall rate of placenta accreta has been reported to range from 1 in 2500 pregnancies to (more recently) 1 in 111 pregnancies.[69] The increasing rate of placenta accreta is thought to be caused by the rising rate of cesarean births. Reports of placenta accreta are also thought to vary based on how the diagnosis is made, with some providers or institutions over- or under-reporting its incidence.

If the placenta is completely adherent, minimal bleeding usually occurs. If it is partially separated or partially adherent, there will likely be more bleeding, which may or may not be visible. If placenta accreta is suspected due to a retained and adherent placenta, physician consultation and in-hospital care are necessary. A hysterectomy, while leaving the placenta intact, may be the necessary treatment.

## Postpartum Hemorrhage

Postpartum hemorrhage is termed *early* or *primary* when it occurs within the first 24 hours postpartum; in contrast, it is described as *late*, *delayed*, or *secondary* when it occurs after 24 hours and up to 12 weeks postpartum.[41] PPH is defined as a cumulative blood loss of greater or equal to 1000 mL, regardless of mode of birth, or blood loss of any amount accompanied by signs or symptoms of hypovolemia within 24 hours of birth.[41] However, blood loss of 500 mL or greater during a vaginal birth should be considered a warning sign, and should trigger investigation of its source and close monitoring of the birthing person. It is important

for the midwife to keep in mind that a change in vital signs does not occur until considerable blood loss has occurred, so early recognition is critical.[41] Care of the person with late PPH—a much less common condition—focuses on assuring hemodynamic stability and correcting the suspected cause of the hemorrhage.[72]

Signs and symptoms of *hypovolemia* can be used to define PPH. Because symptoms such as hypotension and tachycardia appear only after approximately 25% of the total blood volume is lost,[41] these developments are not a sensitive indicator that the midwife can use to identify PPH in the early stages, when the excessive bleeding needs to be recognized and controlled effectively. In clinical practice, if blood loss is not measured quantitatively, PPH is a subjective assessment of an estimated blood loss that threatens hemodynamic stability. It is important to initiate steps to control postpartum bleeding *before* the blood loss reaches any of these thresholds. Early action in the presence of excessive bleeding may prevent an actual hemorrhage. In addition, even in the absence of visible bleeding exceeding 500 mL, any postpartum person experiencing signs of hypovolemia should be assessed for excessive blood loss.

Internationally, PPH is a leading cause of perinatal mortality. The incidence of early PPH—and especially severe hemorrhage requiring blood transfusion—has markedly increased in the last several years in many developed nations, including the United States.[71] Although many factors are involved in the increasing incidence of PPH, a significant proportion of this increase is associated with more frequent use of oxytocin for labor augmentation or induction and the increased rate of cesarean section birth.[71]

In the United States, PPH occurs in 2% to 3% of all births, but is the cause of 20% of all perinatal deaths.[71] Most importantly, more than half of all perinatal deaths attributed to hemorrhage are preventable. In developed nations where adequate resources are available, these deaths are mostly attributed to failure to coordinate the management of this emergency.[73] However, persistent racial and ethnic disparities in PPH exist in the United States. Collaborative quality improvement strategies have been effective in reducing the rates of severe maternal morbidity due to hemorrhage in all races and in reducing this health disparity between Black and white birthing people.[74]

Identification of risk factors, preventive measures, and early detection and management can mitigate the adverse consequences of this PPH. Over the last several years, use of simulation, clinical guidelines, bundles, and checklists has improved how care teams respond to and manage a range of emergencies, including PPH. Adherence to guidelines for managing PPH has lowered the incidence of severe perinatal morbidity by 20% and across all racial and ethnic groups.[73,74] A list of these resources is included at the end of this chapter.[75,76]

## Causes of Postpartum Hemorrhage

Table 31-5 lists the most common causes of early PPH, along with a mnemonic (tone, tissue, trauma, thrombin) that can be used as a memory prompt.[47,76–78] Uterine atony and retained placental fragments are the causes of approximately 80% of all cases of

| Table 31-5 | The "Four Ts" Mnemonic for Causes of Immediate Postpartum Hemorrhage | | |
|---|---|---|---|
| **Cause** | | **Etiology** | **Clinical Presentation** |
| **Tone** | | ~70% | Bright red bleeding, clots, boggy or soft uterus |
| Overdistended uterus—large fetus, multifetal gestation, polyhydramnios | | | |
| Prolonged labor (all stages) | | | |
| Rapid labor | | | |
| Oxytocin-induced or -augmented labor | | | |
| High parity | | | |
| Postpartum hemorrhage with previous birth | | | |
| Chorioamnionitis | | | |
| Poorly perfused myometrium—hypotension | | | |
| Medications such as magnesium sulfate, nifedipine, and some general anesthetics | | | |
| Uterine abnormalities such as fibroids | | | |
| **Tissue, Retained** | | ~20% | Bright red bleeding, clots, boggy or soft uterus |
| Avulsed cotyledon, succenturiate lobe | | | |
| Abnormal placentation—accreta, increta, percreta | | | |
| Retained blood clots | | | |
| **Trauma** | | ~10% | Multiple presentations |
| Episiotomy, especially mediolateral | | | Bright red bleeding, firm uterine fundus |
| Hematoma | | | Hematomas: intense pain at site of bleeding |
| Lacerations of perineum, vagina, or cervix | | | |
| Ruptured uterus | | | Bright red bleeding firm uterine fundus |
| Uterine inversion | | | Shock greater than expected from estimated blood loss |
| **Thrombin** | | ~1% | Excessive bleeding |
| Coagulopathies | | | |
| Acquired coagulopathies such as placental abruption, amniotic fluid embolism, disseminated intravascular coagulation, HELLP syndrome (i.e., hemolysis, elevated liver enzymes, and low platelet count), stillbirth, or sepsis | | | |
| Congenital coagulation defects such as von Willebrand's disease | | | |
| Therapeutic anticoagulation (e.g. low-molecular weight heparin) | | | |

Based on Rani PR, Begum J. Recent advances in the management of major postpartum hemorrhage: a review. *J Clin Diagnost Res.* 2017;11(2):QE01-QE05. doi:10.7860/JCDR/2017/22659.946377; Evensen A, Anderson JM, Fontaine P. Postpartum hemorrhage: prevention and treatment. *Am Fam Physician.* 2017;95(7):442-449.

| Table 31-6 | **Stages of Hemorrhagic Shock** | | | |
|---|---|---|---|---|
| | **Compensated PPH** | **Mild PPH** | **Moderate PPH** | **Severe PPH** |
| Blood volume loss (mL) | < 1000 | 1000–1500 | 1500–2000 | ≥ 2000 |
| Percentage of blood volume lost (%) | 10–15 | 15–30 | 30–40 | ≥ 40 |
| Heart rate (beats/min) | < 100 | > 100 | ≥ 120 | ≥ 140 |
| Systolic blood pressure (mm Hg) | Normal | Normal | Hypotension | Profound hypotension |
| Pulse pressure | Normal or increased | Narrowed | Narrowed | Narrowed |
| Respiratory rate (breaths/min) | 14–20 | 20–30 | 30–40 | > 40 |
| Urine output (mL/hr) | ≥ 30 | 20–30 | 5–15 | Slight or anuria |
| Mental status | Normal | Weakness, sweating, agitation or mild anxiety | Restless, pallor, extremities cool to touch | Air hunger, collapse, lethargy |

Abbreviation: PPH, postpartum hemorrhage.
Based on Arafeh J, Gregory K, Main E, Lyndon A. Definition, early recognition and rapid response using triggers: CMQCC obstetric hemorrhage toolkit. 2015. https://www.cmqcc.org/resource/ob-hem-definition-early-recognition-and-rapid-response-using-triggers. Accessed October 3, 2021.

early PPH.[41,74,76] Late PPH is most often caused by retained placental fragments, infection, coagulopathies, or subinvolution at the placental site.[41]

Many strategies have been used to identify people who are at risk for excessive blood loss. Stratifying birthing people into low-, medium-, and high-risk groups is valuable as a guide for anticipatory preparation. Even so, most PPH events occur in people who have no risk factors.[41,73,76]

### Stages of Postpartum Hemorrhage

As shown in Table 31-6, symptoms of hypovolemia usually parallel the amount of blood lost. Thus, PPH can be categorized as compensated, mild, moderate, or severe depending on the individual's symptoms and the amount of blood loss.[75] Birthing persons who are already volume depleted, such as those with preeclampsia, may decompensate more rapidly.

The first physiologic compensation that occurs when blood loss is excessive is systemic vasoconstriction, which is clinically evident as a narrowed pulse pressure. Thus, decreases in pulse pressure (the difference between the systolic and diastolic blood pressures in a single measurement) are a better vital sign to initially monitor when bleeding becomes excessive than is pulse or absolute blood pressure. Systolic blood pressure begins to fall and pulse rises after 15% to 25% of the total blood volume is lost.

Hypotension and tachycardia are relatively late signs of hemorrhage.

### Complications of Postpartum Hemorrhage

Postpartum hemorrhage can result in anemia, hypotension, and, in severe cases, hypovolemic shock that can lead to disseminated intravascular coagulation (DIC), adult respiratory distress syndrome (ARDS), and Sheehan syndrome.

DIC is a consumptive coagulopathy that results in depletion of platelets and coagulation factors. Its etiology is widespread activation of the clotting and fibrolytic systems. This cascade of events is stimulated by circulatory exposure to large amounts of tissue factor, which is present in the placenta. The result is uncontrolled bleeding. Recent studies of PPH have found that DIC occurs earlier than previously thought.[77] Early treatment of DIC can significantly improve perinatal outcomes. Evaluation of coagulation studies is part of the initial response to PPH, and transfusion protocols for PPH recommend treating DIC as soon as it is determined to be a significant risk.

ARDS and Sheehan syndrome are rare complications of PPH. ARDS results from damage to the endothelial cells in the pulmonary vasculature that causes fluid to leak into the alveoli, producing respiratory distress. Postpartum pituitary infarction (Sheehan syndrome) is the result of pituitary necrosis.[41,79] The pituitary is perfused via venous pressure, which makes it vulnerable to ischemia and damage in the presence of hypotension. The most common initial symptom of postpartum pituitary infarction is lack of milk production. Amenorrhea, adrenal insufficiency, hyponatremia, and hypoglycemia are additional complications of pituitary hypofunction.

### Strategies to Prevent Postpartum Hemorrhage and Minimize Adverse Effects

Strategies to minimize the adverse effects of PPH include correcting anemia preconceptionally or in the prenatal period, eliminating routine episiotomies, and avoiding genital tract lacerations.[78] The best prevention strategy during the third stage of labor is active management of the third stage, starting with administration of a uterotonic agent during or immediately following the birth of the infant.[13] Table 31-7 lists recommended preparations to implement for birthing people at a moderate or high risk of early hemorrhage.

## Management Steps for Treating Postpartum Hemorrhage

The Partnership for Maternal Safety, a national workgroup, developed a Maternal Safety Consensus Bundle to reduce severe maternal morbidity from PPH.[77] This bundle was organized into four action domains: Readiness, Recognition and Prevention, Response, and Reporting and System Learning.[80] A treatment bundle, developed for the same purpose, focuses on care when PPH is identified.[81] These bundles complement each other, but the Maternal Safety Consensus Bundle is more comprehensive.

The Readiness domain focuses on the necessity for every birth facility to have a mechanism for early identification and early treatment to prevent delays and serious morbidity. This domain includes the availability of a hemorrhage cart with necessary supplies, immediate access to uterotonic medications, the development of a response team with clear processes, protocols for emergency blood transfusion, and unit-based education including simulation and debriefing. Standard procedures that are practiced in simulations or rehearsals can improve the response time when a real PPH occurs.[74,75,80]

The Recognition and Prevention domain addresses the assessment of hemorrhage risk for every birthing person, measurement of cumulative blood loss using quantitative methods, and the administration of prophylactic oxytocin during the third stage of labor, except in the case of a person experiencing

| Table 31-7 | Management Plan for a Person at Moderate or High Risk for Postpartum Hemorrhage |
| --- | --- |

1. Provide anticipatory guidance to the pregnant person and their significant other/family (with the person's permission).

2. Choose the birth site based on the risk assessment and availability of staff and resources.

3. Prepare a plan of care and communicate it to all healthcare team members, including nursing and anesthesia staff, when a person is in labor. Regular meetings of the entire healthcare staff for a particular shift, or huddles, are encouraged as an intervention to improve communication around postpartum hemorrhage preparations. A physician may be alerted when the person enters labor based on the level of risk.

4. A prepared hemorrhage cart should be immediately accessible, such as outside the room for the person at risk for postpartum hemorrhage.

5. Plan to quantify blood lost during birth and postpartum care.

6. Based on the person's risk, the plan of care for the person in labor may include the following steps:

   a. Order a blood type and screen or type and cross-match for blood if needed.

   b. Initiate a large-bore (at least 18 gauge) intravenous line during labor for rapid access.

   c. Catheterize the person's bladder if it is full and the person is unable to void, as a full bladder may impede postpartum uterine contraction effectiveness.

   d. Consider pain management methods that will support the steps undertaken to manage postpartum hemorrhage, and plan with the person early in labor.

   e. Administer a uterotonic agent with the release of the neonate's anterior shoulder, assuming there is assurance that a second fetus does not exist.

   f. Use a method to measure blood lost quantitatively.

7. If hemorrhage occurs, proceed to the steps outlined in the *Management of Immediate Postpartum Hemorrhage* appendix.

physiologic birth (depending on the birthing person's informed choice). A combination of bimanual compression and uterotonic drugs will control bleeding in the vast majority of people with PPH. If management steps are initiated rapidly, excessive blood loss can be avoided. An interprofessional team should be called to address the emergency if the hemorrhage continues despite bimanual compression and use of uterotonic drugs, or if the person has signs of hypovolemia. The use of agreed-upon vital sign "triggers" that signal the need for more aggressive treatment can help standardize management of PPH and minimize morbidity. Many facilities use the Maternal Early Warning Signs Protocol, which has been endorsed by multiple perinatal organizations.[82] For example, triggers that could signal the need to initiate a hemorrhage protocol could be maternal pulse more than 120 beats per minute, estimated blood loss more than 500 mL, or systolic blood pressure less than 90 mm Hg. The team that responds to such emergencies commonly includes an anesthesia provider, an obstetric physician, and additional nursing staff. Once the hemorrhage is controlled, close postpartum surveillance is maintained until bleeding is minimal and the person is stable.

The Response domain for every hemorrhage includes a detailed management plan with stepwise response to blood loss and warning signs. WHO recommends the development of formal protocols for prevention and treatment of PPH,[11] although no specific protocol has been established as best practice. The second component is to provide support for the laboring person, families, and the healthcare team. Many sources delineate sequential steps the midwife should follow when managing a PPH.[75,77] In addition, the midwife can find some excellent flowcharts that institutions use to guide management of a PPH. Evidence-based flowcharts and pocket algorithms that can be used to help manage obstetric hemorrhage and improve outcomes are available and examples are listed in the Resources section at the end of this chapter.

The Reporting and System Learning domain focuses on system improvements that should be implemented by every birth site to support teams as they review and improve their processes after a hemorrhage. A culture of briefings, huddles, and debriefings can establish a climate of safety and provide for team preparations and support. Formal multidisciplinary, interprofessional reviews of serious hemorrhage events provide an opportunity to identify system issues that could be improved for future cases. Goals are to provide rapid evaluation of use of the agreed-upon bundles, decrease the frequency of severe hemorrhages, and reduce morbidity related to PPH.

Table 31-8 summarizes the doses, contraindications, and side effects of the uterotonic agents commonly used to treat PPH.[83-86] Oxytocin (Pitocin) is considered the first-line uterotonic. If the hemorrhage does not resolve with its use, second-line drugs—such as methylergonovine maleate (Methergine) or tranexamic acid (TXA)—are administered. TXA, a fibrinolytic agent, is an important new tool in efforts to improve maternal morbidity and mortality outcomes of PPH.[87] In a meta-analysis of randomized controlled trials ($N = 14,363$ birthing people), the use of TXA for the treatment of PPH decreased the risk of hysterectomy without increasing the risk of thrombotic events. The recommended dosage of TXA is 1 gram intravenously over 10 minutes (add a 1-gram vial to 100 mL of normal saline and administer over 10 minutes) soon after a PPH is diagnosed (within 3 hours) and a repeat dose of 1 gram (in the same manner) if bleeding continues after 30 minutes.[87,88]

The *Management of Immediate Postpartum Hemorrhage* appendix lists the steps recommended for managing a PPH, and the *Intrauterine Exploration* appendix reviews the steps taken to explore the intrauterine cavity if needed.[41,78,89–91]

## Hematoma

Although uterine atony is the most common reason for PPH, damage to blood vessels, or hematomas, may also result in PPH. When they occur in association with childbirth, they are most likely to become apparent during the intrapartum or postpartum periods. The most common locations for hematomas are (1) the vulva, (2) the vagina, and (3) the retroperitoneum.[78] The types of hematomas and their initial presentation are described in more detail in the *Genital Tract Injury: Immediate Postpartum Inspection of the Vulva, Perineum, Vagina, and Cervix* appendix in the *Second Stage of Labor and Birth* chapter and in the *Postpartum Complications* chapter.

If the pain is severe, the hematoma is increasing rapidly, or signs of hypovolemia develop, emergency measures are needed. If the person is giving birth in an out-of-hospital setting, emergency transport is begun. The midwife's consulting physician and anesthesia staff should be notified and immediate assistance requested. The midwife should not incise the hematoma without additional aid because of the potential for hemorrhage. Measures to initiate intravenous fluid volume replacement and possible blood transfusion should be begun while waiting for the healthcare team.

## Rare Emergency Complications

If a newly postpartum person experiences respiratory impairment, cardiovascular collapse, altered

| Table 31-8 | Uterotonic Treatment of Immediate Postpartum Hemorrhage Due to Uterine Atony | | | |
|---|---|---|---|---|
| **Drug: Generic (Brand)** | **Dose and Route** | **Contraindications** | **Side Effects** | **Clinical Considerations** |
| **First-Line Therapies** | | | | |
| Oxytocin (Pitocin) | 10–40 U in 250 or 500 mL of normal saline or lactated Ringer's solution *OR* 10 U IM injection | Hypersensitivity | Cramping Large doses can cause hyponatremia | Onset of action: 2–3 minutes Effective in 15–30 minutes Duration of action: 2–3 hours if given IM or 1 hour if given IV Rapid infusion of an undiluted bolus can cause hypotension and cardiac collapse |
| **Second-Line Therapies** | | | | |
| Methylergono- vine maleate (Methergine) | 0.2 mg IM May repeat in 5 minutes Thereafter every 2–4 hours | Hypertension, preeclampsia Do not give IV secondary to risk of sudden vasospasm and hypertensive or cerebrovascular accident | Cramping Nausea, vomiting Hypertension, seizure, headache | It is recommended that the person's blood pressure be taken prior to administration Onset of action: 2–5 minutes Peak plasma concentration: 20–30 minutes Plasma half-life: 3–4 hours People with coronary artery disease may have increased risk for myocardial infarction FDA black box warning to avoid breastfeeding for 12 hours following the last dose of methylergonovine maleate, although data suggest effects on the newborn including tachycardia, vomiting, diarrhea, and agitation are associated with longer courses of administration May affect serum prolactin levels and milk production |
| Carboprost tromethamine or 15 methyl prostaglandin $F_{2\alpha}$ analogue (Hemabate) | 250 mcg IM May repeat every 15–90 minutes, up to 8 doses | Asthma or active cardiac, pulmonary, renal, or hepatic disease | Nausea, vomiting, diarrhea, bronchospasm, hypertension Pyrexia is common | FDA black box warning to use recommended doses only and in a hospital setting as well as to avoid breastfeeding for the first 12 hours of the newborn's life Peak serum concentration: 30 minutes Less effective than methylergonovine |
| Dinoprostone (Prostin $E_2$) | 20 mg vaginal or rectal suppository May repeat every 2 hours | Hypotension Cardiac disease | Nausea, vomiting, and diarrhea Pyrexia is common | FDA black box warning to use recommended doses only and in a hospital setting Onset of action: 10 minutes |
| Misoprostol (Cytotec) | 600–800 mcg sublingual or 800–1000 mcg per rectum; 1 dose | | Nausea, vomiting, diarrhea, abdominal pain, shivering Pyrexia can occur with higher doses | Onset of action: 3–5 minutes Peak concentration: 30 minutes following sublingual administration; 40–60 minutes following rectal administration |

*(continues)*

| Table 31-8 | Uterotonic Treatment of Immediate Postpartum Hemorrhage Due to Uterine Atony (*continued*) | | | |
|---|---|---|---|---|
| **Drug: Generic (Brand)** | **Dose and Route** | **Contraindications** | **Side Effects** | **Clinical Considerations** |
| Tranexamic acid (Cyklokapron) | 1 g IV diluted in 100 mL of normal can be repeated after 30 minutes | Preexisting active thromboembolic disorder, disseminated intravascular coagulation, active coagulopathy, renal failure, placement of a coronary or vascular stent within 6 months to 1 year, acute subarachnoid hemorrhage | Mild gastrointestinal signs | Peak plasma concentration immediate, then decreases until hour 6<br><br>Half-life: 2 hours |

Abbreviations: FDA, U.S. Food and Drug Administration; IM, intramuscular; IV, intravenous.
Modified with permission from Lowe N, Openshaw M, King TL. Labor. In: Brucker MC, King TL, eds. *Pharmacology for Women's Health*. Burlington, MA: Jones & Bartlett Learning; 2017:1088; WOMAN Trial Collaborators. Effect of early tranexamic acid administration on mortality, hysterectomy, and other morbidities in women with post-partum haemorrhage (WOMAN): an international, randomised, double-blind, placebo-controlled trial. *Lancet*. 2017 May 27;389(10084):2105-2116. doi:10.1016/S0140-6736(17)30638-4.

mental status, or loss of consciousness, emergency measures are indicated. Differential diagnoses include pulmonary embolus, anaphylactoid syndrome of pregnancy (i.e., amniotic fluid embolus), septic shock, peripartum cardiomyopathy, and atypical eclampsia, among others. Sudden and rapid deterioration of the birthing person necessitates a quick response. Initial management steps for any postpartum emergency are listed in the *Sudden Postpartum Cardiovascular or Neurologic Emergencies* appendix.[92]

Life support measures focusing on adequate oxygenation are important regardless of the cause of the emergency. Once the emergency team is in place, the midwife plays an important role in communicating the birthing person's past history, including the labor and birth; reviewing how the emergency presented; and identifying which management steps have been implemented. Finally, maintaining communication with the family members to keep them informed is a critical component of the management of any perinatal emergency that a midwife can perform.

Clinical tools to identify maternal early warning signs (MEWS) of a perinatal emergency include bundles, protocols, and checklists.[93–95] The purpose of these tools is to promote interprofessional and patient-centered care so as to reduce preventable morbidity and mortality. While the components of MEWS tools vary, they all include a list of triggers that identify at-risk patients in need of further

attention as well as a protocol for necessary action. Postpartum MEWS tools are only just starting to undergo a review to determine their association with clinical outcomes. One barrier to the acceptance of these tools is the need to individualize them based on each institution's model of care, local patient population, and institutional structure and functions.[94] Midwives are critical members of the interprofessional team and should engage in local efforts to develop, implement, and evaluate institutional protocols.

## Processing Rare Adverse Emergencies

Midwives can experience post-traumatic stress disorder and a variety of negative feelings following a traumatic birth or an adverse emergency.[96–99] The impact of one trauma or a collective body of traumatic events over time can diminish the midwife's self-confidence and clinical judgment as well as impede relationships with future patients and colleagues.[97,99] Strategies to minimize the negative impacts of birth trauma on midwives include a supportive environment for debriefing among the healthcare team, collegial peer support, and follow-up care for the patients, when possible.[97,98] Organizations often have employee assistance programs that offer healthcare workers an opportunity to process their work-related stress. Promotion of self-care will help support the necessary emotional and professional well-being of midwives over their career, particularly following rare adverse emergencies.

## Conclusion

The third stage of labor is a critical period in the formation of each new family. Attention to prevention, early identification, and treatment of perinatal complications can mitigate the potential long-term effects of third-stage complications. Witnessing the welcome of a newborn into a family is a sweet reward for the midwife. No matter how hard the midwife may have worked to assist the birthing person and their significant others through the labor and birth, complimenting the birthing person and stressing their accomplishment is a gift the midwife can offer in return.

## Resources

| Organization | Description |
| --- | --- |
| California Maternal Quality Care Collaborative (CMQCC) | Collaborative of researchers and stakeholder organizations that analyzes data and quality improvement initiatives to end preventable morbidity, mortality, and racial disparities in maternity care in California. This organization is a leader in the publication of guidelines for managing postpartum hemorrhage, preventing cesarean birth, and treatment of preeclampsia. The website has multiple resources, slide sets, toolkits, and flowcharts for managing postpartum hemorrhage. |
| Council on Patient Safety in Women's Health Care | Collaborative of national professional organizations that works to improve safe care through multidisciplinary collaboration. Teams in this organization create and disseminate safety bundles. |

## References

1. GBD 2015 Maternal Mortality Collaborators. Global, regional and national levels of maternal mortality, 1990–2015: a systematic analysis of the Global Burden of Disease study 2015. *Lancet.* 2016;388:1775-1812.

2. Moore ER, Bergman N, Anderson GC, Medley N. Early skin-to-skin contact for mothers and their healthy newborn infants. *Cochrane Database Syst Rev.* 2016;11:CD003519. doi:10.1002/14651858.CD003519.pub4.

3. Edwards HM, Svare JA, Wikkelsø AJ, et al. The increasing role of a retained placenta in postpartum blood loss: a cohort study. *Arch Gynecol Obstet.* 2019;299(3):733-740.

4. Frolova AI, Stout MJ, Tuuli MG, et al. Duration of the third stage of labor and risk of postpartum hemorrhage. *Obstet Gynecol.* 2016;127:951-956.

5. Perlman NC, Carusi DA. Retained placenta after vaginal delivery: risk factors and management. *Int J Womens Health.* 2019;11:527.

6. van Ast M, Goedhart MM, Luttmer R, et al. The duration of the third stage in relation to postpartum hemorrhage. *Birth.* 2019;46:602-607.

7. Soltani H, Hutchon DR, Poulose TA. Timing of prophylactic uterotonics for the third stage of labour after vaginal birth. *Cochrane Database Syst Rev.* 2010;8:CD006173. doi:10.1002/14651858.CD006173.pub2.

8. Magann EF, Evans S, Chauhan SP, et al. The length of the third stage of labor and the risk of postpartum hemorrhage. *Obstet Gynecol.* 2005;105:290-293.

9. Dombrowski MP, Bottoms SF, Saleh AA, et al. Third stage of labor: analysis of duration and clinical practice. *Am J Obstet Gynecol.* 1995;172:1279-1284.

10. Cummings KF, Helmich MS, Ounpraseuth ST, et al. The third stage of labour in the extremely obese parturient. *J Obstet Gynaecol Can.* 2018;40:1148-1153. doi:10.1016/j.jogc.2017.12.008.

11. World Health Organization. WHO recommendations for the prevention and treatment of postpartum haemorrhage. 2012. https://apps.who.int/iris/bitstream/handle/10665/75411/9789241548502_eng.pdf;jsessionid=5A4E37F01A029452EB4BDEA22C2A7C0E?sequence=1. Accessed October 1, 2021.

12. Schorn MN. Uterine activity during the third stage of labor. *J Midwifery Womens Health.* 2012;57:151-155.

13. Begley CM, Gyte GM, Devane D, et al. Active versus expectant management for women in the third stage of labour. *Cochrane Database Syst Rev.* 2019;2(2):CD007412. doi:10.1002/14651858.CD007412.pub5.

14. Schorn MN. Management terminology during the third stage of labor. *J Midwifery Womens Health.* 2020;65:301-305.

15. Fahy K, Hastie C, Bisits A, et al. Holistic physiological care compared with active management of the third stage of labour for women at low risk of postpartum haemorrhage: a cohort study. *Women Birth.* 2010;23:146-152.

16. Kearney L, Reed R, Kynn M, et al. Third stage of labour management practices: a secondary analysis of a prospective cohort study of Australian women and their associated outcomes. *Midwifery.* 2019;75:110-116. doi:10.1016/j.midw.2019.05.001.

17. Schorn MN, Minnick A, Donaghey B. An exploration of how midwives and physicians manage the third stage of labor in the United States. *J Midwifery Womens Health.* 2015;60:187-198.

18. Tan WM, Klein MC, Saxell L, et al. How do physicians and midwives manage the third stage of labor? *Birth*. 2008;35:220-229.

19. International Confederation of Midwives; International Federation of Gynaecologists and Obstetricians. Joint statement: management of the third stage of labour to prevent post-partum haemorrhage. *J Midwifery Womens Health*. 2004;49(1):76-77. doi:10.1016/j.jmwh.2003.11.005.

20. Erickson EN, Lee CS, Grose E, Emeis C. Physiologic childbirth and active management of the third stage of labor: a latent class model of risk for postpartum hemorrhage. *Birth*. 2019;46:69-79. doi:10.1111/birt.12384.

21. Schorn MN, Dietrich MS, Donaghey B, Minnick AF. US physician and midwife adherence to active management of the third stage of labor international recommendations. *J Midwifery Womens Health*. 2017;62:58-67.

22. Erickson EN, Lee CS, Emeis CL. Role of prophylactic oxytocin in the third stage of labor: physiologic versus pharmacologically influenced labor and birth. *J Midwifery Womens Health*. 2017;62:418-424. doi:10.1111/jmwh.12620.

23. Chen X, Li X, Chang Y, et al. Effect and safety of timing of cord clamping on neonatal hematocrit values and clinical outcomes in term infants: a randomized controlled trial. *J Perinatol*. 2018;38:251-257. doi:10.1038/s41372-017-0001-y.

24. Katariya D, Swain D, Singh S, Satapathy A. The effect of different timings of delayed cord clamping of term infants on maternal and newborn outcomes in normal vaginal deliveries. *Cureus*. 2021;13:e17169. doi:10.7759/cureus.17169.

25. McDonald SJ, Middleton P. Effect of timing of umbilical cord clamping of term infants on maternal and neonatal outcomes. *Cochrane Database Syst Rev*. 2008;2:CD004074. doi:10.1002/14651858.CD004074.pub2. Update in: *Cochrane Database Syst Rev*. 2013;7:CD004074. PMID: 18425897.

26. Qian Y, Lu Q, Shao H, et al. Timing of umbilical cord clamping and neonatal jaundice in singleton term pregnancy. *Early Hum Dev*. 2020;142:104948. doi:10.1016/j.earlhumdev.2019.104948.

27. Govind N. Prophylactic oxytocin for the third stage of labour to prevent postpartum haemorrhage: a Cochrane review summary. *Int J Nurs Stud*. 2021;121:103712. doi:10.1016/j.ijnurstu.2020.103712.

28. Salati JA, Leathersich SJ, Williams MJ, et al. Prophylactic oxytocin for the third stage of labour to prevent postpartum haemorrhage. *Cochrane Database Syst Rev*. 2019;4(4):CD001808. doi:10.1002/14651858.CD001808.pub3.

29. Charles D, Anger H, Dabash R, et al. Intramuscular injection, intravenous infusion, and intravenous bolus of oxytocin in the third stage of labor for prevention of postpartum hemorrhage: a three-arm randomized control trial. *BMC Pregnancy Childbirth*. 2019;19:38. doi:10.1186/s12884-019-2181-2.

30. Oladapo OT, Okusanya BO, Abalos E, et al. Intravenous versus intramuscular prophylactic oxytocin for the third stage of labour. *Cochrane Database Syst Rev*. 2020;11(11):CD009332. doi:10.1002/14651858.CD009332.pub4.

31. Soltani H, Hutchon DR, Poulose TA. Timing of prophylactic uterotonics for the third stage of labour after vaginal birth. *Cochrane Database Syst Rev*. 2010;8:CD006173. doi:10.1002/14651858.CD006173.pub2.

32. Yaju Y, Kataoka Y, Eto H, et al. Prophylactic interventions after delivery of placenta for reducing bleeding during the postnatal period. *Cochrane Database Syst Rev*. 2013;11:CD009328.

33. Yildirim D, Ozyurek SE. Intramuscular oxytocin administration before vs. after placental delivery for the prevention of postpartum hemorrhage: a randomized controlled prospective trial. *Eur J Obstet Gynecol Reprod Biol*. 2018;224:47-51. doi:10.1016/j.ejogrb.2018.03.012.

34. Du Y, Ye M, Zheng F. Active management of the third stage of labor with and without controlled cord traction: a systematic review and meta-analysis of randomized controlled trials. *Acta Obstet Gynecol Scand*. 2014;93:626-633. doi:10.1111/aogs.12424.

35. Hofmeyr GJ, Mshweshwe NT, Gülmezoglu AM. Controlled cord traction for the third stage of labour. *Cochrane Database Syst Rev*. 2015;1:CD008020. doi:10.1002/14651858.CD008020.pub2.

36. Wu HL, Chen XW, Wang P, Wang QM. Effects of placental cord drainage in the third stage of labour: a meta-analysis. *Sci Rep*. 2017;7:7067. doi:10.1038/s41598-017-07722-7.

37. Soltani H, Poulose TA, Hutchon DR. Placental cord drainage after vaginal delivery as part of the management of the third stage of labour. *Cochrane Database Syst Rev*. 2011;9:CD004665. doi:10.1002/14651858.CD004665.pub3.

38. Chen M, Chang Q, Duan T, et al. Uterine massage to reduce blood loss after vaginal delivery: a randomized controlled trial. *Obstet Gynecol*. 2013;122(2 Pt 1):290-295. doi:10.1097/AOG.0b013e3182999085.

39. Hofmeyr GJ, Abdel-Aleem H, Abdel-Aleem MA. Uterine massage for preventing postpartum haemorrhage. *Cochrane Database Syst Rev*. 2013;7:CD006431. doi:10.1002/14651858.CD006431.pub3.

40. Menard MK, Main EK, Currigan SM. Executive summary of the reVITALize initiative. *Obstet Gynecol*. 2014;124:150-153.

41. American College of Obstetricians and Gynecologists. ACOG Practice Bulletin No. 183: postpartum hemorrhage. *Obstet Gynecol*. 2017;130:e168-e186.

42. Andrikopoulou M, D'Alton ME. Postpartum hemorrhage: early identification challenges. *Semin Perinatol.* 2019;43(1):11-17. doi:10.1053/j.semperi.2018.11.003.

43. Diaz V, Abalos E, Carroli G. Methods for blood loss estimation after vaginal birth. *Cochrane Database Syst Rev.* 2018;9(9):CD010980. doi:10.1002/14651858. CD010980.pub2.

44. Natrella M, Di Naro E, Loverro M, et al. The more you lose the more you miss: accuracy of postpartum blood loss visual estimation: a systematic review of the literature. *J Matern Fetal Neonatal Med.* 2018;31: 106-115. doi:10.1080/14767058.2016.1274302.

45. Schorn MN. Measurement of blood loss: review of the literature. *J Midwifery Womens Health.* 2010; 55:20-27.

46. American College of Obstetricians and Gynecologists. ACOG Committee Opinion No. 794: quantitative blood loss in obstetric hemorrhage. *Obstet Gynecol.* 2019;134:e150-e156. doi:10.1097 /AOG.0000000000003564.

47. Lyndon A, Lagrew D, Shields L, et al., eds. *Improving Health Care Response to Obstetric Hemorrhage: California Maternal Quality Care Collaborative Toolkit to Transform Maternity Care.* Version 2. California Maternal Quality Care Collaborative; March 24, 2015. https://www.cmqcc.org/resource /obstetric-hemorrhage-20-toolkit. Accessed October 2, 2021.

48. Neiman E, Austin E, Tan A, et al. Outcomes of waterbirth in a US hospital-based midwifery practice: a retrospective cohort study of water immersion during labor and birth. *J Midwifery Womens Health.* 2020;65(2):216-223. doi:10.1111/jmwh.13033.

49. Palmer J. Estimating blood loss in an inflatable birth pool. *Pregnancy: Birth & Beyond.* 2020. https://www .pregnancy.com.au/estimating-blood-loss-in-an -inflatable-birth-pool/. Accessed December 26, 2021.

50. Prates LA, Timm MS, Wilhelm LA, et al. Being born at home is natural: care rituals for home birth. *Rev Bras Enferm.* 2018;71(suppl 3):1247-1256. doi:10.1590/0034-7167-2017-0541.

51. Buckley SJ. Placenta rituals and folklore from around the world. *Midwifery Today Int Midwife.* 2006;80:58-59.

52. Burns E. More than clinical waste? Placenta rituals among Australian home-birthing women. *J Perinat Educ.* 2014;23:41-49.

53. Cole M. Placenta medicine as a galactogogue: tradition or trend?. *Clin Lact.* 2014;5:116-122.

54. Farr A, Chervenak FA, McCullough LB, et al. Human placentophagy: a review. *Am J Obstet Gynecol.* 2018;218:401.e1-401.e11. doi:10.1016/j .ajog.2017.08.016.

55. Joseph R, Giovinazzo M, Brown M. A literature review on the practice of placentophagia. *Nurs Womens Health.* 2016;20:476-483. doi:10.1016/j .nwh.2016.08.005.

56. Marraccini ME, Gorman KS. Exploring placentophagy in humans: problems and recommendations. *J Midwifery Womens Health.* 2015;60:371-379.

57. Langston C, Kaplan C, Macpherson T, et al. Practice guideline for examination of the placenta: developed by the Placental Pathology Practice Guideline Development Task Force of the College of American Pathologists. *Arch Pathol Lab Med.* 1997;121: 449-476.

58. Graham N, Heazell AEP. When the fetus goes still and the birth is tragic: the role of the placenta in stillbirths. *Obstet Gynecol Clin North Am.* 2020;47: 183-196. doi:10.1016/j.ogc.2019.10.005.

59. American College of Obstetricians and Gynecologists, Society for Maternal–Fetal Medicine. Management of stillbirth: Obstetric Care Consensus No. 10. *Obstet Gynecol.* 2020;135:e110-e132. doi:10.1097/ AOG.0000000000003719.

60. Cypher RL. Placental pathology and liability: a window to fetal health? *J Perinat Neonatal Nurs.* 2020;34: 294-296. doi:10.1097/JPN.0000000000000514.

61. Mittal N, Byard RW, Dahlstrom JE. A practical guide to placental examination for forensic pathologists. *Forensic Sci Med Pathol.* 2020;16(2):295-312. doi:10.1007/s12024-019-00214-2. Erratum in: *Forensic Sci Med Pathol.* January 8, 2020. PMID: 31873913.

62. Whitaker AK, Chen BA. Society of family planning guidelines: postplacental insertion of intrauterine devices. *Contraception.* 2018;97:2-13. doi:10.1016/j .contraception.2017.09.014.

63. Favilli A, Tosto V, Ceccobelli M, et al. Risk factors for non-adherent retained placenta after vaginal delivery: a systematic review. *BMC Pregnancy Childbirth.* 2021;21:268. doi:10.1186/s12884-021-03721-9.

64. Magann EF, Doherty DA, Briery CM, et al. Obstetric characteristics for a prolonged third stage of labor and risk for postpartum hemorrhage. *Gynecol Obstet Invest.* 2008;65:201-205. doi:10.1159/000112227.

65. Royal Women's Hospital. The third stage of labour—management. 2020. https://thewomens.r.worldssl. net/images/uploads/downloadable-records/clinical -guidelines/third-stage-labour-management-guideline_ 280720.pdf. Accessed December 26, 2021.

66. Patrick HS, Mitra A, Rosen T, et al. Pharmacologic intervention for the management of retained placenta: a systematic review and meta-analysis of randomized trials. *Am J Obstet Gynecol.* 2020;223(3):447. e1-447.e19. doi:10.1016/j.ajog.2020.06.044.

67. Wendel MP, Shnaekel KL, Magann EF. Uterine inversion: a review of a life-threatening obstetrical emergency. *Obstet Gynecol Surv.* 2018;73:411-417. doi:10.1097/OGX.0000000000000580.

68. Coad SL, Dahlgren LKS, Hutcheon JA. Risks and consequences of puerperal uterine inversion in the United States, 2004 through 2013. *Am J Obstet Gynecol*. 2017. doi:10.1016/j.ajog.2017.05.018.

69. Duzyj CM, Cooper A, Mhatre M, et al. Placenta accreta: a spectrum of predictable risk, diagnosis, and morbidity. *Am J Perinatol*. 2019;36:1031-1038. doi:10.1055/s-0038-1676111.

70. Carusi DA. The placenta accreta spectrum: epidemiology and risk factors. *Clin Obstet Gynecol*. 2018;61:733-742. doi:10.1097/GRF.0000000000000391.

71. Kramer MS, Berg C, Abenhaim H, et al. Incidence, risk factors, and temporal trends in severe postpartum hemorrhage. *Am J Obstet Gynecol*. 2013;209(449):449.e1-449.e7.

72. Bienstock JL, Eke AC, Hueppchen NA. Postpartum hemorrhage. *N Engl J Med*. 2021;384(17):1635-1645. doi:10.1056/NEJMra1513247.

73. Main EK, Cape V, Abreo A, et al. Reduction of severe maternal morbidity from hemorrhage using a state perinatal quality collaborative. *Am J Obstet Gynecol*. 2017;216:298.e1-298.e11.

74. Main EK, Chang SC, Dhurjati R, et al. Reduction in racial disparities in severe maternal morbidity from hemorrhage in a large-scale quality improvement collaborative. *Am J Obstet Gynecol*. 2020;223:123.e1-123.e14. doi:10.1016/j.ajog.2020.01.026.

75. Arafeh J, Gregory K, Main E, Lyndon A. Definition, early recognition and rapid response using triggers: CMQCC obstetric hemorrhage toolkit. 2015. https://www.cmqcc.org/resource/ob-hem-definition-early-recognition-and-rapid-response-using-triggers. Accessed October 3, 2021.

76. Merriam AA, Wright JD, Siddiq Z, et al. Risk for postpartum hemorrhage, transfusion, and hemorrhage-related morbidity at low, moderate, and high volume hospitals. *J Matern Fetal Neonatal Med*. 2018;31(8):1025-1034.

77. Rani PR, Begum J. Recent advances in the management of major postpartum hemorrhage: a review. *J Clin Diagnost Res*. 2017;11(2):QE01-QE05. doi:10.7860/JCDR/2017/22659.9463.

78. Evensen A, Anderson JM, Fontaine P. Postpartum hemorrhage: prevention and treatment. *Am Fam Physician*. 2017;95:442-449.

79. Matsuzaki S, Endo M, Ueda Y, et al. A case of acute Sheehan's syndrome and literature review: a rare but life-threatening complication of postpartum hemorrhage. *BMC Pregnancy Childbirth*. 2017;17:188. doi:10.1186/s12884-017-1380-y.

80. Main EK, Goffman D, Scavone BM, et al. National partnership for maternal safety consensus bundle on obstetric hemorrhage. *J Midwifery Womens Health*. 2015;60(4):458-464. doi:10.1111/jmwh.12345. Erratum in: *J Midwifery Womens Health*. 2015;60(6):789.

81. Bohren MA, Lorencatto F, Coomarasamy A, et al. Formative research to design an implementation strategy for a postpartum hemorrhage initial response treatment bundle (E-MOTIVE): study protocol. *Reprod Health*. 2021;18(1):149. doi:10.1186/s12978-021-01162-3.

82. Mhyre JM, D'Oria R, Hameed AB, et al. The maternal early warning criteria: a proposal from the national partnership for maternal safety. *J Obstet Gynecol Neonatal Nurs*. 2014;43(6):771-779. doi:10.1111/1552-6909.12504.

83. Gallos ID, Papadopoulou A, Man R, et al. Uterotonic agents for preventing postpartum haemorrhage: a network meta-analysis. *Cochrane Database of Syst Rev*. 2018;2018(12). doi:10.1002/14651858.CD011689.pub3

84. Lowe N, Openshaw M, King TL. Labor. In: Brucker MC, King TL, eds. *Pharmacology for Women's Health*. Burlington, MA: Jones & Bartlett Learning; 2017:1088.

85. WOMAN Trial Collaborators. Effect of early tranexamic acid administration on mortality, hysterectomy, and other morbidities in women with post-partum haemorrhage (WOMAN): an international, randomised, double-blind, placebo-controlled trial. *Lancet*. 2017. pii:S0140-6736(17)30638-4.

86. Vallera C, Choi LO, Cha CM, Hong RW. Uterotonic medications: oxytocin, methylergonovine, carboprost, misoprostol. *Anesthesiol Clin*. 2017;35:207-219.

87. Della Corte L, Saccone G, Locci M, et al. Tranexamic acid for treatment of primary postpartum hemorrhage after vaginal delivery: a systematic review and meta-analysis of randomized controlled trials. *J Matern Fetal Neonatal Med*. 2020;33(5):869-874. doi:10.1080/14767058.2018.1500544.

88. American College of Obstetricians and Gynecologists. Obstetric hemorrhage checklist. Revised September 2020. https://www.acog.org/-/media/project/acog/acogorg/files/forms/districts/smi-ob-hemorrhage-bundle-hemorrhage-checklist.pdf.

89. Chandraharan E, Krishna A. Diagnosis and management of postpartum haemorrhage. *BMJ*. 2017;358:j3875. doi:10.1136/bmj.j3875.

90. Ring L, Landau R. Postpartum hemorrhage: anesthesia management. *Semin Perinatol*. 2019;43:35-43. doi:10.1053/j.semperi.2018.11.007.

91. Watkins EJ, Stem K. Postpartum hemorrhage. *J Am Acad PA*. 2020;33:29-33. doi:10.1097/01.JAA.0000657164.11635.93.

92. Dubbs SB, Tewelde SZ. Cardiovascular catastrophes in the obstetric population. *Emerg Med Clin North Am*. 2015;33:483-500.

93. Blumenthal EA, Hooshvar N, McQuade M, McNulty J. A validation study of maternal early warning systems: a retrospective cohort study. *Am J Perinatol*. 2019;36:1106-1114. doi:10.1055/s-0039-1681097.

94. Arora KS, Shields LE, Grobman WA, et al. Triggers, bundles, protocols, and checklists: what every maternal care provider needs to know. *Am J Obstet Gynecol*. 2016;214:444-451. doi:10.1016/j.ajog.2015.10.011.

95. Zuckerwise LC, Lipkind HS. Maternal early warning systems: towards reducing preventable maternal mortality and severe maternal morbidity through improved clinical surveillance and responsiveness. *Semin Perinatol*. 2017;41:161-165. doi:10.1053/j.semperi.2017.03.005.

96. Aydın R, Aktaş S. Midwives' experiences of traumatic births: a systematic review and meta-synthesis. *Eur J Midwifery*. 2021;5:31. doi:10.18332/ejm/138197.

97. Minooee S, Cummins A, Foureur M, Travaglia J. Catastrophic thinking: is it the legacy of traumatic births? Midwives' experiences of shoulder dystocia complicated births. *Women Birth*. 2021;34:e38-e46. doi:10.1016/j.wombi.2020.08.008.

98. Minooee S, Cummins A, Sims DJ, et al. Scoping review of the impact of birth trauma on clinical decisions of midwives. *J Eval Clin Pract*. 2020;26:1270-1279. doi:10.1111/jep.13335.

99. Toohill J, Fenwick J, Sidebotham M, et al. Trauma and fear in Australian midwives. *Women Birth*. 2019;32:64-71. doi:10.1016/j.wombi.2018.04.003.

# 31A

# Management of the Third Stage of Labor

MAVIS N. SCHORN

## History

- Previous birth complications during the third stage, including postpartum hemorrhage (PPH)
- Risk factors for PPH
- Course of this labor and birth
- Maternal requests for specific management in the third stage of labor

## Physical Examination

- Birthing person's response to birth
- Vital signs stable
- Continuing evaluation of any previous significant findings
- Evaluation of new findings—for example, nausea is unusual in the third stage
- Evaluation of progress of the third stage, including signs of placental separation
- Continual assessment of bleeding

## Management Steps

These steps include components of both physiologic management and active management of the third stage of labor. Individual situations may require alterations in the order of individual steps.

1. Following birth, maintain or reinstate a calm environment to reduce anxiety and facilitate management of normal progress and treatment of perinatal complications if they occur.

2. Communicate the next steps and reassurance to the birthing person.

3. Place the newborn in skin-to-skin contact on the birthing person's abdomen or arrange to have the newborn placed skin to skin with a person whom the birthing person designates for this initial period with the infant.

4. Check the newborn's heart rate by palpating at the base of the umbilical cord and abdomen. If the heart rate is faster than 100 beats per minute, the newborn is breathing, and there are no obvious abnormalities, no intervention is needed.

5. Continue to observe the neonatal transition to extrauterine life while the newborn is in skin-to-skin contact. Note that the midwife conducting the birth has a primary responsibility to the birthing person during the third stage of labor, not to the newborn.

6. Administer or request administration of a uterotonic agent, if not already given during birth of the anterior shoulder (optional depending on the birthing person's risk for postpartum hemorrhage, policies, and amount of bleeding present).

7. Consider upright positioning, which uses gravity to assist with placental expulsion, if feasible.

8. If cord blood gases are not indicated, two clamps are needed:

   a. Clamp the cord with two clamps placed close together near the newborn's umbilicus after at least 1 to 3 minutes or when the cord stops pulsating or appears drained of blood. See the *Umbilical Cord Clamping at Birth* appendix for more information.

b. Cut the cord between the two clamps or guide the partner, other support person, or birthing person to do this.

9. If cord blood gases are indicated, four clamps are needed:

a. Place an initial clamp on the cord near the birthing person's introitus.

b. Place two clamps in close approximation to each other on the cord distal (toward the newborn's umbilicus) to the first clamp.

c. Cut the cord (or have another person cut it) between the last two clamps, and place the newborn on the birthing person's abdomen or hand off the newborn to another provider as indicated.

d. Place a fourth clamp close to the first clamp that was placed near the birthing person's introitus, and cut the cord between these two last clamps. There is now a sealed double-clamped section of cord that can be used to obtain cord blood gases (**Figure 31A-1**).

e. Obtain a sample of blood from the umbilical artery first, and then a sample from one of the umbilical veins, in a heparinized syringe, marking each syringe correctly as from the artery or the vein. Once the syringe is capped, the blood is stable for up to 30 minutes before the blood gas measurement has to be obtained.

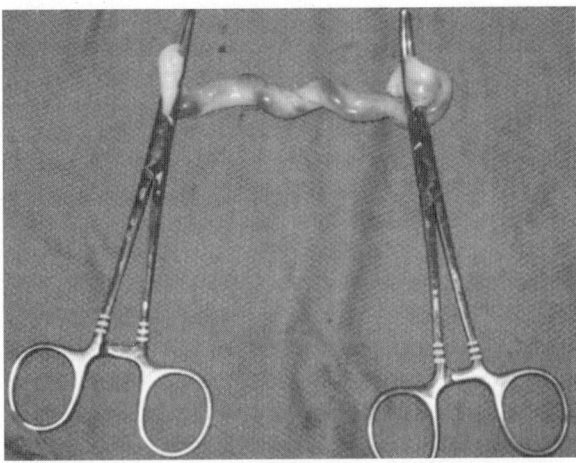

**Figure 31A-1** Double-clamped cord.
Photograph courtesy of Tekoa L. King, CNM, MPH.

(Interpretation of cord gases is discussed in the *Umbilical Cord Gas Technique and Interpretation* appendix.)

10. Inspect the cut end of the umbilical cord and count the number of umbilical vessels. See the *Inspection of the Umbilical Cord, Placenta, and Membranes* appendix for more information.

11. Open the clamp nearest the birthing person's introitus and allow blood from the placenta to fill a non-heparinized blood collection tube. If the end of the cord is visibly covered with maternal blood, it is good practice to clean the cord before inserting it into the collection tube to aid in visibility and reduce the amount of maternal blood mixed with neonatal blood for analysis. Approximately 5 to 10 mL is needed. This blood will be used to determine the type and Rh status of the newborn. Do not milk the cord, as tissue thromboplastin can interfere with the analysis.

12. Observe for signs of placental separation (Table 31-1). Do not massage the uterus before placental separation. Massaging the uterus prior to complete separation may increase uterine bleeding or lead to incomplete expulsion of the placenta.

13. Guard the uterus by placing a hand suprapubically, anterior to the uterine fundus, to assess for uterine position in the abdomen and to prevent uterine inversion as the placenta is expelled.

14. Determine whether the placenta has separated:

a. Use the Brandt–Andrews maneuver (Figure 31A-2). Apply slight downward pressure just above the pelvic brim with the hand that is guarding the uterus, while holding the cord taut with the other hand. If the placenta is still in the uterus, the cord will retract as the uterus is displaced upward into the abdomen by pressure from the abdominal hand. If the placenta has separated and is in the vagina, upward displacement of the uterus will not cause the cord to retract, and additional cord traction can be safely provided while maintaining abdominal counter-traction.

b. Another method of checking for placental location is to slide one finger (using sterile gloves) beside the umbilical cord

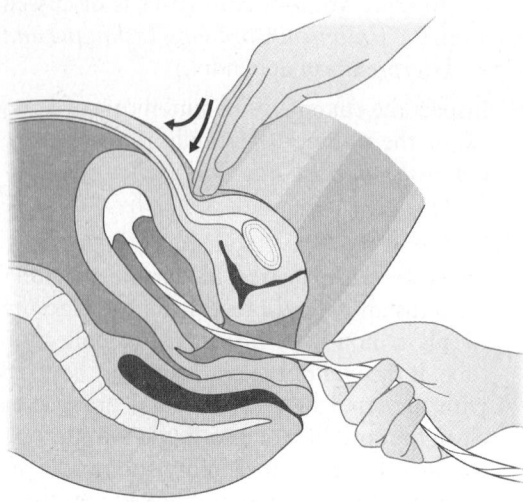

**Figure 31A-2** Brandt–Andrews maneuver.

into the vagina. If the placenta is in the vagina, it will be felt by the tip of the finger. The cord insertion into the placenta feels somewhat like an inverted umbrella. If the cord goes past the cervix, the placenta has not been expelled from the uterus. If the placenta is palpated in the vagina, additional traction can be safely performed.

15. Once the placenta has separated, the birthing person may spontaneously expel it by pushing. The midwife can also use a combination of the Brandt–Andrews maneuver and controlled cord traction to facilitate its expulsion.

16. Cord traction should *not* be performed without guarding the uterus, as this maneuver may result in an avulsed cord or inverted uterus.

17. Grasp the placenta with both hands as it is being expelled. Slowly guide the placenta out, perhaps following the curve of the pelvis to allow the membranes to follow the same path and not tear. If there appear to be more membranes than are immediately expelled, continue to hold the placenta and either twist it slowly or grasp the membranes with a ring forceps to gently extract the membranes—a process commonly known as "teasing" out the membranes.

18. Palpate the fundus abdominally to assess if the fundus is firm. Routine vigorous massage to stimulate uterine contraction has not been shown to decrease the incidence of hemorrhage. Such massage may be indicated to express clots through the cervix if excessive bleeding is present, but it is not indicated if the estimated blood loss is normal.

19. Inspect the cord, placenta, and membranes as described in the *Inspection of the Umbilical Cord, Placenta, and Membranes* appendix (Table 31-3).

20. Show the placenta to the birthing person and family if they are interested.

21. Count instruments, gauze, and sharps, retaining gauze for quantified blood loss measurement.

22. Measure or weigh blood loss.

23. Weigh the placenta.

24. Send the placenta for pathology evaluation if indicated.

# 31B

# Inspection of the Umbilical Cord, Placenta, and Membranes

MAVIS N. SCHORN

Inspection of the umbilical cord, placenta, and membranes is performed as soon as the birthing person and newborn are stable and comfortable. Any abnormal findings are documented in the health records. In some situations, a photograph may be of value for documentation.

## Inspection of the Umbilical Cord

### Count the Number of Vessels

Wipe off the cut end with a gauze or towel if needed. Apply pressure; the apertures of the vessels will be visible. If vessels have collapsed, reclamp and recut the cord, then look for the vessels at the site of the new cut (Figure 31B-1).

Three vessels should be visible: two small arteries and one large vein. Any two-vessel cord should

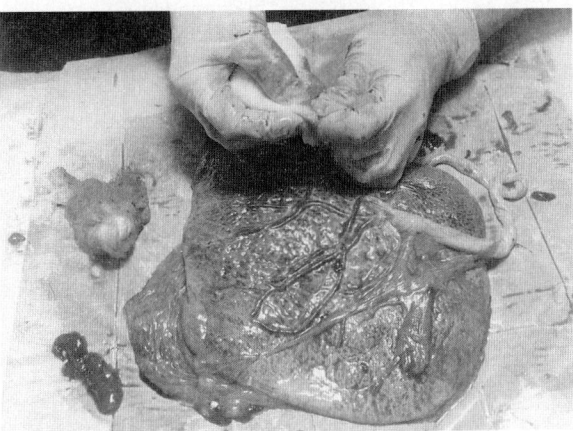

**Figure 31B-1** Counting the number of cord vessels.
Photograph courtesy of Carrie Klima, CNM, PhD.

be submitted for pathology examination, and neonatal providers should be informed.

### Measure the Length of the Cord

If the cord appears abnormally long or short, it should be measured. Remember to include the length of cord cut off the newborn's end when the cord was clamped and cut.

The normal length of a term umbilical cord is approximately 55 to 60 centimeters (range: 30 to 90 centimeters). A long cord, more than 75 centimeters, is associated with knots and fetal entanglement. Short cords, less than 32 centimeters, may be associated with limited fetal movement.

### Inspect the Cord for Abnormalities

Look for knots, hematomas, tumors, cysts, edema, and the amount of Wharton's jelly (Figure 31B-2). The normal width of an umbilical cord is 1 to 2 cm. The width is affected by the amount of Wharton's jelly.

### Inspect the Cord Insertion Site

Observe the insertion site for where the cord inserts in relation to the body of the placenta—central, eccentric, or marginal (Battledore placenta). Determine whether the cord is inserted directly into the placenta or is attached by exposed vessels (velamentous cord insertion) (Figure 31B-3). Centric and eccentric (off-center) insertions are variations of normal; however, velamentous and marginal insertions are unusual and associated with a risk of

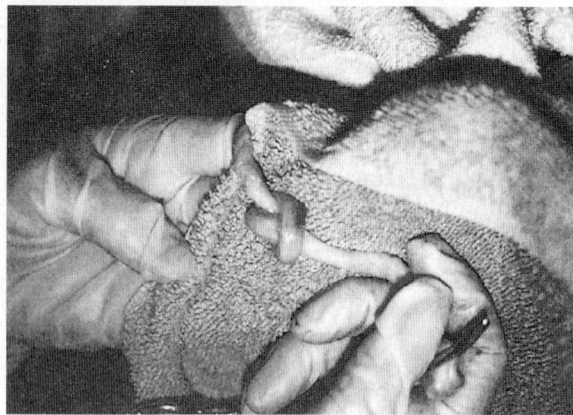

**Figure 31B-2** True knot in the umbilical cord.
Photograph courtesy of Carrie Klima, CNM, PhD.

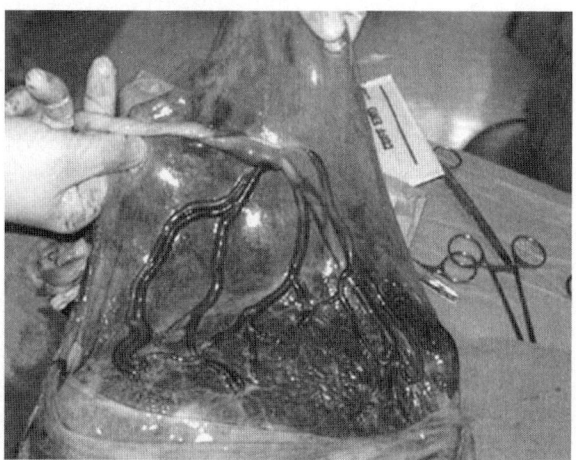

**Figure 31B-3** Velamentous insertion of the umbilical cord.
Photograph courtesy of Tekoa L. King, CNM, MPH.

vasa previa should one of these vessels tear when the membranes rupture.

## Inspection of the Placenta

### Inspect the Placenta for Color, Shape, Size, and Consistency

Lay the placenta flat on a surface. Look at the fetal and uterine sides. If necessary, invert the membranes to see both surfaces.

The placental shape is usually round to slightly oval and approximately 2 to 3 centimeters in thickness. The fetal surface is smooth. The uterine surface is usually smooth with indentations at the edges of cotyledons, but may have gritty white areas of calcification. Generally, the quantity of calcifications has no clinical importance. A pale placenta is associated with immature neonates and anemia.

With extended exposure to meconium, a placenta may be stained green.

### Inspect the Smooth, Shiny Fetal Side of the Placenta

Inspect for distribution of vessels from the umbilical cord over the surface of the placenta. The fetal blood vessels traverse the fetal surface of the placenta from the cord insertion toward the placental margin before turning into the parenchyma, toward the uterine surface. Inspect for cysts and to determine whether this is an extrachorial placenta (either a placenta circumvallata or a placenta marginata). If necessary, invert the membranes to visualize the entire fetal surface. In addition, examine the fetal surface closely for torn or intact blood vessels leading into the membranes so as to identify a missing or intact succenturiate (accessory) lobe.

### Inspect the Uterine Side

Examine the placental margin for torn blood vessels leading into the membranes to look for evidence of a succenturiate lobe. A cotyledon missing from the main placental mass is identified by a defect in the placental mass with a rough surface where it tore away/avulsed or by a torn vessel at the edge of the placenta. This must be differentiated from a simple tear in the placenta without loss of tissue, which also leaves a rough surface. Differentiation can be achieved by holding the placenta, uterine surface up, so that the cotyledons fall into place against each other (Figure 31B-4). A missing cotyledon is then evident because, as in a jigsaw puzzle, the surrounding pieces will not fit together smoothly. Observe for infarcts, cysts, tumors, and edema.

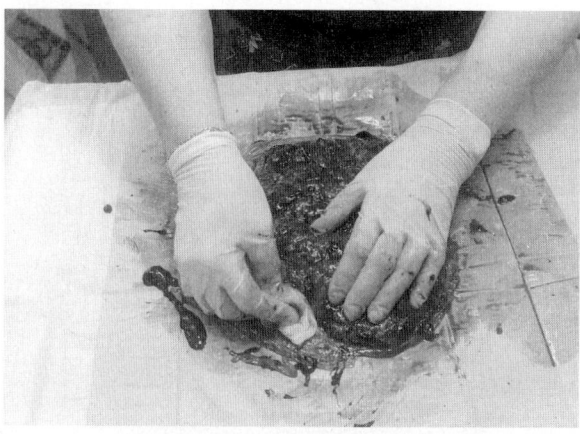

**Figure 31B-4** Midwife examining the uterine side of the placenta. The placenta is intact.
Photograph courtesy of Carrie Klima, CNM, PhD.

**Measure and Weigh the Placenta**

Measuring and weighing of the placenta are usually dictated by policy and are not always routinely performed. A term placenta usually weighs between 400 and 4600 grams. Regardless of the policy in place, if the placenta appears to be of abnormal size, weighing and referring for pathology examination are indicated. This information is then recorded in the health record for both the birthing person and the newborn.

## Inspection of the Membranes

Place the placenta uterine side down, place a hand inside the membranes on the fetal surface of the placenta, and then hold the membranes up to simulate the sac they once were (**Figure 31B-5**). If the membranes are ragged and do not form a sac, they may be incomplete. If a portion of the membranes is missing, membranes may still be within the uterus, although this is not a sensitive indicator of retained membranes.

When inspection and documentation are complete, the placenta should be disposed of appropriately. In some cases, families may wish to keep

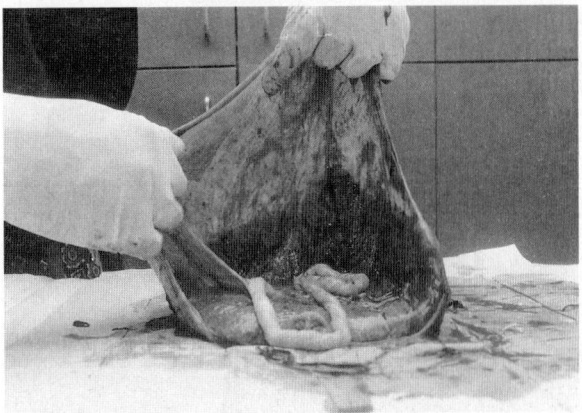

**Figure 31B-5** Midwife examining the fetal side of the placenta. The membranes are incomplete.
Photograph courtesy of Carrie Klima, CNM, PhD.

this organ for culturally appropriate disposal, such as planting in their gardens. Others may desire to make impressions of it for a type of placental art. However, midwives should be aware that the placenta contains body fluids and should be treated with universal precautions.

# APPENDIX

# 31C

# Postplacental Intrauterine Device Insertion and Removal

MELICIA ESCOBAR AND SIGNEY OLSON

## Introduction

Intrauterine devices, a form of long-acting reversible contraceptive (LARC) agent, are safe for contraceptive and noncontraceptive usage among postpartum patients when inserted postplacentally into the uterus after birth. Intrauterine devices can be referred to by several different terms and abbreviations: intrauterine device (IUD), intrauterine contraceptive device (IUCD), intrauterine contraception (UC), and intrauterine system (IUS). For the purposes of this appendix, the terms "intrauterine device" and "IUD" will be used throughout. Of the five different brands of IUDs currently available in the United States, three are appropriate for postplacental insertion: the copper version (copper IUD) and two IUDs containing 52 mg of levonorgestrel (LNG-IUD). More information about the effectiveness and use of these devices in the postplacental period is found in the *Fertility, Family Building, and Contraception*; *Nonhormonal Contraception*; and *Hormonal Contraception* chapters. For more information on IUD insertion and removal outside of the postplacental period, see the *Intrauterine Device Insertion and Removal* appendix.

This appendix can be used as a guide for insertion of an IUD during the postplacental period. Note that the LNG-IUD can be used in the treatment of women with menorrhagia; more information about this noncontraceptive usage is found in the *Menstrual Cycle Abnormalities* chapter.

## Advancing Reproductive Justice

In advance of IUD insertion, the clinician should examine personal biases toward contraceptive options, as this is essential to providing evidence-based information that is free of judgment.[1] Additionally, a discussion with the patient using shared decision making should be undertaken to determine optimal insertion timing. In cases where individuals have limited access to care, postplacental IUD insertion can serve as a means of improving patient reproductive rights. However, midwives should be aware that the United States has a history of reproductive coercion, especially the provision of contraceptives to impair the reproductive potential of individuals from marginalized groups. This long-acting method requires a healthcare visit to discontinue and should not be placed unless the individual desires the method, understands its potential side effects, and knows how it can be removed.

## Counseling About Postplacental IUD Insertion

Ideally, individuals should receive counseling about postpartum contraceptive options prenatally. A thorough reproductive life plan and health history, health education, contraindications, risks, contraceptive and noncontraceptive benefits, side effects, and adverse effects are reviewed as part of the shared decision-making process.[1-7] Specific to postplacental IUD insertion, counseling should include a discussion of risks and benefits related to the higher rate of expulsion, signs and symptoms of insertion, and possible need for a back-up method if expulsion occurs. These topics are presented briefly in this appendix along with key information to inform the discussion around expulsion. The reader is referred to the *Hormonal Contraceptives* chapter, which includes resources and references, for a more detailed description of health counseling prior to IUD insertion.

A written consent form granting permission to the clinician for IUD insertion, signed by the patient either on paper or by electronic means, is part of the shared decision making and legal informed consent. Health education should include the costs involved with IUD insertion. Although the initial cost may be higher than for other contraceptive methods, the IUD becomes cost neutral after 3 years of continuous use and has the added cost savings associated with reduction in unintended pregnancies.[6,7] Although most state Medicaid programs now offer guidance for postplacental IUD reimbursement, there is variability with regard to how it is reimbursed and variability of its coverage among private insurers.[8] For those individuals without coverage, some financial support for IUD use may be available directly through the pharmaceutical companies, their associated philanthropic programs, or LARC programs within the institution.

### Contraindications for Postplacental IUD Insertion

Similar to interval IUD insertion occurring outside of the postpartum period, the initial step prior to consideration of an intrauterine device is to determine if the patient has any potential contraindications as listed in the *Hormonal Contraception* chapter. Particularly relevant to postplacental IUD insertion, among most individuals of reproductive age, including adolescents, there are limited contraindications for either LNG or copper IUDs. Puerperal sepsis is an absolute contraindication, while uterine infection and ongoing PPH have also been identified as contraindications.[3,4,9]

### Risks and Benefits Associated with Postplacental IUD Insertion

The benefits of postplacental IUDs include improved contraception continuance rates, decreased rates of short-interval birth, increased access to individuals who would otherwise lose access postpartum, and a cost-effective way to prevent unplanned pregnancy.[10–12] With continued long-term use, IUDs confer the same benefits as with interval placement. There are also some potential risks that can be mitigated with care upon insertion and access to ongoing contraceptive care.

### Uterine Perforation and Infection

While perforation and infection of the uterus at the time of postplacental IUD insertion are theoretical risks, studies looking at these events have not found this to be an issue.[13] Any person demonstrating symptoms of bleeding or shock post insertion should be transferred to an appropriate care facility for prompt treatment.

### Expulsion

The risk of IUD expulsion is higher among individuals after postplacental insertion as compared to those after interval insertion (20% to 27% compared to 0% to 4.4%).[14] Timing, method of birth, and device type may play a role. Immediate insertion within 10 minutes of birth, as opposed to placement from 10 minutes to discharge, can limit the risk of expulsion (10% versus 29.7%).[15] Expulsion rates have been found to be higher after vaginal birth (19% to 30%) as compared to cesarean birth (3% to 20%) and the same or higher with insertion of LNG-IUDs as compared to copper IUDs (no difference or 17% versus 4%).[13,16–18] Access to contraceptive care for replacement or removal positively impacts rates of continued use in the event of expulsion or malposition.[19] The risk of expulsion must be weighed against the known benefits and be placed in the context of the individual and their reproductive health goals through shared decision making. It should not be the sole reason for limiting this option.

### Side Effects and Adverse Effects Associated with Postplacental IUDs

As with interval insertion of LNG or copper IUDs, myths and misconceptions are best addressed during pre-insertion counseling.[9] Side effects associated with continued use, primarily changed vaginal bleeding patterns, should be reviewed.

There exists debate in the literature with regard to the impact and safety of LNG-IUDs related to breast/chestfeeding initiation, milk supply, and continuation. The U.S. Medical Eligibility Criteria (MEC) recognize that the potential advantages outweigh the theoretical risks and assign a Category 2 rating to this usage.[4] Earlier findings suggested that immediate postpartum IUD insertion does not impact initiation, although continuation rates and rates of exclusively breastfeeding/chestfeeding among infants may be lower among this group.[20] A more recent study, however, found no significant impact among healthy breastfeeding/chestfeeding individuals.[21] In light of the theoretical risk, breastfeeding/chestfeeding goals should be incorporated into the shared decision-making process.

### Choice of an IUD

Several IUDs are currently available in the United States. Both the copper and 52-mg LNG IUDs are appropriate for postplacental insertion, provide highly effective contraception, can be identified on ultrasound if needed, and are easily reversible. Nevertheless, in the context of continued use of the IUD, certain differences between these options must be taken into consideration to determine the most suitable choice for a particular individual. A detailed description can be found in the *Hormonal Contraception* and *Nonhormonal Contraception* chapters.

### Timing of IUD Insertion

Insertion of an IUD in the immediate postpartum period is becoming more common in the United States in an effort to increase patient convenience and reduce unplanned pregnancies.[14,22] While postplacental insertion (i.e., within 10 minutes of birth) may be favored due to the open state of the cervical os, insertion in the early postpartum period (i.e., more than 10 minutes to 72 hours through 1 week after birth) is also reasonable and may be advantageous in situations where postplacental insertion may be prohibitive (e.g., in the setting of immediate PPH).[23] Through shared decision making, timing of insertion can be determined in partnership with the birthing person and should include consideration of access to contraception during and after the postpartum period.

## Postplacental IUD Insertion

Postplacental IUD insertion can be done effectively using either the forceps or manual techniques regardless of device type. The choice of technique should be guided by clinician competency and comfort, the state of the cervix, and, most importantly, the comfort of the patient.

Multiple resources for IUD insertion procedures exist online, including video recordings that can help the clinician review the process.[24] In addition, the U.S. Food and Drug Administration (FDA)–approved prescribing information and package label for each device include insertion instructions and images. The following steps for insertion are general guidelines and cannot replace hands-on experiences.

### Premedication

The need for premedication prior to postplacental insertion will depend on the patient's comfort and needs. If epidural analgesia is already in place, it may be continued through insertion. For those individuals who do not and require additional comfort measures, nitrous oxide may be effective.[14,25] While typically unnecessary, local anesthesia for a cervical block or perineal laceration can be kept at the ready.

### Required Equipment for IUD Insertion

*General equipment* includes the following items:

- Fresh sterile gloves of appropriate size (i.e., ideally separate from those used during the birth)
- Sterile water-impermeable gown
- Sterile speculum or retractors
- Adequate lighting for visualization
- Antiseptic solution (povidone–iodine or 4% chlorhexidine gluconate)
- Sterile field
- Sterile drapes
- IUD
- Two sterile ring forceps
- Sharp, long, curved scissors (optional if strings are left long)
- Bedside ultrasound (confirmation of placement optional)

The IUD of choice may be placed on the field or handed to the clinician by an assistant. If resources allow, a secondary IUD may be available should contamination occur with the first one.

### Key Points for Insertion

1. After engaging in shared decision making, the patient should have signed legal consent for documentation and verification of understanding of the procedure when they were not under the effects of systemic opioids.

2. The patient should be reassured that the procedure can be stopped at any time should they make this request.

3. Optimally, the clinician should have another individual available to assist with the procedure.

4. The patient should be in a physical position that prioritizes their comfort and safety during the procedure. Analgesia can be administered as appropriate.

5. Palpate the fundus and assess the uterus for position.

6. The insertion is begun using sterile technique and new sterile gloves (not the ones used during the birth) should be donned immediately prior to the procedure.

7. The cervix and vagina can be swabbed with the antiseptic.

8. While performing these actions, the clinician should be mindful of the patient's comfort.

9. At this point, the steps for the insertion vary based on technique. However, for all IUDs, the clinician must maintain scrupulous sterile technique. The device is not opened until it has been deemed appropriate for immediate insertion.

## Postplacental Insertion of an IUD After Vaginal Birth

Again, placement of an IUD in the postplacental postpartum period is contraindicated for patients with uterine infection (e.g., peripartum chorioamnionitis or endometritis) or puerperal sepsis.[22] Alternative methods of contraception should be offered and placement of the IUD deferred in such a case. As with any contraceptive method, a patient should be engaged in shared decision making and the decision should be made prior to labor.

## Ring Forceps Technique

1. Ensure that the device is placed within 10 minutes of the birth of the placenta.

2. Clean the external genitalia and apply sterile drapes over the abdomen and under the buttocks.

3. Retraction of the vagina with a gloved hand, speculum, or retractor may be performed if visualization is necessary.

4. Swab the cervix and vagina with an antiseptic if desired; similarly, analgesia can be administered as appropriate.

5. Using a ring forceps, stabilize the cervix by grasping the anterior lip.

6. Remove the IUD from the inserter and, with a second ring forceps, grasp the device by the vertical arm, with the horizontal arms slightly outside the ring but on the same plane. When grasping the device, be sure to do so firmly without completely locking the teeth so as not to damage the device (Figure 31C-1).

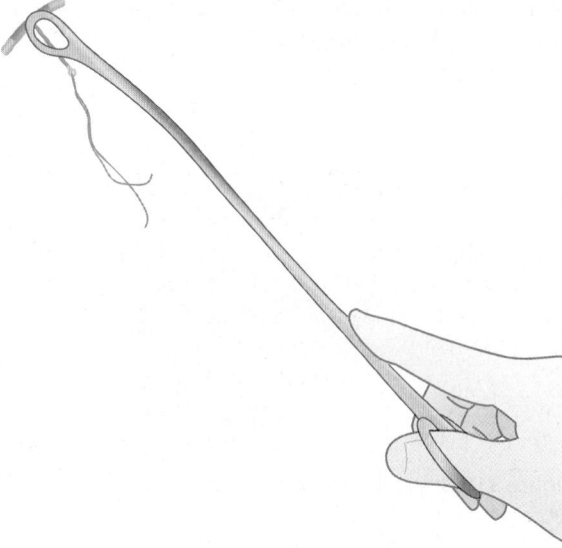

**Figure 31C-1** Grasping the intrauterine device with ring forceps.

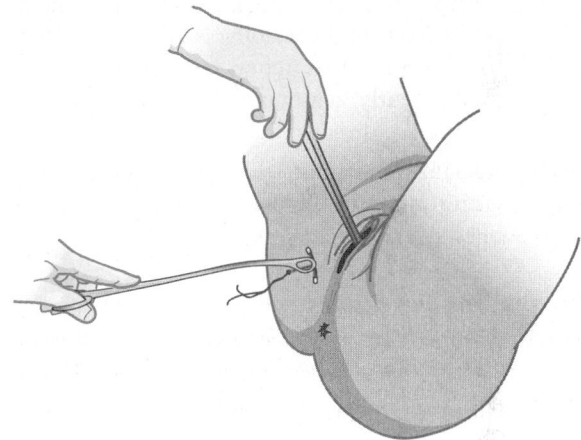

**Figure 31C-2** Inserting the intrauterine device with ring forceps while placing traction on the cervix.

7. Cut the strings to approximately 10 centimeters in length.

8. Apply gentle traction to the ring forceps to stabilize the cervix.

9. Insert the device through the cervix and into the lower uterine segment (**Figure 31C-2**).

10. With the clinician's nondominant hand placed on the fundus to stabilize the uterus, advance the device to the uterine fundus, with ring forceps still grasping it, in an upward angle toward the umbilicus (**Figure 31C-3**).

11. If desired, confirm that the device is in place using ultrasound guidance.

12. Once in the fundus, release the device and remove the ring forceps by opening the

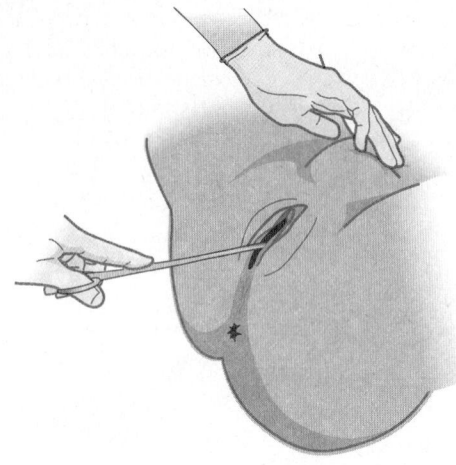

**Figure 31C-3** Stabilizing the uterus while placing the intrauterine device in the fundus.

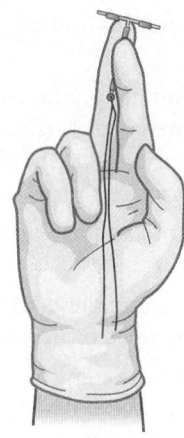

**Figure 31C-4** Grasping the intrauterine device prior to manual insertion.

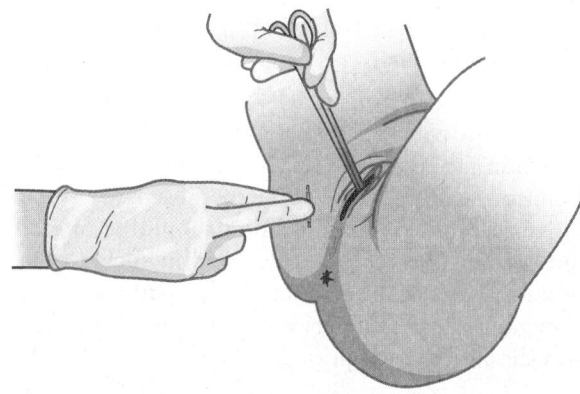

**Figure 31C-5** Manually inserting the intrauterine device with a retractor in place if needed.

forceps slightly, rotating the instrument 90 degrees, and carefully sweeping laterally to withdraw. This action reduces the risk of inadvertently removing the new device by pulling the threads.

13. Visualize or palpate the cervix, examine for laceration, and remove the ring forceps applied to the cervix.

## Manual Technique

1. Ensure that the device is placed within 10 minutes of when the placenta is expelled.

2. Clean the external genitalia with warm water and apply sterile drapes over the abdomen and under the buttocks.

3. Swab the cervix and vagina with the antiseptic if desired; similarly, analgesia can be administered as appropriate.

4. Visualize the cervix with a gloved hand, speculum, or retractor.

5. Remove the IUD from the inserter and grasp the vertical rod between the index and middle fingers of the dominant hand, noting the plane of the horizontal arms (**Figure 31C-4**).

6. Cut the strings to approximately 10 centimeters in length.

7. Insert the device through the cervix (**Figure 31C-5**).

8. With the clinician's nondominant hand placed fundally to stabilize the uterus, advance the device to the uterine fundus manually at an upward angle toward the

umbilicus, following the curve of the uterine cavity (**Figure 31C-6**).

9. If desired, confirm that the device is in place using ultrasound.

10. Release the IUD and carefully remove the dominant hand from the uterus and vagina, while avoiding dislodging the device or inadvertently applying traction on the threads.

## Health Education

After postplacental insertion of an IUD, health education is similar to that for interval insertion. The information to be provided includes signs associated with expulsion, displacement, perforation, heavy uterine bleeding, or new-onset uterine or abdominal pain.[1] Discomfort or heavy bleeding in the postpartum period that persists after corrective measures are taken may be associated with expulsion or displacement. A pelvic exam can be done to

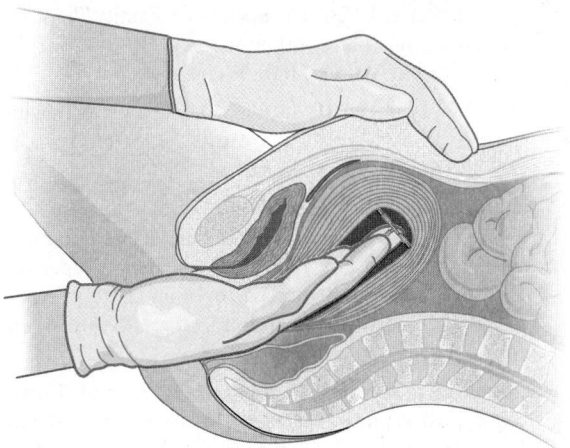

**Figure 31C-6** Stabilizing the uterus while manually placing the intrauterine device in the fundus.

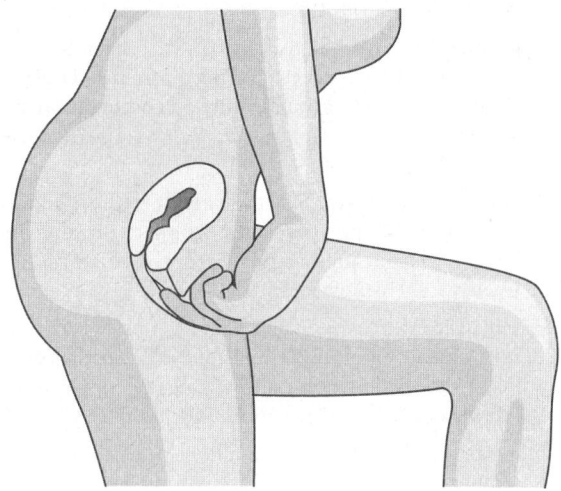

**Figure 31C-7** How to feel for intrauterine device threads or strings.

evaluate IUD placement, prior to discharge or at a follow-up visit.

Teaching about how to feel for and identify the threads in the vagina is also warranted (**Figure 31C-7**). A sample IUD with strings the woman can feel may be used as a teaching aid. Any significant variations—such as unusual lengthening of the strings, which may indicate nonfundal placement, or feeling any part of the plastic of the device through the cervix—should be reported, as these findings may suggest partial expulsion of the IUD.

Patients should be counseled that the theoretical risk of deep vein thrombosis is low (i.e., Category 1 for copper IUDs and Category 2 for LNG-IUDs) despite the hypercoagulable state that is present postpartum.[4]

The mnemonic "PAINS" is often shared after IUD insertion as an easy-to-use reminder of potentially significant deviations that should be reported (Table 12-15). In all cases, individuals with IUDs should be encouraged to contact their provider with questions or concerns, although most do not experience major side effects. With continued use, among the most common side effects of all IUDs are menstrual irregularities. In some people, especially those using a copper IUD, dysmenorrhea or heavy bleeding may occur; the use of nonsteroidal anti-inflammatory drugs (NSAIDs) provides relief from either or both of these symptoms. Conversely, people using an LNG-containing IUD may experience decreased menstrual flow or amenorrhea. However, sudden amenorrhea for any person with an IUD may be suggestive of pregnancy, and they should be evaluated for this condition.

Finally, a plan for removal consistent with the life span of the device should be made in accordance with the package insert. Although a 2- to 6-week postpartum visit offers an opportunity to check in with the individual about potential symptoms and side effects they may be experiencing after IUD placement, a separate, earlier follow-up visit specifically for IUD assessment is not necessary.[3]

### Follow-Up Care

At scheduled postpartum visits, any concerns may be addressed. A speculum exam can be performed to confirm that the threads are visible and to trim them if needed. Using sharp scissors, strings may be trimmed to a length of approximately 3 centimeters from the external os. If the patient's body size and habitus or physical mobility warrant it, the clinician may cut the IUD threads longer than 3 centimeters to assure that they can easily feel them. The device may be replaced at the time of expiration or if device placement is altered and strings readjusted if needed, which promotes long-term IUD use.

If strings are not visible at the postpartum follow-up visit, a thin forceps, such as foreign body forceps, or an IUD extractor hook can be used to gently draw out the strings or a uterine sound can be used to check for placement of the device. If it is unclear whether expulsion has occurred, an ultrasound may be conducted to assess for placement. If needed, a back-up method of contraception should be discussed using shared decision making. If the IUD has been expelled or is no longer desired, alternative contraceptive or family building methods may be discussed at this time.

## Removal of an IUD

Common reasons cited for requesting removal of an IUD include desire for a pregnancy, unresolved or troublesome side effects of menstrual irregularities, establishment of menopause, or end of duration of effectiveness. The removal procedure is the same for all of the IUDs and is addressed in the *Intrauterine Device Insertion and Removal* appendix.

## References

1. Dole DM, Martin J. What nurses need to know about immediate postpartum initiation of long-acting reversible contraception. *Nurs Womens Health*. 2017;21(3):186-195.

2. Callegari LS, Aiken AR, Dehlendorf C, et al. Addressing potential pitfalls of reproductive life planning with patient-centered counseling. *Am J Obstet Gynecol*. 2017;216(2):129-134.

3. Curtis KM, Jatlaoui TC, Tepper NK, et al. U.S. selected practice recommendations for contraceptive use, 2016. *MMWR Recomm Rep*. 2016;65(RR-4):1-66.

4. Curtis KM, Tepper NK, Jatlaoui TC, et al. U.S. medical eligibility criteria for contraceptive use, 2016. *MMWR Recomm Rep*. 2016;65(RR-3):1-104.

5. American College of Obstetricians and Gynecologists. Adolescents and long-acting reversible contraception: implants and intrauterine devices. ACOG Committee Opinion No. 539. *Obstet Gynecol*. 2014;120;983-938.

6. Trussell J, Hassan F, Lowin J, et al. Achieving cost-neutrality with long-acting reversible contraceptive methods. *Contraception*. 2015;91(1):49-56.

7. Bearak JM, Finer LB, Jerman J, Kavanaugh ML. Changes in out-of-pocket costs for hormonal IUDs after implementation of the Affordable Care Act: an analysis of insurance benefit inquiries. *Contraception*. 2016;93(2):139-144.

8. American College of Obstetricians & Gynecologists. Medicaid reimbursement for postpartum LARC in the hospital setting. https://www.acog.org/programs /long-acting-reversible-contraception-larc/activities -initiatives/medicaid-reimbursement-for-postpartum -larc. Updated June 30, 2020. Accessed October 15, 2021.

9. American College of Obstetricians and Gynecologists. Long-acting reversible contraception: implants and intrauterine devices. ACOG Practice Bulletin No. 186. *Obstet Gynecol*. 2017 (reaffirmed 2021); 130(5):e251-e269.

10. Moniz MH, Roosevelt L, Crissman HP, et al. Immediate postpartum contraception: a survey needs assessment of a national sample of midwives. *J Midwifery Womens Health*. 2017;62(5):538-544.

11. Whitaker AK, Chen BA. Society of Family Planning guidelines: postplacental insertion of intrauterine devices. *Contraception*. 2018;97(1):2-13.

12. Woo VG, Lundeen T, Matula S, Milstein A. Achieving higher-value obstetrical care. *Am J Obstet Gynecol*. 2017;216(3):250.e1-205.e14.

13. Blumenthal PD, Lerma K, Bhamrah R, Singh S; Dedicated PPIUD Inserter Working Group. Comparative safety and efficacy of a dedicated postpartum IUD inserter versus forceps for immediate postpartum IUD insertion: a randomized trial. *Contraception*. 2018;98(3):215-219.

14. Lopez LM, Bernholc A, Hubacher D, et al. Immediate postpartum insertion of intrauterine device for contraception. *Cochrane Database Syst Rev*. 2015;6:CD003036.

15. Jatlaoui TC, Whiteman MK, Jeng G, et al. Intrauterine device expulsion after postpartum placement: a systematic review and meta-analysis. *Obstet Gynecol*. 2018;132(4):895.

16. Blumenthal PD, Chakraborty NM, Prager S, et al. Programmatic experience of postpartum IUD use in Zambia: an observational study on continuation and satisfaction. *Eur J Contracept Reprod Health Care*. 2016;21(5):356-360.

17. Gurney EP, Sonalkar S, McAllister A, et al. Six-month expulsion of postplacental copper intrauterine devices placed after vaginal delivery. *Am J Obstet Gynecol*. 2018;219(2):183.e1-183.e9.

18. Hinz EK, Murthy A, Wang B, et al. A prospective cohort study comparing expulsion after postplacental insertion: the levonorgestrel versus the copper intrauterine device. *Contraception*. 2019;100(2):101-105.

19. Strasser J, Borkowski L, Couillard M, et al. Access to removal of long-acting reversible contraceptive methods is an essential component of high-quality contraceptive care. *Womens Health Issues*. 2017;27(3): 253-255.

20. Chen BA, Reeves MF, Creinin MD, Schwarz EB. Postplacental or delayed levonorgestrel intrauterine device insertion and breastfeeding duration. *Contraception*. 2011;84(5):499-504.

21. Turok DK, Leeman L, Sanders JN, et al. Immediate postpartum levonorgestrel intrauterine device insertion and breastfeeding outcomes: a noninferiority randomized controlled trial. *Am J Obstet Gynecol*. 2017;217(6):665.e1-665.e8.

22. American College of Obstetricians and Gynecologists. Immediate postpartum long-acting reversible contraception. Committee Opinion No. 670. *Obstet Gynecol*. 2016 (reaffirmed 2020);128:e32-e37.

23. Escobar M, Shearin S. Immediate postpartum contraception: intrauterine device insertion. *J Midwifery Womens Health*. 2019;64(4):481-487.

24. American College of Obstetricians and Gynecologists. LARC video series. https://www.acog.org/programs/long-acting-reversible-contraception-larc/video-series. Updated 2021. Accessed October 16, 2021.

25. Berlit S, Tuschy B, Brade J, et al. Effectiveness of nitrous oxide for postpartum perineal repair: a randomised controlled trial. *Eur J Obstet Gynecol Reprod Biol.* 2013;170(2):329-332.

APPENDIX

# 31D

# Manual Removal of the Placenta

MAVIS N. SCHORN

A retained placenta occurs in approximately 0.5% to 4.8% of women who have a vaginal birth.[1] Although there is no clear consensus on the length of time necessary for an unexpelled placenta to warrant the diagnosis of retained placenta, the World Health Organization considers the placenta to be retained if it remains unexpelled for longer than 30 minutes, but recommends waiting another 30 minutes before manually removing the placenta unless the birthing person is actively bleeding.[2] In the United States, the placenta is generally considered to be retained if not expelled at 30 minutes after the birth, and manual removal is recommended between 30 and 60 minutes if the birthing person has no signs of overt or concealed bleeding.

## History

Retained placenta is defined by a prolonged time since birth of the infant.

## Physical Examination

- Progress of the third stage of labor is evaluated, including signs of placental separation.
- Continual assessment of bleeding: Active bleeding may be apparent in the presence of an unexpelled placenta, even if the time since birth is not prolonged. Active bleeding requires prompt intervention.

## Management Steps

1. Explain to the birthing person and others/family in attendance (with the birthing person's permission) the problem and the steps needed to resolve the problem.

2. Discuss options of pain management, such as opioids, redosing of an epidural, and/or nitrous oxide.

3. Alert the birth team (e.g., birth assistant, nurses) regarding the problem and plan for manual removal. Based on the birth site, another provider (e.g., physician, other midwife) with more experience may be immediately available and consulted as appropriate.

4. If an intravenous line is not already in place, insert one using a large-bore (at least 18-gauge) needle, in case a hemorrhage occurs and intravenous fluids are needed.

5. Verify that the newborn is being cared for appropriately. If the birthing person is holding the neonate, ask another responsible individual to hold the infant or place the newborn in a safe site.

6. Catheterize the birthing person's bladder as needed, as a full bladder may impede the effective uterine contractions needed after placental removal.

7. Change gloves or put on second pair so that the procedure is as sterile as possible. Gloves of a regular length can be used, but a longer length that overlaps a sterile gown may provide more protection from body fluids.

8. Reduce the diameter of the hand by squeezing the extended fingers close together, and gently insert one hand slowly and steadily through the vagina and past the cervix. The entire hand is inserted to facilitate the ability to perform the procedure. Once inserted, the hand should not be removed until the procedure is complete. Repeated insertion and

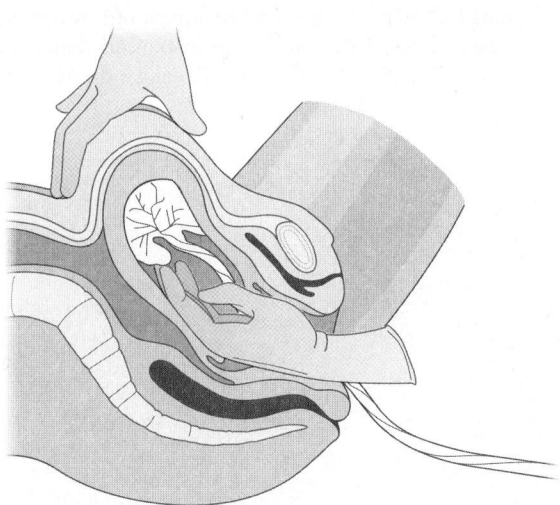

**Figure 31D-1** Manual removal of the placenta.

removal of the hand increases pain and risk of infection for the birthing person.

9. Using the internal hand, sweep the margin of the placenta to find any area of separation. Once a point of separation is found, rotate the hand so the back of the hand is next to the uterine wall. This placement results in the hand being in a cup-like position and minimizes the risk of inadvertent uterine rupture.

10. Insinuate the fingers between the placenta and the uterus to establish a line of cleavage. Separate the placenta by sweeping back and forth from side to side, sweeping through the decidua with the outer edge of the hand, fingertips, and first finger (**Figure 31D-1**).

11. Separate the entire placenta before attempting to extract it. If uncertain whether the placenta is totally separated, sweep the uterine wall again, feeling for and separating any remaining areas of attachment. Extraction while a section remains adherent increases the birthing person's risk of uterine inversion.

12. *Stop* the attempt to remove the placenta if it or its components are adherent. This finding is suggestive of a placental abnormality such as a placenta accreta. Immediate consultation/referral with a physician is required at this point.

13. Extract the placenta slowly after ascertaining that the placenta is not adherent; simultaneously continue to use the external hand to maintain fundal contraction. Ideally, the external hand moves from the birthing person's abdomen to the introitus to guide the expulsion while the internal hand stays internal until the procedure is complete. Placental membranes and clots may need to be removed. Avoiding or minimizing the number of times the internal hand must reenter the vagina and uterus decreases the birthing person's discomfort and risk of infection.

14. Membranes may need to be slowly teased out, as described in the *Management of Third Stage of Labor* appendix.

15. The placenta should be carefully inspected, as described in the *Inspection of the Umbilical Cord, Placenta, and Membranes* appendix. If the placenta does not appear complete, consider performing a uterine exploration to remove any retained tissue (*Intrauterine Exploration* appendix).

16. Maintain uterine contractility through uterine massage (as needed) and administration of a uterotonic agent. Continue close observation to rule out uterine atony.

17. After the placenta is removed:

    a. Count all sponges or laps that were used during the birth and ensure all sponges and laps have been removed from the uterus and vagina.

    b. Continue to observe for blood loss and signs of infection.

    c. For birthing people who are Rh negative, a fetal blood screen may be needed to determine if additional RhoGAM is needed.

    d. If the birthing person experienced excessive blood loss, assess their response by repeated laboratory evaluations, including hemoglobin or hematocrit values, and the person's symptoms during the first 24 to 72 hours postpartum. Because tolerance of blood loss is contingent upon many factors, some people will be symptomatic (e.g., syncope) at higher levels than others. Management, including blood transfusions, will need to be individualized.

    e. Antibiotic therapy is controversial and strong evidence is lacking to either support or refute its use. Individualization is indicated, and consultation may be a reasonable action.

    f. Document all procedures and the birthing person's response. Include consultations/referrals if appropriate.

## References

1. Favilli A, Tosto V, Ceccobelli M, et al. Risk factors for non-adherent retained placenta after vaginal delivery: a systematic review. *BMC Pregnancy Childbirth*. 2021;21:268. doi:10.1186/s12884-021-03721-9.

2. World Health Organization. WHO recommendations for the prevention and treatment of postpartum haemorrhage. 2012. http://apps.who.int/iris/bitstream /10665/75411/1/9789241548502_eng .pdf. Accessed October 2, 2021.

APPENDIX

# 31E

# Initial Management of Uterine Inversion

MAVIS N. SCHORN

A uterine inversion is an emergency. When a uterine inversion occurs, the risk for postpartum hemorrhage (PPH) and disseminated intravascular coagulation (DIC) is high. The uterus may need to be repositioned when the birthing person is under general anesthesia. The most common symptom of uterine inversion is rapid shock in the birthing person. Treatment for shock should be instituted immediately, even before symptoms become evident.

1. Inform the nurse or other birth assistant of the diagnosis. Request emergency obstetrician and anesthesiology consultation and additional nursing support. Initiate emergency transfer steps if the birth has occurred in an out-of-hospital setting.

2. Have a family member or someone else hold the newborn.

3. Explain to the birthing person and others in attendance that the uterus is inverted and briefly describe the steps needed to reposition the uterus.

4. Attempt to reposition the uterus immediately. Repositioning will be more successful if attempted as soon as the inversion is recognized and before the lower uterine segment and cervix contract to form a constriction ring.

   a. Do *not* remove the placenta if still attached. Removing the placenta while the uterus is inverted will increase the blood loss and increase the risk of complications.

   b. Manual repositioning is accomplished by placing the entire dominant hand in the vagina.

      i. Initially place the fingertips on the sides of where the uterus has turned on itself so that the inverted fundus is in the palm of the hand (Figure 31E-1).

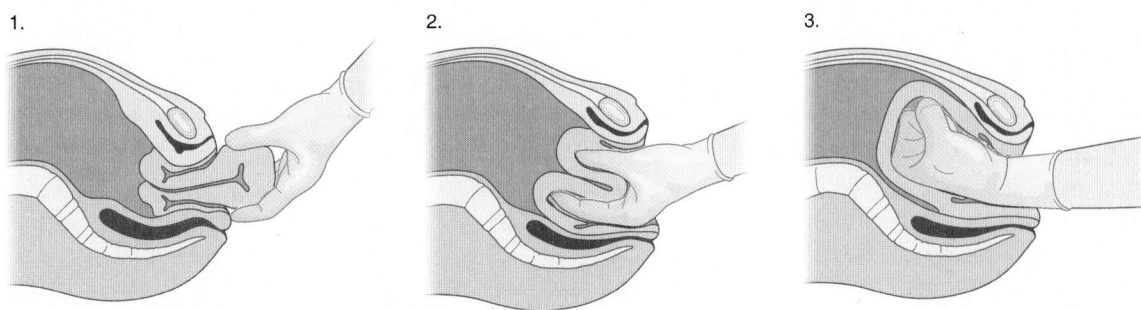

1.     2.     3.

**Figure 31E-1** Repositioning uterine inversion.

1381

ii. Apply pressure with the palm of the hand on the fundus and with the fingertips on the uterine walls. Gently walk or slide the fingertips up the uterine walls so the fundus is folded back into its original position. Take care not to puncture or rupture the soft uterine wall.

c. Hold the fundus in place by forming the hand into a fist while waiting for the uterus to contract around the fisted hand. This puts tension on the uterine ligaments, which keeps the uterus in place, and the fist forms a ball that does not allow the fundus to fold in on itself.

d. Keep the hand in the uterus until a consulting physician is present and can take over the maneuver, even if it appears that the inversion has been corrected.

e. Use the abdominal hand to guard the uterus so it is lifted out of the pelvis, above the level of the symphysis, and hold in this position for several minutes.

5. Simultaneously:

a. Have the birthing person assume Trendelenburg position.

b. Ask that an intravenous line be placed with a large-bore needle.

c. Discontinue uterotonics until the uterus is replaced.

d. Evaluate for signs of shock.

e. Request operating room and team preparation.

f. Request blood type and cross-match for 2 units of packed red blood cells, or initiate the PPH protocol if one is in place.

g. Initiate quantitative evaluation of blood loss.

APPENDIX

# 31F

# Management of Immediate Postpartum Hemorrhage

MAVIS N. SCHORN

## Introduction

The management of a person who is bleeding excessively during or immediately after the third stage of labor depends on the severity of bleeding, whether the placenta has been expelled, and the available resources. The steps listed in this appendix detail the process of assessing and managing care of a person who has just expelled the placenta and whose bleeding is brisk but not life threatening. In practice, management will be customized for the birthing person and the situation. For example, if the individual is hemorrhaging and the uterus is not firm, bimanual compression may be indicated as the first response. Conversely, if the bleeding is less severe, the midwife may check for lacerations before other steps are taken. Similarly, if the placenta is not expelled, the first step will be manual removal of the placenta.

Multiple algorithms are available that outline the recommended management steps for a person who is hemorrhaging after birth. Midwives are encouraged to know all possible management responses so that the response may be individualized as appropriate. Quantitative blood loss is the preferred method of determining the amount of blood lost during the third stage of labor and during/following a hemorrhage.

## Management Steps

1. Maintain or reinstate a calm environment to reduce anxiety and facilitate management.

2. Palpate the person's uterus, as approximately 80% of immediate postpartum hemorrhages (PPH) occur secondary to uterine atony.

3. Order a uterotonic, if one has not yet been administered. Uterotonic administration and external uterine massage may be the only interventions necessary.

4. If bleeding continues, proceed to the next steps. If there is a standardized PPH protocol, request its initiation.

5. Request an additional (second) nurse if available.

6. Explain to the birthing person and others/family in attendance (with permission) that vaginal bleeding is excessive and describe the steps needed to resolve the problem.

7. Have a family member or other responsible adult hold the newborn. Alternatively, place the newborn in a safe site under observation.

8. Consult with other members of the perinatal healthcare team, including an anesthesiology provider and an obstetric physician, if bleeding continues unabated. At this point, depending on the amount and rate of bleeding, ask for another practitioner to come to the bedside, or if in an out-of-hospital setting, initiate emergency transport.

9. Rule out bleeding from a laceration by efficiently performing an examination of the perineum, vulva, vagina, and cervix. Suture any active bleeding vessels appropriately.

10. If bleeding is not secondary to a laceration or the uterus is atonic, proceed to the next steps.

11. Catheterize the birthing person's bladder so a full bladder will not interfere with uterine contractility.

12. Order a uterotonic agent, if one was not administered earlier with release of the anterior shoulder of the newborn. Oxytocin (Pitocin) is the most commonly used agent, either 10 to 80 units in 250 to 500 mL solution administered intravenously at a rapid rate (500 mL/hour), titrated to uterine tone, or 10 units given intramuscularly while intravenous access with a large-bore (usually 18-gauge) needle is initiated. If a uterotonic agent was administered with the birth of the neonate, consider a second agent (e.g., methylergonovine [Methergine] 15-methyl PG-F$_{2a}$ [Hemabate]). Table 31-8 identifies the doses, routes of administration, and side effects of uterotonic drugs used to treat PPH. Continue administration of additional uterotonic agents to treat uterine atony.

13. If bleeding continues after the previous steps have been taken and the person is in an out-of-hospital site, commence with an emergency transfer to a hospital. If the excessive bleeding is controlled quickly, the transfer can be canceled if the person has normal vital signs and feels well.

14. If bleeding continues, initiate a second intravenous line with normal saline in preparation for blood transfusion and maintenance of intravascular volume.

15. Verify that an anesthesia provider and an obstetric physician have been called; while waiting for emergency services arrival, proceed to the following steps.

16. Initiate *bimanual compression* (Figure 31F-1) of the person's uterus to treat uterine atony.

    a. Extend the fingers of one hand and squeeze the extended fingers close together, gently insert this hand into the vagina, and close the fingers into a fist as the hand enters the vagina.

    b. Position the fist, palmar side up, into the anterior fornix.

    c. Direct pressure to the lower uterine segment and uterine corpus by applying pressure inward and upward against the anterior wall of the uterus.

    d. Simultaneously, place the other hand externally on the abdomen and grasp the uterus between the two hands.

    e. Apply pressure to the uterus trapped between the two hands by massaging it using pressure directed against the posterior

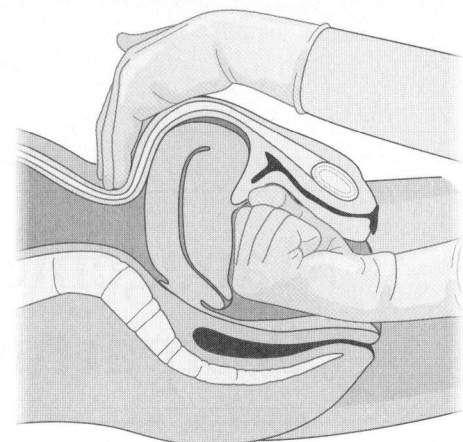

**Figure 31F-1** Bimanual compression.

wall of the uterus, primarily in the area of the fundus and corpus of the uterus with the abdominal hand. This compression places direct pressure on the bleeding uterine vessels while stimulating the uterus to contract, an action that will also provide continuous compression.

    f. Continue bimanual compression until bleeding is controlled and uterine atony is resolved. The effectiveness of this intervention can be ascertained by momentarily releasing the pressure on the uterus and evaluating uterine consistency and bleeding at that moment.

    g. Be aware that atony may seem to be resolved before it actually is, so bimanual compression should not be discontinued until the uterus is firm for several minutes. Removal of the hand and reinsertion increases pain/discomfort and risk of infection.

    h. If bimanual compression stimulates a response but uterine atony does not resolve, continue compression until a physician is present and joint decisions can be made.

17. If in a hospital, the blood bank should be notified and type and cross-match for 2 units prepared.

18. Prepare for the massive transfusion protocol (**Figure 31F-2**).[1]

19. Administer tranexamic acid (TXA) 1 g added to 100 mL normal saline and administer intravenously over 10 minutes.[2]

20. While waiting for a surgeon/obstetrician, engage other essential healthcare team members

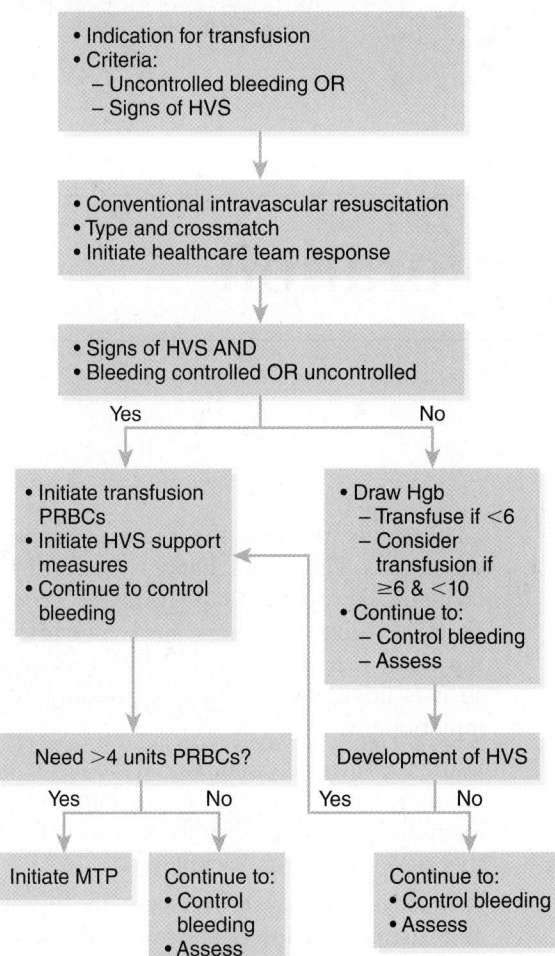

**Figure 31F-2** Massive transfusion protocol algorithm.
Abbreviations: Hgb, hemoglobin; HVS, hypovolemic shock; MTP, massive transfusion protocol; PRBCs, packed red blood cells.
Reproduced with permission from Schorn MN, Phillippi JC. Volume replacement following severe postpartum hemorrhage. *J Midwifery Womens Health*. 2014 May-Jun;59(3):336-343. doi:10.1111 /jmwh.12186. Epub 2014 Apr 21. PMID: 24751109.

such as anesthesia personnel, nursing leadership, and other experienced providers available.

21. If retained products of conception are suspected to be the cause of the bleeding, proceed to performing an intrauterine exploration as detailed in the *Intrauterine Exploration* appendix. Additional anesthesia or pain management methods may be needed at this point.

22. If the preceding measures have not controlled the bleeding, insert a Bakri balloon or Jada System into the uterus to compress the blood vessels and control bleeding.[3,4]

23. After bleeding has been controlled, discuss and explain the situation to the person and their family, as the person desires.

24. Continue to collect the blood lost and calculate the total loss both during the acute hemorrhage and 12 to 24 hours postpartum.

25. Assess the person's response to PPH by repeat laboratory evaluations, including hemoglobin or hematocrit values, and by monitoring the birthing person's symptoms during the first 24 to 72 hours postpartum. Because tolerance of blood loss is contingent upon many factors, some people will be symptomatic (e.g., syncope) at different hemoglobin levels than others. Management, including blood transfusions, will need to be individualized.

26. Antibiotic therapy following uterine exploration is controversial, and strong evidence is lacking to either support or refute its use. Individualization is indicated, and consultation may be a reasonable action.

27. Document all procedures and the person's responses. Include any consultations and referrals if appropriate.

28. Once the hemorrhage is resolved, provide time for the birthing person and family to ask questions and process what occurred. This may need to occur at several times.

29. A constructive debrief with all the healthcare team is also warranted.

## References

1. Schorn MN, Phillippi JC. Volume replacement following severe postpartum hemorrhage. *J Midwifery Womens Health*. 2014;59(3):336-343. doi:10.1111 /jmwh.12186.

2. Della Corte L, Saccone G, Locci M, et al. Tranexamic acid for treatment of primary postpartum hemorrhage after vaginal delivery: a systematic review and meta-analysis of randomized controlled trials. *J Matern Fetal Neonatal Med*. 2020;33(5):869-874. doi:10.1080/14767058.2018.1500544.

3. Suarez S, Conde-Agudelo A, Borovac-Pinheiro A, et al. Uterine balloon tamponade for the treatment of postpartum hemorrhage: a systematic review and meta-analysis. *Am J Obstet Gynecol*. 2020;222(4):293. e1-293.e52. doi:10.1016/j.ajog.2019.11.1287.

4. D'Alton M, Rood K, Simhan H, Goffman D. Profile of the Jada® System: the vacuum-induced hemorrhage control device for treating abnormal postpartum uterine bleeding and postpartum hemorrhage. *Expert Rev Med Devices*. 2021;18(9):849-853. doi:10.1080/17434440.2021.1962288.

A P P E N D I X

# 31G

# Intrauterine Exploration

MAVIS N. SCHORN

To perform an intrauterine exploration:

1. Quickly explain to the birthing person the need for the procedure and what it entails. Get consent for the procedure.

2. Request additional healthcare staff and assistance if you have not requested this already. Consider whether additional pain relief is necessary and can be obtained in a timely manner given the rate of blood loss.

3. Change gloves or put on second pair so that the procedure is as sterile as possible. Gloves of a regular length can be used, but a longer length that overlaps a sterile gown provides more protection from body fluids.

4. Wrap one gauze sponge (e.g., 4 × 4) around two or four fingers, with the thumb stabilizing the gauze against the side of the first finger. The rougher surface of the gauze tends to be an effective modality to pick up placental fragments, ragged membranes, or blood clots. Use only one gauze so that it can easily be accounted for and to minimize the risk of leaving a gauze pad in the uterus or vagina.

5. Place the external hand on the birthing person's abdomen and grasp their uterus in a similar manner to that performed during bimanual compression, thereby stabilizing the organ.

6. Reduce the diameter of the internal hand by squeezing the extended fingers close together, and gently insert this hand slowly and steadily through the vagina and past the cervix. The entire hand is inserted to facilitate the ability to perform the procedure. Multiple insertions and removals of the hand increase pain and infection risk, so it is advisable to proceed carefully and intentionally.

7. Using the internal hand, sweep the inside of the uterus with the back of the hand while maintaining contact with the uterine wall so that the entire cavity is explored.

8. Remove the hand slowly from the uterus and vagina, and unwrap, assess, and discard the gauze. If uncertain whether all the tissue was removed, repeat the procedure once for any remaining tissue or clots.

9. Maintain uterine contractility through uterine massage and administration of a uterotonic agent. Continue close observation to rule out uterine atony. An extended recovery period may be indicated.

10. Count the number of gauzes used and confirm that none remains in the vagina or uterus.

11. *Stop* the procedure at any time if portions of the placenta are felt to be adherent. This finding is suggestive of a placental abnormality such as placenta accreta. Immediate consultation/referral with a physician is required at this point, and preparation of the operating room team is indicated.

APPENDIX

# 31H

# Sudden Postpartum Cardiovascular or Neurologic Emergencies

MAVIS N. SCHORN

## Physical Examination

- Level of consciousness and orientation of the birthing person
- Presence of an unremitting headache, agitation, or confusion
- Vital signs, including temperature
- Oxygenation ($O_2$ saturation)
- Skin color
- Shortness of breath
- Pain score
- Evaluation of new findings (i.e., bleeding from unexpected sites)
- Continue monitoring uterine tone, vaginal bleeding, and urine output

If a newly postpartum person experiences respiratory impairment, cardiovascular collapse, altered mental status, or loss of consciousness, emergency measures are indicated.[1-4]

## Management

- Initiate measures to obtain emergency assistance. If out of the hospital, implement the emergency transport protocol. If in the hospital, call for an emergency response team. Emergency response teams vary but should include an anesthetist/anesthesiologist, an obstetric physician provider, and an additional nurse.[1]

- Initiate a large-bore (18-gauge or larger) intravenous line if not already in place. If already in place, ensure its patency, and consider placing a second line.
- Provide calm explanations to the birthing person and friends or family who are present.
- Assign someone to provide care to the neonate.
- Administer crystalloid, 0.9% sodium chloride, or lactated Ringer's solution rapidly if the person is hypotensive.
- Normal saline is the fluid of choice for a second line to allow for blood administration.
- Apply oxygen at a 10 to 12 L/min flow rate via a nonrebreather face mask.
- Obtain blood pressure, pulse, temperature, and oxygen saturation levels frequently. If blood pressure is maintained, do not overload the person with intravenous fluids—fluid overload can contribute to pulmonary edema.
- Be prepared to initiate cardiopulmonary resuscitation. Prepare for and assist with intubation and ventilation if needed.
- Position the person in semi-Fowler's position.
- Order arterial blood gases, complete blood count, platelet count, fibrinogen, partial thromboplastin time, blood type and cross-match for 2 units of red blood cells, and chest X ray.

- Catheterize the bladder with an indwelling Foley catheter that drains to a urometer so output is monitored accurately.
- Depending on the clinical evaluation, laboratory and additional diagnostic studies to consider include[1-4]:
  - Complete blood count
  - Type and screen or type and cross-match if bleeding
  - Complete metabolic panel
  - Magnesium level
  - Electrocardiogram (EKG), particularly in the presence of tachycardia, bradycardia, or chest pain
  - Computed tomography (CT) angiogram or perfusion scan in patients with acute chest pain
  - Chest X ray if the patient is short of breath, particularly if preeclamptic
  - Echocardiogram

### References

1. Arora KS, Shields LE, Grobman WA, et al. Triggers, bundles, protocols, and checklists: what every maternal care provider needs to know. *Am J Obstet Gynecol.* 2016;214:444-451. doi:10.1016/j.ajog.2015.10.011.
2. Blumenthal EA, Hooshvar N, McQuade M, McNulty J. A validation study of maternal early warning systems: a retrospective cohort study. *Am J Perinatol.* 2019;36:1106-1114. doi:10.1055/s-0039-1681097.
3. Dubbs SB, Tewelde SZ. Cardiovascular catastrophes in the obstetric population. *Emerg Med Clin North Am.* 2015;33:483-500.
4. Zuckerwise LC, Lipkind HS. Maternal early warning systems: towards reducing preventable maternal mortality and severe maternal morbidity through improved clinical surveillance and responsiveness. *Semin Perinatol.* 2017;41:161-165. doi:10.1053/j.semperi.2017.03.005.

C H A P T E R

# 32

# Birth in the Home and Birth Center

ALEXIS DUNN AMORE AND NIKIA D. GRAYSON

*Special thanks to Marsha E. Jackson and Alice J. Bailes, who contributed
to the previous version of this chapter.*

## Introduction

Birth is profoundly affected by the environment in which it takes place. Ideally, every laboring person and the team that supports and facilitates the birth process will work together in an environment that is most comfortable and safe for the birthing family. For many individuals, families, and providers, that safe and comfortable place to give birth is in the home or birth center, sometimes known as community birth. Pregnant people have the right to choose where they give birth, and midwives serve as important advocates during that decision-making process.

The midwife who works in the home or birth center has an opportunity to develop the hands-on, low-tech skills that are the hallmarks of midwifery. Expertise in and fascination with normal birth make midwives keenly aware of the pregnant person and their natural ability to complete the birth process. Although midwives in all settings finely tune their perception and interpersonal skills to amplify pregnant persons' ability to give birth, the opportunity to use these skills is increased in the home and birth center environments. The individuals who give birth in these settings are active in creating their own support network that enables them to optimize their health, and to give birth safely, effectively, and with great satisfaction. Table 32-1 outlines essential elements for home and birth center births.

This chapter describes how the midwife works with those pregnant persons who choose home or birth center as the preferred birth site, highlights the importance of grounding community birth within a reproductive justice framework, and presents evidence-based guidelines for safe practice in these settings.

## Background

Until the mid-nineteenth century, healing arts in the United States were home-based, do-it-yourself types of assistance and included a variety of approaches.[1] Pregnant people in the United States anticipated giving birth at home, using their own power, without surgical or medical interventions. Surrounded by community attendants, birthing people were the central figure during a social childbirth.[1,2] Attendants transmitted supportive midwifery skills, through direct empirical experience and apprenticeship.

As the twentieth century dawned, industrialization and urbanization had powerful effects in disrupting social organization and family life, and negatively affecting public health.[3] As midwifery became professionalized, midwives introduced education programs with home-based clinical practices and founded, owned, and staffed practices in both homes and birth centers. The data on the outcomes associated with these midwifery practices revealed good outcomes for midwife-attended births.[4]

Over the course of the twentieth century, a variety of physician-led and social campaigns that promoted physician care in hospitals for childbirth tipped public opinion toward birth in the hospital, where midwives were not permitted to practice. Additionally, the passing of laws governing professional standards for midwifery practice coupled with the rise in medicalized childbirth resulted in a systematic elimination of the Indigenous, Black, and immigrant midwife experts who served as the foundation of midwifery practice.[5–7] The details of how this happened varied by region, state, and locality. A variety of racist reports, campaigns, and laws led to the elimination of traditional midwifery practice by

| Table 32-1 | Essential Elements of Birth Center and Home Births |
|---|---|

The birthing person desires a birth center birth or home birth

Shared decision making in the client–midwife partnership

Informed consent obtained by the midwife and pregnancy team throughout pregnancy and birth

Clear recognition of the autonomy of the birthing person and the birthing family

Privacy available to the laboring person

Encouragement of family participation guided by the laboring person's wishes

Promotion of physiologic birth

Minimal use of unnecessary interventions

Skilled personnel and equipment provided by the midwife and birthing team

Collaborative relationship with the community's healthcare system

community midwives, and a new model of perinatal care began to take root in the United States.[8]

By the late 1940s and early 1950s, most births in the United States occurred in hospitals, although individuals from marginalized populations were often excluded from hospitals either explicitly or by cost. Pain medications sedated women during childbirth, and families were separated during and after the birth process. In the late 1950s and 1960s, a consumer backlash occurred, as many childbearing families rejected the hospital environment as too confining and disempowering. In turn, consumers, midwives, and some physicians began work to return birth to the home.[9,10]

The birth center concept was the culmination of an idea that had been evolving informally for many years. Some midwives may have preferred not to travel, or a laboring person may not have had a suitable home in which to give birth. In such cases, midwives or groups of midwives would designate a separate area of their home or a separate structure in which to attend births. Later, consumers who perceived hospital policies as too restrictive, yet did not want to give birth in their own homes, began to search for an alternative. Midwives were also in search of a place to attend physiologic births. The National Association of Childbearing Centers (NACC), now the American Association of Birth Centers (AABC), was established in 1983; this organization sought to create standards and promote a model facility integrated with the healthcare

system, in which "low-tech, high-touch" care could be accessed.[11,12]

Some hospitals today advertise their labor and delivery suite as a birth center or as an alternative birthing center. These labels can be confusing, as they may be used to refer to both in-hospital and out-of-hospital centers. The birth centers discussed in this chapter are either freestanding facilities or, if within a hospital, are physically separate from the main hospital labor and delivery area (alongside midwifery unit [AMU]).[13] In most cases, they are administratively autonomous units and have specific policies and procedures for operating both the facility and the program for the low-risk childbearing families they serve.

## Comparison of Home and Birth Center Services

Both home and birth center practices share philosophical and administrative characteristics. The primary difference between them is that birth in a birth center occurs within the professional's territory, to which the pregnant person comes, whereas a home birth occurs within the pregnant person's territory, to which the midwife goes.[14] Thus, the balance of power in each setting is different.

In the pregnant person's home, the midwife and the assistant are the guests, and the pregnant person is the host. Because the midwife is the one who travels, labor, birth, and postpartum care are not disturbed. Travel can cause intense discomfort to a person in active labor or incur the risk of giving birth en route. When families give birth at home, there is little interruption in family routines for adults as well as for children, and bonding is uninterrupted. Between 2004 and 2017, the United States saw a doubling of both home births (from 0.56% to 0.99%) and birth center births (from 0.23% to 0.52%). These births currently represent 1.61% of all births in the United States.[15] Prior to the COVID-19 pandemic, fewer than 2% of people in the United States chose to give birth at home or in a birth center.[15] The pandemic, however, increased the demand for community birthing options.[16] As yet, no data are available to confirm the magnitude of this rise.[17]

Among those who access birth services in community settings in the United States, non-Hispanic white pregnant people represent the highest percentage of individuals who choose to give birth in a community setting, accounting for 81% of the births from 2004 to 2017. Although community birth is desired by many, multiple barriers to this care exist that are unequally carried by people of color, including limited coverage of community birth care by Medicaid, expensive out-of-pocket fees for people who are uninsured, and limited access to midwives of color in community settings.[18] The reproductive justice movement advocates for the recognition of bodily autonomy and the right to have a sacred and safe pregnancy and birth experience in whatever setting the person chooses.[19] With their focus on the importance of each person's agency and autonomy, homes and birth centers are optimal settings that embody reproductive justice principles. Thus, community birth provides many individuals, but especially those who are Indigenous and persons of color, with the cultural, emotional, and mental safety they need to give birth without fear, especially in the face of widespread reports of disparities in pregnancy outcomes linked to structural racism.[20] However, structural changes to increase insurance coverage of community birth options for all pregnant people and increase the supply of midwives of color in these settings are needed for the benefits of community birth care to be available to all persons who desire this model of care.

The birth center concept is a replicable model that has become a well-recognized choice for families. According to the AABC:

> The birth center is a homelike facility, existing within a healthcare system with a program of care designed in the wellness model of pregnancy and birth. Birth centers are guided by principles of prevention, sensitivity, safety, appropriate medical intervention, and cost-effectiveness. Birth centers provide family-centered care for healthy women before, during, and after normal pregnancy, labor, and birth.[21]

The Commission for the Accreditation of Birth Centers (CABC) provides a mechanism for external review of birth centers, which in turn gives guidance to professionals planning and practicing in birth centers.[22] Accreditation may enhance both family and practitioner confidence in the birth center choice. There is no comparable agency for home birth.

## Safety During Birth in Home and Birth Center Settings

To preserve safety at home and in the birth center, it is necessary to adhere to some essential principles:[1,23,24]

1. The pregnant person must be committed to actively partnering with their midwife and birth team. When persons are healthy and are experiencing low-risk, healthy pregnancy, they increase their chances for good outcomes for labor and birth. Some health problems preclude a home birth or birth center plan.

2. The place of birth must be planned before the onset of labor. Adequate planning for the place of birth includes determination that the person's health and the pregnancy are low risk and healthy when labor begins, and that family preparations for appropriate support are in place.

3. The midwife must be skilled and able to assess health status appropriately, provide vigilant care, and manage emergency complications should they occur. In addition to assisting with health promotion in the prenatal period, a midwife skilled in caring for pregnant people at home or in a birth center is vigilant in observation, communication, data collection, and care. This vigilance identifies both reassuring signs and deviations from normal. If problems occur or persist at any time during the prenatal, intrapartum, or postpartum period, the midwife acts to correct the problem or, if necessary, works to stabilize the condition and transfers the client to hospital-based care.

4. There is a system in place to access consultation, hospitalization, and emergency transport. Clinical practice guidelines outline indications for consultation and a mechanism for transport to a hospital-based system. The midwife has established relationships with hospital-based practitioners to assure a smooth transition into the hospital should a transfer be indicated.

## Outcomes of Birth in Home and Birth Centers

Data collection and research related to the safety and outcomes of home and birth center births have been conducted in many developed nations using a variety of research methods and populations.[25–30] Studies in the United States have demonstrated that planned home and birth center births for well persons who are at term with a singleton fetus in vertex presentation, and who are experiencing a low-risk pregnancy, are at least as safe as—and, in some cases, safer than—births for their counterparts taking place in the hospital.[27,31] However, neonatal outcomes for well persons in U.S. community birth settings can be worse than those for similar people giving birth in hospital settings—especially if hospital care is available with a midwife.[32,33]

Analysis of this research is complex given the differing populations, risk status, provider type, and study methods included in the various investigations. Moreover, the geographic area where community birth occurs often has significant implications for the integration of midwifery care within the local healthcare system;[34,35] in U.S. regions with low midwifery integration, transfer delays and variations in community birth protocols can result in poor perinatal outcomes compared to hospital births or community births internationally or in other areas of the United States.

### Outcomes for the Birthing Person

Outcomes among low-risk persons who give birth at home or in a birth center are good, and generally better than the outcomes of those matched for demographic characteristics and provider type who give birth in a hospital.[31,36–38] Rates of obstetric interventions and cesarean birth are lower for persons who begin their labors planning to give birth in a community setting. A recent Center for Medicare and Medicaid Innovation report (2013–2017) of Medicaid beneficiaries enrolled in the AABC Strong Start for Mothers and Newborns Initiative ($n = 6424$) found that the overall cesarean section rate among AABC sites was 12.3% compared to the national rate of 31.9%; additionally, the primary cesarean rate was significantly lower in the group (8.7%) compared to 21.8% nationally.[31]

Similarly, in a large meta-analysis of studies from across the world ($N = 16$ studies, 500,000 labors), Reitsma and colleagues compared maternal outcomes and birth interventions, finding that pregnant people intending to give birth at home were 40% less likely to deliver by cesarean section compared to those birthing in a hospital ($n = 6$ studies; odds ratio [OR], 0.58; 95% CI, 0.44–0.71). They also found that people intending to give birth at home were 55% less likely to have an episiotomy ($n = 6$ studies; OR, 0.45 95% CI, 0.28–0.73) and 40% less likely to experience a third- or fourth-degree perineal tear ($n = 5$ studies; OR, 0.57; 95% CI, 0.43–0.75).[27] The data did not include any maternal deaths, and the pooled results for postpartum hemorrhage risk showed that this complication was less likely in a community setting

(OR, 0.66; 95% CI, 0.54– 0.80) compared to hospital birth. These findings were supported by a 2018 international meta-analysis,[38] where researchers saw three times higher odds of vaginal birth for pregnant people planning to deliver at home (OR, 2.93; 95% CI, 2.1–4.03) and two times higher odds of vaginal delivery in birth centers (OR, 2.12; 95% CI, 1.54–2.92) compared to pregnant people planning hospital-based birth. Additionally, those reviewers saw a less severe odds of postpartum hemorrhage (blood loss greater than 1000 mL) in planned home births (OR, 0.73; 95% CI, 0.55–0.96), but no difference in that risk for birth center births, compared to hospital births.

Together, these findings suggest that the birth center and community birth settings for low-risk birthing individuals desiring these locations of birth are associated with quality care that reduces the risk for selected maternal health outcomes compared to hospital birth.

### Neonatal Outcomes

The rates of many adverse perinatal outcomes are consistently lower in birth center and community birth settings compared to hospital settings.[15,31] However, the research findings with regard to newborn outcomes in home and birth center settings vary, and the clinical significance of these findings remains somewhat controversial. Most of the research in this area is observational, which often means that researchers must take advantage of data from birth certificate or clinical data sets to compare outcomes between birth settings. As a result, different groups of researchers are likely to report outcome measures using varied definitions. For example, some groups, such as the Centers for Disease Control and Prevention's National Center for Health Statistics, define neonatal death as the death of a fetus or infant from age 0 to 7 days, whereas others have used neonatal mortality rates that include only live births and count deaths up to 28 days of life.[33] Despite these limitations, there is a growing body of literature in this area that should be used when counseling patients about their options regarding place of birth.[39]

When freestanding birth centers are compared to hospital settings, low-risk individuals appear to have increased risk for neonatal mortality, especially if they are nulliparous, are older than age 35 years, or give birth at more than 42 weeks' gestation.[33,39,40] However, as mentioned earlier, geographic variations exist in people's risk for perinatal mortality. For example, in a 2018 systematic review of studies from six developed nations including the United States, Phillippi et al. ($N = 17$ studies;

$n = 84,500$ low-risk birthing people) identified no increased risk of neonatal mortality in birth centers compared to hospital settings.[33] By contrast, in a large birth certificate review comparing freestanding birth center to hospital birth across the United States between 2016 and 2019 ($N = 9,894,978$), researchers saw a nearly four-fold increase in neonatal mortality among birth center births.[39] Neonates born in U.S. birth centers also had a two-fold increase in neonatal seizures compared to hospital births in that study.

Outcomes of home births are also difficult to assess due to differences in research design and geographic variations between studies. However, it appears that in U.S. geographic settings where midwifery care and community birth are well integrated into the larger healthcare system, rates of neonatal mortality are low ($0.19/1000$) and do not differ for planned home birth versus birth center birth.[41] As with birth center births, nulliparous individuals choosing a planned home birth have higher risks of perinatal morbidity compared to multiparous individuals. In the United States, Snowden et al. identified an increase in the perinatal death rate (which includes both stillbirths and neonatal deaths) associated with planned home birth compared to hospital birth ($3.9/1000$ and $1.8/1000$, respectively).[42] Overall, most studies of home birth in the United States and other developed nations have found a small but persistent increased risk of adverse neonatal outcomes associated with home birth, primarily in nulliparous women, although the absolute increase in risk is quite low.

Professional organizations have conflicting positions regarding the safety of birth in community settings. The American College of Nurse-Midwives (ACNM) states that birth at home can be safe for essentially well individuals who experience an uncomplicated pregnancy and have assistance from a qualified provider.[43,44] The World Health Organization's position is similar in recommending that persons who are medically at low risk can choose home birth if they are attended by a skilled provider and have plans for transfer to a higher level of care if needed.[45] By contrast, the American College of Obstetricians and Gynecologists (ACOG) supports hospitals and birthing centers as the safest sites for birth, but states that its members respect pregnant individuals' right to make an informed choice about their planned birth site.[46] What is often lost in these professional recommendations is the importance of patient autonomy. Some individuals are primarily motivated to find care that is congruent with their values rather than supported by national safety statistics.[47] In other developed countries, evidence shows that community birth can be a safe option for both the birthing person and their neonate if safety protocols are standardized, team members are trained consistent with the International Confederation of Midwives standards, and transfer to a hospital occurs quickly and easily when unplanned complications arise.[34]

## Essential Elements of Birth Center and Home Birth

### Shared Decision Making

Shared decision making is an inherent component of midwifery care and reproductive justice, but the process of shared decision making assumes an even more prominent role in the home or birth center setting. Early in the clinical relationship, the midwife introduces the concept of working in a client–midwife partnership, in which each party has a unique set of responsibilities. By partnering with clients, midwives can center the care around each pregnant person's values and lived experiences. It is especially important to utilize community-informed models of perinatal care to ensure equity in experiences and health outcomes among Black birthing communities.[48] For example, a full-scope, comprehensive reproductive health center located in Memphis, Tennessee, was recently expanded to meet community needs based on assessment and community activism. Shaping and implementing initiatives to address factors related to structural and obstetric racism and the impact on clinical care are key to creating safe experiences and improving outcomes.

### Authority, Centrality, and Privacy

Everyone has the right to own their births (e.g., to have bodily autonomy surrounding their experience) and to choose those with whom they wish to share their experience. The birthing person should be encouraged to select the birth location and attendants who will create a personal feeling of safety, while recognizing that this decision can be changed as needed. Although family wishes and finances may play a part in the decision, the birthing person should be the ultimate authority for birth location selection. Even in the small and intimate environments provided in the home or birth center, it is necessary to respect the authority and autonomy of the birthing person to make their own choices and expect that their preferences will be honored. At home or in a birth center, the birthing person should be surrounded by only the people whom they choose, thereby meeting their needs for privacy or companionship.[49] In this personalized milieu, distracting events are minimized, increasing the laboring individual's centrality.

With the explicit recognition of their authority in the home and birth center settings, laboring persons feel a sense of control over their birth's environment, management, and outcome. Their confidence in their providers' approach to care grows during the prenatal period, so the only surprises encountered in labor are the ones that labor brings. The pregnant person and their family should carefully choose who they will have as a part of their support team. Choosing people who are supportive of their decision to have a community birth is important. When all members focus only on the pregnant person's needs, the team may offer their skills, presence, and support for the all-important task of giving birth.

At home or in a birth center, the environment communicates an expectation of the promotion of physiologic birth. The laboring person's natural efforts are respected, and all who work with them are dedicated to the concept that birth is normal. It is expected that the laboring person has the ability to give birth, and that they can do so with physical, social, and psychological support. They are not attached to equipment designed to do the job for them. They are free to move around and to be in any position they choose. A walk outdoors can invigorate them, occupy their attention, and promote labor progress. Hydrotherapy can be used to promote relaxation.

The private labor environment also helps the laboring person feel safe. They can make sounds without fear of being overheard by strangers close by. They have their own clothes to wear or not wear as they see fit. Familiar food and drink that they and their family have provided are available to keep them well nourished and hydrated. Moreover, whether at home or in the birth center, new parents and their newborns are less likely to encounter pathogenic bacteria and invasive procedures, thereby reducing the risk of nosocomial infection.

In such a setting, emphasis is placed on labor as dynamic, progressing rapidly at some times and slowly at others. Ebbs and flows are expected. Encouraging activity to promote progress and quieting the environment to promote rest are simple tasks. At home or in the birth center, attention can be focused on addressing the laboring person's needs, enabling them to progress or rest, expecting and accommodating plateaus of progress.

## Client–Midwife Relationships

In every setting, the relationship between the midwife and the client is vital. In the home and birth center, it is particularly important to specify the roles that each participant assumes as they share responsibility and work together in a partnership based on mutual trust. Pregnant people choose an attendant intentionally, searching for a good fit, and seeking a collaborative, nonhierarchical relationship that will respect their goals. Goals and criteria for what constitute safe variations are clearly delineated. Collectively, along with the individual's support system, all team members share responsibility for both the process of care and the outcome. Working in this way, all promote clear and ongoing communication throughout perinatal care.

Midwives who choose home and birth center practice need a clear sense of their own strengths and limitations. They must be comfortable with sharing power and occupying a role that is not central in the birthing process. This requirement challenges midwives to sharpen their communication skills, be open to discovering how to expand flexibility, and know how to set and explain evidence-based limits and boundaries. When a person plans to give birth in the home or the birth center, it is easier for them to see the connections between their actions and the outcomes. Their responsibilities for care are also clear, including recognition that their actions can make a difference.

Midwives who work in home and birth center settings must be able to identify philosophical gaps between themselves and their clients, and strategize to resolve them. These midwives must also feel comfortable taking a guiding role in the client–midwife partnership. Each midwife must be assertive when describing the limits of their practice in the home or birth center environments.

## Midwife–Consultant Relationships

When variations in the client's health state require consultation, collaboration, or referral, midwives need links to the community's healthcare system that they can activate to ensure high-quality perinatal care. These relationships can promote a smooth continuation of care and reduce the fragmentation that is often experienced when managing care with multiple providers. Consultation can be provided by family physicians or obstetricians who work as solo practitioners, a group practice, several different practices, or the staff employed by the hospital. Some midwives who attend home and birth center births maintain hospital privileges, facilitating seamless transfer into the hospital when necessary. Other home birth and birth center midwives elect not to have hospital privileges, but maintain consultative relationships with physicians or with hospital-based midwives. For the midwife without hospital privileges, establishing a consultation agreement with hospital-based midwifery practices affords a means of access to the hospital and fosters a collegial relationship among midwives. Clients appreciate this arrangement because even if they transfer to the hospital, they still may have their birth attended by a midwife.

Before negotiations with a consulting practice take place, the midwife should write clinical practice guidelines and identify those situations for which consultation, collaboration, or referral would be needed. These guidelines are *not* a supervisory agreement. Many states have passed legislation repealing the requirement that midwives have written collaborative practice agreements with physicians or hospitals. Although writing guidelines is important, midwives and consultants must build a relationship based on open communication, mutual trust, and respect. Most consulting services do not see clients prenatally unless a problem is identified, but the pregnant person may still want to meet with the consultant and should be encouraged to do so if desired.

## Prenatal Care

During prenatal visits, the midwife works to enhance the pregnant person's self-confidence and self-reliance. By giving reassurance regarding the normalcy of pregnancy's changes, and by communicating faith in the ability to give birth, the midwife assists the pregnant person in amplifying their strengths and minimizing limitations that have the potential to influence the pregnancy and birth process. Empowerment and giving voice to pregnant people is essential to effective and safe prenatal care.

### Introduction to the Practice

At the first prenatal visit, the midwife orients the family and introduces them to the services and philosophy of the practice. The midwife actively engages the pregnant individual and their chosen support network in a discussion focused on identifying the unique needs of both the individual and the family unit. This conversation is conducted via a shared decision-making process, which places the needs of the pregnant person and family at the center of the care model. It can be a challenge to have these discussions while maintaining the family's confidence in the birth process, particularly when working with people who are disproportionately at risk for experiencing disparities in perinatal health outcomes. In all cases, it is important for the midwife to take the time to listen to concerns, validate the pregnant person's perspective, and develop a tailored plan of care to ensure that safety and trust are the foundation of the care model.

Ongoing communication and exploration of concerns should occur throughout the perinatal care process to build trust and establish rapport and safety with the client. In this way, self-care is fostered, good decision making takes place, and the pregnant person and their family are actively engaged throughout the experience.[49,50] The midwife reviews the strong commitment to health promotion, to keeping birth normal, and to using non-pharmacologic comfort measures for childbirth. This visit also provides an opportunity for both the pregnant person and the midwife to assess their abilities to work together as a team. It is important that adequate time be allotted to cover all of these tasks.

### Client Responsibilities During Pregnancy

As part of the introductory visit, the midwife provides an overview of the pregnant person's tasks to promote optimal health and maximize the likelihood of having a healthy pregnancy, with labor and birth occurring in the birth site of choice. Basic health promotion includes good nutrition, adequate rest and exercise, stress reduction, keeping scheduled appointments, and avoiding drugs, alcohol, and smoking. The pregnant person's responsibilities also include assuring the participation of a support partner who will take primary responsibility to be available during pregnancy, labor and birth, and the postpartum period. When small children will be present at the birth, an adult other than the primary support partner must be available to care for them.

Other expectations introduced during the initial visit will be addressed again later in the pregnancy, including breastfeeding/chestfeeding preparation, attending childbirth education classes, learning about the hospital transfer location, gathering birth supplies, and arranging for the services of a pediatric healthcare provider. Individuals may also be required to meet with the consultant service during the pregnancy, depending on the practice's guidelines.

## Midwife Responsibilities During Pregnancy

The midwife's responsibilities are outlined during the initial visit so that the patient and family understand the midwife's role. The midwife explains the concept of working in a client–midwife partnership, with each partner having a separate set of responsibilities that are equally important for achieving optimal outcomes. Throughout perinatal care, the midwife provides education, guidance, and health care, with particular emphasis on signs of normalcy and deviations from normal. These client–provider interactions should be respectful and inclusive of all pregnant populations. The midwife makes 24-hour midwifery on-call services available. Finally, the midwife describes the referral and transport services available.

## Selection of the Birth Site

The advantages and disadvantages of all available birth site options are reviewed in detail during the first prenatal visit so that the pregnant individual and midwife can work together in considering the best birth setting, delineating what can and cannot be done in each site. When discussing birth site options, both positive and negative aspects of each site are explored. An understanding of the individual's motivation for the choice of birth location will enable the midwife and the pregnant person to work together more effectively. The attitudes and concerns of the support partner and/or family should also be included in this discussion.

Factors influencing the choice of birth setting may include the philosophy of the pregnant person, beliefs of the support network and the caregivers, preferences regarding technology, feelings about previous birth experiences, societal and family considerations, financial concerns, and individual health status and risk factors. The low-risk pregnant person should be reminded that this decision is theirs to make.

## Safety Criteria and Transfer to Hospital-Based Care

The issue of possible transfer of care if a complication occurs should be addressed at the initial visit and reviewed as needed during subsequent visits. These discussions include a review of the midwife–consultant relationships, hospital privileges, and planned sites for transfer if needed. Problems that can develop during pregnancy, labor, or birth, or in the immediate postpartum period, and their frequency of occurrence should be reviewed with the pregnant person and their family. It is helpful if the midwife has access to up-to-date statistics on the practice's rate of transfer by parity and stage of labor to share during these conversations. The importance of self-care and early intervention to promote health should be reemphasized. The midwife reviews the pregnant person's health needs to ensure the choice of an appropriate birth site, making the pregnant person aware that some health conditions are best addressed in the hospital. Table 32-2 lists conditions that may be present before pregnancy or may become evident during pregnancy, which suggest planning birth in a hospital setting is indicated.[43] Table 32-3 identifies conditions that may develop during labor, birth, and the immediate postpartum period and require transfer to a hospital setting.[43]

The midwife's clinical judgment, skills, and resources influence decision making regarding the optimal birth setting for a pregnant individual. This assessment includes an evaluation of safety by the midwife. If the midwife feels the selected birth location is unsafe, the pregnant person does not have documented prenatal care, or hospital resources are geographically too distant, a hospital setting should be recommended. The midwife has ultimate responsibility for connecting their clients to the rest of the healthcare system, even though some pregnant people may arrange or lay the groundwork for consultation or hospital services.

Although emergencies may occur in any birth setting, they are rare in the home and in the birth center.[37,42,51,52] All pregnant people need to explore their feelings regarding the possibility of a negative birth outcome regardless of their planned birth setting. They may not be ready to discuss this very sensitive issue in depth at the initial visit. Instead, introducing this subject during the first visit and revisiting it during subsequent prenatal visits is the best way to make sure this topic is fully explored.

## Financial Considerations

There are many different payer options for financing prenatal and birth services. Financial arrangements must be clear for both self-pay and insured clients, and discussed openly by all responsible parties. Clients who choose to use private insurance for their prenatal care and community birth should check with their insurance plan about coverage, deductibles, and any other costs they may incur. A written payment plan should be reviewed and signed, which includes insurance information and a schedule for payments. Although an out-of-hospital birth may be less expensive if everything remains normal, it may be more expensive than a planned

| Table 32-2 | Conditions That Are Indications for Planned Hospital Birth[a,b] |
|---|---|

**Prior Pregnancy Conditions**

Previous stillbirth or neonatal death related to an intrapartum event

Primary postpartum hemorrhage requiring additional procedures[c]

Shoulder dystocia with resulting injury

**Current Pregnancy Conditions**

Active preterm labor (before 37 0/7 weeks' gestation) or preterm, prelabor rupture of membranes

Chronic or gestational hypertension

Evidence of congenital fetal anomalies requiring immediate assessment and/or management by a neonatal specialist

Fetal growth restriction less than the 5th percentile

Insulin-dependent diabetes or gestational diabetes requiring pharmacologic management

Malpresentation: breech, transverse lie

Need for pharmacologic induction of labor

Post-term pregnancy > 41 6/7 weeks' gestation

Multifetal gestation

Oligohydramnios with additional complicating factors

Polyhydramnios

Placenta previa in the third trimester

Placental abruption

Preeclampsia

Rh isoimmunization

**Medical Conditions**

Evidence of active infection with hepatitis, human immunodeficiency virus, genital herpes, syphilis, or tuberculosis

Psychiatric conditions that may affect intrapartum care management, the pregnant person, or neonatal transition following birth

Substantial medical conditions that have required acute medical supervision during the pregnancy and that could impact the birth, such as cardiac disease, epilepsy, thromboembolic disease, or hemoglobinopathy

Substance use/dependence

[a] This list is not exhaustive.

[b] Other obstetric or medical conditions may occur during pregnancy that warrant consultation, collaboration, or referral to determine the optimal site for the birth. Risk assessment for an individual may vary based on their prior medical, surgical, and obstetric history as well as resources available for hospital access within their community. Individual midwifery practice guidelines and/or client and/or midwife discretion will affect shared decision making about the selection of site of birth, and this process will be documented.

[c] Such as Bakri balloon, dilation and curettage, transfusion, and manual removal of placenta.

Reproduced with permission from American College of Nurse-Midwives. Clinical Bulletin No. 14: midwifery provision of home birth services. *J Midwifery Womens Health*. 2015;61(1):127-133.

hospital birth if complications arise. If a transfer to a hospital becomes necessary, the pregnant person may incur other costs in addition to the midwifery services that they obtained.

Pregnant people of color, persons who are uninsured, and those with Medicaid coverage for their perinatal care are the least likely to be afforded the option of having a community birth due to lack of coverage by public insurance and the inability to pay out of pocket.[53] These barriers create disparities by race, ethnicity, insurance coverage, and wealth to options in birth care that cause many pregnant

| Table 32-3 | Intrapartum, Postpartum, and Newborn Conditions That Are Indications for Transfer from Community Birth Setting to a Hospital[a] |
|---|---|
| **Intrapartum Indications[b]** | |
| Malpresentation: breech, transverse lie identified during labor | |
| Development of signs or symptoms of gestational hypertension or preeclampsia | |
| Evidence of chorioamnionitis/intra-amniotic infection | |
| Evidence of fetal intolerance of labor or persistent Category II fetal heart tones that are unresponsive to intrauterine resuscitation when birth is not imminent or in the presence of meconium | |
| Need for pharmacologic augmentation of labor | |
| Signs of placental abruption or unexplained increased vaginal bleeding | |
| **Postpartum Indications** | |
| Management of lacerations beyond the expertise of the attending midwife | |
| Postpartum hemorrhage unresponsive to initial treatments | |
| Retained placenta | |
| Unexplained vaginal bleeding | |
| **Newborn Indications** | |
| Unstable health status (e.g., unable to discharge to parental care; resuscitation; congenital abnormality requiring evaluation) | |

[a] Other obstetric or medical conditions may occur that warrant consultation, collaboration, or referral to determine the optimal site for the birth. Risk assessment for an individual may vary based on their prior medical, surgical, and obstetric history as well as resources available for hospital access within their community. Individual midwifery practice guidelines and/or client and/or midwife discretion will affect shared decision making about the selection of site of birth, and this process will be documented.

[b] When birth is imminent, careful consideration of the potential effect of transport on best practice management must be a priority consideration.

Reproduced with permission from American College of Nurse-Midwives. Clinical bulletin no. 14: midwifery provision of home birth services. *J Midwifery Women's Health.* 2015;61(1):127–133.

people to lose their autonomy and feel forced into perinatal care where they feel unsafe.

### Initial Prenatal Visit

At the initial visit, it is especially important in home and birth center practice for the midwife to assess the client for predictors of health outcomes that might be evident in the history and physical examination (see Table 32-2). Records from other healthcare providers should be requested if needed. Once this information is obtained, an appropriate birth site may be selected. The pregnant person and the midwife can identify factors that have the potential to develop into problems. Instituting prevention strategies early increases the likelihood that the client will successfully give birth in the chosen birth site.

### Calculation of an Accurate Due Date

Particular attention is paid to calculation of an accurate due date, because for most home and birth center practices there is a 5-week window of safety for the planned birth. A pregnancy is designated as full term from 37 weeks' gestation until 41 6/7 weeks' gestation. Births occurring at less than 37 weeks' gestation or more than 41 6/7 weeks' gestation are considered to be more safely accomplished in the hospital. When labor occurs before 37 weeks' gestation, the infant may not be adequately mature. In such a case, the client in preterm labor is referred to the hospital, where staff and technology can give appropriate support to the newborn if needed. Likewise, individuals who begin labor after 41 6/7 weeks of pregnancy are at increased risk for meconium staining and variant fetal heart rate patterns during labor, both of which are associated with morbidity and mortality.[54]

### Return Visits

During each return visit, the client and the midwife identify reassuring signs of normalcy or identify problems through an interim history, physical examination, and laboratory and adjunctive studies. In the role of educator, the home and birth center midwife teaches the client about symptoms that could indicate a complication. In this way, the client is empowered to take a primary role in the early identification of problems, allowing for early intervention. For a pregnant client to remain a candidate for a home or birth center birth, it is especially vital to intervene early, before uncorrectable problems develop. For example, if a client exhibits symptoms of dehydration early in labor, the midwife may recommend intravenous fluids to restore hydration and promote optimal health for birth. Clients should know that if specific complications arise, the increased risk associated with giving birth in a community setting can require a change in care setting; this knowledge can be a powerful motivator for clients to engage in and remain consistent in achieving health promotion goals.

### The Family's Preparation for Birth and the Postpartum Period

Planning for birth and the immediate postpartum period requires considerable time, thought, and energy. Additional preparation on the part of the family is required when birth occurs at home or in a birth center. Table 32-4 outlines key aspects of family responsibilities in preparing for childbirth and the postpartum period. More details regarding the development of a postpartum care plan to address the unique needs of the fourth trimester are provided later in this chapter.

As the due date nears, childbirth classes can help the client and their primary support partner learn about and focus on the upcoming birth. The classes that are most helpful include information about labor and birth progress, emphasize the power of inner strength, and are presented by an instructor who is knowledgeable about home and birth center births. The instructor communicates confidence that unmedicated birth is possible, given that pharmaceutical options are limited in the home or birth center. Clients should be educated on techniques focused on enhancing comfort and relaxation, options available to alleviate pain, and therapies available to augment the labor progress if indicated. Be

| Table 32-4 | The Family's Preparation for Birth and Postpartum |
|---|---|
| Continuing commitment to a jointly created plan of perinatal care | |
| Informing the midwife of any life changes | |
| Reading material focused on perinatal and health promotion activities | |
| Attending childbirth education classes with an educator familiar with community birth practices | |
| Writing an intrapartum birth plan that considers individual desires and preferences appropriate to the patient's health status at the time of birth | |
| Addressing fears and impacts of past trauma and abuse | |
| Preparing prenatally for breastfeeding/chestfeeding and pediatric care | |
| Preparing invited participants for their roles and responsibilities | |
| Preparing siblings for their participation | |
| Paying fees for care and/or conveying insurance information | |
| Collecting and organizing specified supplies | |
| Preparing a clean and open space for home birth | |
| Arranging for pet safety and care at the time of labor and birth | |
| Obtaining an infant car seat and assuring proper installation | |
| Making an accurate, detailed map to the home or checking global positioning system (GPS) accessibility | |
| Visiting an obstetric consultant and other specialists, if needed | |
| Knowing the route to the hospital or birth center | |
| Arranging doula participation if desired | |

aware that childbirth classes located in hospitals are often intended as an orientation to the hospital system and prepare the woman for labor and birth in that setting.

Writing a birth plan gives pregnant clients and their partners an opportunity to discuss what is important to them for their birth. These plans detail preferences about the environment, social interaction, comfort measures, pain management, support people, and medical procedures. Pregnant individuals and their partners identify the persons who will be present at the birth, the specific duties they may have, the role of siblings, religious or spiritual observances, and planned events with family and friends. Birth plans also describe coping measures learned from previous births, desired positions for labor and birth, and preferences for privacy and company at various points in labor. Plans for music, photography, and audio and/or video recording may be outlined.

To promote realistic thinking about possible transfer of care, families can be encouraged to write a hospital birth plan in addition to a home or birth center birth plan. This plan focuses on preferences regarding interventions and parental or family contact with the newborn in the presence of necessary medical interventions.

Most home and birth center practices anticipate that clients will breastfeed/chestfeed their infants except in extenuating circumstances. Breastfeeding/chestfeeding is an important safety factor for individuals giving birth in homes or birth centers. Breastfeeding/chestfeeding helps to keep the uterus contracted, thereby helping to control bleeding postpartum after the birth attendants leave the home or the family is discharged from the birth center. La Leche League and other support groups are invaluable resources for prenatal breastfeeding/chestfeeding preparation and support. If problems are encountered in this area, lactation consultants can be very helpful.

Persons who will be present for the birth also require preparation. If children will be present, they need to be prepared for birth events, including sights and sounds. The children must be cared for by a designated adult other than the birth partner, so the client and their partner can give their complete attention to managing labor. The designated adult's primary responsibility is attending to the children's needs and the client preferences at the time of the birth. This individual's plans for attendance at the birth may change as the children's or the client's needs change. Adults designated to care for the children should be prepared to leave the birth room if necessary. The children's support person also commits to caring for the children continuously until the client or the partner returns from the hospital if a transfer becomes necessary during or after the birth.

The people attending the birth should be selected carefully. It should be made clear that people invited to attend the birth may be asked to leave if the client seems to be distracted by their presence. Some participants may have fears about out-of-hospital births. Addressing their fears before the birth may change attitudes, and their attendance at the birth can be a transformative experience.

For clients who plan to give birth in a birth center, bags should be packed and supplies ready by 36 weeks' gestation. Supplies needed for home birth should be organized by 36 weeks' gestation and kept in or close to the room in which the woman intends to give birth. For more detail on the supplies needed, see the *Supplies for Birth in the Home and Birth Center* appendix.

### Prenatal Home Visit

A home visit by the midwife or the assistant at approximately 36 weeks' gestation can provide assurance that the family is ready for the birth. For home birth, a relatively clean house and pet care are obvious responsibilities of the family. Plans for cord blood preservation, placenta encapsulation, or other requested services are discussed during this home visit. If a water birth is planned, the midwife reminds the family to test the hot water tank capacity before labor begins, to assure that all faucet/hose attachments are at hand and functioning properly, and to troubleshoot for any leaks.

An emergency plan and important telephone numbers should be posted in the birthing room and in the pregnant person's chart. The family should make a "practice run" to the backup hospital to ensure that they know the location of parking, and the point at which to enter the building should a transfer become necessary. The car that will be used for emergency transportation needs to be in good repair and have adequate fuel to get to the hospital. Having hospital admission forms completed online or a completed paper copy in the chart before labor begins will decrease stress if a transfer to the hospital becomes necessary.

## The Intrapartum Period at Home or in the Birth Center

During the intrapartum period, the midwife's role is to be the guardian of both the birth environment and the pregnant person's energy. The laboring person depends on the midwife's ability to assess for and promote physiologic birth. The midwife's ongoing presence provides physical and psychological labor support, using simple interventions only when necessary. Should any complication occur, the midwife must have the skills needed to manage, stabilize, and in many cases resolve the situation, utilizing other resources if indicated (e.g., professional guidelines, emergency services, consulting providers). If complications cannot be resolved in the home or birth center setting, the midwife must have a plan to implement a transfer to the hospital.

The assistant provides support and technical labor, birth, and postpartum skills. Essential skills for the assistant include evaluation of the laboring person's physical and emotional status during labor;

the ability to monitor adult, fetal, and newborn vital signs; and certification in both adult cardiopulmonary resuscitation (CPR) and the Neonatal Resuscitation Program (NRP). In addition, the assistant should be able to provide support with lactation and postpartum care. It is not necessary for the assistant to be a healthcare professional: Childbirth educators, lactation counselors, and doulas may also possess the additional skills needed. AABC offers a birth assistant training that encompasses evidence-based learning to assist with labor, birth, and the immediate postpartum period.

The equipment needed to assist with community birth is simple. Each time the midwife and their team attend a birth, they review the individual's chart and birth plan to focus attention on the individual needs. They organize and check the equipment (see the *Supplies for Birth in the Home and Birth Center* appendix) and review the skills needed to address any specific health issues. **Figure 32-1** shows the equipment needed for basic newborn resuscitation.

When labor begins, the family contacts the midwife who is the primary attendant and is responsible for coordinating care. During this initial labor call, the midwife gathers data about how the pregnant person is experiencing labor, their needs, and their support systems. The midwife, the laboring person, and their support network review choices and make appropriate management plans, considering the laboring person's perceptions and history. Plans may include a decision for the midwife to meet the pregnant person for additional assessment. Maintaining contact with the midwife may be all that is necessary during the early phases of labor.

If the laboring person is comfortable at home and has the support they need, they may want to continue their normal activities of daily living while emphasizing hydration, nutrition, and increased rest. A variety of food choices should be provided by the family for the laboring person, guests, and the professional staff. All persons attending the birth should bring positive energy and support and not be a distraction. Friends and family may come to help with final preparation and management of other household activities, freeing the pregnant person and their primary support partner to focus on the labor.

In preparation for labor and birth, the bed can be "double-made" to protect the mattress. The bed can be made with a full set of linen and then completely covered with a plastic mattress cover, a drop cloth, or a shower curtain. A clean old sheet is placed on top of the plastic so that the bed may be used as desired for labor or birth. When the birth is

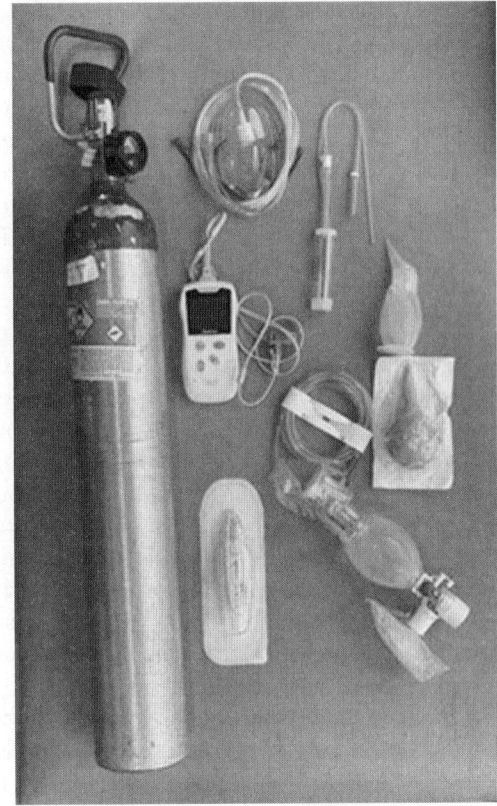

**Figure 32-1** Examples of newborn resuscitation equipment necessary for a home birth: oxygen tank, oxygen saturation monitor, adult oxygen face mask, DeLee suction, bulb syringe, self-inflating bag and mask, and laryngeal mask airway. See the *Supplies for Birth in the Home and Birth Center* appendix for more items.
Note: The American Heart Association and American Academy of Pediatrics' Newborn Resuscitation Program algorithm (not shown) is available on a small card and can be used to guide the resuscitation process.
Photo courtesy of Nikia Grayson.

completed, it is a simple matter to remove the top sheet and the plastic. Clean linen is then in place for the postpartum period.

The midwife or the assistant can perform the first physical assessment of labor in the home, the birth center, or the midwife's office. The initial assessment should include a review of the prenatal record, a physical examination to assess the fetal presentation, vital signs of the pregnant person and fetus, uterine contractions, and the pregnant person's response to labor. If membranes are not ruptured, a pelvic examination might be part of the initial physical assessment to document cervical dilation, verify the presenting part, or provide information that the pregnant person requests.

The time frame in which the midwife should be in close or continuous attendance can vary as labor progresses. As labor becomes active, the midwife and/ or the assistant will be present to assess maternal well-being and fetal heart tones using intermittent ausculatation.[55] The midwife or the assistant also may augment the birth partner's support measures, give reassurance, and guide the laboring person to conserve their energy. The laboring person is free to move around and assume any position they choose. The midwife may suggest positions that promote comfort, encourage progress, and maintain fetal well-being.

During the second stage of labor, it is not unusual for the laboring person to continue to change positions, moving from the bed to other locations within the home or birth center. The midwife must be alert, flexible, and able to anticipate the laboring person's movements. Sterile instruments should be placed on a portable sterile surface, allowing the midwife to move while following the laboring person's lead. If the laboring person is reluctant to change position, the midwife may use persuasive communication to suggest positions that will facilitate the birth.

As the fetal head emerges, the laboring person and/or their partner might reach down to complete the birth. The newborn is immediately placed on the birthing person's abdomen or breast (**Figure 32-2**). Within the first few seconds after birth, the midwife or assistant will do a quick evaluation of newborn well-being, assessing the newborn's muscle tone, cord pulsations, and respiratory effort, and then assign a 1-minute Apgar score. The midwife and the assistant continue frequent newborn assessment for the first hour after birth. The newborn is kept in skin-to-skin contact with the parent and covered with warm dry blankets, supporting newborn thermoregulation. The midwife is responsible for directing the assistant's care and continuing to observe the newborn for a successful transition from intrauterine to extrauterine life.

It is normal for some newborns to latch on immediately for their first feeding. Other newborns are more interested in exploring the change in their environment—looking, listening, nuzzling, licking, and taking their time to find the nipple and latch on. While the midwife is attentive to the progress of the third stage of labor, the assistant monitors the newborn's vital signs without disturbing family–infant bonding. The newborn can remain skin-to-skin in the birthing person's arms while the assistant checks the vital signs every 30 minutes, or more frequently as indicated. Welcoming the newborn can take place as the family has planned. Siblings are often present at the birth, or they can be invited in when the parent wishes.

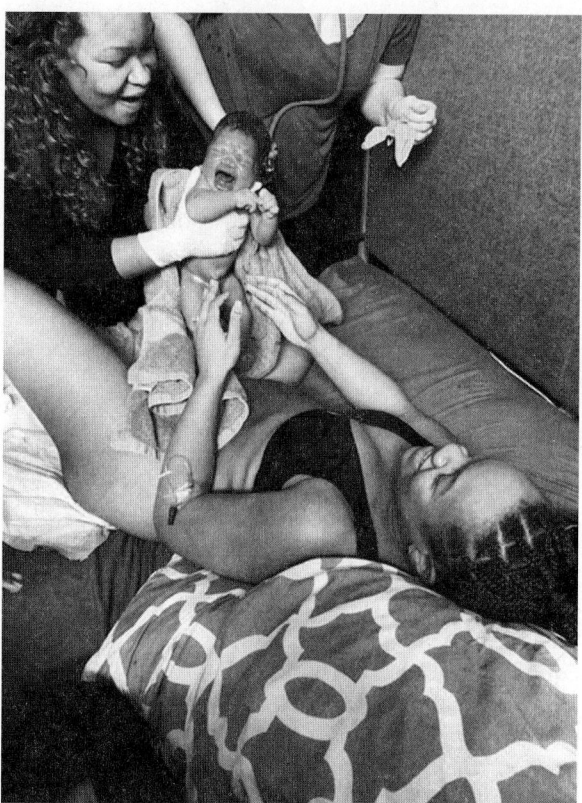

**Figure 32-2** Home birth.
Photo courtesy of Nikia Grayson.

Birth of the placenta is usually unhurried. If the laboring person needs or chooses to do so, they may squat or sit on the toilet to facilitate the completion of the third stage. The midwife may dispose of the placenta through a hazardous waste company. Some families desire to keep their placenta to bury under a plant; other families may arrange for the placenta to be dried and encapsulated.

## The Early Postpartum Period and Follow-Up

The first 2 to 4 hours postpartum is a special time for the parents, family, and friends to welcome and bond with the newborn. The midwife and the assistant are participants during this time of welcome. Once the birthing individual's and newborn's vital signs are within normal limits, breastfeeding/chestfeeding is established, and the amount of lochia, uterine position, and uterine consistency indicate the uterus is contracted, the midwife can leave the birthing room to facilitate a period of privacy and continued bonding time for the family. In some cases, eye prophylaxis and vitamin K administration are delayed until after this initial period of family bonding. Some families make an informed choice to waive these newborn procedures; however, it is recommended that the benefits of these procedures are discussed prenatally and encouraged during the postpartum period. Perineal suturing, if necessary, can be delayed an hour if there is no bleeding from the wound; alternatively, it may be done immediately, according to the client's preference.

While bonding continues, the midwife can attend to the usual responsibility of documenting the birth. It is not unusual for the midwife to spend this period on tasks typically accomplished in the hospital by nursing, secretarial, housekeeping, and dietary staff. The midwife and the assistant ensure proper nourishment for the client, help with breastfeeding/chestfeeding, assist the client to shower and void, wash the instruments, and put the birth site in order. Quite often, family and friends who have attended the birth as guests become helpers during this postpartum family time.

As long as the newborn is adapting to life outside the uterus well, the physical examination is usually done after a period of bonding according to the family's preference. The midwife performs a complete newborn physical examination, while ensuring the baby stays thermoneutral. This examination provides an opportunity for teaching, as it usually takes place in the client's bed and may be performed in the presence of excited children greeting the new sibling. Family members often participate in weighing, measuring, and dressing the newborn in the midst of friends taking photographs and a great deal of socializing and celebration. At a birth center, the family stays for at least 4 hours following the birth, and typically 6 to 12 hours; the need for longer observation often necessitates transport. At a home birth, the midwife and assistant stay until the postpartum person has appropriate lochia and is able to void and eat, and the newborn has transitioned well to extrauterine life and had at least one good feeding.

After the midwife departs the home or the family leaves the birth center, it is recommended that the newborn and postpartum person stay close together to aid in temperature stabilization, enhance parent–newborn communication, and stimulate milk production. A newborn bath may be delayed for the first 24 to 48 hours after birth. The couplet should be assessed in the first 2 days either at a home or office visit or via a telephone assessment. The midwife assesses breastfeeding/chestfeeding, the developing family relationships, adequacy of help in the home, infant caretaking abilities, and follow-up

appointments with the newborn's healthcare provider at this visit. In addition, the dried blood spot test for metabolic disorders, hearing screen, and pulse oximetry for the assessment of congenital heart conditions are performed after 24 hours of life. Assessment of the postpartum individual should include the items discussed in the *Postpartum Care* chapter.

During the subsequent postpartum recovery period, the family may be seen in the midwife's office to evaluate uterine involution and other postpartum, infant, or family needs. This process should be ongoing and tailored to the client's individual needs; however, an initial assessment should be conducted within 3 weeks of birth to ensure that appropriate care is provided and that the postpartum transition is occurring successfully. A postpartum care plan should detail topics such as care team contact information, postpartum visit schedule, reproductive plans, mental health management, nutrition, self-care activities, and newborn care. A comprehensive postpartum assessment, as discussed in the *Postpartum Care* chapter, should occur between 4 and 12 weeks postpartum to ensure that recovery and support are provided in these key areas and that any complications and health issues from the pregnancy are being managed appropriately.[56]

## Framework for Clinical Management

Management strategies for selected clinical situations in the home and birth center can be divided into three categories: preventive, non-urgent, and emergency. In-labor transfer rates to hospital-based care for clients planning to give birth at home or in a birth center range from approximately 7% to 30%.[28,29,41] The likelihood of transfer depends on multiple factors in addition to birthing individual or fetal clinical status, including distance to the collaborating hospital and collaborative protocols. Of those individuals who begin labor at home or at a birth center, the majority ultimately give birth at their preferred site.[51] The most common reasons for transfer to a hospital during labor are lack of progress in labor (40% of transfers) and desire for pain relief medications often accompanied by exhaustion (20.5% of transfers).[51] Due to their increased labor duration, nulliparous people are more likely to have an intrapartum hospital transfer than are multiparous people.[41] Postpartum transfer occurs for approximately 1.5% of clients who give birth at home, and neonatal transfer occurs for approximately 1% of newborns.[51] Postpartum transfer rates from birth centers are similar, with 2.5% of clients requiring transfer postpartum and 2.6% of newborns requiring transfer.[37] Most transports for hospital care are nonemergent. When Stapleton et al. reviewed transfers in a national birth center study (*n* = 13,030), they found that emergency transfer was required for fewer than 1% of clients who gave birth in a birth center.[37]

Preventive management is the first line of defense to maintain safety during any birth. Ideally, health promotion during the antepartum period will succeed in bringing a well pregnant person with a healthy pregnancy to term. Safety is most effectively maintained when strategies to promote health are actively implemented. Early identification of deviations from normal should ideally be non-urgent, then resolved with consultation and collaboration. Urgent emergency situations may require referral in addition to consultation and/or collaborative care. If the midwife determines that more personnel and complex technologies are needed, previously arranged plans are implemented to ensure transfer of care to a hospital-based system.[22,37,43] During this transfer, the midwife must utilize excellent decision-making and clinical skills, and promote good communication among all parties involved—the midwife, the birthing individual, the family, and the consulting practice. Communication with the receiving clinicians is enhanced with a verbal report, along with a concise, complete health record.

## Management of Non-urgent Clinical Situations
### Prolonged Labor

Prolonged labor with exhaustion in nulliparous pregnant individuals is the most common reason for transfer of a client from home or a birth center to the hospital. The most important preventive intervention by the midwife for prolonged labor is to support the client's efficient use of energy during labor. Adequate hydration and ingestion of nutritional sources of energy are essential. The midwife can encourage periods of rest when labor ebbs.

When slow progress becomes a concern, it must be clearly understood that oxytocin (Pitocin), an agent used for augmentation of labor, is not administered in the home or birth center. If labor progression cannot be accomplished by means of upright positions, adequate hydration, nutritional support, or nipple stimulation, then a hospital transfer is indicated.

Sometimes when labor continues without progress, the client becomes too fatigued to cope with labor pain, and strategies for nonpharmacologic pain relief are no longer effective. In these cases, a

transfer to the hospital is indicated. A non-urgent transfer may take place in the family car as long as the birthing individual's vital signs and fetal heart rate are reassuring. Clients transferred for prolonged labor with their first birth can usually complete subsequent births at home or in birth center settings.

### Prolonged Rupture of Membranes

In cases of prolonged rupture of the membranes, regular monitoring for signs of infection is critical. The precise time limit set before transfer to the hospital becomes necessary will depend on the midwife's preferences, the client's preferences, and negotiations with the healthcare system, including consideration of maternity care and neonatal community standards of care. The midwife should avoid vaginal examinations whenever possible, and discourage the laboring individual from introducing anything into their vagina. To encourage regular uterine contractions, the midwife can consider interventions such as ambulation, nipple stimulation, and castor oil, although more studies are needed to evaluate the effectiveness of these interventions.[57-60]

### Group B Streptococcus Colonization

Individuals who have vaginal colonization with group B *Streptococcus* (GBS) can give birth safely at home or in a birth center. If intravenous antibiotic prophylaxis is indicated, the antibiotic can be administered in these settings. In birth centers, infants born to GBS-colonized individuals often have a longer postpartum stay. Individuals who are colonized with GBS should make follow-up plans prenatally with their pediatric care provider for the neonate's care. Families can be taught to monitor and record the newborn's vital signs, enabling them to convey information about the newborn's health to the pediatric care provider within 12 to 48 hours after birth.

### Meconium Staining

If meconium appears at any time after rupture of the membranes, the color, consistency, and amount of the meconium should be evaluated. Notification of the consultant depends on the consultation agreement and the characteristics of the meconium. However, amniotic fluid with thick meconium indicates that the client should be transferred to the hospital before the birth, if there is adequate time to do so safely. The presence of thick, undiluted meconium can indicate a breech presentation.

In the absence of thick meconium, it is appropriate to proceed with birth in the home or birth center if the fetal heart rate has normal characteristics and labor is progressing. Before a decision is made concerning the best place for birth, the midwife should engage in a shared decision-making discussion with the client and support partner regarding the midwife's assessment, possible consequences of meconium aspiration, and treatment options both in and out of the hospital. The content of this conversation should be documented in the labor record. If the decision is made to remain at home or in the birth center for the birth, adequate suction and other resuscitation equipment should be available.

### Vaginal Birth After Cesarean Birth

Many persons who experience a cesarean birth are interested in avoiding another cesarean in their next pregnancy. However, across large geographic expanses of the United States, local hospitals with vaginal birth after cesarean (VBAC) services are not available.[40,51] In addition, some pregnant persons who had a prior cesarean birth come to their next pregnancy feeling traumatized by their prior birth experience, wishing to avoid hospitals where they may have experienced poor treatment, loss of autonomy, or poor communication.[61] As a result of these factors, VBAC rates in the United States over the past few decades have decreased in hospitals and increased in community birth settings.[15,62] There are both risks and benefits for the laboring person and their fetus of either a labor after cesarean (LAC) or an elective repeat cesarean birth (ERCB), as reviewed in the *Pregnancy-Related Conditions* chapter. Thus, the decision about which type of birth to have can be a complicated one for families.

Limited data indicate that approximately 87% of people who give birth at home or in a birth center and who have had a previous cesarean birth will experience a vaginal birth—a rate that is higher than the 74% successful VBAC rate among persons who plan a VBAC in a hospital setting.[63–65] Although VBAC can be more successful in out-of-hospital settings, pregnant people who labor after a prior cesarean birth also have an increased risk for uterine rupture that is especially difficult to manage in community intrapartum settings.[32,63] This complication has consequences for the fetus and newborn as well. In a large cohort of pregnant people who planned a home birth with ($n = 1052$) versus those without a prior cesarean ($n = 12,092$), Cox and colleagues found an almost four-fold increase in fetal and neonatal mortality in the prior cesarean birth group (4.74/1000 births versus 1.24/1000 births; $P \leq$ 0.05).[63] In another study, researchers identified an eight-fold increase in neonatal seizures associated with home birth compared to hospital birth among people with a prior cesarean (adjusted odds ratio [aOR], 8.53; 95% CI, 2.87–25.4; 0.19% versus 0.02%, respectively).[64]

In community settings where VBAC is offered, it is important that the midwife discuss these outcomes with prospective clients, taking care to differentiate between relative and absolute risks. Birth at home after a previous cesarean birth with no prior vaginal births is among the conditions associated with the highest perinatal mortality (10.2/1000 pregnancies)—a rate that is similar to the perinatal death rates for breech presentation (16.8/1000 pregnancies), twin gestation (14.5/1000 pregnancies), and preeclampsia (16.1/1000 pregnancies).[32] Increased perinatal morbidity and mortality in home versus hospital settings for pregnant people attempting to give birth vaginally have also been found by other investigators.[63,64,66] Based on this evidence of perinatal harm associated with a first VBAC in home or birth center settings, it is better for these clients' labor and birth to occur in a hospital.

Perinatal risks associated with VBAC are lower for the pregnant person with a prior vaginal birth. For example, during a planned community birth, the absolute risk of perinatal death for a pregnant person with a previous cesarean birth and at least one prior vaginal birth is lower than the perinatal death rate for a nulliparous person (1.27/1000 pregnancies versus 3.43/1000 pregnancies, respectively).[32] Thus, having a prior vaginal birth confers a significant reduction in the risk for adverse outcomes, which means that these pregnant people can consider community birth as an option to hospital care. Both ACNM and AABC advocate that pregnant people with a prior cesarean birth have access to VBAC, regardless of their geographic location, including the option to have their labor and birth occur in a birth center for those who are good candidates following proper assessment.[67,68]

### Management of Emergency Clinical Situations
### Variant Fetal Heart Rate Patterns

Concerning fetal heart rate patterns, such as recurrent late decelerations or tachycardia, that do not resolve with supportive measures such as increased hydration or position changes, indicate that the fetus is at increased risk for developing metabolic acidemia. In these cases, a transfer to the hospital by ambulance is indicated. Similarly, if at any point during the labor, the midwife feels a need to monitor the fetus more closely than is possible with intermittent use of the fetoscope or Doppler ultrasound, the laboring person should be moved to the hospital. Continuous intrapartum use of electronic fetal monitors is beyond the scope of AABC's standards.

## Malpresentation: Breech Presentation

Pregnant people diagnosed prenatally with a fetus in breech presentation or other malpresentation should be engaged in a shared decision-making discussion about external cephalic version, planned hospitalization for vaginal breech birth, or cesarean birth. Breech presentation at the onset of labor is an indication for hospitalization, given the increased risk for adverse newborn outcomes.[32] Rarely, a person in labor at home or in the birth center may present with a fetus in breech presentation that was not previously detected. If the birth is imminent, the midwife should manage the breech birth in place, but call 911 for extra personnel and transport resources should they be needed. Emergency maneuvers for breech birth are discussed in the *Breech Birth* appendix.

## Postpartum Hemorrhage

Postpartum hemorrhage requiring transport is rare, occurring in only 0.2% of home births and 2.4% of birth center births.[37] Researchers report that in low-risk groups of laboring people, rates of postpartum hemorrhage are higher in hospitals compared to community settings.[26]

If a pregnant person has a prenatal hematocrit level of less than 30% or a hemoglobin level of less than 10 g/dL, they may be unable to tolerate even a normal postpartum blood loss. In this circumstance, prenatal transfer to hospital-based care may be considered as a precaution. After birth, if postpartum bleeding is excessive at home or in a birth center and is attributed to uterine atony, intravenous volume expanders with added oxytocin can be initiated. In addition, the midwife can give oxytocin intramuscularly, methylergonovine maleate (Methergine) intramuscularly or orally, and/or misoprostol (Cytotec) orally or rectally per standard protocols for drug, dosage, and timing. Tranexamic acid (TXA) can also be given within the first 3 hours after birth to reduce bleeding. TXA can be administered intravenously, or orally when intravenous administration is not possible. Oral methylergonovine maleate can be used short periods postpartum to provide extra support against further bleeding at home or following birth center discharge in people who had slightly excessive blood loss immediately following birth. However, midwives using this medication

should carefully consider if it is safe for the patient and avoid its use in the presence of maternal hypertension. If more than one dose is given, the birthing person should avoid breastfeeding/chestfeeding for 12 hours following the last dose to avoid neonatal complications such as vomiting and diarrhea. Methylergonovine maleate can also decrease the birthing person's milk supply.

If immediate or delayed postpartum blood loss results in symptoms of hypovolemia such as dizziness, weakness, or difficulty in ambulation, transfer to hospital-based care is needed because blood and blood products are not available in home and birth center settings. If the birthing person is stabilized at home but subsequently experiences symptoms of hypovolemia or delayed milk production, they may require hospitalization for evaluation and treatment. It is important to remember that people giving birth at home or in a birth center will not have continuous professional postpartum support beyond 3 to 12 hours postpartum.

## Newborn Complications

Neonatal resuscitation is rarely needed when a well person experiences a healthy pregnancy, has an unmedicated and uncomplicated intrapartum course,[44] and has an uncomplicated birth at home or in a birth center. Nevertheless, as noted earlier, neonatal resuscitation is a critical skill for both the midwife and a second qualified person who attend home and birth center births. When a need for resuscitation arises in these settings, both the laboring person and the newborn may need medical support at the same time, so having two qualified providers present is essential. In the large majority of cases, the resuscitation equipment and skills provided by home and birth center midwives are usually successful in stimulating the newborn's respiratory effort. If this does not occur, the goal is to stabilize the newborn and provide adequate oxygenation until transport to a neonatal intensive care unit is completed.

## Transfer to Hospital-Based Care

As noted earlier, transfer from the home or birth center to the hospital is sometimes necessary. Intrapartum transfer is stressful for all concerned—the family, the midwife, and the hospital receiving the family—and good communication among everyone involved is critical. Notifying the receiving providers as far in advance as possible will help the transfer go smoothly and enable the laboring person to get the care they need in a timely fashion.[69] Management of complications that may occur during labor, birth, or the early postpartum period depends on written clinical practice guidelines, characteristics of the client and their support system, the network of health system support, and the midwife's clinical skill set.[43] Other factors that influence decision making may include the midwife's level of experience, the pregnant person's and family's reluctance to allow transfer, distance to the hospital, and road conditions.

The transfer summary is a simple, easy-to-use form that conveys pertinent data to the receiving staff (Figure 32-3). It is also a quality management tool that enables accurate statistical collection of practice data.

In most situations, the problem necessitating transfer is identified as it develops over time. When a hospital transfer becomes necessary, the pregnant person who had planned a home or birth center birth must cope with two concerns: worrying about their health and/or their fetus/newborn's health, and experiencing the feelings (perhaps grief) associated with the loss of their planned home or birth center birth. The client and their family may be disappointed, and sometimes they may blame the midwife for their difficult situation.

Providing anticipatory guidance during prenatal visits can reduce the family's distress if transport becomes a reality. Reminding families late in pregnancy of the possibility that transfer could be necessary, reviewing practice statistics, and describing actual transport experiences may be helpful. Discussion may include a review of not only the decision-making process, but also consultation

Name_____

| Date | Time | |
|------|------|---|
| | | Reason for transfer: |
| | | Review with client and family: |
| | | Name of consultant: |
| | | Name of hospital: |
| | | Consultation and plan: |
| | | Transport called (if applicable): |
| | | Arrival of transport vehicle (if applicable): |
| | | Mode of transport: |
| | | Mother: T ____ P ____ R ____ BP ____ Condition ____ |
| | | Baby: FHT ____ T ____ P ____ R ____ Condition ____ |
| | | Departure from home/birth center (circle one) |
| | | Arrival at hospital/accompanied by: |
| | | Receiving provider: |
| | | Type of intervention: |
| | | Initiation of treatment: |
| | | Birth information:    SVD      Inst. Asst. C/S  Apgar ___/___ |
| | | Outcome summary: |
| | | CNM departure from hospital: |
| | | Breastfeeding status: |
| | | Release for hospital records sent: |
| | | Hospital records received: |

Signature _____

Figure 32-3 Transfer summary.
© BirthCare & Women's Health, Ltd. Reprinted by permission.

services, the trip to the hospital, and the admission process. The pregnant person and their family need help to understand that if they are going to the hospital, it is because they need interventions.

During the process of shared decision making at the first visit, and again around 36 weeks' gestation, the client should be made aware of the possibility of complications that might affect the birth, including that their fetus/newborn could be injured or die during the birth process. Although most people hesitate to focus on this frightening issue, the pregnant person needs to ask themselves what they would do and how they would cope. They also need to explore how they would respond to family or friends who may not have been supportive of their decision to give birth away from a hospital. In such circumstances, the midwife needs to be prepared to offer additional support and counseling for the pregnant person and their family. Some clients, as well as the practitioners who serve them, may benefit from professional counseling to process unexpected outcomes.

### Promoting a Smooth Transfer of Care

Best practice guidelines for transferring from a planned home birth to a hospital setting have been developed by the Home Birth Summit.[69] These guidelines include model practices for midwives and receiving hospital staff as well as recommendations for policy development.[69]

Management dilemmas may occur particularly if the pregnant person's birth plan or desires conflict with accepted medical community standards. It may be difficult to convince a consultant to implement a plan that may be safe, but unpopular in the medical community. Both the midwife and the consultant may be caught in the middle. Families may pressure their midwife to continue care despite complications that arise during the labor or birth. This conundrum has the potential to threaten the relationship with the consultant, and it can create a climate of disrespect at the hospital that could cause clinical harm for that family. Such a choice also has the potential to negatively affect the home or birth center practice, creating barriers for clients and the practitioners who serve them and, therefore, adversely affecting future birth options in the community. Many times, a midwife may be tempted to be led by the heart instead of the head. Wish management does not work. Learning to say "no" is not just important—it is critical. Midwives must be brutally honest with themselves and not be pressured by clients to practice outside of their clinical practice guidelines and circle of

safety. Care must be taken not to jeopardize the entire practice for one client.

## Business Aspects of Home and Birth Center Settings

The number of birth centers in the United States is on the rise. AABC reports that as of 2020, there were 384 freestanding birth centers in the United States—a 97% increase since 2010.[12] The legal status of home birth and birth center settings varies on a state-by-state basis, however. In a few states, it is illegal for midwives to attend home births. Furthermore, the regulatory requirements that must be met by midwives who attend home births vary by state, as do regulations for birth centers. Midwives practicing in the United States are encouraged to investigate the legal requirements for home birth and birth center operation in the states in which they live and practice. ACNM and the National Association of Certified Professional Midwives (NACPM) have staff specializing in professional services and legislative liaisons to keep members aware of practice and political issues. AABC also has staff who can assist midwives who plan to open and operate birth centers. To break down barriers, safeguard the profession, and protect the healthcare rights of pregnant people and their families, home and birth center midwives have to be both alert and proactive.

All midwifery practices need to address business and regulatory issues. Many of the same professional and legal documents that are necessary when starting a hospital practice are also necessary for a home or birth center practice. Birth centers and home birth practices are often midwifery owned and operated. A self-employed independent midwife has more control over clinical, business, and administrative decisions. These practices tend to be small, minimizing bureaucracy and simplifying communication and policy. Such a small organization is more responsive to the needs of the clients, the family, and the midwife when compared to a larger institution. On the downside, self-employment usually involves much more responsibility, time demands, and financial risk for the self-employed person.[49]

Administrative support is helpful for a home or birth center practice, so that the midwife can continue providing clinical services. The person in charge of billing and collections is key to the practice's financial survival. Their interpersonal skills and commitment to the practice help keep the service financially sound. Salaries for clinical staff should amount to approximately 50% of the income generated by the practice. Even in established practices, it is not uncommon for home birth or birth center midwives to have lower salaries than their hospital-based colleagues.

Many home birth and birth center midwives are participating providers on health insurance panels and are reimbursed by Medicaid. Some insurance companies require accreditation through CABC for birth center–based midwives to become participating providers. ACNM has developed materials to help midwives develop the business and negotiation skills needed to sustain a successful practice.

Financial arrangements with consulting practices should be clear. Consultants may decide not to charge a consultation fee to the midwife for providing services, but rather charge the pregnant person only for services actually rendered. By assuring that the client pays the consulting practice promptly, the midwife fosters a good midwife–consultant relationship. Sometimes when consultants serve home and birth center practices, they may benefit from referrals not only from the midwifery practice, but also from client networks and sympathetic childbirth educators. Conversely, hospital-based colleagues may refuse cross-coverage for the consultants.

A system for data collection and analysis should be put in place before a practice opens. Accurate data collection and analysis facilitates evaluation, quality management, validation of effective practice, peer review, and research. Practice data should be collected regularly and analyzed at least annually. ACNM, AABC, and Midwives Alliance of North America (MANA) have web-based data collection applications. When presented clearly and succinctly, statistics can also serve as a public relations tool conveying important information to families about outcomes and transfers.

Midwives working in home and birth center practices need to be astutely aware of who wields power. These midwives are practicing outside of the mainstream maternity system. Although they likely work with less bureaucracy and more clinical freedom, their practice is subject to increased scrutiny, and they lack the protective institutional layer that a hospital may provide. ACNM and AABC have staff specializing in professional services and legislative liaisons to keep members aware of practice and political issues.

## Conclusion

Midwifery as a profession was developed within the community context. Whether in the home or birth center environment, midwives utilize the key resources of time, place, and social connection while

also promoting authority, centrality, and privacy for the birthing families in their care. Within the home and birth center environment, utilizing national standards coupled with a framework of reproductive justice to promote safety and ensure optimal health outcomes for pregnant people and their infants is critical (Table 32-5). Key aspects to consider

| Table 32-5 | Resources Supporting the Development of Birth Centers and Community Birth Settings |
|---|---|
| **Organization/Author** | **Description** |
| American Association of Birth Centers (AABC) | Provides information about birth centers, position statements, information on standards for birth centers, and resources for health outcomes in birth centers. |
| Commission for Accreditation of Birth Centers (CABC) | Provides information on which birth centers are CABC accredited and requirements for accreditation. |
| JJ Way BIPOC–created Group Prenatal Care Model The JJ Way. Commonsense Childbirth Inc. | The Group Prenatal Care Model focuses on reducing disparities and improving outcomes through use of the midwifery model of care. Trainings for providers, institutions, and communities are provided. |
| Midwives Alliance of North America (MANA) | Professional organization for certified professional midwives and midwives who care for women exclusively at home or in birth centers. |
| Black Mamas Matter Alliance (BMMA) | Organization focused on advocacy, research, and advancing care for Black maternal health, rights, and justice. |
| National Association to Advance Black Birth (NAABB) | Organization that aims to increase the number of midwives and doulas of color. Initiatives are focused on building the workforce capacity in the Black community. |
| Birth Center Equity.org | Organization that focuses on developing and sustaining birth centers to serve Black, Indigenous, and people of color. |

during this evaluation include addressing sources of structural and obstetric racism within care settings, avoiding interpersonal interactions that promote racism and bias, and ensuring that service offerings allow for every person to have access to accessible, appropriate, and affordable care options.[48]

Birthing families deserve to feel safe and supported during the birthing process. Midwives in the community setting often have more freedom to offer one-to-one care and to be a continuous presence during labor. The midwife carefully selects interventions with the birthing family and utilizes them only when the pregnant person needs them and without interrupting the flow of labor. Being aware of and encouraging changes during the labor, birth, and postpartum process that are individually tailored, culturally appropriate, and free from bias and prejudice are essential tasks of the midwife in the community setting.

## References

1. Litoff JB. *American Midwives 1860 to the Present.* Westport, CT: Praeger; 1978.

2. Wertz R, Wertz D. *Lying-In: A History of Childbirth in America.* New Haven, CT: Yale University Press; 1989.

3. Neiderud CJ. How urbanization affects the epidemiology of emerging infectious diseases. *Infect Ecol Epidemiol.* 2015;5:27060. doi:10.3402/iee.v5.27060.

4. Laird MD. Report of the Maternity Center Association Clinic, New York, 1931–1951. *Am J Obstet Gynecol.* 1955;69(1):178-184. doi:10.1016/s0002-9378(16)37927-3.

5. Kobrin FE. The American midwife controversy: a crisis of professsionalization. *Bull Hist Med.* 1966;40(4):350-363.

6. Brodsky PL. Where have all the midwives gone? *J Perinat Educ.* 2008;17(4):48-51. doi:10.1624/105812408x324912.

7. Craven C, Glatzel M. Downplaying difference: historical accounts of African American midwives and contemporary struggles for midwifery. *Feminist Studies.* 2010;36(2):330-358.

8. Bonaparte A. Physicians' discourse for establishing authoritative knowledge in birthing work and reducing the presence of the granny midwife: physicians' authoritative knowledge in birthing work. *J Hist Sociol.* 2014;28. doi:10.1111/johs.12045.

9. Kline W. Back to bed: from hospital to home obstetrics in the city of Chicago. *J Hist Med Allied Sci.* 2018;73(1):29-51. doi:10.1093/jhmas/jrx055.

10. Ventre F. Lay midwifery. I. The lay midwife. *J Nurse Midwifery.* 1978;22(4):32-35. doi:10.1016/0091-2182(78)90088-5.

11. Phillippi JC, Alliman J, Bauer K. The American Association of Birth Centers: history, membership, and current initiatives. *J Midwifery Womens Health.* 2009;54(5):387-392. doi:10.1016/j.jmwh.2008.12.009.

12. Ernst K, Bauer K. Birth centers in the United States. American Association of Birth Centers. https://cdn.ymaws.com/www.birthcenters.org/resource/collection/028792A7-808D-4BC7-9A0F-FB038B434B91/Birth_Centers_in_the_United_States__2020_.pdf. Accessed October 12, 2021.

13. Commission for Accreditation of Birth Centers. Benefits of AMU accreditation. https://birthcenteraccreditation.org/benefits-of-amu-accreditation/. Accessed November 16, 2021.

14. Varney H. *Varney's Midwifery.* 3rd ed. Sudbury, MA: Jones and Bartlett; 1997.

15. MacDorman MF, Declercq E. Trends and state variations in out-of-hospital births in the United States, 2004–2017. *Birth.* 2019;46(2):279-288. doi:10.1111/birt.12411.

16. Davis-Floyd R, Gutschow K, Schwartz DA. Pregnancy, birth and the COVID-19 pandemic in the United States. *Med Anthropol.* 2020;39(5):413-427. doi:10.1080/01459740.2020.1761804.

17. Daviss BA, Anderson DA, Johnson KC. Pivoting to childbirth at home or in freestanding birth centers in the US during COVID-19: safety, economics and logistics. *Front Sociol.* 2021;6:618210. doi:10.3389/fsoc.2021.618210.

18. Hardeman RR, Karbeah J, Almanza J, Kozhimannil KB. Roots Community Birth Center: a culturally-centered care model for improving value and equity in childbirth. *Healthc (Amst).* 2020;8(1):100367. doi:10.1016/j.hjdsi.2019.100367.

19. Green CL, Perez SL, Walker A, et al. The cycle to respectful care: a qualitative approach to the creation of an actionable framework to address maternal outcome disparities. *Int J Environ Res Public Health.* 2021;18(9). doi:10.3390/ijerph18094933.

20. National Heart, Lung and Blood Institute, National Institutes of Health. Systemic racism, a key risk factor for maternal death and illness. https://www.nhlbi.nih.gov/news/2021/systemic-racism-key-risk-factor-maternal-death-and-illness. Published April 26, 2021. Accessed November 16, 2021.

21. Ernst KB, Bauer K. The birth center experience. https://cdn.ymaws.com/www.birthcenters.org/resource/collection/028792A7-808D-4BC7-9A0F-FB038B434B91/The_Birth_Center_Experience.pdf. Accessed October 17, 2021.

22. Commission for Accreditation of Birth Centers. What does accreditation mean? https://birthcenteraccreditation.org/accreditation-is-the-mark-of-quality/. Accessed October 17, 2021.

23. Jackson ME, Bailes AJ. Home birth with certified nurse-midwife attendants in the United States: an

overview. *J Nurse Midwifery*. 1995;40(6):493-507. doi:10.1016/0091-2182(95)00059-3.

24. Sakala C, Corry M. *Evidence-Based Maternity Care: What It Is and What It Can Achieve.* New York, NY: Milbank Memorial Fund. https://www.national partnership.org/our-work/resources/health-care /maternity/evidence-based-maternity-care.pdf.

25. Li Y, Townend J, Rowe R, et al. Perinatal and maternal outcomes in planned home and obstetric unit births in women at "higher risk" of complications: secondary analysis of the Birthplace national prospective cohort study. *BJOG*. 2015;122(5): 741-753. doi:10.1111/1471-0528.13283.

26. Hutton EK, Cappelletti A, Reitsma AH, et al. Outcomes associated with planned place of birth among women with low-risk pregnancies. *CMAJ*. 2016;188(5):e80-e90. doi:10.1503/cmaj.150564.

27. Reitsma A, Simioni J, Brunton G, et al. Maternal outcomes and birth interventions among women who begin labour intending to give birth at home compared to women of low obstetrical risk who intend to give birth in hospital: a systematic review and meta-analyses. *E Clin Med*. 2020;21:100319. doi:10.1016/j.eclinm.2020.100319.

28. Brocklehurst P, Hardy P, Hollowell J, et al. Perinatal and maternal outcomes by planned place of birth for healthy women with low risk pregnancies: the Birthplace in England national prospective cohort study. *BMJ*. 2011;343:d7400. doi:10.1136/bmj.d7400.

29. Janssen PA, Saxell L, Page LA, et al. Outcomes of planned home birth with registered midwife versus planned hospital birth with midwife or physician. *CMAJ*. 2009;181(6-7):377-383. doi:10.1503/cmaj .081869.

30. De Jonge A, van der Goes BY, Ravelli AC, et al. Perinatal mortality and morbidity in a nationwide cohort of 529,688 low-risk planned home and hospital births. *BJOG*. 2009;116(9):1177-1184. doi:10.1111/j.1471-0528.2009.02175.x.

31. Alliman J, Stapleton SR, Wright J, et al. Strong Start in birth centers: socio-demographic characteristics, care processes, and outcomes for mothers and newborns. *Birth*. 2019;46(2):234-243. doi:10.1111 /birt.12433.

32. Bovbjerg ML, Cheyney M, Brown J, et al. Perspectives on risk: assessment of risk profiles and outcomes among women planning community birth in the United States. *Birth*. 2017;44(3):209-221. doi:10.1111/birt.12288.

33. Phillippi JC, Danhausen K, Alliman J, Phillippi RD. Neonatal outcomes in the birth center setting: a systematic review. *J Midwifery Womens Health*. 2018;63(1):68-89. doi:10.1111/jmwh.12701.

34. National Academies of Sciences, Engineering, and Medicine. The National Academies Collection: reports funded by National Institutes of Health. In: Backes EP, Scrimshaw SC, eds. *Birth Settings in America: Outcomes, Quality, Access, and Choice.* Washington, DC: National Academies Press; 2020.

35. Vedam S, Stoll K, MacDorman M, et al. Mapping integration of midwives across the United States: impact on access, equity, and outcomes. *PLoS One*. 2018;13(2):e0192523. doi:10.1371/journal .pone.0192523.

36. Cheng YW, Snowden JM, King TL, Caughey AB. Selected perinatal outcomes associated with planned home births in the United States. *Am J Obstet Gynecol*. 2013;209(4):325.e1-325.e8. doi:10.1016/j .ajog.2013.06.022.

37. Stapleton SR, Osborne C, Illuzzi J. Outcomes of care in birth centers: demonstration of a durable model. *J Midwifery Womens Health*. 2013;58(1):3-14. doi:10.1111/jmwh.12003.

38. Scarf VL, Rossiter C, Vedam S, et al. Maternal and perinatal outcomes by planned place of birth among women with low-risk pregnancies in high-income countries: a systematic review and meta-analysis. *Midwifery*. 2018;62:240-255. doi:10.1016/j.midw .2018.03.024.

39. Grünebaum A, McCullough LB, Bornstein E, et al. Neonatal outcomes of births in freestanding birth centers and hospitals in the United States, 2016–2019. *Am J Obstet Gynecol*. July 1, 2021. doi:10.1016/j .ajog.2021.06.093.

40. Gottvall K, Grunewald C, Waldenström U. Safety of birth centre care: perinatal mortality over a 10-year period. *BJOG*. 2004;111(1):71-78. doi:10.1046/j.1471-0528.2003.00017.x.

41. Nethery E, Schummers L, Levine A, et al. Birth outcomes for planned home and licensed freestanding birth center births in Washington State. *Obstet Gynecol*. 2021;138(5):693-702. doi:10.1097 /aog.0000000000004578.

42. Snowden JM, Tilden EL, Snyder J, et al. Planned out-of-hospital birth and birth outcomes. *N Engl J Med*. 2015;373(27):2642-2653. doi:10.1056/ NEJMsa1501738.

43. American College of Nurse Midwives. Midwifery provision of home birth services. *J Midwifery Womens Health*. 2016;61(1):127-133. doi:10.1111/jmwh.12431.

44. American College of Nurse Midwives. Position statement: planned home birth. https://www.midwife .org/acnm/files/ACNMLibraryData/UPLOAD FILENAME/000000000251/Planned-Home-Birth -Dec-2016.pdf. Accessed October 17, 2021.

45. World Health Organization. Care in normal birth: a practical guide. Technical Working Group, World Health Organization. *Birth*. 1997;24(2):121-123.

46. Committee on Obstetric Practice. Committee Opinion No. 697: planned home birth. *Obstet Gynecol*. 2017;129(4):e117-e122. doi:10.1097/aog .0000000000002024.

47. Phillippi JC. Community birth: the value of collaboration. *Obstet Gynecol.* 2021;138(5):691-692. doi:10.1097/aog.0000000000004583.

48. Julian Z, Robles D, Whetstone S, et al. Community-informed models of perinatal and reproductive health services provision: a justice-centered paradigm toward equity among Black birthing communities. *Semin Perinatol.* 2020;44(5):151267. doi:10.1016/j.semperi.2020.151267.

49. Bailes A. *The Home Birth Practice Manual.* 3rd ed. Silver Spring, MD: American College of Nurse Midwives; 2016.

50. Begley K, Daly D, Panda S, Begley C. Shared decision-making in maternity care: acknowledging and overcoming epistemic defeaters. *J Eval Clin Pract.* 2019;25(6):1113-1120. doi:10.1111/jep.13243.

51. Cheyney M, Bovbjerg M, Everson C, et al. Outcomes of care for 16,924 planned home births in the United States: the Midwives Alliance of North America Statistics Project, 2004 to 2009. *J Midwifery Womens Health.* 2014;59(1):17-27. doi:10.1111/jmwh.12172.

52. Hutton EK, Reitsma A, Simioni J, et al. Perinatal or neonatal mortality among women who intend at the onset of labour to give birth at home compared to women of low obstetrical risk who intend to give birth in hospital: a systematic review and meta-analyses. *E Clin Med.* 2019;14:59-70. doi:10.1016/j.eclinm.2019.07.005.

53. Thompson D. Midwives and pregnant women of color: why we need to understand intersectional changes in midwifery to reclaim home birth. *Columbia J Race Law.* 2016;6:27-36.

54. Murphy PA, Fullerton J. Outcomes of intended home births in nurse-midwifery practice: a prospective descriptive study. *Obstet Gynecol.* 1998;92(3):461-470. doi:10.1016/s0029-7844(98)00182-3.

55. American College of Nurse Midwives. Intermittent auscultation for intrapartum fetal heart rate surveillance. *J Midwifery Womens Health.* 2015; 60(5):626-632. doi:10.1111/jmwh.12372.

56. American College of Obstetrics and Gynecology. ACOG Committee Opinion No. 736: optimizing postpartum care. *Obstet Gynecol.* 2018;131(5):e140-e150. doi:10.1097/aog.0000000000002633.

57. Demirel G, Guler H. The effect of uterine and nipple stimulation on induction with oxytocin and the labor process. *Worldviews Evid Based Nurs.* 2015;12(5):273-280. doi:10.1111/wvn.12116.

58. Mousavi S, Rouhollahi B, Zakariya NA, et al. Evaluating the effect of nipple stimulation during labour on labour progression in term pregnant women. *J Obstet Gynaecol.* 2021:1-5. doi:10.1080/0144361 5.2021.1980515.

59. DeMaria AL, Sundstrom B, Moxley GE, et al. Castor oil as a natural alternative to labor induction: a retrospective descriptive study. *Women Birth.* 2018;31(2):e99-e104. doi:10.1016/j.wombi.2017 .08.001.

60. Gilad R, Hochner H, Savitsky B, et al. Castor oil for induction of labor in post-date pregnancies: a randomized controlled trial. *Women Birth.* 2018;31(1): e26-e31. doi:10.1016/j.wombi.2017.06.010.

61. Keedle H, Schmied V, Burns E, Dahlen HG. Women's reasons for, and experiences of, choosing a home-birth following a caesarean section. *BMC Pregnancy Childbirth.* 2015;15:206. doi:10.1186/s12884-015 -0639-4.

62. Macdorman MF, Declercq E, Mathews TJ, Stotland N. Trends and characteristics of home vaginal birth after cesarean delivery in the United States and selected states. *Obstet Gynecol.* 2012;119(4):737-744. doi:10.1097/AOG.0b013e31824bb050.

63. Cox KJ, Bovbjerg ML, Cheyney M, Leeman LM. Planned home VBAC in the United States, 2004–2009: outcomes, maternity care practices, and implications for shared decision making. *Birth.* 2015;42(4): 299-308. doi:10.1111/birt.12188.

64. Tilden EL, Cheyney M, Guise JM, et al. Vaginal birth after cesarean: neonatal outcomes and United States birth setting. *Am J Obstet Gynecol.* 2017;216(4):403. e1-403.e8. doi:10.1016/j.ajog.2016.12.001.

65. National Institutes of Health Consensus Development conference statement: vaginal birth after cesarean: new insights, March 8–10, 2010. *Obstet Gynecol.* 2010;115(6):1279-1295. doi:10.1097/AOG .0b013e3181e459e5.

66. Ryan GA, Nicholson SM, Morrison JJ. Vaginal birth after caesarean section: current status and where to from here? *Eur J Obstet Gynecol Reprod Biol.* 2018;224:52-57. doi:10.1016/j.ejogrb.2018.02.011.

67. American College of Nurse Midwives. Position statement: vaginal birth after cesarean. https://www.midwife .org/acnm/files/ACNMLibraryData/UPLOADFILE NAME/000000000090/VBAC-PS-FINAL-10-10-17. pdf. Accessed October 17, 2021.

68. American Association of Birth Centers. Clinical bulletin: VBAC-labor & birth after cesarean in the birth center setting. https://cdn.ymaws.com/www .birthcenters.org/resource/resmgr/about_aabc_-_documents/AABC_Clinical_Bulletin_-_VBA.pdf. Accessed October 17, 2021.

69. Home Birth Summit. Best practice guidelines: transfer from planned home birth to hospital. https://www. homebirthsummit.org/wp-content/uploads/2014/03/ HomeBirthSummit_BestPracticeTransferGuidelines. pdf. Accessed October 17, 2021.

APPENDIX

# 32A

---

# Supplies for Birth in the Home and Birth Center

---

ALEXIS DUNN AMORE AND NIKIA D. GRAYSON

*Special thanks to Marsha E. Jackson and Alice J. Bailes, who contributed to the previous version of this appendix.*

## Family Supplies for a Birth Center Birth

Nutritious, easy-to-prepare meals and snacks for the family, any support persons, and birth attendants

Juice, electrolyte drink, tea, and broths that the birthing person enjoys

Comfortable clothing to wear during labor and extra clothing to wear home

Extra pillows

Music

Aromatherapy

Camera and/or video camera

Swim trunks/suit and extra towels for partner when water immersion is anticipated

Entertainment for older children (e.g., books, games, videos)

Nutritious postpartum meal for the new parents and birth attendants

### For the Newborn

Clean thermometer

Receiving blankets

Petroleum jelly

At least five disposable newborn-size diapers and baby wipes

Baby clothing suitable for the weather

Car seat, in place, adjusted to fit the newborn

# Midwife Equipment for Birth at Home or in the Birth Center

## Essential Supplies

### Supplies for Labor and Birth

Current electronic or paper copy of chart
Paper or electronic forms for intrapartum, postpartum, and newborn charting
Birth certificate forms
Blood pressure cuff, stethoscope
Thermometer
Fetoscope/Doppler stethoscope
Gloves (sterile and nonsterile)
Lubricant (sterile and nonsterile)
Antiseptic wash
Urinary catheters
Suture with needles
Local anesthetic, syringes, and needles
Urine dipsticks
pH indicator paper
Intravenous fluids: Ringer's lactate and 5% dextrose in Ringer's lactate, normal saline
Intravenous catheters, long intravenous tubing, tape, antiseptic ointment, gauze pads
Blood collecting supplies: tourniquet, tubes, syringes, needles and Vacutainer
Sharps box and mechanism for hazardous waste disposal
Small oxygen tank, oxygen mask and tubing
Biohazard bags

### Sterile Instruments

Scissors (2 pairs)
Large clamps (Kelly or Rochester-Ochsner)
Needle holder/driver
Ring forceps
Amniohook
Sterile 4 × 4 gauze pads

### Newborn Supplies

Heating pad for baby blankets
Cord clamp or tape
Baby scale
Measuring tape
Vitamin K
Erythromycin ophthalmic ointment

### Neonatal Resuscitation Supplies

See the current edition of the American Academy of Pediatrics and American Heart Association's *Textbook of Neonatal Resuscitation* or other regional textbook for a comprehensive set of supplies.

### Postpartum Hemorrhage Control

Injectable oxytocin (Pitocin)
Injectable and oral methylergonovine maleate (Methergine)
Misoprostol tablets (Cytotec)
Tranexamic acid (TXA)

## Extra Supplies

Adult positive-pressure resuscitation bag and mask
Antibiotics and 150-mL normal saline bags for intravenous administration of antibiotics
Electrolyte replacement drink (e.g., Pedialyte, Gatorade)
Flexible straws
Hot-water bottle
Lidocaine jelly for topical use
Massage roller
Flashlight or other light source
Slow-cooker pot for warm perineal compresses

### Newborn Supplies

Baby footprint stamp
Blood glucose monitoring sticks and/or glucometer
Cotton baby hats
Otoscope/ophthalmoscope

### Personal Supplies

Apron or gown
Change of clothes
Protective eyewear
Toilet articles, personal medications
Mirror
Speculum

### Sterile Instruments

Allis clamps
Culturette
Hemostats
Tissue forceps
Scissors

Based on Bailes A. *The Home Birth Practice Manual*. 3rd ed. Washington, DC: American College of Nurse-Midwives; 2016.

# Postpartum

CHAPTER

# 33

# Anatomy and Physiology of Postpartum

TEKOA L. KING

## Introduction

Physiologically, the postpartum period begins with expulsion of the placenta and continues until the reproductive organs have returned to a nonpregnant state. Historically, the postpartum period was considered to last between 6 and 8 weeks. This time period was based on the average time it takes the uterus to return to a nonpregnant size. The physiologic progression during the postpartum period is not sharply delineated, however, and varies among individuals and with factors such as gestational age at the time of birth. Among breastfeeding/chestfeeding individuals, the anatomy and physiology of the mammary glands will continue to be different than in nonpregnant, nonlactating persons for the duration of lactation and beyond. In addition, pregnancy has some lasting effects on a person's body. Thus, there is no clear consensus on when the postpartum period ends. This chapter reviews the anatomic and physiologic changes that occur in the postpartum period.

## Physiologic Changes Immediately Following Placental Expulsion

A rapid cascade of physiologic changes is initiated immediately following placental expulsion. The mean weight loss from the newborn, amniotic fluid, and placenta at a term birth is approximately 13 pounds. Shivering occurs in as many as 23% to 50% of individuals in the first 30 to 60 minutes following birth.[1,2] Although the cause is unknown, this benign response is not associated with adverse effects.

The uterine muscles contract following birth and in the first postpartum hours. As a result, the uterus can be palpated abdominally as a hard mass in which the fundus is at approximately the level of the umbilicus.[3] First, oxytocin-induced contractions of the myometrial muscles result in a permanent and progressive shortening of the muscle fibers, which reduces the area of placental attachment and mechanically helps the placenta separate. In addition, this shortening and retraction of muscle fibers compresses the maternal arteries that served as the vascular supply to the placenta, which is the primary mechanism of hemostasis in the immediate postpartum period.[4] Uterine atony or inadequate uterine contractions during the first hour following delivery are the most common causes of postpartum hemorrhage.

In addition to uterine muscle contraction, remarkable shifts occur in the cardiovascular system once the placenta separates from the uterine wall. Immediately following placental expulsion, an autotransfusion of 300 to 500 mL of blood is shifted from the intervillous space in the uterus where it filled the maternal/placental unit into the maternal circulation. This dramatic fluid shift increases cardiac output in the birthing person by 60% to 80%.[5-7] Thus, the initial postpartum hours are a period of maternal cardiovascular instability and a time of increased risk for pulmonary edema, cardiac failure, and death, in persons who have preexisting cardiac disease, hypertension, or preeclampsia.[8,9]

Clotting is initiated at the time of placental expulsion and aided by the compression of vessels passing through the myometrium as well as the hypercoagulable state of the coagulation system. This hypercoagulable state, which persists for the first several postpartum weeks, increases the risk for thromboembolic events such as deep vein thrombosis or stroke.

The first hour following birth is also a time of rapid and remarkable neurobiologic changes in the birthing person. Although much of the research on the physiologic transition immediately following birth is based on animal studies, work in humans supports the concept of the first hour postpartum being a "Golden Hour"—that is, events that occur during this time have long-lasting effects. Plasma levels of beta-endorphins and corticosteroids increase significantly during labor and stay elevated for the first several hours postpartum. The progesterone production by the placenta ceases with placental expulsion, which in turn halts suppression of prolactin and oxytocin secretion. These hormones facilitate the initiation of lactation.

Maternal–newborn interactions during the first hours following birth have profound effects on both members of the dyad. Bonding with the infant is facilitated and multiple parameters of newborn function, such as thermoregulation and breastfeeding behaviors, are established following uninterrupted physical contact with the newborn during this period.

## Postpartum Changes in Reproductive Organs

Although the physiologic changes that occur immediately after birth are striking, a person's body continues to adapt to the nonpregnant status in multiple ways for several weeks and months postpartum. Some of these changes involve a simple reestablishment of nonpregnant homeostasis; others are permanent responses to the process of pregnancy, labor, and birth.

### Uterine Involution

Uterine involution is the process of uterine contraction, myometrial cell shrinkage, and reestablishment of the endometrium. Immediately following birth, the uterus at term is approximately 20 centimeters in length, weighs approximately 1 kg, and is in a retroverted position.[10] When well contracted, the uterus is easily identified as a firm, regular, round mass that is slightly mobile. The term uterus involutes by approximately 50% in the first 24 to 48 hours postpartum[10,11] (Figure 33-1). This process takes longer in multiparous individuals than in primiparous individuals, and may also be slower for persons with an intrauterine infection or other health conditions.[12] Abdominal palpation of the uterine fundus in the first 24 to 48 hours after birth

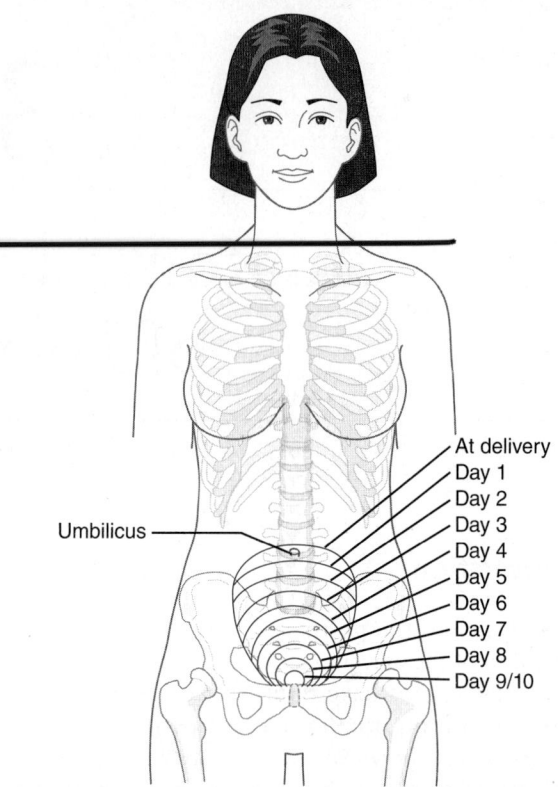

**Figure 33-1** Postpartum involution of the uterus. The fundal height descends toward the pelvis at a rate of approximately 1 centimeter per day.

is a common postpartum assessment used to assist the healthcare provider in detecting inadequate uterine contraction, uterine tenderness, or uterine displacement to the side of the abdomen, which can occur when the individual has a full bladder.

In the first 1 to 2 weeks after a birth, the uterus involutes more slowly than in the initial involution and undergoes a rotation of 100 to 180 degrees along the axis of the internal os, assuming an upright position by postpartum day 7.[3] By the end of the first week postpartum, the uterus weighs approximately 500 grams and may still be palpable above the symphysis pubis.[11] By 10 to 14 days postpartum, the uterus weighs approximately 300 grams; at this point, it has typically resumed its nonpregnant anatomic position in the pelvis, which in most individuals is in an anteverted inclination, and can no longer be palpated abdominally.

During involution, the uterus loses mass secondary to myometrial cell autolysis. The result is a marked decrease in the size—rather than the number—of myometrial cells. Approximately 90% of the excess cellular protein is broken down by proteolytic enzymes that are released by myometrial cells, endothelial cells of the uterine blood vessels, and macrophages.

The uterine decidua is divided into multiple layers (strata) during pregnancy. Postpartum, the placenta separates at the spongy portion of the layer known as the decidua basalis, most of which is detached with the placenta or sloughed off in the early postpartum period. In the second and third postpartum days, the remaining decidua becomes differentiated into two layers, identified as the superficial and basal layers. The basal layer remains intact and gives rise to the new endometrium through proliferation of the remaining glandular and stromal tissues. The superficial layer is formed through leukocyte invasion and protects the desquamated endometrium from infection. This layer becomes necrotic and is sloughed off.

### Lochia

The postpartum vaginal discharge that begins immediately at birth and continues for approximately 4 to 8 weeks is termed lochia. The mean total duration of lochia is 33 days, and the total amount is approximately 200 to 500 mL.[13–15] Lochia is further described as lochia rubra, lochia serosa, and lochia alba based on its changing color. This color results from the changing composition of the tissue that is sloughed and expelled in the postpartum endometrial restoration process. Initially, the lochia consists primarily of blood and decidual tissue; as a result, *lochia rubra* is red or brownish red in color. As the uterine bleeding decreases at approximately 3 to 5 days postpartum, leukocyte infiltration occurs and the placental implantation site undergoes exfoliation. At this point, the discharge contains some blood but primarily consists of wound exudate and leukocytes; therefore, *lochia serosa* is a pinkish brown color. The median duration of lochia serosa is 22 days.[13,14] Some individuals will experience a transient increase in bleeding 7 to 14 days postpartum secondary to sloughing of the placental *eschar* (scab) at the placental site. Toward the end of the uterine involution process, the endometrium has been primarily restored. *Lochia alba* is composed predominantly of leukocytes and some decidual cells and is white or yellowish white in color.

In contrast to the sloughing of the superficial layer of the decidua, the basal layer remains intact and gives rise to the new endometrium through proliferation of the remaining glandular and stromal

tissue. By 1 week postpartum, the endometrial surface has become epithelized; by 2 to 3 weeks postpartum, the endometrium has regenerated and resembles a nonpregnant endometrium, excluding the placental implantation site. The remaining thrombosed vessels at the placental implantation site take approximately 6 weeks to heal through an "exfoliation" process of sloughing infarcted and necrotic tissue, followed by a process of endometrial remodeling.

### Cervical and Vaginal Involution

During labor, the maternal cervix undergoes remodeling to become soft and dilated; it also shortens so that it is not palpable as distinct from the lower uterine segment. The first two stages of remodeling are described in more detail in the *Anatomy and Physiology of Labor and Birth* chapter. During vaginal birth, the cervix may sustain lacerations. Immediately after birth, the cervix may be edematous. However, the cervix begins to reconstitute within the first hours after birth, secondary to expression of several genes that promote reorganization of the cervical matrix and collagen synthesis.[16] Internally, the extracellular matrix is repaired and the epithelial barrier is restored.[17] By the end of the first week postpartum, the endocervical canal has reappeared and the os is only approximately 1 centimeter dilated. The external cervical os usually does not return to its previous nonpregnant form with the dimple shape characteristic of most cervices of nulliparous individuals, but rather takes the form of a slit (Figure 33-2). The cervical endothelium also undergoes remodeling during the postpartum period, which has been associated with a high incidence of spontaneous regression of high-grade cervical intraepithelial lesions.[18]

The vagina is initially edematous and bruised after a vaginal birth and has lost its prepregnant tone and rugae. The vaginal rugae return at approximately 3 to 4 weeks postpartum, but the prepregnant vaginal tone may never be completely restored to the nonpregnant tone present before pregnancy.

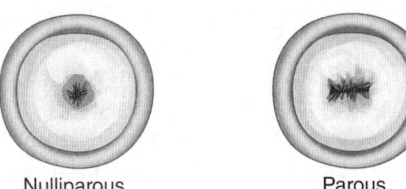

Nulliparous            Parous

**Figure 33-2** Postpartum anatomic changes in the cervix.

The vaginal epithelium is usually healed by 6 to 10 weeks postpartum. During a person's first vaginal birth, the tissue that makes up the hymeneal ring is split into discontinuous tags, also known as hymeneal tags or myrtiform caruncles. The vaginal opening becomes visible, rather than being closed by the labia minora.

### The Pelvic Floor and Urogenital System

The pelvic floor muscles undergo significant stretch during labor and birth.[19] Although many persons experience vaginal birth without complications or damage to the pelvic floor, these muscles can become damaged secondary to excessive stretch. Levator ani avulsion, pelvic organ prolapse, and urinary or anal incontinence can be the result.[20,21] Urogenital organs and structures can also sustain traumatic injury during labor and birth. The passage of the fetus through the pelvis places mechanical pressure on the surrounding organs, muscles, and nerves, but effects from the gravid uterus and hormonal changes of pregnancy cannot easily be disentangled from the effects of second-stage pushing efforts, a large fetal head, or birth-related trauma. That said, very prolonged obstructed labor can cause tissue damage that results in obstetric fistulas.

While some pelvic floor disorders, such as urinary incontinence, become apparent in the postpartum period, some are more likely to occur postmenopausally as estrogen levels decline and striated muscle loses volume and tone. Thus, the independent effects of pregnancy, mode of birth, and aging have made it difficult to determine the exact causality of pelvic floor disorders across the lifespan.[22] Nevertheless, urinary incontinence and dyspareunia are the most common symptoms of pelvic floor dysfunction in the first year postpartum.[23,24] Urinary incontinence, pelvic organ prolapse, and anal incontinence are strongly associated with vaginal birth.[23,25]

In the first 48 hours postpartum, voiding difficulties are common. Physiologic diuresis and urethral edema from second-stage pushing or vaginal birth increase the risk of urinary retention. This risk is increased in persons who have a lack of sensation of urinary fullness secondary to use of regional analgesia during labor. The immediate postpartum days are also associated with an increased risk for developing a urinary tract infection, which can be related to mechanical trauma to the urethra that occurs during vaginal birth, and potential ascending infection. Stress urinary incontinence is relatively common in the first postpartum days, but in most individuals this problem resolves within a few weeks.

Mobility of both the bladder neck and urethral mobility is increased postpartum, and these changes are presumed to be factors contributing to the increased incidence of stress urinary incontinence.[26]

The pelvic floor tissue and levator ani muscles are subject to pressure and mechanical stretching during the second stage of labor, which peaks during the final stages of vaginal birth. As a result, the levator ani muscle can be avulsed, be denervated, or sustain damage to its connective tissue support. It is estimated that approximately 10% to 30% of birthing persons will have levator ani muscle injury following childbirth that is detectable on magnetic resonance imaging (MRI), although the exact incidence of subsequent pelvic organ prolapse related to levator ani damage has not been determined.[27] Perineal tears disrupt the structures within the perineal body and are associated with anal incontinence if the anal sphincter is torn. Anal sphincter tears are associated with anal incontinence, even when repaired.

Sexual activity is resumed by approximately half of postpartum individuals by 5 to 6 weeks after birth, but dyspareunia is reported by 41% to 83% of individuals in the first 2 to 3 months postpartum and can be present in a minority of persons as long as a year after birth.[20,28] The physiologic etiology of dyspareunia can be directly related to muscle damage, scar tissue, and healing, as well as the effects of low levels of estrogen and high levels of prolactin on vaginal tone. Other factors such as breastfeeding, changing identity, loss of time for intimacy, decreased sexual desire, and sleep deprivation may also be contributing factors that have varying degrees of influence for different individuals.

## Wound Healing

Identification, categorization, and repair of perineal and vaginal lacerations are described in the appendices of the *Second Stage of Labor and Birth* chapter. The wound healing process is divided into three phases: hemostasis and inflammation, granulation and proliferation, and remodeling.[29]

### Hemostasis and Inflammation

The hemostatic process begins immediately at the time of injury and continues for a few days. First, platelets adhere to damaged tissue and combine to form a platelet plug. Fibrinogen is attracted to this platelet plug, where it is subsequently cleaved into fibrin via the action of thrombin. Fibrin is an elastic, insoluble protein that forms an interlacing fibrous network that stabilizes the area of blood vessel injury. Platelets also release growth factors that call fibroblasts to migrate to the damaged area, as well as cytokines that mediate the initial inflammatory response.

The inflammatory response begins within the first 6 to 8 hours following the perineal injury. Polymorphonuclear neutrophils (PMNs) from blood vessels in and surrounding the injured area migrate to the area of injury. These white blood cells work to rid the area of bacteria, damaged cells, and cell debris. The PMNs also assist in recruiting monocytes to the area, which then differentiate into macrophages and cleanse the area of foreign cells as well as damaged and dead cells via the process of phagocytosis. After approximately 3 or 4 days, in addition to their work in ridding the area of debris and foreign and dead cells, the macrophages begin to release key growth factors that trigger the growth of new tissue. During this phase, the affected person may experience swelling, burning, or pruritus in the area in which the laceration occurred.

### Granulation and Proliferation

Approximately 5 to 7 days after the original injury, the fibroblasts that were recruited in the initial inflammatory response migrate to the area of the wound and begin to lay down the extracellular matrix and collagenous tissue in the area that will serve as the "framework" or scaffold for the rebuilding of the new tissue. Revascularization (angiogenesis) is essential to feed the new (granulation) tissue with nutrients and oxygen. New vessels arise as branches from intact vessels in the area. Regrowth of the epithelial layer occurs as epithelial cells migrate to this layer from the edges of the injured area or from adjacent tissues. This process can take up to 4 to 5 weeks.

As the granulation tissue grows to fill the wound, the area will take on a red or pebbled pink appearance, particularly if the tissue is healing via secondary intention (not approximated by sutures). This new tissue is highly vascular and friable. As part of health education, the patient should be advised to keep the area clean and to blot the area dry after urinating/defecating or after washing. Blotting is preferred instead of wiping, to avoid damaging this new tissue. Individuals who have sutures in place should be made aware that, depending on the suturing material, it may take 6 weeks or longer for the sutures to be fully absorbed.

### Remodeling

During the last phase of wound healing, the collagen tissue undergoes remodeling to become similar to the prebirth tissue; this phase can last for years. Many of the new blood vessels created during the proliferative stage of wound healing begin to regress. Wound contracture occurs secondary to the action of specialized contractile fibroblasts known as myofibroblasts. The collagen scar tissue, and particularly the initial scar tissue that has not undergone remodeling, will feel thicker and less distensible—a change that may contribute to postpartum dyspareunia. As the healing process continues, some individuals describe the scar tissue as transitioning from feeling painful to feeling numb. With time, the tissue is likely to regain most of its elasticity and sensation. The scar tissue is not as strong or elastic as normal tissue, however, and there is an increased risk of lacerations along the scar tissue with subsequent births.

## Postpartum Physiology of Nonreproductive Organs

Pregnancy results in anatomic and/or physiologic changes in every organ system of the body, all of which are altered again during the puerperium (Table 33-1).[7,30–36] These physiologic changes may disappear over time, depending on the organ involved and the underlying health of the individual. Because of their importance and profound changes, the postpartum changes that affect the cardiovascular and endocrine systems are described in detail.

### Cardiovascular and Hematologic Changes

Following the dramatic changes in blood volume and cardiac output that occur immediately after placental expulsion, maternal blood volume slowly increases over the first few postpartum days secondary to mobilization of extracellular fluid back into the individual's circulation. The increased blood volume helps compensate for the normal blood loss of parturition. Subsequently, blood volume declines to prepregnant levels over a period of approximately 2 weeks. Normal return of cardiovascular function depends in part on the physiologic diuresis that occurs in the first week postpartum. Without normal excretion of the extracellular fluid into the intravascular system, there is an increased risk of pulmonary edema, particularly among individuals with cardiac disease or preeclampsia.

The increase in cardiac stroke volume that first occurs during pregnancy and then again in the initial postpartum period leads to a temporary increase in the size of the left atrium of the heart.[33] This physiologic ventricular hypertrophy resolves more slowly

| Table 33-1 | Postpartum Maternal Physiologic Adaptations | |
|---|---|---|
| **Postpartum Change** | **Timing of Return to Nonpregnant Status** | **Clinical Implications** |
| **Cardiovascular** | | |
| Auto-transfusion of 300–500 mL of blood volume secondary to removal of the placenta, shifting of extracellular fluid into the intravascular system, and release of the pregnancy-induced pressure on the inferior vena cava. | Immediate | Individuals with hypertension, preeclampsia, or cardiac disease have an increased risk for pulmonary edema or cardiac failure in the first 24–48 hours postpartum. |
| Cardiac volume and stroke volume increase. Pulse increases by 15%, blood pressure remains unchanged. | | |
| Cardiac output is increased by 80% secondary to the increased flow of blood back to the heart from the loss of the uteroplacental circulation, decreased pressure from the pregnant uterus, and mobilization of extracellular fluid. Stroke volume increases correspondingly. | Cardiac output increases during the first 48 hours after birth, then slowly returns to normal by 6–12 weeks postpartum. | Individuals with some types of structural cardiac disorders are at increased risk for cardiac failure, pulmonary edema, and other cardiac abnormalities such as cardiomyopathy during the first week postpartum.[31,33] |
| Plasma volume slowly returns to nonpregnant values. | Elevated 10% to 15% at 2 weeks postpartum; returns to prepregnant volume by 6 weeks. | Individuals have a natural diuresis and diaphoresis in the initial postpartum period. Physiologic anemia of pregnancy resolves by 6 weeks postpartum. |
| **Hematologic and Coagulation Indices** | | |
| WBC levels normalize. | 6 days | WBCs are significantly elevated in labor and gradually return to normal in the puerperium, which can make it difficult to use a WBC count as an accurate indication of infection. |
| Coagulation factors normalize. | 4–6 weeks | An increased risk for thromboembolic events is present for the first several weeks postpartum. |
| Platelet function normalizes. | 12 weeks | Platelet count remains in the normal range postpartum.[30] |
| **Respiratory** | | |
| Removal of the weight of the gravid uterus at birth relieves intra-abdominal pressure and allows for elevation of the diaphragm, so that normal excursion of the diaphragm is reestablished. Respiratory rate and oxygen saturation are normally consistent with nonpregnant reference ranges.[34] | Immediate | The dyspnea related to pregnancy usually resolves rapidly after birth. Therefore, complaints of shortness of breath or chest pain in the postpartum period should be evaluated immediately, especially because of the increased risk of thromboembolic events in the postpartum period. |
| Decrease in tidal volume back to normal. | Immediate | |
| Loss of placental progesterone production, a mediator of many respiratory changes of pregnancy, leads to a rapid return of normal nonpregnant respiratory parameters. | | |

| Postpartum Change | Timing of Return to Nonpregnant Status | Clinical Implications |
| --- | --- | --- |
| Residual volume and expiratory reserve volume that were decreased during pregnancy return to nonpregnant values. | Residual volume returns immediately; expiratory reserve volume takes several months to return to nonpregnant values. | |
| **Renal** | | |
| Gradual return to nonpregnant values of GFR, renal plasma flow, plasma creatinine, BUN, and creatinine clearance, all of which were altered during pregnancy. | 2–3 months postpartum | Alterations in measures of renal function may reflect normal pregnancy-related changes that have not returned to nonpregnant levels. |
| Mild proteinuria may develop in the first few postpartum days. | 3–5 days | New-onset proteinuria may be related to normal postpartum changes. However, evaluation for preeclampsia should occur if new-onset proteinuria is noted in the first 2–3 weeks postpartum. |
| Natriuresis (sodium excretion) and diuresis (increased urine production) lead to a decrease in blood volume, causing it to return to nonpregnant levels. | 3 weeks or less | Oxytocin promotes reabsorption of water. The decrease in oxytocin contributes to postpartum diuresis. Urine production on postpartum days 2–5 can reach 3000 mL. In addition to increased urine production, many individuals will experience episodes of diaphoresis in the first postpartum week. |
| Gradual return of bladder tone and normal size and function of the bladder, ureters, and renal pelvis, all of which were dilated during pregnancy. | 6–8 weeks, although it may take longer | Pregnancy-related changes in bladder and ureter morphology and birth-related trauma to the urethra can lead to an increased risk of urinary tract infections and urinary retention during the postpartum period. Urinary stress incontinence may persist postpartum.[32] |
| **Hepatic** | | |
| Liver function indices (AST, ALT, LDH) that increased during labor return to normal. | 3 weeks or less | Interpretation of liver function tests drawn in the postpartum period must reflect the knowledge that pregnancy-related changes and/or labor effects on hepatic indices may not have returned to nonpregnant levels. |
| Alkaline phosphate, which increased during pregnancy, returns to normal. | 6 weeks | |
| **Gastrointestinal** | | |
| Gastric tone and motility remain decreased for 2–3 days postpartum. | Bowel movements resume 2–3 days postpartum; normal GI function and bowel patterns return in 1–2 weeks postpartum. | Decreased GI motility in the postpartum period can lead to abdominal distension, constipation, and, in severe cases, ileus. |

*(continues)*

| Table 33-1 | Postpartum Maternal Physiologic Adaptations (*continued*) | |
|---|---|---|
| **Postpartum Change** | **Timing of Return to Nonpregnant Status** | **Clinical Implications** |
| **Musculoskeletal** | | |
| Ligaments and muscles are lax, so the abdominal wall remains soft and flaccid in the immediate postpartum. Separation of the rectus muscle (diastasis recti abdominis) may be present. | Variable | The recovery of abdominal muscular tone and resolution of diastasis recti abdominis are somewhat related to activity/exercise. |
| Muscles and associated tissues that were stretched during childbirth gradually regain tone. | Variable, but can take months to years | Stretching and injury of the pelvic and perineal musculature and associated structures increase the risk of urinary and anal incontinence as well as pelvic organ prolapse. Prevention of these complications includes avoidance of episiotomy and performance of postpartum pelvic exercises. |
| **Integument (Skin and Hair)** | | |
| Hyperpigmentation (including linea nigra and melasma), striae gravidarum (stretch marks), varicosities, and other skin changes of pregnancy fade or regress. | 6 months or less | Many skin changes do not disappear completely. Striae commonly progress from red to silvery white in color in approximately 3 months. |
| With the return of estrogen levels to nonpregnant levels, hair growth slows and follicles enter into a hair-shedding phase, which results in a period of alopecia or postpartum telogen effluvium. | Normal hair growth is reestablished by 4–6 months postpartum for most individuals. | Reports of hair loss in individuals in the postpartum period are common, and the provider can offer reassurance. Individuals with excessive hair loss leading to bald patches or with hair loss lasting longer than 6 months should be evaluated for thyroid dysfunction or nutritional deviations. |
| **Metabolism** | | |
| Demand for nutrients and hormone levels drop abruptly. Maternal metabolism of nutrients begins to return to normal. Maternal insulin resistance seen during pregnancy begins to resolve shortly after removal of the placenta. | Fasting glucose plasma levels and plasma free fatty acid levels return to prepregnant levels in the first 3–5 days for individuals with normal glucose metabolism in pregnancy; triglyceride levels normalize within 2–3 weeks. | Insulin resistance resolves nearly immediately following birth, which may require medication adjustment for individuals with Class A2, GDM. Maternal glucose values should be back to nonpregnant values by 6 weeks postpartum. |
| The increase in intestinal calcium absorption seen during pregnancy resolves to nonpregnant levels of calcium absorption. | 6 weeks in nonlactating individuals | In individuals who are lactating, increased calcium is needed for milk production, which occurs via increased reabsorption of calcium from the skeleton. This process is associated with a reversible decrease in maternal bone density. |

| Postpartum Change | Timing of Return to Nonpregnant Status | Clinical Implications |
|---|---|---|
| **Endocrine** | | |
| Thyroid hormones: The thyroid-binding globulin level decreases, which leads to a drop in $T_3$ and $T_4$. | First 3–4 days | After giving birth, individuals are at increased risk for Graves' disease, postpartum thyroiditis, and thyroid storm. |
| FSH and LH levels are low. | 2 weeks<br>Nonpregnant values return by 4–6 weeks in nonlactating individuals. | Ovulation is highly unlikely in the first 2 weeks postpartum. Return of FSH and LH levels to normal is related to lactation status; ovulation occurs earlier among non-breastfeeding/chestfeeding individuals than among those who lactate. |
| Prolactin and oxytocin | Fall to normal nonpregnant values in 7–14 days if not lactating | Pituitary disorders can cause an alteration in prolactin levels that interfere with lactogenesis. |

Abbreviations: ALT, alanine aminotransferase; AST, aspartate aminotransferase; BUN, blood urea nitrogen; FSH, follicle-stimulating hormone; GDM, gestational diabetes; GFR, glomerular filtration rate; GI, gastrointestinal; LDH, lactic dehydrogenase; LH, luteinizing hormone; RV, residual volume; WBC, white blood cell.

than the increase in stroke volume and cardiac output. Left ventricular size does not return to normal until approximately 6 months postpartum.[33]

The blood loss that occurs during birth causes a marked decrease in red blood cell (RBC) volume. In addition, a period of hemodilution arises in the first postpartum week as interstitial fluid is shifted into the individual's circulation. The loss of RBCs combined with this hemodilution results in a decrease in hemoglobin and hematocrit in the first postpartum week. These normal physiologic events can make it difficult to use a hemoglobin or hematocrit value to assess for anemia during this transition. Both hemoglobin and hematocrit values gradually return to their prepregnant values over a 4- to 6-week period as plasma volumes and RBC production return to normal.

### Coagulation and Hemostasis

During pregnancy, changes in the coagulation and fibrolytic systems promote coagulation via increased platelet activity, decreased fibrinolysis, and increased production of coagulation factors. This "hypercoagulable" state encourages and supports adequate coagulation at the placental attachment site and protects against hemorrhage following birth. In brief, during pregnancy (and particularly in the third trimester), production of a number of clotting factors (I, II, VII, VIII, IX, and XII) increases, whereas production of factors that prevent clotting, such as protein S and activated protein C, decreases.[37] Postpartum, the balance of clotting and anticlotting factors present promotes coagulation of the sheared maternal vessels at the placental attachment site. However, while the clotting factors are protective against hemorrhage, they also predispose postpartum individuals to thromboembolic events.[38] The relative proportions of coagulation factors appear to return to their nonpregnant levels by 3 weeks postpartum, but certain clotting cofactor, such as protein S, may not return to normal levels until 8 weeks postpartum or later.[39] Thus, the risk for thromboembolic events such as deep vein thrombosis and stroke remains elevated throughout the postpartum period.

An additional factor that contributes to the increased risk of thromboembolic events postpartum is the delay in return to nonpregnant vascular capacitance. Under the influence of progesterone during pregnancy, distensibility throughout the vascular system increases to accommodate the larger cardiovascular load. Venous capacitance resolves more slowly in the first several postpartum weeks when compared to the total blood volume, which places the individual at risk for venous stasis.[40] The higher blood volume normalizes before the vessel capacity decreases. Thus, the continuing hypercoagulable state increases the risk for deep vein thrombosis. Individuals with vascular damage, such as can result from hypertension or preeclampsia, are at higher risk of this complication.

## Neuroendocrine Changes

An abrupt drop in the blood levels of multiple hormones—including human placental lactogen (hPL), human chorionic gonadotropin (hCG), estrogen, and progesterone—occurs when the placenta is expelled. This event sets in motion a series of endocrine alterations, including changes in thyroid hormone levels, glucose and lipid metabolism, and the initiation of lactogenesis II. With the exception of postpartum thyroiditis, most of the hormone levels that change postpartum gradually return to nonpregnant levels and are not associated with alterations in physiologic function. However, it has been theorized that some of these dramatic hormonal fluctuations may be associated with the development of postpartum mood disorders secondary to the temporal relationship between hormonal changes and the emergence of mood disorders postpartum.[41] More recent research has also looked at the role of postpartum hormones in the development of maternal caregiving behaviors.

Thyroid dysfunction is more common in the postpartum period than in other times during an individual's life.[42] As circulating levels of estrogen decrease in the initial postpartum period, the thyroid-binding globulin level (which was elevated in pregnancy) also drops. This change, in turn, leads to less production of triiodothyronine ($T_3$) and thyroxine ($T_4$) and a gradual return to nonpregnant thyroid function. Postpartum thyroiditis—a thyroid disorder that manifests during the first postpartum year—is thought to be an autoimmune disorder that is unmasked in the postpartum period due to the rebound in immunologic function following pregnancy.[43] In approximately 23% of individuals, thyroid dysfunction that develops postpartum will become permanent.[43]

Several of the normal postpartum hormonal changes may contribute to the development of postpartum mood and psychotic disorders. Studies that have evaluated the link between postpartum changes in thyroid hormone levels and postpartum depression have yielded contradictory results and, in general, have not identified a consistent link.[44] Estrogen receptors, however, are ubiquitous throughout the brain. The sudden drop in estrogen levels following birth could contribute to dysregulation of the dopamine pathways—a dysregulation that is associated with postpartum depression. Although estrogen withdrawal and estrogen instability are associated with an increased incidence of mood disorders at several different phases across the lifespan,[45] absolute estrogen levels are not reliably related to the onset of postpartum depression and estrogen replacement is not well researched as a treatment for this mental health condition. In short, postpartum mood and psychotic disorders are multifactorial. For example, postpartum is a time of sleep disruption, which has also been associated with changes in brain function. Although a robust body of research has assessed the factors that contribute to perinatal mood disorders, the findings in this area are considered preliminary. In general, though, it appears that integrated models that include biologic, psychosocial, and cultural factors have the most promise in capturing the complexity of these conditions.

The neuroendocrine changes that facilitate maternal–newborn bonding and caregiving behaviors are also likely related to the sudden shift in hormonal homeostasis, and particularly with regard to the effects of oxytocin, a hormone that reaches high levels during labor and the initial stage of lactation.[46,48] Oxytocin is well known as the hormone that causes uterine contractions during labor and milk secretion during lactation, but it also plays many other complex roles in the body. Notably, it has been called the "tend and befriend" hormone, reflecting its association with a calming effect on the lactating person, stabilization of maternal blood pressure, lower cortisol levels, increase in trust and facial recognition, and decrease in anxiety and aggressive behaviors.[47,48] Oxytocin activates parts of the brain related to bonding and empathy, which are often referred to as prosocial and maternal bonding behaviors.

Although most of the research on postpartum neural plasticity and caregiving behavior is based on animal studies, human studies have documented anatomic changes in the maternal brain that support the concept of postpartum neural plasticity.[49] For example, oxytocin receptors are abundant in the amygdala, which is larger in size postpartum. The amygdala is active in the motivation–reward circuit and facilitates feelings of pleasure that occur in response to infant stimuli. These responses become stronger caregiving behaviors as they are integrated into the natural stimuli–reward circuit. Similarly, postpartum neural plasticity occurs in the circuits that cause anxiety, so that a parent learns to respond to infant distress with caregiving rather than avoiding behavior. This effect of oxytocin is referred to as buffering stress reactivity.[46]

## Resumption of Pituitary Function and of Menstruation and Ovulation

Throughout pregnancy, the hypothalamic–pituitary–ovarian (HPO) axis is suppressed and, as a result, production of follicle-stimulating hormone (FSH) and luteinizing hormone (LH) is diminished. Following birth, FSH and LH levels remain low for the first 2 weeks postpartum, but then rise gradually. Ovarian production of estrogen and progesterone, therefore, also remains low during the first few postpartum weeks.

Pituitary function returns to nonpregnant levels by 4 to 6 weeks postpartum. However, return of nonpregnant levels and release patterns of gonadotropin-releasing hormone (GnRH), FSH, and LH secretion are related directly to lactation status. In breastfeeding/chestfeeding individuals, the return of ovulation and menstruation varies and reflects both the duration and the frequency of breastfeeding/chestfeeding. Elevated levels of prolactin, along with other endocrine alterations related to frequent and regular infant suckling, disrupt the pulsatile release of GnRH, which in turn suppresses the LH surge. This cascade of events culminates in the suppression of ovulation. This breastfeeding-related suppression of ovulation and menstruation is referred to as *lactational amenorrhea*.

In nonlactating individuals, the return of ovulation occurs sometime between postpartum days 45 and 94.[36] As many as 70% of these ovulations may be fertile, and in 20% to 70% of individuals, ovulation precedes the first menses.[36] Therefore, appropriate contraceptive counseling and provision of appropriate contraceptives is essential for postpartum individuals since many—particularly those who are not breastfeeding—may ovulate and be fertile prior to their first postpartum visit. For individuals who desire to defer another pregnancy for a period of time, timely initiation of their chosen method of contraception is an important management intervention.

## Weight Loss in the Postpartum Period

Weight loss following pregnancy is a common concern for birthing persons. Aside from the immediate weight loss that occurs directly related to the birth of the newborn, expulsion of the placenta, and loss of fluid in the first postpartum week, the physiology of weight loss does not appear to differ in the postpartum period from the physiology of weight loss at other times in a person's life.[50] Furthermore, studies indicate that pregnancy weight retention is not a significant determinant of excessive weight. A study of 7000 individuals who were followed from the beginning of one pregnancy to the beginning of the next pregnancy found that the average increase in weight between the first pregnancy and the next was 3.4 kg.[51] In recognition that humans tend to gain weight as they get older, additional studies that controlled for age found an increase of only 0.3 to 0.5 kg between pregnancies.[51] These findings suggest that interventions to reduce rates of maternal obesity should focus not only on the loss of weight gained in pregnancy, but also on primary prevention of obesity and weight management at a preconceptional visit.

## Anatomy and Physiology of Lactation

Ramsay's ultrasound studies of lactating breasts "in action" profoundly changed our knowledge of the process of milk production and release.[52,53] The parenchyma includes the milk ducts—structures that have been described as "tangled tree roots." Random and intertwined, the milk ducts often intersect as they reach the nipple–areolar complex. The 9 to 10 ducts open onto the surface of the nipple and the lobular alveolar structure. The "lactiferous sinuses," found where the ducts terminate under the nipple, are no longer considered to be distinct anatomic structures. The stroma includes the connective tissue, fat (adipose) tissue, blood vessels, lymphatics, and suspensory ligaments of the breasts (Cooper's ligaments). The glandular tissues (lactocytes, alveoli, and supporting structures) where milk is formed are interspersed throughout the breast, with more than 65% of the glandular tissues being located in a 30-mm radius from the base of the nipple.[52] During lactation, the breast weighs, on average, 600 to 800 grams.

The functional milk-making unit is the alveolus. The lactocytes—that is, the alveolar epithelial cells—convert nutrients from the maternal circulation into various milk components and secrete milk into the lumen of the alveolar sac (Figure 33-3). The alveoli are surrounded by myoepithelial cells that contract under the influence of oxytocin, causing milk to be released into the ductules and ducts and to move toward the nipple. The sebaceous glands (Montgomery glands) just under the areola secrete volatile compounds that elicit specific infant behaviors, including increased sleepiness, head turning, and appetite response; the secretion of these compounds has been proposed as one of the stimuli that promote the so-called breast crawl, which refers to the observation that the newborn may spontaneously crawl toward the breast after birth if placed in skin-to-skin contact on the birthing person's abdomen and chest.[54]

## Lactogenesis

Lactogenesis—that is, the ability to secrete milk—occurs in four stages (Table 33-2). *Lactogenesis I* (secretory initiation) starts during the second half of pregnancy, whereas *lactogenesis II* (secretory activation) occurs in the first postpartum days. *Lactogenesis III* refers to the time when lactation is fully established. *Lactogenesis IV* refers to the mammary gland involution that occurs when breastfeeding ceases.

### *Lactogenesis I: Development During Pregnancy*

By the end of the first trimester, the alveoli epithelial cells (lactocytes) begin secreting proteins and

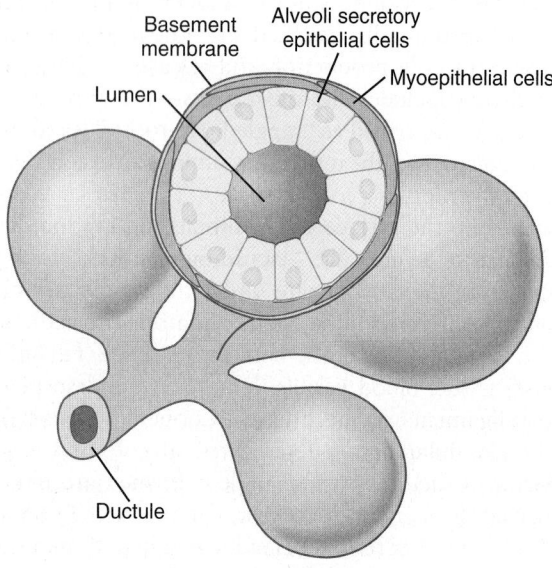

**Figure 33-3** Anatomy of the alveoli of the breast.

fat (colostrum), placental lactogen, progesterone, estrogen, and prolactin. In the second and third trimesters, the duct system expands, and the number and activity of the lobules increase. Veins become increasingly visible on the skin surface of the breast, and individuals may observe some colostrum leaking from their nipples. By 16 to 18 weeks' gestation, colostrum secretion has begun in preparation for the subsequent onset of copious secretion of milk. Patterns of breast growth during pregnancy vary and are unrelated to the pregnant person's nutritional status.

### *Lactogenesis II: Onset of Copious Milk Production*

The sudden drop in the plasma progesterone level that occurs once the placenta is expelled triggers the second stage of lactogenesis, which features the onset of copious milk secretion ("milk coming in") and the subsequent delivery of milk to the newborn. Specifically, the rapid fall in the progesterone level triggers mammary epithelial cells in the alveoli to become lactocytes.[55] The lactose secretion in the lactocytes, in combination with osmosis of fluid from the interstitial spaces, causes milk volume to rapidly increase, beginning approximately 30 to 40 hours after birth.

Lactogenesis II involves both milk synthesis and milk ejection/release (or milk production), with at least two different hormones working in tandem to coordinate these functions. Suckling stimulates the secretion of prolactin by the anterior pituitary. Plasma concentrations of prolactin increase rapidly once suckling starts. The increased prolactin level,

| Table 33-2 | Stages of Lactogenesis | |
|---|---|---|
| **Stage** | **Description** | **When This Stage Occurs** |
| Lactogenesis I | Cytologic and enzymatic differentiation of alveolar cells; uptake of the substrates for milk begins; colostrum production begins with small fat droplets and proteins. | Begins at approximately 16 weeks' gestation and continues through a few days or even weeks after birth. |
| Lactogenesis II | Lactose secretion begins and fluid volume increases. Colostrum is essentially diluted by lactose and fluids, becoming "mature" milk. | Occurs approximately 30–72 hours postpartum; may be delayed as long as 96 hours after cesarean birth. |
| Lactogenesis III | Ongoing copious secretion of milk in response to milk removal from the breast by the infant or other means. | Ongoing until weaning and involution. |
| Lactogenesis IV | Involution of mammary gland and apoptosis of alveolar cells. | Begins when milk removal from the breast diminishes or ends. Some milk may be produced for many weeks or longer after overt production ends. |

in turn, initiates milk secretion by the lactocyte cells. Suckling stimulates a neural feedback response that causes the posterior pituitary to release oxytocin, which causes the myoepithelial cells to contract, ejecting the milk from the alveoli and lobules into the ducts. Removal of milk from the alveoli then allows for further milk production. The alveoli stop producing milk when the alveoli are engorged and the lactocytes are flattened.[56]

The composition of human milk is one of the more fascinating aspects of this biology, as it varies according to the individual infant's needs. Human milk is a highly bioactive fluid and considered the ideal food for newborns and infants up to 6 months of age. It contains a complex array of molecules that have multiple functions, including, but not limited to, immune factors that provide passive immunization for the infant, calories, and nutrients. But human milk also contains factors that inhibit inflammation and stimulate the development of the infant microbiome.[57] The primary components of human milk are lactose, oligosaccharides, fats, proteins, minerals, and other bioactive agents such as immune globulins that provide passive immunization. Other components include neutrophils, lymphocytes, epithelial cells, and macrophages. The macrophages are capable of pinocytosis and chemotaxis, while the lymphocytes direct some immune reactions and development of cell-mediated immunity in the infant.

The initial milk produced in the first 48 to 72 hours following birth is called colostrum. Compared to mature milk, colostrum has higher levels of protein, immune factors, growth factors, lactoferrin, and leucocytes, but lower levels of lactose.[58] It is followed by the appearance of transitional milk when production becomes more copious. During this period, the lactating person may report "engorgement" and the breasts will be firm and warm to the touch. Engorgement is a combination of the alveoli filling with milk, interstitial tissue edema, and increased blood flow that occurs as lactogenesis II is occurring. This physiologic engorgement typically resolves spontaneously in 24 to 48 hours, leaving the breasts larger and lactating but no longer edematous or warm. By 5 to 6 days postpartum, mature milk is produced.

Several risk factors may lead to failed lactogenesis, insufficient milk production, and delayed onset of lactogenesis II beyond 72 hours postpartum. As a whole, these disorders can be categorized as preglandular, glandular, and postglandular causes. Obesity, diabetes, polycystic ovary syndrome, and other biologic conditions that are associated with increased androgen levels are preglandular causes of delayed lactogensis.[59-62] These conditions are associated with increased levels of hormones that result in an impaired response to prolactin, although the exact mechanisms are not fully understood. Delayed onset of lactogenesis II is also associated with cesarean birth, retained placental fragments, ovarian theca lutein cysts, hypothyroidism, certain types of breast surgery, and severe maternal anemia.[62] The actual etiology of delayed lactogenesis II may also be multifactorial. For example, individuals with obesity are at higher risk for receiving interventions that delay lactogenesis, such as cesarean birth.[60]

Although infant or postglandular factors such as prematurity or newborn illness that disallows early suckling can negatively affect the normal onset of lactogenesis II, early milk expression (within 1 to 2 hours after birth) can ameliorate this situation and provide nutrition for the infant. Newborns with an ineffective or weak suck, palate abnormalities, tongue-tie, and congenital heart defects may not be able to effectively remove colostrum. When the infant has any of these conditions, it is recommended that expression of milk begin within the first 1 to 2 hours postpartum to support the onset of lactogenesis II.

### Lactogenesis III: Ongoing Milk Synthesis

Lactogenesis III, also known as galactopoiesis, comprises the ongoing maintenance of milk production, which includes a switch to autocrine or local control of lactation once lactation is fully established. The mechanism is as follows: Nipple stimulation via infant suckling triggers prolactin release from the anterior pituitary and stimulates the hypothalamus to produce oxytocin, which is released from the posterior pituitary.[63] Prolactin stimulates the lactocytes to produce milk, and oxytocin stimulates contraction of the myoepithelial cells surrounding the alveoli, which causes milk ejection into the lactiferous ducts (Figure 33-4). Oxytocin is also released through sensory pathways when the lactating parent sees, feels, touches, smells, or hears stimuli that remind them of the infant and breastfeeding.[64]

In addition, milk removal stimulates milk synthesis. If milk is not removed from the breast, secretion first slows and then ceases over a period of days.[63,65] When the milk is not removed, inflammatory pressure causes synthesis and release of a milk protein known as the feedback inhibitor of lactation. This protein downregulates the cell surface prolactin receptors on the lactocytes.[66] In this way, the rate of milk synthesis and the total daily amount of milk produced are closely related to the degree of

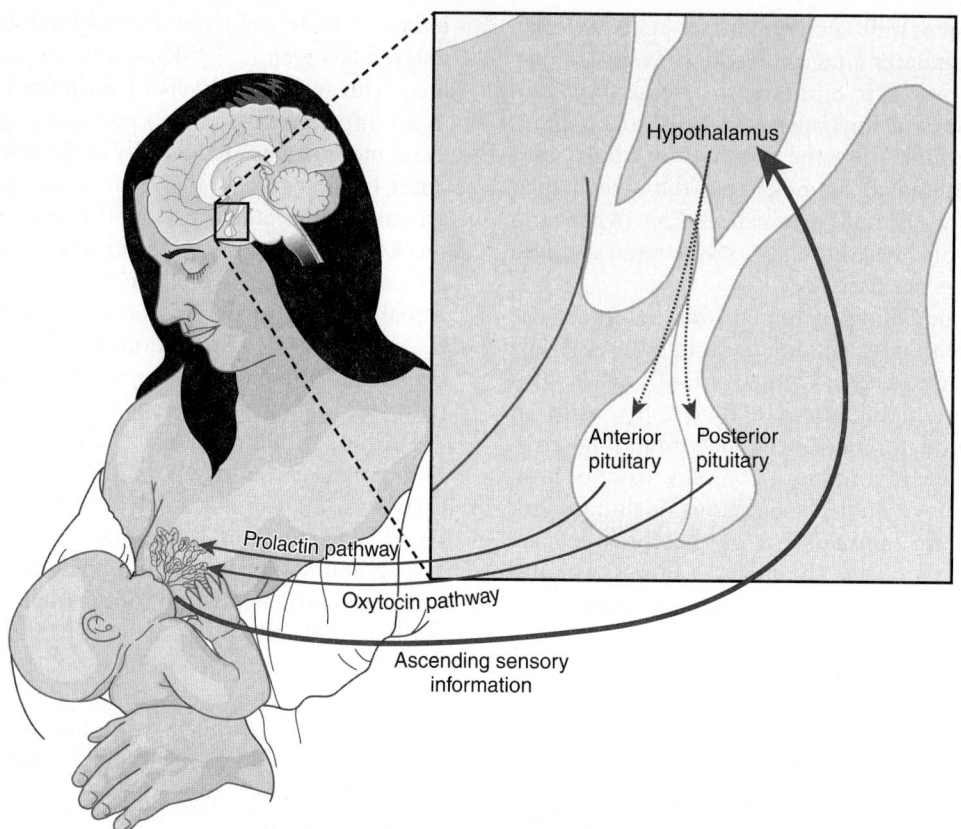

**Figure 33-4** Autocrine control of lactation: Infant suckling triggers a nerve impulse that terminates in the hypothalamus. The hypothalamus then (1) manufactures oxytocin and signals the anterior pituitary to release oxytocin and (2) signals the anterior pituitary to release prolactin. Oxytocin is released first, so the myometrial cells around the alveoli contract and eject premade milk. Prolactin initiates formation of milk.

"emptiness" of the breast, such that milk production varies during the day and night, and from one breast to the other.[67]

In brief, breastfeeding/chestfeeding has important short-term and substantial long-term benefits for the health of the newborn and infant. Some of these benefits reflect physiologic actions of human milk, whereas others are more likely to be indirect effects of the maternal–infant interactions. The interested reader is referred to the *Infant Feeding and Lactation* chapter for more in-depth reviews of the benefits of breastfeeding/chestfeeding.

### Lactogenesis IV: Involution

The process of mammary involution occurs after lactation ceases. Most of the anatomic studies of mammary involution have been performed on mice, so the exact chain of physiologic events that occur in humans is not definitively known.[68] When the infant no longer suckles at the breast, prolactin levels fall in the lactating individual and the effects of prolactin

on breast milk production end. The early stages of involution appear to be reversible if suckling resumes. Otherwise, the mammary gland involutes, or regresses through the process of mammary epithelial cell apoptosis (cell self-destruction). Any remaining secretion is absorbed, and adipose tissue from the lactocytes is redeposited within the breast. In most cases, involution takes approximately 6 weeks after milk removal ceases, although the human breast never fully returns to its prepregnant condition.[68] Gradual weaning invokes a different process of inhibition of lactation and mammary involution that does not involve acute milk stasis, wherein a progressive autocrine inhibition of milk production occurs in response to gradually decreased intake by the infant.[68]

Regardless of whether a person breastfeeds their child, some of the mammary epithelium that was produced during pregnancy is retained. The breasts, therefore, never return to their prepregnant state.

Some persons may choose to reestablish lactation. Relactation and induced breastfeeding may be desirable for an ill child or an adopted infant, for example. This process involves stimulating the breasts via infant suckling or pumping frequently. Relactation has been achieved with varying degrees of success, but can be an important method of supporting infants at risk of illness or malnutrition. Relactation is supported by the World Health Organization.[69]

## Conclusion

The postpartum period is a time of remarkable and rapid physiologic adjustments. Knowledge of postpartum physiology is necessary to determine the difference between normal and abnormal progression during this period. The postpartum period is also associated with significant risks for maternal morbidity and mortality, most of which can be prevented via close observation, identification of warning signs, and clinical care when needed. Moreover, although the vast majority of individuals have a normal course of recovery following childbirth, these physiologic changes can be uncomfortable or even distressing to persons who are not prepared for them. A person's ability to complete the important tasks of bonding and caring for a newborn—or, in the case of a stillbirth or other loss, the tasks of grieving and healing—is affected to a significant degree by their physical well-being. In turn, the individual's physical well-being can influence their risk for developing postpartum depression, post-traumatic stress disorder, or another perinatal mood disorder. The postpartum period is a profound role transition and life-changing event that cannot be fully described via a review of anatomic and physiologic changes.

## References

1. Benson MD, Haney E, Dinsmoor M, Beaumont JL. Shaking rigors in parturients. *J Reprod Med.* 2008; 53(9):685-690.

2. Ravid D, Gidoni Y, Bruchim I, et al. Postpartum chills phenomenon: is it a feto-maternal transfusion reaction? *Acta Obstet Gynecol Scand.* 2001;80(2): 149-151.

3. Diniz CP, Araujo Júnior E, Lima MM, et al. Ultrasound and Doppler assessment of uterus during puerperium after normal delivery. *J Matern Fetal Neonatal Med.* 2014;27(18):1905-1911.

4. Weydert JA, Benda JA. Subinvolution of the placental site as an anatomic cause of postpartum uterine bleeding: a review. *Arch Pathol Lab Med.* 2006;130: 1538-1542.

5. Ouzounian JG, Elkayam U. Physiologic changes during normal pregnancy and delivery. *Cardiol Clin.* 2012;30(3):317-329.

6. Wang N, Shen X, Zhang G, et al. Cerebrovascular disease in pregnancy and puerperium: perspectives from neuroradiologists. *Quant Imaging Med Surg.* 2021;11(2):838-851.

7. Tan EK, Tan EL. Alterations in physiology and anatomy during pregnancy. *Best Pract Res Clin Obstet Gynaecol.* 2013;27(6):791-802.

8. Sanghavi M, Rutherford JD. Cardiovascular physiology of pregnancy. *Circulation.* 2014;130(12):1003-1008.

9. Ambrožič J, Lučovnik M, Prokšelj K, et al. Dynamic changes in cardiac function before and early postdelivery in women with severe preeclampsia. *J Hypertens.* 2020;38(7):1367-1374.

10. Langer JE, Oliver ER, Lev-Toaff AS, Coleman BG. Imaging of the female pelvis through the life cycle. *Radiographics.* 2012;32(6):1575-1597.

11. Gonzalo-Carballes M, Ríos-Vives MÁ, Fierro EC, et al. A pictorial review of postpartum complications. *Radiographics.* 2020;40(7):2117-2141.

12. Paliulyte V, Drasutiene GS, Ramasauskaite D, et al. Physiological uterine involution in primiparous and multiparous women: ultrasound study. *Obstet Gynecol Int.* 2017;2017:6739345.

13. Chi C, Bapir M, Lee CA, Kadir RA. Puerperal loss (lochia) in women with or without inherited bleeding disorders. *Am J Obstet Gynecol.* 2010;203(1):56. e1-56.e5.

14. Fletcher S, Grotegut CA, James AH. Lochia patterns among normal women: a systematic review. *J Womens Health (Larchmt).* 2012;21(12):1290-1294.

15. Sherman D, Lurie S, Frenkel E, et al. Characteristics of normal lochia. *Am J Perinatol.* 1999;16(8):399-402.

16. Mahendroo M. Cervical remodeling in term and preterm birth: insights from an animal model. *Reproduction.* 2012;143(4):429-438.

17. Timmons BC, Mahendroo M. Processes regulating cervical ripening differ from cervical dilation and postpartum repair: insights from gene expression studies. *Reprod Sci.* 2007;14(8 suppl):53-62.

18. Ueda Y, Enomoto T, Miyatake T, et al. Postpartum outcome of cervical intraepithelial neoplasia in pregnant women determined by route of delivery. *Reprod Sci.* 2009;16(11):1034-1039.

19. Lien KC, Mooney B, DeLancey JO, Ashton-Miller JA. Levator ani muscle stretch induced by simulated vaginal birth. *Obstet Gynecol.* 2004;103(1):31-40.

20. Rogers RG, Leeman LL. Postpartum genitourinary changes. *Urol Clin North Am.* 2007;34(1):13-21.

21. Urbankova I, Grohregin K, Hanacek J, et al. The effect of the first vaginal birth on pelvic floor anatomy and dysfunction. *Int Urogynecol J.* 2019;30(10):1689-1696.

22. Hallock JL, Handa VL. The epidemiology of pelvic floor disorders and childbirth: an update. *Obstet Gynecol Clin North Am.* 2016;43(1):1-13.

23. Barca JA, Bravo C, Pintado-Recarte MP, et al. Pelvic floor morbidity following vaginal delivery versus cesarean delivery: systematic review and meta-analysis. *J Clin Med*. 2021;10(8):1652.

24. Huber M, Malers E, Tunón K. Pelvic floor dysfunction one year after first childbirth in relation to perineal tear severity. *Sci Rep*. 2021;11(1):12560.

25. Memon H, Handa VL. Pelvic floor disorders following vaginal or cesarean delivery. *Curr Opin Obstet Gynecol*. 2012;24(5):349-354.

26. Panayi D, Khullar V. Urogynaecological problems in pregnancy and postpartum sequelae. *Curr Opin Obstet Gynecol*. 2009;21(1):97-100.

27. Caudwell-Hall J, Kamisan Atan I, Guzman Rojas R, et al. Atraumatic normal vaginal delivery: how many women get what they want? *Am J Obstet Gynecol*. 2018;219(4):379.e1-379.e8.

28. Leeman LM, Rogers RG. Sex after childbirth: postpartum sexual function. *Obstet Gynecol*. 2012;119(3): 647-655.

29. Almadani YH, Vorstenbosch J, Davison PG, Murphy AM. Wound healing: a comprehensive review. *Semin Plast Surg*. 2021;35(3):141-144.

30. Hellgren M. Hemostasis during normal pregnancy and puerperium. *Semin Thromb Hemost*. 2003;29(2): 125-130.

31. Umazume T, Yamada T, Yamada S, et al. Morphofunctional cardiac changes in pregnant women: associations with biomarkers. *Open Heart*. 2018;5(2): e000850.

32. Wang K, Xu X, Jia G, Jiang H. Risk factors for postpartum stress urinary incontinence: a systematic review and meta-analysis. *Reprod Sci*. 2020;27(12):2129-2145.

33. Ramlakhan KP, Johnson MR, Roos-Hesselink JW. Pregnancy and cardiovascular disease. *Nat Rev Cardiol*. 2020;17(11):718-731.

34. Green LJ, Pullon R, Mackillop LH, et al. Postpartum-specific vital sign reference ranges. *Obstet Gynecol*. 2021;137(2):295-304.

35. Gaberšček S, Zaletel K. Thyroid physiology and autoimmunity in pregnancy and after delivery. *Expert Rev Clin Immunol*. 2011;7(5):697-706.

36. Glasier JE. A return of ovulation and menses in postpartum nonlactating women: a systematic review. *Obstet Gynecol*. 2011;117:657-662.

37. O'Riordan MN, Higgins JR. Haemostasis in normal and abnormal pregnancy. *Best Pract Res Clin Obstet Gynaecol*. 2003;17(3):385-396.

38. Marik PE, Plante LA. Venous thromboembolic disease and pregnancy. *N Engl J Med*. 2008;359:2025-2033.

39. Saha P, Stott D, Atalla R. Haemostatic changes in the puerperium 6 weeks postpartum (HIP study): implication for maternal thromboembolism. *BJOG*. 2009;116(12):1602-1612.

40. Skudder PA Jr, Farrington DT, Weld E, Putman C. Venous dysfunction of late pregnancy persists after delivery. *J Cardiovasc Surg*. 1990;31(6):748-752.

41. Yu Y, Liang HF, Chen J, et al. Postpartum depression: current status and possible identification using biomarkers. *Front Psychiatry*. 2021;12:620371.

42. Amino N, Arata N. Thyroid dysfunction following pregnancy and implications for breastfeeding. *Best Pract Res Clin Endocrinol Metab*. 2020;34(4): 101438.

43. Alexander EK, Pearce EN, Brent GA, et al. 2017 guidelines of the American Thyroid Association for the diagnosis and management of thyroid disease during pregnancy and the postpartum. *Thyroid*. 2017; 27(3):315-389.

44. Le Donne M, Mento C, Settineri S, et al. Postpartum mood disorders and thyroid autoimmunity. *Front Endocr*. 2017;8:9.

45. Douma SL, Husband C, O'Donnell ME, et al. Estrogen-related mood disorders: reproductive life cycle factors. *ANS Adv Nurs Sci*. 2005;28(4):364-375.

46. Bell AF, Erickson EN, Carter CS. Beyond labor: the role of natural and synthetic oxytocin in the transition to motherhood. *J Midwifery Womens Health*. 2014;59(1):35-42.

47. Olza I, Uvnas-Moberg K, Ekström-Bergström A, et al. Birth as a neuro-psycho-social event: an integrative model of maternal experiences and their relation to neurohormonal events during childbirth. *PLoS One*. 2020;15(7):e0230992.

48. Galbally M, Lewis AJ, Ijzendoorn M, Permezel M. The role of oxytocin in mother–infant relations: a systematic review of human studies. *Harv Rev Psychiatry*. 2011;19(1):1-14.

49. Kim P, Strathearn L, Swain JE. The maternal brain and its plasticity in humans. *Horm Behav*. 2016;77: 113-123.

50. Schauberger CW, Rooney BL, Brimer LM. Factors that influence weight loss in the puerperium. *Obstet Gynecol*. 1992;79(3):424-429.

51. Gore SA, Brown DM, Smith West D. The role of postpartum weight retention in obesity among women: a review of the evidence. *Ann Behav Med*. 2003; 26(2):149-159.

52. Ramsay DT, Kent JC, Hartmann RA, Hartmann PE. Anatomy of the lactating human breast redefined with ultrasound imaging. *J Anat*. 2005;206(6):525-534.

53. Geddes DT. Inside the lactating breast: the latest anatomy research. *J Midwifery Womens Health*. 2007;52(6):556-563.

54. Doucet S, Soussignan R, Sagot P, et al. The secretion of areolar (Montgomerys') glands from lactating women elicits selective, unconditional responses in neonates. *PLoS One*. 2009;4(10):e7579.doi: 10 .1371/journal.pone.0007579.

55. Truchet S, Honvo-Houéto E. Physiology of milk secretion. *Best Pract Res Clin Endocrinol Metab*. 2017; 31(4):367-384.

56. Buhimschi CS. Endocrinology of lactation. *Obstet Gynecol Clin North Am*. 2004;31(4):963-979.

57. Andreas NJ, Kampmann B, Mehring Le-Doare K. Human breast milk: a review on its composition and bioactivity. *Early Hum Dev*. 2015;91(11):629-635.

58. Ballard O, Morrow AL. Human milk composition: nutrients and bioactive factors. *Pediatr Clin North Am*. 2013;60(1):49-74.

59. Lind JN, Perrine CG, Li R. Relationship between use of labor pain medications and delayed onset of lactation. *J Hum Lactat*. 2014;30(2):167-173.

60. Jevitt C, Hernandez L, Goer M. Lactation complicated by obesity. *J Midwifery Womens Health* 2007; 52(6):606-613.

61. Hurst NM. Recognizing and treating delayed or failed lactogenesis II. *J Midwifery Womens Health*. 2007;52(6):588-594.

62. Farah E, Barger MK, Klima C, et al. Impaired lactation: review of delayed lactogenesis and insufficient lactation. *J Midwifery Womens Health*. 2021; 66(5):631-640.

63. Kent JC. How breastfeeding works. *J Midwifery Womens Health*. 2007;52(6):564-570.

64. Stuebe AM, Grewen K, Meltzer-Brody S. Association between maternal mood and oxytocin response to breastfeeding. *J Womens Health (Larchmt)*. 2013; 22(4):352-61. doi:10.1089/jwh.2012.3768.

65. Kent JC, Mitoulas LR, Cregan MD, et al. Volume and frequency of breastfeedings and fat content of breast milk throughout the day. *Pediatrics*. 2006; 117(3):e387-e395.

66. Wilde CJ, Addey CV, Bryson JM, et al. Autocrine regulation of milk secretion. *Biochem Soc Symp*. 1998; 63:81-90.

67. Neville MC, Allen JC, Archer PC, et al. Studies in human lactation: milk volume and nutrient composition during weaning and lactogenesis. *Am J Clin Nutr*. 1991;54(1):81-92.

68. McNally S, Stein T. Overview of mammary gland development: a comparison of mouse and human. *Methods Molec Biol*. 2017;1501:1-17.

69. Hormann E, Savage F. *Relactation: A Review of Experience and Recommendations for Practice*. World Health Organization; 1998. https://apps.who.int/iris/handle/10665/65020. Accessed May 10, 2023.

CHAPTER

# 34

# Postpartum Care

ABIGAIL HOWE-HEYMAN

*The editors acknowledge Ira Kantrowitz-Gordon, who was the author of this chapter in the previous edition.*

## Introduction

The end of pregnancy initiates physiologic changes, as many organ systems return to their nonpregnant states. The uterus involutes, cardiac output and blood volume decrease, and estrogen and progesterone levels fall. Lactogenesis II begins and may continue for years in patients who choose to breastfeed/chestfeed. Yet the postpartum period is so much more than just these physical changes—birth transforms the social and emotional context for the postpartum patient and family.

### Definition of the Postpartum Period

Pregnancy ends with the birth of the placenta and membranes; the postpartum period then begins. Traditionally the postpartum period, or puerperium, has been defined as lasting 6 weeks. This is a somewhat arbitrary—and an arguably short—time frame for the transition to parenting. The American College of Obstetricians and Gynecologists (ACOG) has made the case that the postpartum period should be redefined as lasting 12 weeks, considering the time a "fourth trimester"—a label that acknowledges the important physical, emotional, and social changes experienced by the postpartum patient.[1]

With the arrival of the newborn, parents assume new roles both within the family and in the community. For many families, employment status may change for one or both parents. As legal and social definitions of family have expanded in recent decades, recognition that there are considerable variations in a family's adjustment after childbirth has become more widespread. Despite the significance of these changes, patients and families often receive less attention and support during the postpartum period than they did during pregnancy and the intrapartum period. Consequently, the postpartum period is a time of both opportunity and challenges to health.

### Postpartum Care in the United States

Traditionally, postpartum care in the United States has consisted of an office visit with the prenatal care provider at 4 to 6 weeks postpartum. A notable exception has been the group care model, such as the CenteringPregnancy, in which families have a group reunion at 1 to 2 months postpartum. In the traditional model, after hospital discharge, many patients do not have contact with their healthcare provider until the 6-week postpartum office visit, and as many as 40% of patients do not attend this visit.[1] There has been a recent move to shift the approach to postpartum care to an ongoing process, rather than a single encounter, in which patients' individual needs are addressed by a well-defined provider. ACOG recommends that an initial assessment be conducted by phone or in person within the first 3 weeks postpartum.[1] This initial assessment will then dictate the subsequent care and visits, concluding with a wellness visit no later than 12 weeks after birth.[1] However, this proposed approach to care is not supported by the current reimbursement policies of most insurance providers, which generally reimburse providers for one postpartum visit, or may include payment as part of the global fee for antepartum, intrapartum, and postpartum care.

In developed countries, there is a wide variation in the amount of financial support provided to individuals after childbirth. In the United States, unpaid parental leave is guaranteed for 12 weeks under the Family and Medical Leave Act (FMLA), but only approximately 56% of U.S. employees are eligible for this job protection.[2] The conditions for employment that make an employee eligible for FMLA protections frequently exclude non-native English speakers, individuals of color, low-income workers, and those who are not college-educated.[3] For many families, taking time off in the postpartum period places the family at significant financial risk. Few states and jurisdictions provide paid family leave, and among those, most pay only a fraction of the employee's usual pay.[4] The economic challenges faced by the majority of postpartum families in the United States stand in contrast to the situation in most other developed countries, where paid leave extends from 6 weeks (e.g., Portugal) to longer than 2 years (e.g., Estonia and Finland).[5] In many countries, there is also a similar range of paid leave for the birthing person's partner.[5]

A growing body of literature has correlated the availability of paid family leave with improved outcomes for the postpartum patient and the infant. Paid family leave has been associated with improved parental mental health, improved parenting skills, improved mental health for children, and decreased neonatal mortality.[6–8] Midwives can use these scientific data to assist in their communication with lawmakers as they serve as advocates for postpartum families in the public policy arena.

### Racial Bias and Health Disparities in Postpartum Care

Significant differences in postpartum health outcomes exist between racial and ethnic groups in the United States. Non-Latinx Black patients have a three to four times greater risk of death in the perinatal period as compared to white postpartum patients.[9] Beyond mortality, Black and Native American patients are also more likely to experience complications from pregnancy compared with white patients, regardless of their socioeconomic status and comorbidities.[9] Structural racism that has led to inequity in health care, social conditions, and access to resources is the root cause of these disparities.[10] Additionally, inequities in the quality of care provided in hospitals that serve mainly Black and Latinx patients is another driver of poor postpartum outcomes.[11,12] This difficult history of racial bias has led to mistrust of the healthcare system among many families of color, which can result in delays in seeking care and ambivalence toward treatment plans.[9] Interventions to mitigate the impact of racial bias on postpartum outcomes range from policy changes that focus on the underlying problems of racial inequity to grassroots programs that provide culturally sensitive care to patients of color.[13,14]

## Cultural Perspectives of the Postpartum Period

The first essential perspective for provision of effective postpartum care is understanding the patient in their social and cultural context so that the care provided is culturally sensitive. Throughout history, in all parts of the world, and across cultures, the postpartum period has been acknowledged as a special or vulnerable time during which women follow distinct rituals. Many of these rituals and traditions are gender-based and may not apply to nonbinary individuals or those who do not parent after giving birth, but for individuals with strong cultural ties, these practices may be foundational to how they perceive their needs in the postpartum period.

Mexican American immigrant families may practice the *cuarentena*, or 40 days of postpartum recovery.[15] During this time, the woman's body is considered open and vulnerable to illness. Practices to protect the woman include sexual abstinence, wrapping the abdomen in tight garments (*fajas*), avoiding strong foods and cold substances, staying warm, and remaining at home as much as possible.[15]

In many parts of Asia, the new mother remains at home and rests for 30 to 40 days after giving birth—a period of confinement often referred to as "doing the month." In most Asian cultures, this period of prolonged rest is intended to protect the woman from exposure to illness, build back strength, and prevent infection. In some countries, such as Nepal, Bangladesh, Papua New Guinea, and Pakistan, the main purpose of isolation is to protect others from the woman's "polluted" state.[16] Women are considered vulnerable to infection due to a loss of heat during the birth, leading to an imbalance between hot and cold forces in their bodies. The primary treatment for this heat loss is heat therapy. In countries such as Cambodia, Laos, Vietnam, China, and Malaysia, women stay wrapped in blankets for several days or weeks and may also use heat lamps, hot compresses, or steam to further restore heat. Additionally, in many cultures, women may eat special foods, avoid showering, and stay in bed. Sexual abstinence is practiced for 30 to 40 days. In some Asian cultures, there is a restriction on household chores, reading, eating or drinking while standing, or experiencing strong emotions.[16]

The postpartum cultural practices in Turkey share some similarities with those of Asian and Latin cultures, such as wrapping the woman's abdomen and providing support for 40 days. Additionally, practices to ward off an evil fairy who may cause harm to the woman and infant are common and include the exchange of sewing needles between postpartum women, the placement of needles under the pillow of the woman and infant, and the wearing of red ribbons.[17]

Some Jewish patients may adhere to religious laws regarding postpartum practices, though these will vary considerably by the patient's level of observance. Religiously observant Jews adhere to practices that pertain to intimacy, diet, and observation of the Sabbath, as well as laws that are specific to the postpartum period. In religious practice, men and women are not allowed to touch until 7 days after the cessation of vaginal bleeding. Given the wide variety of religious observance in the Jewish community, it is important that the midwife communicate openly with the family about their practices.[18]

When a patient is geographically distant from their extended family, it may be difficult to maintain cultural practices.[9] Knowledge about other cultures and practices is a necessary beginning for midwives, but it is also important to incorporate this knowledge into clinical practice with curiosity and humility, so that patients and families are treated as *they* wish to be treated. To accomplish this balancing act requires an ongoing process of clinical inquiry and communication with patients to provide care that is culturally congruent—that is, care that fits with the family's values and meanings.[19,20] Questions that can help the midwife conduct a cultural assessment are listed in Table 34-1. Resources for providing culturally congruent midwifery care can be found at the end of this chapter.

### Beyond Sexuality and Gender

Parenting has traditionally been a gendered, socially constructed experience. Lesbian, gay, bisexual, queer (LGBQ), and transgender and gender-nonconforming (TGNC) parents may have different psychosocial experiences of childbirth, and recent research has found that the transition can be especially challenging for trans families.[21] These families may experience difficulty interacting with the healthcare system due to gendered and heterocentric practices in language use and history forms, discriminatory practices, and lack of support from the extended family.[22] Transgender men may experience the physical aspects of childbirth differently than do other parents.[23] The highly gendered environment of a postpartum hospital unit can be uncomfortable for trans men as well.[24] The midwife should use an approach of cultural humility and inquiry in caring for trans parents and use language that supports their preferred pronouns and gender identity.[25] Additionally, assumptions about

| Table 34-1 | Postpartum Cultural Assessment |
|---|---|

Consider the following questions when caring for patients and families postpartum:

- Is the postpartum period viewed as a normal physiologic process, a wellness experience, a time of vulnerability and risk, or a state of illness? What does the postpartum experience mean to the patient?
- Is the postpartum period a time for privacy or socialization?
- What kinds of support are the new family given during the postpartum period, and who gives that support?
- Are there culturally expected practices during the postpartum period regarding diet, nutrition, treatments (including pharmacologic therapies), and activity?
- What precautions or restrictions are necessary during the postpartum period?
- How is postpartum pain managed?
- What are the patterns regarding care of the infant and relationships within the nuclear and extended families? Are there expected patterns for feeding and caring for the infant?

gender-based parenting roles may not be valid. Lesbian couples may not identify with the cultural expectations that are traditionally placed on mothers and in some couples, both parents may choose to breastfeed.[26] Due to the additional stresses facing these families, a supportive environment, healthcare team, and social network are important for birth and postpartum care. General healthcare issues germane for LGBT and TGNC individuals are briefly reviewed in the *Context of Individuals Seeking Midwifery Care* and *Gender-Affirming Care* chapters.

## The First Hour Postpartum: The Fourth Stage of Labor

The term *fourth stage of labor* refers to the first postpartum hour following placental expulsion. Immediately following the expulsion of the placenta, a number of changes occur in the postpartum patient as the physical and emotional stresses of labor and birth resolve and postpartum recovery and bonding begin. Close observation and frequent assessment as described in the *Management of the Fourth Stage of Labor Following Vaginal Birth* appendix are needed during the fourth stage of labor, as this is a time of both physical vulnerability to emergent complications and heightened sensitivity as the patient and family are introduced to the newborn. This section presents a brief overview of parental–infant behaviors during the initial postpartum hours and evidence-based practices that support attachment and the formation of the family.

### Parental–Infant Bonding and Attachment

The theory that there is a biologically determined critical period immediately after birth during which parent–infant bonding takes place was first proposed by Klaus and Kennell in the 1970s.[27] Their work was completed within the context of the time and focused on gendered parenting and mothering, specifically. These researchers found that skin-to-skin contact between the woman and her newborn in the first hour after birth resulted in more attachment behavior by a woman toward her infant up to a month after birth. This seminal work by Klaus and Kennell set the stage for the plethora of subsequent research that has profoundly influenced the care of newborns and families in the postpartum period. Emotional attachment between parents and their newborn has lifelong implications.

During the fourth stage of labor, postpartum patients experience profound physical and psychological changes as they recover from the act of giving birth in the setting of an intense hormonal milieu and first meet the newborn. Partners, grandparents, siblings, and other family members or support persons present at a birth also experience heightened awareness and possible psychological vulnerability. Factors such as a traumatic birth, previous life traumas, or newborn illness can all influence an individual's response to childbirth, attachment to the newborn, and development of identity and role as a parent or primary caretaker. It is important to remember that the midwife's perception of a traumatic birth and the patient's perception of a traumatic birth may differ and may not be tied to the health of the patient or infant. Addressing the patient's perceptions and feelings during this time can help facilitate the bonding process.

Definitions of parent–infant attachment and bonding (or more often referred to in the literature as the gendered term *mother–infant attachment*) have historically included concepts such as bonding, love, attachment, or an instinctual connection. Although the terms are frequently used interchangeably, the most widely accepted definition of attachment is the connection of the newborn to the parent, while bonding is considered the connection of the parent to the infant.[28] The initial development of a

relationship between parents and a newborn takes many forms; the response of one parent may differ from the other. More importantly, the process is bidirectional and includes a great deal of interactive and reciprocal behaviors. The newborn's primary behavior is seeking physical proximity, using all their senses to connect with the birthing parent.[29,30] The parent's (or other primary caregiver's) behavior demonstrates responsiveness to the newborn's cues. For example, animal and human studies of attachment in the first postpartum hour have found that healthy newborn infants undergo a predictable series of behaviors immediately after birth, including crawling toward the breast, rooting and suckling, and looking at the parent's face. It is theorized that this behavior is stimulated by parental odor, taste, and voice recognition.[30]

Goulet et al. used concept analysis methodology to examine the vast literature on attachment to develop a clearer understanding and definition of this process.[18] In their analysis, these authors identified three key attributes in the mutual relationship between mothers and newborns:

- *Proximity.* Physical closeness allows interaction with multiple senses (e.g., hearing, touch, sight, and smell), facilitates a strong emotional connection, and creates an awareness of the infant's individuality and needs that are different from the parent's needs.

- *Reciprocity.* Parents and newborns interact in a responsive and adaptive manner. Parents become sensitive to the infant's cues and body language in their caregiving. The infant contributes to the interaction by reinforcing the parents' behaviors.

- *Commitment.* Feeling and acting responsibly to ensure the safety, growth, and development of the infant place the infant in a central position in the family and identify the parenting role as an important part of the adult's identity.[18]

Somewhat more recently, Kinsey and Hupcey conducted a concept analysis to review the literature regarding maternal–infant bonding, specifically considering maternal behaviors and actions.[28] The authors identified three key concepts in the research on bonding:

- *Promotion of maternal–infant bonding.* The most commonly identified factors that promote bonding in the postpartum period are pre-pregnancy bonding; support in labor;

physical proximity between the mother and infant after birth; breastfeeding; rooming-in; infant crying, visual tracking, and smiling; and the mother's attitude and level of expectations about parenting.

- *Hindrance of maternal–infant bonding.* The most frequently cited reason for poor bonding was physical or emotional separation of the mother and infant around the time of birth. Causes of physical separation include preterm birth, maternal incarceration, non-vaginal birth, traumatic birth, or physical complications experienced by the mother. Emotional separation can occur in the case of a traumatic event around the time of the birth; unwanted pregnancies; or disappointments and frustrations around infant gender, appearance, or behaviors, such as fussiness or sleep problems.

- *Outcomes of maternal–infant bonding.* The main outcomes of maternal–infant bonding noted in the review were improved parenting skills, improved survival and development of the infant, and improved later attachments for the child. One author found that strong maternal–infant bonding may prolong breastfeeding duration. The outcomes of poor bonding have been suggested to be an increased risk of child abuse and neglect and behavioral problems in the child.

A recent review of the literature explored the relationship between oxytocin levels and bonding.[31] Most of the studies found a positive correlation between parent–infant contact and oxytocin levels in the mother and in the father. Increased maternal oxytocin levels were significantly related to bonding behaviors in the mother such as eye contact, engagement, and synchrony, and paternal oxytocin levels increased following father–infant contact. Additionally, infant oxytocin levels were found to be correlated with maternal oxytocin level.[31] Although this review still relied on gendered research, the inclusion of mothers and fathers may indicate that the findings could be applicable to parent–infant bonding relationships regardless of gender.

Most of the research on bonding and attachment has been conducted exclusively on women, with little research conducted on LGBQ or TGNC families, so the findings may not be generalizable to all individuals. Additionally, the underlying premise that this sensitive period is necessary for the maternal–newborn relationship has been criticized. Attachment bonds form over time and involve a complex interplay of neural circuitry, hormones such as oxytocin, and interactive behavior.[32] Overemphasis on the first hour may be harmful in situations where it is missed, such as when the medical condition of the patient or the newborn requires physical separation of this dyad. Fortunately, there are countless opportunities to develop attachment, as demonstrated by parents who adopt children at a variety of ages. Ongoing reciprocal responses, strengthening of the relationship, and changing roles are processes that occur throughout life, including during the postpartum period.

Caregiver interventions during the fourth stage of labor, including those related to medical, psychosocial, and environmental conditions, can either facilitate or interfere with these important processes. Despite incomplete knowledge about the exact neurobiology involved in parental adaptation, a great deal of research has been conducted that has identified short-term and long-term effects of specific care practices such as skin-to-skin contact and early breastfeeding/chestfeeding with newborn self-latching.

### Early Continuous Skin-to-Skin Contact

Early skin-to-skin contact involves placing a naked newborn prone on the patient's abdomen or chest immediately or soon after birth. The infant is dried and the area of the infant's body that is not touching the patient's skin is covered with a blanket to assist in maintaining warmth. A cap may be applied to the dried head of the newborn to assist with temperature maintenance. The vital signs of the newborn and postpartum patient are monitored with the infant on the patient's chest. Other procedures are delayed for at least 1 hour or until after the first successful breastfeeding/chestfeeding.

Continuous parental–newborn contact and skin-to-skin touching have been found to improve bonding, support newborn thermoregulation, reduce stress in the parent and newborn, reduce the newborn's pain response, and increase the initiation, duration, and exclusivity of breastfeeding/chestfeeding.[33] Moore et al. conducted a meta-analysis of 46 randomized controlled trials (RCTs) of early skin-to-skin contact ($n = 3850$ mother–infant dyads) and found that skin-to-skin contact improved breastfeeding/chestfeeding duration at 1 to 4 months (relative risk [RR], 1.24; 95% confidence interval [CI], 1.07–1.43), although differences in study methodology and risks of bias cast some doubt on the strength of these findings.[34] Positive trends in improved summary scores for maternal affectionate love/touch, maternal attachment behavior, and shorter duration of infant crying were also noted in the group that experienced early skin-to-skin contact.[21]

For patients who have cesarean births, skin-to-skin contact should be supported in the operating room as soon as possible. Improved breastfeeding/chestfeeding exclusivity and duration have been associated with skin-to-skin contact after cesarean birth.[35] In the first 2 hours after cesarean birth (Figure 34-1), neonates who were held in skin-to-skin contact with the father demonstrated less crying, became calmer, and were more drowsy than newborns left in a crib.[36]

As noted earlier, oxytocin appears to play an important role in bonding and attachment, and skin-to-skin contact is one mediator of oxytocin release. Increased oxytocin levels in infants have been demonstrated after skin-to-skin care following preterm birth[37] and cesarean birth,[38] which suggests a physiologic mechanism for increased attachment and breastfeeding success in these contexts.

Oxytocin levels in parents have been shown to correlate with affectionate behaviors and touch at 6 months postpartum.[34]

Skin-to-skin contact after birth has also been associated with other health benefits. Newborns who experience skin-to-skin care may have lower salivary cortisol levels when compared to infants who do not share skin-to-skin contact immediately after birth.[39] Decreased parental anxiety levels and improved parent–infant interaction have also been noted. Given the strength of these findings, hospitals in the United States are increasingly instituting skin-to-skin contact immediately after birth for all patients, including in the operating room and recovery room following a cesarean birth.[40]

When healthy term infants are placed in skin-to-skin contact during the first hours following birth, they frequently crawl and find the areola by themselves, and most will initiate suckling spontaneously.[29] Supporting newborn interaction with the parents may enhance newborns' ability to self-regulate their behavior over the long term (i.e., improved sleep, social-interactive behavior, and language development).[29] The wide-ranging positive effects of unrestricted parental–newborn contact reinforce the importance of protecting the family in the first hours after birth from unnecessary intervention.

### Inclusion of Significant Others

Involvement of the patient's partner, newborn's parent, or other support persons during the fourth stage of labor has been found to help the patient during the postpartum period, increase the partner's emotional involvement with the neonate,[41] and increase the sense of security experienced by the partner.[42] Men and lesbian partners have expressed feeling helpless, useless, anxious, out of place, and vulnerable during birth; including family members in the experience is an important component of family-centered midwifery care.[43–45]

For all these reasons, it is important to assess and address the partner's needs during the fourth stage of labor to facilitate the transition to parenthood. Strategies include anticipatory guidance and explanations to the patient and family. Support via midwifery presence and information has been found to enhance the birth experience of the partner.[46] Engaging partners in activities such as cutting the cord and skin-to-skin contact has been found to enhance their emotional involvement with the neonate.[41] Additional activities may include encouraging continued support for the patient during required genital tract repair, engaging in observation of the neonatal transition, and assisting with initial breastfeeding/chestfeeding.

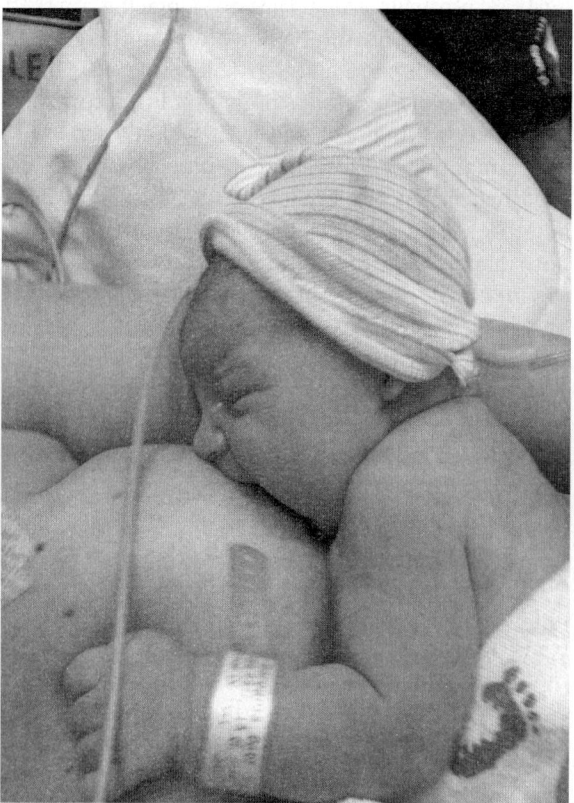

**Figure 34-1** Skin-to-skin contact and breastfeeding immediately after cesarean birth.
Courtesy of Tekoa L. King, CNM, MPH.

### Early Breastfeeding/Chestfeeding

Evidence that breastfeeding improves health outcomes for breastfeeding patients and their infants is overwhelming; this evidence is reviewed in detail in the *Infant Feeding and Lactation* chapter. Initiation of breastfeeding/chestfeeding in the first few hours after birth is recommended, as the infant is alert and awake during this time. Skin-to-skin contact promotes early lactation success.[34] If the patient and neonate must be separated for medical reasons, skin-to-skin contact in the intensive care nursery, early effective breast milk expression, and support from peers and staff can be implemented and are very important to the promotion of breastfeeding/chestfeeding in neonatal units.[47]

## Initial Postpartum Period

The first 72 hours after birth is labeled as the early puerperium period. The frequency with which the midwife evaluates the patient and newborn during this period will vary depending on the birth setting and individual circumstances. In most settings, the midwife assesses the postpartum patient at least once daily. Each visit includes a chart review; interval history, including physical, psychological, and emotional changes since the birth; physical examination; and observation of family interactions. Care of postpartum patients during this period includes treatment of pain and common discomforts, immunizations as needed, and health education.

### Health Record Review

The patient's prenatal record and record of labor and birth are reviewed prior to all postpartum examinations. A review of the infant's status is part of this pre-assessment because the newborn's health status may directly influence the management plan for the postpartum patient. A review of the health record includes assessment of the patient's vital signs, laboratory results, medication use, and comments from other caregivers. Previous orders and progress notes are reviewed as well. Medications that were temporarily stopped during the pregnancy or labor should be evaluated and a decision made about restarting them.

Time elapsed since birth, in hours or days, is ascertained to identify expected physical findings. When entering notes in the health record, it is important to indicate precise time information. For example, postpartum day 1 may denote that the patient is within 24 hours postpartum or between 24 to 48 hours postpartum. Since indicating postpartum days may generate confusion based on the time of birth and calendar days, specifying how many *hours* have elapsed since the birth is preferred.

### Interval History

The initial assessment of the patient's physical well-being starts with eliciting information about bleeding, nutrition, bladder and bowel function, activity level, mood, and a description of pain or discomfort if present. Information about the infant feeding method, infant behavior, and sleep–wake cycles should be collected even if the midwife is not the primary provider for the newborn. Assessment of parent–newborn interactions and the parents' skill and comfort in handling the newborn can also be done at this time. Examples of criteria for assessment of parent–newborn interactions are listed in Table 34-2.[36] Cultural factors need to be considered when evaluating these interactions.[37]

### Physical Examination

The physical examination focuses on the physiologic changes that occur after birth, and includes assessment of the heart, lungs, breasts, uterine fundus, abdomen, perineum and anus, and lower extremities. The postpartum examination procedure with expected findings is detailed in the *History and Physical Examination During the Early Postpartum Period* appendix.

| Table 34-2 | Clinical Assessment of Parent's Interaction with Newborn |
|---|---|

**Gaze:** Looks at newborn's face during interactions and uses a range of facial expressions.

**Touch:** Demonstrates gentle touch to care for newborn or to express affection (e.g., hug, cradle).

**Talk:** Positive and loving communication with newborn through speech, song, or high-pitched voice.

**Affect:** Expresses positive emotions regarding newborn.

**Responsiveness:** Responds to newborn's cues and behavior.

Based on Feldman R, Eidelman AI. Direct and indirect effects of breast milk on the neurobehavioral and cognitive development of premature infants. *Dev Psychobiol.* 2003;43(2):109-19. doi: 10.1002/dev.10126; Fowles ER, Horowitz JA. Clinical assessment of mothering during infancy. *J Obstet Gynecol Neonatal Nurs.* 2006;35(5):662-670.

## Care of the Patient in the Early Postpartum Period

Midwifery interventions will stem from the subjective and objective assessment findings in the health history and physical examination. Specific components of care for patients during the early puerperium will vary based on the patient's needs and location of birth.

For midwives practicing in hospital settings, routine or standing orders for the first postpartum days are used as a standard template for all patients, but it is imperative that clinicians tailor their orders to the specific needs of each patient. Orders may be individualized—for example, by modifying pain management routines, discontinuing intravenous fluids, or requesting a referral to a lactation consultation. The midwife should ensure that the topics outlined in Table 34-3 are addressed in written orders, or that they are considered in the care of patients delivering in community birth settings.[48,49] In community birth settings, many of the same plans of care will be in place, but there may be more flexibility around routines. Care plans should be tailored to the needs of the patient and family, the proximity of the midwife to the patient, the availability of support persons, and the accessibility of emergency care should it be needed.

### Rhesus Alloimmunization

Most patients experience a small transfer of fetal blood into their circulation (fetal–maternal or fetal–parental hemorrhage) during childbirth, primarily at the time of placental separation. If the fetal blood type is Rh D positive and the postpartum patient's blood type is Rh D negative, the fetal red blood cells that enter the patient's circulation are identified as a foreign antigen. The fetal cells stimulate an immune response (alloimmunization) that produces immunoglobulin M (IgM) and immunoglobulin G (IgG) antibodies, which are directed against Rh D–positive red blood cells. In a subsequent pregnancy with a Rh D–positive fetus, these antibodies can cross the placenta and bind to fetal red blood cells, causing hemolytic disease of the fetus and newborn.

Anti-D immune globulin (RhoGAM) is a hyperimmune plasma derivative that binds fetal Rh D–positive cells and prevents the patient's production of anti-D antibodies.[50] Administration of anti-D immune globulin within 72 hours following birth reduces the risk of alloimmunization from 13% to 16% to approximately 0.5% to 1.8% and is therefore recommended for all Rh D–negative patients who have a newborn with Rh D–positive blood who are not already sensitized.[50]

The newborn's blood type usually is tested on a small sample from the umbilical cord. If blood typing of the newborn's cord blood is not available, the benefits of Rh immune globulin administration to Rh D–negative postpartum patients outweigh the theoretical risks of unnecessary administration. Administration after 72 hours may be protective, and anti-D immune globulin should be given even up to 28 days after the birth.[50] Because anti-D immune globulin is a blood product, it has theoretical risks of infection; however, current technologies screen the product for all known viruses, such as human immunodeficiency virus (HIV). Midwives should discuss its benefits and risks carefully with their patients, especially with those who object to the use of blood products.

The standard 300-mcg dose of anti-D immune globulin is sufficient to treat a fetal–parental hemorrhage containing 15 mL of red blood cells or 30 mL of whole blood. Excessive fetal–parental hemorrhage, defined as exceeding 30 mL of Rh D–positive fetal whole blood, occurs in approximately 2 to 3 per 1000 births. It is important to know when this event has occurred, because additional anti-D immune globulin will be needed if the amount of hemorrhage is larger than 30 mL of whole blood. Therefore, a qualitative rosette assay (fetal bleed screen) is performed on the birthing patient's blood as a screening test after the birth to ascertain whether Rh D–positive blood is detectable in the patient's blood. If the rosette assay is positive, a quantitative Kleihauer–Betke test is performed to determine the amount of fetal hemoglobin present. In some facilities, a Kleihauer–Betke test is the only test ordered because it entails the quantitative measurement of fetal red blood cells in the patient's blood; the test results are used to determine if and how much additional Rh immune globulin should be administered.[50]

### Immunizations

The early postpartum period provides an opportunity to vaccinate new parents against several infections, and vaccines can be administered according to the same schedule as the general population. Given the high percentage of postpartum patients who do not continue with care, this may be the last face-to-face interaction that the patient has with a healthcare provider in the coming months or years. Midwives should use this postpartum moment to promote wellness and the primary prevention of disease.

Postpartum patients should receive all recommended vaccines that were not administered during pregnancy, including coronavirus disease 2019

| Table 34-3 | Postpartum Orders and Plans |
| --- | --- |
| **Topic** | **Details/Options** |
| Fundal checks | After the first 2 hours after birth, should be done approximately every 4 hours for the first 24 hours after birth (by either a clinician or the patient) |
| Laboratory tests | Hemoglobin and hematocrit if symptoms of anemia or hypovolemia, history of EBL > 500 mL, or prenatal anemia; white blood cell count if infection is suspected; Rh screen of the newborn if the patient is Rh negative |
| Perineal care | Ice packs, topical medications, peri-bottle, and sitz-bath; high-fiber diet for patients with disrupted anal sphincters |
| Inability to void | Peppermint oil essence in commode or toilet, catheterization if necessary |
| Breast/chest care | Assist with positioning and latch to prevent nipple trauma and engorgement; apply cool or warm compresses or expressed breast milk for nipple soreness; manual expression or breast pump, hot or cold packs, cool green cabbage leaves for engorgement; supportive bra for patients who are not breastfeeding/chestfeeding |
| Prevention of venous thrombosis | Consider prophylaxis for high-risk patients (history of previous venous thromboembolic event, sickle cell disease, obesity, smoking, cesarean birth, postpartum hemorrhage) especially if not ambulating soon after birth |
| Pain management | Acetaminophen, ibuprofen, or diclofenac suppositories for routine afterpains, perineal pain, nipple pain, or pain from engorgement; multimodal pain strategies for patients who have had cesarean births |
| Hydration | Oral hydration preferred; should specify when to discontinue any intravenous hydration |
| Nutrition | Consider food allergies, cultural preferences, and diabetes |
| Activity level | Generally unrestricted; first time out of bed with assistance after epidural anesthesia, cesarean birth, or postpartum hemorrhage |
| Routine postpartum medications | Rho (D) immune globulin if needed, vitamins and iron, stool softeners or laxatives, analgesics, immunizations, and sleep medications as needed |
| Preexisting medications | Continue or reinstate medications used prenatally, such as thyroid replacement and antidepressants, per the plan that was made prenatally. Consult with a physician colleague as indicated. |
| Immunizations | All recommended vaccines that were not administered during pregnancy should be administered, including rubella and varicella; smallpox vaccine is not recommended; all members of the newborn's household should be vaccinated, especially for Tdap, influenza, and COVID-19. |
| Contraception | Prescription for self-administered contraceptives; DMPA, IUD, or implant placement, or tubal sterilization in selected clients |
| Mood and emotional well-being | Screen for postpartum depression and anxiety with a validated instrument; screen for tobacco use; screen for substance use; follow-up on preexisting mental health disorders; refer as appropriate |
| Discharge from immediate postpartum care | Depends on family readiness and status of newborn |
| Follow-up | Check in by phone, telehealth, or in office between 3 days and 3 weeks; ensure that patient has a phone number of a healthcare provider to contact for concerns about themselves or their newborn |

Abbreviations: COVID-19, coronavirus disease 2019; DMPA, depot medroxyprogesterone acetate; EBL, estimated blood loss; IUD, intrauterine device; Rh, Rhesus factor; Tdap, tetanus–diphtheria–acellular pertussis.

Based on Berens P. Overview of the postpartum period: normal physiology and routine maternal care. *UpToDate*. https://www.uptodate.com/contents/overview-of-the-postpartum-period-normal-physiology-and-routine-maternal-care. Updated May 9, 2023. Accessed May 13, 2023; Spencer J. Common problems of breastfeeding and weaning. *UpToDate*. https://www.uptodate.com/contents/common-problems-of-breastfeeding-and-weaning. Updated March 29, 2023. Accessed May 13, 2023.

(COVID-19), influenza, MMR (measles/mumps/rubella), varicella, Tdap (tetanus/diphtheria/acellular pertussis), and human papillomavirus (HPV). These vaccines are not contraindicated with breastfeeding/chestfeeding. Smallpox vaccine is not recommended in the postpartum period. Additionally, all members of the newborn's household should be vaccinated, especially for COVID-19, Tdap, and influenza, to help protect the newborn from illnesses for which they are too young to be vaccinated.[48]

## Common Discomforts in the Early Postpartum Period

Many patients experience pain and fatigue in the early postpartum period. Pain can occur secondary to perineal lacerations or abdominal incisions, breast/chest pain from engorgement, nipple trauma related to infant suckling, uterine contractions/afterpains, and hemorrhoids. Unmitigated pain can interfere with a patient's ability to care for their infant, delay recovery, and increase the risk for postpartum depression and for persistent pain.[51]

### *Treatment of Pain in the Early Postpartum Period*

***Nonpharmacologic Pain Management.*** Nonpharmacologic options are often tailored to the type of pain that the patient is experiencing.[52] Perineal pain can be managed with cold compresses applied for up to 30 minutes every 60 to 90 minutes for the first 24 to 48 hours.[53] Warm compresses applied for up to 30 minutes every 60 to 90 minutes may also be soothing for some patients beginning 48 hours after the birth.[52] Anecdotally, some patients find comfort from sitz baths with lavender essential oils, comfrey, rosemary, or shepherd's purse, through there is little contemporary research to support their use.[52]

Breast/chest pain from engorgement can be treated with cold compresses applied up to 30 minutes every 60 to 90 minutes or cabbage leaves applied for 20 minutes up to 3 times a day.[54] The best method for preventing nipple pain is to have an effective latch. Once nipple trauma has occurred, expressed breast milk and gel packs can be effective for pain relief.[55]

One effective intervention for afterpains is hydrotherapy through submersion in a tub.[56] Other anecdotal nonpharmacologic methods for managing afterpains include heating pads, warm packs, or ice packs.[52]

***Pharmacologic Pain Management.*** Individual medications are usually chosen based on the severity of pain, mechanism of action, any known drug allergies, side effects of the medications (including potential for dependence), and compatibility with breastfeeding/chestfeeding. Recent Cochrane reviews have found that ibuprofen[57] and acetaminophen[58] are very effective at managing postpartum perineal pain, and that both of these medications are more effective than opioids in managing involution pain.[59] In selecting pain medications, midwives should be mindful of the risk of dependency on opioids, as the opioid misuse epidemic has reached emergency levels in the United States.[60] The risk of misuse increases with longer durations of therapy.

Midwives must also consider that racial disparities in medication management in the postpartum period exist. In one recent study examining pain management in the postpartum period, both non-Hispanic Black patients and Hispanic patients were significantly more likely than non-Hispanic white patients to report a pain score of 5/10 or higher. However, Hispanic and non-Hispanic Black patients had lower odds of receiving opioid pain prescriptions on hospital discharge than non-Hispanic white patients.[61] The significance of the correlation of higher pain scores in the Hispanic and non-Hispanic Black patients with lower rates of opioid prescriptions could indicate either that the Hispanic and non-Hispanic Black patients were underprescribed or that the non-Hispanic white patients were over-prescribed—but in either case a clear racial disparity in the management of postpartum pain was demonstrated. It is also worth noting that the opioid crisis has had a relatively greater impact on non-Hispanic white communities in the United States.[62,63]

Given the wide variability in postpartum pain, an individualized stepwise approach using a multimodal strategy is recommended.[51,64] Medications that are commonly prescribed to treat pain during the early puerperium are listed in Table 34-4.[48,51,65]

Patients who have experienced an uncomplicated vaginal birth should not require medication stronger than acetaminophen (Tylenol) 325 to 1000 mg every 4 to 6 hours or ibuprofen (Advil) 600 mg taken orally every 6 hours for uterine cramping and nipple pain. If these medications are not adequate to manage a patient's pain, the midwife should explore the possibility that the pain is coming from another source, especially a vulvar or vaginal hematoma. Occasionally, perineal pain may require a short-term course of opioids if there has been significant trauma or a repair of a laceration or episiotomy.[48]

Nonsteroidal anti-inflammatory drugs (NSAIDs) appear to be more effective than acetaminophen or aspirin, probably because NSAIDs have both

| Table 34-4 | Medications Commonly Prescribed to Treat Pain in the Early Postpartum Period | | | |
|---|---|---|---|---|
| **Drug: Generic (Brand)** | **Formulations** | **Indications and Dose** | **Clinical Considerations** | **Lactation** |
| Acetaminophen (Tylenol) | 325, 500, 650 mg | *Mild to moderate pain* 325–1000 mg every 4–6 hours | Maximum: 4000 mg/day acetaminophen from all sources Can be hepatotoxic in large doses. Use with caution in patients with liver disease. | Enters human milk but is considered compatible with lactation by the ABM |
| Ibuprofen (Motrin, Advil) | 200, 400, 600 mg | *Mild to moderate pain* 400–800 mg every 6–8 hours | Take with food Maximum: 3200 mg/day May increase risk of cardiovascular thrombotic events, myocardial infarction, and stroke All NSAIDs have a ceiling effect such that larger doses do not increase pain relief | Considered safe by the ABM due to short half-life Do not administer to lactating parent of an infant with ductal-dependent cardiac lesion. |
| Ketorolac (Toradol) | IM: 15, 30, 60 mg PO: 10 mg Should not be given PO as initial dose | *Short-term treatment for moderately severe postoperative pain* 60 mg IM × 1 dose, then first PO dose can be 20 mg, followed by 10 mg PO every 4–6 hours | Reduces postoperative opioid use Maximum: 40 mg/day Total combined duration of use of IV or IM and PO dosing should not exceed 5 days Do not use for patients with renal impairment Do not shorten dosing interval to less than 4 hours Side effects include peptic ulcers, cardiovascular thrombotic events, and inhibited platelet function | Use with caution, though likely to have low concentration in human milk when used for a limited time |
| Acetaminophen/ codeine (Tylenol No. 3) | 300/30 mg | *Moderate to severe pain not managed with NSAIDS or acetaminophen* Tylenol No. 3 every 4–6 hours | Take with food Total acetaminophen dosage from all sources should be considered May cause excessive sedation in patients and newborns who are rapid metabolizers | **FDA advisory to avoid codeine in breastfeeding/ chestfeeding patients.** Patients with genetic variations in cytochrome CYP2D6 can transfer a high level of metabolites in human milk that can lead to excessive infant sedation and fatal overdose. If needed, use smallest effective dose for less than 4 days. Observe infant closely. |

*(continues)*

| Table 34-4 | Medications Commonly Prescribed to Treat Pain in the Early Postpartum Period (*continued*) | | | |
|---|---|---|---|---|
| **Drug: Generic (Brand)** | **Formulations** | **Indications and Dose** | **Clinical Considerations** | **Lactation** |
| Hydrocodone/ acetaminophen (Norco) | Hydrocodone/ acetaminophen combination as 5/325 mg, 7.5/325 mg, or 10/325 mg | *Moderate to severe pain not managed with alternative methods*<br><br>1–2 tablets of 5/325 every 4–6 hours<br><br>1 tablet of 7.5/325 or 10/325 every 4–6 hours | Maximum: 4 g/day acetaminophen from all sources<br><br>Do not exceed 8 5/325 tablets in 24 hours.<br><br>Do not exceed 6 7.5/325 or 10/325 tablets in 24 hours<br><br>May cause excessive sedation in patients and newborns who are rapid metabolizers | Hydrocodone is partially metabolized by CYP2D6 to more potent metabolites. Use caution and advise close observation of the infant. |
| Hydrocodone/ acetaminophen (Vicodin) | Hydrocodone/ acetaminophen combination as 5/300 mg, 7.5/300 mg, or 10/300 mg | *Moderate to severe pain not managed with alternative methods*<br><br>1–2 tablets every 4–6 hours | Maximum: 4 g/day acetaminophen from all sources<br><br>May cause excessive sedation in patients and newborns who are rapid metabolizers | Hydrocodone is partially metabolized by CYP2D6 to more potent metabolites. Use caution and advise close observation of the infant. |
| Oxycodone HCl/acetaminophen (Percocet) | Oxycodone HCl/ acetaminophen combination as 2.5/325 mg, 5/325mg, 7.5/325 mg, or 10/325 mg | *Moderate to severe pain not managed with alternative methods*<br><br>2.5/325 mg tablets 2 tablets every 6 hours<br><br>5/325 mg, 7.5/325 mg, or 10/325 mg tablets 1 tablet every 6 hours | Maximum: 4 g/day acetaminophen from all sources | Oxycodone is partially metabolized by CYP2D6 to more potent metabolites. Use caution and advise close observation of the infant. |
| Hydromorphone (Dilaudid) | Oral liquid (usual dose)<br><br>Immediate-release tablet | 2.5–10 mg liquid every 3–6 hours<br><br>2–4 mg immediate-release tablet every 4–6 hours | Maximum: 4 g/day acetaminophen from all sources | Preferred by the AAP, as hydromorphone has limited transport to human milk and poor bioavailability in infants |

Abbreviations: AAP, American Academy of Pediatricians; ABM, Academy of Breastfeeding Medicine; FDA, Food and Drug Administration; HCl, hydrochloride; IM, intramuscular; NSAIDs, nonsteroidal anti-inflammatory drugs; PO, oral.

Based on ACOG Committee Opinion No. 742: postpartum pain management; *Obstet Gynecol.* 2018;132(1):e35-e43. doi:10.1097 /AOG.0000000000002683; Berens P. Overview of the postpartum period: normal physiology and routine maternal care. *UpToDate.* https://www.uptodate.com/contents/overview-of-the-postpartum-period-normal-physiology-and-routine-maternal-care. Updated May 9, 2023. Accessed May 13, 2023; Fahey JO. Best practices in management of postpartum pain. *J Perinat Neonat Nurs.* 2017;31(2):126-136.

analgesic and anti-inflammatory effects.[51] NSAIDs have a ceiling effect, which means that increasing the dose beyond a certain point will increase the incidence of side effects but does not increase the analgesic effect. The ceiling dose for ibuprofen appears to be approximately 400 mg per dose. NSAIDs transfer into human milk in very small amounts and are considered safe for lactating patients.

For patients who need stronger pain relief, ketorolac (Toradol) or opioids may be considered. Opioids should be used only after applying a stepwise approach to pain management that uses nonpharmacologic and combined acetaminophen and NSAIDS. Caution is required when selecting an opioid for breastfeeding/chestfeeding patients.[51] The active metabolite of codeine and tramadol is morphine, which is lipophilic and crosses into human milk. Individuals who have a genetic polymorphism that involves duplication of the enzyme CPY2D6 are ultra-rapid metabolizers of drugs such as codeine and tramadol that are metabolized by CYP2D6. The frequency of CYP2D6 ultra-rapid metabolizers varies by genetic ancestry. Overall, in the United States, the prevalence is 4% to 5%.[51] Only 0.5% of people with Chinese ancestry have duplicates of this enzyme, but the prevalence is as high as 29% in people of Ethiopian descent.[51] Although genomic tests that can detect this status are available commercially, they are costly and not recommended for general screening.

There have been multiple cases of infants who experienced excessive sedation and respiratory depression after being exposed to high levels of metabolites in human milk and one report of an infant death.[66,67] This has led to a Food and Drug Administration (FDA) warning that codeine and tramadol are not recommended when breastfeeding due to the risk of serious adverse reactions in breastfed infants.[66] The FDA guidance did not address the use of hydrocodone and oxycodone, but these two opioids are also partially metabolized by CYP2D6. Hydromorphone, morphine, and fentanyl are not metabolized by CYP2D6. Because of this, ACOG,[51] the American Academy of Pediatrics (AAP),[68] and the Academy of Breastfeeding Medicine (ABM)[69] recommend hydromorphone, morphine, or fentanyl as preferred options when opioid analgesia is necessary.

### Breast/Chest Engorgement

Primary breast/chest engorgement may occur as lactogenesis II starts. This stage begins between 48 and 72 hours after birth in most patients, but may be slightly delayed in primiparous patients and in patients who have had cesarean births.[49] It is theorized that engorgement of the breasts/chest is due to a combination of milk accumulation and interstitial edema of the breast caused by a drop in progesterone levels with the birth of the placenta.[49] Engorgement occurs as the milk supply increases and lasts approximately 1 to 7 days.[48] The breasts/chest become distended, tense, and tender to the touch. The skin is warm to the touch, with visible veins, and is taut across the breasts/chest. The nipples are firmer and may become difficult for the infant to grasp. Although engorgement is not an inflammatory process, the increased metabolism associated with milk production may cause a mildly elevated temperature. However, a fever of 38.0°C (100.4°F) or higher suggests the presence of mastitis or another infection, as discussed in the *Postpartum Complications*

chapter. Patients who begin breastfeeding/chestfeeding immediately after birth, nurse frequently on both sides, and avoid the use of supplements or pumping to express milk for bottle-feeding, are less likely to experience painful engorgement.

Effective treatments for engorgement should focus on removing milk from the breasts/chest. The first step in managing engorgement is to evaluate and assist with positioning and infant latch. If the areola is also engorged, manual expression of small amounts of milk will soften the breast and ease the ability of the infant to latch. Other methods include using a pump in a limited way so as not to overstimulate the breast/chest and increase milk production, and applying pressure toward the chest wall, which may soften the edema and allow the infant to latch.[49] Supportive measures have not been well studied, but a Cochrane review suggested that cabbage leaves, cold gel packs, herbal compresses (ginger, cactus, aloe, and hollyhock), and massage may reduce discomfort from engorgement as well as breast/chest hardness.[70]

When a patient is not breastfeeding/chestfeeding, comfort measures for engorgement are targeted toward pain relief and cessation of milk production. There are no medications approved for lactation suppression in the United States. Nevertheless, several strategies may be implemented to help with the discomfort and inhibit milk production: the use of good breast/chest support by a supportive bra, avoidance of breast/chest stimulation, application of ice packs, and the use of analgesics.[48] No attempt should be made to express milk, either manually or by using heat, as this will promote milk ejection (i.e., the let-down reflex) and further milk production. For example, the patient should avoid standing in a warm shower and letting the water run over the breasts/chest. When using ice for comfort, caution should be used to not apply the ice directly to the skin. Engorgement will improve within 24 to 48 hours, although the presence of milk may take several weeks to resolve completely. For transgender men who do not chestfeed, anticipatory guidance around engorgement and lactation should occur in pregnancy and again in the early puerperium to address both the physical discomfort of engorgement and the potential for gender dysphoria related to lactogenesis.[71]

### Nipple Pain

Sore nipples are very common in the initial days postpartum. The midwife should differentiate between nipple sensitivity and nipple injury. Normal sensitivity usually lasts 30 seconds to 1 minute after the first few suckles at the breast/chest and typically diminishes by the fourth postpartum day and resolves by the seventh day. This differs from nipple pain caused by trauma, which will persist at the same or an increasing level throughout the time that the infant is suckling. If the patient describes nipple sensitivity, acetaminophen or ibuprofen can be used before feeding to reduce discomfort. Nipple toughening has not been shown to be effective in treating nipple sensitivity and should not be recommended.[49]

Nipple pain caused by trauma can lead to discontinuation of breastfeeding/chestfeeding if untreated. Nipple injury is most commonly caused by poor positioning and latch-on, so the management of nipple pain should begin by assessing the patient's breastfeeding/chestfeeding technique, providing guidance, and referring the patient to a lactation consultant when needed. The infant should also be assessed for mechanical feeding problems and referred as necessary for treatment.[49]

Injured nipples should be treated with moist wound healing principles, and bacitracin or mupirocin can be applied to cracked or abraded nipples to prevent infection. A nonstick pad should also be used to prevent the nipple from sticking to the pad or bra. If the nipples appear to be infected, a culture of the drainage should be collected to check for bacterial or candidal infection.[49] Assessment, diagnosis, and treatment of nipple pain are reviewed in more detail in the *Infant Feeding and Lactation* chapter.

Cool or warm compresses, application of expressed human milk, and mild analgesics such as acetaminophen or ibuprofen may also provide comfort. Anhydrous lanolin has historically been recommended for treatment of nipple pain and nipple trauma, although little evidence supports effectiveness. Other traditional remedies, such as honey and vitamin E, are potentially dangerous for infants and should not be used.[49]

### Uterine Cramping

Uterine cramping postpartum, commonly referred to as *afterpains*, is caused by the continuing sequential contraction and relaxation of the uterus. Painful cramping is more common in multiparous patients and occurs most often during breastfeeding/chestfeeding in the first few days after birth. Infant suckling stimulates secretion of oxytocin by the posterior pituitary, which then causes the uterus to contract. Having an empty bladder will lessen uterine cramping because a full bladder displaces the uterus upward, which is associated with more painful contractions. Use of heating pads or lying prone with a pillow or blanket roll under the lower abdomen also may relieve the discomfort of afterbirth pains. NSAIDs are generally very effective for treating uterine cramping and are generally needed for 48 to 72 hours at most.[48]

### Perineal Pain

Perineal pain can be treated with nonpharmacologic topical agents, oral analgesics, or topical anesthetics. A helpful toileting technique includes rinsing with warm water from a peri-bottle during urination, wiping front to back, and patting any incision area dry, instead of rubbing or wiping. If perineal discomfort does not progressively improve with time, reexamination should be performed to rule out pathology, including infection.

Ice packs or cold gel packs may be useful for reducing swelling and numbing the perineum in the first 24 hours. All ice packs should be wrapped in a soft covering, with the absorbent side out, for protection against freezing injury; they should not be applied for more than 20 minutes. A recent review demonstrated no significant benefits of using cooling agents, despite their frequent use.[53] Witch hazel compresses may be applied to the perineum or anal area and held in place by the sanitary pad. A 4 × 4 gauze soaked in witch hazel or a ready-to-use commercial witch hazel product may be used. There are no studies that have evaluated the effectiveness of witch hazel. Topical anesthetic sprays and creams have not been shown to be effective, and research has not been conducted to evaluate the long-term effects of topical anesthetics.[72]

When analgesics are needed for perineal pain, NSAIDs provide effective pain relief for most patients. Opioid analgesics should be reserved for patients whose pain is not well controlled with moderate doses of an NSAID.[51] The constipation that can be caused by opioids can exacerbate perineal pain.

### Hemorrhoids and Constipation

Pushing during the second stage of labor can cause hemorrhoids to become edematous and traumatized. Some common comfort measures for patients with hemorrhoids include ice packs/warm water compresses, sitz baths (with either warm or cold water per patient comfort), and hemorrhoidal medications such as hydrocortisone suppositories or creams, analgesic sprays, and witch hazel pads. The nonpharmacologic comfort techniques may be used in combination, except that cold and warm options should not be used during the same time span.

In addition, a mild stool softener can prevent painful bowel movements that occur when the stool is hard. Increased fluid intake and a high-fiber diet also will promote normal function. Stool softeners or laxatives should be discontinued if the stools become too soft or liquid. Suppositories should be avoided if the patient has sustained a third- or fourth-degree laceration.

### Thrombosis Prevention

The increased risk of thrombosis that is present in pregnancy persists into the immediate postpartum period, as the altered coagulation factors and venous stasis that began in pregnancy slowly diminish over the first 6 weeks after birth.[73] Thrombi can occur in all patients, but some patients—such as those with a prior history of a thromboembolic event or a thrombophilia—are at high risk. For patients with no history of a venous thromboembolism, surveillance for symptoms is adequate. For patients with no history of a venous thromboembolism but with multiple risk factors such as a first-degree relative with a history of thrombotic episode, obesity, prolonged immobility, or cesarean birth, prophylactic anticoagulation therapy may be appropriate. Currently, there is not one standard protocol to guide clinicians in determining exactly which patients should receive prophylactic anticoagulation medications, but prophylaxis in high-risk patients should be considered for 6 to 8 weeks postpartum.[74]

### Postoperative Care Following Cesarean Birth

While the goals of postpartum care are similar after cesarean birth, some unique circumstances must be considered. In the immediate postoperative period, vital signs, uterine tone, and bleeding are monitored quite frequently. The risk of hemorrhage (intraabdominal or vaginal) is highest during this initial period. Typically, nursing, anesthesia, and surgical staff care for patients during this period. Care activities are directed toward preventing complications such as deep vein thrombosis, ileus, and endometritis. Common postpartum complications associated with cesarean birth are reviewed in the *Postpartum Complications* chapter.

### Thrombosis Prevention

The risk of thrombotic events after cesarean birth is 246 per 100,000, which is significantly higher than the risk following vaginal birth of 165 per 100,000. This increased risk may be related to the patient's immobility after surgery. Strategies to mitigate this risk include use of pneumatic compression devices until the patient is fully ambulating and initiation of early ambulation. Some patients are considered to be at even higher risk of thrombotic events following cesarean birth, including those with a history of previous venous thromboembolism (VTE), thrombophilias, body mass index (BMI) greater than 35 kg/m$^2$, and two or more less-prominent risk factors such as postpartum hemorrhage, hypertension, obesity, heart disease, sickle cell disease, and preeclampsia.[75] Early ambulation should be encouraged as soon as the effects of the anesthesia have worn off—usually within 4 hours.[76]

### Nutrition

Two meta-analyses have found that early intake of oral fluids and food after cesarean birth is well tolerated and is not associated with gastrointestinal discomfort.[77,78] Early, unrestricted oral intake after cesarean birth may accelerate the return of gastrointestinal function, as does chewing gum three times a day for 15 minutes.[76] Bowel sounds should be audible within 12 to 24 hours after surgery.

### Prevention of Infection

Prophylactic antibiotic therapy is unnecessary after cesarean birth if a single antibiotic dose was administered during the surgical procedure. Patients who were receiving group B *Streptococcus* (GBS) prophylaxis will similarly have this treatment discontinued immediately after surgery. However, if the patient develops chorioamnionitis during labor, antibiotics should be continued or switched to ampicillin–sulbactam until the patient is afebrile for 24 hours.[75]

### Anemia

Postpartum anemia is more likely after a cesarean birth because the typical average blood loss with cesarean birth is 1000 mL. There is little evidence to support routine testing for anemia in the postpartum period, and the treatment of anemia in the postpartum period is based mainly on clinical experience and standing protocol. However, it is reasonable to treat any symptomatic patient for anemia with supplemental iron for 6 to 8 weeks.[79] Treatment of iron-deficiency anemia is reviewed in the *Medical Complications in Pregnancy* chapter.

### Pain Management

Strategies for pain control after surgery may vary and should consider the principles of pain management discussed earlier. The goal is to transition the patient to oral pain medications by the time of discharge.

NSAIDs and acetaminophen should be considered as part of a multimodal pain strategy for postoperative pain and can be used in conjunction with low-dose, low-potency, and short-acting opioids as part of a stepwise approach to pain management.[64] Midwives should take care to prescribe an appropriate quantity of opioid medications—that is, to avoid both over-prescribing and under-prescribing. Research has found that the median number of opioids prescribed to patients after a cesarean birth is 40 tablets and the median number consumed is 20 tablets.[80] Because approximately 1 in every 300 opioid-naïve patients prescribed opioids after cesarean becomes a persistent user, it is important to use shared decision making to individualize the type of drug and amount ordered in discharge prescriptions.[51] Providing around-the-clock NSAIDs and acetaminophen with opioids prescribed as needed is recommended as a method to reduce opioid exposure.[64] Splitting doses—which involves providing half of the intended opioid dose and then reevaluating for sufficient pain relief—is another method to provide pain relief while avoiding unnecessary exposure to opioids.[64]

Complementary therapies may also be useful for patients experiencing pain after a cesarean birth. Some evidence indicates that acupuncture or acupressure, aromatherapy, electromagnetic therapy, massage, music, relaxation, and transcutaneous electrical nerve stimulation (TENS) for up to 24 hours may all help to reduce post-cesarean pain.[79]

### Wound Healing

By 48 hours after surgery, the surgical wound develops a thin epithelial layer that serves as a barrier to bacteria and foreign bodies. The surgical dressing can be removed 6 to 24 hours after surgery, with the dressing removed slowly, in the direction of hair growth, at an angle of 150 degrees to the skin.[76] Staples are usually removed from a transverse wound 4 to 6 days after surgery, but can stay in for as long as 10 days in patients at high risk for poor wound healing, such as patients with obesity or diabetes. Staples in a vertical wound should not be removed before 5 days after surgery. Typically, patients are advised to avoid showering for 48 hours after surgery, but there is no evidence that it is harmful to shower in the first 48 hours if the wound is closed.[76]

### Activity

Patients are usually advised to lift nothing heavier than the infant and to avoid other activities that may put excessive strain on the surgical site. Heavy lifting and lifting from a squat increase intra-abdominal pressure and theoretically can place pressure on the healing surgical wound. There is little research to support this theory, but it is prudent for patients to avoid heavy lifting for 1 to 2 weeks after surgery.[76] Driving should be avoided while patients are taking opioids for pain management and if the patient experiences pain while conducting the normal actions of a driver such as twisting and leaning. Exercise can slowly resume as tolerated.[76]

### Discharge Instructions

A patient usually is discharged from a hospital, assuming no major complications, approximately 48 to 72 hours after the cesarean birth. In addition to postpartum care planning and education provided to all patients, health education for patients who have had a cesarean birth should include warning signs for surgical-site infections as well as all other post-birth warning signs.

### Postoperative Care Following Tubal Sterilization

Postpartum tubal sterilization is usually performed the day after a vaginal birth or during a cesarean birth. When a tubal sterilization is planned, the patient will be asked to discontinue all oral intake for 6 to 8 hours prior to the sterilization procedure. If an epidural was used during labor or birth, the epidural catheter will be retained in place and used during the sterilization procedure. Typically, the surgical incisions for tubal sterilization are small, dressed with simple adhesive bandages, and require no special postoperative care. No additional restrictions or instructions are needed for the postpartum tubal sterilization. Additional information regarding types of sterilization and health education can be found in the *Nonhormonal Contraception* chapter.

### Early Postpartum Education

The postpartum period can be an exciting time, but there is also the potential for patients and families to feel detached from care and alone as they face the physical, mental, and social challenges of healing and caring for a newborn. In a recent survey, one in four postpartum patients did not have a point of contact in the case of concerns regarding their own health or that of their infant.[81] More than one-half of perinatal deaths occur after the birth of an infant, a statistic that belies the traditional hands-off approach to postpartum care in the United States.[1] Considering the high rate of morbidity and mortality in the early postpartum period, it is essential that patients are well informed about warning signs and know what to do and who to contact should they experience any of these symptoms. Ideally, postpartum education begins prenatally, so that the patient and family have time to plan and make informed decisions about support, infant feeding, and newborn care. ACOG recommends that a postpartum care plan be developed during the prenatal period and then reviewed and updated after the birth.[1] The suggested components of the postpartum care plan are presented in Table 34-5.

An important part of the postpartum care plan is defining the postpartum care team. Documentation of this information helps the patient and family know who to contact and how to reach them for a variety of potential concerns and questions that may arise in the postpartum period. The care plan should include contact information for all members of the team and should identify who to call for which types of problems that may arise. Members of

the postpartum care team may include the perinatal care provider, infant's healthcare provider, primary care provider, lactation consultant, care coordinator, home visitor, and specialist providers.[1]

Health education in the early puerperium is prioritized and targeted to the needs of each patient and family. Assessing the parents' learning needs is the first step. Assumptions may be misleading, such as expecting that a multiparous patient already has a wealth of knowledge about recommended infant care or that a primiparous patient is unfamiliar with personal or neonatal care. It may be helpful to focus on essential topics in discussions, then supplement that verbal health education with written materials or electronic sources and provide contact information for further help in the community. Including available family members in postpartum teaching may maximize the benefits. Recommended patient education topics are listed in Table 34-6. Discomforts specific to breastfeeding/chestfeeding (nipple tenderness and

| Table 34-5 | Postpartum Care Plan |
|---|---|
| **Element** | **Components** |
| Care team | Name, phone number, and office or clinic address for each member of the care team |
| Postpartum visits | Time, date, and location for postpartum visit(s); phone number to call to schedule or reschedule appointments |
| Infant feeding plan | Intended method of infant feeding, resources for community support (e.g., WIC, lactation support, new parents' groups), return-to-work resources |
| Reproductive life plan and contraception | Desired number of children and timing of next pregnancy |
| | Method of contraception, instructions for when to initiate, effectiveness, potential adverse effects, and care team member to contact with questions |
| Pregnancy complications | Pregnancy complications and recommended follow-up or test results (e.g., glucose screening for gestational diabetes, blood pressure check for gestational hypertension), as well as risk reduction recommendations for any future pregnancies |
| Adverse pregnancy outcomes associated with ASCVD | Patients who experienced adverse pregnancy outcomes associated with ASCVD (preterm birth, gestational diabetes, or hypertensive disorders of pregnancy) will need baseline ASCVD risk assessment, as well as discussion of need for ongoing annual assessment and need for ASCVD prevention over their lifetime. |
| Mental health | Anticipatory guidance regarding signs and symptoms of perinatal depression or anxiety; management recommendations for birthing persons with anxiety, depression, or other psychiatric issues identified during pregnancy or in the postpartum period |
| Postpartum problems | Recommendations for management of postpartum problems (i.e., pelvic floor exercises for stress urinary incontinence, water-based lubricant for dyspareunia) |
| Chronic health problems | Treatment plan for ongoing physical and mental health conditions and the care team member responsible for follow-up |

Abbreviations: ASCVD, atherosclerotic cardiovascular disease; WIC, Special Supplemental Nutrition Program for Women, Infants, and Children.

Reproduced from ACOG Committee Opinion No. 736: optimizing postpartum care. *Obstet Gynecol.* 2018;131(5):e140-e150. doi:10.1097/AOG.0000000000002633.

| Table 34-6 | Early Postpartum Education Topics |
|---|---|

**Physical Care**

Breast care during breastfeeding and engorgement

Perineal care and pelvic floor exercises (Kegel)

Cesarean surgical wound care

Hygiene, including tub bath or shower as preferred

Chronic disease management

Pain management

Signs and symptoms of postpartum complications

Sleep and fatigue

Activity, exercise, and nutrition

Contraception, sexuality, and birth spacing

**Mental Health**

Signs and symptoms of postpartum depression and anxiety

Smoking

Substance use

Follow-up for preexisting mental health disorders

**Relational Care**

Asking for help

Emotional self-care

Transitional family relationships

Sibling rivalry

Intimate-partner violence

**Safety**

Motor vehicle safety (seatbelts)

Gun safety

Based on ACOG Committee Opinion No. 736: optimizing postpartum care. *Obstet Gynecol.* 2018;131(5):e140-e150. doi:10.1097/AOG.0000000000002633.

| Table 34-7 | Postpartum Signs of Complications |
|---|---|

Headache

Dizziness or fainting

Changes in vision

Excessive vaginal bleeding (bleeding that saturates a peripad in 1 hour or less)

Fever of 100.4°F (38°C) or chills

Extreme swelling of face or hands

Trouble breathing

Severe nausea and vomiting

Chest pain or fast-beating heart

New or worsening perineal or pelvic pain

Pain with urination

Redness, heat, firmness, or pain in one or both breasts

Calf pain, heat, or swelling

Overwhelming tiredness

Loss of connection with reality

Marked changes in mood—thoughts of self-harm or harming infant

Adapted from Centers for Disease Control and Prevention. Urgent maternal warning signs. https://www.cdc.gov /hearher/maternal-warning-signs/index.html. Last reviewed November 17, 2022. Accessed May 13, 2023.

to access care. Patients should also be educated in self-advocacy so that their symptoms are not dismissed or ignored in the early stages of these disorders.[82] When presenting for emergency care outside of the perinatal setting, patients should be advised to emphasize that they are in the postpartum period. Important signs of complications for the postpartum patient are listed in Table 34-7.[83] Signs of complications in the newborn are reviewed in the *Neonatal Care* chapter.

### Pelvic Floor Exercises

Traditionally, teaching patients to perform pelvic floor exercises (also known as Kegel exercises) is another strategy for promoting long-term perineal comfort and strength. However, a recent Cochrane review found limited evidence that performing pelvic floor exercises in the postpartum period has an effect on urinary incontinence.[84] There is some support for the idea that pelvic floor exercise improves sexual function postpartum.[85] The patient may tighten the perineum, drawing it up and in and maintaining this contracted state while moving in bed or moving to a chair. For strengthening muscle tone, the exercises can be done in sets of 10,

cracked nipples) are discussed in the *Infant Feeding and Lactation* chapter.

Considering the severe health consequences of complications in the postpartum period, the midwife should give ample time for reviewing the signs and symptoms of postpartum complications. While most postpartum patients will not experience these symptoms, the implications of untreated preeclampsia, thromboembolism, sepsis, and postpartum mood disorders are devastating. Education about the early warning signs of these conditions should be emphasized, as well as guidance regarding how repeatedly tightening and relaxing the muscles for 5 to 10 seconds. It is helpful to repeat these sets two to three times daily—a regimen that will avoid direct pressure to the sensitive areas. If the patient has undergone a mediolateral episiotomy, tightening the muscles when performing Kegel exercises pulls on the posterior end of the suture line because the incision interrupts muscles diagonally and may be too uncomfortable to perform until the perineum is healed.

### Sexuality Postpartum

There is wide variation in the time after childbirth that postpartum individuals resume sexual activity with their partners, as well as cultural variations in prescribed waiting times. Factors that are correlated with less sexual activity and dyspareunia include operative vaginal delivery, episiotomy, third- and fourth-degree lacerations, and negative birth experiences.[86] Other circumstances that may interfere with postpartum sexuality are reduced privacy, increased interruptions, and fatigue. There is no scientific basis for the traditional recommendation to delay sexual activity until the 6-week postpartum examination. Instead, a more nuanced approach is that the patient should wait until they feel comfortable and ready to resume sexual activity. Additional recommendations include using water-based vaginal lubrication, particularly if the patient is lactating; trying alternative positions for comfort during penetrative vaginal intercourse; and engaging in other sexual and nonsexual forms of intimacy.

### Contraception

The early postpartum period is an opportune time to explore contraceptive plans with the patient. While sexual activity may be far from the mind of the patient who has recently given birth, as many as 50% of patients will have initiated sexual activity by the time they return to a clinic for the traditional postpartum examination at 6 weeks.[87] In patients who are not breastfeeding/chestfeeding, ovulation can return as soon as 25 days after birth.[48] In breastfeeding/chestfeeding patients, the return of ovulatory cycles varies a great deal, depending on the duration and frequency of breastfeeding/chestfeeding. For patients who breastfeed/chestfeed exclusively without supplements, around the clock, and remain amenorrheic, the risk of unplanned pregnancy is less than 5% in the first 6 months.[48]

It is best to open the discussion with an inquiry regarding the patient's desire for future pregnancy and perceived need for contraception. This is an important time to discuss pregnancy spacing and the impact of shorter interpregnancy intervals on perinatal and neonatal health. The World Health Organization (WHO) and ACOG recommend that patients should be counseled to avoid interpregnancy intervals of less than 6 months.[88] Shared decision making and individualized care are foundational to the discussion of postpartum contraception, as each patient's circumstances will differ. Elements of the conversation should include the patient's reproductive life plan, contraception characteristics (e.g., efficacy, cost, convenience, tolerability of side effects, and compatibility with lactation), a review of medical comorbidities, and plans for breastfeeding/chestfeeding.[88] Table 34-8 lists questions that can be used to guide counseling of breastfeeding/chestfeeding patients about hormonal contraception.[89]

Sterilization of either partner is an option for families that do not want another pregnancy. Sterilization of the postpartum patient via bilateral tubal sterilization can occur in the 24 to 48 hours after the birth in the case of a vaginal birth in a hospital and at the time of surgery in the case of a cesarean birth. Counseling regarding sterilization should occur prenatally to ensure that the patient has a full understanding of the permanency of this choice. Even with prenatal discussion and consent, the decision to undergo sterilization should be reaffirmed prior to the procedure. Additional options include tubal sterilization after the postpartum period or vasectomy, which provides permanent sterilization for partners who produce sperm.[88]

Insertion of an intrauterine device (IUD) may be performed safely after birth of the placenta, although expulsion rates are higher than if insertion is performed earlier than 4 weeks postpartum. A copper or progestin-only IUD may be used, based on the patient's preferences.[88]

Progestin-only forms of contraception are generally considered to be safe for healthy postpartum patients, as their benefits outweigh their risks.[90] The long-acting progestin-only implants, etonogestrel (Nexplanon) and levonorgestrel (Jadelle and Sino-implant [II]), can be inserted any time after the birth, as can a progestin-only IUD. Short-acting progestin-only options, including depot medroxyprogesterone acetate (DMPA) and progestin-only oral contraceptives, may be offered at the time of postpartum discharge. Some research suggests that DMPA may have an impact on milk production, and WHO advises against its use in breastfeeding/chestfeeding patients who are less than 6 weeks postpartum.[91] The Centers for Disease Control and Prevention (CDC) guidelines state that there are not

| Table 34-8 | Questions for Counseling Breastfeeding/Chestfeeding Patients About Hormonal Contraception |
|---|---|

**Readiness**

Are you interested in contraception? Is this a good time for you to talk about contraception?

**Breastfeeding/Chestfeeding**

How important to you is breastfeeding/chestfeeding your baby?

How long would you like to breastfeed/chestfeed your baby?

Who supports your decision on how to feed your baby?

Are there any barriers for meeting your breastfeeding/chestfeeding goals?

How would getting pregnant again fit with your breastfeeding/chestfeeding goals?

**Sexuality**

Are you sexually active with someone who can get you pregnant (produces sperm)?

When might you resume sexual activity after giving birth?

Do you have any questions or concerns about sex after giving birth?

**Reproductive Plans**

Are you interested in getting pregnant again in the future?

Have you heard recommendations on how long to wait between pregnancies? What is ideal for you?

Is it important to you to avoid another pregnancy right now?

How would you feel if you were to get pregnant sooner than you desired?

How would your family and support people react to your pregnancy?

**Contraception**

What has your experience been with contraceptives in the past? What worked well for you?

What characteristics of contraceptive methods are important for you?

What have you heard about breastfeeding/chestfeeding and contraception? Are you worried about contraception reducing your milk supply?

Do you have any questions about contraceptive methods?

Based on Bryant AG, Lyerly AD, DeVane-Johnson S, et al. Hormonal contraception, breastfeeding and bedside advocacy: the case for patient-centered care. *Contraception.* 2019;99(2):73-76. doi:10.1016/j.contraception.2018.10.011; Bullington BW, Sata A, Arora KS. Shared Decision-Making: The Way Forward for Postpartum Contraceptive Counseling. *Open Access J Contracept.* 2022;25;13:121-129. doi: 10.2147/OAJC.S360833.

enough data to recommend against DMPA in the immediate postpartum period.[90]

There have been some concerns regarding progestin-only contraception. One study found a 2- to 3-fold increased risk of postpartum depression in patients who had received DMPA in the immediate postpartum period as compared to those who had not.[92] A systematic review did not find other evidence to support this conclusion, however.[93] Another concern is the postpartum use of the progestin-only pill (POP) by Latinx patients who had gestational diabetes. In a study of 904 Latinx patients, POP use was associated with an almost 3 times greater risk of developing type 2 diabetes within 2 years relative to use of nonhormonal or combined hormonal contraceptives (adjusted RR, 2.87; 95% CI, 1.57–5.27). This risk increased with the duration of uninterrupted use.[90] Additional studies of DMPA in this population found an increased risk of developing diabetes, especially for breastfeeding/chestfeeding patients, though this increase was not statistically significant.[90]

Because the postpartum period is a time of hypercoagulation, CDC guidelines state that estrogen-containing methods, or combined hormonal contraception, pose an unacceptable health risk and should not be used in the first 21 days of the postpartum period. Combined hormonal contraception is not recommended until at least 30 days postpartum (for patients without a risk factor for venous thrombus events) or 42 days in all patients, when the benefits of pregnancy prevention outweigh the risks of adverse reactions.[94]

According to the U.S. Medical Eligibility Criteria,[90] lactation is not a contraindication to the use of any contraceptive options. Other authorities warn against the use of combined hormonal contraceptives such as oral contraceptive pills, patches, and vaginal rings because of concerns that these contraceptive methods might reduce milk supply.[95] For similar reasons, they recommend delaying use of high-dose progestins such as DMPA for several weeks.

## Mid-Postpartum Period

Historically, the defined endpoint of the puerperium is 6 weeks—a benchmark likely chosen because by that time the uterus has completed its involution to the nonpregnant state. Traditionally, patients have not been seen for a healthcare visit during the time between discharge and 6 weeks postpartum. However, as many as 5% of patients may experience complications during the mid-postpartum period,[96] and more than half of pregnancy-related deaths occur after the birth of the infant.[1] Complications that can occur during the mid-postpartum period include stroke, postpartum depression, infection, lactation difficulties, or the exacerbation of chronic conditions.[1] Even in the absence of severe complications, many patients experience physical challenges

in the mid-postpartum period such as urinary incontinence, pain, heavy bleeding, and exhaustion.[81] In light of this, ACOG[1] and WHO[97] recommend providing increased monitoring and care for all postpartum patients, with a special emphasis placed on continuity of care for patients at high risk for complications.

### Care During the First Six Weeks Postpartum

Contact with a midwife or other healthcare provider during the first 6 weeks postpartum is beneficial for all patients and especially necessary for some high-risk patients.[97] Patients with severe hypertension should be seen for a blood pressure check within 72 hours of discharge from the hospital, and all other patients with hypertensive disorders should be seen no later than 7 to 10 days after discharge.[1] Postoperative patients and other high-risk patients may need to be seen 1 week after discharge. However, all patients will benefit from ongoing contact with their midwife or care provider, and interval care should be considered for all postpartum patients.

Interval care during this period can be performed in several ways. Some midwives make telephone calls, some do home visits, and others see the patient and/or infant for an office visit. In addition, some midwives may work with nurses or train birth assistants to initiate the telephone calls or perform the home visits. Many midwives combine these activities depending on the needs of the patient, infant, and family. Telehealth is another effective option for many postpartum visits, as it saves the family the burden of traveling to an office, particularly for those families who live remote from their provider or who are juggling childcare and work responsibilities.[98] Face-to-face visits either at home or in an office are recommended for patients who had hypertension, a cesarean birth or complicated perineal laceration, breastfeeding difficulties, and chronic medical conditions, and for any patient who has an identified risk for developing postpartum depression.[1] Regardless of the modality used for the visit, all postpartum patients should have contact with their midwives within the first 3 weeks postpartum. Some patients will need to be seen sooner than 3 weeks, and some may require multiple interactions with the midwife to address health concerns.

#### Phone Calls

Using a telephone call to assess the parent–infant dyad's well-being allows the midwife to triage for emergent problems that might require a trip to the office, the pediatric provider's office, or even the emergency department. Telephone calls are frequently made the day after the birth or the day after the patient returns home from the birth center or hospital, and again a few days later. During the telephone call, the midwife screens for problems by asking about both parental and infant well-being. A comprehensive assessment of the patient's condition by telephone may include obtaining a self-report of physical and emotional well-being, breastfeeding/chestfeeding success, and coping with the significant family changes associated with childbirth. The midwife should ask about the presence of signs or symptoms for postpartum complications. At-home blood pressure monitors can be used for blood pressure checks over the telephone, as well. Content to be covered in this phone call is listed in Table 34-9.

The telephone call also provides an opportunity to check on the newborn's condition, regardless of whether the midwife is the primary healthcare provider for the newborn. This conversation can be an important opportunity to triage for adequacy of infant feeding and signs of hyperbilirubinemia, infection, or heart disease. Assessment of the newborn is also conducted in this phone call. Details of this assessment can be found in the *Neonatal Care* chapter.

### Telehealth

Telehealth technology includes teleconferencing and SMS/text messaging. In recent years, patients and providers have grown more accustomed to use of this modality for convenient communication, and a growing body of literature supports its effectiveness.[98,99] Teleconferencing can be used in lieu of telephone visits and allows for the midwife and patient to see each other and for the midwife to visualize some physical concerns. Targeted text messaging has been associated with exclusive breastfeeding and potentially improved mortality in the postpartum period.[100] Telehealth technology can also be used to monitor high-risk patients. Remote blood pressure monitoring for patients with a history of hypertension has been found to be an effective way of identifying hypertension in the postpartum period.[101–103] Mental health can also be managed through telehealth in the postpartum period.[104] As this technology continues to expand and grow, midwives may find that telehealth visits are a way to provide continuity of care without placing a burden on patients to travel to the office during the postpartum period.

### Home Visits

A home visit involves the same evaluations as does a telephone call or telehealth visit, but also allows

| Table 34-9 | Postpartum Telephone Call: Postpartum Assessment |
|---|---|
| **System** | **Assessment** |
| General | Food and fluid intake |
| | Sleep quality and quantity |
| | Fever or chills |
| | Headaches |
| Breasts/chest | Breast engorgement, nipple condition, pain, masses |
| | Progression from colostrum to milk |
| | Feeding frequency and success |
| Abdomen | Abdominal pain, cramping, epigastric pain |
| | Bowel function, constipation, incontinence |
| | Urinary pain or incontinence, urgency |
| Pelvis | Lochia amount, color, and odor |
| | Perineal pain, swelling, or redness |
| | Hemorrhoids |
| Lower extremities | Edema, pain, redness, varicosities |
| Adjustment | Emotional changes (postpartum blues or depression) |
| | Coping with life changes and response to newborn |
| | Social support and help with household chores |
| | Physical activity level |
| | Abdominal and perineal exercises |
| | Family adjustment to newborn |
| | Confidence in infant care |
| Chronic conditions | Change in signs and symptoms |
| | Medication changes |
| | Follow-up with specialist |

the midwife to observe the patient's responses to the infant's needs and cues, the parent–newborn interaction, the place of the newborn in the home's social environment, and resources in the home (e.g., plumbing, water supply, refrigeration, air conditioning/heat, window screens, supplies for baby care). A home visit may also include a brief physical examination of the patient and newborn. Postpartum home visits are standard in many areas of the world and are recommended by WHO in the first week postpartum for all patients.[97] Nurse home visiting programs such as the Nurse–Family Partnership and other universal home visiting programs[105] can be another resource for postpartum patients.

### Office Visit

In-person assessments are recommended for postpartum patients who had hypertension, are facing breastfeeding challenges, are at high risk for postpartum depression, or have chronic medical conditions. These visits frequently occur in an office, although many of these areas can also be addressed through a home visit or telehealth visit. A standard 2-week in-person visit is another way to maintain continuity of care for all patients and conforms to the ACOG and WHO recommendations for care in the postpartum period.

*Standard Two-Week Postpartum Visit.* Assessments performed at a 2-week visit focus on expected physical, physiologic, and psychological changes in the postpartum period. Particular attention should be paid to how well the patient is coping and an assessment for postpartum depression. A targeted physical examination may be performed as indicated.

If the patient brings the infant to the 2-week visit, the midwife can observe the patient's interaction with the infant and responsiveness to the infant's needs and cues. Every contact with a new parent is an opportunity to highlight the developmental capabilities of the infant and to discuss safety, infant stimulation, and parenting skills. This is also a good time to verify that the infant either has already seen or has an appointment to see a pediatric healthcare provider and to discuss the need for these visits and for immunizations. Some midwives also provide pediatric care for the infant up to 1 month old. An overview of newborn care is provided in the *Neonatal Care* chapter.

For breastfeeding/chestfeeding patients, the 2-week visit also can be used as a time to support effective infant feeding and target any problems. If the patient needs to select a contraceptive method, the 2-week visit is an excellent opportunity to review available options. Many couples will choose to begin sexual intercourse shortly after the lochia resolves, if not before, and patients who are not breastfeeding/chestfeeding may ovulate before a routine postpartum physical is performed at 4 to 6 weeks.

*High-Risk Patients and Office Visits.* Patients with hypertensive disorders of pregnancy should be seen no later than 7 to 10 days postpartum, and those with severe hypertension should be seen within 72 hours of discharge.[1] In-person visits can also be helpful for assessing perineal or cesarean wound healing and assessing a patient for postpartum depression. The timing of these visits is less prescribed, however, than the timing of visits for patients with hypertension.

### Comprehensive Postpartum Visit

The exact timing of the postpartum examination is flexible and may be done as early as 4 weeks after the birth and as late as 12 weeks. The timing of this visit should be tailored to the patient's needs and may relate to the individual's return to work, overall health, or changing insurance status. This visit serves as the transition from perinatal care to ongoing wellness care. It should not be considered a "parting visit" or an "all-clear sign," but rather a transitional visit that bridges the perinatal period with the patient's ongoing physical, emotional, and social needs.[1] Viewed in this way, the postpartum examination will include each of the elements described here, plus the recommended screening and counseling provided during a wellness visit as described in the *Health Promotion Across the Lifespan* chapter.

The comprehensive postpartum visit consists of a comprehensive history, physical examination, and pelvic examination, as outlined in the *Introduction to Sexual, Reproductive, and Primary Care* chapter. Available records of prenatal, intrapartum, and postpartum care during this pregnancy should be reviewed. A description of the procedure for this postpartum visit is presented in the *History and Physical Examination During the Postpartum Period* appendix. Topics that should be addressed during this visit are listed in Table 34-10.[74–80]

### Management Plans

A review of the prenatal record will identify conditions from the pregnancy that have not resolved. For example, a patient may need follow-up care for an ovarian or renal cyst identified by ultrasound during the pregnancy. Based on the scope of the midwife's practice, follow-up care should be arranged within the service or by referral to another primary care provider. Screening for postpartum depression is recommended for all patients who attend a postpartum visit.[106–108]

Based on the history and physical examination, the midwife may be asked to complete an authorization for parental leave or return to employment. Proper evaluation should include an understanding of the type of work that the patient performs. Midwives

| Table 34-10 | Topics for Comprehensive Postpartum Visit | |
|---|---|---|
| **Topic** | **Discussion** | **Follow Up** |
| Debrief pregnancy and birth | Provide an opportunity for the patient to share their experience and ask any questions they have about the birth. | Referral for counseling as needed. |
| | Discussion around birth trauma, if experienced. | Stillbirth or miscarriage: Visit for review of autopsy findings, emotional support, bereavement counseling, as needed. |
| | | Placental pathology reports should be reviewed and discussed. |
| Postpartum experience | Assess for urinary or fecal incontinence. | Refer to physical therapy/ urogynecologist as needed. |
| | Assess for perineal or cesarean incision pain and address normal versus prolonged recovery. | |
| | Provide specific guidance regarding physical activity, exercise, and weight. | |
| | Discuss coping options for fatigue and sleep disruption. | |
| | Resumption of sexual activity, normal healing following birth, and strategies for improving postpartum sexual experiences. | |
| | Resumption of employment, if applicable. | |
| Mental health | Use a validated screening tool for postpartum mood disorders that includes screening for anxiety and depression. | Provide resources for support groups. |
| | Screen for tobacco and substance use and discuss relapse risk. | Refer, as needed, for tobacco use, substance use, and mental health care. |
| | Follow up on pre-pregnancy mental health issues. | Continuation of medications for substance use and mental health care needs. |
| Infant care (if applicable) | Ask about feelings on parenting/adoption. | Social support agencies. |
| | Ask about infant health since birth. | Postpartum doula services. |
| | Infant feeding method and updated teaching, if feeding method has changed. | Pediatric care, if not established. |
| | Ensure infant has a pediatric care home. | Provide information on local vaccination clinics for family members and infant caregivers. |
| | Childcare strategy | |
| | Discuss immediate family and caregiver vaccination needs. | |
| | Assess material needs such as housing, diapers, food. | |
| | Advise patient to seek assistance from family and support person to assist with infant care. | |
| Breastfeeding/ chestfeeding (if applicable) | Assess comfort and confidence. | Referral to lactation specialist, La Leche League, as needed. |
| | Assess breastfeeding/chestfeeding associated pain. | |
| | Review legal rights regarding breastfeeding/ chestfeeding and milk expression at school and work. | |
| Reproductive planning | Assess for desire for future pregnancies. | Provide contraception as desired. |
| | An interpregnancy interval of at least 6 months (ideally at least 18 months) is recommended. | Discuss availability of emergency contraception. |
| | After cesarean birth, interbirth interval of at least 18 months reduces risk of uterine rupture. | |
| | For patients who chose to use contraception, establish a plan and review the method's effectiveness, instructions, and side effects. Ensure contraception method is compatible with chronic disease conditions. | |

| Topic | Discussion | Follow Up |
|---|---|---|
| Chronic disease management | Review of chronic conditions needing ongoing care.<br><br>Review abnormal screenings or findings from before and during pregnancy.<br><br>Review medications for chronic conditions and evaluate use in breastfeeding/chestfeeding if needed.<br><br>If the patient had complications such as gestational diabetes, hypertensive disorders, or preterm birth, counsel that these conditions increase the lifetime risk for cardiometabolic disease.<br><br>Review health behaviors that may improve long-term outcomes.<br><br>Discuss screening frequency based personal and family risk factors for chronic disease. | Gestational diabetes: Order fasting plasma glucose or 75-g, 2-hour glucose tolerance test.<br><br>Hypertension, obesity, diabetes, renal disease, preterm birth, abnormal cervical cytology screening, uterine or ovarian cysts: Plan for follow-up as indicated.<br><br>Ensure a plan for follow up care is established at an accessible location consistent with insurance or financial needs. |
| Resumption of primary care | Review vaccination history.<br><br>Review schedule of preventative care and screening based on age as well as personal and family medical history. | Provide vaccinations or referral, as needed.<br><br>Perform routine wellness care, such as cervical cytology screening, as needed.<br><br>At the end of the postpartum visit, the patient should have an accessible primary care provider (compatible with insurance or financial needs) identified and should understand appropriate timing of the next visit. |

Based on ACOG Committee Opinion No. 736: optimizing postpartum care. *Obstet Gynecol*. 2018;131(5): e140-e150. doi:10.1097/AOG.0000000000002633; American College of Nurse-Midwives and the National Association of Nurse Practitioners in Women's Health; American College of Obstetricians and Gynecologists and the Society for Maternal–Fetal Medicine, Louis JM, Bryant A, Ramos D, Stuebe A, Blackwell SC. Interpregnancy Care. *Am J Obstet Gynecol*. 2019;220(1):B2-B18. doi: 10.1016/j.ajog.2018.11.1098. Epub 2018 Dec 20. PMID: 30579872.

can advocate for patients who desire to continue breastfeeding/chestfeeding after returning to work and to offer guidance on strategies to continue lactation.

Patients who need contraception should receive necessary prescriptions, appointments, and education. It is not necessary to wait for menses to resume before starting oral contraceptives or inserting an IUD. If the patient has engaged in unprotected penile–vaginal intercourse, use of emergency contraception and/or urine pregnancy testing after 2 weeks of abstinence or condoms can reasonably ensure that the patient is not pregnant. The postpartum visit is also an good time to discuss future plans for pregnancy and to provide preconception counseling.

Nutrition and exercise are topics of great importance to many individuals. By 6 weeks postpartum, most patients should be physically ready to resume regular exercise routines, in addition to abdominal and pelvic floor exercises to restore tone to those muscle groups most impacted by pregnancy and childbirth. According to the Physical Activity Guidelines for Americans, adults should get at least 150 minutes of moderate exercise per week.[109] It may be advisable to gradually increase activity to this level

of exercise when reinitiating activity postpartum. Pelvic floor exercises, abdominal strengthening exercises, and aerobic exercise are all recommended in the postpartum period.[110] Based on limited evidence, aerobic activity in breastfeeding/chestfeeding individuals has been shown to improve cardiovascular health without having an impact on milk production or infant growth.[111] Patients should be advised to feed their infants prior to engaging in exercise for comfort while exercising and to ensure that they are staying well hydrated.[110] Additional recommendations for physical activity can be found in the *Health Promotion Across the Lifespan* chapter.

Many patients desire weight loss to return to their pre-pregnancy weight or to achieve another weight goal. The best way to achieve these goals is through a combination of healthy nutrition and exercise and by identifying what constitutes a healthful weight goal based on BMI and other factors. Patients should be cautioned against rapid weight loss postpartum; a useful reminder is that it took 9 months to gain the weight, so it may take at least the same amount of time to lose it. A detailed discussion of dietary recommendations can be found in the *Nutrition* chapter.

### Adjusting to Parenthood

The comprehensive postpartum visit is also a time to observe the transition to parenting and parent–infant attachment and bonding. Midwifery assessment of the process of becoming a parent requires three discrete evaluations: (1) observation of parent–infant interactions to determine how well attachment is progressing, (2) a review of the patient's environment to identify supports and factors that may impede progress, and (3) a formal assessment for signs of postpartum mood disorders.

The postpartum period can bring about many conflicting feelings for new parents as they juggle new responsibilities and feelings of fatigue, being overwhelmed, loss of control, loss of identity, and lonliness.[112,113] Patients' reports of their needs during the postpartum period consistently refer to four items: (1) more information about their infant, (2) psychological support, (3) a need to share the experience, and (4) practical or material help.[81,113,114] These four items provide a good framework for midwifery assessment of the adjustment to parenting.

Postpartum mood disorders such as anxiety, post-traumatic stress disorder (PTSD), and depression are highly correlated with preexisting and prenatal mental health conditions. Additionally, many patients without a previous mental health history will develop postpartum mood disorders; it is estimated that as many 13% of postpartum patients report postpartum depression, and the rate is as high as 20% in some high-risk groups.[115] Untreated postpartum mood disorders can have a lasting impact on the physical, mental, and emotion health of the postpartum patient and the infant.[115] Mood disorders can also interfere with establishment of a parent–infant bond and should be considered whenever the midwife has concerns about attachment and bonding. A detailed review of postpartum mood disorders and ways to screen for them is presented in the *Mental Health Conditions* chapter, where the reader will also find information about preexisting mental health conditions and prenatal mental health conditions that can have an impact on the postpartum transition.

### Debriefing the Birth/Birth Trauma

A review of the pregnancy, birth, and immediate postpartum period should be included in the comprehensive postpartum visit. This is the moment for the patient and family to ask questions, talk about their feelings, and get clarity regarding any complications or health concerns that may have occurred. Complications should be discussed with consideration of their possible impact on future pregnancies,

and placental pathology reports should be reviewed, as appropriate.[1]

The events of childbirth are difficult to predict and often do not match the patient's birth plan. Differences between the planned labor and birth and the reality may include use of analgesia or anesthesia, mode of delivery, and the quality of support provided in labor. For some families, the experience goes beyond disappointment, as the parents must grieve after a trauma or loss. Examples of losses include stillbirth or early neonatal death, loss of fertility after an emergency hysterectomy, the discovery of congenital birth defects, voluntary or involuntary relinquishment of the newborn to adoptive parents or the legal system, and admission to the neonatal intensive care unit. Patients' grief reactions to these outcomes will be unique to their specific circumstances, coping strategies, and social support.

Regardless of the clinician's interpretation of the events surrounding the birth, some patients may experience birth as a traumatic event. This interpretation is personal; trauma results in distress and psychological disturbance that are unrelated to the physical events occurring at the time of birth.[116] A traumatic birth places a patient at risk for PTSD. In the Listening to Mothers II national survey of childbirth, 9% of participants met the diagnostic criteria for PTSD, and 18% of participants experienced significant levels of post-traumatic stress symptoms 7 to 18 months after childbirth.[81]

In most situations involving fearful events, the act of listening is by itself therapeutic. After listening to patients describe their experiences of birth during the early postpartum period and validating their feelings, midwives may identify those who could benefit from formal counseling after traumatic birth. There are mixed results from randomized trials of debriefing after traumatic birth in reducing symptoms of PTSD or postpartum depression.[117] Because patients' perceptions of their birth experience may differ from the midwife's perception, the first step in identifying a traumatic birth is to openly ask each postpartum patient about their feelings about their birth. Several validated tools, such as the Wijma Delivery Expectancy/Experience Questionnaire (version B)[118] and the Delivery Satisfaction Scale,[119] can be used to guide the discussion. Addressing and treating PTSD early in the postpartum period can help to prevent more severe cases of PTSD, which can have lasting effects on the patient's health and well-being.[117]

### Smoking

In the United States, the prevalence of smoking has declined in the past decade, both in the general population and among pregnant individuals. In 2010, 9.2% of pregnant Americans smoked; by 2017, this rate was down to 6.9%.[120] However, for those patients who did smoke and stopped smoking in pregnancy, the rate of relapse is high. Some studies have shown that 40% of individuals who stop smoking in pregnancy relapse in the first 6 months postpartum, and 90% relapse in the first year.[121,122] Younger patients and those whose partners smoke are at higher risk of relapse.[123]

There is a growing body of research regarding the use of pharmacotherapeutics to prevent relapse in the general population,[124] but very little research has specifically focused on preventing smoking relapse in postpartum and breastfeeding/chestfeeding patients.[125] Although the most effective treatment to prevent relapse in the general population is varenicline,[124] this medication is not recommended with breastfeeding/chestfeeding as it is postulated that it may be excreted in breast milk.[125]

Midwives should offer patients information about available community programs for maintaining abstinence and educate them on the important health benefits of not smoking for themselves and their children. Additional information about strategies used for smoking cessation can be found in the *Health Promotion Across the Lifespan* chapter.

### Substance Use

Substance use and substance use disorder can present in many ways and affect a diverse group of postpartum patients. Midwives may encounter patients with dependence on a variety of substances, including alcohol, cannabis, opioids, and other substances. In 2018, approximately 8 million Americans aged 12 or older had a substance use disorder related to their use of alcohol or other substances.[126] As part of the transition from perinatal care to wellness care, midwives should screen all postpartum adults for unhealthy drug use at the comprehensive postpartum visit, regardless of risk factors.[127] A variety of screening tools exist, though none is specifically targeted for postpartum patients. As with all healthcare screening, these tools do not diagnose substance use disorder, but simply identify those persons who should be referred for a diagnostic assessment.

For opioid users, the postpartum period is one of increased risk for fatal and nonfatal overdose, with the incidence of such events increasing from 3.3 per 100,000 person-days in the third trimester to 12.3 per 100,000 person-days in the 7 to 12 months after birth.[128] The postpartum period is stressful for all patients, but particularly for those with a history of

substance use disorder, increasing the risk of relapse or increased use. Notably, a lack of access to care related to the loss of insurance and fewer programs targeted at postpartum patients versus pregnant patients may lead to an increased risk of relapse. Additionally, patients whose infants are experiencing neonatal opioid withdrawal syndrome may experience shame and stigma that increases their likelihood of relapse. Hormonal changes in the postpartum period may also influence the effectiveness of medications used to manage opioid use disorder.[128] The highest risk of overdose among opioid users in the postpartum period occurs after 6 months, when studies have found that as many as 56% of patients discontinue pharmacotherapy.[128,129]

Heavy episodic drinking is a frequent pattern of alcohol use in individuals of childbearing age and is associated with numerous adverse effects, including unintended pregnancies, unintentional injuries, suicide attempts, and sexually transmitted infections.[130] Rates of heavy episodic drinking have increased in the United States over the past decades, with approximately 36% of pregnant and postpartum individuals engaging in such behavior in 2012–2013.[130] Alcohol use in breastfeeding/chestfeeding individuals is quite common, with 12% to 83% of these patients reporting alcohol consumption.[131] Alcohol can pass readily into human milk at parallel concentrations to the patient's blood alcohol concentration. Alcohol is associated with decreased oxytocin and affects prolactin production as well. There appears to be a relationship between beer consumption and milk supply, but use of non-alcoholic beer has also been found to increase prolactin levels—suggesting that it may be malt or barley that influences prolactin levels, rather than the beer itself.[132] Moderate alcohol use with breastfeeding/chestfeeding, such as one drink per day with a meal, is unlikely to harm an infant, so long as the patient waits approximately 2 to 2.5 hours after drinking to breastfeed/chestfeed the infant. Nursing sooner than that can affect the infant's behavior. Heavy drinking by a breastfeeding/chestfeeding parent can cause serious adverse effects for the infant and can have a negative impact on let-down.[132]

The legalization of cannabis in many states has resulted in changing social perceptions of its use, and perceptions of its safety. However, as with alcohol and smoking, the legality of a substance does not change its impact on the postpartum patient's health. In the United States, 6.8% of postpartum patients report using cannabis.[133] Some may feel that using cannabis is safe, or that it may be helpful with managing postpartum physical and mental symptoms.[134] Patients have also reported a lack of clear communication from their providers regarding the safety of cannabis in the postpartum period.[134-136]

The main psychoactive component of cannabis, tetrahydrocannabinol (THC), is excreted into human milk in small quantities; the duration of detection of THC in milk has been found to range from 6 days to 6 weeks.[137] Short-term effects on an infant exposed to THC in milk may include delayed motor development, as well as sedation, growth delay, low tone, and poor sucking.[138] There are insufficient data regarding the long-term effects of THC on infants, so its use should be avoided. Cannabis should also not be used in the vicinity of the infant, as infants can be exposed to the effects of secondhand cannabis smoke.[137]

It is important for the midwife to participate in the ongoing identification of patients with substance use disorder through the use of validated tools, as well as to provide support and referrals for specialized care as necessary.[139] Care of patients with substance use disorder is reviewed in the *Mental Health Conditions* chapter. Patients affected by substance use disorder often experience negative healthcare encounters in the perinatal period that can prevent them from seeking help and support.[140] Advocating for more care options for this marginalized population is an important role for the midwife. The criminalization of drug use and the severe consequences of separation of parent and infant in some states may act as a deterrent to patients seeking assistance. Midwives should discourage the separation of parents and infants solely on the basis of suspected or confirmed substance use, and in states where midwives are mandated reporters, they should lobby lawmakers to rescind punitive laws that inhibit the treatment of substance use disorders.[139]

## Special Considerations

### Adolescents

Becoming a parent at a young age may have negative consequences for both the adolescent and the infant. Adolescents in the postpartum period are more likely than their peers who delay pregnancy to experience postpartum depression, lower self-esteem, substance use, and poverty. Further, adolescent parents are less likely to attain higher levels of education and are more likely to experience intimate-partner violence than their peers.[141]

A variety of programs exist for providing care to adolescent patients postpartum. The goals of these programs usually include improvement of the individual's parenting skills, provision of social support, support for educational attainment, and prevention of repeat pregnancy through the use of contraception. Programs may be provided in the home, in the community or school, or in clinics.

Adolescents have high rates of repeat pregnancy, with 25% of teen parents becoming pregnant again within 1 year of birth and 35% within 2 years.[141] Repeat teen pregnancies account for 20% of all teen births in the United States.[141] Teens who have a second pregnancy in their adolescence have even greater risks of poor perinatal outcomes, including preterm birth and stillbirth.[141] Therefore, it is imperative that the midwife help the postpartum adolescent select a form of contraception that the patient will use, taking into consideration cultural barriers, cost, side effects, and failure rates. This is also a time to review the importance of safe sex for the prevention of sexually transmitted infections. Long-acting reversible contraception (LARC) is the preferred method of contraception for this population if the patient is willing to consider these methods.[142]

### Transgender Men

Transgender men may have a very different postpartum experience than cisgender women. Ideally, the midwife and the pregnant transgender man will have planned during pregnancy for postpartum care and decision making. Care considerations include increasing the sensitivity and support from the care team in the hospital, birth center, or home; decisions on whether to feed the infant with human milk or substitutes; and the timing of resumption of testosterone therapy.

Transgender men may be more comfortable with referring to lactation as *chestfeeding* rather than *breastfeeding*.[71] Transgender men may have had chest surgery such as bilateral mastectomy that reduced or eliminated their ability to lactate. Others may have delayed such surgery until after childbearing or decided not to have surgery. Transgender men may have varying comfort with lactation because of its association with female body function.[24]

Some transgender men may elect to postpone resumption of testosterone therapy until after weaning. Whether or not the transgender man chooses to lactate, there is no research to suggest the optimal timing for resumption of testosterone therapy. A recent case study of a lactating transgender man receiving gender-affirming testosterone found that the parent's serum testosterone rose with testosterone therapy, as would be expected. Milk testosterone concentrations also increased to a maximum concentration of 35.9 ng/dL when the parent was on a dose of 80 mg subcutaneous testosterone weekly. The calculated relative infant dose remained less than 1%, the infant's serum testosterone remained undetectable, and the infant did not display any observable side effects. The parent did not notice any change in the child's feeding patterns or milk supply.[143]

Transgender men whose sexual partners can produce sperm may need contraception, regardless of their use of testosterone.[144] Anticipating these clinical decisions and communicating openly and respectfully will allow the midwife to provide individualized care for transgender men and their families.

## Infant in the Neonatal Intensive Care Unit

Prematurity is the most likely reason for a newborn to need intensive care, as approximately 10% of all newborns born in the United States are born preterm.[145] Other reasons for neonatal intensive care unit (NICU) admission include hyperbilirubinemia, hypoglycemia, infection, meconium aspiration, birth asphyxia, congenital anomalies, and respiratory distress. Having an infant in the NICU can interfere with parental–newborn attachment. Many factors may potentially hinder attachment when an infant is in the NICU, including restricted access to the newborn, difficulty in reading the infant's cues, and inability to commit one's time exclusively to the newborn once the parent is at home. The hospitalization of a newborn is associated with high rates of post-traumatic stress, feelings of guilt and shame, high levels of stress, anxiety, and symptoms of depression.[146] Breastfeeding the hospitalized infant is particularly a challenge when the infant is premature and lacks the neuromuscular development to successfully suckle.

Midwives can do much to support these families when the focus of the healthcare team turns toward the fragile infant. Support for the establishment and continuation of breastfeeding/chestfeeding includes initiating pumping with a hospital-grade mechanical pump within 6 hours of the birth and continuing to pump milk at least six times per day. Midwives may advocate for parents to be able to hold their ill infants in skin-to-skin contact even with monitors and ventilation equipment in place.[147,148] Consultation with mental health professionals on the NICU unit and participation in peer-to-peer support have been found to be effective in helping new

parents manage the stress of having an infant in the NICU.[149] Parents should be monitored for psychological consequences of the infant hospitalization, with attention being paid to their emotional health.

## Relinquishment/Adoption of an Infant

Patients may relinquish the care of their infant voluntarily through adoption or surrogacy, or involuntarily through the legal system. Under these circumstances, midwives might be involved in the care of the birth parents, the adoptive or receiving parents, and/or the newborn. The circumstances around the adoption or removal of the infant and emotional reactions are complex and unique to each family.

Support for the patient who gives birth includes providing psychosocial support, therapeutic communication, follow-up services, and advocacy. The midwife can talk with the patient about their emotions in a nonjudgmental way, validating their feelings and acknowledging that their feelings may be conflicted. As the patient's advocate, the midwife can ensure that the decision to relinquish an infant for adoption was not coercive except under the condition of legal removal by child protective services. Referrals to social workers and counselors may be offered to address ongoing issues of grief and visitation.

As primary care providers, midwives may also be in the position of caring for families who adopt an infant. The decision to adopt often follows failed attempts at getting pregnant and possibly multiple miscarriages. Thus, the emotional reaction to adoption can be complex, as these parents struggle with a sense of legitimacy as parents and fear that the infant will be returned to the biologic parents.[150] Postpartum depression is possible among individuals who become parents by adoption, as they experience stressors similar to those faced by individuals who have given birth. Parents who adopt will likely have educational needs about infant care and may attempt to initiate lactation. Referral to resources and support groups for adoptive families may be helpful. Laws regarding adoption vary according to jurisdiction, so midwives should be aware of credible agencies and attorneys in this field.

## Individuals in Prison

Incarceration presents another circumstance in which the infant will be separated from the parent during the postpartum period. This group of individuals presents special challenges for the provision of postpartum care due to the likelihood of separation of the infant from the parent when the patient returns to the prison. Many postpartum incarcerated patients experience loneliness and depression due to separation from their infants and often fear losing custody of their infants as a result of their incarceration. These patients are already at high risk of mental illness and substance use, putting them at higher risk for mental illness in the postpartum period.[151]

Prison nurseries, in which infants are housed with their incarcerated parents, represent an alternative to the forced separation of infants from their parents, but relatively few of these special units are available. These settings also support breastfeeding/chestfeeding the infant, which has inherent health benefits for the patient and infant.[151,152] When prison nurseries are unavailable, community-based residential parenting programs and placement of the infant with relatives are options for continuing the care of the infant within the family.

Midwives can advocate for these families and coordinate with prison healthcare providers to provide comprehensive perinatal and postpartum care. When providing care to patients who are prisoners, it is important to maintain privacy while in the presence of guards and to avoid the use of restraints or shackles for safety and respect.

## Conclusion

The puerperium is a time of great physical and psychological change. Midwives can provide effective care by attending to patients in the context of their environment, family, and culture. The postpartum period is not just the end of the childbearing year, but also the beginning of the nonpregnant phase of the patient's life, and continuity of care continues to be important. The repercussions of severe complications, while rare, are devastating for the patient's and family's health, and the midwife should remain vigilant in assessing for the development of new or worsening health conditions. There is also a need to address the high rates of problems such as incontinence, dyspareunia, and depression that can be the consequences of otherwise normal pregnancy and childbirth. By moving beyond the care of individuals, midwives can address the health of postpartum families in general through advocacy at the system level. In the context of rising healthcare costs and the desire to increase healthcare access to the underserved, there will be new challenges and opportunities for promoting the health of families.

## Resources

| Organization | Description |
|---|---|
| Postpartum Support International (PSI) | PSI has a mission of support, education, advocacy, and research for people living with mental illness. |
| Postpartum Progress | Focuses on raising awareness, reducing stigma, providing social support, and connecting patients to help for perinatal mood and anxiety disorders such as postpartum depression. |
| Centers for Disease Control and Prevention (CDC) | Focuses on prevention of pregnancy-related deaths by sharing potentially lifesaving messages about urgent warning signs in a variety of languages. |
| Ethnomed | Information on health care and cultures organized by clinical topic, culture, and language. Includes information for practitioners and patients. |
| U.S. Medical Eligibility Criteria for Contraceptive Use | Recommendations for contraception for postpartum patients, including differences based on breastfeeding/chestfeeding status. |

## References

1. ACOG Committee Opinion No. 736: optimizing postpartum care. *Obstet Gynecol*. 2018;131(5): e140-e150. doi:10.1097/AOG.0000000000002633.

2. Brown S, Herr J, Roy R, Klerman JA. Employee and worksite perspectives of the Family and Medical Leave Act: executive summary for results from the 2018 surveys. https://www.dol.gov/sites/dolgov/files /OASP/evaluation/pdf/WHD_FMLA2018Survey Results_ExecutiveSummary_Aug2020.pdf. Published 2020. Accessed August 28, 2021.

3. Flores JC. 12 months, 12 weeks, 1250 hours, 75 miles, and 50 employees: why the numbers of the FMLA don't add up for new parents of color and low-wage workers. *University of San Francisco Law Review*. 2020;54(2):313-337.

4. National Partnership for Women and Families. State paid family and medical leave insurance laws. https:// www.nationalpartnership.org/our-work/resources /economic-justice/paid-leave/state-paid-family-leave -laws.pdf. Published October 2022. Accessed May 13, 2023.

5. Organisation for Economic Co-operation and Development. OECD family database. https://www.oecd.org /els/soc/PF2_1_Parental_leave_systems.pdf. Updated December 2022. Accessed May 13, 2023.

6. Bullinger LR. The effect of paid family leave on infant and parental health in the United States. *J Health Econ.* 2019;66:101-116. doi:10.1016/j.jhealeco.2019.05.006.

7. Irish AM, White JS, Modrek S, Hamad R. Paid family leave and mental health in the U.S.: a quasi-experimental study of state policies. *Am J Prev Med.* 2021;61(2):182-191. doi:10.1016/j.amepre.2021.03.018.

8. Montoya-Williams D, Passarella M, Lorch SA. The impact of paid family leave in the United States on birth outcomes and mortality in the first year of life. *Health Serv Res.* 2020 Oct;55(Suppl 2):807-814. doi: 10.1111/1475-6773.13288. Epub 2020 Apr 5.

9. Collier AY, Molina RL. Maternal mortality in the United States: updates on trends, causes, and solutions. *Neoreviews.* 2019;20(10):e561-e574. doi:10.1542/neo.20-10-e561.

10. Prather C, Fuller TR, Marshall KJ, Jeffries WLT. The impact of racism on the sexual and reproductive health of African American women. *J Womens Health (Larchmt).* 2016;25(7):664-671. doi:10.1089/jwh.2015.5637.

11. Howell EA, Egorova NN, Balbierz A, et al. Site of delivery contribution to Black–white severe maternal morbidity disparity. *Am J Obstet Gynecol.* 2016;215(2):143-152. doi:10.1016/j.ajog.2016.05.007.

12. Howell EA, Egorova NN, Janevic T, et al. Severe maternal morbidity among Hispanic women in New York City: investigation of health disparities. *Obstet Gynecol.* 2017;129(2):285-294. doi:10.1097/aog.0000000000001864.

13. Howell EA, Padrón NA, Beane SJ, et al. Delivery and payment redesign to reduce disparities in high risk postpartum care. *Matern Child Health J.* 2017;21(3):432-438. doi:10.1007/s10995-016-2221-8.

14. Howell EA, Zeitlin J. Improving hospital quality to reduce disparities in severe maternal morbidity and mortality. *Semin Perinatol.* 2017;41(5):266-272. doi:10.1053/j.semperi.2017.04.002.

15. Dennis C-L, Fung K, Grigoriadis S, et al. Traditional postpartum practices and rituals: a qualitative systematic review. *Women's Health.* 2007;3(4):487-502. doi:10.2217/17455057.3.4.487.

16. Withers M, Kharazmi N, Lim E. Traditional beliefs and practices in pregnancy, childbirth and postpartum: a review of the evidence from Asian countries. *Midwifery.* 2018;56:158-170. doi:10.1016/j.midw.2017.10.019.

17. Altuntuğ K, Anık Y, Ege E. Traditional practices of mothers in the postpartum period: evidence from Turkey. *Afr J Reprod Health.* 2018;22(1):94-102.

18. Noble A, Rom M, Newsome-Wicks M, et al. Jewish laws, customs, and practice in labor, delivery, and postpartum Care. *J Transcult Nurs.* 2009;20(3):323-333. doi:10.1177/1043659609334930.

19. Grigoriadis S, Erlick Robinson G, Fung K, et al. Traditional postpartum practices and rituals: clinical implications. *Can J Psychiatry.* 2009;54(12):834-840. doi:10.1177/070674370905401206.

20. Coast E, Jones E, Lattof SR, Portela A. Effectiveness of interventions to provide culturally appropriate maternity care in increasing uptake of skilled maternity care: a systematic review. *Health Policy Plan.* 2016;31(10):1479-1491. doi:10.1093/heapol/czw065.

21. Hafford-Letchfield T, Cocker C, Rutter D, et al. What do we know about transgender parenting? Findings from a systematic review. *Health Soc Care Comm.* 2019;27(5):1111-1125. doi:10.1111/hsc.12759.

22. Casey LS, Reisner SL, Findling MG, et al. Discrimination in the United States: experiences of lesbian, gay, bisexual, transgender, and queer Americans. *Health Serv Res.* 2019;54(suppl 2):1454-1466. doi:10.1111/1475-6773.13229.

23. Ellis SA, Wojnar DM, Pettinato M. Conception, pregnancy, and birth experiences of male and gender variant gestational parents: it's how we could have a family. *J Midwifery Womens Health.* 2015;60(1):62-69.

24. MacLean LR-D. Preconception, pregnancy, birthing, and lactation needs of transgender men. *Nurs Womens Health.* 2021;25(2):129-138. doi:10.1016/j.nwh.2021.01.006.

25. McCann E, Brown M, Hollins-Martin C, et al. The views and experiences of LGBTQ+ people regarding midwifery care: a systematic review of the international evidence. *Midwifery.* 2021;103:103102. doi:10.1016/j.midw.2021.103102.

26. Kahalon R, Preis H, Shilo G, Benyamini Y. Maternal expectations among pregnant women from single, lesbian, and heterosexual parented families. *J Fam Iss.* 2021;42(4):863-880.

27. Klaus MH, Kennell JH. *Maternal–Infant Bonding: The Impact of Early Separation or Loss on Family Development.* St. Louis, MO: Mosby; 1976.

28. Bicking Kinsey C, Hupcey JE. State of the science of maternal–infant bonding: a principle-based concept analysis. *Midwifery.* 2013;29(12):1314-1320. doi:10.1016/j.midw.2012.12.019.

29. Widstrom AM, Lilja G, Aaltomaa-Michalias P, et al. Newborn behaviour to locate the breast when skin-to-skin: a possible method for enabling early self-regulation. *Acta Paediatr.* 2011;100(1):79-85. doi:10.1111/j.1651-2227.2010.01983.x.

30. Widström AM, Brimdyr K, Svensson K, et al. A plausible pathway of imprinted behaviors: skin-to-skin actions of the newborn immediately after birth follow the order of fetal development and intrauterine training

of movements. *Med Hypotheses.* 2020;134:109432. doi:10.1016/j.mehy.2019.109432.

31. Scatliffe N, Casavant S, Vittner D, Cong X. Oxytocin and early parent–infant interactions: a systematic review. *Int J Nurs Sci.* 2019;6(4):445-453. doi:10.1016/j.ijnss.2019.09.009.

32. Kim P. Human maternal brain plasticity: adaptation to parenting. *New Dir Child Adolesc Dev.* 2016; 2016(153):47-58. doi:10.1002/cad.20168.

33. Cleveland L, Hill CM, Pulse WS, et al. Systematic review of skin-to-skin care for full-term, healthy newborns. *J Obstet Gynecol Neonatal Nurs.* 2017;46(6): 857-869. https://doi.org/10.1016/j.jogn.2017.08.005.

34. Moore ER, Bergman N, Anderson GC, Medley N. Early skin-to-skin contact for mothers and their healthy newborn infants. *Cochrane Database Syst Rev.* 2016;11:CD003519. doi:10.1002/14651858. CD003519.pub4.

35. Guala A, Boscardini L, Visentin R, et al. Skin-to-skin contact in cesarean birth and duration of breastfeeding: a cohort study. *Sci World J.* 2017;2017:1940756. doi:10.1155/2017/1940756.

36. Erlandsson K, Dsilna A, Fagerberg I, Christensson K. Skin-to-skin care with the father after cesarean birth and its effect on newborn crying and prefeeding behavior. *Birth.* 2007;34(2):105-114. doi:10.1111 /j.1523-536X.2007.00162.x.

37. Vittner D, Butler S, Smith K, et al. Parent engagement correlates with parent and preterm infant oxytocin release during skin-to-skin contact. *Adv Neonatal Care.* 2019;19(1):73-79. doi:10.1097/anc .0000000000000558.

38. Yuksel B, Ital I, Balaban O, et al. Immediate breastfeeding and skin-to-skin contact during cesarean section decreases maternal oxidative stress: a prospective randomized case-controlled study. *J Matern Fetal Neonatal Med.* 2016;29(16):2691-2696. doi: 10.3109/14767058.2015.1101447.

39. Vittner D, McGrath J, Robinson J, et al. Increase in oxytocin from skin-to-skin contact enhances development of parent–infant relationship. *Biol Res Nurs.* 2018;20(1):54-62.doi:10.1177/1099800417735633.

40. Schorn MN, Moore E, Spetalnick BM, Morad A. Implementing family-centered cesarean birth. *J Midwifery Womens Health.* 2015;60(6):682-690. doi:10.1111/jmwh.12400.

41. Vischer LC, Heun X, Steetskamp J, et al. Birth experience from the perspective of the fathers. *Arch Gynecol Obstet.* 2020;302(5):1297-1303. doi:10 .1007/s00404-020-05714-z.

42. Persson EK, Fridlund B, Kvist LJ, Dykes AK. Fathers' sense of security during the first postnatal week: a qualitative interview study in Sweden. *Midwifery.* 2012;28(5):e697-e704. doi:10.1016/j.midw .2011.08.010.

43. Steen M, Downe S, Bamford N, Edozien L. Not-patient and not-visitor: a metasynthesis fathers' encounters with pregnancy, birth and maternity care. *Midwifery.* 2012;28(4):362-371. doi:10.1016/j.midw .2011.06.009.

44. McKelvey MM. The other mother: a narrative analysis of the postpartum experiences of nonbirth lesbian mothers. *Adv Nurs Sci.* 2014;37(2):101-116. doi:10.1097/ANS.0000000000000022.

45. Wojnar DM, Katzenmeyer A. Experiences of preconception, pregnancy, and new motherhood for lesbian nonbiological mothers. *J Obstet Gynecol Neonatal Nurs.* 2014;43(1):50-60. doi:10.1111/1552 -6909.12270.

46. Hildingsson I, Cederlof L, Widen S. Fathers' birth experience in relation to midwifery care. *Women Birth.* 2011;24(3):129-136. doi:10.1016/j.wombi.2010 .12.003.

47. Renfrew MJ, Dyson L, McCormick F, et al. Breastfeeding promotion for infants in neonatal units: a systematic review. *Child Care Health Dev.* 2010;36(2):165-178. doi:10.1111/j.1365-2214.2009.01018.x.

48. Berens P. Overview of the postpartum period: normal physiology and routine maternal care. *UpToDate.* https://www.uptodate.com/contents/overview-of -the-postpartum-period-normal-physiology-and -routine-maternal-care. Updated May 9, 2023. Accessed May 13, 2023.

49. Spencer J. Common problems of breastfeeding and weaning. *UpToDate.* https://www.uptodate.com /contents/common-problems-of-breastfeeding-and -weaning. Updated March 29, 2023. Accessed May 13, 2023.

50. Practice Bulletin No. 181: prevention of Rh D alloimmunization. *Obstet Gynecol.* 2017;130(2):e57-e70. doi:10.1097/aog.0000000000002232.

51. ACOG Committee Opinion No. 742: postpartum pain management. *Obstet Gynecol.* 2018;132(1): e35-e43. doi:10.1097/aog.0000000000002683.

52. Eshkevari L, Trout KK, Damore J. Management of postpartum pain. *J Midwifery Womens Health.* 2013;58(6):622-631. https://doi.org/10.1111/jmwh .12129.

53. East CE, Dorward EDF, Whale RE, Liu J. Local cooling for relieving pain from perineal trauma sustained during childbirth. *Cochrane Database Syst Rev.* 2020; 10. doi:10.1002/14651858.CD006304.pub4.

54. Roberts KL, Reiter M, Schuster D. A comparison of chilled and room temperature cabbage leaves in treating breast engorgement. *J Hum Lact.* 1995;11(3): 191-194. doi:10.1177/089033449501100319.

55. Dodd V, Chalmers C. Comparing the use of hydrogel dressings to lanolin ointment with lactating mothers. *J Obstet Gynecol Neonatal Nurs.* 2003;32(4): 486-494. doi:10.1177/0884217503255098.

56. Batten M, Stevenson E, Zimmermann D, Isaacs C. Implementation of a hydrotherapy protocol to improve postpartum pain management. *J Midwifery Womens Health*. 2017;62(2):210-214. doi:10.1111/jmwh.12580.

57. Wuytack F, Smith V, Cleary BJ. Oral non–steroidal anti–inflammatory drugs (single dose) for perineal pain in the early postpartum period. *Cochrane Database Syst Rev*. 2021;1. doi:10.1002/14651858.CD011352.pub3.

58. Abalos E, Sguassero Y, Gyte GML. Paracetamol/acetaminophen (single administration) for perineal pain in the early postpartum period. *Cochrane Database Syst Rev*. 2021;1. doi:10.1002/14651858.CD008407.pub3.

59. Deussen AR, Ashwood P, Martis R, et al. Relief of pain due to uterine cramping/involution after birth. *Cochrane Database Syst Rev*. 2020;10. doi:10.1002/14651858.CD004908.pub3.

60. Azar A. Renewal of determination that a public health emergency exists. Public Health Emergency. https://www.phe.gov/emergency/news/healthactions/phe/Pages/opioid-17jul2019.aspx. Published July 17, 2019. Accessed May 13, 2023.

61. Badreldin N, Grobman WA, Yee LM. Racial disparities in postpartum pain management. *Obstet Gynecol*. 2019;134(6):1147-1153. doi:10.1097/aog.0000000000003561.

62. Groenewald CB, Rabbitts JA, Hansen EE, Palermo TM. Racial differences in opioid prescribing for children in the United States. *Pain*. 2018;159(10):2050-2057. doi:10.1097/j.pain.0000000000001290.

63. Friedman J, Kim D, Schneberk T, et al. Assessment of racial/ethnic and income disparities in the prescription of opioids and other controlled medications in California. *JAMA Intern Med*. 2019;179(4):469-476. doi:10.1001/jamainternmed.2018.6721.

64. American College of Obstetricians and Gynecologists' Committee on Clinical Consensus–Obstetrics. Pharmacologic stepwise multimodal approach for postpartum pain management: ACOG Clinical Consensus No. 1. *Obstet Gynecol*. 2021;138(3):507-517. doi:10.1097/aog.0000000000004517.

65. Fahey JO. Best practices in panagement of postpartum pain. *J Perinat Neonatal Nurs*. 2017;31(2):126-136. doi:10.1097/jpn.0000000000000241.

66. U.S. Food and Drug Administration. FDA drug safety communication: FDA restricts use of prescription codeine pain and cough medicines and tramadol pain medicines in children; recommends against use in breastfeeding women. https://www.fda.gov/drugs/drug-safety-and-availability/fda-drug-safety-communication-fda-restricts-use-prescription-codeine-pain-and-cough-medicines-and. Published April 20, 2017. Accessed Spetember 4, 2021.

67. Koren G, Cairns J, Chitayat D, et al. Pharmacogenetics of morphine poisoning in a breastfed neonate of a codeine-prescribed mother. *Lancet*. 2006;368(9536):704. doi:10.1016/S0140-6736(06)69255-6.

68. Sachs HC, Committee on Drugs. The transfer of drugs and therapeutics into human breast milk: an update on selected topics. *Pediatrics*. 2013;132(3):e796-e809. doi:10.1542/peds.2013-1985.

69. Martin E, Vickers B, Landau R, Reece-Stremtan S. ABM Clinical Protocol #28: peripartum analgesia and anesthesia for the breastfeeding mother. *Breastfeed Med*. 2018;13(3):164-171. doi:10.1089/bfm.2018.29087.ejm.

70. Zakarija-Grkovic I, Stewart F. Treatments for breast engorgement during lactation. *Cochrane Database Syst Rev*. 2020;9:CD006946. doi:10.1002/14651858.CD006946.pub4.

71. García-Acosta JM, San Juan-Valdivia RM, Fernández-Martínez AD, et al. Trans pregnancy and lactation: a literature review from a nursing perspective. *Int J Environ Res Public Health*. 2019;17(1). Doi:10.3390/ijerph17010044.

72. Hedayati H, Parsons J, Crowther CA. Topically applied anaesthetics for treating perineal pain after childbirth. *Cochrane Database Syst Rev*. 2005;2. doi:10.1002/14651858.CD004223.pub2.

73. Malhotra A, Weinberger SE. Deep vein thrombosis in pregnancy: epidemiology, pathogenesis, and diagnosis. *UpToDate*. https://www.uptodate.com/contents/deep-vein-thrombosis-in-pregnancy-epidemiology-pathogenesis-and-diagnosis. Updated October 3, 2022. Accessed May 13, 2023.

74. ACOG Practice Bulletin No. 196: thromboembolism in pregnancy. *Obstet Gynecol*. 2018;132(1):e1-e17. doi:10.1097/aog.0000000000002706.

75. Berghella V. Cesarean birth: preoperative planning and patient preparation. *UpToDate*. https://www.uptodate.com/contents/cesarean-birth-preoperative-planning-and-patient-preparation. Updated January 31, 2023. Accessed May 13, 2023.

76. Berghella V. Cesarean birth: postoperative care, complications, and long-term sequelae. *UpToDate*. https://www.uptodate.com/contents/cesarean-birth-postoperative-care-complications-and-long-term-sequelae. Updated April 5, 2023. Accessed May 13, 2023.

77. Hsu YY, Hung HY, Chang SC, Chang YJ. Early oral intake and gastrointestinal function after cesarean delivery: a systematic review and meta-analysis. *Obstet Gynecol*. 2013;121(6):1327-1334. doi:10.1097/AOG.0b013e318293698c.

78. Huang H, Wang H, He M. Early oral feeding compared with delayed oral feeding after cesarean section: a meta-analysis. *J Matern Fetal Neonatal Med*. 2016;29(3):423-429. doi:10.3109/14767058.2014.1002765.

79. Auerbach M. Anemia in pregnancy. *UpToDate.* https://www.uptodate.com/contents/anemia-in-pregnancy. Updated May 1, 2023. Accessed May 13, 2023.

80. Bateman BT, Cole NM, Maeda A, et al. Patterns of opioid prescription and use after cesarean delivery. *Obstet Gynecol.* 2017;130(1):29-35. doi:10.1097/AOG.0000000000002093.

81. Declercq E, Sakala C, Corry M, et al. *Listening to Mothers III: New Mothers Speak Out.* New York, NY: Childbirth Connection; 2013.

82. ACOG Practice Bulletin No. 202: gestational hypertension and preeclampsia. *Obstet Gynecol.* 2019;133(1):1. doi:10.1097/AOG.0000000000003018.

83. Centers for Disease Control and Prevention. Urgent maternal warning signs. https://www.cdc.gov/hearher/maternal-warning-signs/index.html. Last reviewed November 17, 2022. Accessed May 13, 2023.

84. Woodley SJ, Lawrenson P, Boyle R, et al. Pelvic floor muscle training for preventing and treating urinary and faecal incontinence in antenatal and postnatal women. *Cochrane Database Syst Rev.* 2020;5. doi:10.1002/14651858.CD007471.pub4.

85. Citak N, Cam C, Arslan H, et al. Postpartum sexual function of women and the effects of early pelvic floor muscle exercises. *Acta Obstet Gynecol Scand.* 2010;89(6):817-822. doi:10.3109/00016341003801623.

86. Handelzalts JE, Levy S, Peled Y, et al. Mode of delivery, childbirth experience and postpartum sexuality. *Arch Gynecol Obstet.* 2018;297(4):927-932. doi:10.1007/s00404-018-4693-9.

87. Lopez LM, Hiller JE, Grimes DA. Postpartum education for contraception: a systematic review. *Obstet Gynecol Surv.* 2010;65(5):325-331. doi:10.1097/OGX.0b013e3181e57127.

88. Sonalkar S, Moody S. Postpartum contraception: counseling and methods. *UpToDate.* https://www.uptodate.com/contents/contraception-postpartum-counseling-and-methods. Updated August 15, 2022. Accessed May 13, 2023.

89. Bryant AG, Lyerly AD, DeVane-Johnson S, et al. Hormonal contraception, breastfeeding and bedside advocacy: the case for patient-centered care. *Contraception.* 2019;99(2):73-76. doi:10.1016/j.contraception.2018.10.011.

90. Curtis KM, Tepper NK, Jatlaoui TC, et al. U.S. medical eligibility criteria for contraceptive use, 2016. *MMWR Recomm Rep.* 2016;65(3):1-103. doi:10.15585/mmwr.rr6503a1.

91. World Health Organization. *Medical eligibilty criteria for contraceptive use.* http://apps.who.int/iris/bitstream/handle/10665/181468/9789241549158_eng.pdf?sequence=9. 2015. Accessed September 5, 2021.

92. Singata-Madliki M, Hofmeyr GJ, Lawrie TA. The effect of depot medroxyprogesterone acetate on postnatal depression: a randomised controlled trial. *J Fam Plann Reprod Health Care.* 2016;42(3):171-176. doi:10.1136/jfprhc-2015-101334.

93. Ti A, Curtis KM. Postpartum hormonal contraception use and incidence of postpartum depression: a systematic review. *Eur J Contracept Reprod Health Care.* 2019;24(2):109-116. doi:10.1080/13625187.2019.1569610.

94. Tepper NK, Curtis KM, Cox S, Whiteman MK. Update to U.S. medical eligibility criteria for contraceptive use, 2016: updated recommendations for the use of contraception among women at high risk for HIV infection. *MMWR.* 2020;69(14):405-410. doi:10.15585/mmwr.mm6914a3.

95. Contraceptives, oral, combined. *Drugs and Lactation Database (LactMed).* National Library of Medicine; 2006. https://www.ncbi.nlm.nih.gov/books/NBK501295/.

96. Brousseau EC, Danilack V, Cai F, Matteson KA. Emergency department visits for postpartum complications. *J Womens Health (Larchmt).* 2018;27(3):253-257. doi:10.1089/jwh.2016.6309.

97. World Health Organization. *WHO Recommendations on Postnatal Care of the Mother and Newborn.* Geneva, Switzerland: World Health Organization; 2014.

98. Brown HL, DeNicola N. Telehealth in maternity care. *Obstet Gynecol Clin North Am.* 2020;47(3):497-502. doi:10.1016/j.ogc.2020.05.003.

99. Goldstein KM, Gierisch JM, Zullig LL, et al. VA evidence-based synthesis program reports. In: *Telehealth Services Designed for Women: An Evidence Map.* Washington, DC: Department of Veterans Affairs; 2017.

100. Palmer MJ, Henschke N, Bergman H, et al. Targeted client communication via mobile devices for improving maternal, neonatal, and child health. *Cochrane Database Syst Rev.* 2020;8. doi:10.1002/14651858.CD013679.

101. Hauspurg A, Lemon LS, Quinn BA, et al. A postpartum remote hypertension monitoring protocol implemented at the hospital level. *Obstet Gynecol.* 2019;134(4):685-691. doi:10.1097/aog.0000000000003479.

102. Thomas NA, Drewry A, Racine Passmore S, et al. Patient perceptions, opinions and satisfaction of telehealth with remote blood pressure monitoring postpartum. *BMC Pregn Childbirth.* 2021;21(1):153. doi:10.1186/s12884-021-03632-9.

103. Hoppe KK, Thomas N, Zernick M, et al. Telehealth with remote blood pressure monitoring compared with standard care for postpartum hypertension. *Am J Obstet Gynecol.* 2020;223(4):585-588. doi:10.1016/j.ajog.2020.05.027.

104. Hussain-Shamsy N, Shah A, Vigod SN, et al. Mobile health for perinatal depression and anxiety: scoping review. *J Med Internet Res.* 2020;22(4):e17011. doi:10.2196/17011.

105. Handler A, Zimmermann K, Dominik B, Garland CE. Universal early home visiting: a strategy for reaching all postpartum women. *Matern Child Health J.* 2019;23(10):1414-1423. doi:10.1007/s10995-019 -02794-5.

106. ACOG Committee Opinion No. 757: screening for perinatal depression. *Obstet Gynecol.* 2018; 132(5):e208-e212. doi:10.1097/AOG.0000000000 002927.

107. Kroska EB, Stowe ZN. Postpartum depression: identification and treatment in the clinic setting. *Obstet Gynecol Clin North Am.* 2020;47(3): 409-419. doi:10.1016/j.ogc.2020.05.001.

108. Learman LA. Screening for depression in pregnancy and the postpartum period. *Clin Obstet Gynecol.* 2018;61(3):525-532. doi:10.1097/GRF.000000000 0000359.

109. *Physical Activity Guidelines for Americans.* 2nd ed. Washington, DC: U.S. Department of Health and Human Services; 2018. https://health.gov/sites /default/files/2019-09/Physical_Activity_Guidelines _2nd_edition.pdf. Accessed May 13, 2023.

110. ACOG Committee Opinion, Number 804: physical activity and exercise during pregnancy and the postpartum period. *Obstet Gynecol.* 2020;135(4): e178-e188. doi:10.1097/aog.0000000000003772.

111. Cary GB, Quinn TJ. Exercise and lactation: are they compatible? *Can J Appl Physiol.* 2001;26(1):55-75. doi:10.1139/h01-004.

112. Javadifar N, Majlesi F, Nikbakht A, et al. Journey to motherhood in the first year after child birth. *J Fam Reprod Health.* 2016;10(3):146-153.

113. Slomian J, Reginster JY, Emonts P, Bruyère O. Identifying maternal needs following childbirth: comparison between pregnant women and recent mothers. *BMC Pregn Childbirth.* 2021;21(1):405. doi:10.1186/s12884-021-03858-7.

114. Slomian J, Emonts P, Vigneron L, et al. Identifying maternal needs following childbirth: a qualitative study among mothers, fathers and professionals. *BMC Pregn Childbirth.* 2017;17(1):213. doi:10.1186/s12884-017-1398-1.

115. Bauman BL, Ko JY, Cox S, et al. Vital signs: postpartum depressive symptoms and provider discussions about perinatal depression—United States, 2018. *MMWR.* 2020;69(19):575-581. doi:10.15585/mmwr .mm6919a2.

116. Watson K, White C, Hall H, Hewitt A. Women's experiences of birth trauma: a scoping review. *Women Birth.* 2021;34(5):417-424. doi:10.1016/j .wombi.2020.09.016.

117. de Graaff LF, Honig A, van Pampus MG, Stramrood CAI. Preventing post-traumatic stress disorder following childbirth and traumatic birth experiences: a systematic review. *Acta Obstet Gynecol Scand.* 2018;97(6):648-656. doi:10.1111/aogs.13291.

118. Wijma K, Wijma B, Zar M. Psychometric aspects of the W-DEQ; a new questionnaire for the measurement of fear of childbirth. *J Psychosom Obstet Gynaecol.* 1998;19(2):84-97. doi:10.3109/01674829809048501.

119. Rouhe H, Salmela-Aro K, Toivanen R, et al. Obstetric outcome after intervention for severe fear of childbirth in nulliparous women: randomised trial. *BJOG.* 2013;120(1):75-84. doi:10.1111/1471-0528 .12011.

120. Azagba S, Manzione L, Shan L, King J. Trends in smoking during pregnancy by socioeconomic characteristics in the United States, 2010–2017. *BMC Pregn Childbirth.* 2020;20(1):52. doi:10.1186 /s12884-020-2748-y.

121. Tong VT, Dietz PM, Morrow B, et al. Trends in smoking before, during, and after pregnancy— Pregnancy Risk Assessment Monitoring System, United States, 40 sites, 2000–2010. *MMWR Surveill Summ.* 2013;62(6):1-19.

122. Mullen PD. How can more smoking suspension during pregnancy become lifelong abstinence? Lessons learned about predictors, interventions, and gaps in our accumulated knowledge. *Nicotine Tob Res.* 2004;6(suppl 2):S217-S238. doi:10.1080/1462 2200410001669150.

123. Kia F, Tosun N, Carlson S, Allen S. Examining characteristics associated with quitting smoking during pregnancy and relapse postpartum. *Addict Behav.* 2018;78:114-119. doi:10.1016/j.addbeh.2017.11 .011.

124. Livingstone-Banks J, Norris E, Hartmann-Boyce J, et al. Relapse prevention interventions for smoking cessation. *Cochrane Database Syst Rev.* 2019;10. doi:10.1002/14651858.CD003999.pub6.

125. Baraona LK, Lovelace D, Daniels JL, McDaniel L. Tobacco harms, nicotine pharmacology, and pharmacologic tobacco cessation interventions for women. *J Midwifery Womens Health.* 2017;62(3):253-269. doi:10.1111/jmwh.12616.

126. Substance Abuse and Mental Health Services Administration. Key substance use and mental health indicators in the United States: results from the 2018 National Survey on Drug Use and Health. https:// www.samhsa.gov/data/sites/default/files/cbhsq -reports/NSDUHNationalFindingsReport2018 /NSDUHNationalFindingsReport2018.pdf. 2019. Accessed September 13, 2021.

127. U.S. Preventive Services Task Force. Screening for unhealthy drug use: US Preventive Services Task Force recommendation statement. *JAMA.* 2020; 323(22):2301-2309. doi:10.1001/jama.2020.8020.

128. Schiff DM, Nielsen T, Terplan M, et al. Fatal and nonfatal overdose among pregnant and postpartum women in Massachusetts. *Obstet Gynecol.* 2018; 132(2):466-474. doi:10.1097/aog.000000000000 2734.

129. Wilder C, Lewis D, Winhusen T. Medication-assisted treatment discontinuation in pregnant and postpartum women with opioid use disorder. *Drug Alcohol Depend.* 2015;149:225-231. doi:10.1016/j .drugalcdep.2015.02.012.

130. Tebeka S, De Premorel Higgons A, Dubertret C, Le Strat Y. Changes in alcohol use and heavy episodic drinking in U.S. women of childbearing-age and peripartum between 2001–2002 and 2012–2013. *Addict Behav.* 2020;107:106389. doi:10.1016/j .addbeh.2020.106389.

131. Gibson L, Porter M. Drinking or smoking while breastfeeding and later cognition in children. *Pediatrics.* 2018;142(2):e20174266. doi:10.1542/peds .2017-4266.

132. Anderson PO. Alcohol use during breastfeeding. *Breastfeed Med.* 2018;13(5):315-317. doi:10.1089 /bfm.2018.0053.

133. Allen AM, Jung AM, Alexander AC, et al. Cannabis use and stressful life events during the perinatal period: cross-sectional results from Pregnancy Risk Assessment Monitoring System (PRAMS) data, 2016. *Addiction.* 2020;115(9):1707-1716. doi:10.1111/add.15003.

134. Barbosa-Leiker C, Burduli E, Smith CL, et al. Daily cannabis use during pregnancy and postpartum in a state with legalized recreational cannabis. *J Addict Med.* 2020;14(6):467-474. doi:10.1097 /adm.0000000000000625.

135. Bayrampour H, Zahradnik M, Lisonkova S, Janssen P. Women's perspectives about cannabis use during pregnancy and the postpartum period: an integrative review. *Prev Med.* 2019;119:17-23. doi:10.1016/j.ypmed.2018.12.002.

136. Young-Wolff KC, Gali K, Sarovar V, et al. Women's questions about perinatal cannabis use and health care providers' responses. *J Womens Health (Larchmt).* 2020;29(7):919-926. doi:10.1089/jwh .2019.8112.

137. Cannabis. *Drugs and Lactation Database (LactMed).* National Library of Medicine; 2006. https:// www.ncbi.nlm.nih.gov/books/NBK501587/.

138. Navarrete F, García-Gutiérrez MS, Gasparyan A, et al. Cannabis use in pregnant and breastfeeding women: behavioral and neurobiological consequences. *Front Psychiatry.* 2020;11:586447. doi:10.3389/fpsyt .2020.586447.

139. Committee Opinion No. 711: opioid use and opioid use disorder in pregnancy. *Obstet Gynecol.* 2017; 130(2):e81-e94. doi:10.1097/aog.000000000000 2235.

140. Renbarger KM, Shieh C, Moorman M, et al. Health care encounters of pregnant and postpartum women with substance use disorders. *West J Nurs Res.* 2020; 42(8):612-628. doi:10.1177/0193945919893372.

141. Leftwich HK, Alves MV. Adolescent pregnancy. *Pediatr Clin North Am.* 2017;64(2):381-388. doi: 10.1016/j.pcl.2016.11.007.

142. Allen S, Barlow E. Long-acting reversible contraception: an essential guide for pediatric primary care providers. *Pediatr Clin North Am.* 2017;64(2): 359-369. https://doi.org/10.1016/j.pcl.2016.11.014.

143. Oberhelman-Eaton S, Chang A, Gonzalez C, et al. Initiation of gender-affirming testosterone therapy in a lactating transgender man. *J Hum Lact.* 2021: 8903344211037646. doi:10.1177/089033442110 37646.

144. Light A, Wang LF, Zeymo A, Gomez-Lobo V. Family planning and contraception use in transgender men. *Contraception.* 2018;98(4):266-269. doi:10.1016/j .contraception.2018.06.006.

145. Martin J, Hamilton B, Osterman M, Driscoll A. Births: final data for 2019. *Natl Vital Stat Rep.* 2021;70. https://www.cdc.gov/nchs/data/nvsr/nvsr70 /nvsr70-02-508.pdf. Accessed September 13, 2021.

146. Roque ATF, Lasiuk GC, Radünz V, Hegadoren K. Scoping review of the mental health of parents of infants in the NICU. *J Obstet Gynecol Neonatal Nurs.* 2017;46(4):576-587. doi:10.1016/j.jogn.2017 .02.005.

147. Craig JW, Glick C, Phillips R, et al. Recommendations for involving the family in developmental care of the NICU baby. *J Perinatol.* 2015;35(suppl 1): S5-S8. doi:10.1038/jp.2015.142.

148. Haward MF, Lantos J, Janvier A, POST Group. Helping parents cope in the NICU. *Pediatrics.* 2020; 145(6):e20193567. doi:10.1542/peds.2019-3567.

149. Treyvaud K, Spittle A, Anderson PJ, O'Brien K. A multilayered approach is needed in the NICU to support parents after the preterm birth of their infant. *Early Hum Dev.* 2019;139:104838. doi:10.1016/j .earlhumdev.2019.104838.

150. Foli KJ, Hebdon M, Lim E, South SC. Transitions of adoptive parents: a longitudinal mixed methods analysis. *Arch Psychiatr Nurs.* 2017;31(5):483-492. doi:10.1016/j.apnu.2017.06.007.

151. Paynter MJ, Drake EK, Cassidy C, Snelgrove-Clarke E. Maternal health outcomes for incarcerated women: a scoping review. *J Clin Nurs.* 2019;28(11-12): 2046-2060. doi:10.1111/jocn.14837.

152. Kwarteng-Amaning V, Svoboda J, Bachynsky N, Linthicum L. An alternative to mother and infants behind bars: How one prison nursery program impacted attachment and nurturing for mothers who gave birth while incarcerated. *J Perinat Neonatal Nurs.* 2019;33(2):116-125. doi:10.1097/jpn.000000 0000000398.

# A P P E N D I X

# 34A

---

# Management of the Fourth Stage of Labor Following Vaginal Birth

ABIGAIL HOWE-HEYMAN

*The editors acknowledge Ira Kantrowitz-Gordon, who was the author of this appendix in the previous edition.*

---

## Physical Examination and Management

### Vital Signs

Check the patient's vital signs every 5 to 15 minutes. If the patient's condition or bleeding pattern changes, assess vital signs more frequently.

### Bleeding

The majority of postpartum hemorrhages occur during the fourth stage of labor. Evaluate vaginal bleeding every 5 to 15 minutes immediately after birth of the newborn or more frequently as indicated by changes in the patient's condition and bleeding pattern.

### Uterus

Evaluate the uterus for position and tone every 5 to 15 minutes if there is no excessive bleeding that suggests a need for more frequent evaluation.

- *Position.* Assess the uterus by abdominal palpation; it is usually midline in the middle of the abdomen, between the symphysis pubis and the umbilicus. If the uterus is above the umbilicus or significantly deviated to one side of the umbilicus, blood clots may be filling in the uterus or the uterus may be displaced by a full bladder. Emptying of the bladder should be considered, followed by fundal massage and administration of uterotonics if the uterus remains displaced.

- *Tone.* The uterus should be firm to the touch and immediately identifiable. A soft, boggy uterus that is difficult to palpate is not well contracted. Gentle massage of the uterus through the abdomen can promote uterine contraction and should be performed if the uterus is not firm. Assess for postpartum hemorrhage and the presence of blood or clots in the uterus if the uterus does not become firm following abdominal massage. Re-inspect the placenta and membranes to note any missing tissue that may be retained in the uterus. Consider the use of oxytocin followed by additional uterotonic medications if the uterus does not remain firm.

### Bladder

Assess the bladder immediately after the third stage and at least 30 minutes after birth for distension and urinary retention. Review the time of the last void or catheterization, palpate for tenderness or distension, and consider a bladder scan. A distended bladder can cause increased uterine bleeding, since the uterus is unable to contract when the bladder is full and displacing it. A patient who has not received regional anesthesia usually can void spontaneously. If the patient has had regional anesthesia, they may need urinary catheterization to empty the bladder.

### Perineum

Inspect the vagina and perineum for lacerations, bruising, or early hematoma formation immediately after the conclusion of the third stage of labor. Edema or bruising at the introitus or throughout the perineal area should be noted and documented. Repair lacerations as needed. Inspection of the cervix is indicated only if a cervical laceration is suspected.

## Additional Assessments and Care Practices

- Encourage skin-to-skin placement of the newborn following birth, which allows patients to notice when the newborn is beginning to root.

- Help the patient into a position to promote newborn latch if planning to breastfeed/chestfeed.

- Count any needles used to ensure that all sharps are disposed of safely. Remove any sharps from the sterile field.

- Count any gauze used to ensure that no gauze is inadvertently left in the vagina.

- Clean the patient and replace bed sheets and blankets as needed.

- A perineal pad or ice pack may be placed against the perineum to reduce edema and provide pain relief. An ice pack may be placed next to the perineum intermittently for the first 24 hours after birth.

- Assess for comfort. A short period of tremor not associated with infection can be common in the fourth stage of labor and can be relieved with warm blankets, reassurance, and relaxation techniques.

- Provide a nonsteroidal anti-inflammatory drug (NSAID) for pain relief and prevention of perineal swelling and pain.

- Assess intake and encourage intake of oral fluids and a meal if all vital signs and bleeding are stable.

- Promote and support family bonding.

APPENDIX

# 34B

# History and Physical Examination During the Postpartum Period

ABIGAIL HOWE-HEYMAN

*The editors acknowledge Ira Kantrowitz-Gordon, who was the author of this appendix in the previous edition.*

The needs of the postpartum patient change over the course of the postpartum period. Given this reality, this appendix presents the care of the postpartum patient in the early postpartum period, the mid-postpartum period, and the comprehensive postpartum visit.

## Early Postpartum Care (0 to 3 Days)

As in all encounters with patients, as assessment begins with a review of the patient's health record, to identify any new issues that may have arisen since the patient's last contact with the midwife (Table 34B-1).

After the chart review, an interval history is conducted (Table 34B-2), focusing on the patient's priorities and concerns, and then moving into education and anticipatory guidance, as appropriate.

Physical examinations during the immediate postpartum period, like any examination, begin with performing a personal greeting, ascertaining if the moment is an appropriate time for the examination, and adapting the environment to provide comfort and privacy. Throughout the examination, the midwife can integrate teaching, and provide anticipatory guidance. Table 34B-3 summarizes the procedure for a postpartum physical examination. The order of the exam may be modified to meet the patient's comfort and to minimize position changes, but all areas should be assessed. Table 34B-4 provides an example of a SOAP note for documentation of a visit during the early postpartum period.

| Table 34B-1 | Elements of Chart Review in the Early Postpartum Period |
|---|---|
| **Category** | **Specific Information to Review** |
| Visits with clinicians | Review notes from midwives, nurses, medical team, consultants, lactation consultants, social workers, and other members of the interdisciplinary team. |
| Vital signs | Review vital signs over the course of the postpartum period, making note of any abnormalities or trends. |
| Flow sheets | Review input and output, blood loss, and any other objective data that have been collected over the postpartum period. |
| Lab values | Review complete blood count, rubella, coronavirus disease 2019 (COVID-19), blood type, and human immunodeficiency virus (HIV) test results. |
| Newborn lab values | Review cord blood type and fetal cell screen. |
| Medications | Review pre-pregnancy and prenatal medications and their resumption in the postpartum period. Review pain medication use in the postpartum period. |

| Table 34B-2 | Interval History in the Early Postpartum Period |
|---|---|
| **Category** | **Specific Information to Review** |
| Healthcare encounters | Communication with consultants |
| Adjustment | Thoughts on and questions about the labor and birth |
| | Emotional changes |
| | Physical activity level |
| | Confidence in newborn care |
| General physical health | Food and fluid intake |
| | Sleep quality and quantity |
| | Pain and medication use |
| | Fever or chills |
| | Headaches with description if present |
| Breasts/chest | Breast/chest filling, engorgement, nipple condition, pain, masses |
| | Latch assessment |
| | Signs of satiety |
| | Feeding frequency and success |
| Abdomen | Abdominal pain, cramping, epigastric pain |
| Gastrointestinal | Bowel function, frequency of bowel movements, constipation, incontinence |
| Urinary | Urinary pain or incontinence, urgency |
| Ano-genital | Lochia amount, color, and odor |
| | Episodes of excessive bleeding |
| | Perineal pain, swelling, or redness |
| | Hemorrhoids |
| Lower extremities | Edema, pain, redness, varicosities |
| Chronic conditions | Change in signs or symptoms |
| | Medication changes |
| | Follow-up with specialist |
| Contraception | Contraceptive desired and timing for initiation |
| | Past contraceptive experience |
| Exercise | Pelvic floor exercises |
| | Resumption of activity |
| Mental health | Signs or symptoms of postpartum mood disorder |
| | Resumption of mental health medications |
| Postoperative issues | Pain management |
| | Ambulation or use of pneumatic compression devices |
| Hypertension follow-up for patients with history of hypertensive disorders of pregnancy | Headache |
| | Visual disturbances |
| | Nausea/vomiting |
| | Epigastric pain |
| | Medications for hypertension and seizure prevention |

| Table 34B-3 | Postpartum Physical Examination in the Early Postpartum Period: Procedure and Expected Findings | | |
|---|---|---|---|
| | **Procedure** | **Expected Findings** | **Signs of Possible Complications** |
| General | Observe general affect, mobility, and signs of pain or splinting. | Tired, ambulatory without assistance, repeating birth events, usually happy | Inability to ambulate without assistance; sad or teary; reporting pain |
| Vital signs | Assess temperature, blood pressure, pulse, and respiratory rate. | Temperature: normal or low-grade elevation | Temperature: > 38°C (100.4°F) |
| | | Blood pressure: returns to patient's pre-pregnancy baseline | Blood pressure: higher than 140/90 mm Hg or lower than 85/60 mm Hg |
| | | Pulse: 65–80 beats/min at rest | Pulse: higher than 100 beats/min |
| | | Respirations: 12–16 breaths/min at rest | |
| Neurologic | | Oriented to person, place, and time | Disorientation |
| | | Not in apparent pain | Excessively sedated or somnolent, unable to easily awaken |
| | | Normal movements and speech | Excessive or unexplained pain or restlessness |
| | | Normal reflexes | Headache that has sudden onset, is severe, is unresolved with acetaminophen or ibuprofen, or is positional, resolving while lying flat. |
| Skin | Assessed throughout the exam | No immediate changes. | Pallor |
| | | Hyperpigmentation may be retained but will fade with time. Striae, spider nevi, capillary hemangiomas, varicosities, and skin tags regress but may not completely disappear. | Reactions to tape on back or arms |
| | | | Atypical bruising |
| | | Presence of an intravenous or epidural catheter should be noted. | |
| Cardiovascular | The examination of the heart and lungs during the puerperium is performed in the same manner as when the patient is not pregnant. Auscultate the heart (rate, rhythm, cardiac sounds). <br> • Systolic ejection murmur persists past the first week of puerperium in 20% of patients. <br> • Heart rate decreases to the nonpregnant level within 10 days postpartum. | No chest pain. Some patients feel heartbeat increasing with minimal activity. <br> Regular rate and rhythm | Tachycardia |

*(continues)*

| Table 34B-3 | Postpartum Physical Examination in the Early Postpartum Period: Procedure and Expected Findings (*continued*) | | |
|---|---|---|---|
| | **Procedure** | **Expected Findings** | **Signs of Possible Complications** |
| Lungs/pulmonary | Auscultate the lungs and percuss as appropriate (the midwife may assist the patient to a sitting position for evaluation of the inferior lobes).<br>• Respiratory rate decreases to the nonpregnant rate within the first postpartum week. | No shortness of breath or difficulty breathing<br>Clear to auscultation | Shortness of breath<br>Adventitious sounds<br>Diminished breath sounds or crackles in the lung base suggest pulmonary edema or pneumonia. |
| Breasts/chest[a] | Observe breasts/chest for symmetry.<br>• Palpate to assess engorgement if present.<br>• Palpate axilla to assess for accessory mammary tissue.<br>• Inspect the nipple epithelium for erythema, bruising, petechiae, and cracks or bleeding.<br>• Observe the integrity of the areola and inspect for blisters or cracks. | Neonate is nursing frequently with a good latch. Shows signs of satiety such as relaxed head and face; appears content.<br>Nipples sore, but not painful<br>Colostrum for 3–5 days<br>Soft for 1–2 days; some fullness beginning days 3–5<br>Soft swelling in the axilla may be evidence of accessory mammary tissue that can cause discomfort, but is otherwise benign | Neonate is not latching well or frequently. Agitated or unsettled between feeds.<br>Painful nipples<br>No breast/chest filling by days 4–5<br>Nipples: flat, inverted, cracked, bruised, blistered, or bleeding<br>Breasts/chest: erythema, engorged |
| Abdomen/gastrointestinal | Assess bowel sounds.<br>Postoperative patients: Examine surgical incision, using REEDA to evaluate healing.[b] | Eating and drinking without difficulty.<br>Bowel movements usually return after 2–3 days.<br>Nontender, nondistended; bowel sounds present; muscle tone is decreased<br>Postoperative patients: Incision is dry and intact, no diffuse erythema, no exudate. | Nausea or vomiting, abdominal pain, constipation, or diarrhea<br>Distended, tender, or no bowel sounds<br>Postoperative patients: Erythema, purulent drainage, foul odor. |
| Abdomen—diastasis recti | Request that the patient lift their head onto their chest while the midwife simultaneously palpates the center of the abdomen to assess the degree of separation of the rectus abdominis (rectus diastasis). Determine the size of the separation in centimeters or fingerbreadths for later documentation. | Diastasis recti is an expected finding. | |
| Fundus | Position the patient in supine position.<br>Palpate the fundus abdominally and verify its location.<br>Immediately after birth, the fundus is several centimeters below the umbilicus. | Fundus firm, nontender, midline, height normal for postpartum day<br>Uterine contractions/cramping particularly with nursing | Increasing fundal height, deviation from midline, or tender to palpation |

| | Procedure | Expected Findings | Signs of Possible Complications |
|---|---|---|---|
| | About 12 hours after the birth, the fundus rises to just above or below the umbilicus.<br><br>The fundus recedes by approximately 1 cm/day for the first week.<br><br>Deviations may exist if the patient is at extremes of height or weight. | | |
| Urinary | Palpate the suprapubic area to rule out distended bladder.<br>• There is a high index of suspicion that the bladder is full if the uterus is displaced upward and to one side.<br>Assess for urinary retention and symptoms of infection.<br>Assess for CVAT. | Voiding spontaneously, diuresis, and natriuresis normal, especially between days 2 and 5<br><br>Mild external burning, some retention and/or incontinence, and lack of sensation or urge to void are common in the first 2 days postpartum if the patient had epidural analgesia, an operative vaginal birth, or extensive perineal trauma, but should resolve rapidly.<br><br>Tender or sore at area of repair<br><br>Bladder: nondistended—not palpable | Pelvic pressure or pain increasing<br><br>Persistent retention or incontinence<br><br>Bladder: distended<br><br>Costovertebral angle tenderness |
| Lower extremities | Observe for unilateral calf tenderness, erythema, or swelling that may suggest deep vein thrombosis.[c]<br><br>If one calf is larger, measure the difference in circumference in centimeters. | No pain<br><br>Generalized muscle soreness<br><br>Edema is common<br><br>Reflexes normal | Pain, aching, or swelling, particularly in one leg<br><br>Deep calf tenderness, one calf larger in circumference than the other, heat, varicosities that are erythematous and/or painful on palpation |
| Perineum | Because it is likely that the midwife will come in contact with body fluids, most clinicians defer examination of the perineum until after assessment of the patient's extremities. Then don nonsterile gloves.<br>• Obtain adequate visualization with good lighting (using a flashlight or penlight as needed).<br>• Ask the patient to lie on their side:<br>  ◆ Choose the side based on the patient's comfort and the layout of the room.<br>  ◆ A lateral view and gentle elevation of the upper buttocks allow visualization of the posterior aspect of the repair and the anus. | Perineum: mild erythema, edema, or bruising may be present<br><br>Repair: approximated without drainage<br><br>Lochia: amount decreasing, color, odor | Perineum: increasing tenderness, erythema, edema, bruising<br><br>Laceration repair: separation of repair, suppuration, or excessive edema, signs of hematoma<br><br>Lochia: increase over previous amount, malodor, clots, soaked or overflowing pads |

*(continues)*

| Table 34B-3 | **Postpartum Physical Examination in the Early Postpartum Period: Procedure and Expected Findings** (*continued*) | | |
|---|---|---|---|
| | **Procedure** | **Expected Findings** | **Signs of Possible Complications** |
| | • Observe the patient for discomfort throughout the examination.<br>• Consider use of a large mirror to show the patient the perineum if they desire.<br>• If laceration or episiotomy is present, inspect the full length of the suture line using the REEDA scale for later documentation.[b]<br>  ◆ If signs of a hematoma are present, use a gloved hand to palpate gently with thumb and forefinger to distinguish between normal edema and hematoma. Signs of hematoma include unilateral labial swelling, black/blueish area of erythema, report of vaginal or rectal pressure, or sudden onset of severe pain.<br>• Evaluate lochia on a sanitary pad, observing the color and extent of saturation and noting the length of time since the pad was changed. | | |
| Anus | Assess for presence or absence of hemorrhoids.<br>• If needed, discard the soiled pad and provide a new one to the patient.<br>Discard used gloves, and perform hand hygiene. | Normal in appearance<br>Hemorrhoids: pink, soft, mildly tender | Hemorrhoids: deep blue/purple, firm, very painful |
| Laboratory values[1] | Hemoglobin and hematocrit testing should be individualized to the patient.<br>Hemoglobin testing is recommended for patients with:<br>• Prenatal anemia<br>• History of postpartum hemorrhage<br>• Symptoms of anemia (lightheadedness, dizziness, shortness of breath<br>• Estimated quantitative blood loss of ≥ 500 mL | Hemoglobin decreases slightly in the first 24 hours after birth, then plateaus for 4 days, followed by a slow rise to day 14.<br>WBC count falls to 6000–10,000/mm$^3$, then returns to normal values by 6 days. | A 500-mL blood loss will usually result in approximately a 1-g reduction in hemoglobin or 3% reduction in hematocrit.<br>These values return to normal by 4–6 weeks postpartum. |

| Procedure | Expected Findings | Signs of Possible Complications |
|---|---|---|
| WBC and differential tests should be ordered only when there is a clinical suspicion of infection.<br><br>Review the patient's blood type and the newborn's blood type. | If the patient is Rh negative and the newborn is Rh positive:<br><br>• Review the screening test for fetomaternal bleeding.<br><br>• The rosette test is a qualitative test to identify fetomaternal bleeding.<br><br>With a negative rosette test, the standard dose (300 mcg) of anti-D immune globulin should be given within 72 hours of the birth. | If the rosette test is positive, a quantitative fetal cell assay (Kleinhauer–Betke) test should be ordered to determine the appropriate dosage of anti-D immune globulin.<br><br>The percentage of fetal RBCs determined by the fetal cell assay is multiplied by 50 to estimate the volume of the fetomaternal hemorrhage.<br><br>The volume is then divided by 30 to determine the number of vials of anti-D immune globulin that should be administered. Consultation with a blood bank pathologist is recommended to calculate the total dose. |

Abbreviations: CVAT, costovertebral angle for tenderness; RBCs, red blood cells; REEDA, redness, ecchymosis, edema, discharge/drainage, and approximation; WBC, white blood cell.

[a] During the phases of lactogenesis, the breast/chest consistency may be soft, filling (i.e., tense, increasing firmness, slightly enlarged), or engorged (i.e., enlarged, hard, reddened, shiny; skin temperature elevated; painful, dilated veins).

[b] The REEDA scale provides a mnemonic for documentation of healing lacerations or incisions. This midwife-developed instrument was created to provide a standard description of perineal healing, but today it is used widely for documentation of any healing incision. Although a scoring system has been used with this scale in the past, today most midwives use descriptors for each component.[2]

[c] Evaluation of the extremities has previously included foot dorsiflexion (Homan's sign) to assess for deep vein thrombosis (DVT). This test is not diagnostic and could theoretically loosen a thrombus that might be present. Therefore, Homan's sign is no longer recommended. DVT is increased 60-fold in the first 3 months postpartum compared with patients who are not pregnant or postpartum.[3] Other signs that are more predictive of DVT than a positive Homan's sign include unilateral calf tenderness, erythema, and swelling.

| Table 34B-4 | Sample SOAP Note for the Early Postpartum Visit |
|---|---|

32-year-old cis female G3P1011 patient at 14 hours post-elective repeat cesarean birth with estimated blood loss of 1200 mL. Pregnancy complicated by gestational hypertension. Breastfeeding.

Current pain management regimen:

• Received one dose of ketorolac 60 mg IM immediately after surgery

• Acetaminophen 1000 mg every 6 hours

• Ibuprofen 800 mg every 6 hours—beginning at 12 hours after ketorolac administration

• Hydromorphone immediate-release tablet 2 mg every 4–6 hours as needed. Patient has taken one dose at 13 hours postpartum.

S:

• General: Reports slept well overnight, woke at 5 A.M. when baby cried, partner at bedside, assisting with newborn care. Has been out of bed to the bathroom × 2, No hallway ambulation yet. Started regular diet last night—well tolerated. Pain 3/10 at rest, 5/10 with ambulation; patient is satisfied with pain management regimen.

• Breasts: Reports infant breastfeeding every 2–3 hours, no nipple tenderness or pain with latch. States infant seems satisfied after feeding with periods of rest between feeding sessions. Using football hold due to postsurgical pain.

• Abdomen: Denies epigastric pain, nausea/vomiting.

• GI: + flatus, no bowel movement, some bloating.

(continues)

| Table 34B-4 | Sample SOAP Note for the Early Postpartum Visit (*continued*) |
|---|---|

- GU: Voiding every 2–3 hours since Foley removal at 6 hours post surgery.
- Ano-genital: Reports scant lochia rubra, changing pads with every void. No perineal pain, no hemorrhoids.
- Lower extremities: +2 pitting edema, no erythema, no pain.
- Neuro: Denies headache, no visual changes.

**O:**

- Labs: hemoglobin/hematocrit: 10.6/ 30.3; white blood cells: 18,000; platelets: 160,000. A+ blood type.
- General: Well-appearing, interacting with infant and partner, excited for visit by older sibling today.
- VS: Blood pressure, 138/85; pulse, 72; respiratory rate, 16; temperature, 97.4°F.
- Neuro: Alert and oriented × 3, deep tendon reflexes 2+.
- Skin: Slight pallor, good skin turgor. IV catheter w/heparin lock in right hand.
- CV: Heart: regular rate and rhythm, no murmurs.
- Lungs: Clear to auscultation bilaterally.
- Breasts: Soft, nipples intact, no bruising. Observed infant breastfeeding—noted good latch, audible swallow.
- Abdomen: Soft, nondistended. + bowel sounds in all four quadrants. Incision dry and intact, no erythema, no exudate. Staples in place. Dressing removed. Diastasis recti = 2 fingerbreadths.
- Fundus: Firm at umbilicus. Midline.
- GU: Bladder nonpalpable abdominally, no costovertebral angle tenderness.
- Ano-genital: Scant lochia rubra, no perineal swelling or pain, no hemorrhoids.

**A:** 32 year- old G3P1011 at 14 hours post-cesarean birth with postpartum hemorrhage and history of gestational hypertension, now resolving. Stable. Breastfeeding without complications.

**P:**

- Routine postoperative care.
- Labs: Complete blood count in the morning to evaluate hemoglobin and hematocrit.
- Encouraged frequent ambulation; discussed signs and symptoms of deep vein thrombosis and importance of sequential compression devices when not ambulating.
- Reviewed signs and symptoms of worsening preeclampsia/gestational hypertension and what to do if they occur.
- Reviewed signs and symptoms of postpartum hemorrhage and what to do if they occur.
- Discussed contraception plans. Patient plans to use lactational amenorrhea method for 6 weeks, then will have copper IUD inserted at 6-week postpartum visit.
- Reviewed importance of high-iron diet.
- Medications: Continue with current pain management regimen, prenatal vitamins.
- Will visit again tomorrow. Plan to discharge to home on post-surgical day 3.

## Care in the Mid-Postpartum Period (72 Hours to 4 Weeks)

All patients can benefit from contact with their midwife in the mid-postpartum period, and both the American College of Obstetricians and Gynecologists (ACOG)[4] and the World Health Organization (WHO)[5] strongly recommend that all patients receive care at 7 to 14 days after the birth. Beyond this recommendation, patients at high risk for postpartum complications must be seen during this time as part of their ongoing care. The location and mode of contact can vary from in-person, to telehealth, to telephone contact, based on the patient's individual needs. The components of the interval history in the mid-postpartum period are included in Table 34B-5.

A physical assessment is not necessary for all patients in the mid-postpartum period; instead, the type of physical assessment will be dictated by the patient's needs. For patients without risk factors, education and counseling are frequently sufficient at this time in the puerperium. Table 34B-6 outlines the physical assessment requirements for high-risk patients.

| Table 34B-5 | Interval History in the Mid-Postpartum Period |
|---|---|
| **Category** | **Specific Information to Review** |
| Healthcare encounters | Calls to the midwife or the physician |
| | Visits to the hospital emergency department |
| | Hospital admissions |
| | Communication with consultants |
| Adjustment | Thoughts on and questions about the labor and birth |
| | Emotional changes |
| | Coping with life changes and response to newborn |
| | Social support and help with household chores |
| | Physical activity level |
| | Family adjustment to newborn |
| | Confidence in newborn care |
| | Intimate-partner violence screening |
| General physical health | Food and fluid intake |
| | Sleep quality and quantity |
| | Fever or chills |
| | Headaches with description if present |
| | Medications—for new or chronic conditions and use of prenatal vitamins or iron supplements. |
| Chronic conditions | Change in signs/symptoms |
| | Medication changes |
| | Follow-up with specialist |
| Pain | Pain location |
| | Pain management—nonpharmacologic and pharmacologic |
| Breasts/chest | Breast/chest engorgement, nipple condition, pain, masses |
| | Feeding frequency and success |
| | Latch assessment |
| | Signs of satiety |
| | Comfort with breastfeeding/chestfeeding |
| Abdomen | Abdominal pain, cramping, epigastric pain |
| Gastrointestinal | Bowel function, constipation, incontinence |
| Urinary | Urinary pain or incontinence, urgency |
| Ano-genital | Lochia amount, color, and odor |
| | Resolution of lochia |
| | Episodes of excessive bleeding |
| | Resumption of menses |
| | Perineal pain, swelling, or redness |
| | Hemorrhoids |
| Lower extremities | Edema, pain, redness, varicosities |
| Sexual activity | Resumption of sexual activity |
| | Dyspareunia |
| | Patient's/partner's enjoyment and satisfaction |

*(continues)*

| Table 34B-5 | Interval History in the Mid-Postpartum Period (*continued*) |
|---|---|
| **Category** | **Specific Information to Review** |
| Contraception | Contraceptive desired |
| | Past contraceptive experience |
| | Plan to begin selected contraception if applicable |
| Exercise | Exercise and activities since childbirth |
| | Pelvic floor exercises |
| Mental health | Signs or symptoms of postpartum mood disorder ("baby blues" should resolve by 10–14 days) |
| | Signs or symptoms of postpartum depression such as suicidality or self-harm. |
| | Screening tool score (EPDS, PHQ-9, or PHQ-2) |
| Postoperative issues | Pain at incision site and return of sensation around the site |
| | Signs and symptoms of infection |
| Hypertension follow-up for patients with history of hypertensive disorders of pregnancy | Headache |
| | Visual disturbances |
| | Nausea/vomiting |
| | Epigastric pain |
| | Medications for hypertension |

Abbreviations: EPDS, Edinburgh Postnatal Depression Scale; PHQ-9, Patient Health Questionnaire–9; PHQ-2, Patient Health Questionnaire–2.

| Table 34B-6 | Physical Assessment of High-Risk Patients in the Mid-Postpartum Period | | |
|---|---|---|---|
| | **Procedure** | **Expected Findings** | **Signs of Possible Complications** |
| Patients who had a cesarean birth | Evaluation of surgical incision<br><br>Staple removal 4–6 days after surgery (up to 10 days for patients at risk for wound complications, such as patients with diabetes mellitus or obesity)[6] | Incision is well approximated, no exudate, no redness around the incision.<br><br>Adhesive strips may be applied after staple removal. | Signs of a surgical site infection:[7]<br>• Localized swelling<br>• Warmth<br>• Purulent drainage with or without odor<br>• Wound breakdown and separation<br>• Erythema around the incision<br>• Pain at the incision site<br>• Systemic evidence of an infection (e.g., fever, leukocytosis)<br>  ♦ Not always present with superficial infection<br>• Fever (more common with deep infection)<br>• Increased C-reactive protein or procalcitonin (more common with deep infection) |
| Patients with hypertensive disorders of pregnancy | Blood pressure check[4] (can be done by self-check at home or in the outpatient setting)<br>Severe hypertension: within 72 hours of discharge<br>Non-severe hypertension: no later than 7–10 days after discharge | Systolic blood pressure < 140 mm Hg<br>Diastolic blood pressure < 90 mm Hg | Headache<br>Visual disturbances<br>Nausea/vomiting<br>Epigastric pain<br>Systolic blood pressure ≥ 140 mm Hg<br>Diastolic blood pressure ≥ 90 mm Hg |

## The Comprehensive Postpartum Visit (4 to 12 Weeks)

The comprehensive postpartum visit should be scheduled at a time that works for the patient and their ongoing health. A variety of factors may influence the timing, including the patient's plans for returning to work, their access to transportation and childcare, and their insurance coverage. This visit should be viewed as a transition from postpartum care to wellness care, but is not specifically an "all-clear."[4] Such a visit includes a complete assessment of the patient's physical, mental, and social health. Table 34B-7 reviews the interval history for this visit.

The physical examination should include elements that are specific to the postpartum period as well as elements of the annual wellness exam (see *The Physical Examination* appendix). This is the opportunity to assess any complications that arose during the pregnancy, birth, and immediate postpartum period as well as to provide a baseline assessment for the patient's transition to wellness care. A review of the typical physical assessment findings is included in Table 34B-8.

### Laboratory Tests at the Comprehensive Postpartum Visit

Laboratory assessments may be required at the comprehensive postpartum visit based on the patient's history, as indicated in Table 34B-9. Since the postpartum visit marks the end of the childbearing year as well as the continuation of health promotion across the lifespan, recommended screening and counseling for health maintenance, as described in the *Health Promotion Across the Lifespan* chapter, should be provided as indicated.

| Table 34B-7 | Interval History at the Comprehensive Postpartum Visit |
|---|---|
| **Category** | **Specific Information to Review** |
| Healthcare encounters | Calls to the midwife or the physician |
| | Visits to the hospital emergency department |
| | Hospital admissions |
| Review of pregnancy and birth | Provide an opportunity for the patient to share their experience and ask any questions they have about the birth. |
| | Discussion around birth trauma, and available resources. |
| Review of pregnancy-related complications | If the patient had complications such as gestational diabetes, hypertensive disorders, or preterm birth, they should be counseled that these conditions increase the lifetime risk for cardiometabolic disease and the need for follow-up. |
| | Stillbirth or miscarriage: Review of autopsy findings, emotional support, bereavement counseling as needed. |
| | Placental pathology reports should be reviewed with the patient. |
| General physical health | Food and fluid intake |
| | Sleep quality and quantity/fatigue |
| | Medications—for new or chronic conditions and use of prenatal vitamins or iron supplements |
| Adjustment | Emotional changes |
| | Coping with life changes and response to newborn |
| | Social support and help with household chores |
| | Physical activity level |
| | Abdominal and perineal exercises |
| | Family adjustment to newborn |
| | Confidence in infant care |
| Breasts/chest | Breast/chest engorgement, nipple condition, pain, masses |
| | Milk supply |
| | Feeding frequency and success |
| | Comfort and confidence with breastfeeding/chestfeeding |

*(continues)*

| Table 34B-7 | Interval History at the Comprehensive Postpartum Visit (*continued*) |
|---|---|
| **Category** | **Specific Information to Review** |
| Gastrointestinal | Bowel function, constipation, fecal incontinence |
| Urinary | Urinary pain or incontinence, urgency |
| Ano-genital | Lochia—timing of cessation |
| | Resumption of menses |
| | Perineal pain, swelling, or redness |
| | Hemorrhoids |
| Lower extremities | Edema, varicosities |
| Chronic conditions | Change in signs/symptoms |
| | Medication changes |
| | Follow-up with specialist |
| Sexual activity | Resumption of sexual activity and number of times |
| | Dyspareunia |
| | Patient's/partner's enjoyment and satisfaction |
| Contraception | Contraceptive used or desired |
| | Past contraceptive experience |
| | Reproductive life plan/discussion of interpregnancy intervals > 18 months |
| Exercise | Exercise and activities since childbirth |
| | Pelvic floor exercises |
| Mental health | Signs or symptoms of postpartum mood disorder |
| | Follow-up on preexisting mental health disorders |
| Vaccination history | Review vaccination record |
| Wellness screening | Review screening test history such as Pap test, screening for sexually transmitted infection |
| | Tobacco screening |
| | Substance use screening |

| Table 34B-8 | Physical Examination at the Comprehensive Postpartum Visit: Procedure and Expected Findings | | |
|---|---|---|---|
| | **Procedure** | **Expected Findings** | **Signs of Possible Complications** |
| General | Observe general affect, mobility, and signs of pain or splinting. | Tired, ambulatory without assistance, repeating birth events, usually happy | Inability to ambulate without assistance; sad or teary; reporting pain |
| Vital signs | Assess temperature, blood pressure, pulse, and respiratory rate. | Temperature: normal Blood pressure: returns to patient's pre-pregnancy baseline Pulse: 65–80 beats/min at rest Respirations: 12–16 breaths/min at rest | Temperature: > 38°C (100.4°F) Blood pressure: higher than 140/90 mm Hg or lower than 85/60 mm Hg Pulse: higher than 100 beats/min |

| | Procedure | Expected Findings | Signs of Possible Complications |
|---|---|---|---|
| Cardiovascular | Auscultate the heart (rate, rhythm, cardiac sounds). | Regular rate and rhythm | Chest pain, palpitations<br>Tachycardia |
| Lungs/pulmonary | Auscultate the lungs, and percuss as appropriate. | No shortness of breath or difficulty breathing<br>Clear to auscultation | Shortness of breath<br>Adventitious sounds |
| Breasts/chest[a] | Observe breasts/chest for symmetry.<br>• Palpate to assess engorgement and whether any plugged milk ducts are present.<br>• Palpate axilla to assess for accessory mammary tissue.<br>• Inspect the nipple epithelium for erythema, bruising, petechiae, and cracks or bleeding.<br>• Observe the integrity of the areola and inspect for blisters or cracks.<br>• If the patient is not breastfeeding/chestfeeding, breast/chest tissue has returned to pre-pregnancy state.<br>• If the patient is breastfeeding/chestfeeding, verify adequate bra support. | Neonate is nursing frequently with a good latch<br>Breasts/chest are soft when empty and full prior to feeding | Neonate is not latching well or frequently<br>Painful nipples<br>Nipples: flat, inverted, cracked, bruised, blistered, or bleeding<br>Breasts/chest: erythema, engorged |
| Abdomen/gastrointestinal | Light and deep abdominal palpation<br>Assessment of diastasis recti | Eating and drinking without difficulty<br>Bowel movements normal<br>Abdomen: nontender, nondistended; diastasis recti is an expected finding<br>Uterus: nonpalpable in the abdomen<br>Surgical scar, if present, is approximated and dry without evidence of infection | Nausea or vomiting, abdominal pain, constipation, or diarrhea<br>Abdomen: distended, tender<br>Surgical scar not approximated, surrounded by an area of redness, or discharge present |
| Urinary | Assess for urinary retention and symptoms of infection.<br>Assess for CVAT. | Voiding spontaneously, slight urinary leakage with cough or sneeze is typical<br>Bladder: nondistended—not palpable, nontender | Persistent urinary incontinence<br>Persistent retention or incontinence<br>Bladder: distended or tender, visible urinary incontinence<br>CVAT tenderness |

*(continues)*

| Table 34B-8 | Physical Examination at the Comprehensive Postpartum Visit: Procedure and Expected Findings (*continued*) | | |
|---|---|---|---|
| | **Procedure** | **Expected Findings** | **Signs of Possible Complications** |
| Perineum | Examine perineum for healing of any lacerations. Observe for granulation tissue. | Well-healed, nontender<br>Repair: approximated | Tender, poorly approximated, pink granulation tissue |
| Vagina and cervix | A speculum examination is not necessary unless a Pap test is indicated.<br>If an intrauterine device was inserted immediately postpartum, inspect for the presence of strings during the speculum exam. | Cervix closed, nontender, parous if had labored, no evidence of cervical lacerations<br>Uterus, nontender to palpation, return to nonpregnant shape and size | Cervix tender<br>Uterus tender |
| Anus | Assess for presence or absence of hemorrhoids. | Normal in appearance<br>Hemorrhoids: pink and reduce spontaneously | Hemorrhoids: large or deep blue/purple—consider surgical consult |
| Skin | | Normal color<br>Without bruising<br>No immediate changes<br>Hyperpigmentation may be retained but will fade with time. Striae, spider nevi, capillary hemangiomas, varicosities, and skin tags regress but may not completely disappear. | |

Abbreviation: CVAT, costovertebral angle tenderness.

| Table 34B-9 | Potential Postpartum Laboratory Tests | | |
|---|---|---|---|
| **Laboratory Tests** | **Indications** | **Timing** | **Normal Range** |
| Hemoglobin (Hgb) or hematocrit (Hct) | Prenatal anemia, postpartum hemorrhage, cesarean birth | At least 4 weeks postpartum unless symptomatic of acute anemia | Hgb $\geq$ 12 g/dL<br>Hct $\geq$ 36% |
| Thyroid-stimulating hormone (TSH) | Current or recent thyroid disease, history of postpartum thyroiditis, enlarged thyroid, symptoms of postpartum depression | 6 weeks, 3 months, and 6 months postpartum | TSH: 0.4–5.0 mU/L |
| Cervical cytology[8] | 21–29 years of age: screening for cervical cancer every 3 years with cervical cytology<br>30–65 years of age: screening every 3 years with cervical cytology alone, every 5 years with high-risk human papillomavirus (hrHPV) testing alone, or every 5 years with hrHPV testing in combination with cytology (cotesting). (See the *Malignant and Chronic Gynecologic Disorders* chapter for more information.) | After perineal and vulvar healing is complete | Negative for intraepithelial lesion or malignancy |

| Laboratory Tests | Indications | Timing | Normal Range |
|---|---|---|---|
| Sexually transmitted infection screening (gonorrhea, chlamydia, syphilis, human immunodeficiency virus) | All sexually active patients younger than 25 years and patients age 25 years and older with a history of sexually transmitted infections, unprotected sexual intercourse, multiple sexual partners in past 12 months | Annually and within 3 months of past infection | Negative |
| 2-hour 75-g glucose challenge | Gestational diabetes<br>Also screen patients age 35 years and older with a BMI of 30 or higher | 6–12 weeks postpartum and annually thereafter | Fasting glucose < 100 mg/dL<br>2-hour glucose < 140 mg/dL |
| **Additional Screening Recommended for Health Maintenance** | | | |
| Alcohol misuse | Screen all patients using a validated screening tool and provide counseling and education as described in the *Health Promotion Across the Lifespan* chapter. | | |
| Depression | Screen all patients using a validated screening tool and provide management as described in the *Mental Health Conditions* and *Postpartum Complications* chapters. | | |
| Intimate-partner violence | Screen all patients using a validated screening tool as described in the *Health Promotion Across the Lifespan* chapter. | | |
| Lipid disorders | Screen patients age 40 years and older using nonfasting or fasting total cholesterol, LDL-C, and HDL-C. | | |
| Tobacco use | Screen all patients using a validated screening tool and provide counseling and education as described in the *Health Promotion Across the Lifespan* chapter. | | |

Abbreviations: BMI, body mass index; HDL-C, high-density lipoprotein cholesterol; LDL-C, low-density lipoprotein cholesterol.

## References

1. Berens P. Overview of the postpartum period: normal physiology and routine maternal care. *UpToDate.* https://www.uptodate.com/contents/overview-of-the-postpartum-period-normal-physiology-and-routine-maternal-care. Published May 9, 2023. Accessed May 15, 2023.

2. Davidson N. REEDA: evaluating postpartum healing. *J Nurse Midwifery.* 1974;19(2):6-8.

3. Pomp ER, Lenselink AM, Rosendaal FR, Doggen CJ. Pregnancy, the postpartum period and prothrombotic defects: risk of venous thrombosis in the MEGA study. *J Thromb Haemost.* 2008;6(4):632-637. doi:10.1111/j.1538-7836.2008.02921.x.

4. ACOG Committee Opinion No. 736: optimizing postpartum care. *Obstet Gynecol.* 2018;131(5):e140-e150. doi:10.1097/AOG.0000000000002633.

5. World Health Organization. *WHO Recommendations on Postnatal Care of the Mother and Newborn.* Geneva, Switzerland: World Health Organization; 2014.

6. Berghella V. Cesarean birth: postoperative care, complications, and long-term sequelae. *UpToDate.* https://www.uptodate.com/contents/cesarean-birth-postoperative-care-complications-and-long-term-sequelae. Published April 5, 2023. Accessed May 15, 2023.

7. Evans HL, Hedrick TL. Overview of the evaluation and management of surgical site infection. *UpToDate.* https://www.uptodate.com/contents/overview-of-the-evaluation-and-management-of-surgical-site-infection/print. Published April 1, 2022. Accessed May 15, 2023.

8. U.S. Preventive Services Task Force. Screening for cervical cancer: US Preventive Services Task Force recommendation statement. *JAMA.* 2018;320(7):674-686. doi:10.1001/jama.2018.10897.

# CHAPTER 35

# Postpartum Complications

DEBORAH KARSNITZ AND LINDA MCDANIEL

## Introduction

As beautifully stated in the campaign by the Centers for Disease Control and Prevention, "Hear Her." It is imperative to listen carefully to everyone who has given birth. Take time to hear their story and give them room to voice concerns.[1] Most postpartum individuals experience a healthy postpartum recovery (puerperium) while discovering the subtle but extraordinary capabilities of the newborn. Occasionally, however, complications arise that must be recognized and managed promptly. In the United States, more than 700 lives are lost each year from pregnancy or postpartum complications and even more individuals have lifelong health consequences from such complications. Many of these catastrophic consequences could be prevented.

Approximately 70% of pregnancy-related deaths occur on the day of birth or in the early postpartum period.[2] Historically, infection and hemorrhage were the leading causes of postpartum mortality. With the advent of antibiotics, the most frequent causes of death have changed, such that throughout the twentieth century, hemorrhage, hypertension, and thromboembolism were the three leading causes of maternal mortality and morbidity.[2] Today, however, pregnant individuals are more likely to be older and have chronic health conditions compared to their counterparts in previous generations. The incidence of obesity and cesarean birth has also increased. In the United States, cardiovascular conditions, cardiomyopathy, infection, and hemorrhage are the leading causes of pregnancy-related mortality.[3] More than 60% of deaths related to pregnancy are preventable.[1] Most significant, there are large racial disparities in rates of severe maternal morbidity and mortality. Historically, care guidelines have recognized that

individuals who identify as Black, American Indian, and Alaska Native are at increased risk; however, it is increasingly acknowledged that these disparities have roots in racism, inequities in healthcare access, and social determinants of health. It is critical for healthcare providers to broaden their view to incorporate these causes of increased maternal morbidity and mortality. Through increased awareness, healthcare providers can participate in organizational improvements geared toward reducing these disparities.[4] At the individual level of care, midwives are uniquely poised to listen to their patients, recognize signs and symptoms of severe maternal morbidity, and "hear" them during the postpartum period.[5]

Communication is a key element of effective health care and integral to prompt treatment and recovery when a complication occurs. To facilitate recognition of postpartum complications, the post-birth warning signs developed by the Association of Women's Health, Obstetric, and Neonatal Nurses (AWHONN) are a useful tool for healthcare providers and patients.[6] Postpartum individuals are encouraged to communicate any of the signs in Table 35-1 to their healthcare provider, and providers should respond promptly when individuals voice these concerns.[6]

Many postpartum complications can be managed independently by midwives, some require nonurgent consultation with physician colleagues, and rarely complications require an immediate and team-based response to prevent morbidity and mortality. While some consultation patterns are unique to the midwifery practice or birth location, there is a movement in the United States to standardize the signs and symptoms that require immediate response. Maternal early warning signs (MEWS) are the same in the postpartum period as

| Table 35-1 | Post-Birth Warning Signs for Patients |
|---|---|
| **P** | Pain in the chest |
| **O** | Obstructed breathing or shortness of breath |
| **S** | Seizures |
| **T** | Thoughts of hurting yourself or someone else |
| **B** | Bleeding that is soaking through one pad per hour, or blood clots the size of an egg or larger |
| **I** | Incision (or laceration) that is not healing |
| **R** | Red or swollen leg or arm that is painful to touch |
| **T** | Temperature of 38°C (100.4°F) or higher |
| **H** | Headache that does not improve, even after taking medicine, or a bad headache with visual changes |

Reprinted with permission from the Association of Women's Health, Obstetric and Neonatal Nurses (AWHONN) (www.awhonn.org). Copyright AWHONN.

in the intrapartum period. See the *Complications During Labor and Birth* chapter for detailed information. Certain symptoms require immediate and team-based intervention, even prior to knowing the exact causal diagnosis.

This chapter presents complications that can occur postpartum, after the fourth stage of labor, and that affect the reproductive tract organs. Urinary retention—an early postpartum complication that rarely causes significant morbidity—is described first. Management of uncomplicated urinary retention is within the midwifery scope of practice. A review of complications associated with severe maternal morbidity or mortality, such as bleeding (e.g., secondary hemorrhage and hematoma), wound complications (seroma, hematoma, dehiscence, and infection), cardiomyopathy, preeclampsia/eclampsia, and thromboembolism, follows. Conditions less often seen in clinical practice, such as postpartum thyroid disorders, are presented toward the end of the chapter. The chapter concludes with a brief overview of postpartum considerations associated with opioid use. Immediate postpartum hemorrhage, which occurs during the third stage of labor or in the first hours after birth, is reviewed in the *Third Stage of Labor* chapter. Postpartum mood and anxiety disorders are discussed in the *Mental Health Conditions* chapter, and breastfeeding/chestfeeding complications such as mastitis are reviewed in the *Infant Feeding and Lactation* chapter.

## Urinary Retention

Postpartum urinary retention can present as an overt problem, the inability to void spontaneously within 6 hours after birth, or as a covert problem, wherein the individual can void but has a residual bladder volume of more than 150 mL. Urinary retention is a common event, with a reported prevalence that ranges from 1.7% to 17.9%; the wide range of estimates is most likely due to variations in definition and reporting.[7] Risk factors include epidural analgesia, instrumental birth, perineal injury, prolonged labor, high birth weight, primiparity, and previous cesarean birth.[7,8] Potential causes of urinary retention include slow recovery of sensation after epidural anesthesia, excessive vulvar edema that compresses the urethra, trauma and edema of the bladder neck, and injured bladder innervation. Although long-term adverse effects are rare, urinary retention increases the risk of urinary tract infection (UTI) and bladder dysfunction in the short term. Likewise, in the short term, urinary retention can increase uterine bleeding after birth. Urinary retention is distinct from urinary incontinence, a relatively common, though often transient, concern during the first year postpartum. Urinary incontinence is discussed in the *Malignant and Chronic Gynecologic Disorders* and *Postpartum Care* chapters.

Postpartum urinary retention should be suspected when an individual has not urinated in 6 hours, there is palpable bladder above the symphysis pubis on abdominal examination, the uterine fundus is displaced upward and to the side of the midline, or a full bladder is identified on ultrasound. Initially, noninvasive methods should be implemented to help the individual urinate. Such measures include maintaining privacy, early and frequent ambulation, adequate analgesia, warm-water immersion, placement of a few drops of peppermint oil in the toilet water or bedpan, and the sound of running water. Although little research evidence supports the effectiveness of these strategies, they are not harmful. However, if these measures are not immediately successful, urinary catheterization should be used to empty the bladder. Urinary stasis is a risk factor for UTI and needs to be resolved soon once it is diagnosed.

Urinary retention is usually diagnosed clinically based on the subjective inability to void and/or abdominal examination to palpate a full bladder. Individuals who have a palpable full bladder but who are able to void spontaneously should have the amount of voided urine measured; the individual should then be reassessed immediately after voiding to rule out covert postpartum urinary retention. Ultrasound or post-void catheterization can be used to diagnose covert postpartum urinary retention. The treatment for covert postpartum urinary retention is catheterization.

In general, intermittent catheterization is associated with less risk of a catheter-associated UTI than placement of an indwelling catheter for individuals with bladder-emptying dysfunction. If an indwelling catheter is used, it should be maintained for the shortest period possible.[7] In this situation, a common approach is to leave the indwelling catheter in place overnight, to be removed in the morning. If the individual is unable to urinate the next day, it may be necessary to leave the catheter in place for a longer period.

Although 150 mL is commonly used as the criterion for diagnosing covert urinary retention, there is no evidence that this cutoff value reflects an increased risk for adverse outcomes. Mulder et al. found that following vaginal birth ($n = 439$), the mean post-residual bladder volume was 140 mL, and that the majority of individuals with a post-residual volume greater than 150 mL were able to empty their bladder spontaneously by the fourth postpartum day.[9,10] Therefore, reliance on the 150 mL criterion may result in a higher rate of indwelling catheter use than is necessary. Given the lack of clear evidence for a specific post-residual amount that is associated with adverse effects, the choice of intermittent versus indwelling catheterization should be individualized to the needs and preferences of the individual.

Figure 35-1 provides a sample algorithm for management of an individual who has postpartum

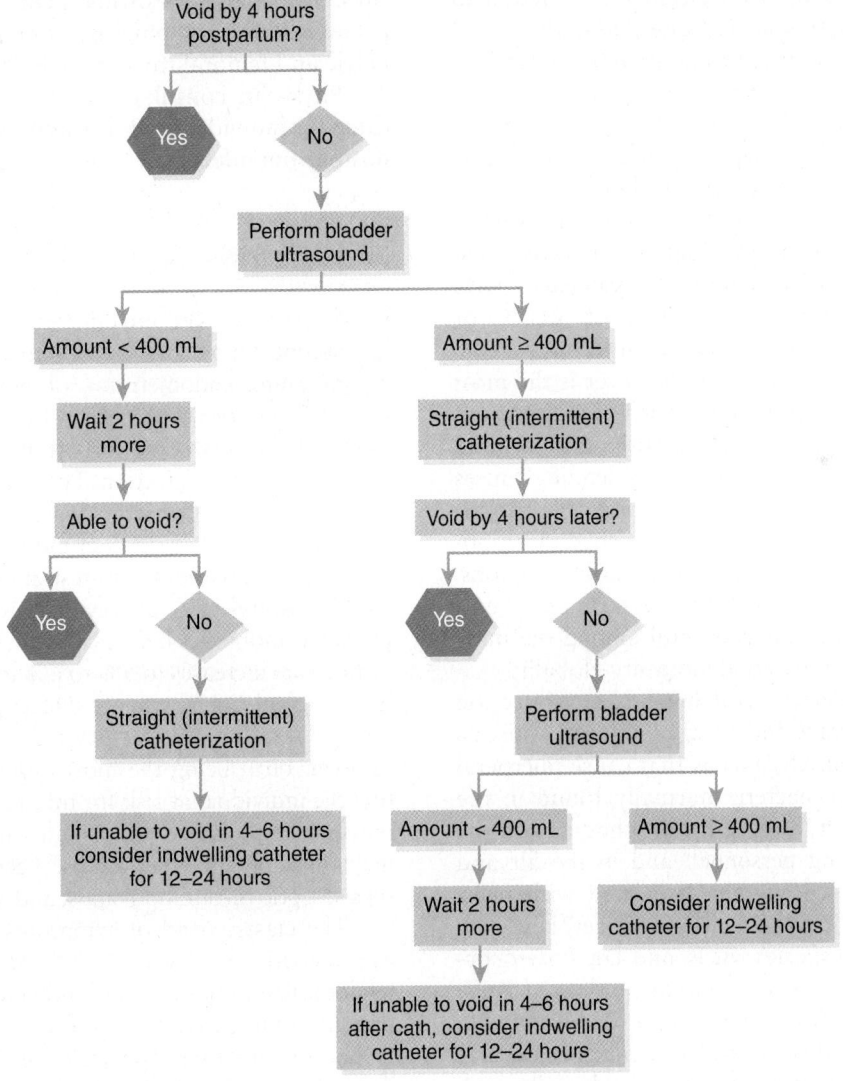

**Figure 35-1** Sample algorithm for assessment of voiding and management of urinary retention following vaginal birth.

urinary retention. Institutional guidelines will dictate the cutoff values for each step in this algorithm. If an individual is able to successfully void after catheterization, they should be assessed for adequate urinary output for the next two or three occasions to evaluate whether retention is still experienced to some degree.

## Puerperal Fever and Puerperal Infection

Puerperal pyrexia or fever is defined as a temperature of 38.0°C (100.4°F) or higher, occurring on any two of the first 10 days postpartum excluding the first 24 hours. The first postpartum 24-hour period is excluded because a mild transient temperature elevation can develop as a physiologic reaction to childbirth during this span of time. Similarly, a brief temperature elevation of less than 38.0°C occasionally occurs with the onset of milk production 3 to 5 days after birth.

Infection during pregnancy and postpartum is one of the leading causes of morbidity and is responsible for more than 12% of all deaths in pregnant and postpartum individuals.[11] The three most common differential diagnoses associated with postpartum temperature elevations of 38.0°C or more are endometritis, wound infections (e.g., surgical-site infection), and UTIs. Fever is the most common concern reported postpartum. Postpartum infections—specifically, endometritis and wound infection—are the second and third leading causes of hospital readmissions.[12] Less commonly, postpartum fever can be caused by septic pelvic thrombophlebitis, transfusion reactions, or drug reactions. Despite the availability of effective antibiotic therapies, puerperal infections are still among the most frequent causes of maternal mortality globally.

Puerperal infection is defined as any infection in the genital tract following childbirth, miscarriage, or abortion. Organisms that cause puerperal infections include bacteria normally found in the lower genital tract, bowel, or nasopharynx; on the hands of attending personnel; and in the air and dust. Organisms commonly associated with puerperal infection include gram-positive aerobes, such as *Streptococcus* species (A, B, and D), *Enterococcus*, and *Staphylococcus aureus* and *epidermis*; gram-negative aerobes, such as *Escherichia coli*, *Klebsiella*, *Enterobacter*, and *Proteus* species; and gram-variable organisms, such as *Gardnerella vaginalis*. A fever of 39.0°C or higher that develops within 24 hours after a cesarean birth can indicate a group A *Streptococcus* infection. Anaerobes associated with puerperal infection include *Peptostreptococcus*, *Peptococcus*, *Bacteroides* species, *Clostridium*, and *Fusobacterium*. Other organisms implicated in puerperal infection include *Mycoplasma*, *Chlamydia*, and *Neisseria gonorrhoeae*.

In addition to an elevated temperature, signs and symptoms of puerperal infection include general malaise, pain, chills, increased pulse, abdominal pain, and malodorous lochia. Because symptoms of puerperal infection are often generalized, the differential diagnosis includes appendicitis, pyelonephritis, and pneumonia. It is important to consider the possibility of extended infections. These infections originate from a localized infection and extend via the path of venous circulation or the lymphatic system to produce bacterial infection in more distant sites. Extended sites of puerperal infection include pelvic cellulitis, salpingitis, oophoritis, peritonitis, pelvic and femoral thrombophlebitis, and sepsis.

Physician consultation and/or referral is indicated for individuals who require evaluation for any postpartum infection.

## Endometritis

Endometritis or endomyometritis is an infection of the uterine lining anywhere within the uterus (i.e., myometrium, endometrium, or both). Endometritis typically develops within 2 to 4 days postpartum or as late as 2 to 6 weeks postpartum and can be either a mild or a severe infection. This type of infection occurs in 1% to 2% of individuals following a vaginal birth, approximately 27% of individuals who have a cesarean birth without administration of prophylactic antibiotics, and 11% of individuals who are given prophylactic antibiotics before cesarean birth.[13,14] The infection rate increases to 5% to 6% in individuals who have vaginal births when risk factors are present.[13] Table 35-2 lists risk factors for endometritis, with cesarean birth being the most important factor putting the individual at risk for this infection.[13] Adverse outcomes associated with endometritis (if not treated) include salpingitis, peritonitis, necrotizing fasciitis, sepsis, septic thrombophlebitis, and death.

The classic triad of symptoms associated with endometritis is fever, tachycardia, and uterine tenderness/suprapubic pain. Individuals can also experience chills, malaise, hypotension, foul-smelling lochia, or anorexia. The onset of symptoms varies depending on the infectious organism.

Evaluation includes physical examination to rule out other sources of infection, such as pneumonia,

| Table 35-2 | Risk Factors for Postpartum Endometritis |
|---|---|
| **Bacterial Colonization** | |
| Bacterial vaginosis | |
| Group A or B *Streptococcus* | |
| *Chlamydia trachomatis* | |
| *Mycoplasmas hominis* | |
| *Ureaplasma urealyticum* | |
| **Postpartum Individual** | |
| Obesity | |
| Diabetes | |
| Severe anemia | |
| Human immunodeficiency virus (HIV) infection | |
| Young age | |
| Nulliparity | |
| **Pregnancy** | |
| Preterm birth | |
| Post-term pregnancy | |
| **Labor** | |
| Chorioamnionitis | |
| Internal monitoring | |
| Meconium staining (thick) | |
| Prolonged labor | |
| Prolonged rupture of membranes | |
| Operative vaginal birth | |
| Cesarean birth | |
| Manual removal of the placenta | |

mastitis, pyelonephritis, or surgical-site infection. A urine culture can rule out pyelonephritis, and a chest X ray may be indicated to rule out pneumonia. Endometrial cultures are not obtained because uncontaminated cultures are difficult to obtain. Blood cultures are not routinely recommended in persons without severe illness because most individuals respond well to empiric therapy. Although diagnostic ultrasound can help rule out other diagnoses such as infected hematoma, retained products of conception, or unidentified abscess, it is not always helpful because the findings will likely show normal variants that occur in the postpartum period. Thus, the diagnosis is generally clinical and based on ruling out other sources of infection.

Consultation should be obtained rapidly for any individual who has signs or symptoms that indicate they are at risk for severe morbidity, such as hypotension, tachypnea, oxygen saturation of less than 95%, shortness of breath, or any MEWS.

Most endometrial infections are polymicrobial in nature, and frequently include a combination of aerobes and anaerobes from the genital tract. Broad-spectrum antibiotics are the treatment of choice, with several regimens available. Individuals who present with signs and symptoms of mild endometritis—for example, a low-grade fever, mild abdominal pain, or foul-smelling lochia—several days after a vaginal birth may be offered oral antibiotics. Treatment consists of the same antibiotics as are used for pelvic inflammatory disease, doxycycline and metronidazole; these medications are not contraindicated while breastfeeding/chestfeeding as long as the duration of treatment is less than 3 weeks. Other options include amoxicillin-clavulanate; levofloxacin and metronidazole can be used as well. Levofloxacin is not recommended while breastfeeding/chestfeeding.[13,14] Intramuscular regimens are available for individuals in low-resource settings where intravenous treatment is not available.

When individuals have moderate to severe infection, evidenced by persistent fever, severe abdominal pain, or symptoms of sepsis, the gold-standard treatment is intravenous clindamycin (Cleocin) and gentamicin (Garamycin) administered until the person is afebrile for 24 to 48 hours.[13] Most individuals with moderate to severe cases respond to intravenous treatment within 48 to 72 hours and do not require follow-up with oral antibiotics, although oral antibiotics may be recommended for individuals with acute bacteremia.

If the individual is still febrile after 48 to 72 hours of antibiotics, the most likely problem is resistant organisms such as *Enterococcus*. In this situation, physician consultation and referral are indicated, as the choice of antibiotic depends on multiple factors, including the possibility of other differential diagnoses such as pelvic abscess. A change of antibiotic regimen typically resolves the infection.

### Prevention of Endometritis

Reducing cesarean birth rates would significantly lower the rate of postpartum endometritis. Likewise, judicious perinatal practice—that is, prenatal treatment of infections, limiting the number of vaginal examinations during labor, avoiding artificial rupture of membranes, and minimal intrauterine exploration after birth—can decrease the risk of an individual developing infection postpartum.

One dose of antimicrobial therapy, administered within 60 minutes before the start of cesarean surgery, significantly reduces the incidence of endometritis; thus, this has become standard practice in the United States.[14] Vaginal cleansing with chlorhexidine prior to cesarean surgery also reduces the incidence of endometritis.[15] Manual removal of the placenta should be reserved for when conservative measures, such as gentle, controlled cord traction, have failed.

## Wound Complications

Wound complications include infections or dehiscence in a repaired perineal laceration or episiotomy following a vaginal birth, as well as surgical-site complications such as seroma, hematoma, dehiscence, and infections in an abdominal incision following a cesarean birth. Wound complications are one of the most common reasons for postpartum emergency department visits or hospital readmission.[16]

Common pathogens associated with wound infections include *S. aureus*, *Streptococcus*, and both aerobic and anaerobic bacilli. The signs and symptoms of infection are similar for both abdominal and perineal wounds. Individuals usually experience a low-grade temperature, seldom greater than 38.3°C (100.9°F). Localized pain and edema are accompanied by red and inflamed repair edges. Exudate and wound separation or dehiscence can occur as well. Perineal wound infections are often accompanied by dysuria.[13]

### Perineal Wound Infection and Laceration Dehiscence

Infection or dehiscence in a perineal laceration or episiotomy repair is generally confined to the skin and subcutaneous tissue. The treatment includes removal of sutures, as well as opening, debriding, and cleansing the wound to allow the area to heal by granulation. Physician consultation is indicated. Antibiotics may be administered if cellulitis is present. Most perineal wound infections are not repaired again unless a third- or fourth-degree perineal extension is present. A reduction in the incidence of wound infections has been reported with the administration of prophylactic antimicrobial agents when a third- or fourth-degree laceration occurs.[17]

### Surgical-Site Complications

Midwives frequently collaborate in the care of individuals who have a cesarean birth, so they need knowledge of expected findings during recovery from this surgery and signs of surgical complications. Abdominal surgical-site infections following cesarean birth usually appear 4 to 7 days after the procedure.

A seroma is a collection of fluid (serum) that appears under the surgical incision. Clear fluid can leak from the incision, and the incision can appear swollen around the edges. Seromas generally do not need to be treated, but are observed carefully to make sure they do not become too large. Occasionally the skin incision is opened in a small area to allow the fluid to drain and/or a drainage tube can be placed temporarily.[18] Similarly, small hematomas usually reabsorb without intervention, but larger ones may require evacuation of the clot. Both seromas and hematomas increase the individual's risk of infection. Once such a complication is identified, physician consultation is indicated, and the surgical incision is reassessed frequently until it is determined that the seroma or hematoma is not increasing in size.

Surgical-site infections can require treatment with antibiotics and occasionally drainage. Culture of exudates is not usually required. Reclosure of an abdominal wound may be indicated if dehiscence occurs. Depending on the degree of infection and dehiscence, management may include daily debridement, wound packing, judicious antibiotic treatment, and drainage if necessary. Physician consultation or referral is indicated. If a fever lasts for 3 or more days, the individual should be evaluated for complications such as sepsis, septic pelvic thrombophlebitis, abscess, and septic shock.

Many techniques can be implemented to help prevent surgical-site infections. Basic measures include attention to hand washing prior to touching the area and ensuring that only sterile or very clean dressings or cloths touch the wound. In addition to strategies used to prevent endometritis, such as use of prophylactic antibiotics, other techniques include shaving with clippers, skin cleansing with chlorhexidine (rather than iodine), and skin closure with sutures rather than staples.[18]

## Urinary Tract Infection: Pyelonephritis

During the postpartum period, individuals can be at increased risk for UTIs for several reasons, including pregnancy-induced dilation of the urethra and ureters, gestational diabetes, cesarean birth, operative vaginal birth, trauma to the urethra during birth, urinary retention, and bladder catheterization.[19] The organisms responsible for UTIs during the puerperium are similar to those observed in nonpregnant individuals—namely, *Escherichia coli* (which accounts for 80% to 90% of such UTIs), *Proteus mirabilis*, and *Klebsiella pneumoniae*. The incidence of UTI typically peaks at 6 to 7 days postpartum.[19]

UTIs may cause urinary frequency, urgency, dysuria, and, occasionally, lower abdominal pain. Pyelonephritis is characterized by low-grade fever, flank pain, costovertebral angle tenderness (CVAT), nausea, and vomiting. In contrast, postpartum individuals with upper or lower tract UTIs often present with fever and generalized symptoms without dysuria, frequency, or urgency. Therefore, any individual with a fever postpartum should be evaluated for UTI.

Definitive diagnosis of UTI is made by culture of a clean-catch or catheter urine specimen that reveals a significant number of a single type of bacteria. Management of UTI and pyelonephritis during the postpartum period is the same as that in primary care outside of pregnancy. Note, however, that nitrofurantoin is not the optimal postpartum treatment option. Prompt diagnosis and treatment can prevent further complications. Both UTI and pyelonephritis are common diagnoses when postpartum individuals are readmitted for sepsis.[20]

## COVID-19 During Postpartum

Severe acute respiratory syndrome coronavirus-2 (SARS-CoV-2), a novel coronavirus commonly referred to as COVID-19, is a potentially deadly illness that has been responsible for countless fatalities throughout the world. Initially identified in China in 2019, COVID-19 evolved and spread, causing a worldwide pandemic. This multisystem disease varies in its effects and outcomes, but has significantly affected vulnerable populations. Emerging science focuses on treatments and preventive strategies, such as masking, limiting visitors, and vaccines. Pregnancy and postpartum have been particularly troubling for many individuals as they weigh decisions about receiving the relatively new vaccines for COVID-19.

Once preventive vaccines became available, only about 30% of individuals received the vaccine during pregnancy. The risk for developing postpartum COVID-19 is similar to that for the general population. Obesity, gestational diabetes, and other illnesses may also increase the risk for severe illness.[21] Individuals with symptomatic COVID-19 are at an increased risk for more severe illness or fatality.[21] A joint statement released in August 2021

between the American College of Obstetricians and Gynecologists (ACOG), American College of Nurse-Midwives (ACNM), American Association of Pediatrics (AAP), and many other national healthcare organizations strongly recommended vaccination against COVID-19 for all individuals who are pregnant, planning to become pregnant, recently pregnant, or lactating.[21]

While COVID-19 during postpartum can be transmitted by respiratory droplets, it has not currently been shown to be transmitted in human milk.[22] Individuals testing positive for COVID-19 can choose to express milk or breastfeed/chestfeed while using precautions such as hand washing and masking during this process.[22]

## Postpartum Bleeding Complications

After immediate postpartum hemorrhage, the two bleeding complications most frequently observed in the postpartum period are genital tract hematomas and secondary (late) postpartum hemorrhage. Fortunately, neither is a common occurrence. Postpartum hemorrhage (PPH) is classified as primary or secondary. Primary hemorrhage occurs within the first 24 hours and is reviewed in the *Third Stage of Labor* chapter. Secondary (late) PPH occurs between 24 hours and 6 to 12 weeks postpartum.[23]

### Genital Tract Hematomas

A hematoma is a localized collection of extravasated blood that is usually clotted. The dangers associated with its development include hemorrhage, anemia, and infection. The incidence of postpartum hematoma varies from 1 per 500 to 1 per 12,500 births; this condition is most often the result of trauma from instrumental birth or episiotomy.[24] A hematoma arises following spontaneous or traumatic rupture of a blood vessel. Development occurs most often during birth or within a few hours after the birth. The most commonly seen postpartum hematomas can be classified anatomically as vulvar, vulvovaginal, or paravaginal (see Figures 3 and 4 in the *Genital Tract Injury: Immediate Postpartum Inspection of the Vulva, Perineum, Vagina, and Cervix* appendix). Because postpartum hematomas vary in size from small to large, some may be overlooked, which could account for the variations in incidence estimates.

Risk factors for postpartum hematoma formation include operative vaginal birth and unrepaired laceration of a torn blood vessel, which can occur during injection of local anesthesia or during repair of a perineal or vaginal laceration. Failure to achieve hemostasis or ligate torn vessels above the vaginal apex prior to repairing an episiotomy or laceration also increases the risk of hematoma formation. Other risk factors include primiparity, multiple gestation, large fetal weight, preeclampsia, coagulopathies, vulvovaginal varicosities, and prolonged second-stage labor.[24]

Signs and symptoms of vulvar or vaginal hematomas include (1) perineal, vaginal, bladder, or rectal pressure and severe pain; (2) a tense, fluctuant swelling; and (3) bluish or blue-black discoloration of tissue. The characteristic presentation of a hematoma is extreme pain out of proportion to the expected amount of discomfort and pain for that time period, and pain that develops quite rapidly in the first 2 to 6 hours after birth.[23] Individuals who have received epidural analgesia may report a sudden onset of rectal pressure as the only symptom.

Presenting signs and symptoms of a hematoma more internal than the vulva or vagina include lateral uterine pain sensitive to palpation, extension of pain into the flank, a painful swelling identified on high rectal examination or ultrasound, a ridge of tissue just above the pelvic brim extending laterally (i.e., the edge of the swollen broad ligament), and possibly abdominal distension. Subperitoneal hematoma formation—a rare occurrence following vaginal birth—leads to unrestricted bleeding and is typically not recognized until the individual experiences hypovolemic shock.

Vulvar hematomas are the most easily recognizable genital tract hematomas, while vaginal hematomas are generally identifiable with careful inspection and palpation of the vagina and cervix. Small and moderate-sized hematomas can be spontaneously absorbed and managed expectantly. If a vulvar hematoma is small and visible, the edges can be demarcated with a pen, and it can be observed frequently to determine whether it is enlarging.

If the hematoma is large or possibly continuing to grow (which indicates active bleeding within the hematoma space), a complete blood count should be ordered as soon as the hematoma is identified, and an intravenous line started. Vital signs should be monitored frequently to observe for signs of shock, and pain medication prescribed as needed. A physician should be consulted. Management might include monitoring hematocrit levels, vaginal packing to produce counterpressure, or an incision to evacuate blood and blood clots and ensure closure of the cavity. The individual with a diagnosis of a hematoma may also need other interventions, such as interventional radiology, blood replacement, or antibiotics.

## Secondary Postpartum Hemorrhage

Approximately 1% of individuals experience secondary PPH, with most of these cases occurring within the first 2 weeks postpartum.[23] However, secondary PPH should be considered in any postpartum individual with excessive bleeding that is soaking through one pad per hour, or blood clots the size of an egg or larger that occur more than 24 hours and up to 12 weeks after birth. Common causes of secondary PPH include uterine subinvolution at the placental site, retained placental fragments or membranes, infection, and inherited clotting factor deficiency such as von Willebrand's disease (VWD).[25,26] Less common causes include carcinoma, aneurysms, and arteriovenous malformations. Primary PPH is a known risk factor for secondary PPH.[27]

## Uterine Subinvolution

The process of uterine involution involves anatomic changes in the size and shape of the uterus as well as physiologic changes in the endometrial cavity that include restoration of the altered spiral arteries that supported the placenta. For the uterus to involute appropriately, the uterus must contract, phagocytosis occurs, myometrial cells undergo autolysis, and epithelial cells regenerate and proliferate. The endometrial arteries regain their elasticity, shrink, and coil, and the cytotrophoblasts that invaded the endometrial decidua disappear.[28] By approximately 2 weeks postpartum, the uterus can no longer be palpated abdominally, though involution is not typically complete until 6 weeks after birth. When the uterus does not return to its prepregnant size and position within the expected time frame, the term *uterine subinvolution* is used.

The process of involution may be hampered by various factors—most commonly, retained placental fragments, leiomyomas, or infection. Subinvolution of the placental site occurs when the uteroplacental arteries (modified spiral arteries during pregnancy) do not remodel normally. Abnormal thrombi formation alters normal physiologic processes, causing inadequate sloughing and inhibiting regeneration of the endothelial lining.[28] Retained placenta products inhibit contraction of the blood vessels at the placental attachment site. New-onset bleeding or hemorrhage as a result of placental-site subinvolution most often occurs during the second postpartum week; it can present as an increase or return of lochia rubra (i.e., dark or bright red blood).[28] Interruption of involution can also occur when maternal activity is excessive; the direct etiology is not clear, but it is postulated that excessive activity might slow the healing process, although no direct evidence supports this theory.

## Diagnosis and Management of Postpartum Bleeding

The progress of normal postpartum lochia is described in the *Postpartum Care* chapter. The differential diagnosis for abnormal postpartum bleeding initially includes placental subinvolution, retained placental fragments, and endometritis. Management depends on the briskness and amount of bleeding and whether the individual is hemodynamically stable. Individuals who experience a sudden, severe delayed PPH will often present to the emergency department for care. They may need acute care to support their hemodynamic stability.

Elements of the individual's history that can help establish a diagnosis are listed in Table 35-3. Bimanual pelvic examination findings may include a soft, tender uterus that is larger than expected for the postpartum week. Because retained placental fragments can cause endometritis, however, it is not always easy to differentiate between retained placental fragments and endometritis based on physical examination. Signs of endometritis also include malodorous lochia, tenderness or pain in the adnexa on movement of the uterus, and cervical motion tenderness elicited during a vaginal examination.

| Table 35-3 | Evaluation of Postpartum Bleeding |
|---|---|
| **Evaluation** | **Clinical Considerations** |
| Review of health record from recent birth (mode of birth, third stage abnormalities, placental inspection) | Retained placental fragments are more common after a vaginal birth; endometritis is more common after cesarean birth |
| History of heavy menstrual bleeding or primary postpartum hemorrhage | History of heavy menstrual bleeding or previous postpartum hemorrhage can indicate the presence of a coagulopathy |
| Current medications | Medications that may predispose the individual to uterine bleeding such as anticoagulants and uterine relaxants |
| History of vaginal penetration or trauma | Possible new vaginal laceration |
| Symptoms of infection | Endometritis may present with fever, pain, and malodorous lochia |

If retained placental fragments are suspected, ultrasound is indicated. Note that ultrasound does not always provide definitive results, and it might not differentiate between placental fragments and blood clots.[13] Consultation and team-based care are appropriate for these individuals. Uterine curettage may be performed.

If the bleeding is heavier than usual but not markedly so, the individual is stable, the uterus has the expected size and shape, and there is no indication of infection or retained placental fragments, then outpatient treatment may begin with ergonovine (Ergotrate) or methylergonovine (Methergine), 0.2 mg by mouth, every 3 to 4 hours for 24 to 48 hours. Breastfeeding/chestfeeding individuals should refrain from breastfeeding/chestfeeding for at least 12 hours after the last dose of methylergonovine. Individuals taking either of these uterotonic agents should be informed that cramping can increase and bleeding should decrease during the course of therapy.

Physician consultation should be obtained if bleeding is saturating more than one pad in an hour, the individual has signs of infection, or other abnormal findings are noted in the history and physical examination. For example, a history of heavy menstrual bleeding or previous PPH may indicate VWD, as does the timing of a hemorrhage that occurs between 2 to 5 days postpartum. Preliminary laboratory evaluation includes a complete blood count with platelets, activated partial thromboplastin time (aPTT), prothrombin time, and fibrinogen levels.[26] The initial evaluation is not directed at diagnosing this disease, but rather at ruling out other causes of bleeding. Another test that can aid the diagnosis is beta human chorionic gonadotropin (beta-hCG).

Although different subtypes of VWD are possible, 80% of cases identified during the postpartum period are due to decreased levels of factor VIII. Management depends on the specific subtype. Levels of clotting factors, including factor VIII, increase during pregnancy, which usually provides protection from bleeding and consequently is not a concern until approximately 2 days postpartum, when clotting factors and factor VIII levels decrease.[25,26] PPH risk secondary to VWD persists for as long as 4 months postpartum. Approximately 50% of individuals with a diagnosis of VWD are likely to experience a postpartum hemorrhage.[26] Individuals with known VWD will require a personalized care plan depending on blood loss, peripartum complications, and other risk factors for thrombosis.[27] Consultation is appropriate for planning for both immediate and long-term care.

If infection is present, administration of broad-spectrum antibiotics such as ampicillin–sulbactam (Unasyn) or cefoxitin (Mefoxin) is recommended. If chlamydia is suspected, doxycycline 100 mg twice daily for 7 days or azithromycin 1 g orally (one dose) should be added to the regimen.[29] Concerns have been raised about possible infant dental staining with use of tetracyclines, but evidence shows that this harm is minimized with short-term use.[30] Antibiotics can be administered intravenously or orally depending on the severity of the individual's symptoms.

## Preeclampsia and Eclampsia

Hypertensive disorders of pregnancy (HDP) can extend beyond the antepartum or intrapartum periods or occur as new-onset conditions in the postpartum period.[31] HDP are among the leading causes of severe maternal morbidity and mortality.[31] Incidence of HDP has increased significantly during the past decade.[32] Cerebral hemorrhage, pulmonary edema, renal failure, hepatic rupture, and death are potential complications associated with hypertensive disorders. Early identification and prompt treatment can significantly reduce the incidence of these complications.[31,32]

Blood pressure may be transiently elevated postpartum secondary to administration of intravenous fluids or medications, but the presence of neurologic, cardiac, or gastrointestinal symptoms suggests a more serious underlying pathology.[31,33] The differential diagnosis in such cases includes persistence of gestational hypertension or preeclampsia, HELLP (hemolysis, elevated liver enzymes, and low platelet count) syndrome, chronic hypertension, new-onset preeclampsia, and, more rarely, cerebral vasoconstriction syndrome, cerebral vascular accident, or hemolytic uremic syndrome.[31,33]

Postpartum preeclampsia often presents more subtly than the onset of preeclampsia during the prenatal period. Neurologic indicators (e.g., visual disturbance, headache), nausea, and vomiting appear more frequently during postpartum-onset preeclampsia compared to the prenatal-onset or intrapartum-onset condition.[33,34] Hypertension and proteinuria are not always present in postpartum preeclampsia. New-onset late postpartum preeclampsia/eclampsia generally occurs after 48 hours postpartum and prior to 6 weeks postpartum.[33,35]

Maternal blood pressure normally decreases for the first 48 hours postpartum, but then individuals with preeclampsia will experience an increase to a peak at 3 to 6 days postpartum.[33,34,36] Thus, individuals who develop postpartum preeclampsia are often at home when this condition manifests. Early recognition is key to preventing eclampsia or worsening of the individual's condition, which is why all individuals should be educated about the signs and symptoms of postpartum preeclampsia prior to being discharged from immediate birth care.[31,36] In addition, individuals who had preeclampsia during pregnancy and received antihypertensive medication prior to or after giving birth should have their blood pressure checked within 3 to 7 days after birth. If they were not given antihypertensive medication, they should have their blood pressures checked within 7 to 14 days after birth.[33]

Midwives often work with physician colleagues to care for individuals who have hypertension postpartum. Patients who have mild hypertension (140–150 mm Hg systolic and 90–100 mm Hg diastolic) without any other signs or symptoms of pathology are likely to be treated with oral antihypertensive agents that are compatible with lactation such as labetalol, hydralazine, and nifedipine.

Blood pressure measurements exceeding 140/90 mm Hg require immediate assessment for further symptoms. The consensus bundle for severe hypertension during pregnancy and postpartum developed by the National Partnership for Maternal Safety calls for every perinatal unit to have a protocol that includes notification of a physician or the primary care provider if the individual's systolic blood pressure is 160 mm Hg or higher or the diastolic blood pressure is 110 mm Hg or higher for two measurements within 15 minutes.[36] If an individual being evaluated by a midwife presents with hypertension in these ranges, physician consultation and referral should be obtained quickly. Treatment should begin as soon as possible, often using preestablished guidelines; medication should be initiated within 60 minutes following the second elevated reading.

## Hemorrhagic Stroke

Hemorrhagic stroke is the most common type of stroke during pregnancy and postpartum and can lead to pregnancy-related mortality. Risk is highest during the third trimester and until 6 weeks postpartum.[37] The most common causes of hemorrhagic stroke are preeclampsia/eclampsia, arteriovenous malformations, and aneurysms. Other risk factors include chronic hypertension, hypertensive disorder of pregnancy, coagulopathy, smoking, advanced age, heart disease, diabetes, infection, cesarean birth, and stressors associated with racism and social determinants of health.[37] The rate for stroke during the postpartum period is 14.7 cases per 100,000 post-birth individuals.[37]

Most hospital readmissions for stroke occur within the first 10 days postpartum. Warning signs include an unrelenting headache not relieved by medication, headache with visual changes, seizure, or focal neurologic deficits.[37] Depending on the part of the brain affected, some individuals can experience hallucinations or delusions.[38] Physician management is required and includes control of blood pressure and treatment of the underlying condition.[37]

## Peripartum Cardiomyopathy

Traditionally, cardiac disorders have not been a common complication among pregnant or postpartum individuals. Today, however, cardiovascular disorders account for 15.5% of pregnancy-related deaths in the United States, and cardiomyopathy accounts for 11% of such deaths.[11]

Peripartum cardiomyopathy (PPCM) is a relatively uncommon condition in which an individual develops new heart failure during the last few weeks of pregnancy or in the first 6 months postpartum and there is no other identifiable cause.[39,40] Regionally within the United States and worldwide, large variations are noted in the incidence of this condition.

For the midwife, care for an individual with PPCM is limited to prompt referral to an appropriate specialist or interdisciplinary care team, preferably including a cardiologist experienced in treating patients with heart failure.[41] Although care and management of an individual with PPCM are not within the scope of midwifery practice, being able to recognize and refer early can be beneficial for individuals, as it is sometimes possible for the heart to recover some of its lost function.[39]

The etiology of PPCM remains unknown.[40] Risk factors for this condition include chronic hypertension, preeclampsia, multiple gestation, teenage pregnancy, advanced maternal age, family history of heart failure, and use of tocolytics during pregnancy.[40] One challenge in diagnosing PPCM is that the symptoms are very similar to the normal symptoms seen during pregnancy and in preeclampsia.[40,41] Specifically, fatigue, shortness of breath, edema, and weight gain are symptoms of both PPCM and normal pregnancy. However, the symptoms most commonly associated with PPCM are persistent; they include marked shortness of breath, orthopnea, tachycardia, palpitations, chest pain, cough, and edema.[40]

To warrant a diagnosis of PPCM, the symptoms of heart failure must present either in the last month of pregnancy or up to 6 months after birth, the heart ejection fraction (EF) must be less than 45%, and no other etiologies can be present that might cause heart failure with a diminished ejection fraction.[40]

Physical examination can reveal crackles in the bases of the lungs, pitting edema, jugular vein distension, a galloping heart sound, or laterally shifted point of maximum impulse when auscultating the heart.[39] The definitive diagnosis of PPCM is made by echocardiogram, but a 12-lead electrocardiogram showing either signs of left ventricular hypertrophy or ST-T wave abnormalities, or a markedly elevated beta natriuretic peptide (BNP) blood test, indicates a strong likelihood of PPCM.[39]

Although PPCM can become evident during the last few weeks of pregnancy, the majority of individuals with this condition are diagnosed in the postpartum period.[40] This pattern might indicate that features of PPCM are present during pregnancy, but that individuals seek help only when symptoms such as shortness of breath and fatigue do not resolve postpartum.

Individuals with PPCM often require dietary modifications, fluid restriction, and a medication regimen to control their condition. It is unclear why some individuals regain their ejection fraction and others do not, but evidence suggests that an ejection fraction that remains greater than 30% for the course of the illness is a key component.[42] In extreme cases, heart transplantation or a surgically implanted mechanical ventricular assist device may be needed for survival.[43]

Vigilance is needed on the part of the midwife to recognize and refer postpartum individuals suspected of having PPCM. Access to appropriate postpartum contraception is important, as affected individuals have an increased risk of recurrence of PPCM. Nevertheless, this condition is not an absolute contraindication to pregnancy, provided that the ejection fraction has recovered to baseline.

## Postpartum Thrombophlebitis and Thromboembolism

Postpartum thrombophlebitis is defined as inflammation of a vein accompanied by formation of a thrombosis (blood clot). Thrombophlebitis can occur in both superficial and deep veins. Thrombosis is more common in individuals with varicosities and in individuals who are perhaps genetically susceptible to vein-wall relaxation and venous stasis.

Venous thromboembolism (VTE) is defined is defined as the development of a blood clot in the vein that can be classified as a deep vein thrombosis (DVT) or pulmonary embolism (PE). DVT can form in the leg, thigh, pelvis, or arm. When a DVT is dislodged, the clot can travel to the lungs, causing PE.

Pulmonary embolism remains a leading cause of morbidity and mortality in the United States.[2,44] During the postpartum period, 1 in 2000 individuals will be diagnosed with venous thrombosis and embolism.[45] Results from the Nationwide Inpatient Sample revealed a 40% decrease of DVT from cesarean birth between 2004 to 2014.[45] However, there was no decrease in PE from cesarean birth from this same time frame. Likewise, risk for DVT and pulmonary embolism from vaginal birth did not significantly change.[45] Many thromboembolic events can be anticipated or prevented.[46]

Risk assessment for VTE should begin prior to pregnancy or prenatally. Subsequently, follow-up risk assessment should occur during the intrapartum period and up to 6 weeks postpartum and include a review of the items in Table 35-4.[45] Studies indicate individuals have a 20 to 37 times higher rate of VTE during the first 6 weeks postpartum compared to nonpregnant individuals, with the highest risk being noted during the first 3 weeks postpartum.[45]

Three important physiologic changes in pregnancy and postpartum increase the risk of thrombosis formation (previously known as Virchow's triad): (1) stasis of blood, (2) hypercoagulability, and (3) vascular trauma. Venous-wall relaxation resulting from the effects of progesterone and pressure on the veins by the gravid uterus fosters venous stasis. Pregnancy is also a hypercoagulable state, and this state persists throughout the early postpartum period. Venous-wall inflammation and endothelial damage secondary to distension, in the setting of this hypercoagulable state, predisposes the individual to thrombus formation.[47] Prolonged venous compression during positioning for labor or birth can contribute to the problem as well. Cesarean birth is also considered a risk factor for thrombosis; thus, mechanical thromboprophylaxis, such as alternating compression devices, is recommended before and after cesarean birth.

Guidelines vary among professional organizations regarding prophylactic treatment for VTE. There is consensus, however, that high-risk individuals with prior VTE events and certain

| Table 35-4 | Risk Factors for Venous Thrombosis |
|---|---|
| **Individual History–Related Risks** | |

Obesity

Smoking

Age > 35 years

History of thrombosis

Inherited thrombophilias

Antiphospholipid antibody syndrome

Sickle cell disease

Heart disease

Diabetes

Immobility (paraplegia)

History of postpartum hemorrhage

**Pregnancy-Related Risks**

Hypercoagulable state

Venous stasis

Multiple pregnancy

Higher parity

Preeclampsia

Antepartum hospitalizations

**Labor- and Birth-Related Risks**

Operative vaginal birth

Cesarean birth

Infection

Vascular trauma

Immobilization

Postpartum hemorrhage

Preterm birth

Stillbirth

Immediate postpartum period

Based on Friedman AM. Obstetric venous thromboembolism prophylaxis, risk factors and outcomes. *Curr Opin Obstet Gynecol.* 2021;33(5):384-390. doi:10.1097/GCO.0000000000000733; American College of Obstetricians and Gynecologists. ACOG Practice Bulletin No. 196: thromboembolism in pregnancy. *Obstet Gynecol.* 2018;132:e1-e17.

thrombophilias should receive prophylaxis. Many sources agree that thromboprophylaxis should be individualized according to risk.[46,47]

DVT is more common in the left lower extremity (accounting for 70% to 80% of cases), presumably due to compression of the left iliac vein from the gravid uterus and the crossing of the right iliac artery, as well as the nearly 50%

decreased blood flow to the lower extremities.[47] Individuals with a body mass index (BMI) of 30 or greater are at higher risk for postpartum and postsurgical thrombus formation than individuals with lower BMIs; this risk also increases as BMI increases.[45,47] Under no circumstances should the individual's leg be massaged when thrombophlebitis in this location is suspected. Physician management is necessary.

Risk factors for postpartum thrombophlebitis are summarized in Table 35-4, and the signs and symptoms of superficial thrombophlebitis, DVT, and PE are summarized in Table 35-5.[47–49] DVT presents as unilateral edema and an increase in leg circumference. Tenderness and a feeling of warmth

| Table 35-5 | Signs and Symptoms of Superficial Thrombophlebitis Versus Deep Vein Thrombosis and Pulmonary Embolism |
|---|---|
| **Condition** | **Signs and Symptoms** |
| Superficial thrombophlebitis | Inflammation at the site |
| | Leg pain |
| | Localized heat |
| | Palpation of a knot or cord, tenderness |
| Deep vein thrombosis | Abrupt onset with leg pain worsening with motion or when standing |
| | Generalized edema of ankle, leg, or calf |
| | Mild tachycardia and possible slight elevation in temperature |
| | Pain with calf pressure |
| | Tenderness along course of involved vessel with possible palpable cord |
| Pulmonary embolism | Dyspnea |
| | Leg edema |
| | Tachycardia |
| | Chest pain |

Based on American College of Obstetricians and Gynecologists. ACOG Practice Bulletin No. 196: thromboembolism in pregnancy. *Obstet Gynecol.* 2018;132:e1-e17; Bennett A, Chunilal S. Diagnosis and management of deep vein thrombosis and pulmonary embolism in pregnancy. *Semin Thromb Hemost.* 2016;42:760-773; Petersen EE, Davis NL, Goodman D, et al. Vital signs: pregnancy-related deaths, United States, 2011–2015, and strategies for prevention, 13 states, 2013–2017. *Morb Mortal Wkly Rep.* 2019;68(18):423-429.

can be noted over the affected veins. Superficial thrombophlebitis is more localized in appearance, but it can be difficult to distinguish between the two conditions based on physical examination.

The differential diagnosis includes superficial thrombophlebitis versus deep vein thrombosis, muscle strain or trauma, ruptured cyst, vasculitis, and lymphedema. Compression ultrasound is the primary diagnostic test, with or without color Doppler imaging.[50] Diagnostic ultrasound is indicated for DVT as well as for superficial thrombophlebitis to rule out underlying DVT. Laboratory analysis includes high-sensitivity D-dimer studies, which measure fibrin degradation. However, D-dimer values often do not return to prepregnant levels until 4 to 5 weeks postpartum. Diagnosis for PE includes D-dimer testing and computed tomography pulmonary angiography (CTPA).[44]

Elicitation of Homan's sign (pain on dorsiflexion of the foot) was once thought to be a diagnostic sign of DVT. A positive Homan's sign may, in fact, indicate DVT—but it could also indicate a strained calf muscle. This sign is present in fewer than one-third of individuals who have a confirmed DVT. Conversely, a negative Homan's sign does not rule out DVT. Furthermore, eliciting Homan's sign could disturb a thrombosis; thus, this test is no longer recommended for evaluation of leg pain in the postpartum period.

Management differs significantly for superficial thrombophlebitis and DVT. Treatment of superficial thrombophlebitis includes leg rest, elevation of the affected extremity, supportive stockings, and non-steroidal anti-inflammatory drug (NSAID) analgesia as needed. Treatment for DVT includes these same elements, with the addition of anticoagulants. Ambulation should occur gradually as tolerated. Anticoagulation therapy is usually continued for at least 6 months or longer if needed. Warfarin (Coumadin) is considered safe during lactation. Physician referral is indicated for management of DVT and PE.

### Pulmonary Embolism

The greatest risk associated with thrombophlebitis is PE.[44] This is true for individuals who develop DVT, whereas PE is unlikely in individuals who have a superficial thrombophlebitis. Tachypnea, dyspnea, leg edema, and sudden-onset, sharp chest pain are the symptoms most commonly associated with PE. Sudden onset of these symptoms requires urgent evaluation. Many other, less specific symptoms can be present, including altered lung and heart sounds and apprehension as the individual's blood oxygen level decreases. Vigilant assessment is imperative for early identification. PE is considered an emergent condition and is best treated with a team-based approach.

## Thyroiditis and Thyroid Storm

Some postpartum thyroid disorders can occur slowly and present with subtle symptoms; others may develop suddenly as a marked illness. These disorders can occur anytime during the first postpartum year, so symptoms can be remote from childbirth and not identified as a postpartum complication. Postpartum thyroid disease can be particularly difficult to recognize, as symptoms are similar to those commonly encountered in the postpartum period: lack of energy, sleep difficulties, appetite changes, weight changes, memory difficulty, and depressed affect. These symptoms are also found in individuals with postpartum mood disorders, as discussed in the *Mental Health Conditions* chapter. Postpartum thyroid dysfunction has been associated with postpartum depression.[51] Thyroid illness and mood disorder symptoms are so similar that thyroid-stimulating hormone (TSH) screening is an initial step in the evaluation of postpartum mood disorders.

### Postpartum Thyroiditis

Postpartum thyroiditis is an autoimmune thyroiditis that can present as (1) transient hypothyroidism, (2) transient hyperthyroidism, or (3) hyperthyroidism followed by hypothyroidism and then recovery.[52,53] Reported incidence of this condition ranges from 1.1% to 16.7%.[54] Individuals at increased risk for postpartum thyroiditis include those with gestational diabetes, autoimmune disorders such as type 1 diabetes, previous thyroid dysfunction, and history of thyroid disorders.[52,54] Although most individuals recover and are euthyroid within 1 year, a small proportion remain hypothyroid and need long-term replacement therapy.

The clinical course of postpartum thyroiditis starts with thyroid inflammation that damages thyroid follicles. These changes result in excessive thyroid hormone release ($T_3$ and $T_4$) leading to hyperthyroidism, which is then followed by transient hypothyroidism once the stores of thyroid hormone are exhausted. Ultimately, the inflammation subsides and thyroid hormone synthesis resumes. The hyperthyroid phase typically occurs around 3 months postpartum and resolves spontaneously within 2 to 3 months.

Signs and symptoms of postpartum thyroiditis resemble common postpartum recovery symptoms. In addition, there is usually no recognizable pain or swelling of the thyroid. Common symptoms of postpartum thyroiditis depend on the phase (hyper or hypo) of the illness. Table 35-6 compares and contrasts common signs and symptoms of both the hyperthyroidism and hypothyroidism phases of the illness.[53,55]

Because thyroiditis does not manifest until later in the postpartum period, its symptoms can go unnoticed in either phase of the disorder and misdiagnosis can occur. In the hyperthyroid phase, low levels of TSH, the presence of thyroid peroxidase antibodies, and a lack of TSH receptor antibodies suggest the diagnosis of postpartum thyroiditis. In the hypothyroid phase, an elevated TSH level and a positive test for antithyroid peroxidase antibodies are pathognomonic for this disorder. Postpartum depression and anxiety have similar symptoms, however, and should be included in the differential diagnosis. Individuals experiencing thyroiditis can have symptoms that can mimic psychosis.

Treatment depends on the degree of symptoms. If symptoms are mild, no treatment will be instituted. If symptoms of hyperthyroidism are bothersome, beta blockers are the usual treatment of choice, whereas thyroid supplementation with levothyroxine (Synthroid) is prescribed for hypothyroid symptoms.[54,56] While physician consultation or management is indicated for hyperthyroidism, midwives often manage hypothyroid symptoms independently. There is no consensus on criteria for treatment, dose of medication, or duration of

| Table 35-6 | Signs and Symptoms of Postpartum Thyroiditis | |
|---|---|---|
| **Condition** | **Timing** | **Signs and Symptoms** |
| Hyperthyroid | 1–4 months postpartum | Anxiety, fatigue, goiter, heat intolerance/ sweats, insomnia, irritability, weight loss |
| Hypothyroid | 4–8 months postpartum | Constipation, depression, dry skin, fatigue, goiter, impaired concentration |

Based on American College of Obstetricians and Gynecologists. Practice Bulletin No. 223: thyroid disease in pregnancy. *Obstet Gynecol.* 2020;135:261-274; Korevaar T, Medici M, Visser T, et al. Thyroid disease in pregnancy: new insights in diagnosis and clinical management. *Nat Rev Endocrinol.* 2017;13:610-622. https://doi.org/10.1038/nrendo.2017.93.

treatment for postpartum thyroid disorders but endocrinology specialists can be helpful in determining a long-term plan of care.

### Thyroid Storm

Thyroid storm, also known as clinical thyrotoxicosis, is a rare, life-threatening, acute exacerbation of hyperthyroidism. It occurs earlier than thyroiditis (usually during the first month postpartum) and is distinguished by an abrupt onset of symptoms. This disorder, which results from overproduction of thyroid hormone, is characterized by the sudden onset of a hypermetabolic state. Signs and symptoms include nausea and vomiting, diarrhea, fever ($> 41°C$ [105°F]), tachycardia, and tremor. Potential outcomes include dehydration, seizures, coma, and death if the thyroid storm goes untreated. Increased $T_4$ levels can lead to cardiomyopathy and heart failure.[57]

The diagnosis of thyroid storm is based on symptoms and presentation Treatment is initiated prior to obtaining the results of confirmatory laboratory studies. Individuals in thyroid storm usually present to an emergency department acutely ill and may initially be assumed to have preeclampsia. The presence of altered mental changes and hyperpyrexia distinguish thyroid storm from postpartum preeclampsia or eclampsia.[53,57] Individuals in thyroid storm need to be hospitalized for intensive care management.

## Postdural Puncture Headache (Spinal Headache/Wet Tap)

Postpartum headache can be mild to severe and complicate quality of life during the early puerperal period. Early identification of its cause is crucial to appropriate treatment and relief. A common cause of headaches during the first few days postpartum is postdural puncture headache (PDPH), which can occur after administration of neuraxial anesthesia, commonly used during epidural or spinal anesthetic procedures. This complication occurs when cerebrospinal fluid leaks through a hole in the dura at the site of the epidural or spinal procedure. Although not considered a complication of significance in the past, evidence now suggests that PDPH is associated with both acute and chronic effects.[58]

Acute PDPH most often occurs within 5 days post procedure. Most individuals experience a severe or dull headache in the frontal or occipital area, sometimes associated with nausea, neck pain, or tinnitus. PDPH is often identified when the pain worsens while the individual is in the upright position but improves significantly when the person is supine. Standard treatment for PDPH has been an epidural blood patch, using blood from the patient to patch the offending hole in the dura. A blood patch is successful 85% of the time. Sequelae of PDPH included the potential for interruption of interactions with the newborn, delay in breastfeeding/chestfeeding, increased hospital stay, hospital readmission, and overall dissatisfaction.[58] Although most headaches or other associated symptoms resolve, some individuals with PDPH report persistent headaches for up to 18 months postpartum or that are chronically recurrent.[59]

Recently, severe sequelae such as subdural hematoma (SDH) and cerebral venous sinus thrombosis (CVST) have been associated with PDPH.[59] Symptoms of SDH include headache, nausea, emesis, and cranial nerve palsies. If the bleeding is slow, cognitive impairment, lightheadedness, somnolence, or seizures can occur. Treatment of SDH usually requires surgical intervention. Symptoms of CVST also include headache, visual disturbance, seizure, or neurologic deficits. These symptoms are emergency warning signs, and a team-based approach to care should be initiated immediately and intensive care begun even as diagnostic testing is ongoing. Diagnostics include computed tomography or magnetic resonance venogram. Anticoagulants are the most common treatment for CVST.[58]

Along with the usual symptoms experienced from PDPH, clinicians should be vigilant for reports of unusual or severe "thunderclap" headaches, concomitant hypertension, neurologic deficits, headaches that increase while lying down, or awakening with a headache. These symptoms could indicate stroke and warrant immediate collaborative intensive care. Counseling should include specific symptomatology that requires immediate follow-up along with how to get medical help quickly if the symptoms occur.

## Substance Use Disorder

Substance use disorders are a global issue whose rates are increasing.[60] Often individuals with substance use disorders undergo much scrutiny and stigmatization, which can be a barrier to obtaining adequate care during pregnancy.[61] Some individuals may receive treatment or abstain from substances during pregnancy but relapse during the postpartum period. Continuation of treatment and medications for opioid use disorder is important in the postpartum period and beyond. Individuals treated with methadone or buprenorphine should follow up with their prescriber to adjust medication dosages postpartum. Leading causes of postpartum death include mental health disorders and overdose, so ongoing care can be life-saving. Referral to new locations for treatment may be needed if an individual has been receiving care at a perinatal-specific clinic.

Opioid use disorder is of particular concern when managing postpartum pain. Adequate pain management is important for establishing a parental bond, self-care, reducing the risk of postpartum depression, and preventing substance use disorder relapse.[60,62] Individuals who have a vaginal birth typically do not have the same pain management challenges as those who have a cesarean birth. For individuals who have had cesarean births, a stepwise approach to pain management should be used, including a combination of oral and parenteral opioids, acetaminophen, or anti-inflammatory medications.[60,62] These individuals need healthcare providers who are trusting and compassionate to assist them with pain management, establishing a parental bond, breastfeeding/chestfeeding, and addressing their concerns about possible involvement of state or local authorities. Also, this trusting relationship can help them to explore different coping and treatment modalities to care for themselves and their families.[61]

## Conclusion

Midwives should be astute in assessing the normal physiology of the puerperium, readily recognize pathologic processes, and be prepared to initiate early treatment and prevent worsening illness. Midwives often initiate diagnosis and treatment of postpartum complications, recognizing when it is appropriate to consult, collaborate, or refer, thereby reducing first-line morbidity and mortality. Knowledge of nationally recognized warning symptoms and vital signs standards as well as local guidelines for emergency team notification are important in ensuring rapid intervention when needed. While physicians will medically manage some complications, the midwife will continue to manage other aspects of the individual's postpartum course and adjustments to ensure continuity of care. Person-centered care includes taking time to explain diagnoses and debrief the individual and family following emergencies. Thus, midwifery care of individuals who have experienced postpartum complications includes provision of person-centered and medically

appropriate contraception and ensuring the individual has ongoing primary care for chronic conditions to improve long-term health outcomes

### Resources

| Organization | Description |
|---|---|
| California Maternal Quality Care Collaborative (CMQCC) | Preeclampsia toolkit |
| Centers for Disease Control and Prevention (CDC) | Guideline for the Prevention of Surgical Site Infection, 2017 |
| Centers for Disease Control and Prevention (CDC) | Hear Her campaign |
| Global Library of Women's Medicine (GLOWM) | Management of secondary postpartum hemorrhage |
| Council on Patient Safety in Women's Health Care | Maternal venous thromboembolism |
| Substance Abuse and Mental Health Services Administration (SAMHSA) | Substance use disorder information |

### References

1. Centers for Disease Control and Prevention. Reproductive health: Hear Her campaign. https://www.cdc.gov/hearher/?gclid=EAIaIQobChMIj_Wvut-18gIVhozICh2CeAYhEAAYASAAEgJqpPD_BwE. Accessed August 16, 2021.

2. Murphy SL, Xu J, Kochanek KD, et al. Deaths: final data for 2018. *Nat Vital Stat Rep.* 2021;69(13).

3. Collier AY, Molina RL. Maternal mortality in the United States: updates on trends, causes, and solutions. *Neoreviews.* 2019;20(10):e561-e574. doi:10.1542/neo.20-10-e561.

4. Yacoubian C. *Scaling NLP in healthcare: who are the winners? Linguamatics.* https://www.linguamatics.com/solutions/social-determinants-health-sdoh?gclid=CjwKCAjwhaaKBhBcEiwA8acsHONLknlYGUREGonfFcaULNnLzRss60Ec38SwHlU5vQ5vMdDd8BBOdxoCUC8QAvD_BwE. Published August 31, 2021. Accessed September 21, 2021.

5. Kramer MR, Strahan AE, Preslar J, et al. Changing the conversation: applying a health equity framework to maternal mortality reviews. *Am J Obstet Gynecol.* 2019;221(6):609.E1-609.E9. https://doi.org/10.1016/j.ajog.2019.08.057.

6. Association of Women's Health, Obstetric and Neonatal Nurses. Post-birth warning signs. https://www.awhonn.org/education/hospital-products/post-birth-warning-signs-education-program/. Updated 2021. Accessed October 24, 2022.

7. Ain Q, Shetty N, Supriya K. Postpartum urinary retention and its associated obstetric risk factors among women undergoing vaginal delivery in tertiary care hospital. *J Gynecol Obstet Hum Reprod*. 2021;50(2):101837. doi:10.1016/j.jogoh.2020.101837.

8. Biurrun GP, Gonzalez-Doza E, Fernandez C, Corona AF. Postpartum urinary retention and related risk factors. *Urology*. 2020;143:97-102. doi:10.1016/j.urology.2020.03.061.

9. Mulder FEM, Rengerink KO, van der Post JAM, et al. Delivery-related risk factors for covert postpartum urinary retention after vaginal delivery. *Int Urogynecol J*. 2016;27:55-60.

10. Mulder FE, Hakvoort RA, de Bruin JP, et al. Long-term micturition problems of asymptomatic postpartum urinary retention: a prospective case-control study. *Int Urogynecol J*. 2018. doi:10.1007/s00192-017-3457-6.

11. Centers for Disease Control and Prevention. Pregnancy Mortality Surveillance System: causes of pregnancy-related deaths. https://www.cdc.gov/reproductivehealth/maternal-mortality/pregnancy-mortality-surveillance-system.htm. Accessed August 18, 2021.

12. Black CM, Vesco KK, Mehta V, et al. Hospital readmission following delivery with and without severe maternal morbidity. *J Womens Health*. 2021. doi:10.1089/jwh.2020.8815.

13. Taylor M, Pillarisetty LS. Endometritis. In: *StatPearls*. Treasure Island, FL: StatPearls Publishing; January 2021. https://www.ncbi.nlm.nih.gov/books/NBK553124/. Updated April 4, 2021. Accessed October 24, 2022.

14. ACOG Practice Bulletin No. 199: use of prophylactic antibiotics in labor and delivery. *Obstet Gynecol*. 2018;132(3):e103-e119. doi:10.1097/AOG.0000000000002833.

15. Haas DM, Morgan S, Contreras K, Kimball S. Vaginal preparation with antiseptic solution before cesarean section for preventing postoperative infections. *Cochrane Database Syst Rev*. 2020;4:CD007892. doi:10.1002/14651858.CD007892.pub7.

16. Patel S, Rodriguez AN, Macias DA, et al. A gap in care: postpartum women presenting to the emergency room and getting readmitted. *Am J Perinatol*. 2020;37(14):1385-1392. doi:10.1055/s-0040-1712170.

17. Liabsuetrakul T, Choobun T, Peeyananjarassri K, Islam QM. Antibiotic prophylaxis for operative vaginal delivery. *Cochrane Database Syst Rev*. 2020;3:CD004455. doi:10.1002/14651858.CD004455.pub5.

18. Kawakita T, Landy HJ. Surgical site infections after cesarean delivery: epidemiology, prevention and treatment. *Matern Health Neonat Perinatol*. 2017;3:12. doi:10.1186/s40748-017-0051-.

19. Axelsson D, Brynhildsen J, Blomberg M. Postpartum infection in relation to maternal characteristics, obstetric interventions and complications. *J Perinat Med*. 2018;46(3):271-278.

20. Foeller ME, Sie L, Foeller TM, et al. Risk factors for maternal readmission with sepsis. *Am J Perinatol*. 2020;37(5):453-460. doi:10.1055/s-0039-1696721.

21. Hill J, Patrick HS, Ananth CV, et al. Obstetrical outcomes and follow-up for patients with asymptomatic COVID-19 at delivery: a multicenter prospective cohort study. *Am J Obstet Gynecol MFM*. 2021;3(6):100454. https://doi.org/10.1016/j.ajogmf.2021.100454.

22. Centers for Disease Control and Prevention. Covid-19: care for breastfeeding people: interim guidance on breastfeeding and breast milk feeds in the context of Covid-19. https://www.cdc.gov/coronavirus/2019-ncov/hcp/care-for-breastfeeding-women.html. Published 2021.

23. American College of Obstetricians and Gynecologists. Practice Bulletin No. 183: postpartum hemorrhage. *Obstet Gynecol*. 2017;130(4):e168-e186.

24. İskender C, Topçu H, Timur H, et al. Evaluation of risk factors in women with puerperal genital hematomas. *J Matern Fetal Neonatal Med*. 2016;29(9):1435-1439. doi:10.3109/14767058.2015.1051018.

25. O'Brien SH, Stanek JR, Kaur D, et al. Laboratory monitoring during pregnancy and post-partum hemorrhage in women with von Willebrand disease. *J Thromb Haemost*. 2020;18:604-608.

26. American College of Obstetricians and Gynecologists. Committee Opinion No. 580: von Willebrand disease in women. *Obstet Gynecol*. 2013;122:1368-1373. Reaffirmed 2021.

27. Byrne B, Ryan K, Lavin M. Current challenges in the peripartum management of women with von Willebrand disease. *Semin Thromb Hemost*. 2021;47:217-228.

28. Schrey-Petersen S, Tauscher A, Dathan-Stumpf A, Stepan H. Diseases and complications of the puerperium. *Dtsch Arztebl Int*. 2021;118:436-446. doi:10.3238/arztebl.m2021.0168.

29. Centers for Disease Control and Prevention. Chlamydial infections. https://www.cdc.gov/std/treatment-guidelines/chlamydia.htm. Accessed June 27, 2022.

30. Drugs and Lactation Database (LactMed). *Doxycycline*. Bethesda, MD: National Library of Medicine; January 18, 2021. https://www.ncbi.nlm.nih.gov/books/NBK500561/. Accessed October 24, 2022.

31. Gestational hypertension and preeclampsia. *Obstet Gynecol*. 2020;135(6):e237-e260. doi:10.1097/AOG.0000000000003891.

32. Wang W, Xie X, Yuan T, et al. Epidemiological trends of maternal hypertensive disorders of pregnancy at the global, regional, and national levels: a population-based study. *BMC Pregnancy*

*Childbirth.* 2021;21:364. https://doi.org/10.1186/s12884-021-03809-2.

33. Folk D. Hypertensive disorders of pregnancy: overview and current recommendations. *J Midwifery Womens Health.* (2018);63(3):289-300.

34. Redman EK, Hauspurg A, Hubel CA, et al. Clinical course, associated factors, and blood pressure profile of delayed-onset postpartum preeclampsia. *Obstet Gynecol.* 2019;134(5):995-1001. doi:10.1097/AOG.0000000000003508.

35. Takaoka S, Ishii K, Taguchi T, et al. Clinical features and antenatal risk factors for postpartum-onset hypertensive disorders. *Hypertens Pregnancy.* 2016;35(1):22-31. doi:10.3109/10641955.2015.1100308.

36. Bernstein PS, Martin JN, Barton JR, et al. Consensus bundle on severe hypertension during pregnancy and the postpartum period. *J Midwifery Womens Health.* 2017;62(4):493-501.

37. Camargo EC, Singhal AB. Stroke in pregnancy: a multidisciplinary approach. *Obstet Gynecol Clin North Am.* 2021;48:75-96. https://doi.org/10.1016/j.ogc.2020.11.004.

38. Joyce EM. Organic psychosis: the pathobiology and treatment of delusions. *CNS Neurosci Ther.* 2018;24:598-603.

39. Bauersachs J, Konig T, van der Meer P, et al. Pathophysiology, diagnosis and management of peripartum cardiomyopathy: a position statement from the Heart Failure Association of the European Society of Cardiology Study Group on peripartum cardiomyopathy. *Eur J Heart Failure.* 2019;21(7):827-843.

40. Iorgoveanu C, Zaghloul A, Ashwath M. Peripartum cardiomyopathy: a review. *Heart Failure Rev.* 2021;26:1287-1296.

41. Fowler K, Schafer D, Sica M, et al. Peripartum cardiomyopathy (PPCM): interdisciplinary coordination for a complex patient population. *Heart Lung.* 2017;46(3):212-213.

42. Elkayam U, Habakuk O. The search for a crystal ball to predict early recovery from peripartum cardiomyopathy? *JACC: Heart Failure.* 2016;4(5):389-391.

43. Hamdan R, Nassar P, Zein A, et al. Peripartum cardiomyopathy, place of drug therapy, assist devices, and outcome after left ventricular assistance. *J Crit Care.* 2017;37:185-188.

44. Elgendy IY, Gad MM, Mansoor H, et al. Acute pulmonary embolism during pregnancy and puerperium: national trends and in-hospital outcomes. *Mayo Clin Proc.* 2021;96(8):2102-2113. https://doi.org/10.1016/j.mayocp.2021.01.015.

45. Friedman AM. Obstetric venous thromboembolism prophylaxis, risk factors and outcomes. *Curr Opin Obstet Gynecol.* 2021;33(5):384-390. doi:10.1097/GCO.0000000000000733.

46. D'Alton ME, Friedman AM, Smiley RM, et al. National Partnership for Maternal Safety: consensus bundle on venous thromboembolism. *J Midwifery Womens Health.* 2016;61(5):649-657.

47. American College of Obstetricians and Gynecologists. ACOG Practice Bulletin No. 196: thromboembolism in pregnancy. *Obstet Gynecol.* 2018;132:e1-e17.

48. Bennett A, Chunilal S. Diagnosis and management of deep vein thrombosis and pulmonary embolism in pregnancy. *Semin Thromb Hemost.* 2016;42:760-773.

49. Petersen EE, Davis NL, Goodman D, et al. Vital signs: pregnancy-related deaths, United States, 2011–2015, and strategies for prevention, 13 states, 2013–2017. *Morb Mortal Wkly Rep.* 2019;68(18):423-429.

50. Stevens SM, Woller SC, Baumann Kreuziger L, et al. Executive summary: antithrombotic therapy for VTE disease: second update of the CHEST guideline and expert panel report, *Chest.* 2021. https://doi.org/10.1016/j.chest.2021.07.056.

51. LeDonne M, Mento C, Settineri S, et al. Postpartum mood disorders and thyroid autoimmunity. *Front Endocrinol (Lausanne).* 2017;8:91. doi:10.3389/fendo.2017.00091.

52. Alexander EK, Pearce EN, Brent GA, et al. 2017 guidelines of the American Thyroid Association for the diagnosis and management of thyroid disease during pregnancy and the postpartum. *Thyroid.* 2017;27(3):315-389. http://online.liebertpub.com/doi/pdf/10.1089/thy.2016.0457. Accessed September 29, 2021.

53. American College of Obstetricians and Gynecologists. Practice Bulletin No. 223: thyroid disease in pregnancy. *Obstet Gynecol.* 2020;135:261-274.

54. Rad NS, Deluxe L. Postpartum thyroiditis. In: *StatPearls.* Treasure Island, FL: StatPearls Publishing; January 2021. https://www.ncbi.nlm.nih.gov/books/NBK557646/. Updated June 20, 2021. Accessed October 24, 2022.

55. Korevaar T, Medici M, Visser T, et al. Thyroid disease in pregnancy: new insights in diagnosis and clinical management. *Nat Rev Endocrinol.* 2017;13:610-622. https://doi.org/10.1038/nrendo.2017.93.

56. Epp R, Malcolm J, Jolin-Dahel K, et al. Postpartum thyroiditis. *BMJ.* 2021;372:n495. doi:10.1136/bmj.n495.

57. Pearce EN. Management of thyrotoxicosis: preconception, pregnancy, and the postpartum period. *Endocr Pract.* 2018;25:62-68.

58. Joudi N, Ansari J. Postpartum headaches after epidural or spinal anesthesia. *Curr Opin Obstet Gynecol.* 2021;33:94-99.

59. Guglielminotti J, Landau R, Li G. Major neurologic complications associated with postdural puncture headache in obstetrics: a retrospective cohort study. *Anesth Analg.* 2019;129(5):1328-1336. doi:10.1213 /ANE.0000000000004336.

60. American College of Obstetricians and Gynecologists. Opioid use and opioid use disorder in pregnancy: Committee Opinion No. 711. *Obstet Gynecol.* 2017a;130(2):488-489.

61. Mahoney K, Reich W, Urbanek S. Substance abuse disorder: prenatal, intrapartum and postpartum care. *MCN Am J Matern Child Nurs.* 2019;44(5): 284-288.

62. American College of Obstetricians and Gynecologists. Postpartum pain management: Committee Opinion No. 742. *Obstet Gynecol.* 2018;132(1): 252-253.

# VII

# Newborn

**Section Editor**

PAM REIS

CHAPTER

# 36

# Anatomy and Physiology of the Newborn

TRACEY BELL AND PAMELA J. REIS

*The editors acknowledge Celia M. Jevitt, who was the author of this chapter in the previous edition.*

## Introduction

The first few moments and hours of extrauterine life are among the most dynamic of any that occur during the entire life cycle. At birth, the newborn moves from complete dependence to physiologic independence. Some organs, such as the lungs, make rapid changes that are fully accomplished within days of birth. Other organ systems, such as the hepatic system, take longer to convert to extrauterine function. Overall, the transition to extrauterine life is an ongoing process and part of a continuum that starts with conception and extends through infancy.

The extrauterine transition can be profoundly influenced by prenatal factors as well as intrapartum events. At each birth, the midwife considers prenatal or intrapartum factors that could cause compromise in the first extrauterine hours of newborn life. Events during conception and the prenatal period that can cause compromise include congenital malformations, genetic disorders, prenatal infections (especially viral), fetal growth restriction, prematurity or postmaturity, chronic diseases (such as cardiac, renal, and hepatic disease and diabetes), the residual effects of environmental or workplace teratogens, and substance use by the birth parent. Labor and birth events that can adversely influence the extrauterine transition include prolonged labor, intrapartum fever, hypoxic uterine conditions, birth trauma, infection, fetal passage of meconium, fetal or intrapartum blood loss, use of medications during labor, difficult or operative birth, and any condition resulting in excessive blood loss. Accurate risk prediction is essential for selection of the appropriate site and personnel for the birth.

The most dramatic and rapid extrauterine transitions that happen immediately after birth occur in four areas: the respiratory system, the circulatory system, thermoregulation, and glucose metabolism. These four areas of transition are interdependent; failure of one can lead to impairment of others, and all must occur successfully for the neonatal transition to proceed smoothly. In utero, an infant is in a state of relative hypoxia with mild acidosis; if this state is not gently corrected after birth, the transition process will be hampered. Barriers to smooth transition can be noted during labor and birth and may be reflected in umbilical cord gases measurements.

In the first few hours of life, newborns experience numerous physiologic changes. After transitioning from the uterine environment to extrauterine life, infants continue to experience many shifts. The first 30 to 60 minutes after birth is a period of reactivity characterized by a state of being awake and alert, with a period during which infants display their strongest suck. During this period, neonates demonstrate transient tachypnea and periodic breathing as cardiovascular and respiratory adaptations persist. A period of relative inactivity occurs 2 to 3 hours after birth. It is during this time that infants demonstrate a stabilized heart rate and respiratory pattern if the transition process is occurring without compromise. Most newborns will have fully transitioned to extrauterine life by 4 to 6 hours of age, though some cardiac changes occur later.

## Respiratory Changes

Prior to birth, the fetus receives oxygen from the birth parent's circulation through the placenta and umbilical vein. Lung development progresses through distinct stages during gestation.[1] Initially, the airways develop into branches, as do the pulmonary capillaries, although the two systems are separated by a mesenchyme. Terminal alveolar sacs appear during the second canalicular stage, between 16 and 24 weeks' gestation. The third saccular stage occurs between approximately 28 and 36 weeks' gestation; during this period, the space between the pulmonary capillaries and the alveoli diminishes so that capillaries are in direct contact with the alveolar basement membrane.

During the third stage, primitive alveoli develop and become lined with two types of alveolar cells, type I and type II epithelial cells. Gas exchange occurs across the very thin type I cells. Interspersed within this cell population are cuboidal-shaped type II epithelial alveolar cells that produce and store surfactant. Surfactant is the complex phospholipid that lines the alveoli and keeps them partially open during exhalation through its surface-acting properties. The lungs of full-term infants contain more surfactant in the type II cells than is the case in adult lungs, and they are ready to release the surfactant at the onset of labor.[2] The alveolar period starts at 36 weeks' gestation and continues throughout childhood. During this period, more alveoli form, creating a larger surface area for gas exchange. Approximately one-third of the 300 million alveoli are mature at birth; the rest mature after birth.

The primary events that occur in the lung after birth are (1) clearance of alveolar fluid, (2) lung expansion, and (3) circulatory changes that increase pulmonary perfusion. Prior to labor, the fetal lungs are full of fluid, which is secreted in type II alveolar cells into the alveolar space as a secondary effect of chloride ion secretion. The term fetus begins to experience a decrease in lung fluid in the days before labor, which in turn reduces the amount of fluid that needs to be cleared during the neonate's initial respirations. Clearance of alveolar fluid is facilitated by increased production and activity of epithelial sodium channels (ENaCs). When the ENaCs become active, sodium ($Na^+$) ions enter the cell from the fetal lung fluid and are actively extruded from the cell into the interstitial space. This process creates an electrochemical gradient that lung fluid and chloride ($Cl^-$) ions follow, which results in clearing the alveoli of lung fluid (Figure 36-1).[3] During labor, fetal plasma levels of catecholamines and cortisol

increase; these hormones further stimulate reabsorption of lung fluid during labor by up-regulating the genes that produce ENaCs.[3,4] This overall process causes the lungs to change from active fluid secretion to active fluid absorption. Also during this time, the lung begins to secrete more surfactant.[2]

Activation of ENaCs is correlated with gestational age. This process is further supported after birth through the infant's increased oxygenation status. Preterm and near-term infants have less activation of ENaCs after birth and more lung fluid compared to term newborns, which increases the incidence of respiratory distress in these neonates.[4]

Figure 36-1 depicts the physiology of fetal lung fluid changes after birth. Sodium enters the cell through the apical surface of both alveolar type I (AT-I) and AT-II cells via amiloride-sensitive ENaCs, both highly selective channels and nonselective channels, and via cyclic nucleotide gated channels (CNGC) (seen only in AT-I cells). Electroneutrality is conserved with chloride movement through the cystic fibrosis transmembrane conductance regulator (CFTR), through chloride channels in AT-I and AT-II cells, or paracellularly through tight junctions. The increase in cell sodium levels stimulates $Na^+$, $K^+$-ATPase activity on the basolateral aspect of the cell membrane, which drives out three sodium ions in exchange for two potassium ions, a process that can be blocked by the cardiac glycoside ouabain. If the net ion movement is from the apical surface to the interstitium, an osmotic gradient is created, which in turn directs water transport in the same direction, either through aquaporins or by diffusion.

The squeezing of the thorax that occurs in the last minutes of second stage labor, when the fetus is in the birth canal, helps extrude some upper airway fluid, although this effect is small.[5,6] Neonates who are delivered by cesarean, especially in the absence of labor, do not experience all processes that contribute to diminution of lung fluid and have an increased risk for transient tachypnea of the newborn (TTN) or respiratory distress syndrome (RDS). It is hypothesized that preterm infants have less mature $Na^+$ transport channels, leading to ineffective fetal lung fluid clearance. Furthermore, the transition from fluid secretion to absorption is augmented by labor; thus, in cases of planned cesarean birth without onset of labor, this process is hindered.

Despite decades of investigation, the phenomena that stimulate the neonate to take the first breath are only partly understood. Several biochemical and mechanical events have been implicated in these processes. For example, the relative hypoxia of the end of labor and the physical stimuli to which

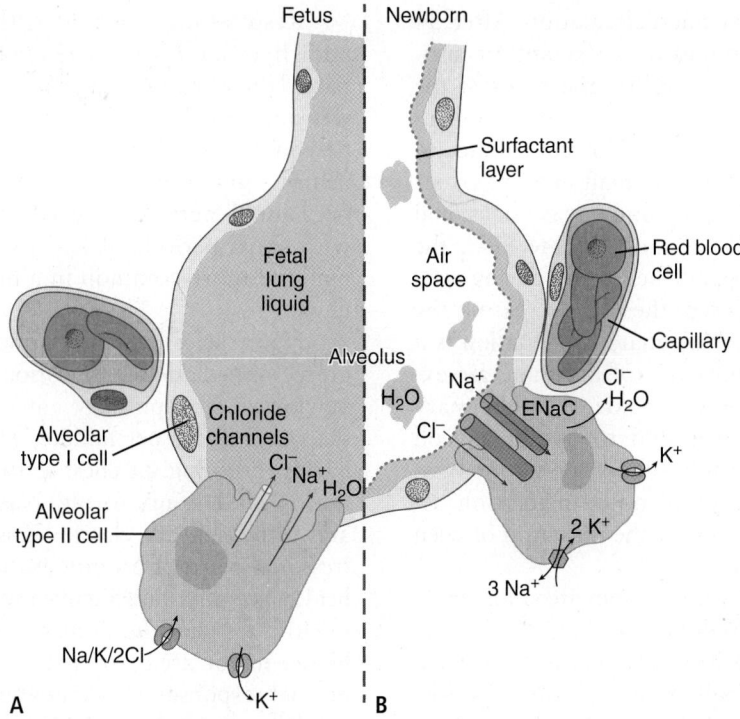

**Figure 36-1** Clearance of alveolar fluid at birth. **A.** Fetal alveoli: $Cl^-$ is actively excreted by the type II alveolar cell. $Na^+$ and water follow passively, so that fluid is secreted into the alveolar space. **B.** Newborn alveoli: Epithelial sodium channels (ENaCs) up-regulate in the apical surface of the alveolar cell. $Na^+$ enters the cell through the ENaCs. The increase in cell Na stimulates Na, $K^+$-ATPase activity on the basolateral aspect of the cell membrane, which drives out three $Na^+$ ions in exchange for two $K^+$ ions. When the net ion movement is from the apical surface to the interstitium, an osmotic gradient is created, directing water in the same direction via either aquaporins or diffusion. This process empties the alveolar fluid into the interstitial space and pulmonary circulation.
Abbreviations: $Cl^-$, chloride; ENaCs, epithelial sodium channels; $H_2O$, water; $K^+$, potassium, $Na^+$, sodium.
Based on Keene SD, Bland RD, Jain L. Lung fluid balance in developing lungs and its role in neonatal transition. In: Oh W, Baum, M, Polin, RA, eds. *Nephrology and Fluid/Electrolyte Physiology: Neonatology Questions and Controversies.* 3rd ed. Philadelphia, PA: Elsevier; 2019:225-236.

the neonate is exposed, such as cold, gravity, pain, light, and noise, cause excitation of the respiratory center. The release of thoracic pressure and rebound chest expansion at birth may help stimulate respirations. With the first breath, fluid filling the mouth and trachea is partially released, and air begins to fill the tracheal column. The first active breaths set in motion a seamless chain of events that (1) assist with the conversion from fetal to adult circulation, (2) further empty the lungs of liquid, (3) establish neonatal lung volume and the characteristics of pulmonary function in the newborn, and (4) decrease pulmonary artery pressure.

When the head is born, mucus drains from the nares and mouth. Many newborns gasp and cry at this time. With the first few breaths, room air starts to fill the large airways of the neonate's trachea and bronchi. Fetal lung fluid remaining in the alveoli is pushed to the lung periphery, where it is absorbed. The first few breaths require more pressure or effort because room air is flowing into a fluid-filled space of approximately 50 cm $H_2O$).[7] Newborns who are exhausted and compromised by the birth process may need assistance in clearing fluid and mucus from the upper airway. Use of a suctioning device such as a bulb syringe or wall suction should be limited to situations in which the newborn's respiratory efforts are diminished or the infant has excessive secretions that they are unable to handle.[8]

All alveoli expand with air over time. The maximum function of alveoli is realized in the presence of adequate surfactant and adequate blood flow through the pulmonary microcirculation. After 34 weeks' gestation, quantities of surfactant are usually adequate to help to stabilize the walls of the alveoli so that they do not collapse onto themselves at the end of each respiration. This contributes to the fetal lungs maintaining a small amount of air at the end of each breath, known as functional residual capacity (FRC). With adequate FRC, the pressure needed to expand the alveoli during subsequent breaths is reduced, thereby decreasing the workload of breathing. Adequate oxygenation is a critical factor in *maintenance* of adequate air exchange. In the presence of hypoxia, the pulmonary vasculature vasoconstricts and oxygen in alveoli cannot be transported into blood vessels for oxygenation of other areas of the body. In addition, severe hypoxemia can suppress the initiation of even the first breath.[2]

If the initial breaths are of adequate volume and pressure, they help establish the neonate's FRC. Crying has been found to have a functional purpose.[9] In a crying neonate, expiration is slowed by resistance from the narrowed glottis, which helps maintain end-expiratory pressure within the lungs. The muscles of the diaphragm also slow the rate of lung deflation. Control of expiration ensures a slower lung deflation, which in turn minimizes the chance of alveolar collapse and loss of FRC.

Continuation of breathing occurs due to central brain stem activity and the actions of specialized cells within the carotid body. In the term newborn, chemoreceptors in the carotid body initiate increases in ventilatory effort in response to acidosis and hypercapnia, and decreases in ventilatory effort in response to hypocapnia. It is also hypothesized that certain prenatal hormones inhibit respirations, so that when the umbilical cord is clamped, those hormone influences are lost.[2]

Respirations fluctuate—they are not stable and rhythmic for an extended period in the neonate. Newborn respirations may sound noisy and wet during this period of transition. Additionally, newborns often experience short periods of apnea or sighing.[10] Lack of a persistent rhythm and occasional periodic breathing (irregular rhythm with short periods of apnea) are considered normal and more common in a near-term or preterm newborn.

Nevertheless, certain abnormal responses require immediate identification and action in the newborn. A respiratory rate consistently greater than 60 breaths per minute, with or without nasal flaring, grunting, or chest retractions, is clearly abnormal at 2 hours of life. Nasal flaring, grunting, and retracting are classic signs of respiratory distress and warrant prompt evaluation by a pediatric healthcare provider. Significant episodes of periodic breathing signal the need for medical intervention before major apnea occurs. Other normal and abnormal responses are summarized in Table 36-1.

When a newborn needs resuscitation and respiratory support, room air (21%)—rather than 100% oxygen—should be used as the initial treatment.[11] The switch to 100% oxygen should be made only if room air is not sufficient. This increase should be gradual and should be titrated using saturations. Although historically 100% oxygen has been used for respiratory resuscitation, it is now known that 100% oxygen can create free oxygen radicals that exacerbate reperfusion injury and decrease cerebral perfusion. Therefore, room air is preferred in neonates. Evidence has demonstrated that healthy, term infants should have saturations ranging from 60% to 90% in the first 5 minutes of life, with incremental increases occurring with each passing minute (Figure 36-2).

| Table 36-1 | Normal and Abnormal Respiratory Characteristics in the Newborn After 10 Minutes of Age | |
|---|---|---|
| **Characteristic** | **Normal** | **Abnormal** |
| Respiratory rate | 40–60 breaths/minute | < 30 breaths/minute or sustained > 60 breaths/minute; periodic breathing or apnea |
| Diaphragm | Diaphragmatic and abdominal breathing | Grunting with every expiration |
| Nasal | Obligate nasal breather | Nasal flaring with every breath |
| Chest | No retractions | Visible suprasternal or subcostal retraction with breaths |
| Pulse oximetry | 95–100% | Less than 95% |

## Circulatory Changes

The blood flow from the placenta stops with the clamping of the umbilical cord. This action eliminates the parental supply of oxygen to the newborn and triggers a subsequent series of reactions. These reactions are complemented by those occurring in the lungs in response to the first breath.

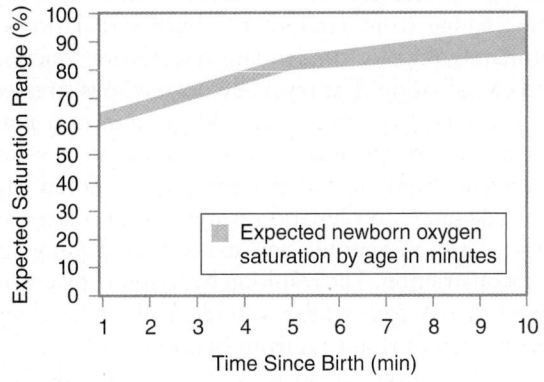

**Figure 36-2** Expected newborn oxygen saturation by age in minutes.

The fetal circulation is characterized by three shunts: (1) the foramen ovale, (2) the ductus arteriosus, and (3) the ductus venosus (**Figure 36-3**). Because the lungs are a closed, fluid-filled organ, they need minimal blood flow; therefore, the pulmonary circulation has high vascular resistance. Pulmonary blood flow is estimated to be approximately 8% of fetal cardiac output. Oxygenated blood bypasses the lungs by flowing through a shunt within the fetal heart known as the foramen ovale, the opening between the right and left atria, and then into the descending aorta. In the second shunt, blood in the right ventricle does not flow far into the pulmonary arteries because of the high-pressure pulmonary vasculature, but rather flows through the shunt known as the ductus arteriosus directly into the descending aorta. Placental prostaglandin, prostacyclin, and low oxygen tension keep the ductus arteriosus open.[12] The third fetal shunt, the ductus venosus, connects the umbilical vein to the inferior vena cava, which allows a portion of fetal blood to bypass the circulation through the liver.

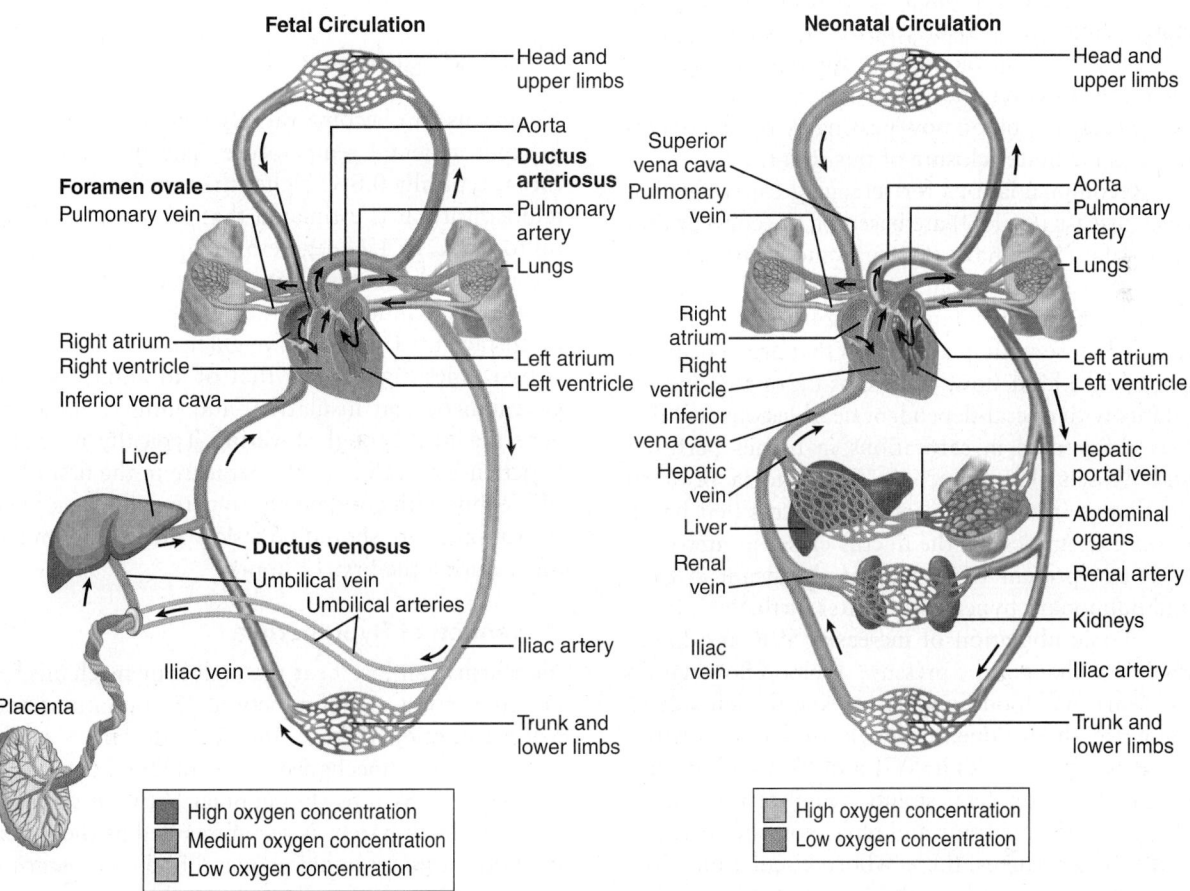

**Figure 36-3** Fetal and neonatal circulation.

Clamping the umbilical cord shuts down the low-pressure system that characterizes the fetal–placental circulatory unit so that the newborn circulatory system becomes an independent, closed system. The immediate effect of cord-clamping is a rise in systemic vascular resistance (SVR). Most importantly, this rise occurs at the same time that the newborn takes their initial breaths. The oxygen in those breaths and expansion of the lung cause the pulmonary vasculature to relax and open. Pulmonary vasculature resistance (PVR) decreases just as SVR increases, and this shift in pressure, in combination with closure of the ductus arteriosus, encourages blood flow into the pulmonary system. Pulmonary vascular resistance continues to decrease over the first 24 hours of life. A transitional period ensues during which kinked pulmonary vessels straighten, which decreases resistance to blood flow. Over time, the development of elongated and thinner cell walls also increases vessel flexibility.[13]

At birth, oxygen tension in the newborn rises, and placental prostaglandins and prostacyclin no longer enter the system via the umbilical vein. This causes constriction of the ductus arteriosus. Within 48 to 72 hours, the ductus arteriosus functionally closes. Anatomic closure, however, can take days to weeks to occur. Blood from the right ventricle is then able to enter the pulmonary circulation, and the oxygenated blood now passing by the ductus arteriosus facilitates closure of this shunt.

Recommendations for screening for congenital heart disease (CCHD) are based on the concept that most infants will have closure of the ductus arteriosus within 24 to 48 hours after birth. This screening is required for all infants after 24 hours of life to identify those with heart lesions that are dependent on ductal blood flow. With closure of the ductus, infants with ductal-dependent heart lesions will display differences in saturations in tissues perfused with vessels that branch from the aorta prior to the ductus (right hand) and post ductus (left hand, lower extremities). If the ductus closes in utero, infants can present with signs of significant distress and pulmonary hypertension after birth.[14]

The combination of increased SVR and lower PVR also changes the pressure of blood flow within the heart. As blood flow increases in the left side of the heart, the foramen ovale closes due to pressure changes. The changes in SVR and PVR and the closure of the three fetal shunts complete the radical changes in the anatomy and physiology of the heart. After these changes, the newborn circulation is the same as that found in children and adults—that is, deoxygenated blood enters the neonatal heart, becomes fully oxygenated in the lungs, and is distributed to all other body tissues.

Clinical evidence of these tremendous changes in circulation is manifested in the moments after birth as increasingly pink color, normal heart rate, and strong pulses. Although newborn cardiopulmonary changes are not anatomically complete for weeks, the functional closure of the foramen ovale and the ductus arteriosus occurs soon after birth. The change from fetal to newborn circulation is intimately related to adequate respiratory function and oxygenation. The term newborn who is stressed by hypoxia, hypoglycemia, cold, or infection may not make the transition smoothly and can develop persistent pulmonary hypertension.[5] As noted earlier, adequate oxygenation supports decreases in PVR, whereas hypoxia can exacerbate pulmonary vasoconstriction. The resulting hypoxemia places an infant at risk for metabolic acidosis. Peripheral vasoconstriction resulting from hypothermia can also lead to metabolic acidosis. Metabolic acidosis is a contributor to pulmonary vasoconstriction, which leads to a cycle of hypoxia, vasoconstriction, tissue hypoperfusion, and further metabolic acidosis.

## Thermoregulation

Newborns can become rapidly stressed by changes in environmental temperature. The fetal temperature is typically 0.6°C higher than the birth parent's temperature. It is estimated that an infant can lose up to 0.5°C to 1°C degree of temperature per minute after birth. Factors that contribute to heat loss in newborns include their large surface area (the ratio of surface area to body weight ratio in a neonate is two times higher than that of an adult), limited subcutaneous fat insulation, and limited ability to generate heat through shivering. Typically, neonates experience a decline in temperature in the first hour of life, but with good newborn care and physiologic transition, there should be a slow incline in temperature during the first 12 hours.[15]

### Prevention of Hypothermia

Newborns can lose heat through four mechanisms: (1) convection, (2) conduction, (3) radiation, and (4) evaporation (Figure 36-4). Furthermore, when more than one mechanism is available, heat loss is accentuated. Skin-to-skin contact between the neonate and birth parent is recommended as the initial method for maintaining neonatal body temperature for healthy term infants.[16] Skin-to-skin contact minimizes heat loss via conduction and results in better

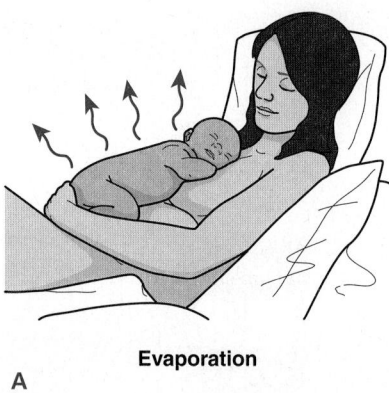

**Evaporation**

A

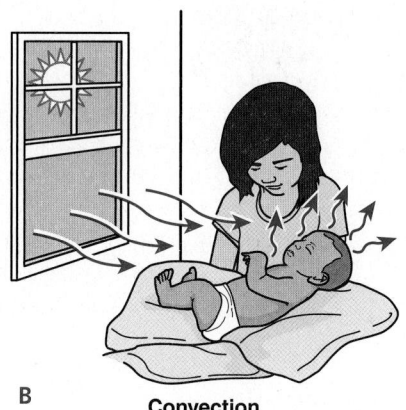

B

**Convection**

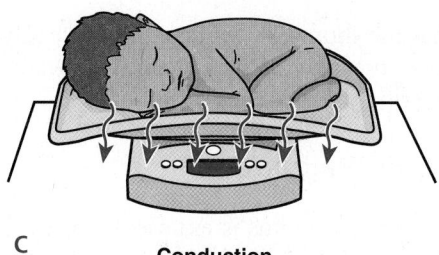

C

**Conduction**

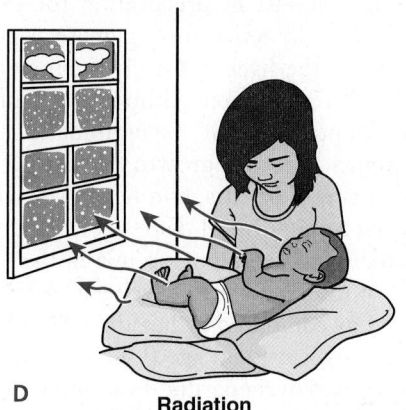

D

**Radiation**

**Figure 36-4** Mechanisms of newborn heat loss. **A.** Evaporation. **B.** Convection. **C.** Conduction. **D.** Radiation.

short-term temperature stability than bundling or placing the neonate under a warmer. This approach should be the first line of treatment for hypothermia, especially in low-resource environments.[17,18] To minimize the effects of heat loss from evaporation, all wet linens should be promptly removed from the infant's vicinity. While the infant is on the birth parent's chest for skin to skin, careful attention to prevention of heat loss via convection should be avoided by limiting draft exposure to both the parent and infant.

## Coping with Cold Stress

Neonates can create heat in three ways: voluntary muscle activity, shivering, and nonshivering thermogenesis. Muscle activity can generate heat but is of limited benefit in increasing temperature, even in term infants with sufficient muscle strength. Nonshivering thermogenesis can increase heat production for a limited amount of time, ranging from minutes to a few hours.[15] Shivering in term neonates is very rare and is typically seen only in those with the most severe cold stress.

Nonshivering thermogenesis refers to utilization of brown fat for heat production. Brown adipose tissue contains more lipids, mitochondria, and capillaries than does white adipose tissue. The primary purpose of brown adipose tissue is to generate heat; such tissue is a nonrenewable resource for the newborn. Brown adipose tissue is found in and around the upper spine, the clavicles and sternum, the kidneys, and major blood vessels. The amount of brown adipose tissue depends on gestational age, with this tissue being relatively sparse in growth-restricted newborns and preterm infants. Brown fat development does not begin until 25 to 28 weeks' gestation.

Creation of heat through utilization of brown adipose stores starts at birth, with a surge of catecholamines and withdrawal of placental prostaglandin and adenosine. The cold stimulus of leaving the birth parent's warm body triggers activity in the newborn hypothalamus, including release of norepinephrine that leads to oxidation of lipids stored in brown adipose tissue and subsequent production of heat.[19] Through the mediation of glucose and glycogen, brown adipose cells convert multiple small intracellular fat vacuoles into heat energy. The heat that is produced via this mechanism warms the blood before it circulates to peripheral areas of the neonate's body and ensures a stable temperature for other biochemical reactions.[20] Nonshivering thermogenesis uses glucose, however, so it places the infant at risk for metabolic acidosis. In a newborn

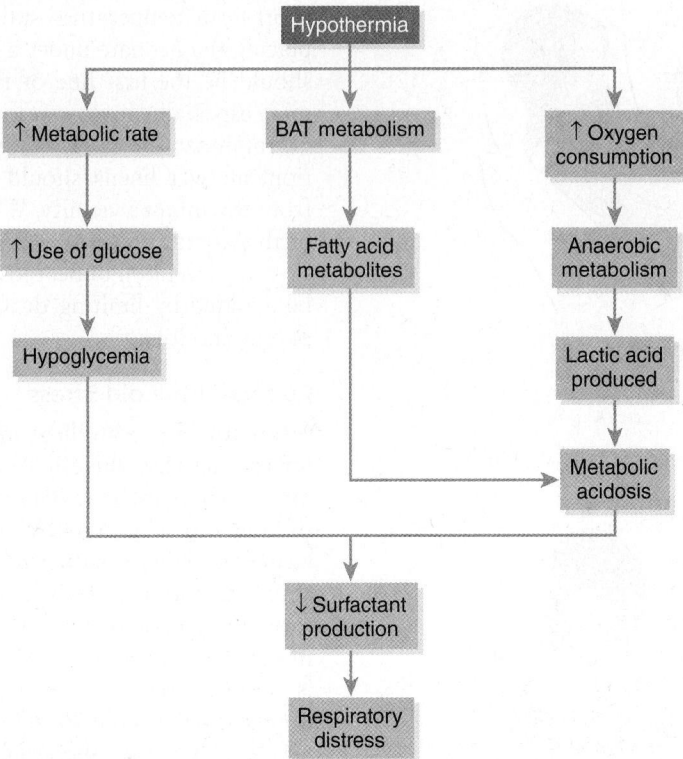

**Figure 36-5** Hypothermia in the newborn.
Abbreviation: BAT, brown adipose tissue.

experiencing hypoglycemia or thyroid dysfunction, the use of brown adipose stores does not proceed efficiently.

The sequelae of heat loss in the neonate can cascade quickly into hypoglycemia, hypoxia, acidosis, and respiratory distress (Figure 36-5). Pulmonary vasoconstriction occurs during hypothermia, leading to hypoxia, which then causes respiratory distress. The body of the term infant will attempt to prevent heat loss by initiating peripheral vasoconstriction. This vasoconstriction can lead to hypoxemia with resulting lactic acid production and metabolic acidosis. These adverse effects are also consequences of the increased metabolic demands that result from the newborn's attempts to create a neutral thermal zone. With hypoxia, metabolic acidosis, and hypoglycemia, the infant becomes at risk for development of pulmonary hypertension.

The World Health Organization defines hypothermia as a core temperature less than 36.5°C (97.7°F).[21] Clinical symptoms of hypothermia may be subtle and include a low core temperature and cold skin, pale skin, pallor, hypotonia, lethargy or irritability, poor feeding or vomiting, tachypnea, and an increased heart rate.[21,22] Any newborn who is

hypothermic should be evaluated for hypoglycemia because of the high caloric demands associated with nonshivering thermogenesis.[22]

## Metabolic Regulation

Prior to birth, the fetus is exposed to a nearly constant blood glucose supply; the levels of glucose in fetal blood are approximately 60% to 70% of the birth parent's levels. In preparation for extrauterine life, the healthy fetus stores glucose as glycogen, particularly in the liver. Most glycogen storage occurs in the third trimester. Although any infant can develop symptomatic or asymptomatic hypoglycemia, infants who are growth restricted, preterm infants, post-term infants, and newborns who have experienced some form of distress prior to birth are at particular risk for hypoglycemia in the newborn period.[23] In these neonates, glycogen stores may be diminished as compared to healthy term newborns. The large for gestational age (LGA) neonate is also at risk for hypoglycemia due to a different mechanism, which involves increased calorie consumption to maintain body temperature. This mechanism occurs in LGA infants independent of the birth parent's diabetes status, with the newborn's risk increasing as birth weight increases.[24] In addition, infants with more than one risk variable have an even higher risk for developing hypoglycemia.

Infants born to a birthing parent with diabetes are at increased risk for developing hypoglycemia secondary to transient hyperinsulinemia. In utero, the fetus responds to the gestational parent's glucose levels by secreting insulin. Upon clamping of the umbilical cord, the birth parent's glucose supply ceases abruptly, but the newborn's secretion of insulin continues. In the first hours after birth, such an infant is at increased risk for significant hypoglycemia and should be monitored closely.

The moment the cord stops pulsating or is clamped, newborns must find a way to maintain a serum glucose level sufficient for optimal brain function. Blood glucose levels initially fall to a nadir at approximately 1 to 2 hours after birth. The physiologic low occurs at approximately 1 to 1.5 hours after birth, with levels subsequently stabilizing at 3 to 4 hours of age. The American Academy of Pediatrics states that healthy term infants may have glucose levels as low as 30 mg/dL in the first 1 to 2 hours of life, but those levels should be greater than 45 mg/dL by 12 hours of life.[25]

Controversy exists regarding glucose monitoring and the optimal level that would define euglycemia, including at what time the newborn's glucose levels should be assessed after birth. Studies have demonstrated no harm from transient levels of hypoglycemia during the initial physiologic transitional period.[26] Researchers have also noted that further study is needed to determine normal blood glucose levels for exclusively breastfed newborns.

Healthy newborns maintain blood glucose levels in one of three ways: (1) utilization of breast milk or a substitute; (2) utilization of glycogen stores (glycogenolysis); or (3) creation of glucose (gluconeogenesis). They generate glucose at a rate of approximately 4 to 8 milligrams per kilogram of body weight per minute. Newborns should be encouraged to feed as soon as they show interest after birth. Indeed, many newborns are active feeders during the first period of reactivity. This is an ideal time to imprint the infant with the physiologic tasks of breastfeeding. Newborns who are exhausted or stressed from long labor may show minimal interest in feeding; consequently, they are at increased risk for hypoglycemia.

Newborns who cannot ingest adequate nutrition will create glucose from glycogen. Gluconeogenesis in the liver will maintain a state of euglycemia until oral intake is improved.[6] Although it is possible for newborns to create glucose from fats or proteins, this process of gluconeogenesis is inefficient and creates many undesirable metabolic by-products. However, glycogenolysis can occur only if the infant has adequate stores of glycogen. Infants who are preterm or small for gestational age have decreased amounts of glycogen stores and will deplete them quickly.

Routine blood glucose testing of term newborns after an uncomplicated birth and without risk factors is not recommended.[27,28] Nevertheless, all newborns should be monitored for signs of hypoglycemia. Hypoglycemia may at first be asymptomatic. Symptoms, when they occur, can be nonspecific and include jitteriness, cyanosis, apnea, weak cry, lethargy, limpness, and refusal to feed. Means of preventing hypoglycemia include identifying risk factors, early recognition of infants who may be at higher risk, and appropriate monitoring. Although a glucose level that signifies danger and would be widely acceptable in all settings has not been identified, it is known that long-term sequelae of persistent and symptomatic hypoglycemia include damage to the occipital area of the brain manifesting as seizures, intellectual disability, and attention-deficit disorder.[29] Damage to the brain is exacerbated when the hypoglycemia is accompanied by neonatal asphyxia.

## Hematologic Changes

Normal values for term newborns' blood components are listed in Table 36-2. Newborn blood cell indices vary by weeks of gestation, vaginal birth, and cesarean birth without labor.[30,31] In response to hypoxia, a fetus will exhibit increased erythropoiesis. At birth, newborns have higher hemoglobin and hematocrit levels compared to adults. Typically, hematocrit will increase after birth, peak at around 2 hours of life, and stabilize by 12 hours of life.[32] Neonatal blood contains both fetal hemoglobin (HbF), which contains two alpha subunits and two gamma subunits, and adult hemoglobin (HbA), which contains two alpha subunits and two beta subunits. HbF has a higher affinity for oxygen than does HbA, is more stable in an acidic environment, and has a shorter life span. After birth, HbA gradually replaces HbF. HbF comprises less than 1% of total hemoglobin after 6 months of life.[33] Because HbF breaks down faster than it can be replaced through erythropoiesis, newborns experience a physiologic anemia approximately 6 to 8 weeks after birth. The life span of the neonatal erythrocyte is about 70 days.[34] Hemoglobin levels decrease slowly

| Table 36-2 | Hematologic Values for a Full-Term Newborn | |
|---|---|
| **Component** | **Optimal Range** |
| Hemoglobin concentration | 14.0–20.0 g/dL |
| RBC count | 4,200,000–5,800,000/mm³ |
| Hematocrit | 43–63% |
| Mean cell diameter | 8.0–8.3 μm |
| MCV | 100–120 μm³ |
| MCH | 32–40 pg |
| MCHC | 30–34% |
| Reticulocyte count | 3–7% |
| Nucleated red blood cell count | 200–600/mm³ |
| White blood cell count | 10,000–30,000/mm³ |
| Granulocytes | 40–80% |
| Lymphocytes | 20–40% |
| Monocytes | 3–10% |
| Platelet count | 150,000–350,000/mm³ |
| Serum iron concentration | 125–225 mcg/dL |
| Total iron-binding capacity | 150–350 mcg/dL |

Abbreviations: MCH, mean corpuscular hemoglobin; MCHC, mean corpuscular hemoglobin concentration; MCV, mean corpuscular volume; RBC, red blood cell.

over the first 7 to 9 weeks after birth, reaching an average of 12.0 g/dL by 2 months of age.

## Effects of Cord-Clamping

The initial hemoglobin/hematocrit values in newborns can be influenced by the timing of cord-clamping and the newborn's position immediately after birth. Delay in clamping the umbilical cord after birth allows for passive placental transfusion, which increases the neonate's blood volume.[35] The physiology of delayed cord-clamping is reviewed in the *Umbilical Cord-Clamping at Birth* appendix in the *Second Stage of Labor and Birth* chapter. When placental transfusion continues for several minutes after birth owing to delayed cord-clamping, it delivers approximately 30% more blood volume and 50% more iron-rich blood cells compared to immediate clamping.[35] Delaying

cord-clamping has several benefits: (1) The neonate receives a bolus of oxygenated blood during the first breaths; (2) the volume expansion promotes pulmonary capillary perfusion in the newborn; (3) the more rapid achievement of adequate oxygenation leads to closure of fetal structures such as the ductus arteriosus; and (4) the infant has a decreased risk of iron-deficiency anemia at 4 to 6 months of life.[35–38] Delaying cord-clamping until cord pulsation ceases has been shown to be safe and is recommended to increase neonatal iron storage at birth, despite this practice being associated with a slightly increased risk for hyperbilirubinemia.[39,40] The difference in the risk for hyperbilirubinemia associated with delayed versus immediate cord-clamping has not been shown to be statistically significant, and no difference has been noted in the need for phototherapy.

To support the physiologic transfusion that occurs over the first minutes of life, the newborn ideally will be placed on the birth parent's abdomen (skin-to-skin) with the cord intact. This position promotes modest amounts of blood flow to the newborn without the potential danger of a forced and large bolus of blood. It also allows for thermoregulation control. By 5 minutes, most of the blood flow from the cord to the neonate is usually accomplished.

## Red Blood Cells and Hyperbilirubinemia

Newborn red blood cells (RBCs) have a short life span of 70 to 80 days, on average, compared to the average adult RBC life span of 120 days. In addition to experiencing faster breakdown of their RBCs, infants have higher hematocrit levels at birth when compared to adults. During the process of RBC breakdown, heme is converted into biliverdin, which is then turned into bilirubin. The rapid cell turnover creates by-products of cell breakdown that must be metabolized, including bilirubin. Bilirubin is transported by albumin to the liver, binds with glucuronate, and is conjugated from a fat-soluble to a water-soluble molecule. In newborns, the activity of the protein uridine diphosphate glucuronosyltransferase (UGT), which helps to conjugate bilirubin and prepare it for excretion, is reduced, so this process in the liver is impaired at birth. Rapid RBC turnover and this reduced activity of UGT are the two factors most responsible for the physiologic jaundice seen in many newborns.[41] In conjunction with these two factors, delayed clearance because of decreased enteral intake and subsequent meconium passage also influence development of hyperbilirubinemia. Supporting early and frequent feeding (more than 8 times per day) can improve bilirubin clearance.

It is estimated that approximately 80% of term and preterm infants will develop physiologic jaundice in the first 7 days of life. Total serum bilirubin peaks at approximately 3 to 5 days of postnatal life in term infants. Approximately 96% of term newborns will have a total serum bilirubin of less than 17 mg/dL at 96 hours of age; levels higher than this concentration are considered a risk for the development of neurotoxicity.[41] Preterm infants have a greater risk for hyperbilirubinemia requiring treatment. Significant jaundice before postnatal day 3 may be pathologic, and any visible jaundice in the first 24 hours of life is of significant concern. There is a correspondingly high reticulocyte count in newborns, reflecting the high rate of formation of new RBCs.

Exposing the newborn's skin to light, known as phototherapy, causes photochemical reactions that improve bilirubin excretion. The threshold at which phototherapy is recommended depends on the newborn's gestational age, hours since birth, and risk factors for hyperbilirubinemia neurotoxicity as phototherapy has some associated risks.

### White Blood Cells

The average white blood cell (WBC) level in newborns ranges from 10,000 to 26,000 cells/mm$^3$. Further elevation in WBC counts may occur in normal newborns during the first 24 hours of life, with levels gradually decreasing over the next 3 to 5 days. Because of these physiologic shifts, it is more useful to focus on neutrophils as a marker for infection. Limits for normal neutrophil shifts in term newborns reflect a normal peak of 28,500 cells/mm$^3$ at 8 hours of age and 13,000 cells/mm$^3$ at 72 hours.[42] Labor, meconium aspiration, prolonged periods of crying, and intrapartum fever can cause a shift upward in neutrophil count.

### Platelets and Clotting Factors

Prothrombin time, thrombin time, and partial thromboplastin time are slightly prolonged in the neonatal period. Platelet counts in newborns should be within the same range as adult values. Levels lower than 150,000 cells/mm$^3$ should prompt further medical evaluation. However, platelet aggregation can vary in term newborns. In the first month of life, there is an overall deficiency of many clotting factors that are dependent on vitamin K.

Vitamin K is a fat-soluble vitamin that is required for production of functional forms of factors II, VII, IX, and X. Infants are born with low stores of vitamin K and may have insufficient dietary intake following birth, especially if fed exclusively human milk. In children and adults, microbes that are part of the intestinal flora provide vitamin K, but the intestinal flora of exclusively breastfed infants does not contain the same number of vitamin K-producing microbes.

Vitamin K–deficiency bleeding (VKDB) is defined as a bleeding disorder in which coagulation rapidly responds to vitamin K supplementation.[43] Classical VKDB occurs between 24 hours and 7 days of life, and is commonly associated with delayed or insufficient feeding. Infants may present with bruises, gastrointestinal blood loss, or bleeding from the umbilicus and puncture sites. Blood loss can range from mild to significant, including intracranial hemorrhage. Late VKDB occurs between 2 to 12 weeks of life, and is associated with exclusive breastfeeding. Generally, the clinical presentation is severe, with a 50% incidence of intracranial hemorrhage and a 20% mortality rate. To prevent bleeding related to vitamin K deficiency, it is customary to give newborns supplementary vitamin K after birth. (See the *Neonatal Care* chapter.) The most common route of administration for vitamin K is intramuscular, as studies have not demonstrated a reliably effective oral vitamin K dose.[44,45]

## The Newborn Immune System

The neonatal immune system is immature in several ways, including having incomplete physical and chemical barriers in the gastrointestinal system, limited and delayed secretory immunoglobulin A (IgA) production, incomplete complement cascade function, and decreased anti-inflammatory mechanisms within the respiratory and gastrointestinal tract. This functional immaturity renders the neonate vulnerable to many infections and allergic responses. Innate immunity is the primary line of defense for the neonate.[46]

### Innate Immunity

Innate immunity consists of both cellular and noncellular first responders to infection. Examples of innate immunity include (1) the barrier protection offered by the skin, mucous membranes, and intestinal mucosa; (2) the sieve-like action of the respiratory passages; (3) the colonization of skin and intestines with protective microbes; (4) the chemical protection offered by the acidic environment of the stomach; and (5) the actions of breast milk that support neonatal innate immune function.

The skin and mucous membranes of the neonate become colonized as the fetus passes through the vaginal canal. The vernix caseosa contains a variety of antimicrobial proteins and peptides (APPs) and forms a "microbial shield" on the newborn's body.[47,48] The presence of vernix also moistens the skin and increases its acidity, which inhibits growth of pathogenic bacteria.[49] The inflammatory skin reaction of normal newborns called erythema toxicum or "newborn rash" contains the antimicrobial peptide LL-37, indicating that this skin condition may be a manifestation of bacterial colonization.[46,48]

Colostrum that is ingested in the first few days of life and human milk consumed in the first month of life are powerful stimulants of an infant's innate immune response. Human milk contains bioactive substances that facilitate development of the immune system. In the infant's gastrointestinal tract, human milk inhibits the binding of many toxins, inhibits inflammatory responses, and facilitates colonization of commensal bacteria that will make up the microbiome.[50] In addition, human milk influences the expression of immune signaling genes in intestinal epithelial cells. These toll-like receptors (TLRs) play a central role in immune signaling by recognizing patterns of pathogen-associated molecular signals.[50]

Innate immunity is also provided at the cellular level. Three cell types—polymorphonuclear neutrophils (PMNs), monocytes, and macrophages—act through phagocytosis to engulf and destroy foreign antigens. These PMNs will eventually become the primary phagocytes in the defense of the host. In neonates, however, PMNs are compromised in their ability to mobilize, move in the right direction, and adhere to inflammatory sites.[48,51] While the numbers of these neutrophils are not deficient in neonates, their chemotaxis and opsonization is inadequate.

Chemotaxis refers to the organized movement of a phagocytic cell, or its ability to travel throughout the body. Opsonization is the alteration, or "marking," of the cell surface of a foreign microbe or antigen; it promotes the destruction of foreign cells. The immaturity of chemotaxis and opsonization in the newborn decreases the effectiveness of the phagocytic response and leads to one of the main weaknesses of the neonatal immune system—the inability to localize infection. Thus, the risk for systemic infection is higher in newborns than in older children and adults. In turn, newborn infections can rapidly lead to sepsis.

The innate immune system includes numerous noncellular proteins, such as complement molecules, acute-phase reactants, cytokines, chemokines, coagulation proteins, and vasoactive substances. The process of phagocytosis is enhanced if foreign cells are prepared for identification and destruction by complement components. Natural killer (NK) cells also contribute to innate immunity. However, their function is compromised in neonates, as these NK cells have limited cytolytic ability.[52]

Signs of infection can be subtle in newborns. Changes in activity, tone, color, or feeding, for example, may be difficult to recognize in newborns in the early stages of an infection. In addition, lack of fever does not exclude the possibility of infection. Many infants with an infection will present with hypothermia rather than hyperthermia. More information on care of infants with suspected infection can be found in the *Neonatal Care* chapter.

## Adaptive Immunity

Adaptive immunity is the acquired response to specific pathogens. It is divided into two components: cellular and antibody-mediated (humoral) immunity. Cellular adaptive immunity is modulated through T-cell and B-cell lymphocytes. T cells have two main roles: destroying infected cells and secreting cytokines, which aid in the differentiation of B cells into plasma cells. T cells are found in high levels in the newborn, but are slow to respond and require increased stimuli to generate their activity compared to later in life.[51] The T cells that develop immunologic memory—CD8 and CD4 cells—are present in low levels in the neonate; their populations increase slowly throughout childhood. T cells do not offer significant protection in the neonatal period; their protective effects typically become evident only 4 to 6 weeks after birth, when newborns have been exposed to various antigens.[53]

The activation of the antibody-mediated B cells is dependent on T-cell activity. Because of diminished T-cell functionality in the newborn, B-cell responses are also deficient in newborns, having a delayed onset and shorter duration. Bacteria, however, can trigger B-cell development. Recent evidence indicates that B cells are activated by the birth parent's intestinal bacteria during early newborn intestinal colonization.

## Passive Immunity

Neonates are born with passive immunity to viruses and bacteria owing to transplacental passage of immunoglobulin G (IgG) from the birth parent.

Antibodies, including those from vaccination of the pregnant person, pass transplacentally to the fetus during the last trimester of pregnancy and continue to protect the infant for the first few months of life.[51] Newborns are dependent on this form of passive immunity until approximately 6 months of age, when significant amounts of IgG are finally produced. Other immunoglobulins, such as IgM and IgA, are larger in size than IgG and do not cross the placenta. Breast milk, however, contains a significant amount of secretory IgA that protect the infant from microbes in the birth parent's intestinal tract.

Over time, infants gradually begin to produce adequate circulating antibodies of the IgG class. This process notably takes an extended period of time, which means that mounting a full antibody response to a foreign antigen is not possible until well into early childhood.

In summary, because of a variety of deficiencies in both natural and acquired immunity, neonates are highly vulnerable to infection. Neonates' response to infection is sluggish and inadequate, predisposing them to systemic rather than localized infections. Vaginal birth and breastfeeding help establish healthy microbial colonization that persists throughout infancy. Breastfeeding has additional direct and indirect mechanisms that support and stimulate development of immunity in the newborn.

## The Newborn Gastrointestinal Tract

The gastrointestinal system in term newborns exhibits varying levels of maturity. Prior to birth, the term fetus exhibits sucking and swallowing motions in utero. Mature gag and cough reflexes are intact at birth. Most term infants, barring neurologic compromise, can suck, swallow, and breathe in an organized manner shortly after birth. Meconium, although sterile, contains debris from the amniotic fluid.

The ability of term newborns to ingest and digest exogenous food sources is limited due to varying amounts of digestive enzymes and hormones in all portions of the gastrointestinal tract. In particular, newborns are less able to digest proteins and fats than are adults. Carbohydrate absorption is relatively efficient but still less efficient than in adults. Newborns are particularly efficient in absorbing monosaccharides, such as glucose, if the amount of glucose is not too much.

The cardiac sphincter—the juncture of the lower esophagus and the stomach—is incomplete at birth, which contributes to frequent regurgitation of stomach contents in newborns and young infants. The capacity of the stomach itself is limited, holding less than 30 mL in a term newborn. A literature review by Bergman estimated that the term infant stomach could hold 20 mL.[54] However, the actual volume of the newborn stomach remains controversial. Instead of relying solely on stomach volume as a nutritional metric, consideration should be given to the physiologic aspect of milk production and the infant's ability to digest milk.[54,55]

A newborn's intestines are relatively immature because prior to birth, this organ is semi-dormant. The normal extrauterine transition includes a striking increase in blood flow and a decrease in vascular resistance that result in increased blood flow to the newborn's rapidly growing intestines.[56] The underlying intestinal musculature is thinner and less efficient in newborns than in adults, resulting in unpredictable peristaltic waves. The folds and villi of the intestinal wall are not fully developed, and the epithelial cells lining a newborn's small intestine do not have the rapid cell turnover that promotes highly effective absorption. This immaturity of the intestinal epithelium affects the intestine's protection from harmful substances, and decreased vascular resistance increases the risk of hypoxic damage.[56]

During early infancy, newborns face the substantial task of "gut closure," the process by which the epithelial surfaces of the intestine become impermeable to antigens. Prior to gut closure, infants are vulnerable to bacterial and viral infections as well as to allergenic stimulation through intestinal absorption of large molecules.

Among the defenses present in the gastrointestinal tract are the chemical barriers of increased acidity, the digestive enzymes that break down large molecules, and secretory IgA that lines the small intestine. Secretory IgA dampens inappropriate immune activation and binds with harmful antigens.[57,58] In breastfed newborns, the birth parent's secretory IgA restricts immune activation and bacterial attachments.[56] Unlike other types of immunoglobulins, secretory IgA is not systemically absorbed and works at the local level in the intestine.[59]

The beginning of oral feedings stimulates the intestinal lining to mature through promotion of rapid cell turnover and production of microvillus enzymes such as amylase, trypsin, and pancreatic lipase. All enteral feedings, even in very small amounts, lead to helpful surges in gastrointestinal trophic factors, mainly hormones that lead to full maturation in functioning.[60] The newborn's colon conserves water less efficiently than an adult's colon does, which predisposes the newborn to complications from water loss. This makes a diarrheal illness potentially life-threatening in a young infant.

## The Newborn Microbiome

In humans, the entire gastrointestinal tract serves as a component of the natural immune system, which collectively represents a system of defense for the host. Ongoing research on biologic parent and newborn microbiomes is replacing former theories of newborn bacterial colonization. Microbiomes flourish on the skin, in the mouth, and in the gut, and appear to influence digestion, the immune system, endocrine function, and possibly neurologic signaling.[61] At birth, the rapid colonization of the sterile fetal intestine with commensal bacteria performs valuable functions and prevents pathogenic bacteria from dominating this microbiota.

Following vaginal birth, the first colonization for the newborn is with vaginal bacteria. Following a cesarean birth, the first colonization is with bacteria from the operating room environment. Thus, after birth, the intestinal epithelium is exposed to a large and diverse population of microbes. This exposure results in the creation of an effective barrier against harmful bacteria in a process known as mucosal host–microbial homeostasis. The initial mucosal host–microbial interaction begins with development of an intestinal microbiota that recognizes healthy bacteria and repels harmful ones.[57] These microorganisms also assist in digestion and breakdown of toxins, and the synthesis of vitamins and other nutrients.

Many factors have the potential to change neonatal microbiomes, such as perinatal stress and diet, antibiotic exposure, cesarean birth, and infant diet. Differences between preterm and term neonate microbiomes have been demonstrated as well as differences in the microbiomes of newborns born vaginally and by cesarean birth, breastfed and human milk substitute–fed neonates, and between those exposed to antibiotics before and after birth. Research about ideal ways to seed the neonatal microbiome is ongoing. The outcomes of emerging research are not conclusive enough at the present time to affect current newborn care practices.[61]

## The Renal System

The renal systems of term newborns have both structural and functional immaturity, most of which resolves spontaneously during the first month of life.[62] The majority of nephrogenesis occurs in the third trimester, with approximately 80% of nephrons formed by the end of 36 weeks' gestation.[63] The newborn kidney has less renal blood flow and a lower glomerular filtration rate (GFR) compared to that of an adult. Due to this lower GFR and the relative state of poor fluid intake in the first few days of life, the recommended time for a postnatal renal ultrasound is after the first week of life.[64] Tubular function in newborns is immature, which can lead to large sodium losses and other electrolyte imbalances.[65] Newborns are unable to concentrate urine very well, which is reflected in a low specific gravity and osmolality of their urine. All of these renal limitations are accentuated in the preterm infant. Aspects of renal functional immaturity are typically problematic only for sick or stressed newborns, especially if they require intravenous fluids or medications that further tax their immature renal system.[65]

Newborns excrete a small quantity of urine in the first 48 hours of life, often as little as 30 to 60 mL. The urine excreted by newborns should not contain protein or blood. Large amounts of cellular debris may indicate injury to or irritation of the renal system. It can be difficult to decipher renal function based on laboratory values since the infant after birth has a serum creatinine that is equivalent to the creatinine of the birth parent. This value will typically decrease in the first week of life.

## The Integumentary System

At birth, infants have immature skin barrier function, although function improves with increasing gestational age. The epidermal layer serves as a barrier to chemical irritants as well as mechanical trauma or damage. In addition to offering physical protection, the skin assists with thermoregulation after birth. In utero, the fetal skin is protected by vernix caseosa, an oily yellow or white substance consisting of skin cells, proteins, and secretions from the sebaceous glands. The amount of vernix increases during the third trimester but gradually diminishes as the infant nears term. After birth, vernix continues to provide protection for the newborn. Evidence suggests that vernix assists in thermoregulation, prevention of infection, and in moisturizing the skin.[66,67] The newborn's skin is more alkaline than that of older persons, and vernix has been suggested as the mechanism by which the skin maintains therapeutic pH levels. Recent research supports delayed bathing for most infants, typically until after 6 to 24 hours of life. However, for infants with infectious concerns, such as those whose birth parent is HIV-positive, the risks for acquiring infection outweigh the benefits of delayed bathing; thus, these infants should be bathed immediately after they have demonstrated cardiovascular stability.[68]

## Sensory Development

The infant's senses begin developing in utero in response to various stimuli.[69] The first to develop is the tactile sense in response to stimulation, as evidenced by the grasping and rooting noted in the first trimester.

At birth, term infants' vision extends only up to 25 centimeters. As they have limited ability to focus, discordant movements of the eye muscles may also be noted.

Function of the auditory system is noted at 25 weeks' gestation. At 25 to 27 weeks' gestation, the fetus develops functional hearing.[70,71] Further development of the auditory system requires external stimulation including speech and music.

Smell is developed in the uterus by fetal exposure to amniotic fluid. The biologic parent's diet can familiarize the fetus through swallowed amniotic fluid and help the fetus recognize the smell of the biologic parent. Studies have shown that infants at 5 to 6 days old prefer a breast pad with their birth parents' scent when compared to unused pads.[72]

Development of taste is less studied. Fetuses are known to swallow amniotic fluid, however, so it is hypothesized that taste is developed in the womb as well. Neonates can differentiate between bitter, sour, and sweet, and show a preference for sweet substances.

Development of these senses prior to birth contributes to the importance of skin-to-skin contact following birth. The infant can sense the birth parent's touch, hear the parent's voice, initially smell, and then subsequently taste colostrum as part of normal transition to extrauterine life.[70,71,73]

## Conclusion

Newborn physiology encompasses fascinating, dynamic, and rapidly changing systems that both protect the newborn during adjustment to extrauterine life and exhibit significant vulnerabilities to certain stressors such as cold and infection. Basic knowledge of newborn physiology can help midwives develop evidence-based plans of care for newborns.

## References

1. Laudy JA, Wladimiroff JW. The fetal lung 1: developmental aspects. *Ultrasound Obstet Gynecol.* 2000;16(3):284-290.

2. Hillman NH, Kallapur SG, Jobe AH. Physiology of transition from intrauterine to extrauterine life. *Clin Perinatol.* 2012;39(4):769-783. doi:10.1016/j.clp.2012.09.009.

3. Keene SD, Bland RD, Jain L. Lung fluid balance in developing lungs and its role in neonatal transition. In: Oh W, Baum M, Polin RA, eds. *Nephrology and Fluid/Electrolyte Physiology: Neonatology Questions and Controversies.* 3rd ed. Philadelphia, PA: Elsevier; 2019:225-236.

4. O'Brodovich HM. Immature epithelial Na+ channel expression is one of the pathogenetic mechanisms leading to human neonatal respiratory distress syndrome. *Proc Assoc Am Physicians.* 1996;108(5):345-355.

5. Swanson J, Sinkin R. Transition from fetus to newborn. *Pediatr Clin North Am.* 2015;62:329-343.

6. Morton S, Brodsky D. Fetal physiology and the transition to extrauterine life. *Clin Perinatol.* 2016;43:395-407.

7. Vyas H, Field D, Milner AD, Hopkin IE. Determinants of the first inspiratory volume and functional residual capacity at birth. *Pediatr Pulmonol.* 1986;2:189-193.

8. Evans M. Does medical evidence support routine oronasopharyngeal suction at delivery? *J Okla State Med Assoc.* 2016;109(4-5):140-142.

9. Te Pas AB, Wong C, Kamlin CF, et al. Breathing patterns in preterm and term infants immediately after birth. *Pediatr Res.* 2009;3(65):352-356.

10. MacLean J, Fitzgerald D, Waters K. Development changes in sleep and breathing across infancy and childhood. *Paediatr Resp Rev.* 2015;16:276-284.

11. Wyckoff MH, Aziz K, Escobedo MB, et al. Part 13: neonatal resuscitation: 2015 American Heart Association guidelines update for cardiopulmonary resuscitation and emergency cardiovascular care. *Circulation.* 2015;132(18 suppl 2):S543-S560.

12. Backer CL, Eltayeb O, Monge MC, et al. Shunt lesions part I: patent ductus arteriosus, atrial septal defect, ventricular septal defect, and atrioventricular septal defect. *Pediatr Crit Care Med.* 2016;17(8S1):S302-S309.

13. Lakshminrushimha S, Sauqstad OD. The fetal circulation, pathophysiology of hypoxemic respiratory failure and pulmonary hypertension in neonates and the role of oxygen therapy. *J Perinatol.* 2016;36(S2):S3-S11.

14. Ishida H, Kawazu Y, Kayatani F, Inamura N. Prognostic factors of premature closure of the ductus arteriosus in utero: a systematic literature review. *Cardiol Young.* 2017;27(4):634-638. doi:10.1017/S1047951116000871.

15. Walker VP. Newborn evaluation. In: Gleason CA, Juul SE, eds. *Avery's Diseases of the Newborn.* Philadelphia, PA: Elsevier; 2018.

16. Association for Women's Health, Obstetric and Neonatal Nurses. Immediate and sustained skin-to-skin contact for the healthy term newborn after with AWHONN Practice Brief Number 5. *JOGN.* 2016;45(6):842-844.

17. Lunze K, Hamer DH. Thermal protection of the newborn in resource-limited environments. *J Perinatol.* 2012;32(5):317-324.

18. World Health Organization, United Nations Population Fund, World Bank, United Nations Children's Fund's. *Pregnancy, Childbirth, Postpartum and Newborn Care: A Guide for Essential Practice.* 3rd ed. Geneva, Switzerland: World Health Organization; 2015. https://apps.who.int/iris/handle/10665/249580. Accessed October 24, 2022.

19. Ravussin E, Galgani JE. The implication of brown adipose tissue for humans. *Annu Rev Nutr.* 2012;31(1): 33-47.

20. Tews D, Wabitsch M. Renaissance of brown adipose tissue. *Hormone Res Pediatr.* 2011;75:231-239.

21. World Health Organization. WHO_RHT_MSM_97.2 _Thermal protection of the Newborn.pdf. Published 1997. https://apps.who.int/iris/bitstream /handle/10665/63986/WHO?sequence=1. Accessed November 5, 2022.

22. Soll RF. Heat loss prevention in neonates. *J Perinatol.* 2008;28(suppl 1):S57-S59.

23. Rozance PJ. Management and outcome of neonatal hypoglycemia. *UpToDate.* https://www-uptodate-com .ckmproxy.vumc.org/contents/management-and-outcome-of-neonatal-hypoglycemia?search= Management%20and%20outcome%20of%20neonatal%20hypoglycemia&source=search_result& selectedTitle=1~71&usage_type=default&display _rank=1. Accessed March 6, 2022.

24. Weissmann-Brenner A, Simchen MJ, Zilberberg E, et al. Maternal and neonatal outcomes of large for gestational age pregnancies. *Acta Obstet Gynecol Scand.* 2012;91(7):844-849.

25. Committee on Fetus and Newborn, Adamkin DH. Postnatal glucose homeostasis in late-preterm and term infants. *Pediatrics.* 2011;127(3):575-579. doi:10.1542/peds.2010-3851.

26. Rozance PJ, Hay WW. Hypoglycemia in newborn infants: features associated with adverse outcomes. *Biol Neonate.* 2006;90(2):74-86. doi:10.1159/000091948.

27. Adamkin D. Metabolic screening and postnatal glucose homeostasis in the newborn. *Pediatr Clin North Am.* 2015;62:385-409.

28. Stanley C, Rozance PJ, Thornton PS, et al. Re-evaluating "transitional neonatal hypoglycemia": mechanism and implications for management. *J Pediatr.* 2015;166(6):1520-1525.

29. Jobe A. Transitional neonatal hypoglycemia. *J Pediatr.* 2015;166(6):1329-1332.

30. Henry E, Christensen R. Reference intervals in neonatal hematology. *Clin Perinatol.* 2015;42:483-497.

31. Christensen RD, Henry E, Jopling J, Wiedmeier SE. The CBC: reference ranges for neonates. *Semin Perinatol.* 2009;33:3-11.

32. Polin RA, Abman SH, Rowitch DH, et al. Developmental erythropoiesis. In: *Fetal and Neonatal Physiology.* Polin RA, Abman SH, Rowitch DH, et al., eds. Philadelphia, PA: Elsevier; 2017.

33. Diab Y, Luchtman-Jones L. Hematologic and oncologic problems in the fetus and neonate. In: Martin RJ, Fanaroff AA, Walsh MC, eds. *Fanaroff and Martin's Neonatal Perinatal Medicine Diseases of the Fetus and Infant.* Philadelphia, PA: Mosby Elsevier; 2015:1294-1394.

34. Riviere D, McKinlay CJD, Bloomfield FH. Adaptation for life after birth: a review of neonatal physiology. *Anaesth Intens Care Med.* 2017;18(2):59-67. doi:10.1016/j.mpaic.2016.11.008.

35. Katheria AC, Lakshminrusimha S, Rabe H, et al. Placental transfusion: a review. *J Perinatol.* 2017;37(2): 105-111.

36. McDonald SJ, Middleton P, Dowswell T, Morris PS. Effect of timing of umbilical cord clamping of term infants on maternal and neonatal outcomes. *Cochrane Database Syst Rev.* 2013;7:CD004074. doi:10.1002/14651858 .CD004074.pub3.

37. Mercer JS, Skovgaard RL. Neonatal transitional physiology: a new paradigm. *J Perinatal Neonatal Nurs.* 2002;15(4):56-75.

38. Chaparro CM. Timing of umbilical cord clamping: effect on iron endowment of the newborn and later iron status. *Nutr Rev.* 2011;69:S30-S36.

39. McDonald SJ, Middleton P, Dowswell T, Morris PS. Effect of timing of umbilical cord clamping of term infants on maternal and neonatal outcomes. *Evid Based Child Health.* 2014;9(2):303-397.

40. Yang S, Duffy JY, Johnston R, et al. Association of a delayed cord-clamping protocol with hyperbilirubinemia in term neonates. *Obstet Gynecol.* 2019;133(4): 754-761. doi:10.1097/AOG.0000000000003172.

41. Muchowski KE. Evaluation and treatment of neonatal hyperbilirubinemia. *Am Fam Physician.* 2014;89(11):873-878.

42. Prosser A, Hibbert J, Strunk T, et al. Phagocytosis of neonatal pathogens by peripheral blood neutrophils and monocytes from newborn preterm and term infants. *Pediatr Res.* 2013;74(5):503-510.

43. Lippi G, Franchini M. Vitamin K in neonates: facts and myths. *Blood Transfus.* 2011;9(1):4-9. doi:10.2450/2010.0034-10.

44. Phillippi J, Holley SL, Morad A, Collins MR. Prevention of vitamin K deficiency bleeding. *J Midwifery Womens Health.* 2016;51(5):632-636.

45. Ipema HJ. Use of oral vitamin K for prevention of late vitamin K deficiency bleeding in neonates when injectable vitamin K is not available. *Ann Pharmacother.* 2012;46(6):879-893.

46. Gil A, Kenney L, Mishra R, et al. Vaccination and heterologous immunity: educating the immune system. *Trans R Soc Trop Med Hyg.* 2015;109:62-69.

47. Tollin M, Bergsson G, Kai-Larsen Y, et al. Vernix caseosa as a multi-component defence system based on polypeptides, lipids and their interactions. *Cell Molecul Life Sci.* 2005;62(19):2390-2399.

48. Kumar S, Bhat B. Distinct mechanisms of the newborn innate immunity. *Immunol Lett.* 2016;173:42-54.

49. Visscher M, Narendran V. Vernix caseosa: formation and functions. *Newborn Infant Nurs Rev.* 2014;14(4):142-146. doi:10.1053/j.nainr.2014.10.005.

50. He Y, Lawlor NT, Newburg DS. Human milk components modulate toll-like receptor–mediated inflammation. *Adv Nutr.* 2016;7(1):102-111.

51. Ygberg S, Nilsson A. The developing immune system: from foetus to toddler. *Acta Paediatr.* 2012;101(2):120-127.

52. Lee Y, Lin S. Neonatal natural killer cell function: relevance to antiviral immune defense. *Clin Devel Immunol.* 2013;2013:427696. doi:10.1155/2013/427696.

53. Lusyati S, Hulzebos CV, Zandvoort J, Sauer PJ. Levels of 25 cytokines in the first seven days of life in newborn infants. *BMC Res Notes.* 2013;2013;6:547. doi:10.1186/1756-0500-6-547.

54. Bergman NJ. Neonatal stomach volume and physiology suggest feeding at 1-h intervals. *Acta Paediatr.* 2013;102(8):773-777. doi:10.1111/apa.12291.

55. Spangler AK, Randenberg AL, Brenner MG, Howett M. Belly models as teaching tools: what is their utility? *J Hum Lact.* 2008;24(2):199-205. doi:10.1177/0890334408316079.

56. Walker A. Intestinal colonization and programming of the intestinal immune response. *J Clin Gastroenterol.* 2014;48(S1):S8-S11.

57. Nuriel-Ohayon M, Neuman H, Koren O. Microbial changes during pregnancy, birth and infancy. *Front Microbiol.* 2016;14(7):1031.

58. Turfkruyer M, Verehasselt V. Breast milk and its impact on maturation of the neonatal immune system. *Curr Opin Infect Dis.* 2015;28(3);199-206.

59. Harris NL, Spoerri I, Schopfer JF, et al. Mechanisms of neonatal mucosal antibody protection. *J Immunol.* 2006;177(9):6256-6262.

60. Neu J. Gastrointestinal maturation and implications for infant feeding. *Early Hum Develop.* 2007;83:767-775.

61. Yang I, Corwin E, Brennan P, et al. The infant microbiome: implications for infant health and neurocognitive development. *Nurs Res.* 2016;65(1):76-88.

62. Saint-Faust M, Boubred F, Simeoni U. Renal development and neonatal adaptation. *Am J Perinatol.* 2014;31(9):773-780.

63. Faa G, Gerosa C, Fanni D, et al. Marked interindividual variability in renal maturation of preterm infants: lessons from autopsy. *J Matern Fetal Neonatal Med.* 2010;23(suppl 3):129-133. doi:10.3109/14767058.20 10.510646.

64. Wiener JS, O'Hara SM. Optimal timing of initial postnatal ultrasonography in newborns with prenatal hydronephrosis. *J Urol.* 2002;168(4 pt 2):1826-1829. doi:10.1097/01.ju.0000030859.88692.dd.

65. Sulemnji M, Vakili K. Neonatal renal physiology. *Semin Pediatr Surg.* 2013;22:195-198.

66. Lund C. Bathing and beyond: current bathing controversies for newborn infants. *Adv Neonatal Care.* 2016;16(suppl 5S):S13-S20. doi:10.1097 /ANC.0000000000000336.

67. Oranges T, Dini V, Romanelli M. Skin physiology of the neonate and infant: clinical implications. *Adv Wound Care (New Rochelle).* 2015;4(10):587-595. doi:10.1089/wound.2015.0642.

68. Brogan J, Rapkin G. Implementing evidence-based neonatal skin care with parent-performed, delayed immersion baths. *Nurs Womens Health.* 2017;21(6):442-450. doi:10.1016/j.nwh.2017.10.009.

69. Bremner AJ, Spence C. The development of tactile perception. *Adv Child Dev Behav.* 2017;52:227-268. doi:10.1016/bs.acdb.2016.12.002.

70. Clark-Gambelunghe MB, Clark DA. Sensory development. *Pediatr Clin North Am.* 2015;62(2):367-384. doi:10.1016/j.pcl.2014.11.003.

71. Graven SN, Browne JV. Auditory development in the fetus and infant. *Newborn Infant Nurs Rev.* 2008;8(4):187-193. doi:10.1053/j.nainr.2008.10.010.

72. Varendi H, Porter RH, Winberg J. Attractiveness of amniotic fluid odor: evidence of prenatal olfactory learning? *Acta Paediatr.* 1996;85(10):1223-1227. doi:10.1111/j.1651-2227.1996.tb18233.x.

73. Moore ER, Bergman N, Anderson GC, Medley N. Early skin-to-skin contact for mothers and their healthy newborn infants. *Cochrane Database Syst Rev.* 2016;11(11):CD003519. Published November 25, 2016. doi:10.1002/14651858.CD003519.pub4.

CHAPTER

# 37

# Infant Feeding and Lactation

ROBYN SCHAFER, STEPHANIE DEVANE-JOHNSON, MELISSA G. DAVIS, AND JULIA C. PHILLIPPI

*The editors acknowledge Linda J. Smith, Tekoa L. King, and Cecilia M. Jevitt, who were the authors of this chapter in the previous edition.*

## Introduction

Newborn and infant feeding decisions affect neonatal, maternal, and familial health. These decisions are based on many different factors including personal experience and beliefs, socioeconomic and cultural influences, and the advice of healthcare providers. Midwives are uniquely positioned to support individuals and families in meeting their infant feeding goals by, for example, reducing barriers to breastfeeding initiation and continuation. Globally, breastfeeding is recognized as the optimal feeding method for newborns and postpartum individuals, and midwives play an important role in enabling breastfeeding and lactation success. Midwives are a valuable part of the healthcare team in promoting breastfeeding, providing lactation support, and advancing public health goals for human milk feeding. This chapter focuses on midwifery scope of practice for feeding for the healthy, term, singleton newborn and infant, with an emphasis on maternal health in lactation and breastfeeding. Infant feeding for neonates or infants who are ill, preterm, or part of multiple gestations presents unique challenges and can be managed by midwives in collaboration with pediatric and lactation care providers; however, such care is beyond the scope of this text.

## Terminology

As in all areas of health care, it is important to acknowledge the power of language in infant feeding and lactation and its influence on thought and action, especially as it relates to structural inequality and health disparities. The terms used throughout this chapter reflect the distinction, historically unacknowledged in health care, between lactation, breastfeeding, and human milk feeding. *Lactation* refers to the biologic production of human milk. *Breastfeeding* is infant feeding of one's own human milk directly at the breast. Some individuals such as transgender men, gender-nonconforming individuals, or persons with breast dysphoria may prefer alternative terms such as *chestfeeding*, nursing, lactating, or feeding.[1] *Human milk feeding* describes the provision of human milk to the neonate whether directly through breastfeeding or indirectly following milk expression, such as with a bottle, spoon, syringe, cup, or supplemental feeding system. Definitions of key terms related to infant feeding and lactation are provided in Table 37-1.

The language used in this chapter strives to be inclusive and nonjudgmental, recognizing that individuals who lactate, breastfeed/chestfeed, or otherwise feed their infants with human milk or human milk substitutes have diverse identities and relationships with infant feeding. This terminology also aims to be anatomically accurate to ensure clarity of meaning. For example, from an anatomic perspective, all humans (regardless of sex assigned at birth or gender identity) have breasts and breast tissue. Some individuals may prefer to use the term "chest" to refer to this area of the body, and use of the patient's preferred language is encouraged in the clinical context of a direct patient encounter. However, the terms "breast" and "chest" are not interchangeable in a medical context: A documented "chest mass" has a distinctly different meaning than a "breast mass." The use of precise terminology avoids confusion and facilitates timely and appropriate clinical care. Therefore, the term "breast" is used throughout the chapter to refer to this glandular organ, in distinction from the chest—the thoracic region it overlays.

| Table 37-1 | Terminology in Infant Feeding and Lactation |
|---|---|
| **Term** | **Definition** |
| Breastfeeding | Feeding of one's own human milk directly at the breast |
| Chestfeeding | Alternative term for "breastfeeding," which, along with terms such as nursing, feeding, or bodyfeeding, may be preferred by transgender and gender-nonconforming individuals[1] |
| Human milk | Milk produced by human mammary glands; may be commonly referred to as "breast milk," "mother's milk," "donor milk," or "expressed milk" |
| Human milk feeding | Feeding of human milk through a variety of methods, including directly at the breast or indirectly following milk expression |
| Human milk substitute | A milk or product (i.e., concentrate or powder) specifically designed or marketed for infant feeding; may be commonly referred to as "formula" |
| Lactation | Biologic production of human milk |
| Milk expression | Purposeful removal of human milk from the breast; commonly referred to "pumping" or "hand expression" |

Similarly, the term "maternal" may be used in this chapter to designate the gestational and lactating parent, since no gender-neutral replacement has yet gained widespread acceptance other than the term "parental," which may be confused with reference to a co-parent or nongestational parent who may also be lactating, breastfeeding/chestfeeding, human milk feeding, or providing human milk substitutes to the neonate.[2] The use of the term "maternal" in no way is meant to exclude individuals with gender-diverse identities who gestate and lactate but do not consider themselves to be mothers.

Where used in the original research, gendered language has been retained to avoid homogenizing the effects of research findings among cisgendered individuals onto those with diverse gender identities, thereby masking potential distinctions between these populations and the need for future research. The authors recognize that some individuals may find degendered language alienating and/or insufficient for capturing the relational nature of infant feeding. Midwives are encouraged to adapt their language in clinical practice to reflect the identity, preferences, and comfort of their clients and their families.

## Overview of Infant Feeding Practices

Human milk is widely recognized as the optimal form of nutrition for neonates, and lactation and breastfeeding have numerous benefits for maternal, neonatal, infant, and child health; society; and the environment (Table 37-2). The promotion of breastfeeding initiation, exclusive human milk feeding for the first 6 months of life, and continued human milk feeding as long as mutually desired, up to 2 years of age or beyond (along with complementary infant foods), are recommended by the American Academy of Pediatrics (AAP) and World Health Organization (WHO) to maximize nutritional and non-nutritional benefits.[3] It is unclear from the research whether the benefits historically associated with lactation and breastfeeding are related to the consumption of human milk and/or other aspects of breastfeeding such as parent–infant interactions.

Although lactation and breastfeeding should be promoted from a public health perspective, some individuals may not be able to or may choose not to breastfeed or provide human milk to their infant, and some may opt to feed their infant a combination of human milk and human milk substitutes. Many cultural, behavioral, relational, environmental, historical, social, and socioeconomic factors influence infant feeding decisions. Healthcare providers, perinatal care practices, and access to lactation and education and support also affect infant feeding choice. Each individual/family is best positioned to make an informed choice about infant feeding methods and goals based on their unique needs and circumstances. Providers should aim to support the optimal health and overall well-being of the neonate, lactating person, and family unit. A patient-centered care approach is useful to support parents and caregivers in making informed infant feeding decisions. It is important to approach these conversations with a nonjudgmental attitude. Communication techniques from motivational interviewing and shared decision making may be helpful. Individuals and families should be informed about the numerous health benefits of human milk feeding for both children and lactating individuals, and clinicians should be respectful of patients' values and preferences regarding infant feeding practices.

Despite the well-established benefits of breastfeeding, breastfeeding rates remain below public

| Table 37-2 | Benefits of Lactation and Breastfeeding Compared to Human Milk Substitutes |
|---|---|
| **Neonatal/Pediatric** | **Maternal/For the Lactating Person** |
| Lower risk of:<br>• Infant mortality<br>• Acute illness and infectious disease, including:<br>  ♦ Lower respiratory tract infections<br>  ♦ Otitis media<br>  ♦ Sudden infant death syndrome (SIDS)<br>• Gastrointestinal dysfunction and disease<br>  ♦ Gastroenteritis<br>  ♦ Diarrhea<br>  ♦ Inflammatory bowel disease<br>• Chronic conditions, including:<br>  ♦ Type 1 and type 2 diabetes<br>  ♦ Leukemia<br>  ♦ Childhood obesity<br>  ♦ Asthma<br>  ♦ Eczema<br>  ♦ Malocclusion and dental caries<br>Improvements in:<br>• Neurodevelopmental outcomes<br>• Gut microbiome | Lower risk of:<br>• Breast, ovarian, and endometrial cancer<br>• Excessive postpartum blood loss<br>• Type 2 diabetes<br>• Hypertension and cardiovascular disease<br>Improvements in:<br>• Pregnancy spacing (interpregnancy interval)<br><br>**Economic and Environmental**<br><br>Positive effects on:<br>• Healthcare costs (associated with deceased perinatal morbidity and mortality)<br>• Economic productivity and less workplace absence<br>• Environmental safety and sustainability (compared to manufacturing, delivery, and disposal of human milk substitutes and use of water)<br>• Family financial savings (compared to purchasing human milk substitutes) |

Based on Meek JY, Noble L, American Academy of Pediatrics Section on Breastfeeding. Breastfeeding and the use of human milk. *Pediatrics*. 2022;e2022057988; Bartick MC, Schwarz EB, Green BD, et al. Suboptimal breastfeeding in the United States: maternal and pediatric health outcomes and costs. *Matern Child Nutr*. 2017;13(1):e12366; Pereyra-Elías R, Quigley MA, Carson C. To what extent does confounding explain the association between breastfeeding duration and cognitive development up to age 14? Findings from the UK Millennium Cohort Study. *PLoS One*. 2022;17(5):e0267326; Rameez RM, Sadana D, Kaur S, et al. Association of maternal lactation with diabetes and hypertension: a systematic review and meta-analysis. *JAMA Netw Open*. 2019;2(10):e1913401; Victora CG, Bahl R, Barros AJD, et al. Breastfeeding in the 21st century: epidemiology, mechanisms, and lifelong effect. *Lancet*. 2016;387(10017):475-490.

health goals. According to the 2020 Centers for Disease Control and Prevention's (CDC) Breastfeeding Report Card, only 84.1% of U.S. infants were breastfed at any point, with 25.6% of infants being exclusively breastfed at 6 months of age, and nearly 1 in 5 breastfed newborns receiving supplementation with human milk substitutes before 2 days of age.[4] Not breastfeeding is associated with negative health effects in children, childbearing individuals, and society, including increased risk of childhood infections, breast cancers, and chronic health conditions, and economic losses totaling more than $300 billion annually worldwide.[5,6]

Significant disparities in lactation and breastfeeding rates have been identified based on race, ethnicity, level of parental education, and socioeconomic status. For example, based on the latest CDC data, 66% of Black mothers initiate breastfeeding compared to 82% of non-Hispanic white mothers.[4] Why the disproportionately low rates of breastfeeding among African American women (compared to Hispanic and non-Hispanic white women) occur is poorly understood; this lack of understanding in turn has limited the development of interventions that are able to successfully eliminate disparities. A growing body of research suggests that powerful sociocultural factors impact Black women's perspectives and decisions on infant feeding. In addition, Black women who opt to breastfeed/chestfeed report receiving less support for overcoming common barriers immediately following birth. Long-term rates of breastfeeding continuation in Black women may also reflect societal and structural barriers such as poor employer support.[4]

Lack of support for breastfeeding/chestfeeding has been reported by individuals from many marginalized and minoritized groups, including religious minorities, sexual and gender minorities, and individuals receiving treatment for substance use disorders, among many others. Age and body size have also been associated with decreased breastfeeding/chestfeeding support. Efforts to identify and rectify disparities in breastfeeding/chestfeeding rates are often hampered by lack of data, as many characteristics associated with implicit and explicit biases are not captured on vital statistics forms or in electronic health records.

It is also important to acknowledge social, historical, and cultural influences on breastfeeding. These include the medicalization of childbirth, mistrust of the pregnant or lactating body, and sexualization of female breasts. Sociohistorical factors that influence health beliefs and decisions include thoughts, attitudes, and traditions; these are personally experienced or relayed via oral histories that have been passed down and integrated into families and communities.[7] The trauma of colonialism, enslavement, and systemic oppression disrupted a culture of breastfeeding, leading to lower rates of lactation and breastfeeding in affected communities.[8] Similarly, the use of "wet nurses" created lasting stigmatization of breastfeeding, as did aggressive marketing of human milk substitutes. Historical perinatal and neonatal care practices such as maternal sedation and infant separation continue to influence current practices related to lactation and breastfeeding initiation and exclusivity. Healthcare worker bias has also contributed to postpartum individuals not being able to reach their infant feeding goals. Efforts to improve lactation and breastfeeding rates cannot ignore these critical barriers to success and must take a holistic perspective to address lactation and breastfeeding goals and disparities.

It should also be acknowledged that historically, the focus of research, policy, and clinical practice in lactation and breastfeeding was on achieving higher rates of breastfeeding initiation, duration, and exclusivity. While these are certainly worthwhile public health goals, midwives should approach care related to lactation and breastfeeding from a person-centered lens and define positive lactation and breastfeeding outcomes based on the preferences and goals of the lactating individual and their family. In other words, positive or "successful" lactation and breastfeeding outcomes should not be defined solely by the quantity of breastmilk produced and ingested, but rather from a more holistic understanding of health optimization including positive child and familial relationships, mental health, satisfaction with infant feeding, parental self-efficacy, and socioeconomic stability in meeting infants' nutritional needs.[9]

## Efforts to Increase Rates of Lactation and Breastfeeding

Due to the numerous health, social, and environmental benefits of breastfeeding, the *Healthy People 2030* initiative aims to increase lactation and breastfeeding exclusivity and duration, with its goals including 42.4% of infants being exclusively human milk fed through 6 months of age and 54.1% still receiving human milk at 1 year of age.[10] Federal support for human milk feeding echoes multiple position statements and recommendations from professional health organizations, including the U.S. Preventive Services Task Force, CDC, AAP, American College of Nurse-Midwives, and American College of Obstetricians and Gynecologists. See the Resources section for more details.

Most childbearing individuals are able to produce sufficient human milk, and most neonates have the innate ability to breastfeed. However, the physiologic processes of lactation and breastfeeding initiation and the continuation of breastfeeding or human milk feeding are often hindered by cultural and structural barriers. To improve breastfeeding and human milk feeding rates, changes are needed to improve perinatal care practices, healthcare provider education, and breastfeeding and lactation education and support. Structural and policy changes are also necessary to create environments that are supportive and enabling of breastfeeding and lactation. For example, enforcement of the International Code of Marketing of Breast-Milk Substitutes, adopted by WHO in 1981, would improve outcomes by reducing harmful marketing of human milk substitutes. Greater adoption of the WHO/UNICEF Baby-Friendly Hospital Initiative and its Ten Steps to Successful Breastfeeding (Table 37-3) would increase the provision of breastfeeding-friendly care practices in healthcare settings. (Note that Table 37-3 uses the original wording of the document, which is not inclusive of all lactating people.) Trained, community-based peer counselors play an important role in improving human milk feeding rates, especially among historically minoritized and vulnerable populations.[11]

Moreover, there is a need for widespread worksite lactation programs and "family-friendly" employment policies to improve human milk feeding duration and exclusivity.[12] Lack of paid parental

| Table 37-3 | Ten Steps to Successful Breastfeeding from the WHO/UNICEF Baby-Friendly Hospital Initiative |
|---|---|

**Critical Management Procedures**

1a. Comply fully with the International Code of Marketing of Breast-Milk Substitutes and relevant World Health Assembly resolutions.

1b. Have a written infant feeding policy that is routinely communicated to staff and parents.

1c. Establish ongoing monitoring and data-management systems.

2. Ensure that staff have sufficient knowledge, competence, and skills to support breastfeeding.

**Key Clinical Practices**

3. Discuss the importance and management of breastfeeding with pregnant women and their families.

4. Facilitate immediate and uninterrupted skin-to-skin contact and support mothers to initiate breastfeeding as soon as possible after birth.

5. Support mothers to initiate and maintain breastfeeding and manage common difficulties.

6. Do not provide breastfed newborns any food or fluids other than breast milk, unless medically indicated.

7. Enable mothers and their infants to remain together and to practice rooming-in 24 hours a day.

8. Support mothers to recognize and respond to their infants' cues for feeding.

9. Counsel mothers on the use and risks of feeding bottles, teats, and pacifiers.

10. Coordinate discharge so that parents and their infants have timely access to ongoing support and care.

Reproduced with permission of World Health Organization. Ten Steps to Successful Breastfeeding–revised 2018 version, accessed 6/15/22. https://www.who.int/teams/nutrition-and-food-safety/food-and-nutrition-actions-in-health-systems/ten-steps-to-successful-breastfeeding.

leave is a major barrier to breastfeeding and human milk feeding continuation, and disproportionately affects people of color and low-income populations.[13] A workplace culture supportive of lactation with accommodations for milk expression such as protected breaks with access to a comfortable location for milk expression can increase the duration of human milk feeding. Efforts to better understand and address those factors, which contribute to breastfeeding disparities in people of color, are also critical to improve health equity.

Increasing the breastfeeding rate among Black individuals will contribute to overall health equity. As noted earlier, the disproportionately low rates of breastfeeding among Black women (compared to Hispanic and non-Hispanic white women) are poorly understood, which limits the development of interventions to eliminate disparities. Bringing attention to any cultural and historical influences that impact decisions whether to breastfeed may create a context in which individuals will be motivated to breastfeed and successful in their infant feeding goals.

## Composition of Human Milk

Human milk production is a physiologic process known as lactogenesis. In the second phase of lactogenesis (secretory activation), an increase in milk production occurs in response to a rapid drop in the postpartum person's progesterone level following delivery of the placenta. This process typically occurs 2 or 3 days postpartum. Foundational concepts for lactogenesis and the anatomy and physiology related to breasts, lactation, breastfeeding, and newborn feeding are presented elsewhere in the text (see the chapters *Anatomy and Physiology of the Reproductive System*, *Anatomy and Physiology of Postpartum*, and *Physical Assessment of the Newborn*).

Human milk is an individual-specific biofluid that contains multiple bioactive, cellular, and nutritional ingredients (Figure 37-1). Its composition is dynamic and changes over time, in both the short and long term. Approximately 80% of the content of human milk is water. The other 20% consists of a wide range of substances, including numerous bioactive agents that protect and facilitate many aspects of infant health and development:[14–16]

- Macronutrients: The primary macronutrients in human milk are carbohydrates (predominately lactose), milk fat (lipids), proteins such as whey and casein, and minerals including calcium and phosphorus.
- Micronutrients: Vitamin D and vitamin K are present in constitutionally low levels. Other vitamins vary based on the diet of the lactating individual.
- Bioactive agents: Substances in human milk that can inhibit inflammation and induce

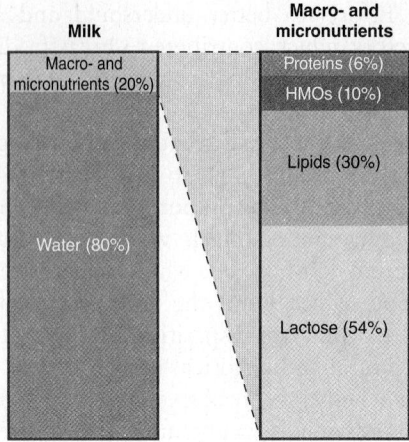

**Figure 37-1** Composition of human milk.
Abbreviation: HMOs, human milk oligosaccharides.
Note: Although the percentages of various constituents vary over time and even during the course of a single breastfeeding session, more than 200 individual bioactive substances have been identified in human milk.

antibody responses include growth factors, cells involved in immune response (macrophages, T cells, lymphocytes, leukocytes), cytokines, immunoglobulins (predominately IgA, but also IgG and IgM), and oligosaccharides.

There is considerable variability in the composition of human milk, as it is affected by a multitude of factors, including the stage of lactation, gestational age at birth, time of day, and environmental factors. The lipid component of human milk is the most variable in terms of concentration. Human milk undergoes a continuum of changes to form mature milk, which is commonly divided into three stages: colostrum (prenatal onset of lactogenesis II), transitional milk (2 to 5 days after birth), and mature milk (lactogenesis II and III). Colostrum contains relatively large quantities of protein and less lactose compared to mature milk. This liquid also contains large quantities of secretory immunoglobulins (IgA), oligosaccharides, and growth hormones. Based on these components, it is theorized that the primary role of colostrum is immunologic rather than nutritional, because the immunoglobulins in colostrum provide passive immunity that protects the infant in several ways. Compared to mature milk, both colostrum and transitional milk have more calories in the form of fat and carbohydrates. Transitional milk is not a discrete entity per se, but rather is the milk produced as colostrum changes to mature milk.

Approximately 24 hours before lactogenesis II becomes clinically evident, the content of lactate and citrate in milk increases, while lesser amounts of sodium and chloride are present. Signs of lactogenesis II include breast fullness, tingling and hardness, leaking, and change of milk color from yellow/creamy to blue/watery.

Mature milk is thinner than transitional milk and has a higher water content. Mature milk is subdivided into foremilk and hindmilk. The foremilk that appears at the beginning of a feed has more carbohydrates, whereas the hindmilk that appears near the end of the feeding session has more fat and lipids.[15] Once lactation is established, lactating individuals produce approximately 700 to 800 mL of breast milk per day, although this amount can vary considerably.

## Peripartum Factors Affecting Lactation and Breastfeeding

Care practices during pregnancy, labor, birth, and postpartum can affect lactogenesis, breastfeeding initiation, self-efficacy, and human milk feeding continuation. Support for early initiation of breastfeeding aligns with the consensus midwifery and WHO breastfeeding recommendations for early initiation of breastfeeding (within 1 hour after birth).[17] Practices that support physiologic birth, self-efficacy, and early breastfeeding initiation are associated with positive lactation and breastfeeding outcomes (Table 37-4). Peripartum interventions can disrupt the normal, physiologic processes of lactation and breastfeeding initiation and lead to delays in feeding, lethargy or pain, and diminished breast-seeking and breastfeeding instincts and behaviors.

Healthcare providers' lactation and breastfeeding/chestfeeding education and support should occur throughout perinatal care of the pregnant person and family, starting in preconception care or antenatal counseling. Taking a person-centered care approach, providers should discuss infant feeding with pregnant patients and encourage them to pursue lactation and breastfeeding/chestfeeding. For individuals with risk factors for lactation or feeding difficulties, antepartum assessment and management of these conditions and collaboration with a lactation specialist can increase lactation and breastfeeding/chestfeeding success.

Intrapartum care practices supportive of breastfeeding/chestfeeding include the continuous presence of a labor support person, which is associated with increased breastfeeding initiation.[18]

| Table 37-4 | Peripartum Care Practices That Support Lactation and Breastfeeding |
|---|---|
| Prenatal breastfeeding counseling and education | |
| Assessment for risk factors and referral to a lactation specialist as indicated | |
| Continuous labor support | |
| Spontaneous vaginal birth | |
| Skin-to-skin care | |
| Delaying routine neonatal procedures until breastfeeding is established | |
| Lactation support | |
| Avoidance of oral suctioning and supplemental feeding unless indicated | |
| Judicious approach to pacifier use | |

Data from Holmes AV, McLeod AY, Bunik M. ABM Clinical Protocol #5: peripartum breastfeeding management for the healthy mother and infant at term, revision 2013. *Breastfeeding Med.* 2013;8(6): 469–473.

Systematic reviews have not provided conclusive evidence about the effects of epidural anesthesia on lactation, breastfeeding initiation, or human milk feeding duration.[19] Similarly, there are no conclusive data regarding the effects of exogenous oxytocin for labor induction or augmentation on breastfeeding outcomes.[20] Administration of high amounts of intravenous fluids to the birthing person during labor can lead to volume expansion and concerns about excessive neonatal weight loss, resulting in supplementation that disrupts the establishment and exclusivity of breastfeeding. Longer labors are associated with delayed breastfeeding initiation, although this may be due to underlying medical complications or maternal/neonatal fatigue.

Both operative and surgical births are risk factors for complications with lactation and breastfeeding. Vacuum- or forceps-assisted births have the potential to cause neonatal birth trauma and pain, facial or cranial asymmetries, or torticollis, leading to impaired suckling and neonatal breastfeeding reflexes.[21] Cesarean birth has been linked with lower rates of breastfeeding in several studies, although it is not known if the surgery itself or the underlying indications for surgery are the most important factors. Delayed breastfeeding initiation is common following surgical birth, and both postsurgical pain

and incisional pain can increase discomfort in common breastfeeding positions. Excessive blood loss during childbirth or postpartum can lead to delayed lactogenesis II and challenges in producing an adequate milk supply.

## Physiologic Breastfeeding Initiation

In the absence of interventions, a healthy, term neonate placed on the abdomen or chest of the postpartum person will go through a predictable sequence of instinctive behaviors focused on breast-seeking and suckling.[22] This sequence is outlined in Table 37-5. Interventions in the immediate postpartum can disrupt this process. One of the most beneficial care practices to facilitate this newborn sequence and early initiation of breastfeeding is immediate, continuous, and uninterrupted skin-to-skin care.

In skin-to-skin care, the postpartum person is placed into a semi-prone position, and the healthy newborn is placed on their chest or abdomen immediately following birth. The newborn is dried and remains naked in a prone position, in direct skin-to-skin contact with the postpartum person, often covered by a warm blanket. The newborn ideally would remain in skin-to-skin contact for at least 1 hour after birth or until breastfeeding has been initiated.

Skin-to-skin care helps to facilitate the physiologic neonatal transition to extrauterine life and is positively associated with breastfeeding initiation, exclusivity, and duration (without distinction between breastfeeding and human milk feeding).[23] Dyads who experience skin-to-skin care postpartum also demonstrate higher scores on measures of breastfeeding effectiveness.[23] The AAP recommends that healthy, term neonates receive skin-to-skin care in the absence of interventions or any separation from the birthing parent until the conclusion of the initial breastfeeding session. When circumstances permit, skin-to-skin care is also beneficial for preterm infants. Precautions should be taken to supervise skin-to-skin care, especially when the gestational parent is using opioid analgesia, to ensure neonatal safety and prevent sudden unexpected postnatal collapse associated with neonatal asphyxiation or entrapment.[24]

Infant bonding and the normal sequence of neonatal breast-seeking and feeding behaviors are protected by delaying routine newborn procedures until after the first feeding session. Unnecessary neonatal suctioning should be avoided. Moreover, separation of the infant from the lactating parent in the

| Table 37-5 | Sequence of Newborn Behaviors | |
|---|---|---|
| **Stage** | **Newborn Behavior** | |
| 1. Birth cry | Intense crying just after birth | |
| 2. Relaxation | Rest/recovery with no activity of mouth, head, body, or limbs | |
| 3. Awakening | Begins to show signs of activity such as head thrusts and lateral movements, small movements of shoulders and limbs | |
| 4. Activity | Moves limbs and head in more determined movements, rooting activity, "pushing" with limbs without shifting body | |
| 5. Crawling | "Pushing" (stepping reflex), which results in shifting of the newborn's body | |
| 6. Resting | Rests with some activity such as mouth activity, sucks on hand | |
| 7. Familiarization | Has reached the areola/nipple with mouth positioned to brush and lick areola | |
| 8. Suckling | Suckling on the nipple | |
| 9. Sleeping | Closes eyes, sleeps | |

Based on from Widström A-M, Lilja G, Aaltomaa-Michalias P, et al. Newborn behaviour to locate the breast when skin-to-skin: a possible method for enabling early self-regulation. *Acta Paediatr*. 2011;100:79-85 and Widström A, Brimdyr K, Svensson K, Cadwell K, Nissen E. Skin-to-skin contact the first hour after birth, underlying implications and clinical practice. *Acta Pædiatr*. 2019;108(7):1192-1204. doi:10.1111/apa.14754.

early postpartum period can interfere with lactation and breastfeeding success. Keeping the newborn together with the postpartum person ("rooming-in") in perinatal care facilitates the establishment of lactation and breastfeeding/chestfeeding as parents learn and respond to infant feeding cues. However, research has not demonstrated a positive effect of rooming-in on breastfeeding duration compared to nursery-based care.[25]

The approach to lactation support also influences lactation and feeding outcomes. In the absence of interventions and in an environment supportive of breastfeeding/chestfeeding, many dyads can initiate breastfeeding/chestfeeding independently (Figure 37-2). When support is necessary, providers should aim to provide encouragement rather than direction, helping parents recognize signs of readiness and breast-seeking behaviors in the newborn, and offering reassurance and suggestions in a way that maximizes parental confidence and breastfeeding self-efficacy.[26]

## When Breastfeeding/Chestfeeding Is Not Possible

In some situations, neonates may not be able to feed directly at the breast. These include the presence of underlying medical conditions or separation from the lactating parent for prolonged periods of time (such as for neonatal intensive care admission). When neonates are not able to breastfeed/chestfeed in the immediate postpartum but lactation and human milk feeding are desired, interventions are needed to establish or maintain lactation and provide human milk to the neonate. In these situations, lactating individuals may be encouraged and supported in milk expression and indirect human milk feeding using a spoon, syringe, cup, or bottle (as discussed later in this chapter). Strategies to establish the human milk supply include the expression of colostrum in the first hour after birth, education about "hands-on" breast stimulation and expression techniques, and encouragement to express milk at regular 3- to 4-hour intervals. In the immediate postpartum period, hand expression has been found to be as effective or more effective than expression with a breast pump. When lactating individuals experience a perinatal loss, they may still be provided with lactation support, as expression and donation of human milk have been shown to benefit some individuals in coping with loss.[27] Whenever complications arise with initiation of neonatal feeding, team-based care involving lactation consultants and neonatal care providers is important in supporting lactation and optimizing neonatal health.

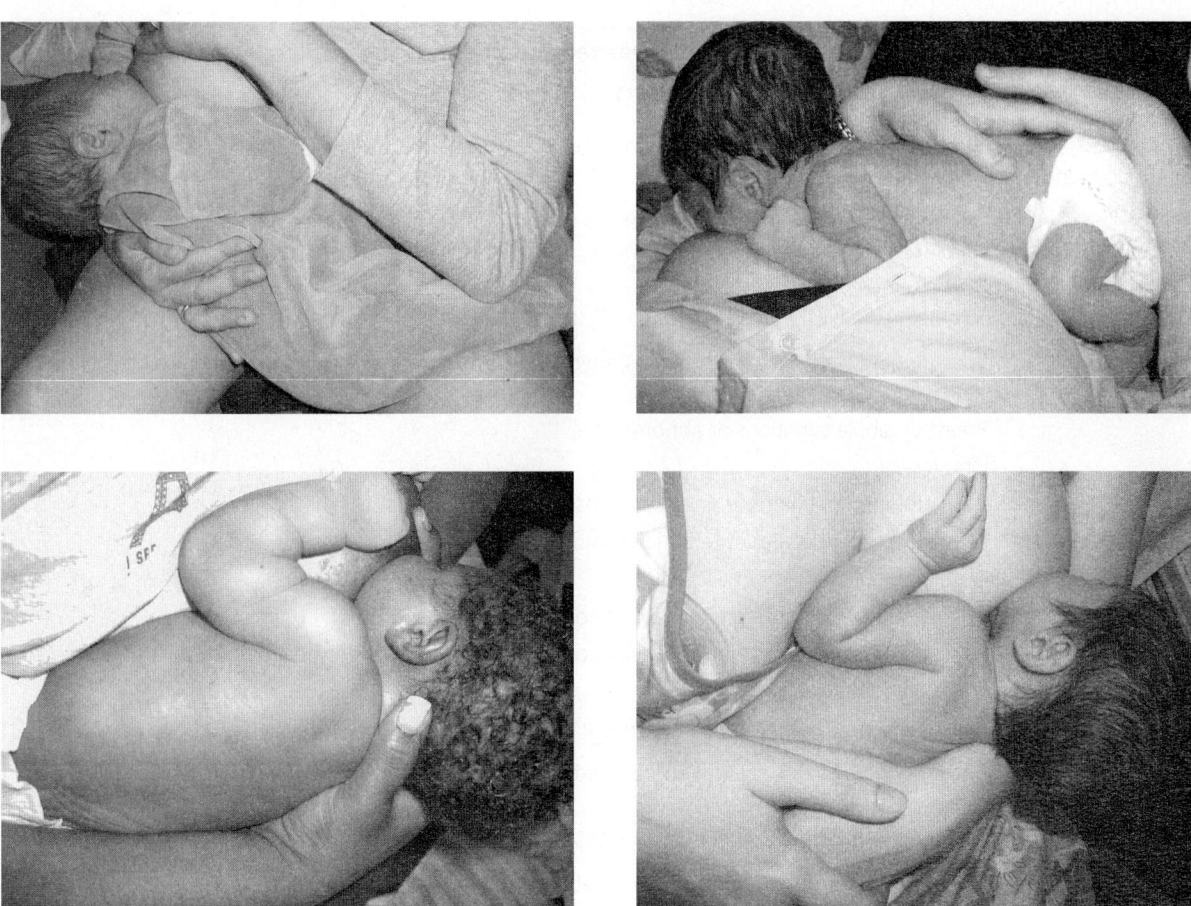

**Figure 37-2** Physiologic breastfeeding initiation.
Reproduced from Genna, CW Supporting Sucking Skills in Breastfeeding Infants. 3rd ed. Burlington, MA: Jones & Bartlett Learning; 2016. Courtesy of Catherine Watson Genna, BS, IBCLC.

## Health Assessment for Lactation and Breastfeeding

Health assessment for lactation and breastfeeding takes place throughout the perinatal period, beginning in the preconception or antepartum period. A comprehensive and person-centered, trauma-informed care approach should include a detailed health history and a targeted physical examination of both the lactating person and the neonate. Observation of a feeding or milk expression session is also useful to prevent or diagnose complications. Individualized counseling for health promotion and education is essential to help lactating and breastfeeding dyads reach their infant feeding goals.

### Health History

Lactation and breastfeeding are dependent on the dynamic relationship between the lactating person and the child and are affected by both internal and external factors. Therefore, a comprehensive health history is necessary to identify risk factors for lactation or breastfeeding complications. Table 37-6 presents factors that should be considered as part of a health assessment for lactation and breastfeeding. Many individuals who present with risk factors for lactation or breastfeeding complications will be able to successfully breastfeed or produce a sufficient milk supply. However, they may benefit from early interventions, including preventive measures, education and counseling, and lactation support, to help them reach their infant feeding goals and prevent infant complications associated with inadequate intake.

While most lactating individuals are able to produce a sufficient milk supply, several conditions are associated with impaired lactation due to delayed lactogenesis (beyond 72 hours after birth) or insufficient milk production. These include underlying endocrine dysfunction that inhibits physiologic hormonal responses (e.g., to stress), diabetes, obesity, thyroid dysfunction, polycystic ovary syndrome, ovarian theca

| Table 37-6 | Health History for Lactation and Breastfeeding/Chestfeeding |
| --- | --- |
| **Component** | **Targeted Aspects of Health History** |
| Individual preferences and concerns | Attitude toward lactation and breastfeeding |
| | Infant feeding goals |
| | Any individual concerns or circumstances that may affect breastfeeding, milk expression, or milk supply (e.g., perceived milk supply, infant fussiness, return to work, desire for partner to participate in infant feeding) |
| | Targeted review of symptoms and characteristics of chief concern(s) |
| Medical history | Endocrine dysfunction (e.g., diabetes, thyroid disease, polycystic ovary syndrome, isolated prolactin deficiency) |
| | Breast or nipple variations or abnormalities |
| | Obesity |
| | Dermatologic conditions (e.g., eczema, psoriasis) |
| | Musculoskeletal conditions (e.g., joint, muscle, or back pain) |
| | Autoimmune conditions |
| | Circulatory conditions (e.g., Raynaud syndrome) |
| | Pain disorders (e.g., migraines, irritable bowel syndrome, dysmenorrhea, dyspareunia) |
| | Hospitalizations |
| | Extremes in age (adolescent or advanced) |
| Surgical history | Breast surgery (e.g., reduction/augmentation, biopsies, mastectomy, lumpectomy, nipple piercing, abscesses) |
| | Obstetric surgery (e.g., dilation and curettage, cesarean birth) |
| Family history | Genetic disorders such as chromosomal abnormalities or phenylketonuria |
| | Family breastfeeding/lactation history |
| | Breast cancer |
| | Children with congenital anomalies |
| Social history | Partnership status |
| | Social support |
| | Environmental exposures |
| | Financial stability |
| | Nutritional status |
| Psychiatric history | Depression |
| | Anxiety |
| | Stress |
| | History of trauma |
| | Body dysphoria |
| | Eating disorders |
| Perinatal history | Current pregnancy status |
| | Single or multiple gestation |
| | Breast changes in size, color, or sensitivity in pregnancy |
| | Weight gain/loss in pregnancy |
| | Results of prenatal testing and fetal assessment |
| | Presence of any abnormalities on ultrasound (including theca lutein ovarian cysts) |

| Component | Targeted Aspects of Health History |
|---|---|
| Intrapartum history | Length of labor |
| | Mode of birth |
| | Anesthesia or analgesia |
| | Complications and interventions |
| | Neonatal transition, need for resuscitation, and Apgar scores |
| | Birth weight |
| | Placental abnormalities, including manual or surgical removal |
| | Postpartum blood loss and need for blood transfusion |
| Reproductive history | Pregnancy history (gravidity, parity, termination, abortion) |
| | Infertility or conception by assisted reproductive technology |
| Lactation and breastfeeding history | Exposure to (familiarity with) breastfeeding |
| | Experience of breastfeeding initiation |
| | Previous and current lactation and/or breastfeeding experience and duration |
| | Feeding patterns (frequency, duration, and one or both breasts) |
| | Milk expression patterns (method, frequency, and quantity expressed) |
| | Assessment of milk supply including experience of engorgement and sensations of breast fullness |
| | Concerns with lactation or breastfeeding |
| | Use of supplementation with human milk or human milk substitutes |
| Immunization history | Immunization status |
| Sleep history | Level of fatigue |
| | Quality and quantity of sleep |
| Medications, herbs, or substances | Medications used during pregnancy |
| | Current medication, herbal supplementation, or substance use |
| | Contraceptive plan during lactation |
| Allergies | Known allergies or sensitives |
| Neonatal behaviors | Feeding, sleeping, voiding, and stooling patterns |
| | Stool consistency |
| | Fussiness, crying, or colic |
| | Use of pacifiers |
| Neonatal complications and medical conditions | Low birth weight or large for gestational age |
| | Twins or high-order multiples |
| | Prematurity or early term birth |
| | Gastrointestinal conditions |
| | Musculoskeletal conditions |
| | Hyperbilirubinemia |
| | Hypoglycemia |
| | Chromosomal abnormalities |
| | Neuromotor delays or impairment |
| | Abnormalities of the oral cavity |
| | Candidiasis (oral or diaper area) |
| | Medication use |

lutein cysts, retained placental fragments, and postpartum pituitary infarction (formally known as Sheehan syndrome).[28] In addition, anatomic variations or abnormalities of the breast/nipple (e.g., insufficient glandular tissue or complications from surgical procedures) or the neonate's oral cavity (e.g., cleft lip or palate), as well as some musculoskeletal conditions (e.g., hypotonia or torticollis), place the dyad at increased risk for lactation or breastfeeding difficulties. Individuals who underwent cesarean surgery may experience discomfort and difficulty with breastfeeding initiation and can benefit from additional lactation support. Musculoskeletal conditions of the lactating person or neonate may also present challenges to feeding comfortably at the breast.

Many individuals with a history of breast surgery can successfully lactate and breastfeed, although it is recommended that they closely monitor their infant for adequate growth and signs of satiety to determine the need for supplementation. Early engagement with peer counselors and breastfeeding support groups is especially helpful to increase breastfeeding self-efficacy for those individuals who lack social support or familiarity with lactation or breastfeeding. Psychotherapeutic and social support interventions are also especially important for lactating individuals with peripartum depression, as there is a negative correlation between depressive symptoms and human milk feeding duration.

## Contraindications to Breastfeeding and Human Milk Feeding

Few true contraindications to breastfeeding and human milk feeding exist, as outlined in Table 37-7. The only neonatal contraindication to human milk feeding is classic galactosemia, a rare genetic metabolic disorder that is included in routine newborn screening programs.

Contraindicated conditions of the lactating individual are (1) infection with human T-cell lymphotropic virus (type I or type II), (2) suspected or confirmed Ebola virus disease, and (3) use of illicit street drugs such as PCP (phencyclidine) or cocaine. (However, lactating individuals taking methadone or buprenorphine as part of a supervised program with negative screening for drug use may provide their human milk for infant feeding.) Human immunodeficiency virus (HIV) can be transmitted through breast milk. If a lactating person with HIV is on antiretroviral therapy (ART) and has a

| Table 37-7 | Contraindications to Feeding at the Breast or Human Milk Feeding | | |
|---|---|---|---|
| **Condition(s)** | | **Breastfeeding** | **Human Milk Feeding** |
| **Conditions of the Lactating Individual** | | | |
| • Human immunodeficiency virus infection in the United States in the absence of antiretroviral therapy (ART) and suppressed viral load* <br> • Human T-lymphotropic virus infection (Type I or II) <br> • Use of illicit drugs <br> • Suspected or confirmed Ebola virus disease | | Contraindicated | Contraindicated |
| • Untreated brucellosis <br> • Use of contraindicated mediations or exposure to radioactive pharmaceuticals <br> • Active herpes simplex virus infection with lesions on the breast <br> • Mpox virus infection (symptomatic or in medically indicated isolation) | | Temporarily suspended *(May resume when it is determined to be clinically safe)* | Temporarily suspended *(May resume when it is determined to be clinically safe)* |
| • Untreated active tuberculosis <br> • Active varicella that developed around the time of birth (between 5 days prior to 2 days following birth) | | Contraindicated | Permitted |
| **Conditions of the Neonate** | | | |
| • Classic galactosemia | | Contraindicated | Contraindicated |

* Note: Individuals with HIV and detectable viral loads who choose to breastfeed should be provided guidance on neonatal HIV prophylaxis and testing and assistance to achieve and sustain viral suppression.

Data from Centers for Disease Control and Prevention. Contraindications to breastfeeding or feeding expressed breast milk to infants. https://www.cdc.gov/breastfeeding/breastfeeding-special-circumstances/contraindications-to-breastfeeding.html. Published 2023. Accessed December 16, 2023.

sustained, undetectable viral load, the risk of transmission through breastfeeding is less than 1%. For individuals with detectable viral loads who wish to breastfeed, consultation with an expert or the National Perinatal HIV/AIDS hotline (1-888-448-8764) is recommended. In certain settings without safe infant feeding alternatives, WHO recommends that lactating persons with HIV breastfeed and continue ART to reduce risk of HIV transmission. Lactating persons with untreated brucellosis or active herpes simplex lesions on the breast should not use their human milk for infant feeding until it is determined to be clinically safe. Temporary suspension of human milk feeding of their own milk may also be necessary for lactating individuals who are exposed to certain radioactive pharmaceuticals or contraindicated medications (as discussed later in this chapter). Although expressed milk may be provided from individuals who have active, untreated tuberculous or active varicella around the time of birth (5 days prior or 2 days following birth), these individuals should not feed their infants directly at the breast due to risk of transmission. Contraindicated drugs and substances are discussed in the "Medications, Herbs, and Substances in Lactation" section later in this chapter.

Lactating individuals with suspected or confirmed COVID-19 or those who are not fully vaccinated and have been in close contact with someone who has COVID-19 may continue to breastfeed and/or provide their milk to a neonate with some precautions. The best available research suggests that the SARS-CoV-2 virus (responsible for COVID-19) is not likely to be transmitted in human milk, so there are no restrictions on feeding of human milk from COVID-positive lactating individuals. However, COVID-positive individuals should follow current guidelines regarding quarantine or isolation and wear a mask when breastfeeding or expressing milk. Hand washing and sanitizing of breast pumps and infant feeding items are also recommended. The breastfed neonate of an individual with suspected or confirmed COVID-19 who is not fully vaccinated is considered a close contact and should follow quarantine guidelines during the lactating person's period of isolation and quarantine.[29]

### Physical Examination

Although it is not possible to predict lactation or breastfeeding complications based on physical examination alone, assessments of the breasts and of the neonate can identify conditions that place the dyad at increased risk for complications. For example, widely spaced tubular or triangular breasts may be an indication of insufficient glandular tissue (breast hypoplasia), resulting in an inability to produce a full milk supply, and a short, tight lingual frenulum (neonatal ankyloglossia) may restrict the mobility of the neonate's tongue and cause nipple injury. Table 37-8 presents key components of the targeted physical examination for lactation and breastfeeding complications.

Physical examination for lactation begins with a general impression of well-being of the lactating person, including their mood, affect, and response to the newborn. Individuals experiencing extreme stress, fatigue, anxiety, or depressive symptoms may require collaborative, team-based care to reach their infant feeding goals. Similarly, individuals with a body mass index (BMI) greater than 30 are at increased risk for delayed lactogenesis and early cessation of breastfeeding and may benefit from additional lactation support.[30] Persons with large, pendulous breasts may also benefit from recommendations for positioning, such as use of a semi-reclined or breast-supported position to achieve a comfortable latch.

Physical assessment of the lactating breast includes inspection and palpation. Although the size, shape, symmetry, and spacing of the breasts do not indicate an ability to breastfeed or produce an adequate milk supply, this assessment may reveal potential risk factors or complications. For example, as insufficient glandular tissue (breast hypoplasia) is often associated with impaired lactation. Accessory or supernumerary breast tissue or nipples may be present along the embryonic mammary ridge (milk line) (as discussed in the *Anatomy and Physiology of the Reproductive System* chapter) and become enlarged during lactogenesis II. Palpation techniques are useful to assess for tissue density, masses, warmth, and tenderness to differentiate breast conditions such as engorgement, plugged ducts, mastitis, galactoceles, and other breast conditions unrelated to lactation.

Nipple size and shape can vary widely. Most nipples protrude slightly at rest and become erect when stimulated (Figure 37-3). Nipples that are exceptionally large, flat, retracted, or inverted may be more challenging for infants to effectively grasp for breastfeeding. When these anatomic variations lead to lactation or breastfeeding complications, a variety of interventions—such as nipple shields, breast shields, or use of products to evert the nipple—can be used to obtain an effective latch. Nipples that are misshapen, compressed, or blanched after feeding, when associated with pain or insufficient lactation, likely indicate an ineffective latch. Nipple cracks, fissures, or ulcerations are potential sources of bacterial infection and should be addressed. A plugged nipple pore can result in a raised, white bump on the tip of the nipple (bleb). Dermatoses or cutaneous infections can cause alterations in skin color and the condition

| Table 37-8 | Physical Examination for Lactation and Newborn Feeding | | |
|---|---|---|---|
| **Component of Examination** | **Targeted Assessments** | **Component of Examination** | **Targeted Assessments** |
| **Lactating Individual** | | **Neonate** | |
| General | Posture | General | Gestational age assessment |
| | Fatigue | | Singleton/multiple gestation |
| | Psychosocial: mood, confidence, anxiety, response to newborn | | Birth weight and current weight |
| | Weight | | Respiratory pattern |
| | Pallor | | Muscle tone and posture |
| Breasts | Size, shape, symmetry, and spacing | | Alertness and level of arousal |
| | | | Skin color and turgor |
| | Presence of scars | | Medical complications (e.g., hypoglycemia, jaundice, cardiac or respiratory complications) |
| | Engorgement, edema, or fullness | | |
| | Location of extra-mammary breast tissue | | Neurologic complications or neurodevelopmental delay |
| | Tissue density, masses, or abscesses | Head and neck | Range of motion |
| | Tenderness, pain, or sensitivity | | Symmetry (facial, cranial, mandibular) |
| | Color (i.e., erythema, ecchymosis) and warmth | | Position/tilt |
| | | | Signs of trauma |
| | Skin turgor | | Jaw position (i.e., extension or recession) |
| | Dermatologic conditions | | Adenoid size |
| Nipples | Location | | Nasal congestion |
| | Eversion | Oral cavity | Lips: blisters, frenulum, cleft lip |
| | Size | | Mouth: color, lesions, mucous membranes, gape |
| | Shape/compression/edema | | Palate: height, shape, cleft palate |
| | Color (vasoconstriction) | | Tongue: size, shape, position, mobility, extension |
| | Skin integrity (e.g., cracks, abrasions, blisters, blebs) | | Signs of infection (oral candidiasis) |
| | Discharge | Digital suck examination | Strength |
| | | | Coordination |

of the nipple–areolar complex. These conditions and other common complications with lactation and breastfeeding are discussed in greater detail in the "Assessment and Management of Common Lactation Concerns" section later in this chapter.

Targeted physical examination of the newborn for concerns related to infant feeding focuses on the head, neck, and oral cavity. Visual inspection of the head can identify neonates at risk for feeding complications due to birth trauma; musculoskeletal conditions that limit range of motion, such as torticollis (unilateral tension or shortening of the sternocleidomastoid muscle of the neck); and anatomic variations that impact latch or suck, such as micrognathia, cleft

lip/palate, or facial, cranial, or mandibular asymmetry. Palpation of the oral cavity is important to assess tongue mobility and extension. Digital suck examination using a gloved finger inserted into the neonate's mouth can be useful to assess for neuromuscular conditions that affect suck strength and coordination. Despite the trend toward more diagnosis and treatment of ankyloglossia ("tongue-tie" due to a short, thick, or tight lingual frenulum) in breastfeeding infants, the Academy of Breastfeeding Medicine (ABM) does not recommend routine examination of the frenulum as part of the initial physical examination for breastfeeding due to a lack of high-quality evidence supporting interventions.[31] Finally,

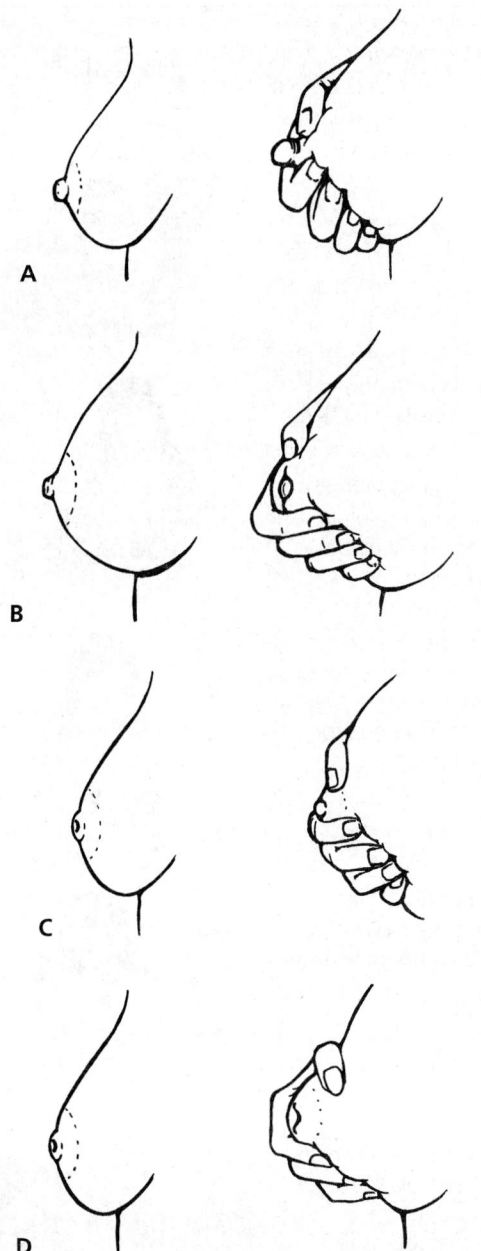

**Figure 37-3** Nipple response to stimulation. **A.** Protraction. **B.** Retraction. **C.** Eversion of inverted-appearing nipple. **D.** Inversion. Reproduced from Wambach, K & Spencer, B *Breastfeeding and Human Lactation* 6th ed. Burlington, MA: Jones & Bartlett Learning; 2019.

neonatal assessment includes evaluation for signs of adequate milk intake, such as voiding and stooling patterns and weight gain, as discussed in the "Signs of Adequate Feeding" section later in the chapter.

## Observation of Breastfeeding or Milk Expression Session

The final component of health assessment for the lactating individual or breastfeeding dyad is an observation of a breastfeeding session. For individuals who are experiencing problems with lactation related to milk expression, observation of a pumping or hand expression session can useful. Lactation specialists may use any of several validated instruments to comprehensively assess breastfeeding behaviors, skills, and mechanics. For primary care providers with limited time to perform a breastfeeding assessment in the clinical setting, the focus is on identifying common concerns with positioning, latch, and suckling that may cause pain or inadequate milk transfer.

### Positioning

Dyads can breastfeed in any position that is comfortable to the lactating person and results in a comfortable latch and effective milk transfer. Common positions for breastfeeding are depicted in Table 37-9.[32] Regardless of the position used, the newborn should be positioned so that their body is well aligned for attachment to the breast and swallowing, most commonly with the neonate's abdomen toward the lactating person's chest, chin against the breast, nose tilted up into a "sniffing position," and mouth open with a wide gape (Figure 37-4).

### Latch

It is important that the infant has a deep latch onto the breast to both facilitate effective milk removal and avoid causing nipple pain or trauma. Many factors influence the ability to obtain a deep latch, including situational and breast and neonatal anatomic factors (as outlined earlier). When the infant latches on deeply, the nipple is drawn into the mouth near the junction of the hard and soft palates, allowing the infant to form a seal around the nipple using the tongue, lips, and cheeks. This allows for effective suckling and avoids compressing or injuring the nipple. In an effective latch, the neonate's lips are flanged outward, positioned slightly off-center on the breast, with the chin touching the breast and the nose free (see Table 37-10). The infant's body should be well supported, and the lactating person should be comfortable.

If the lactating person is experiencing nipple pain, it typically signals that infant has an ineffective or shallow latch. Compression of the nipple and milk ducts in a shallow latch can cause nipple trauma and ineffective milk transfer. A nipple that appears misshapen or compressed after breastfeeding is likely an indication of a shallow latch.

Lactating persons may be concerned when the neonate's nose is buried in the breast and may

| Table 37-9 | Common Positions for Breastfeeding | | |
|---|---|---|---|
| **Position** | **Description** | **Considerations** | **Illustration** |
| Semi-reclining ("laid back")[32] | Lactating person is semi-reclined with the newborn prone in contact with the chest and abdomen. | Gravity and skin-to-skin contact supports neonatal instinctive breastfeeding behaviors.<br><br>Comfortable position for the lactating person but requires a sitting area with sufficient size and back support to enable a semi-reclined position. | |
| Cradle | Lactating person sits upright with the newborn in side-lying position supported by the same-side arm. | Generally comfortable and commonly used position, especially after the first few weeks.<br><br>May require pillows or supports to lift the baby up to nipple height or can result in uncomfortable positioning and shoulder tension for the lactating person. | |
| Cross-cradle | Similar to cradle position, the lactating person sits upright with the newborn in side-lying position supported by the parent's opposite-side arm. | Provides more stability for the infant's upper body and head, so may be useful for nursing a small or preterm newborn. May require pillows or additional supports for optimal comfort and positioning. | |
| Football or clutch (underarm) | Lactating person sits upright with the newborn supine, feet pointed toward the maternal back, and body wrapped along the parental side, supported by the same-side arm. | Post-cesarean birth, this positions the neonate's body away from the incision to minimize pain. May not be ergonomic with larger newborns. | |
| Side-lying, or "recovery" position | Lactating person lies on their side with the newborn side-lying facing the breast. | Allows the lactating person to lie down and rest. Precautions should be in place in case they fall asleep while breastfeeding. May be difficult for some newborns to effectively latch in this position in the first few days/weeks of life. | |

Modified from International Lactation Consultant Association; Mannel R, Martens PJ, Walker M, eds. *Core Curriculum for Lactation Consultant Practice*. 3rd ed. Burlington, MA: Jones & Bartlett; 2013.

attempt to pull back their breast or depress the breast tissue to clear the infant's nose. However, this behavior can disrupt an effective latch. Parents should be reassured that healthy, term neonates can breathe comfortably with their nose touching the breast and will instinctively release the nipple and pull back from breast to breathe through their mouths if the nose is truly blocked. If parents are still concerned that the infant cannot breathe, it may be helpful to raise the infant so that the chin is positioned closer to the breast to create more space between the infant's nose and the breast.

### Suckling and Swallowing

Effective breastfeeding has a visible and audible rhythm, driven by the infant's ability to coordinate

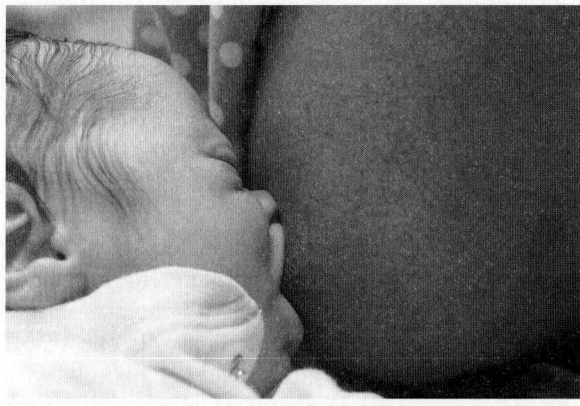

**Figure 37-4** Optimal positioning at the breast.
© lostinbids/E+/Getty Images.

| Table 37-10 | Signs of an Effective Latch |
| --- | --- |
| Lips flanged outward | |
| Asymmetrical (slightly off-center) position on the breast | |
| Abdomen facing toward the lactating person's abdomen/chest | |
| Chin touching the lactating breast | |

suck, swallow, and breathe actions.[33] As part of the breastfeeding assessment, it is useful to observe the sucking pattern and listen for swallowing. At the start of a feed, there is a faster suck–swallow–breathe rhythm, with the infant taking several sucks before swallowing and breathing. When the milk ejection reflex (milk "let-down") occurs, milk flows more rapidly, and the infant suckling pattern adjusts in response to the faster milk flow. Most lactating persons experience multiple ejection reflexes per feeding session, although they may not perceive them. Infants who show signs of fatigue and slow down their sucking actions before the breast is emptied may benefit from the lactating person using their hands to compress the breast and stimulate milk flow.

### Additional Assessments

Additional components of breastfeeding observation include parent–infant interaction, infant's behavior at the breast, and any signs of pain in the lactating individual. At the conclusion of a feed, examination of the shape and color of the nipple is useful to diagnose potential complications such

as shallow latch or vasospasm. Finally, at the conclusion of a feed, the infant should be observed for signs of satiety. Following an effective breastfeeding session, the newborn often will release the breast, relax the hand and facial muscles, close the mouth, and rest comfortably.

### Observation of Milk Expression

Observation of a milk expression session will vary based on the method of expression. For hand or manual expression, the focus is on evaluation and effectiveness of technique. For pumping, assessment will include the size and fit of breast shields or flanges and the dynamics of pumping such as the type of pump, level of suction, and cycle frequency. Observation of pumping also includes evaluation for signs of trauma or pain, quantity of expressed milk, and duration of pumping session.[34]

## Anticipatory Guidance for Human Milk Feeding

Providing education and support for human milk feeding can increase parental efficacy and enable early identification of complications. Health education and promotion of newborn feeding and lactation can help parents to recognize and respond to early newborn feeding cues, have realistic expectations for feeding frequency, and assess signs of effective and adequate infant feeding. Anticipatory guidance is especially important since breastfeeding self-efficacy is a major modifiable determinant of breastfeeding exclusivity and duration.[35]

A bra is not a requirement for successful breastfeeding/chestfeeding but can be used for comfort and support as needed. Common guidance includes information about avoidance of tight-fitting bras or chest binders during lactation to avoid compressing the breast tissue and potentially increasing the risk of lactational mastitis.

### Newborn Feeding Cues

Parents should be encouraged to observe their newborns for signs that they are ready to feed and to recognize and respond to early hunger cues. A healthy term, exclusively human milk-fed newborn will wake and show signs of readiness to feed at least 8 to 12 times a day. Early signs of hunger include small movements around the mouth such as moving the hand to the mouth, smacking or licking the lips, thrusting the tongue, or opening and closing the mouth. As hunger grows, the newborn's activity increases, as evidenced by head turning; rooting; sucking on lips, hands, or fingers; or making soft noises. Clenched fingers and fists and flexed arms and legs also indicate hunger. Agitation, crying, and forceful head movements seeking the breast are late signs of hunger.

The ideal level of arousal and activity for breastfeeding is state of calm alertness. Newborns who are agitated and crying may need to be soothed before they can effectively latch on to the breast, and newborns who are overly sleepy may benefit from gentle stimulation.

### Feeding Patterns

Breastfed infants feed frequently, typically 8 to 12 times during a 24-hour period. Infants fed human milk substitutes feed slightly less frequently than human milk-fed infants. While the milk supply is being established, it is recommended to feed "on demand," led by the newborn's signs of hunger. This newborn-led feeding approach typically results in feeding every 1.5 to 3 hours. Frequent milk removal is the most important mechanism regulating ongoing breast milk synthesis, so it is not recommended that newborns go more than 4 hours between feeds, even overnight. Once infants get older, they may go longer periods between feedings and adapt to a scheduled feeding pattern. Some infants tend to have a pattern of paired or cluster feeds—that is, two or more feeds with short periods of sleep or a quiet alert state between feeding cues.

There is no set amount of time at the breast required to achieve an adequate feed. Lactating persons should be encouraged to "watch the baby, not the clock" and assess for signs of satiety. In the first month, the newborn stomach capacity is less than 1 ounce, and newborns need approximately 20 to 24 ounces of human milk per day.[36] Commercially available visual aids demonstrating graphic depictions of the stomach capacity of infants as they grow may be a helpful teaching tool.

### Signs of Adequate Feeding

Because it is difficult to determine the amount of milk a newborn consumes at the breast, it is important to provide anticipatory guidance regarding signs of adequate intake. Physiologic changes in the lactating individual, newborn elimination patterns, and newborn weight loss or gain are useful indicators of effective and adequate feeding. Knowing what to expect can help parents feel more confident that breastfeeding is going well or allow for early intervention when milk intake is inadequate to prevent further complications.

When lactation is effective, the lactating individual will notice physiologic changes. On the first day postpartum, they may feel uterine cramping at the onset of a feeding due to the increase in oxytocin that results from nipple stimulation. On days 2 to 5 postpartum, changes in the breast such as increases in fullness, firmness, and size and the presence of colostrum with manual or mechanical expression are signs of milk production increasing from effective stimulation. Following a feeding, the breasts should feel softer and less heavy. There may also be visible changes in the color and consistency of milk with the transition from colostrum to mature milk with effective feeding within 1 to 2 weeks of life.

Newborn elimination patterns, including the quantity of wet and soiled diapers, the color and consistency of stool, and the frequency of voids/stools, are helpful indicators of adequate intake (Table 37-11). A general guideline is that the newborn should have one wet diaper and one dirty diaper for each day of age in the first few days of life. Newborns may void only a few times in the first days after birth before lactogenesis is established. Once breastfeeding is established, infants who are receiving sufficient nutrition will void frequently, approximately 6 to 8 times per day.[36] Breastfed infants may have stools after every feeding. Any neonate who presents with insufficient voids or stools or shows symptoms of dehydration (e.g., dry mucous membranes, depressed anterior fontanel, loss of skin turgo should be evaluated immediately.[37]

Excessive neonatal weight loss or insufficient weight gain may indicate inadequate milk intake. Concerns about neonatal weight contribute to higher rates of supplementation with human milk substitutes and shorter breastfeeding duration.[38] In the first few days of life, newborns are expected to lose weight; indeed, they may lose as much as 10% of their birth weight. Exclusively breastfed neonates born by cesarean are more likely to experience weight loss greater than 10%.[39] The newborn who is exclusively breastfed should begin gaining weight by day 4 of life with the onset of lactogenesis II. Delayed lactogenesis (discussed later in this chapter) is a risk factor for inadequate milk production and excessive neonatal weight loss.[40] When appropriate, assessment of neonatal weight before and after a breastfeeding session on a reliable scale may be used to determine the amount of milk ingested during a breastfeeding session. Newborns should regain their birth weight by 10 to 14 days of life.

Weight gain for newborns consuming human milk substitutes is discussed in greater detail in

| Table 37-11 | Signs of Adequate Feeding: Newborn Elimination Patterns | | | |
|---|---|---|---|---|
| Age (in Days of Life) | Quantity Voids (Wet Diapers) | Quantity Stools (Dirty Diapers) | Stool Quality | Weight Loss or Gain |
| 1 | 1 | 1 | Black, tarry | < 5% loss (from birth weight) |
| 2 | 2–3 | 1–2 | Greenish black, softening | < 5% loss (from birth weight) |
| 3 | 3–4 | 3–4 | Greenish yellow, soft | ≤ 8–10% loss (from birth weight) |
| 4 | ≥ 4–6 | ≥ 4 large (10 small) | Yellow, loose or watery | < 10% (from birth weight) |
| 5+ | ≥ 6 | ≥ 4 | Yellow, seedy | Gaining 0.5 to 1 ounce (15–30 g) per day |

Adapted from Walker M. *Breastfeeding Management for the Clinician: Using the Evidence.* 4th ed. Burlington, MA: Jones & Bartlett Learning; 2016.

the "Human Milk Substitutes" section later in this chapter. Providers can use the Newborn Weight Tool (Newt; included in the Resources at the end of this chapter) to identify newborn weight loss that warrants further evaluation. Collaboration with pediatric care providers is recommended if concerns arise about excessive weight loss (greater than 7% to 10% of birth weight in the first 48 hours of life or greater than 75th percentile for age and mode of delivery based on the Newt tool) or insufficient weight gain.

## Medications, Herbs, and Substances in Lactation

Most, though not all, over-the-counter and prescription medications are compatible with human milk feeding.[41] Even though most drugs are excreted into human milk, the amount ingested by the neonate is usually very small and unlikely to pose significant risks. All medications should be reviewed on an individual basis to determine their safety for infant feeding and potential for adverse effects on lactation. The National Library of Medicine's Drugs and Lactation Database (LactMed; listed in the Resources section at the end of this chapter) is a free online reference regarding the transfer of drugs and other chemicals into human milk, evidence on possible adverse effects, and recommendations for alternative therapies.

To guide individuals in making an informed choice about use of medications while lactating, the known benefits of human milk feeding should be weighed against the benefits of medication use, risks of drug exposure, and infant feeding goals. The drug dosage, duration of use, and pharmacokinetic and chemical properties determine the amount that is excreted into human milk and absorbed by the child. The child's age is also a consideration for two reasons. First, newborns are at increased risk of adverse events from drug exposure compared to older human milk–fed infants.[41] Second, in the first 7 to 10 days postpartum, large gaps exist between alveolar cells in the breast. These gaps allow for easier easy transfer of immunoglobulins, lymphocytes, and proteins into human milk. Transfer of drugs into milk is also greater during this time. As mature milk develops, alveolar cells swell and the intracellular gaps shrink, decreasing drug transfer to the human milk–fed infant.

The principles of prescribing and the basic pharmacokinetic and pharmacodynamic considerations for medications are important to understand when assessing medication use during lactation. Drugs that are more highly protein-bound, have large molecular weights, lack ionization, or have low lipid solubility are transferred into human milk at low rates. Drugs that move from plasma to tissue rapidly have lower rates of diffusion into human milk due to their reduced concentration in plasma.

The method of calculating breast milk concentrations of drugs that is the most clinically useful is the relative infant dose (RID). The RID is the maximum percentage of the maternal dose that the infant consumes assuming a milk intake of approximately 150 mL per kilogram of body weight per day and a standard therapeutic adult dose. An RID of less than 10% is considered safe for healthy term infants.[41] To limit neonatal drug exposure, lactating individuals can be advised to take any medications after breastfeeding or expressing milk.

Fortunately, most drugs are compatible with lactation and breastfeeding. Although more research is needed regarding many agents, drug transfer is rarely a reason to discontinue breastfeeding or human milk feeding. Providers should seek out the most current and reliable information when counseling individuals about drug safety in lactation. General guidelines for medication use during lactation are outlined in Table 37-12.

The need for a particular medication to maintain the health of the lactating individual is an important consideration in discussions about medication use during lactation. Some individuals may need permission to prioritize their health when making infant feeding decisions. Continuation of medications for chronic conditions may benefit the infant in both the short and long terms as a result of having a healthier parent.

Newborns born to pregnant individuals receiving medication therapy (methadone or buprenorphine) for opioid use disorder have fewer symptoms of neonatal opioid withdrawal syndrome (NOWS) if they consume breast milk from their gestational parent who is continuing treatment than if they are fed a human milk substitute. Therefore, breastfeeding/chestfeeding is encouraged for lactating individuals receiving medication therapy for opioid dependence.

While a few medications are incompatible with breastfeeding, lactating individuals can often receive needed treatments through careful selection of the medication as well as modification of the feeding or dosing schedule to ensure infant safety.

| Table 37-12 | General Guidelines for Medication Use During Lactation |
|---|---|

It is rare that a medication is a reason to discontinue lactation or breastfeeding.

Use pharmaceuticals only when necessary.

Use the smallest therapeutic dose for the shortest time that is effective.

Whenever possible, choose an agent with a short half-life, an agent with a relative infant dose that is less than 10%, and an agent that is not delivered by sustained release.

Arrange the timing of drug dosing so that the medication is given immediately after breastfeeding or expressing milk, or before the neonate has a long sleep period.

If the drug is contraindicated for infant exposure, expressing and discarding the milk may be necessary.

## Drugs That Affect Milk Production

A few drugs are known to suppress milk production, including pseudoephedrine, nicotine, testosterone, ergot-derived dopamine agonists (i.e., bromocriptine and cabergoline), and high levels of alcohol and estrogen.[42] Estrogen-containing contraceptive products with less than 30 micrograms of estrogen are considered safe for use in lactation and are unlikely to affect milk supply; current CDC guidelines for contraception during lactation are described in the *Postpartum Care* chapter. Use of pharmacologic treatments for lactation suppression in the first week postpartum is not recommended due to insufficient evidence regarding their effectiveness and potential adverse effects; however, they may be useful in cases of hyperlactation (as discussed later in this chapter).[43,44] Nonpharmacologic approaches to lactation suppression are presented in the "Continuation or Cessation of Lactation" section later in this chapter.

*Galactagogues* are medications or other substances used to increase or maintain adequate milk supply. These therapies have been used in many situations, including when individuals feel they have a suboptimal milk supply or are looking to induce or restart lactation. Dopamine antagonists such as domperidone and metoclopramide are known to increase prolactin secretion and have been used as galactagogues. However, high-quality evidence that supports the efficacy of these medications is lacking, and they have potential to cause adverse effects including cardiac arrhythmias and gastrointestinal distress.[45] Although prolactin is essential for lactation, human milk production is a complex interaction of internal and external factors, and there is no evidence of a direct correlation between prolactin levels and milk production after lactation has been established.

Despite widespread use of herbal supplements such as fenugreek, goat's rue, blessed thistle, and shatavari as galactagogues, there is very limited research to support their effectiveness or safety. Caution is recommended with use of herbal preparations, as these products are not standardized, may be contaminated, and have the potential for adverse interactions with other drugs.[45] Beer is also used as a galactagogue in some cultures. While the consumption of hops in beer may have some benefit on lactation, these gains are outweighed by the negative effects of alcohol consumption on milk synthesis.

More research about potential galactagogues is needed. At this time, the best recommendation for individuals aiming to increase milk supply is frequent and thorough milk removal.

### Nicotine, Alcohol, and Marijuana

Nicotine, alcohol, and marijuana used by a lactating person all transfer into that individual's human milk. Nicotine decreases milk production and is associated with a shorter duration of breastfeeding. It also adversely affects milk composition, taste, and protective properties.[46] Neonates exposed to secondhand smoke are at increased risk of sudden infant death syndrome (SIDS), respiratory illness, and ear infections.[46] Counseling and support for tobacco cessation should be provided to lactating persons, and pharmacologic therapies may be used during lactation if needed.[47] Current CDC recommendations are that individuals who use tobacco products should breastfeed and provide their human milk to their infants even if they continue to use nicotine products. Lactating individuals using nicotine should take protective measures to avoid neonatal secondhand smoke exposure, and should use nicotine products immediately after breastfeeding or milk expression to reduce drug ingestion.

Alcohol diffuses easily into breast milk, such that concentrations approximate the maternal blood alcohol level about 30 to 60 minutes after the lactating person consumes alcohol. Current recommendations are that moderate alcohol consumption (one drink per day) by the lactating individual is unlikely to be harmful to the neonate, but that the lactating individual should wait at least 2 to 2.5 hours after consuming alcohol to breastfeed or express milk to minimize neonatal exposure and potential adverse effects on neonatal behavior.[48] There is no need to express and dispose of milk (colloquially, "pump and dump") after alcohol consumption; doing so will not affect rates of alcohol transfer into human milk.

Marijuana is lipophilic and easily accumulates in human milk. Moderate amounts of its active ingredient, delta-9-tetrahydrocannabinol (THC), have been found in human milk.[49] As yet, there are few longitudinal studies of neonatal marijuana exposure from affected human milk; however, extrapolation of data following in utero exposure and data on the effects of marijuana on adult brains suggest potential for neurodevelopmental delays.[49] Similar to the case for tobacco, secondhand marijuana smoke is a risk factor for SIDS. Current professional recommendations are to abstain from using any marijuana products during lactation and to avoid neonatal secondhand smoke exposure.[50]

## Nutrition During Lactation

Lactating individuals have unique nutritional considerations in areas such as caloric intake, ingestion of specific nutrients to benefit the human milk–fed child, and avoidance of substances that may negatively affect milk synthesis or cause adverse effects for the human milk–fed child. As always, an individualized approach to nutritional counseling is essential, while recognizing that access to food, socioeconomic status, cultural considerations, and personal preferences strongly influence dietary and nutritional decisions. Individuals with nutritional risk factors such as a history of bariatric surgery or a severely restricted diet may benefit from referral to a nutritionist or dietician for specialized counseling. The recommended daily reference intakes for nonlactating individuals for macronutrients, micronutrients, and vitamins are listed in the *Nutrition* chapter.

### Caloric Intake

Most lactating individuals can produce milk of sufficient volume and nutritional quality to support healthy infant growth, regardless of their diet.[51] However, due to the increased energy demands involved in lactation, the nutritional status and body weight of the lactating individual may be affected by insufficient caloric intake. The U.S. Department of Agriculture (USDA) and the U.S. Department of Health and Human Services (DHHS) recommend that lactating persons consume an additional 330 to 400 kilocalories (kcal) per day over the amount consumed prior to pregnancy (approximately 2000 to 2800 kcal per day).[52] The specific recommendation for caloric intake is affected by the lactating person's age, BMI, level of activity, extent of lactation, and amount of milk expression. The Dietary Reference Intakes calculator (listed in the Resources section at the end of the chapter) from the Health and Medicine Division of the National Academies of Sciences, Engineering, and Medicine is a useful tool to help clinicians calculate individual daily nutrient recommendations during lactation.

Many individuals believe that lactation is associated with increased postpartum weight loss. This relationship has not been well defined by scientific research, however, and weight loss among lactating individuals is highly variable.[53] After lactation has been established, lactating individuals can safely achieve gradual weight loss through a reduction of their caloric intake by 500 kcal/day with moderate exercise without affecting milk production.[54] Guidelines for postpartum exercise and weight loss are no different for lactating persons than for nonlactating postpartum individuals. Milk supply does not appear to be affected by moderate variations in diet or level of activity, but instead is associated with the frequency of breast stimulation and milk expression. Long-term dietary restrictions such as severe diets or prolonged fasting can affect milk supply; consideration should be given to balance this concern against cultural or religious practices for individualized decision making.

### Nutritional Supplementation

Routine nutritional supplementation is not necessary for the lactating individual, as nutritional needs in lactation can be met through consumption of a healthy, well-balanced, and varied diet. Specific daily intake recommendations are outlined in the USDA and DHHS guidelines.[52] Recommendations to continue prenatal vitamins during lactation without consideration of the individual's diet may result in excessive intake of iron and folic acid and insufficient intake of choline and iodine; the latter are essential nutrients during lactation. Daily recommended intake of these micronutrients is 550 milligrams of choline (found in dairy and animal- and plant-based proteins) and 290 micrograms of iodine (most commonly found in iodized table salt). Nutritional counseling during lactation should be individualized based on the needs and diet of each client.

Increased intake of calcium is not recommended, despite the temporary loss of bone density associated with lactation, as bone mass recovers spontaneously after lactation cessation. There is also insufficient evidence to support routine supplementation of docosahexaenoic acid (DHA) fatty acids during lactation.[55] However, individuals with limited animal product consumption, such as those following vegan or strict vegetarian diets, should evaluate their diet for sufficient sources of fatty acids in addition to vitamin $B_{12}$–fortified foods and use nutritional supplementation as indicated to meet daily recommended intake values. Individuals with severely restrictive diets, preexisting anemia, or conditions that affect their nutritional status should take supplements as appropriate to ensure they are meeting the nutritional goals for lactation.

The vitamin D content of human milk reflects the lactating individual's vitamin D status, and most human milk contains low amounts of vitamin D. As discussed in the *Neonatal Care* chapter, the AAP recommends routine supplementation of 10 micrograms (400 IU) of vitamin D daily for human milk–fed newborns.[56] However, research has not conclusively shown that such supplementation reduces the risk of vitamin D deficiency in these infants.[57] High-dose vitamin D supplementation ($\geq$ 4000 IU/day) for the lactating individual has been shown to result in similar infant vitamin D levels as infant supplementation with 400 IU/day, but the overall benefit of this supplementation and its effects on bone health are unclear.[57]

### Recommendations for Dietary Restrictions

As during pregnancy, while moderate fish consumption is beneficial, mercury exposure is a concern with certain types of seafood in lactation (see the *Nutrition* chapter). Thus, lactating individuals should avoid consuming fish containing high levels of mercury. Limiting daily caffeine intake to two to three cups of coffee (or less than 300 milligrams per day) is recommended to avoid disruptions in newborn sleep and mood from overstimulation. There is insufficient evidence to recommend against consumption of artificial sweeteners during lactation, although they do transfer into human milk at low levels. Consumption of alcohol was discussed earlier, in the "Nicotine, Alcohol, and Marijuana" section.

## Human Milk Expression and Storage

There are many reasons why lactating individuals might need or want to express their milk, such as separation from the infant, as is common with a return to work or school. Breast stimulation and milk removal can be achieved through use of a manual or electric breast pump or by hand expression. Expressed milk can then be provided to the neonate indirectly using bottles or other infant feeding methods (e.g., syringe, dropper, cup, or supplemental nursing system) or stored for later use. This section provides information and anticipatory guidance for the expression and collection, storage, and preparation of human milk.

### Breast Pumps

Many different types of breast pumps may be used for milk expression. The selection of a breast pump should be guided by the preferences and intended use of the lactating individual. Two basic categories of breast pumps are distinguished: manual (hand-operated) and electric. Manual pumps are the most affordable and easy to carry, but they may take more time and effort to empty the breast than is the case with electric pumps. Manual pumps are typically recommended for occasional use or situations where an electric breast pump may not be convenient or feasible.

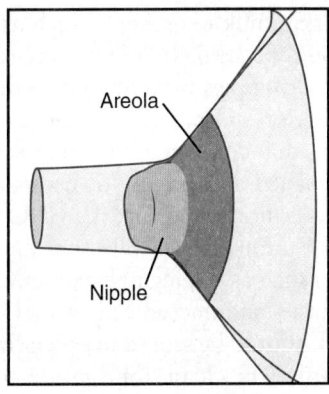
**Flange too small**

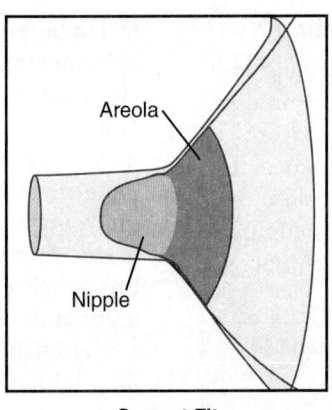
**Correct Fit**

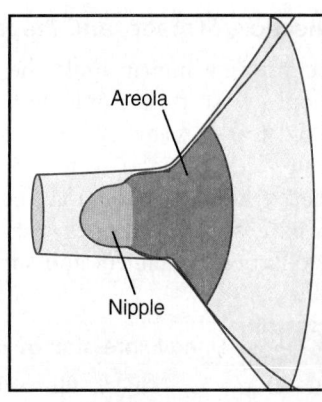
**Flange too large**

**Figure 37-5** Flange fit for a breast pump.

Electric pumps are often preferred for more frequent use or during longer periods of separation. These pumps are programmed to mimic infant suckling patterns and can generally express a greater volume of milk more quickly than a manual pump can. Double-electric breast pumps can also be used to express milk from both breasts simultaneously. However, personal electric pumps are more expensive, heavy, difficult to transport, and noisy compared to manual pumps, and they require a battery or access to an electrical outlet for use. Hospital-grade (multiuser) pumps are a type of electric pump that provides strong stimulation to increase supply; they are most commonly used in hospitals or rented for outpatient use in situations that pose challenges to lactation, such as separation from a premature newborn.

For lactating individuals planning to return to work or school away from their infant, it may be beneficial to start expressing milk for a few weeks prior that return, to gain familiarity with the process and accumulate a supply of expressed milk for infant feeding. To maintain an adequate supply over prolonged or recurrent separation, lactating individuals should plan to pump or express milk to match their child's feeding patterns and milk consumption (most commonly about every 3 hours). In accordance with federal law under the Fair Labor Standards Act, many employers are required to provide break time and a private space for employees to express milk for up to 1 year after birth.

When lactation complications arise with breast pump use, it may be useful for the healthcare provider or lactation specialist to observe a pumping session. This assessment can help to ensure that the breast pump flanges fit appropriately (Figure 37-5). A flange that is too small can compress the breast or rub against the nipple, leading to inadequate expression and nipple injury. Similarly, a flange that is too large will result in a weak seal and reduced milk flow. Accessories such as pumping bras or bands can be used to hold the flange in place and allow for hand use while pumping.

Electric pumps should be set to a vacuum level that optimizes milk yield without causing discomfort through excessive suctioning. For individuals who have difficulty achieving "let-down" (milk ejection reflex) with a pump, the use of warm compresses, breast and nipple stimulation, relaxation and imagery techniques, or audiovisual reminders of the infant may be helpful.[58] The duration of a pumping session depends on individual characteristics, but the breast should be fully emptied at the end of a session for optimal milk supply stimulation and to ensure the expressed milk has the maximum fat content. Breast massage or hand expression can be used to assist with thorough milk removal.

### Hand Expression

Milk may also be expressed by hand, without a pump. This method of milk expression is especially effective in the first few days after birth. It can also be used for antepartum colostrum collection, during lactation in combination with pumping, when a pump is not available, or when lactating individuals experience difficulty achieving let-down with a pump. Milk from hand expression can be collected in a variety of clean containers, such as a spoon, tube, funnel, or bowl; it can then be provided directly to the infant or transferred into a storage container for later use. Prior to hand expression, it may be helpful to stimulate the breasts through gentle massage. The steps for hand expression are described in Table 37-13. An organization with an online educational video on hand expression is provided in the Resources section at the end of the chapter.

## Milk Collection, Storage, and Preparation

Prior to expressing human milk, the lactating individual should wash their hands with soap and water to avoid transmission of bacteria or viruses to the neonate.[59] If soap and water are not available, alcohol-based hand sanitizer may be substituted.[60] Any milk expression accessories such as pump parts or milk collection containers and surfaces that will be contacted during milk expression (such as knobs or counters) should be cleaned. It is not necessary to clean the breasts or nipples prior to milk expression. Following completion of milk expression, any products or containers that contacted human milk should be thoroughly cleaned and dried. For neonates who are younger than 3 months of age, the CDC recommends daily sterilization of milk collection equipment through methods such as boiling or steam-cleaning in accordance with the manufacturer's instructions.

Human milk should be stored in specialized human milk containers or clean, food-grade containers. Research is ongoing about optimal container characteristics to maintain the beneficial properties of human milk and facilitate ease of use. Current evidence supports use of glass and polypropylene containers with tight-fitting lids over use of flexible polyethylene bags.[59] Plastic that contains bisphenol A (BPA) should be avoided due to the potential for endocrine disruption in the neonate. The ABM also recommends caution regarding plastic containing bisphenol S, a BPA alternative.[59]

A variety of factors—such as milk volume, temperature, and environmental stability—affect the safety of human milk storage. National guidelines differ slightly on temperatures for milk storage. According to the CDC guidelines, freshly expressed human milk can be safely stored up to 4 hours at room temperature, up to 4 days in the refrigerator, or for 6 to 12 months in the freezer (Table 37-14).[60] There is limited research about human milk kept cool by ice or cold packs in cooler containers, but it has been suggested to be safe for consumption if kept at a temperature lower than 15°C (60°F) for no more than 24 hours. Human milk should not be stored in the door of a refrigerator or freezer to avoid temperature fluctuations from the door opening and closing. Once thawed, human milk should not be refrozen. Storing human milk in small increments can reduce waste of thawed milk. It is recommended to cool freshly

| Table 37-13 | Hand Expression of Human Milk |
|---|---|
| **Technique** | **Illustration** |
| 1. Position the hand behind the areola while making a "C" shape with the thumb and fingers. | 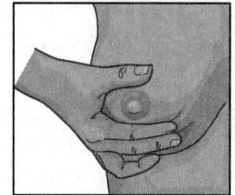 |
| 2. Press the fingers and thumb back toward the chest wall. | 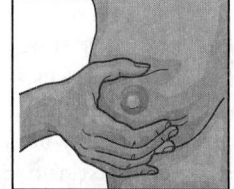 |
| 3. Compress the breast by rolling the fingers and thumb toward the nipple. | 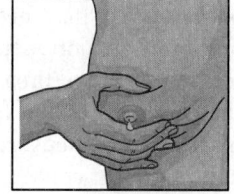 |
| 4. Release the compression to allow for milk expression. Repeat the process rhythmically, until desired or milk flow ceases. | 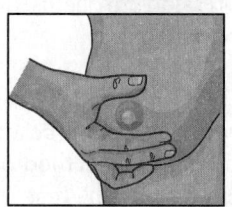 |

| Table 37-14 | Human Milk Storage Guidelines: Maximum Recommended Storage Duration | | |
|---|---|---|---|
| | **Storage Location and Temperature** | | |
| **Type of Human Milk** | **Room Temperature** 16–29°C (60–85°F) | **Refrigerator** 4°C (40°F) | **Freezer** < –4°C (25°F) |
| Freshly expressed | 4 hours | 4 days | 6 months (optimal) to 12 months (acceptable) |
| Thawed (previously frozen) | 2 hours | 1 day (24 hours) | Thawed human milk should never be refrozen. |

Data from Eglash A, Simon L. ABM Clinical Protocol #8: human milk storage information for home use for full-term infants, revised 2017. *Breastfeed Med.* 2017;12(7):390-395; Centers for Disease Control and Prevention. Proper storage and preparation of breast milk. https://www.cdc.gov/breastfeeding/recommendations/handling_breastmilk.htm. Accessed January 24, 2022.

expressed milk before adding it to a container with previously cooled or frozen milk to avoid warming or thawing the previously stored milk. It is useful to label the milk with the date of the expression so that the oldest acceptable milk can be used first.

Infants can be fed expressed human milk through a variety of methods, such as bottles and cups. For premature or young newborns, a dropper, syringe, or spoon may be used for this purpose. Human milk can also be provided through a feeding tube at the breast as part of a supplemental nursing system to provide supplementation while stimulating milk production. Freshly expressed human milk requires no preparation for infant feeding. Because milk quality degrades over time, freshly expressed milk should be provided instead of refrigerated or frozen milk when it is available.

Refrigerated or cooled human milk does not have to be warmed before feeding and may be served cold. However, some infants who are used to the lukewarm temperature of milk from the breast may prefer warmed milk. To warm human milk, the sealed milk storage container should be placed in a container of warm (not hot) water or held under a stream of warm running water for several minutes. To ensure the milk is not too hot for the infant, the person feeding the infant may check the temperature by putting a few drops on their wrist. Human milk should never be warmed directly on a stove or in a microwave to avoid overheating or unevenly heating the milk and decreasing the milk's protective properties.

Frozen milk must be thawed before use. Human milk can be thawed overnight in a refrigerator or using the technique for warming cooled milk. Thawed milk should be used within 24 hours and should never be refrozen (Table 37-14). Milk that was previously frozen and thawed should be left at room temperature for no more than 2 hours.

Regardless of whether human milk is freshly expressed, cooled, or frozen and thawed, bacterial contamination of partially consumed milk is a concern.[60] Once an infant has partially fed from human milk in a bottle or cup, bacteria from the infant's mouth will enter the milk. The CDC recommends using leftover milk from a partial feeding within 2 hours and disposing of any remaining milk after that time.

## Continuation or Cessation of Lactation

When to discontinue breastfeeding or human milk expression is a very individualized decision. There are no limits on the amount of time a dyad should breastfeed or a child should consume human milk.

Human milk continues to provide valuable nutrition and health benefits after complementary foods are introduced at about 6 months of age and into toddlerhood. In 2022, the AAP extended its recommendation for breastfeeding from 1 year to "as long as mutually desired . . . for 2 years or beyond,"[3] which aligns with WHO guidelines.

Infant feeding decisions, including breastfeeding or human milk feeding duration, are influenced by healthcare providers' attitudes and behaviors, and individuals who breastfeed beyond 1 year have reported feeling stigmatized by their providers.[61,62] Healthcare providers should examine their own potential biases toward extended breastfeeding duration, approach history taking regarding lactation and breastfeeding from a nonjudgmental perspective, and normalize longer-term lactation and breastfeeding with patients.[63]

Breastfeeding, lactation, and human milk expression can continue safely during a subsequent pregnancy.[64] Pregnant individuals who are breastfeeding or expressing milk may experience breast tenderness, nipple soreness, or a decrease in milk supply. When patients with lactational amenorrhea present with these concerns, pregnancy testing should be considered.[65] Individuals who wish to continue lactation into pregnancy should be provided with nutritional counseling about ways to meet the caloric demands of both pregnancy and lactation. Theoretical concerns that oxytocin from nipple stimulation with breastfeeding or milk expression could lead to increased rates of pregnancy loss or preterm labor has not been supported by the research.[65] Due to changes in the taste of human milk in pregnancy, some older children spontaneously wean from, decrease, or temporarily discontinue breastfeeding or human milk consumption. Near the end of pregnancy, milk composition transitions from mature milk to colostrum. The older child can continue breastfeeding or, when desired, resume in the postpartum period and feed "in tandem" with the newborn. When the parent is breastfeeding both a newborn and an older child, the newborn should be fed first at each feeding to ensure adequate milk intake.[66]

When a lactating individual or breastfeeding dyad decides to discontinue lactation or breastfeeding, gradual weaning is recommended to avoid breast engorgement. If abrupt cessation of lactation is required, interventions such as application of cold compresses to the breast, wearing of a tight-fitting bra to reduce breast stimulation, minimal milk expression (typically hand expression) to decrease discomfort without triggering excess milk production, and oral analgesics can minimize discomfort.

Children naturally wean themselves at different ages, gradually showing less interest in breastfeeding and more interest in solid foods.[67] Occasionally, a lactating individual who wishes to continue may find that a child is suddenly uninterested in breastfeeding (commonly referred to as a "nursing strike"); this behavior is most likely temporary. When the lactating person decides to wean but the child remains interested in breastfeeding, strategies such as decreasing the frequency and duration of breastfeeding sessions, avoiding common breastfeeding situational triggers, and offering alternative bonding activities may be helpful. Breastfeeding support groups or lactation specialists can be valuable resources to help lactating parents deal with these situations and other common challenges of breastfeeding and weaning.

## Human Milk Substitutes

In countries with safe water supplies and intact infrastructure, safe human milk substitutes are available for parents who opt not to or cannot provide human milk to their infants. While breastfeeding/chestfeeding and reliance on human milk should be encouraged, substitutes are also available that can provide adequate nutrition and fluids for infant growth and development. (In this section, the term *human or breast milk substitute* is used interchangeably with *infant formula*.) WHO and UNICEF have long-standing guidelines surrounding marketing of these substitutes and provide guidance to birth facilities for methods to support provision of human milk. However, some parents need to or prefer to feed their infant with a human milk substitute, and midwives should support those parents, without passing judgment on their feeding decisions.

In selecting a human milk substitute, parents should be instructed to only use products that have been approved as infant nutrition by a national organization, such as the Food and Drug Administration (FDA) in the United States and Health Canada in Canada. In addition, they should use the products as directed on the label. Over and under dilution can lead to nutritional and electrolyte imbalances. Nonprocessed animal milks (such as pure cow milk or goat milk) are not appropriate human milk substitutes as they do not contain all needed nutrients. Unpasteurized (raw) animal milks can expose infants to dangerous microbes.

Human milk substitutes include a protein base, lipids, a carbohydrate source, and additional vitamins and nutrients such as iron, vitamin K, calcium, magnesium, and phosphorus.[68] Infant formula should be produced in commercial factories that meet strict standards for the content of the milk and the cleanliness of the facility.[69] Three main base proteins are used to produce formulas: cow milk protein, soy, and protein hydrolysate (Table 37-15).[68]

Cow milk–based infant formulas with iron are the ideal starting formula for healthy, term infants. These formulas are usually well tolerated and carry a lower cost than soy-based or protein hydrolysate formulations. Specialized cow milk–based formulas are available for infants with special needs. For example, lactose-free formula can be used if an infant is suspected of having an allergy to lactose, and anti-reflux formulas are available; infants need a comprehensive assessment to rule out health conditions prior to use of these formulas.

Soy milk–based formulas should be selected for infants with galactosemia or congenital lactose intolerance. This type of human milk substitute can also be used during and for a brief time after

| Table 37-15 | **Major Types of Human Milk Substitutes** | | |
|---|---|---|---|
| **Type of Human Milk Substitute** | **Protein Source** | **Carbohydrate** | **Considerations** |
| Cow milk–based | Casein and whey proteins derived from cow milk | Lactose | Appropriate selection for most infants |
| Soy-based | Soy | Corn-based | Appropriate for infants with congenital lactose deficiency and galactosemia |
| | | | More expensive than cow milk–based products |
| Protein hydrolysate | Extensively hydrolyzed proteins derived from cow milk | Corn or sucrose-based | Appropriate for infants with cow milk protein or other allergy |
| | | | More expensive than cow milk–based or soy-based milks |

a diarrheal illness in infants older than 2 months. Soy-based infant formulas are popular, despite lack of pediatric recommendations for their use and their increased cost compared to cow milk–based formulas. Research has not supported the contention that they improve colic or fussiness better than parent/caregiver counseling on measures to console infants. Soy-based formulas are often promoted as being vegan for families where this is an important consideration; however, soy-based formulas do use lanolin for their vitamin D source.

Protein hydrolysate formulas are made with extensively hydrolyzed proteins that are smaller and easier to digest than unhydrolyzed cow milk or soy proteins. These products are more expensive than the other types of formulas, so they are usually reserved for infants who do not tolerate other, more common formulas due to allergies or underlying medical conditions.

Many infant formula brands advertise the addition or removal of various ingredients; however, these changes are not always supported by evidence and may be associated with additional cost. Regardless of which protein is used as the base for the product, iron should be included in the infant formula. The standard amount of iron in infant formula is 12 mg/dL. While low-iron formulations are available at retail stores, the vast majority of infants need the standard amount of iron to avoid iron-deficiency anemia. Docosahexaenoic acid or arachidonic acid (a fatty acid) may be added to some brands, but per a Cochrane review, there is not enough evidence to support inclusion of these supplements in infant formula as a way to improve infant health.[70]

Most infant formulas provide 20 calories per ounce, similar to human milk. However, some versions intended for use by preterm infants provide more calories, calcium, and phosphorus per ounce. "Preterm" formula has 24 calories per ounce, is distributed only in ready-to-feed bottles, and is not usually found in stores; this formulation is used only until the infant reaches approximately 4 pounds or 34 weeks' gestation. "Enriched" formula that contains 22 calories per ounce is used for infants born preterm and can be purchased in retail stores. There is no set weight or gestational age for when infants using an enriched formula should switch to regular infant formula, and studies have not found these formulations improve long-term growth and development.

### Selection of a Human Milk Substitute

In general, healthy, term infants who need a human milk substitute should be given a standard, FDA-approved, cow milk–based infant formula with

iron.[68] Major retail stores use the state-level Special Supplemental Nutrition Program for Women, Infants, and Children (WIC) selections to decide which infant formulas will be made available in those stores. Initial selection of a formula from the state's WIC list can decrease the need for a family to change infant formulas later for access reasons. While it is ideal to use the same brand and type of infant formula over time to decrease gastrointestinal changes and infant taste-based refusal, families may safely switch brands of infant formula if needed.

### Forms of Approved Infant Formulas

There are three main concentrations of infant formula that remain shelf stable without refrigeration until opened. Any concentration is acceptable, and parents can switch between types without the infant having any problems. The decision of which form to use is up to the parent; the availability of safe water, cost, and access to refrigeration are important considerations.

The process used to reconstitute the infant formula should follow the guidelines printed on the package. These ratios are mostly standardized (as shown in Table 37-16), but not all brands around the world use this standard. Too much water or too much concentrate can cause electrolyte disturbances and major health problems. Newborns do not need any additional water beyond that used in reconstitution.

Ready-to-feed formula does not require dilution with safe water. Once the package is opened, it will need refrigeration, and the opened product should be used in a timely manner as directed on the package, usually within 24 hours. Concentrated formula requires reconstitution in a 1:1 ratio with safe water. Once the container is opened, it needs to be refrigerated and used within the time frame noted on the package. Powdered infant formula,

| Table 37-16 | Forms of Infant Formula | |
|---|---|---|
| Concentration | Reconstitution | Comments |
| Ready-to-feed | None needed | Most expensive; Does not require water |
| Concentrated | 1 part concentrate to 1 part water | Requires a safe water source |
| Powdered | 1 level scoop to 2 oz or 60 mL of water | Least expensive; Requires a safe water source |

once opened, can remain at room temperature for about 1 month. Powdered formula is the least expensive of the concentrations but requires a larger volume of safe water.

### Water Source

Only water that is free from dangerous microbes and contaminants should be used for reconstitution of concentrated and powdered human milk substitutes.[71] It can be difficult for individuals to know if the water and sewer infrastructure is sufficient to ensure water safety, and water testing can be expensive. The local health department or utility system can provide information on the safety of the municipal water supply.[71]

Municipal water supplies are usually tested for microbial contamination and lead, and are safe for consumption by infants with functioning immune systems. However, in some geographic locations the municipal water is not safe to drink, and local water supplies can be temporarily contaminated with either microbes or chemical contaminants. Boiling water can kill microbes, but does not decrease the presence of contaminants such as lead or chemicals. In areas where the water supply is not safe, families can obtain water from someone they know with a safe water source or purchase water. Both bottled and distilled water are acceptable for reconstitution of infant formula. Bottled water is often packaged municipal tap water. Distilled water is created through boiling of water and collecting the condensation; it is more expensive than bottled water.

About one in six households in the United States uses a well for their water supply.[71] Wells on private property may have little to no required testing. Wells can be contaminated by microorganisms or chemical pollutants. Fecal contamination is the most common source of microbial contamination and can cause severe illness in newborns and infants.[71] Common chemical well contaminants include volatile organic compounds and pesticides, which are found in about one-third of tested wells. High levels of nitrites in well water can cause infants to develop methemoglobinemia (MetHb), a life-threatening blood disorder.[71] Well water should be tested for nitrites and coliform bacteria prior to using it to reconstitute a human milk substitute. If the parents or caregiver are unable to get their water tested, they should use water from a safe source for all infant feeding needs.

Even when the source of water is known to be safe, the pipes of houses can contain lead that leaches into water. Lead in household and municipal pipes occurs more often in housing built before 1986. Local utility companies may be able to test household water for lead. Some strategies for decreasing the amount of lead in water used for infant feeding include using only cold water from the pipes and running the water for several minutes prior to using the water for consumption.

### Items for Bottle-Feeding

Most infants are fed human milk substitutes in specially designed infant feeding bottles, although cup feeding and spoon feeding are also possible. A variety of styles of bottles and nipples are available. None is superior to the others, though infants may have preferences for one type or shape over another. Nipples have different sizes of openings that affect the flow; preterm and newborn sizes are appropriate starting sizes for newborns. Special nipples are offered for newborns with oral and facial differences, and these infants can benefit from being evaluated by a feeding specialist soon after birth. Bottles also come in several different shapes and sizes; smaller sizes can be easier to use with newborns. Some plastic bottles may contain bisphenol A (BPA) and should be avoided; bottles that are clear plastic, made from polycarbonate, or have the recycling number 7 are more likely to contain BPA.

Bottles and nipples should be washed and rinsed thoroughly before the first use and after each use. Bottles and nipples can be placed in the dishwasher if they do not contain BPA. Sterilization of nipples and bottles is not needed for infants with functioning immune systems.[72] Before each use, nipples should be inspected to ensure they are without tears or debris.

### Recommendations for Bottle-Feeding

Parents should use the same infant hunger cues for beginning bottle-feeding as for beginning breastfeeding/chestfeeding. Infants can be held in a variety of positions for bottle-feeding. The infant should be held throughout the feeding and benefits from interaction with the person feeding them. This moment provides time for developmentally appropriate interactions similar to those that occur with breastfeeding. Bottle-propping does not promote this type of development and creates choking risks.

The nipple can be introduced gently into the infant's mouth when open or slightly open and gently held there as the infant begins to taste and suck. The newborn will have an easier time drinking if their head is a neutral position or slightly extended. Keeping the infant's head slightly higher than their body can be beneficial. Healthy newborns receiving their first feeding from a bottle usually accept the appropriate-sized nipple without problem and rarely struggle to suck and swallow the human milk substitute. If the infant chokes, gags, or turns away, feeding should paused, with the nipple being pulled back or out of the mouth and the infant's position adjusted to be more upright. Feeding can resume when the infant shows signs of readiness. Some infants benefit from burping, but not all infants swallow air during feeding.

Infants should be allowed time to consume the infant formula; most feedings are completed within 20 minutes. While newborns usually drink 2 to 3 ounces (60 to 90 mL) per feeding and feed every 2 to 3 hours, feedings should be sensitive to the infant and the caregiver should not require a well infant to consume a predetermined amount of formula at a feeding. Formula remaining in a bottle after a feeding should be discarded. Infants should not be put to sleep with a bottle to prevent later tooth decay.

Some individuals or families may choose to do a combination feeding method, both breastfeeding and providing expressed milk or human milk substitutes. If this feeding approach is desired, it is best to wait until lactation has been established to introduce an artificial nipple. Infants who have experience feeding at the breast may have expectations for how feeding occurs. For these infants, strategies to improve acceptance of an artificial nipple have been suggested, but no singular evidence-based approach is recommended, as each infant is unique. Strategies that may be helpful include having someone other than the lactating parent introduce a bottle when the infant is showing early hunger cues. Placing the infant in an upright, outward-facing position (not facing the chest as with breastfeeding) can also improve acceptance. A nipple with a wide base may be more acceptable to the infant as it may mimic sensations of feeding at the breast.

### Elimination Patterns for Infants Who Receive Human Milk Substitutes

Urination patterns for newborns who are exclusively fed human milk substitutes should meet or exceed the amounts of voids and stools for human milk–fed infants. The timing and consistency of stools is different between infants fed exclusively human milk and those receiving human milk substitutes, in part because of differences in the intestinal microbiome. Supplementation or change to infant formula cause a gradual change in the frequency of stools. Stools occur 1 to 8 times a day in the first week and then decrease to 4 or fewer times per day until around 8 weeks of age.[72] Stools of infants receiving infant formula are usually yellow or green in color and thicker than stools of infants receiving

only human milk; they also have a stronger and less sweet odor. Constipation is more common in infants fed human milk substitutes than those receiving only human milk.

## Diverse Human Milk Feeding Situations

Midwives may care for patients in diverse human milk feeding situations such as induced lactation, human milk sharing, and lactation in transgender and nonbinary persons. Midwives should be prepared to provide appropriate counseling and anticipatory guidance to support diverse individuals and families in meeting their infant feeding goals. Consultation with lactation consultants or specialists may also be appropriate.

### Induced Lactation

*Induced lactation* is the process of stimulating milk production in an individual who has not recently been pregnant or is not currently lactating, such as nongestational parents, same-sex partners, or transgender women. The quantify of human milk produced following induced lactation is typically not sufficient to adequately meet neonatal nutritional needs but may be combined with other infant feeding methods including supplemental feeding at the breast.[73] Research about best practices for inducing lactation, including lactation in transgender women, is ongoing.[74] Often, it involves a combination of pharmacologic and nonpharmacologic interventions including hormone therapy, galactagogues, and breast and nipple stimulation over a period of several months.[73,75,76] Similar interventions may be useful to facilitate relactation—that is, stimulation of milk production in an individual who previously lactated and recently stopped.

### Human Milk Sharing

The provision of human milk from sources other than the gestational and lactating parent is called *milk sharing*. Milk sharing is a growing and somewhat controversial practice.[77] Most frequently, milk sharing occurs when individuals or families cannot produce or access sufficient human milk for their child and so use pasteurized *donor milk* from human milk banks, Internet- or community-based milk-sharing networks, or a known milk donor. It also includes alloparental situations such as *co-lactation* or cross-nursing ("wet nursing") with known individuals such as a lactating co-parent, family member, or caregiver, a practice that is normative in some cultures and communities.[77]

The use of donor milk that has been screened and pasteurized is not controversial and is supported by the AAP for use in neonatal intensive care units and other settings.[78] Comprehensively screened and pasteurized donor milk may be obtained safely from nonprofit milk banks such as those accredited by the Human Milk Banking Association of North America in the United States and Canada. Additional information about accredited human milk banks is provided in the Resources section at the end of the chapter.

In addition, Internet- and community-based networks exist to support informal milk sharing between donors and recipients. Informal sharing of milk is controversial, given its potential benefits and risks due to the lack of screening and oversight. The U.S. FDA and the AAP discourage community- and Internet-based human milk sharing based on the potential for milk contamination and spread of illness from inadequate or unsafe milk screening, collection, and storage practices.[78,79] The ABM takes a more nuanced position on milk sharing, advocating against Internet-based milk-sharing networks or use of milk from an anonymous donor, but recognizing that individual circumstances around community-based milk sharing vary widely and are best determined by the donor and parent or caregiver of the milk recipient. The ABM position statement, *Informal Breast Milk Sharing for the Term Health Infant*, encourages healthcare providers to help individuals or families considering informal milk sharing evaluate the potential risks and benefits and make informed choices for their individual situation; it also provides guidance for clinicians regarding medical screening of potential milk donors and safe milk handling practices.[80]

### Transgender and Nonbinary Individuals

Transgender and nonbinary individuals may experience unique challenges in lactation related to body or gender dysphoria and social and structural barriers due to discrimination and stigmatization.[76,81] Complications may also arise from gender-affirming therapies or interventions. For example, hormonal therapy can affect breast tissue development and human milk production, and individuals who chestbind or underwent surgical procedures to the breasts (commonly referred to as "top surgery") may experience difficulty achieving an effective latch or producing an adequate supply to meet the infant's nutritional needs.[1] Transmen or gender-nonbinary individuals who are lactating and wish to resume testosterone therapy or chest-binding following pregnancy should be made aware of the suppressive effect of these interventions on milk production. Transwomen who underwent augmentation mammoplasty and wish to breastfeed or express milk may wish to consider induced lactation (discussed earlier). Individualized counseling is necessary for gender-diverse individuals to guide informed choices that support optimal neonatal, parental, and familial health.

## Assessment and Management of Common Lactation Concerns

Approximately 60% of lactating individuals report not being able to reach their infant feeding goals, with many stopping breastfeeding or human milk expression due to complications associated with lactation and breastfeeding.[82] Midwives play an important role in helping lactating individuals overcome these challenges, preventing further complications in lactation and breastfeeding, reducing barriers (especially among historically disadvantaged or vulnerable populations), and protecting overall health. This section reviews midwifery care for assessment and management of the most common lactation-related concerns.

### Psychosocial Concerns

Many lactating individuals fail to meet their goals for lactation and breastfeeding due to psychosocial concerns. Anxiety, depression, mood disorders, and other mental health concerns in lactating persons should be addressed comprehensively, as with any nonlactating individual; appropriate treatment should not be withheld due to lactation status. The unique hormonal shifts associated with lactation or stress of infant feeding can affect maternal mental health. For example, approximately 9% of lactating individuals experience dysphoric milk ejection reflex (D-MER), an abrupt dysphoria that occurs with the milk ejection reflex ("let-down") and spontaneously resolves within a few minutes.[83] Assessment and management of postpartum mood and anxiety disorders are discussed in greater detail in the *Postpartum Complications* chapter. The focus of this section is on widespread psychosocial concerns that affect lactating and breastfeeding cessation—namely, low self-efficacy and a lack of social and/or workplace support.

Low lactation/breastfeeding self-efficacy is one of the most common challenges in lactation and breastfeeding initiation. Many lactating individuals lack confidence in their ability to breastfeed or produce human milk that is adequate in quantity or quality for their newborn. This perceived insufficient milk supply is widely acknowledged as the major reason for early lactation and breastfeeding cessation and is strongly correlated with low breastfeeding self-efficacy.[84,85] Lactating individuals with low self-efficacy may interpret normal newborn or infant fussiness, feeding frequency, or ease of achieving an effective comfortable latch as a "failure" of their ability to lactate/breastfeed successfully and an indication for supplementation. When the infant receives supplementation, this reduces breast stimulation and milk removal and, correspondingly, decreases milk synthesis, thereby creating a self-fulfilling prophecy.[84] Increased anxiety or stress can also impair the milk ejection reflex and increase perception of breastfeeding-related pain, reinforcing negative breastfeeding experiences. Lactation-related stress may also stem from a lack of social and/or workplace support, often conflated with fatigue or feelings of inconvenience, which are significant factors in lactation and breastfeeding discontinuation.[86] Conversely, high breastfeeding self-efficacy and levels of support are positively correlated with increased breastfeeding duration.

Healthcare provider support for lactation and breastfeeding has been shown to positively affect breastfeeding outcomes.[87] Psychosocial concerns can be assessed and addressed at numerous points along the care continuum, from preconception through postpartum and beyond, in the primary care of lactating persons. Providing education and anticipatory guidance about breastfeeding and human milk feeding and ongoing lactation support can help to alleviate psychosocial concerns. Lactating persons should be encouraged to increase physical contact (especially skin-to-skin) and bonding activities with their infant. They should also be urged to focus on recognizing, differentiating, and responding to infant cues, so that not every cry is interpreted as hunger. Lactation support groups and peer counselors can be especially beneficial in supporting individuals through these challenges, boosting self-efficacy, and normalizing the lactation/breastfeeding experience. Workplace interventions such as a dedicated space for milk expression, supported breaks, and organizational policies supportive of breastfeeding and milk expression have been shown to positively affect duration of human milk feeding and self-efficacy in attaining infant feeding goals.[88,89] Policy and community-based interventions may be especially beneficial for populations with lactation and breastfeeding health disparities.[90,91]

When exclusive or continued breastfeeding or human milk feeding is exacerbating psychosocial issues or causing undue stress to the lactating person, providers should be open to a discussion that explores their infant feeding goals and possible alternatives to meet the newborn's nutritional needs without negatively affecting parental self-efficacy. For example, individuals who are exclusively breastfeeding may wish to start expressing their milk so that someone else can take over a few feedings. A combination feeding approach incorporating both a human milk substitute and breastfeeding or human milk feeding may also be appropriate in some circumstances. Some individuals may decide to discontinue lactation or breastfeeding, and they should be reassured that breastfeeding or providing human milk for their infant is just one of the many ways they can support their child's overall health and well-being. Healthcare providers should be sure to approach psychosocial concerns from a place of cultural humility and person-centered care. Lactating individuals should never be made to feel guilty for their infant feeding choices or prioritization of their own needs and values over breastfeeding initiation, exclusivity, or duration.

### Impaired Lactation

Human milk synthesis is the result of a complex interplay of numerous internal and external factors. The physiologic process of lactation is regulated by several hormones and feedback pathways, as outlined in the *Anatomy and Physiology of Postpartum* chapter. Most lactating individuals are able to produce adequate human milk to meet infant feeding requirements, but approximately 1 in 20 will experience impaired lactation.[28] The two most common forms of impaired lactation are delayed lactogenesis and low milk supply. Of note, negative terms such as "failed lactogenesis" or "insufficient" or "inadequate" milk supply may be found in the literature. Such terminology does not reflect positive and respectful communication[92] and can be disempowering, leading to negative effects on parental self-efficacy, relationship with the infant, and lactation/breastfeeding duration.[9]

At onset of lactation/breastfeeding, impaired lactation may stem from underlying anatomic or physiologic factors that result in delayed onset of lactogenesis II. Lactogenesis is triggered by a rapid drop in progesterone levels following placental expulsion and is maintained by the presence of elevated prolactin levels. A delay in lactogenesis is associated with increased supplementation with human milk substitutes and shorter breastfeeding duration.[93] The clinical definition of *delayed lactogenesis* is the

| Table 37-17 | Risk Factors for Impaired Lactation |
|---|---|
| **Category** | **Risk Factors** |
| Hormonal factors (preglandular) | Thyroid dysfunction |
| | Diabetes mellitus |
| | Obesity |
| | Polycystic ovary syndrome |
| | Retained placental fragments |
| | Postpartum pituitary necrosis |
| | Ovarian theca lutein cysts |
| | Pregnancy |
| Anatomic factors (glandular) | Breast surgery |
| | Mammary hypoplasia |
| External factors (postglandular) | Adverse effects of medication |
| | Tobacco use |
| | Insufficient milk removal |
| | Cesarean birth |
| | Preterm birth |

Data from Farah E, Barger MK, Klima C, et al. Impaired lactation: review of delayed lactogenesis and insufficient lactation. *J Midwifery Womens Health*. 2021;66:631-640. doi:10.1111/jmwh.13274; Hurst NM. Recognizing and treating delayed or failed lactogenesis II. *J Midwifery Womens Health*. 2007;52(6):588-594; Walker M. *Breastfeeding Management for the Clinician: Using the Evidence*. 4th ed. Burlington, MA: Jones & Bartlett Learning; 2016.

lack of a transition from colostrum to mature milk and a concurrent increase in human milk production within 72 hours after birth. However, research has shown that variations in normal human physiologic lactogenesis actually extend beyond that time, with 20% of all lactating persons and 44% of primiparous individuals meeting the criteria for delayed lactogenesis using this clinical definition.[28]

When lactogenesis is delayed beyond the normal time frame, many potential underlying causes may be involved. These include underlying physiologic or hormonal (preglandular) factors such as endocrine dysfunction or ovarian theca lutein cysts, anatomic (glandular) factors such as insufficient glandular tissue or complications from breast surgery, and external (postglandular) factors such as side effects from medication or neonatal factors (Table 37-17).[94]

Once lactation and breastfeeding have been established, some individuals experience impaired lactation as a low milk supply despite sufficient stimulation and drainage of the breasts. Low milk supply may be caused by complications affecting milk production (as discussed earlier) but is more commonly caused by infrequent or incomplete milk removal or an increase in infant demand (such as with a growth spurt). In the absence of internal factors, milk production is governed by milk removal. When the breast is full, a complex interplay between serotonin and possibly other bioactive factors (previously termed feedback inhibitors of lactation) inhibits mammary function and slows milk production.[95] When the breast is empty, milk is produced more quickly and in greater quantities. Therefore, although optimal management of impaired lactation depends on the specific cause, increased breast stimulation with thorough and frequent emptying of the breast is often useful to stimulate milk synthesis. If low milk supply persists despite frequent and thorough milk removal, use of herbal or pharmacologic treatments (galactagogues) to increase supply may be considered using a shared decision-making approach; however, such treatments should not be used routinely due to a lack of research supporting their efficacy and safety.

Impaired lactation cannot be determined based on the presence of risk factors or physical examination. Diagnosis can be made only through an assessment of milk production and associated markers such as neonatal satiety and growth. A detailed history and observation of breastfeeding or milk expression session are useful to identify potential causal factors. Close assessment for adequate neonatal hydration and weight gain is important, and supplementation may be necessary.

### Hyperlactation

Once breastfeeding is established after an initial period of engorgement from 1 to 2 weeks postpartum, milk production is typically regulated by milk removal to align with the needs of the healthy, growing infant. Occasionally, milk supply exceeds the quantity required for infant demand, based on international standards of normal infant nutritional needs. This overproduction of milk is termed *hyperlactation* or hypergalactia, or colloquially, "oversupply."

Homeostasis in human milk synthesis is regulated by four key factors: (1) the amount of mammary glandular tissue, (2) the extent of alveolar distension, (3) the frequency and extent of milk removal, and (4) complex neuroendocrine pathways.[95] Hyperlactation results from dysregulation of one of these factors, most commonly overstimulation of the breasts, such as when an individual is both regularly expressing milk and fully breastfeeding. Historically, hyperlactation was thought to be caused by pathologic conditions associated with hyperprolactinemia such as pituitary adenomas and prolactinomas. However, recent evidence has not supported this association, and laboratory testing and pituitary imaging tests for hyperlactation are no longer recommended.[95]

Clinical symptoms of hyperlactation are present in both the lactating person and the infant. In the lactating individual, signs and symptoms include overfull and/or leaking breasts, breast pain, persistent breast engorgement, recurrent plugged ducts or mastitis, and a forceful milk ejection reflex, potentially causing the infant to bite the nipple, gag, cough, or choke at the breast.[95,96] The infant may present with excessive infant weight gain, difficulty with sustained latch, breast refusal, and gastrointestinal symptoms such as reflux and large, frothy, green stools.[95,96] Lactating individuals experiencing hyperlactation are at increased risk for plugged ducts, mastitis, and early cessation of breastfeeding due to pain and difficulty with infant latch.

Management for hyperlactation focuses on breastfeeding or milk expression interventions to reduce breast stimulation and milk synthesis, such as single-sided or "block" feedings (removing milk from only breast per session), laid-back or side-lying positioning (to minimize gravitational effects), and limiting milk expression (to avoid triggering milk synthesis).[95,96] These interventions may be used in conjunction with cold compresses and/or herbal or pharmacologic treatments to suppress milk production (Table 37-18). Pharmacologic treatments should be reserved for situations in which nonpharmacologic approaches have not been sufficiently effective.

### Engorgement

*Engorgement* describes breast fullness and firmness that is associated with pain or discomfort in lactation. It is typically bilateral and is not accompanied by systemic symptoms such as fever or myalgia. Primary engorgement occurs at the onset of lactogenesis II as the result of a combination of interstitial edema and hyperemia. Generally, onset of primary engorgement is 3 to 5 days postpartum, with spontaneous resolution within 48 hours. Secondary engorgement can occur at any time during lactation that milk is not emptied in sufficient quantity or with sufficient frequency from the breast. Secondary engorgement requires intervention to restore homeostasis of milk production, as discussed in the "Hyperlactation" section, to avoid progression to inflammatory mastitis or acute bacterial mastitis (discussed later in this section).

| Table 37-18 | Herbal and Pharmacologic Treatments to Reduce Milk Supply |
|---|---|
| **Pharmaceuticals** | |
| Pseudoephedrine | |
| Estrogen | |
| **Herbs** | |
| Sage | |
| Peppermint | |
| Chasteberry | |
| Jasmine | |

Data from Johnson HM, Eglash A, Mitchell KB, et al. ABM Clinical Protocol #32: management of hyperlactation. *Breastfeeding Med.* 2020;15(3):129-134.

The goals of treatment for primary engorgement are to facilitate infant latch and decrease maternal discomfort. Recommendations for breastfeeding individuals include more frequent and effective breastfeeding, avoidance of excess breast stimulation, minimal hand expression for relief, avoidance of pumping, reverse-pressure softening (i.e., applying gentle pressure to edematous tissue) to facilitate latch, and cold compresses and acetaminophen or ibuprofen for reduction of pain and inflammation.[97] There is insufficient evidence to support complementary and alternative therapies for treatment of engorgement such as herbal compresses, gua sha (breast massage or scraping therapy), or acupuncture.[98] Historically, application of cold cabbage leaves was recommended; however, research has found that cabbage leaves have no additional benefit over cold packs and pose a potential risk for transmission of *Listeria* bacteria.[97]

### Ductal Narrowing and Nipple Blebs

*Ductal narrowing* is the inflammation and narrowing of the milk ducts resulting from focal milk stasis. This condition is commonly referred to as having a "plugged duct"; however, this term is somewhat misleading, as the physiologic and anatomic characteristics of milk ducts make it impossible for only a single duct to be obstructed. Ductal narrowing presents as a focused area of induration or congested breast tissue that is often palpable and tender. Mild erythema may be present, but systemic symptoms such as fever or malaise (characteristic of mastitis) are absent. Along with restriction of milk flow in the ducts, obstruction may occur in the nipple pore ducts. This presents as a white bleb on the nipple, commonly referred to as a "milk blister."

Both ductal narrowing and nipple blebs often resolve spontaneously within 48 hours. When interventions are necessary, treatment focuses on relieving the obstruction and restoring milk flow. In addition to more frequent and effective breastfeeding or milk expression, application of heat or warm water soaks and gentle, focused massage behind the area of obstruction may be used to relieve congestion. Aggressive massage or squeezing may result in trauma and should be avoided. For nipple blebs, olive oil may be applied to the nipple to soften the tissue and remove the obstruction.[99] When these techniques are unsuccessful, a sterile needle may be used to open the pore and facilitate drainage.

### Galactoceles

If unresolved, ductal narrowing can result in an obstructed milk flow that collects and forms a milk retention cyst known as a *galactocele*. Galactoceles present as firm breast masses of fluctuating size, ranging from 1 to 10 cm or larger. Their size varies based on the time of day, duration since onset, and proximity in time to breastfeeding or milk expression.[97] Galactoceles may be tender but are not associated with erythema, severe pain, or systemic symptoms such as fever or malaise. They are more commonly experienced during the weaning phase of breastfeeding or human milk feeding. Diagnosis is made by ultrasound imaging and may be confirmed by aspiration. Based on severity of symptoms, galactoceles may be managed with surgical excision and/or drainage.

### Mastitis

The term *mastitis* refers to inflammation of the mammary gland and encompasses a spectrum of clinical conditions ranging from subacute inflammation to severe infection.[97] Lactational mastitis results from hyperlactation and/or milk dysbiosis (disruption of the milk microbiome) that progresses to ductal narrowing and stromal breast edema and then to inflammatory mastitis. If unresolved, this condition may worsen to become acute bacterial mastitis, a breast abscess, or, in rare cases, septicemia. Mastitis occurs in as many as 1 in 5 lactating individuals, with the highest incidence in the first 4 weeks postpartum.[100] Risk factors for mastitis include hyperlactation, nipple trauma, and the presence of other

difficulties in lactation and/or breastfeeding.[100] Although milk stasis is commonly thought to be the cause of mastitis, this relationship has not been proven, and research into dysbiosis is evolving.[97]

*Inflammatory mastitis* is characterized by two key clinical symptoms: (1) localized inflammation of the breast associated with pain, erythema, and warmth; and (2) fever and/or other systemic symptoms such as tachycardia, myalgia, chills, and malaise. Prompt recognition and intervention are critical to halt worsening progression to more complicated clinical conditions in the mastitis spectrum. If the condition persists longer than 24 hours or progresses in severity, bacterial mastitis can develop.

*Bacterial mastitis* is characterized by moderate to severe erythema and induration, which can spread to other quadrants of the breast. Systemic symptoms may also increase in severity, and axillary lymphadenopathy may be present. In severe cases, the lactating person may develop *phlegmons*, acute areas of inflammation and firm but fluctuating complex fluid collections in the breast tissue.[97] As symptoms progress, these collections may become infected and form a lactational *abscess*, which presents as a palpable collection of fluid (pus) in a localized area of the breast marked by severe induration, erythema, and tenderness. By the time mastitis reaches the breast abscess stage, the body may have isolated the infectious process, resulting in resolution of systemic symptoms (though they may recur).

Due to the wide spectrum of conditions encompassed by the diagnosis of mastitis, there are no widely accepted clinical criteria for diagnosis or initiation of treatment. Diagnosis is made based on the clinical presentation, and appropriate management depends on the severity and duration of symptoms. Routine laboratory testing including human milk culture is not recommended. In severe cases, ultrasound imaging may be used to aid diagnosis and management of a breast abscess. Table 37-19 presents conditions along the mastitis spectrum to guide differential diagnosis and treatment decisions.

Conservative and supportive measure are often all that are necessary to treat mastitis when it is recognized in early stages. Unless symptoms are severe or persistent, initial management of inflammatory mastitis focuses on breastfeeding or expressing milk on demand and comfort measures to reduce pain and edema. If direct infant breastfeeding is possible, milk expression (including breast pump use) and thorough emptying of the breasts are discouraged, as this may overstimulate the breast. Psychosocial support, such as increased opportunities for rest and

| Table 37-19 | Mastitis Spectrum: Differential Diagnoses | | |
|---|---|---|---|
| Condition | Breast Symptoms | Systemic Symptoms (e.g., fever, chills, myalgia, tachycardia) | Management |
| Engorgement | Breast fullness, edema, and pain, typically bilateral | Absent | Comfort measures Cold compresses |
| Ductal narrowing ("plugged ducts") | Focal area of breast induration or congested breast tissue, may have mild erythema | Absent | Milk removal Gentle massage Heat application |
| Galactocele | Firm, fluctuant breast mass following ductal narrowing; most common during weaning | Absent | Consultation for surgical management |
| Inflammatory mastitis | Focal area of breast edema, erythema, and pain | Present | Feeding on demand Comfort measures Patient self-management |
| Bacterial mastitis | Moderate to severe breast erythema and induration | Present > 24 hours | Antibiotic therapy |
| Breast abscess | Moderate to severe breast erythema and induration with a palpable, fluctuant breast mass | Absent or present | Consultation for surgical management |

stress reduction, is also useful to facilitate resolution of symptoms.[97] Therapeutic ultrasound may be performed to reduce inflammation and relieve edema. There are mixed findings regarding the role of probiotics in preventing or treating inflammatory mastitis, and research in this area is ongoing.

Providers should be cautious so that they do not overtreat inflammatory mastitis. Antibiotics are not recommended for inflammatory mastitis as they can increase dysbiosis, risk for bacterial mastitis, and antibiotic resistance. If the initial measures do not resolve symptoms within 24 hours or if symptoms worsen, evaluation by the midwife or another healthcare provider is recommended.

Once mastitis has progressed to the bacterial mastitis phase, antibiotics are recommended for treatment. *Staphylococcus* and *Streptococcus* are the pathogens most commonly associated with bacterial mastitis. Preferred antibiotics are shown in Table 37-20. First-line antibiotic therapy is dicloxacillin or flucloxacillin; alternatively, cephalexin may be used.[97] Second-line options are clindamycin 300 mg 4 times daily or trimethoprim–sulfamethoxazole double-strength 2 times daily.[97] Regardless of the agent and dosage, a 10- to 14-day course is recommended.

Lactating individuals should be reassured that the infection is not contagious to the infant

| Table 37-20 | Antibiotics Used to Treat Bacterial Mastitis |
|---|---|
| **First-Line Agents (10- to 14-day treatment)** | |
| Dicloxacillin or flucloxacillin 500 mg 4 times daily | |
| Cephalexin 500 mg 4 times daily | |
| **Second-Line Agents (10- to 14-day treatment)** | |
| Clindamycin 300 mg 4 times daily | |
| Trimethoprim–sulfamethoxazole double-strength 2 times daily | |

and there is no need to interrupt or discontinue breastfeeding or human milk feeding. The milk of the affected breast is safe for infant consumption and should not be expressed and discarded. Management of a breast abscess requires surgical aspiration or drainage; collaboration or referral is warranted.

## Persistent Pain

In addition to mastitis, a range of complications can cause persistent pain during lactation. Persistent pain is one of the major causes of early cessation of breastfeeding and is experienced by as many as

| Table 37-21 | Conditions Associated with Persistent Pain During Lactation | |
|---|---|---|
| **Condition** | **Clinical Presentation** | **Initial Management** |
| Nipple injury | Visible signs of nipple or soft tissue damage (i.e., erythema, edema, cracks, abrasions, or blisters) | Identification of source of nipple trauma<br>Optimization of breastfeeding or milk expression technique<br>Wound healing |
| Dermatoses | Typical of the presentation of the dermatosis in other areas of the body | Identification and reduction of exposure to potential irritants or triggers<br>Topical emollient and/or steroid ointment |
| Superficial bacterial infection | Persistent nipple cracks or fissures<br>Cellulitis | Skin, wound, or milk culture<br>Targeted topical (i.e., mupirocin or bacitracin) or oral or oral antibiotics (i.e., cephalosporin or penicillinase-resistant penicillin) |
| Cutaneous candidal infection | Nipple appears pink, shiny, or flaky<br>Burning, radiating pain out of proportion to the clinical findings | Consider alternative etiologies of pain<br>Topical antifungal ointment or cream (miconazole and clotrimazole) on nipples, plus nystatin suspension or miconazole oral gel for infant's mouth |
| Vasospasm | Shooting or burning pain<br>Nipple blanching and color changes | Application of heat (warm compresses or heating pads); avoidance of cold exposure |

Based on Berens P, Eglash A, Malloy M, Steube AM. ABM Clinical Protocol #26: persistent pain with breastfeeding. *Breastfeed Med.* 2016;11:46-53.

1 in 5 lactating individuals.[34] While mastitis affects the breast, other causes of persistent pain in lactation typically affect the nipple–areolar complex. The most common etiologies for pain other than mastitis are nipple injury, dermatoses, infection, and vasospasm. A thorough, targeted history and assessment are essential to guide diagnosis. Table 37-21 outlines key characteristics of the clinical presentation and management of these conditions.

Mild to moderate breast tenderness and transient nipple soreness can be normal in the immediate postpartum period during an initial period of adjustment and physiologic engorgement. However, severe, persistent, or worsening pain is not normal and requires intervention. Clinical evaluation is warranted for any pain associated with breastfeeding or milk expression that is severe in intensity, lasts beyond an initial 30 seconds into a breastfeeding or milk expression session, persists beyond 2 weeks' duration, is present between feedings, or is associated with nipple injury.

Prompt recognition and treatment are essential to support lactating individuals and families in reaching their infant feeding goals. Initial interventions focus on assessment and optimization of breastfeeding or milk expression technique. Targeted management will depend on the underlying cause of persistent pain. Research has demonstrated a correlation between persistent pain in lactation and functional pain syndromes and peripartum mood and anxiety disorders, reinforcing the importance of screening, psychosocial support, and close follow-up for the mental health of the lactating individual who presents with persistent pain.

### Nipple Injury

Differentiation of nipple injury from nipple soreness or sensitivity is based on the severity and duration of symptoms. Nipple soreness or sensitivity is the result of physiologic and anatomic adjustments to the onset of breastfeeding, milk expression, or milk ejection reflex; it typically resolves within 30 to 60 minutes after breastfeeding or expression initiation. Incidence is highest in the first 3 to 4 days postpartum, and resolution of symptoms typically occurs by 7 to 10 days postpartum. Nipple soreness or sensitivity can be alleviated with breastfeeding education and support focused on reassurance, comfort measures, and optimization of breastfeeding or milk expression technique. Research has shown that application of glycerin gel dressings, lanolin, expressed breast milk, or a compounded medication containing mupirocin, miconazole, and hydrocortisone (commonly referred to as "all-purpose nipple ointment" or APNO) is ineffective in alleviating nipple pain.[101]

Nipple injury is characterized by persistent or severe pain and/or visible signs of nipple trauma such as erythema, edema, cracks, abrasions, or blisters. The most common causes of nipple injury are suboptimal breastfeeding or milk expression technique. In breastfeeding, the most likely causes are maternal or neonatal factors leading to shallow infant latch or disorganized infant suck, both of which lead to nipple compression, friction, and damage. With milk expression, nipple trauma can arise from breast pump misuse including ill-fitting flanges, excessive suction, or extended pumping duration. Dermatoses (discussed later in this section), exposure to irritants, and infant or toddler biting are other potential causes of nipple damage. Although most infants with ankyloglossia ("tongue-tie") can breastfeed without difficulty, a severely restricted sublingual frenulum may cause nipple pain and damage. Physical examination of the lactating person and neonate and observation of a breastfeeding or milk expression session can help to identify potential causal factors for targeted management.

When cracks or abrasions appear on the nipple, best practices for wound healing should be followed to promote healing and prevent infection. Comfort measures such as use of NSAIDs or acetaminophen and application of cool compresses can be implemented to alleviate pain and are safe during lactation. Some providers recommend using a topical antibiotic ointment such as mupirocin or bacitracin, covered by a nonstick barrier such as gauze or a plastic breast shield to prevent the affected area from adhering to breast pads, bras, or clothing. However, topical antibiotics have not been shown to be effective in improving symptoms and may cause complications from disruption of the microbiome or epithelial overhydration leading to moisture-associated skin damage.[101,102]

### Dermatoses

Dermatologic conditions such as atopic or contact dermatitis and psoriasis can also cause persistent pain during lactation. These conditions are most often visualized on the areola and can be diagnosed based on the clinical presentation. Findings from a focused health assessment that includes a history of dermatologic conditions or exposure to potential irritants and a physical examination can guide the differential diagnosis of breast and nipple dermatoses. Assessment and management of dermatoses of the breast and nipple follow the steps for all dermatoses.

Although the condition is rare, midwives should consider the potential for mammary Paget's disease, a type of breast cancer that causes eczema-like skin changes to the breast and nipple and warrants referral. The use of topical emollients, antibiotics, or low/medium-strength steroid ointment as indicated is safe with breastfeeding/chestfeeding; however, it is recommended that these agents be applied immediately after feeding and removed from the nipple and/or areola prior to feeding to minimize neonatal ingestion. If symptoms do not respond to initial treatment, consultation with a dermatologist is indicated.

### Superficial Infection

Nipple and breast pain may also be caused by viral, bacterial, or fungal infections. Viral infections such as herpes simplex and herpes zoster can occur on the breasts and/or nipples. Diagnosis and management of these conditions are the same as when they occur in nonlactating persons or in other regions of the body.

Superficial bacterial infection most commonly occurs due to secondary *Staphylococcus aureus* infection of damaged skin around the nipple–areolar complex. The clinical presentation of superficial bacterial infection is characterized by persistent nipple cracks or lesions, which may be weeping, yellow, or crusted, often with cellulitis. Skin, milk, or wound cultures can guide diagnosis and treatment recommendations. Application of topical antibiotic ointments (e.g., mupirocin or bacitracin) has not been shown to improve pain symptoms or prevent development of mastitis compared to expectant management.[101,103] Oral antibiotics such as a cephalosporin or penicillinase-resistant penicillin may be beneficial, although it unclear if this outcome is primarily due to their anti-inflammatory effect.[103]

Diagnosis of candidal infection of the breast/nipple during lactation has changed dramatically in recent years and is controversial. Recent research has reached the conclusion that breastfeeding dyads are being overdiagnosed and overtreated for candidal infections.[104–106] Previously, it was generally accepted that infection with *Candida* (most commonly *C. albicans*) often caused persistent pain in lactation. This condition, termed "mammary candidiasis," was characterized by shooting, stabbing, or radiating breast pain between feeds, often presenting with a nipple that was pink, shiny, or flaky. Antifungal agents were commonly prescribed for both the lactating individual and the infant. However, recent scientific research has called this diagnosis into question, as evidence has not shown a clear association between candidal infection and pain symptoms. *Candida* may be more prevalent in the human milk samples of symptomatic individuals; however, many asymptomatic, healthy individuals also have *Candida* on their breasts and nipples and in their human milk, and many symptomatic individuals do not.[105,107,108] Some researchers have proposed abandoning the diagnosis of "mammary candidiasis" entirely, in favor of "subacute mastitis" or "mammary dysbiosis."[105,106]

The use of antifungal treatments for pain symptoms is also unsupported by research, as antifungals have been shown to be no more effective than expectant management and are not without adverse effects.[104] Because antifungal agents have both antimicrobial and anti-inflammatory effects, these treatments may provide temporary relief of symptoms even in the absence of a fungal infection.[106] The effects of overtreatment are unknown, and research into the microbiomes of human milk, the infant's gut, and the lactating person's skin and the role of dysbiosis in persistent pain during lactation is ongoing. Until further information is available, clinicians should exercise caution in diagnosing and treating candidal infections as part of responsible antifungal stewardship.

Evaluation for suspected candidal infection should include a thorough history and examination exploring other potential etiologies of pain. Risk factors for candidiasis include recent antibiotic use and concurrent neonatal candidal infection. Initial interventions should include support for optimizing breastfeeding or milk expression technique and addressing any identified impediments. When other potential causes of pain have been ruled out or clear dermatologic evidence of infection is present, human milk culture and pharmacologic treatment may be appropriate. Treatment options include topical miconazole or clotrimazole, and oral fluconazole for refractory cases. Research supporting cotreatment of the neonate with oral nystatin suspension in the absence evidence of oral candidiasis is lacking, but the practice is still commonplace. Gentian violet is no longer recommended when other alternatives are available due its potential for carcinogenic effects, allergic sensitization, and tattooing of the skin.

### Vasospasm

Nipple vasospasm (formerly "Raynaud syndrome") is a common cause of pain during lactation, experienced by as many as 1 in 5 lactating individuals.[109]

Vasospasm results from constriction of peripheral blood vessels following exposure to cold. Risk factors include a history of Raynaud's phenomenon or cold sensitivity and nipple injury. Clinical features of vasospasm include pain of the nipple–areolar complex that may radiate deep into the chest and nipple blanching or purple discoloration, sometimes following a triphasic pattern of blanching, erythema, and cyanosis (colloquially, "red, white, and blue"). Diagnosis may be made through clinical observation of the nipple following breastfeeding or milk expression.

Management of vasospasm aims to achieve thermoregulation through avoidance of cold exposure and application of heat. Breastfeeding or expressing milk in a warm area, wearing warm clothing, and applying warm packs to the nipple–areolar complex may minimize symptoms. In severe cases, treatment with 30 to 60 mg of sustained-release daily nifedipine for 2 weeks may be used to relieve symptoms.

## Conclusion

This chapter has provided an overview of infant feeding practices, public health initiatives to increase rates of lactation and breastfeeding, and guidance for supporting individuals and families in achieving their infant feeding goals. Midwives should provide peripartum care that facilitates lactation and breastfeeding success by avoiding unnecessary interventions and maternal–infant separation. Targeted health history taking and physical assessment approaches are useful to identify risk factors and guide the differential diagnosis. The midwife's role in health education and promotion is especially important in infant feeding to enable lactating individuals to reach their infant feeding goals and ensure that neonates' nutritional needs are met. Anticipatory guidance and supportive care for breastfeeding initiation, human milk expression and storage, the continuation or cessation of lactation, and the feeding of human milk substitutes can reduce barriers to success and prevent complications. When complications do arise in breastfeeding/chestfeeding or lactation, the midwife is a valuable member of the healthcare team in diagnosing and managing complications, preventing early cessation of lactation and breastfeeding/chestfeeding, and advancing maternal, neonatal, and familial health. The benefits of lactation and human milk feeding last a lifetime, and midwives can facilitate these lasting positive outcomes.

## Resources

| Organization | Description |
|---|---|
| Academy of Breastfeeding Medicine (ABM) | Protocols in English, Spanish, and other languages for key topics in lactation and breastfeeding medicine |
| Baby-Friendly Hospital Initiative (BFHI) | Baby-Friendly USA is the accrediting body for the BFHI in the United States. |
| Black Mothers' Breastfeeding Association | Nonprofit organization dedicated to reducing racial inequities in lactation and breastfeeding support for Black families |
| Centers for Disease Control and Prevention (CDC) | U.S. breastfeeding data, policies, and information for healthcare consumers and professionals |
| Global Health Media | The breastfeeding series from Global Health Media provides videos on normal breastfeeding as well as common problems. Videos include people from a variety of settings around the world and focus on low-cost, low-resource solutions. |
| Human Milk Banking Association of North America (HMBANA) | Guidelines for establishing a milk bank and locations of milk banks in the United States and Canada |
| International Breastfeeding Centre | Breastfeeding and lactation videos |
| International Lactation Consultant Association (ILCA) | Directory of lactation consultants (IBCLCs) and continuing education opportunities |
| Kelly Mom | Consumer-oriented website with breastfeeding and lactation education, including an article on transgender parents and breastfeeding/chestfeeding by Trever MacDonald |
| La Leche League International (LLLI) | Community-based support for lactation and breastfeeding |
| LactMed (National Library of Medicine) | Drugs and lactation database that covers medication use during lactation |
| Office on Women's Health (OWH) | Resource for lactating individuals returning to work |
| Organization of Teratology Information Specialists (OTIS) | MotherToBaby service provides fact sheets and counseling about medications and other exposures during pregnancy and lactation |
| Penn State Health Children's Hospital (Newt) | Newt: Newborn Weight Tool |
| Stanford Medicine: Hand Expression | Video of hand expression technique |
| U.S. Breastfeeding Committee (USBC) | Coalition of professional, educational, and governmental organizations that publishes core competencies on breastfeeding for healthcare professionals |
| U.S. Department of Agriculture, Center for Nutrition Policy and Promotion | MyPlate: nutritional needs while breastfeeding |
| U.S. Department of Agriculture | Dietary Reference Intakes calculator for healthcare professionals |
| World Health Organization | International Code of Marketing of Breast-Milk Substitutes |
| ZipMilk | Database of lactation support providers |

## References

1. MacDonald TK. Lactation care for transgender and non-binary patients: empowering clients and avoiding aversives. *J Hum Lact.* 2019;35:223-226.

2. Bartick M, Stehel EK, Calhoun SL, et al. Academy of Breastfeeding Medicine position statement and guideline: infant feeding and lactation-related language and gender. *Breastfeed Med.* 2021;16:587-590.

3. Meek JY, Noble L, Section on Breastfeeding. Breastfeeding and the use of human milk. *Pediatrics.* 2022:e2022057988.

4. Centers for Diease Control and Prevention, Division of Nutrition, Physical Activity, and Obesity. *Breastfeeding Report Card: United States 2020.* https://www.cdc.gov/breastfeeding/pdf/2022-Breastfeeding-Report-Card-H.pdf. Accessed November 5, 2022.

5. Victora CG, Bahl R, Barros AJD, et al. Breastfeeding in the 21st century: epidemiology, mechanisms, and lifelong effect. *Lancet.* 2016;387:475-490.

6. Rollins NC, Bhandari N, Hajeebhoy N, et al. Why invest, and what it will take to improve breastfeeding practices? *Lancet.* 2016;387:491-504.

7. DeVane-Johnson S, Woods-Giscombé C, Thoyre S, et al. Integrative literature review of factors related to breastfeeding in African American women: evidence for a potential paradigm shift. *J Hum Lact.* 2017;33:435-447.

8. Tomori C. Overcoming barriers to breastfeeding. *Best Pract Res Clin Obstet Gynaecol.* 2022;83: 60-71.

9. Edwards R. An exploration of maternal satisfaction with breastfeeding as a clinically relevant measure of breastfeeding success. *J Hum Lact.* 2017; 34:93-96.

10. U.S. Department of Health and Human Services. Healthy People 2030: nutrition and healthy eating. https://health.gov/healthypeople/objectives-and-data/browse-objectives/nutrition-and-healthy-eating. Accessed June 15, 2022.

11. McFadden A, Gavine A, Renfrew MJ, et al. Support for healthy breastfeeding mothers with healthy term babies. *Cochrane Database Syst Rev.* 2017;2(2):CD001141.

12. Pérez-Escamilla R. Breastfeeding in the 21st century: how we can make it work. *Soc Sci Med.* 2020;244:112331.

13. Goodman JM, Williams C, Dow WH. Racial/ethnic inequities in paid parental leave access. *Health Equity.* 2021;5:738-749.

14. Ballard O, Morrow AL. Human milk composition: nutrients and bioactive factors. *Pediatr Clin.* 2013;60:49-74.

15. Andreas NJ, Kampmann B, Mehring Le-Doare K. Human breast milk: a review on its composition and bioactivity. *Early Hum Dev.* 2015;91:629-635.

16. Gomez-Gallego C, Garcia-Mantrana I, Salminen S, Collado MC. The human milk microbiome and factors influencing its composition and activity. *Semin Fetal Neonatal Med.* 2016;21:400-405.

17. American College of Nurse-Midwives, Midwives Alliance of North America, National Association of Certified Professional Midwives. Supporting healthy and normal physiologic childbirth: a consensus statement. *J Midwifery Womens Health.* 2012;57:529-532.

18. Acquaye SN, Spatz DL. An integrative review: the role of the doula in breastfeeding initiation and duration. *J Perinat Educ.* 2021;30:29-47.

19. French CA, Cong X, Chung KS. Labor epidural analgesia and breastfeeding: a systematic review. *J Hum Lact.* 2016;32:507-520.

20. Erickson EN, Emeis CL. Breastfeeding outcomes after oxytocin use during childbirth: an integrative review. *J Midwifery Womens Health.* 2017;62:397-417.

21. Smith LJ, Kroeger M. *Impact of Birthing Practices on Breastfeeding.* 2nd ed. Sudbury, MA: Jones and Bartlett; 2010.

22. Widström AM, Lilja G, Aaltomaa-Michalias P, et al. Newborn behaviour to locate the breast when skin-to-skin: a possible method for enabling early self-regulation. *Acta Paediatr.* 2011;100:79-85.

23. Moore ER, Bergman N, Anderson GC, Medley N. Early skin-to-skin contact for mothers and their healthy newborn infants. *Cochrane Database Syst Rev.* 2016;11(11):CD003519.

24. Feldman-Winter L, Goldsmith JP, Committee on Fetus and Newborn, Task Force on Sudden Infant Death Syndrome. Safe sleep and skin-to-skin care in the neonatal period for healthy term newborns. *Pediatrics.* 2016;138:e20161889.

25. Ng CA, Ho JJ, Lee ZH. The effect of rooming-in on duration of breastfeeding: a systematic review of randomised and non-randomised prospective controlled studies. *PLoS One.* 2019;14:e0215869.

26. Schafer R, Genna CW. Physiologic breastfeeding: a contemporary approach to breastfeeding initiation. *J Midwifery Womens Health.* 2015;60:546-553.

27. Fernández-Medina IM, Jiménez-Lasserrotte MdM, Ruíz-Fernández MD, et al. Milk donation following a perinatal loss: a phenomenological study. *J Midwifery Womens Health.* 2022;67(4):463-469.

28. Farah E, Barger MK, Klima C, et al. Impaired lactation: review of delayed lactogenesis and insufficient lactation. *J Midwifery Womens Health.* 2021;66:631-640.

29. Centers for Disease Control and Prevention. Care for breastfeeding people: interim guidance on breastfeeding and breast milk feeds in the context of COVID-19. https://www.cdc.gov/coronavirus/2019-ncov/hcp/care-for-breastfeeding-women.html. Published 2021. Accessed June 21, 2022.

30. Jevitt C, Hernandez I, Groër M. Lactation complicated by overweight and obesity: supporting the mother and newborn. *J Midwifery Womens Health.* 2007;52:606-613.

31. LeFort Y, Evans A, Livingstone V, et al. Academy of Breastfeeding Medicine position statement on ankyloglossia in breastfeeding dyads. *Breastfeed Med.* 2021;16:278-281.

32. Colson SD, Meek JH, Hawdon JM. Optimal positions for the release of primitive neonatal reflexes stimulating breastfeeding. *Early Hum Dev.* 2008;84:441-449.

33. Sakalidis VS, Geddes DT. Suck–swallow–breathe dynamics in breastfed infants. *J Hum Lact.* 2016;32:201-211; quiz 393-395.

34. Berens P, Eglash A, Malloy M, Steube AM. ABM Clinical Protocol #26: persistent pain with breastfeeding. *Breastfeed Med.* 2016;11:46-53.

35. Chipojola R, Chiu H-Y, Huda MH, et al. Effectiveness of theory-based educational interventions on breastfeeding self-efficacy and exclusive breastfeeding: a systematic review and meta-analysis. *Int J Nurs Stud.* 2020;109:1075.

36. Nommsen-Rivers LA, Heinig MJ, Cohen RJ, Dewey KG. Newborn wet and soiled diaper counts and timing of onset of lactation as indicators of breastfeeding inadequacy. *J Hum Lact.* 2008;24:27-33.

37. Feldman-Winter L, Kellams A, Peter-Wohl S, et al. Evidence-based updates on the first week of exclusive breastfeeding among infants ≥ 35 weeks. *Pediatrics.* 2020;145:e20183696.

38. DiTomasso D, Cloud M. Systematic review of expected weight changes after birth for full-term, breastfed newborns. *J Obstet Gynecol Neonatal Nurs.* 2019;48:593-603.

39. Flaherman VJ, Schaefer EW, Kuzniewicz MW, et al. Early weight loss nomograms for exclusively breastfed newborns. *Pediatrics.* 2015;135:e16-e23.

40. Dewey KG, Nommsen-Rivers LA, Heinig MJ, Cohen RJ. Risk factors for suboptimal infant breastfeeding behavior, delayed onset of lactation, and excess neonatal weight loss. *Pediatrics.* 2003;112:607-619.

41. Sachs HC, Committee on Drugs, Frattarelli DAC, et al. The transfer of drugs and therapeutics into human breast milk: an update on selected topics. *Pediatrics.* 2013;132:e796-e809.

42. National Library of Medicine. Contraceptives, oral, combined. https://www.ncbi.nlm.nih.gov/books/NBK501295/. Reviewed June 21, 2021. Accessed June 27, 2022.

43. Oladapo OT, Fawole B. Treatments for suppression of lactation. *Cochrane Database Syst Rev.* 2012;9(9):CD005937.

44. Johnson HM, Eglash A, Mitchell KB, et al. ABM Clinical Protocol #32: management of hyperlactation. *Breastfeed Med.* 2020;15:129-134.

45. Brodribb W. ABM Clinical Protocol #9: use of galactogogues in initiating or augmenting maternal milk production, second revision 2018. *Breastfeed Med.* 2018;13:307-314.

46. Napierala M, Mazela J, Merritt TA, Florek E. Tobacco smoking and breastfeeding: effect on the lactation process, breast milk composition and infant development: a critical review. *Environ Res.* 2016;151:321-338.

47. Reece-Stremtan S, Marinelli KA. ABM Clinical Protocol #21: guidelines for breastfeeding and substance use or substance use disorder, revised 2015. *Breastfeed Med.* 2015;10:135-141.

48. Anderson PO. Alcohol use during breastfeeding. *Breastfeed Med.* 2018;13:315-317.

49. Foeller ME, Lyell DJ. Marijuana use in pregnancy: concerns in an evolving era. *J Midwifery Womens Health.* 2017;62:363-367.

50. American College of Obstetricians and Gynecologists Committee on Obstetric Practice. Committee Opinion Summary No. 722: marijuana use during pregnancy and lactation. *Obstet Gynecol.* 2017;130:931-932.

51. Minato T, Nomura K, Asakura H, et al. Maternal undernutrition and breast milk macronutrient content are not associated with weight in breastfed infants at 1 and 3 months after delivery. *Int J Environ Res Public Health.* 2019;16(18);3315.

52. U.S. Department of Agriculture, U.S. Department of Health and Human Services. *Dietary Guidelines for Americans, 2020–2025.* 9th ed. http:dietaryguidelines.gov. Published 2020. Accessed November 11, 2022.

53. Neville CE, McKinley MC, Holmes VA, et al. The relationship between breastfeeding and postpartum weight change: a systematic review and critical evaluation. *Int J Obesity.* 2014;38:577-590.

54. Lovelady C. Balancing exercise and food intake with lactation to promote post-partum weight loss. *Proc Nutr Soc.* 2011;70:181-184.

55. Delgado-Noguera MF, Calvache JA, Bonfill Cosp X, et al. Supplementation with long chain polyunsaturated fatty acids (LCPUFA) to breastfeeding mothers for improving child growth and development. *Cochrane Database Syst Rev.* 2015;2015(7):CD007901.

56. Wagner CL, Greer FR, Section on Breastfeeding, Committee on Nutrition. Prevention of rickets and vitamin D deficiency in infants, children, and adolescents. *Pediatrics.* 2008;122:1142-1152.

57. Tan ML, Abrams SA, Osborn DA. Vitamin D supplementation for term breastfed infants to prevent vitamin D deficiency and improve bone health. *Cochrane Database Syst Rev.* 2020;12(12):CD013046.

58. Becker GE, Smith HA, Cooney F. Methods of milk expression for lactating women. *Cochrane Database Syst Rev.* 2016;12(12):CD01304.

59. Eglash A, Simon L. ABM Clinical Protocol #8: human milk storage information for home use for full-term infants, revised 2017. *Breastfeed Med.* 2017;12:390-395.

60. Centers for Disease Control and Prevention. Proper storage and preparation of breast milk. https://www.cdc.gov/breastfeeding/recommendations/handling_breastmilk.htm. Published 2022. Accessed June 28, 2022.

61. DiGirolamo AM, Grummer-Strawn LM, Fein SB. Do perceived attitudes of physicians and hospital staff affect breastfeeding decisions? *Birth.* 2003;30:94-100.

62. Cockerham-Colas L, Geer L, Benker K, Joseph MA. Exploring and influencing the knowledge and attitudes of health professionals towards extended breastfeeding. *Breastfeed Med.* 2012;7:143-150.

63. Dowling S, Brown A. An exploration of the experiences of mothers who breastfeed long-term: what are the issues and why does it matter? *Breastfeed Med.* 2012;8:45-52.

64. López-Fernández G, Barrios M, Goberna-Tricas J, Gómez-Benito J. Breastfeeding during pregnancy: a systematic review. *Women Birth.* 2017;30:e292-e300.

65. American College of Obstetricians and Gynecologists. Committee Opinion No. 756: optimizing support for breastfeeding as part of obstetric practice. *Obstet Gynecol.* 2018;132:e187-e196.

66. Madarshahian F, Hassanabadi M. A comparative study of breastfeeding during pregnancy: impact on maternal and newborn outcomes. *J Nurs Res.* 2012;20:74-80.

67. Dettwyler KA. When to wean: biological versus cultural perspectives. *Clin Obstet Gynecol.* 2004;47(3): 712-723.

68. O'Connor NR. Infant formula. *Am Fam Physician.* 2009;79:565-570.

69. Koletzko B, Baker S, Cleghorn G, et al. Global standard for the composition of infant formula: recommendations of an ESPGHAN coordinated international expert group. *J Pediatr Gastroenterol Nutr.* 2005;41:584-599.

70. Osborn DA, Sinn JKH, Jones LJ. Infant formulas containing hydrolysed protein for prevention of allergic disease. *Cochrane Database Syst Rev.* 2018;10(10): CD003664.

71. Committee on Environmental Health, Committee on Infectious Diseases. Drinking water from private wells and risks to children. *Pediatrics.* 2009;123:1599-1605.

72. Schmitt B. *Bottle-Feeding (Formula) Questions: Pediatric Patient Education.* American Itasca, IL: Academy of Pediatrics; 2021.

73. Wittig SL, Spatz DL. Induced lactation: gaining a better understanding. *MCN Am J Matern Child Nurs.* 2008;33(2):76-81.

74. Reisman T, Goldstein Z. Case report: induced lactation in a transgender woman. *Transgender Health.* 2018;3:24-26.

75. Cazorla-Ortiz G, Obregón-Guitérrez N, Rozas-Garcia MR, Goberna-Tricas J. Methods and success factors of induced lactation: a scoping review. *J Hum Lact.* 2020;36:739-749.

76. Ferri RL, Rosen-Carole CB, Jackson J, et al. ABM Clinical Protocol #33: lactation care for lesbian, gay, bisexual, transgender, queer, questioning, plus patients. *Breastfeed Med.* 2020;15:284-293.

77. Palmquist AEL, Doehler K. Human milk sharing practices in the U.S. *Matern Child Nutr.* 2016;12:278-290.

78. Committee on Nutrition, Section on Breastfeeding, Committee on Fetus and Newborn, et al. Donor human milk for the high-risk infant: preparation, safety, and usage options in the United States. *Pediatrics.* 2017;139:e20163440.

79. U.S. Food and Drug Administration. Use of donor human milk. https://www.fda.gov/science-research /pediatrics/use-donor-human-milk. Published 2018. Accessed June 29, 2022.

80. Sriraman NK, Evans AE, Lawrence R, Noble L. Academy of Breastfeeding Medicine's 2017 position statement on informal breast milk sharing for the term healthy infant. *Breastfeed Med.* 2018;13:2-4.

81. Chetwynd EM, Facelli V. Lactation support for LGBTQIA+ families. *J Hum Lact.* 2019;35:244-247.

82. Odom EC, Li R, Scanlon KS, et al. Reasons for earlier than desired cessation of breastfeeding. *Pediatrics.* 2013;131:e726-e732.

83. Ureño TL, Berry-Cabán CS, Adams A, et al. Dysphoric milk ejection reflex: a descriptive study. *Breastfeed Med.* 2019;14:666-673.

84. Huang Y, Liu Y, Yu X-Y, Zeng T-Y. The rates and factors of perceived insufficient milk supply: a systematic review. *Matern Child Nutr.* 2022;18:e13255.

85. Gatti L. Maternal perceptions of insufficient milk supply in breastfeeding. *J Nurs Scholarsh.* 2008;40:355-363.

86. Brown CR, Dodds L, Legge A, et al. Factors influencing the reasons why mothers stop breastfeeding. *Can J Public Health.* 2014;105:e179-e185.

87. Balogun OO, O'Sullivan EJ, McFadden A, et al. Interventions for promoting the initiation of breastfeeding. *Cochrane Database Syst Rev.* 2016;11:CD001688.

88. Vilar-Compte M, Hernández-Cordero S, Ancira-Moreno M, et al. Breastfeeding at the workplace: a systematic review of interventions to improve workplace environments to facilitate breastfeeding among working women. *Int J Equity Health.* 2021; 20:110.

89. Wallenborn JT, Perera RA, Wheeler DC, et al. Workplace support and breastfeeding duration: the mediating effect of breastfeeding intention and self-efficacy. *Birth.* 2019;46:121-128.

90. Gyamfi A, O'Neill B, Henderson WA, Lucas R. Black/ African American breastfeeding experience: cultural, sociological, and health dimensions through an equity lens. *Breastfeed Med.* 2021;16:103-111.

91. Segura-Pérez S, Hromi-Fiedler A, Adnew M, et al. Impact of breastfeeding interventions among United States minority women on breastfeeding outcomes: a systematic review. *Int J Equity Health.* 2021; 20:72.

92. Vimalesvaran S, Ireland J, Khashu M. Mind your language: respectful language within maternity services. *Lancet.* 2021;397:859-861.

93. Preusting I, Brumley J, Odibo L, et al. Obesity as a predictor of delayed lactogenesis II. *J Hum Lact.* 2017;33:684-691.

94. Neville MC, Morton J. Physiology and endocrine changes underlying human lactogenesis II. *J Nutr.* 2001;131:3005S-3008S.

95. Johnson HM, Eglash A, Mitchell KB, et al. ABM Clinical Protocol #32: management of hyperlactation. *Breastfeed Med.* 2020;15:129-134.

96. Trimeloni L, Spencer J. Diagnosis and management of breast milk oversupply. *J Am Board Fam Med.* 2016;29:139.

97. Mitchell KB, Johnson HM, Rodríguez JM, et al. Academy of Breastfeeding Medicine Clinical Protocol #36: the mastitis spectrum, revised 2022. *Breastfeed Med.* 2022;17:360-376.

98. Zakarija-Grkovic I, Stewart F. Treatments for breast engorgement during lactation. *Cochrane Database Syst Rev.* 2020;9:CD006946.

99. Obermeyer S, Shiehzadegan S. Case report of the management of milk blebs. *J Obstet Gynecol Neonatal Nurs.* 2022;51:83-88.

100. Wilson E, Woodd SL, Benova L. Incidence of and risk factors for lactational mastitis: a systematic review. *J Hum Lact.* 2020;36:673-686.

101. Dennis CL, Jackson K, Watson J. Interventions for treating painful nipples among breastfeeding women. *Cochrane Database Syst Rev.* 2014;12(12):CD007366.

102. Douglas P. Re-thinking lactation-related nipple pain and damage. *Womens Health.* 2022;18:17455057221087865.

103. Crepinsek MA, Taylor EA, Michener K, Stewart F. Interventions for preventing mastitis after childbirth. *Cochrane Database Syst Rev.* 2020;9(9):CD007239.

104. Douglas P. Overdiagnosis and overtreatment of nipple and breast candidiasis: a review of the relationship between diagnoses of mammary candidiasis and *Candida albicans* in breastfeeding women. *Womens Health (Lond).* 2021;17:17455065211031480.

105. Jiménez E, Arroyo R, Cárdenas N, et al. Mammary candidiasis: a medical condition without scientific evidence? *PLoS One.* 2017;12:e0181071.

106. Betts RC, Johnson HM, Eglash A, Mitchell KB. It's not yeast: retrospective cohort study of lactating women with persistent nipple and breast pain. *Breastfeed Med.* 2020;16:318-324.

107. Kaski K, Kvist LJ. Deep breast pain during lactation: a case-control study in Sweden investigating the role of *Candida albicans*. *Int Breastfeed J.* 2018;13:21.

108. Hale TW, Bateman TL, Finkelman MA, Berens PD. The absence of *Candida albicans* in milk samples of women with clinical symptoms of ductal candidiasis. *Breastfeed Med.* 2009;4:57-61.

109. Anderson JE, Held N, Wright K. Raynaud's phenomenon of the nipple: a treatable cause of painful breastfeeding. *Pediatrics.* 2004;113:e360-e364.

CHAPTER

# 38

# Physical Assessment of the Newborn

PAMELA J. REIS AND TRACEY BELL

*The editors acknowledge Cecilia M. Jevitt, who was the author of this chapter in the previous edition. The authors would like to thank Julia Phillippi for her assistance with this chapter.*

## Introduction

Midwives often provide the initial assessments of newborn health. Assessment of fetal well-being leads into neonatal assessment at the time of birth and continues until care for the newborn is assumed by another provider. Since midwives are present at birth, they are well positioned to provide early neonatal care. Newborn assessment often focuses on differentiation of healthy newborns who are transitioning well to extrauterine life from those who need additional interventions or health care.

The complete newborn assessment includes three parts: (1) a thorough history, (2) the gestational age assessment, and (3) the physical examination. Based on the results of this examination, the midwife can determine a newborn's level of wellness and identify potential or existing problems to create a plan of care appropriate for the newborn and family. This chapter reviews the basic newborn examination; a guide to the content and findings of the newborn physical examination is provided in the *Physical Examination Findings of Healthy Newborn Infants* appendix. Information about care of the newborn in the first month of life is provided in the *Infant Feeding and Lactation* and *Neonatal Care* chapters.

Knowledge of genetic inheritance, genomics, fetal development, and the effects of chronic and perinatal conditions on fetal well-being makes it clear that the neonatal transition to extrauterine life is affected by many variables. An accurate history of these variables is a critical piece of the full assessment of the newborn. Prior to starting a physical examination and gestational age assessment, the antenatal records, intrapartum records, and neonatal records should be reviewed; obtaining an interval history since birth from the parent(s) may also be needed.

The goal in examination of the newborn is to maximize the amount of information gathered while minimizing the distress incurred by the newborn and parents. It is best to examine the newborn approximately 1 hour after a feeding, when the infant is most likely to be content. The examination should be performed in an environment with proper lighting, cleanliness, and warmth. All equipment needed for the examination should be organized before beginning the examination, including gestational age and physical examination forms (or access to an electronic health record), a measuring tape and growth charts, a stethoscope, and an ophthalmoscope. Familiarity with the correct use of this equipment and guidelines for accurate measurement is essential.

Typically, the first step in the examination is quiet observation. Many key parts of the exam can be accomplished just by careful observation. The observation may even be begun while talking with the newborn's parent(s) or caregiver(s). Prior to making physical contact with the newborn, the goal and purpose of the examination is explained to the caregiver and/or family members, and permission to handle the newborn is obtained. After proper hand washing, the midwife typically dons nonsterile gloves to perform the examination, especially in hospital settings or if the infant has not been bathed. During the examination, information can be offered to the parents about the findings of the examination or guidance on normal newborn care.

The general order of the examination should be modified based on the infant's status at the time of the examination. For example, if the infant is asleep or in a quiet alert phase, collect information that benefits from this status—specifically, assessment of the heart and respiratory system. Once these data are collected, more potentially invasive examination techniques can follow.

## Perinatal History

The perinatal health record is a vital source of essential information for anticipatory guidance and care of the newborn infant. Items of importance to gather in the history that inform care of the newborn include environmental and genetic factors, social history, medical and perinatal history, and neonatal factors, including intrapartum events and gestational age assessment. Information about perinatal events that may influence newborn outcomes is obtained through chart review and interviews with the birth parent and possibly other members of the newborn's family. An interval history that includes feeding and elimination is important if the exam is not being conducted immediately after birth.[1]

### Environmental and Genetic Influences

Genetic disorders are classified as monogenetic, multifactorial, and chromosomal. For more information on inheritance, see the *Assessment for Genetic and Fetal Abnormalities* chapter. "Red flags" in the genetic history include recurrent pregnancy loss, one or more family members who died at a young age, or family members who died from unexplained causes or known genetic disorders. A comprehensive family history should include a three-generation account of the health status of family members, to be updated as new diagnoses are received.[1]

Environmental factors that influence the health of fetuses and newborns include occupational exposure of the birth parents or family members to hazardous materials, poor air quality in the home or community, acute toxic substance releases, unsafe drinking water, exposure to paints and solvents (including lead-based products), and exposure to infectious agents. The National Environmental Public Health Tracking Network has published a tracking tool that covers data on environmental hazards, health effects, and population health. Data can be extrapolated based on location through interactive maps, tables, and charts.[2]

### Social and Support Systems

The social environment is a key determinant of a newborn's current and future health.[3] Aspects of the social history include obtaining a list of everyone living in the household, an assessment of the household environment, and screening for interpersonal violence, substance use (including the use of tobacco or vaping products and risk of secondhand smoke exposure), and mental health disorders (including stress and depression). Access to support systems, such as transportation and child care, should be assessed. In addition, inquiring about food insecurity and access to healthy food options should be part of the support systems assessment. Inquiring about the health and well-being of the children living in the home with the newborn is also important, including their immunization status, overall health, and the presence of patterns of behaviors or physical manifestations that would suggest the need for referrals or support. Obtain consent from the individual before processing any such referrals.

### Birth Parent Health and Perinatal History

Many perinatal risk factors that result in adverse neonatal outcomes can be identified prior to birth. Table 38-1 lists antenatal tests that should be reviewed in the perinatal record as part of the newborn assessment.[4,5] Since some pregnancies are conceived with donor eggs, the table differentiates risks that are related to the birthing parent and the genetic parent.

A wide variety of medical, prenatal, and intrapartum conditions can adversely affect the newborn's health and well-being. Table 38-2 lists some of the medical conditions and fetal and newborn implications that may be associated with those conditions.[4-13]

### Intrapartum and Neonatal History Immediately After Birth

Often several hours elapse between the birth and the physical exam to allow for skin-to-skin contact, feeding, and thermoregulation. Data from the intrapartum and immediate neonatal period that inform the care of the newborn infant include the birth parent's status in labor, such as significant blood loss, fever, prolonged rupture of membranes, and chorioamnionitis. Fetal conditions leading to the need for resuscitation at birth include abnormal or indeterminate fetal heart rate tracing, malpresentation, meconium-stained amniotic fluid, and administration of narcotics shortly before birth.[1] The "Golden Minute" is the first minute of life during which initial steps to resuscitate the infant should be successful in the prevention of hypoxia and asphyxia.[14] If resuscitation was required, a careful assessment

| Table 38-1 | Perinatal Tests Reviewed in Assessment of the Newborn | |
|---|---|---|
| **Type of Screening or Testing** | **Perinatal Screening and Testing** | **Neonatal Implications** |
| Birthing parent blood type and neonatal blood type | ABO blood type and Rhesus (Rh) type, antibody screen for isoimmunization of the birthing parent. Note if antepartum Rho(D) immune globulin was administered. | ABO incompatibility<br>Rh incompatibility<br>Hydrops |
| Group B *Streptococcus* (GBS) colonization of the birthing parent | GBS colonization can be detected in urine or through routine screening. Results of vagino-rectal screening are most accurate within 5 weeks of birth. | If the birthing parent did not receive adequate GBS treatment: Newborns should be evaluated for sepsis risk using assessment tools provided by the American Academy of Pediatrics.[4] |
| Perinatal infections in the birthing parent | Assess if antenatal and intrapartum testing was consistent with CDC guidelines[5] and treatment or prophylaxis was appropriately provided if indicated for the following:<br>• Hepatitis B<br>• Hepatitis C<br>• *Chlamydia trachomatis*<br>• *Neisseria gonorrhoeae*<br>• Human immunodeficiency virus (HIV)<br>• Syphilis<br>• Herpes simplex infection<br>• Human papilloma virus lesions | Inadequate screening and treatment prior to birth may mean additional neonatal screening is indicated.<br>If the birth parent had evidence of infection, follow CDC guidance on neonatal care[5] |
| Genetic parent carrier screening | Sickle cell<br>Thalassemias<br>Cystic fibrosis | Carrier testing of the genetic parent(s) or testing of the newborn may be warranted depending on the clinical presentation, More information can be found in the *Assessment for Genetic and Fetal Abnormalities* chapter. |
| Fetal screening | Screening and testing for chromosomal anomalies and disorders of development such as open neural tube defects | If abnormalities were identified, consultation with and evaluation by neonatal specialists is needed, ideally prior to birth to develop a plan for care. |
| Fetal ultrasound | Fetal survey for morphology, amniotic fluid volume, gestational age; anomalies (kidney, heart, limb, gastrointestinal, genitourinary, neurologic) | If abnormalities were identified, consultation with and evaluation by neonatal specialists is needed, ideally prior to birth to develop a plan for care. |
| Substance use by the birthing parent | Screening may be conducted prenatally or on neonatal specimens such as cord blood or stool. (In some states positive results have legal implications for the parent-newborn dyad.) | Neonatal consultation is indicated to assess for and treat neonatal withdrawal. |

Abbreviation: CDC, Centers for Disease Control and Prevention.

of the type and duration of resuscitation should be noted, as well as the Apgar scores, infant response to resuscitation, and cord blood gas results. If the infant has been weighed, given medications, or had laboratory tests since birth, this information should also be noted.[15]

Following birth, newborns progress through a predictable sequence of events signifying successful transition to extrauterine life, such as robust crying followed by a period of relaxation, opening the eyes and moving the mouth, nursing and suckling, and becoming quiet and falling asleep.[16] The presence

| Table 38-2 | Neonatal Complications Associated with Selected Medical Conditions of the Birthing Parent |
|---|---|
| **Factor** | **Possible Newborn Effects** |
| **Medical Conditions** | |
| Cardiac disease | Chronic intrauterine hypoxia |
| Diabetes (type 1, type 2, or gestational)[a] | Neonatal risks are directly related to the onset, duration, and degree of glucose dysregulation in the birth parent.[6] Risks include congenital anomalies; stillbirth; perinatal asphyxia; fetal growth restriction; large for gestational age; polyhydramnios; birth injury, especially brachial plexus injury following shoulder dystocia; polycythemia; hyperbilirubinemia; hypoglycemia; and respiratory distress.[7] Long-term: The infant has an increased risk of diabetes, obesity, and metabolic syndrome.[7] |
| Hypertensive disorders[a] | Neonatal risks are directly related to the onset, duration, and degree of the birth parent's hypertension. Neonatal complications include fetal growth restriction, prematurity, abruptio placentae, stillbirth, and respiratory distress. Intrapartum use of magnesium sulfate increases the risk of needing neonatal resuscitation at birth.[5] |
| Renal disease | Prematurity, fetal growth restriction |
| Rh or other isoimmunization | Anemia, jaundice, hydrops fetalis |
| Seizure disorder requiring anticonvulsant therapy | Increased risk for congenital anomalies associated with some anticonvulsant drugs. Seizure disorder may independently increase the risk for numerous newborn morbidities including stillbirth, preterm birth, placental abruption, and preeclampsia.[8] |
| Sexually transmitted infections | The infant may need treatment if the birth parent has a current infection. In utero exposure to syphilis is associated with infant skeletal abnormalities.[2] |
| Substance use | Neonatal risks depend on the substance type and length and type of treatment. Neonatal opioid withdrawal syndrome is possible; an evaluation should be performed post delivery. |
| **Prenatal Conditions** | |
| Infection/bacterial colonization | Perinatal transmission of many infections is possible. |
| Oligohydramnios | Fetal growth restriction, amniotic band defects, dehydration syndromes, neonatal kidney/bladder abnormalities |
| Polyhydramnios | Neonatal kidney problems, tracheoesophageal fistula, bowel obstruction, other congenital anomalies |
| Size–dates discrepancy | Fetal growth restriction, macrosomia, birth trauma |
| **Perinatal Events** | |
| Medication use | Intrauterine exposure to some medications may affect neonatal transition to extrauterine life. |
| Antenatal vaccination | Vaccination during pregnancy can cause transplacental passage of antibodies. Key vaccines recommended for neonatal protection include the vaccine against COVID-19 and the tetanus toxoid, reduced diphtheria toxoid, and acellular pertussis (Tdap) vaccine. |
| Abnormal presentation or position of fetus | Birth trauma, brachial plexus injury, hip dysplasia (breech presentation) |
| Acute fetal bradycardia (e.g., placental abruption, uterine rupture, prolapsed cord) | Intrauterine fetal demise, neonatal encephalopathy, neonatal hypovolemia, metabolic acidemia at birth (base excess [pH > 12]), cerebral palsy[b 9] |
| Cesarean birth | Fetal laceration, transient respiratory distress |
| Fetal intolerance of labor | Increased risk for needing neonatal resuscitation at birth, metabolic acidemia at birth (base excess [pH > 12]), neonatal encephalopathy[9] |

| Factor | Possible Newborn Effects |
|---|---|
| Intra-amniotic infection or fever in labor | Neonatal sepsis |
| Meconium-stained fluid | Meconium aspiration syndrome |
| Preterm birth | Neonatal risks are related to the degree of prematurity and antenatal corticosteroids. Steroids administered prior to birth can decrease rates of respiratory distress, mortality, and morbidities. Selected problems include both short-term and long-term morbidities such as neonatal intensive care unit admission, respiratory distress syndrome, intraventricular hemorrhage, and cerebral palsy.[10,11] |
| Prolonged rupture of membranes, term or preterm | Neonatal sepsis |
| Postdates birth (> 42 weeks' gestation) | Postmaturity syndrome, meconium aspiration syndrome, neonatal intensive care unit admission[12] |
| Operative vaginal birth: vacuum or forceps | Vacuum: cephalohematoma, intracranial hemorrhage, subgaleal hemorrhage, retinal hemorrhage, shoulder dystocia<br>Forceps: bruising, skull fracture, facial nerve palsy, intracranial hemorrhage, subgaleal hemorrhage[13] |
| Shoulder dystocia | Brachial plexus injury, fractured clavicle |

[a] Neonatal risks associated with diabetes and hypertensive disorders of pregnancy range from minimal to severe. Infants born to individuals with diet-controlled gestational diabetes only, or mild chronic hypertension that does not require treatment, are less likely to have severe adverse effects. Hematologic outcomes related to hypertension are usually exacerbated in infants with growth restriction.

[b] Birth asphyxia has been associated with increased risk for development of cerebral palsy, but outcomes are improved with use of therapeutic hypothermia in cases of moderate–severe asphyxia.

of these behaviors following birth should be documented in the medical record. Behaviors that are indicative of a pathologic extrauterine transition include respiratory distress, temperature instability, hypoxemia, and hypoglycemia.[16]

### Interval History Since Last Examination

If time has elapsed since the birth or the last examination, obtaining an interval history is appropriate. This history includes a review of any laboratory results, weight, and medication administration since birth. Important events to ask parents about include sleep–wake cycles, feeding behaviors and frequency, and elimination—both wet diapers and bowel movements, including their color. (Diapers that contain gel are very absorbent and can make it difficult for parents to know when they are wet; a tissue in the diaper can be used to determine when urination has taken place.) Discussion of incorporation of the infant into the larger family is also helpful in assessment. The history should include exposure of children and other individuals in the home to illnesses that may affect the fetus/neonate such as varicella, cytomegalovirus, parvovirus, coronavirus, or other viral illnesses.

## Initial Rapid Physical Assessment and Apgar Scoring

An initial brief examination of the newborn is performed immediately after birth. Although not considered a formal physical examination, many important assessments are made during the evaluation that takes place in the first minute of life before a formal Apgar score is awarded. While the newborn is placed on the birth parent's abdomen or remains in the midwife's hands, the midwife focuses on identifying various neonatal parameters of health such as tone, color, and heart rate (which can be palpated on the umbilical cord), as well as any obvious birth injuries or congenital abnormalities. In addition, the physiologic responses of the newborn and the corresponding parental behaviors are observed, all while maintaining vigilance regarding the birthing parent's well-being. If required, resuscitation is initiated before the 1-minute Apgar score is determined.[15]

The second assessment of the neonate includes assignment of the Apgar score, preferably by someone other than the person attending the birth to avoid bias and ensure proper identification of any

**Apgar Score**                                                                            Gestational age _____ weeks

| Sign | 0 | 1 | 2 | 1 minute | 5 minute | 10 minute | 15 minute | 20 minute |
|------|---|---|---|----------|----------|-----------|-----------|-----------|
| Color | Blue or pale | Acrocyanotic | Completely pink | | | | | |
| Heart rate | Absent | <100 minute | >100 minute | | | | | |
| Reflex irritability | No response | Grimace | Cry or active withdrawal | | | | | |
| Muscle tone | Limp | Some flexion | Active motion | | | | | |
| Respiration | Absent | Weak cry; Hypoventilation | Good; Crying | | | | | |
| | | | Total | | | | | |

| Comments: | Resuscitation | | | | | |
|-----------|---------------|---|---|---|---|---|
| | Minutes | 1 | 5 | 10 | 15 | 20 |
| | Oxygen | | | | | |
| | PPV/NCPAP | | | | | |
| | ETT | | | | | |
| | Chest compressions | | | | | |
| | Epinephrine | | | | | |

**Figure 38-1** The expanded Apgar score form.
Legend: ETT, endotracheal intubation; NCPAP, nasal continuous positive airway pressure; PPV, positive-pressure ventilation.
Used with permission from: American Academy of Pediatrics Committee on Fetus and Newborn, American College of Obstetricians and Gynecologists Committee on Obstetric Practice, Watterberg KL, Aucott S, Benitz WE, et al. The Apgar score. *Pediatrics.* 2015;136(4):819-822.

abnormal findings. The Apgar newborn scoring system was devised during the mid-twentieth century by Virginia Apgar, an anesthesiologist who was interested in assessing the effects of intrapartum anesthesia and analgesia on the newborn infant at a time when heavy sedation during labor and birth was common.[15] The Apgar score is not used to guide resuscitation, but rather is an expression of how well the newborn has adapted to extrauterine life.

The Apgar scoring system uses five components to assess the newborn's transition to extrauterine life.[15] These five components assess cardiovascular and circulatory status, lung function, and neuromuscular integrity. A score of 7–10 denotes a vigorous neonate, a newborn with a score of 4–6 is associated with focused resuscitation efforts, and a newborn with a score of 3 or less requires intensive resuscitation procedures. Several years after the scoring system was published, an acronym was devised using Virginia Apgar's surname. Some professionals remember the scoring system as Appearance, Pulse, Grimace, Activity, and Respirations (APGAR).

If the infant transitions well to extrauterine life, the traditional Apgar score is sufficient, but if resuscitation is needed, the expanded Agar score should be used.[15] The expanded version of the Apgar score, shown in Figure 38-1, notes valuable information about resuscitation measures.

The Apgar score may be misinterpreted as an assessment used to detect the presence of perinatal asphyxia. Although some components of the Apgar score are related to prebirth acid–base balance, this score is not a reliable measure of perinatal asphyxia, though it can be used to determine if umbilical cord gases should be collected. Apgar scores are an indicator of resuscitation success and should be obtained every 5 minutes if neonatal resuscitation efforts are ongoing or the score is less than 7.[15]

## Gestational Age Assessment

Gestational age assessment guides early postnatal care and is part of the infant birth certificate; a standardized examination should be conducted at least once. Key components of both the gestational age assessment and the physical examination can be accomplished by observation alone. If the newborn is ill, minimal touching and handling will allow the infant to conserve oxygen and glucose.

Standardized forms for gestational assessment entered into widespread use after the publication of research by Dubowitz and colleagues in 1970, which described a detailed examination of gestational age–related newborn attributes.[17] The Dubowitz examination combined assessment of both physical and neurologic characteristics seen at various gestational ages. In 1979, Ballard published a simplified method for assessing gestational age based on physical examination and neuromuscular assessment.[18] The Ballard Score, based on the work of Dubowitz and others, involves less handling of newborns, and primarily relies on a quiet, rested newborn for accurate results. The scale was revised in 1991 to assess extremely premature newborns more accurately and to provide more precise parameters for assessing term newborns.[19] The revised scale, known as the New Ballard Score, has become the universally accepted scale to assess newborn gestational age.

The New Ballard Score is accurate within a range of 2 weeks and can determine the gestational age of newborns as early as 20 weeks. This test is standardized and best performed by a trained examiner. The technique for performing this examination is discussed further in the *Physical Examination Findings of Healthy Newborn Infants* appendix. Researchers have found that prior knowledge of the obstetric assessment of gestational age does not bias the examiner who is determining the New Ballard Score.[20] The New Ballard Score has been validated as a reliable clinical tool until day 7 of postnatal life of the moderate preterm infant, with the neurologic signs being more reliable than the physical exam alone.[21] This score does have limitations, however. Most notably, it may overestimate gestational age compared with ultrasound or last menstrual period for infants with a lower birth weight or earlier gestational age, including newborns whose birth parents received prenatal corticosteroid therapy.[22]

The New Ballard Score test takes approximately 2 or 3 minutes to perform, and results should be recorded directly on the standardized form, either written or in the electronic medical record. It is best to record findings as the assessment is made, rather than rely on memory. After scores for each category of physical and neuromuscular maturity have been assigned, they are summed, and the aggregate score is plotted to obtain gestational age.

The scoring criteria for both the neuromuscular evaluation and the assessment of physical maturity are included in the *Physical Examination Findings of Healthy Newborn Infants* appendix. Accurate assessment using the New Ballard Score requires practice, and new examiners should have their examinations validated by an experienced examiner

for several gestational age assessments with infants of different gestational ages.

### Gestational Age Categories

When the physical maturity score and the neuromuscular maturity score on the New Ballard Score form are added together, the sum yields a gestational age determination. Using this clinical information as well as available pregnancy dating, the newborn is then classified into one of the categories shown in Table 38-3.[23-26] Classification of infants by size related to their gestational age allows for identification of potential adverse conditions and a more individualized plan of care. Midwives may be involved in collaborative care of late preterm newborns (34 to 36 6/7 weeks' gestation) or provide anticipatory guidance to their birth parents. Late preterm infants are at higher risk for respiratory problems, hyperbilirubinemia, feeding difficulty, hypoglycemia, temperature instability, sepsis, intraventricular hemorrhage, and long-term neurodevelopmental outcomes than are term infants.[26]

### Small, Appropriate, and Large for Gestational Age

It is possible to estimate newborn health risks solely based on gestational age. By comparison, a more sophisticated relationship exists between gestational age and birth weight.[26] Within each of the categories of gestational age, there are a range of birth weights. The extremes of accelerated and diminished growth are associated with certain newborn problems and predispositions.

| Table 38-3 | Categorization of Gestational Age |
| --- | --- |
| **Preterm: less than 37 weeks' gestation** | |
| *Extreme preterm*: 27 6/7 or less weeks' gestation | |
| *Moderate-severe preterm*: 28 to 33 6/7 weeks' gestation | |
| *Late preterm*: 34 0/7 to 36 6/7 weeks' gestation | |
| **Term: 37 to 42 completed weeks' gestation** | |
| *Early term*: 37 0/7 through 38 6/7 weeks' gestation | |
| *Full term*: 39 0/7 through 40 6/7 weeks' gestation | |
| *Late term*: 41 0/7 through 41 6/7 weeks' gestation | |
| **Post-term: 42 weeks' gestation and beyond** | |

Data from American College of Obstetricians and Gynecologists. ReVITALize: obstetric data definitions. https://www.acog.org/practice-management/health-it-and-clinical-informatics/revitalize-obstetrics-data-definitions. Published 2014. Accessed January 29, 2022.

| Table 38-4 | Categorization of Birth Weight |
|---|---|
| **Categorization** | **Definition** |
| Small for gestational age (SGA) | Birth weight below the 10th percentile for the estimated gestational age |
| Appropriate for gestational age (AGA) | Birth weight between the 10th and 90th percentiles for estimated gestational age |
| Large for gestational age (LGA) | Birth weight greater than the 90th percentile for gestational age |
| Macrosomia | Birth weight that exceeds > 4000 grams regardless of gestation |

At any gestational age, birth weights vary according to the birth parent's anthropometric characteristics, gestational weight gain, and sociodemographic factors leading to preterm birth and low birth weight.[27] Thus, there is no international standard for what would be considered as "normal" birth weights for specific gestational ages. Instead, percentiles in relationship to a specified population are used for assessment of birth weight. The categorization of birth weight by gestational age is shown in Table 38-4.[28,29]

Infants who are small and large for gestational age, or who have macrosomia, are at risk for hypoglycemia. They need additional assessment and can benefit from support for feeding. Infants who are small for gestational age are more susceptible to hypothermia compared with those who are appropriate weight or large for gestational age.

## Physical Examination of the Newborn

The physical examination of the newborn is intended to identify physical variations, malformations, and overall health of the newborn. During the examination of the newborn, the four basic techniques of physical examination—inspection, palpation, auscultation, and percussion—are used. The complete examination involves multiple components: anthropomorphic measurements, assessment of body systems, and assessment for birth defects and birth injuries. A thorough examination enables the midwife to assess the newborn's overall health and needs.

When documenting findings, the examiner should describe their findings, noting any variations present, and avoid use of the phrase "within normal limits." Many newborn physical and behavioral variations fall within the range of what could be considered as "normal." Thus, specific terms and descriptions for newborn characteristics should be used where appropriate.

### Approach to the Examination

Most textbooks and physical examination records discuss an examination procedure that proceeds from head to toe. Strict adherence to the order of assessment is not necessary as long as all components are performed. For example, if the newborn is quiet or sleeping, it is appropriate to start the hands-on examination with auscultation of heart, lung, and bowel sounds and palpation of the femoral pulses. In an awake, alert newborn, the examiner may check the red reflex first.[30] A crying newborn presents an opportunity to inspect the mouth and throat. Be aware that excessive handling can over-stimulate the newborn. The newborn may be calmed during an examination by being given something to suck on if the birth parent gives permission.

### Anthropomorphic Measurements

Anthropomorphic measurements include the infant's length, as well as the chest and head circumferences. The newborn body has a unique appearance. For most infants, the head circumference is larger than the chest circumference and the abdomen is protuberant (Figure 38-2). Measurements should be performed using a standardized

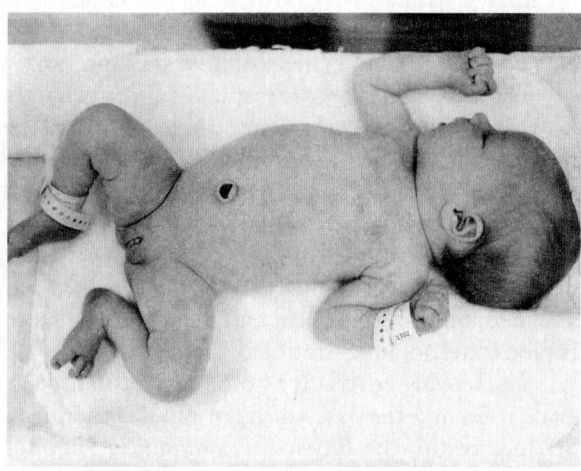

**Figure 38-2** A term infant, size appropriate for gestational age, with appropriate tone and body proportions.

technique. Newborn measurements vary by gestational age, sex, and parental genetic and anthropometric characteristics. Using correct measurement standards can prevent unnecessary testing for newborns incorrectly categorized as small or large for gestational age.

The newborn length is most accurately assessed if the newborn's head is flush against a firm surface. A mark often is made on the table paper to designate the top of the neonate's head. The newborn's legs are then gently extended, and a mark is made on the table paper where the heels rest when the legs are completely extended. After the newborn is moved, the distance between the mark from the top of the head and the mark placed at the heel is measured and documented in centimeters.

The newborn head circumference is measured around the head at the level of the occiput, parietal bosses, and just above the eyebrows. This measurement may decrease in the first week of life as caput succedaneum, cephalohematoma, or soft facial tissue swelling from birth recedes. The chest circumference is measured under the arms and across the nipple line. Disposable, paper tape is often used for these measurements; care should be taken to avoid pulling the tape across the skin to avoid paper cuts.

The newborn's weight should be assessed on a scale, with a drape being placed between the newborn and the metal or plastic. This covering prevents conductive heat loss and minimizes infection from cross-contamination. The scale should be calibrated to account for the weight of the drape. The newborn should be undressed with no diaper.

## Comprehensive Physical Exam

Details of a comprehensive physical exam are discussed in the *Physical Examination Findings of Healthy Newborn Infants* appendix. This appendix includes needed components of the exam as well as typical findings.

## Assessment of Systems

During a comprehensive assessment, the midwife is both assessing individual components, as described in the *Physical Examination Findings of Healthy Newborn Infants* appendix, and using information obtained through this examination as evidence of the functioning of various newborn organ systems, including the respiratory, cardiac, gastrointestinal, renal, and sensory systems. Assessment of each system for physiologic transition or abnormalities yields exam findings that, when grouped together, provide information about the system as a whole.

### Respiratory System

Respiratory system function is demonstrated by several components of the newborn physical exam. The presence of a strong and clear cry at least once after birth is a good indicator of breathing. Healthy newborns have at least a few initial cries and then usually cry intermittently or when uncomfortable. With adequate respirations, there should be no central cyanosis, and the skin is usually pink. Pulse oximetry is used to assess the adequacy of ventilation for neonates requiring resuscitation.

Infants are obligate nose breathers to allow for breastfeeding. Each nare should be assessed for patency through gentle manual occlusion while the infant is not crying. If the infant opens their mouth to breathe, further assessment is needed.

Auscultation with a neonatal-size stethoscope to assess respiratory rate and lung sounds provides valuable information. Newborn respirations can be regular, or they can consist of several strong breaths followed by a pause of up to 20 seconds, a pattern known as periodic breathing, which usually disappears within the first week after birth for term infants. Auscultation should include six areas on both sides of the chest, and the results compared for the two lungs. However, since the chest of the infant is so small and the chest wall has less subcutaneous fat, it can be difficult to localize sounds. Physiologic lung sounds change rapidly in the first hours of life. In the first minutes after birth, crackles and other adventitious sounds are more common as newborns clear their airways of fluid and mucus, but should decrease rapidly. Persistent adventitious sounds in a newborn who is not transitioning well should be investigated further.

The work of newborn breathing can be assessed through observation of the newborn's nares for flaring, listening for expiratory grunting, and inspection of the newborn's chest for retractions. When they are having difficulty breathing, newborns are often unable to successfully breastfeed and may require assessment for hypoglycemia. Inspection of the abdomen also provides insight into the respiratory system. A scaphoid abdominal contour is suggestive of a diaphragmatic hernia and impaired lung volume.

## Cardiac System

Cardiac function is assessed through observation of the infant's color, auscultation of heart sounds, and bilateral palpation of pulses, as well as pulse oximetry testing. Assessment of newborn color is a gross examination that provides a rapid assessment. While valuable in the first assessments of the transition to extrauterine life, pink color is not a reliable indicator of cardiac function, as infant skin color varies according to genetic heritage, room lighting, and temperature. In addition, newborns with life-threatening cardiac defects can appear pink because central cyanosis may not be visible until the arterial oxygen levels are less than 85%.[1] Central cyanosis of the body or mouth, viewed with adequate lighting, is a good indicator of a poor transition to extrauterine life and warrants immediate investigation and, if the cyanosis does not rapidly resolve with intervention, rapid referral. Cyanosis of only the hands and feet, known as acrocyanosis, is common in the first few days of life and does not require any further investigation.

While the infant is quiet, the heart should be auscultated for rate and rhythm; any irregularities need further investigation and consultation with pediatric providers. Heart sounds should be auscultated initially over both sides of the chest to rule out dextrocardia (placement of the heart on the right instead of the left side of the chest), and then over the aortic, pulmonic, tricuspid, and mitral valves. Murmurs are more frequent in newborns during the transition to extrauterine life. If the infant is otherwise asymptomatic, is transitioning well to extrauterine life, and has a normal pulse oximetry reading, routine consultation with pediatric providers is all that is needed. Infants with murmurs that are louder than grade I or that persist after 48 hours of life, as well as neonates with a murmur and any additional examination findings suggestive of poor cardiac function, need a referral for additional assessment. Ejection clicks within the first 24 hours after birth are common and do not require further investigation, but need evaluation if present more than 24 hours after birth.

Pulses provide information about cardiac output and should be palpated bilaterally. Weak pulses can be an indicator of poor cardiac function. Weak femoral pulses are an indicator of decreased aortic blood flow and require further investigation. The abdominal exam also provides information useful in cardiac assessment: An enlarged liver that is 3 or more centimeters below the right costal margin is indicative of cardiac problems and requires referral. Cardiac abnormalities are often part of larger genetic or developmental syndromes. Infants with one major abnormality, such as cleft palate, or several minor abnormalities need careful cardiac assessment by an experienced provider due to their increased risk of cardiac defects.

Pulse oximetry is an important, noninvasive component of routine assessment for critical congenital cardiac defects in newborns; in some states, these results are reported as part of a larger newborn testing program. The ideal time for screening is after 24 hours of life. Earlier screening is acceptable if the infant is being discharged from the birth facility, but can fail to detect some critical congenital defects that would be apparent in later screening.[1] More information is provided in the "Routine Newborn Screening" section later in this chapter.

## Renal and Genitourinary System

Assessment of the renal system includes review of any prenatal ultrasound results, as many renal structural abnormalities are detected prenatally. The amount of amniotic fluid is one of the first indicators of renal function, as it consists primarily of fetal urine; absent or very low levels of amniotic fluid are concerning for renal abnormalities. Neonatal voiding also provides reassurance of some kidney function.

During the physical examination, bimanual abdominal palpation is used to assess the neonatal kidneys. Enlarged kidneys or abdominal masses warrant further investigation for polycystic kidneys. Abnormalities of the ear are associated with renal defects as well. Neonates with any findings suggestive of renal defects can benefit from additional assessment from specialists.

Ambiguous genitalia can be a sign of life-threatening adrenal disorders and should prompt immediate referral to specialist-level care. However, small changes in the shape of genitalia, and hypospadias on the glans, warrant a nonurgent referral to a pediatrician for further assessment.

## Gastrointestinal System

Gastrointestinal function is assessed through amniotic fluid volume and observation of the infant's ability to handle their secretions, feed, and excrete meconium as well as through the physical examination of the abdomen. Physical inspection of the lips and oral cavity, including visualization of the uvula, is part of the assessment of this system.

Newborns with prenatal polyhydramnios, excessive oral secretions, choking with feeding, or vomiting of bile can have tracheal or esophageal atresia or other gastrointestinal abnormalities and need further evaluation without delay. Newborns usually have their first meconium stool within 24 hours after birth. Failure to pass meconium by 48 hours post birth is associated with an imperforate anus or other abnormalities and needs additional pediatric evaluation. In the absence of concerning findings, catheters do not need to be passed into the infant's stomach or items inserted into the anus to test for patency.

An intact lip and palate, normal feeding, the presence of bowel sounds, and a lack of abdominal masses or defects are all reassuring findings. Hernias are fairly common in newborns. If they are small, soft, and easily reduced, they can be assessed and monitored by the pediatric provider at the first well-child visit. In contrast, hernias that are large, tense, or unable to be reduced need more immediate assessment by a specialist.

### Neurologic System

The procedure for assessing reflexes, cranial nerves, and sensory responses is integrated into the overall physical examination as outlined in the *Physical Examination Findings of Healthy Newborn Infants* appendix. The neurologic examination assesses the integrity of the nervous system. Both diminished (hypo) and accentuated (hyper) responses are cause for concern. Diminished responses can result from congenital nerve hypoplasia, damage to sensory or motor pathways, or infection. Diminished or accentuated responses to stimulation can also reflect a central neurologic deficit.

Observation of the newborn provides valuable information. The overall tone of the infant is important to assess in light of the gestational age. Overall tone increases with gestational age and can be assessed by observing the infant's resting posture and response to handling. Newborns with tone inappropriate for their gestational age need further evaluation.

Newborns exhibits two general types of reflexes: *proprioceptive* and *exteroceptive*. *Proprioceptive* reflexes include gross motor reflexes such as the Moro reflex, which can be checked at any time. Complete absence or asymmetry of any of these reflexes is cause for alarm. *Exteroceptive* reflexes are best evoked when the infant is quiet and alert, as they are stimulated by light touch. They include the rooting, grasping, plantar, and superficial abdominal reflexes.

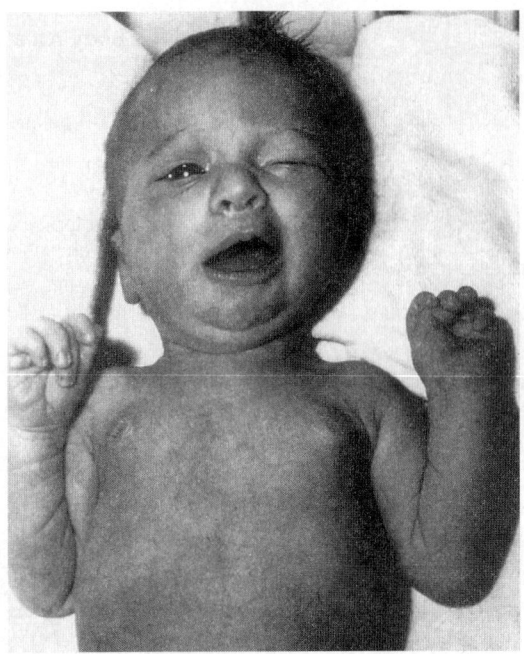

**Figure 38-3** Facial nerve paralysis.

An absent or diminished response to an elicited reflex may be an indication of a variety of conditions.[31] Sometimes a reflex is partial or diminished because of newborn depression secondary to medications or other causes. In other cases, responses may not be optimal because the sensory pathway conducting the stimulation has been damaged owing to a spinal or central nervous system lesion. Sometimes a reflex cannot be elicited because of temporary motor nerve damage that prevents the muscles in the affected area from responding to stimulation, such as a weak palmar grasp after a breech delivery or facial nerve paralysis following a forceps delivery (Figure 38-3). Sometimes damage is permanent, as in some brachial plexus injuries and spinal cord defects. The loss of a previously strong reflex in the first month of life is cause for alarm and should be reported promptly to a pediatric provider. Absent, markedly diminished, or accentuated reflexes and asymmetrical reflexes should be noted on the physical examination form, and consultation with a pediatric provider about further testing and follow-up is indicated.

Reflexes are elicited as part of the physical examination (Table 38-5) and are described in detail in the *Physical Examination Findings of Healthy Newborn Infants* appendix. The plantar reflex is shown in Figure 38-4 and the Babinski reflex is depicted in Figure 38-5.

| Table 38-5 | Newborn Reflexes by Body Area |
| --- | --- |
| **Newborn Body Area** | **Reflexes** |
| Eyes | Pupillary reflex, doll's eye reflex, blink reflex (the red reflex is not neurologic) |
| Upper extremities | Palmar grasp reflex |
| Lower extremities | Patellar reflex, plantar reflex, Babinski reflex |
| Torso | Anal wink, tonic neck reflex, Gallant reflex |

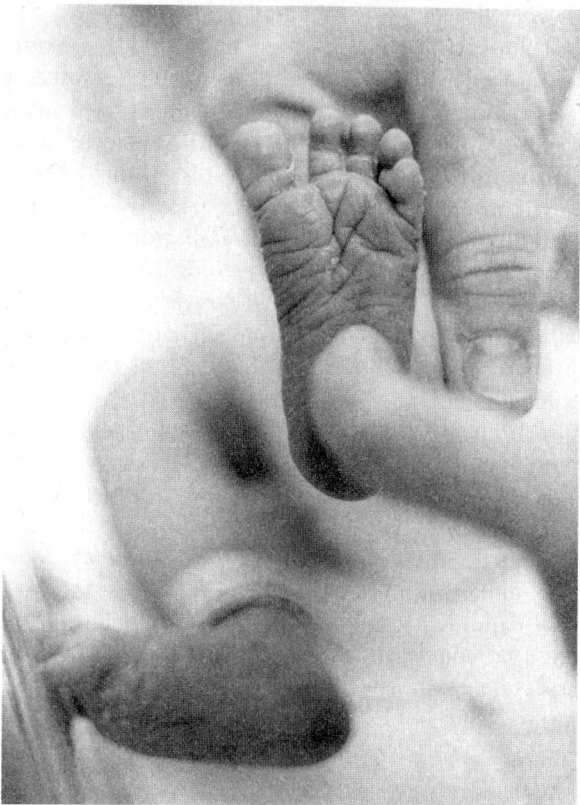

**Figure 38-5** Babinski reflex.

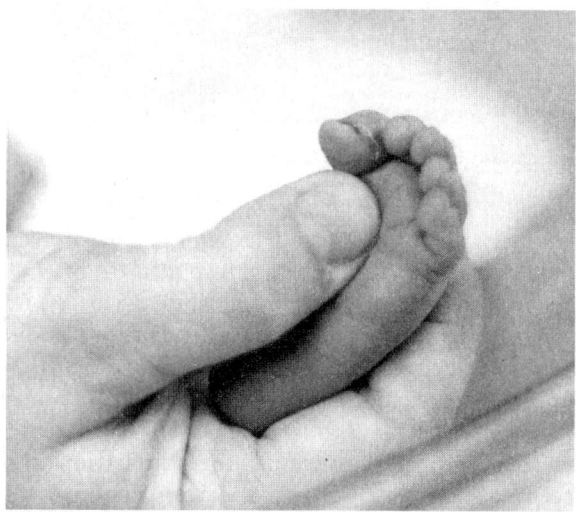

**Figure 38-4** Plantar reflex.

One of the most widely used evaluations of the neurologic status of the newborn is elicitation of the Moro reflex, also known as the embracing reflex. As is true for other primitive reflexes, the Moro reflex is mediated by the brain stem and becomes apparent at approximately 25 to 26 weeks' gestational age.[32] Once thought to reflect an infant's effort to cling to or "embrace" its caregiver, this reflex is now more commonly seen as an involuntary motor response meant to protect the infant from sudden changes in body displacements.[32] In healthy term infants, the response is symmetrical and disappears by 6 months of age.[31-32] The Moro reflex consists predominantly of abduction and extension of the arms with hands open, and the thumb and index finger semi-flexed to form a "C". Leg movements may occur, but they are not as uniform as the arm movements. With return of the arms toward the body, the infant either relaxes or cries.

As one of the primary primitive reflexes, any deviations found in the Moro reflex necessitate a pediatric consultation at a minimum and possibly a full neurologic work-up, especially if deviations in other reflexes are also found. Absence of the Moro reflex may indicate the presence of intracranial lesions. Asymmetrical responses may indicate birth injury involving the brachial plexus, clavicle, or humerus.

During the neurologic examination, evaluations can made of the newborn's sensory responses, such as response to touch and visual stimuli. For example, poor or absent response to oral or auditory stimulation may indicate nerve damage.

### Musculoskeletal System

The musculoskeletal system is assessed throughout the physical examination and includes the hands, feet, and spine as well as overall muscular mobility and function. While muscular tone is often an expression of gestational age and neurologic factors, the range of motion of the muscles can demonstrate structural factors. If the first examination occurs within the first few hours of birth, the muscles and joints may be found to naturally assume their previous in utero positions. For example, infants with frank breech presentations often have extended legs. However, the joints should retain the ability to move through the full range of motion with gentle pressure. If a full range of motion is not possible, further assessment is needed. The appearance of the newborn's feet may also be affected by in utero positioning. If the foot cannot be gently moved into a typical position, this finding should be non-urgently communicated to the pediatric care provider. [24]

Assessment for congenital hip dysplasia includes several components, symmetry of gluteal folds, and changes in the location of the femur head with abduction (Ortolani maneuver) and adduction of the thighs (Barlow maneuver). Any concerning findings should be communicated to the pediatric provider for additional assessment.[24]

Abnormalities of the limbs and digits, including webbing and polydactyly, should be noted. These conditions can be isolated abnormalities, may reflect genetic factors, and may be evidence of a larger syndrome. In particular, bilateral malformations are more likely to be associated with a larger syndrome.

The newborn's skin and appearance of the spine should be inspected down the full length to the coccyx. Any variations in the appearance of the spine need further assessment.[32] Any open defects need immediate intervention and referral, as described in the *Neonatal Care* chapter.

### Sensory System

The infant's response to stimuli provides evidence of both sensation and a responsive neurologic system, as just described. While it is not possible to definitively diagnose sensory losses in newborn infants, screening for potential loss of senses can identify possible abnormalities. Two key areas of assessment include vision and hearing.

*Vision.* Newborn vision is assessed through observing the infant's response to visual stimulation and the doll's eyes reflex as described in the *Physical Examination Findings of Healthy Newborns* appendix. In addition, the physical exam of the eye assesses for congenital cataracts that can affect vision and may be part of a larger genetic or developmental syndrome. The red reflex should be assessed with each comprehensive physical exam using an ophthalmoscope set to "0" magnification power. The exact hue of the red reflex varies by genetic heritage, but should be reddish (not white) and symmetrical in both eyes.[33] The red reflex provides information about the pathway from the pupil to the ocular fundus. Abnormalities can result from cataracts, glaucoma, retinoblastomas, and other retinal and systemic abnormalities. Lack of a red reflex or visualization of any reflection of white instead of red during this exam warrants specialist referral within a few days. [33]

*Hearing* Assessment of hearing sensation includes noting the infant's response to sound, inspection of the ear, and noninvasive hearing screening. In the United States, universal hearing screening is advocated for all infants younger than the age of 1 month.[1] Approximately half of children with hearing loss have no identifiable risk factors; thus, risk-based screening for hearing loss has been problematic. Universal screening has been found to be useful, and newborns with identified hearing conditions have benefited from early intervention and have fewer communication disorders.[34] Hearing screening is discussed in the "Routine Newborn Screening" section later in this chapter.

### Assessment for Birth-Related Physical Variations and Injuries

Birth injuries may occur during a long, protracted labor or a difficult birth. For example, they may be associated with situations in which the fetus is large, or the fetal presentation/position is abnormal. However, they can also occur without an obvious cause. Physical examination findings related to birth trauma may include small scalp abrasions, bruises that correspond to forceps placement along the side of the face, brachial plexus injury to the arm, and fractures of bones, most often the clavicle or extremities.

The skull bones are not fused in newborns; they are somewhat mobile and conform to pressures from the pelvic bones during passage through the vaginal canal. Thus, a newborn skull that appears misshapen is not an unusual finding. Parents can usually be reassured that the skull will assume the typical newborn shape within a few days with no need for intervention.

Possible physical examination findings of the newborn head are depicted in Figure 38-6. There is often a soft tissue swelling (edematous collection of

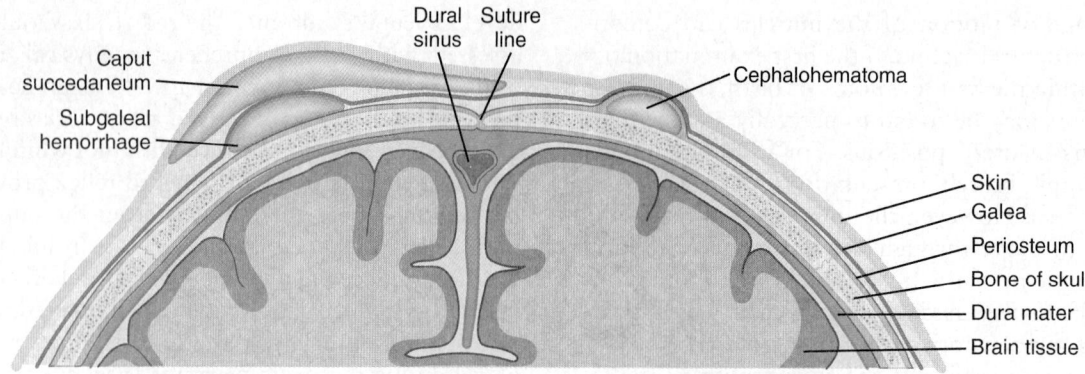

**Figure 38-6** Anatomy of caput succedaneum, cephalohematoma, and subgaleal hemorrhage.

serosanguineous and subcutaneous fluid) called *caput succedaneum* that is visible on the area of the fetal head that was the presenting part. Caput succedaneum has poorly defined margins, may cross suture lines, and is not markedly tense. In contrast, a *cephalohematoma* is a collection of blood under the periosteum of one of the cranial bones, usually the parietal bone. Unlike caput succedaneum or general edema, the blood does not cross the suture lines of the newborn skull because the bleeding is found under the periosteum. Some cephalohematomas occur with linear skull fractures, most of which heal well. A *subgaleal hemorrhage* is an accumulation of blood below the scalp but above the periosteum. It is a rare but life-threatening complication because this space is large and the newborn can lose a large volume of blood quickly. Signs include diffuse swelling in the head that shifts independent of movement, with extension to the eyes, ears, and nape of the neck. In addition, the newborn will display symptoms of shock and hypovolemia.

Facial nerve palsy due to birth trauma results from damage to the facial nerve during birth, and often resolves with a few days to a few months following birth. Signs of facial palsy include asymmetrical movement of the face or little to no movement on the affected side of the face.[35,36]

Injuries to the brachial plexus are not uncommon, occurring in 1 to 3 per 1000 term births. The manifestations of such an injury will depend on which nerve root was injured and the extent of the injury. Breech birth and shoulder dystocia are common risk factors for brachial plexus injury; however, injury can also occur in the absence of risk factors. The nerve roots that supply the brachial plexus—that is, C5 through C8 and T1—are impacted with these injuries. In most cases, damage to the C5 to C6 nerve roots results in Erb or

Duchenne paralysis. With this type of injury, the affected arm is held straight and internally rotated. The elbow may be extended, and the wrist and fingers are flexed. The fingers usually retain function. Damage to the C8 through T1 roots results in Klumpke paralysis, in which the hand may be totally flaccid. In most cases, although nerve function may be temporarily impaired, the prospects for recovery are generally good.[36]

Pressure and manipulation during the birth process is the most common cause of bone fractures. The bones most frequently fractured include the clavicles and the extremities. Signs of bone fracture include swelling, skin discoloration, lack of movement, abnormal positioning, and pain with movement. Crepitus can occasionally be elicited with palpation.[36] Occasionally intrauterine fractures occur, but such findings are often associated with larger disorders. Consultation is needed for further assessment of all suspected fractures.

### Assessment for Birth Defects

Prenatal screening and testing serves as a first line of assessment for anomalies but has limitations. With the routine use of prenatal ultrasound, many physical malformations of the fetus are detected during the prenatal period. However, the accuracy of ultrasonography can be compromised by numerous factors, such as the technician's experience level and the fetal position during the sonogram, which may lead to subtle malformations going undetected. In addition, some conditions are not apparent until after birth or later in infant development.

Variations in physical appearance may be due to inconsequential human variation or familial traits. However, approximately 3% of infants born in the United States have a birth defect. Congenital birth defects are the leading cause of infant deaths in the United States, accounting for 20% of all infant deaths.[37] Birth defects have multifactorial causes, including genetics and alterations during fetal development. See the *Assessment for Genetic and Fetal Abnormalities* chapter for more information.

Minor malformations (Table 38-6), when found in isolation, are most likely simple physical variations in development. However, the presence of three or more malformations is suggestive of a major underlying malformation or congenital syndrome, and requires further evaluation.[38] For example, a widow's peak alone may be due to genetic heritage, but in combination with other minor or major malformations, genetic evaluation is warranted.

Table 38-7 lists physical examination findings related to diagnoses.[38] Early evaluation and intervention can help prevent serious sequelae of malformations such as infection, intestinal perforation, spinal cord injury, intellectual disability, or death.

Newborns with genitalia that express both male and female characteristics in appearance should be immediately referred for consultation with a multidisciplinary, experienced team of experts; such teams are typically found in tertiary care centers. In some instances, intersexual genitalia are associated

| Table 38-6 | Common Benign Malformations Noted on a Newborn Examination in the Absence of Additional Malformations |
|---|---|

Large fontanel

Palpebronasal folds

Multiple or abnormally located hair whorls

Widow's peak

Low posterior hair line

Preauricular tags and pits

Minor ear anomalies: protruding, rotated, low-set

Darwinian tubercle (thickening of the ear's helix at the junction of the upper and lower thirds)

Digital anomalies: clinodactyly (curved finger), camptodactyly (bent finger), syndactyly (webbed finger), polydactyly (extra digit)

Transverse palmar crease

Shawl scrotum (scrotum surrounds penis)

Redundant umbilicus

Widespread nipples

Supernumerary nipples

| Table 38-7 | Neonatal Diagnoses and Findings on Examination |
|---|---|
| **Diagnosis** | **Examination Findings** |
| **Chromosomal Abnormalities** | |
| Trisomy 13 | Polydactyly, cleft palate, scalp defects |
| Trisomy 18 | Finger and joint contracture, webbed neck, "rocker bottom feet" |
| Trisomy 21 | Hypotonia, single palmar crease, increased gap between great toe and other toes, flat mid face |
| Monosomy X (also known as Turner syndrome (45XO) | Loose nuchal skin/webbed neck, lymphedema of the extremities |
| **Autosomal Dominant Disorders with Mendelian Inheritance** | |
| Neurofibromatosis I | Café-au-lait spots (6 or more), bone deformities especially of the tibia |
| **Autosomal Recessive Disorders with Mendelian Inheritance** | |
| Autosomal recessive polycystic kidneys | History of oligohydramnios, enlarged and irregularly-shaped kidneys, high blood pressure |
| Congenital adrenal hyperplasia | Ambiguous genitalia |

*(continues)*

| Table 38-7 | Neonatal Diagnoses and Findings on Examination (*continued*) |
|---|---|
| **Diagnosis** | **Examination Findings** |
| **Disorders with Non-Mendelian Inheritance** | |
| Mitochondrial disorders | Muscle weakness, feeding difficulties, ophthalmoplegia (paralysis or weakness of eye muscles), failure to thrive, seizures |
| Osteogenesis imperfecta | Bone deformities, blue/gray tint to the sclera |
| Prader–Willi syndrome | Hypotonia, poor feeding. genital abnormalities |
| **Diagnoses with multifactorial origins (genetic and developmental/ environmental associations)** | |
| Cleft lip and/or palate | Linear non-junction of the lip and/or hard or soft palates |
| Congenital hip dysplasia | Abnormal movement of the acetabulum when the hip is adducted or abducted, leg length discrepancies, asymmetrical gluteal folds |
| Critical congenital heart defects | Oxygen saturation of <95%, cyanosis, tachypnea, pulmonary edema |
| Diaphragmatic hernia | Respiratory distress, cyanosis, scaphoid abdomen, abnormal chest shape |
| Esophageal atresia | History of polyhydramnios, feeding difficulties including choking when fed small amounts, excessive oral secretions |
| Neural tube defects (spina bifida, anencephaly, encephalocele) | Open or closed defects of the neural tube and the bony structures overlying it including the skull or spine. |
| Talipes equinovarus | Adducted foot that is unable to be moved to midline due to bony abnormalities |
| Urinary tract abnormalities | Anomalies in the location of the urethral opening, most commonly on the glans or ventral side of penile shaft (hypospadias) |
| **Diagnoses primarily related to intrauterine environment** | |
| Intrauterine infection during pregnancy | Findings are dependent on the pathogen and the timing of exposure. Findings can include skull and central nervous system defects, cataracts, hearing abnormalities, and skin manifestations, but may not be apparent at birth. |
| Limb reduction defects | Complete or partial absence or a limb, hand, or foot, bone and soft tissue are not present. |
| Malformations related to teratogen exposure | Dependent on the teratogen and the timing of exposure. Some malformations are not detectable at birth. |
| **Syndromes with multifactorial origins** | |
| Sturge–Weber syndrome | Nevus flammeus (port wine stain) on the trigeminal nerve pathway, seizures may be present |
| VACTERL (vertebral abnormalities, anal atresia, cardiac defects, tracheal-esophageal abnormalities, renal and radial abnormalities, limb abnormalities) association or VATER (vertebral, anal, tracheal, esophageal, and renal) syndrome | Abnormalities of the vertebral column, tracheoesophageal fistula, imperforate anus, limb and heart defects |

Data from Wardinsky T. Visual clues to diagnosis of birth defects and genetic disease. *J Pediatr Health Care.* 1994;8(2):63-73.

with congenital adrenal hyperplasia—a condition that can cause life-threatening dehydration shortly after birth.[39]

Complete assessment of an infant with physical variations should be performed by a multidisciplinary team of experts, which may include neonatologists, geneticists, endocrinologists, and others. Some common abnormalities may be confirmed quickly following birth; in contrast, a comprehensive genetic karyotype analysis may take several weeks to complete. Extensive additional testing may be necessary to evaluate the type and extent of the malformation. When a physical variation of concern is detected, the midwife's role is to obtain consultation and support the family.

## Routine Newborn Screening

Technological developments have increased the ability to screen newborns for diseases and conditions that are life threatening but not apparent at birth.[1] Routine newborn screening began in the 1960s when it became possible to detect phenylketonuria (PKU). Today, newborn screening programs test for a wide variety of conditions.

A standard set of newborn screening tests, known as the core or uniform panel, are mandated across the United States. States manage their own newborn screening programs, however, so differences may arise between states in terms of which tests are included in the screening program. Information about the recommended uniform screening panel recommendations can be found in the Resources section at the end of this chapter.

There is consensus that no test should be included in a state newborn screening program unless treatment for the condition—albeit not necessarily a "cure"—exists.[40] Factors such as financial and family costs associated with false-positive results have been discussed as important considerations when a particular test is being evaluated for inclusion in a state program. Privacy of the newborn's genetic material also has been noted as a concern.[40]

In summary, a variety of screening tests are mandated or available for newborns. Parental education may be included in state newborn screening programs, though midwives may not always be reimbursed by the state for providing this type of health education. Midwives who practice in out-of-hospital settings may either invest in the appropriate equipment for newborn screening or refer new parents to facilities where they can obtain the necessary screening.

A positive screen does not indicate the infant has the condition, but such a result needs further investigation in a timely manner to determine if the infant needs additional care or intervention. There are three main types of early newborn screening: pulse oximetry screening, hearing screening, and the dried blood spot test. All of these tests are time sensitive and usually conducted around 24 hours of age. Results of the pulse oximetry and hearing screens are often reported to the state with submission of the dried blood spot specimen, but healthcare providers should not wait for the state to act on abnormal screening results.

## Pulse Oximetry Screening for Critical Congenital Heart Defects

Pulse oximetry screens for several major and secondary critical congenital heart defects (CCHDs), including hypoplastic left heart syndrome, pulmonary atresia with intact septum, tetralogy of Fallot, coarctation of the aorta, and transposition of the great vessels. Although a number of studies in the early twenty-first century found that pulse oximetry is a good screening method to identify undiagnosed CCHDs among otherwise healthy newborns, the initial research had few participants and a low prevalence of CCHDs.[41-43] However, in a systematic review of more than 400,000 infants published in 2018, pulse oximetry screening for CCHDs was found to be a highly specific and moderately sensitive test for detection of CCHDs with very low false-positive rates. The authors concluded that evidence supports routine screening for CCHDs in asymptomatic newborns before discharge from the birth setting.[43] States with mandatory screening noted a 33% decrease in CCHD-related mortality when compared with states with a nonmandatory screening policy.[44]

A variety of testing algorithms are in use, some of which are mandated by states. In general, testing involves pulse oximetry readings taken from the right hand and foot. The arteries that supply the right hand branch off of the aorta prior to the ductus arteriosus (known as preductal), a common location for cardiac defects. The right foot branches off after the location of the ductus arteriosus (known as postductal). See the *Anatomy and Physiology of the Newborn* chapter for more information. Low pulse oximetry readings in both locations or differences between these two measurements can indicate life-threatening defects. In the normal newborn, oxygenation should be higher than 95% by 24 hours of life, and less than a 2% to 3% difference should be apparent when the pulse oximetry results for the lower extremities (postductal) and the results for the right hand (preductal) are compared.[44]

To screen for CCHDs after 24 hours of life, a pulse oximeter is placed on the newborn's right hand and either foot. If an infant fails screening but has oxygen saturation levels more than 90%, the test can be repeated once. If the infant fails the repeat test, immediate neonatal evaluation with possible cardiac echocardiography is recommended.[44] Infants with abnormal screening results should not be discharged from the birth facility until further assessment is conducted.

### Hearing Screening

Assessment of newborn hearing permits early intervention to improve communication. Hearing screening programs often follow a two-step process, beginning with otoacoustic emissions (OAE) testing in the first few days of life. (The test is difficult to perform within the first few hours of life due to vernix occluding the ear canal, and is best performed at or after 24 hours post birth to allow the ear to dry out.) If a newborn fails the OAE test, an auditory brain stem response (ABR) is conducted. In some sites, both tests are regularly performed. False-positive results occur occasionally, so confirmatory testing by pediatric providers is necessary. Midwives who conduct out-of-hospital births may find the equipment needed is costly; some states provide funding to support equipment purchase. Alternatively, midwives may refer parents to other providers or sites for testing. If an infant does not pass screening, they should have further evaluation by specialists in the weeks following birth.[34]

### Dried Blood Spot Testing

Testing of newborn blood for abnormalities began with testing for PKU, so such testing is often called the PKU test. Many metabolic disorders were added to the screening over time, leading to the test also being known as metabolic screening. However, screening for some nonmetabolic disorders, such as hemoglobinopathies and cystic fibrosis, is now included in many states. A more accurate description is, therefore, dried blood spot screening or, more broadly, newborn screening.

Blood collection should occur after 24 hours of life to allow for detection of key metabolic disorders. Large drops of blood are placed on a special type of paper obtained from the state lab. For best results, collection should be performed by individuals who have received training in newborn blood spot collection. Abnormal screening results are reported to the provider listed on the data collection form and should prompt timely follow-up to allow for rapid diagnosis and intervention if needed. While many of the conditions screened for are rare, early screening results in valuable life-saving information for many infants.

## Conclusion

Midwives are an integral part of the initial newborn assessment process. Rapid determination of neonatal health and the transition to extrauterine life is essential to facilitate the physiologic transition for well infants and to expedite interventions for neonates needing additional support. If abnormalities are discovered, midwives can provide appropriate immediate care, and can consult with or refer to colleagues in the larger healthcare system to ensure subsequent appropriate diagnosis, support, and treatment. All midwives and midwifery practices should have established consultation and referral patterns for newborns that are easily accessed when needed. These plans should take into consideration local availability of resources and personnel, allow for rapid team-based care of struggling infants, and prioritize family-centered care whenever possible.

Many intricacies and nuances are involved in conducting a complete newborn examination. Recognition of normal findings as well as possible deviations is an essential skill for any clinician involved in the care of infants. While many scholarly sources are available for reference and review, they cannot substitute for multiple clinical experiences involving the observation and examination of newborns.

## Resources

| Organization | Description |
| --- | --- |
| New Ballard Score | A comprehensive website can be found at ballardscore.com. This site explains gestational age estimation using the Ballard Score with drawings, photos, and video clips. |
| Global Health Media | The Global Health Media website includes training videos on examination of the newborn, featuring both term and preterm infants. Several videos show common newborn anomalies. |
| National Environmental Public Health Tracking Network | This organization provides data on environmental and hazards, health effects, and population health. Data can be extrapolated based on location through interactive maps, tables, and charts. |
| Stanford Medicine Newborn Nursery | This photo gallery serves as a photographic resource for health professionals who care for newborn infants. |
| Merck Manual for the Professional | This site provides a written overview of a thorough physical exam, as well as providing pictures and diagrams for reference. |
| U.S. Department of Health and Human Services (DHHS) | The DHHS has established Recommended Newborn Screening from the Uniform Screening Panel. |
| Baby's First Test | Detailed information on newborn screening for healthcare professionals and parents. Provides detailed lists of required screenings by state as well as information on disorders detected by screening. |

## References

1. AAP Committee on Fetus and Newborn, ACOG Committee on Obstetric Practice. *Guidelines for Perinatal Care*. 7th ed. Elk Village, IL: American Academy of Pediatrics Books; 2017. doi.org/10.1542/9781610020886

2. Centers for Disease Control and Prevention. National Environmental Public Health Tracking Network. https://ephtracking.cdc.gov/. Updated 2021. Accessed January 29, 2022.

3. Pierce MC, Kaczor K, Thompson R. Bringing back the social history. *Pediatr Clin North Am.* 2014;61(5):889-905. doi:10.1016/j.pcl.2014.06.010.

4. Puopolo KM, Lynfield R, Cummings JJ; Committee on Fetus and Newborn; Committee on Infectious Diseases. Management of infants at risk for group B streptococcal disease [published correction appears in *Pediatrics.* 2019 Oct;144(4):]. *Pediatrics.* 2019;144(2):e20191881. doi:10.1542/peds.2019-1881.

5. Workowski KA, Bachmann LH, Chan PA. Sexually transmitted infections treatment guidelines. *MMWR Recommendations and Reports.* 2021;70(4):1-187.

6. Farrar D, Simmonds M, Bryant M, et al. Hyperglycaemia and risk of adverse perinatal outcomes: systematic review and meta-analysis. *BMJ.* 2016;354:i4694.

7. Mitanchez D, Yzydorczyk C, Siddeek B, et al. The offspring of the diabetic mother: short- and long-term implications. *Best Pract Res Clin Obstet Gynaecol.* 2015;29:256-259.

8. Razaz N, Tomson T, Wikström AK, Cnattingius S. Association between pregnancy and perinatal outcomes among women with epilepsy. *JAMA Neurol.* 2017;74(8):983-991.

9. Fahey JO. The recognition and management of intrapartum fetal heart rate emergencies: beyond definitions and classifications. *J Midwifery Womens Health.* 2014;59(6):616-623.

10. Manuck TA, Rice MM, Bailit JL, et al.; Eunice Kennedy Shriver National Institute of Child Health and Human Development, Maternal–Fetal Medicine Units Network. Preterm neonatal morbidity and mortality by gestational age: a contemporary cohort. *Am J Obstet Gynecol.* 2016;215(1):103.e1-103.e14.

11. Tucker J, McGuire W. Epidemiology of preterm birth. *BMJ.* 2004;329(7467):675-678.

12. American College of Obstetricians and Gynecologists. Practice Bulletin No. 146: management of late-term and postterm pregnancies. *Obstet Gynecol.* 201;124(2 pt 1):390-396.

13. Caughey AB, Sandberg PL, Zlatnik MG, et al. Forceps compared with vacuum: rates of neonatal and maternal morbidity. *Obstet Gynecol.* 2005;106(5 pt 1):908-912.

14. Perlman JM, Wyllie J, Kattwinkel J, et al. Part 7: neonatal resuscitation: 2015 International Consensus on Cardiopulmonary Resuscitation and Emergency Cardiovascular Care Science with treatment recommendations. *Circulation.* 2015;132(suppl 1):S204-S241.

15. American Academy of Pediatrics Committee on Fetus and Newborn, American College of Obstetricians and Gynecologists Committee on Obstetric Practice;

Watterberg KL, Aucott S, Benitz WE, et al. The Apgar score. *Pediatrics*. 2015;136(4):819-822

16. Shaw-Battista J, Gardner SL. Newborn transition: the journey from fetal to extrauterine life. In: Snell BJ, Gardner SL, eds. *Care of the Well Newborn*. Burlington, MA: Jones & Bartlett Learning; 2017:69-100.

17. Dubowitz L, Dubowitz V, Goldberg C. Clinical assessment of gestational age in the newborn infant. *Pediatrics*. 1970;77:1-10.

18. Ballard J, Novak K, Driver M. A simplified score for assessment of fetal maturation of newly born infants. *J Pediatr*. 1979;95(5 pt 1):769-774.

19. Ballard J, Khoury J, Wedig K, et al. New Ballard Score, expanded to include extremely premature infants. *J Pediatr*. 1991;119(3):417-423.

20. Smith LN, Dayal VH, Monga M. Prior knowledge of obstetrical gestational age and possible bias of Ballard Score. *Obstet Gynecol*. 1999;93(5):712-714.

21. Sasidharan K, Dutta S, Narang A. Validity of New Ballard Score until 7th day of postnatal life in moderately preterm neonates. *Arch Dis Child Fetal Neonatal Ed*. 2009;94:39-44.

22. Donovan EF, Tyson JE, Ehrenkranz RA, et al.; National Institute of Child Health and Human Development, Neonatal Research Network. Inaccuracy of Ballard Scores before 28 weeks' gestation. *J Pediatr*. 1999;135(2 pt 1):147-152.

23. American College of Obstetricians and Gynecologists. reVITALize: obstetric data definitions. https://www.acog.org/practice-management/health-it-and-clinical-informatics/revitalize-obstetrics-data-definitions. Published 2014. Accessed January 29, 2022.

24. Boucher, N, Marvicsin, D, Gardner, SL. Physical examination, interventions, and referrals. In: Snell BJ, Gardner SL, eds. *Care of the Well Newborn*. Burlington, MA: Jones & Bartlett Learning; 2017: 101-134.

25. Karnati S, Kollikonda S, Abu-Shaweesh J. Late preterm infants: changing trends and continuing challenges. *Intl J Pediatr Adolesc Med*. 2020; 7:36-44.

26. Engle WA. A recommendation for the definition of "late preterm" (new term) and the birth weight-gestational age classification system. *Semin Perinatol*. 2006;30(1):2-7.

27. Morisaki N, Kawachi I, Oken E, et al. Social and anthropometric factors explaining racial/ethnical differences in birth weight in the United States. *Sci Rep*. 2017;7:46657. https://doi.org/10.1038/srep46657.

28. Cunningham FG, Leveno KJ, Bloom SL et al. Chapter 42: preterm birth. In: Cunningham FG, Leveno KJ, Bloom SL, et al., eds. *Williams Obstetrics*. 25th ed. New York, NY: McGraw-Hill; 2018. https://accessmedicine.mhmedical.com/content.aspx?book

id=1918&sectionid=185085160. Accessed January 29, 2022.

29. Cunningham FG, Leveno KJ, Bloom SL, et al. Chapter 44: fetal-growth disorders. In: Cunningham FG, Leveno KJ, Bloom SL, et al., eds. *Williams Obstetrics*. 25th ed. New York, NY: McGraw-Hill; 2018. https://accessmedicine.mhmedical.com/content.aspx?sectionid=171807435&bookid=1918#185086063. Accessed January 29, 2022.

30. Cagini C, Tosi G, Stracci F, et al. Red reflex examination in neonates: evaluation of 3 years of screening. *Int Ophthalmol*. 2016;7. [Epub ahead of print]. doi:10.10007/s10792-016-0393-2.

31. Hawes J, Bernardo S, Wilson D. The neonatal neurological examination: improving understanding and performance. *Neonatal Netw*. 2020;39(3):116-128.

32. Lewis M. A comprehensive newborn examination: part II. Skin trunk, extremities, neurologic. *Am Fam Physician*. 2014;90(5):297-302.

33. American Academy of Pediatrics. Red reflex examination in neonates, infants, and children. *Pediatrics*. 2008;122(6):1401-1404.

34. Harlor AD, Bower C, Committee on Practice and Ambulatory Medicine, Section on Otolaryngology–Head and Neck Surgery. Hearing assessment in infants and children: recommendations beyond neonatal screening. *Pediatrics*. 2009;124(4):1252-1263.

35. Harbert MJ, Pardo AC. Neonatal nervous system trauma. In: Swaiman KF, Ashwal S, Ferriero DM, et al., eds. *Swaiman's Pediatric Neurology: Principles and Practice*. 6th ed. Philadelphia, PA: Elsevier; 2017:chap 21.

36. Cunningham FG, Leveno KJ, Bloom SL, et al. Chapter 33: diseases and injuries of the term newborn. In: Cunningham FG, Leveno KJ, Bloom SL, et al., eds. *Williams Obstetrics*. 25th ed. New York, NY: McGraw-Hill; 2018. https://accessmedicine.mhmedical.com/content.aspx?sectionid=185053901&bookid=1918#185054047. Accessed January 29, 2022.

37. Centers for Disease Control and Prevention. Data & statistics on birth defects. https://www.cdc.gov/ncbddd/birthdefects/data.html. Updated 2020. Accessed January 29, 2022.

38. Wardinsky T. Visual clues to diagnosis of birth defects and genetic disease. *J Pediatr Health Care*. 1994;8(2):63-73.

39. Hughes IA, Houk C, Ahmed SF; LWPES/ESPE Consensus Group, et al. Consensus statement on management of intersex disorders *Arch Dis Child*. 2006;91:554-563.

40. Kemper AR, Green NS, Calonge N, et al. Decision-making process for conditions nominated to the recommended uniform screening panel: statement of the US Department of Health and Human Services

Secretary's Advisory Committee on Heritable Disorders in Newborns and Children. *Genetics in Medicine.* 2014 Feb;16(2):183-187.

41. Ewer AK. Review of pulse oximetry screening for critical congenital heart defects in newborn infants. *Curr Opin Cardiol.* 2013;28(2):92-96.

42. Ewer AK, Middleton LF, Furnston AT, et al. Pulse oximetry screening for congenital heart defects in newborn infants. *Lancet.* 2011;378:785-794.

43. Plana MN, Zamora J, Suresh G, et al. Pulse oximetry screening for critical congenital heart defects. *Cochrane Database Syst Rev.* 2018;3(3):CD011912. Published 2018 Mar 1. doi:10.1002/14651858. CD011912.pub2.

44. Martin GR, Ewer AK, Gaviglio A, et al. Updated strategies for pulse oximetry screening for critical congenital heart disease. *Pediatrics.* 2020;146(1):e20191650. doi:10.1542/peds.2019-1650.

# 38A

---

# Physical Examination Findings of Healthy Newborn Infants

---

TRACEY BELL

*The editors acknowledge Cecilia M. Jevitt, who was the author of this appendix in the previous edition.*

Infants should have a brief, immediate assessment within moments of birth while they rest on their parent's chest. If the newborn is term, has good tone, and is breathing or crying, the infant should remain skin-to-skin, ideally on the chest of the birthing parent. As long as the infant continues to demonstrate signs indicative of a successful transition to extrauterine life, the parent's chest is the ideal thermoneutral location for at least the first hour after birth. The ideal time for the initial comprehensive physical examination is after the first hour and following at least one breastfeeding/chestfeeding (if applicable). Delaying the examination for at least 1 hour helps with thermoregulation, but the midwife should still ensure the infant can remain warm throughout the exam; this may require adjustment of the room temperature.

The midwife should gather and arrange cleaned supplies and charting aids prior to beginning the exam.

## Supplies

Thermoneutral environment or blankets to keep the newborn warm

Flat surface for the examination

Gloves if the infant has not been bathed

Scale

Measuring tape

Stethoscope (neonatal size)

Otoscope/ophthalmoscope

Access to guides as a prompt

Method of recording examination findings (avoid contamination)

## Gestational Age Assessment

Gestational age is determined using data from the parent's menstrual history or fertility treatment, any prenatal ultrasounds, and the clinical assessment of gestational age.[1] The Ballard assessment provides a reliable method to clinically assess gestational age following birth. Basic assessment findings and scoring are shown in Figure 38A-1.[2] More information and videos describing techniques are included in the References section of the chapter.

NEUROMUSCULAR MATURITY

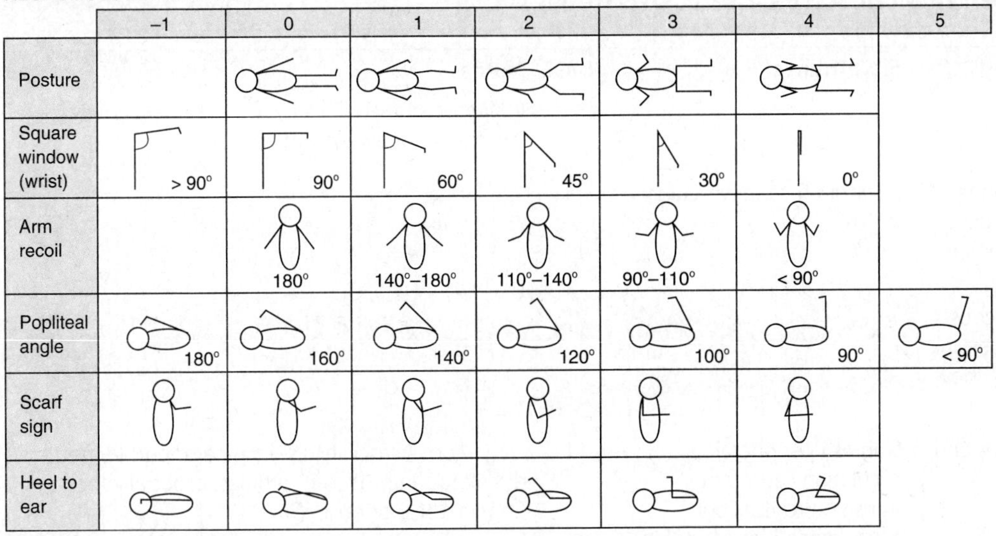

| | −1 | 0 | 1 | 2 | 3 | 4 | 5 |
|---|---|---|---|---|---|---|---|
| Posture | | | | | | | |
| Square window (wrist) | > 90° | 90° | 60° | 45° | 30° | 0° | |
| Arm recoil | | 180° | 140°–180° | 110°–140° | 90°–110° | < 90° | |
| Popliteal angle | 180° | 160° | 140° | 120° | 100° | 90° | < 90° |
| Scarf sign | | | | | | | |
| Heel to ear | | | | | | | |

PHYSICAL MATURITY

| | | | | | | | |
|---|---|---|---|---|---|---|---|
| Skin | Sticky, friable, transparent | Gelatinous, red, translucent | Smooth, pink, visible veins | Superficial peeling and/or rash, few veins | Cracking, pale areas, rare veins | Parchment, deep cracking, no vessels | Leathery, cracked, wrinkled |
| Lanugo | None | Sparse | Abundant | Thinning | Bald areas | Mostly bald | |
| Plantar surface | Heel-toe 40–50 mm: −1 < 40 mm: −2 | > 50 mm, no crease | Faint red marks | Anterior transverse crease only | Creases anterior two-thirds | Creases over entire sole | |
| Breast | Imperceptible | Barely perceptible | Flat areola, no bud | Stippled areola, 1–2 mm bud | Raised areola, 3–4 mm bud | Full areola, 5–10 mm bud | |
| Eye/Ear | Lids fused loosely: −1 tightly: −2 | Lids open; pinna flat, stays folded | Slightly curved pinna, soft, slow recoil | Well-curved pinna, soft but ready recoil | Pinna formed and firm, instant recoil | Thick cartilage, ear stiff | |
| Genitals (male) | Scrotum flat, smooth | Scrotum empty, faint rugae | Testes in upper canal, rare rugae | Testes descending, few rugae | Testes down, good rugae | Testes pendulous, deep rugae | |
| Genitals (female) | Clitoris prominent, labia flat | Clitoris prominent, labia minora small | Clitoris prominent, labia minora enlarged | Labia majora and minora equally prominent | Labia majora large, labia minora small | Labia majora cover clitoris and labia minora | |

MATURITY RATING

| Score | Weeks |
|---|---|
| −10 | 20 |
| −5 | 22 |
| 0 | 24 |
| 5 | 26 |
| 10 | 28 |
| 15 | 30 |
| 20 | 32 |
| 25 | 34 |
| 30 | 36 |
| 35 | 38 |
| 40 | 40 |
| 45 | 42 |
| 50 | 44 |

**Figure 38A-1** The New Ballard Score (NBS).
Reproduced with permission from Ballard J, Khoury J, Wedig K, et al. New Ballard Score, expanded to include extremely premature infants. *J Pediatr.* 1991;119:417.

## Comprehensive Physical Assessment of The Newborn

| Findings | Significance | MOE | Notes |
|---|---|---|---|
| **Color** | | | Indicative of overall status of infant, especially cardiopulmonary system |
| In infants of light-skinned parents: Body and mucous membranes should be pink | Reassuring cardiovascular status | I | |
| In infants of dark-skinned parents: Mucous membranes should be pink and body should not show signs of cyanosis | | | |
| Acrocyanosis of hands and feet during first 24 hours of life | Sluggish peripheral circulation caused by transition to the cool extrauterine life; normal in the first 24 hours | I | *Definition:* Acrocyanosis—a blue or purple mottled discoloration of the extremities, especially the fingers, toes, or nose |
| Reddish hue | Adjustment in oxygen levels in the extrauterine environment; polycythemia | I | Especially noted immediately after birth |
| Ecchymosis | Pressure over the presenting part or from forceps or vacuum, causing bruising and trapping of blood in external tissue layers | I | *Definition:* Ecchymosis—the escape of blood into the tissues from ruptured blood vessels marked by a livid black-and-blue or purple spot or area<br>*Technique:* To differentiate between cyanosis and ecchymosis, apply pressure to darkened area; a cyanotic area will blanch, an ecchymotic area will remain dark |
| Slate gray nevus over buttocks, with possible extension to sacral region and scapular | Hyperpigmentation | I | *Normal variation*, especially if found in dark-skinned infants; careful documentation is warranted to avoid later confusion with bruising and concern for child maltreatment |
| Visible jaundice after first 24 hours of age, receding by day 5 | Physiologic jaundice | I | *Definition:* Physiologic jaundice—transition of blood supply to liver, increased RBC count with decreased life span of cells, decreased plasma protein level, and decreased glucuronyl transferase that aids in bilirubin conjugation<br>Jaundice is visible when bilirubin level > 5 mg/dL<br>*Prematurity:* Peak in jaundice may occur later (typically days 5–7) |
| Jaundice within the first 24 hours, duration more than 8 days in term infant and 14 days in preterm infant | Pathologic jaundice | I | Careful family history looking for history of jaundice, liver disease, and blood type incompatibility. Birth parent illness or certain medications may also interfere with binding of bilirubin to albumin. |
| **General Appearance** | | | |
| Well formed and rounded, with presence of subcutaneous tissue<br>No obvious anomalies | Good nutritional status; generally healthy | I | Indicative of nutritional status, infant maturity, and general well-being |

| Findings | Significance | MOE | Notes |
|---|---|---|---|
| Vernix | Increases with gestational age until close to term then decreases | I | *Definition:* Vernix—a pasty covering, consisting chiefly of dead cells and sebaceous secretions, which protects the skin of the fetus |
| Lanugo | Decreases with gestational age | I | *Definition:* Lanugo—a dense cottony or downy growth of hair; specifically, the soft downy hair that covers the fetus of some mammals to act as protectant<br><br>*Technique (NBS):* Evaluate lanugo on the back with a direct light to get a clear assessment of amount and distribution |

**Posture**

| Findings | Significance | MOE | Notes |
|---|---|---|---|
| Newborn position:<br>• Fists clenched<br>• Arms adducted, flexed<br>• Hips abducted<br>• Knees flexed<br>• Flexion moves upward to arms<br>• Spinal column straight<br>Movement:<br>• Spontaneous, symmetrical, may be slightly tremulous<br>• Flexion and extension should be equal bilaterally | Full-term newborn activity | I<br><br><br><br>I | *Technique (NBS):* With the infant supine and quiet, score as indicated on Figure 38A-1<br>Normal resting position for term infant—flexion<br>*Prematurity:* "Frog position" of legs; normal resting position—extension<br>*Definition:* Tremulous—jerky motions, unequal movement<br>*Prematurity:* No movement or asymmetrical, irregular, tremulous |

**Muscle Strength and Tone**

| Findings | Significance | MOE | Notes |
|---|---|---|---|
| Strength and tone: Strong | May be full term | I | *Prematurity:* Strength and tone weak, hypotonia, or flaccid |
| Palmar grasp: Strong | Good overall strength and equal bilaterally present in hands and feet | I | *Prematurity:* Palmar grasp weak |

**Alertness and Cry**

| Findings | Significance | MOE | Notes |
|---|---|---|---|
| Mood:<br>• Ranges from quiet to alert<br>• Consolable when upset | Normal newborn activity | I | *Prematurity:* Not easily aroused, not very alert<br>*Variation on normal:* Persistent irritability or inconsolable with swaddling and containment |
| Cry: Strong and vigorous | Able to generate strong respirations | I | *Variation on normal:* High pitched, hoarse, or weak; inspiratory stridor—can be associated with obstruction or stenosis of glottic structure |
| Moro (embracing) reflex:<br>• Symmetrical<br>• Disappears by 2–4 months | | I/Pa | *Definition:* Consists predominantly of abduction and extension of the arms with hands open and the thumb and index finger semi-flexed to form a "C". Leg movements may occur, but they are not as uniform as the arm movements. With return of the arms toward the body, the infant either relaxes or cries. |

*(continues)*

| Findings | Significance | MOE | Notes |
|---|---|---|---|
| | | | *Technique:* Acceptable ways to elicit a Moro reflex include the following:<br><br>• While the newborn is in a semi-sitting position, allow the infant to fall backward onto the examiner's open hand from an angle of 30 degrees<br>• While holding the infant in a horizontal position with both hands, quickly lower the infant approximately 10–20 cm and come to sudden halt |
| **Cardiopulmonary System** | | | |
| Respiratory effort:<br>• Easy, unlabored rhythm<br>• May be irregular, but periods of apnea < 15 seconds<br>Abdominal breathing | No respiratory distress or difficulty | I | *Variations:*<br><br>• Grunting—glottis closed during inspiration to increase end-expiratory pressure; grunting with every breath warrants further evaluation<br>• Nasal flaring—widening of nostrils with inspiration to reduce resistance<br>• Retractions—intended to increase air flow; can be noted in various rib locations, with more than one location of retractions visible being indicative of worsening respiratory distress |
| Respiratory rate: 40–60 breaths/min | Normal rate | I | *Variation on normal:* Tachypnea in cesarean section or in full-term infants; may be transient from retention of lung fluid; may have mild tachypnea (60–80 breaths/min) for the first 6 hours of life; normal transition when no other signs of increased work of breathing present *and* normal oxygen saturations<br><br>*Prematurity:* Periodic breathing may be normal; apnea (cessation of respirations for > 15 seconds accompanied by duskiness, cyanosis); respiratory rate > 60 breaths/min |
| Thorax: Symmetrical excursion | Normal respiratory pattern | I | *Definition:* Excursion—one complete movement of expansion and contraction of the lungs and their membranes (as in breathing) |
| Anteroposterior diameter: Normal | Normal respiratory pattern | I | |
| Breath sounds:<br>• Clear<br>• Equal bilaterally, anteriorly, and posteriorly<br>• Occasional rales in first 24 hours | Clear lung fields | A | *Variation on normal:* Occasional rales may be present the first few hours after birth because of residual fetal lung fluid; no color changes, increased work of breathing (grunting, retractions, or nasal flaring), or cyanosis should accompany this finding |

| Findings | Significance | MOE | Notes |
|---|---|---|---|
| Heart rate:<br>• 100–160 bpm<br>• Regular rate and rhythm<br>• Without murmurs or only initial slight murmur | Normal cardiac rhythm without significant abnormalities | A | *Variation on normal:* Initial, slight murmur, usually heard at left sternal border or above apical pulse; may persist until the ductus arteriosus closes; murmur persisting past the first 24 hours of life warrants further evaluation<br><br>*Term infants*: May have low resting heart rate (may drop to 80 bpm with sleep) but rate should increase with stimulation<br><br>*Prematurity:* Bradycardia < 100 bpm or sustained tachycardia > 160 bpm; Grade II/VI murmur |
| Cranium/abdomen: No bruit<br>Apical pulse: At fourth or fifth intercostal space, mid-clavicular line, left anterior chest | No arteriovenous malformation<br><br>Normal position of cardiac pulse; no shifting; without cardiomegaly | Pa/A | *Definition:* Bruit—any of several generally abnormal sounds heard on auscultation<br><br>*Variation on normal*: Point of maximum impulse at the fourth intercostal space just right of the mid-clavicular line may be shifted to the right during the first few hours of life |
| Thrill: None present after first few hours of life | No increased cardiac activity | Pa | *Definition:* Thrill—an abnormal fine tremor or vibration in the respiratory or circulatory systems felt on palpation |
| Blood pressure:<br>• Normal values vary depending on gestational age and birth weight<br>• > 2 kg: Systolic 35–75 mm Hg; diastolic 20–50 mm Hg; measurement of BP in all four extremities if concern for congenital heart disease, persistent murmur, or difficulty obtaining BP—all four extremities should be equal | Normal cardiac output; good circulation; possibly no cardiac defect | Pa | If upper extremity BP > lower extremity BP, concern for possible cardiac defect (coarctation of aorta or interrupted aortic arch) and need for emergent referral<br><br>Must use appropriate-size cuff to prevent erroneous measurements (cuff too small—hypertensive values) |
| Tympany: Not increased over lung fields | Normal lung field borders | Pe | *Definition:* Tympany—a resonant sound heard in percussion; not commonly performed in newborns |
| **Skin** | | | |
| Moist<br>Warm to touch<br>No peeling, wrinkles, edematous or shiny/taut skin | Normal, well hydrated | I | *Technique (NBS):* With the infant supine and quiet, score as indicated on Figure 38A-1<br><br>*Variation on normal* (unless other abnormal findings are also present): Nevus flammeus (if noted on face around trigeminal nerve, consider further evaluation); meconium staining; petechiae (if diffuse, consider checking platelet count); skin tags<br><br>*Prematurity:* Gelatinous with visible veins (transparent skin and visible veins disappear with increasing gestational age)<br><br>*Postmaturity:* Dry, peeling, cracked |

*(continues)*

| Findings | Significance | MOE | Notes |
|---|---|---|---|
| Vernix: Present | Increases with gestational age until close to term then decreases | I | *Prematurity:* No vernix |
| Lanugo: Scant | Full term<br>Decreases with gestational age | I | *Prematurity:* Abundant lanugo |
| Milia | Common in newborns | I | *Definition:* Milia—a small, pearly, firm, non-inflammatory elevation of the skin due to retention of keratin in an oil gland duct blocked by a thin layer of epithelium; commonly noted on nose, forehead, and chin |
| Erythema toxicum | Newborn rash over body, most prevalent within 48 hours of life, but may present as late as 7–10 days | I | *Definition:* Small raised erythematous rash; under microscopic staining predominately eosinophils<br>*Prematurity:* Less common in infants < 34 weeks, so consider other causes if noted |
| Mottling | May be normal reaction to immaturity of organ systems, if infant is of normal temperature, without color changes or bradycardia | I | *Definition:* splotching or blots of color and pallor |
| Transient neonatal pustular melanosis | Benign condition, starts in utero | I | Three stages: Pustules, ruptured vesiculopustules with scaling, and hyperpigmented macules |
| Temperature:<br>• Warm<br>• Axillary temperature 36.5–37.0°C | Normal range | P | *Prematurity:* Temperature may be cool (< 35.5°C) or warm (> 37°C) |

| **Head** | | | |
|---|---|---|---|
| Normocephalic in proportion to body (head circumference for average full-term newborn is 32–37 cm) | Normal | I | |
| Molding: Cranial distortion lasting < 5–7 days | Excessive pressure on cranium during vaginal delivery | I | |
| Sutures | Palpate by pressing thumbs on either side of bone of suture and then the other side | I/Pa | *Variations:* Overriding sutures—excessive pressure on cranium during vaginal delivery<br>If unable to palpate mobile sutures, consider further evaluation for craniosynostosis |
| Caput succedaneum | Edematous region of scalp extending over suture lines, resulting from pressure on the presenting part during vaginal delivery | I | Important to differentiate between caput, cephalohematoma, and subgaleal hemorrhage |

| Findings | Significance | MOE | Notes |
|---|---|---|---|
| Head lag: ≥ 10 degrees in full-term infant<br>Able to support head | Head lag: Decreases with maturity | I | *Technique:* Pull newborn up, supporting the arms, from supine to sitting position; grade degree of head lag by position of head in relationship to trunk<br>*Prematurity:* Head lag > 10 degrees; little or no support of head |
| Hair distribution: Over top of head, with single strands identifiable | Full term | I | *Abnormal:* Multiple hair whorls or whorls in atypical locations (especially low on the posterior skull) warrant further evaluation as they can be associated with brain abnormalities<br>*Prematurity:* Fine, fuzzy, may be over entire head |
| Without masses or soft areas over skull bones | Normal | Pa | *Variation on normal:* Masses or soft areas such as craniotabes over parietal bones may be normal if no abnormality is present<br>*Definition:* Craniotabes—thinning and softening of the infantile skull in spots; "ping pong ball" skull (may be associated with vitamin D deficiency in utero) |
| Bruit: None | Normal | A | |
| **Fontanels** | | | |
| Anterior fontanel:<br>• Open until 24 months<br>• Diamond shaped<br>• Approximately 0.6–3.6 cm across (measurement should be done diagonally); found at intersection of metopic, coronal, and sagittal sutures | Normal<br>Evaluate if flat or bulging; palpate with infant in upright, sitting position | I/A | *Variations:* Large anterior fontanel can be seen with hypothyroidism; sunken fontanel associated with dehydration |
| Posterior fontanel:<br>• Approximate closure by 2–3 months of life<br>• Triangle shaped<br>• Approximately 5-cm diameter (measurement should be done diagonally)<br>• Found along sagittal and lambdoidal suture lines | Normal—flat<br>May be closed at birth | I/A | |

*(continues)*

| Findings | Significance | MOE | Notes |
|---|---|---|---|
| **Oral Cavity** | | | |
| Mouth:<br>• Midline on face, symmetrical without drooping or slanting unilaterally with crying or other movement of mouth<br>• Shape and size in proportion with face<br>• Mucous membranes: Moist, pink | Normal<br>Well hydrated and oxygenated | I | Assess for presence of natal teeth; if present and loose, will need referral to pediatric dentist for removal to minimize risk of aspiration |
| Chin: Shape and size in proportion with face | Normal | I | *Variation:* Small, recessed chin or jaw associated with genetic syndromes, concern for airway compromise |
| Lips: Completely formed, pink, moist | Normal | I | |
| Palate: No arching; hard and soft palates intact | Normal | I/Pa | *Variation:* Cleft palate can interfere with feeding and nutrition; a cleft can be an isolated birth defect, but further evaluation is warranted if other malformation are noted |
| Tongue:<br>• Size in proportion with mouth<br>• Midline | Normal<br>No neurologic dysfunction | I | *Variation on normal:* Ankyloglossia—tight frenulum; may warrant frenulectomy if it interferes with feeding |
| Uvula: Midline rises with crying | Normal function of glossopharyngeal and vagus nerves | I | |
| Gag reflex: Present | Normal neurologic function of glossopharyngeal and vagus nerves | I | *Physiology:* Reflexes generally develop from head to toe during gestation |
| Sucking reflex: Present and strong | Normal maturity and intact hypoglossal nerve | I | *Technique:* Offer non-latex gloved finger or nipple to test<br>*Prematurity:* May be absent |
| Rooting reflex: Present | Normal maturity and intact trigeminal nerve | I | *Technique:* When cheek is stroked, infant turns toward stroking<br>*Prematurity:* May be absent |
| Salivation: Without excess | Normal | I | *Variation:* Excessive secretions can be seen with esophageal atresia |
| **Nose** | | | |
| Position: Midline | Normal | I | |
| Nares: Bilaterally present | Intact | I | |
| Nares: Patent | Normal | I | *Technique:* Occlude the neonate's nostrils one at a time while holding the mouth closed; infant should be able to breathe through one side at a time; passing a catheter into newborn's nares, one at a time, also demonstrates patency |

| Findings | Significance | MOE | Notes |
|---|---|---|---|
| Nares: Grimace or cry in response to strong odors passed under nose | Normal; intact olfactory nerve | I | |
| Nares: Breathing detected bilaterally | Patent | A | *Technique:* With a stethoscope, auscultate for breathing one side at a time |
| **Eyes** | | | |
| • Eye distance: Distance between eyes (approximately 2.5 cm) | Normal | I | |
| Sclera: Clear | Normal; scleral hemorrhages with normal vaginal delivery with usual resolution within 7–10 days | I | *Variation on normal*: Yellow sclera— jaundice, exudates—conjunctivitis<br>*Prematurity:* Bluish tint |
| Conjunctiva: Clear | Normal | I | |
| Iris: Colored evenly, bilaterally | Normal; generally dark gray, blue, or brown, with final color acquired at about 6 months of age | I | *Variation on normal:* Brushfield's spots (these gold flecks may be normal if not found with other anomalies) |
| Pupils: Equal bilaterally and reactive to light | Normal; intact oculomotor nerve | I | *Technique:* Examination is done in a darkened room with penlight or flashlight; if done with a newborn in an incubator or in the nursery, shield the infant's eyes as much as possible |
| Cornea: Clear | Normal; intact | I | *Prematurity:* Hazy |
| Lacrimal duct: Patent | Normal; tear formation does not occur until 2–3 months of age | I | *Definition:* Lacrimal duct—any of several small ducts that carry tears from the lacrimal gland to the fornix of the conjunctiva |
| Blink reflex: Reactive | Intact optic nerve | I | *Technique:* Responds to bright light |
| Red reflex: Present | Lens intact and clear; reddish hue reflected | I | *Technique:* Hold a direct ophthalmoscope close to the examiner's eye, with the ophthalmoscope lens power set at 0. In a darkened room, the ophthalmoscope light should then be projected onto both eyes of the child from approximately 18 inches away. To be considered normal, a red reflex should emanate from both eyes and be symmetrical in character.[3]<br>*Variation on normal:* Transient opacity from mucus in the tear film that is mobile and completely disappears with blinking<br>*Abnormal:* White reflex indicative of opacity of lens; suggestive of cataract, retinoblastoma, or glaucoma; requires urgent referral |
| Eyelids: Without edema, ptosis, or palpebronasal folds | Normal: Intact oculomotor nerve; eyelid edema normal in the first few days after delivery | I | *Definition:* Ptosis—drooping of the upper eyelid<br>*Definition:* Palpebronasal fold—prolongation of a fold of the skin of the upper eyelid over the inner angle or both angles of the eye; palpebronasal folds can be normal but if other malformations noted, the infant should be evaluated closely for possible trisomy |

*(continues)*

| Findings | Significance | MOE | Notes |
|---|---|---|---|
| Doll's-eye response: Present | Normal: Intact trochlear, abducens, and oculomotor nerves | I | *Technique:* With the infant in supine position, turn the head from one side to the other; eyes move to the side opposite the side to which the head is turned |
| Eye position: Without slant | Normal | I | *Variation on normal:* Eye upslanting if the outer canthus of the eye is higher than the inner canthus |
| **Ears** | | | |
| Position: In straight line with eyes; vertical angle that is greater than straight vertical line; without slant | Normal | I | |
| Skin tags: Absent | Normal | I | |
| Ear pits | Normal; may be familial | I | *Variation on normal:* Hypothesized to be embryologic remnants of first branchial cleft or arch; may communicate with inner ear or brain |
| Cartilage formation: Well-curved pinna, sturdy, stiff cartilage, instant recoil | Normal | I/Pa | *Technique:* Palpate the entire pinna of the ear for the presence of cartilage; recoil scored as in Figure 38A<br><br>*Prematurity:* Cartilage flattened or folded with slow recoil |
| Hearing: Neonate responds to sound | Normal; intact auditory nerve | I | *Technique:* See newborn screening section in the *Physical Assessment of the Newborn* chapter.<br><br>Universal hearing screen recommended for all infants |
| Otoscopic examination:<br>• Umbo (cone) of light present, pearl-gray tympanic membrane may have vernix<br>• Membrane is movable without bulging | Normal; intact ear without infection | I | *Technique:* This examination is frequently omitted because the ear canal is often obstructed with vernix and hair; the technique is difficult to perform and may be potentially harmful if the examiner is not skilled; ear should be pulled down and back for examination |
| **Neck** | | | |
| Shape: Symmetrical | Normal | I | *Variation on normal:* Asymmetrical shape may be due to fetal position in utero |
| Head:<br>• Turns from side to side equally, full range of joint motion<br>• Shape symmetrical | Normal | I | *Variations:* Shortening of sternocleidomastoid muscle leading to head turned toward the affected side—torticollis; typically treated with physical therapy |
| Length: Short, without excessive skin | Normal | I | |

| Findings | Significance | MOE | Notes |
|---|---|---|---|
| Tonic neck reflex: Asymmetrical and present but decreases | Normal | I | *Technique:* Observe spontaneously or place the infant in supine position; turn the head to one side with the body restrained; extremities on the side to which the head is turned are extended, but extremities on the other side are flexed; newborn's attempt to right the head when turned to the side tests the accessory nerve<br>*Prematurity:* May be asymmetrical and strongly present |
| Thyroid: Midline | Normal; may be difficult to palpate unless enlarged | P | |
| Lymph nodes: Not palpable | Normal | P | |
| Masses: None | Normal | P | *Variation:* Cystic hygroma-fluctuant mass that transilluminates well, present laterally or over the clavicle, most noted neck mass |
| Carotid: Pulse rate strong and regular | Normal cardiac and circulatory function | P | *Technique:* Do not massage the carotid artery or neck, as this action can result in reflex bradycardia |
| Clavicles:<br>• Even and without "lumps" along bones<br>• Symmetrical | No fractures | P | *Abnormal:* Signs of fracture may not be evident for weeks |
| **Abdomen and Thorax** | | | |
| Chest circumference: 30–35 cm | Average for full-term neonate; typically head circumference is 2 cm larger than chest | I | *Prematurity:* Chest circumference < 30 cm |
| Diaphragm: Equal excursion | Normal | I | |
| Ribs: Symmetrical | Normal | I | |
| Breast: Nipple spacing on line without extra nipples | Normal | I | *Variation on normal:* Extra nipple |
| Areola: Raised and without discharge | Full term | I | *Variations on normal:* Flat areola, discharge, or hypertrophy may be due to birth parent's hormonal influence<br>*Prematurity:* Flat areola and/or discharge |
| Abdomen: Rounded, contoured, symmetrical | Normal | I | *Technique:* To document distension accurately, measure the abdominal girth every 4 hours to detect changes<br>*Prematurity:* Abdominal edema or distension may be present<br>*Abnormal:* Scaphoid abdomen, when the abdomen dips down instead of being full and rounded, is a sign of diaphragmatic hernia |

*(continues)*

| Findings | Significance | MOE | Notes |
|---|---|---|---|
| Umbilical cord:<br>• 3 vessels (2 arteries, 1 vein)<br>• Bluish white color | Normal | I | *Variation on normal:* 2 vessels (1 artery, 1 vein) |
| Abdominal musculature: Strong | Normal | I | *Variation:* Hypertonicity may indicate pain |
| Peristaltic waves: Not visible | Normal bowel activity | I | |
| Bowel sounds: Present | Normal; should be audible within 15 minutes after birth | A | |
| Abdomen: No bruit | Normal | A | |
| Renal: No bruit | Normal | A | |
| Xiphoid process: Present | Normal; intact | Pa | |
| Ribs: Without masses or crepitus | Intact, without defects or "air leaks" | Pa | *Definition:* Crepitus—grating or crackling sound or sensation (like that produced by the fractured ends of a bone moving against each other) |
| Breast tissue: 1 cm | Normal: Full term | Pa | *Technique (NBS):* Palpate to accurately assess breast tissue<br>*Prematurity:* Breast tissue may be < 1 cm and as little as 5 mm |
| Abdomen:<br>• Soft<br>• Nontender<br>• Without masses | Normal | Pa | *Prematurity:* Separation of abdomino-rectus muscles (diastasis recti) is common |
| Kidneys:<br>• 4.5–5 cm in length<br>• Right kidney lower than left<br>• Found in abdomen and posteriorly in lumbar or flank area | Normal | Pa | *Technique:* Palpate with the newborn's legs flexed in a fetal position to relax the infant<br>Enlarged or irregularly shaped kidneys suggest polycystic kidneys |
| Liver:<br>• Sharp edge palpated 1–2 cm below right costal margin<br>• Firm | Normal | Pa | *Technique:* Begin above the right iliac crest; palpate in progressively caudal fashion depressing 1–2 cm and not lifting hands completely off abdomen<br>A liver more than 3 cm below the costal margin is associated with cardiac problems; further evaluation is needed |
| Spleen: Typically not palpable | Normal | Pa | *Abnormal:* More than 1 cm below the costal margin is enlarged; further evaluation warranted |
| Bladder: Not distended | Normal kidney and urinary tract system | Pa | *Technique:* Be sure to evaluate immediately post void or may be falsely evaluated as distension |
| Groin:<br>• Femoral pulse rate strong and regular bilaterally<br>• No hernias or masses | Normal | Pa | Decreased or absent femoral pulses warrant immediate consultation for possible cardiac defect<br>*Abnormal:* Bulge in inguinal or femoral area—hernia; will need surgical evaluation |

| Findings | Significance | MOE | Notes |
|---|---|---|---|
| Gastric bubble:<br>• Just below left costal margin and toward midline<br>• Tympanic | Normal | Pe | |
| Abdomen: Tympanic except dull over liver, spleen, and bladder | Normal liver, spleen, bladder, no masses (indicated by dullness) | Pe | *Technique:* Be sure to examine post void; typically not performed in neonates |
| **Genitourinary Tract, Female** | | | |
| Labia majora: Present and extend beyond labia minora | Full term | I | *Technique (NBS):* With the infant supine and quiet, part of the gestational age assessment - score as indicated on Figure 38A-1<br>*Prematurity:* Labia majora smaller than labia minora |
| Labia minora: Present and well formed | Full term | I | *Technique (NBS):* With the infant supine and quiet, score as indicated on Figure 38A-1<br>*Prematurity:* Labia minora larger than labia majora |
| Clitoris: Present, may be enlarged | Full term | I | *Technique (NBS):* With the infant supine and quiet, score as indicated in Figure 38A, also part of the gestational age assessment<br>*Prematurity:* May also be enlarged |
| Urethral meatus: Present in front of vaginal orifice | Normal | I | |
| Vagina: Patent with or without white discharge | Normal | I | *Variation on normal:* Slight bleeding related to birth parent's hormonal influence |
| Perineum: Smooth | Normal | I | *Abnormal:* Abnormal spacing between vaginal, urethral, and anal openings can be associated with anomalies of genitourinary system |
| Anus: Midline, patent | Normal | I | *Technique:* Digital exam or instrument insertion to assess patency is *not* recommended; most term infants will stool within 48 hours; without other concerning symptoms more extensive evaluation for patency not recommended |
| Anal wink: Present | Normal sphincter | I | *Technique:* Light stroking of anal area produces constriction of sphincter |
| **Genitourinary Tract, Male** | | | |
| Penis:<br>• Straight<br>• Proportionate to body<br>• Length: 2.8–4.3 cm | Normal | I | |
| Urinary meatus:<br>• Midline<br>• At tip of glans | Normal | I | *Technique:* Visualize urethral meatus on tip of penis; do *not* forcefully retract the prepuce. If circumcised, also check for edema or bleeding. |
| Urinary stream: Straight from penis | Normal urinary pattern | I | First void should occur within 24 hours after birth |

*(continues)*

| Findings | Significance | MOE | Notes |
|---|---|---|---|
| Testes and scrotum: Full, numerous rugae | Full term | I | *Technique (NBS):* With the infant supine and quiet, score as indicated on Figure 38A-1<br><br>*Prematurity:* Testes and scrotum may be flaccid, smooth, or with few rugae |
| Pigmentation: Dark | Normal | I | |
| Perineum: Smooth | Normal | I | |
| Anus:<br>• Midline<br>• Patent | Normal | I | *Technique:* Digital exam or instrument insertion to assess patency is *not* recommended; most term infants will stool within 48 hours; without other concerning symptoms, more extensive evaluation for patency not recommended |
| Anal wink: Present | Normal sphincter | I | *Technique:* Light stroking of anal area produces constriction of sphincter |
| Testes: Descended on at least one side; 1.4–1.6 cm | Full term | Pa | *Variation on normal:* Undescended testes<br><br>*Prematurity:* Testes not palpable, though they may be found high in the inguinal canal; descent into inguinal canal at 28–30 weeks |
| **Upper Extremities** | | | |
| Length:<br>• In proportion to each other<br>• Lower extremities and body symmetrical | Normal | I | |
| Full range of joint motion, including:<br>• Abduction<br>• Adduction<br>• Internal and external rotation<br>• Flexion<br>• Extension as applicable to joint | Normal | I | *Physiology:* Full flexion of upper extremities comes with maturity<br><br>*Prematurity:*<br>Limited range of joint motion<br>Limited range of flexion |
| **Upper Extremities** | | | |
| Shoulder: Full range of motion and flexion | Normal | I | |
| Clavicles: Full range of motion and flexion | Normal | I | |
| Elbow: Full range of motion and flexion | Normal | I | *Variation on normal:* Limited range of motion or flexion of the elbow may be related to fetal position in utero |

| Findings | Significance | MOE | Notes |
|---|---|---|---|
| Wrist: Square window test | Normal | I | *Technique (NBS):* Test for square window by flexing the infant's wrist on the forearm, then measure the angle according to gestational examination chart (i.e., 0-degree angle for term neonate); exert pressure sufficient to get as much flexion as possible |
| | | | *Variation on normal:* Limited range of motion or flexion of the wrist may be due to fetal position in utero |
| | | | *Prematurity:* |
| | | | • Limited range of motion or flexion of the wrist |
| | | | • Square window angle > 0 degrees |
| Hand–grasp reflex: Present, strong, equal bilaterally | Normal; maturity | I | *Variation on normal:* Weak, absent, or unequal grasp reflex may be due to fetal position in utero |
| | | | *Prematurity:* Hand–grasp reflex may be weak or absent, or unequal bilaterally |
| Scarf sign: Elbow short of midline | Maturity | I | *Technique (NBS):* With the infant supine, take the infant's hand and draw it across the neck and as far across the opposite shoulder as possible. Assist the elbow by lifting it across the body. Observe the position of the elbow to the chest. Grade the position according to the gestational chart. |
| | | | *Prematurity:* Scarf sign—elbow beyond midline |
| Arm recoil | Maturity | I | *Technique (NBS):* With the infant supine, fully flex the forearm for 5 seconds, then fully extend by pulling the hands, and release; recoil time is graded |
| | | | *Prematurity:* Arm recoil—slow |
| Palm: two palmar creases | Normal | I | *Definition:* Single palmar crease—a deep crease extending across the palm that results from the fusion of the two normally occurring horizontal palmar creases; can be found in in individuals with trisomy 21 especially when combined with incurved little finger and low-set thumb |
| Fingers:<br>• 10 digits and without webbing<br>• Equal spacing | Normal | I | *Variations:*<br>• Polydactyly—supernumerary digits; most common placement is postaxial; strong family history<br>• Brachydactyly—shortened digit; usually benign if isolated finding<br>• Syndactyly—fusion of the digits, most noted between third and fourth fingers |
| Carpals and metacarpals:<br>• Present<br>• Equal bilaterally | No fractures; bone formation normal | I | |
| Nails: Extend beyond nailbeds | Normal; full term | I | |

*(continues)*

| Findings | Significance | MOE | Notes |
|---|---|---|---|
| Nailbeds:<br>• Pink<br>• Brisk capillary refill (< 3 seconds)<br>• Equal bilaterally | Normal peripheral perfusion, normal oxygenation | Pa | |
| **Upper Extremeties** | | | |
| Clavicles:<br>• Symmetrical<br>• Without fractures or pain | Normal | Pa | |
| Humerus, radius, and ulna:<br>• Present<br>• Symmetrical<br>• Without fractures | Normal bone formation | Pa | |
| Pulses:<br>• Brachial and radial strong and equal bilaterally<br>• Brachial and radial strong and equal in comparison with femoral pulses | Good peripheral perfusion, without obvious cardiac defects | Pa | |
| **Lower Extremities** | | | |
| Legs:<br>• Length in proportion to body<br>• Equal bilaterally<br>• Limbs straight | Normal extremity length | I | |
| Toes:<br>• 10 digits<br>• Without webbing<br>• Equal spacing | Normal | I | *Variations:* Syndactyly—fusion of the digits, most noted between second and third toes |
| Feet: Straight | Normal | I | *Variations on normal:*<br>Valgus (turned outward) or varus (turned inward) position of the foot may be related to fetal position in utero and usually resolves<br>Pedal edema may be due to pressure exerted by fetal position in utero |
| Ankle dorsiflexion: 0-degree angle | Maturity | I | *Technique:* Foot is flexed back on ankle, then angle between foot and ankle is measured<br>*Prematurity:* Ankle dorsiflexion angle > 0 degrees; may be up to 90 degrees in very premature neonates |

| Findings | Significance | MOE | Notes |
|---|---|---|---|
| Popliteal angle: < 90 degrees | Maturity | I | *Technique (NBS):* With the infant supine and the pelvis flat on the examining surface, the leg is flexed on the thigh and the thigh fully flexed using one hand; with the other hand, the leg is then extended<br><br>*Prematurity:* Popliteal angle: > 90 degrees and < 180 degrees in very immature infant |
| Heel-to-ear maneuver | Maturity | | *Technique (NBS):* With the infant supine, hold the infant's foot with one hand and move it as near to the head as possible without forcing it; keep the pelvis flat on the examining surface. The heel will not reach the ear but only near the shoulder area in a full-term infant.<br><br>*Prematurity:* The heel reaches the ear, or just short of the ear |
| Nails: Extend to end of nailbed | Normal; maturity | I | *Prematurity:* Nails do not extend to end of nailbed |
| Nailbeds:<br>• Pink<br>• Brisk capillary refill (< 3 seconds) | Good peripheral perfusion | I/Pa | |
| Plantar creases: Cover the sole of foot | Maturity | I | *Technique (NBS):* With the infant supine and quiet, score as indicated on Figure 38A-1<br><br>*Prematurity:* Plantar creases are few or cover only the anterior third of the sole of the foot |
| Buttocks: Creases symmetrical | Normal hips without evidence of dislocation | I | |
| Fibula, tibia, trochanter, and femur:<br>• Present<br>• Equal bilaterally | No fractures; bone formation normal | Pa | |
| Tarsals and metatarsals:<br>• Present<br>• Equal bilaterally | No fractures; bone formation normal | Pa | |
| Full range of joint motion (includes abduction, adduction, internal and external rotation, flexion, and extension as applicable to respective joints of legs, knees, ankles, feet, and toes) | Normal; maturity | Pa | *Prematurity:* Limited range of joint motion; flexion of legs, knees, ankles, feet, and toes is limited |
| Hips: Without clicks and full range of joint motion | Normal range of joint motion and no clicks | Pa | *Technique:* Ortolani's maneuver—flex the newborn's hips and knees, then abduct and adduct the hip to detect a slipping of the hip out of the acetabulum or an uneven motion unilaterally<br><br>*Technique:* Barlow's maneuver—flex the newborn's hips and knees, then place a finger on the femur and trochanter, put the hip through full range of joint motion, and listen for an audible click |

*(continues)*

| Findings | Significance | MOE | Notes |
|---|---|---|---|
| Knee jerk or patellar reflex:<br>• Present<br>• Symmetrical | Normal; mature | Pa | *Prematurity:* Knee jerk or patellar reflex absent, weak, or asymmetrical |
| Flexor plantar reflex:<br>• Present<br>• Symmetrical | Normal; mature | Pa | *Technique:* Stroking the lateral part of the sole of the foot produces plantar flexion of the big toe; often there is also flexion and adduction of the other toes<br><br>*Prematurity:* Plantar reflex absent, weak, or asymmetrical |
| Extensor plantar (Babinski) reflex:<br>• Present<br>• Symmetrical | Normal; mature | Pa | *Technique:* When the sole of the foot is firmly stroked, the big toe extends (bends back toward the top of the foot) and the other toes fan out; this is a normal reflex up to about 2 years of age |
| **Back** | | | |
| Spinal column: Straight | Normal alignment | I | *Variation on normal:* A curved spinal column should gradually resolve if it results from fetal positioning while in utero |
| No visible deviations or defects | Intact | I | *Abnormal:* A pilonidal dimple—containing hair nested or a cyst; needs further investigation |
| Vertebrae: Present, without enlargement or pain | Normal spinal column | Pa | |
| Anus: See genitourinary tract | | Pa | |
| Buttocks: See lower extremities | | Pa | |

Abbreviations: A, auscultation; BP, blood pressure; I, inspection; MOE, method of evaluation; NBS, New Ballard Score; Pa, palpation; Pe, percussion; RBC, red blood cell.

Based on American Academy of Pediatrics, Section on Ophthalmology, American Association for Pediatric Ophthalmology and Strabismus, et al. Red reflex examination in neonates, infants, and children. *Pediatrics.* 2008;122:1401-1404; Tappero EP, Honeyfield ME. *Physical Assessment of the Newborn: A Comprehensive Approach to the Art of Physical Examination.* 6th ed. New York, NY: Springer; 2019; Boucher N, Marvicsin D, Gardner SL. Physical examination, interventions, and referrals. In: Snell BJ, Gardner S, eds. *Care of the Well Newborn.* Burlington, MA: Jones & Bartlett Learning; 2017:101-134.

## References

1. American Academy of Pediatrics, American College Obstetricians and Gynecologists. *Guidelines for Perinatal Care.* 8th ed. Elk Grove Village, IL: American Acadamy of Pediatrics; 2017.

2. Ballard J, Khoury J, Wedig K, et al. New Ballard Score, expanded to include extremely premature infants. *J Pediatr.* 1991;119(3):417-423.

CHAPTER

# 39

# Neonatal Care

PAMELA J. REIS AND TRACEY BELL

*The editors acknowledge Cecilia M. Jevitt, who was the author of this chapter in the previous edition. The authors would like to thank Julia Phillippi for her edits to this edition.*

## Introduction

The role of the midwife in caring for the neonate during the first 28 days of life varies markedly across practices and settings. In some settings, midwives provide very little care once the newborn leaves the birthing room. In others, midwives continue care of the birth parent and newborn throughout the first several weeks of life. The 2020 ACNM *Core Competencies for Basic Midwifery Practice* affirm that midwives should have the knowledge, skills, and abilities to independently manage the care of well neonates up to 28 days of life.[1] Parents often call their midwife with questions related to the care and well-being of their newborn. Therefore, knowledge of typical newborn behaviors and signs of newborn disorders is an important component of practice for all midwives. During the first few hours after birth, newborns must successfully navigate the physiologic transition from an intrauterine environment to an extrauterine one. This process is described in the *Anatomy and Physiology of the Newborn* chapter. Information about the newborn examination is presented in the *Physical Assessment of the Newborn* chapter. This chapter reviews newborn care through the first month of life.

## The First Golden Hour

The concept of the Golden Hour originated in the care of trauma victims, for whom the first 60 minutes of care tended to predict death or survival. Today this term can also be applied to the important hours and actions immediately after birth.[2] Initial rapid assessment of the newborn should follow guidelines published by the American Academy of Pediatrics. This initial gross assessment focuses on the newborn's color, tone, respirations, heart rate, and response to stimulation.

Term newborns who are transitioning well to extrauterine life, as evidenced by crying or breathing, good tone, and a heart rate more than 100 beats per minute, should be placed skin-to-skin on their parent's chest, dried, and supported with gentle, physiologic support. The birthing person can determine where the newborn should be placed ahead of the birth. If the individual is not parenting, they may prefer the infant to go directly to the parents. Once the cord is cut, anyone selected by the birthing person can provide skin-to-skin care, though if breastfeeding/chestfeeding is planned, it is best provided by the person who will nurse the baby.

Infants who are not transitioning well immediately after birth, as evidenced by gasping, apnea, and a low heart rate, should receive care according to national standards. In the United States, resuscitation care is as outlined in the American Academy of Pediatrics' *Guidelines for Neonatal Resuscitation*. The Apgar score can be assigned at 1 minute and 5 minutes after birth (see the *Physical Assessment of the Newborn* chapter) but should not guide resuscitation decisions. If clinically indicated, umbilical artery blood gases may be drawn during the period immediately after birth. See the *Umbilical Cord Gas Technique and Interpretation* appendix for more information. Also, if the parents have requested cord blood banking, cord blood for this purpose is collected at this time.

## Newborn Assessment and Care in the First Hours After Birth

For decades, immediate cord-clamping and placement of the infant on a warmer for evaluation and examination by healthcare professionals was the standard of practice. However, several well-conducted studies disputed the need for immediate evaluation and separation from the birthing parent during the first hour after birth.[3]

### Skin-to-Skin Contact

Placing the newborn on the parent's bare chest or abdomen provides several advantages. While on the chest, the infant can be dried and stimulated, Apgar scores assigned, and the initial assessment completed. Early skin-to-skin contact (SSC), also known as kangaroo care, has many theoretical benefits for both the infant and the birthing parent. During the drying process, the parent's warmth assists with neonatal thermoregulation. In addition, early prolonged SSC has been shown to lead to a longer period of exclusive breastfeeding and less crying among newborns when compared to infants who were separated from their parent immediately after birth.[4] Other potential advantages of SSC are presumed to be the establishment of a trusting relationship between the birth parent and child at a sensitive period, although long-term studies of the "sensitive period" hypothesis have not conclusively demonstrated that SSC improves parent–infant bonding over time. Increased oxytocin release has been noted with SSC as well. If an infant requires assistance at birth during the transition period, an effort should be made to get the infant back to the birthing parent as soon as possible to initiate SSC.

### Delayed Umbilical Cord-Clamping

For the well-transitioning newborn, the umbilical cord can be left intact for several minutes before being clamped and cut. The midwife can perform this task, or the birthing parent's partner or designated support person may cut the cord between two clamps. Delayed cord-clamping, as described in the *Umbilical Cord-Clamping at Birth* appendix, allows for blood in the umbilical and placental circulation to be physiologically transfused to the newborn and is recommended for all newborns.[5-8] Although professional association guidelines differ, evidence indicates that a delay of 3 to 5 minutes is optimal for the newborn.[9-12] The current recommendation from the American Academy of Pediatrics is to delay umbilical cord clamping for at least 30 to 60 seconds for most vigorous term and preterm infants.[12] The benefits and procedure for delayed cord-clamping are reviewed in the *Umbilical Cord-Clamping at Birth* appendix.

### Neonatal Hypothermia Prevention

Newborns are predisposed to developing hypothermia because of their large surface area per unit of body weight compared to adults. As discussed in the *Anatomy and Physiology of the Newborn* chapter, brown fat is the major site for production of heat in neonates and serves as the circulatory route for heat production, or nonshivering thermogenesis. The most crucial period for development of hypothermia is immediately after birth, as the infant is transitioning from a wet environment to a sometimes cold and drafty setting. Hypothermia is associated with depression of the central nervous system, hypoglycemia, metabolic acidosis, respiratory distress, pulmonary vasoconstriction, and decreased peripheral perfusion. The newborn is at higher risk for hypothermia following hypoxic, hypoglycemic, or other stressful episodes.

The practice of SSC provides the best source of heat for the newborn and can prevent hypothermia.[3,4] It has also been found to be at least equivalent to incubators for rewarming infants who already have experienced chilling,[13] and has additional benefits in facilitating breastfeeding initiation.[14] Table 39-1 lists other methods used to prevent hypothermia.

| Table 39-1 | Interventions to Prevent Newborn Hypothermia |
|---|---|
| Prewarm the newborn resuscitation area. | |
| Set the birth room temperature at 23.9°C (75°F). | |
| Prewarm any blankets, hats, or clothing prior to the birth. | |
| Place the newborn in skin-to-skin contact immediately after birth. | |
| Gently dry the newborn after birth, and then immediately replace wet blankets with dry ones. | |
| Do not evaluate the newborn on wet sheets or towels. | |
| Postpone the newborn's bath until newborn temperature has been stable for minimum 2 hours. | |
| Place the newborn care areas away from windows, outside walls, and doorways. | |
| Keep the newborn's head covered and body well wrapped. | |

Maintaining the temperature of the birth room at 25°C to 28°C (77°F to 82.4°F) is recommended by the World Health Organization (WHO).[13] Covering the newborn's head with a stockinet cap after initial drying is conventional care because the head has a large surface area from which heat can be lost. A warm, dry blanket can be tented over the newborn's head while the newborn is in SSC with the birth parent and will assist in thermostabilization. In addition, during SSC, thermoregulation is enhanced through a process of thermal synchrony with the birthing parent (the parent's chest skin temperature warms up in response to a cold infant and cools down if the infant is too warm).

The newborn's temperature can be assessed at various sites of the body with different types of thermometers. Historically, rectal temperatures were commonly measured in newborns, but this technique had some notable disadvantages: The rectal temperature can remain high after the core temperature drops; it can be affected by the presence of stool; and rectal perforation is possible. Therefore, rectal temperatures are no longer recommended. Axillary temperatures are normally in the range of 36.5°C to 37.5°C (97.7°F to 99.0°F) but may be falsely elevated in a cold-stressed infant due to metabolism of brown adipose tissue. Abdominal skin temperature is normally in the range of 36°C to 36.5°C (96.8°F to 97.7°F). Infrared tympanic thermometers (2 seconds in the ear) can be used to measure temperature but are the least reliable method in a newborn.

Noncontinuous temperature assessment will be accurate only if the thermometer remains in place for an adequate amount of time. If temperature is assessed with an abdominal skin sensor, the sensor must be in good contact with the skin and covered with a reflective shield. Skin temperatures should be slightly lower than core temperatures. The goal is to maintain skin temperature between 36.5°C and 37.5°C (97.7°F and 99.0°F) after birth.

### Neonatal Hypoglycemia: Prevention and Assessment

In the first 2 hours post birth, a newborn's blood glucose level normally falls to a nadir, which can be as low as 30 mg/dL. In utero, the fetus has a continuous supply of glucose, and the fetal glucose level is approximately 70% to 80% of the birth parent's glucose level. After birth, the newborn must adapt to the change from this continuous supply to an intermittent supply through feedings with breast milk or breast milk substitutes. Blood glucose levels may remain slightly low for several days, though the newborn will typically remain asymptomatic. Because there is a great deal of individual variability in blood glucose levels associated with clinical symptoms of hypoglycemia, no specific blood glucose value that defines hypoglycemia has been published.[14,15]

Despite the definitional controversy, newborns are at increased risk for hypoglycemia and specific risk factors have been identified. Specifically, newborns born to birth parents who have diabetes, who are preterm, and who are small for gestational age are at increased risk for hypoglycemia. Common symptoms of hypoglycemia include jitteriness, irritability, lethargy, or poor feeding. Blood glucose levels obtained by heel stick can be of value in diagnosing hypoglycemia. In general, glucose levels should be greater than 45 mg/dL after the first 12 hours of life.[15,16]

Early and frequent feeding is an important preventive measure that protects most newborns from developing clinical hypoglycemia. The exact degree of hypoglycemia that requires human milk or human milk substitute feeding, or intravenous administration of glucose, depends on other clinical factors, such as feeding ability, weight, and risk factors for hypoglycemia. Hypoglycemia can be easily treated; in extreme circumstances, prolonged hypoglycemia is associated with neurodevelopmental delays.

Evaluation of hypoglycemia is done through capillary blood sampling. However, bedside glucometers are known to vary, with the greatest variation noted at low values. It is recommended that values noted to be low on rapid-test glucometers be confirmed with a laboratory specimen. However, if the initial results are low, treatment should not be delayed while awaiting repeat results.[17]

The newborn's heel should be prewarmed prior to obtaining the capillary specimen.[18,19] When performing this blood test, care should be taken to avoid puncturing sensitive structures on the back of the heel (**Figure 39-1**). Use of an automated blood collection device may cause less trauma and lead to more successful sample collection results than use of manual lancets and squeezing the heel, which creates hemolysis.[18] To prevent infection, the infant's heel should be cleansed with antiseptic, followed by sterile water, and allowed to air dry. Alcohol should be avoided, as it is drying and can leave residue. Newborn discomfort may be diminished by swaddling, being held in the arms of the neonate's parent or other family member, and non-nutritive sucking.

Any glucose level below the recommended threshold for normal requires intervention. Feeding the infant is the first step. A repeat glucose test is

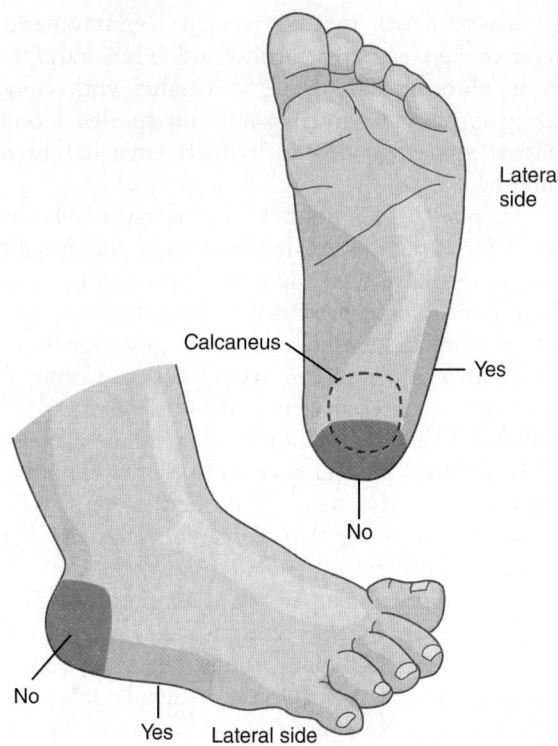

Lateral side

Calcaneus

Yes

No

No

Yes    Lateral side

**Figure 39-1** Anatomic landmarks for heel sticks.

performed 30 minutes after feeding. If the low value is confirmed, pediatric consultation is needed, and treatment is indicated. It is recommended that infants at increased risk have feeds initiated within the first hour of life with subsequent feedings every 2 to 3 hours, and preprandial glucose checks for the first 24 hours of life.

Venous samples can be analyzed using either whole blood or plasma (serum). Samples should be chilled during transport to the laboratory. Most laboratories report the plasma result, which will be close to 15% higher than a sample run on whole blood. Thus, it is important to know the testing method and reference ranges used by a particular laboratory to accurately interpret the results.

### Initial Newborn Prophylaxis Treatments

Two prophylactic treatments are recommended for newborns within the first 4 hours of life: ophthalmic treatment for prevention of ophthalmia neonatorum and administration of vitamin K to prevent hemorrhagic disease of the newborn.

### *Ophthalmic Treatments*

Eye prophylaxis is pharmacologic treatment originally intended to prevent blindness associated with undiagnosed perinatal *Neisseria gonorrhoeae*

infection. Today in the United States, neonatal conjunctivitis (also known as ophthalmia neonatorum) is more commonly caused by *Chlamydia trachomatis*, although infection with *N. gonorrhoeae* is more likely to cause loss of vision.[20–22] Screening and treatment of the birthing person during pregnancy is the first step in prevention of blindness caused by chlamydia or gonorrhea but does not guarantee that reinfection will not occur at the time of birth.

The risk that an infant will acquire conjunctivitis is 20% to 50% if the parent is infected when they give birth. Neonatal conjunctivitis due to *C. trachomatis* infection usually becomes symptomatic 5 to 14 days after birth but can present earlier.[22] Conjunctivitis due to *N. gonorrhoeae* infection becomes symptomatic in infants at 1 to 5 days after birth.[22,23] Infants with suspected *C. trachomatis* or *N. gonorrhoeae* infection need a referral and will likely receive systemic antibiotic treatment.

In the past, silver nitrate or tetracyclines were used as treatments to prevent colonization leading to conjunctivitis or blindness. Neither product is currently available in the United States. Erythromycin 0.5% ophthalmic ointment is the Centers for Disease Control and Prevention's (CDC) recommended agent for neonatal ocular prophylaxis throughout the United States. Its effectiveness against *N. gonorrhoeae* and *C. trachomatis* conjunctivitis is well documented.[22] A small percentage of infants may develop chemical conjunctivitis after eye prophylaxis, which typically resolves spontaneously within 24 to 48 hours. Though not common in the United States, povidone-iodine is widely used around the world for prevention of colonization with *N. gonorrhoeae*. A Cochrane review of high-, middle-, and low-income countries found that newborns given ophthalmic prophylaxis were less likely to have conjunctivitis at 1 month of age compared to infants not given prophylaxis.[23]

The CDC recommends that prophylaxis be administered as soon after birth as possible. The medication is placed on each of the lower conjunctival sacs and spread with gentle massage of the eyelids. The excess ointment can be wiped away after 1 minute, but the eyes should not be irrigated, as that practice can reduce the efficacy of the prophylaxis.[22]

### *Prophylactic Administration of Vitamin K*

Vitamin K is a fat-soluble vitamin that is required for the body's production of functional forms of factors II, VII, IX, and X. For adults, most vitamin K is obtained from the intestinal flora. Infants are born with low stores of vitamin K and have insufficient intake following birth, especially if fed exclusively human milk.

Vitamin K–deficiency bleeding (VKDB) is a bleeding disorder in which coagulation rapidly responds to vitamin K supplementation. Classical VKDB occurs between 24 hours and 7 days of life and is commonly associated with delayed or insufficient feeding. Infants may present with bruises, gastrointestinal blood loss, or bleeding from the umbilicus and puncture sites. Blood loss can range from mild to significant, including intracranial hemorrhage. Prothrombin time, thrombin time, and partial thromboplastin time are slightly prolonged in the neonatal period. Late VKDB occurs between 2 to 12 weeks of life and is associated with exclusive breastfeeding. Generally, the clinical presentation is severe, with a 50% incidence of intracranial hemorrhage and a 20% mortality rate.[24,25]

To prevent bleeding related to vitamin K deficiency, it is customary to give newborns supplementary vitamin K after birth. The most common route of administration for vitamin K is intramuscular, as studies have not demonstrated a reliably effective oral vitamin K dose.[24,25] As there are many common myths about vitamin K prophylaxis, parents should be referred to evidence-based sources, such as the CDC, to assist them in understanding the need for and preferred administration of vitamin K.

### Cord Treatments

For decades, treatment of the umbilical cord stump was initiated immediately or shortly after birth. Various antiseptic solutions were used for this purpose, including rubbing alcohol, iodine, goldenseal, and echinacea. Currently, evidence suggests that best practice is to simply keep the area clean and dry. If the umbilical area becomes soiled with urine or stool, cleansing with plain water is sufficient. A Cochrane systematic review found that newborns with umbilical cord stumps treated with antiseptic solutions were no more or less likely to develop omphalitis when compared to neonates who received no treatment or placebo.[26]

Cord care practices vary worldwide and employ a variety of substances applied to the umbilical stump.[27,28] WHO recommends daily chlorhexidine as a cord treatment during the first week of life for newborns born at home in settings with high neonatal mortality.[29] Clean, dry cord care is recommended for newborns born in health facilities, and at home in settings with low neonatal mortality.[29] In

all birth and outpatient settings, signs of infection of the umbilical cord or site, including discharge, foul odor, and inflammation of the cord site, should be promptly assessed and treated as described later in this chapter.

## The First Hours: The Newborn with a Health Condition

The wide availability of fetal screening and testing means that parents and care providers often have time to plan for infants with health conditions. However, prenatal assessments of fetal morphology do not detect congenital anomalies in all cases. When a newborn presents with an unexpected health problem, the midwife identifies deviations from normal and initiates transfer to pediatric care. A critical component of this process is communicating the extent and urgency of pediatric intervention required.

### Newborn Conditions Requiring Non-urgent Pediatric Consultation

Addressing a single (isolated) abnormality that does not impair the transition to extrauterine life and is not associated with other abnormalities can often wait until the neonate's regular care provider or a regional specialist can see the infant. If the newborn has two or more minor abnormalities, the likelihood of a major disorder is increased, and the infant should be evaluated by a pediatric specialist more rapidly. A poor transition to extrauterine life in these infants may indicates that more urgent assessment is needed.

Common findings on a newborn examination that, in isolation in a well-transitioning newborn, require a non-urgent consultation include hypospadias, extra digits without other evidence of a syndromic disorders, unilateral malformations of the ear pinna, unilateral malformations of the shape of a limb or foot, and hearing screening failures.

### Newborn Conditions Requiring Consultation in the First Hours or Days of Life

Some physical variations found on a newborn exam are associated with long-term health outcomes or may be indicative of a larger syndrome or genetic disorder, but do not require immediate attention if the infant is transitioning well. These infants can be supported and monitored, remaining with their parent(s) in the original birth facility while they await additional assessment. Some examples of conditions requiring pediatric consultation within the first few hours or days of life are described in this section. Since many disorders first become apparent in the newborn period, the midwife should err on the side of caution, asking for pediatric consultation if a morphologic defect or risk factor for poor transition to extra-uterine life is identified.

### Malformations Affecting Function

Any malformations that affect bodily function need timely assessment by a pediatric provider, and the rapidity of assessment depends on the potential for disruption of the neonate's transition to extrauterine life. Gentle support while remaining skin-to-skin with a parent may facilitate the physiologic transition for newborns with many minor abnormalities. For example, infants with a cleft lip may struggle with feeding, but may be successful if left skin-to-skin and given gentle assistance with positioning.

### Musculoskeletal Concerns

Management of bone fractures includes obtaining a pediatric consultation and splinting. If a clavicle or arm fracture is suspected, parents can be assured that newborn bones usually heal well and quickly. The assessment of the fractured extremity will include evaluation for potential nerve injury.

Infants with isolated and unilateral limb malformations can receive supportive care until additional assessment can occur. Care for congenital hip dysplasia can also be delayed until morning or a pediatric consultant is available.

### Evidence of Syndrome or Risk Factors in a Well-Transitioning Newborn

Infants with two or more minor abnormalities or one major abnormality (as described in the *Physical Assessment of the Newborn* chapter) who are breathing well, with a normal heart rate, and feeding without difficulty, can also remain with their parents with additional monitoring until consultation can be obtained. These infants need prompt assessment but do not require urgent, specialist-level care. Examples include newborns with bilateral malformations such as webbed digits and ear abnormalities. Infants with an abnormal red reflex, especially white coloration instead of red, need prompt evaluation due to the risk of retinoblastoma. With a normal transition to extrauterine life, including good feeding, assessment can be delayed until after the first hours of life.

### Newborn Conditions Requiring Urgent Referral to Specialist Care

Often life-threatening conditions are known about prior to birth and a team is present to immediately assist with specialized neonatal care. However, some life-threatening congenital conditions do not become known until the moment of birth or soon afterward. For these newborns, a plan for care must be rapidly developed and implemented. In the United States, most areas have a regional center that can provide care and accept referrals of sick newborns; infants may need to be transferred to a regional center to have access to specialists and appropriate diagnostic equipment.

### Cardiac Conditions

Cardiac conditions in newborns result from a variety of causes and mimic other conditions such as respiratory disease and sepsis. Pulse oximetry is advocated for all infants after the first 24 hours of life and can be used to identify such anomalies.[30,31] Some newborns will quickly demonstrate signs of an underlying structural congenital heart defect. These defects may affect the heart valves, the walls between the atria and the ventricles, or the heart muscle itself.

Primary signs of heart disease include central cyanosis, murmurs, and other cardiac sounds.[31] Depending on the defect, pulses may be either bounding or diminished. Pulses can vary in intensity from the upper to lower extremities. Similarly, based on the defect, a loud murmur may be present at birth or may not be heard until 1 to 2 weeks after birth. The cyanosis of heart disease may be present over the entire body, which differentiates this condition from the peripheral cyanosis that is often found in healthy newborns shortly after birth, or the acrocyanosis that may persist for the first 24 to 48 hours. For infants with a ventral septal defect, oxygenated blood crosses over the opening in the septum and recirculates through the lungs. In this case, cyanosis may not be present, and a murmur may not be heard until the infant reaches 2 or more weeks of age, when the compensatory measure of increased pulmonary vascular resistance diminishes and more blood flows from the left side to the right side of the heart. This shift is characteristic of a large defect and may be associated with a subtle onset of congestive heart failure evidenced by tachypnea, feeding problems, and failure to thrive. A parent may describe troubling symptoms during a postpartum visit or during calls about breastfeeding. In infants with smaller ventricular septal defects, a systolic murmur is heard soon after birth; a small defect rarely leads to congestive heart failure.

Some newborns will not make the transition from intrauterine to extrauterine circulation without intervention. In these neonates, pulmonary resistance remains so high that blood flow through the newborn lungs is decreased. This relatively rare phenomenon results in persistent pulmonary hypertension (formerly called persistent fetal circulation). Signs include cyanosis, tachypnea, nasal flaring, and intercostal retractions. Because of the high level of resistance from the lungs, the ductus arteriosus and the foramen ovale may stay open with subsequent right-to-left shunting. In this case, peripheral pulses will be bounding, the precordium will be active, and a murmur will be heard.[32]

Midwifery management of newborns with acute signs of heart disease includes immediate consultation with the pediatric team and supportive care for resulting respiratory distress. The newborn's heart rate and respiratory rate are constantly monitored. If heart disease is suspected, the blood arterial oxygen saturation in the right hand can be compared to that of a lower extremity. In persistent pulmonary hypertension, the saturation is lower in the descending aorta. Warm, humidified oxygen is provided at high concentrations, as oxygen is a potent vasodilator and may help decrease pulmonary vascular resistance. When the newborn has a cardiac defect, however, even high concentrations of oxygen may not lead to normal cardiorespiratory function. If the newborn is tachypneic, oral feedings are withheld. The metabolic demands of respiratory distress will predispose newborns to hypoglycemia.

### Respiratory Conditions

Symptoms of respiratory dysregulation are the most widely encountered abnormal finding in newborns. Common pulmonary causes of neonatal respiratory distress in term infants include pneumothorax, aspiration of meconium, neonatal pneumonia, and transient tachypnea of the newborn (Table 39-2). Signs of respiratory distress include tachypnea (more than 60 breaths/min), nasal flaring, retractions of intercostal muscles or the sternum if severe, or grunting. Cyanosis, rales, or rhonchi are possible. Central cyanosis (of the trunk, lips, tongue, and oral mucous membranes) is a sign of serious compromise of hemoglobin oxygen saturation and requires supplemental oxygen.

If a newborn is having respiratory distress, continued monitoring of the heart rate, respiratory rate, and oxygen saturations are necessary while awaiting pediatric consultation or transport. To assess the oxygen level, use continuous pulse oximetry. This method computes arterial oxygen saturation ($SaO_2$), with an acceptable level being between 92% and 95% after the first 10 minutes of life. If possible, check the newborn's blood pressure.

| Table 39-2 | Common Neonatal Respiratory Conditions |
|---|---|
| **Condition** | **Comments** |
| Transient tachypnea of newborn (TTN) results from a prolonged period of transitioning from fluid-filled to air-filled lungs. | TTN lasts 48 to 72 hours with spontaneous resolution, although newborns may need supplemental oxygen and assistance with feedings. Generally, infants with TTN are monitored in the hospital until the condition resolves. |
| Meconium aspiration that can result in pneumonitis, hypoxia, respiratory failure, and persistent pulmonary hypertension. | Can require support ranging from a nasal cannula to mechanical ventilation and occasionally extracorporeal membrane oxygenation (ECMO). |
| Neonatal pneumonia caused by bacteria, viruses, or other microorganisms. | Antimicrobial agents and supportive therapy. |
| Pneumothorax (unilateral or bilateral), often after mechanical ventilation and overdistension. | Small pneumothoraxes may resolve spontaneously; a large pneumothorax compromising cardiac output is an emergency. |
| Congenital anomalies causing airway obstruction or pulmonary obstruction. | Infant may need immediate intervention and may require surgical intervention once stabilized. |
| Respiratory distress due to sepsis. | Evaluate for risk factors and other signs of sepsis such as temperature variations, poor feeding, and lethargy. Sepsis calculators can be helpful in assessment. |

### Facial Palsy and Brachial Plexus Injuries

Palsies and plexus conditions are generally categorized as birth injuries and traditionally have been assumed to be associated with an event such as shoulder dystocia. Sometimes injury may occur in utero, such that parents and professionals are surprised when a child is born with a palsy or injury after an uneventful labor and birth.[33–35]

Injuries to the face include bruising from forceps or facial palsy caused by forceps or pressure from the birth parent's sacrum. Consultation will be needed for infants with persistent palsy, and use of lubricating eye drops may be a necessary if the infant is unable to close the eyelids.

Injuries to the brachial plexus may occur prenatally or during a birth when traction is applied to the neck.[34,35] Such injuries can occur during breech births, during births involving shoulder dystocia, or following an operative vaginal birth.

Management includes referral to occupational and physical therapy as well as consultation with the pediatric team. Physical and occupational therapy should begin as soon as possible. Parents are encouraged to minimize handling the affected extremity for the first week of life because of pain and swelling involved. If there is concern for bony injury, immobilization of the extremity is recommended. Parents can be reassured that in most newborns, paralysis disappears in 3 to 6 months, with initial improvement becoming evident within a few weeks.

Injuries to nerve roots higher in the brachial plexus (C3 to C5) can cause significant respiratory compromise because of paralysis of the phrenic nerve and diaphragmatic compromise. Newborns with this type of nerve injury can be observed to take very shallow breaths with limited respiratory excursion and need aggressive respiratory support after birth. When injuries do not respond to 6 months of physical therapy, surgical repairs are often attempted. In most cases, infants have complete recovery, but residual damage can persist, especially with injuries in the higher cervical regions.[34,35]

### Cephalohematoma, Subgaleal Hemorrhage, Intracranial Hemorrhage, and Skull Fractures

Traumatic birth injuries to the head include cephalohematoma, subgaleal hematoma, intracranial hemorrhage, scalp abrasions, retinal hemorrhage, and skull fractures.[36] Cephalohematomas and small scalp abrasions occur in approximately 10% of newborns who are born by vacuum extraction.[36] Cephalohematomas can also occur during a spontaneous vaginal birth, although the incidence of such injuries is much lower under this condition. More severe cranial hemorrhages are often associated with use of forceps or vacuum births.

Pediatric support is needed urgently if symptoms of a subgaleal hemorrhage are present. With a severe subgaleal hemorrhage, a newborn can experience rapid blood loss, with potentially loss of their entire blood volume into the subgaleal space. Infants with subgaleal hemorrhage will present with increasing head circumference and a fluctuant mass that crosses suture lines. The edema may be significant, extending from the scalp down into the eyes, ears, and neck. Symptoms of intracranial hemorrhage generally appear a few hours after birth and include irritability, apnea, poor feeding, lethargy, and possibly a bulging fontanel.

A clear sign of a skull fracture is a depressed area of the skull, particularly over the parietal bones. An area of skull depression increases the likelihood that fragments of skull bone have penetrated through the dura, the covering of the brain. Management includes careful positioning of the newborn on the side opposite of the affected area and consultation with the pediatric team, who will order imaging tests.

### Abdominal Wall Defects

Abdominal wall defects are subdivided into gastroschisis and omphalocele, both of which have unclear etiologies.[37,38] *Gastroschisis* is a condition that develops between weeks 4 and 10 of gestation, in which protrusion of the bowel occurs through an abdominal wall defect. As a result of the bowel being exposed to amniotic fluid throughout the pregnancy, at birth the bowel may be matted or dilated. The prevalence of gastroschisis is increasing, and its incidence in the United States is now 3.8 per 10,000 live births.[37]

In an *omphalocele*, the abdominal organs are external to the infant's body, but are covered by peritoneal membrane that protects the intestines from exposure to amniotic fluid and, after birth, ambient air. In such a case, there is a high likelihood of infection, hypothermia, and dehydration because of the large surface area that is exposed. An omphalocele is one of the most common anterior abdominal wall defects. Concurrent gastrointestinal, genitourinary, chromosomal, musculoskeletal, and central nervous system anomalies are common in infants with this condition—that is, about 40% to 80% of cases will have at least one concurrent anomaly.[38]

Management of newborns with an abdominal wall defect requires an immediate call for pediatric assistance and transport to a tertiary pediatric hospital or unit. The newborn is placed in a radiant warmer in as sterile an environment as possible. With birth of the newborn and recognition of the defect, the exposed bowel needs to be protected. The current recommendation is to place the infant in either a plastic bag or plastic wrap.[37–40] Wrapping the defect in sterile gauze is no longer recommended since the gauze can further exacerbate matting of the bowel. In addition, careful attention to positioning is needed to prevent kinking and decreased perfusion to the intestines; right-sided positioning is preferred. Shortly after birth, a gastric tube is inserted to decompress the intestines. The infant is not given enteral feedings. Immediate administration of intravenous fluids is needed since rapid and significant insensible water loss via evaporative losses from the exposed bowel can occur.

### Neural Tube Defects

The two most common neural tube defects are meningocele and meningomyelocele (also called spina bifida).[41,42] A *meningocele* is a defect in the spinal cord with protrusion of the meninges and cerebrospinal fluid into the subcutaneous tissue. The skin is usually intact. With a *meningomyelocele*, the vertebra is defective, and the spinal cord and spinal roots are externally located in a meningeal sac. Meningomyeloceles are usually found in the lower spine, lumbar, and sacral areas. The principles for immediate management of spinal cord defects are similar to those described for abdominal wall defects: application of a sterile, warm saline dressing with a dry sterile overwrap; thermoregulation; and fluid maintenance. In addition, the infant is positioned prone and fecal contamination is scrupulously avoided. With both abdominal wall and neural tube defects, sterile gloves should be used when handling the area.[41,42]

### Diaphragmatic Hernia

Diaphragmatic hernias are surgical emergencies in the newborn, because herniation of abdominal contents into the chest cavity in utero may have resulted in pulmonary hypoplasia.[43] Diaphragmatic hernias are usually unilateral, typically on the left side. The degree of respiratory distress is directly related to the amount of lung tissue that has been compromised. In some newborns, the herniation is so severe that lung growth has been stunted, if any occurred, on the affected side. Signs of diaphragmatic hernia include a scaphoid abdomen, barrel-shaped chest, decreased left-sided breath sounds, heart sounds on the right side, and severe respiratory distress at birth due to pulmonary hypoplasia. Skilled pediatric care must be sought immediately, as these infants need immediate intubation in cases of compromising respiratory distress. Infants with this defect should not receive bag and mask ventilation, as this intervention can further compromise the affected lung if the intestines become distended with air.

### Congenital and Acquired Newborn Infections

Newborns may present with infection acquired either in utero or during the intrapartum or immediate postpartum period.[44] The immune system of newborns is immature (as discussed in the *Anatomy and Physiology of the Newborn* chapter), which means that infections can rapidly progress to sepsis. Management depends on the pathogen and transmissibility of the pathogenic agent, but may include isolation of the infant from other newborns and from pregnant healthcare workers until the pathogen is identified. Typically, the birth parent and infant can be isolated together.

Two neonatal infections that are initially localized include conjunctivitis and infection of the umbilical cord. Conjunctivitis, which manifests as discharge from the eye along with localized redness, can be related to post-birth contact with normal skin flora or pathogens. Ophthalmia and conjunctivitis can also be signs of vertical transmission of maternal infection, such as gonorrhea and chlamydia, to the neonate. Symptoms of eye infections should be promptly investigated to ensure rapid local and systemic treatment as needed.

Infections starting with or near the umbilical cord are a major cause of neonatal morbidity and mortality in some geographic areas. The umbilical cord tissue is susceptible to infection when it comes into contact with bacteria or other pathogens, especially when the cord stays moist. *Staphylococcus aureus* is the most common causal organism. Infections of the umbilical cord tissue and the surrounding area can rapidly progress from the cord itself to the abdominal wall, and then to systemic infection and sepsis. Signs of infection, such as an unhealthy-looking umbilical cord with a foul odor or discharge from the cord or stump and inflammation or infection of the skin and tissues surrounding the umbilicus, should receive prompt assessment and treatment in concert with specialists.[1]

Rapid assessment of potential infections is important as part of sepsis prevention and treatment. Risk factors for early-onset sepsis include: preterm birth, increasing duration of rupture of membranes, maternal fever, chorioamnionitis, inadequate treatment for group B *Streptococcus,* and lack of intrapartum antibiotic administration.[45] Common bacterial pathogens in neonatal sepsis acquired in utero and during the intrapartum and postpartum period include group B *Streptococcus, Escherichia coli,* and *Listeria monocytogenes.*[45] Table 39-3 lists symptoms of neonatal sepsis, but symptoms often appear only after infection is systemic. If sepsis is suspected, immediate consultation is indicated because the immature immune system of newborns can become quickly overwhelmed by infection.

If in utero infection acquisition is suspected, cord blood is saved for further testing. Depending on the pathogen, infants with congenitally acquired infections may manifest a variety of symptoms, such as growth restriction, pathologic jaundice, rash, petechiae, skin lesions, congenital cataracts, hepatosplenomegaly, microcephaly, seizures, and lymphadenopathy.[44,45] Laboratory testing may reveal abnormal liver, kidney, and hematologic function. The effects of the infection will vary according to the timing of fetal exposure and the severity of the infection.

The TORCH acronym has been used to describe five congenital infections that have similar presentations: Toxoplasmosis, Other (syphilis), Rubella,

| Table 39-3 | Signs of Neonatal Sepsis |
|---|---|
| Lethargy | |
| Poor feeding | |
| Temperature instability (hypothermia or hyperthermia) | |
| Respiratory distress or apnea | |
| Abdominal distension | |
| Pallor | |
| Cyanosis | |
| Evidence of poor circulation with cool extremities | |
| Vomiting and/or abnormal stool pattern | |
| Jaundice | |
| Hypoglycemia | |
| Jitteriness or seizures | |

Based on AAP Committee on Fetus and Newborn, ACOG Committee on Obstetric Practice. *Guidelines for Perinatal Care.* 7th ed. Elk Village, IL: American Academy of Pediatrics Books; 2017. doi.org/10.1542/9781610020886; Mukhopadhyay S, Eichenwald EC, Puopolo KM. Neonatal early-onset sepsis evaluations among well-appearing infants: projected impact of changes in CDC GBS guidelines. *J Perinatol.* 2013;33(3):198-205.

Cytomegalovirus, and Herpes simplex virus. However, there are other well-known causes of in utero infection, such as enteroviruses, varicella-zoster virus, parvovirus B19, and Zika virus.[44] While the presence of immunoglobulin M (IgM) antibodies in cord blood can help to confirm a suspected viral infection, it is rare that IgM antibodies are present at birth to aid in diagnosis. Often the diagnosis of congenital infection does not become clear until the infant is older. Treatment in the newborn period is commonly based on symptoms.

### Signs of Neurologic Compromise

The most common sign of neurologic compromise in the newborn period is seizure activity. Neonatal seizures have many etiologies, ranging from hypoglycemia to neonatal encephalopathy.[46] Treatment is based on the underlying cause of the seizure. Prognosis is also related to the etiology more than the seizure activity itself, unless seizures are prolonged or frequent. In rare cases, a congenital abnormality of the brain may be present. In the older newborn, seizures can be an indicator of an inborn error of metabolism.[46]

Newborns may present with evidence of various types of seizure activity, including subclinical manifestations that present as subtle changes in vital signs.[46,47] Signs of seizures may include sucking motions, chewing, bicycling of limbs, drooling, apnea, lip smacking, deviation of the eyes, and eyelid fluttering, which present as short, repetitive bursts of activity. Such repetitive behavioral patterns can be observed during a newborn examination. Because there is an association between hypoglycemia and seizure activity, a point-of-care glucose screening is recommended when seizure activity is suspected. Because of the risk of apnea, the newborn with possible seizure activity is carefully monitored for cessation of respirations.

Current treatment for newborns with seizures due to hypoxia–ischemic encephalopathy (HIE) includes therapeutic hypothermia or brain cooling, which should be initiated soon after birth.[46,47] Infants with HIE typically have injury to the brain occurring either intrapartum or in utero, so if certain risk factors are present (e.g., perinatal asphyxia, cardiorespiratory depression, and need for resuscitation after birth), the midwife should maintain a narrower window of suspicion.

Other types of seizures (multifocal, focal) are less common in newborns. Signs of these types of seizures include movement of one limb with progression to other limbs or movement of both limbs on one side of the body. These movements can be confused with nonpathologic jitteriness related to neurologic immaturity. To differentiate between the two, gentle steady pressure should be applied to the extremity. In the case of seizure activity, the movement of the extremity would persist, whereas with jitteriness the movement will stop.

### Gastrointestinal Defects

Tracheoesophageal fistula and esophageal atresia are not visible on physical examination. However, signs such as excess salivation, respiratory distress, coughing with feedings, and difficulty swallowing will be present. If an esophageal fistula is suspected, a referral to a specialist is needed for diagnosis and nutritional stabilization. Tracheoesophageal fistula and esophageal atresia often occur together; however, esophageal atresia can also occur independently.[48]

A variety of congenital defects can lead to intestinal obstruction in the newborn. Among these are malrotation and midgut volvulus, meconium plugs, meconium ileus, Hirschsprung disease (megacolon), and imperforate anus. The major diagnostic signs of all these anomalies are bile-stained emesis, abdominal distension, and failure to pass stool. Significant abdominal distension will be present if the newborn has meconium ileus, meconium plug, and Hirschsprung disease.[49,50] Newborns with these symptoms must be evaluated immediately by a pediatric provider, as the causative conditions can be surgical emergencies. In the case of bilious emesis, the infant should be immediately put on NPO (nothing by mouth) status and consultation with a pediatric provider arranged. If neglected, any of these defects can lead to intestinal perforation and death.

### Genitourinary Defects

Many types and causes of genitourinary malformations are possible, which have a wide range of effects on function. Renal anomalies, such as fetal renal pyelectasis and pelviectasis, can be discovered with ultrasound, and there may already be a plan within the chart for postnatal care of infants in such cases. For infants with newly suspected renal abnormalities, urgent consultation with a specialist is indicated.[51]

Infants with ambiguous genitalia need an immediate referral to a specialist, as this condition is associated with congenital adrenal hyperplasia and the inability to regulate salts and fluids. These infants will undergo blood tests, genetic testing, and imaging. It may take time to get a definitive diagnosis and plan; during this time, the midwife can support the parents and use gender-neutral terms for the infant.[2, 52]

## The First Days: Common Newborn Behavior

Parental advice from professionals, websites, social media, and even family often presumes that all newborns act similarly. Of course, each neonate is an individual—and all information, especially about behavior, should be viewed in that light. The midwife can help parents develop realistic expectations about common newborn behaviors during the newborn period.

### Sleep and Wake States

Newborns are in a period of behavioral instability. By the time parents figure out a pattern of newborn behavior, that pattern will have changed. A good rule of thumb for the first month of life is "There is no pattern."

Newborns' activities can be organized into two major categories of behavior: periods of waking and periods of sleeping. Waking states include crying, considerable motor activity, alertness, and drowsiness. Sleep states include active (light) sleep and deep sleep. Table 39-4 summarizes these states, along with their implications for care.[52–54]

During the first month of life, the percentage of time spent in each of these states changes. Healthy newborns spend as much as 60% of their time sleeping. However, much of this sleep takes the form of short naps. As the first month of life progresses, newborns shift away from active (light) sleep and toward more extended periods of deep sleep. Similarly, there is a shift in the waking states toward an increase in alertness.

### Sensory Capabilities

Sensory capabilities are strongly related to gestational age. Dramatic increases in the sensory stimulation that occur just after birth can lead to neonatal exhaustion, evidenced as fussiness or aversion. Crying infants and fatigued parturients are frequently encountered in tandem.[52,54]

At term, the healthy newborn has an ability to fix on and track objects visually for up to 25 centimeters from their eyes.[53] Many studies have shown a strong newborn preference for patterns of stripes. During the first month of life, however, newborns become preferentially interested in patterns with

| Table 39-4 | **Infant Behavioral States** | | | | |
|---|---|---|---|---|---|
| **State** | **Appearance** | **Eye/Facial Movements** | **Breathing** | **Response to Stimuli** | **Implications** |
| **Sleep States** | | | | | |
| Quiet sleep (deep sleep) | Essentially still with occasional startle | Eyes closed, no spontaneous movements | Smooth and regular | Only responds to intense stimuli | Avoid trying to feed at this time; will lead to frustration<br><br>Active growth hormones are released during this state |
| Active sleep (light sleep/REM sleep) | A few body movements; sucking movements may occur | REM<br><br>Fluttering of eyes with occasional smiling or crying sounds | Irregular | More responsive to hunger and handling than in quiet sleep; if stimulated, may return to active sleep, then progress to quiet sleep or arousal | Highest proportion of newborn sleep; brain growth and differentiation occur during this time<br><br>Usually occurs before arousal<br><br>Although may provide evidence of hunger, will not eat well in this state |
| **Awake States** | | | | | |
| Drowsy | Activity varies | Eyes may open and close or dull and heavy lidded<br><br>Although often no facial movement, may smile or make sounds | Irregular | Will respond to stimuli, although response may be delayed | To promote awakening, provide stimulation such as visual, auditory, or sucking stimuli |
| Quiet alert | Minimal movements | Eyes widen<br><br>Face appears bright and attentive | Regular | Very responsive | Often occurs immediately after nonmedicated birth and can be positive for parent–child interactions<br><br>As infant ages, spends more time in this state<br><br>Good state in which to feed and play with infant |
| Alert, fussy | Jerking, disorganized movements | Eyes are open, but appearance is more dull<br><br>Although often no facial movement, may smile or make sounds | Irregular | Transitional state to crying; fussiness with too much stimulation | More sensitive to stimuli (e.g., hunger, handling)<br><br>May move into crying state<br><br>If fatigued, may move into drowsy or sleep state |

| State | Appearance | Eye/Facial Movements | Breathing | Response to Stimuli | Implications |
|-------|-----------|----------------------|-----------|---------------------|--------------|
| Crying | Increased body movements, often with darkening skin tones | Eyes may be open or closed Grimaces | More irregular than other states | Communication of hunger, pain, discomfort, tiredness | Sometimes crying infants can self-console May need swaddling, cuddling, or other measures to resolve crying |

Abbreviation: REM, rapid eye movement.

Based on Blackburn S, Bakewell-Sachs S. *Understanding the Behavior of Term Infants*. White Plains, NY: March of Dimes Birth Defects Foundation. http://www.marchofdimes.com/nursing/modnemedia/othermedia/states.pdf. Accessed July 12, 2017.

contours that resemble the human face. The ability to see in color is limited at first, so newborns respond well to black-and-white patterns or bold colors like red. Newborns in the alert behavioral state will spend several minutes staring at patterns.

Newborns can discriminate among distinctive odors.[54] For example, a newborn can discriminate between the odor of the birthing parent's breast pad and the odors of breast pads from other nursing people. Newborns react strongly to variations in taste and show a strong preference for sweet liquids.

Newborns have acute hearing and can localize sound in the environment. They can discriminate finely among sounds and show a preference for actual voices as opposed to synthesized voices. By the end of 1 month, neonates prefer sounds with a pattern that resembles speech.

Prior to birth, the fetus experienced touch in the form of the shifting amniotic fluid. At birth, the newborn is dry for the first time and is subject to many and varied forms of touch. The ability of the newborn to respond to touch is well demonstrated with the elicitation of the various exteroceptive reflexes such as rooting, grasping, abdominal reflexes, and spinal curving.

### Regulation of Behavior

Infants may convey their ability or inability to engage by exhibiting a variety of neurobehavioral cues. For example, stability and engagement cues include sucking, smiling, feeding posture, flexion of arms and legs, searching for a sound, facial eye-to-eye contact, and normal vital signs. Distress cues in newborns include crying, grimacing, startled or jerky movements, changes in skin color and turgor, grunting, arching, tachypnea or bradycardia, jitteriness, flaccidity or tremors, and vomiting, frequent regurgitation, or stooling.[54]

Caregivers play a critical role in brain development by interacting and helping the infant regulate the stress response system. The caregiver interprets behavioral cues and responds with visual, vocal, and physical interactions that provide feedback to the infant. Each infant has a unique ability to react to stimulation presented by the environment and personal bodily functions. Infants vary in their responses to these stimuli, but generally learn best in the alert state.

On occasion, a midwife may recommend to parents that the Brazelton Neonatal Behavioral Assessment Scale (NBAS) be performed.[55] This test generates a picture of the infant's communication through responses to stimuli and neurologic reflexes. The results are then used to help parents interpret their newborn's behaviors. The NBAS is standardized and can be reliably administered only by a trained examiner. Testing begins with the newborn in a sleeping state. Repeated stimulations are offered, and the examiner observes how the newborn adjusts to the stimuli. The behavioral components of the NBAS assess the infant's ability to perform the six tasks listed in Table 39-5.[54]

Several other assessment instruments address infant behaviors and development. For example, the Denver Developmental Screening Test (Denver Scale) assesses children from birth to age 6 years. Like the NBAS, this test observes the actions of the child and can assist in identifying conditions suggestive of neurologic compromise. The Broussard Neonatal Perception Inventory explores how parents perceive their infants and assesses the attachment of the birth parent to child.[55] Several other assessments exist, but most—if not all—are intended as screening tools and not diagnostic instruments.

| Table 39-5 | Behavioral Components of the Brazelton Neonatal Behavioral Assessment Scale |
|---|---|
| Organization of behavioral state | |
| Decrease in motor activity to cope with sensory input | |
| Ability to become alert and oriented to auditory and visual stimuli | |
| Interaction with a caregiver through cuddling | |
| Ability for self-consoling | |
| Habituation to repeated stimulation | |

Based on Brazelton TB, Nugent JK. *Neonatal Behavioral Assessment Scale.* 4th ed. London: Mac Keith Press; 2011.

## The First Days of Life: Care of the Well Neonate

### Feeding

The *Infant Feeding and Lactation* chapter provides an overview of methods of feeding and establishment of breastfeeding or chestfeeding.

### Newborn Bathing

The World Health Organization (WHO) recommends delaying bathing for up to 24 hours after birth, but at least a minimum of 6 hours.[29] This delay is intended to ensure that the infant has successfully transitioned to extrauterine life and is at minimal risk for development of hypothermia after the bath. Furthermore, research supports that leaving vernix on the infant's skin as opposed to implementing prompt bathing can be beneficial in thermoregulation and establishing breastfeeding. Several studies have found that water alone is as effective as mild soaps in cleansing infants.[56] Antimicrobial soaps tend to be harsh on newborn skin and can impair the formation of a healthy skin microbiome; thus, they should be avoided.[56-58] More rigorous dermatologic studies are needed to clarify the effects that the various bathing methods have on neonatal skin integrity and hydration.

### Newborn Vaccination and Vitamin Supplementation

#### Hepatitis B Vaccine

Vaccination of newborns against hepatitis B within the first 12 hours of life has been recommended in the United States for more than 30 years. The schedule for hepatitis B immunization of infants varies based on the birth parent's status. If the birth parent is positive for hepatitis B surface antigen (HBsAg), the infant should receive both hepatitis B vaccine (HBV) and hepatitis B immune globulin (HBIG) within the first 12 hours of birth.[59] These injections are administered at separate injection sites. Although most states require obstetric providers to screen pregnant individuals for hepatitis B, occasionally a birthing person may present for care with an unknown HBsAg status. If HBsAg status is unknown, the birthing person should be tested as soon as possible after admission. If the parent is found to be HBsAg positive, the infant should receive HBIG as soon as possible but no later than age 7 days.[59]

Table 39-6 summarizes the CDC recommendations based on whether the birth parent has a negative, positive, or unknown HBsAg test.[59] According to the CDC, approved vaccines contain 10 to 40 mcg of HBsAg protein per milliliter; they do not contain thimerosal. Only a single-antigen HBV is used for the birth dose. The HBV series consists of either three or four injections, based on the type of HBV used. In some parts of the world, a combination vaccine including vaccination against hepatitis B, diphtheria, tetanus, pertussis, and influenza is administered during the first year of life.[59]

Some parents decline HBV for their infants. This decision reflects parental autonomy, although evidence supports the advantages of primary prevention of disease through immunization, as discussed in the *Health Promotion Across the Lifespan* chapter. However, for birth parents who are HBsAg positive, there are distinct risks to the infant regarding the development of chronic hepatitis B and potentially fatal hepatic carcinoma or cirrhosis. Thus, the ethical concerns in such situations are more complex, and the family can be best served with a full discussion of the risks and benefits associated with the disease and with vaccination.[60]

### Vitamin D Supplementation

All infants exclusively receiving human milk or a mixture of human milk and human milk substitutes should receive a nutritional supplement of 400 IU of vitamin D daily, beginning in the first few days of life. Parents should receive specific instructions on administration of the prescribed supplement to ensure correct dosing.[61]

### Circumcision

In the United States, circumcising male newborns became prevalent in the 1950s. A complex set of religious, cultural, and family traditions contribute to the decision about circumcision. The types

| Table 39-6 | Hepatitis B Vaccine Schedules for Term Newborn Infants, by Birth Parent Hepatitis B Surface Antigen Status | | | |
|---|---|---|---|---|
| **Single-Antigen Vaccine** | | **Single-Antigen + Combination Vaccine** | | |
| **Dose** | **Age** | **Dose** | **Age** | |
| **HBsAg Positive** | | | | |
| 1[a] | Birth (≤ 12 hours) | 1[a] | Birth (≤ 12 hours) | |
| HBIG[b] | Birth (≤ 12 hours) | HBIG | Birth (≤ 12 hours) | |
| 2 | 1–2 months | 2 | 2 months | |
| 3 | 6 months | 3 | 4 months | |
| | | 4[c] | 6 months (Pediarix) or 12–15 months (Comvax) | |
| **HBsAg Unknown[d]** | | | | |
| 1[a] | Birth (≤ 12 hours) | 1[a] | Birth (≤ 12 hours) | |
| 2 | 1–2 months | 2 | 2 months | |
| 3[c] | 6 months | 3 | 4 months | |
| | | 4[c] | 6 months (Pediarix) or 12–15 months (Comvax) | |
| **HBsAg Negative** | | | | |
| 1[a,e] | Birth (before discharge) | 1[a,e] | Birth (before discharge) | |
| 2 | 1–2 months | 2 | 2 months | |
| 3[c] | 6 months | 3 | 4 months | |
| | | 4[c] | 6 months (Pediarix) or 12–15 months (Comvax) | |

Abbreviations: HBIG, hepatitis B immune globulin; HBsAg, hepatitis B surface antigen.

[a] Recombivax HB or Engerix-B should be used for the birth dose. Comvax and Pediarix cannot be administered at birth or before age 6 weeks.
[b] Hepatitis B immune globulin (0.5 mL) is administered intramuscularly in a separate site from the vaccine.
[c] The final dose in the vaccine series should not be administered before age 24 weeks (164 days).
[d] Birth parents should have blood drawn and tested for HBsAg as soon as possible after admission for delivery; if is found to be HBsAg positive, the infant should receive HBIG as soon as possible, but no later than 7 days of age.
[e] On a case-by-case basis and only in rare circumstances, the first dose may be delayed until after hospital discharge for an infant who weighs 2000 g or more and whose birth parent is HBsAg negative. When such a decision is made, an order to withhold the birth dose and a copy of the original laboratory report indicating that HBsAg was negative during the pregnancy should be placed in the infant's medical record.

Data from Schillie S, Vellozzi C, Reingold A, et al. Prevention of hepatitis B virus infection in the United States: recommendations of the Advisory Committee on Immunization Practices. *MMWR Recomm Rep* 2018;67(No. RR-1):1–31. http://dx.doi.org/10.15585/mmwr.rr6701a1external icon.

of practitioners that perform circumcision vary. In many sites, obstetricians are responsible for this procedure; in others, pediatric or neonatal providers or a family physician may perform the procedure. If the reason for the procedure is religious, a cleric such as a rabbi or a midwife who also is a mohel may perform the circumcision. Circumcision is not a core competency in midwifery education and practice, but midwives practicing in the United States can learn and offer this procedure as an advanced procedure following the recommended steps outlined in the *ACNM Standards for the Practice of Midwifery*.

The circumcision procedure involves the surgical removal of adhesions, retraction, and removal of the foreskin covering the glans of the penis (prepuce). The procedure typically occurs in a hospital or within the first 2 weeks of life as a religious ceremony. Analgesia is indicated for the newborn. Complications from circumcision are uncommon but can be serious, with the most common being infection and bleeding. Although the foreskin of newborns is rarely able to be retracted, within the first few years the foreskin can be spontaneously retracted for most male children who are not circumcised.

The contemporary rationale for circumcision is a source of controversy. Arguments exist both for and against male circumcision, although the true benefits and hazards are relatively rarely cited.[62] Proponents of circumcision note that circumcised males experience lower incidence of medical problems including cancer of the penis, urinary tract infection (UTI), and sexually transmitted infections (STIs). Cancer of the penis is an unusual malignancy, especially in the cooler climates of the Northern Hemisphere. UTIs are similarly uncommon in infants. Several studies have found a positive correlation between men who were uncircumcised and increased incidence of STIs, including human immunodeficiency virus (HIV), although other contributing factors such as social determinants of health and sexual practices have confounded the association, especially in higher-income countries. Routinely circumcising newborns does prevent the small percentage of individuals with phimosis (inability to retract the foreskin) from developing problems with edema and inflammation of the glans, and male circumcision has not been demonstrated to interfere with reproductive function of the penis.[63]

For some, this topic inspires passionate debate, in which male circumcision is likened to female circumcision or genital mutilation. Opponents of circumcision maintain that modern sanitary conditions in the United States diminish the need for this procedure and argue that the procedure is a painful violation of a nonconsenting infant that removes a functional body part. Parents who choose not to circumcise their child are taught normal anatomy and development of the penis. As the child matures, they will be taught to retract the foreskin gently while bathing to clear any collection of smegma. Parents are counseled not to retract the foreskin forcefully, as the resultant irritation and edema may cause further adhesions.

Just as conflicting opinions have arisen in the general population regarding circumcision, so the American Academy of Pediatrics (AAP) has issued statements on this practice that have varied over the years. Based on research studies from 2005 to 2010, the most recent AAP statement notes that the health benefits of circumcision outweigh the risks and supports access to the procedure for families who choose it.[63] A critical component of this statement is the informed desire of families. Information about circumcision should be included in prenatal care, giving parents and their families adequate time to make this decision. Some healthcare practices

develop their own culturally sensitive documents to help individuals with this decision.

## Conditions That Influence Newborn Care

### Birth Parent with HIV Infection

HIV infection is a major perinatal threat. In the late 1990s, a major breakthrough occurred when a study found that treatment of newborns born to HIV-positive birth parents with zidovudine (AZT, Retrovir) reduced the newborn's risk of developing the infection.[64] In 2013, it was reported that a newborn with evidence of HIV shortly after birth was treated with a short course of multiple antiviral agents and later found to be free of infection.[65] Currently, treatment of newborns born to individuals with HIV is recommended. A newborn whose birth parent has HIV should be treated by a pediatric provider with expertise in this area. One crucial point regarding care of infants born to HIV-positive birth parents is that they must be bathed as soon as possible after birth. If any injections are given, the site needs to be cleansed thoroughly.[66]

In the United States, it is recommended that HIV-positive individuals not breastfeed their infants because the virus is transmitted through breast milk. However, in areas where safe breast milk substitutes are lacking, the risks of HIV must be weighed against the risks of newborn diarrhea and nutritional deficits associated with human milk substitute feeding; thus, the recommendation to breastfeed is more complex in such locations.[67]

### Birth Parent Colonized with Group B *Streptococcus*

Group B *Streptococcus* (GBS) infection is a leading cause of neonatal sepsis in the United States. If the birth parent is colonized with GBS, vertical transmission to the newborn occurs for approximately 50% of newborns. Without treatment during labor, 1% to 2% of newborns born to birth parents who are colonized with GBS will develop newborn sepsis.[68] Because newborn sepsis carries a significant risk of morbidity and mortality, efforts to prevent GBS-related newborn disease are a standard part of perinatal care in the United States.

Intrapartum GBS prophylaxis is recommended if antepartum GBS cultures were positive or if other risk factors are present. The infant born at 35 weeks or later gestation whose birth parent received adequate intrapartum GBS prophylaxis—defined as administration of penicillin G, ampicillin, or cefazolin

4 or more hours before birth—can receive routine newborn care in the absence of symptoms or other risk factors.[69]

If the birth parent has a stated allergy to penicillin, allergy testing is recommended to confirm the allergy, and antimicrobial susceptibility testing should be performed prenatally to select an appropriate second-line agent for prophylaxis. If susceptibility testing has not been performed, intrapartum prophylaxis is deemed incomplete, and the infant will require serial physical examinations and vital signs monitoring for 36 to 48 hours.[69]

Newborns who have signs of clinical illness should be promptly evaluated, and care of these newborns is often provided in consultation with specialist providers. Neonatal sepsis calculators can be useful in determining the risk for sepsis. Blood cultures and empiric antibiotics are often included in the care of these newborns.[69]

## Birth Parent with Gestational and Pregestational Diabetes Mellitus

Individuals with gestational or pregestational diabetes mellitus (DM) are at increased risk for having newborns with growth abnormalities (macrosomia or fetal growth restriction), congenital anomalies, birth injuries, respiratory distress, polycythemia, and metabolic disturbances including hypoglycemia. Newborn hypoglycemia may result from a temporary condition of hyperinsulinemia, which develops in response to intrauterine hyperglycemia from exogenous glucose provided through the placental circulation and diminished endogenous glucose production after birth. The risk of neonatal complications depends on the time of onset of DM, the degree of the birth parent's hyperglycemia, the length of fetal exposure to hyperglycemia, and the severity of the birth parent's disease.[70]

Because of the risk of hypoglycemia, early feeding is essential. SSC and immediate breastfeeding/chestfeeding have been shown to decrease the risk of hypoglycemia. Asymptomatic infants should be screened within the first 4 hours of life.[70,71] Consultation with a member of the pediatric team is needed for newborns with abnormal blood glucose levels, and administration of intravenous fluids may be indicated.

## Birth Parent with Substance Use

The term *substance exposure*, when used in reference to a newborn, covers a wide variety of substances. Many attempts have been made to quantify the effects on the fetus and newborn following in utero exposure to substances such as nicotine, alcohol, and opioid and non-opioid drugs. A major limitation of studies that have examined prenatal substance exposure is polysubstance use. In addition, substances vary in terms of the additives they contain and their level of purity. Confounding and concurrent conditions, such as malnutrition, poverty, and chronic stress, also have a negative and interdependent effect on the fetus and newborn.

Newborns who have had significant exposure to a teratogenic or fetotoxic agent during pregnancy may be small for gestational age and have dysmorphic physical characteristics. Neonatal signs of withdrawal include a wide spectrum of physiologic and neurobehavioral symptoms. Any infant suspected of being at risk for neonatal abstinence syndrome or neonatal opioid withdrawal syndrome should be carefully observed for the first 72 hours of life as described next.[72]

### Tobacco and Nicotine Use

There are significant risks to the fetus and neonate associated with tobacco and nicotine use during pregnancy, such as orofacial defects, fetal growth restriction, preterm labor and birth, low birth weight, intrauterine growth restriction, and placenta previa and abruption. Children born to individuals who smoke during pregnancy are at an increased risk of respiratory infections, asthma, infantile colic, bone fractures, sudden unexplained infant death, and childhood obesity.[73] Studies suggest that prenatal nicotine exposure contributes to adverse behavioral and cognitive outcomes.[73]

### Alcohol

Newborns born to individuals who ingest alcohol can suffer serious and irreversible sequelae. Ethanol readily crosses the placenta, so fetal exposure to alcohol can be significant. Fetal consequences of prenatal alcohol consumption are characterized as a continuum, with two terms being used to describe the extent of the harm: fetal alcohol syndrome (FAS) and fetal alcohol spectrum disorders (FASD). FASD encompasses FAS but also includes individuals with milder effects of fetotoxicity. FAS and FASD are the most common nonheritable causes of intellectual disability.[74]

The signs of FAS may not be obvious during the newborn period. However, newborns exhibiting signs of FAS may have dysmorphic facial characteristics, central nervous system dysfunction, and neurobehavioral impairment. The manifestations of FASD in newborns are subtle, then become more pronounced when the child is older. The type and level of impairment vary with the timing and dose of exposure. If physical or behavioral signs that are possibly indicative of FAS or FASD are noted, consultation with a pediatric team is necessary. Growth deficiency is a common manifestation of FAS and FASD, and behavioral impairments can present a challenge for parents and other caregivers.[74-76]

### Perinatal Opioid Use Disorder

Opioid use disorder (OUD) during pregnancy has had a profound impact on pregnant individuals throughout the United States. The crisis of opioid use disorder during pregnancy is compounded by the fact that significant barriers exist for pregnant persons who want to access evidence-based therapies for OUD such as methadone or buprenorphine. Rural communities are disproportionally impacted by OUD.

Opioid use in pregnancy can lead to a withdrawal syndrome in newborns called neonatal opioid withdrawal syndrome (NOWS), a term used by federal agencies including the Food and Drug Administration. NOWS is specific to neonatal withdrawal from opioids, whereas neonatal abstinence syndrome (NAS) is a more general term for neonatal withdrawal that includes non-opioid exposures. Recent evidence suggests that most in utero drug exposures involve opioids or opioids in combination with other substances.[72]

Assessment of newborns with NOWS includes a thorough history from the pregnant person about substance use, adverse childhood experiences, past and present traumatic and violent experiences, mental health status, and infectious diseases, including hepatitis C and HIV. The needs of the family and the living environment should also be assessed.

Newborns with NOWS can present with signs of central nervous system irritability, gastrointestinal dysfunction (vomiting and diarrhea), or autonomic nervous system lability such as sweating, yawning, tachypnea, or nasal stuffiness. Treatment of newborns who have been chronically exposed to opioids in utero often includes toxicology testing, ideally in meconium (since meconium testing provides information about a longer window of time during the pregnancy), and observation for at least 72 hours to monitor for withdrawal. Note that testing of newborns can have legal ramifications and may be controversial.

There is little evidence to inform decisions about observation periods, and excess monitoring could result in prolonged separation of the infant and birth parent. Nonpharmacologic care such as a dimly lit environment or swaddling may be helpful for infants who are not severely impacted. The goals of pharmacotherapy for infants with severe NOWS are to improve clinical signs and minimize complications from withdrawal. The first line of pharmacologic therapy for NOWS is morphine.[72]

The birth parent can be an integral member of the team if the Eat, Sleep, Console (ESC) method is utilized for neonatal management. In this regimen, caregivers are encouraged to stay with the infant and maximize the use of nonpharmacologic efforts (swaddling, SSC, calm environment). If the newborn is eating appropriately, sleeping more than 1 hour, and can be consoled within 10 minutes, no further intervention is necessary. The ESC method has been shown to decrease parent–child separation, need for administration of medications for withdrawal symptoms, length of hospital stay, and healthcare costs.[77,78] Other treatment considerations include providing adequate caloric and nutritional support and holistic and supportive care by a knowledgeable pediatric team.

Breastfeeding/chestfeeding is safe for individuals taking methadone and buprenorphine and may reduce the clinical signs of NOWS in their infants. Both drugs are excreted in breast milk in small concentrations.[72] Individuals with OUD may have co-morbidities; individuals with HIV in high-income countries should not breastfeed, and those who are positive for hepatitis C virus and have bleeding or cracked nipples should not breastfeed. Be aware that sudden cessation or discontinuation of breastfeeding by individuals on methadone or buprenorphine can result in infant withdrawal.

Discharge teaching should include a discussion of withdrawal symptoms and ways to seek help if symptoms worsen or become difficult to manage. Newborns with prenatal substance exposure are at risk for sleep-related unexplained deaths, so instructions on safe sleeping should be provided.

### Neonatal Jaundice

Neonatal jaundice is the most common cause of newborn hospital readmission. As many as 60% to 80% of newborns present with clinically evident jaundice.[79,80] Management of jaundice depends on whether the etiology is a physiologic or pathologic process and on the infant's bilirubin levels according to gestational age and time since birth. Table 39-7 provides a list of signs and symptoms that can help the midwife distinguish physiologic jaundice from pathologic jaundice.[79-81]

In 1999, an hour-specific bilirubin nomogram was first published for evaluation of total serum bilirubin (TSB) in newborns born at 35 weeks' gestation or later.[82] Figure 39-2 is an updated version of the nomogram published in 2021 by Bahr and colleagues.[83] Unlike the original nomogram, the updated version

| Table 39-7 | Newborn Jaundice |
|---|---|
| **Type of Jaundice** | **Signs and Symptoms** |
| Physiologic jaundice | Jaundice appears between 24 and 72 hours of age |
| | Peaks between days 4 and 5 for term infants and by day 7 for preterm infants |
| | Disappears by 10 to 14 days of life |
| Pathologic jaundice | Jaundice is visible during first 24 hours after birth |
| | Peak levels are higher than the expected ranges |
| | Clinical jaundice is present beyond 2 weeks of age |
| Breastfeeding and breast milk jaundice (suboptimal intake hyperbilirubinemia) | Jaundice usually appears between 24 to 72 hours of age |
| | Peaks by days 5 to 15 of life |
| | Typically disappears by the third week of life |
| Hemolytic jaundice | Most common causes are Rh hemolytic disease, ABO incompatibility, glucose-6-phosphate dehydrogenase (G-6-PD) deficiency, and minor blood group incompatibility |
| | Severe jaundice can appear in the first 24 hours of life and requires referral for a pathologic jaundice work-up and neonatal intensive care |

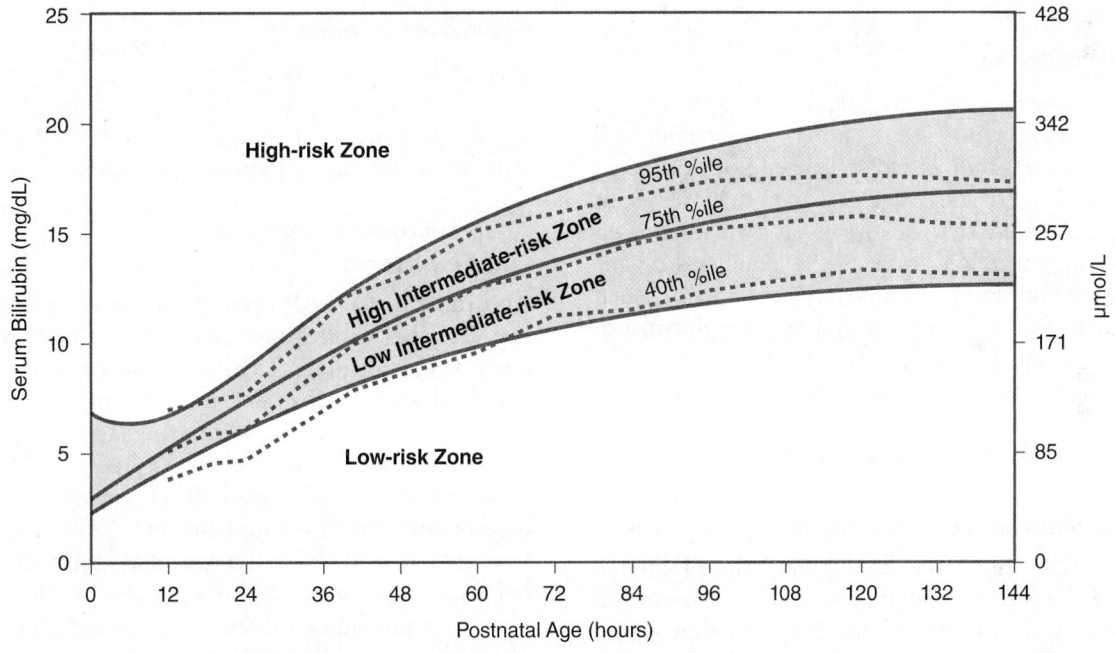

**Figure 39-2** The new neonatal bilirubin nomogram (solid lines) with the 1999 Bhutani nomogram superimposed in the dashed lines. Used with permission.
Reproduced with permission from Bahr TM, Henry E, Christensen RD, Minton SD, Bhutani VK. A new hour-specific serum bilirubin nomogram for neonates ≥35 weeks of gestation. *J Pediatr.* 2021;236:28-33.e1.

considers TSB values obtained from a sample of more than 400,000 infants born at 35 weeks' gestation or later within the first 12 hours of life.

### Physiologic Jaundice

Newborn physiologic jaundice is the result of bilirubin deposits in the dermis. More detailed information is provided in the *Anatomy and Physiology of the Newborn* chapter. Bilirubin levels rise during the first few days after birth, secondary to three aspects of newborn physiology:

- Newborns have more red blood cell volume than adults, and neonatal red blood cells have a shorter lifespan. As fetal red blood cells break down so that fetal hemoglobin can be replaced with adult hemoglobin, heme catabolism produces bilirubin as a by-product.

- Bilirubin must be converted from an unconjugated (indirect), non-water-soluble form to a conjugated (direct), water-soluble form so that it can be excreted through urine and stool. The hepatic metabolism pathway that conjugates bilirubin is immature in the newborn and is not fully effective for several weeks of life.

- Conjugated bilirubin must be broken down further by intestinal bacteria so that it can be excreted. Because the newborn gastrointestinal tract is not as densely colonized as adults, conjugated bilirubin is reabsorbed and recirculated via the enterohepatic system to a greater extent than occurs in adults.

Physiologic jaundice is the result of increased production of bilirubin at a time when elimination is delayed.

### Breast Milk Jaundice

Approximately 20% to 30% of infants in the United States who receive mostly breast milk will develop breast milk jaundice. The etiology of breast milk jaundice is not well understood; however, it is hypothesized that factors in human milk itself or genetic mutations increase the likelihood of this phenomenon. Human milk or genetic factors, such as mutations of the uridine diphosphate glucuronosyltransferase (bilirubin-UGT) enzyme gene code, which is key to conjugation of bilirubin with the hepatocyte, result in decreased excretion of bilirubin and the development of jaundice.[82]

### Assessment of Neonatal Jaundice

The AAP's Subcommittee on Hyperbilirubinemia recommends that all infants be routinely monitored for the development of jaundice, and that established protocols be put in place for assessing and managing jaundice. Protocols should include when transcutaneous bilirubin (TcB) and TSB levels are to be obtained. Infants who are breastfed should be fed at least 8 to 12 times per day for the first several days of life to prevent dehydration and exacerbation of jaundice. Furthermore, before discharge, every newborn should be assessed for their risk of developing severe hyperbilirubinemia, and protocols should be established for minimizing this risk. Parents should be provided with written and verbal information at discharge that includes a clear explanation of jaundice and how to monitor jaundice in

| Table 39-8 | Newborn Discharge Age and Suggested Jaundice Follow-Up | |
|---|---|
| **Age at Discharge** | **Follow-up needed (Age in Days)** |
| <24 hours | 3 days |
| 24–47 hours | 4 days |
| 48–72 hours | 5 days |

Adapted from: American Academy of Pediatrics, Subcommittee on Hyperbilirubinemia. Management of hyperbilirubinemia in the newborn infant 35 or more weeks of gestation. *Pediatrics.* 2004;114:297-316

their infant. Follow-up for monitoring of jaundice is described in Table 39-8.[84]

Several online hyperbilirubinemia risk calculators, such as the BiliTool mentioned in the Resources section, are freely available for use by clinicians.

### Hyperbilirubinemia

Hyperbilirubinemia is defined as a rise in total serum bilirubin above the 95th percentile for age during the first week of life.[79,80,83–85] Table 39-9 lists risk factors for severe hyperbilirubinemia.

### Acute Bilirubin Encephalopathy and Kernicterus

According to the AAP, acute bilirubin encephalopathy describes central nervous system effects stemming from bilirubin toxicity to the basal ganglia and brainstem nuclei. The term *kernicterus* refers to the chronic and long-term sequelae of bilirubin toxicity, which can include cerebral palsy, auditory dysfunction, dental enamel dysplasia, oculomotor defects, and cognitive impediments. Clinical manifestations of acute bilirubin encephalopathy include lethargy, hypotonia, and poor suck in the early phase, progressing to drowsiness, stupor, hypertonia, shrill cry, inability to feed, apnea, fever, seizures, coma, and death in the advanced phase. Hypertonia can be manifested as arching of the neck (retrocollis) and trunk (opisthotonos). In the advanced phase, the central nervous system damage may be irreversible.[84]

### Phototherapy

Phototherapy is an effective treatment for newborn jaundice and has vastly reduced the number of exchange transfusions required to treat infants with hyperbilirubinemia.[84–86] The light from phototherapy converts bilirubin to a less lipophilic substrate

| Table 39-9 | Risk factors for Severe Hyperbilirubinemia |
|---|---|

**Known at Birth**

Lower gestational ages (increasing risk as gestational age decreases)

Parent or sibling who needed jaundice treatment

Genetic relative with inherited blood disorders (e.g. glucose-6-phosphate dehydrogenase (G6PD) deficiency)

East Asian genetic heritage

Perinatal asphyxia

Acidosis

Positive antibody screen in the birthing parent

Macrosomia following parental gestational diabetes

Trisomy 21 (Down syndrome)

**Newborn Conditions Developing After Birth**

Positive direct anti-globulin test

Inadequate milk intake (breast-feeding <8 times in 24 hours or excessive weight loss)

Cephalohematoma or significant bruising

Sepsis diagnosis

Clinical instability in the past 24 hours

Jaundice in the first 24 hours of life

Hemolytic disease of any type

Rapidly increasing total serum bilirubin (TSB) or transcutaneous bilirubin (TcB) measurement

Predischarge TSB or TcB measurement near the threshold to begin phototherapy

Albumin <3.0 mg/dL

Adapted from Maisels MJ, Bhutani VK, Bogen D, Newman TB, Stark AR, Watchko JF. Hyperbilirubinemia in the newborn Infant ≥35 weeks' gestation: an update with clarifications. *Pediatrics.* 2009;124(4):1193-1198. doi:10.1542/peds.2009-032985; Kemper A, Newman TB, Slaughter JL, et al. Clinical practice guideline revision: management of hyperbilirubinemia in the newborn infant 35 or more weeks of gestation. *Pediatrics.* 2022;150(3):e2022058859.

in newborns that can be more easily excreted. The efficacy of phototherapy depends on the irradiance of the light source as measured by a radiometer or spectroradiometer. The AAP has issued guidelines for newborn jaundice that are generally followed throughout the United States, especially regarding indications for phototherapy.[84–86] Currently blue, fluorescent lamps or light-emitting diode (LED) lamps have been found to be most effective. The

dose and efficacy of phototherapy are affected by the distance the infant is from the light source and the area of skin exposed.[86]

Phototherapy can be used safely and effectively in home settings, provided bilirubin levels are monitored regularly. Most home phototherapy devices are less efficient than those used in hospitals, but the newer devices with special blue or LED lights are more effective. The use of home phototherapy should be avoided in infants with risk factors for severe or rapidly progressing hyperbilirubinemia. Candidates for home phototherapy are infants with TSB levels of 2 to 3 deciliters below those recommended for hospital phototherapy.[86]

## Discharging the Newborn from Early Newborn Care

Midwives should be confident that parents understand the basics of newborn care, can feed their newborn comfortably, and understand warning signs requiring additional care. Many hospitals and birth settings have specific criteria for discharge, such as passage of urine and stool, a completed physical examination, and two successful feeds.[87] The infant's GBS status and need for treatment may influence the timing of discharge.

Prior to discharge, follow-up for routine newborn care should be scheduled as well as any specialist follow-up needed due to prenatal or postnatal diagnoses. When a newborn is discharged prior to 24 hours from the birth setting, follow-up assessment is recommended for approximately 24 hours later, and arrangements need to be made for newborn screening such as dried blood spot screening, hearing testing, and congenital heart disease screening. Records should be sent to the selected provider office. Transition between providers is facilitated if new parents know that the midwife remains available for questions.

## The First Month: Primary Care of the Newborn

The role of the midwife during the newborn's first month of life varies markedly. In some settings, midwives have little to no formal role in care once the newborn leaves the birthing room. In other settings, midwives will continue care of the birth parent and newborn throughout the first 4 weeks after birth. They work in a collegial relationship with pediatric providers, with well-child care gradually shifting to pediatric or family healthcare providers.

When a midwife is the provider for a newborn during the first 28 days of life, the neonate may be seen in an ambulatory setting, often at the same time the birthing parent is seen for a postpartum examination. The purposes of this visit are four-fold: (1) to monitor growth and development, (2) to identify symptoms of disease, (3) to offer screening measures, and (4) to educate and support the parents. When a caregiver brings a newborn in for a well-child visit, every effort should be made to avoid the infant's exposure to other people, especially anyone who is ill. Whenever possible, caregivers should be escorted into an examination room as soon as they arrive with their child.

The visit starts with a brief interview of the parent(s) or primary caregiver. Particular attention should be paid to unresolved problems related to the birth or the immediate care of the newborn following birth. The midwife should assess the well-being of the parents and look for signs of depression or inability to cope with the demands of the newborn. Inquiries should be made about help in the home, sibling reactions, and reaction of other relatives to the newborn. Emphasis should be placed on the infant's feeding patterns, levels of alertness, elimination patterns, and crying patterns as well as parental coping with parenting demands.

A complete physical examination is performed. During the physical examination, the midwife has an opportunity to observe the parent–newborn relationship. Observing a feeding can also provide valuable insight into the parental–newborn relationship and parenting knowledge.

The greatest part of the initial well-child visit should be spent soliciting parental concerns and offering guidance and anticipatory advice. Any midwife providing well-child care should have clearly established protocols for pediatric consultation or referral of any infant presenting with signs or symptoms of illness.

### Well-Neonate Physical Care in the First Month of Life

Parents have many concerns regarding the physical care of their newborn. Overall, they should be reassured that there is more than one way to approach many aspects of their child's care. Various common conditions about which parents may have concerns are summarized in Table 39-10.

| Table 39-10 | Common Neonatal Conditions and Parental Concerns in the First Month of Life | |
|---|---|---|
| **Conditions/Questions** | **Comments** | **Treatments/Advice** |
| **Skin Conditions** | | |
| Simple diaper dermatitis | Flat, reddened areas | Gentle cleaning with water |
| | Minimal skinfold involvement | Frequent diaper changes |
| | Neonate may demonstrate distress during cleaning/diaper changes | Use of protectants (e.g., zinc oxide) |
| Diaper dermatitis due to fungal infection | Usually due to *Candida albicans* | Topical antifungals (e.g., miconazole) |
| | Confluent erythematous lesions | Topical steroids (e.g., hydrocortisone) |
| | Often lesions remote from the main area (satellite lesions) | |
| | Painful to the neonate, even when not touched | |
| Diaper dermatitis with secondary infection | Usually due to *Staphylococcus* or *Streptococcus* microorganisms | Treatment based on type of microorganism involved |
| | Peeling skin | May require pediatric consultation or referral |
| | Vesicles | |
| | Exudates | |
| Cradle cap | Seborrheic exudates | Gently comb the hair/scalp with oil (e.g., vegetable, olive) |
| | | Remove exudate with shampoo |
| | | Regular shampooing usually resolves the issue |

| Conditions/Questions | Comments | Treatments/Advice |
|---|---|---|
| Erythema toxicum neonatorum and milia | Various eruptions, small vesicles, or generalized rash | These dermatologic conditions are common in the first week of life and will spontaneously resolve.<br><br>No treatment is necessary, and the condition does not appear to be painful to the newborn. Use of topical creams may worsen the condition and lead to neonatal acne.<br><br>Parents can be reassured that this is a normal transient finding in newborns. |
| **Oral Conditions** | | |
| Thrush | Adherent white plaques on the tongue, gums, and/or palate | Oral antifungals; consider topical treatment for the nursing parent as well<br><br>Also rule out mastitis if the individual is breastfeeding |
| Nasal discharge | Discharge may be apparent<br><br>Occasional periods of irregular breathing<br><br>Crusting around the nares may or may not be present | Counsel the parents to avoid bulb syringes; they can cause trauma and edema<br><br>Saline drops<br><br>Differentiate between nasal congestion and apnea (apnea is associated with a low heart rate, pauses of 20 seconds or more); apnea warrants pediatric referral to evaluate for more serious conditions<br><br>Consider viral screening (especially during RSV/flu season) if discharge persists |
| **Behavior** | | |
| "Fussiness" | Crying<br>"Colicky" behavior<br>Difficult to console<br><br>Reasons unknown and likely to be unique to the individual parent–newborn dyad | Multiple suggestions to console an infant—although no research supports that one method is better than another:<br>• Swaddling<br>• Talk with the infant *en face*<br>• Cuddle, reposition, walk, or move with the infant<br>• Attempt to feed or give a pacifier<br>• Reduce environment sensory stimulation<br>*Never shake a newborn!* |
| **Sleep** | | |
| Timing of sleep | Usually sleep 16–18 hours in first few days<br><br>Variation more profound as infant grows, ranging from as few as 8 hours or as much as almost 20 hours by 4 weeks<br><br>Newborns are less governed by circadian rhythms than adults<br><br>Sleep is associated with feeding; more likely to sleep during day | Reassure parents that newborns do not necessarily have days and nights confused<br><br>Most likely will take 12 weeks at least to start sleeping more at night and may take 3–5 months based on melatonin and cortisol production |

*(continues)*

| Table 39-10 | Common Neonatal Conditions and Parental Concerns in the First Month of Life (*continued*) | |
| --- | --- | --- |
| **Conditions/Questions** | **Comments** | **Treatments/Advice** |
| Safe sleep | Newborns who sleep on their backs are less likely to experience sudden infant death syndrome (SIDS)<br><br>Originally part of the national campaign "Back to Sleep"; now termed "Safe Sleep" | Newborns should be placed on their backs for sleep; should sleep on a separate surface (not co-bedding with parents); no stuffed animals, blankets, or pillows in the bed space; prevent exposure to smoking (passive or active); avoid overheating<br><br>Should have "tummy time" or interactions when on abdomen only when the newborn is awake |
| **Feeding**[a] | | |
| Adequate feeding | Newborn should feed multiple times daily (e.g., approximately every 2–4 hours)<br><br>May lose 5–7% of birth weight in first few days of life | Proxy measures for adequate intake include:<br>• Weight gain at end of first week or beginning of the second week (usually 150–200 g per week)<br>• Stools and urine in diapers at least 1–3 times during each of the first few days of life<br>• Once lactation or feeding with human milk substitutes is established, 3–4 stools and 5–6 wet diapers every day<br>• If difficult to ascertain if diaper is wet, place a soft tissue inside the diaper<br>If no bowel movement or urine within 24–48 hours, consult the pediatric provider |
| **Car Safety** | | |
| Car seats | Newborns should travel in a proper-installed, rear-facing car seats with minimal clothing in between the newborn and the car seat straps | Never leave an infant alone in a car<br>Choose a car seat that meets U.S. safety standards (will be marked on the box and tag). Have the car seat installed by or verified by a car seat technician. See the Resources section. |

[a] More details can be found in the *Infant Feeding and Lactation* chapter.

Parents should be reminded that infants do not require a full bath daily and that submersion of the abdomen should wait until after the umbilical cord stump has fallen off. Newborns should have their diaper areas and other areas that collect milk or dirt sponged whenever appropriate, with the area then being completely dried. A full-body bath can be given occasionally when the parent has the time to make it a relaxing event for the newborn. Parents should be instructed to never leave a newborn unattended in the bath. The home water heater should be set at no more than 120°F (49°C) to avoid burns, and the bath water tested by an adult to ensure it is lukewarm prior to placing the baby in the water. The towels, cleanser if needed, and clean clothes should all be organized before starting the bath. Slip-proof bathmats are inexpensive and helpful.

Family members may encourage new parents to dress infants in excessive layers of clothing. A general rule of thumb is to clothe the infant with as many layers as other persons in the room are wearing, plus one layer. Because infants cannot sweat effectively, symptoms of overheating are mainly red skin color, irritability, and body warmth. Eventually, an overheated infant will appear lethargic.

From the earliest moments at home with their newborn, parents should evaluate the environment for safety risks. In the first months of life, these risks are primarily related to falling or becoming stuck in small places such as between the bars on the sides of

| Table 39-11 | Neonatal Signs and Symptoms Requiring Prompt Parental Reporting/Pediatric Referral |
|---|---|
| Danger Signs[a] | Description |
| Temperature instability | Axillary temperature > 37.4°C (99.3°F) or < 36.5°C (97.5°F) |
| Abnormal respirations | Regular retractions, wheezing, grunting, nasal flaring |
| | Tachypnea (> 60 breaths/min) |
| | Apnea: pause in breathing > 20 seconds |
| Infection of umbilicus | Odor, redness, drainage, or bleeding from umbilical stump |
| Infection of eyes | Purulent discharge from eyes, erythema, or edema |
| Jaundice | Icteric changes of eyes, chest, or extremities |
| Gastrointestinal signs | Projectile vomiting |
| | Bile-stained vomit (needs immediate neonatal provider assessment to rule out need for surgical intervention) |
| | No stools/no urination within 24 hours of birth |
| | Taut, swollen abdomen |
| | > 6 stools per 24 hours/bloody or very watery stools |
| General signs of illness | Cough |
| | Poor muscle tone |
| | Sleepiness/refusal to feed/inability to rouse |
| | Poor suck |
| | Neurologic signs such as bulging fontanel, irritability, abnormal reflexes |

[a] This list is not exhaustive. Midwives who provide well-newborn care develop relationships with local pediatric providers to learn preferred consultation routines.

cribs. Parents should follow safe sleep guidance and have the baby sleep on their back in an approved sleep device without any blankets or soft items in the sleep area.

If parents choose to use a pacifier, the pacifier should be cleaned regularly and checked for signs of dirt, mold, or cracks. Pacifiers should never be placed on a cord around the infant's neck because of the risk of strangulation.

Parents should recognize situations in which immediate pediatric care is needed for the newborn. Table 39-11 lists situations in which a pediatric provider should be consulted promptly.

### Psychological Tasks of Early Infancy

During the first months after birth, a profound psychodynamic develops between the infant and the principal caregiver (usually the birth parent). The infant is performing the psychological task of differentiation—identifying as a separate being in relation to other beings. A growing body of research implicates the hormone oxytocin in the initiation and maintenance of human attachment behaviors.[88]

The brain is a target organ for oxytocin activity, as it is known to contain oxytocin receptors. Although most literature refers to "maternal–infant" attachment, it is important to be cognizant of other possible "secure bases" for infants, including parents, grandparents, or others who are primary caregivers. In discussions with the newborn's primary caregivers, the midwife can explain the critical importance of response to infant cues.

## Conclusion

Midwives often provide early neonatal care, including care during the first Golden Hour, the first neonatal assessment at birth, and as part of ongoing care of the parent–infant dyad. Even in areas where pediatric care is quickly assumed by other professionals, the relationship between a midwife and a birthing parent and family often means that as questions arise about the infant, the midwife may be the first person to be called. Through their acceptance of this responsibility, midwives have an integral role in caring for the health of future generations.

## Resources

| Organization or Resource | Description |
|---|---|
| American Academy of Pediatrics (AAP) | The AAP provides policy statements and practice guidelines, such as guidelines for delayed cord-clamping and breastfeeding. |
| BiliTool | This interactive website uses existing nomograms to allow clinicians to input the age of the newborn in hours and total bilirubin levels to generate estimates of risk for hyperbilirubinemia. |
| Office on Women's Health (OWH) | The OWH's website contains information on newborn care for new parents, including bathing, feeding, car seat safety, circumcision care, and sudden infant death syndrome (SIDS) prevention. |
| Global Health Media | Training videos on neonatal breathing difficulties and umbilical cord infections. These training videos are based on standards of care described in *Care of the Newborn Reference Manual*, Save the Children, 2004; *Managing Newborn Problems*, World Health Organization, 2003; and *Integrated Management of Childhood Illnesses Chart Booklet*, World Health Organization, 2011. |
| National Highway Traffic Safety Administration | The website maintained by this federal agency can assist with determining which type of car seat is appropriate as well as providing recommendations for approved car seat testing sites. |
| Safe Sleep | The American Academy of Pediatrics has a Safe Sleep Toolkit available.<br><br>The Eunice Kennedy Shriver National Institute of Child Health and Human Development has several resources related to its Safe to Sleep campaign. |

## References

1. American College of Nurse-Midwives. *Core Competencies for Basic Midwifery Practice*. Silver Spring, MD: American College of Nurse-Midwives; 2020.

2. Sharma D, Pradeep Sharma P, Sweta Shastri S. Golden 60 minutes of newborn's life: part 2: term neonate. *J Matern Fetal Neonatal Med.* 2016;29:1-6.

3. Moore ER, Bergman N, Anderson G, Medley N. Early skin-to-skin contact for mothers and their healthy newborn infants. *Cochrane Database Syst Rev.* 2016;5:CD003519. doi:10.1002/14651858.CD003519.pub4.

4. American Academy of Pediatrics. Delayed umbilical cord clamping after birth. *Pediatrics.* 2017;139(6). doi:10.1542/peds.2017-0957.

5. World Health Organization. *Guideline: Delayed Umbilical Cord Clamping for Improved Maternal and Infant Health and Nutrition Outcomes.* Geneva, Switzerland: World Health Organization; 2014.

6. American College of Obstetricians and Gynecologists. ACOG Committee Opinion No. 814: delayed umbilical cord clamping after birth. *Obstet Gynecol.* 2020;136:e100-e106.

7. American College of Nurse-Midwives. *Position Statement: Delayed Umbilical Cord Clamping.* Washington, DC: American College of Nurse Midwives; 2014. https://www.midwife.org/ACNM/files/ACNMLibraryData/UPLOADFILENAME/000000000290/Delayed-Umbilical-Cord-Clamping-May-2014.pdf. Accessed February 20, 2022.

8. McDonald SJ, Middleton P, Dowsell T, Morris P. Effect of timing of umbilical cord clamping of term infants on maternal and neonatal outcomes. *Cochrane Database Syst Rev.* 2013;2:CD004074. doi:10.1002/14651858.CD004074.pub3.

9. Mercer JS, Erickson-Owens DA, Collins J, et al. Effects of delayed cord clamping on residual placental blood volume, hemoglobin and bilirubin levels in term infants: a randomized controlled trial. *J Perinatol.* 2017;37(3):260-264.

10. Katheria AC, Lakshminrusimha S, Rabe H, et al. Placental transfusion: a review. *J Perinatol.* 2017;37(2):105-111.

11. Rabe H, Diaz-Rossello JL, Duley L, Dowswell T. Effect of timing of umbilical cord clamping and other strategies to influence placental transfusion at preterm birth on maternal and infant outcomes. *Cochrane Database Syst Rev.* 2012;8:CD003248. doi:10.1002/14651858.CD003248.pub3.

12. Delayed umbilical cord clamping after birth. *Pediatrics.* 2017;139(6):e20170957. doi:10.1542/peds.2017-0957.

13. World Health Organization, Department of Reproductive Health and Research. *Thermal Protection of the Newborn. A Practical Guide.* Geneva, Switzerland: World Health Organization; 1997.

14. Rozance PJ, Hay WW Jr. New approaches to management of neonatal hypoglycemia. *Matern Health Neonatol Perinatol.* 2016;2:3. doi:10.1186/s40748-016-0031-z.

15. Thompson-Branch A, Havranek T. Neonatal hypoglycemia. *Pediatr Rev.* 2017;38(4):147-157.

16. Adamkin DH. Postnatal glucose homeostasis in late-preterm and term infants. In: *Neonatal Care: A Compendium of AAP Clinical Practice Guidelines*

*and Policies.* 2019; 317-321. doi:10.1542/9781610023047-part06-postnatal_glucose.

17. Folk L. Guide to capillary heelstick blood sampling in infants. *Adv Neonatal Care.* 2007;7(4):171-178.

18. Morrow C, Hidinger A, Wilkinson-Faulk D. Reducing neonatal pain during routine heel lance procedures. *Am J Matern Child Nurs.* 2010;35(6):346-354.

19. Yin T, Yang L, Lee TY, et al. Development of atraumatic heel-stick procedures by combined treatment with non-nutritive sucking, oral sucrose, and facilitated tucking: a randomized, controlled trial. *Int J Nurs Stud.* 2015;52(8):1288-1299.

20. Makker K, Nassar GN, Kaufman EJ. Neonatal conjunctivitis. In: *StatPearls.* Treasure Island, FL: StatPearls Publishing; updated July 21, 2021. https://www.ncbi.nlm.nih.gov/books/NBK441840/. Accessed February 20, 2022.

21. Centers for Disease Control and Prevention. Gonococcal infections among neonates. https://www.cdc.gov/std/treatment-guidelines/gonorrhea-neonates.htm. Published 2021. Accessed February 20, 2022.

22. Neonatal ophthalmia. In: *Red Book: 2021–2024 Report of the Committee on Infectious Diseases.* American Academy of Pediatrics; 2021:1023-1026.

23. Kapoor VS, Evans JR, Vedula SS. Interventions for preventing ophthalmia neonatorum. *Cochrane Database Syst Rev.* 2020;9:CD001862. doi:10.1002/14651858.CD001862.pub4.

24. Lippi G, Franchini M. Vitamin K in neonates: facts and myths. *Blood Transfus.* 2011;9(1):4-9. doi:10.2450/2010.0034-10.

25. Phillippi J, Holley S, Morad A, Collins M. Prevention of vitamin K deficiency bleeding. *J Midwifery Womens Health.* 2016;61(5):632-636.

26. Sinha A, Sazawal S, Pradhan A, et al. Chlorhexidine skin or cord care for prevention of mortality and infections in neonates. *Cochrane Database Syst Rev.* 2015;3:CD007835. doi:10.1002/14651858.CD007835.pub2.

27. Stewart D, Benitz W. Umbilical cord care in the newborn infant. *Pediatrics.* 2016;138(3):e20162149.

28. Coffey PS, Brown SC. Umbilical cord-care practices in low- and middle-income countries: a systematic review. *BMC Pregnancy Childbirth.* 2017;17. https://doi.org/10.1186/s12884-017-1250-7.

29. World Health Organization. *WHO Recommendations on Newborn Health: Guidelines Approved by the WHO Guidelines Review Committee.* Geneva, Switzerland: World Health Organization; updated May 2017.

30. Newborn Screening Authoring Committee. Newborn screening expands: recommendations for pediatricians and medical homes: implications for the system. *Pediatrics.* 2008;121(1):192-217. doi:10.1542/peds.2007-3021.

31. Fillips DJ, Bucciarelli RL. Cardiac evaluation of the newborn. *Pediatr Clin North Am.* 2015;62(2):471-489.

32. Jain A, McNamara PJ. Persistent pulmonary hypertension of the newborn: advances in diagnosis and treatment. *Semin Fetal Neonatal Med.* 2015;20(4):262-271.

33. Yan LJ. Neonatal brachial plexus palsy: management and prognostic features. *Semin Perinatol.* 2014;38(4):222-234.

34. Govindan M, Burrows H. Neonatal brachial plexus injury. *Pediatr Rev.* 2019;40(9):494-496.

35. Doumouchtsis SK, Arulkumaran S. Head injuries after instrumental vaginal deliveries. *Curr Opin Obstet Gynecol.* 2006;18(2):129-134.

36. Akangire G, Carter, B. Birth injuries in neonates. *Pediatr Rev.* 2016;37(11):451-462.

37. Verla MA, Style CC, Olutoye OO. Prenatal diagnosis and management of omphalocele. *Semin Pediatr Surg.* 2019;28(2):84-88.

38. Marven S, Owen A. Contemporary postnatal surgical management strategies for congenital abdominal wall defects. *Semin Pediatr Surg.* 2008;17(4):222-235.

39. Slater BJ, Pimpalwar A. Abdominal wall defects. *NeoReviews.* 2020;21(6):e383-e391.

40. DeJong P, Adams N, Mann R, et al. Management of lumbosacral myelomeningocele. *Eplasty.* 2016;16:ic51.

41. Meningocele. In: *StatPearls.* Treasure Island, FL: StatPearls Publishing; December 17, 2021. https://www.statpearls.com/articlelibrary/viewarticle/24971/.

42. Lu VM, Niazi TN. Pediatric spinal cord diseases. *Pediatr Rev.* 2021; 42(9):486-99.

43. Tovar J. Congenital diaphragmatic hernia. *Ophanet J Rare Dis.* 2012;7(1). doi:10.1186/1750-1172-7-18.

44. Neu N, Duchon J, Zachariah P. TORCH infections. *Clin Perinatol.* 2015;42(1):77-103.

45. Kuzniewicz MW, Puopolo KM, Fischer A, et al. A quantitative, risk-based approach to the management of neonatal early-onset sepsis. *JAMA Pediatr.* 2017 Apr 1;171(4):365-371.

46. American College of Obstetricians and Gynecologists, Task Force on Neonatal Encephalopathy. *Neonatal Encephalopathy and Neurologic Outcome.* 2nd ed. Washington, DC: American College of Obstetricians and Gynecologists; 2014 (reaffirmed 2019).

47. Martinello K, Hart AR, Yap S, et al. Management and investigation of neonatal encephalopathy: 2017 update. *Arch Dis Child Fetal Neonatal Ed.* 2017;102:F346-F358.

48. Morris MW, Blewett CJ. Tracheoesophageal fistula. *NeoReviews.* 2017;18(8):e472-9.

49. Lotfollahzadeh S, Taherian M, Anand S. Hirschsprung disease. In: *StatPearls.* Treasure Island, FL: StatPearls

Publishing; updated December 3, 2021. https://www.ncbi.nlm.nih.gov/books/NBK562142/. Accessed October 7, 2022.

50. Yasir M, Kumaraswamy AG, Rentea RM. Meconium plug syndrome. In: *StatPearls*. Treasure Island, FL: StatPearls Publishing; updated August 12, 2021. https://www.ncbi.nlm.nih.gov/books/NBK562320/. Accessed October 7, 2022.

51. Vricella GJ, Coplen DE. Neonatal urogenital issues: evaluation and management. *NeoReviews*. 2017;18(6):e372-85.

52. Clark-Gambelunghe M, Clark D. Sensory development. *Pediatr Clin North Am*. 2015;62(2):367-384.

53. Winberg J. Mother and newborn baby: mutual regulation of physiology and behavior: a selective review. *Dev Psychobiol*. 2005;47(3):217-222.

54. Brazelton TB, Nugent JK. *Neonatal Behavioral Assessment Scale*. 4th ed. London, UK: Mac Keith Press; 2011.

55. Povedrano MCA, Noto IS, Pinhiero MDS, Guinsburg R. Mothers' perceptions and expectations regarding their newborn infants: the use of Broussard's Neonatal Perception Inventory. *Rev Paul Pediatr*. 2011;29(2):239-244.

56. Ness MJ, Davis DMR, Care WA. Neonatal skin care: a concise review. *Int J Dermatol*. 2013;52:14-22.

57. Lavender T, Bedwell C, Roberts SA, et al. Randomized, controlled trial evaluating a baby wash product on skin barrier function in healthy, term neonates. *J Obstet Gynecol Neonatal Nurs*. 2013;42(2):203-214.

58. Blume-Peytavi U, Hauser M, Stamatas GN, et al. Skin care practices for newborns and infants: review of the clinical evidence for best practices. *Pediatr Dermatol*. 2012;29(1):1-14.

59. Schillie S, Vellozzi C, Reingold A, et al. Prevention of hepatitis B virus infection in the United States: recommendations of the Advisory Committee on Immunization Practices. *MMWR Recomm Rep*. 2018;67(RR-1):1-31. http://dx.doi.org/10.15585/mmwr.rr6701a1.

60. Isaacs D, Kilham HA, Alexander S, et al. Ethical issues in preventing mother-to child transmission of hepatitis B by immunisation. *Vaccine*. 2011;29(37):6159-6162.

61. Wagner CL, Greer FR; American Academy of Pediatrics Section on Breastfeeding; American Academy of Pediatrics Committee on Nutrition. Prevention of rickets and vitamin D deficiency in infants, children, and adolescents [published correction appears in *Pediatrics*. 2009;123(1):197]. *Pediatrics*. 2008;122(5):1142–1152.

62. Mielke R. Counseling parents who are considering newborn male circumcision. *J Midwifery Womens Health*. 2013;58(6):671-682. [Erratum: *J Midwifery Womens Health*. 2014;59(2):225.]

63. Blank S, Brady M, Buerk E, et al.; Task Force on Circumcision. Circumcision policy statement. *Pediatrics*. 2012;130(3):585-586. doi:10.1542/peds.2012-1989.

64. Sperling RS, Shapiro DE, Coombs RW, et al. Maternal viral load, zidovudine treatment, and the risk of transmission of human immunodeficiency virus type 1 from mother to infant. Pediatric AIDS Clinical Trials Group, Protocol 076 Study Group. *N Engl J Med*. 1996;335(22):1621-1629.

65. Cohen J. HIV/AIDS: early treatment may have cured infant of HIV infection. *Science*. 2013;339(6124):1134.

66. Human immunodeficiency virus infection. In: *Red Book: 2021–2024 Report of the Committee on Infectious Diseases*. Elk Grove Village, IL: American Academy of Pediatrics; 2021.

67. World Health Organization, United Nations Children's Fund. *Guideline: Updates on HIV and Infant Feeding: The Duration of Breastfeeding, and Support from Health Services to Improve Feeding Practices Among Mothers Living with HIV*. Geneva, Switzerland: World Health Organization; 2016.

68. Prevention of group B streptococcal early-onset disease in newborns: ACOG Committee Opinion, Number 797. *Obstet Gynecol*. 2020;135(2):e51-e72. [Published correction appears in *Obstet Gynecol*. 2020;135(4):978-979.] doi:10.1097/AOG.0000000000003668.

69. Puopolo KM, Lynfield R, Cummings JJ; AAP Committee on Fetus and Newborn, AAP Committee on Infectious Diseases. Management of infants at risk for group B streptococcal disease. *Pediatrics*. 2019;144(2):e20191881.

70. Sutton DM, Han CS, Werner EF. Diabetes mellitus in pregnancy. *NeoReviews*. 2017;18(1):e33-e43. https://doi.org/10.1542/neo.18-1-e33.

71. Thompson-Branch A, Havranek T. Neonatal hypoglycemia. *Pediatr Rev*. 2017;38(4):147-157. https://doi.org/10.1542/pir.2016-0063.

72. Patrick SW, Barfield WD, Poindexter BB;, AAP Committee on Fetus and Newborn, Committee on Substance Use and Prevention. Neonatal opioid withdrawal syndrome. *Pediatrics*. 2020;146(5):e2020029074.

73. Tobacco and nicotine cessation during pregnancy: ACOG Committee Opinion, Number 807. *Obstet Gynecol*. 2020;135(5):e221-e229. doi:10.1097/AOG.0000000000003822.

74. Denny L, Coles S, Blitz R. Fetal alcohol syndrome and fetal alcohol spectrum disorders. *Am Fam Physician*. 2017;96(8):515-522.

75. Dejong K, Olyaei A, Lo JO. Alcohol use in pregnancy. *Clin Obstet Gynecol*. 2019;62(1):142-155. doi:10.1097/GRF.0000000000000414.

76. American College of Obstetricians and Gynecologists. At-risk drinking and alcohol dependence: obstetric and gynecologic implications. Committee Opinion, Number 496. *Obstet Gynecol.* 2011;118:383-388.

77. Grossman MR, Berkwitt AK, Osborn RR, et al. An initiative to improve the quality of care of infants with neonatal abstinence syndrome. *Pediatrics.* 2017;139(6):e20163360.

78. Grisham LM, Stephen MM, Coykendall MR, et al. Eat, sleep, console approach: a family-centered model for the treatment of neonatal abstinence syndrome. *Adv Neonatal Care.* 2019;19(2):138-144.

79. Mitra S, Rennie J. Neonatal jaundice: aetiology, diagnosis and treatment. *Br J Hosp Med (Lond).* 2017;78(12):699-704.

80. Ullah S, Rahman K, Hedayati M. Hyperbilirubinemia in neonates: types, causes, clinical examinations, preventive measures and treatments: a narrative review article. *Iran J Public Health.* 2016;45(5):558-568.

81. Bratton S, Cantu RM, Stern M. Breast milk jaundice. In: *StatPearls.* Treasure Island, FL: StatPearls Publishing; updated September 6, 2021. https://www.ncbi.nlm.nih.gov/books/NBK537334/. Accessed October 7, 2022.

82. Bhutani VK, Johnson L, Sivieri EM. Predictive ability of a predischarge hour-specific serum bilirubin for subsequent significant hyperbilirubinemia in healthy term and near-term newborns. *Pediatrics.* 1999;103(1):6-14.

83. Bahr TM, Henry E, Christensen RD, et al. A new hour-specific serum bilirubin nomogram for neonates ≥35 weeks of gestation. *J Pediatr.* 2021;236:28-33.

84. American Academy of Pediatrics, Subcommittee on Hyperbilirubinemia. Management of hyperbilirubinemia in the newborn infant 35 or more weeks of gestation. *Pediatrics.* 2004;114:297-316.

85. Maisels MJ, Bhutani VK, Bogen D, et al. Hyperbilirubinemia in the newborn infant ≥35 weeks' gestation: an update with clarifications. *Pediatrics.* 2009;124(4):1193-1198. doi:10.1542/peds.2009-0329.

86. Maisels MJ, McDonagh AF. Phototherapy for neonatal jaundice. *N Engl J Med.* 2008;358(9):920-928. doi:10.1056/NEJMct0708376.

87. Watterberg KL, Aucott S, Benitz WE, et al.; Committee on Fetus and Newborn. Hospital stay for healthy term newborn infants. *Pediatrics.* 2015;135(5):948-953. doi:10.1542/peds.2015-0699.

88. Szymanska M, Schneider M, Chateau-Smith C, et al. Psychophysiological effects of oxytocin on parent–child interactions: a literature review on oxytocin and parent–child interactions. *Psychiatry Clin Neurosci.* June 2, 2017. [Epub ahead of print]. doi:10.1111/pcn.12544.

# A

# Chapter Alignment with ACNM Core Competencies and ICM Essential Competencies

## Introduction

To ensure safe practice, national and international midwifery organizations have established documents detailing the foundational knowledge, skills, and behaviors needed for safe entry into independent midwifery practice. These documents are used to sculpt the content of educational programs, are valuable in studying for certification, and may be incorporated into state and local practice standards as they express the expected skill set of all new midwives.

Globally, the International Confederation of Midwives (ICM) publishes the *Essential Competencies for Basic Midwifery Practice*; at the time of publication, this document had been most recently updated in 2019. Countries often have their own specific documents that use the *Essential Competencies* as a foundation and add other knowledge or skills needed for country-specific practice. As an example, the American College

of Nurse-Midwives (ACNM) publishes the *Core Competencies for Basic Midwifery Practice*. Last published in 2020, this document is updated approximately every 5 years. The Accreditation Commission for Midwifery Education (ACME) requires that all accredited educational programs include each of the ACNM *Core Competencies* within their curricula. Other competencies for North America are listed in the *Resources on the History of Midwifery* appendix.

Since the ICM *Essential Competencies* and the ACNM *Core Competencies for Basic Midwifery Practice* encompass the required knowledge and skills needed for entry-level midwifery practice, they are useful to both learners and educators. We have mapped the contents of this edition to ACNM and ICM competencies, as shown here. Chapters that are new to this edition or have been substantially revised from the previous edition are noted in the table with footnotes.

| Chapter | Chapter Name | ACNM *Core Competencies* (2020) | ICM *Essential Competencies* (2019) |
|---|---|---|---|
| Chapter 1[a] | Context of Individuals Seeking Midwifery Care | I D, E, I, K, L, N, O<br>II A, B, F, G, H, J | 1e, h, j, m |
| Chapter 2 | Professional Midwifery Today | I (all)<br>II (all) | 1a, b, c, f |
| Appendix 2A[b] | Interpreting Published Research Data with a Clinical Midwifery Lens | Same as Chapter 2 | |
| Appendix 2B | Reproductive Health Statistics | IV D, H, J | 1d |

| Chapter | Chapter Name | ACNM *Core Competencies* (2020) | ICM *Essential Competencies* (2019) |
|---|---|---|---|
| Appendix 2C[a] | Global Health: An Overview of Practicalities and Practice | II (all) | 1a, b, c, d, e, f, g, h |
| Appendix 2D[a] | Resources on the History of Midwifery | II (all) | - |
| Chapter 3 | Introduction to Sexual, Reproductive, and Primary Care | I D, E, L, N<br>II E, H<br>III (all)<br>IV J | 1a, e, f, g, h, j, k, l, m |
| Appendix 3A | Standard and Specific Transmission-Based Precautions | Same as Chapter 3 | |
| Appendix 3B | Collecting a Health History | Same as Chapter 3 | |
| Appendix 3C | The Physical Examination | Same as Chapter 3 | |
| Appendix 3D[a] | Breast and Chest Examination | Same as Chapter 3 | |
| Appendix 3E[a] | Pelvic Examination | Same as Chapter 3 | |
| Appendix 3F | Collecting Laboratory Specimens | Same as Chapter 3 | |
| Chapter 4 | Health Promotion Across the Lifespan | I C, D, E, H, I, K, L, N<br>II E, L, K, O, P<br>III A, B, D, E<br>IV G, H<br>V A1, 3, 4, B1a, b, 2, 3, C2, 6, D3–4, E5–6 | 1a, b, d, e, g, h, j, m<br>2a, b, e, f<br>4f |
| Appendix 4A[b] | Skillful Communication to Mitigate Clinician Bias | I C– H, J–L, N, O<br>II A, F, G, H, J, K, M<br>III A, B, C, D, E, F, G<br>IV B, D, E, G, H, J<br>V A1–3, 7, B1, 3, C1, 4, 6, D5, 7, 8, F3, 5, 6, G1, 5 | 1a, b, d, e, g, h, i<br>2a, b, e |
| Appendix 4B | Preconception Care | Same as Chapter 4 | |
| Chapter 5 | Common Conditions in Primary Care | III (all)<br>IV A, B, D, E, F, J<br>V A, B | 1a, c, d, e, f, g, h, j, k, l, m<br>2a, b |
| Chapter 6 | Nutrition | I C, D, E, H, I, K, L, N<br>II E, I, K, O, P<br>III A, B, D, E<br>IV G, H<br>V A1, 3, 4, B1, 2, 3, C2, 6, 3–4, E5–6 | 1a, b, d, e, g |
| Chapter 7 | Mental Health Conditions | I H, I, J, K, M, N, P<br>II F, H<br>III A–G<br>V A2, 3, 4, 5, 6, 7 B3, D 5, 8, 9, F, G | 1a, b, d–h, j–m<br>2b, e, f, g |
| Chapter 8[a] | Anatomy and Physiology of the Reproductive System | IV A, B,<br>V A5a, g | 2a, b |

| Chapter | Chapter Name | ACNM *Core Competencies* (2020) | ICM *Essential Competencies* (2019) |
|---|---|---|---|
| Chapter 9[b] | Sexuality | V A2, 7, C1, 6, 7a, b, F8 | 1e, g, h, j, k, m |
| Chapter 10[a] | Fertility, Family Building, and Contraception | I C– F, J–L, N, P<br><br>II A, F, H, J, K, T<br><br>III<br><br>IV B, C, F, G, H, J<br><br>V A5, B, C | 1b, c, e, g, h, l |
| Appendix 10A | Fertility Awareness Methods | Same as Chapter 10 | 2a, f, i |
| Appendix 10B[b] | Intrauterine Insemination | Same as Chapter 10 | 4f |
| Chapter 11 | Nonhormonal Contraception | I C, E, N<br>V C4 | 1g, 2a, 4f |
| Chapter 12 | Hormonal Contraception | V C4, 8, F8 | 1a, d, g, h, 4a, f |
| Appendix 12A | Intrauterine Device Insertion and Removal | I A, D, L, N, Q<br><br>II K<br><br>III<br><br>IV A<br><br>V F8 | Same as Chapter 12 |
| Appendix 12B[a] | Implant Insertion and Removal | Same as Chapter 12 | |
| Chapter 13[b] | Gender-Affirming Care | I A–Q<br><br>II A–H, J–O, Q, T<br><br>III A–G<br><br>IV A– J<br><br>V A2, 4–7, B2–3, 5–6, C1–6, 8, D2, 4, 7, 9, 10, E5, F3–7 | 1a–h, j–m<br><br>2a, b, e, f, h |
| Chapter 14 | Menopause | I A, C, E, K, L, N<br>IV A, B, E, F<br>V A2, 3, C2, 7a, b, 8 | 1g, j, l |
| Chapter 15 | Menstrual Cycle Abnormalities | I A, B, C, D, M | 1d, l |
| Appendix 15A | Endometrial Biopsy | III A, B, C, D<br>IV D, E, F<br>V C2, 3, 8 | 2b |
| Chapter 16 | Malignant and Chronic Gynecologic Disorders | I H<br><br>II O<br><br>III A–G<br><br>IV A–D<br><br>V A3–6, C1–8 | 1c–e, p<br><br>2<br><br>4a, d |
| Appendix 16A | Fitting a Pessary | Same as Chapter 16 | N/A |
| Appendix 16B[b] | Punch Biopsy | Same as Chapter 16 | N/A |
| Chapter 17 | Breast and Chest Conditions | I A, B, C, D<br>II A, B<br>III A, B, C, D, E, F | 1j, l |
| Chapter 18 | Reproductive Tract and Sexually Transmitted Infections | V A1–7, C5–6 | 1a, d–h, j–l<br><br>2a, b, e |

| Chapter | Chapter Name | ACNM *Core Competencies* (2020) | ICM *Essential Competencies* (2019) |
|---------|--------------|--------------------------------|-------------------------------------|
| Chapter 19 | Anatomy and Physiology of Pregnancy | I A<br>IV A<br>IV F<br>V B, C | 2a, b, d |
| Chapter 20 | Assessment for Genetic and Fetal Abnormalities | III A, B, C, E | 1g, j, l |
| Appendix 20A | Steps in Constructing a Three-Generation Pedigree | V A2, 3, 4<br>V D5, 11 | 2a, b, c, d, e, g |
| Chapter 21 | Prenatal Care | I (all)<br>III (all)<br>IV B, C, D, E, G, J | 1a, c–e, g, h, j–m<br>2 (all) |
| Appendix 21A | Abdominal Examination During Pregnancy | V A1–12 | |
| Chapter 22[b] | Early Pregnancy Loss and Abortion | V D1–3 | 2g, i |
| Chapter 23 | Pregnancy-Related Conditions | V D4, 5, 6, 7, 8, 10, 11, 12 | 1a, d, g, j, l, m<br>2a–h |
| Chapter 24 | Medical Complications in Pregnancy | I C, E, H, J, N, P<br>II F, T<br>III C, D, E, F, G<br>IV A, D, J<br>V A1–6, B3–4, D7–8, D11 | 1c, d, h, j, l<br>2b, c, e, g |
| Chapter 25 | Anatomy and Physiology of Labor and Birth | I A<br>IV A<br>V E1 | 3a |
| Chapter 26 [a] | First Stage of Labor | I A–G, J–M, O–P, Q<br>II A, F–L, N, T<br>III A–G<br>IV D, J<br>V E | 1a, c, d, e, f, g, h, i, j, k, l<br>3 (all) |
| Appendix 26A[b] | Assessment for Diagnosis of Labor | Same as Chapter 26 | |
| Appendix 26B | Assessment and Diagnosis of Rupture of Membranes | Same as Chapter 26 | |
| Appendix 26Ca | Fetal–Pelvic Relationships | Same as Chapter 26 | |
| Chapter 27 | Fetal Assessment During Labor | V E2, 3a, b, c | 3a |
| Appendix 27A | Intermittent Auscultation During Labor | Same as Chapter 27 | |
| Appendix 27B | Fetal Scalp Electrode | Same as Chapter 27 | |
| Appendix 27C[b] | Intrauterine Pressure Catheter | Same as Chapter 27 | |
| Appendix 27D[b] | Umbilical Cord Gas Technique and Interpretation | Same as Chapter 27 | |
| Chapter 28 | Support During Labor | I B–G, K–Q<br>II D, I, T<br>II A–F<br>IV A–F, J<br>V E1–7 | 1a, d–m<br>3a, b<br>4d |

| Chapter | Chapter Name | ACNM *Core Competencies* (2020) | ICM *Essential Competencies* (2019) |
|---------|--------------|----------------------------------|--------------------------------------|
| Appendix 28A | Sterile Water Injections for the Relief of Low Back Pain in Labor | Same as Chapter 28 | |
| Chapter 29 | Second Stage of Labor and Birth | I A–Q<br>II D, I, T<br>II A–F<br>V E1–7 | 1d, e, g, h–j<br>3a, b |
| Appendix 29A | Pudendal Nerve Block | V E6, 7a | Same as Chapter 29 |
| Appendix 29B | Hand Maneuvers for Birth | V E7b | Same as Chapter 29 |
| Appendix 29C | Umbilical Cord-Clamping at Birth | V E7b<br>VI G3b | Same as Chapter 29 |
| Appendix 29D | Genital Tract Injury, Immediate Postpartum Inspection of the Vulva, Perineum, Vagina, and Cervix | V E3, 7e | Same as Chapter 29 |
| Appendix 29E | Local Infiltration for Genital Tract Repair | V E7a, d | Same as Chapter 29 |
| Appendix 29F | Repair of Genital Tract Lacerations and Episiotomy | V E7e | Same as Chapter 29 |
| Chapter 30 | Complications During Labor and Birth | I C–E, G, K–N, P–Q<br>II D, I, T<br>III A–G<br>IV A, D, G, J<br>V A4, 5b, d, 6b, 1, 3, 4, E1–7 | 1a, b, d, e, f, g, h, j, k, l<br>3a, b, d |
| Appendix 30A[b] | Urgent Maneuvers to Shorten Second Stage | Same as Chapter 30 | |
| Appendix 30B | Shoulder Dystocia | Same as Chapter 30 | |
| Appendix 30C | Emergency Interventions for Umbilical Cord Prolapse | Same as Chapter 30 | |
| Appendix 30D | Intrapartum Management of Twin Gestation | Same as Chapter 30 | |
| Appendix 30E | Breech Birth | Same as Chapter 30 | |
| Chapter 31 | Third Stage of Labor | V A, E1–6, F1–2 | 3a, b, 4d |
| Appendix 31A | Management of Third Stage of Labor | Same as Chapter 31 | |
| Appendix 31B | Inspection of the Umbilical Cord, Placenta, and Membranes | Same as Chapter 31 | |
| Appendix 31C[b] | Postplacental IUD Insertion | I A, D, L, N, Q<br>II K<br>III (all)<br>IV A<br>V F8 | 1a, d, e, g, h, 4a, f |
| Appendix 31D | Manual Removal of the Placenta | Same as Chapter 31 | |
| Appendix 31E | Initial Management of Uterine Inversion | Same as Chapter 31 | |
| Appendix 31F | Management of Immediate Postpartum Hemorrhage | Same as Chapter 31 | |
| Appendix 31G | Intrauterine Exploration | Same as Chapter 31 | |
| Appendix 31H | Sudden Postpartum Cardiovascular or Neurologic Emergencies | Same as Chapter 31 | |

| Chapter | Chapter Name | ACNM *Core Competencies* (2020) | ICM *Essential Competencies* (2019) |
|---|---|---|---|
| Chapter 32 | Birth in the Home and Birth Center | I<br>III<br>V E, F<br>IV A, B<br>V A5 | 2h<br>3 |
| Appendix 32a[b] | Supplies for Birth in the Home and Birth Center | Same as Chapter 32 | |
| Chapter 33 | Anatomy and Physiology of Postpartum | IV A<br>V F9 | 2a |
| Chapter 34 | Postpartum Care | I A–Q<br>II E–H<br>III A–G<br>V F1–9 | 1g, h, j, l<br>4a, c, d, f |
| Appendix 34A | Management of the Fourth Stage of Labor Following Vaginal Birth | Same as Chapter 34 | |
| Appendix 34B[a] | History and Physical Examination During the Early Postpartum Period | Same as Chapter 34 | |
| Chapter 35 | Postpartum Complications | I C, D, J, P<br>III A–G<br>V G9 | 1a, d, e, h, l<br>4d |
| Chapter 36 | Anatomy and Physiology of the Newborn | IV A<br>V F6, 7, 9, G1, 3 | 4a, b, c |
| Chapter 37[a] | Infant Feeding and Lactation | V G3a–d, f | 3c<br>4c, e |
| Chapter 38 | Physical Assessment of the Newborn | V G1, G4a–f | 3c, 4b |
| Appendix 38A | Physical Examination Findings of Healthy Newborn Infants | Same as Chapter 38 | |
| Chapter 39[a] | Neonatal Care | I (all)<br>III (all)<br>IV B, C, D<br>V A5, G4c–d, 5 | 3c, 4e |

[a] Major revision from *Varney's Midwifery,* Sixth Edition.
[b] New Chapter for this edition.

# Index